RETINA

RETINA

FOURTH EDITION

Editor-In-Chief
Stephen J. Ryan MD

President, Doheny Eye Institute, Los Angeles, California, USA

Volume One
Basic Science and Inherited Retinal Disease

Edited by
David R. Hinton MD

Tumors
Edited by
Andrew P. Schachat MD

Volume Two
Medical Retina

Edited by
Andrew P. Schachat MD

Volume Three
Surgical Retina

Edited by
C. P. Wilkinson MD

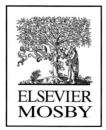

ELSEVIER
MOSBY

Editor-In-Chief
Stephen J. Ryan MD
President, Doheny Eye Institute, Los Angeles, California, USA

RETINA

FOURTH EDITION

Volume Two
Medical Retina

Edited by
Andrew P. Schachat MD
Karl Hagen Professor of Ophthalmology
Johns Hopkins University and Hospital
Baltimore, Maryland
USA

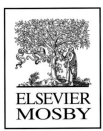

ELSEVIER
MOSBY

MOSBY
An Affiliate of Elsevier

First edition 1989
Second edition 1994
Third edition 2001
Fourth edition 2006

ISBN-13: 978–0–323–02598–0
ISBN-10: 0–323–02598–6

This book is also available as an E-dition package, including access to online updates:
ISBN-13: 978–0–323–04091–4
ISBN-10: 0–323–04091–8

An online version of this book, with updates is also available:
ISBN-13: 978–0–323–04323–6
ISBN-10: 0–323–04323–2

British Library Cataloguing in Publication Data
A catalogue record for this book is available from the British Library

Library of Congress Cataloging in Publication Data
A catalog record for this book is available from the Library of Congress

Notice
Medical knowledge is constantly changing. Standard safety precautions must be followed, but as new research
and clinical experience broaden our knowledge, changes in treatment and drug therapy may become necessary
or appropriate. Readers are advised to check the most current product information provided by the manufacturer
of each drug to be administered to verify the recommended dose, the method and duration of administration, and
contraindications. It is the responsibility of the practitioner, relying on experience and knowledge of the patient,
to determine dosages and the best treatment for each individual patient. Neither the Publisher nor the authors
assumes any liability for any injury and/or damage to persons or property arising from this publication.
The Publisher

Printed in China
Last digit is the print number: 9   8   7   6   5   4   3   2

Working together to grow
libraries in developing countries

www.elsevier.com | www.bookaid.org | www.sabre.org

ELSEVIER   BOOK AID International   Sabre Foundation

Commissioning Editor: **Paul Fam**
Project Development Manager: **Tim Kimber**
Editorial Assistants: **Amy Jane Lewis, Firiel Benson**
Project Manager: **Jessica Thompson**
Design Manager: **Andy Chapman**
Illustration Manager: **Mick Ruddy**
Illustrators: **Tim Hengst, Tim Loughhead and Danny Pyne**
Marketing Manager(s): **Lisa Damico, Gaynor Jones**

Contributors

Thomas M. Aaberg, Jr. MD
Associated Retinal Consultants
Assistant Clinical Professor
Michigan State University
Grand Rapids, Michigan
USA
Chapter 23, Chapter 118, Chapter 140

Mohamed H. Abdel-Rahman MD PhD
Fellow, Clinical Cancer Genetics Program
College of Medicine and Public Health
The Ohio State University
Ohio
USA
Chapter 37

Gary W. Abrams MD
The David Barsky Professor and Chair
Department of Ophthalmology
Kresge Eye Institute
Wayne State University
Detroit, Michigan
USA
Chapter 136, Chapter 142

Anita Agarwal MD
Assistant Professor of Ophthalmology
Retina and Vitreous
Vanderbilt Eye Institute
Nashville, Tennessee
USA
Chapter 23

Everett Ai MD
Director, Ophthalmic Diagnostic Center
California Pacific Medical Center
San Francisco, California
USA
Chapter 51, Chapter 105, Chapter 147

Daniel M. Albert MD MS
Chair Emeritus
F. A. Davis Professor and Lorenz E. Zimmerman
Professor
Department of Ophthalmology and Visual Sciences
University of Wisconsin
Madison, Wisconsin
USA
Chapter 32

Judith Alexander BA
Scheie Eye Institute
University of Philadelphia
Philadelphia, Pennsylvania
USA
Chapter 99

Rajiv Anand MD FRCS FRCOphth
Texas Retina Associates
Associate Professor of Ophthalmology
Dallas, Texas
USA
Chapter 123

Gerasimos Anastassiou MD
Department of Ophthalmology
University Hospital Essen
University of Essen-Duisburg
Germany
Chapter 42

G. William Aylward MD FRCS FRCOphth
Consultant Vitreoretinal Surgeon and Medical
Director
Moorefields Eye Hospital
London
UK
Chapter 121

Mohammed K. Barazi MD
Co-Director, Vitreoretinal Fellowship
The Retina Group of Washington
Sterling, Virginia
USA
Chapter 82

David Bingaman DVM PhD Dipl AVCO
Assistant Director
Retina Discovery Unit
Alcon Research, Ltd.
Fort Worth, Texas
USA
Chapter 5

Alan C. Bird MD FRCS FCOphth
Professor, Department of Clinical Ophthalmology
Institute of Ophthalmology
London
UK
Chapter 54, Chapter 59, Chapter 104

Barbara A. Blodi MD
Associate Professor
Department of Ophthalmology and Visual Sciences
University of Wisconsin
Madison, Wisconsin
USA
Chapter 68

Mark S. Blumenkranz MD
Professor and Chairman
Department of Ophthalmology
Stanford University School of Medicine
Stanford, California
USA
Chapter 21, Chapter 65, Chapter 132

James P. Bolling MD
Associate Professor and Chair
Department of Ophthalmology
Mayo Clinic
Jacksonville, Florida
USA
Chapter 78

Norbert Bornfeld MD
Professor of Ophthalmology
Zentrum fur Augenheilkunde
Universitatsklinikum Essen
Essen
Germany
Chapter 42

Susan B. Bressler MD
The Julia G. Levy Professor of Ophthalmology
The Wilmer Eye Institute
John Hopkins University School of Medicine
Baltimore, Maryland
USA
Chapter 60, Chapter 61

Neil M. Bressler MD
The James P. Gills Professor of Ophthalmology
The Wilmer Eye Institute
The Johns Hopkins University School of Medicine
Baltimore, Maryland
USA
Chapter 60, Chapter 61

Daniel A. Brinton MD
Assistant Clinical Professor
Department of Ophthalmology
University of California - San Francisco
Oakland, California
USA
Chapter 119

Jeremiah Brown, Jr. MS MD
Associate Clinical Professor
Department of Ophthalmology
University of Texas Health Science Center
Ophthalmology Associates of San Antonio
San Antonio, Texas
USA
Chapter 16

Gary C. Brown MD MBA
Director, Retina Service, Wills Eye Hospital
Co-Director, Center for Value-Based Medicine
Professor of Ophthalmology, Jefferson Medical
College
Adjunct Senior Fellow, Leonard Davis Institute of
Health Economics, University of Pennsylvania
Philadelphia
USA
Chapter 46, Chapter 69, Chapter 84

Justin C. Brown MD
Medical and Surgical Retinal Fellow
The Wilmer Eye Institute
Johns Hopkins Hospital
Baltimore, Maryland
USA
Chapter 72

Helmut Buettner MD
Professor of Ophthalmology
Mayo Clinic College of Medicine
Department of Ophthalmology
Mayo Clinic
Rochester, Minnesota
USA
Chapter 30

Serge de Bustros MD
Director, The Retina Center
Munster
Indiana
Associate Professor in Ophthalmology
Rush University Medical Center
Chicago, Illinois
Senior Physician
Illinois Retina Associates
Harvey, Illinois
USA
Chapter 143

Sandra Fraser Byrne MD
Western Carolina Retina Associates
Asheville, North Carolina
USA
Chapter 14

Mark T. Cahill MCh FRCSI(Ophth)
Consultant Ophthalmologist
Vitreo-Retinal Service
Royal Victoria Eye and Ear Hospital
Dublin
Ireland
Chapter 152

Peter A. Campochiaro MD
George S. and Doloris Doré Eccles Professor of
Ophthalmology
The Departments of Ophthalmology and
Neuroscience
The Johns Hopkins University School of Medicine
Baltimore, Maryland
USA
Chapter 131

Ronald E. Carr MD
Professor of Ophthalmology
New York University Medical Center
New York, New York
USA
Chapter 18, Chapter 19

Stanley Chang MD
Edward S Harkness Professor and Chairman
Department of Ophthalmology
College of Physicians and Surgeons
Columbia University
New York
USA
Chapter 127, Chapter 128, Chapter 137

Steve Charles MD
Clinical Professor of Ophthalmology
Department of Ophthalmology
University of Tennessee College of Medicine
Memphis, Tennessee
USA
Chapter 125

Jeannie Chen PhD
Associate Professor
Departments of Ophthalmology, and Cell and
Neurobiology
Keck School of Medicine
University of Southern California
Los Angeles, California
USA
Chapter 8

Clara A. Chen MHS
Epidemiology Unit
Massachusetts Eye and Ear Infirmary
Boston, Massachusetts
USA
Chapter 58

Emily Y. Chew MD
Deputy Director
Division of Epidemiology and Clinical Research
National Eye Institute
National Institutes of Health
Bethesda, Maryland
USA
Chapter 67, Chapter 74, Chapter 76, Chapter 81

Louis J. Chorich III MD
Clinical Assistant Professor
Department of Ophthalmology
The Ohio State University
Columbus, Ohio
USA
Chapter 37

David R. Chow MD FRCS(C)
Assistant Professor
Rush University
Illinois Retina Associates
Harvey, Ilinois
USA
Chapter 143

Antonio P. Ciardella MD
Chief, Department of Ophthalmology
Denver Health Medical Center
Denver, Colorado
USA
Chapter 53, Chapter 63

Thomas A. Ciulla MD
Retina Service
Midwest Eye Institute
Methodist Hospital
Indianapolis
USA
Chapter 5

Gabriel J. Coscas MD
Emeritus Professor of Ophthalmology
Hospital of Creteil
University Paris XII-Val de Marne
Creteil
France
Chapter 62

Alan F. Cruess MD
Professor and Head, District Chief, Capital Health
Department of Ophthalmology and Visual Sciences
Dalhousie University
Halifax, Nova Scotia
Canada
Chapter 25

Lyndon da Cruz MBBS MA FRCOphth, PhD,
FRACO
Consultant Ophthalmic Surgeon
Moorfields Eye Hospital
Vitreo-Retinal Service
London
UK
Chapter 155

Bertil E. Damato MD PhD
Consultant Ophthalmologist and Honorary Professor
Director of Ocular Oncology Service
The Royal Liverpool University Hospital
Liverpool
UK
Chapter 40

Frederick H. Davidorf MD
Martha G and Milton Staub Chair
Department of Ophthalmology
Ohio State University College of Medicine
Columbus, Ohio
USA
Chapter 37

Matthew D. Davis MD
Emeritus Professor of Ophthalmology and Visual
Sciences
University of Wisconsin - Madison
Madison, Wisconsin
USA
Chapter 68

Janet L. Davis MD
Professor of Ophthalmology
Bascom Palmer Eye Institute
University of Miami School of Medicine
Miami, Florida
USA
Chapter 97

August F. Deutman MD
Professor and Chairman
Institute of Ophthalmology
University of Nijmegen
Nijmegen
Netherlands
Chapter 64

Ranjit S. Dhaliwal MD FRCSC FACS
Vitreo Retinal Diseases and Surgery
The Retina Eye Center
Augusta, Georgia
USA
Chapter 28, Chapter 49

Diana V. Do MD
Assistant Professor of Ophthalmology
The Wilmer Eye Institute
The Johns Hopkins University School of Medicine
Baltimore, Maryland
USA
Chapter 18, Chapter 41, Chapter 77, Chapter 88

Pravin U. Dugel MD
Vitreo-Retinal Diseases and Surgery
Retinal Consultants of Arizona
Phoenix, Arizona
USA
Chapter 95, Chapter 139

John D. Earle *MD*
Professor of Oncology and Chairman of
Department of Radiation Oncology
Mayo Clinic
Jacksonville, Florida
USA
Chapter 38

Albert O. Edwards MD PhD
Assistant Professor
Department of Ophthalmology
University of Texas Southwestern Medical Center
Dallas, Texas
USA
Chapter 20

Dean Eliott MD
Director, Retina Service
Associate Professor
Department of Ophthalmology
Kresge Eye Institute
Wayne State University
Detroit, Michigan
USA
Chapter 31, Chapter 142

Geoffrey G. Emerson MD, PhD
Resident
Department of Ophthalmology
The Wilmer Eye Institute
Baltimore, Maryland
USA
Chapter 79

Sharon Fekrat MD
Associate Professor
Vitreoretinal Surgery
Department of Ophthalmology
Duke University Eye Center
Duke University Medical Center
Durham, North Carolina
USA
Chapter 70, Chapter 71, Chapter 79

Steven E. Feldon MD
Chairman, Department of Ophthalmology
Professor of Ophthalmology, Neurology,
Neurological Surgery, and Visual Science
University of Rochester
Director, University of Rochester Eye Institute
New York
USA
Chapter 12

Frederick L. Ferris III MD
Clinical Director and Director
Division of Epidemiology and Clinical Research
National Eye Institute
National Institutes of Health
Bethesda, Maryland
USA
Chapter 67

Stuart L. Fine MD
The William F Norris and George E de Schweinitz
Professor of Ophthalmology
Chairman, Department of Ophthalmology
Director, Scheie Eye Institute
University of Pennsylvania Health System
Philadelphia, Pennsylvania
USA
Chapter 61

Daniel Finkelstein MD
Professor, Department of Ophthalmology
The Wilmer Ophthalmological Institute
Johns Hopkins Hospital
Baltimore, Maryland
USA
Chapter 71

Steven K. Fisher PhD
Professor
Molecular, Cellular and Developmental Biology
Neuroscience Research Institute
University of California Santa Barbara
Santa Barbara, California
USA
Chapter 115

John Flannery PhD
Professor of Vision Science
The Neuroscience Division, Department
of Molecular and Cell Biology
The Helen Wills Neuroscience Institute
University of California Berkeley
Berkeley, California
USA
Chapter 8

James C. Folk MD
Professor, Department of Ophthalmology and
Visual Sciences
The University of Iowa Hospitals and Clinics
Iowa City, Iowa
USA
Chapter 101

Wallace S. Foulds MD ChM DSc (Hon) FRCS
FRCOphth
Emeritus Professor of Ophthalmology
University of Glasgow
UK
Senior Consultant
Singapore Eye Research Institute
Singapore
Chapter 40

Robert N. Frank MD
The Robert S Jampel Professor of Ophthalmology
Professor of Anatomy and Cell Biology
Departments of Ophthalmology and Anatomy
& Cell Biology
Kresge Eye Institute
Wayne State University School of Medicine
Detroit, Michigan
USA
Chapter 66

William R. Freeman MD
Professor of Ophthalmology
Director Jacobs Retina Center
Department of Ophthalmology
University of California San Diego
La Jolla, California
USA
Chapter 92

Martin Friedlander MD PhD
Department of Cell Biology
The Scripps Research Institute
Division of Ophthalmology
Scripps Clinic
La Jolla, California
USA
Chapter 2

Laura J. Frishman PhD
Moores Professor and Associate Dean for
Graduate Studies/Research
College of Optometry
University of Houston
Houston, Texas
USA
Chapter 6

Arthur D. Fu MD
West Coast Retina Medical Group
Department of Ophthalmology
California Pacific Medical Center
San Francisco, California
USA
Chapter 51, Chapter 105, Chapter 147

Gildo Y. Fujii MD PhD
Instructor of Clinical Ophthalmology
Doheny Retina Institute
Doheny Eye Institute
Keck School of Medicine
University of Southern California
Los Angeles, California
USA
Chapter 151, Chapter 156

Ron P. Gallemore MD PhD
Assistant Clinical Professor
Retina-Vitreous Associates Medical Group
Los Angeles, California
USA
Chapter 130

Daniel C. Garibaldi MD
Fellow
Department of Oculoplastic and Reconstructive
Surgery
The Wilmer Eye Institute
Baltimore, Maryland
USA
Chapter 18

Enrique Garcia-Valenzuela MD PhD
Emory University Eye Center
Atlanta, Georgia
USA
Chapter 136

J. Donald M. Gass MD
Fomerly, Professor
Vanderbilt Eye Institute
Vanderbilt University Medical Center
Nashville, Tennessee
USA
Chapter 97

Sandrine Gautier PhD
Product Development Manager
KitoZyme sa
Parc Industriel des Hauts-Sarts
Herstal
Belgium
Chapter 129

Scott Geller PhD
Helen Wills Neuroscience Institute
School of Optometry
University of California Berkeley
Berkeley, California
USA
Chapter 8

Morton F. Goldberg MD
The Joseph Green Professor of Ophthalmology
and Director Emeritus
The Wilmer Eye Institute
Johns Hopkins University School of Medicine
Baltimore, Maryland
USA
Chapter 79

Christine R. Gonzales MD
Assistant Professor of Ophthalmology
Jules Stein Eye Institute
University of California Los Angeles School of
Medicine
Los Angeles, California
USA
Chapter 146

Justin L. Gottlieb MD
Associate Professor
Department of Ophthalmology and Visual Sciences
University of Wisconsin
Madison, Wisconsin
USA
Chapter 32

Evangelos S. Gragoudas MD
Professor of Ophthalmology
Harvard Medical School
Director, Retina Service
Massachusetts Eye and Ear Infirmary
Boston, Massachusetts
USA
Chapter 39

Ronald L. Green MD
Professor
Department of Ophthalmology
Doheny Eye Institute
Los Angeles, California
USA
Chapter 14

W. Richard Green MD
Independent Order of Odd Fellows Professor of
Ophthalmology Professor of Pathology Eye
Pathology Laboratory
The Johns Hopkins University School of Medicine
Baltimore, Maryland
USA
Chapter 3, Chapter 35, Chapter 41, Chapter 114

Zdenek J. Gregor FRCS FRCOphth
Consultant Ophthalmic Surgeon
Moorfields Eye Hospital
London
UK
Chapter 155

Kevin Gregory-Evans MD FRCOphth
Reader in Molecular Ophthalmology and
Consultant Ophthalmologist
Department of Visual Neuroscience
Western Eye Hospital
Imperial College London
London
UK
Chapter 17

Nicole E. Gross MD
Clinical Instructor
New York University Department of Ophthalmology
Manhattan Eye, Ear & Throat Hospital
New York, New York
USA
Chapter 86

Vamsi K. Gullapalli MD
Institute of Ophthalmology and Visual Science
New Jersey Medical School
University of Medicine and Dentistry of New Jersey
Newark, New Jersey
USA
Chapter 153

David R. Guyer MD
Chief Executive Officer
Eyetech Pharmaceuticals Inc
New York, New York
USA
Chapter 3

Robyn Guymer MBBS PhD FRANZCO
Associate Professor
Centre for Eye Research Australia
The University of Melbourne
Melbourne, Victoria
Australia
Chapter 59

Julia A. Haller MD
Katharine Graham Professor of Ophthalmology
Department of Ophthalmology
Johns Hopkins Wilmer Eye Institute
Baltimore, Maryland
USA
Chapter 41, Chapter 77

J. William Harbour MD
Director, Center for Ocular Oncology
Assistant Professor of Ophthalmology
Washington University School of Medicine
St Louis, Missouri
USA
Chapter 22

Joseph B. Harlan, Jr. MD FACS
Assistant Professor
Johns Hopkins University School of Medicine
Director, Vitreo-retinal Surgery
Krieger Eye Institute
Sinai Hospital
Baltimore, Maryland
USA
Chapter 79

Alon Harris MSc PhD
Letzter Professor of Ophthalmology
Professor of Physiology and Biophysics
Department of Ophthalmology
Indiana University School of Medicine
Indianapolis, Indiana
USA
Chapter 5

Mary Elizabeth Hartnett MD FACS
Associate Professor of Ophthalmology
Department of Ophthalmology
University of North Carolina
Chapel Hill, North Carolina
USA
Chapter 116

Michael K. Hartzer PhD
Principal Scientist – Pharmacology
Department of Ophthalmology
William Beaumont Hospital Research Institute
Royal Oak, Michigan
USA
Chapter 132

Barbara S. Hawkins PhD
Professor of Ophthalmology and Epidemiology
The Wilmer Eye Institute
Johns Hopkins University School of Medicine
Baltimore, Maryland
USA
Chapter 44, Chapter 88, Chapter 99

Heinrich Heimann MD
Consultant Ophthalmic Surgeon
St Paul's Eye Unit
Royal Liverpool University Hospital
Liverpool
UK
Chapter 120

David R. Hinton MD
Gavin S. Herbert Professor of Retinal Research
Professor of Pathology and Ophthalmology
Keck School of Medicine
University of Southern California
Los Angeles, California
USA
Chapter 7, Chapter 56

Brad J. Hinz MD FRCSC
Assistant Clinical Professor
University of Alberta
Alberta
Canada
Chapter 24

Stephan Hoffmann MD
Universitätsaugenklinik Leipzig
Leipzig
Germany
Chapter 7

Nancy M. Holekamp MD
Associate Clinical Professor
Department of Ophthalmology and Visual Science
Washington University School of Medicine
Barnes Retina Institute
St. Louis, Missouri
USA
Chapter 150

Gary N. Holland MD
Vernon O Underwood Family Professor of
Ophthalmology
Chief, Cornea-External Ocular Disease and Uveitis
Division
Department of Ophthalmology
David Geffen School of Medicine at UCLA
Jules Stein Eye Institute
Los Angeles, California
USA
Chapter 91, Chapter 94

Carel B. Hoyng MD
Associate Clinical Professor
University Medical Centre St Radboud
Nijmegen
The Netherlands
Chapter 64

Mark S. Humayun MD PhD
Professor of Ophthalmology
Biomedical Engineering and Cell & Neurobiology
Associate Director of Research
Doheny Retina Institute
Department of Ophthalmology
Keck School of Medicine
University of Southern California
Los Angeles, California
USA
Chapter 154

Yasushi Ikuno MD
Assistant Professor
Department of Ophthalmology
Osaka University Medical School
Japan
Chapter 124

Douglas A. Jabs MD MBA
Alan C Woods Professor of Ophthalmology
Professor of Medicine
The Wilmer Eye Institute
Johns Hopkins University School of Medicine
Professor of Epidemiology
Johns Hopkins University Bloomberg School of
Public Health
Baltimore, Maryland
USA
Chapter 75, Chapter 89, Chapter 103

Glenn J. Jaffe MD
Professor of Ophthalmology
Department of Ophthalmology
Duke University
Durham, North Carolina
USA
Chapter 55

Valérie Jallet PhD
Laboratory Manager
Research and Development
Corneal Industie
Pringy
France
Chapter 129

Lee M. Jampol MD
Louis Feinberg Professor and Chairman
Department of Ophthalmology
Feinberg School of Medicine
Northwestern University
Chicago, Illinois
USA
Chapter 102

Leonard Joffe MD FCS(SA) FRCSEdin
Clinical Associate Professor
Department of Ophthalmology
University of Arizona
Retina Associates Southwest PC
Tucson, Arizona
USA
Chapter 29

Robert N. Johnson MD
West Coast Retina Medical Group
Assistant Clinical Professor of Ophthalmology
University of California
San Francisco, California
USA
Chapter 51, Chapter 105, Chapter 147

Daniel P. Joseph MD PhD
Barnes Retina Institute
St. Louis, Missouri
USA
Chapter 149

Eugene de Juan, Jr. MD
Formerly, Chief Executive Officer
Doheny Retina Institute
Professor, Department of Ophthalmology
Keck School of Medicine
University of Southern California
Los Angeles, California
USA
Chapter 126, Chapter 151, Chapter 156

J. Michael Jumper MD
West Coast Retina Medical Group
Retina Service Chief
California Pacific Medical Center
Assistant Clinical Professor
University of California, San Francisco
San Francisco, California
USA
Chapter 51, Chapter 105, Chapter 147

Henry J. Kaplan MD
Professor and Chairman
Department of Ophthalmology and Visual Sciences
University of Louisville
Louisville, Kentucky
USA
Chapter 134

James S. Kelley MD
Assistant Professor
Department of Ophthalmology
John Hopkins University School of Medicine
Baltimore, Maryland
USA
Chapter 110

Mohamad A. Khodair MD PhD
Institute of Ophthalmology and Visual Science
New Jersey Medical School
University of Medicine and Dentistry of New Jersey
Newark, New Jersey
USA
Chapter 153

Bernd Kirchhof MD
Department of Vitreo-retinal Surgery
Center of Ophthalmology
University of Cologne
Cologne
Germany
Chapter 120

Christina M. Klais MD
Retina Fellow
LuEsther T Mertz Retinal Research Center
Manhattan Eye, Ear and Throat Hospital
New York
USA
Chapter 53, Chapter 63

Barbara E. K. Klein MD
Department of Ophthalmology and Visual Sciences
University of Wisconsin Medical School
Madison, Wisconsin
USA
Chapter 85

Ronald Klein MD MPH
Professor, Department of Ophthalmology and
Visual Sciences
University of Wisconsin Medical School
Madison, Wisconsin
USA
Chapter 85

Robert W. Kline PhD
Associate Professor of Radiological Physics
Department of Radiation Oncology
Mayo Clinic
Rochester, Minnesota
USA
Chapter 38

David L. Knox MD
Associate Professor
Department of Ophthalmology
Wilmer Ophthalmological Institute
Baltimore, Maryland
USA
Chapter 96

Brian R. Kosobucki MD
Carolina Retina & Vitreous Consultants
Charlotte, North Carolina
USA
Chapter 92

Allan E. Kreiger MD
Professor, Department of Ophthalmology
The Jules Stein Eye Institute
Los Angeles, California
USA
Chapter 146

Derek Y. Kunimoto MD
Retina Service
Wills Eye Hospital
Philadelphia, Pennsylvania
USA
Chapter 95

Robert Choi Kwun MD
Partner
Retina Associates of Utah
Salt Lake City, Utah
USA
Chapter 128

Rohit R. Lakhanpal MD
Fellow and Clinical Instructor
Vitreoretinal Diseases and Surgery
Cullen Eye Institute
Baylor College of Medicine
Houston, TX
USA
Chapter 154

Linda A. Lam MD
Attending Physician and Clinical Instructor
Retina Group of Washington
Washington Hospital
Washington, DC
USA
Chapter 74

Maurice B. Landers III MD
Professor of Ophthalmology
Department of Ophthalmology
University of North Carolina
Chapel Hill, North Carolina
USA
Chapter 116

Anne Marie Lane MPH
Department of Ophthalmology
Harvard Medical School
Manager
Clinical Research Unit, Retina Service
Massachusetts Eye and Ear Infirmary
Boston, Massachusetts
USA
Chapter 39

Michael S. Lee MD
Assistant Professor
Department of Ophthalmology
Southwestern Medical School
Dallas, Texas
USA
Chapter 142

Henry C. Lee MD
Barnes Retina Institute
Washington University School of Medicine
St. Louis, Missouri
USA
Chapter 150

Hilel Lewis MD
E Bruce and Virginia Chaney Professor
Chairman, Division of Ophthalmology
Director, Cole Eye Institute
The Cleveland Clinic Foundation
Cleveland, Ohio
USA
Chapter 50

Geoffrey P. Lewis PhD
Research Biologist
Neuroscience Research Institute
University of California Santa Barbara
Santa Barbara, California
USA
Chapter 115

Wee-Kiak Lim FRCOphth FRCS(Ed) MMED
Associate Consultant
Ocular Inflammation and Immunology
Singapore National Eye Centre
Singapore
Senior Staff Clinical Fellow
Uveitis and Ocular Immunology
National Eye Institute
Bethesda, Maryland
USA
Chapter 13

Eugene S. Lit MD
East Bay Retina Associates
Oakland, California
USA
Chapter 119

Anat Loewenstein MD
Professor and Chairman
Department of Ophthalmology
Tel-Aviv Sourasky Medical Center
Sackler Faculty of Medicine
Tel-Aviv University
Tel-Aviv
Israel
Chapter 41

José Manuel Lopez MD
Assistant Professor
Harkness Science Institute
New York, New York
USA
Chapter 137

Gerard A. Lutty PhD
Associate Professor
Department of Ophthalmology
Wilmer Ophthalmological Institute
Johns Hopkins Hospital
Baltimore, Maryland
USA
Chapter 79, Chapter 80

Steven Madreperla MD PhD
Retina Associates of New Jersey
Teaneck, New Jersey
USA
Chapter 153

Albert M. Maguire MD
Director, Retina and Vitreous Service
Department of Ophthalmology
Sheie Eye Institute
Univeristy of Pennsylvania
Philadelphia, Pennsylvania
USA
Chapter 83

Martin A. Mainster MD PhD
Luther L Fry Professor and Vice Chairperson
Department of Ophthalmology
Kansas University Medical Center
Kansas City, Missouri
USA
Chapter 109

Nancy C. Mansfield PhD
Family Counselor and Patient Ombudsman
The Retinoblastoma Centre
Childrens Hospital of Los Angeles
Los Angeles, California
USA
Chapter 22

Michael F. Marmor MD
Professor of Ophthalmology
Stanford University Medical Center
Stanford, California
USA
Chapter 112

Bruce J. Martin PhD
Associate Professor of Physiology and Biophysics
Assistant Director
Medical Sciences Program
Indiana University
Bloomington, Indiana
USA
Chapter 5

Stephen C. Massey PhD
Elizabeth Morford Professor and Research Director
Department of Ophthalmology and Visual Science
University of Texas Medical School
Houston, Texas
USA
Chapter 4

Elias C. Mavrofrides MD
Lecturer in Ophthalmology
Florida Retina Institute
Lake Mary, Florida
USA
Chapter 87

Brooks W. McCuen II MD
Robert Machemer Professor, Department of Ophthalmology
Vice Chairman, Department of Ophthalmology
Director, Vitreoretinal Surgery
Duke University Eye Center
Durham, North Carolina
USA
Chapter 130

H. Richard McDonald MD
West Coast Retina Medical Group
Associate Clinical Professor of Ophthalmology
University of California San Francisco
San Francisco, California
USA
Chapter 51, Chapter 105, Chapter 147

Petra Meier MD
Assistant Professor
Klivik und Poliklinik für Augen
Leipzig
Germany
Chapter 145

Shannath L. Merbs MD PhD
Associate Professor
Departments of Ophthalmology and Oncology
The Wilmer Eye Institute
Johns Hopkins University School of Medicine
Baltimore, Maryland
USA
Chapter 35

Travis A. Meredith MD
Chairman, Department of Ophthalmology
Sterling A Barrett Distinguished Professor
University of North Carolina at Chapel Hill
Chapel Hill, North Carolina
USA
Chapter 133

William F. Mieler MD
Professor and Chairman
Department of Ophthalmology and Visual Science
University of Chicago
Chicago, Illinois
USA
Chapter 108

Robert F. Miller MD
Professor
Department of Neuroscience
University of Minnesota
Minneapolis, Minnesota
USA
Chapter 9

Joan W. Miller MD
Henry Willard Williams Professor of Ophthalmology
Chief and Chair, Department of Ophthalmology
Harvard Medical School
Massachusetts Eye and Ear Infirmary
Boston, Massachusetts
USA
Chapter 141

Peter Milne PhD
Associate Professor, Ophthalmic Biophysics Center
Bascom Palmer Eye Institute
University of Miami School of Medicine
Miami, Florida
Department of Atmospheric Chemistry
University of Miami Rosenstiel School of Marine and Atmospheric Science
Key Biscayne, Florida
USA
Chapter 129

Robert A. Mittra MD
Vitreoretinal Surgery PA
Minneapolis St Paul, Minnesota
USA
Chapter 108

Darius M. Moshfeghi MD
Director of Ophthalmic Oncology and Pediatric Vitreoretinal Surgery
Department of Ophthalmology
Stanford University School of Medicine
Stanford, California
Chapter 65

Andrew A. Moshfeghi MD
Lecturer in Ophthalmology
Bascom Palmer Eye Institute
University of Miami Miller School of Medicine
Miami, Florida
USA
Chapter 87

Ala Moshiri PhD
Neurobiology and Behavior Program
Department of Biological Structure
University of Washington
Seattle, Washington
USA
Chapter 1

Prithvi Mruthyunjaya MD
Assistant Professor of Ophthalmology
Duke Eye Center
Durham, North Carolina
USA
Chapter 70

Toshinori Murata MD PhD
Professor and Chairman
Department of Ophthalmology
Shinshu University School of Medicine
Matsumoto
Japan
Chapter 56

A. Linn Murphree MD
Director
The Retinoblastoma Centre
Childrens Hospital of Los Angeles
Los Angeles, California
USA
Chapter 22

Robert P. Murphy MD
The Retina Group of Washington
Fairfax, Virginia
USA
Chapter 74, Chapter 81, Chapter 82

Sumit K. Nanda MD
Clinical Associate Professor
Department of Ophthalmology
University of Oklahoma
Oklahoma City, Oklahoma
USA
Chapter 136

Quan Dong Nguyen MD MSc
Assistant Professor of Ophthalmology
The Wilmer Eye Institute
The Johns Hopkins University School of Medicine
Baltimore, Maryland
USA
Chapter 89, Chapter 103

Robert B. Nussenblatt MD
Chief, Laboratory of Immunology
Intramural Program
National Eye Institute
National Institutes of Health
Bethesda, Maryland
USA
Chapter 13

Michael D. Ober MD
Fellow, Vitreoretinal Surgery
Columbia University College of Physicians and
Surgeons
LuEsther T Mertz Retinal Research Center
Manhattan Eye, Ear, and Throat Hospital
New York, New York
USA
Chapter 53, Chapter 63

Richard R. Ober
Clinical Director
Ophthalmology Section
Southern Arizona Veterans Affairs Health Care
System
Tucson, Arizona
USA
Chapter 73, Chapter 139

Thomas E. Ogden MD PhD
Emeritus Professor of Physiology and Biophysics
Keck School of Medicine
University of Southern California
Los Angeles, California
USA
Chapter 15

Kean T. Oh MD
Assistant Professor of Ophthalmology
Department of Ophthalmology
University of North Carolina
Chapel Hill, North Carolina
USA
Chapter 116

Masahito Ohji MD
Associate Professor
Department of Ophthalmology
Osaka University Medical School
Osaka
Japan
Chapter 124

Karl R. Olsen MD
Clinical Assistant Professor
Retina Vitreous Consultants
University of Pittsburgh Medical School
Pittsburgh, Pennsylvania
USA
Chapter 97

Daniel Palanker MD
Assistant Professor
Department of Ophthalmology
and Hansen Experimental Physics Laboratory
Stanford University
Stanford, California
USA
Chapter 21

Earl A. Palmer MD
Professor
Departments of Ophthalmology and Pediatrics
Casey Eye Institute
Oregon Health and Science University
Portland, Oregon
USA
Chapter 80

Jean-Marie Parel PhD IngETS-G
Henri and Flore Lesieur Chair in Ophthalmology
and Director, Ophthalmic Biophysics Center
Bascom Palmer Eye Institute
University of Miami School of Medicine
Miami, Florida
USA
Chapter 129

Carl H. Park MD
Assistant Professor of Ophthalmology
Thomas Jefferson University
Wills Eye Hospital
Philadelphia, Pennsylvania
USA
Chapter 55

Jonathan E. Pederson MD
Adjunct Professor of Ophthalmology
University of Minnesota
Minneapolis, Minnesota
USA
Chapter 113

Christopher D. Pelzek MD
Partner, Retina-Vitreous Associates
Chicago, Illinois
USA
Chapter 27

Jay S. Pepose MD PhD
Professor of Clinical Ophthalmology and Visual
Sciences
Washington University School of Medicine
St Louis, Missouri
USA
Chapter 93

Dale L. Phelps MD
Professor
Departments of Pediatrics and Ophthalmology
University of Rochester School of Medicine and
Dentistry
Rochester, New York
USA
Chapter 80

Stephen Phillips MD
Carolina Centers for Sight
Murrells Inlet, South Carolina
USA
Chapter 71

Joel Pokorny PhD
Professor
Departments of Ophthalmology and Visual Science
and Psychology
Committee on Computational Neuroscience
University of Chicago
Chicago, Illinois
USA
Chapter 10

Carmen A. Puliafito MD MBA
Chairman
Bascom Palmer Eye Institute
Miami, Florida
USA
Chapter 87

Narsing A. Rao MD
Professor of Ophthalmology and Pathology
Doheny Eye Institute
University of Southern California Los Angeles
Los Angeles, California
USA
*Chapter 57, Chapter 100, Chapter 106,
Chapter 107*

P. Kumar Rao MD
Retina Specialist
Retinal Consultants of Arizona
Phoenix, Arizona
USA
Chapter 107

Franco M. Recchia MD
Assistant Professor
Vanderbilt Eye Institute
Vanderbilt University Medical Center
Nashville, Tennessee
USA
Chapter 140

Thomas A. Reh PhD
Neurobiology and Behavior Program
Department of Biological Structure
University of Washington
Seattle, Washington
USA
Chapter 1

Dennis M. Robertson MD
Professor, Department of Ophthalmology
Mayo Clinic
Rochester, Minnesota
USA
Chapter 38

Joseph E. Robertson, Jr. MD
Professor and Chairman
Casey Eye Institute
Department of Ophthalmology
Portland, Oregon
USA
Chapter 20

Gary S. Rubin PhD
Helen Keller Professor of Ophthalmology
Institute of Ophthalmology
London
UK
Chapter 11

Stephen J. Ryan MD
President
Doheny Eye Institute
Los Angeles, California
USA
Chapter 56, Chapter 100, Chapter 138

Srinivas R. Sadda MD
Assistant Professor
Department of Ophthalmology
Keck School of Medicine
University of Southern California
Los Angeles, California
USA
Chapter 52

Alfredo A. Sadun MD PhD
The Flora Thornton Professor of Ophthalmology
Doheny Eye Institute
Keck School of Medicine
University of Southern California
Los Angeles, California
USA
Chapter 111

José Alain Sahel MD
Professor of Biomedical Sciences
Institute of Ophthalmology
University College London
London, UK
Professor of Ophthalmology
Pierre et Marie Curie University
Chairman, Department of Ophthalmology IV
Centre Hospitalier National d'Ophtalmologie des
Quinze-Vingts
and Department of Vitreoretinal Diseases
Fondation Ophtalmologique
Adolphe de Rothschild
Paris
France
Chapter 32

Maite Sainz de la Maza MD
Associate Professor, Department of
Ophthalmology
Division of Ocular Immunology and Uveitis
Hospital Clinico y Provincial of Barcelona
Barcelona University Central School of Medicine
Barcelona
Spain
Chapter 98

Michael A. Samuel MD
Attending Surgeon, Retina Service
Wills Eye Hospital
Thomas Jefferson University
Philadelphia, Pennsylvannia
USA
Chapter 22

George E. Sanborn MD
Richmond Retinal Associates
Richmond, Virginia
USA
Chapter 47

John P. Sarks FRACO
Honorary Consultant Ophthalmologist
Prince of Wales Hospital
Sydney, New South Wales
Australia
Chapter 60

Shirley H. Sarks MD, FRACO
Honorary Senior Research Associate
Medical Research Institute
Prince of Wales Hospital
Sydney, New South Wales
Australia
Chapter 60

Andrew P. Schachat MD
Karl Hagen Professor of Ophthalmology
Johns Hopkins University and Hospital
Baltimore, Maryland
USA
*Chapter 3, Chapter 24, Chapter 27, Chapter 28,
Chapter 31, Chapter 44, Chapter 45, Chapter 49,
Chapter 50, Chapter 83, Chapter 99*

J. Sebag MD FACS FRCOphth
Professor of Clinical Ophthalmology
Doheny Eye Institute
University of Southern California
California, USA
Chapter 114

Johanna M. Seddon MD ScM
Associate Professor of Ophthalmology and
Epidemiology
Harvard Medical School
Surgeon in Ophthalmology and Director,
Epidemiology Unit
Massachusetts Eye and Ear Infirmary
Boston, Massachusetts
USA
Chapter 33, Chapter 34, Chapter 58

Sanjay Sharma MD
Assistant Professor, Department of Epidemiology
Queen's University
Hotel Dieu Hospital
Kingston, Ontario
Canada
Chapter 25, Chapter 46, Chapter 69, Chapter 84

Val C. Sheffield MD
Professor and Investigator
Department of Pediatrics
Howard Hughes Medical Institute
Iowa City, Iowa
USA
Chapter 16

Carol L. Shields MD
Associate Director, Oncology Service
Wills Eye Hospital
Professor of Ophthalmology
Thomas Jefferson University
Philadelphia
USA
Chapter 26, Chapter 46

Jerry A. Shields MD
Director, Oncology Service
Wills Eye Hospital
Professor of Ophthalmology
Thomas Jefferson University
Philadelphia
USA
Chapter 26, Chapter 29, Chapter 36, Chapter 46

Arun Singh MD
Director, Department of Ophthalmic Oncology
Cole Eye Institute
Cleveland Clinic Foundation
Cleveland, Ohio
USA
Chapter 50

Raymond N. Sjaarda MD
Retina Specialists
Baltimore, Maryland
USA
Chapter 148

Jason S. Slakter MD
Vitreous-Retina-Macula Consultants of New York
Clinical Professor of Ophthalmology
New York University School of Medicine
New York
USA
Chapter 53

Vivianne C. Smith PhD
Emeritus Professor
Department of Ophthalmology Visual Science
The University of Chicago
Chicago, Illinois
USA
Chapter 10

Ronald E. Smith MD
Professor and Chair
Department of Ophthalmology
Keck School of Medicine
University of Southern California
Los Angeles, California
USA
Chapter 95

Sharon D. Solomon MD
Assistant Professor of Ophthalmology
Vitreo-retinal and Retinal Vascular Services
Wilmer Ophthalmologic Institute
Johns Hopkins University School of Medicine
Baltimore, Maryland
USA
Chapter 99

Gisele Soubrane MD PhD FEBO
Professor and Chair
Clinique Ophthalmologique Universitaire de Creteil
University Paris XII-Val de Marne
Creteil
France
Chapter 62

Rand Spencer MD
Clinical Associate Professor
University of Texas Southwestern Medical School
Dallas, Texas
USA
Chapter 80

Paul Sternberg, Jr. MD
GW Hale Professor and Chair
Vanderbilt Eye Institute
Nashville, Tennessee
USA
Chapter 23, Chapter 140

Jay M. Stewart MD
Clinical Instructor in Ophthalmology
Doheny Retina Institute
Los Angeles, California
USA
Chapter 126

Edwin M. Stone MD PhD
Professor of Ophthalmology
The Carver College of Medicine
HHMI Investigator, Howard Hughes Medical
Institute
The University of Iowa
Iowa City, Iowa
USA
Chapter 16

Ilene K. Sugino MA
Institute of Ophthalmology and Visual Science
New Jersey Medical School
University of Medicine and Dentistry
Newark, New Jersey
USA
Chapter 153

Janet S. Sunness MD
Medical Director
Hoover Vision Services
Greater Baltimore Medical Center
Townson, Maryland
USA
Chapter 18, Chapter 19, Chapter 72

Yasuo Tano MD
Professor and Chairman
Department of Ophthalmology
Osaka University Medical School
Osaka
Japan
Chapter 124

William S. Tasman MD
Ophthalmologist-in-Chief
Wills Eye Hospital
Professor and Chairman
Department of Ophthalmology
Jefferson Medical College
Philadelphia, Pennsylvania
USA
Chapter 123

Matthew A. Thomas MD
Associate Clinical Professor of Ophthalmology
Department of Ophthalmology and Visual Sciences
Washington University
Barnes Retina Institute
St. Louis, Missouri
USA
Chapter 149

John T. Thompson MD
Partner, Retina Specialists and
Assistant Professor
The Wilmer Institute
The Johns Hopkins University
Baltimore, Maryland
USA
Chapter 117, Chapter 135, Chapter 148

Jennifer E. Thorne MD
Assistant Professor of Ophthalmology
Division of Ocular Immunology
Wilmer Eye Institute
The Johns Hopkins University
Baltimore, Maryland
USA
Chapter 75

Gabriele Thumann MD
Department of Ophthalmology
University of Cologne
Cologne
Germany
Chapter 7

Cynthia A. Toth MD
Associate Professor of Ophthalmology and
Biomedical Engineering
Duke University Eye Center
Durham, North Carolina
USA
Chapter 152

Michael T. Trese MD
Associate Retinal Consultant
Clinical Professor of Biomedical Sciences
Eye Research Institute
Oakland University
Royal Oak, Michigan
USA
Chapter 144

Linda M. Tsai MD
Assistant Professor
Department of Ophthalmology and Visual Sciences
Washington University
St Louis, Missouri
USA
Chapter 102

Patricia L. Turner MD
Department of Ophthalmology
University of Kansas Medical Center
Kansas City, Kansas
USA
Chapter 109

Timothy H. Tweito MD
Clinical Assistant Professor
Department of Ophthalmology
The Ohio State University School of Medicine
Columbus, Ohio
USA
Chapter 37

Paul G. Updike MS
Instructor
Department of Ophthalmology
Keck School of Medicine
University of Southern California
Los Angeles, California
USA
Chapter 52

Russell N. Van Gelder MD PhD
Associate Professor
Department of Ophthalmology and Visual Sciences
Department of Molecular Biology and
Pharmacology
Washington University School of Medicine
St Louis, Missouri
USA
Chapter 93, Chapter 134

Janneke J. C. van Lith-Verhoeven MD PhD
Department of Ophthalmology
UMCN St Radboud
Netherlands
Chapter 64

Jean D. Vaudaux MD
Department of Ophthalmology
Jules Gonin Eye Hospital
Lausanne University
Lausanne
Switzerland
Chapter 91

Franck Villain PhD
Assistant Professor
Department of Biomedical Engineering
University of Miami College of Engineering
Coral Gables, Florida
and Scientific Director
Corneal SA,
Paris
France
Chapter 129

Albert T. Vitale MD
Associate Professor
Department of Ophthalmology and Visual Sciences
John A Moran Eye Center
Salt Lake City, Utah
USA
Chapter 98

Jonathan D. Walker MD
Clinical Assistant Professor
Indiana University School of Medicine
Fort Wayne, Indiana
USA
Chapter 101

Alexander C. Walsh MD
Assistant Professor
Doheny Eye Institute
Keck School of Medicine
University of Southern California
Los Angeles, California
USA
Chapter 52

Hao Wang MD MA
Institute of Ophthalmology and Visual Science
New Jersey Medical School
University of Medicine and Dentistry
Newark, New Jersey
USA
Chapter 153

Andrew R.Webster MA FRCOphth MD
Honorary Consultant Ophthalmologist
Moorfields Eye Hospital
London
UK
Chapter 16

James D. Weiland PhD
Assistant Professor of Ophthalmology and
Biomedical Engineering
Doheny Eye Institute
Keck School of Medicine
University of Southern California
Los Angeles, California
USA
Chapter 154

John J. Weiter MD PhD
Associate Clinical Professor in Ophthalmology
Harvard Medical School
Associate Clinical Professor in Ophthalmology
Tufts University School of Medicine
Retina Specialists of Boston
Boston, Massachusetts
USA
Chapter 21

Richard G. Weleber MD
Professor of Ophthalmology and Molecular and
Medical Genetics
Casey Eye Institute
Oregon Health Sciences University
Portland, Oregon
USA
Chapter 17

Moody D. Wharam, Jr. MD FACR
Willard and Lillian Hackerman
Professor of Radiation Oncology
Department of Radiation Oncology and Molecular
Radiation Sciences
Sidney Kimmel Comprehensive Cancer Center
Johns Hopkins University
Baltimore, Maryland
USA
Chapter 45

A. Jeffrey Whitehead MD
Ophthalmology Fellow of Retina
University of Wisconsin
Madison, Wisconsin
USA
Chapter 149

Peter Wiedemann MD
Professor and Chair
Augenklinik
UniversitatKinkum Leipzig
Leipzig
Germany
Chapter 145

C. P. Wilkinson MD
Chairman
Department of Ophthalmology,
Greater Baltimore Medical Center
Professor, Department of Ophthalmology
Johns Hopkins University School of Medicine
Baltimore, Maryland
USA
Chapter 90, Chapter 122

George A. Williams MD
Chair, Department of Ophthalmology
Director, Beaumont Eye Institute
Royal Oak, Michigan
USA
Chapter 118

James K. V. Willson MD
Director, Harold C Simmonds Comprehensive
Cancer Center
University of Texas Southwestern Medical Center
Dallas, Texas
USA
Chapter 43

David J. Wilson MD
Professor, Department of Ophthalmology
Director, Christensen Eye Pathology Laboratory
Oregon Health and Sciences University
Casey Eye Institute
Portland, Orgeon
USA
Chapter 48

Peter H. Win MD
Resident
Department of Ophthalmology
Mayo Clinic
Rochester, Minnesota
USA
Chapter 139

Lawrence A. Yannuzzi MD
Vitreous-Retina-Macula Consultants of New York
New York, New York
USA
Chapter 53, Chapter 63, Chapter 86

Young Hee Yoon MD
Professor, Department of Ophthalmology
Asan Medical Center
University of Ulsan, College of Medicine
Seoul
Korea
Chapter 138

Tara A. Young MD
Retina Division
Co-Director Ophthalmic Oncology Center
Jules Stein Eye Institute
University of California, Los Angeles
Los Angeles, California
USA
Chapter 33, Chapter 34, Chapter 141

Marco A. Zarbin MD PhD FACS
Professor and Chair
Institute of Ophthalmology and Visual Science
New Jersey Medical School
University of Medicine and Dentistry
Newark, New Jersey
USA
Chapter 153

Kang Zhang MD PhD
Assistant Professor of Ophthalmology
University of Utah School of Medicine
Salt Lake City, Utah
USA
Chapter 18

Dedication

The fourth edition of *Retina* is dedicated to all of the clinicians and scientists who have contributed to the education of medical students, residents, and fellows.

The second edition included a special dedication to

Ronald G. Michels (1942-1991),

who was vitally involved in the planning of the original edition and in the recruitment of our initial team of editors and authors. Ron was an enthusiastic and talented leader in vitreoretinal surgery, and his teaching efforts had a major impact on the other editors of *Retina* and on ophthalmology. We will always be thankful for the privilege of having known and worked with Ron.

For the third edition, we offered an additional special dedication to

A. Edward Maumenee (1913-1998),

who was a true giant who influenced virtually every field and subspecialty in ophthalmology. Although most of his later contributions involved anterior segment surgery, his original observations regarding macular degeneration provided a basis for subsequent clinical and research investigations in this area. Most important, as a gifted teacher, relentless investigator, and valued mentor, Ed inspired the editors and may authors of this textbook, as well as a multitude of academicians and clinicians around the world.

For the fourth edition, we add a special dedication to

Arnall Patz

who was an editor of the original edition. Arnall was a true pioneer and leader in the establishment of the field of medical retina. He founded the Retinal Vascular Center at the Wilmer Institute and, subsequently, he became the Director of the Wilmer Institute. He trained many of today's leaders in the field and many contributing authors to *Retina*. Arnall is an inspiration for the multitude of retinal specialists around the world.

Foreword

Each year, more than 1 200 000 articles in 16 000 journals produced by 2 000 publishers present new information in the biomedical and technological sciences related to medicine. Relevant to the retina, a crescendo of discovery has revealed the intricate cell biology and molecular engineering that create, maintain and regulate neuronal, glial and vascular cells. Paradoxically, from the vast quantity of new information and seemingly disconnected facts emerge the rational explanations of retinal function and the molecular pathophysiology of retinal disease.

Technological progress in physical sciences and applications of mathematics have advanced retinal information management, biometric devices and imaging capabilities. Also reflecting progress are the burgeoning prowess of micromechanical surgical systems, computerized laser therapy and precisely tailored molecular agents. Cumulatively, biology and technology are altering clinical assessment of the retina and therapeutic intervention at a meteoric pace.

In *Retina*, Stephen J. Ryan and Co-Editors present an encyclopaedic distillation of basic biology and diagnostic-therapeutic intervention. Volume I depicts biology, inherited disease and oncology. Volume II contains a cohesive treatise on medical retina with emphasis on inflammatory, vascular and metabolic disease. Surgical therapy of the retina, the subject of Volume III, includes sections on management of retinal detachment, utilization of surgical adjuncts and treatment of ocular trauma.

Substantively enhancing *Retina*, authors for the individual chapters are recognized authorities. As a result, the chapters present factual information as well as an overriding expert perspective. Throughout the three volumes, each chapter is complete "packet." However, like the separate "Kleinrock packets" that convey pieces of information on the Internet, the message of *Retina* is truly complete when the packets of basic, medical and surgical information are joined in a seamless continuum.

Bradley R. Straatsma
Jules Stein Eye Institute
University of California at Los Angeles
2005

Preface

Retinal specialists, both clinicians and scientists, share a common fascination with the retina, a truly unique tissue. The retina forms the anatomic and physiologic basis for the gift of sight and supplies over 30% of the sensory input to the brain. These three volumes summarize current knowledge about the retina. Chapter topics range from fundamental concepts of molecular biology and genetics to the principles of pharmacologic and surgical therapy. Volume I includes the basic science research that provides the foundation for our understanding of the pathogenesis of retinal disease and includes reviews of genetics, ultrasonography, and inherited retinal disorders including retinitis pigmentosa. The second part of volume I deals with ocular oncology. Volume II describes medical conditions of the retina, including major diseases affecting the macula and retinal vasculature. There is a particular emphasis on macular degeneration and diabetic retinopathy and many other common diseases. Volume III addresses surgical diseases of the vitreous and retina. Cell biology of various disease states and the principles of surgical treatment are emphasized.

Many of us believe that the human retina is not only essential to sight and the most accessible aspect of the brain for neuroscience, but, in addition, may be the most beautiful tissue in nature. We hope the reader will enjoy and appreciate the figures which illustrate the text.

The 156 chapters are authored by internationally recognized leaders in visual science, ophthalmology, and vitreoretinal surgery and provide a thorough compilation of our current knowledge about the retina. However, the field of retina is so broad and the evolution of knowledge so rapid that the work cannot be comprehensive. The information is current at the time of printing. Fortunately, research is constantly expanding our knowledge of these topics.

We have a series of 18 new chapters reflecting our advances in the sciences, technology and clinical medicine as applied to our specialty – the retina. In addition to these 18 new chapters, we have welcomed new contributing authors to this edition and we particularly appreciate the updated current chapters provided by colleagues who have contributed to the previous editions.

As a multiauthored text, there are multiple literary styles. The editors have worked to provide a level of conformity and scientific balance without sacrificing the originality and style of the individual authors. A distinctive and attractive feature of *Retina* is the diversity of its many outstanding contributors in addition to their leadership in the field.

The editors gratefully acknowledge the support of the faculties and staff of The Wilmer Eye Institute and the Doheny Eye Institute who contributed greatly to the completion of this project. Others who contributed substantially to the quality of these volumes include Timothy Hengst, whose artistic talent is displayed in the illustrations. We thank office staffs of the individual authors and editors and, in particular, Sharon Henry and Joy Roque, who contributed tremendously to this effort.

S.J.R
D.R.H
A.P.S
C.P.W
2005

Contents

Volume 2

Medical Retina

Volume 3

Surgical Retina

Fluorescein Angiography: Basic Principles and Interpretation

Robert N. Johnson
H. Richard McDonald
Everett Ai
J. Michael Jumper
Arthur D. Fu

For over 35 years, fundus photography and fluorescein angiography have been extremely valuable for expanding our knowledge of the anatomy, pathology, and pathophysiology of the retina and choroid, and have aided the diagnosis and monitoring of the treatment of retinal vascular and macular diseases. Initially, fluorescein angiography was used primarily as a laboratory and clinical research tool; only later was it used for diagnosis of fundus diseases. Although fluorescein angiography now fulfills many roles, it is most often used as a guide to laser treatment of retinal vascular and choroidal diseases, and as a means of evaluating that treatment. An understanding and an ability to interpret a fluorescein angiogram is essential in order to accurately evaluate, diagnose, and treat patients with retinal vascular and macular disease.

The first part of this chapter discusses the basic principles of fluorescein angiography and the equipment and techniques needed to produce a high-quality angiogram. Potential side effects and complications of fluorescein injection are also discussed. The second part focuses on the interpretation of fluorescein angiography, including fundus anatomy and histology, the normal fluorescein angiogram, and abnormal fundus fluorescence.

BASIC PRINCIPLES

In order to understand fluorescein angiography, one must have knowledge of fluorescence. Likewise, to understand fluorescence, one must know the principles of luminescence.

Luminescence is the emission of light from any source other than high temperature. Luminescence occurs when energy in the form of electromagnetic radiation is absorbed and then re-emitted at another frequency. When light energy is absorbed into a luminescent material, free electrons are elevated into higher energy states. This energy is then re-emitted by spontaneous decay of the electrons into their lower energy states. When this decay occurs in the visible spectrum, it is called luminescence. Luminescence, therefore, always entails a shift from a shorter wavelength to a longer wavelength. The shorter wavelengths represent higher energy; the longer wavelengths, lower energy.

Fluorescence is luminescence that is maintained only by continuous excitation. In other words, excitation at one wavelength occurs and is emitted immediately through a longer wavelength. Emission stops at once when the excitation stops. Fluorescence thus does not have an afterglow. A typical example of fluores-

cence is television. In the television tube, the excitation radiation is the electron beam from the cathode-ray tube. This beam excites the phosphors of the screen, which re-emit the beam as a glow that constitutes a television picture.

Sodium fluorescein is a hydrocarbon that responds to light energy between 465 and 490 nm and will fluoresce at a wavelength of 520 to 530 nm. The excitation wavelength, the type that is absorbed and changed, is blue; the resultant fluorescence, or emitted wavelength, is green-yellow. If blue light between 465 to 490 nm is directed to unbound sodium fluorescein, it will emit a light that appears green-yellow (520 to 530 nm).

This is a fundamental principle of fluorescein angiography. In the procedure, the patient, whose eyes have been dilated, is seated behind the fundus camera in which a blue filter has been placed in front of the flash. Fluorescein is then injected intravenously. Eighty percent of the fluorescein becomes bound to protein and is not available for fluorescence, but 20% remains free in the bloodstream and is available for fluorescence. The blue flash of the fundus camera excites the unbound fluorescein within the blood vessels or the fluorescein that has leaked out of the blood vessels. The blue filter shields out (reflects or absorbs) all other light and allows through only the blue excitation light. The blue light then changes those structures in the eye containing fluorescein to green-yellow light at 520 to 530 nm. In addition, blue light is reflected off the fundus structures that do not contain fluorescein. The blue reflected light and the green-yellow fluorescent light are directed back toward the film of the fundus camera. Just in front of the film a filter is placed that allows the green-yellow fluorescent light through but keeps out the blue reflected light. Therefore, the only light that penetrates the filter is true fluorescent light (Fig. 51-1).

Pseudofluorescence occurs when nonfluorescent light passes through the entire filter system. If green-yellow light penetrates the original blue filter, it will pass through the entire system. If blue light reflected from nonfluorescent fundus structures penetrates the green-yellow filter, pseudofluorescence will occur (Fig. 51-2). Pseudofluorescence, i.e. fake fluorescence, causes nonfluorescent structures to appear fluorescent. It can confuse the physician interpreting the fluorescein angiogram and lead him or her to think that certain fundus structures or materials are fluorescing when they are not. Pseudofluorescence also causes decreased contrast, as well as decreased resolution. Because fluorescein angiography

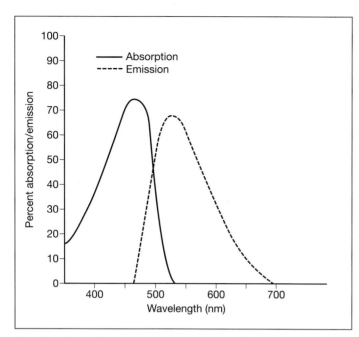

Fig. 51-1 Absorption and emission curves of sodium fluorescein dye. The peak absorption (excitation) is at 420 to 430 nm (blue light). The peak emission occurs at 465 to 590 nm (yellow-green light).

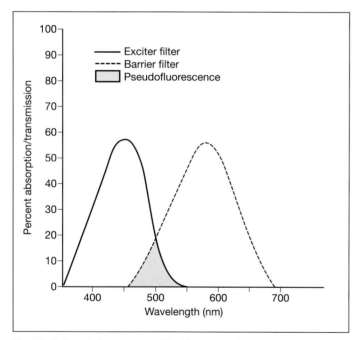

Fig. 51-2 Pseudofluorescence. The blue exciter filter overlaps into the yellow-green zone, and the yellow-green barrier filter overlaps into the blue zone. The combination results in pseudofluorescence.

is done with black-and-white film, the nonfluorescent or pseudofluorescent light appears as a background illumination. The background illumination from pseudofluorescence is especially heightened if there are white areas of the fundus, such as highly reflective, hard exudates. It is important that pseudofluorescence be avoided. Therefore, the excitation (blue) and barrier (green-

yellow) filters should be carefully matched so that there is a minimal overlap of light between them.

Sodium fluorescein, Na orange-red crystalline hydrocarbon ($C_{20}H_{12}O_5Na$), has a low molecular weight (376.27 daltons) and readily diffuses through most of the body fluids and through the choriocapillaris, but it does not diffuse through the retinal vascular endothelium or the pigment epithelium. Fluorescein is eliminated by the liver and kidneys within 24 hours, although traces may be found in the body for up to a week after injection. Retention may increase if renal function is impaired. The skin will have a yellowish tinge for a few hours following injection, and the urine will take on a characteristic yellow-orange color for most of the first day following injection.

EQUIPMENT

Because fluorescein angiography is a highly technical form of ophthalmic photography, it requires sophisticated equipment. We currently utilize both digital and film angiography.

The equipment and materials needed for film-based angiography are the following:

1. Fundus camera and auxiliary equipment.
2. Two camera backs (one with motor drive and a timer).
3. Matched fluorescein filters (barrier and exciter).
4. 35-mm black-and-white film.
5. 35-mm color film.
6. 23-gauge scalp-vein needle.
7. 5-ml syringe.
8. 5 ml of 10% fluorescein solution.
9. 20-gauge, 1½ inch needle to draw the dye.
10. Armrest for fluorescein injection.
11. Tourniquet.
12. Alcohol swabs.
13. Bandage.
14. Standard emergency equipment.

Camera and auxiliary equipment

A fundus camera should be easy to use, dependable, and capable of producing an excellent angiogram. Reliable service is an important consideration when selecting a fundus camera. The currently available brands of fundus cameras have many intricate mechanical and electrical components, and the physician must have a dependable source of servicing.

Most of the various brands of fundus cameras currently available for fluorescein angiography will produce well-resolved photographs when the media are clear, though some cameras are superior to others. Only a few yield well-resolved photographs when the photographic situation is not ideal, such as with a small pupil, hazy media, poor circulation, irregular or extreme refractive problems, or an uncooperative patient.

Cameras differ in the degree of fundus area included in the photographs. Most fundus cameras can take 30-degree photographs, which are extremely useful for highly magnified, well-resolved macular detail. Some cameras can also take 60-degree (or more) photographs that are reasonably well resolved, but the

60-degree format is most useful for fundus problems in which the pathology includes a large area of the fundus. The 30-degree camera is essential for macular problems, especially when laser treatment is to be done, as with background diabetic retinopathy, branch vein occlusion, or choroidal neovascularization.

Flash unit and power pack

The power pack should recharge rapidly enough to allow angiophotographs to be taken at a rate of one every 1 or 1½ seconds. Although, in most cases, photographs taken at 2-second intervals are satisfactory, it is useful to have the option of more rapid-sequence photography.

In our experience, we have found, however, the power pack to be a very fragile component. Because we depend on quick, reliable angiograms, we have a second power pack in reserve. It takes only minutes to remove and replace the inoperable power pack. An alternative power pack saves the physician the expense of a second camera.

Camera backs

Two 35-mm camera backs should be available: one with color film for regular color fundus photography and one with black-and-white film for fluorescein angiography. The latter camera should be equipped with a motor drive and timer (Fig. 51-3). Because of their many electrical and mechanical parts, when cameras are used a great deal they can break down, becoming jammed, not flash appropriately, or overflash. Backup cameras are essential in any busy angiography unit.

Motor drive

Although an optional accessory, a motor-driven camera has two important advantages. First, the motor drive advances the film automatically without the photographer having to move the camera, alter its position, or change its alignment. Second, the motor drive

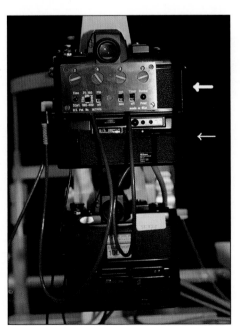

Fig. 51-3 Two camera backs. The top camera back, for black-and-white film for fluorescein angiography, is equipped with a motor drive (small arrow) and a timer that marks the film (large arrow). The lower camera is for color fundus photography.

advances the film rapidly. This is particularly important during the initial phase of the angiogram when dye begins to enter the eye (transit phase) and the photographs should be taken no more than 2 seconds apart.

Timer

A timer in a data-back records on each frame the exact length of time from the beginning of the fluorescein injection to the particular frame. In many cases, the specific timing of fluorescein filling is not an important issue, but in other situations, as when there is a question of reduced arterial perfusion pressure, a timer is indispensable.

Stereophotography

Some cameras are equipped with an optional accessory, a stereo separator. The separator automatically shoots stereophotographic pairs. Many consider this attachment a luxury, and the photographer must be reasonably skilled and experienced to use it properly. Another reservation is that it is unnecessary for every photograph in the angiographic study needs to belong to a stereo pair. If there is at least one good stereo pair of fluorescein photographs for each important fundus structure, sufficient information will be available to determine the histopathologic locations of various angiographic abnormalities.

Matched fluorescein filters

Fluorescein angiography uses both exciter and barrier filters. The exciter filter must transmit blue light at 465 to 490 nm, the absorption peak of fluorescein excitation. The barrier filter transmits light at 525 to 530 nm, the fluorescent, or emitted, peak of fluorescein. The filters should allow maximal transmission of light in the proper spectral range to achieve a good image without the use of an excessively powerful flash unit. Most new cameras come with filters. When choosing a camera, one should request the transmission curves of the filter combination to be sure that no significant overlap exists. In cases where there is overlap, pseudofluorescence will result.

After several years, filters become thin, emitting more light and increasing the incidence and degree of pseudofluorescence. The clinician should always check the control photograph of each angiogram for excessive pseudofluorescence. When pseudofluorescence reduces the quality of the angiophotograph, the filters should be replaced.

Light sources (viewing bulb and flash strobe)

These bulbs burn out, but it is easy to replace them. A supply of each should always be kept on hand (Fig. 51-4).

Film

The most frequently used film in the United States for fluorescein angiography is Tri-X black-and-white film (TX 135-36, ISO 400). Black-and-white film with an ASA of 400 is sufficiently light-sensitive to compensate for camera flash units that are not excessively powerful.

For color fundus photography, we use Kodak Ektachrome 100.

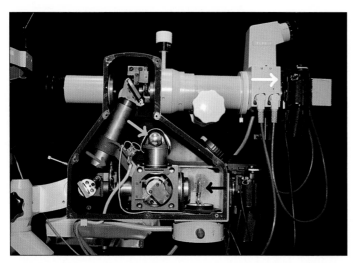

Fig. 51-4 Fundus camera with side-wall removed to view inside parts. Yellow arrow, Viewing bulb; black arrow, flash bulb; red arrow, exciter filter wheel. The light from the flash goes through the system in this photograph from right to left. The light is reflected off a mirror and travels upward to another mirror; it is then reflected to the left, into the patient's eye. From there it is reflected directly to the right of the fluorescein camera back (white arrow).

Developing the film

Developing time of the black-and-white film depends on the power of the strobe and the temperature concentration and type of developing solution. The lower the flash power and the longer the developing time, the higher will be the contrast of the film. However, the longer the developing time, the longer the photographer must spend in the darkroom. Also, with increased contrast, resolution is decreased.

In our laboratory, we have switched to an automated developer. This improves work flow, and allows the photographer to continue photographing rather than monitoring the process of developing the film (Fig. 51-5).

Printing

After the film is developed, the negatives can be contact-printed onto either film (transparency) or paper (print). Contacts are

made by cutting and arranging the roll of 36 frames onto six rows of six frames each (Fig. 51-6). On the negatives, fluorescence appears black, and on positive film or paper it is white. The negative, contact print, and positive transparency can each be interpreted, or "read," with a magnifying lens or stereo viewer instead of enlarging individual photographic frames of the angiogram. The enlarged photographs are impressive, but the process is time-consuming and expensive and the enlargements are unnecessary for the purpose of diagnosis.

Positive transparencies are valuable for making 35-mm slides to use for projection. In our laboratory, we use Kodak Kodalith film type 3, no. 2556, for positive transparencies. Individual frames can be cut from the 8 × 10 contact sheet of Kodalith film and mounted onto 35-mm slide mounts for projection.

To make contact prints, we use Agfa-Gevaert Rapidoprint or Kodak Ektamatic SC paper with a stabilization processor. In the absence of a stabilization processor, standard black-and-white enlarging paper can be used.

Fluorescein solution

Solutions containing 500 mg of fluorescein are available in vials of 10 ml of 5% fluorescein or 5 ml of 10% fluorescein. Also available are 3 ml of 25% fluorescein solution (750 mg). The greater the volume, the longer the injection time will be, the smaller the volume, the more likely a significant percentage of fluorescein will remain in the venous dead space between the arm and the heart (see "Injecting the fluorescein," p. 880). For this reason, we prefer 5 ml of 10% solution (500 mg fluorescein).

TECHNIQUE

Aligning camera and photographing

To align the fundus camera properly, the photographer must first assess the "field of the eye." The camera is equipped with a joystick with which the photographer can adjust the camera laterally and for depth. The camera is also equipped with a knob for vertical

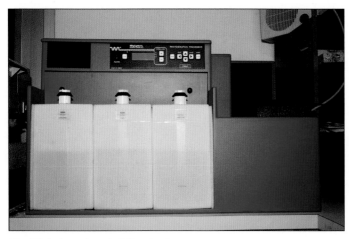

Fig. 51-5 An automated film developer.

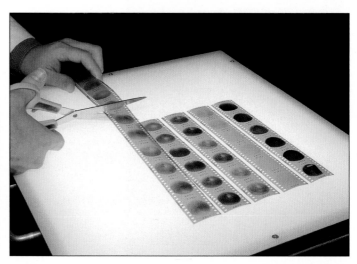

Fig. 51-6 Cutting the negatives. The negatives are cut into rows of six frames, unless doing so would break-up a stereo pair. In that case, a row should be cut after five frames.

adjustment. The photographer finds the red fundus reflex, which is an even, round sharply defined pink or red light reflex. If the camera is too close to the eye, a hazy, poorly contrasted photograph will result. If the camera is too far away, a bright, crescent-shaped light reflex will appear at the edge of the viewing screen, or a bright spot will appear at its center.

The photographer moves the camera from side to side to ascertain the width of the pupil and the focusing peculiarities of the particular cornea and lens. The photographer studies the eye through the camera lens, moving the camera back and forth, and up and down, looking for fundus details (e.g. retinal blood vessels). The photographer then determines the single best position from which to photograph (Figs 51-7 and 51-8).

Occasionally, the patient will have a peculiar corneal reflex or a central lens opacity, and the usual procedure of aligning the camera through the central axis of the eye may not be possible. Moving the camera slightly off axis may help improve focus and resolution.

Any abnormalities, such as an unusual light reflex or a poorly resolved image, which the photographer sees through the camera system, will appear on the photograph. If the ophthalmoscopic view seen through the camera is not optimal, the photograph will not be optimal (Fig. 51-9). If the view is optimal, well-aligned, in focus, and without reflexes, the photograph *can* be optimal. A helpful concept for the photographer is "what you see is what you get (or worse, never better)."

Focusing

Achieving perfect focus is a major factor in the photographic process. The eyepiece crosshairs and the fundus details must both

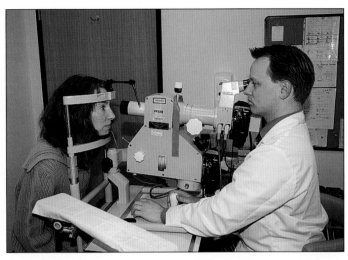

Fig. 51-8 The patient's head is kept steady in the chinrest and headrest of the fundus camera. The photographer aligns the fundus camera and focuses on the patient's right fundus. Each is in a comfortable position, which facilitates the stability necessary to achieve a good fluorescein angiogram.

be in sharp focus to obtain a well-resolved photograph. The proper position of the eyepiece is determined by the refractive error of the photographer and the degree to which he or she accommodates while focusing the camera.

The photographer first turns the eyepiece counterclockwise (toward the plus, or hyperopic, range) to relax his own accommodation. This will cause the crosshairs to blur. The photographer then turns the eyepiece slowly clockwise to bring the crosshairs into sharp focus. The eyepiece is focused properly when the crosshairs appear sharp and clear (Fig. 51-10). They must remain perfectly clear while the photographer focuses on the fundus with the camera's focusing detail. With experience, the photographer becomes expert in adjusting the eyepiece and in keeping the crosshairs in focus throughout the entire photographic sequence.

The best position for the eyepiece is the point at which the crosshairs are in focus while the photographer's accommodation is relaxed. Photographers learn to relax accommodation by keeping both eyes open. The photographer focuses the eyepiece with one eye and, with the other eye, keeps a distant object, such as the eye chart, in sharp focus. This skill may be difficult for technicians without ophthalmic training, but it is seldom impossible to learn.

Keeping the crosshairs in sharp focus, the photographer then turns the focusing dial on the camera to focus the fundus detail. Some photographers focus the crosshairs just once at the beginning of each day and control their accommodation throughout the day. This is not a good idea because the photographer's accommodation may change during a photographic session; the photographer should be aware of this possibility and regularly check and readjust the eyepiece for focus. With the camera properly aligned and focused, the photographer is ready to start the preliminary photographs and angiograms.

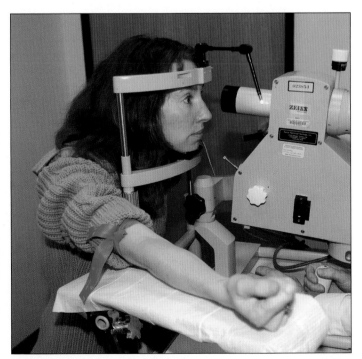

Fig. 51-7 The patient's arm rests on an adjustable armrest that is elevated so that the patient's arm is at or above the level of her heart. The armrest also facilitates easy placement of the intravenous needle and injection of fluorescein.

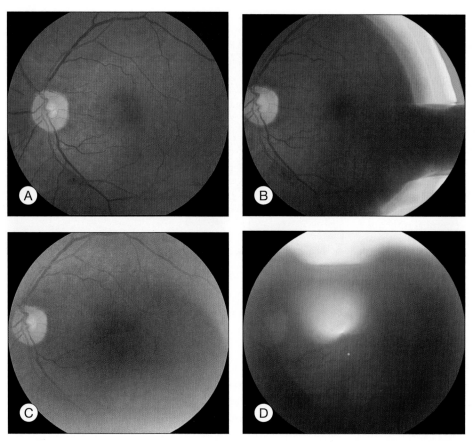

Fig. 51-9 Fundus photograph and reflexes. A, Photograph of right fundus without reflexes. The camera was properly aligned and focused. B, In this case the camera was placed at the proper distance from the fundus but was placed too far to one side (to the right), which allowed the bright white arc reflex on the right side. C, The saturation of the fundus details is poor. In this case the camera was in proper alignment but was placed too close to the patient's eye. D, Note the bright reflex in the photograph. The camera was properly aligned but was placed too far from the patient's eye.

Digital angiography

The resolution of digital angiography has improved substantially and currently it functions for us as an excellent and convenient alternative to film. The instantaneous imaging facilitates prompt diagnosis and management of retinal disorders. Digital angiography offers several advantages including the instantaneous availability of the angiogram, and the avoidance of the equipment and time necessary to develop film. Moreover, digital angiography facilitates discussions with the patient concerning their condition and possible treatment options. Also, digital angiography facilitates training of ophthalmic personnel. We have found that it is useful

to stay in the room during the initial frames of the angiogram to ensure that the desired pathology is photographed. Any changes can be promptly made, and the photographer can also learn from this instantaneous feedback. Digital angiography, however, necessitates a larger initial investment of money. Also, some artifacts can occur. Specifically, some areas may appear overly hyperfluorescent due to limited dynamic range of the chip in the digital camera. This has improved significantly, but one needs to be aware of this possibility when interpreting a digital angiogram.

Using stereophotography

Stereophotography separates, photographically, the tissues of the eye for the observer. Stereo fluorescein angiography facilitates interpretation by separating in depth the retinal and choroidal circulation. Stereo angiography is considered absolutely essential by many authorities in certain situations. The photographic protocol for the Macular Photocoagulation Study required stereo fluorescein angiography. Without well-resolved stereo images, interpretation of angiograms with, for instance, choroidal neovascularization associated with age-related macular degeneration, can be extremely difficult, some may even argue, impossible. On the other hand, stereophotography, although extremely helpful in cases difficult to interpret, is not always absolutely necessary because other fundus features and characteristics usually indicate the level at which abnormal fluorescence is located.

Adequate stereo photographs can be achieved with a pupillary dilation of 4 mm, although dilation of 6 mm or more is best. The

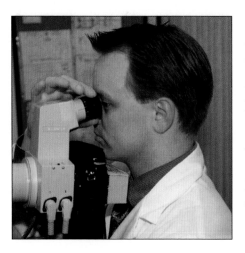

Fig. 51-10 The photographer focuses the eyepiece of the camera by initially turning the eyepiece counterclockwise, then clockwise, and stopping when it is in exact focus. The photographer must be sure that the eyepiece crosshairs remain in perfect focus throughout the photographic procedure.

first photograph of any stereo pair is taken with the camera positioned as far to the photographer's right (the patient's left) of the pupil's center as possible (of course, without inducing reflexes). The second photograph of the stereo pair is taken with the camera held as far to the photographer's left (the patient's right) of the pupil's center as possible. This order is extremely important because the photographs are taken and positioned on the film so that the angiogram is read from right to left. Thus, the first photograph in the stereo sequence will appear on the right on the contact sheet to correspond with the interpreter's right eye; the second is printed on the left for his or her left eye. It follows, then, that the first view of a stereo pair should be taken from the photographer's right, followed by a view from the left.

Because the roll of 35-mm film with the 36 frames is usually cut into six rows of six frames each, care must be taken not to make a cut between a stereo pair (i.e. when the right stereo view is at the end of a row and the left stereo view is at the beginning of the next row). Reading the stereo pairs on the negatives, contact print, or computer monitor (Fig. 51-11) is done with magnifying lenses (+6 D to l2 D) in front of each eye.

Photographing the periphery

Photographing the peripheral retina with a standard 30-degree fundus camera demands precision and skills acquired only after many hours of practice. Problems with patient position and camera alignment and focus are compounded by marginal corneal astigmatism, unsteadiness of patient fixation, light reflexes, and awkward camera placement. All steps necessary for taking posterior photographs, such as alignment and focusing, must be employed to achieve good peripheral fundus photography. The Zeiss camera comes with an astigmatic dial to help neutralize the induced astigmatism. A tilt mechanism, now standard on most cameras, helps position the camera for extreme superior and inferior peripheral photography (Fig. 51-12).

During photography of the periphery, the patient will tend to turn or move his or her head. Unsatisfactory photographs caused by the movement of the head away from the camera or to the side can be avoided if the photographer is alert to these possibilities and takes the necessary steps to prevent them. On the whole, achieving good peripheral photographs depends on photographic skill, of course, but also on patience on the part of both photographer and patient.

Informing the patient

An important step toward a successful angiogram is to inform the patient about the procedure. An informed patient is generally less anxious and more cooperative than one who is unsure of the situation. Some institutions routinely provide a consent form to be signed by patients who are to have angiograms. This practice, however, cannot replace the physician freely informing the patient about the procedure, potential complications and answering all questions.

The patient should be told that the eyes will be dilated, that sodium fluorescein will be injected in a vein in the arm or back of the hand, and that photographs will be taken. The patient should be assured that the flash is a harmless, bright light (not an X-ray) and that fluorescein dye is safe. The patient should be told that injection of the dye can cause complications but that such occurrences are rare. If the patient requests further details about complications, the physician is obligated to supply the information.

Positioning the patient

Before the patient is seated at the camera, the photographer makes sure that the front lens is free of any dirt or dust. The lens should always be covered by a lens cap when the camera is not in use. The front of the lens should be kept clean using chloroform and a tightly rolled rod of lens tissue. To clean the lens, begin at the center and rotate out to the periphery.

The patient is positioned at the camera with the chin in the chinrest and the forehead against the head bar. Because the most common cause of poor fluorescein photographs is involuntary movement of the patient's head, the photographer should prepare and make adjustment for this before the fluorescein is injected. The photographer should aim and focus the camera on the specific

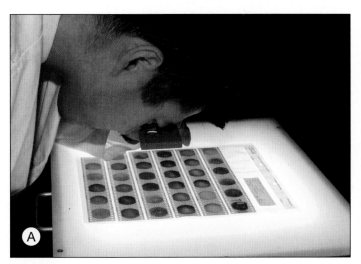
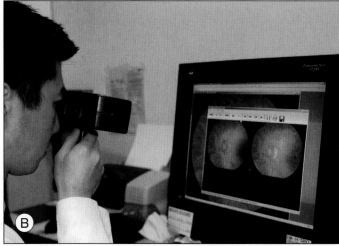

Fig. 51-11 Reading stereo pairs. A, Reading the negatives of the angiogram. B, Reading a stereo pair of digital angiograms. The special viewer allows the observer to focus both images. This software is Ophthalmic Imaging Systems.

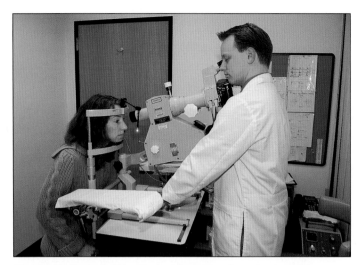

Fig. 51-12 Photographing the periphery. The tilt mechanism of the camera allows the back of the camera to be lifted up (tilted to aim downward) for photography of the inferior periphery. The same tilt mechanism can be used to bring the camera far down (tilted to aim upward) to take pictures of the superior periphery. In photographing the inferior periphery, the photographer must sometimes stand. The photographer or an assistant needs to lift the patient's upper lid in order to properly view the inferior periphery.

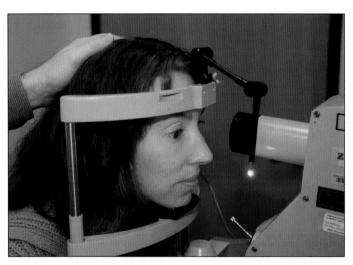

Fig. 51-13 An assistant holds the patient's head as a reminder to the patient to keep his or her chin in the chinrest and forehead against the bar.

area of primary interest, at the same time noting the patient's responses. If the photographer finds that the camera must continually be moved closer to the patient while aligning it or taking preliminary photographs, or if reflexes suddenly appear in the view even though the camera is steady, then the patient's head has moved away from the chinrest. If so, the photographer can make some adjustment before injecting the fluorescein dye. Sometimes having an assistant hold the patient's head in the chinrest is helpful (Fig. 51-13). The photographer may either lower the entire camera and chinrest or raise the patient's chair. This causes the patient to lean forward in the chinrest and against the forehead bar, making it more difficult for the patient to pull back.

Before photography begins, and between shots, the photographer may ask the patient to blink several times. This usually makes the patient more comfortable, and also moistens the cornea and keeps it clear. When the pictures are actually being shot, the patient should be instructed to blink as infrequently as possible.

During the procedure, the photographer should talk to the patient frequently, informing the patient of the progress of the testing, and assuring him or her that all is going well. Explanation and reinforcement help produce better photographs.

Injecting the fluorescein

The color stereoscopic fundus photographs are taken first, before the fluorescein is injected. For injection, we recommend a syringe with a 23-gauge scalp-vein needle (Fig. 51-14). The scalp-vein needle has several advantages: it is small enough to enter most visible veins, and an intravenous opening is then available in the event of an emergency. Once in the vein, it requires no further attention, and although it can be taped in place, there is usually no need to do so. Whenever an antecubital vein is not visible or accessible, the vein in the back of the hand or radial (thumb) side of the wrist can usually be used for injection. Injecting the fluorescein into a hand or wrist vein increases the circulation time by a few seconds, but this seldom makes any difference.

Injection of the fluorescein is coordinated with the photographic process and is done after the first six photographs (identification, red-free, and control photographs; see next section) have been taken. With the needle in place, angiography can begin. By a predetermined, preferably silent signal such as a nod of the head, the photographer indicates to the physician to begin injecting fluorescein. The photographer starts the timer on the camera simultaneously with the start of injection and takes one photograph. This frame will show zero time on the photograph. In this way, the time from the beginning of injection is recorded on each subsequent angiographic photograph. When the injection is finished, the photographer may take another picture, which will show how long the injection took.

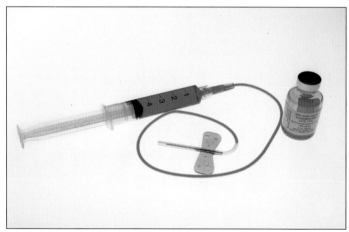

Fig. 51-14 Ten percent fluorescein solution, 5-ml syringe, and 23-gauge scalp-vein needle.

A rapid injection of 2 or 3 seconds delivers a high concentration of fluorescein to the bloodstream for a short time and probably yields somewhat better photographs than does a slower injection. However, the more rapid the injection, the greater is the incidence of nausea from the highly concentrated bolus of fluorescein. For this reason a slower injection (4–6 seconds) is preferable; the photographs will still be of good quality. Because some fluorescein dye will remain in the tubing, the scalp-vein needle should have short, rather than long, tubing to ensure that more of the dye will be injected.

Developing a photographic plan

To photograph and print the fluorescein angiogram, we suggest the following comprehensive plan, designed to yield maximal angiographic information from each fundus and to facilitate a thorough and complete interpretation (Fig. 51-15). Although most angiograms will be complete by following this procedure, there will be exceptions. When abnormalities occur in areas other than the macula and disc, or when laser treatment evaluation is done following an angiogram of only the treated eye, this plan must be modified. A second plan for diabetic retinopathy is discussed in the next section.

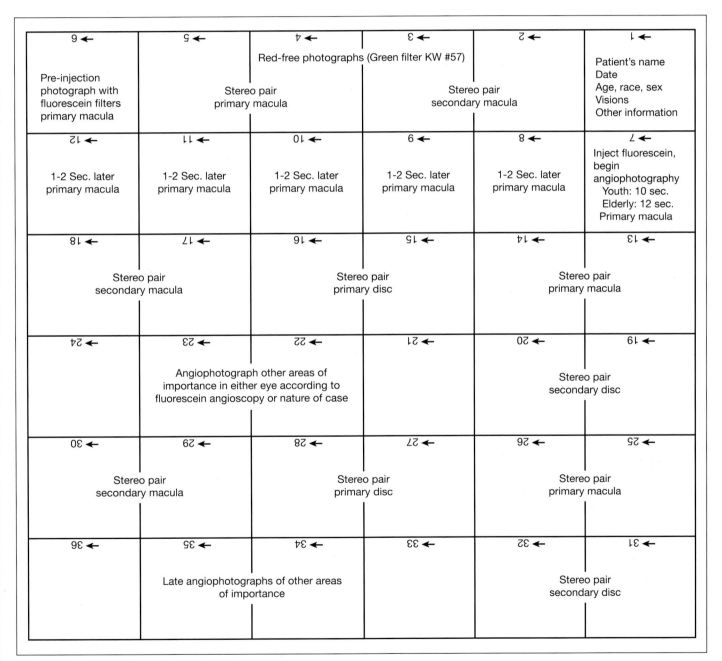

Fig. 51-15 Photographic plan for fluorescein angiography of macular disease. The numbers indicating each of the 36 frames are printed upside down because the fundus camera inverts the image of the fundus, and in order to read the angiogram upright, the film is printed with the frame numbers upside down.

Because the roll of 35-mm negative film used for fluorescein angiography has 36 frames, it is convenient to think of the photograph session in terms of six rows of six frames each. Thus frame 1 will appear in the upper right-hand corner and frame 36 in the lower left-hand corner. The angiogram is read from right to left and from top to bottom.

The first frame of the angiographic series, located in the upper right-hand corner of the assembled contact print, is the identification photograph. This frame includes the patient's name, the date of the angiogram, and other pertinent data (e.g. vision of each eye, patient number, name of referring doctor). For this photograph the photographer switches the camera's diopter knob to the plus (+) position, inserts a green (red-free) filter, and takes a close-up photograph of this information, using the strobe at its lowest power level. The diopter is then switched back to refocusing to the patient's eye. This frame is followed by red-free stereoscopic photographs recording the ophthalmoscopic changes. Stereoscopic views of the primary eye should be included as the fourth and fifth photographs. The sixth frame is taken with the fluorescein filters in place but before fluorescein injection. This "control" photograph checks the dual-filter system for autofluorescence and pseudofluorescence.

At this point the fluorescein injection is begun. The needle is inserted in a vein in the patient's arm, and with a silent signal (as previously mentioned), the photographer turns on the timer simultaneously with the beginning of the injection. Because it is important to observe the site of the needle tip for extravasation of fluorescein, the lights are turned off only at the end of the injection (Fig. 51-16). An alternative method is to turn the lights off after the needle has been inserted in the vein. The person injecting can hold a hand light to observe the fluorescein flow into the vein to be sure extravasation is not occurring. With the lights off, the photographer can become dark-adapted, which allows him or her to be better able to see the flow of fluorescein into the fundus as it occurs. So as not to miss the appearance of fluorescein as it

enters the fundus, the photographer should begin taking the initial-transit fluorescein photographs 8 seconds after the beginning of the injection of the dye if the patient is young and 12 seconds after injection for older patients. This is done so that these early photographs will not miss the appearance of fluorescein as it enters the fundus. Then, at intervals of 1½ to 2 seconds, approximately six photographs should be taken in succession. Costly, sophisticated, photoelectric power units available with current fundus cameras provide fast recharging for rapid sequential photographic capability. These strong power packs are useful as investigative tools but are rarely necessary in most clinical situations, because photographs taken as often as every second are not usually necessary.

If the photographer does not see fluorescein entering and filling the retinal vessels while the six initial-transit photographs are taken, he or she must continue to photograph the fundus until filling takes place and should also check to see why no fluorescein is present. Sometimes, raising the arm into which the fluorescein was injected improves venous flow to the heart and brings fluorescein to the eye.

After the first six initial-transit photographs and approximately 20 to 30 seconds after injection, with sufficient fluorescein concentration in the eye, the photographer should take a stereoscopic pair of photographs of the primary area of interest, followed by a stereoscopic pair of other pertinent areas. For example, in the suggested photographic plan, after stereophotographs of the right macula are taken, stereophotographs of the right disc are taken. The photographer should then photograph in stereo the macula and disc of the fellow eye.

At this point, approximately 1 minute will have elapsed from the time fluorescein was injected. Angioscopy, the viewing of fluorescein in the eye with an ophthalmoscope, can now be performed to see if any other abnormal hyperfluorescent or hypofluorescent areas should be photographed. Angioscopy can be done with either the fundus camera, which is an excellent ophthalmoscope, or with an indirect ophthalmoscope.

The photographer can easily perform camera angioscopy by instructing the patient to follow the fixation light with one eye while the photographer uses the camera and its blue-filtered light to view the patient's other eye. The best way to perform angioscopy with the indirect ophthalmoscope is with a blue exciter filter attachment. A useful filter for this purpose is the Kodak Wratten No. 47, which is easily inserted into a ring on the direct ophthalmoscope and placed in front of its light. The blue light illuminates the patient's fundus and excites the fluorescein in the fundus. The viewer can see the yellow-green fluorescein-containing structures against the blue light reflected off the nonfluorescent structures. A yellow barrier filter, Kodak Wratten No. 12 or No. 15, placed over the eyepieces or on a pair of glasses, eliminates the reflected blue light and allows only the yellowish-green fluorescing light to be seen. Angioscopy can be performed adequately, however, without the use of a barrier filter.

Sometimes the angiogram may be done in a hospital laboratory, where an ophthalmologist is not available and where neither the photographer nor the person giving the injection is trained to perform angioscopy. In this case, the ophthalmologist may perform

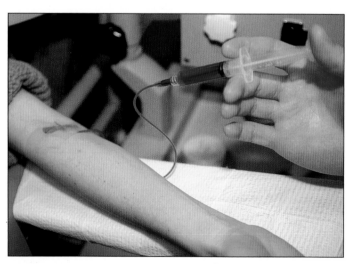

Fig. 51-16 After the needle is placed in the vein, the person injecting closely watches the injection site so as to be sure extravasation is not occurring. A handheld penlight, or a head mounted flashlight (such as used for hiking) can be used to monitor the injection site if the room lights are turned out.

angioscopy a day or so before the angiogram and then instruct the photographers as to exactly which areas should be photographed. Angioscopy will indicate all the abnormalities of the fundus that can be photographed, and other abnormal areas beyond the scope of the camera can be noted in the patient's record. Late-stage angiographs, preferably in stereo, are taken of the pertinent areas of each eye. It is important to photograph both discs and maculas and any other areas of abnormal fluorescence and to note any areas that could not be photographed. This will ensure that the interpreter will have adequate information for a complete interpretation of the angiogram.

The entire photographic process lasts from 5 to 10 minutes. Angiophotographs taken more than 10 minutes after injection are usually not necessary. In some cases of CSR, or other rare situations, angiophotographs taken longer than 10 minutes following injection are helpful. At the end of the session the patient should be reminded that the urine will be discolored for about a day.

In the event of a technical difficulty, such as camera breakdown, repeat fluorescein injection or photography can be carried out with satisfactory results after a waiting period of 30 to 60 minutes.

Interpretation is facilitated by following a specific photographic plan. The plan we have suggested will allow the fluorescein angiogram to yield all the information necessary to make a proper and thorough interpretation.

Box 51-1 provides a checklist of important steps in the fluorescein angiography procedure.

Diabetic retinopathy

The following is an alternative photographic plan for the study of diabetic retinopathy (Fig. 51-17).

The first six photographs follow the plan for macular disease except that the stereo pair may be of each macula, each disc, or the disc and macula combined. The second six (initial-transit) photographs all replicate the plan for macular disease except that the photographs all may again be of macula, disc, or macula and disc. Photographs 13 to 16 are as in the original plan, i.e. stereo pairs of the primary macula and primary disc.

With photograph 17 the plan changes. Rather than stereo pairs of macula and disc of the fellow eye, the next four photographs are of the nasal, superior, temporal, and inferior quadrants, respectively, of the primary eye under study. For the purpose of orientation, interpretation, and uniformity, the nasal, superior, and inferior photographs are taken with the edge of the disc at the edge of the photograph and the temporal photograph with the fovea at the edge of the photograph. Photographs 21 to 24 are the stereo pairs of the macula and disc of the secondary eye; photographs 25 to 28, the nasal, superior, temporal, and inferior quadrants, respectively, of the secondary eye. The late photographs (29–36) are stereo pairs of the primary macula and disc, followed by the secondary macula and disc. This plan yields maximal information about proliferative or preproliferative diabetic retinopathy, and only one roll of film is necessary for the entire angiogram.

Finally, it is not only very useful but actually both essential and extremely cost-effective for the physician to indicate specifically what areas of each or which fundus to photograph (Fig. 51-18).

Box 51-1 Checklist for fluorescein angiography

1. Inform patient about fluorescein angiography. Obtain verbal or written informed consent.
2. Dilate patient's pupil
3. Prepare fluorescein solution, scalp-vein needle, and syringe
4. Prepare fundus camera
   - Clean front lens
   - Load color and black-and-white film into two camera backs
   - Focus eyepiece crosshairs
5. Take identification photograph, which includes patient's name, the date, and other data (number of fluorescein angiogram, patient's vision of right eye and left eye, referring physician, etc.)
6. Position patient for alignment, focus, and comfort
7. Align and focus camera
8. Complete color photography
9. Switch to camera with black-and-white film for fluorescein photography
10. Take red-free photographs (frames 2–5)
11. Insert scalp-vein needle
12. Simultaneously start timer from zero and inject fluorescein dye
13. Take preinjection color photographs; shoot at exact start of injection as timer is turned on and shoot second shot at exact finish of injection (length of time of injection is automatically recorded)
14. Start fluorescein photograph 8 seconds after the start of injection in young patients and 12 seconds in older patients
15. Follow fluorescein angiography plan
16. When photography is done, reassure patient that all went well and remind him or her that the urine will be discolored for a day or so. Have patient wait an additional 20 minutes for observation for possible reactions to fluorescein

---

The photographer should be directed as to where to start the angiogram and what other areas to photograph. He or she should know all of the issues that are important for each specific angiogram. Color film and its processing are extremely expensive, so it is most cost-effective for the photographer to be instructed as to how many color slides to take of each area. It is most efficient to use a photographic instruction slip that indicates the specific number of color photographs to take of each area, where to start the angiogram, what the diagnosis is, and any other information about the patient or fundus that are pertinent to the photographic process. Of course, digital color and angiograms avoid the issue of cost, and can insure that the necessary information is obtained. Duplicate photos can be easily deleted, so as to avoid unnecessary computer storage of images.

Various side effects and complications can occur with fluorescein injection (Box 51-2). The prepared physician will have at hand equipment necessary to manage these problems as well as an emergency plan in place.

A serious complication of the injection is *extravasation of the fluorescein* under the skin. This can be extremely painful and may result in a number of uncomfortable symptoms. Necrosis and sloughing of the skin may occur, although this is extremely rare. Superficial phlebitis has also been noted. A subcutaneous granuloma has occurred in a few patients after fluorescein extravasation.

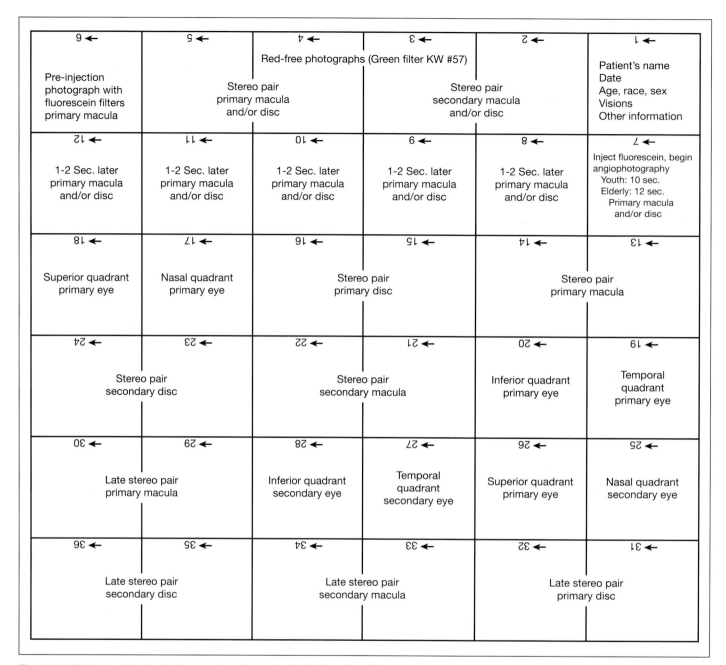

← 6	← 5	← 4	← 3	← 2	← 1
Pre-injection photograph with fluorescein filters primary macula	Stereo pair primary macula and/or disc	Red-free photographs (Green filter KW #57) Stereo pair primary macula and/or disc	Stereo pair secondary macula and/or disc	Stereo pair secondary macula and/or disc	Patient's name Date Age, race, sex Visions Other information
← 12	← 11	← 10	← 9	← 8	← 7
1-2 Sec. later primary macula and/or disc	1-2 Sec. later primary macula and/or disc	1-2 Sec. later primary macula and/or disc	1-2 Sec. later primary macula and/or disc	1-2 Sec. later primary macula and/or disc	Inject fluorescein, begin angiophotography Youth: 10 sec. Elderly: 12 sec. Primary macula and/or disc
← 18	← 17	← 16	← 15	← 14	← 13
Superior quadrant primary eye	Nasal quadrant primary eye	Stereo pair primary disc	Stereo pair primary disc	Stereo pair primary macula	Stereo pair primary macula
← 24	← 23	← 22	← 21	← 20	← 19
Stereo pair secondary disc	Stereo pair secondary disc	Stereo pair secondary macula	Stereo pair secondary macula	Inferior quadrant primary eye	Temporal quadrant primary eye
← 30	← 29	← 28	← 27	← 26	← 25
Late stereo pair primary macula	Late stereo pair primary macula	Inferior quadrant secondary eye	Temporal quadrant secondary eye	Superior quadrant primary eye	Nasal quadrant secondary eye
← 36	← 35	← 34	← 33	← 32	← 31
Late stereo pair secondary disc	Late stereo pair secondary disc	Late stereo pair secondary macula	Late stereo pair secondary macula	Late stereo pair primary disc	Late stereo pair primary disc

Fig. 51-17 Photographic plan for fluorescein angiography of diabetic retinopathy.

In each instance, however, the granuloma has been small, cosmetically invisible, and painless. Toxic neuritis caused by infiltration of extravasated fluorescein along a nerve in the antecubital area can result in considerable pain for up to a few hours. The application of an ice pack at the site of extravasation may help relieve pain. For extremely painful reactions an injection of a local anesthetic at the site of extravasation is very effective but rarely necessary.

When extravasation occurs, the physician must decide whether or not to continue angiography. Extravasation may occur immediately, and thus the serum concentration of the fluorescein will be insufficient for angiography. In this case it is usually best to place the needle in another vein and reinject a full dose of fluorescein,

starting the process again from the beginning. Occasionally, only a small amount of fluorescein is extravasated at the end of the injection. In this case photography can continue without stopping or reinjecting.

A common cause of extravasation is the use of a large, long needle directly attached to a syringe. It is difficult to hold the syringe steady while the injection is being given. For this and other reasons we have discussed earlier, a scalp-vein needle attached to a syringe by a flexible tube is the best choice for this procedure. Also, the patient's own blood can be drawn back into the tubing of the scalp-vein needle, with the blood going all the way up to but not into the syringe. When it is time to inject, the person giving the injection can look at the tip of the needle to ensure

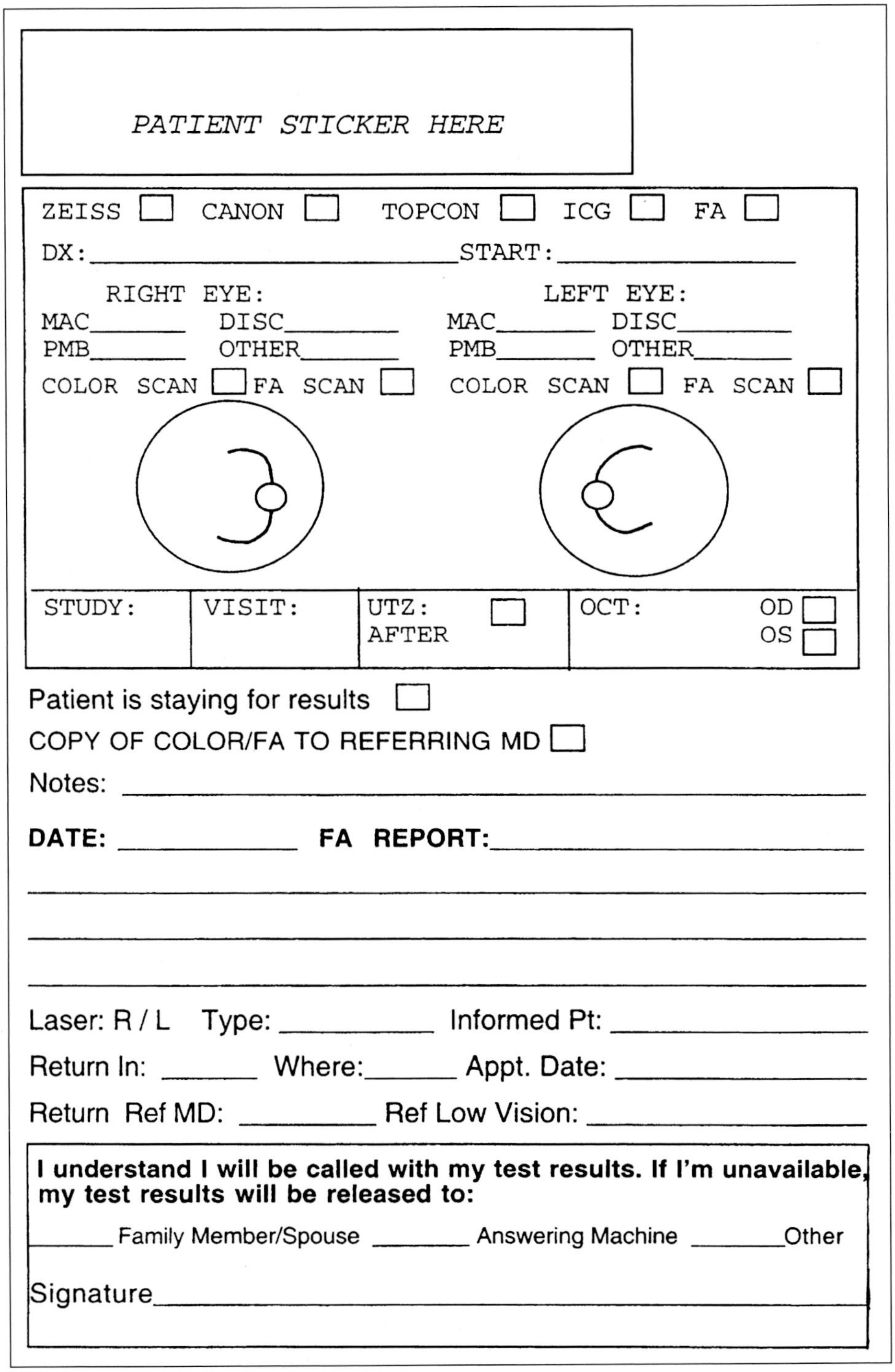

PATIENT STICKER HERE

ZEISS ☐   CANON ☐   TOPCON ☐   ICG ☐   FA ☐

DX:_____START:_____

RIGHT EYE: LEFT EYE:

MAC_____   DISC_____   MAC_____   DISC_____
PMB_____   OTHER_____   PMB_____   OTHER_____

COLOR SCAN ☐ FA SCAN ☐   COLOR SCAN ☐ FA SCAN ☐

| STUDY: | VISIT: | UTZ: ☐ AFTER | OCT: | OD ☐ OS ☐ |

Patient is staying for results ☐

COPY OF COLOR/FA TO REFERRING MD ☐

Notes: _____

DATE: _____ **FA REPORT:**_____

_____

_____

_____

Laser: R / L   Type: _____   Informed Pt: _____

Return In: _____   Where:_____   Appt. Date: _____

Return Ref MD: _____   Ref Low Vision: _____

I understand I will be called with my test results. If I'm unavailable, my test results will be released to:

_____ Family Member/Spouse _____ Answering Machine _____Other

Signature_____

Fig. 51-18 Photographic request form. In the top portion of the form patient identifying information is placed. The visual acuity of each eye can be written in this area. The physician indicates the number of color photographs required for each area in the fundus. The physician also indicates the diagnosis because experienced photographers will know which type of photographs to take for each particular diagnosis. The physician also indicates in which location of the fundus the initial-transit phase of the angiogram should take place or, in other words, where the photographer should start the angiogram. We use these forms to facilitate patient flow. If a patient needs to have other testing done, for instance, optical coherence tomography, it is indicated on the form. Also, we indicate if the patient is staying for the results, or will be contacted later. When film angiography is done, and the results read later, the interpretation and message for the patient is recorded. In this way, the nurse can contact the patient with the results.

that extravasation has not occurred. If it has, the patient's own blood is extravasated, and little chance of complication exists if the injection is stopped at this point so that no fluorescein is injected.

It is always important to watch for extravasation at the beginning of the injection so that, should it occur, the process can be halted; thus only a minimal amount of fluorescein will have been injected and extravasated. The amount of extravasated fluorescein can be minimized by slow injection and constant observation of the needle with a handheld light or if injection is done before turning off the room lights.

Nausea is the most frequent side effect of fluorescein injection, occurring in about 5% of patients. It is most likely to occur in patients under 50 years of age or when fluorescein is injected rapidly. When nausea occurs, it usually begins approximately 30 seconds after injection, lasts for 2 to 3 minutes, and disappears slowly.

Vomiting occurs infrequently, affecting only 0.3% to 0.4% of patients. When it does occur, it usually begins 40 to 50 seconds

> **Box 51-2** Side effects and complications of fluorescein injection
>
> Extravasation and local tissue necrosis
> Inadvertent arterial injection
> Nausea
> Vomiting
> Vasovagal reaction (circulatory shock, myocardial infarction)
> Allergic reaction, anaphylaxis (hives and itching, respiratory problems, laryngeal edema, bronchospasm)
> Nerve palsy
> Neurologic problems (tonic–clonic seizures)
> Thrombophlebitis
> Pyrexia
> Death

after injection. By this time most of the initial-transit photographs of the angiogram will have been taken. A receptacle and tissues should be available in case vomiting does occur. When patients experience nausea or vomiting, they must be reassured that the unpleasant and uncomfortable feeling will subside rapidly. Photographs can be taken after the vomiting episode has passed. A slower, more gradual injection may help to avoid vomiting.

Patients who have previously experienced nausea or vomiting from fluorescein injection may be given an oral dose of 25 to 50 mg of promethazine hydrochloride (Phenergan) by mouth approximately 1 hour before injection. Promethazine has proved to be helpful in preventing or lessening the severity of nausea or vomiting. We have recently found that we can also reduce the incidence of nausea by warming the vial of fluorescein to body temperature and drawing it into the syringe through a needle with a Millipore filter. Restriction of food and water for 4 hours before the fluorescein injection may reduce the incidence of vomiting; an empty stomach may prevent vomiting but will not affect nausea. If the patient still has a tendency to vomit despite taking all these measures, a lesser amount of fluorescein can be given and injected more slowly if the photographic results will not be compromised.

Vasovagal attacks occur much less frequently during fluorescein angiography than does nausea and are probably caused more by patient anxiety than by the actual injection of fluorescein. We have even seen vasovagal attacks when the patient sees the needle or immediately after the skin has been penetrated by the needle but before the injection has begun. Occasionally a vasovagal reaction will cause a patient to faint, but consciousness is regained within a few minutes. If early symptoms of a vasovagal episode are noted, smelling salts will usually reverse the reaction. The photographer must be alert for signs of fainting because the patient could be injured if he or she falls.

Shock and syncope (more severe vasovagal reaction) consist of bradycardia, hypotension, reduced cardiovascular perfusion, sweating, and the sense of feeling cold.

If the photographer and person injecting see that the patient is getting "shocky" or lightheaded, the patient should be allowed to bend over or lie down with the feet elevated. The patient's blood pressure and pulse should be carefully monitored.

It is important to differentiate this from *anaphylaxis*, in which hypotension, tachycardia, bronchospasm, hives, and itching occur.

Hives and *itching* are the most frequent allergic reactions, occurring 2 to 15 minutes after the fluorescein injection. Although hives usually disappear within a few hours, an antihistamine, such as diphenhydramine hydrochloride (Benadryl), may be administered intravenously for an immediate response. Bronchospasm and even anaphylaxis are other reactions that have been reported, but these are extremely rare. Epinephrine, systemic steroids, aminophylline, and pressor agents should be available to treat bronchospasm or any other allergic or anaphylactic reactions. Other equipment that should be readily available in the event of a severe vasovagal or anaphylactic reaction are oxygen, a sphygmomanometer, a stethoscope, and a device to provide an airway. The skilled photographer observes each patient carefully and is alert to any scratching, wheezing, or difficulty in breathing that the patient may experience after injection.

There are a few published and unpublished reports of death following intravenous fluorescein injection. The mechanism may be a severe allergic reaction or a hypotensive episode induced by a vasovagal reaction in a patient with pre-existing cardiac or cerebral vascular disease. The cause of death in each case may have been coincidental. Acute pulmonary edema following fluorescein injection has also been reported. We have also seen a delayed hypersensitivity reaction occurring approximately 48 hours later with a diffuse rash and fever.

There are no known contraindications to fluorescein injections in patients with a history of heart disease, cardiac arrhythmia, or cardiac pacemakers. Although there have been no reports of fetal complications from fluorescein injection during pregnancy, it is current practice to avoid angiography in women who are pregnant, especially those in the first trimester.

Fluorescein angiography is a relatively safe procedure with serious side effects occurring rarely. Nevertheless, prior preparation with availability of appropriate emergency equipment, and an emergency plan, is imperative. All involved staff should be familiar with the location of the equipment as well as their role as indicated by the emergency care plan (Preferred Practice Pattern, American Academy of Ophthalmology, Age-Related Macular Degeneration).

INTERPRETATION

FUNDUS ANATOMY AND HISTOLOGY

Fluorescein angiography has greatly increased our knowledge of retinal and choroidal circulatory physiology and fundus pathology. This clinical and research tool facilitates the in vivo study of histopathologic characteristics of fundus disease. Before the advent of fluorescein angiography, conditions such as pigment epithelial detachment, cystoid retinal edema, and subretinal neovascularization could be evaluated and understood only histologically. Now they are widely appreciated and recognized clinically. Because fluorescein angiography graphically demonstrates fundus pathophysiology, and because we rely on histologic points of reference when we interpret a fluorescein angiogram, a thorough knowledge of the anatomy of the fundus and its microscopic layers is necessary to correctly interpret fluorescein angiograms. Therefore, to interpret a fluorescein angiogram, it is essential to understand the microscopic layers of the fundus, i.e. the histology.

A logical place to begin this study is at the vitreous. In its normal state, and in a normal angiogram, the vitreous is clear and non-fluorescent. However, when it contains opacities that block the view of retinal and choroidal fluorescence, hypofluorescence occurs. The vitreous is also an important point of reference when intraocular inflammation or retinal neovascularization is present. In these cases fluorescein leaks into the vitreous, causing fluffy fluorescence as fluorescein molecules disperse into fluid vitreous and vitreous gel.

For the purpose of fluorescein angiographic interpretation, it is convenient to divide the sensory retina into two layers: the inner vascular half and the outer half, which is avascular. The *inner vascular half* extends from the internal limiting membrane to the inner nuclear layer. This portion of the retina contains the retinal blood vessels, which are located in two separate planes: the larger retinal arteries and veins are located in the nerve fiber layer; the retinal capillaries are located in the inner nuclear layer. In a well-focused stereoscopic fluorescein angiogram, these two vascular layers can be seen as distinct planes in the retina. An extremely important fluorescein angiographic concept is that normal retinal blood vessels are impermeable to fluorescein leakage; i.e. fluorescein flows through the normal retinal vessels without leakage into the retina.

The *outer avascular half* of the sensory retina consists of the outer plexiform layer, the outer nuclear layer, and the rods and cones. The outer plexiform layer is the primary interstitial space in the retina. When the retina becomes edematous, it is in this layer that fluid accumulates, causing cystoid spaces. Deep retinal hemorrhages and exudates (lipid deposits) may also be deposited in the outer plexiform layer.

The rods and cones are very loosely attached to the pigment epithelium, especially in the macular region, while the pigment epithelium is very firmly attached to Bruch's membrane. In fluorescein angiographic interpretation the pigment epithelium is an extremely important tissue because it prevents fluorescein leakage from the choroid and blocks, to a greater or lesser extent, visualization of choroidal fluorescence.

Bruch's membrane separates the pigment epithelium from the choriocapillaris, which is permeable to fluorescein. Fluorescein passes freely from the choriocapillaris and diffuses through Bruch's membrane up to, but not into, the pigment epithelium. Beneath the choriocapillaris are the larger choroidal vessels, which are impermeable to fluorescein. Melanocytes are dispersed throughout the choroid but are most heavily concentrated in the lamina fusca, the thin layer between the choroid and sclera. The sclera lies beneath the choroidal vessels.

The ophthalmic artery gives rise usually to two main posterior ciliary arteries: the lateral and medial. However, three posterior ciliary arteries may be present, in which case the medial artery is the one usually duplicated less frequently. In rare instances there may be a superior posterior ciliary artery.

The posterior ciliary arteries supply the lateral and medial halves of the disc and choroid. During angiography a vertical zone of slightly delayed filling may be seen passing through the papillomacular region, including the disc. Occasionally, there is an oblique orientation to this supply or even a superoinferior distribution. This border between the main posterior ciliary arteries has been termed the *watershed zone*, where patchy choroidal filling can often be seen on fluorescein angiograms.

Each main posterior ciliary artery divides into numerous short arteries and one long artery. On the temporal side the short posterior ciliary arteries supply small, variously sized, wedge-shaped choroidal segments, whose apices are centered near the macula. The lateral long posterior ciliary artery passes obliquely through the sclera. It supplies a wedge of choroid that begins temporal to the macular region and participates in the formation of the greater circle of the iris.

The choriocapillaris is made up of discrete units called *lobules*, thought to be approximately one fourth to one half of a disc diameter in size. The center of each lobule is fed by a precapillary arteriole (terminal choroidal arteriole), which comes from a short posterior ciliary artery. Each lobule functions independently in the normal state. It has been assumed that angiographic zones of delayed or patchy choroidal filling gradually fill in a transverse fashion, with one lobule spilling over into another. Careful inspection, however, indicates that these filling defects generally remain the same size, indicating a delayed filling from a posterior origin (its own arteriolar feeder). In the abnormal state, as when a choroidal vascular occlusion occurs, there is a freely connecting "spilling over" of blood flow from well-perfused choroid to the occluded area.

Around the margin of each lobule is a ring of postcapillary venules that drain each lobule. These postcapillary venules drain into the vortex veins, which drain the entire choroid. There are usually four vortex veins, and each functions as a well-defined quadrantic segmental drainage system for the entire uvea. In the case of a posterior ciliary artery obstruction, this occluded portion of the choroid can fill by a retrograde mechanism from an adjacent posterior ciliary artery by way of the choroidal venous system. This mechanism may provide adequate nourishment to prevent extensive ischemic changes until the occluded artery reopens.

Knowledge of each of these layers of the fundus is important in understanding fundus histopathology. The following six areas, however, are more important than others in interpretation of abnormal fundus fluorescence:

1. Preretinal area, where contraction from an epiretinal membrane may influence the retinal circulation and where hemorrhage may be located.
2. Vascular layers of the sensory retina, both superficial and deep.
3. Avascular portion of the sensory retina, particularly the outer plexiform layer, the principal site of intraretinal edema and exudate.
4. Retinal pigment epithelium, which has the potential for many manifestations, including proliferation, depigmentation, hyperpigmentation, and detachment.

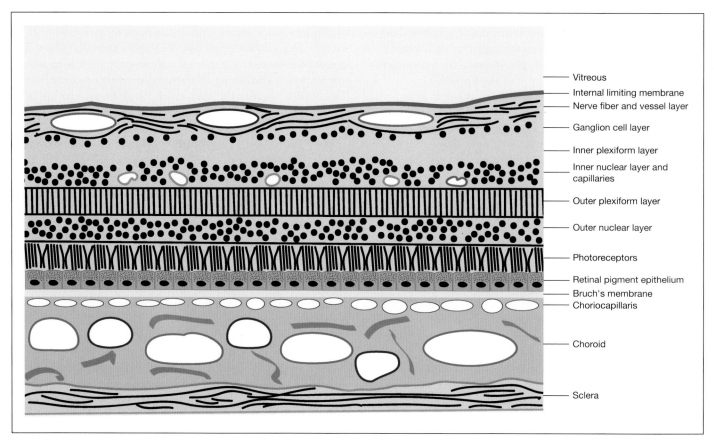

Vitreous
Internal limiting membrane
Nerve fiber and vessel layer
Ganglion cell layer
Inner plexiform layer
Inner nuclear layer and capillaries
Outer plexiform layer
Outer nuclear layer
Photoreceptors
Retinal pigment epithelium
Bruch's membrane
Choriocapillaris
Choroid
Sclera

Fig. 51-19 Modified schematic drawing of a microscopic section of retina, pigment epithelium, and choroid.

5. Choroidal circulation, including the choriocapillaris and the large choroidal vessels.
6. Sclera, which lies beneath the choroid.

Throughout this chapter a modified schematic drawing relates various fluorescein angiographic abnormalities to fundus histopathologic changes (Fig. 51-19). The size and proportion of these various layers have been modified to include various pathologic manifestations and to illustrate the effects of these abnormalities on the angiogram. Because of its importance and various pathologic changes, the pigment epithelium is drawn to a larger scale in relation to other fundus structures. The retinal and choroidal vessels are drawn larger and more numerous than they appear in a normal histopathologic section to emphasize the contribution of circulatory pathophysiologic interpretation.

Two specialized areas of the fundus warrant more detailed discussion: the macula (Fig. 51-20) and the optic nerve head. The fovea is the center of the *macula* and contains only four layers of the retina: the internal limiting membrane, the outer plexiform layer, the outer nuclear layer, and the rods and cones. No intermediate layers exist between the internal limiting membrane and the outer plexiform layer in the fovea, which in the macula is oblique. This is an important factor in understanding the stellate appearance of cystoid edema in the macula as opposed to the honeycomb appearance of cystoid edema outside the macula.

Beyond the macular region the outer plexiform layer is perpendicular rather than oblique.

The pigment epithelial cells in the macula are more columnar and have a greater concentration of melanin and lipofuscin granules than in the remainder of the fundus. Xanthophyll is present in the fovea, located probably in the outer plexiform layer. These differences in pigmentation are the chief factors responsible for producing the characteristic dark zone in the macular region on normal angiograms. The absence of retinal vessels in the fovea (i.e. the perifoveal capillary-free zone), in most cases approximately 400 to 500 μm in diameter in the center of the fovea, is another cause of the dark appearance of the macula.

The *optic nerve head*, or *disc*, is the other highly specialized tissue of the posterior pole. The disc is fed by two circulatory systems: the retinal vascular system and the posterior ciliary vascular system. Widespread anastomotic channels exist between the posterior ciliary vasculature and the optic nerve retinal vasculature. These are available and become exaggerated in certain pathologic conditions. The disc is made up of many layers of nerve fibers and glial supporting columns that contain the large retinal vessels.

The central retinal artery arises from the ophthalmic artery in close proximity to the main posterior ciliary arteries. In about 45% of the population, the central retinal artery and the medial posterior ciliary artery arise from a common trunk. In 12% of persons the central retinal artery originates from the ciliary artery. Therefore, it is impossible to have a choroidal infarction, anterior ischemic

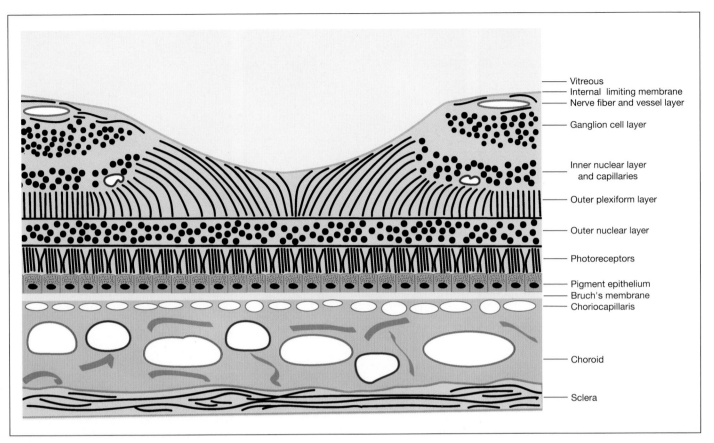

— Vitreous
— Internal limiting membrane
— Nerve fiber and vessel layer

— Ganglion cell layer

— Inner nuclear layer
  and capillaries

— Outer plexiform layer

— Outer nuclear layer

— Photoreceptors

— Pigment epithelium
— Bruch's membrane
— Choriocapillaris

— Choroid

— Sclera

Fig. 51-20 Modified schematic drawing of a microscopic section of the macula.

optic neuropathy, and a central retinal artery occlusion all due to a single site of obstruction.

The central retinal artery provides a major source of blood supply to the axial portion of the anterior orbital portion of the optic nerve. In the intraneural or axial course, short centrifugal branches arise but usually end a short distance behind the lamina cribrosa. There are then no further branches from the central retinal artery until it reaches the retina. If a cilioretinal artery is present, it supplies the corresponding segment of the disc.

The peripapillary nerve fiber layer is supplied by small, recurrent branches from the retinal arterioles at the peripapillary region. Emanating from these arterioles at the disc are the radial papillary capillaries. These capillaries are rather straight and long, have few anastomoses, and lie in the superficial portion of the peripapillary nerve fiber layer. The capillaries to the disc are continuous with these retinal peripapillary capillaries.

The short posterior ciliary arteries, or the recurrent branches from the peripapillary choroid, supply the retrolaminar portion of the optic nerve. The laminar cribrosa portion of the nerve is supplied by centripetal branches of the short posterior ciliary arteries. In this region a partial, or rarely a complete, Zinn's vascular circle is occasionally found. The prelaminar portion is supplied by centripetal branches from the peripapillary choroid.

Because most of the disc is fed by the ciliary system, fluorescein appears simultaneously at the optic nerve head and the choroid and before it is apparent in the retinal arteries.

The main venous drainage of the disc is into the central retinal vein. The prelaminar portion empties into both the central retinal vein and the peripapillary choroid, thus providing potential collateral drainage in the case of obstruction of the central retinal vein behind the lamina cribrosa. Such large dilated collaterals are frequently seen following central retinal vein occlusion and are called *retinociliary veins*. Some mistakenly call them "opticociliary shunts," a misnomer because they are not true shunts (defined as a congenital artery that empties into a vein and that skips the capillary bed, sometimes part of the Wyburn–Mason syndrome), and they are not "optico" because they emanate from the retina. They are, most accurately, retinovenous to ciliovenous collaterals.

In summary, fluorescein angiography provides an in vivo understanding of the histopathologic and pathophysiologic changes of various fundus abnormalities. Therefore, an anatomic and, more specifically, a histologic understanding of important fundus landmarks are essential to fluorescein angiographic interpretation.

NORMAL FLUORESCEIN ANGIOGRAM

The normal fluorescein angiogram is distinguished by certain specific characteristics. Knowledge of these characteristics provides an essential frame of reference for interpreting abnormal fluorescein angiograms.

In the normal fluorescein angiogram (Fig. 51-21), the first true fluorescence begins to show in the choroid approximately 10 to 12 seconds after injection in young patients (e.g. adolescents) and

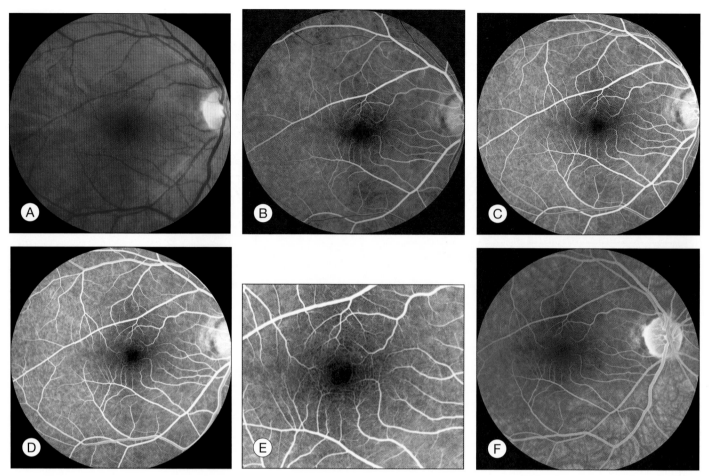

Fig. 51-21 Normal fluorescein angiogram of right disc and macula taken with a digital Topcon camera. A, Color photograph shows normal macula, fovea, and retinal vessels. B, Early arterial phase of the fluorescein angiogram. Note the ground-glass fluorescence of the choriocapillaris. There is very little fluorescence in the retinal veins. Just the margins of the veins are fluorescent. Occasionally, the choriocapillaris will initially fill incompletely, which has been termed patchy choroidal filling. This is not pathologic when not prolonged for more than a few seconds. C, One or two seconds later. Note the laminar fluorescence of the veins has become still thicker. The dark hypofluorescent line in the veins represents blood flow that is not yet fluorescent; it is coming from the periphery and takes longer to fluoresce. Note the very fine capillaries around the perifoveal capillary net. Note the dark macula. D, Mid arteriovenous-phase fluorescein angiogram. The retinal arteries and veins are almost completely filled. E, A high magnification view of the foveal vessels. Good focus and a more darkly pigmented eye can achieve excellent resolution of these vessels. F, Late arteriovenous-phase fluorescein angiogram showing the disc. Again, there is diffuse fluorescence of the choriocapillaris. The arteries and veins have completely filled. There is normal optic nerve fluorescence.

12 to 15 seconds after injection in older patients. Fluorescence can appear even earlier than 8 seconds in very young patients. The choroid occasionally begins to fluoresce 1 or 2 seconds before the initial filling of the central retinal artery. Early choroidal fluorescence is faint, patchy, and irregularly scattered throughout the posterior fundus. It is interspersed with scattered islands of delayed fluorescein filling. This early phase is referred to as the *choroidal flush*. When adjacent areas of choroidal filling and nonfilling are quite distinct, the pattern is designated as *patchy choroidal filling*.

Within the next 10 seconds (approximately 20–25 seconds after injection), the angiogram becomes very bright for about 5 seconds because of the extreme choroidal fluorescence. Choroidal fluorescence, however, is not visible in the macula because of the taller, more pigmented epithelium present in the fovea (retina). Therefore, the macula remains dark throughout the angiogram.

If a cilioretinal artery is present, it usually begins to fluoresce as the choroid fluoresces, rather than as the retina fluoresces. Within 1 to 3 seconds after choroidal fluorescence is visible, or approximately 10 to 15 seconds after injection, the central retinal artery begins to fluoresce. The less dense the concentration of pigment in the pigment epithelium, the greater the time will be between the visibility of the choroidal fluorescence and the filling of the retinal vessels. The lighter pigment presents less interference to choroidal fluorescence, allowing it to be evident earlier in its filling phase. With a more densely pigmented pigment epithelium, the blockage-barrier effect is greater. Therefore, choroidal fluorescence appears somewhat later because a greater concentration of fluorescein is required to overcome the increased density of the pigment epithelial barrier.

Because no barrier exists in front of the retinal vessels, the patient's pigmentation has no effect on the visibility of the retinal vessels, although the degree of pigmentation does affect the contrast of the angiophotographs. The darker the pigment epithelium, the less visible the choroidal fluorescence will be and the greater the contrast of the retinal vascular fluorescence; i.e. the better they stand out. The lighter the pigment epithelium, the more visible the choroidal fluorescence will be and the less the contrast of the fluorescence from the retinal vessels.

After the central retinal artery begins to fill, the fluorescein flows into the retinal arteries, then into the precapillary arterioles, the capillaries, the postcapillary venules, and finally the retinal veins. Because the fluorescein from the venules enters the veins along their walls, the flow of fluorescein in the veins is laminar. Because vascular flow is faster in the center of a lumen (tube) than on the sides, the fluorescein seems to stick to the sides, creating the laminar pattern of retinal venous flow. The dark (nonfluorescent) central lamina is nonfluorescent blood that comes from the periphery, which takes longer to fluoresce because of its more distant location.

In the next 5 to 10 seconds, fluorescence of the two parallel laminae along the walls of the retinal veins becomes thicker. At the junction of two veins, the inner lamina of each vein may merge. This creates three laminae: one in the center and one on each side of the vein. As fluorescein filling increases in the veins, the laminae eventually enlarge and meet, resulting in complete fluorescence of the retinal veins.

Fluorescence of the disc emanates from the posterior ciliary vascular system, both from the edge of the disc and from the tissue between the center and the circumference of the disc. Filling also comes from the capillaries of the central retinal artery on the surface of the disc. Because healthy disc tissue contains many capillaries, the disc becomes fairly hyperfluorescent on the angiogram.

The perifoveal capillary net cannot always be seen on the fluorescein angiogram. It can be seen best in young patients with clear ocular media about 20 to 25 seconds after a rapid fluorescein injection. This is called the "peak" phase of the fluorescein angiogram. The photographer should be aware of this phase and be sure not to miss it by shooting as rapidly as possible as the fluorescein concentration increases, and by continuing to shoot rapidly until the concentration of fluorescein begins to decrease.

Approximately 30 seconds after injection, the first high-concentration flush of fluorescein begins to empty from the choroidal and retinal circulations. Recirculation phases follow, during which fluorescein in a lower concentration continues to pass through the circulation of the fundus.

Generally, 3 to 5 minutes after injection, the choroidal and retinal vasculatures slowly begin to empty of fluorescein and become gray. The vessels of most normal patients almost completely empty of fluorescein in approximately 10 minutes. The large choroidal vessels and the retinal vessels do not leak fluorescein. However, because of large gaps in its endothelium, the choriocapillaris does leak fluorescein. The extravasated fluorescein diffuses through the choroidal tissue, Bruch's membrane, and sclera. Leakage of fluorescein with retention in tissues is designated as *staining*. In the later phase of the angiogram, staining of Bruch's membrane, the choroid, and especially the sclera may be visible

if the pigment epithelium is lightly pigmented. The disc and adjacent visible sclera remain hyperfluorescent because of staining. When the retinal pigment epithelium is especially lightly pigmented, the large choroidal vessels can be seen in silhouette against the fluorescent (fluorescein-stained) sclera. The lamina cribrosa within the disc also remains hyperfluorescent because of staining. This depends on the cup-to-disc ratio and the presence of any visible sclera, such as occurs within a conus adjacent to the disc. The edge of the disc stains from the adjacent choriocapillaris, which normally leaks.

To summarize, the angiogram is initially dark; choroidal and retinal filling is seen 10 to 15 seconds after fluorescein injection. The retinal and choroidal vasculatures fill maximally about 20 to 30 seconds after injection. Late angiophotographs show fluorescence of the choroid and sclera (if the pigment epithelium is light) and fluorescence of the optic cup and the edge of the disc, but otherwise the fundus is dark (nonfluorescent in the late phase).

ABNORMAL FLUORESCEIN ANGIOGRAM

The purpose of this section is to offer a schema by which the interpretation of the fluorescein angiogram follows a simple and logical progression. The first step is to recognize areas of abnormal fluorescence and determine if they are hypofluorescent or hyperfluorescent (Fig. 51-22).

Hypofluorescence

Hypofluorescence is a reduction or absence of normal fluorescence, whereas *hyperfluorescence* is abnormally excessive fluorescence. A systematic series of decisions follows this initial differentiation to arrive at a proper diagnosis. These decisions relate to (1) the anatomic location of various abnormalities; (2) the quality and quantity of the abnormal fluorescence; and (3) other unique characteristics, as indicated in the schematic chart.

Hypofluorescence is any abnormally dark area on the positive print of an angiogram. There are two possible causes of hypofluorescence: blocked fluorescence or a vascular filling defect.

Blocked fluorescence is sometimes referred to as *masked*, *obscured*, or *negative fluorescence* or *transmission decrease*. Each of these terms indicates a reduction or absence of normal retinal or choroidal fluorescence because of a tissue or fluid barrier located anterior to the respective retinal or choroidal circulation. For example, blood in the vitreous or a layer of blood in front of the retina obscures the view of the retinal and choroidal circulations and therefore blocks fundus fluorescence from these tissue. Hemorrhage that lies under the retina or retinal pigment epithelium, but in front of the choroidal circulation, does not obstruct visibility of the retinal circulation but does block the view of the choroidal circulation. Therefore the approximate histologic location of blocking material can be determined by the presence or absence of visibility of one or both fundus circulations.

Fluorescein is present but cannot be seen in blocked fluorescence. With vascular filling defects, however, fluorescein cannot be seen because it is not present.

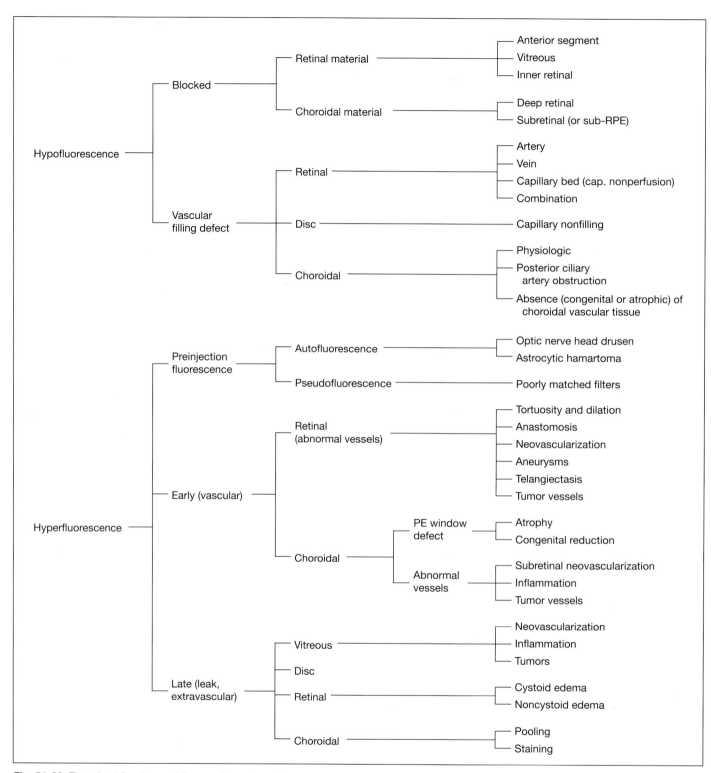

Fig. 51-22 Flow sheet for abnormal fluorescein angiography.

The key to differentiating blocked fluorescence from a vascular filling defect is to correlate the hypofluorescence on the angiogram with the ophthalmoscopic view. If there is material visible ophthalmoscopically that corresponds in size, shape, and location to the hypofluorescence on the angiogram, then blocked fluorescence is present. If there is no corresponding material on the color photograph, then it must be assumed that fluorescein has not perfused the vessels and that the hypofluorescence is caused by a vascular filling defect.

Hypofluorescence resulting from a vascular filling defect occurs when either of the two fundus circulations is not perfusing normally. This is caused by an absence of the vascular tissue or by a complete or partial obstruction of the particular vessels. In these situations an absence or delay of fluorescence of the involved vessels will occur. This type of hypofluorescence has a pattern that follows the geographic distribution of the vessels involved. Although the ophthalmoscopic picture will demonstrate the material blocking fluorescence, it may show nothing if the hypofluorescence is the result of a vascular filling defect.

To summarize, after an area of hypofluorescence is recognized, one must refer to the ophthalmoscopic photograph to determine the cause. If material is visible ophthalmoscopically and corresponds to the area of hypofluorescence, this is blocked fluorescence. If no corresponding blocking material exists, the hypofluorescence is therefore a vascular filling defect.

Anatomic location of hypofluorescence

After determining the cause of the hypofluorescence, the next step is (1) to determine the anatomic location of the material that is blocking fluorescence; or (2) to determine which of the two fundus circulations is involved in the filling defect. Blocking material affects the retinal and choroidal circulations if it is located in front of the retina. The material blocks only the choroidal circulation if it is located beneath the retinal circulation and in front of the choroid. Similarly, vascular filling defects occur in either the retinal or the choroidal vasculature or in the vessels of the optic nerve head.

Blocked retinal fluorescence

Blocked retinal vascular hypofluorescence is caused by anything that reduces media clarity. An opacification in front of the retinal vessels, involving the cornea, anterior chamber, iris, lens, vitreous, or the most anterior portion of the retina or disc will produce hypofluorescence.

The further the opacification is in front of the fundus, the less it will block fluorescence and the more it will affect the overall quality of the photographs. The closer the material is to the fundus, the more it will block, causing hypofluorescent images on the angiogram. Any material that blocks retinal vascular fluorescence will, of course, block choroidal fluorescence as well.

Any anterior segment material, such as a corneal opacity, anterior chamber haziness, or lens opacity, obscuring the view of the ocular fundus will result in an angiogram of reduced brilliance, contrast, and resolution. This affects the quality of the angiogram and is, in a sense, a type of blocked fluorescence.

Many conditions of the vitreous produce a hazy medium, which prevents visualizing fundus detail. The most common vitreous opacity to cause blockage is hemorrhage. Whether diffusely dispersed in the vitreous gel or more densely accumulated, vitreous hemorrhage reduces or completely blocks fundus fluorescence. In addition to hemorrhage, media haze may be caused by a variety of opacifications, e.g. asteroid hyalosis, vitreous condensation resulting from vitreous degenerative disease, inflammatory debris, vitreous membranes, or opacification secondary to amyloidosis.

When anterior segment and vitreous opacities are present, the angiogram may be of higher resolution and quality than the color photograph. This is because the light scattered from the nonfluorescing opacities is not transmitted through the barrier filter and therefore has no effect on the angiographic photograph.

Any translucent or opacified material in the retina or in the nerve fiber layer will block fluorescence from both planes of retinal vessels as well as from the choroidal vessels. The large retinal vessels and precapillary arterioles are located in the nerve fiber layer in the anterior plane of the retina. The capillaries and postcapillary venules are located deeper in the retina, in the inner nuclear layer. If a blocking material lies in front of the nerve fiber layer, it will block both planes of retinal vessels (Fig. 51-23). However, if the material lies beneath the nerve fiber layer but within or in front of the inner nuclear layer (where the smaller retinal vessels are located), it will block only the retinal capillaries (and choroidal vessels), leaving the view of the large retinal vessels unobstructed. If a blocking material lies deeper than the retinal vascular structures, deep to the inner nuclear layer, it will not block the vessels but will block the choroidal vascular fluorescence. In other words, deep intraretinal blocking material, such as hemorrhage or exudate, will not obstruct retinal vascular fluorescence, since the retinal vessels are located in the inner half of the retina (Fig. 51-24).

Therefore, one can determine the location of a retinal abnormality, such as hemorrhage, by the vessels that are blocked by it and by the fluorescence of the vessels that are not blocked.

The most common cause of blocked retinal vascular fluorescence is hemorrhage. Subinternal limiting membrane hemorrhage blocks fluorescence of all underlying retinal vessels and choroidal vasculature. Nerve fiber layer hemorrhage, which is usually flame-shaped, will block the smaller retinal vessels lying deeper in the retina but will only partially block the larger retinal vessels in the nerve fiber layer. Blockage from hemorrhage is usually complete, as opposed to the partial blockage caused by the myelinated nerve fibers.

Various retinal vascular (arteriolar) occlusive diseases may cause white ischemic thickening (nerve fiber edema), which results in some opacification of the retina and blockage of the remaining retinal vascular and choroidal fluorescence. Conditions such as arterial occlusion in hypertension or Purtscher's retinopathy cause enough intracellular "cloudy" swelling and opacification to block fluorescence. It should be noted that because there is occlusion in this type of hypofluorescence, the hypofluorescence is caused partly by the vascular filling defect. However, the opacified ischemic retina effectively blocks fluorescence from underlying retinal and choroidal vasculature.

In summary, the concept of blocked retinal vascular hypofluorescence is fairly easy to understand and to identify on the angiogram. When the retinal vessels do not fluoresce, the ophthalmoscopic view should be studied to determine if blocking material is located in front of the retinal vessels. If blocking material is present, the next step is to determine its anatomic location.

Blocked choroidal fluorescence

Hypofluorescence caused by blocked choroidal vasculature occurs when fluid, exudate, hemorrhage, pigment, scar, and

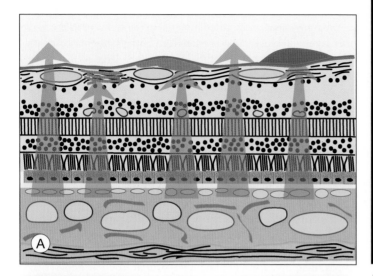

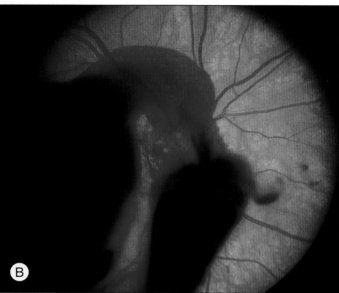

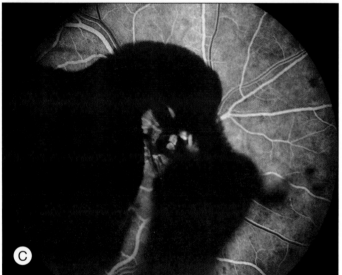

Fig. 51-23 Preretinal hemorrhage causing hypofluorescence–blockage of all retinal and choroidal fluorescence. A, Schematic drawing of subhyaloid (right), subinternal limiting membrane (central), and nerve fiber layer (left) hemorrhages. Each hemorrhage lies in front of the retinal, and therefore choroidal, vasculature, causing hypofluorescence–blocked fluorescence. B, Color photograph of the right disc showing substantial preretinal hemorrhage. C, Fluorescein angiogram of the right disc showing hypofluorescence caused by blockage caused by the preretinal hemorrhage. COMMENT: All fluorescence of the fundus is blocked because the hemorrhage lies in front of the retinal vasculature.

inflammatory material, accumulates in front of the choroidal vasculature and deep to the retinal vasculature (Fig. 51-25).

Deep retinal material

Materials deposited in the deep retina that cause blockage of choroidal fluorescence are fluid, hard exudate, hemorrhage, and pigment.

When fluid accumulates in the deep retina, it has a predilection for the tissue of least resistance, the outer plexiform layer. Deposition of edema fluid, originating from leaking retinal vessels or migrating from subretinal space into the retina most frequently occur in the outer plexiform layer. When the fluid reaches a certain volume, it tends to form spaces or pockets between compressed nerve and Müller's fibers, which are pushed aside in the process. This pattern of fluid accumulation in the outer plexiform layer is called *cystoid retinal edema*. *Noncystoid retinal edema* occurs when the volume of extracellular fluid is insufficient to produce pockets or spaces in the outer plexiform layer or other

layers of the retina. A significant amount of retinal edema, whether cystoid or noncystoid, especially if turbid or containing lipid-laden macrophages, will partially block choroidal fluorescence in the early phase of the fluorescein angiogram. Later in the angiogram, retinal edema fluoresces. Intraretinal hard exudates and lipid-laden macrophages, usually located in the outer plexiform layer, partially block choroidal fluorescence. When retinal vessels bleed, the blood can be deposited anywhere in the retina. When the blood is located deep to the retinal vessels beneath the inner nuclear layer, retinal vascular fluorescence will be visible, whereas choroidal fluorescence will be blocked.

Subretinal material

Any opaque or translucent substance located beneath the retina but in front of the choroid will block fluorescence of the choroidal vasculature but will not block retinal vascular fluorescence (Fig. 51-25). Blood located under the retina will cause complete blockage of choroidal fluorescence, with the retinal fluorescence showing

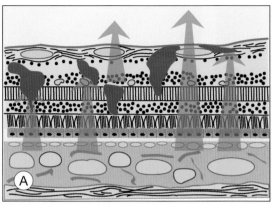 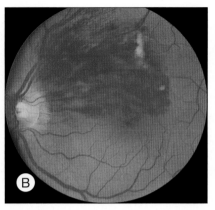 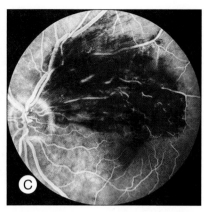

Fig. 51-24 Intraretinal hemorrhages causing hypofluorescence–blockage. A, Schematic of retina showing hemorrhages located in most of the layers of the retina from the internal limiting membrane to the outer nuclear layer. B, Color photograph of left macula shows primarily flame-shaped hemorrhages superonasal to the fovea due to a branch vein occlusion. C, Fluorescein angiogram of left macula shows that the hemorrhage causes irregular hypofluorescent blockage. The flame-shaped hemorrhage located in the nerve fiber layer blocks all the retinal vasculature. Where the hemorrhage is deeper or thinner, retinal vessels can be seen. Hemorrhages that do not block retinal capillary fluorescence can be located deeper to the capillary layer, which is in the inner nuclear layer. COMMENT: Once the determination of hypofluorescent blockage is made, an anatomic localization of the blocking material can be made by determining which normally fluorescent structures can be seen and which are being blocked.

through normally. Subretinal hemorrhage will appear red, and subpigment epithelial hemorrhage will appear dark. Subretinal hemorrhage is generally scalloped with somewhat irregular margins, whereas subpigment epithelial hemorrhage is often quite round and well-demarcated (Fig. 51-25).

Accumulated pigment (melanin and lipofuscin) from diseased retinal pigment epithelium causes blocked choroidal fluorescence. Any hyperpigmentation of the pigment epithelium will cause blocked choroidal fluorescence (Fig. 51-26). Xanthophyll, the pigment present in the outer layers of the fovea, blocks choroidal fluorescence by selectively absorbing the blue exciting light, which results in less fluorescence. Finally, a choroidal nevus may block much of the choroidal fluorescence (Fig. 51-27) and will especially block the later hyperfluorescent staining of the sclera. The choriocapillaris may be seen normally over the nevus.

To summarize, various materials located in the deep retinal layers, or beneath the retina, block choroidal fluorescence and will be evident ophthalmoscopically. These materials result from a variety of disease processes.

Vascular filling defect

The second cause of abnormal hypofluorescence is vascular filling defect. With blocked fluorescence, the fluorescein is present in the circulations of the fundus but is not visible because a tissue or fluid barrier conceals it. With vascular filling defect, fluorescein cannot be seen because it is not present. Since fluorescein reaches the retina and choroid by way of vessels, lack of the fluorescein dye in either vascular system indicates an obstructive problem or a lack of vessels, i.e. a vascular filling defect.

As previously indicated, when a hypofluorescent area is seen on an angiogram, the best way to differentiate blocked fluorescence from a vascular filling defect is to compare the angiogram with the ophthalmoscopic picture. When blood, pigment, or exudate can be seen ophthalmoscopically corresponding to the area of

hypofluorescence, the material is causing blocked fluorescence. When no material is visible ophthalmoscopically (on the color photograph), one must assume that fluorescein has not perfused the vessels and the abnormal hypofluorescence is caused by a vascular filling defect. In some instances both forms of hypofluorescent mechanisms play a role simultaneously, as with retinal arteriolar occlusion, when the retina is not only not perfused (vascular filling defect) but is ischemic and therefore white and opaque, causing blocked fluorescence.

Vascular filling defects result from vascular obstruction, atrophy, or absence (congenital or otherwise) of vessels. Any of these conditions can be total or partial. When the obstruction is complete (occlusion) or the vascular tissue is atrophied completely, the hypofluorescence is complete and lasts throughout the angiogram. When the obstruction is only partial or the vascular tissue is not entirely atrophied, the vascular fluorescein filling is delayed or reduced relative to corresponding areas that fill normally. Whatever the cause of a partial vascular filing defect, hypofluorescence will be seen in the early phases of the angiogram but may not persist throughout the entire angiogram. Some vascular filling, although delayed or reduced, will eventually occur.

Once it is determined that a vascular filling defect is the cause of an area of hypofluorescence, the next step is to determine which of the retinal, disc, or choroidal vessels are involved. A vascular filling defect of the disc is easy to discern angiographically. Determining whether a vascular filling defect is retinal or choroidal can be more difficult. Since retinal vessels are normally present, however, the absence of retinal vessels is usually readily apparent. If, on the other hand, a vascular filling defect is found but the retinal vessels are full and visible, the hypofluorescence must be choroidal in origin. Stereoscopic angiophotographs allow one to distinguish between the planes of the retina and choroid, and enable exact determination of the location of the hypofluorescence.

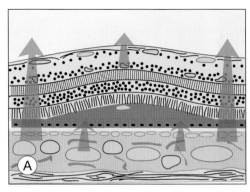 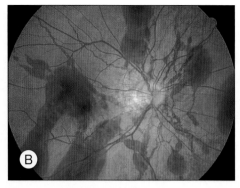 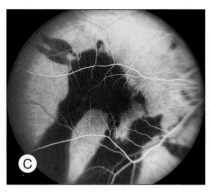

Fig. 51-25 Subretinal hemorrhage causing hypofluorescence, i.e. blockage of choroidal fluorescence. A, Schematic of retina with subretinal hemorrhage (blood located between photoreceptors and pigment epithelium). B, Color photograph of right macula showing large scattered areas of subretinal hemorrhage. C, Fluorescein angiogram of right macula shows marked hypofluorescence caused by blocked choroidal fluorescence (the retinal vessels are visible) that is due to the subretinal hemorrhage. COMMENT: The subretinal hemorrhage completely obscures fluorescence from the choroid. The retinal vessels are clearly seen overlying the subretinal hemorrhage. This is a case of pseudoxanthomum elasticum with subretinal hemorrhage occurring as a result of trauma.

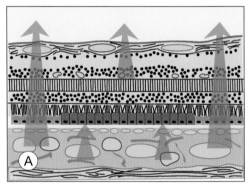 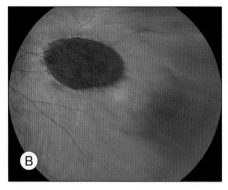 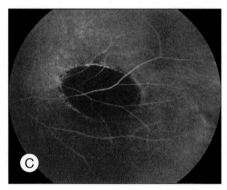

Fig. 51-26 Hypertrophy of the retinal pigment epithelium (RPE). A, Schematic showing hypertrophic pigment epithelial cells. B, Color photograph of the inferior fundus shows a well-demarcated hyperpigmented lesion. C, Fluorescein angiogram of the same area shows marked hypofluorescence of the choroid resulting from blocked fluorescence. COMMENT: This patient has congenital hypertrophy of the retinal pigment epithelium. The marked hypertrophy of the retinal pigment epithelium allows normal retinal fluorescence but completely blocked choroidal fluorescence.

Retinal vascular filling defect

If a retinal vascular filling defect is present, the clinician then considers whether the defect results from obstruction of a retinal artery or vein, capillary bed, or any combination of these. Distinguishing the cause of the obstruction is not difficult because the fluorescein angiographic process is dynamic and timed. When nonfilling of a specific retinal vessel occurs, it is easy to differentiate an arterial occlusion from a venous occlusion because the retinal arteries fill first, then the retinal capillary bed, followed by the retinal veins. In addition, retinal vascular filling defects can be localized by tracing the course of a particular vessel, these defects correspond anatomically to the normal distribution of the retinal vasculature (Figs 51-28 and 51-29).

Thus, retinal vascular filling defects result from a variety of disease processes, but most are commonly associated with atherosclerosis and diabetes.

Vascular filling defects of the disc

Vascular filling defects of the disc occur because of the failure of the capillaries of the optic nerve head to fill. This failure can

result because of a congenital absence of disc tissue, as in an optic pit (Fig. 51-30) or optic nerve head coloboma; because of atrophy of the disc tissue and its vasculature, as in optic atrophy; or because of vascular occlusion, as in an ischemic optic neuropathy. Each condition is characterized by early hypofluorescence caused by nonfilling and late hyperfluorescence resulting from staining of the involved tissue.

Choroidal vascular filling defect

The normal choroidal vasculature is usually difficult to document with fluorescein angiography because of the pigment epithelial barrier. When chronic choroidal vascular filling defects exist, the pigment epithelium is often secondarily depigmented or atrophied. In these cases, the hypofluorescence caused by a vascular filling abnormality of the choroid and choriocapillaris can be documented angiographically.

When choroidal vessels do not fill, dark patches of hypofluorescence beneath the retina appear early in the angiogram. The distribution and morphology of the hypofluorescence vary according to the disease process. Because the choroidal circulation is

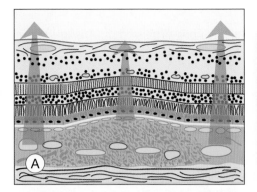

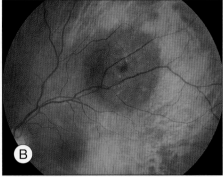

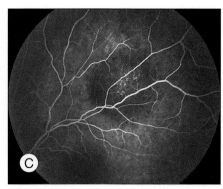

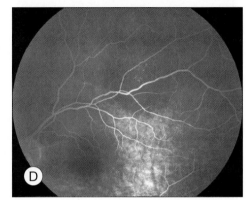

Fig. 51-27 Choroidal nevus hypofluorescence–blockage. A, Schematic drawing of retina, showing choroidal nevus. B, Color photograph of nevus. C, Arteriovenous-phase fluorescein angiogram shows hypofluorescence corresponding to the area of the nevus. D, Later arteriovenous-phase fluorescein angiogram shows that the nevus is still hypofluorescent. The choriocapillaris overlying the nevus is hypofluorescent as well. COMMENT: This patient showed blockage of choroidal fluorescence from the nevus. The later phase fluorescein angiogram showed that the choriocapillaris was involved as well.

completely separate from the retinal circulation, choroidal vascular filling defects do not correlate with the retinal vascular distribution. If the choriocapillaris is absent and the large choroidal vessels are still present, the choroidal and retinal vessels will fluoresce, but hypofluorescent gaps will appear because of the loss of the diffuse "ground-glass" fluorescence from the choriocapillaris (Fig. 51-31). When the choroidal vasculature does not fill such as occurs with total occlusion or atrophy, hypofluorescence occurs early in the angiogram. The hypofluorescence remains throughout the late stages of the procedure, although leakage from surrounding areas of normal choriocapillaris extends into the occluded area. When sufficient leakage occurs, the sclera retains fluorescein (stains) late in the angiogram. When the involved area is large and the leakage is minimal, the hypofluorescence remains throughout the later stages.

A normal physiologic condition exists in many patients in which the choroid fills in a patchy manner. Areas adjacent to the foci that are filling show early hypofluorescence but eventually fill normally, usually 2 to 5 seconds later. This has been termed *patchy choroidal filling*, and it is the most common form of choroidal vascular filling defect. This form of filling follows a pattern in which the short posterior ciliary arteries enter the eye perpendicularly through the sclera. These vessels then feed the choriocapillaris lobules.

The prechoriocapillaris arterioles and lobules are end, or terminal, vessels demonstrating no anastomoses with adjacent choriocapillaris arterioles or lobules. Each choriocapillaris lobule is connected to adjacent lobules on the venous, or emptying, side of the circulation. Fluorescence in each choriocapillaris segment or lobule is in the form of a round, irregular, or hexagonal patch. When some of the channels fill late, a heterogeneous filling pattern results. The choriocapillaris fills most areas, whereas dark hypofluorescent patches are present in other areas. These dark areas are lobules from separate end channels that are not filled simultaneously with adjacent choriocapillaris lobules. They are filled in a delayed fashion by the single feeder choroidal arteriole.

In general, vascular filling defects of the choroid are caused by obstructive disorders or absence of tissue and have the following fluorescein angiographic characteristics: (1) normal retinal vascular flow; (2) depigmentation of the pigment epithelium; (3) reduction of choroidal blood flow; and (4) hypofluorescence in the early phases of angiography caused by loss of the normal ground-glass choriocapillaris fluorescence. In some conditions the large choroidal vessels are also absent, resulting in total early hypofluorescence in the affected area, with scleral staining only on the circumference of the lesion because of the adjacent patent choriocapillaris. Choroidal vascular defects result from a variety of disease processes (Figs 51-32 and 51-33).

Hyperfluorescence

Hyperfluorescence is any abnormally light area on the positive print of an angiogram, i.e. an area showing fluorescence in excess of what would be expected on a normal angiogram. There are four possible causes of abnormal hyperfluorescence: (1) pre-injection fluorescence; (2) transmitted fluorescence; (3) abnormal vessels; and (4) leakage. The appearance of fluorescence depends in part on the relationship of its appearance to the timing of the fluorescein injection.

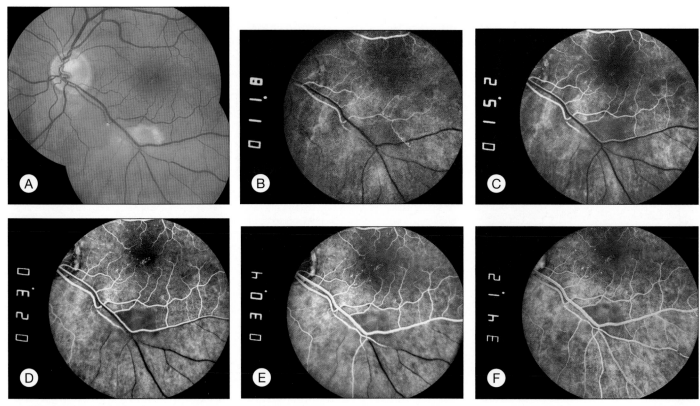

Fig. 51-28 Branch retinal artery occlusion. A, Color photograph showing areas of retinal whitening inferior to the macula. Note the Hollenhorst plaque at the site of the occluded retinal arteriole. B, At 11 seconds after the fluorescein has been injected, a hypofluorescent area is seen below the macula. Also, note the abrupt cessation of fluorescein dye in the occluded arteriole. C–E, The fluorescein frames between 15 and 30 seconds show that fluorescein dye has advanced a short distance beyond the Hollenhorst plaque indicating the presence of some flow through this area. The branch arteriole has not filled completely, although an adjacent vein already has laminar filling of fluorescein from the normally perfused adjacent retina. E, In the late phases of the angiogram, the arteriole is filled, though its caliber is somewhat irregular.

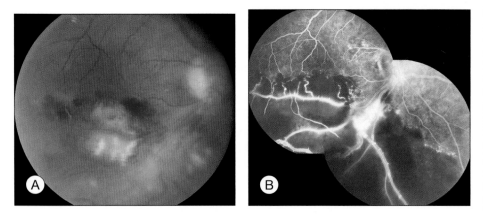

Fig. 51-29 Retinal branch vein occlusion. A, Color photograph of the right macula and disc. There are areas of retinal hemorrhage and retinal whitening and cotton-wool spots. B, The fluorescein angiogram of the right disc and macula shows normal fluorescence of the superior portion of the macula. The inferior portion shows substantial hypofluorescence due to retinal capillary nonperfusion. The very bright hyperfluorescent areas are due to neovascularization. COMMENT: This patient had a very ischemic inferotemporal branch retinal vein occlusion of the right eye. This was a severe occlusion as evidenced by closure of large areas of the capillary bed. The hypofluorescence was caused not only by vascular filling defect but also by the nonperfused retina, which becomes partially opaque and caused hypofluorescence of the choroid. (In other words, there was blockage of choroidal fluorescence by the opaque retina, which was caused by the retinal capillary nonperfusion.)

Preinjection fluorescence is hyperfluorescence that can be seen before fluorescein is injected and is caused by structures that naturally fluoresce (autofluorescence) or by poorly matched filters (pseudofluorescence).

Transmitted fluorescence and *abnormal vascular fluorescence* occur in the early or vascular stage of the angiogram, when fluorescein fills patent blood vessels. Transmitted fluorescence appears when fluorescein fills the normal choriocapillaris but is more

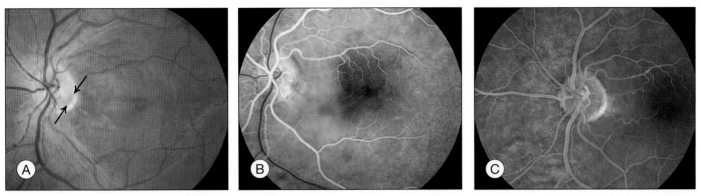

Fig. 51-30 Optic pit and sensory macula detachment. A, Color photograph of left macula. Note the dark area of the optic pit (arrows). Cystic edema is present in the macula secondary to the macula schisis detachment from the optic pit. B, Early arteriovenous-phase fluorescein angiogram shows hypofluorescence of the disc in the area of the pit due to absence of tissue and vessels. C, In the late arteriovenous-phase fluorescein angiogram, the dark (hypofluorescent) area of the pit is evident.

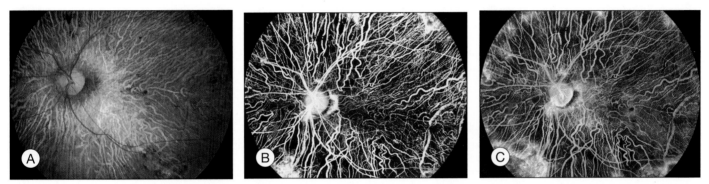

Fig. 51-31 Advance choroideremia. A, Color photograph of the left disc and macula. The large choroidal vasculature can be seen as pale irregular lines. There are some dark patches of pigment located in the macula and around the disc. B, Early arteriovenous-phase fluorescein angiogram of the left disc and macula. The large choroidal vessels can be seen filling as can the retinal arteries. The choriocapillaris is not seen. C, Late arteriovenous phase fluorescein angiogram. The large choroidal vessels and retinal vessels can be seen, but the choriocapillaris (usually seen as ground-glass fluorescence) is not seen except in the far edges of the view. COMMENT: This patient had an advanced stage of choroideremia that resulted in a total loss of RPE and choriocapillaris in most areas of the fundus. The ground-glass choroidal fluorescence was absent from most areas. The large choroidal vessels could be seen. The large choroidal vessels do not leak fluorescein, and therefore the sclera did not stain in these areas. The retinal pigment epithelium and choriocapillaris were partially intact in a few areas. These can be seen in far extremes where there is some mild ground-glass appearance.

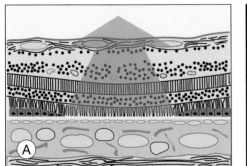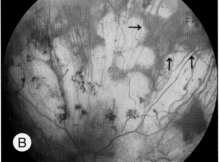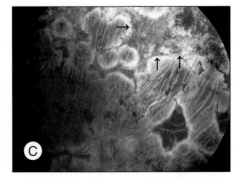

Fig. 51-32 Choroideremia. A, Schematic of retina shows loss of pigment epithelium, choriocapillaris and some of the outer retina (especially photoreceptors). B, Color photograph of left superior retina showing areas of severe atrophy and areas of more intact retinal pigment epithelium (arrows). C, The arteriovenous-phase fluorescein angiogram shows normal fluorescence of the retinal arteries. Large choroidal vessels can be seen in some areas and the ground-glass fluorescence of the choriocapillaris (arrows) in other areas where the retinal pigment epithelium and choriocapillaris are more intact. COMMENT: This patient had severe atrophy of the retinal pigment epithelium and choriocapillaris. Large choroidal vessels could be seen causing hypofluorescence in relationship to absence of ground-glass choroidal fluorescence. Some areas of choriocapillaris remained and showed normal hyperfluorescence (perhaps increased hyperfluorescence caused by loss of overlying retinal pigment epithelium).

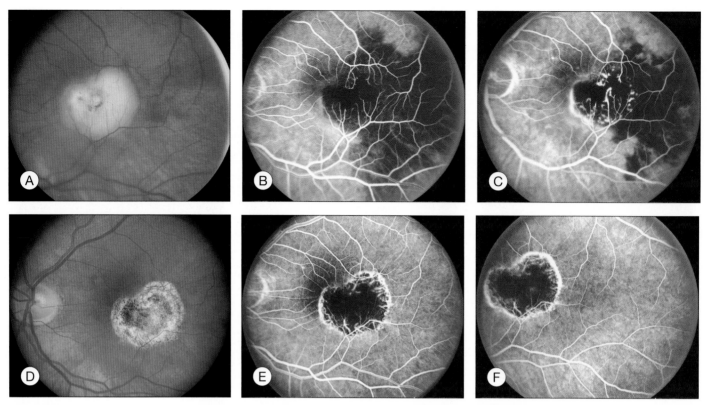

Fig. 51-33 Choroidal occlusion secondary to laser photocoagulation. A, Left macula. Color photograph shows laser photocoagulation treatment of subfoveal subretinal neovascularization. B, The early arteriovenous-phase fluorescein angiogram of the left macula shows hypofluorescence of the macula and a large area temporally. The macula hypofluorescence corresponds to the laser treatment area, which included the overlying retinal vessels; note the closure of the retinal vessels in the treated area. The large area of hypofluorescence temporally represents an area of choroidal occlusion secondary to the laser burn. C, Later-phase fluorescein angiogram shows continued hypofluorescence of the area temporal to the macula and some early leakage from the retinal vessels in the laser treated area. D, Color photograph of the left macula four months later shows an atrophic laser burn with some hyperpigmentation. The pigment epithelium temporal to the macula appears normal. E, Laser lesion centrally shows hypofluorescence that is due partly to hyperpigmentation but mostly to closure of choriocapillaris and choroid. The area of previous occlusion temporal to this lesion now shows normal ground-glass choroidal fluorescence. F, Fluorescein angiogram temporal to the left macula shows normal choriocapillaris filling. COMMENT: This patient had laser treatment of an area of subfoveal subretinal neovascularization. The laser burn caused closure of the choroid in the area of the burn as well as temporary closure of choroidal vessels temporally. Short posterior ciliary arteries and choroidal arteries from the area of the laser burn to the area temporal must have been obstructed by the laser but later reopened. The overlying pigment epithelium temporal to the laser lesion was not affected by the choroidal closure.

noticeable when there is reduced pigment in the pigment epithelium or loss of retinal pigment epithelium. This is designated *pigment epithelial window defect.*

When abnormal retinal, disc, or choroidal vessels are present and fill with fluorescein, hyperfluorescence occurs. This type of hyperfluorescence, abnormal vascular fluorescence, is also seen in the early or vascular phase of the angiography.

Hyperfluorescence caused by *leakage* is seen predominantly in the later, or extravascular, phase of angiography. In this phase fluorescein has emptied from normal and abnormal vessels. Any significant fluorescein that remains in the eye is fluorescein that has escaped or leaked from vascular or tissue barriers and is thus extravascular.

Therefore, to ascertain the type of hyperfluorescence, one must determine the time at which the hyperfluorescence appears in relation to when the fluorescein was injected. Once the hyperfluorescence is determined to be caused by preinjection fluores-

cence, transmitted fluorescence, the presence of abnormal vessels, or by leakage, the next step is to determine the anatomic location of the hyperfluorescence. Abnormal blood vessels may come from the retina and disc or from the choroid. Leakage can occur in the vitreous, disc, retina, or choroid.

Preinjection fluorescence

Each angiographic study should include one photograph of the fundus taken with the fluorescein filters in place and before fluorescein is injected. This exposure is called the preinjection or control fluorescein photograph. In normal situations this photograph is totally dark; it is completely hypofluorescent. When the photograph is not dark, autofluorescence or pseudofluorescence is present. The conditions that cause autofluorescence occur infrequently, and the filter problems that produce pseudofluorescence have, in recent years, been minimized by the development of more precisely matched filter systems.

Autofluorescence

Autofluorescence is the emission of fluorescent light from ocular structures in the absence of sodium fluorescein. Conditions that cause autofluorescence are optic nerve head drusen and astrocytic hamartoma.

Pseudofluorescence occurs when the blue exciter and green barrier filters overlap. The blue filter overlaps into the green range, allowing the passage of green light, or the green barrier filter overlaps into the blue range, which allows the passage of blue light (see Fig. 51-2). The overlapping light passes through the system, reflects off highly reflective surfaces (light-colored or white structures), and stimulates the film. This reflected nonfluorescent light is called pseudofluorescence (Fig. 51-34).

Conditions that tend to produce pseudofluorescence include any light colored or white (reflective) fundus change (e.g. sclera, exudate, scar tissue, myelinated nerve fibers, foreign body).

Currently, fluorescein angiographic filters are usually very well matched; overlap is minimal, so pseudofluorescence is faint and rarely a major problem. But filters do tend to get thin with time. The frequent flashes of light from the fundus camera wear them down, and most filter pairs eventually allow pseudofluorescence. Therefore, depending on frequency of use, fluorescein filters must be changed occasionally. Our experience indicates that change is required approximately every 5 years.

Transmitted fluorescence (pigment epithelial window defect)

This fluorescence is an accentuation of the visibility of normal choroidal fluorescence. Transmitted fluorescence occurs when fluorescence from the choroidal vasculature appears to be increased because of the absence of pigment in the pigment epithelium, which normally forms a visual barrier to choroidal fluorescence. The major cause of pigment epithelial window defect is atrophy of the pigment epithelium (Figs 51-35 to 51-39).

When the pigment epithelium is dense, choroidal fluorescence is not clearly visible because the pigment blocks the view of the choroid and acts as a barrier to fluorescein. The density of the pigment determines the degree to which transmission of the normal choroidal fluorescence is blocked. The visibility of choroidal fluorescence is inversely proportional to the concentration of pigment in the pigment epithelium. If the pigment epithelium contains less than the normal amount of pigment or is defective, the choriocapillaris appears to fluoresce more brightly. The presence of hyperfluorescence caused by a defect in the pigment epithelium depends on the state of both the pigment epithelium and the choriocapillaris. The choriocapillaris must be intact for a depigmented area of the pigment epithelium to be apparent. If the choriocapillaris does not fill, a depigmented area of the pigment epithelium does not fluoresce.

Transmitted fluorescence has the following four basic characteristics:

1. Appears early in angiography, coincidental with choroidal filling.
2. Increases in intensity as dye concentration increases in the choroid.
3. Does not increase in size or shape during the later phases of angiography.

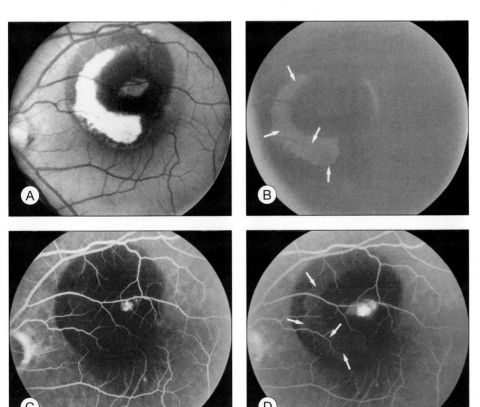

Fig. 51-34 Pseudofluorescence. A, Red-free photograph of left macula. Note the dark subretinal hemorrhage and the pale C-shaped lesion in the upper part of the macula. This very light, pale lesion was an area of dehemoglobinized blood. B, This photograph was taken with the fluorescein filters in place but before fluorescein injection. Note that the pale dehemoglobinized blood appears to fluoresce very faintly (arrows). C, Arteriovenous-phase fluorescein angiogram shows hypofluorescence caused by the large area of subretinal blood. D, Late-phase fluorescein angiogram shows hypofluorescence caused by the large patch of subretinal blood. The dehemoglobinized blood appears to fluoresce very faintly (arrows). COMMENT: This is pseudofluorescence – the light was not true fluorescence. The filters were thin and allowed reflected light through the filter system.

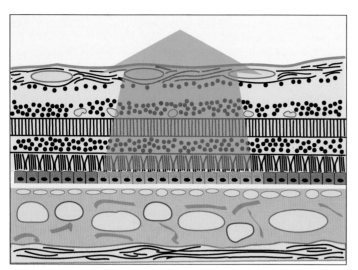

Fig. 51-35 Pigment epithelial window defect. This schematic of the retina shows that the pigment epithelium in the center of the section is less pigmented than the normal pigment epithelium. This allows the normal increased visibility of the choroidal and choriocapillaris fluorescence; i.e. this pathologic condition would create a typical pigment epithelial window defect.

4. Tends to fade and sometimes disappear as the choroid empties of dye at the end of angiography.

In short, transmitted fluorescence appears, peaks early, and fades late without changing size or shape, as would any normal vascular fluorescence. When pigment epithelial depigmentation is extensive, late fluorescein staining of the choroid and sclera may be visible, although it is less intense than the fluorescence of the window defect.

Abnormal retinal and disc vessels

Abnormal vascular fluorescence occurs when abnormal vessels are present. Such pathologic vessels may be in the retina, on the disc, or at the level of the choroid. Normal and abnormal retinal and disc vessels are clearly visible on the angiogram because no barrier obscures them from view. Gross abnormalities of the retinal and disc vasculature and subtle microvascular changes that cannot be appreciated adequately by ophthalmoscopic examination will be well defined and easily distinguished by fluorescein angiography. These changes in the retinal vasculature can be classified into six morphologic categories: (1) tortuosity and dilation (Figs 51-39, 51-42); (2) aneurysms (Figs 51-40, 51-42); (3) neovascularization (Fig. 51-41); (4) anastomosis (Fig. 51-42); (5) telangiectasis (Fig. 51-43); and (6) tumor vessels (Figs 51-44 and 51-45).

All these changes can be viewed in the early (vascular) phases of angiography. Later, as the vessels empty, some of these vascular abnormalities will leak fluorescein, whereas others will not.

Vascular abnormalities of the retina and disc are readily apparent on the fluorescein angiogram. The changes are characterized by early vascular-appearing hyperfluorescence. Each of the six morphologic types indicates specific disease processes that aid the clinician in making a diagnosis, determining the degree of the distinct pathologic process, and understanding the pathophysiology of retinal vascular disease.

Abnormal choroidal vessels

Abnormal vessels that may be present under the retina and originate from the choroid are subretinal neovascularization and vessels within a tumor. When subretinal neovascularization is present, the early angiogram often shows a lacy, irregular, and nodular hyperfluorescence (Figs 51-46 and 51-47). With a choroidal tumor, the abnormal hyperfluorescence is similar early vascular-type fluorescence, although it may be coarser, as seen in choroidal hemangioma (Fig. 51-48) and malignant melanoma (Fig. 51-49).

Leak

Fluorescence of the retinal and choroidal vessels begins to diminish about 40 to 60 seconds after injection. Fluorescein empties almost completely from the retinal and choroidal vasculature about 10 to 15 minutes after injection. Any fluorescence

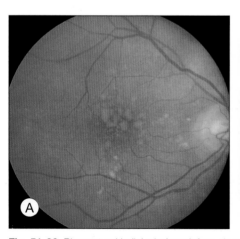
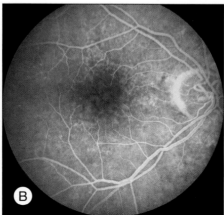
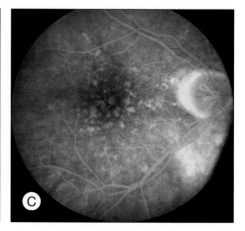

Fig. 51-36 Pigment epithelial window defect, drusen and atrophy. A, Color photograph; right macula shows multiple drusen. B, Arteriovenous-phase fluorescein angiogram shows early hyperfluorescence in the areas of the drusen. C, Late fluorescein angiogram shows some mild increase in the fluorescence. COMMENT: The drusen have created some thinning of the retinal pigment epithelium, producing some early hyperfluorescence. The slight increase in fluorescence in the later phases of the angiogram is due to fluorescein staining of the drusen material.

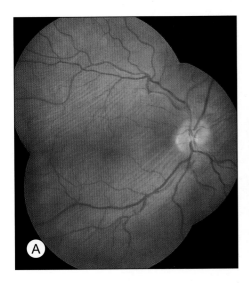

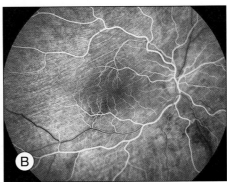

Fig. 51-37 Pigment epithelial window defect: choroidal folds. A, Color photograph of right disc and macula. Note the pale lines (choroidal folds) scattered throughout the posterior pole. B, Arteriovenous-phase fluorescein angiogram of the disc and macula. There are hyperfluorescent lines corresponding to the folds and adjacent hypofluorescent lines noted throughout the macula and surrounding the disc. COMMENT: This patient had idiopathic pigment epithelial folds. The hyperfluorescent lines are thought to be the hills of the folds, in the apices of which the pigment epithelium is thinned, allowing hyperfluorescence in the early phases of the fluorescein angiogram (pigment epithelial window defect). The dark lines are thought to be the valleys of the folds, with an increase in pigmentation causing blockage of choroidal fluorescence. Choroidal folds represent a type of pigment epithelial window defect with early vascular fluorescence and late fading of fluorescence.

that remains in the fundus after the retinal and choroidal vessels have emptied of fluorescein is extravascular fluorescence and represents leakage.

There are four types of late extravascular hyperfluorescent leakage that occur in the normal eye. They are (1) fluorescence of the disc margins from the surrounding choriocapillaris; (2) fluorescence of the lamina cribrosa; (3) fluorescence of the sclera at the disc margin if the retinal pigment epithelium terminates away from the disc, as in an optic crescent; and (4) fluorescence of the sclera when the pigment epithelium is lightly pigmented. These are the only forms of late hyperfluorescence or leakage that can be considered "normal." Any other hyperfluorescence observed 15 minutes after the fluorescein injection represents extravascular fluorescein and is referred to as *leakage*.

Either or both of the two vascular systems of the fundus can produce abnormal late hyperfluorescence (leakage) if defects are present in their respective barriers to fluorescein. The barrier to fluorescein leakage from the retinal vessels is the retinal vascular endothelium. The barrier to leakage from the choroidal circulation is the retinal pigment epithelium. An abnormality of the retinal vascular endothelium can result in permeability to fluorescein and leakage of fluorescein into the retinal tissue. Similarly, an abnormality of the pigment epithelium can result in permeability to fluorescein, and fluorescein will leak from the choroidal tissue through the pigment epithelium. Abnormal late hyperfluorescence of the choroid, however, can occur without damage to the pigment epithelium, as in cellular infiltrates of the choroid that occur in choroidal inflammation or tumor.

There are two other types of late abnormal fluorescence: one type occurs when fluorescein enters the vitreous; the other occurs when fluorescein leaks into the optic nerve head.

Vitreous leak

Leakage of fluorescein into the vitreous creates a diffuse white haze in the late phase of the fluorescein angiogram. In some instances the haze is generalized and evenly dispersed, while in other cases the white haze is localized.

Leakage of fluorescein into the vitreous is due to three major causes: (1) neovascularization growing from the retinal vessels onto the surface of the retina or disc or into the vitreous cavity; (2) intraocular inflammation; and (3) intraocular tumors.

Vitreous hyperfluorescence secondary to retinal neovascularization is usually localized and appears as a cotton-ball type of fluorescence surrounding the neovascularization (Fig. 51-41B). The vitreous fluorescence secondary to intraocular inflammation is often generalized, giving a diffuse white haze to the vitreous because of generalized leakage of fluorescein from the iris and ciliary body. The vitreous fluorescence secondary to tumors is most often localized over the tumor.

Disc leak

The optic nerve head normally has some fluorescein leakage (late hyperfluorescence) as a result of staining of the lamina cribrosa and the surrounding margins of the disc (from the normally leaking peripapillary choriocapillaries). The difference between normal and abnormal leakage at the disc may be subtle.

Papilledema and optic disc edema

Papilledema is swelling of the optic nerve head secondary to increased intracranial pressure. Edema of the optic disc is defined as swelling of the optic nerve head secondary to local or systemic causes (Fig. 51-50). The angiogram is similar in each case, demonstrating leakage associated with swelling of the optic nerve head. In the early phases of the angiogram, dilation of the capillaries on the optic nerve head may be seen; in the late angiogram, the dilated vessels leak, resulting in a fuzzy fluorescence of the disc margin.

Retinal leak

In the late stages of the normal angiogram, the retinal vessels have emptied of fluorescein and the retina is dark. Any late retinal

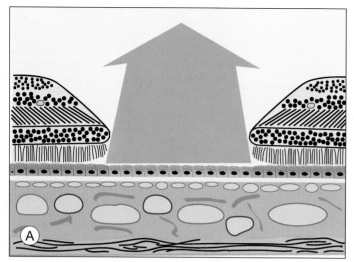

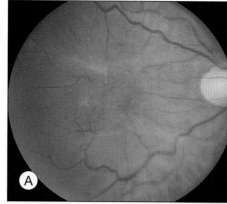

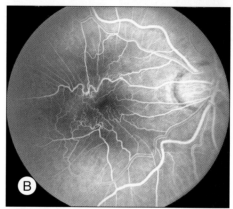

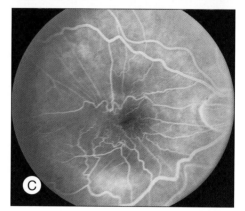

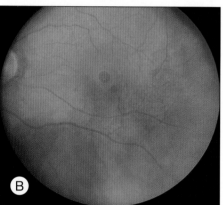

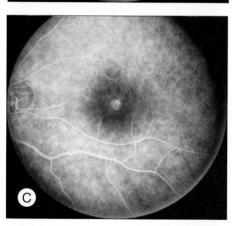

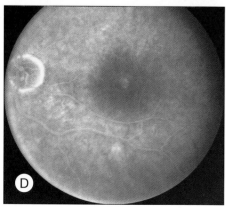

Fig. 51-38 Pigment epithelial window defect: macular hole. A, Schematic drawing of macula showing loss of entire central foveal tissue. The pigment epithelium is depigmented, and thinned. B, Color photograph of the left macula. This patient has a macular hole. Note the dark foveal center where the hole is present. There is a surrounding light ring where the sensory retina around the hole is elevated. C, Arteriovenous-phase fluorescein angiogram shows hyperfluorescence within the macular hole. D, Later phase of the fluorescein angiogram shows fading of the hyperfluorescence within the macular hole. COMMENT: This patient had a complete (through-and-through) macular hole. The choriocapillaris was intact. Therefore the angiogram showed normal fluorescence of the choriocapillaris (early hyperfluorescence within the center of the fovea) and fading in the late phases – a true retinal pigment epithelial window defect.

Fig. 51-39 Abnormal retinal vessels, tortuosity, and dilation: internal limiting membrane contraction. A, Color photograph of right macula shows a white-gray membrane overlying the right macula producing contraction of the retina and tortuosity of the retinal vessels. B, Arteriovenous-phase fluorescein angiogram shows marked irregularity and tortuosity of the retinal vessels in association with the preretinal membrane (macular pucker). C, Late-phase fluorescein angiogram shows the markedly irregular retinal vessels. Minimal leakage is present, though in some cases, traction of this degree produces marked leakage (Fig. 51-54). COMMENT: This is tortuosity and dilation, a type of abnormal retinal vascular fluorescence. It is caused by the mechanical traction of an epiretinal membrane.

hyperfluorescence is abnormal and indicates leakage of retinal vessels. When the leakage is severe, the extracellular fluid may flow into cystic pockets, and the angiogram will show fluorescence of the cystic spaces. Fluorescein flows out of the patent retinal vessels to lie in pools in the cystoid spaces or stains the edematous (noncystic) retinal tissue. Cystoid retinal edema is apparent as the fluorescein pools in small loculated pockets. In the macula, cystoid edema takes on a stellate appearance (Fig. 51-51); elsewhere in the retina, it has a honeycombed appearance (Fig. 51-52). Fluorescent staining of noncystoid edema is diffuse, irregular, and not confined to well-demarcated spaces (Figs 51-53 and 51-54).

The amount of fluorescein leakage depends on the dysfunction of the retinal vascular endothelium (Fig. 51-54). When leakage is not pronounced, the cystoid spaces fill slowly and become visible

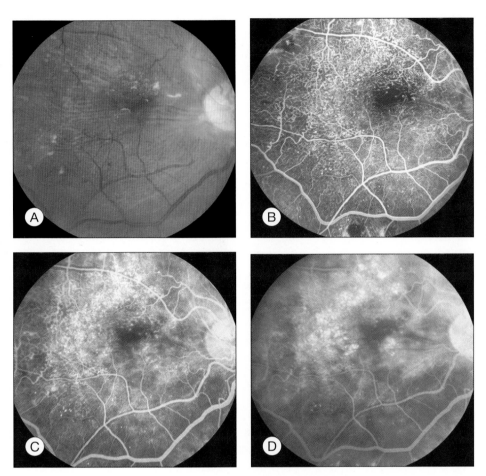

Fig. 51-40 Retinal telangiectasis and microaneurysms secondary to diabetic retinopathy. A, Color photograph of right macula showing retinal exudate, retinal striae, and irregularly dilated retinal vessels (telangiectasis). B, Arteriovenous-phase fluorescein angiogram shows extensive hyperfluorescence of the many numerous microaneurysms, and telangiectatic retinal vessels. C, Later arteriovenous-phase fluorescein angiogram showing leakage of many of these vessels. D, Late-phase fluorescein angiogram of right macula shows multiple, circular areas of hyperfluorescence due to extensive cystoid edema. COMMENT: This patient had significant retinal microvascular changes due to diabetic retinopathy.

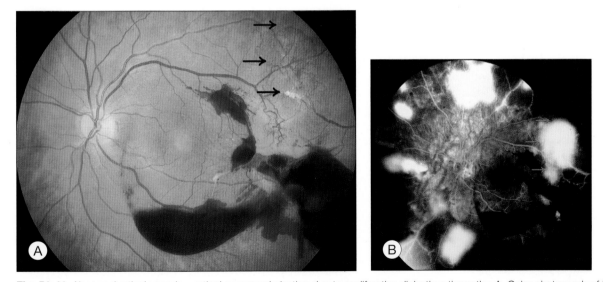

Fig. 51-41 Abnormal retinal vessels – retinal neovascularization due to proliferative diabetic retinopathy. A, Color photograph of left disc and macula. There is a large preretinal hemorrhage, and a large frond of irregular tortuous vessels superotemporal to the macula (arrows). These vessels lie on the surface of the retina. B, Late arteriovenous-phase fluorescein angiogram montage shows significant leakage of the neovascularization into the vitreous seen in the color photograph (red arrows) as well as multiple other areas of leakage due to neovascularization. COMMENT: This patient had severe proliferative diabetic retinopathy with extensive and multiple areas of neovascularization. The vessels fluoresce early (vascular fluorescence) and leak late. This is very typical of retinal or disc neovascularization.

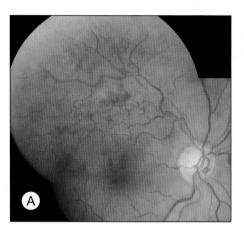

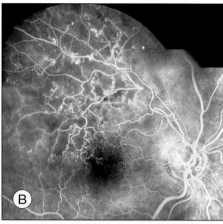

Fig. 51-42 Abnormal retinal vascular fluorescence: retinal vascular microaneurysms, telangiectasis and anastomoses. A, Color photograph of right eye shows numerous telangiectatic retinal vessels due to a superotemporal branch vein occlusion. B, Arteriovenous-phase fluorescein angiogram shows multiple areas of smaller and larger microaneurysms and telangiectasis. Several small venous–venous anastomoses can be seen just temporal to the macula. The venous system of the occluded area has collateralized with patent vessels in uninvolved areas.

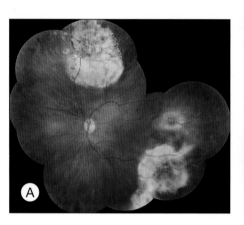

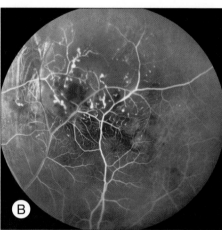

Fig. 51-43 Abnormal retinal vessels: telangiectasis. A, Color montage of left eye demonstrating severe areas of exudation, dilated and telangiectatic vessels. The retina is very edematous. B, Arteriovenous-phase fluorescein angiogram of the superior of retinal telangiectasis shows marked irregularity of the retinal vasculature. There are areas of capillary nonperfusion, telangiectasis, and tortuosity. COMMENT: This patient had Coats' disease with a markedly abnormal retinal capillary bed, including telangiectasis and dilated vessels.

only late in angiography. When this occurs, the area of cystoid retinal edema may be somewhat hypofluorescent early in the angiogram because the fluid in these spaces acts as a barrier and blocks the underlying choroidal fluorescence. When there is heavy fluorescein leakage, the cystoid spaces fill rapidly, in some cases within a minute after injection. The large confluent cysts seen with severe cystoid macular edema may fill late in the angiogram. The large retinal vessels can also leak. This is called perivascular staining and is seen in three distinct situation: inflammation (indicating a perivasculitis); traction (severe pulling on a large retinal vessel, Fig. 51-54); and occlusion. When a large retinal vessel is partially occluded, or when it traverses an area of occlusion (and capillary nonperfusion), it will leak (Fig. 51-55).

Choroidal leak

Late hyperfluorescence under the retina can be classified as either pooling or staining (Fig. 51-56). *Pooling* is defined as leakage of fluorescein into a distinct anatomic space; *staining* is leakage of fluorescein diffused into tissue.

Fluorescein pools in the spaces created by detachment of the sensory retina from the pigment epithelium or in the space created by detachment of the pigment epithelium from Bruch's membrane. The posterior layer of the sensory retina is made up of rods and cones that are loosely attached to the pigment epithelium.

When a sensory retinal detachment occurs, the detached segment separates with little force, forming a very gradual angle at the point of attachment to the pigment epithelium. Because of this narrow angle, the exact limits of a sensory retinal detachment are difficult to locate ophthalmoscopically or by slit-lamp biomicroscopy.

Depending on the specific disease, the late angiogram may or may not portray the full fluorescent filling of the subretinal fluid. For example, in central serous chorioretinopathy the leakage is gradual, and fluorescence of the subsensory retinal fluid will not be complete. In other conditions, such as subretinal neovascularization, fluorescein leakage is profuse, and the subsensory fluid often completely fluoresces (Fig. 51-57).

In contrast to the attachment of the sensory retina, the basement membrane of the pigment epithelium adheres firmly to the collagenous fibers of Bruch's membrane. The firm adhesion and wide angle of detachment make it easy to discern a pigment epithelial detachment ophthalmoscopically. Occasionally a light-orange ring appears around the periphery of a pigment epithelial detachment, further facilitating identification (Fig. 51-58).

The differences in the adherence and the angle of detachment between a sensory retinal detachment and a pigment epithelial detachment result in specific differences in fluorescent pooling

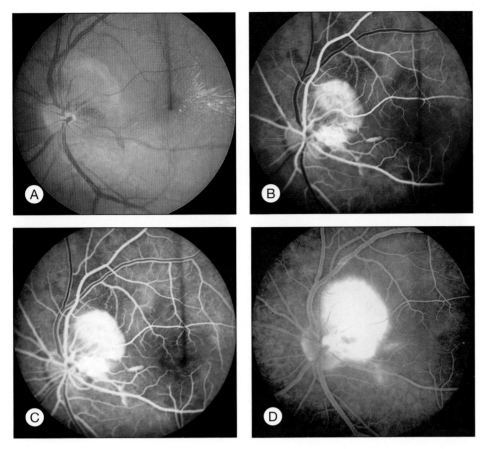

Fig. 51-44 Abnormal retinal vessels: tumor–retinal angioma as part of von Hippel's disease. A, Color photograph of left disc shows hard exudate in the macula. A very vascular, slightly elevated orange-reddish mass is present under the retina on the superotemporal border of the disc. B, Early arterial-phase fluorescein angiogram shows marked fluorescence of the mass. C, Midarteriovenous-phase fluorescein angiogram shows an increased fluorescence of the mass. Note that the hard exudate causes hypofluorescent blockage of the choroid. D, Late-phase fluorescein angiogram shows leakage of fluorescein within the mass. COMMENT: This patient had a peripapillary exophytic retinal angioma. It was very vascular and fluoresced readily with normal retinal fluorescence. It leaked late.

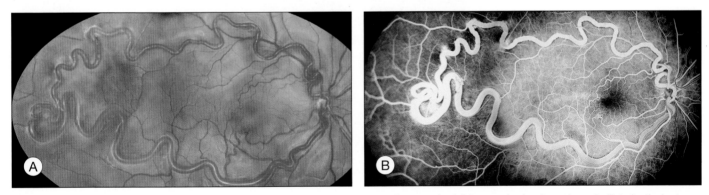

Fig. 51-45 Arteriovenous malformation – Wyburn–Mason type. A, Color montage photograph of right macula showing enlarged, dilated retinal artery, with direct connection to draining vein. There is no intervening capillary bed. B, Fluorescein angiogram showing marked hyperfluorescence of the abnormal, dilated retinal artery and vein. Two smaller arteriovenous malformations appear to be present; one just above the macula, and the other just below.

patterns. The hyperfluorescent pooling of a sensory retinal detachment tends to fade gradually toward the site where the sensory retina is attached. This makes fluorescein angiographic determination of the extent of a sensory retinal detachment difficult. In contrast, the hyperfluorescent pooling under a pigment epithelial detachment extends to the edges of the detachment, making the entire detachment and its margins hyperfluorescent and clearly discernible.

Pooling of fluorescein under a sensory retinal detachment in central serous retinopathy takes place slowly, since the dye passes through one or more points of leakage in the defective pigment epithelium (Fig. 51-56). When leakage comes from subretinal neovascularization (Fig. 51-57) or a tumor (Fig. 51-49), it is more rapid and complete. When the pigment epithelium is detached from Bruch's membrane, fluorescein passes freely and rapidly through Bruch's membrane from the choriocapillaris into the subpigment epithelial space (Fig. 51-58).

In some cases of central serous chorioretinopathy, there is an associated pigment epithelial detachment, and pooling under each (sensory retinal detachment and the pigment epithelial

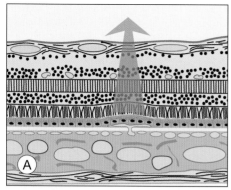

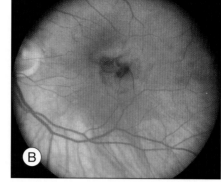

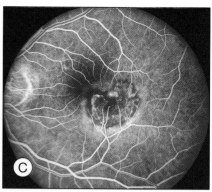

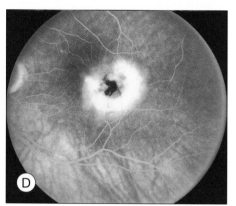

Fig. 51-46 Abnormal choroidal vessels: subretinal neovascularization. A, Schematic view of the retina shows a small break in Bruch's membrane, with a fine proliferation of capillaries through the break dissecting under and lifting up the pigment epithelium. There is a shallow sensory retinal detachment. B, Color photograph of the left macula. There is a dirty-gray membrane involving the central macula. Note the small area of subretinal hemorrhage. There is a shallow sensory retinal detachment. C, The arteriovenous-phase fluorescein angiogram shows fine, lacy, irregular hyperfluorescence corresponding to a small, fine patch of subretinal neovascularization. D, Late-phase fluorescein angiogram shows leakage of these vessels into the subpigment epithelial and subretinal spaces. COMMENT: This patient had a small patch of subretinal neovascularization involving the central fovea. The angiogram shows typical, early vascular fluorescence (in a nodular, irregular, lace-like fashion) and late hyperfluorescent leakage.

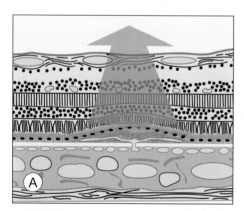

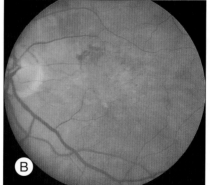

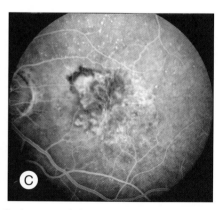

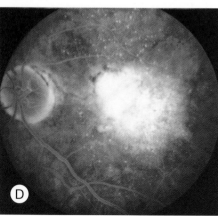

Fig. 51-47 Abnormal choroidal vessels: subretinal neovascularization. A, Schematic drawing of retina shows vascular proliferation from the choriocapillaris dissecting under the pigment epithelium, with associated fibrous tissue. The pigment epithelium has become thinned and the sensory retina detached. B, Color photograph of left macula shows some hemorrhage and a light gray membrane on the nasal side of the macula. C, Early arteriovenous-phase fluorescein angiogram shows irregular hyperfluorescence in the nasal macula. This is a flat patch of vessels that have proliferated from choriocapillaris under the pigment epithelium. There is also some attenuation of the retinal pigment epithelium extending through the macula producing some hyperfluorescence under the macula. D, Late-phase fluorescein angiogram shows leakage of the patch of subretinal neovascularization. Most of the fluorescence is pooling of fluorescein under the sensory retinal detachment. COMMENT: This patient had a patch of subretinal neovascularization that fluoresced early with the vascular phase of the angiogram (typical for subretinal neovascularization) and leaked late. Actually, "subretinal neovascularization" is a misnomer because the new vessels are initially located in the subpigment epithelial space.

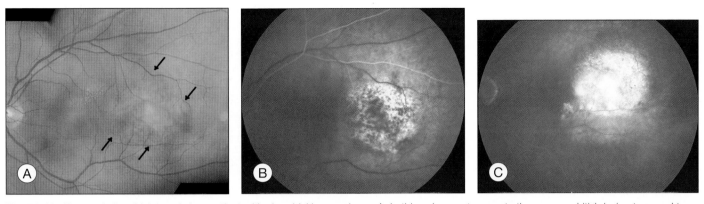

Fig. 51-48 Abnormal choroidal vessels in a patient with choroidal hemangioma. A, In this color montage, note the orange-whitish lesion temporal to the macula (arrows). There is a shallow sensory retinal detachment and exudate. B, Arteriovenous-phase fluorescein angiogram shows prominent hyperfluorescence in this area demonstrating the tumor vessels. C, Late-phase fluorescein angiogram shows marked leakage in this area. COMMENT: This patient had a choroidal hemangioma, which is a very vascularized choroidal mass. The vascularity in this mass causes the marked hyperfluorescence and leakage.

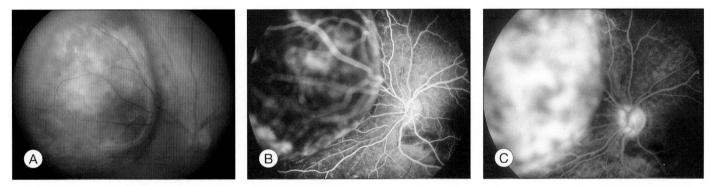

Fig. 51-49 Abnormal choroidal vascular fluorescence due to malignant melanoma. A, Wide-angle color photograph of right eye. Note the darkly pigmented mass nasally. B, Arteriovenous-phase fluorescein angiogram of the mass shows filling of the retinal vessels, as well as vessels within the melanoma. This has been termed the "double-circulation" seen in larger melanomas. C, Late-phase fluorescein angiogram shows significant leakage from these vessels within the melanoma. COMMENT: This patient had a medium-sized choroidal malignant melanoma. The angiogram shows the vascularity that can be evident in thicker melanomas.

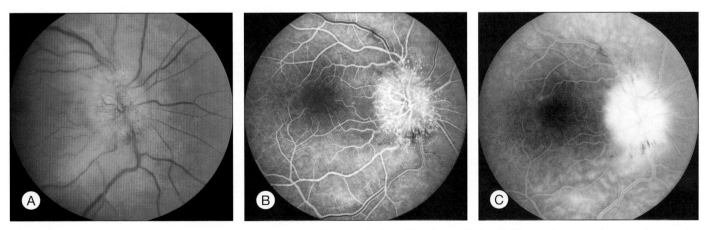

Fig. 51-50 Disc leakage. A, Color photograph of right optic nerve. Note the dilation of the disc capillaries. B, The arteriovenous phase angiogram of the right disc and macula shows the hyperfluorescence due to these dilated disc capillaries. C, The late phase of the angiogram shows significant leakage from these dilated optic disc capillaries. COMMENT: This patient had a papillopathy related to diabetes. This produced significant dilation of the disc capillaries. The leakage from this abnormal disc is quite obvious.

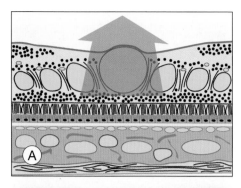

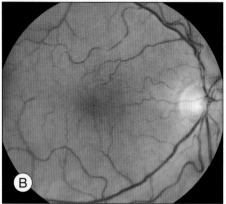

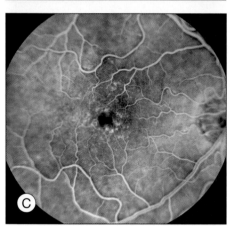

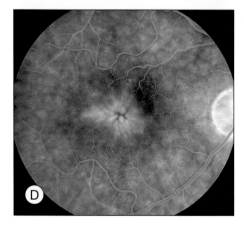

Fig. 51-51 Retinal leak: cystoid macular edema. A, Schematic drawing of the macula shows large cystic spaces in the outer plexiform layer. B, Color photograph of right macula that shows some fine dilation of the perifoveal capillaries. C, Early arteriovenous-phase fluorescein angiogram shows some dilation of the fine capillary network around the fovea. D, Late-phase fluorescein angiogram shows hyperfluorescence filling the cystic spaces. Note the stellate appearance of the cystoid macular edema. The stellate pattern is due to the oblique orientation of the outer plexiform layer in the fovea. COMMENT: This patient had late hyperfluorescence, i.e. leakage, into the retina that was severe enough to create cystic spaces. This is very typical cystoid macular edema. The cystoid edema in this case occurred following uncomplicated cataract surgery.

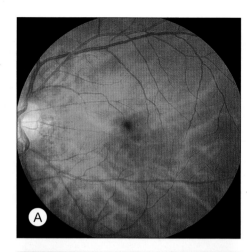

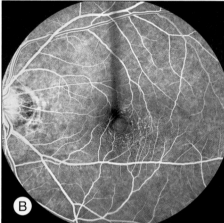

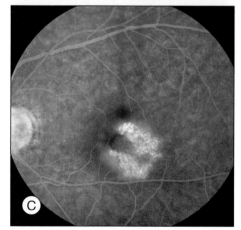

Fig. 51-52 Retinal leakage: cystoid retinal edema. A, Color photograph of the left macula shows some dilation of the perifoveal capillaries. B, Arteriovenous-phase fluorescein angiogram shows well-defined telangiectatic perifoveal vessels. C, Late-phase fluorescein angiogram shows leakage from these vessels. In the center of the macula, the leakage is in stellate cystic pockets, and just outside the macula, temporally, the leakage has taken a honeycomb form. COMMENT: This patient had leakage of telangiectatic vessels into the retina, and the leakage formed cystoid spaces. Cystoid edema in the center of the macula takes on a stellate form because of the oblique nature of the outer plexiform layer. The cystic spaces take on a honeycomb form in nonmacular areas of the retina because of the perpendicular nature of the fibers of the outer plexiform layer.

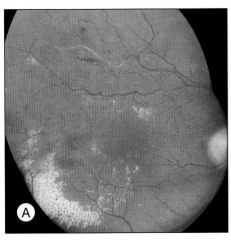
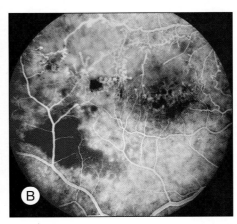
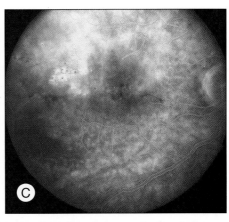

Fig. 51-53 Retinal leakage, severe noncystoid edema. Branch vein occlusion. A, Color montage of right macula and superotemporal retina shows multiple retinal hemorrhages, exudates, dilated and telangiectatic vessels, and a sheathed arteriole superiorly due to a retinal branch vein occlusion. B, Arteriovenous-phase fluorescein angiogram of the right macula shows the vascular abnormalities associated with the branch vein occlusion. C, Late-phase fluorescein angiogram shows diffuse leakage of the fluorescein dye. COMMENT: This patient had generalized leakage of the retinal vascular bed in the distribution of the blocked branch vein. The leakage was not yet severe enough, however, to form cystic spaces. Late hyperfluorescence indicates leakage, and this fluorescence is located in the retina; thus this was retinal edema.

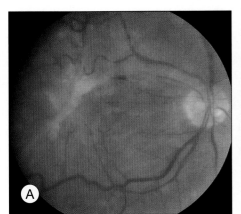
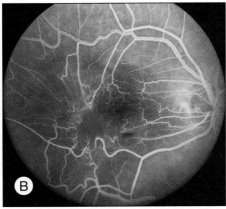
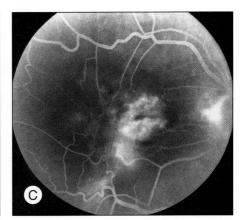

Fig. 51-54 Late hyperfluorescence, retinal leakage: severe epiretinal membrane contraction. A, Color photograph of right macula showing thick epiretinal membrane overlying the macula and producing severe traction and contraction of the retina and vessels. B, Arteriovenous-phase fluorescein angiogram shows that the retinal vasculature is tortuous and irregular. C, Late arteriovenous-phase fluorescein angiogram shows leakage from the retinal vessels temporally. COMMENT: The marked preretinal membrane caused sufficient traction on the retina to result in marked retinal vascular leakage.

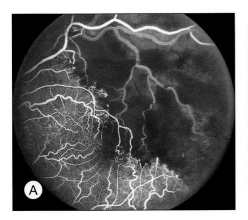
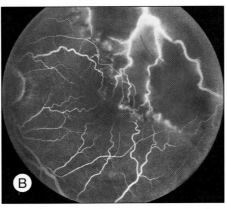

Fig. 51-55 Retinal leakage–perivascular staining. A, In this arteriovenous phase fluorescein angiogram of the left macula, note the severe nonperfusion superotemporally. B, Late-phase fluorescein angiogram shows perivascular staining (leakage) from the large retinal vessels that are traversing the large area of capillary nonperfusion. COMMENT: Whenever a large retinal vessel (artery or vein) is perfused but traverses an area of capillary nonperfusion, ischemic retinal factors will act adversely on the endothelium of the large vessel and cause it to leak. This is called perivascular staining. Perivascular staining also occurs with traction or inflammation.

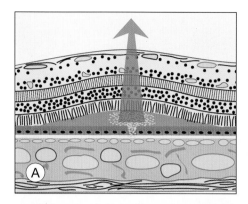

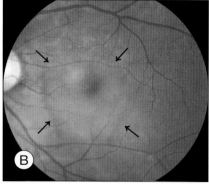

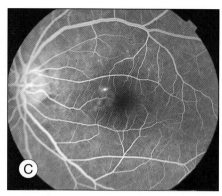

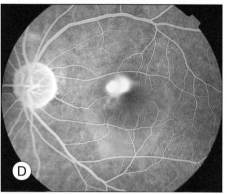

Fig. 51-56 Late hyperfluorescence, subretinal pooling: central serous chorioretinopathy. A, Schematic drawing of retina shows a sensory retinal detachment. There is a break in the pigment epithelium. Fluorescein flows from the choriocapillaris through Bruch's membrane, through the break in pigment epithelium to the subretinal space, under the detached retina. B, Color photograph of left macula shows a shallow sensory detachment (arrows). Just superonasal to the fovea is a small white area with a gray center. The fluorescein angiogram will reveal that this is the area of the leak. C, Arteriovenous-phase fluorescein angiogram shows a hyperfluorescent spot that was seen on stereoangiography to be leakage of fluorescein coming from the pigment epithelium. D, Late-phase fluorescein angiogram shows that the spot of pigment epithelial leakage has enlarged and become fuzzy. This is the release of fluorescein molecules into the fluid under the detached sensory retina. COMMENT: This patient had central serous chorioretinopathy. There was a break in the pigment epithelium that allowed leakage of fluorescein through it into the subretinal space. Late hyperfluorescence means leakage, and in this case, there is pooling of fluorescein under the detached retina.

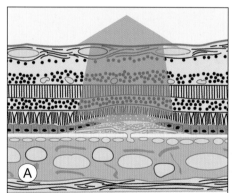

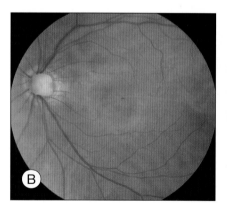

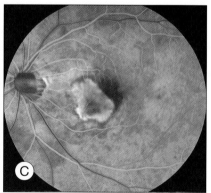

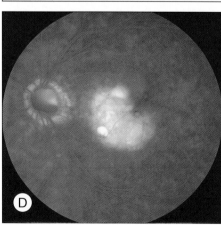

Fig. 51-57 Late hyperfluorescence, leakage, and pooling under the sensory retina caused by subretinal neovascularization, resulting in a sensory retinal detachment. A, Schematic of the retina showing that the retina has detached (photoreceptors are separated from pigment epithelium). Vessels have proliferated from the choriocapillaris through Bruch's membrane. There is a fibrovascular scar involving the pigment epithelium and the sensory retina is detached. B, Color photograph of left macula shows a pale gray lesion in the nasal portion of the macula with some overlying hemorrhage. C, Arteriovenous-phase fluorescein angiogram shows a patch of subretinal neovascularization nasal to the fovea; this is evidenced by the lacy, irregular, nodular hyperfluorescence in this area. D, Late-phase fluorescein angiogram shows fuzzy fluorescence. There is pooling of fluorescein under the detached retina. COMMENT: This patient had a patch of subretinal neovascularization with a great deal of leakage, causing a sensory detachment. The early angiogram showed the vascular nature of the lesion and the late angiogram, the leakage and pooling under the subretinal space.

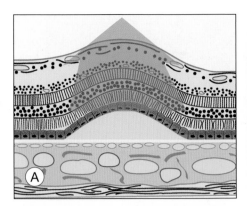

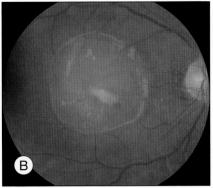

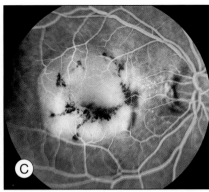

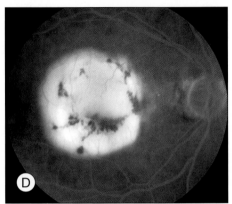

Fig. 51-58 Late hyperfluorescent pooling under the pigment epithelium–pigment, epithelial detachment. A, Schematic drawing of retina shows detached pigment epithelium and fluorescein dye pooling in this space – the pigment epithelium is separated from Bruch's membrane. Because the attachment of the pigment epithelium to Bruch's membrane is quite firm, the angle of detachment is quite large. B, Color photograph of right macula shows a round detachment of the pigment epithelium. C, Early arteriovenous-phase fluorescein angiogram shows early fluorescence from the area of detachment pigment epithelium. D, Late angiogram of right macula shows well-demarcated hyperfluorescent pooling of fluorescein under the detached pigment epithelium. COMMENT: Fluorescein flows freely through Bruch's membrane and stops at the pigment epithelium. When the pigment epithelium is detached, the fluorescein flows right through Bruch's membrane into the space made by the detached pigment epithelium. Therefore a pigment epithelial detachment fluoresces evenly and slowly (like a light bulb on a rheostat) and shows intense hyperfluorescent pooling that is well-demarcated (indicating its well-defined angle of attachment) late in the angiogram.

detachment) is evident. Occasionally, the edge of a pigment epithelial detachment may tear, or "rip," and allow fluorescein dye to pass freely into the subretinal space (Fig. 51-59). Drusen may also show late hyperfluorescence similar to that seen with a pigment epithelial detachment (Fig. 51-60). In some cases of pigment epithelial detachment, especially in older patients, subretinal neovascularization is also present. This combination of subretinal neovascularization and pigment epithelial detachment results in an interesting angiogram that can be challenging to interpret (Fig. 51-61).

In summary, late hyperfluorescence beneath the retina should first be distinguished as pooling of fluorescein into a space or as tissue staining with fluorescein. When pooling is present, one must determine whether a sensory retinal or a pigment epithelial detachment is present. Similarly, if staining is present, one must find out whether the tissue involved is the retinal pigment epithelium and Bruch's membrane, choroid, or sclera. From this anatomic determination a more specific diagnosis can be determined.

Staining
Staining refers to leakage of fluorescein into tissue or material and is contrasted with pooling of the fluorescein into an anatomic space. Many abnormal subretinal structures and materials can retain fluorescein and demonstrate later hyperfluorescent staining.

Drusen   The most common form of staining occurs with drusen. Most drusen hyperfluoresce early in the angiogram because choroidal fluorescence is transmitted through defects in the pigment epithelium overlying the drusen (Fig. 51-36). Fluorescence from most small drusen diminishes as the dye leaves the choroidal circulation. However, some larger drusen display later hyperfluorescence or staining (Fig. 51-60). The larger the drusen, the more likely they will retain fluorescein and staining will occur. When drusen are large and have smooth edges, the late staining on the angiogram is similar in appearance to that of pooling of fluorescein under a pigment epithelial detachment. In many cases it is difficult, if not impossible, to differentiate large drusen from small pigment epithelial detachments: they have a similar ophthalmoscopic, fluorescein angiographic, and even microscopic appearance.

Scar   Scar tissue retains fluorescein and usually demonstrates well-demarcated hyperfluorescence because little, if any, fluid surrounds the scar. Later in the healing process, when only a few vessels remain, the early angiogram is hypofluorescent because of the paucity of vessels and blockage by the scar tissue. The most commonly seen scar tissue is the disciform scar, which is the end stage of subretinal neovascularization. Scarring is also seen following numerous other insults to the pigment epithelium and choroid, especially inflammation (Fig. 51-62).

Sclera   In several situations the sclera is visible ophthalmoscopically and exhibits late hyperfluorescent staining on fluorescein angiography. Scleral staining is best seen when the retinal pigment epithelium is very pale (as in a blonde patient) or when the choriocapillaris is fully intact. When the choriocapillaris is not intact, fluorescein staining of the sclera can occur from the edges

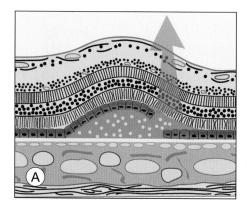

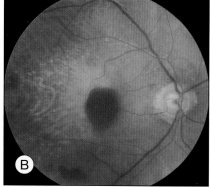

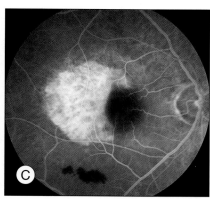

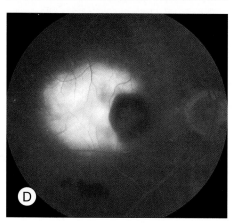

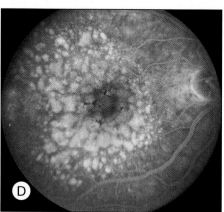

Fig. 51-59 Late hyperfluorescence under the retina – leakage from the choroid due to a retinal pigment epithelial rip. A, Schematic of a pigment epithelial detachment that has developed a tear along one edge. The barrier function of the pigment epithelium is lost and fluorescein dye can diffuse easily and rapidly in the subretinal space. B, Color photograph of right macula showing a round dark area under the fovea, and light (depigmented) area extending temporally. In the inferior portion of the macula, some subretinal hemorrhage is seen. C, Early arteriovenous-phase fluorescein angiogram shows bright hyperfluorescence of the depigmented area temporally, and hypofluorescence under the fovea as well as inferiorly in the area of the subretinal blood. D, Late phase fluorescein angiogram shows pooling of fluorescein under the retina where the dye has been able to freely diffuse through Bruch's membrane in the sensory retinal detachment. COMMENT: This patient developed a tear of pigment epithelial detachment. The dark area of under the fovea is where the pigment epithelium has rolled-up after tearing away from the area temporally. The area temporal to the macula appears light due to absence of the retinal pigment epithelium in this area. Since the retinal pigment epithelial barrier is absent in this area, the dye diffuses readily and rapidly into overlying sensory retinal detachment producing late pooling of fluorescein.

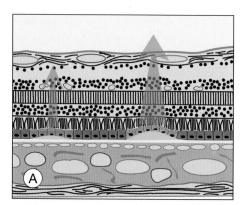

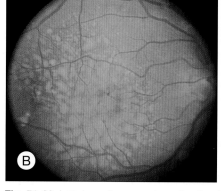

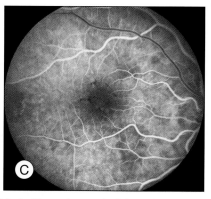

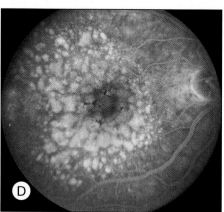

Fig. 51-60 Late hyperfluorescent pooling (or staining) of large drusen. A, Schematic section of retina shows a smaller and larger detachment of pigment epithelium. Drusen deposit between the pigment epithelium and Bruch's membrane and lift the pigment epithelium up, forming small or large pigment epithelial detachments, depending on the size of the drusen. B, Color photograph of right macula shows multiple, pale, round, and variably-sized drusen. C, Arteriovenous-phase fluorescein angiogram shows minimal early hyperfluorescence of the drusen. D, Late fluorescein angiogram shows marked hyperfluorescence of the drusen. The larger drusen take longer for the hyperfluorescence to develop. COMMENT: The larger the drusen, the more like pigment epithelial detachments they are, and therefore the more likely it is that they will show pooling of fluorescein (or staining of the drusen material).

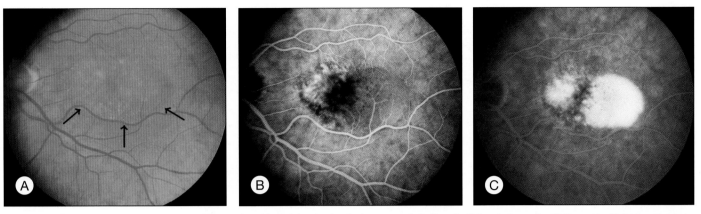

Fig. 51-61 Pigment epithelial detachment with associated (suspicious) subretinal neovascularization. A, Color photograph of left macula. Note the pigment epithelial detachment temporally and sensory retinal detachment overlying this and extending nasally (arrows). B, Arteriovenous-phase fluorescein angiogram shows early hyperfluorescence of the area of choroidal neovascularization nasally, and less intense hyperfluorescence of the pigment epithelial detachment temporally. C, Late-phase fluorescein angiogram of left macula shows that the fluorescence of the pigment epithelial detachment temporally has increased significantly, and fuzzy fluorescence from the area of choroidal neovascularization nasally. COMMENT: This patient had an irregularly shaped pigment epithelial detachment which is a sign of possible choroidal neovascularization. The irregular, fuzzy hyperfluorescence that nasally is due to this area of occult choroidal neovascularization.

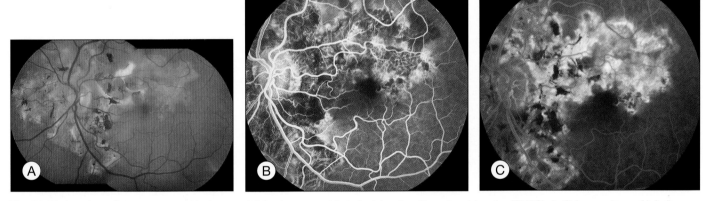

Fig. 51-62 Late hyperfluorescence and leakage – staining in geographic helicoid peripapillary choroidopathy (GHPC). A, Color montage of left disc and macula shows large geographic areas of atrophy of pigment epithelium and choriocapillaris. There is some hyperplasia of the pigment epithelium noted as hyperpigmentation (especially in the macula and papillomacular bundle). Some fibrous scar tissue is present. B, Arteriovenous-phase fluorescein angiogram shows that the geographic lesions are mostly hypofluorescent; they are caused by loss of pigment epithelium and choriocapillaris. Note the large choroidal vessels can be seen within these lesions, indicating that the pigment epithelium and choriocapillaris are both gone. There is some hyperfluorescence along the edges of the geographic lesions. The pigment epithelial hyperplasia causes blocked fluorescence. C, Late fluorescein angiogram of left macula shows hyperfluorescent staining along the edges of the geographic lesion. COMMENT: This patient had GHPC; inflammation of choroid and pigment epithelium resulted in a loss of the pigment epithelium and choriocapillaris and some of the choroid. The angiogram showed that only large choroidal vessels remained within these lesions. The choriocapillaris was intact, however, in the normal tissue adjacent to the geographic atrophic tissue. The normal choriocapillaris leaked into the atrophic area in a horizontal fashion, causing late hyperfluorescence of areas of scar tissue and some scleral staining.

of the atrophic area where fluorescein leaks from the intact choriocapillaris inward toward the atrophy (Fig. 51-62).

In conditions such as physiologically light-colored (blonde) fundus or in myopia, the choriocapillaris is usually sufficient to stain the sclera completely. After the choroidal vessels have emptied of fluorescein in the later phases of angiography, the large hypofluorescent choroidal vessels will appear as dark lines in silhouette against the stained sclera.

When a loss of choroid and choriocapillaris has occurred, there is a consequent diminution of fluorescein flow in the choroid.

When this occurs, the sclera stains with fluorescein only from adjacent normal patent choriocapillaris vasculature. These vessels stain the sclera on the borders of the lesion because the dye tends to diffuse toward the center of the lesion. The entire lesion may not stain if the distance from the edge of the sclera is more than 1 mm. When the choriocapillaris is intact or the lesion is not expansive, the sclera will stain completely.

In summary, late hyperfluorescence beneath the retina should first be distinguished as pooling of fluorescein into a space or as tissue stained with fluorescein. When pooling is present, it must be determined whether a sensory retinal or a pigment epithelium detachment is present. Similarly, if staining is present, it must be determined whether the tissue involved is the retinal pigment epithelium and Bruch's membrane, choroid, or sclera. From this anatomic differentiation, a more specific diagnosis can be determined.

Acknowledgment

This work was supported by the Retina Research Fund of St. Mary's Medical Center, San Francisco.

BIBLIOGRAPHY

1. DeLori F, Ben-Sira I, Trempe C. Fluorescein angiography with an optimized filter combination. Am J Ophthalmol 1976; 82:559–566.
2. Gass JD. Stereoscopic atlas of macular disease: diagnosis and treatment, 4th edn. St. Louis: Mosby-Year Book; 1997.
3. Gitter KA, Schatz H, Yannuzzi LA et al. Laser photocoagulation of retinal disease. San Francisco: Pacific Medical Press; 1988.
4. Hyvärien L, Hochleimer BF. Filter systems in fluorescein angiography. Int Ophthalmol Clin 1974; 14:49–61.
5. Justice J Jr, ed. Ophthalmic photography. Boston: Little Brown; 1982.
6. Kelly SJ. Autofluorescence of drusen of the optic nerve head. Arch Ophthalmol 1974; 92:263–264.
7. LaPiano FG, Penner R. Anaphylactoid reaction to intravenously administered fluorescein. Arch Ophthalmol 1968; 79:161–162.
8. Levacy R, Justice J, Jr. Adverse reactions to intravenous fluorescein. Int Ophthalmol Clin 1976; 16:53–61.
9. Novotny HR, Alvis DL. A method of photographing fluorescence in circulating blood in the human retina. Circulation 1961; 24:82–86.
10. Rabb MF, Burton TC, Schatz H et al. Fluorescein angiography of the fundus: a schematic approach to interpretation. Surv Ophthalmol 1978; 11:387–403.
11. Schatz H. Flow sheet for the interpretation of fluorescein angiograms. Arch Ophthalmol 1976; 94:687.
12. Schatz H. Sloughing of skin following fluorescein extravasation. Ann Ophthalmol 1978; 10:625.
13. Schatz H. Laser treatment of fundus disease: a comprehensive text and composite slide collection. San Anselmo, CA: Pacific Medical Press; 1980.
14. Schatz H. Three-way adjustable armrest for fluorescein angiography. Am J Ophthalmol 1982; 93:244.
15. Schatz H. Essential fluorescein angiography: a compendium of 100 classic cases. San Anselmo, CA: Pacific Medical Press; 1983.
16. Schatz H, Burton TC, Yannuzzi LA et al. Interpretation of fundus fluorescein angiography. St Louis: Mosby-Year Book; 1978.
17. Schatz H, Farkas WS. Nausea from fluorescein angiography. Am J Ophthalmol 1982; 93:370–371.
18. Schatz H, George T, Liu HJ et al. Color fluorescein angiography: its clinical role. Trans Am Acad Ophthalmol Otolaryngol 1973; 77:254–259.
19. Stein MR, Parker CW. Reactions following intravenous fluorescein. Am J Ophthalmol 1971; 72:861–868.
20. Berkow JW et al., eds. Fluorescein angiography. San Francisco: American Academy of Ophthalmology; 1991.
21. Yannuzzi LA, Rohrer KT, Tindel LJ et al. Fluorescein angiography complication survey. Ophthalmology 1986; 93:611–617.
22. Patz A, Finkelstein D, Fine SL et al. The role of fluorescein angiography in national collaborative studies. Ophthalmology 1986; 93:1466–1470.
23. Friberg TR, Rehkopf PG, Warnicki JW et al. Use of directly acquired digital fundus and fluorescein angiographic images in the diagnosis of retinal disease. Retina 1987; 7:246–251.
24. Watson AP, Rosen ES. Oral fluorescein angiography: reassessment of its relative safety and evaluation of optimum conditions with use of capsules. Br J Ophthalmol 1990; 74:458–461.
25. Mimoun G, Soubrane G, Coscas G. Clinical experience with digitized fluorescein angiography. Int Ophthalmol 1991; 15:41–46.
26. Clark TM, Freeman WR, Goldbaum MH. Digital overlay of fluorescein angiograms and fundus images for treatment of subretinal neovascularization, Retina 12: 1992; 118–126.
27. Johnson RN, McDonald HR, Schatz H. Rash, fever, and chills after intravenous fluorescein angiography. Am J Ophthalmol 1998; 126:837–838.
28. Lee PP, Yang JC, Schachat AP. Is informed consent needed for fluorescein angiography? Arch Ophthalmol 1993; 111:327–330.

Chapter

52

Quantitative Fluorescein Angiography

Alexander C. Walsh
Paul G. Updike
Srinivas R. Sadda

0INTRODUCTION

Since its original description by Flocks et al. in 1959[1], MacLean et al.[2] in 1960 and Novotny and Alvis[3] in 1961, fluorescein angiography has served as an invaluable tool for the diagnosis and management of numerous retinal diseases. As discussed in Chapter 51, various patterns of hyper and hypofluorescence visible by angiography have been correlated with specific disease states and have been used for disease staging. For instance, in neovascular age-related macular degeneration (AMD), choroidal neovascularization (CNV) has been recognized to have occult and classic patterns of fluorescein leakage. These patterns of fluorescence have been shown to correlate with clinical outcomes and response to therapy in a number of large randomized clinical trials, such as the Macular Photocoagulation Study (MPS),[4,5] Treatment of Age-related macular degeneration with Photodynamic therapy (TAP),[6–8] and Verteporfin in Photodyamic Therapy (VIP) studies.[9] Similarly, in the Early Treatment Diabetic Retinopathy Study,[10] certain angiographic patterns were found to be predictive of diabetic retinopathy progression. Although these landmark studies illustrated the value of fluorescein angiography and cemented its critical role in current clinical practice, they may not have fully extracted the valuable data contained in these angiographic images.

Over the last half of the 20th century, there has been a dramatic quantitative revolution in medicine. Subjective, qualitative measures of disease activity have been replaced with objective, precise measurements which have allowed physicians to more accurately diagnose and follow their patients. As an example, internists, instead of simply telling their patients that they have "mild" or "severe" osteoporosis, are now able to precisely quantify bone density, allowing earlier detection of osteoporosis and improved monitoring of response to therapy.

Ophthalmology has appeared to lag behind other areas of medicine in embracing this quantitative revolution. In particular, with respect to fluorescein angiography, there has been little change in the angiographic procedure since its original description. Imaging equipment has improved in an evolutionary, rather than revolutionary, fashion. Interpretation of angiographic images has remained largely subjective, with only a handful of semi-quantitative parameters currently used to describe fundus lesions. The development of high-resolution digital fundus imaging systems, high-resolution film scanners, and high-speed computing,

however, has now made complete and objective quantification of fluorescein angiographic findings feasible. This chapter highlights the limitations of current subjective methods of fluorescein interpretation, outlines the major steps in quantitative fluorescein analysis, and summarizes the current state-of-the-art in the field.

SUBJECTIVE, QUALITATIVE FLUORESCEIN ANGIOGRAM INTERPRETATION

Current techniques and principles utilized in the interpretation of fluorescein angiograms are described in Chapter 51. The interpreter or grader studies the entire sequence of angiographic frames, as well as color and red-free images, to identify all relevant normal and abnormal structures in the image set. The patterns of fluorescence and changes in fluorescence intensity of the various structures in the image set are important parameters that assist in the evaluation of the images. The interpreter mentally corrects, when possible, for variations and deficiencies in the image set, such as irregularities in lighting, poor focus, artifacts, alterations in field of view or magnification, differences in injected fluorescein dye volume, systemic vascular variations, low contrast, and missing angiographic phases. These "mental corrections" are intuitive, imprecise, and dependent in part on experience. Ultimately, the grader identifies and classifies various structures by comparing the lesion of interest with similar named entities previously encountered by the grader in his or her training or experience. As the classification system is ultimately finite, the grader is faced with the challenge of assigning the "best-fit" label to the lesion of interest, often using subjective prefixes (such as "questionable" or "probable") to reflect the level of diagnostic uncertainty. This level of diagnostic uncertainty or degree of discrepancy between the lesion of interest and the "ideal" or "prototypical" lesion is not precisely quantified by the grader. Consequently, existing qualitative methods of angiographic interpretation have the potential to inappropriately "lump" together entities which are angiographically (and perhaps pathophysiologically) distinct, and to "split" lesions that are actually similar.

Given these potentially significant drawbacks, why are subjective methods of angiogram interpretation widely accepted as the standard for clinical practice? One obvious reason is the previous reliance on analog (film-based) angiographic images which precluded significant post-capture processing and mathematical analysis without first scanning the images into a digital format. The most important justification for the use of subjective, qualitative fluorescein analysis, however, as noted above, was the successful application of these methods in landmark ophthalmic clinical trials. For example, clinical experts of the Macular Photocoagulation Study group,[4,5] devised definitions for angiographic lesions, such as classic CNV (defined as a bright uniform area of hyperfluorescence which appeared early in the transit and leaked in the mid and late phases of the angiogram), which the investigators surmised may have clinical predictive value based on their previous experience. For other studies, such as the Diabetic Retinopathy Study (DRS)[11] and the ETDRS,[10] clinical experts established subjective and qualitative definitions of disease lesions of varying severity, utilizing "standard" photographs to illustrate prototypical lesions. In both examples, although the definitions were subjective and to some extent arbitrary, the subsequent clinical studies demonstrated that the defined entities correlated with disease outcomes. For instance, neovascularization of the disk greater than Standard Photograph 10A was found to be associated with an increased risk for severe vision loss in the DRS.[11] Similarly, in the TAP study, the relative amount of classic CNV was found to correlate with clinical response to photodynamic therapy.[6–8]

Although the use of subjective methods of angiogram analysis in clinical studies would appear to be valid, the extrapolation of these methods to general clinical practice may be more tenuous. For the large-scale clinical studies, centralized expert photographic reading centers were established to interpret the retinal images. These reading centers employed extensively trained dedicated image graders, rigorous interpretation protocols, and quality control procedures to enhance reproducibility and reliability of the grading process. The realities of clinical practice preclude the implementation of such rigorous methods to the interpretative process, and may compromise the accuracy of routine interpretations relative to the clinical trial standard. Indeed, Kaiser and coworkers[12] observed considerable variability among angiogram interpretation, even among clinical trial investigators. Such variability raises significant concerns regarding the potential inappropriate application of clinical trial results to clinical practice. For example, if a treatment such as photodynamic therapy is only proven to be beneficial for certain subtypes of lesions, misinterpretation of the lesion (relative to the reading center standard) by the clinician may result in exposure of the patient to the risks of the treatment without any benefit. There is also the additional financial burden imposed on the patient and/or the health care system as a result of inadequate testing and unnecessary treatments. Concerns regarding the variability of the interpretative process have compelled several third party payers to employ the use of expert consultants to review fluorescein angiograms prior to authorizing photodynamic therapy treatment.

SUBJECTIVE, SEMI-QUANTITATIVE PARAMETERS OF ANGIOGRAPHIC LESIONS

Despite the qualitative nature of existing methods of fluorescein angiogram interpretation, several semi-quantitative parameters have been developed by centralized reading centers for use in clinical trials. For choroidal neovascular lesions, two spatial parameters, the greatest linear dimension (GLD) and the lesion area have been described.[6] The GLD theoretically provides a precise measurement of the longest linear extent of the lesion and is usually expressed in millimeters. However, the accuracy of the GLD depends on the ability of the clinician to identify the borders of the lesion correctly and to identify the dimension which yields the largest measurement. These determinations are, of course, subjective and consequently, the GLD is a semi-quantitative measure at best. The measurement of lesion area, as assessed in prior clinical trials, is similarly imprecise. In the MPS studies, a unit area (or "one MPS disk area") was defined as a circle with a diameter (d) of 1.5 mm (and area of $\pi(d/2)^2$, or about 1.77 mm^2). Based on this definition, the diameters for circles of various unit areas can be readily derived. The lesion area was defined as the smallest circle which could completely encompass the lesion, after mentally "folding" the lesion as needed, such that the lesion occupied as compact (i.e. circular) a shape as possible. Thus, lesions in clinical trials were classified into size categories and changes in size over time were defined as progression to the next size category. Such a categorical system, however, allowed lesions which differed in size by as much as 1.77 mm^2 (one unit disk area) to be included in the same category, and was potentially insensitive to changes in lesion size of a similar amount. The use of this qualitative, categorical system was necessitated by the availability of film angiograms as the clinical trial standard. The advent of digital imaging technology, however, provides the clinician with the ability to trace the lesion borders and more precisely calculate lesion area. Unfortunately, as with GLD, the accuracy of these measurements still depends on the correct identification of the lesion and its borders. Consequently, existing measures of the spatial properties of fundus lesions are subjective and semi-quantitative at best. Given the subjective nature of these measurements, comparisons of these measurements over time are fraught with a further degree of uncertainty.

Another semi-quantitative parameter obtained with current analysis methods is the lesion number. In the Age Related Eye Diseases Study, the number of drusen present in the macula was used as one criterion to assist the grader in classification of non-neovascular AMD severity.[13,14] Similarly, in the DRS, the numbers of microaneurysms and intraretinal hemorrhages present in retinal images were used to help determine the severity of diabetic retinopathy.[15] Subsequent investigators have further demonstrated the potential importance of microaneurysm counts in monitoring the progression of diabetic retinopathy.[16–18] Precise determinations of lesion number, however, are labor intensive, impractical for clinical use, and are ultimately dependent on the accurate identification of all similar lesions.

In spite of the widespread use of these various spatial or anatomic parameters, functional parameters quantifying fluorescein leakage have not been well-established. The Wisconsin Photographic Reading Center has developed a method for assessing leakage in retinal vasculopathies associated with macular edema, but the technique is ultimately qualitative and limited to a few levels or categories.[10] Furthermore, similar to assessment of lesion number, this method may be challenging to apply in general clinical practice.

VALIDATION OF SUBJECTIVE FLUORESCEIN ANGIOGRAPHIC PARAMETERS

Despite the limitations inherent in the subjective nature of existing methods of FA interpretation, these techniques have been validated in multiple, large-scale clinical trials. As an example, although the definition of classic CNV is subjective, the importance of recognizing this lesion type has been firmly established by the TAP investigation.[19] Patients with predominantly classic CNV lesions were found to benefit from treatment, whereas patients with large minimally classic lesions did not. Moreover, quality control procedures developed at the central photographic reading center confirmed that the defined lesions could be identified reproducibly by trained graders.[19]

Similarly, the importance of semi-quantitative measures such as lesion area has also been established by these same studies. Retrospective analysis of the TAP and VIP studies demonstrated that non-predominantly classic CNV lesions smaller than 6 MPS disk areas (in particular, lesions <4 MPS) appeared to benefit from treatment, whereas larger lesions did not.[20]

A reliance on subjectively derived parameters for assessment of retinal diseases, however, introduces a potentially concerning ascertainment bias. Only those features identified by the clinical trial expert as being relevant are evaluated and correlated with clinical outcomes. However, it is possible that other unidentified factors may be of greater significance. The previously described TAP and VIP studies are good examples, as lesion size was initially underestimated as an important predictor of response to treatment.[20] Complete quantification and analysis of retinal images could permit a more objective determination of the lesion features and parameters which demonstrate the greatest correlation with clinical outcomes.

FACTORS HINDERING THE TRANSITION FROM QUALITATIVE TO QUANTITATIVE FLUORESCEIN ANALYSIS

Reliance on analog (film) image capture techniques has been an important factor limiting the extent of quantitative information that can be extracted. The relatively low-resolution (and consequently limited stereopsis) and limited color depth of the first-generation, digital charged-coupled devices (CCDs) discouraged investigators from employing this technology in clinical trials. As a comparison, these early sensors had fewer than 1 million pixels (i.e. 1 megapixel) of information while photographic film is believed to have resolution that exceeds 10 million pixels and superior color depth.[21] And although quantitative data can be extracted from film through digitization, this scanning process is time-consuming and introduces noise and artifacts into the image data.

Advances in digital imaging, such as the development of high-resolution (i.e. >6 megapixel and higher) sensors, have made further quantification feasible. An enormous amount of data, however, is an attendant consequence of such high-resolution images. Concomitant advances in computing technology and processor speed have allowed researchers in retinal image analysis to begin to cope with this potential problem.

Another limitation which has hindered the development of quantitative fluorescein angiographic analysis is a lack of sophistication in image processing technologies. Fundus images can be compromised by a variety of aberrations that may interfere with data analysis. Precise quantification requires that these aberrations be corrected in a reproducible fashion without distorting the native data or introducing inappropriate bias.

POTENTIAL SIGNIFICANCE OF RETINAL IMAGE QUANTIFICATION

The quantitative analysis of retinal images carries a number of potential advantages. Quantitative assessment of images may allow the generation of objective, numerical definitions of various fundus lesions. These numerical definitions may allow more precise and reproducible recognition of retinal disease phenotypes which can be of value to researchers who are correlating these observations with disease genotypes in an effort to better understand disease mechanisms.

Quantitative assessment also lends itself to the development of automated methods of image analysis. Automated analysis of fluorescein angiograms may help narrow the gap between image interpretation in clinical trials versus clinical practice. Quantitative analysis and precise measurement of disease parameters will increase the sensitivity for the detection of subtle changes in disease activity over time. This may allow for the earlier detection of a response to treatment, and a more rapid and efficient assessment of the efficacy of new therapies.

RATIONAL APPROACHES TO QUANTIFYING RETINAL IMAGES

The development of an objective, quantitative system requires a rational, comprehensive approach. Ideally, the technology should be developed as a *diagnostic tool* to completely describe various features of retinal disease accurately and reproducibly, rather than as a *screening tool* to detect the presence or absence of disease. A relevant example to illustrate this concept is computed tomography (CT) scanning technology. The CT scan was developed as a diagnostic tool to better visualize and describe the features of various structures within the body in normal health and disease. Once the radiologic characteristics of various structures were defined and verified to be accurate and detectable, CT scanning was then employed for the screening and detection of diseases such as cancer and pulmonary embolus.

Currently, numerous efforts are underway to develop screening technologies for the detection of diabetic retinopathy.[22–25] These investigations may benefit from the primary development of validated quantitative methods prior to the creation of definitive screening and/or staging tools. Using the human grading process as a guide, software algorithms should be designed to generate objective, reproducible results. The ultimate proof and optimization of such a system will come from well-controlled clinical studies.

HISTORY

Initial attempts at quantitative fluorescein angiography came soon after its first clinical application more than forty years ago.[2] In 1965, Hickam and Frayser[26] studied mean retinal circulation times using a technique known as densitometry. A densitometer is a device that measures the light-stopping power of exposed and processed photographic film. Their approach was based on the hypothesis that changes in intravascular fluorescence should be proportional to blood flow and could be measured by determining changes in the density of the photographic film exposed during the angiogram. In their study, they showed that oxygen and nitroglycerin prolonged retinal circulation times while carbon dioxide shortened them. Other investigators used similar techniques based on dye dilution curves[27] to examine retinal blood flow in hypertension and anemia,[28] glaucoma,[29–31] and diabetes.[32] Subsequent technological advances also provided better instrumentation for the quantification of fluorescence intensity with procedures such as microdensitometry,[28,33,34] fluorophotometry,[35–37] video angiography,[38–43] and scanning laser ophthalmoscopy.[44–47]

Retinal blood flow can be described in many ways.[48] Commonly used parameters include mean circulation time (MCT), arteriovenous passage time (AVP), mean dye velocity (MDV) and segmental retinal blood flow (SBF).[36] Patients with nonproliferative diabetic retinopathy have been shown to have increased SBF,[49] AVP,[50] and MCT[43] when compared to normal patients using fluorescein angiography. Arend and coworkers studied diabetic patients using SLO and found reductions in capillary blood cell velocities and an increase in perifoveal intercapillary areas.[51] In contrast, Blair et al. only observed a difference in MCT for proliferative disease.[36]

The use of fluorescein angiography for the study of retinal circulation has been mostly supplanted by modern technologies such as laser Doppler velocimetry.[48] However, the early attempts at retinal blood flow quantification raised important questions that spawned the modern era of quantitative fluorescein angiography. In 1983, Akita and Kuga summarized many of the important problems that were to be encountered in the coming decades.[52] These problems, known well in the field of computer vision, can be separated into six main categories as they apply to quantitative fluorescein angiography:

- Image selection
- Image preprocessing
- Image segmentation
- Image registration
- Feature classification
- Feature quantification.

Due to the magnitude and complexity of the total endeavor, a comprehensive solution to all of these problems has not been found. Many investigators have dealt with individual steps as isolated tasks. Small, uncontrolled studies have been performed but few large-scale trials of any developed technologies have been conducted. An economy of scale may exist in developing robust solutions for multiple problems at once. In fact, as will be discussed in subsequent sections of this chapter, the solution to one problem may be identical to the solutions for others.

IMAGE SELECTION

Image quality assessment

Variability in the quality of fluorescein angiograms may affect the accuracy of their interpretation. Patient movement, blinking or improper positioning, camera optics, poor focus, inadequate or heterogeneous illumination, reflections and media opacities, poor quality sensors, and missing frames all affect a reader's ability to arrive at a diagnosis. One screening study for diabetic retinopathy found that up to 15% of submitted images were ungradable because of image quality.[53] In order to improve the accuracy of angiographic assessments, graders concentrate on the highest quality frames in a series. This task comes naturally to human beings who have spent a lifetime looking at personal and professional photographs and developing their own internal sense of "image quality," but computers are not designed to interpret images based on symbolic content and thus, have a very primitive capacity for assessing image quality.

Image quality assessment (IQA) is a context-specific task that is dependent on the photographic medium (i.e. color photography or fluorescein angiography) as well as the subject matter. For instance, the criteria used to rate a color image may differ greatly from those used to evaluate a black and white angiogram frame. Furthermore, an image that is adequate for the evaluation of glaucoma may not be an appropriate image for the assessment of diabetic retinopathy.

Since quality assessment is one of the first steps in the process of interpreting a fluorescein angiogram, an automated method of performing this task would be desirable for the development of an autonomous, objective angiogram interpretation system. Unfortunately, the current gold standard for image quality assessment, human interpretation, is time-consuming and subjective. In published studies, human graders have chosen images for subsequent computerized analysis. Although this could be implemented in a larger-scale analysis program, it would introduce human bias into an otherwise objective system and is far from an automated solution. A more objective method would be to train computers to accurately assess image quality and choose images that provide the highest quality results. However, the development of such an objective model has eluded researchers for decades.[54–57]

One problem encountered when training computers to rate image quality lies in the inherent subjectivity of human assessments. Human descriptors of image quality are context-sensitive, crude, and non-linear. Interpreters may find it difficult to distinguish image focus from contrast, to accurately quantify irregular lighting, or to rate any parameter on a robust linear scale. This inconsistency and nonlinearity, especially between graders, introduces potential noise into correlations with objective, global image parameters such as mean intensity or edge strength.[58] Furthermore, there is no reason to assume that a reader's personal preferences should necessarily reflect the best data for objective analysis. For instance, a human grader, whose perception of luminance is affected by the local environment, may prefer a high-key image with exaggerated brightness and contrast. This same image, however, may be judged as unnecessarily degenerate or biased for a computer that responds linearly to intensity values. A trained grader's symbolic understanding of an image also enhances their ability to assess its context-specific quality. For instance, an image with poor focus or lighting in the fovea might be rejected by a grader who is evaluating a subfoveal lesion. A computer, which has no implicit understanding of this area as a region of interest, might assess the overall parameters of the same image as adequate and give the frame a passing grade.

Most published work on ophthalmic image quality assessment has been performed on color fundus images. Hayashi et al. used the absence of prominent edges as a means of identifying poorly focused images.[59] In addition, they used the presence of numerous lesions detected both on a monochrome image as well as its inverse image as a criterion for exclusion. Other groups have used small sets of subjectively desirable images chosen by a human observer to develop "ideal" image parameters. The same calculations performed on a new set of images could then be compared against these ideal values to determine the quality of the new image set. Lee and Wang rated color images based on brightness, contrast, and signal-to-noise ratio.[60] From a subset of 20 "desired" images, they derived ideal histograms that were then used to calculate quality (Q) indices for new images. Lalonde and Gagnon took this one step further by analyzing local histograms instead of global functions and incorporating edge magnitude assessments.[61,62] Their ideal set was made up of fewer than forty images and the resultant classification was categorized as "good", "fair" or "bad". Neither group presented data comparing their calculated ratings against subjective human assessments.

A continuous image quality function may be more useful in clinical practice than a function that separates images into broad categories such as "good" or "bad."[63] Immediate feedback to ophthalmic photographers with a continuous image grading scale (i.e. 0–100) may provide a method of improving captured clinical image data. Individual grades reflecting specific aspects of the image (e.g. focus, lighting, etc.) might also allow photographers to actively improve their photographic technique. Proper identification of the parameters that discriminate between good and bad photographs may also allow for useful linear correlations with global or local image characteristics that reflect parameters such as focus, contrast, lighting, exposure and artifacts.[64] Finally, continuous input functions based on source data may enable calculations of confidence values in subsequent quantitative assessments.

The ultimate proof of an image quality metric for the purposes of quantitative fluorescein angiography may only be possible after validating the final output of the entire system. In this context, the highest quality images will be defined as those frames that provide the most accurate, reproducible quantitative evaluations. As with current reading center assessments, this will require extensive testing and validation in clinical trials.

Frame selection

In addition to considering the individual quality of each image, human interpreters must also select the frames that accurately represent the pathology depicted in the study. The results of this subjective task depend on the training of the reader as well as knowledge of the patient's physiology and the pathophysiology of the disease. Selecting frames based only on the time elapsed since intravenous injection may be prone to errors due to variations in the speed and amount of injected fluorescein dye as well as the patient's vascular anatomy and perfusion rate. Therefore, the amount of fluorescence at a given time may not be constant between patients or between visits. Because of this temporal variability, the *degree* of intravascular fluorescence may be a more useful marker of angiographic phase since it is independent of absolute time.[65] On the other hand, certain pathologic states, such as retinal venous occlusive disease, may cause significant temporal alterations in the progression of intravascular fluorescence which must also be recognized by any effective quantification system.

Dye dilution curves suggest that changes in fluorescence over time are nonlinear.[27] Therefore, the interval between selected frames need not be constant. Frames may be chosen at frequent intervals early in the course of an angiogram (e.g. the transit phase) when the changes in fluorescence are rapid and less frequently later in the study when fluorescence changes are slower. Rapid, regular image capture, as occurs with video-rate scanning laser ophthalmoscopy systems, in the later stages of an angiogram may result in large amounts of redundant data (since many frames may look exactly the same). Elimination of these redundant frames may therefore save computational time for a computer-based system without affecting the recognition of characteristic fluorescence patterns for each structure.

Identification of the vascular phase represented in a given image is a complex task that requires many human decisions. Although human intervention at this stage may still be required, it may eventually be possible to train computers to automatically perform this challenging job. After first automatically detecting the retinal vasculature, the intensity of fluorescence within the vessels could be calculated and fit to a standard dye dilution curve. By locating the position of this image along the curve of decaying fluorescence, the computer may be able to automatically and objectively determine the phase of fluorescein transit.[27] Once the phases have been delineated, a well-designed IQA system could then select the best frame in each phase to use in subsequent quantitative analysis. Again, validation of such a system would only come after demonstrating reproducible end results.

IMAGE PREPROCESSING

The human visual system is remarkably adept at eliminating noise and compensating for differences in exposure (overall brightness or darkness), contrast (rate of change of intensity) and shading (uniformity or nonuniformity of lighting) between angiographic images. Expert graders intuitively extract the salient features of images – often despite large amounts of image degradation. Computers, on the other hand, often use simpler, larger-scale parameters to describe image data. Local variations in image characteristics such as shading or contrast can perturb these simple, global descriptors. Preprocessing is the stage where image deficiencies are corrected to optimize the quantitative output of the system. The identification of undesirable image characteristics is currently completed by human graders, and all images tend to be subjected to the same preprocessing manipulation regardless of their quality. Automated assessment of image deficiencies with a robust image quality metric would allow for normalization of only those parameters that are aberrant. This objective process might minimize the data manipulation currently required prior to objective quantification.

Noise

An unavoidable aspect of image capture systems is the presence of small but noticeable variations in the true intensity at each pixel. Film-based systems are subject to small amounts of noise artifact during exposure. However, larger errors may be accumulated during the development process and can become quite marked if the film negatives are scanned into a digital image format. Digital images do not undergo this same generational degradation since they do not need to be developed or scanned. However, depending on the type of sensor used, a large amount of noise can be introduced into the image data during acquisition. Traditionally, high quality CCDs (charge-coupled devices) introduce the smallest amount of noise while earlier models of CMOS (complementary metal oxide semiconductor) sensors typically introduced a larger amount. Errors can be minimized by accurately modeling the response of the sensor in the dark (known as dark file correction) and by sophisticated signal processing algorithms. In fact, understanding the type of noise that may perturb native image data is essential in the development of effective noise reduction algorithms.

Most image noise is high in frequency and low in amplitude. Therefore, it is imperceptible to many human observers. Unfortunately, these fine perturbations in image values are noticeable to computer algorithms and may result in erroneous feature detections or omissions. Various methods have been implemented to deal with this problem. The simplest method is to smooth the data by averaging all intensities within a specified neighborhood (or kernel) around the pixel of interest.[58,66,67] Weighted averages, using a two-dimensional Gaussian function, are also useful since they place more importance on the center of the local region than on the edges.[68] Median filters use the same local neighborhood approach, but find the median value in the group instead of calculating the average of all values.[69–71]

An optimal smoothing algorithm would remove only artifactual noise without attenuating true image data. Unfortunately, this is an unobtainable goal. The techniques discussed above require the choice of an arbitrary neighborhood and technique for smoothing. Averaging intensities over a large region results in loss of fine structural detail while utilizing smaller zones of data may not remove all of the noise. Fourier-based techniques may allow for the identification of specific frequency ranges, but have not been widely implemented. Today, the most effective method of noise reduction for quantitative fundus imaging may be in the proper choice of hardware. Selection of a high quality, low-noise digital sensor may greatly reduce the need for post-processing which can distort the underlying data.

Contrast

This term is typically used to describe the brightness ratio of light and dark areas in an image, although it is independent of the actual range of intensities. The importance of this parameter can be appreciated by looking at an image's frequency histogram (Fig. 52-1). This graph depicts the number of occurrences of a given intensity value in each channel of an image. It demonstrates not only the range of values, but also the distribution of intensities within an image. The term "high contrast" is used when few, widely distributed intensity levels are used to describe the objects contained in the image (Fig. 52-1d). Because these images may also have exaggerated feature edges, this characteristic may be confused with precise focus. An extreme example of high contrast is a black and white image where there are no gray levels. "Low contrast" is the term used when the intensity changes between objects are very small. Although these images may appear to be "washed out," they often contain fine gradations of intensities that richly describe angiographic features. In fundus photography, contrast tends to decrease towards the periphery of the image aperture and is often at its maximum near the optic nerve.[24]

Linear contrast stretching is the name given to the global technique of enlarging the range of intensities in an image to equal the total (or desired) range available.[72] Late phase angiograms are often plagued by limited fluorescence, poor contrast and limited dynamic range. In these images, the differences between the most fluorescent structure and the least fluorescent structure is often much less than in prior frames. To the computer, this may cause areas of leakage (increasing hyperfluorescence) to appear to be decreasing in fluorescence due to the contracted dynamic range. On the other hand, artificially expanding the image contrast may cause features with decreasing fluorescence to appear to be increasing. Therefore, if global contrast expansion is to be implemented at all, it should probably incorporate information on the expected dynamic range for each phase of an angiogram.

A more sophisticated and common way of improving global contrast balance in an image is to perform histogram equalization where pixel intensities across the whole image are reassigned so that the resultant image will have a uniform distribution of intensities (Fig. 52-1e). This technique has been employed by a number of investigators to account for differences in lighting and to improve edge details.[68,73–79]

Contrast can also be described as the ability to differentiate an object from its background. Although humans may be able to perceive differences in intensity as small as 2%, larger differences are certainly preferable to distinguish a feature from its environment. These gradients between an object and its surroundings are not necessarily constant across an image. Contrast, therefore, can be considered as a local phenomenon and may need to be modified with a technique known as local contrast enhancement.[72] This process, which enhances image details and can be applied in an iterative fashion, evaluates the mean and variance of intensity values within a given area and expands the intensities in poorly illuminated regions where contrast is often limited.[24,63,80,81] It can also be applied in the spectral domain with a 2D wavelet transform.[82] Unfortunately, local manipulation of intensity values within one frame of a fluorescein angiogram may cause the detection of artificial, erroneous changes in fluorescence when compared to adjacent frames.

Exposure

Ophthalmic photographers may change a camera's exposure setting several times during an angiogram to account for changes in fundus fluorescence. This fluctuation in lighting does not significantly affect human interpreters but, as discussed above, it can wreak havoc on computerized quantitative analysis if it is not properly neutralized. For example, if the overall exposure of each frame in a fluorescein angiogram were decreased successively throughout the study, features with increasing

fluorescence might appear to have stable fluorescence to a computer. If left uncorrected, this might alter the computer's ability to correctly identify these features.

Finding a proper baseline for exposure correction is challenging. Ideally, the timing of each frame, volume of dye injected and the perfusion rate of the subject should all be considered in order to fit the angiogram to a dye dilution curve.[27] However, simpler methods are usually applied. Phillips and colleagues used a straightforward method of adjusting the gray levels of the first frame in each angiogram to the same level.[83,84] They then assumed that the fluorescence would decay linearly with time and quantified macular edema by subtracting an early angiographic frame from a late frame.[83] Cree et al. estimated expected fluorescence using an exponential decay curve.[85] Hipwell and coworkers tested the most advanced approach by modeling fluorescence as a gamma-variate and second order polynomial that predicts the initial appearance of fluorescein followed by a subsequent recirculation phase.[86]

Alternatively, angiographic frames can be normalized to a feature with predictable fluorescence characteristics. Background fluorescence is an obvious candidate but since it can be corrupted by varying amounts of extravascular hyperfluorescence, it may be difficult to detect reproducibly. All other structures in the human fundus are subject to disease states that alter their fluorescence patterns. Therefore, combinations of data from different structure types will likely be necessary to reliably reconstruct exposure patterns in angiograms.

Shading

Although all photographic lenses cause some degree of darkening, or vignetting, towards the edge of the lens aperture, flash fundus photography is subject to an even greater degree of lighting variability within each image. Two different views of

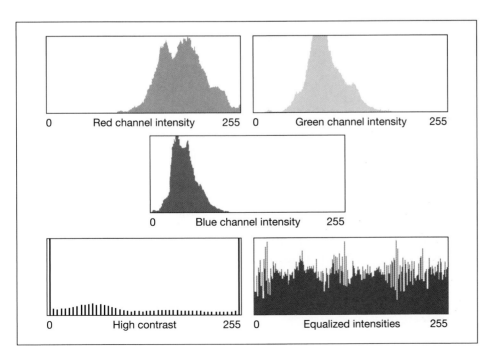

Fig. 52-1 Frequency histograms. Frequency of occurrence for intensity levels in the red, green and blue channels across a typical color fundus image. Examples of frequency histograms for images with increased contrast and after histogram equalization.

the same region may result in different reflectance patterns due to variations in the incidence of light rays reflected off of the spherical fundus surface.[87] The flash filament and the patient's reaction to the bright stimulus may both produce large areas of heterogeneous illumination or artifact. Scanning laser ophthalmoscopy may be less prone to these types of image corruption since it is a low-light, laser-based system.

Modeling of the illumination and sensor irregularities inherent in an image acquisition system with a "flood" image is one method of reducing irregular scene illumination.[86,88] These calibration images are obtained prior to placing the subject in the camera or scanner aperture and can be subtracted from subsequent frames to remove the intrinsic noise in the acquisition system. Although this provides a small, but accurate, correction of lighting variation, it requires empiric flood data for every image set and does not account for the principal causes of lighting irregularity.

Correction for irregular scene lighting in flash fundus photography, also called shade correction, is a major challenge in image preprocessing. To better understand accepted approaches, it may be helpful to decompose observed images into two mid-level, intrinsic components: the reflectance image and the illumination image.[89] The former is made up of the true image data that describes the subject matter (in this case, the fundus) while the latter describes the degradation to the ideal image that happens due to irregular lighting, artifacts, etc. (Fig. 52-2). Subtracting[85,86,88,90–96] or dividing[70,97–99] the illumination image into the original image yields an estimation of the true image data (i.e. the reflectance image). The challenge is to remove the irregular illumination data from the original image without removing any true structure information. For instance, blocked fluorescence in the fovea is a consistent, normal finding that is part of the true reflectance function. It must not be attenuated or mistaken for shading variations that occur due to lighting irregularities, media opacities, etc.

Much work on illumination approximation has been done in color imaging. For instance, the red, green, blue (RGB) color space can be transformed to a hue, saturation, intensity (HSI) space. The shade-corrected image can then be approximated by removing or neutralizing the intensity (I) parameter prior to transforming back to the RGB color space.[59,81,100] Tappen and coworkers implemented various classifiers in a Generalized Belief Propagation Algorithm to derive shading and reflectance images from a single image.[101] Averaging or filtering of multiple images of the same scene over time may also allow one to distinguish between consistent image features and those variations that are simply due to lighting heterogeneity.[102,103] Unfortunately, many of these techniques are not applicable to standard 8 bit black and white angiography where the data degenerates from 16.7 million colors to 256 shades of gray, and where variation in intensity is anticipated and necessary.

In general, lighting irregularities in fluorescein angiograms appear as gradual changes in shading that increase towards one or all edges of the circular aperture. Many approximations of the illumination image have been attempted using large-scale versions of smoothing functions. Mean[91,92,94,96] and median[58,70,86,88,90,93,98,99,104–107] filters based on large neighborhoods of points are commonly implemented as a means of estimating the ambient lighting in an image. Gaussian filters can also be used and may be faster to calculate.[95] The size of the filter kernel used in these approaches should approximate the size of the lighting irregularity and be larger than the largest feature size of interest (which is not always known). Kernels that are too large in size result in inadequate approximations of the illumination image and residual lighting problems. On the other hand, kernels that are too small may cause attenuation and smoothing of the reflectance data.

Homomorphic filtering in the frequency and spatial domains can be used to separate low frequency illumination data from the underlying reflectance data. Both Lee[108] and Rapantzikos[79] used this technique on fundus images, but others[85] have questioned its ability to preserve fluorescent features such as leakage. Feature-based methods of lighting correction have also been attempted. Wang and coworkers developed a bicubic approximation based on vessel intensities in color images to normalize illumination while still preserving the signal-to-noise ratio.[109] Cree et al developed a more fundamental approach based on variations in background fluorescence.[85] They detected the fovea in early angiogram phases, masked it, and fit control points in the remaining image space to a third-degree polynomial to approximate illumination. Leistritz and colleagues identified areas of background for illumination estimation by separating the image into sub-windows and detecting areas of low variance.[110] Finally, Wang and coworkers implemented an

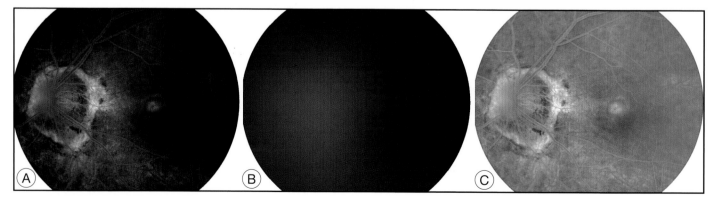

Fig. 52-2 Intrinsic images. Original image (A) decomposed into estimated illumination image (B) and reflectance image (C).

exponential brightening routine that had its maximal effect on the darkest areas in a color image.[111]

Color and grayscale

The "bit depth" of an image or camera reflects the number of different intensities that can be represented per channel. Since each bit can only be a 0 or 1, an 8-bit image is only capable of storing 256 (2^8) different intensities per channel while a 12-bit image can contain 4096 intensities (2^{12}). In computer memory, color images are usually expressed as the combination of intensities in three channels – red, green and blue. The relative ratios of these intensities are responsible for our perception of color. Therefore, a 3-channel, 8-bit color image (also called a 24-bit image) can render 16.7 million (2^{24}) different colors. Image processing can occur using any combination of these channels. However, better color separation of certain structures may be possible with mathematical functions that transform data to other color spaces such as hue, saturation and intensity (HSI)[59,81,100,112] or YIQ[113] (commonly used in television broadcasting). One such space popularized by Goldbaum et al,[114] is called a spherical color space and has been used by several investigators.[111,113] Grayscale images, including fluorescein angiograms, are produced when the values in all color channels are identical. Therefore, angiographic images are limited in their intensity resolution to the number of bits in a single channel (i.e. 10-bit). This is the primary reason why high bit depth (i.e. 10- or 12-bit) fluorescein sensors are preferable to standard 8-bit cameras.

IMAGE SEGMENTATION

Images are stored in computer memory as millions of independent points of data (pixels) that have an assigned position in the image as well as an assigned brightness or intensity. Segmentation is the term used to describe the process of separating pixels into non-overlapping, homogenous, contiguous regions, such as drusen or vessels, which share common characteristics such as color or texture. Features in an image can be defined by the edges that circumscribe them, the pixels that fill them or a combination of both. Accordingly, segmentation usually involves the application of one of two processes: (1) distinguishing different regions by the edges (or dissimilarities) that separate them; or (2) building connected regions which are related according to a similarity measure such as intensity.[116]

So why has a universal solution to this problem evaded computer scientists? Why must unique algorithms be developed for each application of this technique? The answer lies in the differences between human and computer-based segmentation. As stated above, a pure segmentation routine should define an object without attempting to identify it. Human beings, on the other hand, combine the processes of segmentation and classification. Our knowledge of what we expect to see alters our perception of what is truly there. For example, a quick glance at a patient's fundus might initially reveal the optic nerve, vessels, fovea and scattered drusen. Upon closer inspection, one may actually discover that each drusen is made up of relatively discrete areas that happen to be confluent. This process of human perception reveals two of the aspects of human segmentation that differ from computer-based segmentation: context and scale. And since these factors differ with each application, a universal solution to the problem of image segmentation may never be found.

Human observers have expectations of what should be present in a fundus image based on their training and on *a priori* knowledge of retinal anatomy and pathophysiologic processes. This contextual bias allows examiners to combine the processes of feature delineation and identification. Unfortunately, computers do not inherently possess the same contextual knowledge. Therefore, it should not be surprising that computer-based segmentation algorithms produce results that differ greatly from our expectations.

The algorithms discussed below are not pure segmentation routines. They are hybrid algorithms that combine segmentation with implicit classification to encourage the computer to see things the way that human examiners see them. The penalty for this efficiency is the uncertainty of false-positive detections. For example, the algorithms that are designed to detect the optic nerve implicitly classify *any* outlined object as optic nerve. This necessitates the use of substantial post-processing classification in some routines.

The perception of scale is another variable that differs between human and computer-based segmentation processes. Without prior knowledge of the scale of an image, a computer-based algorithm trained with 30-degree photos might incorrectly identify the optic nerve in a 50-degree image as a patch of exudate or drusen. It will be evident from the discussion below that another major challenge for image segmentation routines is to produce coherent regions that make contextual sense on multiple scales.

As mentioned previously, two major approaches to image segmentation are based on dissimilarity and similarity. The slope of intensity change between pixels or regions (also called "edge" or "boundary" detection or a "first derivative" approximation) demonstrates the dissimilarity of the adjacent areas. Similarity between pixels, on the other hand, can be assessed in many ways including the use of thresholding, clustering or statistical methods such as principle component analysis. With these techniques, similarities in color or texture are detected among pixels regardless of their position. In medical imaging, however, knowledge of the anatomy of biologic structures suggests that adjacent pixels in an image are likely to belong to the same structure. Therefore, algorithms that account for position, called region-growing algorithms, have been developed and are commonly used. These routines look for similarity by starting at a central "seed" point and moving outwards in a regimented fashion to all connected, similar neighboring pixels. Since they don't require discretely circumscribed features, this technique is often used to segment biologic structures with indistinct borders. Various combinations of edge detection and region-growing have also been developed.[116]

Image segmentation techniques are referred to as "bottom-up" if each pixel is treated as an independent entity and similarity assessments to neighboring pixels are performed without any assumption of the desired result. "Top-down" techniques, on the other hand, incorporate higher level knowledge such as anatomical information. In the following section, individual image processing techniques used in segmentation will be introduced in the context of the anatomic goals of their application. We will begin with a discussion of techniques used to detect normal anatomic features and continue with the delineation of pathologic findings in disease. Much of this work has been done in color imaging but is still relevant to a discussion of quantitative fluorescein angiography. Therefore, where applicable, techniques used in color imaging will be discussed first, followed by approaches also used in angiography.

Optic disc

The optic nerve has many distinct features that can be used for its detection. It can often be located in a predictable portion of the frame.[117,118] In color images, its yellow hue is frequently responsible for the brightest and most saturated pixels in the image.[52,66,92,112,115,117–119] The prominent, dark blood vessels present on the surface of the optic nerve also cause a large amount of local variation in pixel intensity – a characteristic that has been exploited by various groups.[81,100,120] A statistical model of this variation, based on principle component analysis, was recently shown to detect the optic nerve in 99% of the 89 images tested.[121] Other promising approaches based on these intensity characteristics include clustering,[117] watershed transformation,[122] blood vessel convergence,[52,123] detection of the long axis of an ellipse fit to the vascular arbor,[124] and detection of the vertical orientation of the blood vessels at the optic nerve.[115,125]

Various combinations of these features can be incorporated into a template that can be compared across the entire image to find the best match.[24,126,127] Special kinds of templates, based on a distance measure known as the Hausdorff distance[128,129] or on a wavelet function known as Daubechies wavelet transform,[84] have also been used to locate the optic disc.[62,118] These templates may be sensitive to apparent changes in the size of the optic nerve due to variations in magnification and zoom. Therefore, several investigators have explored multi-scale, pyramidal decomposition approaches for optic disc detection.[53,62,77]

The detection of edges, or rapid changes in intensity, is a fundamental problem in image processing.[130,131] Boundaries between structures can be approximated in a continuous fashion by estimating the slope, or first derivative, of the image intensity. In addition to providing the magnitude of the intensity change, the first derivative also provides directional information that can guide feature boundary tracking. Unfortunately, pixels in a fundus image are discrete and are not part of a continuous function. Therefore, they do not have true derivatives. However, the first derivative can be estimated by looking at a local neighborhood of adjacent pixels (e.g.. in a 3×3 area) or by fitting a complex surface to the data.

Several mathematical operators, such as the Sobel, Prewitt and Roberts filters, generate first derivative approximations that are unidirectional (i.e. emphasize either horizontal or vertical edges) but can be combined to produce an overall map of multidirectional edges in an image (Fig. 52-3a–c). To recover meaningful boundaries, a global or local threshold is usually selected to define the minimum acceptable value that characterizes an edge. Selection of this threshold can be aided by the use of a histogram of local edge strengths. Nevertheless, it is ultimately an arbitrary task that results in either false detections or false omissions – especially in low-contrast images with low signal-to-noise ratios. Since false detections occur due to image noise, their frequency can be reduced by smoothing an image. However, this causes a proportional increase in the frequency of false omissions.

Another common problem encountered in edge detection is that the boundaries that appear to be so continuous to the human eye actually contain many gaps and holes (Fig. 52-3d). Various edge detectors, including the well-known Canny edge detector[132] and algorithms with "momentum," have been developed to ameliorate this problem. The Canny edge detector uses both an upper and a lower threshold for edge strength as well as an additional hysteresis step to achieve superior results in many cases.

Estimates of the second derivative (slope of the first derivative) can be calculated using the Laplacian operator. A subsequent zero-crossing detector can then be used to locate edge points.[133] As with other edge detectors, this operator is very sensitive to image noise and does not necessarily produce continuous lines around a feature (Fig. 52-3d). In 1980, Marr and Hildreth suggested that the human visual system may detect some edges by exploiting the differences between images smoothed with functions of varying sizes.[134] This idea led to the creation of a unique derivation of the Laplacian operator that incorporates smoothing – the so-called Laplacian-of-Gaussian or LoG function. This scale-dependent, noise-resistant operator produces sign changes at feature edges and has the peculiar benefit of always producing closed figures. Unfortunately, it often overestimates the locations of structure boundaries. Refinements, such as the PLUS operator, have been investigated to ameliorate this problem.[135]

Because of its sharp margins, the optic nerve can frequently be detected in both color and angiographic frames using the Sobel edge detector.[66,77,84,93,136] Candidate points generated with this operator can be fit to a circle[117,119] or an ellipse[66,84,93,112,137] using a Hough transform. The center of the optic disc can be approximated by finding the center of this circle. This center point can then be used as an initiation point for a special structure, known as an active contour or genetic snake, which can refine the outline of the optic nerve.[77,113,120,121,126,127,138] First proposed by Kass,[139] these parametric curves are energy-minimizing contours that move iteratively in image space and are subject to both internal (i.e. elastic) and external (i.e. image-derived) forces. Various methods, such as simulated annealing or a popular external force field called the Gradient Vector Flow Model,[140] must often be used to keep active contours from settling into undesirable local minimum configurations.[113,126,138,141] Unfortunately, the peripapillary vessels cause degradation of

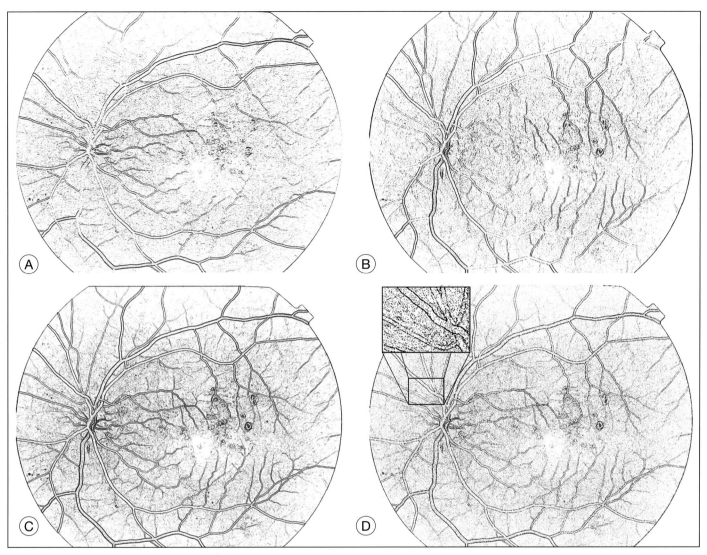

Fig. 52-3 Edge detection. Results of horizontal Sobel (A), vertical Sobel (B), combined Sobel (C) and Laplacian edge detectors (D). Inset shows edge discontinuities.

this gradient vector image and so, they are usually removed prior to initializing the contour. Despite encouraging results from many investigators, this process still requires accurate initialization (gross detection of the nerve) and can produce suboptimal results in patients with significant peripapillary atrophy.

Vessels

Blood vessels are a consistent feature in almost every fundus photograph. Accordingly, the development of an accurate, robust, multimodal vessel detector is a highly sought-after priority in ophthalmic image processing research. Their predictable structure helps to orient both the viewer and the computer. The relative consistency of their position and configuration over time is useful for temporal image registration.

Various diseases, such as hypertension, diabetic retinopathy and vaso-occlusive disease, often cause detectable structural changes in vessels. Finally, the development of augmented reality instruments to aid in the performance of surgical procedures will most likely rely on vascular registration features.[142–149]

Retinal vessel segmentation routines can be split into two main categories: detection and tracking. Detection schemes are "bottom-up" approaches that make few initial assumptions about the global structure of the vascular tree. They may utilize either edge-finding or region-growing algorithms and work on both color images and angiograms. However, they frequently traverse the entire image to find all candidate regions. Moreover, the detection thresholds that result in adequate sensitivity often require a great deal of post-processing classification to remove false-positives. Vessel tracking routines, on the other hand, require less post-processing but are very sensitive to initialization.[124,150–159] As "top-down" algorithms, they rely on several anatomic assumptions: (1) vessels are connected; (2) vessels converge on the optic nerve; and (3) vessels bifurcate consistently. From a starting point on a vessel, they iteratively scan for neighboring pixels likely to be part of the same vessel based on similarity measures such as color[160] or dissimilarity measures such as the antiparallel edges of vessel walls, which can be used as a method of steering the routine. Although these algorithms can work on color images or angiograms, failure to initialize the process on a good candidate vessel may result in failure. Can and coworkers developed an interesting method of increasing the likelihood of appropriate vessel initiation.[151] They identified potential vessel seed points by scanning the image for local extremes of intensity but controlled the distribution of these seed points by dividing the image into a grid pattern. Subsequent investigators have tested algorithms based on this approach.[154–156] One group reported excellent feature detection and alignment on more than 4000 color image pairs.[154]

Another obvious approach to the detection of fundus blood vessels is to attempt to recognize their boundaries *de novo* with edge detection. Sobel,[115,161–164] Prewitt[165] and Kirsch[121,136] edge detectors have all been studied for vascular recognition. Some success has also been achieved with both Canny edge detection[62,81,100] and the LoG operator.[167,168] McInerney and Terzopoulos performed limited testing of active contours, or T-snakes, on vessels from fluorescein angiograms.[169] In general, boundary-finding techniques can be used with both color and angiographic images and can also be incorporated into both top-down and bottom-up algorithms. However, inconsistent edge strengths, confusion at vessel crossings and bifurcations, and problems during the laminar flow phase of angiography have led many investigators to consider other options.

Blood vessels are relatively homogenous in composition and intensity. In addition, the brightness of a vessel is typically quite different from the average intensity of color and angiographic images. Therefore, the other major approach to retinal vessel detection is the recognition of the body of the vessel instead of its edges. Routines of this type utilize information about brightness, shape and texture to recognize regions that resemble blood vessels. Once all vessel candidates have been identified, sophisticated classification schemes can be used to identify true vessels and remove imposters.

With good lighting correction, a simple method of object detection, called thresholding, can be utilized. As the name implies, an arbitrary brightness level is defined that divides all pixels in an image (or in a local area) into two groups. In the case of a fluorescein angiogram, the brighter pixels would be labeled as "vessel" and the darker group would be labeled as "nonvessel." Decreasing the threshold will cause nonvessel objects to be falsely detected. Conversely, increasing the threshold will result in the loss of true vessel segments that happen to be darker than other vessels segments. Several investigators have used such routines in conjunction with post-processing to remove false-positives.[69,170,171] For instance, Tamura took advantage of the linear nature of blood vessels to identify

and exclude them prior to the quantification of fluorescein leakage in angiograms.[172] Unfortunately, due to differences in fluorescence and lighting irregularities, a global threshold with appropriate sensitivity and specificity for detecting vessels across the entire image is unlikely to occur. This has led to the development of adaptive thresholding algorithms that can monitor local contrast and intensity distributions to determine the appropriate local threshold.[137,167] In addition, Jiang and Mojon have tested a promising technique of multi-threshold probing to find curvilinear features that resemble vessels.[173]

Due to the unique linear shape of retinal blood vessels, special filters, called morphological operators,[174,175] can be used for vessel detection. Although a complete discussion of this topic is beyond the scope of this text, it is useful to understand that morphological operators modify the intensity of image pixels based on the shape of the features that surround them. The shape of the structuring element that is passed across the image defines the logical or Minkowski arithmetic that is computed for each pixel. Basic operations include dilation, which tends to increase the size of objects and erosion, which decreases the size of bright areas. More complex calculations, such as opening, closing, and thinning, can be developed based on these primitive operators.[98,167,176–178]

In order to detect blood vessels, a linear structuring element can be passed across the image in multiple orientations. This so-called "top-hat" transformation excludes small, round features like microaneurysms and enhances vessels in angiograms. It has been used by many investigators either for vessel detection or for subsequent subtraction of the vessels from the image.[90,105,167,168,179–181] Unfortunately, these structuring elements are scale-dependent and therefore, must match the approximate size of the retinal vasculature. This condition causes further difficulties at bifurcation points where the vessel width effectively increases. One additional operator, called the Duda Road operator, was used by Goldbaum et al. for vessel detection due to the relative homogeneity of the vessel and its adjacent regions.[125]

Another method of identifying candidate blood vessels relies on a technique similar to morphological processing called matched filtering. Simply put, passing a matched filter across an image and performing cross-correlation calculations will generate peaks wherever the underlying image data mimics the shape of the filter. For example, a linear increase and decrease in pixel intensity somewhere in an image could be detected by a filter containing a linear increase and decrease in intensity of a similar scale. As with morphological filters, matched filters are directional and scale-dependent. However, they have proven to be very useful for retinal vessel detection.

In order to determine the optimal shape for a matched filter that detects blood vessels, one must accurately model the empirical intensity distribution encountered across fundus vessels. Iliasova et al. investigated different cross-sectional models and even accounted for the central light reflex.[182] Although they concluded that vessels are best modeled with an exponential-power distribution, Kaupp et al. were able to use a simpler rectangular distribution to successfully detect vessels.[177]

In 1989, Chaudhuri et al. hypothesized that the intensity distribution across a retinal blood vessel most closely resembles a Gaussian function.[183] They developed a technique using numerous, rotated, matched filters that has been widely used by a large proportion of subsequent investigators over the last decade. Drawbacks to this technique include extensive computational time and relative difficulty with vessel bifurcations.

A number of advanced techniques for vessel detection have been attempted by other investigators. Staal and coworkers detected intensity extrema across the image to approximate "ridges."[184] They then used convex sets and nearest neighbor classifiers to identify the ridges that belonged to linear vessel segments. Chutatape et al. compared the performance of Extended Kalman Filters to standard Gaussian matched filters.[185] Aleynikov et al.[186] compared invariant moments[187] and multiresolution wavelet decomposition for vessel detection in color images. Leandro[167] investigated Morlet wavelets while Lee[166] and Tan[188] both performed energy spectrum analysis. Clustering approaches have been attempted by Hsu,[93] Tolias[117] and Wang[189] while Simo[190] implemented another kind of statistical approach based on Bayesian methods and Markov Random Fields. Finally, Sinthanyothin entered data from a Canny edge detector into a multilayer perceptron neural network to classify potential features as blood vessel segments.[81,100]

Fovea

The fovea is an important and reliable landmark in many retinal images. Precise localization of the foveal center is desirable when assessing diseases that affect visual acuity, such as diabetic macular edema, and when selecting the appropriate treatment for choroidal neovascularization. Although there are gross anatomic definitions of its location, the most common method of foveal identification is visual estimation by a human observer. This works well in eyes with limited pathologic changes in the macula. However, with the progressive retinal pigment epithelial alterations and distortion of retinal anatomy that can occur in advanced disease states, accurate identification of the foveal center may become virtually impossible for a human grader. The use of a sophisticated mathematical model of the foveal center based on invariant landmarks such as the optic nerve and vasculature would have obvious advantages in this situation.

The predictable, continuous gradient of pigmentation in a normal human fovea has led most investigators to treat foveolar identification as a segmentation problem instead of a point localization problem. In color images, the yellowish macular pigment has a low intensity in the blue channel. Since it also exists in a relatively avascular area, the foveola can be located by searching a region of interest for the darkest group of pixels using thresholds, clustering or template matching.[62,81,112,125,137] The location of the region of interest can be estimated using traditional distance relationships between the fovea and optic nerve. Alternatively, Li and coworkers grossly located this area as the center of a parabola with the optic nerve at the apex and the vessels defining the parabola contour.[121] This foveal center was then used as the center of a polar coordinate system for subsequent retinal analysis.

Identification of the foveal avascular zone (FAZ) using fluorescein angiography is a true segmentation problem since it requires the construction of a region comprised of contiguous, homogenous pixels. Two groups have used active contours to outline the boundaries of the avascular zone. Ballerini's technique required manual selection of an initialization point for the genetic snake.[191–193] Gutierrez, on the other hand, found the minimum intensity value in a large-scale Gaussian blur as the starting point for an active contour.[194] Ibanez et al. used Markov chains and Bayesian methods to estimate the position of the FAZ.[195] As with other poorly-demarcated fundus features, however, segmentation of the FAZ is probably not amenable to a boundary detection solution except in the best of cases. Accordingly, Ishaq and coworkers took a different approach by calculating angular momentum and converging on the foveal center with centroids of decreasing size.[196] Although they did not attempt to outline the foveal vascular area, they did calculate the minimum distance to a hyperfluorescent lesion that exceeded a pre-defined intensity threshold. Goldberg and colleagues also attempted to quantify macular ischemia without delineating the FAZ.[197] They separated pixels into four clusters based on fluorescence intensity values and iteratively decided if pixels from the middle two clusters represented perfused or nonperfused retina. As will be discussed later, more sophisticated statistical methods and the use of multiple angiographic frames may provide a better definition of the avascular zone.

Microaneurysms and hemorrhages

These two "red lesions" will be discussed together since they may be confused by automated software. Several studies have indicated that microaneurysm counts or patterns of appearance and disappearance may have some prognostic significance in diabetic retinopathy.[16–18] Unfortunately, accurate counts may be difficult to obtain since clinicians rarely take the time to count each microaneurysm, and color digital images may not be of sufficient resolution or quality to appropriately represent these small lesions. However, as digital sensor resolution improves and nonmydriatic photography becomes more common, there appears to be more interest in studying the detection of microaneurysms and hemorrhages from color images for the purposes of screening for diabetic retinopathy.

The first step in most detection schemes is to remove lighting irregularities that can cause microaneurysms to blend in with their local environment or appear to have too much color variability across the image. The next difficulty is to differentiate these red lesions from the typical red-orange background of the human fundus. Larsen et al. studied 200 eyes of 100 patients using proprietary software that delineated "red lesions" based on the steepness of the gradient between the lesion and its local environment.[198] They reported a sensitivity of 96.7% but a specificity of only 71.4%. They reasoned that, for the purposes of screening, this detection rate would still allow for a reduction in the number of patients that might need to be examined by trained professionals. Hipwell et al used similar logic in their large study of almost 4000 images.[25] They also found a trade-off between sensitivity and specificity with final values of 85% and 76%, respectively, for the detection of patients with retinopathy. Unfortunately, when attempting to maximize both sensitivity and specificity, Usher and colleagues were only able to achieve a sensitivity of 78.9% and specificity of 70.8% for the detection of any retinopathy using their algorithm.[24]

Sinthanyothin[100] and Usher[24] both used a "Moat operator" to differentiate red lesions from the background. However, Sinthanayothin[100] and colleagues improved their false detection rate by excluding blood vessels with a neural network. A back propagation neural network was also tested by Gardner for the detection of pathology consistent with diabetic retinopathy.[76] They subdivided their images into a grid of squares, trained the system based on human observations and then used raw intensity data to determine if any pathology was present in each subwindow. Although sensitivities varied per lesion, overall sensitivity for the detection of retinopathy with this system was 88% with a specificity of 84%. Truitt and colleagues, on the other hand, used an adaptive resonance theory (ART) network and concluded that the information contained in red, green, blue (RGB) images was insufficient to allow proper disease classification.[199]

Various other classification schemes have also been tested with high sensitivity algorithms. Akita and Kuga classified hemorrhages as dark, loop-composable objects.[52] An object was defined as "loop-composable" when its edges curved in the same direction when traced in either a clockwise or counter-clockwise direction. Ege and coworkers used a simple global threshold to identify all candidate lesions and then filtered out false-positives with Bayesian probability, Mahalanobis classifiers and K-nearest neighbor classifiers.[58] Lee et al. developed a unique and promising modification of standard thresholding techniques.[200,201] In this approach, many different thresholds are used to segment features, and the pattern of appearance and growth of features created by this scanning threshold system is used for subsequent lesion classification. The distinct benefits of this algorithm are its relative independence from local contrast and lighting and its multiscale approach. These advantages may allow for lesion identification even for features that vary widely in size and blend in well with their local environment.[200,202] They also implemented a "spider-net" approach to the detection of larger lesions. In this system, radial lines are projected from the foveal center and concentric rings complete the net configuration. Their algorithm was tuned to detect lesions that spanned a square wedge within the spider net instead of a linear portion (as would be seen with a blood vessel).

Hayashi hypothesized that many false-positives and omissions occurred around vessels.[59] In order to remove the confusion between microaneurysms and adjacent vessels, they performed a binary thinning procedure on the vascular tree prior to lesion detection. Hipwell et al.[25] also used a technique on color images that attempts to isolate and remove the vasculature. Developed by Cree[105] for the detection of microaneurysms in fluorescein angiograms, this routine uses a multi-directional, linear, morphologic filter (the "top-hat" transform) to identify vascular structures. The vessels are subtracted from the original image to yield an image of mostly circular features. A Gaussian matched filter is then passed across the image to find areas of maximal response. Region-growing of potential microaneurysms can proceed from these seed points based on several criteria. A final classification test, based on parameters such as size, shape, or intensity distribution, can then be conducted to remove false-positive detections.

Unfortunately, all of these algorithms suffer from the poor signal-to-noise ratio inherent in color fundus images. Investigators have found that difficult trade-offs between sensitivity and specificity must be made when differentiating red lesions from a red-orange background.[24,25] Fluorescein angiography, on the other hand, is a high contrast modality that accentuates even small structures. The large signal-to-noise ratio in this technique putatively makes it a better method for the detection of microaneurysms.[203] Caution must still be used in evaluating only a single frame of an angiogram, though, since some microaneurysms may appear in certain phases of dye transit but not in others.[204]

As with vessel detection, Gaussian matched filters can be used for the detection of small, round microaneurysms that have an intensity distribution which approximates a two-dimensional Gaussian curve.[83,205] Although additional shape criteria can then be used to remove false-positives, a more common approach is to use the "top-hat" transformation prior to using matched filters.[88,90,91,105,106,168,206] As discussed above, this linear morphological operator can be rotated into many different orientations to detect and remove the vascular arbor. With fewer false-positives to sort through, the resulting candidates can be subjected to stringent shape filters to refine these selections. Again, these techniques are highly sensitive to the scale of the object to be detected and an arbitrary threshold must be set for the matched filter response.

Exudates

Exudates are easily detected in color images due to their sharp edges and dissimilarity from the typical red-orange fundus background. However, it is important to distinguish this sign of retinopathy from other yellowish features, such as the optic nerve or drusen, that might be confused with it. Published studies of exudate segmentation have focused on color images since exudates typically have a very faint appearance on fluorescein angiograms. Their ease of detection and their association with sight-threatening macular edema[207,208] have also made exudates attractive targets for many diabetic retinopathy screening development efforts.

More than 20 years ago, Akita detected exudates by applying a circular, "loop-composable" filter to edges extracted from fundus images.[52] More recently, Li et al. combined Canny edge detection with region-growing in a transformed, *Luv* color space to identify exudates.[121] When image lighting irregularities are corrected properly, the unique color composition of exudates allows them to be detected with a simple threshold.[59,68,96,100,111,124,158,164,209,210] Leistritz and coworkers found a particularly good response by thresholding images from a scanning laser ophthalmoscope at a wavelength of 633 nm.[110]

Goldbaum used a slightly different approach by matching a multiscale, bright-object template, which he referred to as a "blob detector," across the image and using a logit classifier to identify potential exudates.[125] Previously, Goldbaum tested Mahalanobis distances to separate similarly colored objects in color space.[114] Due to their unique color composition, clustering pixels in color space with techniques such as c-means or k-means clustering is also a very successful method of identifying areas of exudate.[78,93] However, the significant color overlap between exudates, optic nerve and drusen necessitates the use of additional morphologic filtering with this approach. Other statistical methods, such as linear discriminant analysis and Bayesian probabilities, have also been tested by several groups.[66,111,115,211] Finally, Gardner was able to detect more than 90% of exudates in a small sample of cases with a back propagation neural network operating on subwindowed color images.[76]

Drusen

Like exudates, drusen can be detected in color images due to their dissimilarity from the typical red-orange fundus background. Unlike exudates, drusen may have softer edges, more heterogeneous coloration, and may be more easily seen with fluorescein angiography. Because of this, fluorescein angiograms may actually represent a better gold standard for benchmarking automated drusen detection routines than human interpretations and receiver operator characteristic curves based on color images. Unfortunately, only a few groups have investigated drusen quantification with angiography.

Based on a single, early angiographic frame, Barthes et al. found good agreement between manual detection of drusen by a human grader and automated detection with top-hat transformations and morphological operations.[212] Ben Sbeh and coworkers detected potential drusen centers in angiographic frames with morphologically derived intensity maxima and used adaptive contrast measures with geometric properties such as shape and area to delineate drusen.[104] They then went one step further by temporally registering angiograms to monitor changes in drusen over time. Thaibaoui et al. studied several angiograms containing drusen.[213] They separated image data into three arbitrary classes (background, unknown and drusen) based on gray level intensity distributions. They then used a spatially sensitive, fuzzy classification technique to reclassify pixels in the unknown category as drusen.

Due in part to the need for screening methods for age-related macular degeneration, the majority of development work on drusen detection has taken place using color images. As with many other fundus features, optimal correction of lighting irregularities affords the opportunity to use a simple threshold for drusen delineation. Global,[94] local,[71,99] adaptive,[79,214] and interactive[95] thresholds have all been investigated with moderate success. As they did with exudates, Goldbaum and coworkers used a multiscale, bright-object template followed by a logit classifier to detect drusen.[125] Brandon and Hoover also adopted a multi-scale approach based on Mexican-hat wavelets of different sizes.[215] They reported an 87% drusen detection rate in a study of 119 images.

Clustering has demonstrated utility for drusen detection when combined with excellent shade correction. In 1990, Goldbaum and colleagues discussed the use of Mahalanobis distances to separate drusen in spherical color space.[114] Although they didn't present any experimental results, Hsu and coworkers subsequently discussed the use of the same spherical color space with their clustering system as a method of possible drusen detection.[93]

Leakage

Despite the importance of leakage in the clinical management of the most common causes of blindness, few investigators have successfully addressed the problem of objective leakage quantification. The delineation of areas of leakage on a fluorescein angiogram is as much a classification problem as it is a segmentation problem. Unlike the features discussed previously, there is no objective, defining standard for leakage. And frequently, it cannot easily be differentiated from background fluorescence, vessels or other features. This ambiguity results in diffuse borders that are difficult for human graders to delineate and even more challenging for computerized segmentation algorithms based on edge detection or region-growing to identify.

As a dynamic phenomenon, leakage should best be quantified with information taken from temporally-integrated frames. In 1980, Jaanio and colleagues discussed the advantages of digitally calculating temporal differences in fluorescence using a commercial subtraction angiography system.[216] However, Tamura and coworkers were the first group to publish a feasible algorithm for the actual quantification of fluorescein leakage in the human retina.[172] Despite the primitive computing capabilities of that era, they presented a complex method for image preprocessing, registration, segmentation, classification and quantification of hyperfluorescence. Seven years later, Ishaq et al. described a simpler method that used a single angiographic frame and a fixed threshold to measure the distance from the foveal center to the closest area of hyperfluorescence.[196] It wasn't until 1991 that Phillips and colleagues reported results based on a procedure that advanced the work of Tamura's group.[217,218] In the Phillips algorithm, a late angiographic frame was compared to a frame from the venous portion of the transit phase. After simple image registration was performed, thresholding and region-growing were used to define abnormal areas of hyperfluorescence. The difference in the size of these areas as well as the difference in the gray level intensities contained within the two areas were both calculated. In 1998, Martinez-Costa and colleagues applied a similar technique to patients with vein occlusions.[219] In their study, they developed a more sophisticated registration algorithm and quantified leakage in relation to the foveal center. Finally, Muldrew and coworkers used interactive thresholding to define areas of leakage in serial angiographic frames taken in patients with CNV.[220]

However, the groundbreaking work of Jeffrey Berger was the first to apply so many recent advances in computer science to the methods described by Tamura's group 15 years before. In 1998, he described a system that incorporated geometric and radiometric normalization, temporal intensity analysis and supervised quantification of diseased regions of the fundus.[221] In 2000, Berger and Yoken published the first study in patients with choroidal neovascularization that compared quantitative angiography results from a fully functional software analysis system to clinical observations.[222] This work laid the foundation for the modern era of quantitative fundus imaging.

Unfortunately, Dr Berger's career was cut short by an unexpected illness. Had he been able to continue his research, many of the questions that remain unsolved to this day might have been answered. Fortunately, for those of us who know him mostly from his published work, his ideas and inspiration will live on in the knowledge that he has brought to this field. In the words of Dr Stuart Fine, "His contributions will continue to serve as a beacon that sheds light on the areas in which his insightful publications addressed unsolved problems in vision and ophthalmology."

IMAGE REGISTRATION

Ophthalmic diagnoses often require the evaluation and manipulation of numerous images taken at different times (temporal registration), from different viewpoints (stereoscopic registration) or with different sensors or imaging modalities (multimodal registration). Image registration is the term used to describe the process of superimposing corresponding areas in different images of the same scene. Radiologists have performed this task manually for decades by aligning fiducial markings or clearly-defined anatomic landmarks on X-rays.[223] However, with the advent of digital imaging, a hybrid form of image alignment, called human-interactive registration, has come into widespread clinical use. In this approach, an operator guides computer-based image alignment by manually identifying points in image A that correspond to points in image B. The computer then calculates the mathematical relationship, called the transformation or correspondence function, between these two point sets and "warps" image B onto image A. This process can be used in diagnostic imaging tests, such as digital subtraction angiography, because the human interaction safeguards against catastrophic failure. However, few medical images contain easily identifiable geometric shapes or exact landmark locations. Therefore, inaccuracies can develop when definite, objective landmarks either cannot be identified precisely or do not reflect the true transformation between the two images. In these cases, a computer-based registration system that uses the maximum amount of information from an image may improve the accuracy of alignment. Automated systems such as these are becoming increasingly more useful and important in an era of multimodal, three-dimensional, medical imaging where the shape, size or pose of the subject may change between frames. However, despite decades of active research, custom solutions are still required for most applications since a universal solution for automated image alignment has yet to be discovered.

For the purposes of this discussion, we will divide ophthalmic registration problems into three categories: viewpoint, temporal and multimodal.[224] Viewpoint registration is necessary when aligning two images obtained from different camera poses.

As will be discussed later, the use of high-resolution sensors, stereo photographic technique and the potential for eye movements between frames make this type of registration necessary in many modern fundus imaging systems. Temporal registration refers to the alignment of images separated in time. For example, fluorescein angiograms, although spanning only a short period of time, require registration due to patient and camera movements. The comparison of images taken at different office visits, on the other hand, would be an example of long-term temporal registration. Multimodal registration refers to the alignment of images from different instruments or modalities such as color photography and fluorescein angiography. This problem is becoming increasingly more common in medical imaging due to the wide variety of diagnostic instruments used in clinical practice today.

The scope of the solution required for each of the registration problems listed above can be understood by answering four questions:

1. What type(s) of misalignment is/are anticipated in this scenario?
2. What features exist in common between the images?
3. How do we assess the accuracy of the registration based on these features?
4. How severe can the misalignment be?

Each of these questions will be addressed individually followed by a discussion of specific investigations into three main registration problems that are pertinent to ophthalmology.

Search space

The potential search space for a given registration problem reflects the different types of misalignment that may be encountered between two images. As mentioned previously, the method used to warp one image onto another is referred to as the *transformation function* or model. The *domain* of this function describes its area of operation: *global* models work on the entire image as a whole, while *local* functions operate on only a portion of the image and may need to be implemented in groups to register the entire image.[225] Fortunately, most of the transformation functions investigated for ophthalmic image registration fall into the global category. One complex transformation to be discussed later, elastic registration, is usually modeled as a combination of numerous local functions. However, before we discuss these models, we must answer the question of why our images are misaligned in the first place.

Variations in the camera position (e.g. from stereo acquisition technique), in the position of the chin rest, and in the position of the subject's eye all tend to cause relatively large horizontal movements, somewhat smaller vertical movements, and small rotational differences between images. Causes of magnification or scaling differences between fundus images include changes in the distance between the camera and the patient's eye, wide variations in focusing with a nontelecentric camera, and modifications to the subject's refractive error between visits (i.e. with cataract or refractive surgery). Spherical distortions can be caused by the inherent curvature of the globe, by aberrations from the crystalline lens, or from the aspheric fundus camera lens. Finally, as will be discussed later, departures of the retinal surface from the curvature of the globe (i.e. from subretinal fluid or retinal edema) may cause an irregular type of distortion that requires complex, local modeling to neutralize.

The simplest transformation function, called a translation model (Fig. 52-4), addresses the shifts between images that occur due to eye and camera movements.[41,172,226–229] Since eye and head movements are often accompanied by a torsional component, image rotation should also be considered (Fig. 52-4). The transformation model that incorporates this additional factor is called a *rigid* transform since none of these operations distorts the intrinsic geometry of either image.[73,165,230–233] As mentioned previously, magnification or scaling changes can be induced by variables in the fundus camera and the subject's refractive error (Fig. 52-4). *Similarity* transformations are functions that combine translation, rotation and scaling.[72,86,137,154,234] However, the most common transformation is called the *affine* transformation (Fig. 52-4). It encompasses translation, rotation, scaling and shear and can be approximated in many ways.[98,137,154,168,178,230,235–240]

Despite hypotheses pointing towards higher order aberrations, many investigators have claimed that the linear transformations discussed thus far should be adequate for ophthalmic image registration.[98,239] This may certainly be true for images acquired without stereo technique (i.e. refraining from moving the camera from side to side) or with low-resolution digital sensors that cannot resolve the stereo differences that necessitate higher order transformations. In addition, past investigators who worked in eras of more primitive computing technology may have been forced to use simpler models to perform calculations within a reasonable time frame. However, linear and even global transformations may result in unacceptable levels of misregistration in the era of high-resolution digital sensors.

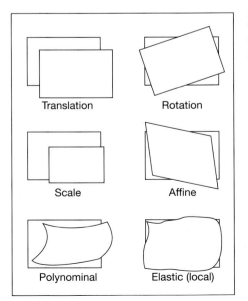

Fig. 52-4
Transformation functions used for image registration.

Translation

Rotation

Scale

Affine

Polynominal

Elastic (local)

Despite limited computational capacity, Jagoe and coworkers implemented a higher-order global model for ophthalmic image registration in 1993.[97] Shin and Berger subsequently presented a compelling argument that polynomial registration should be superior to affine models.[70] Based on our discussion of potential aberrations in fundus imaging, this seems to be a logical conclusion. Higher-order, global transformations (Fig. 52-4) that have been implemented in published algorithms include bilinear,[178,230,237] projective[241] and polynomial functions.[97,170,230,242–245] These global transformations are theoretically capable of modeling most of the potential variability in image alignment hypothesized above. However, as global functions, they cannot accurately account for local elevations or depressions in the retinal surface that cause it to depart from the standard curvature of the globe. Since the optic nerve represents a common structure with these complex, local undulations (Fig. 52-4), a number of groups have tested methods of local, elastic registration in this context.[74,75,246–249] Finally, Stewart and colleagues make the point that a single transformation may not be necessary or even desirable for fundus image alignment.[154] As will be discussed later, initiation with a simple affine model that progresses to a higher order model may prevent distraction of the system that would otherwise result in misregistration.[243]

Feature detection

The detection of features that are present in two or more clinical images is a major challenge in medical image registration. This process comes naturally to human observers who can quickly extract the salient features in a scene. Computers, on the other hand, have a limited symbolic understanding of image content and therefore, struggle with the task of matching structures between images.

The two major approaches to this task are described by the data types used. "Intensity-based" comparisons use raw image data from one image to look for similar patterns in the other image. Although this approach may work well in images with poorly defined structures, it is sensitive to irregularities in lighting, changes due to disease progression, and intensity reversals encountered when comparing red-free images to fluorescein angiograms. Furthermore, it often requires a great deal of computing power. Solutions to this last problem have been presented and offer promise for effective future implementation.

The other major method for finding commonality between images is referred to as "feature-based" comparison since it relies on extracted features instead of raw image data. In this case, the goal of feature extraction is to find salient, distinct, evenly distributed structures that are common to both images and are resistant to image degradation. By distilling the images down to their relevant points, fewer calculations may be required for comparison. This may also result in faster matches with sharper correlation peaks. However, unlike intensity-based methods, the performance of feature-based approaches on images with poorly defined structures may be disappointing.

As discussed in the segmentation section, many techniques can be used for the delineation of ophthalmic structures. Specific features used for fundus image registration include segmented regions,[178,226,228,233,234,237] detected edges,[75,137,165,227,236,241,244,247,250,251] detected points (e.g. vessel bifurcations or crossings),[73,98,170,235,245,252] creases,[232] ridges,[253] and manually-selected registration points.[41,230,218,239] Retinal vessel features are an excellent choice for rapid, rough alignment since they are relatively consistent over time and are present in almost all fundus images. Although Jagoe[252] and Miszalok[254] discuss inconsistencies in vessel position and size, gross misregistration due to this minor variability is likely to be almost imperceptible.

Feature matching based solely on fundus vessels, however, cannot completely describe the transformation required to register ophthalmic images acquired with a stereoscopic technique. Retinal thickening or elevation is a frequent finding in fundus images obtained to evaluate the most common retinal diseases. These pathologic changes cause the surface of the retina to depart from the standard curvature of the globe. Therefore, fundus features in these areas cannot be registered using landmarks from the major retinal vessels that simply approximate the internal curvature of the eye. Unfortunately, clinically relevant elevation or thickening of the retina usually occurs in the most important part of the fundus, the macula, which also happens to be relatively avascular. Without small vessel branches to describe this convoluted, elevated surface, vessel matching algorithms will cause misregistration in the area where it is most unacceptable – the diseased macula. Moreover, in the modern era of high-resolution sensors, viewpoint differences between subretinal structures and inner-retinal structures (like blood vessels) become significant – *even in the absence of retinal elevation* (Fig. 52-5). Therefore, although vessel-based registration is an excellent approximation of the transformation function between two images, it is likely that an additional local, elastic function or multilayered global function will also be required to align areas of retinal elevation as well as important pathologic subretinal structures such as drusen and choroidal neovascularization.

Similarity metric

The identification of areas or features of possible correspondence in each image does not imply that they actually match in any way. An automated registration system must determine how to compare these entities to determine their similarity. This method of comparison is often called a similarity metric. Different similarity metrics may be implemented for the different feature types discussed above.

For intensity-based features, the most common method of determining their similarity is based on a technique known as cross-correlation.[74,75,108,235,236,247–250] In the most common implementation, a small block of pixels (called the template block) is defined in image A. The computer then "slides" this block of pixels across image B to determine the area in image B that best matches this template block. By doing this multiple times, a transformation function of varying complexity can be derived. Unfortunately, this process has many associated problems. Since it relies on image intensities, it is very sensitive to lighting irregularities and white noise. In addition, the template block chosen from image A needs to contain useful, somewhat unique information that compares with image B. If, for instance, a template block composed of a homogenous, gray color is chosen

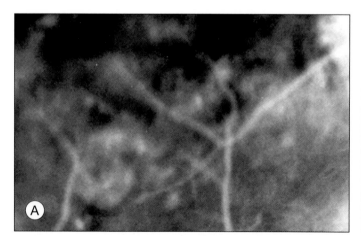

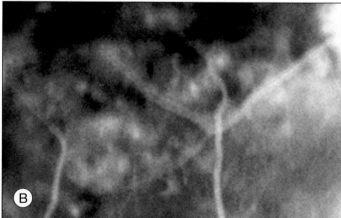

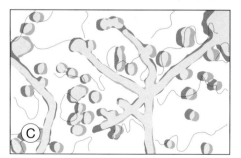

Fig. 52-5 Stereoscopic angiogram frames taken with 1.4 megapixel sensor (A, B). Overlay of two frames: dark gray representing the left view, medium gray representing the right view, and light gray representing areas of commonality (C). Notice that the vessels are relatively stationary while the areas of subretinal hyperfluorescence move in the opposite direction of the camera.

in image A, it might match equally well to many areas of image B that contain a similar flat gray color. This degeneracy of information contained within a template block can lead to many small correlative peaks (instead of one large one) which fails to clearly identify the optimal match location. Finally, the number of required mathematical calculations increases with the square of the size of the template block and with the size of the search space. For this reason, correlation may be more efficiently applied to feature-based methods instead of intensity blocks. This will be discussed further below.

Another common method of determining the similarity of two areas based on their intensity is to use the Fourier transform. A full discussion of this technique is beyond the scope of this chapter, but briefly, the Fourier transform is a way of looking at the frequencies contained within a dataset by describing the data as a series of sine or cosine functions. Phase correlation is an approach based on Fourier transforms that is used to determine the magnitude of the translation offset between two images.[72,86,232,239] Although it is somewhat resistant to lighting irregularities, it is sensitive to white noise and can only be used to account for translation. A variant, known as the power cepstrum, is a homomorphic transformation that is the forward Fourier transform of a spectrum (i.e. the spectrum of a spectrum).[75,231,242,246] It, too, resists lighting variations and can only identify translational offsets. Modifications to the phase correlation algorithm that account for rotation and scaling have also been studied. By performing a log-polar phase correlation at various discrete angles, scale and rotation can be decoupled which then allows for standard phase correlation to identify the magnitude of translation.[72,86,239,242,246] One drawback to this approach is that efficient computation often requires prior knowledge of the center of rotation.

The most promising, recent method developed for intensity-based registration is called mutual information or relative entropy.[234,238,255,256] A full discussion of this topic is also beyond the scope of this chapter. Briefly, however, this approach is based on a measure called *entropy* which reflects the dispersion of a probability distribution. When a sample distribution has a few sharply defined peaks, the entropy is low. When all values in a sample have an equal chance of occurring, entropy is maximized. Minimization of the entropy in the joint histogram of the two images results in image registration.[257] This technique has many distinct advantages over other intensity-based approaches. Unlike correlation techniques, it is very resistant to lighting irregularities, pixel color and noise. Therefore, minimal image preprocessing is required prior to registration. It can find large transformations and deals well with occlusion (disappearance of one feature in the fellow image). In addition, since it views pixel intensities as relative and not absolute values, it works well with multimodal images. In general, it is most effective at finding global, affine transformations that are robust due to the large amounts of data available in the whole image. Much of the statistical power of this approach is lost when attempting to determine an elastic transformation based on the comparison of small local groups of pixels instead of one large sample. Various investigators have

studied methods of ameliorating this problem.[258,259] The statistical nature of mutual information can also cause problems when analyzing image intensities that bridge the gap between discrete and continuous data. And as described in the next section, various strategies may also need to be implemented to keep this algorithm from becoming trapped in a suboptimal solution. Finally, the mutual nature of the calculation occurring between two images may cause difficulty when implementing this technique on long image sequences where all images must be aligned with each other.

In addition to being used for intensity-based comparisons, cross-correlation is a similarity metric that can also be used for the comparison of extracted features.[41,226,232,241] Other mathematical comparisons used for segmented landmarks include: Sequential similarity detection (SSD),[228,233] root mean square error (RMSE),[98,168,236] sum of absolute differences (SAD),[229] measure of match (MOM),[178,237,239] expectation–minimization (EM),[230] Euclidean distance,[73,242] and Hausdorff distance.[251,128,129] Intrinsic properties related to the feature itself, such as the branching angle and number of branching points at each vessel bifurcation, have also been exploited to improve the confidence of the match.[170] In general, feature-based metrics are quicker to calculate than intensity-based similarities because the extracted feature information is distilled into a smaller amount of data. However, the largest contributing factor to the computational cost of this process still comes from the chosen search strategy.

Search strategy

The search for an optimal transformation function may require a substantial amount of computation. In order to minimize calculation time, it is important to choose the most efficient search strategy that approximates the anticipated misregistration between images. For instance, registration of high-speed SLO images of a healthy patient with good fixation might only require small amounts of translational and rotational correction. On the other hand, alignment of images taken years apart in a patient with media opacities and poor fixation may require significant amounts of searching to find the large translation, rotation, scale and higher-order corrections required.

When a search strategy investigates every possible permutation of misalignment based on the transformation model, it is called *exhaustive*.[73,226,227,234,248,249] Although this strategy is reasonable to use for translational misalignment of low-resolution images and can be completed in a finite amount of time with modern processors, it becomes impractical in large images with a prohibitive number of potential permutations of translation, rotation, and scale offsets. An initial, gross approximation of the transformation function can be accomplished more quickly with interactive point selection by the user.[172,230,248] Gross approximations of the registration function can also be achieved automatically by using a Hough transform[168,233,240] or the relative position of easily-recognized, consistent landmarks, such as the optic nerve,[236,242] fovea,[229,242] and vessels.[229,235] Although these techniques reduce computation time by shrinking the area that might contain a potential match, the maximum search space for each pixel still remains an unknown. However, for images grossly registered with at least eight corresponding feature points, a limited search space can be predicted if the epipolar geometry relating the two images can be determined. In these cases, the match for each feature point must exist along a single epipolar line which can then be searched quickly with a simple correlation function.[74] The dense field of corresponding points produced by this process can be used for elastic registration, but may also need to be constrained from improbable geometric transformations by a regularization function.[108] If numerous feature points are known, random sample point matching, especially with a process known as Random Sample Consensus,[260] may also be a useful method for searching small data sets for the optimal consensus of corresponding points.[137]

Improved searching efficiency may be achieved with hierarchical strategies, such as multiresolution or pyramid sampling approaches.[232,238,241,249,261] With these techniques, initial gross alignment is achieved by registering blurred or low-resolution images that contain smaller data sets. As the image resolutions successively increase, refined registration transformations can be calculated quickly without having to search very far for the optimal solution. Other iterative methods, such as simplex,[232,262] error minimization,[236,252] Markov random fields,[73] and closest-point algorithms,[154,245] may also limit the amount of searching required. One very promising approach, known as Dual-Bootstrap ICP, uses a hierarchical estimation algorithm to determine the parameters for successively higher dimensional transformations.[263] This procedure tracks vessels initiated from distributed seed points and simultaneously determines both correspondence and transformation coefficients. In testing on clinical images, the investigators found an overall success rate of only 78.5% but, in most cases, they were able to predict when misregistration had occurred.[264]

When cross-correlation of image intensities is implemented with many search strategies, the algorithm has the potential to get trapped in a local minimum that may not represent the optimal match. Various modifications to standard searching procedures, such as simulated annealing or genetic algorithms, may be useful to avoid this situation and ensure the completion of a comprehensive search.[178,237,238,265]

Registration accuracy

Once the relationship among corresponding feature points in two images has been derived, the resulting transformation function can be used to warp one image into alignment with the other. Since perfect transformation functions are rarely found, registration errors often manifest themselves in the final warping process. To complicate matters further, good objective measures of registration accuracy do not exist. The reason for this is circular: in order to precisely measure registration inaccuracies, one has to know the ideal transformation function required to register the images. But if this optimal transformation function is already known, then there is no need to calculate the image misalignment. Therefore, precise quantification of registration errors can be challenging. Visual inspection, either by flicker testing or interspersing blocks from each image in a checkerboard pattern, is the gold standard for measuring registration

accuracy.[238] Superimposition of vessel centerlines or edges can also be useful.[98] However, this measurement includes errors inherent in the underlying vessel detection algorithm. The sum of differences and measures of match have also been studied.[239] Unfortunately, the intensity variations in fluorescein angiography due to dye transit make these measurement less useful.

Viewpoint registration

Nonrigid image deformations contribute to our perception of stereopsis when viewing paired fundus photographs. As discussed above, this irregular distortion must be neutralized in order to maximize the accuracy of image registration. However, in order to be able to precisely model this deformation, its potential causes must be enumerated. The different viewpoints used to capture stereoscopic fundus images, the lens aberrations inherent in fundus cameras, the natural curvature of the globe, and the abnormal convexity of areas of retinal elevation all contribute to non-rigid image distortions. Proper modeling of these parameters should allow for the development of sophisticated methods for elastic image registration.

Soon after the development of the modern fundus camera, Krakau realized the potential of measuring retinal features with a technique known as stereophotogrammetry.[266,267] Based on simple geometric triangulation, stereophotogrammetry uses the differential shifts of objects imaged from two different camera poses to determine their distance from the camera lens. Since these shifts may be very small, this process is dependent on the resolution of the imaging modality, the movement of the camera, the angular field of view and ultimately, on the resolving power of the subject's eye.[268] Initially, several groups published data based on manual measurements taken from standard film photography.[269,270] Computerized analysis of digitized images was used by subsequent investigators to estimate optic nerve head topography by calculating departures from an affine registration model.[108,248,271,272] In 2000, Berestov outlined a rational process for fundus topographic reconstructions based on epipolar geometry and simple correlation functions.[74]

More recently, the authors presented data demonstrating a strong correlation between stereophotogrammetric fundus topography and optical coherence tomography.[273] In this small study, fundus elevation was estimated by calculating the difference between affine and elastic transformations for angiographic image pairs (Fig. 52-6). The result of these calculations is a vector field with a magnitude that is proportional to the height of the surface being imaged. These data suggest that, with proper modeling of the camera function and optics of the patient's eye, absolute heights of retinal features can be quantified from a single pair of fundus images with an axial resolution of better than 40 microns.

This technique has advantages and disadvantages. It is cheap, repeatable, and independent of patient fixation. It works remotely, retrospectively, and in uncooperative subjects. In addition, it provides exact fundus landmarks for registration with other imaging modalities. However, since it does not detect the level of the retinal pigment epithelium, it cannot calculate retinal thickness. Moreover, it only detects the innermost *visible* retinal

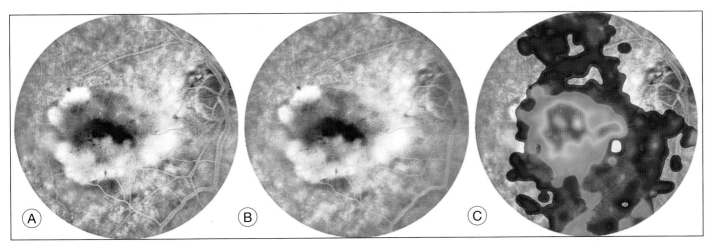

Fig. 52-6 Stereoscopic fundus topography. Stereoscopic angiogram frames digitized from film (A, B) with height map calculated using stereophotogrammetric techniques (C).

layer and neglects areas of homogeneity or transparency. It also does not provide details on intraretinal structures. Nevertheless, the calculation of local image deformations is an essential step in the process of precise image registration. Since this process produces topographic information as a by-product, its clinical utility can remain to be determined in future studies.

Temporal registration

In order for a computer to measure the change in fluorescence of a single feature over time, it must be able to follow the structure (e.g. microaneurysm, drusen, etc.) through each frame of the angiogram. This task is second nature to most human observers, but it presents a major challenge for computers unaccustomed to tracking objects in images. For instance, eye movements during an angiogram may cause the position of structures, such as the optic nerve, to shift between frames. This is of little consequence to a human grader who can easily recognize the new position of the nerve in each frame. However, it poses a problem for computers that cannot reliably recognize the optic nerve in a fundus image. Therefore, in order for a computer to analyze changes in fundus fluorescence, each photograph must be carefully aligned so that corresponding points in each frame, such as the major vessels or optic cup, are collinear.

As mentioned previously, minor errors often occur during the process of registration. Accumulation of these small, pairwise alignment errors in long angiographic sequences can translate into large misalignments between the first and last frames. Therefore, misalignment inaccuracies should be estimated between all images in an angiographic sequence to ensure the global alignment of all frames.[242,245,264] The temporal alignment of fluorescein angiograms is further complicated by changes in the size, shape and intensity of features of interest between frames. Structures that appear and disappear or features that leak and grow irregularly in size all pose a major challenge to computerized analysis. This complicates the application of both intensity and feature-based registration algorithms. Frames that are temporally adjacent may be more easily aligned due to smaller differences in the size and shape of fluorescent areas. However,

these smaller magnitudes of intensity change may result in decreased data precision for subsequent classification.

Multimodal registration

It seems logical to assume that all retinal photographs obtained with a fundus camera should be classified as having originated from the same modality. However, since the intensity values in color photography and fluorescein angiography may be inverted and the structures visible on ICG angiography may not be seen in other modalities, integration of these techniques is considered to be a multimodal registration problem. Alignment of these diagnostic studies with results from newer devices, such as OCT and microperimetry, is a further extension of this same problem.

As discussed previously, intensity-based registration algorithms may have difficulty aligning disparate image types due to intensity inversions or pseudocolor representations. Mutual information, on the other hand, is relatively insensitive to differences in intensity or color. Therefore, it may prove to be a useful technique for this purpose. Feature-based algorithms that utilize distilled, symbolic structures for alignment may also be successful. However, customized segmentation routines will likely be required to detect corresponding features in images from different modalities. The integration of multimodal image data for the purposes of objective lesion quantification will be discussed next.

FEATURE CLASSIFICATION

Classification is the term used to describe the process of identifying pixels or objects that have been discovered in an image. This ability comes naturally to trained observers, but their results are ultimately subjective and may vary over time. The results from computers, on the other hand, are quite objective and repeatable. Therefore, it may be beneficial to train computers to perform this task.

The process of training a computer to automatically recognize fundus lesions is known as supervised classification. It involves three major steps. First, a human grader must manually delineate and classify regions or pixels that comprise a lesion of known identity. Next, generalizations must be made that describe the characteristic features of each lesion. Finally, this data must be compiled into a comprehensive database of all known lesion types. This lesion atlas will be referenced during subsequent unsupervised classification tests when the computer attempts to identify unknown regions or pixels in a newly encountered image set. The adequacy of the feature definitions contained in the atlas can then be determined by studying the accuracy of this unsupervised prediction.

Classification and segmentation routines have closely related objectives. In fact, the segmentation algorithms discussed in this chapter are really hybrid processes that combine segmentation and classification. In its purest form, a segmentation algorithm should delineate an object without trying to identify it. In practice, however, many routines implicitly integrate classification into their process. For instance, algorithms that identify microaneurysms may integrate information about a microaneurysm's color, size and fluorescence characteristics with a segmentation routine that identifies generic, round objects. The implied outcome of this process is that all resulting regions represent microaneurysms. False detections and omissions will obviously occur with these types of algorithms. However, by comparing these automated results to a panel of human graders, sensitivity and specificity values for each approach can be derived.

Based on past experience and training, a human grader identifies features of interest, such as drusen, microaneurysms or veins. By identifying the pixels that comprise each retinal lesion, the human trainer forces the computer to view the fundus in the same way that he or she sees it. A group of pixels identified as a single lesion type by the trainer is called an *information class* (Fig. 52-7). However, these subjectively grouped pixels or regions are frequently heterogeneous and contain too much natural and artificial variation for an untrained computer to perceive as contiguous points. Regions that do make sense to a computer, called *spectral classes* or clusters, tend to be smaller, homogenous subsets of larger groups such as information classes. Therefore, the process of supervised classification involves clumping smaller spectral classes into larger information classes

that will make contextual sense to the viewer when used for unsupervised classification. The smaller, spectral classes also provide a unique opportunity to develop a revised disease classification system. For example, consider a choroidal neovascular membrane that exhibits heterogeneous areas of active leakage as well as older, regressing regions of scarring. Out of practical necessity, a human grader may lump this entire structure into a single CNV category when, in fact, this lesion may better be described by several sub-classified regions. Therefore, the objective, homogenous data contained within these spectral classes may allow for more sophisticated and detailed descriptions of the fundus lesions than is currently possible.

The second step in classification, generalization of image data, can be approached as a pattern recognition task. Several groups have investigated the use of neural networks for the classification of image regions or candidate lesions identified by segmentation routines.[69,76,78,80,81,90,177,186] Although this requires large training sets to produce robust results, it is a very promising approach that deserves further research. Cree and colleagues attempted to manually deduce their own literal morphologic classification criteria to exclude false-positive microaneurysms after segmentation.[105] Unfortunately, this process was laborious even for a small set of images. However, the use of multiple descriptors, such as size, shape and edge strength, in addition to color is a useful method of increasing the specificity of a classification algorithm.

Feature space is the term used to describe the potential characteristics or parameters that define objects contained within it. For instance, if we choose to describe an automobile by its color, weight and length, we have described its "location" in three-dimensional feature space. Similarly, if we describe a pixel in an image by its red, green, and blue intensities, we have also described it in three-dimensional feature space. However, since many pixels in an image may have identical red, green and blue intensities, this description is not unique. The degeneracy in a three-dimensional data set can be improved by adding feature dimensions to increase the specificity of the object description.[274] For example, two pixels with a reddish color may have identical red, green and blue intensities. However, if a fourth dimension is added that describes the aspect ratio (AR) of the object to which they belong, the computer might easily distinguish between the pixel that belongs to a vessel (large AR) and the one that belongs to a hemorrhage (smaller AR). The many frames in an angiogram provide additional dimensions of data that further describe each pixel. This is a distinct advantage of fluorescein angiography over color photography and is the reason why angiographic classification has such potential. In fact, rich definitions of fundus lesions in feature space may form the basis of a quantification system with improved accuracy, objectivity and repeatability when compared to current subjective interpretation procedures.

Several items are important to consider when training a computer to recognize fundus features. First, the regions or pixels delineated by the trainer should be representative of the natural variability of a given lesion type or information class. Including numerous small regions from different areas of the image may

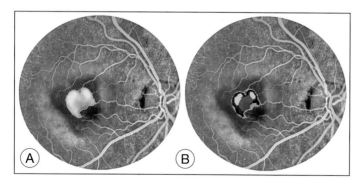

Fig. 52-7 Class comparisons. Leakage identified by viewer (information class) (A) and subdivided by computer into seven spectral classes (B).

sample the innate variability of a lesion type more effectively than outlining a single large region. Second, it is important that ground truth information is communicated to the computer as precisely as possible. For example, angiographic delineation of lesions such as drusen or microaneurysms may be superior to color image identification alone since fluorescein may facilitate the detection of small or subtle lesions.[206,275] Finally, the delineated pixels should reflect the general, underlying distribution of spectral classes within the image and be sufficient in number to support the development of accurate statistical descriptors.

Most of the segmentation routines discussed in this chapter perform calculations on a single image at a time. As a dynamic testing modality, fluorescein angiography contains data that is temporally dispersed across the angiogram sequence. Therefore, a single frame may not adequately capture the wealth of information available to the human interpreter. Angiographic quantification by temporal integration of independently analyzed angiogram frames is a potentially complex process. False detections, false omissions and misidentifications would need to be handled with complicated and arbitrary rules. Furthermore, many structures cannot be reliably classified based on data from a single frame. Therefore, due to the heavy reliance of most segmentation routines on simultaneous classification, many features might be overlooked or misclassified.

Digital subtraction angiography, although unable to integrate data across the entire angiogram, is the first step towards quantitative temporal angiographic analysis.[216,276] Instead of subtracting adjacent frames in an angiogram, Phillips and coworkers tested a variant of this by subtracting a mid-transit frame from a late frame to determine the severity of fluorescein leakage.[218] Martinez-Costa also performed this extended temporal subtraction in patients with vein occlusions.[219]

Dye dilution curves suggest that normal fluorescence should reach a peak and then decrease with time.[27,35,277] Areas of abnormal fluorescence, on the other hand, may increase in brightness with time or simply fail to decrease in intensity as rapidly as normal structures.[218] This property can be exploited with images that have been properly corrected for temporal

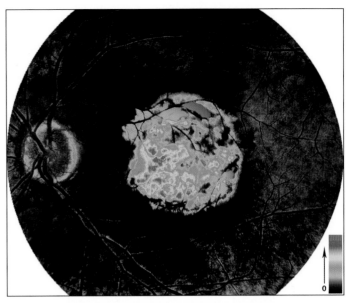

Fig. 52-8 Positive fluorescence quotient (PFQ). Pseudocolor representation of regions of increasing fluorescence after the venous phase of an angiogram. Purple/red indicates areas of greatest increase while blue/black areas show the least change in fluorescence.

exposure variations by calculating the positive fluorescence quotient (PFQ).[278] PFQ quantifies both the area and intensity of regions of interest that increase in fluorescence after the venous phase of an angiogram and is normalized for minor differences in dye volume and exposure by dividing the results by background values (Fig. 52-8). Although this value was found to correlate with vision in a small group of patients with CNV, better quantitative measures are now available.

Human graders use temporal patterns of fluorescence intensity throughout an angiogram to deduce the identity of many fundus features. If digital images are properly prepared and aligned, computers may also be able to accurately extract temporal intensity profiles (TIPs) for every pixel in an image (Fig. 52-9). When combined with color photography, these intensity

Fig. 52-9 Temporal intensity profiles (TIPs).

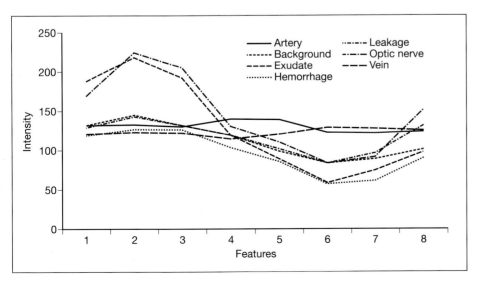

profiles are quite specific for many fundus structures. Pixel-based classification based on this technique may further eliminate the need for independent segmentation algorithms.

As mentioned previously, a great deal of work on vascular flow profiles was done in the 1960s and 1970s using fluorescein angiography and densitometric analysis.[26,30,31] Piccolino and coworkers were the first investigators to publish data demonstrating unique temporal profiles for different structures in age-related macular degeneration.[39] Nagin and colleagues followed soon thereafter with a computerized analysis of the optic nerve and peripapillary retina in two patients with glaucoma.[250] Saito et al. also studied age-related macular degeneration using SLO images.[279] They averaged fluorescence intensities in regions of interest and expressed the results as ratios of lesion intensity versus background fluorescence. However, it wasn't until the work of Berger in the late 1990s that spatial segmentation of fundus features based on characteristic temporal profiles was described.[221] In a short series of papers, he presented a theoretical outline of the process and limited results of fluorescein leakage detection using this algorithm. He subsequently reported on a supervised system of quantification for use in clinical trials that produced a parameter, much like PFQ, that integrated the intensity of fluorescence across the entire lesion (integrated lesion intensity or ILI).[222] Around the same time, Mordon and colleagues used similar temporal profile evaluations to study the fluorescence characteristics of different regions of laser scars in a rabbit model.[280] More recently, Muldrew and Chakravarthy developed a method of distinguishing CNV subtypes based on the size and rate of change of areas of hyperfluorescence.[220]

The authors have recently implemented a fully functional, supervised, quantitative fluorescein angiography system based on the procedural outline described in this chapter (Fig. 52-10). In this system, the subjectivity of lesion delineation is eliminated by objective criteria that accurately guide computer-based decisions on the identity of each pixel in the image. Unlike Berger, we found that the feature space afforded by serial angiographic frames seems to be sufficient to provide unique structure identification.[222] In addition, imprecise segmentation algorithms can be replaced by a single, simple region-growing algorithm that applies to every structure in the image. This simplified, yet highly specific, form of angiographic quantification may provide more repeatable and objective results than standard human interpretation.

FEATURE QUANTIFICATION

Temporal intensity profiles can be used for more than just the classification of individual pixels. The digital quantification of retinal fluorescence presents an entirely new dimension of angiographic information that currently cannot be measured accurately by human graders. Since the complexity of these empirically derived intensity curves may be difficult to model with predictable mathematical equations, simplified parameters can be extracted instead that reveal the underlying trends in fluorescence. In addition, precise, spatial measurements can be

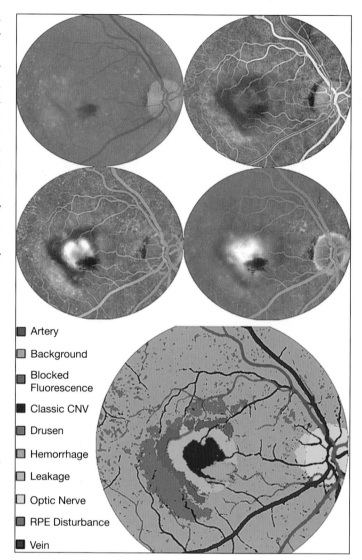

■ Artery
■ Background
■ Blocked Fluorescence
■ Classic CNV
■ Drusen
■ Hemorrhage
■ Leakage
□ Optic Nerve
■ RPE Disturbance
■ Vein

Fig. 52-10 Automated classification. Computer identification of lesion components based on supervised training data.

made from contiguous pixels sharing the same classification. Identical, objective, repeatable techniques can then be used in support of clinical trials, as well as in the clinical practices that execute recommendations from these clinical trials.

One simple parameter that can be calculated from an angiographic sequence is the integral (Fig. 52-11), or sum, of intensity values in every frame.[97,222,226] Differences in lighting and frame number can be accounted for by correcting the data against an area of background fluorescence.[226,278] An advantage of this summation process is that it may emphasize true fluorescence and de-emphasize noise. However, its use for segmentation or classification is limited since many different lesions will have identical intensity integrals and may be indistinguishable. Subtraction techniques have also been investigated.[216,276,278] Sheidow et al. found this technique to be of benefit in approximately half of the cases tested. Sadda and colleagues also found a strong correlation between vision and PFQ.[278] However, lighting and exposure irregularities may cause

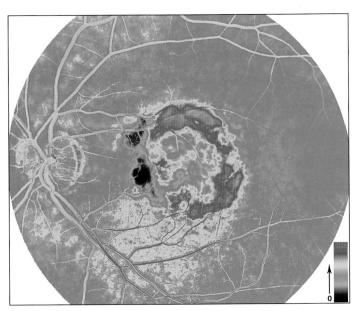

Fig. 52-11 Integral. Summed intensities from aligned angiogram frames displayed in pseudocolor.

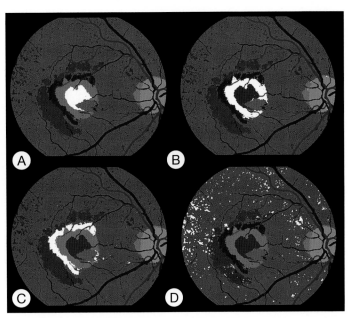

Fig. 52-12 Lesion quantification. Demarcated areas of classic CNV (A), lateral leakage (B), blocked fluorescence (C), and drusen (D). Precise calculations of area, perimeter, lesion number, intensity distributions, etc. can be derived from this.

significant false detections of fluorescence when subtracting adjacent frames. More sophisticated modeling of changes in fluorescence over multiple time scales may ameliorate this problem.

Other parameters that can be extracted from TIPs include time of arrival of dye,[86,277] arterio-venous passage time,[42,281] time to maximum intensity,[42,86,97,277] and rise time.[86,277,281] These data can be graphically presented in three-dimensions[282,283] or with pseudo-colors that represent the magnitude of the calculation at each point.[39] Accurate peaks and troughs may also be detected by modeling these empirically derived data with high order polynomial equations.[86,97] In standard fluorescein angiography, curve fitting can be complicated by poor localization of initial time points (e.g. time of dye arrival) due to irregular frame acquisition.[42] Scanning laser ophthalmoscopy may be superior in this regard since, with an acquisition speed of 20–30 frames per second, it is less likely to miss the precise time of dye arrival.[48] In addition, SLO may provide better lighting stability and exposure homogeneity. Unfortunately, there is a penalty in spatial quantification with SLO sensors that currently have inferior resolutions when compared to those used in modern digital fluorescein angiography systems. Regardless of the system used, many other variables, including the speed of dye injection and the perfusion rate of the patient, may need to be accounted for prior to data interpretation.

A simple region-growing algorithm can produce fundus features with known identities by connecting contiguous pixels that have been similarly classified based on their TIPs (Fig. 52-12). Numerous parameters, including area, perimeter, circularity, edge strength, average intensity and intensity distribution can be calculated for these discrete lesions. When considered as a group, global parameters for each lesion type, such as the number of lesions present and their total area, can be calculated regardless of the number of features detected. For instance, microaneurysm or drusen counts may be predictors of disease progression.[16–18] However, human graders often do not have enough patience or discriminating precision to accurately count these lesions. A quantitative system capable of reproducibly counting lesions may therefore lead to better predictors of disease progression.

Several parameters specific to the retinal vasculature may have importance in diseases such as hypertension and diabetes. Vessel diameters,[41,284–290] segment lengths,[170,177,291,292] branching angles,[202,291] number of vessel branches,[202,291] and tortuosity[157,177,180,289,293] may be useful measurements. Several groups have also studied the fractal nature of retinal vessels.[294–302] However, Hesse[303] has questioned the adequacy of a simple fractal model while Panico and Sterling[304] make the argument that retinal vessels may be space-filling structures instead of fractals. Various measures of venous beading, including distance transform,[166] Fourier-based[171,305,306] and neural network assessments,[307] have been studied by several groups. The accuracy of this calculation, however, depends on adequate image resolution and is sensitive to noise from adjacent pathology. Moreover, due to the subjective nature of the gold-standard clinical definition, development of a scale-independent objective definition has yet to be accomplished.

Finally, in order to maximize quantitative accuracy, an objective fluorescein angiography system must provide feature measurements in universal units that can be used for comparisons in clinical trials. Millimeters and MPS disc areas are common measurements used in reading center assessments. Film-based

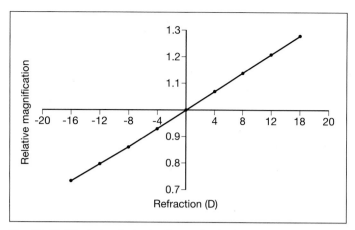

Fig. 52-13 Effect of patient refraction on fundus image magnification using Zeiss telecentric camera (reconstructed from data provided by Bengtsson & Krakau[308]).

analyses require the use of fixed magnification factors or templates to convert photographic measurements to retinal units. However, these conversion factors are less useful when working with digital images comprised of pixels. Moreover, there are significant variables in acquisition, such as the camera type, field of view, and patient refraction, that cannot be accounted for when using a fixed conversion factor. For example, in 1977, Bengtsson and Krakau[308] described approximately a 17% difference in magnification for every 10 diopters of patient refractive error (Fig. 52-13). In this new era of digital imaging, custom conversion factors can now be deduced for each patient and camera system that will standardize the definition of a millimeter of distance on the retinal surface. This more universal measurement may again improve the accuracy of data supplied to clinical trials.

CONCLUSION

The convergence of recent advances in computing and imaging technology affords the opportunity to develop methods for extracting the maximum amount of useful information from fluorescein angiograms. Although it will need extensive testing and validation, a quantitative fluorescein angiography system may improve the speed and accuracy of clinical investigations, improve the precision of disease monitoring, and standardize the clinical application of clinical trials recommendations. A more rational approach to disease classifications may also provide a better understanding of underlying disease processes and a better substrate for the comparison of genomic studies. These same technologies may also lead to better algorithms for automated screening efforts for diabetic retinopathy and age-related macular degeneration.

REFERENCES

1. Flocks M, Miller J, Chao P. Retinal circulation time with the aid of fundus cinephotography. Am J Ophthalmol 1959; 48:3–10.
2. MacLean AL, Maumenee AE. Hemangioma of the choroid. Am J Ophthalmol 1960; 50:3–11.
3. Novotny HR, Alvis DL. A method of photographing fluorescence in circulating blood in the human retina. Circulation 1961; 24:82–86.
4. Macular Photocoagulation Study Group. Subfoveal neovascular lesions in age-related macular degeneration. Guidelines for evaluation and treatment in the macular photocoagulation study. Arch Ophthalmol 1991; 109:1242–1257.
5. Macular Photocoagulation Study Group. Laser photocoagulation of subfoveal neovascular lesions of age-related macular degeneration. Updated findings from two clinical trials. Arch Ophthalmol 1993; 111:1200–1209.
6. Treatment of age-related macular degeneration with photodynamic therapy (TAP) Study Group. Photodynamic therapy of subfoveal choroidal neovascularization in age-related macular degeneration with verteporfin: one-year results of 2 randomized clinical trials – TAP report. Arch Ophthalmol 1999; 117:1329–1345.
7. Bressler NM. Photodynamic therapy of subfoveal choroidal neovascularization in age-related macular degeneration with verteporfin: two-year results of 2 randomized clinical trials – TAP report 2. Arch Ophthalmol 2001; 119:198–207.
8. Bressler NM, Arnold J, Benchaboune M et al. Verteporfin therapy of subfoveal choroidal neovascularization in patients with age-related macular degeneration: additional information regarding baseline lesion composition's impact on vision outcomes – TAP report no. 3. Arch Ophthalmol 2002; 120:1443–1454.
9. Verteporfin in Photodynamic Therapy (VIP) Study Group. Verteporfin therapy of subfoveal choroidal neovascularization in age-related macular degeneration: two-year results of a randomized clinical trial including lesions with occult with no classic choroidal neovascularization – verteporfin in photodynamic therapy report 2. Am J Ophthalmol 2001; 131:541–560.
10. Early Treatment Diabetic Retinopathy Study Research Group. Fluorescein angiographic risk factors for progression of diabetic retinopathy. ETDRS report number 13. Ophthalmology 1991; 98:834–840.
11. The Diabetic Retinopathy Study Research Group. Four risk factors for severe visual loss in diabetic retinopathy. The third report from the Diabetic Retinopathy Study. Arch Ophthalmol 1979; 97:654–655.
12. Kaiser RS, Berger JW, Williams GA et al. Variability in fluorescein angiography interpretation for photodynamic therapy in age-related macular degeneration. Retina 2002; 22:683–690.
13. The Age-related Eye Disease Study Research Group. The Age-related Eye Disease Study (AREDS): design implications. AREDS report no. 1. Control Clin Trials 1999; 20:573–600.
14. The Age-related Eye Disease Study Research Group. A randomized, placebo-controlled, clinical trial of high-dose supplementation with vitamins C and E, beta carotene, and zinc for age-related macular degeneration and vision loss. AREDS report no. 8. Arch Ophthalmol 2001; 119:1417–1436.
15. Early Treatment Diabetic Retinopathy Study Research Group. Fundus photographic risk factors for progression of diabetic retinopathy. ETDRS report number 12. Ophthalmology 1991; 98:823–833.
16. Hellstedt T, Immonen I. Disappearance and formation rates of microaneurysms in early diabetic retinopathy. Br J Ophthalmol 1996; 80:135–139.
17. Klein R, Meuer SM, Moss SE, et al. Retinal microaneurysm counts and 10-year progression of diabetic retinopathy. Arch Ophthalmol 1995; 113:1386–1391.
18. Kohner EM, Sleightholm M. Does microaneurysm count reflect severity of early diabetic retinopathy? Ophthalmology 1986; 93:586–589.
19. Treatment of Age-related Macular Degeneration With Photodynamic Therapy and Verteporfin in Photodynamic Therapy Study Groups. Photodynamic therapy of subfoveal choroidal neovascularization with verteporfin: fluorescein angiographic guidelines for evaluation and treatment. TAP and VIP report no. 2. Arch Ophthalmol 2003; 121:1253–1268.
20. Blinder KJ, Bradley S, Bressler NM et al. Effect of lesion size, visual acuity, and lesion composition on visual acuity change with and without verteporfin therapy for choroidal neovascularization secondary to age-related macular degeneration. TAP and VIP report no. 1. Am J Ophthalmol 2003; 136:407–418.
21. McBroom M. McBroom's camera bluebook: a complete, up-to-date price and buyers guide for new and used cameras, lenses and accessories, 6th edn. Buffalo, New York: Amherst Media, 2000.
22. Teng T, Lefley M, Claremont D. Progress towards automated diabetic ocular screening: a review of image analysis and intelligent systems for diabetic retinopathy. Med Biol Eng Comput 2002; 40:2–13.
23. Larsen N, Godt J, Grunkin M et al. Automated detection of diabetic retinopathy in a fundus photographic screening population. Invest Ophthalmol Vis Sci 2003; 44:767–771.
24. Usher D, Dumskyj M, Himaga M et al. Automated detection of diabetic retinopathy in digital retinal images: a tool for diabetic retinopathy screening. Diabet Med 2004; 21:84–90.
25. Hipwell JH, Strachan F, Olson JA et al. Automated detection of microaneurysms in digital red-free photographs: a diabetic retinopathy screening tool. Diabet Med 2000; 17:588–594.

26. Hickam JB, Frayser R. A photographic method for measuring the mean retinal circulation time using fluorescein. Invest Ophthalmol 1965; 4:876–884.

27. Riva CE, Feke GT, Ben-Sira I. Fluorescein dye-dilution technique and retinal circulation. Am J Physiol 1978; 234:H315–322.

28. Bulpitt CJ, Dollery CT. Estimation of retinal blood flow by measurement of the mean circulation time. Cardiovasc Res 1971; 5:406–412.

29. Boyd TA, Rosen ES. A new method of clinical assessment of an intraocular pressure sensitive ischaemic mechanism in glaucoma. Can J Ophthalmol 1970; 5:12–15.

30. Rosen ES, Boyd TAS. New method of assessing choroidal ischemia in open-angle glaucoma and ocular hypertension. Am J Ophthalmol 1970; 70:912–921.

31. Schwartz B, Fishbein SL, Selles W. Densitometric analysis of blood flow of the optic nerve head in glaucoma. Proc Soc Photo-Optical Instrument Eng 1973; 40:3–10.

32. Kohner EM, Hamilton AM, Saunders SJ et al. The retinal blood flow in diabetes. Diabetologia 1975; 11:27–33.

33. Bulpitt CJ, Kohner EM, Dollery CT. Velocity profiles in the retinal microcirculation. Bibl Anat 1973; 11:448–452.

34. Schwartz B, Kern J. Age, increased ocular and blood pressures, and retinal and disc fluorescein angiogram. Arch Ophthalmol 1980; 98:1980–1986.

35. Ben-Sira I, Riva CE. Fluorophotometric recording of fluorescein dilution curves in human retinal vessels. Invest Ophthalmol 1973; 12:310–312.

36. Blair NP, Feke GT, Morales-Stoppello J et al. Prolongation of the retinal mean circulation time in diabetes. Arch Ophthalmol 1982; 100:764–768.

37. Moses RA. Intraocular blood flow from analysis of angiograms. IOVS 1983; 24:354–360.

38. Fonda S, Bagolini B. Relative photometric measurements of retinal circulation (dromofluorograms): a television technique. Arch Ophthalmol 1977; 95:302–307.

39. Piccolino FC, Zingirian M, Parodi GC. Electronic image analysis in retinal fluoroangiography with one colour plate. Ophthalmologica, Basel 1979; 179:142–147.

40. Piccolino FC, Zingirian M, Parodi GC. Densitometric analysis of macular fluorescein angiography. Ophthalmologica, Basel 1981; 182:171–174.

41. Preussner PR, Richard G, Darrelmann O et al. Quantitative measurement of retinal blood flow in human beings by application of digital image-processing methods to television fluorescein angiograms. Graefes Arch Clin Exp Ophthalmol 1983; 221:110–112.

42. Koyama T, Matsuo N, Shimizu K et al. Retinal circulation times in quantitative fluorescein angiography. Graefes Arch Clin Exp Ophthalmol 1990; 228:442–446.

43. Bursell SE, Clermont AC, Kinsley BT et al. Retinal blood flow changes in patients with insulin-dependent diabetes mellitus and no diabetic retinopathy. IOVS 1996; 37:886–897.

44. Webb RH, Hughes GW. Scanning laser ophthalmoscope. IEEE Trans Biomed Eng 1981; 28:488–492.

45. Lee ET, Rehkopf PG, Warnicki JW et al. A new method for assessment of changes in retinal blood flow. Med Eng Phys 1997; 19:125–130.

46. Yamaji H, Shiraga F, Tsuchida Y et al. Evaluation of arteriovenous crossing sheathotomy for branch retinal vein occlusion by fluorescein videoangiography and image analysis. Am J Ophthalmol 2004; 137:834–841.

47. Mainster MA, Timberlake GT, Webb RH et al. Scanning laser ophthalmoscopy. Clinical applications. Ophthalmology 1982; 89:852–857.

48. Rechtman E, Harris A, Kumar R et al. An update on retinal circulation assessment technologies. Curr Eye Res 2003; 27:329–343.

49. Yoshida A, Feke GT, Morales-Stoppello J et al. Retinal blood flow alterations during progression of diabetic retinopathy. Arch Ophthalmol 1983; 101:225–227.

50. Bertram B, Wolf S, Fiehofer S et al. Retinal circulation times in diabetes mellitus type 1. Br J Ophthalmol 1991; 75:462–465.

51. Arend O, Wolf S, Jung F et al. Retinal microcirculation in patients with diabetes mellitus: dynamic and morphological analysis of perifoveal capillary network. Br J Ophthalmol 1991; 75:514–518.

52. Akita K, Kuga H. A computer method of understanding ocular fundus images. Pattern Recognition 1982; 15:431–443.

53. Liesenfeld B, Kohner E, Piehlmeier W et al. A telemedical approach to the screening of diabetic retinopathy: digital fundus photography. Diabetes Care 2000; 23:345–348.

54. Wang Z, Bovik AC. A universal image quality index. IEEE Signal Process Lett 2002; 9:81–84.

55. Wang Z, Bovik AC. Why is image quality assessment so difficult? IEEE Int Conf Acoustics, Speech, Signal Proc, 2002.

56. Wang Z, Bovik AC, Sheikh HR, Simoncelli EP. Image quality assessment: from error measurement to structural similarity. IEEE Trans Image Process 2004; 13:1–14.

57. Engeldrum PG. Image quality modeling: where are we? IS&T PICS Conference 1999; 251–255.

58. Ege BM, Hejlesen OK, Larsen OV et al. Screening for diabetic retinopathy using computer based image analysis and statistical classification. Comput Methods Programs Biomed 2000; 62:165–175.

59. Hayashi JI, Kunieda T, Cole J et al. A development of computer-aided diagnosis system using fundus images. 7th Int Conf Virtual Syst Multimedia 2001; 429–438.

60. Lee SC, Wang Y. Automatic retinal image quality assessment and enhancement. Proc SPIE 1999; 3661:1581–1590.

61. Lalonde M, Gagnon L, Boucher MC. Automatic visual quality assessment in optical fundus images. Proc Vision Interface 2001; 259–264.

62. Gagnon L, Lalonde M, Beaulieu M et al. Procedure to detect anatomical structures in optical fundus images. Proc SPIE 2001; 4322: 1218–1225.

63. Newsom RS, Sinthanayothin C, Boyce J et al. Clinical evaluation of "local contrast enhancement" for oral fluorescein angiograms. Eye 2000; 14:318–323.

64. Sadda SR, Updike PG, Wong AK et al. Automated assessment of retinal image quality. IOVS 2004; 45:E-Abstract 2809.

65. Berkow JW, Flower RW, Orth DH et al. Fluorescein and indocyanine green angiography: technique and interpretation, 2nd edn. San Francisco: American Academy of Ophthalmology, 1997.

66. Goh KG, Hsu W, Lee ML et al. ADRIS: An automatic diabetic retinal image screening system. In: Cios KJ, ed. Medical data mining and knowledge discovery. Physica (Springer) Verlag 2001; 181–210.

67. Hart WE, Goldbaum MH, Cote B et al. Automated measurement of retinal vascular tortuosity. Proc AMIA Fall Conference 1997; 459–463.

68. Gilchrist J. Analysis of early diabetic retinopathy by computer processing of fundus images – a preliminary study. Ophthalmic Physiol Opt 1987; 7:393–399.

69. Jasiobedzki P, Williams CKI, Lu F. Detecting and reconstructing vascular trees in retinal images. Proc SPIE 1994; 2167:815–825.

70. Shin DS, Kaiser RS, Lee MS et al. Fundus image change analysis: geometric and radiometric normalization. Proc SPIE 1999; 3591: 129–136.

71. Shin DS, Javornik NB, Berger JW. Computer-assisted, interactive fundus image processing for macular drusen quantitation. Ophthalmology 1999; 106:1119–1125.

72. Cideciyan AV. Registration of ocular fundus images by cross-correlation of triple invariant image descriptors. IEEE Eng Med Biol Mag 1995; 14:52–58.

73. Domingo J, Ayala G, Simo A et al. Irregular motion recovery in fluorescein angiograms. Pattern Recognit Lett 1997; 18:805–821.

74. Berestov AL. Stereo fundus photography: automatic evaluation of retinal topography. Proc SPIE 2000; 3957:50–59.

75. Mitra S, Ramirez M, Morales J. Three-dimensional digital mapping of the optic nerve head cupping in glaucoma. Proc SPIE 1992; 1644:237–247.

76. Gardner GG, Keating D, Williamson TH et al. Automatic detection of diabetic retinopathy using an artificial neural network: a screening tool. Br J Ophthalmol 1996; 80:940–944.

77. Morris DT, Donnison C. Identifying the neuroretinal rim boundary using dynamic contours. Image Vis Comput 1999; 17:169–174.

78. Osareh A, Mirmehdi M, Thomas B et al. Automatic recognition of exudative maculopathy using Fuzzy C – means clustering and neural networks. Med Image Understand Anal 2001; 49–52.

79. Rapantzikos K, Zervakis M. Nonlinear enhancement and segmentation algorithm for the detection of age-related macular degeneration (AMD) in human eye's retina. Proc Int Conf Image Processing 2001; 3:1055–1058.

80. Osareh A, Mirmehdi M, Thomas B et al. comparative exudate classification using support vector machines and neural networks. 5th Int Conf Med Image Comput Computer-Assisted Intervent 2002:413–420.

81. Sinthanayothin C, Boyce JF, Cook HL et al. Automated localisation of the optic disc, fovea, and retinal blood vessels from digital colour fundus images. Br J Ophthalmol 1999; 83:902–910.

82. Xu L, Zheng X, Yu Y, Zhang H. Adaptive feature enhancement of retinal vascular images using wavelet-based multiresolution analysis. Proc SPIE 1998; 3545:520–524.

83. Phillips RP, Spencer T, Ross PG et al. Quantification of diabetic maculopathy by digital imaging of the fundus. Eye 1991; 5:130–137.

84. Pallawala PMDS, Hsu W, Lee ML et al. Automated optic disc localization and contour detection using ellipse fitting and wavelet transform. 8th Eur Conf Comp Vision 2004; 139–151.

85. Cree MJ, Olson JA, McHardy KC et al. The preprocessing of retinal images for the detection of fluorescein leakage. Phys Med Biol 1999; 44:293–308.

86. Hipwell JH, Manivannan A, Vieira P et al. Quantifying changes in retinal circulation: the generation of parametric images from fluorescein angiograms. Physiol Meas 1998; 19:165–180.

87. Delori FC, Pflibsen KP. Spectral reflectance of the human ocular fundus. Applied Optics 1989; 28:1061–1077.

88. Spencer T, Olson JA, McHardy KC et al. An image-processing strategy for the segmentation and quantification of microaneurysms in fluorescein angiograms of the ocular fundus. Comput Biomed Res 1996; 29:284–302.

89. Barrow HG, Tenenbaum JM. Recovering intrinsic scene characteristics from images. In: Hanson A, Riseman E, eds. Computer vision systems. New York: Academic Press, 1978.

90. Frame AJ, Undrill PE, Cree MJ et al. A comparison of computer based classification methods applied to the detection of microaneurysms in ophthalmic fluorescein angiograms. Comput Biol Med 1998; 28:225–238.

91. Mendonca AM, Campilho AJ, Nunes JM. Automatic segmentation of microaneurysms in retinal angiograms of diabetic patients. 10th Int Conf Image Analysis Proc 1999; 2:728–733.

92. Hoover A, Goldbaum M. Locating the optic nerve in a retinal image using the fuzzy convergence of the blood vessels. IEEE Trans Med Imaging 2003; 22:951–958.

93. Hsu W, Pallawala PMDS, Lee ML et al. The role of domain knowledge in the detection of retinal hard exudates. Proc IEEE Soc Comp Vision Pattern Recog 2001; 2:246–251.

94. Morgan WH, Cooper RL, Constable IJ et al. Automated extraction and quantification of macular drusen from fundal photographs. Aust NZ J Ophthalmol 1994; 22:7–12.

95. Smith RT, Nagasaki T, Sparrow JR et al. A method of drusen measurement based on the geometry of fundus reflectance. Biomed Eng Online 2003; 18:10.

96. Ward NP, Tomlinson S, Taylor CJ. Image analysis of fundus photographs. The detection and measurement of exudates associated with diabetic retinopathy. Ophthalmology 1989; 96:80–86.

97. Jagoe JR, Arnold J, Blauth C et al. Retinal vessel circulation patterns visualized from a sequence of computer-aligned angiograms. IOVS 1993; 34:2881–2887.

98. Laliberte F, Gagnon L, Sheng Y. Registration and fusion of retinal images – an evaluation study. IEEE Trans Med Imaging 2003; 22:661–673.

99. Kirkpatrick JN, Spencer T, Manivannan A et al. Quantitative image analysis of macular drusen from fundus photographs and scanning laser ophthalmoscope images. Eye 1995; 9:48–55.

100. Sinthanayothin C, Boyce JF, Williamson TH et al. Automated detection of diabetic retinopathy on digital fundus images. Diabet Med 2002; 19:105–112.

101. Tappen MF, Freeman WT, Adelson EH. Recovering intrinsic images from a single image. In: Advances in Neural Information Processing Systems 15 (NIPS). Cambridge, MA: MIT Press, 2003.

102. Tsukada M, Ohta Y. An approach to color constancy using multiple images. Proc Third Int Conf Computer Vision 1990; 385–389.

103. Weiss Y. Deriving intrinsic images from image sequences. Proc Int Conf Computer Vision 2001; 2:68–75.

104. Ben Sbeh Z, Cohen LD, Mimoun G et al. A new approach of geodesic reconstruction for drusen segmentation in eye fundus images. IEEE Trans Med Imaging 2001; 20:1321–1333.

105. Cree MJ, Olson JA, McHardy KC et al. A fully automated comparative microaneurysm digital detection system. Eye 1997; 11:622–628.

106. Cree MJ, Olson JA, McHardy KC et al. Automated microaneurysm detection. IEEE Int Conf on Image Processing 1996; 3:699–702.

107. Jagoe JR, Blauth CI, Smith PL et al. Quantification of retinal damage during cardiopulmonary bypass: comparison by computer and human assessment. IEE Proc Communications, Speech, Vision 1990; 137:170–175.

108. Lee S, Brady M. Integrating stereo and photometric stereo to monitor the development of glaucoma. Image Vision Comput 1991; 9:39–44.

109. Wang Y, Tan W, Lee SC. Illumination normalization of retinal images using sampling and interpolation. Proc SPIE 2001; 4322:500–507.

110. Leistritz L, Schweitzer D. Automated detection and quantification of exudates in retinal images. Proc SPIE 1994; 2298:690–696.

111. Wang H, Hsu W, Goh KG et al. An effective approach to detect lesions in color retinal images. IEEE Comp Soc Conf Comp Vision Pattern Recog 2000; 181–187.

112. Tamura S, Okamoto Y, Yanashima K. Zero-crossing interval correction in tracing eye-fundus blood vessels. Pattern Recognit 1988; 21:227–233.

113. Mendels F, Heneghan C, Thiran JP. Identification of the optic disk boundary in retinal images using active contours. Proc Irish Machine Vision and Image Proc Conf 1999; 103–115.

114. Goldbaum MH, Katz NP, Nelson MR et al. The discrimination of similarly colored objects in computer images of the ocular fundus. IOVS 1990; 31:617–623.

115. Katz N, Goldbaum M, Nelson M et al. An image processing system for automatic retina diagnosis. Proc SPIE 1988; 902:131–137.

116. Chalana V, Costa W, Kim Y. Integrating region growing and edge detection using regularization. Proc SPIE 1995; 2434:262–271.

117. Tolias YA, Panas SM. A fuzzy vessel tracking algorithm for retinal images based on fuzzy clustering. IEEE Trans Med Imaging 1998; 17:263–273.

118. Lalonde M, Beaulieu M, Gagnon L. Fast and robust optic disc detection using pyramidal decomposition and Hausdorff-based template matching. IEEE Trans Med Imaging 2001; 20:1193–1200.

119. Wang Y, Toonen H, Meyer-Ebrecht D. A new method for automatic tracking, measuring blood vessels in retinal image. 12th Int Conf Eng Med Biol Soc 1990; 174–175.

120. Chanwimaluang T, Fan G. An efficient algorithm for extraction of anatomical structures in retinal images. Proc IEEE Internat Conf Image Process 2003; 1:1093–1096.

121. Li H, Chutatape O. Automated feature extraction in color retinal images by a model based approach. IEEE Trans Biomed Eng 2004; 51:246–254.

122. Walter T, Klein JC, Massin P et al. A contribution of image processing to the diagnosis of diabetic retinopathy – detection of exudates in color fundus images of the human retina. IEEE Trans Med Imaging 2002; 21:1236–1243.

123. Hoover A, Kouznetsova V, Goldbaum M. Locating blood vessels in retinal images by piecewise threshold probing of a matched filter response. IEEE Trans Med Imaging 2000; 19:203–210.

124. Kochner B, Schuhmann D, Michaelis M et al. Course tracking and contour extraction of retinal vessels from color fundus photographs: most efficient use of steerable filters for model-based image analysis. Proc SPIE 1998; 3338:755–761.

125. Goldbaum M, Moezzi S, Taylor A et al. Automated diagnosis and image understanding with object extraction, object classification, and inferencing in retinal images. IEEE Int Cong Image Proc 1996; 3:695–698.

126. Osareh A, Mirmehdi M, Thomas B et al. Colour morphology and snakes for optic disc localisation. Med Image Understand Anal 2002; 21–24.

127. Lowell J, Hunter A, Steel D et al. Optic nerve head segmentation. IEEE Trans Med Imaging 2004; 23:256–264.

128. Huttenlocher DP, Klanderman GA, Rucklidge WJ. Comparing images using the Hausdorff distance. IEEE Trans Pattern Anal Machine Intellig 1993; 15:850–863.

129. Rucklidge WJ. Locating objects using the Hausdorff distance. 5th Int Conf Comp Vision 1995; 457–464.

130. Davis L. A survey of edge detection techniques. Computer graphics and image processing. 1975; 4:248–270.

131. Gonzalez RC, Wood RE. Digital image processing. Boston: Addison-Wesley, 1992.

132. Canny J. A computational approach to edge detection. IEEE Trans Pattern Anal Mach Intellig 1986; PAMI-8:679–698.

133. Hildreth EC. The detection of intensity changes by computer and biological vision systems. Computer Vis Graph Image Process 1983; 22:1–27.

134. Marr D, Hildreth EC. Theory of edge detection. Proc R Soc London Ser B 1980; 207:187–217.

135. Verbeek PW, van Vliet LJ. On the location error of curved edges in low-pass filtered 2-D and 3-D images. IEEE Trans Pattern Anal Mach Intellig 1994; 16:726–733.

136. Li H, Chutatape O. Automatic location of optic disk in retinal images. IEEE ICIP 2001; 2:837–840.

137. Pinz A, Bernogger S, Datlinger P et al. Mapping the human retina. IEEE Trans Med Imag 1998; 17:606–619.

138. Agron P. Robust active contours in the context of optic disk boundary extraction. Online course paper, Spring 2003, SUNY Stony Brook.

139. Kass M, Witkin A, Terzopoulos D. Snakes: active contour models. Int J Comp Vision 1987; 1:321–331.

140. Xu C, Prince JL. Snakes, shapes and gradient vector flow. IEEE Trans Image Process 1998; 7:359–369.

141. Storvik G. A Bayesian approach to dynamic contours through stochastic sampling and simulated annealing. IEEE Trans Pattern Anal Mach Intellig 1994; 16:976–986.

142. Becker DE, Turner JN, Tanenbaum H et al. Real-time image processing algorithms for an automated retinal laser surgery system. Proc IEEE 2nd Int Conf Image Proc 1995; 426–429.

143. Barrett SF, Wright CH, Oberg ED et al. Digital imaging-based retinal photocoagulation system. Proc SPIE 1997; 2971:118–128.

144. Markow MS, Rylander G, Welch AJ. Real-time algorithm for retinal tracking. IEEE Trans Biomed Eng 1993; 40:1269–1281.

145. Barrett SF, Jerath M, Rylander III HG et al. Digital tracking and control of retinal images. Optical Eng 1994; 33:150–159.

146. Berger JW, Shin DS. Computer-vision-enabled augmented reality fundus biomicroscopy. Ophthalmology 1999; 106:1935–1941.

147. Berger JW, Madjarov B. Augmented reality fundus biomicroscopy: a working clinical prototype. Arch Ophthalmol 2001; 119:1815–1818.

148. Clark TM, Freeman WR, Goldbaum MH. Digital overlay of fluorescein angiograms and fundus images for treatment of subretinal neovascularization. Retina 1992; 12:118–126.

149. Shen H, Stewart CV, Roysam B et al. Frame-rate spatial referencing based on invariant indexing and alignment with application to online retinal image registration. IEEE Trans Pattern Anal Mach Intellig 2003; 25:379–384.

150. Frame AJ, Undrill PE, Olson JA et al. Structural analysis of retinal vessels. Proc IEEE 6th Int Conf Image Process Applicat 1997; 2:824–827.

151. Can A, Shen H, Turner JN et al. Rapid automated tracing and feature

extraction from retinal fundus images using direct exploratory algorithms. IEEE Trans Informat Technol Biomed 1999; 3:125–138.

152. Gao X, Bharath A, Stanton A et al. A method of vessel tracking for vessel diameter measurement on retinal images. Proc 2001 Int Conf Image Process 2001; 2:881–884.

153. Zhou LA, Rzeszotarski MS, Singerman LJ et al. The detection and quantification of retinopathy using digital angiograms. IEEE Trans Med Imaging 1994; 13:619–626.

154. Stewart CV, Tsai CL, Perera A. A view-based approach to registration: theory and application to vascular image registration. Lecture Notes Comput Sci 2003; 2732:475–486.

155. Shen H, Roysam B, Stewart CV et al. Optimal scheduling of tracing computations for real-time vascular landmark extraction from retinal fundus images. IEEE Trans Inf Tech Biomed 2001; 5:77–91.

156. Englmeier KH, Bichler S, Schmid K et al. Multiresolution retinal vessel tracker based on directional smoothing. Proc SPIE 2002; 4683:230–237.

157. Giansanti R, Boemi M, Fumelli P et al. Quantitative analysis of retinal changes in hypertension. Proc SPIE 1995; 2434:548–556.

158. Zahlmann G, Kochner B, Ugi I et al. Hybrid fuzzy image processing for situation assessment. IEEE Eng Med Biol Mag 2000; 19:76–83.

159. Wallace DK, Jomier J, Aylward SR et al. Computer-automated quantification of plus disease in retinopathy of prematurity. J AAPOS 2003; 7:126–130.

160. Rakotomalala V, Macaire L, Postaire JG et al. Identification of retinal vessels by color image analysis. Mach Graphics Vis 1998; 7:725–742.

161. Becker DE, Can A, Turner JN et al. Image processing algorithms for retinal montage synthesis, mapping, and real-time location determination. IEEE Trans Biomed Eng 1998; 45:105–118.

162. Chapman N, Witt N, Gao X et al. Computer algorithms for the automated measurement of retinal arteriolar diameters. Br J Ophthalmol 2001; 85:74–79.

163. Wang Y, Lee SC. A fast method for automated detection of blood vessels in retinal images. 31st Asilomar Conf Signals, Systems, Computers 1997; 2:1700–1704.

164. Yu JJH, Hung BN, Sun HC. Automatic recognition of retinopathy from retinal images. 12th Int Conf Eng Med Biol Soc 1990; 171–173.

165. Noack J, Sutton D. An algorithm for the fast registration of image sequences obtained with a scanning laser ophthalmoscope. Physics Med Biol 1994; 39:907–915.

166. Lee SC, Wang Y, Tan W. Automated detection of venous beading in retinal images. Proc SPIE 2001; 4322:1365–1372.

167. Leandro JJG, Cesar RM, Jelinek HF. Blood vessels segmentation in retina: preliminary assessment of the mathematical morphology and of the wavelet transform techniques. Proc Brazilian Symp Comp Graphics Image Proc 2001; 84–90.

168. Walter T, Klein JC, Massin P et al. Automatic segmentation and registration of retinal fluorescein angiographies. 1st Int Workshop Comp Assist Fundus Image Anal, 2000.

169. McInerney T, Terzopoulos D. T-snakes: topology adaptive snakes. Med Imag Anal 2000; 4:73–91.

170. Bouaoune Y, Assogba MK, Nunes JC et al. Spatio-temporal characterization of vessel segments applied to retinal angiographic images. Pattern Recognit Lett 2003; 24:607–615.

171. Gregson PH, Shen Z, Scott RC et al. Automated grading of venous beading. Comput Biomed Res 1995; 28:291–304.

172. Tamura S, Tanaka K, Ohmori S et al. Semiautomatic leakage analyzing system for time series fluorescein ocular fundus angiography. Pattern Recognit 1983; 16:149–162.

173. Jiang X, Mojon D. Adaptive local thresholding by verification-based multithreshold probing with application to vessel detection in retinal images. IEEE Trans Pattern Anal Mach Intellig 2003; 25:131–137.

174. Serra J. Introduction to mathematical morphology. Computer Vis Graphics Image Process 1986; 35:283–305.

175. Sternberg SR. Grayscale morphology. Computer Vis Graphics Image Process 1986; 35:333–355.

176. Jasiobedzki P, Macleod D, Taylor CJ. Detection of non-perfused zones in retinal images. IEEE Symp Comp Based Med Syst 1991; 162–169.

177. Kaupp A, Dolemeyer A, Wilzeck R et al. Measuring morphologic properties of the human retinal vessel system using a two-stage image processing approach. Proc IEEE Int Conf Image Proc 1994; 1:431–435.

178. Matsopoulos GK, Mouravliansky NA, Delibasis KK et al. Automatic retinal image registration scheme using global optimization techniques. IEEE Trans Inf Technol Biomed 1999; 3:47–60.

179. Zana F, Klein JC. Robust segmentation of vessels from retinal angiography. Proc Int Conf Digital Signal Proc 1997; 1087–1090.

180. Zana F, Klein JC. Segmentation of vessel-like patterns using mathematical morphology and curvature evaluation. IEEE Trans Image Proc 2001; 10:1010–1019.

181. Fang B, Hsu W, Lee ML. Reconstruction of vascular structures in retinal images. IEEE Int Conf Image Proc 2003; 2:157–160.

182. Iliasova NY, Ustinov AV, Branchevsky SL et al. Methods for estimating geometric parameters of retinal vessels using diagnostic images of fundus. Proc SPIE 1998; 3348:316–325.

183. Chaudhuri S, Chatterjee S, Katz N et al. Detection of blood vessels in retinal images using two-dimensional matched filters. IEEE Trans Medical Imag 1989; 8:263–269.

184. Staal J, Abramoff MD, Niemeijer M et al. Ridge-based vessel segmentation in color images of the retina. IEEE Trans Med Imag 2004; 23:501–509.

185. Chutatape O, Zheng L, Krishnan SM. Retinal blood vessel detection and tracking by matched Gaussian and Kalman filters. Proc 20th Int Conf Eng Med Biol Soc 1998; 20:3144–3149.

186. Aleynikov S, Micheli-Tzanakou E. Classification of retinal damage by a neural network based system. J Med Syst 1998; 22:129–136.

187. Reiss TH. The revised fundamental theorem of moment invariants. IEEE Trans Pattern Analysis Mach Intellig 1991; 13:830–834.

188. Tan W, Wang Y, Lee S. Retinal blood vessel detection using frequency analysis and local-mean-interpolation filters. Proc SPIE 2001; 4322: 1373–1384.

189. Wang L, Bhalerao A. Model based segmentation for retinal fundus images. Proc Scand Conf Image Anal 2003; 422–429.

190. Simo A, de Ves E. Segmentation of macular fluorescein angiographies. A statistical approach. Pattern Recognit 2001; 34:795–809.

191. Ballerini L. Genetic snakes for medical image segmentation. Proc SPIE 1998; 3457:284–295.

192. Ballerini L. Medical image segmentation using genetic snakes. Proc SPIE 1999; 3812:13–23.

193. Ballerini L. Detection and quantification of diabetic retinopathy. Proc SPIE 1999; 3808:213–223.

194. Gutierrez J, Epifanio I, de Ves E et al. An active contour model for the automatic detection of the fovea in fluorescein angiographies. Proc Int Conf Pattern Recognition 2000; 4:312–315.

195. Ibanez MV, Simo A. Bayesian detection of the fovea in eye fundus angiographies. Pattern Recognition Letters 1999; 20:229–240.

196. Ishaq N, Taylor K, Steliou K et al. Extraction of the foveal center and lesion boundary from fundus images. Proc SPIE 1990; 1381:153–159.

197. Goldberg RE, Varma R, Spaeth GL et al. Quantification of progressive diabetic macular non-perfusion. Ophthalmic Surgery 1989; 20:42–45.

198. Larsen M, Godt J, Larsen N et al. Automated detection of fundus photographic red lesions in diabetic retinopathy. IOVS 2003; 44:761–766.

199. Truitt PW, Soliz P, Farnath D, Nemeth S. Utility of color information for segmentation of digital retinal images: neural network-based approach. Proc SPIE 1998; 3338:1470–1481.

200. Lee SC, Wang Y. A general algorithm for recognizing small, vague, imagery-alike objects in a nonuniformly illuminated medical diagnostic image. 32nd Asilomar Conference on Signals, Systems and Computers 1998; 2:941–943.

201. Lee SC, Wang Y, Lee E. A computer algorithm for automated detection and quantification of microaneurysms and hemorrhages (hma's) in color retinal images. Proc SPIE 1999; 3663:61–71.

202. Martinez-Perez ME, Hughes AD, Stanton AV et al. Retinal blood vessel segmentation by means of scale-space analysis and region growing. Med Image Comp Comput Assist Intervent 1999; 90–97.

203. Hellstedt T, Vesti E, Immonen I. Identification of individual microaneurysms: a comparison between fluorescein angiograms and red-free and colour photographs. Graefes Arch Clin Exp Ophthalmol 1996; 234 Suppl 1:S13–17.

204. Jalli PY, Hellstedt TJ, Immonen IJ. Early versus late staining of microaneurysms in fluorescein angiography. Retina 1997; 17:211–215.

205. Spencer T, Phillips RP, Sharp PF et al. Automated detection and quantification of microaneurysms in fluorescein angiograms. Graefes Arch Clin Exp Ophthalmol 1992; 230:36–41.

206. Goatman KA, Cree MJ, Olson JA et al. Automated measurement of microaneurysm turnover. IOVS 2003; 44:5335–5341.

207. Bresnick GH, Mukamel DB, Dickinson JC et al. A screening approach to the surveillance of patients with diabetes for the presence of vision-threatening retinopathy. Ophthalmology 2000; 107:19–24.

208. Kinyoun J, Barton F, Fisher M et al. Detection of diabetic macular edema. Ophthalmoscopy versus photography. Early Treatment Diabetic Retinopathy Study Report no. 5. The ETDRS Research Group. Ophthalmology 1989; 96:746–750.

209. Liu Z, Chutatape O, Kirshnan SM. Automatic image analysis of fundus photograph. Proc 19th Int Conf IEEE Eng Med Biol Soc 1997; 2:524–525.

210. Phillips R, Forrester J, Sharp P. Automated detection and quantification of retinal exudates. Graefes Arch Clin Exp Ophthalmol 1993; 231:90–94.

211. Frame AJ, Undrill PE, Olson JA et al. Texture analysis of retinal neovascularization. IEE Colloquium Pattern Recognition 1997; 5/1–5/6.

212. Barthes A, Conrath J, Rasigni M et al. Mathematical morphology in computerized analysis of angiograms in age-related macular degeneration. Med Phys 2001; 28:2410–2419.

213. Thaibaoui A, Raji A, Bunel P. A fuzzy logic approach to drusen detection in retinal angiographic images. IEEE Int Symp Tech Soc 2000; 748–751.

214. Peli E, Lahav M. Drusen measurement from fundus photographs using computer image analysis. Ophthalmology 1986; 93:1575–1580.

215. Brandon L, Hoover A. Drusen detection in a retinal image using multi-level analysis. Med Image Comp Comput Assist Intervent 2003; 2878: 618–625.

216. Jaanio E, Alanko H, Airaksinen PJ et al. Electronic subtraction method for ophthalmic photography. Ophthalmol (Copenh) 1980; 58:7–13.

217. Phillips RP, Ross PG, Sharp PF et al. Use of temporal information to quantify vascular leakage in fluorescein angiography of the retina. Clin Phys Physiol Meas 1990; 11 Suppl A:81–85.

218. Phillips RP, Ross PG, Tyska M et al. Detection and quantification of hyper-fluorescent leakage by computer analysis of fundus fluorescein angiograms. Graefes Arch Clin Exp Ophthalmol 1991; 229:329–335.

219. Martinez-Costa L, Marco P, Ayala G et al. Macular edema computer-aided evaluation in ocular vein occlusions. Comput Biomed Res 1998; 31:374–384.

220. Muldrew KA, McGivern RC, Stevenson MR et al. Parametric analysis of fluorescein angiograms in choroidal neovascularisation secondary to age-related macular degeneration. IOVS 2004; 45:E-Abstract 2958.

221. Berger JW. Quantitative, spatio-temporal image analysis of fluorescein angiography in age-related macular degeneration. Proc SPIE 1998; 3246:48–53.

222. Berger JW, Yoken J. Computer-assisted quantitation of choroidal neo-vascularization for clinical trials. IOVS 2000; 41:2286–2295.

223. van den Elsen PA, Pol EJD, Viergever MA. Medical image matching – a review with classification. IEEE Eng Med Biol 1993; 12:26–39.

224. Brown LG. A survey of image registration techniques. ACM Comput Surv 1992; 24:325–376.

225. Maintz JB, Viergever MA. A survey of medical image registration. Med Image Anal 1998; 2:1–36.

226. Ballerini L. Integration of retinal image sequences. Proc SPIE 1998; 3460:237–248.

227. Mendonca AM, Campilho AJ, Nunes JM. A new similarity criterion for retinal image registration. Int Conf Image Proc 1994; 696–700.

228. Peli E, Augliere RA, Timberlake GT. Feature-based registration of retinal images. IEEE Trans Med Imag 1987; MI-6:272–278.

229. Yu JJH, Hung BN, Liou CL. Fast algorithm for digital retinal image alignment. Proc Int Conf Eng Med Biol Soc 1989; 11:374–375.

230. Heneghan C, Maguire P, Ryan N et al. Retinal image registration using control points. Proc 20th IEEE Int Symp Biomed Imag 2002; 349–352.

231. Lee DJ, Krile TF, Mitra S. Power cepstrum and spectrum techniques applied to image registration. Appl Opt 1988; 27:1099–1106.

232. Lloret D, Serrat J, Lopez AM et al. Retinal image registration using creases as anatomical landmarks. Proc 15th Int Conf Pattern Recog 2000; 3:203–206.

233. Park J, Keller JM, Gader PD et al. Hough-based registration of retinal images. IEEE Int Conf Sys Man Cybernet 1998; 5:4550–4555.

234. Rosin PL, Marshall D, Morgan JE. Multimodal retinal imaging: new strategies for the detection of glaucoma. Int Conf Image Process 2002; 3:137–140.

235. Goldbaum MH, Kouznetsova V, Cote BL et al. Automated registration of digital ocular fundus images for comparison of lesions. Proc SPIE 1993; 1877:94–99.

236. Hart WE, Goldbaum MH. Registering retinal images using automatically selected control point pairs. IEEE Int Conf on Image Process 1994; 3:576–580.

237. Mouravliansky N, Matsopoulos GK, Delibasis K et al. Automatic retinal registration using global optimization techniques. Proc 20th Int Conf IEEE Eng Med Biol Soc 1998; 2:567–570.

238. Ritter N, Owens R, Cooper J et al. Registration of stereo and temporal images of the retina. IEEE Trans Med Imag 1999; 18:404–418.

239. Ryan N, Heneghan C. Image registration techniques for digital ophthalmic images. Proc Irish Signal and Systems Conf 1999; 301–308.

240. Zana F, Klein JC. A multimodal registration algorithm of eye fundus images using vessels detection and Hough transform. IEEE Trans Med Imag 1999; 18:419–428.

241. Hsu CT, Beuker RA. Multiresolution feature-based image registration. Proc SPIE 2000; 4067:1490–1498.

242. Ege BM, Dahl T, Sondergaard T et al. Automatic registration of ocular fundus images. Presented at the Workshop on Computer Assisted Fundus Image Analysis, Copenhagen, Denmark, 2000.

243. Can A, Stewart CV, Roysam B et al. A feature-based, robust, hierarchical algorithm for registering pairs of images of the curved human retina. IEEE Trans Pattern Anal Mach Intellig 2002; 24:347–364.

244. Jasiobedzki P. Registration of retinal images using adaptive adjacency graphs. Proc VI IEEE Symp Comp Based Med Syst 1993:40–45.

245. Stewart CV, Tsai CL, Roysam B. The dual-bootstrap iterative closest point algorithm with application to retinal image registration. IEEE Trans Med Imag 2003; 22:1379–1394.

246. Corona E, Mitra S, Wilson M et al. Digital stereo image analyzer for generating automated 3-D measures of optic disc deformation in glaucoma. IEEE Trans Med Imag 2002; 21:1244–1253.

247. Dandona L, Quigley HA, Jampel HD. Variability of depth measurements of the optic nerve head and peripapillary retina with computerized image analysis. Arch Ophthalmol 1989; 107:1786–1792.

248. Varma R, Spaeth GL. The PAR IS 2000: a new system for retinal digital image analysis. Ophthalmic Surg 1988; 19:183–192.

249. Yogesan K, Barry CJ, Jitskaia L et al. Software for 3-D visualization/ analysis of optic-disc images. IEEE Eng Med Biol Mag 1999; 18:43–49.

250. Nagin P, Schwartz B, Reynolds G. Measurement of fluorescein angiograms of the optic disc and retina using computerized image analysis. Ophthalmology 1985; 92:547–552.

251. Berger JW, Leventon ME, Hata N et al. Design considerations for a computer-vision-enabled ophthalmic augmented reality environment. Lecture Notes Comput Sci 1997; 1205:399–408.

252. Jagoe JR, Blauth CI, Smith PL et al. Automatic geometrical registration of fluorescein retinal angiograms. Comput Biomed Res 1990; 23:403–409.

253. Maintz JB, van den Elsen PA, Viergever MA. Evaluation of ridge seeking operators for multimodality medical image matching. IEEE Trans Pattern Anal Mach Intellig 1996; 18:353–365.

254. Miszalok VA. Fundus imaging and diagnostic screening for public health. In: Masters BR, ed. Noninvasive diagnostic techniques in ophthalmology. Berlin: Springer-Verlag, 1990; 510–515.

255. Butz T, Thiran JP. Affine registration with feature space mutual information. Med Image Comp Computer-Assist Intervent 2001; 2208:549–556.

256. Maes F, Collignon A, Vandermeulen D et al. Multimodality image registration by maximization of mutual information. IEEE Trans Med Imag 1997; 16:187–198.

257. Pluim JP, Maintz JB, Viergever MA. Mutual-information-based registration of medical images: a survey. IEEE Trans Med Imag 2003; 22: 986–1004.

258. Rueckert D, Clarkson MJ, Hill DLG et al. Non-rigid registration using higher-order mutual information. Proc SPIE 2000; 3979:438–447.

259. Fookes C, Maeder A. Local non-rigid image registration using mutual information. Int Conf Vision Interface 2003; 209–214.

260. Fischler MA, Bolles RC. Random sample consensus: a paradigm for model fitting with applications to image analysis and automated cartography. Comm of the ACM 1981; 24:381–395.

261. Lester H, Arridge SR. A survey of hierarchical non-linear medical image registration. Pattern Recognition 1999; 32:129–149.

262. Cideciyan AV, Jacobson SG, Kemp CM et al. Registration of high-resolution images of the retina. Proc SPIE 1992; 1652:310–322.

263. Can A, Stewart CV, Roysam B et al. A feature-based technique for joint, linear estimation of high-order image-to-mosaic transformations: mosaicing the curved human retina. IEEE Trans Pattern Anal Mach Intellig 2002; 24:412–419.

264. Tsai CL, Majerovics A, Stewart CV et al. Disease-oriented evaluation of dual-bootstrap retinal image registration. Med Image Comp Comput Assist Intervent 2003; 2878:754–761.

265. Mandava VR, Fitzpatrick JM, Pickens DR III. Adaptive search space scaling in digital image registration. IEEE Trans Med Imag 1989; 8:251–262.

266. Krakau CET. A simple apparatus for measuring level differences in the eye ground. Acta Ophthal 1949; 27:263–265.

267. Krakau CET. Papillary protrusion measurements by means of stereo-photographs of the fundus. Acta Ophthal 1956; 34:140–145.

268. Boone BG, de Nicola L, Grabow BE. Reconstruction of surface topography using Fourier phase of structured light. Proc SPIE 1994; 2348: 196–210.

269. Bynke HG, Krakau CE. An improved stereophotographic method for clinical measurements of optic disc protrusion. Acta Ophthalmol (Copenh) 1960; 38:115–118.

270. Crock G, Parel JM. Stereophotogrammetry of fluorescein angiographs in ocular biometrics. Med J Aust 1969; 20:586–590.

271. Kottler MS, Rosenthal AR, Falconer DG. Digital photogrammetry of the optic nervehead. Invest Ophthalmol 1974; 13:116–120.

272. Algazi VR, Keltner JL, Johnson CA. Computer analysis of the optic cup in glaucoma. IOVS 1985; 26:1759–1770.

273. Walsh AC, Sadda SR, Humayun M et al. Three dimensional fundus topographic reconstructions from stereoscopic photographs. Poster at AAO Annual Meeting, Anaheim, CA, 2003.

274. Goldbaum MH, Katz NP, Chaudhuri S et al. Image understanding for automated retinal diagnosis. Proc IEEE Comp Soc Symp Comp Aided Med Care 1989; 756–760.

275. Friberg TR, Lace J, Rosenstock J et al. Retinal microaneurysm counts in diabetic retinopathy: Colour photography versus fluorescein angiography. Can J Ophthalmol 1987; 22:226–229.

276. Sheidow TG, Hooper PL, Bariciak MD. Digital subtraction fluorescein angiography: new technique for evaluating choroidal neovascular membranes. Can J Ophthalmol 1998; 33:180–187.

277. Ciulla TA, Harris A, Kagemann L et al. Choroidal perfusion perturbations in non-neovascular age related macular degeneration. Br J Ophthalmol 2002; 86:209–213.

278. Sadda SR, Walsh AC, Humayun MS et al. The integrated intensity quotient (IIQ) as an adjunctive measure to reading center evaluations of choroidal neovascularization. ASRS Poster, New York, 2003.

279. Saito J, Roxburgh ST, Sutton D et al. A new method of image analysis of fluorescein angiography applied to age-related macular degeneration. Eye 1995; 9:70–76.

280. Mordon S, Desmettre T, Devoisselle JM. Quantitative fluorescein angiography following diode laser retinal photocoagulation. Lasers Surg Med 1999; 24:338–345.

281. Bjarnhall G, Maepea O, Sperber GO et al. Analysis of mean retinal transit time from fluorescein angiography in human eyes: normal values and reproducibility. Acta Ophthalmol Scand 2002; 80:652–655.

282. Teschner S, Noack J, Birngruber R et al. Characterization of leakage activity in exudative chorioretinal disease with three-dimensional confocal angiography. Ophthalmology 2003; 110:687–697.

283. Schmidt-Erfurth U, Teschner S, Noack J et al. Three-dimensional topographic angiography in chorioretinal vascular disease. IOVS 2001; 42:2386–2394.

284. Eaton AM, Hatchell DL. Measurement of retinal blood vessel width using computerized image analysis. IOVS 1988; 29:1258–1264.

285. Gao X, Bharath A, Stanton A et al. Measurement of vessel diameters on retinal images for cardiovascular studies. Proc Med Image Understand Anal, 2001.

286. Gang L, Chutatape O, Krishnan SM. Detection and measurement of retinal vessels in fundus images using amplitude modified second-order Gaussian filter. IEEE Trans Biomed Eng 2002; 49:168–172.

287. Miles FP, Nuttall AL. Matched filter estimation of serial blood vessel diameters from video images. IEEE Trans Med Imag 1993; 12:147–152.

288. Rassam SM, Patel V, Brinchmann-Hansen O et al. Accurate vessel width measurement from fundus photographs' new concept. Br J Ophthalmol 1994; 78:24–29.

289. Swanson C, Cocker KD, Parker KH et al. Semiautomated computer analysis of vessel growth in preterm infants without and with ROP. Br J Ophthalmol 2003; 87:1474–1477.

290. Wu D, Schwartz J, Schwoerer J et al. Retinal blood vessel width measured on color fundus photographs by image analysis. Acta Ophthalmol Scand 1995; 73(Suppl 215):33–40.

291. Martinez-Perez ME, Hughes AD, Stanton AV et al. Retinal vascular tree morphology: a semi-automatic quantification. IEEE Trans Biomed Eng 2002; 49:912–917.

292. Kristinsson JK, Gottfredsdottir MS, Stefansson E. Retinal vessel dilatation and elongation precedes diabetic macular oedema. Br J Ophthalmol 1997; 81:274–278.

293. Hart WE, Goldbaum MH, Cote B et al. Measurement and classification of retinal vascular tortuosity. Int J Med Inform 1999; 53:239.

294. Avakian A, Kalina RE, Sage EH et al. Fractal analysis of region-based vascular change in the normal and non-proliferative diabetic retina. Curr Eye Res 2002; 24:274–280.

295. Cheng SC, Huang YM. A novel approach to diagnose diabetes based on the fractal characteristics of retinal images. IEEE Trans Inf Technol Biomed 2003; 7:163–170.

296. Daxer A. Characterisation of the neovascularisation process in diabetic retinopathy by means of fractal geometry: diagnostic implications. Graefes Arch Clin Exp Ophthalmol 1993; 231:681–686.

297. Daxer A. The fractal geometry of proliferative diabetic retinopathy: implications for the diagnosis and the process of retinal vasculogenesis. Curr Eye Res 1993; 12:1103–1109.

298. Misson GP, Landini G, Murray PI. Fractals and ophthalmology. Lancet 1992; 4:339:872.

299. Mainster MA. The fractal properties of retinal vessels: embryological and clinical implications. Eye 1990; 4:235–241.

300. Family F, Masters BR, Platt DE. Fractal pattern formation in human retinal vessels. Physica D 1989; 38:98–103.

301. Landini G, Misson GP, Murray PI. Fractal analysis of the normal human retinal fluorescein angiogram. Curr Eye Res 1993; 12:23–27.

302. Landini G, Murray PI, Misson GP. Local connected fractal dimensions and lacunarity analyses of 60 degrees fluorescein angiograms. IOVS 1995; 36:2749–2755.

303. Hesse L. Fractal dimension in diabetic retinopathy. Graefes Arch Clin Exp Ophthalmol 1994; 232:447–448.

304. Panico J, Sterling P. Retinal neurons and vessels are not fractal but space-filling. J Comp Neurol 1995 23; 361:479–490.

305. Kozousek V, Shen Z, Gregson P et al. Automated detection and quantification of venous beading using Fourier analysis. Can J Ophthalmol 1992; 27:288–294.

306. Shen Z, Gregson PH, Cheng H et al. Automated grading of venous beading: an algorithm and parallel implementation. Proc SPIE 1991; 1606: 632–640.

307. Yang CW, Ma DJ, Chao SC et al. A computer-aided diagnostic detection system of venous beading in retinal images. Opt Eng 2000; 39:1293–1303.

308. Bengtsson B, Krakau CE. Some essential optical features of the Zeiss fundus camera. Acta Ophthalmol (Copenh) 1977; 55:123–131.

Chapter

53

Diagnostic Indocyanine Green Videoangiography

Christina M. Klais
Michael D. Ober
Antonio P. Ciardella
Lawrence A. Yannuzzi
Jason S. Slakter

Since its introduction in the 1960s, intravenous fluorescein angiography has played a crucial role in the diagnosis and treatment of a variety of retinal diseases.[1] It provides excellent spatial and temporal resolution of the retinal circulation with a high degree of fluorescence efficiency and minimal penetration of the retinal pigment epithelium (RPE). In most eyes, the melanin pigment within the RPE is sufficient to provide contrast for imaging intensely fluorescent retinal capillaries. Unfortunately, there are certain limitations to this technique, particularly with respect to imaging the choroidal circulation secondary to poor transmission of fluorescence through ocular media opacifications, fundus pigmentation, and pathologic manifestations such as serosanguineous fluid (Fig. 53-1), and lipid exudation.

The relatively poor fluorescence efficiency of the indocyanine green (ICG) molecule and its limited ability to produce high-resolution images on infrared film initially restricted its angiographic application; however, ICG has subsequently been found to have several advantages over sodium fluorescein, especially in imaging choroidal vasculature (Fig. 53-2). The emergence of high-resolution infrared digital imaging systems, specifically designed for ICG and a growing awareness of choroidal vascular lesions has led to a resurgence of interest in ICG angiography.[2,3] The applications of ICG angiography continue to grow in number; the full extent of its capabilities is not yet known.

HISTORICAL PERSPECTIVE

Initially used in the photographic industry, ICG was introduced into medicine in 1957.[4] Its first application in medicine was in measuring cardiac output.[5] In 1969, the first attempts at using ICG angiography were performed by Kogure and Choromokos studying cerebral circulation in a dog.[6] The following year, Kogure et al. reported on intra-arterial ICG absorption of the choroid in monkeys.[7] The first human ICG angiogram was of the carotid artery by David and colleagues.[8] In 1971, Hochheimer modified the system for ICG angiography by changing the color film which had been used previously to black-and-white infrared film.[9] In 1972, Flower and Hochheimer performed the first intravenous ICG angiography to image the human choroid.[10] In the following years, Flower and coworkers began a series of studies on primates and humans to evaluate the potential utility

of ICG angiography in the investigation of the normal and pathologic eye.[11-14] They refined the procedure with recommendations for the concentration of the dye and method of injection. Flower also modified the transmission and emission filters to improve the resolution of the choroidal vessels. They eventually found that infrared film lacked the sensitivity to adequately capture low-intensity ICG fluorescence which limited the clinical utility of ICG angiography.

The resolution of ICG angiography was improved in the mid-1980s by Hayashi and coworkers, who developed improved filter combinations with sufficient sensitivity for near-infrared wavelength.[15] They were instrumental in the transition from film to videotape by introducing videoangiography.[16-18] Although the sensitivity of the video camera system was a vast improvement, its inability to study individual images and the potential light toxicity using a 300-watt halogen bulb restricted the duration and quality of the technique.

In 1989, Destro and Puliafito performed ICG angiography with a system very similar to that described by Hayashi.[19] In the same year, the use of scanning laser ophthalmoscope for ICG videoangiography was introduced by Scheider and Schroedel.[20] In 1992, Guyer introduced the use of a 1024 × 1024 line digital imaging system to produce high-resolution ICG angiography.[2] Images were digitized, displayed on a high resolution monitor, and stored on an optical disc, but the system lacked flash synchronization with the video camera. Finally, Yannuzzi and coworkers described a 1024-line resolution system which was synthesized with the appropriate flash synchronization and image storage capability, permitting high-resolution, long-duration ICG angiography.[3]

SPECIAL PROPERTIES OF INDOCYANINE GREEN

Chemical properties

ICG is a sterile, water-soluble tricarbocyanine dye with the empirical formula $C_{43}H_{47}N_2NaO_6S_2$ and molecular weight of 775 daltons.[13] Chemically it is an anhydro-3,3,3',3'-tetramethyl-1-1'-di-(4-sulfobutyl)-4,5,4',5-dibenzoindotricyanine hydroxide sodium salt with both lipophilic and hydrophilic characteristics.

ICG is the product of a complex, synthetic process. Sodium iodine is incorporated to create an ICG lyophilisate which can

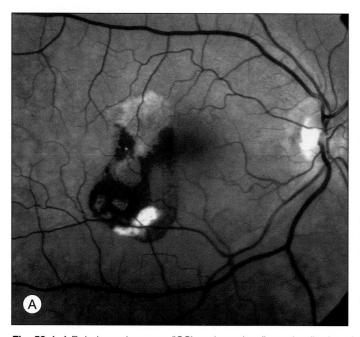

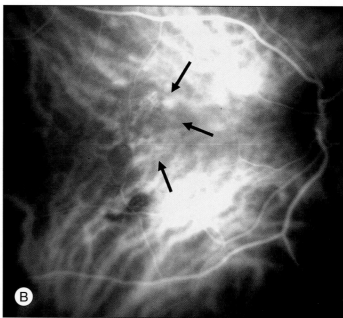

Fig. 53-1 A,B, Indocyanine green (ICG) angiography allows visualization of pathologic conditions through overlying hemorrhages (B) as in this patient with polypoidal choroidal vasculopathy (A). The arrows indicate the polypoidal lesions.

be dissolved in water. Once dissolved, ICG tends to precipitate at high concentration or when mixed in physiologic saline. It is supplied with a solvent consisting of sterile water at pH 5.5–6.5. The final product contains no more than 5% sodium iodine.

Optical properties

ICG absorbs light in the near-infrared range of 790 to 805 nm.[21] The emission spectrum ranges from 770 to 880 nm, peaking at 835 nm. Both absorption and emission spectra are shifted towards shorter wavelength when ICG is in an aqueous solution while the overall intensity of the fluorescence is diminished. Fluorescein angiography does not provide detailed images of the choroidal circulation; the physical characteristics of ICG allow for visualization of the dye through overlying melanin and xanthophyll.[22] It has been demonstrated that the retinal pigment epithelium and choroid absorbs 59% to 75% of blue-green light

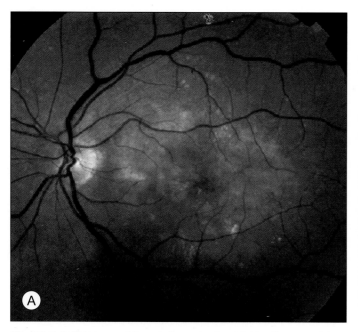

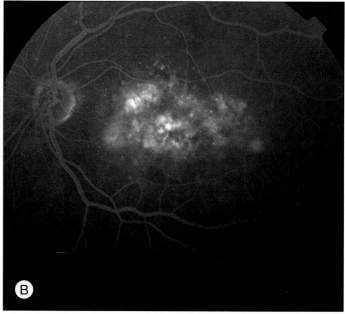

Fig. 53-2 A, This is a red-free photograph of a patient with neovascular age-related macular degeneration. B, C, Early (B) and late (C) phase fluorescein angiograms demonstrate occult choroidal neovascularization without serous PED.

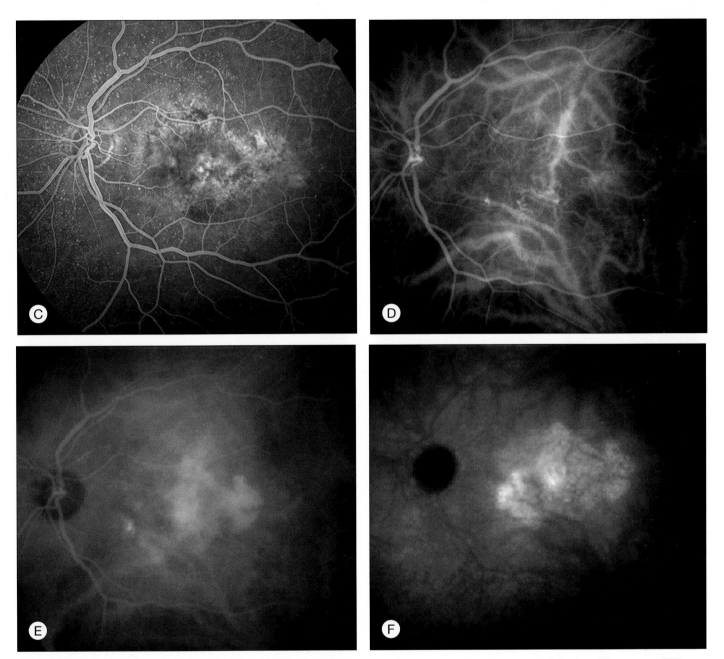

Fig. 53-2—cont'd B, C, Early (B) and late (C) phase fluorescein angiograms demonstrate occult choroidal neovascularization without serous PED. D, E, F, The ICG angiograms show early vascular hyperfluorescence (D) and staining of the abnormal vessels during mid (E) and late (F) phase of the study.

(500 nm) used in fluorescein angiography, but only 21% to 38% of near-infrared light (800 nm) used in ICG angiography. The activity of ICG in the near-infrared light also allows visualization through serosanguineous fluid, shallow hemorrhage, pigment, and lipid exudate. Enhanced imaging of conditions such as choroidal neovascularization and pigment epithelium detachment is the result.

Pharmacokinetics

In vivo, ICG is 98% protein bound because it has both lipophilic and hydrophilic properties. Although it was previously thought to bind primarily to serum albumin,[23] 80% of ICG molecules actually bind to globulins, such as A1-lipoprotein. Therefore, less dye escapes from the fenestrated choroidal vasculature allowing enhanced imaging of choroidal vessels and choroidal lesions.[21] This is in sharp contrast to fluorescein which extravasates rapidly from the choriocapillaris and fluoresces in the extravascular space, thus preventing delineation of choroidal anatomy.

Originally, it was thought that the protein-binding capacity of ICG limited the travel within the choroidal vessel walls. However, it has been demonstrated that ICG dye diffuses through the choroidal stroma during angiography, accumulating within the retinal pigment epithelium cells. It diffuses slowly, staining the choroid within 12 minutes after injection.

The ICG dye is excreted by the liver.[24] It is taken up by hepatic parenchymal cells and secreted into the bile without metabolic alteration or entering enterohepatic circulation.[25] As a result of strong binding to plasma proteins, ICG is not detected in kidney, lungs, and cerebrospinal fluid,[26] nor does it cross the placenta.[27]

Toxicity

Indocyanine green is a relatively safe dye; adverse reactions are rare, and less common than with sodium fluorescein.[28] Mild reactions such as nausea, vomiting, and pruritus occur in 0.15% of patients.[9] There have been isolated reports of vasovagal-type reactions, hypotensive shock, and anaphylactic shock.[29] The dose of ICG administered does not appear to correlate with the presence or severity of adverse reactions. Unlike sodium fluorescein, where extravasation of dye may lead to local tissue reaction and even necrosis of the overlying skin,[30] ICG extravasation is well-tolerated and resolves without complications.

Sterile ICG contains small amounts of iodine and therefore should be used with caution in patients with iodine allergy. It should also be avoided in uremic patients and in those with liver disease where delayed ICG clearance has been described.[31] ICG has not been shown to be harmful to pregnant women or their fetus; however, it is classified as pregnancy category C due to lack of adequate studies. Therefore, there still exists reason for concern.[27] Each angiographic facility should have in place a care plan or an emergency plan.

TECHNIQUE OF INJECTION

Indocyanine green (IC Green; Akorn, Inc., Buffalo Grove, Ill.) should be dissolved in aqueous solvent supplied by the manufacturer and be used within 10 hours after preparation.[32] The standard concentration is 25 mg of ICG dissolved in 5 ml solvent.[33] In patients with poorly dilated pupils or heavily pigmented fundus, the dose of ICG may be increased to 50 mg. For wide-angle angiography, the dosage is increased to 75 mg. Rapid intravenous injection is essential and the injection may be immediately followed by a 5 ml saline flush.

DIGITAL IMAGING SYSTEM

An excitation filter placed over the light source allows only the passage of near-infrared light. This light is absorbed by the ICG molecules in the eye, which in turn emit slightly lower energy light. A barrier filter is used to capture only this light emitted from ICG into the camera by blocking wavelength shorter than 825 nm.

Image acquisition can by produced by standard fundus camera, video camera, or scanning laser ophthalmoscope. The coupling of digital imaging system with an ICG camera enables production of high-resolution (1024-line) images necessary for ICG angiography. Digital imaging systems contain electronic still and video cameras with special antireflective coatings as well as appropriate excitatory and barrier filters. A video camera is mounted in the camera viewfinder and it is connected to a video monitor. The photographer selects the image and activates a trigger which sends the image to the video adapter. The charged coupling device (CCD) camera captures the images and transmits these digitized (1024 × 1024-line resolution) images to a video board within a computer-processing unit. Flash synchronization allows high-resolution image capture and images are displayed on a high-contrast, high-resolution video monitor. Permanent storage is accomplished by downloading to a DVD, CD ROM, or local server.

NEW TECHNIQUES

Recent advances in the technology associated with ICG angiography include real-time, wide-angle,[34] digital subtraction,[35,36] and high-speed angiography.[20,37]

Real-time ICG angiography uses a modified fundus camera with a diode laser illumination system that has an output at 805 nm. This system captures images at 30 frames per second and thus allows for continuous recording. Single frames can be digitized, but the resolution is limited to 640 × 480 pixels.

Wide-angle ICG angiography is achieved with the use of a wide-angle contact lens. Because the lens produces an image lying about 1 cm in front of the lens, the fundus camera is set on "A" or "+" in order to focus on the image plan of the contact lens. This system allows instantaneous imaging of a large fundus area up to 160 degrees of field (Fig. 53-3).[34]

Digital subtraction ICG angiography uses software to eliminate static fluorescence in sequentially acquired images and demonstrates the progression of the dye front within the

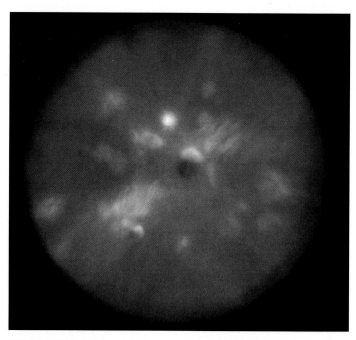

Fig. 53-3 The wide angle indocyanine green (ICG) angiogram of a patient with central serous chorioretinopathy (CSC) illustrates multifocal zones of choroidal hyperpermeability which represent areas of presumed "occult" pigment epithelial detachment (PED) extending far beyond the posterior pole.

choroidal circulation (Fig. 53-4). Pseudocolor imaging of the choroid allows differentiation and identification of choroidal arteries and veins. This technique allows imaging of occult choroidal neovascularization with greater detail and in a shorter period of time than with conventional ICG angiography.[35]

A fundamental problem for any kind of fundus imaging is reflection from interfaces of the ocular media. To obtain high quality fundus images, these reflections must be eliminated. This is achieved by confocal scanning laser ophthalmoscopy (SLO) which separates the illuminating and the imaging beam in the eye, and can be used for high-speed ICG angiography.[38] The SLO can acquire fluorescein angiography images using an argon laser (488 nm), ICG images using an infrared diode laser (795 nm), simultaneous fluorescein angiography and ICG angiography, autofluorescence images, normal fundus reflectance images with green light (514 nm), and images of the nerve fiber layer with infrared light (830 nm). Barrier filters at 500 nm and 810 nm are added to provide a greater efficiency of fluorescent light detection. Single images can be acquired, as well as image sequences with a frame rate up to 30 images per second. Images are digitized in real time with a resolution of 256 × 256 or 512 × 512 pixels. The scanning laser system is able to record the filling phase with great temporal resolution but with a slight loss of spatial resolution.

Recently, three-dimensional confocal angiography has been reported.[39] This system allows for the potential to achieve reliable quantitative and qualitative analysis of defects, exudation, and proliferative vascular lesion.

INDOCYANINE GREEN VIDEOANGIOGRAPHY OF CHORIORETINAL DISORDERS

Age-related macular degeneration

Patz and associates[40] were the first to study choroidal neovascularization (CNV) in age-related macular degeneration (AMD) through ICG angiography (Fig. 53-5). They could resolve only two of 25 CNVs with their early model. Bischoff and Flower[28] studied 100 ICG angiograms of patients with AMD. They found "delayed and/or irregular choroidal filling" in some patients. The significance of this finding is unclear, however, because these authors did not include an age-matched control group. Tortuous choroidal vessels and marked dilation of macular choroidal arteries, often with loop formation, were also observed.

Hayashi and associates found that ICG videoangiography was useful in the detection of CNV.[15,17,18] ICG angiography was able to confirm the FA appearance of CNV in patients with well-defined CNV. It revealed a well-defined neovascularization in 27 eyes with occult CNV by FA. In a subgroup of patients with poorly defined occult CNV, the ICG angiogram, but not the FA, imaged a well-defined CNV in nine of 12 (75%) cases. ICG videoangiography of the other three eyes revealed suspicious areas of neovascularization. These investigators were also the first to show that leakage of ICG from CNV was slow compared to the rapid leakage seen with sodium fluorescein. While the results of these investigators concerning ICG angiographic imaging of occult CNV were promising, the 512-line video monitor and analog tape of their ICG system limited the spatial resolution they could obtain.

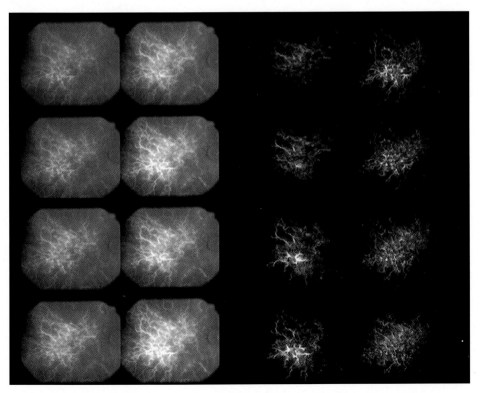

Fig. 53-4 Sequential subtraction of ICG angiogram images from the eye of a normal young male, acquired at 30 IPS using fundus camera optics. The left-hand two columns of images (read from top to bottom) are the original angiogram. The right-hand two columns are the resultant subtracted images; the first image resulted from subtracting the first angiographic image from the second, the second image resulted from subtracting the second angiographic image from the third, etc. (courtesy of Robert Flower.)

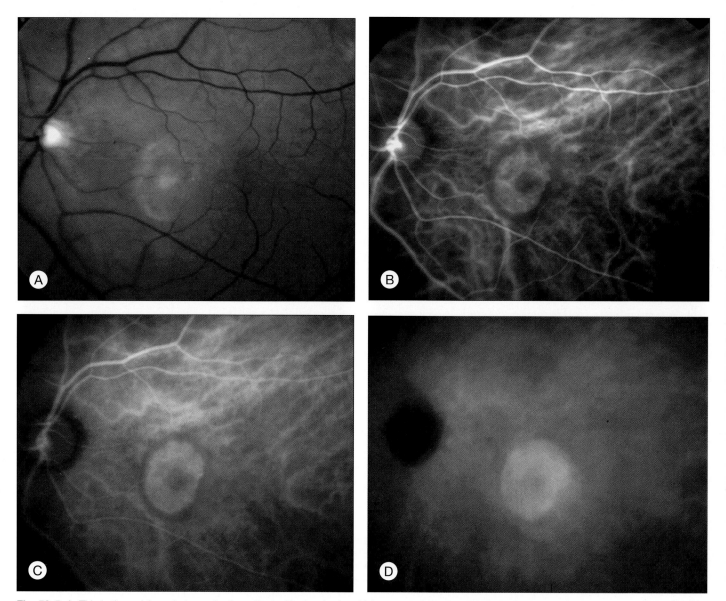

Fig. 53-5 A, This is the red-free photograph of a patient with classic choroidal neovascularization (CNV). B, The early-phase ICG angiogram reveals hyperfluorescence of the CNV. Mid-phase (C) and late-phase ICG angiograms (D) show staining of the hyperfluorescent CNV.

Destro and Puliafito reported that ICG videoangiography was particularly useful in studying occult CNV with overlying hemorrhage and recurrent CNV.[19] Guyer and co-workers used a 1024-line digital imaging system to study patients with occult CNV.[2] These authors reported that ICG angiography is useful in imaging occult CNV and that this technique might allow photocoagulation of otherwise untreatable lesions. Scheider and co-investigators reported enhanced imaging of CNV in a study of 80 patients using the scanning laser ophthalmoscope with ICG angiography.[41]

Yannuzzi and associates[3] have shown that ICG angiography is extremely useful in converting occult CNV into a well-defined pattern of CNV (Fig. 53-6). In their study, 39% of 129 patients with occult CNV were converted to a well-defined CNV based on the information added by ICG angiography. These authors

reported that ICG angiography was especially useful in identifying occult CNV in patients with serous pigment epithelium detachment (PED) or with recurrent CNV (Fig. 53-7).

Yannuzzi et al. studied the ICG angiograms of 235 consecutive AMD patients with occult CNV and associated vascularized PED (V-PED) (Fig. 53-8). These eyes were divided into two groups, depending on the size and delineation of the CNV.[42] Of the 235 eyes, 89 (38%) had a solitary area of neovascularization that was well delineated, no more than one disc diameter in size, and defined as a "hot spot" of focal CNV. The other 146 (62%) eyes had a larger area of neovascularization with variable delineation defined as a plaque CNV.

Guyer and co-authors reported their results on the ICG angiography study of 1000 consecutive eyes with occult CNV diagnosed by FA.[43] They recognized focal spots in 29%

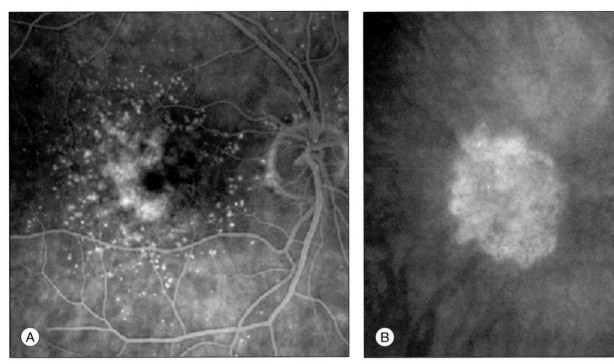

Fig. 53-6 A, Fluorescein angiography reveals occult choroidal neovascularization. B, Late phase ICG angiogram shows a well-defined plaque.

(Fig. 53-9), plaques in 61% consisting 27% of well-defined plaques and 34% of poorly defined plaques (Fig. 53-10) and combination lesions in 8%, consisting of 3% of marginal spots, 4% of overlying spots and 1% of remote spots. A follow-up study of patients with newly diagnosed unilateral occult CNV secondary to AMD showed that the patients tended to develop the same morphologic type of CNV in the fellow eye.[44]

Finally, Lee et al. reported on 15 eyes with surgically excised subfoveal CNV, which underwent preoperative and postoperative ICG angiography. All excised membranes were examined by light microscopy, and all surgically excised ICG-imaged membranes corresponded to sub-RPE and sub-neurosensory retinal CNV.[45]

The above studies demonstrate that ICG angiography is an important adjunctive study to FA in the detection of CNV.

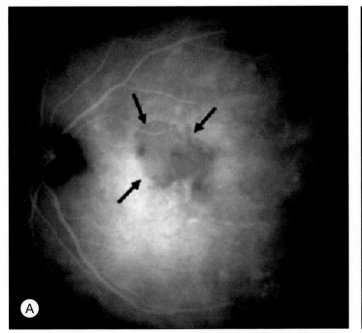
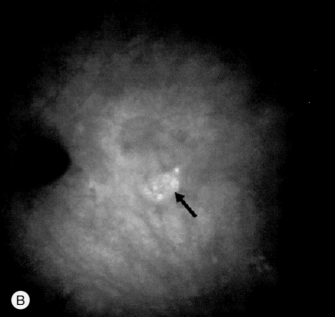

Fig. 53-7 A, Early phase ICG angiogram reveals hypofluorescence (arrows) of serous pigment epithelium detachment (PED) in a patient with age-related macular degeneration. B, Late ICG angiogram shows staining of the abnormal vessels (arrow) and hypofluorescent serous PED.

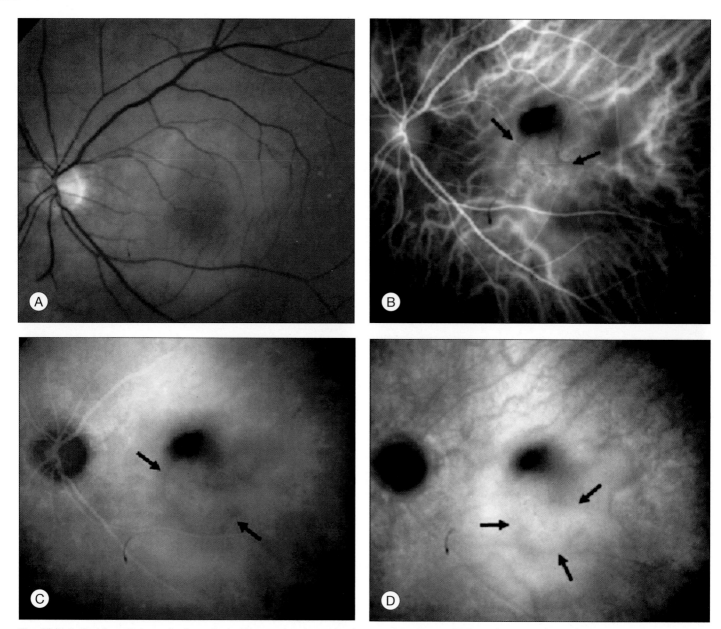

Fig. 53-8 A, Red-free photograph of a patient with age-related macular degeneration shows a PED. B, C, D, All phases of ICG study reveal a well-defined vascularized PED (arrows). A small choroidal nevus superior to the fovea blocks the fluorescence throughout the study.

While FA may image well-defined CNV better than ICG angiography in some cases, ICG videoangiography can enable treatment of about 30% of occult CNV lesions by the detection of well-defined CNV eligible for ICG-guided laser treatment.[46] Thus, the best imaging strategy to detect the CNV is to perform both FA and ICG angiography.

Polypoidal choroidal vasculopathy

Polypoidal choroidal vasculopathy (PCV) is a primary abnormality of the choroidal circulation characterized by an inner choroidal vascular network of vessels ending in an aneurysmal bulge or outward projection, visible clinically as a reddish-orange, spheroid, polyp-like structure (Fig. 53-11).[47] The dis-

order is associated with multiple, recurrent, serosanguineous detachments of the RPE and neurosensory retina secondary to leakage and bleeding from the peculiar choroidal vascular abnormality (Fig. 53-12).[38,48,49] ICG angiography has been used to detect and characterize the PCV abnormality with enhanced sensitivity and specificity.[50–52] The early phase of ICG angiogram shows a distinct network of vessels within the choroid. In patients with juxtapapillary involvement, the vascular channels extend in a radial, arching pattern and are interconnected with the smaller spanning branches that become more evident and more numerous at the edge of the PCV lesion. Larger choroidal vessels of the PCV network begin to fill before retinal vessels. The area within and surrounding the network is relatively hypo-

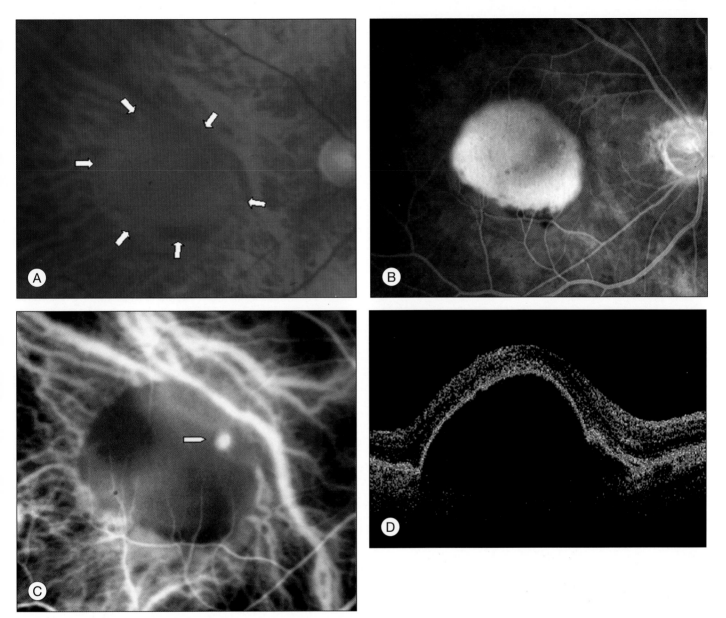

Fig. 53-9 A, Clinical photograph showing a large pigment epithelial detachment (PED) (white arrows) in a patient with focal occult CNV. B, Late-phase fluorescein angiogram illustrating late staining of the PED. C, Early-phase ICG angiogram showing a focal area of abnormal hyperfluorescence (hot spot). D, The OCT confirms a large PED.

fluorescent as compared to the uninvolved choroid (Fig. 53-13). The vessels of the network appear to fill at a slower rate than retinal vessels. Shortly after the network can be identified on the ICG angiogram, small hyperfluorescent "polyps" become visible within the choroids. These polypoidal structures correspond to the reddish, orange choroidal excrescence seen clinically. They appear to leak slowly as the surrounding hypofluorescent area becomes increasingly hyperfluorescent. In the later phase of the angiogram there is uniform disappearance of dye ("washout") from the bulging polypoidal lesions. The late characteristic ICG staining of occult CNV is not seen in the PCV. Polypoidal lesions may be localized in the macular area without any peri-papillary component and it may be formed by a network of small branching vessels ending in polypoidal dilation difficult to image without ICG angiography.

ICG angiography has led to early discovery of polyps in the peripapillary, the macular and the extramacular areas (Fig. 53-14).[52] With the identification of these choroidal polyps, new therapeutic possibilities are being explored, including the use of thermal laser treatment as well as photodynamic therapy.[53]

Retinal angiomatous proliferation

Retinal angiomatous proliferation (RAP) is a distinct subgroup of neovascular AMD.[54] Angiomatous proliferation within the

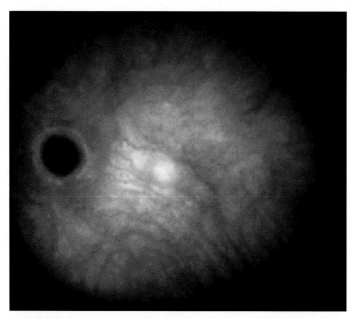

Fig. 53-10 Late phase ICG angiogram reveals an ill-defined plaque with indistinct margins.

retina is the first manifestation of the neovascularized process. Dilated retinal vessels, pre-, intra-, and subretinal hemorrhages, and exudates evolve surrounding the angiomatous proliferation as the process extends into the deep retina and subretinal space. One or more dilated compensatory retinal vessels perfuse and drain the neovascularization, sometimes forming a retinal–retinal anastomosis. FA in these patients usually reveals indistinct staining simulating occult-CNV. ICG angiography is useful to make an accurate diagnosis in most cases. It reveals a focal area of intense hyperfluorescence corresponding to the neovascularization (hot spot) and some late extension of the leakage within the retina from the intraretinal neovascularization (Fig. 53-15). As the intraretinal neovascularization progresses towards the subretinal space and the RPE, the CNV becomes part of the neovascular complex. At this stage there is often clinical and angiographic evidence of a V-PED. ICG angiography is better for imaging the presence of a V-PED because the serous component of the PED remains dark during the study and the vascular component appears as a hot-spot (Fig. 53-16). At this stage, ICG angiography may sometimes be able to image a direct communication between the retinal and the choroidal

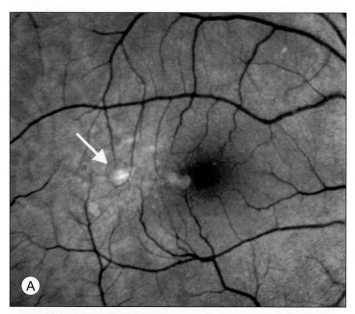

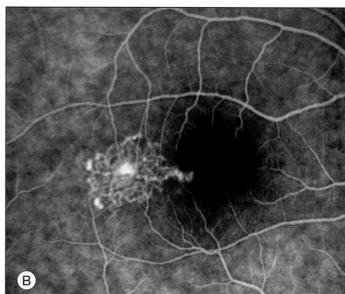

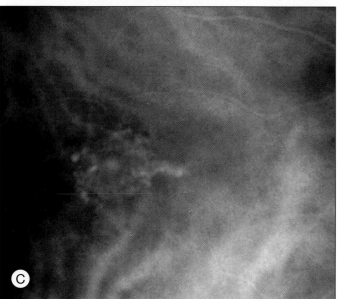

Fig. 53-11 This is a 56-year-old Caucasian male who had three transient episodes of visual disturbance and was diagnosed with CSC. A, Red-free photograph reveals a flat macula overlying multiple, nummular elevations suggestive of small serous PEDs. There is a patch of fibrous metaplasia (arrow) at the center of the lesion. B, Fluorescein angiogram reveals a net of subretinal inner choroidal vessels terminating in aneurysmal or polypoidal lesions. C, Late-phase ICG angiogram confirms the presence of polypoidal vascular abnormality.

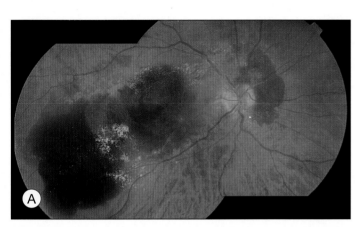

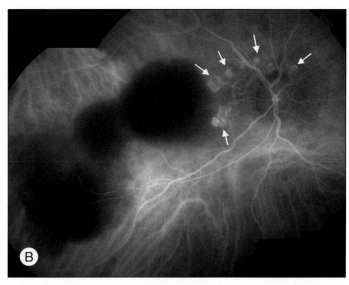

Fig. 53-12 This is a 66-year-old Caucasian male with sudden deterioration of vision in his right eye. A, Color composite photograph shows large subretinal and intraretinal hemorrhages at the posterior pole and surrounding the optic nerve. There are areas with dense lipid exudation. B, Mid-phase ICG angiogram illustrates a large hyperfluorescent area. In the peripapillary area, there is a net of subretinal inner choroidal vessels that terminate in polypoidal lesions (white arrows).

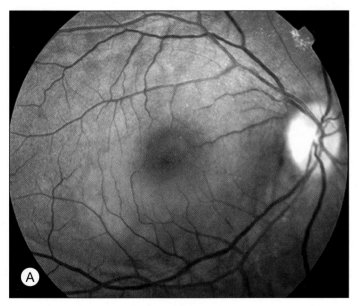

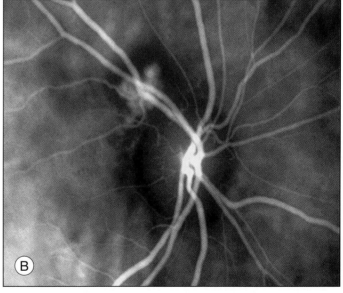

Fig. 53-13 A, Red-free photograph of a 62-year-old female illustrating a neurosensory retinal detachment in the central macula. B, ICG angiogram reveals the presence of a polypoidal choroidal vascular abnormality in the superior temporal juxtapapillary region.

component of the neovascularization to form a retinal-choroidal anastomosis (RCA) (Fig. 53-17).[55]

ICG-GUIDED LASER TREATMENT OF CNV IN ARMD

Patients potentially eligible for thermal laser photocoagulation therapy guided by ICG angiography are those with clinical and fluorescein angiographic evidence of occult CNV (Fig. 53-18). Of the two types of occult CNV that can be identified by ICG study, hot spots and plaques, we recommend direct laser photo-

coagulation of only the hot spots. In fact, the hot spots represent areas of actively leaking neovascularization that can be obliterated by laser photocoagulation in an attempt to eliminate the associated serosanguineous complications, and to stabilize or improve the vision. On the other hand, the plaques seem to represent a thin layer of neovascularization that is not actively leaking, and that may not require laser photocoagulation. This approach has practical considerations. In the case of a lesion combining a hot spot and a plaque and in which the hot spot is at the margin of the plaque (it may extend under the fovea), laser photocoagulation can be applied to the extrafoveal hot

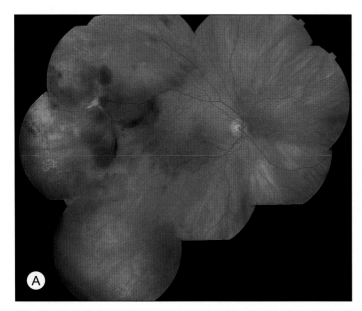
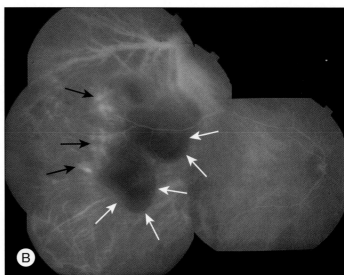

Fig. 53-14 A, Color photograph composite of the fundus of a patient with PCV demonstrates hemorrhagic pigment epithelial detachment (PED) in the temporal periphery and subretinal hemorrhages. Note the subretinal fluid exudation involving the macula. B, ICG angiography composite of the right fundus reveals a cluster of actively leaking polypoidal vessels in the retinal periphery (black arrows). Note the two hemorrhagic PEDs blocking the background fluorescence (white arrows).

spot to spare the foveal area. This treatment approach was successful in obliterating the CNV and stabilizing the vision in 56% of consecutive AMD patients.[45] On the contrary, we have had poor success with the direct laser treatment of hot spots overlying plaques and confluent treatment of the entire plaque.

Two subtypes of hot spots are RCA and polypoidal-type CNV. When RCA is present, the success of laser photocoagulation is negatively influenced by the presence of an associated serous PED. In a small series of patients with RCA and an associated PED laser photocoagulation was successful in closing CNV in only 14% of cases.[56]

Slakter and co-authors performed ICG-guided laser photocoagulation in 79 eyes with occult CNV.[57] Occult CNV was successfully eliminated in a majority of the cases. Visual acuity was stabilized or improved in 29 (66%) of 44 eyes with occult CNV associated with neurosensory retinal elevations, and in 15 (43%) of 35 eyes with occult CNV associated with PED. This study demonstrated that in some cases ICG angiography imaging can successfully guide laser photocoagulation of occult CNV.

A recent study prospectively evaluated 185 consecutive eyes with exudative AMD and a well-delineated area (hot spot or focal area) of hyperfluorescence demonstrated by ICG angiography. All patients were divided into two groups (with PED and without PED). Of the 185 eyes, 99 eyes without PED achieved a 71% rate of obliteration at 6 months and a 48% rate of obliteration at 12 months. Eyes with PED did significantly worse, with an obliteration rate of the CNV of 23% at 12 months. The overall success rate was 36% at 12 months.[58]

The high recurrence rate after laser photocoagulation of occult CNV, particularly when a V-PED is present, may be explained by the peculiar anatomy of the CNV in such cases.

Freund et al. reported that approximately only 13% of patients with CNV secondary to AMD have a classic or well defined extrafoveal choroidal neovascularization by fluorescein angiography that is eligible for laser treatment.[59] With a recurrence rate of approximately 50% following fluorescein angiographic guided laser photocoagulation for classic CNV, only approximately 6.5% of patients will benefit from treatment. The remaining 87% of patients have occult CNV by fluorescein imaging. About 30% of these eyes have a potentially treatable focal spot by ICG angiography. Therefore about one-fourth of all eyes with exudative maculopathy may be treated by the ICG-guided laser photocoagulation. With a success rate of 35%, this means that an additional 9% of patients can be successfully treated using the ICG-guided laser photocoagulation. However, there are still 84.5% of patients who continue to be untreatable or are unsuccessfully treated by thermal laser photocoagulation of CNV.[60]

Costa et al. demonstrated that ICG guided photodynamic therapy with verteporfin was beneficial in eyes with occult subfoveal CNV.[61]

Staurenghi et al. considered a series of 15 patients with subfoveal CNV in whom feeder vessels (FVs) could be clearly detected by means of dynamic ICG angiography but not necessarily by fluorescein angiography (Fig. 53-19).[62] Based on the indications of their pilot study, the authors studied a second series of 16 patients with FVs smaller than 85 microns. Treatment of FV using argon green laser was administered and ICG angiography was performed immediately after treatment, at 2, 7, and 30 days, and then every 3 months to assess FV closure. If a FV appeared patent, it was immediately retreated and the follow-up schedule was started again. The follow-up time ranged from 23 to 34 months for the pilot study, and from 4 to

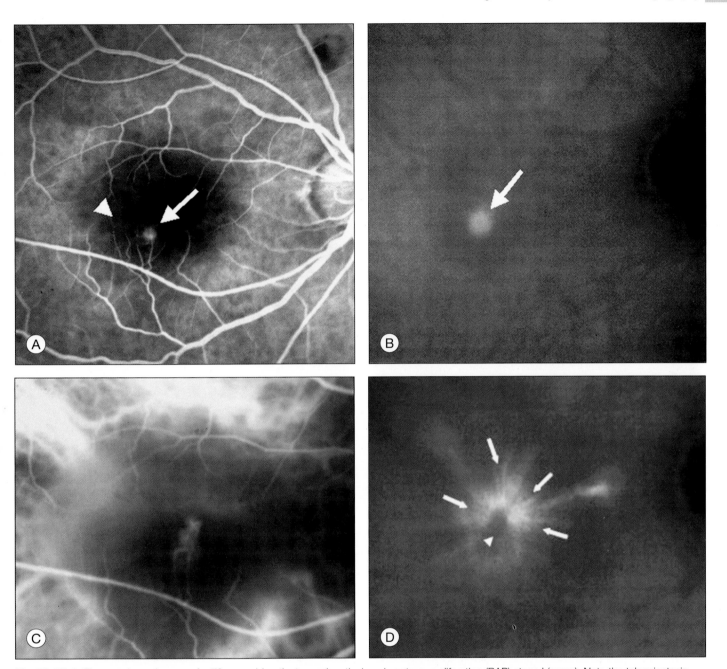

Fig. 53-15 A, Fluorescein angiogram of a 73-year-old patient reveals retinal angiomatous proliferation (RAP) stage I (arrow). Note the telangiectasia surrounding this area (arrowhead). B, ICG angiogram showing a focal area of intense hyperfluorescence (arrow) or so-called "hot spot." C, The ICG angiogram one year later illustrates a retinal–retinal anastomosis and subretinal neovascularization. D, The late-phase ICG angiogram shows intraretinal leakage (arrows) surrounding the fading angiomatous proliferation (arrowhead).

12 months for the second series. In the pilot study, CNV was obliterated after the first treatment in only one patient; five patients needed more than one treatment and obliteration failed in nine patients (40% success rate). The width and the number of the FVs affected the rate of success. The success rate in the second series of 16 patients was higher (75%). The authors concluded that dynamic ICG angiography may detect smaller FVs. It allows controlling the laser effect and initiating immediate retreatment in the case of incomplete FV closure and should be considered mandatory for this type of treatment.

Clinical trials to evaluate the role of ICG guided feeder vessel therapy are ongoing.

CENTRAL SEROUS CHORIORETINOPATHY

The application of ICG angiography to the study of central serous chorioretinopathy (CSC) has expanded our knowledge of the disease.[3,63,64] The common findings in patients with CSC are multifocal areas of hyperfluorescence in the early and mid phases of the study which tend to fade in the late phases (Fig.

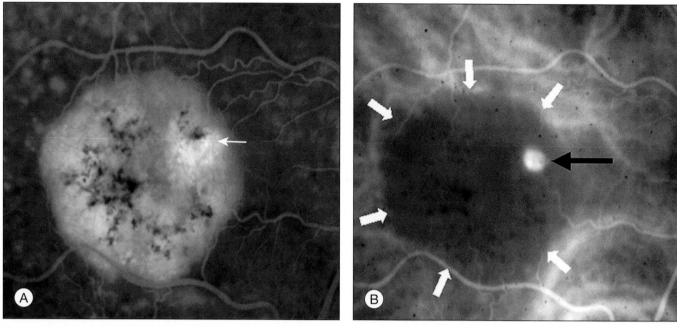

Fig. 53-16 A, The fluorescein angiogram of a patient with stage II (RAP) reveals late staining of a PED. There is an increase in the intensity of fluorescence in the area of the RAP lesion (arrow). B, The ICG angiogram shows hypofluorescence in the area of the PED (white arrows) and a "hot spot" corresponding to the RAP (black arrow).

53-20). Typically, these areas of hyperfluorescence are found not only in corresponding areas of leakage as seen on fluorescein angiography, but also with areas of the fundus that appear clinically and angiographically normal, as well as in the normal fellow eyes. The areas of early hyperfluorescence are believed to represent diffuse choroidal hyperpermeability.

INTRAOCULAR TUMORS

ICG angiography is an important tool in the diagnosis and evaluation of intraocular tumors.[65] Guyer et al. have used ICG angiography to study 40 patients with intraocular tumors and found that certain tumors have characteristic ICG videoangiographic patterns.[66] Pigmented choroidal melanomas block ICG

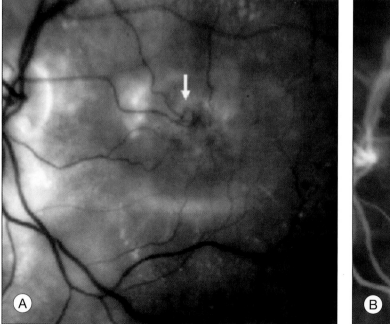

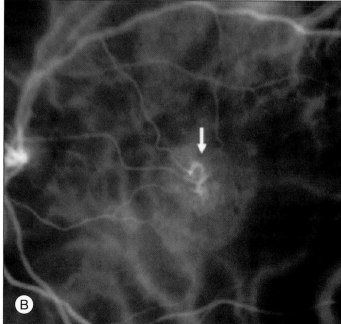

Fig. 53-17 A, Red-free photograph of a patient with retinal angiomatous proliferation demonstrates a retinal choroidal anastomosis (arrow). B, Early ICG angiogram confirms the retinal choroidal anastomosis (arrow).

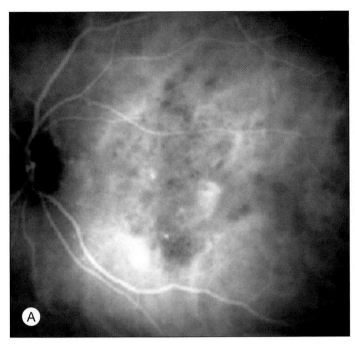

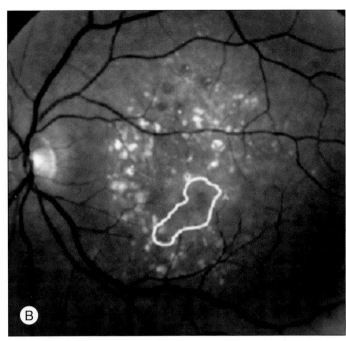

Fig. 53-18 A, This mid-frame indocyanine green (ICG) angiogram showing hyperfluorescence in the macula corresponding to the area of activity within choroidal neovascularization (CNV). B, Corresponding ICG tracing of active CNV applied to a red free photograph which can be displayed during laser treatment for easy reference.

fluorescence because the near-infrared light is absorbed by melanin. The choroidal and tumor vasculature cannot be visualized through dense tumor pigmentation. ICG angiography can distinguish pigmented choroidal melanomas from nonpigmented tumors, such as hemangiomas and osteomas. In our experience, ICG videoangiography cannot distinguish melanomas from other pigmented lesions such as nevi or metastatic cutaneous melanoma. When a pigmented choroidal melanoma thickens or otherwise develops prominent intrinsic vasculature, ICG angiography shows an increase in fluorescence in the late phase.[67]

Marked progressive hyperfluorescence is observed during ICG angiography of choroidal hemangiomas due to the vascu-

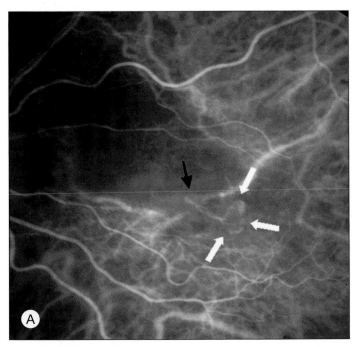

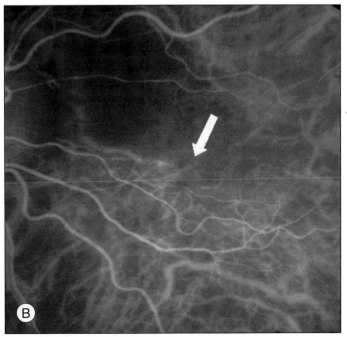

Fig. 53-19 A, High speed angiography of a patient with choroidal neovascularization (white arrows) demonstrates clearly the perfusing and draining feeder vessels (black arrow). b, After focal thermal laser treatment of the feeder vessels ICG angiogram reveals closure of these vessels (arrow).

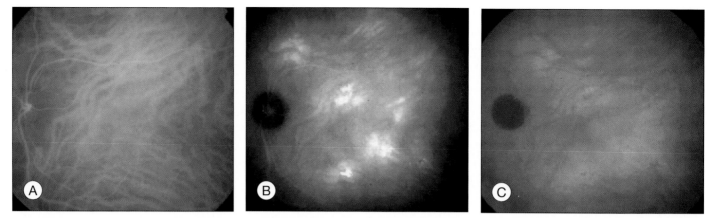

Fig. 53-20 This is a 43-year-old Caucasian female with chronic central serous chorioretinopathy (CSC) in the left eye. A, B, C, Indocyanine green (ICG) angiography is essentially normal in the early phase (A), but reveals multiple patchy areas of hyperfluorescence in the mid phase (B) that fade in the last phase of the study (C).

larity of the lesion.[67,68] A speckled pattern with stellate borders is observed. In early stages of the ICG study, a network of small-caliber vessels is seen. These vessels completely obscure the choroidal pattern. The technique is also useful in evaluating vascular lesions with overlying hemorrhage. ICG, unlike FA, may allow visualization of the tumor through an overlying hemorrhage. Piccolino has developed an interesting technique for studying the vasculature of circumscribed choroidal hemangiomas.[69] ICG angiography of choroidal hemangiomas was performed with artificially increased intraocular pressure to slow down the choroidal circulation and to allow better delineation of the feeding and draining vessels and of the inner circulation of the tumor.

Choroidal metastatic lesions show different pattern on ICG videoangiography depending on vascularity, pigmentation, and primary location of the lesion.[66] In the early study phase, choroidal metastasis shows diffuse, homogenous hypofluorescence. The normal perfusing choroidal pattern can often be visualized underneath. Breast metastasis shows moderate block-age on ICG videoangiography, while metastatic thyroid carcinoma and metastatic bronchial carcinoid tumors show hyperfluorescence. Metastatic skin melanoma shows marked blockage on ICG videoangiography and thus appears indistinguishable from primary choroidal melanoma.[66]

The early ICG phase in choroidal osteomas reveals characteristic small vessels that often leak too quickly to be detected by FA.[70] Variable hypofluorescence is observed in the bony areas. These lesions may show mid to late ICG hyperfluorescence.

Varices of the vortex veins occasionally can be confused with choroidal tumors. Although the diagnosis usually can be made clinically, ICG angiography in these cases shows marked dilation of the vortex veins.[71]

CHORIORETINAL INFLAMMATORY DISEASES

Serpiginous choroidopathy is a rare, progressive condition that appears to affect primarily the inner choroidal and RPE layers

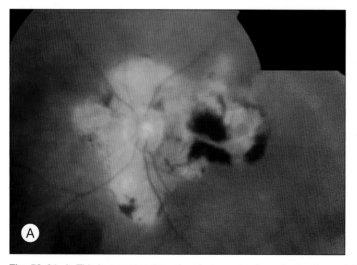

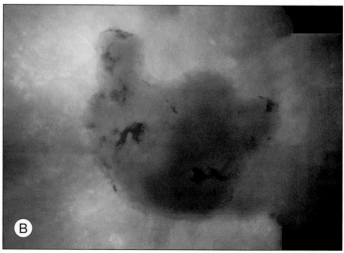

Fig. 53-21 A, This is a composite color photograph of a patient with serpiginous choroidopathy. B, The composite of the indocyanine green (ICG) angiogram reveals a large area of hypofluorescence typical for the acute phase of the disease. The dark pigmented areas represent healed regions.

with secondary retinal involvement, beginning at the optic nerve and advancing centrifugally. The ICG videoangiography typically shows two patterns according also to the stage of the disease.[72] In the acute phase, ICG angiography is characterized by generalized hypofluorescence through all phases of the study. In the subacute stage of the disease, mid- and large-sized choroidal vessels are visualized within the lesions. Persistent delay or nonperfusion of the choriocapillaris and smaller choroidal vessels is noted, giving the area a generalized hypofluorescent appearance but with less distinct margins and a more heterogeneous appearance (Fig. 53-21). This pattern is more typically seen after resolution of acute inflammatory changes and associated edema. In the late phase of the study, lesions present with sharp, well-demarcated borders. This is due to a combination of choroidal perfusion abnormalities as demonstrated on SLO and blockage by inflammatory exudative material, or edema of the RPE and outer retina. In the healed stages, deeper choroidal vessels become better visualized due to the associated development of RPE and choriocapillaris atrophy.

Acute multifocal placoid pigment epitheliopathy (AMPPE) is a syndrome of young adults characterized by the development of multifocal, yellow-white, flat, placoid lesions of the RPE in the posterior pole and midperipheral fundus.[73] The lesions are hypofluorescent by ICG angiography in both early and late phase of the study (Fig. 53-22). The ICG choroidal hypofluorescence in AMPPPE may be due to a partial choroidal vascular occlusion

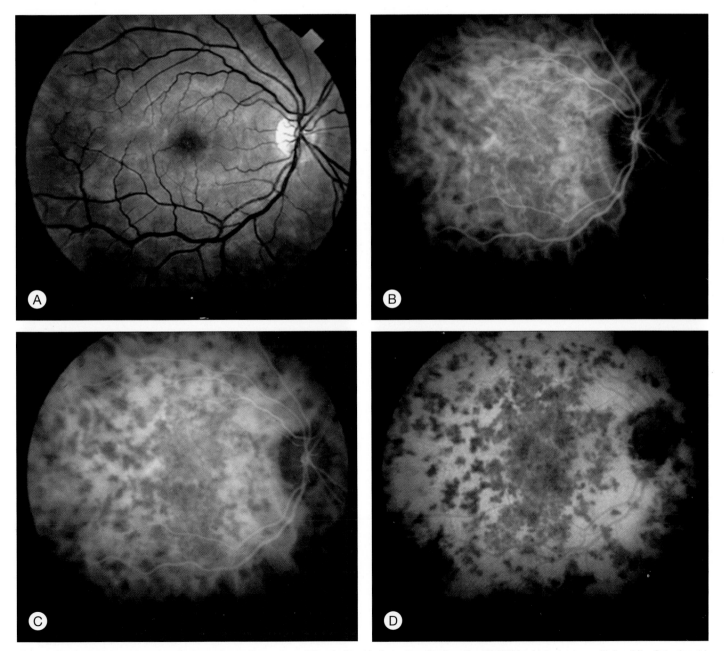

Fig. 53-22 A, Red-free photograph of a patient with acute multifocal placoid pigment epitheliopathy (AMPPE) which shows multiple white, flat, placoid lesions. B, C, D, The lesions are hypofluorescent by ICG angiography in early (B), mid (C), and late (D) phase of the study.

secondary to occlusive vasculitis.[74] ICG study of healed lesions also demonstrates early hypofluorescence and more clearly delineates late choroidal hypofluorescence.

Multiple evanescent white dot syndrome (MEWDS) typically presents with unilateral acute loss of vision in healthy young women. It is a clinical condition of unknown cause, but it is thought to affect primarily the RPE-photoreceptor complex.[75] With ICG, a pattern of hypofluorescent spots throughout the posterior pole and peripheral retina is seen (Fig. 53-23). These hypofluorescent spots appear approximately 10 minutes after dye injection in the mid-ICG phase and persist throughout the remainder of the study. These spots appear larger than the white dots seen clinically, varying in diameter from less than 50 microns to about 500 microns. Many more lesions can easily be identified with ICG angiography than with fundus examination or fluorescence angiography. A ring of hypofluorescence surrounding the optic disc is seen in some cases. In these patients a blind spot enlargement on visual field examination is always

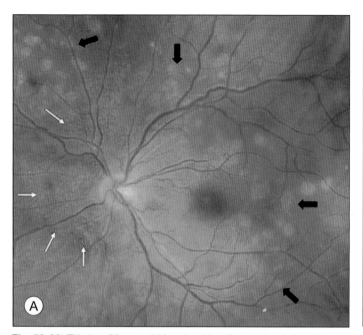
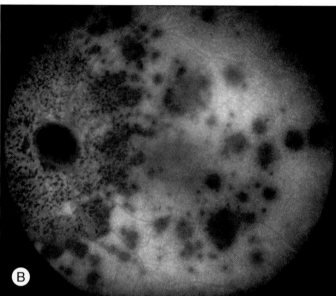

Fig. 53-23 This is a 29-year-old female with unilateral visual disturbance caused by multiple evanescent white dot syndrome (MEWDS). A, The clinical photograph shows multiple round, white to yellow-white spots (black arrows) distributed over the posterior fundus. In the peripapillary region, there are multiple small yellow dots (white arrows). B, The mid-phase ICG reveals multiple large and small hypofluorescent spots in the posterior pole. Note the ring of hypofluorescence surrounding the optic disc.

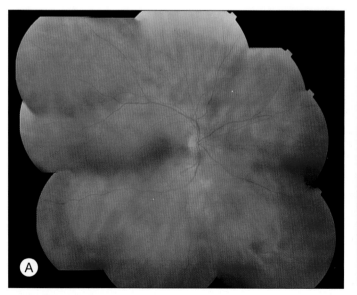
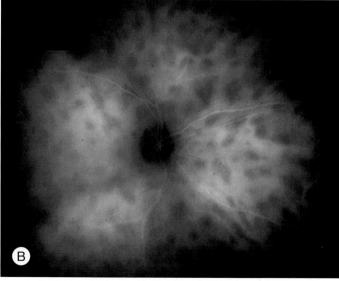

Fig. 53-24 This is a 46-year-old Caucasian female with newly diagnosed birdshot retinochoroidopathy. A, Clinical photograph composite reveals multiple creamy round lesions. B, Mid-phase ICG illustrates multiple hypofluorescent lesions resembling "holes" in the fluorescence of the choriocapillaris.

present. During the convalescent phase, the return of visual function and normalization of the clinical examination does not correlate completely with resolution of the hypofluorescent spots seen on ICG angiography. These findings suggest that MEWDS may result in persistent abnormalities in choroidal circulation even after clinical symptoms disappear.

Birdshot retinochoroidopathy is an uncommon, but potentially serious inflammatory disorder that involves both the choroid and retina. No relation to any systemic disease has been observed, while a strong association with the HLA-A29 class I antigen suggests a genetic predisposition. ICG angiography reveals multiple hypofluorescent lesions resembling "holes" in the fluorescence of the choriocapillaris (Fig. 53-24).[76] These lesions correspond to the clinical creamy lesions. The distribution of the patches follows the larger choroidal vessels. Howe et al. found that ICG angiography detects birdshot lesions more

rapidly than fluorescein angiography and may be of benefit in assessing disease activity.[77]

Multifocal choroiditis (MFC) is an idiopathic choroidal inflammatory disorder with varied presentation and clinical course. Clinical features include "punched out" chorioretinal spots, peripapillary atrophy, peripheral chorioretinal curvilinear lesions, and neovascularized macular degeneration or disciform scar. MFC lesions block fluorescence on ICG videoangiography (Fig. 53-25). Hyperfluorescent foci that do not correlate with lesions seen clinically or by FA can also be observed. These hyperfluorescent areas may represent subclinical foci of choroiditis. Slakter et al. reported on ICG angiography findings in a series of 14 patients with MFC.[78] Fourteen (50%) of the 28 eyes were found to have large hypofluorescent spots in the posterior pole that did not clinically correspond to clinically or fluorescein angiographically detectable lesions. In seven

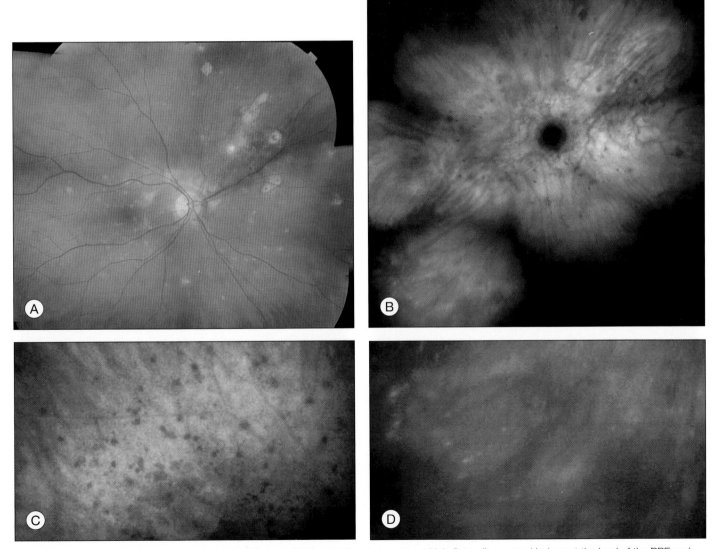

Fig. 53-25 A, Clinical photograph composite of a 35-year-old Hispanic female reveals multiple flat, yellow, round lesions at the level of the RPE and the inner choroid distributed over the posterior pole consistent with the diagnosis of multifocal choroiditis. ICG angiogram composite (B) shows multiple hypofluorescent spots (C) as well as hyperfluorescent foci (D). Note the confluent hypofluorescence surrounding the optic nerve.

eyes exhibiting enlargement of the blind spot on visual field testing, ICG angiography showed confluent hypofluorescence surrounding the optic nerve. The ICG angiogram was useful in evaluating the natural course in two patients with MFC, as well as evaluating the response to oral prednisone treatment in four others. The ICG angiography performed in these patients showed changes correlating with the clinical course. After administration of oral prednisone, the patients were noted to have decreased symptoms and less vitritis on clinical examination. ICG angiography showed a reduction in the size and number of the hypofluorescent spots in three patients with complete resolution of these angiographic lesions in the fourth patient. ICG angiography was also helpful to differentiate MFC from presumed ocular histoplasmosis syndrome which has similar clinical appearance. Patients with MFC clearly have hypofluorescent spots in the posterior pole during periods of relative activity, whereas patients with presumed ocular histoplasmosis syndrome may exhibit focal areas of hyperfluorescence.

CONCLUSIONS

Indocyanine green angiography is a highly specialized technique for imaging choroidal vasculature. It has several advantages over fluorescein angiography including lower toxicity, high protein binding affinity, and infrared fluorescence for better penetration through pigment, serosanguineous fluid and blood. The clinical applications of ICG angiography continue to expand as more experience is gained with current imaging techniques. Further advances in ICG angiography are likely to result from the newer high-speed imaging systems.

REFERENCES

1. Schatz HS, Burton T, Yannuzzi LA et al. Interpretation of fundus fluorescein angiography. St Louis: Mosby-Year Book, 1978.
2. Guyer DR, Puliafito CP, Mones JM et al. Digital indocyanine green angiography in chorioretinal disorders. Ophthalmology 1992; 99:287–291.
3. Yannuzzi LA, Slakter JS, Sorenson JA et al. Digital indocyanine green videoangiography and choroidal neovascularization. Retina 1992; 12:191–223.
4. Fox JJ, Brooker L, Heselstine D et al. A tricarbocyanine dye for continuous recording of dilution curves in the whole blood independent of variations in blood oxygen saturation. Proc Staff Meeting Mayo Clinic 1957; 32:478–484.
5. Fox JJ, Wood EH. Application of dilution curves recorded from the right side of the heart or venous circulation with the aid of a new indicator dye. Proc Mayo Clin 1957; 32:541.
6. Kogure K, Choromokos E. Infrared absorption angiography. J Appl Physiol 1969; 26:154–157.
7. Kogure K, David NJ, Yamanouchi U et al. Infrared absorption angiography of the fundus circulation. Arch Ophthalmol 1970; 83:209–214.
8. David NJ. Infrared absorption angiography. In: Proceedings of the International Symposium on Fluorescein Angiography, Albi. Basel: Karger, 1969; 189–195.
9. Hochheimer BF. Angiography of the retina with indocyanine green. Arch Ophthalmol 1971; 86:564–565.
10. Flower RW, Hochheimer BF. Letter to the editor: Clinical infrared absorption angiography of the choroid. Am J Ophthalmol 1972; 73:458–459.
11. Flower RW. Infrared absorption angiography of the choroid and some observations on the effects of high intraocular pressures. Am J Ophthalmol 1972; 74:600–614.
12. Flower RW, Hochheimer F. A clinical technique and apparatus for simultaneous angiography of the separate retinal and choroidal circulations. Invest Ophthalmol Vis Sci 1973;12:248–261.
13. Patz A, Flower RW, Klein ML et al. Clinical applications of indocyanine green angiography. Doc Ophthalmol Proc Series 1976; 9:245–251.
14. Hyvarinen L, Flower RW. Indocyanine green fluorescence angiography. Arch Ophthalmol 1980; 58:528–538.
15. Hayashi K, DeLaey JJ. Indocyanine green angiography of neovascular membranes. Ophthalmologica 1985; 190:30–39.
16. Hayashi K, Hasegawa Y, Tokoro T. Indocyanine green angiography of central serous chorioretinopathy. Int Ophthalmol 1986; 9:37–41.
17. Hayashi K, Hasegawa Y, Tokoro T et al. Clinical use of indocyanine green angiography in the diagnosis of choroidal neovascular disease. Fortschr Ophthalmol 1988; 85:410–412.
18. Hayashi K, Hasegawa Y, Tokoro T et al. Clinical application of indocyanine green angiography to choroidal neovascularization. Jpn J Ophthalmol 1989; 33:57–65.
19. Destro M, Puliafito CA. Indocyanine green videoangiography of choroidal neovascularization. Ophthalmology 1989; 96:846–853.
20. Scheider A, Schroedel C. High resolution indocyanine green angiography with scanning laser ophthalmoscope. Am J Ophthalmol 1989; 108:458–459.
21. Baker KJ. Binding of sulfobromoophthalein (BSP) sodium and indocyanine green (ICG) by plasma α_1-lipoproteins. Proc Soc Exp Biol Med 1966; 122: 957–963.
22. Geeraets WJ, Berry ER. Ocular spectral characteristics as related to hazards from lasers and other light sources. Am J Ophthalmol 1968; 66:15–20.
23. Cherrick GR, Stein SW, Levy CM et al. Indocyanine green: observations on its physical properties, plasma decay, and hepatic extraction. J Clin Invest 1960; 39:592–596.
24. Caesar J, Sheldon S, Chianduss L et al. The use of indocyanine green in the measurement of hepatic blood flow and as a test for hepatic function. Clin Sci 1961; 21:43–57.
25. Levy CM, Bender J, Silverberg M et al. Physiology of dye extraction by the liver: comparative studies of sulfobromoophthalein and indocyanine green. Ann NY Acad Sci 1963; 111:161–163.
26. Ketterer SG, Wiengand BD. The excretion of indocyanine green and its use in the estimation of hepatic blood flow. Clin Res 1959; 7:71–75.
27. Fineman MS, Maguire JI, Benson WE et al. Safety of indocyanine green angiography during pregnancy. Arch Ophthalmol 2001; 119:353–355.
28. Bischoff PR, Flower RW. Ten years experience with choroidal angiography using indocyanine green dye: a new routine examination or an epilogue? Doc Ophthalmol 1985; 60:235–291.
29. Hope-Ross M, Yannuzzi LA, Gragoudas ES et al. Adverse reactions to indocyanine green. Ophthalmology 1994; 101:529–535.
30. Yannuzzi LA, Rohrer KT, Tindel LJ et al. Fluorescein angiography complication survey. Ophthalmology 1986; 93:611–617.
31. Costa DLL, Huang SA, Orlock DA. Retinal choroidal indocyanine green dye clearance and liver dysfunction. Retina 2003; 23:557–561.
32. Hope-Ross MW. ICG dye: physical and pharmacological properties. In: Yannuzzi LA, Flower RW, Slakter JS, eds. Indocyanine green angiography. Mosby-Year Book, 1997; 46–49.
33. Stango PE, Lim JI, Hamilton P. Indocyanine green angiography in chorioretinal disease: Indications. An evidence-based update. Ophthalmology 2003;110:15–24.
34. Spaide RF, Orlock DA, Herman-Delamazure B et al. Wide-angle indocyanine green angiography. Retina 1998; 18:44–49.
35. Spaide RF, Orlock DA, Yannuzzi LA et al. Digital substraction indocyanine angiography of occult choroidal neovascularization. Ophthalmology 1998; 105:680–688.
36. Matsumoto M, Shiraki K, Obana A. Detection of choroidal neovascularization by subtraction indocyanine green angiography. Osaka City Med J 2003; 49:85–91.
37. Flower RW. Extraction of choroiocapillaris hemodynamic data from ICG fluorescence angiograms. Invest Ophthalmol Vis Sci 1993; 34:2720–2729.
38. Webb RH, Hughes GW, Delori FC. Confocal scanning laser ophthalmoscope. Appl Optics 1987; 26:1492–1499.
39. Teschner S, Noack J, Birngruber R et al. Characterization of leakage activity in exudative chorioretinal disease with three-dimensional confocal angiography. Ophthalmology 2003; 110:687–697.
40. Patz A, Flower RW, Klein ML et al. Clinical applications of indocyanine green angiography. Doc Ophthalmol Proc Series 1976; 9:245–251.
41. Scheider, A, Kaboth A, Neuhauser L. Detection of subretinal neovascularization membranes with indocyanine green and infrared scanning laser ophthalmoscope. Am J Ophthalmol 1992; 113:45–51.
42. Yannuzzi LA, Hope-Ross M, Slakter JS et al. Analysis of vascularized pigment epithelium detachments using indocyanine green videoangiography. Retina 1994; 14:99–113.
43. Guyer DR, Yannuzzi LA, Slakter JS et al. Classification of choroidal neovascularization by digital indocyanine green videoangiography. Ophthalmology 1996; 103:2054–2060.
44. Chang B, Yannuzzi LA, Ladas ID et al. Choroidal neovascularization in second eyes of patients with unilateral exudative age-related macular degeneration. Ophthalmology 1995; 102:1380–1386.
45. Lee BL, Lim JI, Grossniklaus HE. Clinicopathologic features of indocyanine green angiography-imaged, surgically excised choroidal neovascular membranes. Retina 1996; 16:64–69.

46. Guyer DR, Yannuzzi LA, Ladas I et al. Indocyanine green guided laser photocoagulation of focal spots at the edge of plaques of choroidal neovascularization: a pilot study. Arch Ophthalmol 1996; 114:693–697.

47. Yannuzzi LA, Sorenson JS, Spaide RF et al. Idiopathic polypoidal choroidal vasculopathy. Retina 1990; 10:1–8.

48. Guyer DR, Yannuzzi LA, Slakter JS et al. Digital indocyanine-green videoangiography of occult choroidal neovascularization. Ophthalmology 1994; 101:1727–1737.

49. Macular Photocoagulation Study Group. Occult choroidal neovascularization. Influence on visual outcome in patients with age-related macular degeneration. Arch Ophthalmol 1996; 114:400–412.

50. Iida T, Yannuzzi LA, Freund KB et al. Retinal angiopathy and polypoidal choroidal vasculopathy. Retina 2002; 22:455–463.

51. Spaide RF, Yannuzzi LA, Slakter JS et al. Indocyanine green videoangiography of idiopathic polypoidal choroidal vasculopathy. Retina 1995; 15:100–110.

52. Yannuzzi LA, Ciardella AP, Spaide RF et al. The expanding clinical spectrum of idiopathic polypoidal choroidal vasculopathy. Arch Ophthalmol 1999; 115:478–485.

53. Chan WM, Lam DS, Lai TY et al. Photodynamic therapy with verteporfin for symptomatic polypoidal choroidal vasculopathy: one-year results of a prospective case series. Ophthalmology 2004; 111:1576–1584.

54. Yannuzzi LA, Negrao S, Iida T et al. Retinal angiomatous proliferation in age-related macular degeneration. Retina 2001; 21:416–434.

55. Kuhn D, Meunier I, Soubrane G, Coca G. Imaging of chorioretinal anastomoses in vascularized retinal pigment epithelium detachments. Arch Ophthalmol 1995; 113:1392–1396.

56. Slakter JS, Yannuzzi LA, Scheider U et al. Retinal choroidal anastomosis and occult choroidal neovascularization. Ophthalmology 2000; 107:742–753.

57. Slakter JS, Yannuzzi LA, Sorenson JA et al. A pilot study of indocyanine green videoangiography-guided laser photocoagulation of occult choroidal neovascularization in age-related macular degeneration. Arch Ophthalmol 1994; 112:465–472.

58. Schwartz S, Guyer DR, Yannuzzi LA et al. Indocyanine green videoangiography-guided laser photocoagulation of primary occult choroidal neovascularization in age-related macular degeneration. Invest Ophthalmol Vis Sci 1995; 36:186.

59. Freund KB, Yannuzzi LA, Sorenson JA et al. Age-related macular degeneration and choroidal neovascularization. Am J Ophthalmol 1993; 115:786–791.

60. Mandava N, Guyer DR, Yannuzzi LA et al. Indocyanine green videoangiography-guided laser photocoagulation of occult choroidal neovascularization. Ophthal Surg Lasers 1997; 28:844–852.

61. Costa RA, Farah ME, Cardillo JA et al. Photodynamic therapy with indocyanine green for occult subfoveal choroidal neovascularization caused by age-related macular degeneration. Curr Eye Res 2001; 23:271–275.

62. Staurenghi G, Orzalesi N, La Capria A et al. Laser treatment of feeder vessels in subfoveal choroidal neovascular membranes: a revisitation using dynamic indocyanine green angiography. Ophthalmology 1998; 105: 2297–2305.

63. Fernandes LHS, Freund BK, Yannuzzi LA et al. The nature of focal areas of hyperfluorescence or hot spots imaged with indocyanine green angiography. Retina 2002; 22:557–568.

64. Katsimpris J, Donati G, Kapetanios A et al. The value of indocyanine green angiography in detection of central serous chorioretinopathy. Klin Monatsbl Augenheilkd 2001; 218:335–337.

65. Sallet S, Amoakin WM, Lafaut BA et al. Indocyanine green angiography of choroidal tumors. Graefes Arch Clin Exp Ophthalmol 1995; 223:677–689.

66. Guyer DR, Yannuzzi LA, Krupsky S et al. Digital indocyanine green angiography of intraocular tumors. Semin Ophthalmol 1993; 8:224–229.

67. Shields CL, Shields JA, De Potter P. Patterns of indocyanine green videoangiography of choroidal tumors. Br J Ophthalmol 1995; 79:237–245.

68. Gupta M, Singh AD, Rundle PA et al. Efficacy of photodynamic therapy in circumscribed choroidal haemangioma. Eye 2004;18:139–142.

69. Piccolino FC, Borgia L, Zinicola E. Indocyanine green angiography of circumscribed choroidal hemangiomas. Retina 1996; 16:19–28.

70. Kardmas EF, Weiter JJ. Choroidal osteoma. Int Ophthalmol 1997; 37: 171–182.

71. Singh AD, De Potter P, Shields CL et al. Indocyanine green angiography and ultrasonography of a varix of the vortex vein. Arch Ophthalmol 1993; 100:1283–1284.

72. Giovannini A, Ripa E, Scassellati-Sforzolini B et al. Indocyanine green angiography in serpiginous choroidopathy. Eur J Ophthalmol 1996; 6:299–306.

73. Howe LJ, Woon H, Graham EM et al. Choroidal hypoperfusion in acute multifocal posterior placoid pigment epitheliopathy: an indocyanine green angiography study. Ophthalmology 1995; 102:790–798.

74. Park D, Schatz H, McDonald HR et al. Indocyanine green angiography of acute multifocal posterior placoid pigment epitheliopathy. Ophthalmology 1995; 102:1877–1883.

75. Ie D, Glaser BM, Murphy RP et al. Indocyanine green angiography in multiple evanescent white-dot syndrome. Am J Ophthalmol 1994; 117:7–12.

76. Herbort CP, Probst K, Cimino L et al. Differential inflammatory involvement in retina and choroid in birdshot chorioretinopathy. Klin Monatsbl Augenheilkd. 2004;221:351–356.

77. Howe LJ, Stanford MR, Graham EM et al. Choroidal abnormalities in birdshot chorioretinopathy: an indocyanine green angiography study. Eye 1997; 11: 554–559.

78. Slakter JS, Giovannini A, Yannuzzi LA et al. Indocyanine green angiography of multifocal choroiditis. Ophthalmology 1997; 104:1813–1819.

Pathogenesis of Serous Detachment of the Retina and Pigment Epithelium

Alan C. Bird

The mechanisms by which the retina is maintained in apposition to the pigment epithelium, and the pigment epithelium to Bruch's membrane, have not been clearly defined, although many factors have been implicated.

It has been well established that there is water movement from the center of the eye, across the retina toward the choroid.[1] This is due, in part, to constant secretion of fluid into the eye by the ciliary body, causing minor changes in hydrostatic pressure from the center of the eye to the outside. In addition, it has been argued that the high osmotic pressure in the choroid, when compared with that of the vitreous, would cause outward movement of water.[2-5] Also, the retinal pigment epithelium (RPE) is constantly moving ions toward the choroid with associated movement of water.[6] This constant water movement would predictably cause the tissues lining the eye to remain in apposition if these tissues had any resistance, however low, to hydraulic conductivity. It has been demonstrated that the retina has measurable resistance to water flow.[7,8]

It is unlikely that retinal apposition is maintained by active metabolic influences alone in all species; this is manifest by the fact that the retina cannot easily be separated from the RPE, in some animals even several hours after death. This has led to the suggestion that the interphotoreceptor matrix may act as a glue, and structural attachment has been demonstrated around cones.[9]

It is believed that there are structural connections between the RPE and Bruch's membrane. The inner portion of Bruch's membrane is the basement membrane of the pigment epithelial cells, to which the cells adhere. Local electron-dense areas can be seen in this basement membrane, and it is thought that these represent sites of insertion of collagen fibers from the inner collagenous layer of Bruch's membrane into the basement membrane.

Failure of these mechanisms may allow detachment of the neuroretina from the RPE, or of the pigment epithelial basement membrane from the remainder of Bruch's membrane. Our knowledge of the various disorders in which fluid accumulates in these potential cavities is too imprecise to ascribe specific pathogenetic mechanisms to each, although concepts exist to explain observed clinical phenomena. Interestingly, in hypotony, in which it is assumed that water movement across the retina is severely reduced, clinically detectable detachment of the neuroretina from the pigment epithelium is extremely rare; it is much more characteristic under these circumstances for fluid to accumulate within the choroid.

Accumulation of fluid between the neuroretina and pigment epithelium is most commonly associated with a retinal hole; in this instance the subretinal fluid is thought to be derived from the hyaloid cavity, and to enter the subretinal space through the hole. Serous detachment of the neuroretina is observed under two other circumstances. It is a characteristic of central serous retinopathy, which appears to be associated with focal dysfunction of the RPE. Detachment of the retina from the RPE is also seen in primary choroidal disorders such as tumor, choroidal inflammation, and ischemia, and in a variety of other conditions falling into the category of choroidal effusion syndrome. Accumulation of fluid between Bruch's membrane and RPE is seen consistently in only one situation, namely pigment epithelial detachment. This occurs in the young as a manifestation of central serous retinopathy, and in the elderly as a manifestation of age-related macular disease.

CENTRAL SEROUS RETINOPATHY

Albrecht von Graefe[10] described the clinical aspects of central serous retinopathy in 1866, but it was not until 100 years later that Maumenee,[11] utilizing fluorescein angiography, demonstrated that the subretinal fluid was derived from the RPE and presumably originated from the choroid.

During fluorescein angiography, the subretinal space is seen to fill with dye derived from the choroid.[12] The source of fluorescein may appear as a point of hyperfluorescence at the level of the RPE during the early part of the study; fluorescein may then enter the subretinal space as a vertical stream (smokestack), or it may spread evenly and centrifugally. In other cases the source of dye appears to be a pigment epithelial detachment, which becomes hyperfluorescent early and from which is derived the subretinal fluorescein. In a third category of disease named chronic central serous retinopathy, retinal detachment may not be evident clinically, and the hyperfluorescence may appear over a wide area at the level of the RPE. These appearances suggest the possibility of different pathologic processes, yet more than one form of the disorder may be seen in the same patient at different times, or in fellow eyes of the same patient. Most investigators consider these to be different manifestations of the same disorder. The only consistent feature is the increased prevalence of diffuse leakage with chronic disease or with increased number of recurrences.[13]

In the vast majority of patients, the area of serous detachment is limited and the retina is highly elevated. This suggests that detachment is somehow restricted by the adherence of photoreceptor cells to the RPE. In a minority of cases, a shallow track of fluid may be seen derived from the source of fluid, connecting the source to significant detachment of the inferior retina.[14] There is no good explanation as to the difference in distribution of fluid in these two circumstances, although the bilaterality of inferior detachment suggests some specific predisposition to gravitational movement of fluid in these patients.

Although it is clear that RPE cells function abnormally in central serous retinopathy, the nature of the dysfunction is unknown. The RPE has many functions, including maintenance of homeostasis of the extracellular space of the outer retina and prevention of free water movement from choroid to retina. It has been generally considered that central serous retinopathy is caused by loss of this specific metabolic attribute, and that the fluid accumulates in the subretinal space by passive diffusion. This explanation presumes that the hydrostatic pressure in the choroid is higher than in the neuroretina; however, most evidence suggests that the reverse is true.[7]

One surprising aspect of the disorder is the apparent preservation of good suprathreshold receptor function, as manifest by good visual acuity in the acute form of the disease, despite physical separation of the rods and cones from the RPE over months or years. Furthermore, there is no evidence that prolonged detachment causes progressive loss of retinal function, or that there is any correlation between the duration of detachment and the visual prognosis.[13] It can only be assumed that metabolic exchange between the RPE and the photoreceptors is relatively well maintained. This is difficult to reconcile with the concept of a "functional hole" in the RPE layer. It has been shown that threshold function is poor despite relatively good levels of rhodopsin.[15] This apparent loss of transduction gain recovers within 2 weeks of retinal apposition.[15]

These considerations have called into question previous concepts of the pathogenesis of central serous retinopathy. It has been argued that simple loss of the functional integrity of the RPE would not explain the movement of fluid from choroid to the subretinal space, or retention of function over a prolonged period. Spitznas[16] has suggested that this movement could be a result only of reversed polarity of one, or a small population of pigment epithelial cells, so that they move ions from the choroid into the subretinal space actively, with consequent movement of water. The subretinal space would remain closed with respect to other metabolic functions, and thus the exchange of metabolites, such as 11-*cis* retinal, would be relatively unaffected.

Spitznas' hypothesis of the pathogenesis explains many of the observed clinical phenomena in central serous retinopathy, but does not account for the frequent RPE detachment in such cases. It is conceivable that reversed polarity may occur in RPE cells detached from Bruch's membrane, but it does not account for the pigment epithelial detachment itself. There is circumstantial evidence to suggest that detachment of the RPE from Bruch's membrane in the elderly may be due to increased resistance to outward flow at the level of Bruch's membrane[17] (see the section

on pigment epithelial detachment, below). Histopathological studies of central serous retinopathy are few, and to date there is little evidence to imply any changes in Bruch's membrane associated with this disorder.

Of interest is the observation from indocyanine green (ICG) angiography that there is increased accumulation of dye in the inner choroid, both at sites of manifest RPE changes, and at sites where the RPE appears normal on fluorescein angiography.[18] It has been concluded that abnormalities of the choroid may initiate the disorder, but the nature of the relationship between the choroidal changes and RPE disease is not clear. Additional support for the relevance of choroidal disease as being important to the pathogenesis of the disorder is observation of therapeutic benefit of PDT treatment.[19]

In the chronic form of the disease, in which deep detachment of the retina does not occur, there is diffuse dysfunction of the RPE.[20] The nature of the pigment epithelial disease appears to be different from that in acute disease in that the detachment is shallow, and fluorescein diffuses slowly from the choroid into the RPE and subsequently into the subretinal space or the outer retina. Scotopic sensitivity is severely reduced over the entire area of pigment epithelial change, and the visual prognosis is poor when compared with acute disease, although the retinal photoreceptors appear to be viable over this area, at least for a period.[15]

Since the RPE has been identified as the source of subretinal fluid, the precipitating cause of RPE dysfunction has been sought by many investigators. It has been suggested that the RPE metabolic defect may be induced by changes in the choriocapillaris,[21–23] or to a physical defect in Bruch's membrane.[24] Serous retinal detachment has been produced in monkeys by intravascular injection of epinephrine (adrenaline).[25,26] There must be some doubt as to whether there was a significant rise in blood pressure, because the serous detachment of the retina associated with multifocal pigment epithelial disease is also commonly found in association with accelerated hypertension. The authors thought this unlikely since no histopathological changes of hypertension were identified in the eyes, but blood pressure was not evidently monitored during the experiment.

It is well recognized that central serous retinopathy affects men more often than women (in a ratio ranging from 3:1 to 10:1) and reportedly occurs between the ages of 30 and 55 years, although in Europe it is most common at a later age, 40 to 60 years.[25,34,59,99,102] It has also been identified as occurring in those who are "hard driving and tense."[10a,22,27–29] Central serous retinopathy also appears to be associated with hypermetropia.[30] This plus the onset of disease occurring at the time of presbyopia suggests that accommodation may play a role. The disorder affects all races, and is reported to be particularly common in Japan.[31–34] Finally there is evidence that the disorder is associated with corticosteroids either administered in any form or with high endogenous levels.[35–37] The relevance of these various factors to pathogenesis is unknown.

CHOROIDAL VASCULAR DISEASE

There is greater variation in the ophthalmoscopic manifestations of choroidal ischemia than is generally acknowledged. This realization dates from the advent of fluorescein angiography, by which the characteristics of choroidal perfusion have been documented. Usually the choroid fills just before the retina, and this filling occurs in less than 1 s. Delayed perfusion of one well-defined segment of the choroid for as long as 6 s appears to be a feature of some normal eyes, and is a constant feature in certain individuals. Longer delay in perfusion in larger areas of the peripheral choroid and a prolonged filling phase imply defective perfusion.

The concept of focal choroidal infarction would have been difficult to defend at a time when anatomic studies implied that the choriocapillaris was a continuous network of capillaries supplied by many arterioles. However, Dollery and associates[38] showed that, in pigs with increased intraocular pressure, the choriocapillaris filled not as a continuous layer but as a series of dots that later enlarged to become uniform. They concluded that this filling pattern indicated the presence of individual choriocapillaris units. Hayreh[39] demonstrated the lobular pattern of choriocapillaris filling in the posterior pole of normal animals. Scanning electron microscopic examination of corrosion vascular casts has provided further evidence of well-defined capillary units. Lobules of choriocapillaris in the submacular choroid are supplied by short, nonanastomosing precapillary arterioles without functional anastomoses between adjacent capillary units in the normal eye.[40] This lobular arrangement is less well defined in the anterior choroid, in which there is a more direct capillary connection between the arteries and veins.[41]

Considerable deficit of choroidal perfusion is required before there is any clinical manifestation of cell dysfunction. Prolonged reduction in choroidal circulation, as shown by fluorescein angiography examination, is compatible with apparently normal function and absence of any long-term changes in the appearance of the ocular fundus.[42]

Serous detachment of the retina is the most commonly recognized manifestation of choroidal hypoperfusion. It has been described in many forms of vascular disease, including accelerated hypertension,[23,43] toxemia of pregnancy,[44–47] Goodpasture's syndrome,[48] polyarteritis nodosa,[16] thrombotic thrombocytopenic purpura,[49,50] and disseminated intravascular coagulation.[51] For many years, most attention was focused on the retinal vasculature, and it was believed by many that the subretinal fluid was derived from the retina. Subsequent work has shown that there are changes in both the choroid and RPE, and that fluorescein enters the subretinal space from the choroid during angiography. These reports describe multifocal RPE opacification and retinal detachment, but with remarkably little scarring after resolution of the detachment after treatment of the precipitating disorder. It has been suggested that there is sufficient ischemia to cause RPE dysfunction, as manifested by passage of fluid into the abnormal RPE cells or through the RPE into the subretinal space. However, the paucity of fundus change after recovery suggests that there was relatively little cell death in these areas.

The mechanism by which ischemia causes fluid accumulation in the subretinal space is unknown. Results of fluorescein angiographic studies imply that the fluid is derived from the choroid. Therefore, failure to pump water out of the subretinal space alone seems an unlikely cause of the detachment. It is equally unlikely that the fluid passes from the choroid to the subretinal space through nonfunctioning pigment epithelial cells, because the fluid would be passing up a hydrostatic pressure gradient. This is supported by the observation that the removal of RPE during resection of malignant melanoma[52] and presumed RPE cell death due to infarction do not result in detachment.[42] Much more attractive is the concept of reversed or deranged polarity of ion movement by pigment epithelial cells, actively moving fluid into the subretinal space. There is little experimental evidence to support this concept at present, although results of fluorescein angiographic studies imply that the fluid is derived from the choroid.

This situation can be contrasted with infarction of the outer retina in which there is no retinal detachment, and which gives rise to well-defined atrophy of the RPE. Triangular choroidal infarcts of the peripheral choroid in humans have been well documented,[52a,53–55] although fluorescein angiographic studies of such cases during the acute phase have not been reported except after photocoagulation for sickle-cell retinopathy.[55] Central infarcts tend to be smaller and round. The difference in the pattern of infarction may be due to the differences in anatomic arrangement of the choroidal vascular bed between the periphery and the macular areas.[40,41] Many authors have emphasized that the changes within the infarcted area are variable, and that atrophy of the outer retina, RPE, and choriocapillaris may be less extensive than the area of apparent ischemia.

Similar observations have been made in animals after experimental obstruction of the short posterior ciliary arteries, which produces large areas of hypoperfused choroid but only limited infarction.[56,57] It has been argued that rapid restoration of choroidal flow occurred as a result of interarterial bypass channels or of reverse flow within choroidal veins, causing shortening of the period of ischemia,[39,56,58] and consequent reduction of the area of cell death. The possibility that the RPE can survive periods of severe choroidal perfusion deficit could also explain the limited extent of the ophthalmoscopic changes seen under these circumstances. Stern & Ernest[59] injected microspheres into the posterior ciliary arteries. Despite massive embolization of the choroid, only small RPE lesions developed and retinal detachment occurred only in the presence of systemic hypertension.

Together, these observations imply that choroidal ischemia may be more common than has been thought. In some instances the abnormality can be detected only by angiographic examination, and minor disturbance of pigmentation may be the only long-term consequence. If sectorial atrophy is used as the only index of previous choroidal hypoperfusion, many cases will not be detected.

CHOROIDAL INFLAMMATION

It has been shown that clinical changes identical to those seen in generalized vascular disease occur in choroidal inflammatory disease. Some authors[6,60] believe that the RPE disease in placoid pigment epitheliopathy may be due to choroidal perfusion defects on the basis of the choroidal filling patterns on angiography. The behavior characteristics appear to be quite compatible with the concept that mild hypoperfusion may not cause any detectable abnormality of fundus appearance or retinal function, that moderate choroidal ischemia causes passage of fluid through the RPE and consequent retinal detachment, and that retinal detachment does not occur if there is sufficient ischemia to cause cell death.[45,61] Ocular disease may appear to be unilateral despite bilateral choroidal vascular compromise. Patients who have placoid pigment epitheliopathy and retinal detachment when first examined have little scarring after recovery. Placoid pigment epitheliopathy without retinal detachment is followed consistently by well-defined atrophy. Abnormal choroidal perfusion is seen during the recovery phase.

Retinal detachment also characterizes Harada's disease, sympathetic ophthalmia, and scleritis. In these conditions there is inflammatory change in the choroid, with secondary opacification of the RPE. Fluorescein angiography suggests abnormal choroidal perfusion in these diseases, and it is conceivable that the pathogenesis of abnormal fluid movement may be similar to that seen in choroidal ischemia from other causes.

CHOROIDAL EFFUSION SYNDROME

In choroidal effusion syndrome, fluid accumulates between the choroid and the neuroretina in the absence of a retinal hole. It is believed that the fluid is derived from the choroid. There is widespread RPE change in these patients, and fluorescein enters the subretinal space from the choroid during angiographic evaluation. The retinal detachment has the curious characteristic of being mobile and gravity-dependent.[62,63] As the eye is moved, the distribution of detachment changes as rapidly as over a matter of seconds. This can be contrasted with detachment due to retinal hole, in which induced changes in the distribution of subretinal fluid occur over hours, if at all. In the latter case, it is presumed that the fluid is restricted by the normal adhesion of receptor cells to the RPE. If this is correct, it is not clear why such constraints should not be present in choroidal effusion syndromes.

Theories as to the pathogenesis of uveal effusion syndrome are derived from the observation that this disorder occurs more commonly in nanophthalmic eyes in which the sclera is abnormally thick.[63a,64,65] It was considered that the abnormally thick sclera compresses the vortex veins and impedes venous drainage. This concept is supported by a case report of uveal effusion in Hunter syndrome (type IIB mucopolysaccharidosis), in which the scleral thickness is increased by mucopolysaccharide deposition.[66] Further support for this concept is derived from the observation that decompression of the vortex veins may cause the effusion to resolve.[67] It is curious that disorders due to central vein obstruction are well recognized and common, while obstruction of choroidal veins is a novel concept. Many of the anatomic constraints of the central retinal vein that are thought to be important in the pathogenesis of obstruction are shared by the choroidal veins as they exit from the eye. Choroidal effusion has also been described in conditions in which there is raised choroidal venous pressure such as dural arteriovenous fistula.[68]

Choroidal effusion syndromes may also occur in patients without nanophthalmos but with abnormally thick sclera.[69] That surgical thinning of the sclera causes resolution of the detachment led to the alternative proposal that an abnormally thick sclera may represent a barrier to bulk fluid flow out of the eye.[69] It has been suggested that significant volumes of fluid leave the eye normally through the sclera and pass into the orbit,[7] such that the thickened sclera may represent a barrier to this outflow pathway.

CHOROIDAL TUMORS

Choroidal tumors, either primary or secondary, and choroidal hemangiomas cause serous retinal detachment.[70] As with other forms of serous retinal detachment, the cause of abnormal water movement may be failure of the RPE to pump water out of the subretinal space or reversal of RPE orientation, as in central serous retinopathy.

PIGMENT EPITHELIAL DETACHMENT

Originally it was considered likely that RPE detachment in the elderly was induced by weakening of the physical attachment of the RPE to Bruch's membrane by accumulation of debris on the inner surface of Bruch's membrane.[71] The detachment then followed as a result of passive movement of fluid from the choroid through Bruch's membrane into the subpigment epithelial space. This concept is difficult to defend if the hydrostatic pressure in the choroid is no higher than that in the retina.[7]

Alternatively, Gass[72] has postulated that the fluid may be derived from blood vessels that grow on the inner surface of Bruch's membrane. At this site they may be obscured by sub-RPE fluid, such that these vessels may not always be evident by ophthalmoscopy or fluorescein angiographic examinations. Although new vessels are undoubtedly common in these lesions, there is evidence that subpigment epithelial neovascularization is not universal in pigment epithelial detachments.[73–75] In addition, neither of these mechanisms appears to explain fully all the observed phenomena of pigment epithelial detachment. In particular, they do not account for flattening of the detachment after photocoagulation[75a] or for loss of vision following spontaneous flattening.[73]

It has been suggested that the fluid in the subpigment epithelial space may be derived, at least in part, from the RPE rather than from the choroid.[75b] It is widely accepted that fluid crosses the RPE from the neurosensory retina toward Bruch's membrane as a result of active transport of ions, such that some of the fluid must be derived from the pigment epithelium.[76] As Bruch's membrane becomes thicker with age it is predictable that there would be an increase in the resistance to water flow, and it would result in fluid accumulation in the subpigment epithelial space. Furthermore, the resistance to fluid flow may be even more compromised by deposition of nonpolar neutral lipid on the inner surface of Bruch's membrane, thus rendering it hydrophobic.

Some evidence exists to support the hypothesis that there is change in the diffusion characteristics of Bruch's membrane with age. Decreasing hydraulic conductivity of Bruch's membrane with age has been documented.[1,77] Clefts at the inner surface of Bruch's membrane have been ascribed to impedance of fluid flow by "basal linear deposit."[78]

Further support for the concept is derived from laboratory studies which indicate that lipid accumulates in Bruch's membrane with age, and that the ratio of neutral lipids to phospholipids differs from one subject to another. This was shown initially by histochemical staining on frozen sections derived from eye bank eyes.[79] More recently, analysis of the lipid extracted from Bruch's membrane of eye bank eyes from donors of different ages has been undertaken using thin-layer and gas chromatography.[80] It was shown that the lipid extracted increases with the age of the donor, and that the total quantity and ratio of neutral fats to phospholipids varied widely from one specimen to another from donors over the age of 60 years.

There is evidence from fluorescence microscopy that the lipid content of drusen may be identified by fluorescein angiography. Fluorescein was injected intravenously into a patient immediately prior to enucleation for malignant melanoma, and fluorescence microscopy showed that some of the drusen were highly fluorescent while others contained no fluorescein.[17] It was concluded that the former were hydrophilic, allowing the entry of water-soluble dye and that fluorescein may become bound to the polar compounds within the lesion. By contrast, the latter were hydrophobic owing to the presence of neutral lipid so that dye would not enter the tissues and binding would not take place. This conclusion is strengthened by observations made on tissue from donor eyes.[81] A series of macular specimens from human donors older than 65 years of age were examined. In vitro fluorescein binding was recorded microscopically and the presence of fibronectin was sought by immunohistochemistry. The results were correlated with the proportions of phospholipids to neutral fats identified by histochemical and biochemical analysis. It was found that high content of neutral fats was associated with lack of both fluorescein binding and fibronectin, and conversely in those specimens with high proportions of phospholipids, fluorescein binding was strong and fibronectin was present. These findings are compatible with the concept that deposits containing predominantly neutral lipids result in hypofluorescence on fluorescein angiography and confer hydrophobicity, while the presence of polar phospholipids would be indicated clinically by hyperfluorescence and imply hydrophilic properties.

The phenomenon of tearing of the RPE allowed these concepts to be tested clinically. It is believed that RPE detachments that are destined to tear tend to become progressively larger and more highly detached, thereby generating sufficient tangential stress in the detached tissues to cause a rupture.[82–84] This implies that it is in these lesions that the resistance to water flow across Bruch's membrane would be highest. It has been identified that if a tear of the RPE occurs in one eye, there is a high risk for the development of this condition in the fellow eye.[85,86] The drusen in these high-risk fellow eyes show different fluorescein angiographic characteristics than do fellow eyes of macular disciform lesions.[75,87] They are hypofluorescent, which is consistent with the drusen being hydrophobic and limiting entry of fluorescein into the lesion. The proposed hydrophobicity and manifest confluent tendency of such drusen imply that there would be high resistance to water flow at the level of Bruch's membrane in these eyes. These arguments are strengthened by the observation that drusen are

symmetric in number[88] and fluorescence characteristics[89] so that the drusen in the study eye would reflect those which existed previously in the eye with the pigment epithelial detachment.

Furthermore, other clinical observations are in accord with the concept of high lipid content in Bruch's membrane in RPE detachments destined to tear. It has been shown that such lesions show slow appearance of fluorescence on angiographic examination.[82–84] Because fluorescein is water-soluble it would pass slowly through a lipid-laden Bruch's membrane from the choroid into the sub-pigment epithelial space. This mechanism of detachment would also explain some of the clinical behavior of pigment epithelial detachments. Visual loss associated with spontaneous resolution of the detachment[73] could be explained by metabolic failure of the RPE. Reattachment after photocoagulation[75a] could be explained similarly.

Therefore the evidence to date is compatible with detachment of the RPE from Bruch's membrane being initiated by active pumping by the pigment cells in the presence of high resistance to water flow at the level of Bruch's membrane, and that subpigment epithelial neovascularization occurs as a secondary phenomenon. If the RPE is responsible for suppressing vascularity of neighboring structures the separation of pigment epithelium from Bruch's membrane would predictably be followed by growth of blood vessels from the choroid toward the retina. This is not to deny the potential importance of choroidal neovascularization as a determinant of the behavior of pigment epithelial detachments and tears, but does argue against this process as a primary pathogenetic mechanism in such lesions. That the RPE detachment is the primary event, and that subretinal neovascularization occurs as a secondary phenomenon is the sequence of events originally proposed by Gass[71] in his monograph in 1967. Even if subpigment epithelial blood vessels contribute to the detachment, it has been argued that they would not do so unless Bruch's membrane became hydrophobic.[87]

Other clinical phenomena have also been ascribed to decreased conductivity of Bruch's membrane, namely the loss of scotopic sensitivity[75b] and decreased choroidal perfusion.[90] A unifying mechanism has been proposed to explain both the functional loss and choroidal changes. Normal photoreceptor function is dependent on the free diffusion through Bruch's membrane of large-molecule complexes as they pass from the choriocapillaris to the RPE.[64] Predictably, such molecules would not pass freely through a hydrophobic layer of debris, and functional deficit would ensue. The magnitude of change would depend upon the thickness and chemical composition of the material within Bruch's membrane, and would be particularly marked in the presence of a large quantity of neutral fats.[79,80] There is circumstantial evidence that the behavioral characteristics of the choriocapillaris are determined by the RPE,[56,91] and it has been proposed that the diffusible agents from the RPE modulate the choroidal vasculature.[92] If the normal characteristics of the choroidal capillaries are dependent upon a diffusible agent, failure of this agent to reach the choroid would result in the vessels reverting to the more common tubular arrangement of capillary beds.[93] Thus loss of sensitivity, slow dark adaptation, and changes in the choriocapillaris may indicate the presence of diffuse deposits which are sufficiently thick or hydrophobic that metabolic exchange between the choroid and retina is impaired. The observation that geographic atrophy is much more likely to occur in a patient with abnormal choroidal perfusion than in one without this clinical sign, and that sensitivity loss implies threat of an RPE detachment,[94] give direct support to these concepts.

These clinical observations give circumstantial support to the original concept of change in hydraulic conductivity of Bruch's membrane with age and that the effect differs from one subject to another. The functional deficits imply that it is not just water movement that is affected but that there may be global reduction of metabolic exchange between the RPE and choriocapillaris.

Detachment of the RPE is also a characteristic of retinal angiomatous proliferation, a form of late age-related macular disease in which vascular invasion of the outer retina accompanies choroidal neovascularization.[95–97] This occurs in the context of early age-related maculopathy and similar pathogenic mechanisms may pertain. In addition the macular edema may result in increased outward transport of water by the RPE. RPE detachment is also common in polypoidal choroidal vasculopathy.[98–101] In this case there is no evidence that changes in Bruch's membrane are integral to the disorder. It is possible that massive exudation from the vascular complexes may cause the lesion.

REFERENCES

1. Fisher RF. The influence of age on some ocular basement membranes. Eye 1987; 1:184–189.
2. Casswell AG, Gregor ZJ, Bird AC. The surgical management of uveal effusion syndrome. Eye 1987; 1:115–119.
3. Machemer R. The importance of fluid absorption, traction, intraocular currents, and chorioretinal scars in the therapy of rhegmatogenous retinal detachments. Am J Ophthalmol 1984; 98:681–693.
4. Negi A, Marmor MF. The resorption of subretinal fluid after diffuse damage to the retinal pigment epithelium. Invest Ophthalmol Vis Sci 1983; 24:1475–1479.
5. Negi A, Marmor MF. Experimental serous retinal detachment and focal pigment epithelial damage. Arch Ophthalmol 1984; 102:445–449.
6. Van Buskirk EM, Lessell S, Friedman E. Pigmentary epitheliopathy and erythema nodosum. Arch Ophthalmol 1971; 85:369–372.
7. Foulds WS. Clinical significance of trans-scleral fluid transfer. Trans Ophthalmol Soc UK 1976; 96:290–308.
8. Orr G, Goodnight R, Lean JS. Relative permeability of retina and retinal pigment epithelium to the diffusion of tritiated water from vitreous to choroid. Arch Ophthalmol 1986; 104:1678–1680.
9. Hollyfield JG, Varner HH, Rayborn ME et al. Retinal attachment to the pigment epithelium. Linkage through an extracellular sheath surrounding cone photoreceptors. Retina 1989; 9:59–68.
10. Von Graefe A. Uber centrale recidivierende Retinitis. Graefes Arch Opthalmol 1866; 12:211.
10a. Lipowski ZJ. Psychomatic aspects of central serous retinopathy. Psychomatics 1971; 12:398–401.
11. Maumenee AE. Symposium: macular diseases. Pathogenesis. Trans Am Acad Ophthalmol Otolaryngol 1965; 69:691–699.
12. Wessing A. Changing concepts of central serous retinopathy and its treatment. Trans Am Acad Ophthalmol Otolaryngol 1973; 77:275–280.
13. Leaver P, Williams C. Argon laser photocoagulation in the treatment of central serous retinopathy. Br J Ophthalmol 1979; 63:674–677.
14. Gass JDM. Bullous retinal detachment: an unusual manifestation of idiopathic central serous choroidopathy. Am J Ophthalmol 1973; 75:810–821.
15. Chuang EL, Sharp DM, Fitzke FW et al. Retinal dysfunction in central serous retinopathy. Eye 1987; 1:120–125.
16. Spitznas M. Pathogenesis of central serous retinopathy: a new working hypothesis. Graefes Arch Clin Exp Ophthalmol 1986; 224:321–324.
17. Bird AC, Marshall J. Retinal pigment epithelial detachments in the elderly. Trans Ophthalmol Soc UK 1986; 105:674–682.
18. Piccolino FC, Borgia L. Central serous chorioretinopathy and indocyanine green angiography. Retina 1994; 14:231–242.
19. Yannuzzi LA, Slakter JS, Gross NE et al. Indocyanine green angiography-guided photodynamic therapy for treatment of chronic central serous chorioretinopathy: a pilot study. Retina 2003; 23:288–298.
20. Jalkh AE, Jabbour N, Avila MP et al. Retinal pigment epithelium decompensation. I. Clinical features and natural course. Ophthalmology 1984; 91:1544–1548.
21. Ballentyne AJ, Michaelson IC. Textbook of the fundus of the eye. London: E & S Livingstone; 1970.
22. Gass JDM. Pathogenesis of disciform detachment of the neuroepithelium. II. Idiopathic central serous choroidopathy. Am J Ophthalmol 1967; 63:587–615.
23. Klien BA. Ischemic infarcts of the choroid (Elschnig spots): a cause of retinal separation in hypertensive disease with renal insufficiency. A clinical and histopathologic study. Am J Ophthalmol 1968; 66:1069–1074.
24. Leuenberger A, Gasche A. Lichtkoagulation der Retinopathia serosa centralis. Ophthalmologica 1972; 165:368–372.
25. Yoshioka H, Katsume Y. Experimental central serous retinopathy. III. Ultrastructural findings. Jpn J Ophthalmol 1982; 26:397–402.
26. Yoshioka H, Katsume Y, Akune H. Experimental central serous chorioretinopathy. I. Clinical findings. Jpn J Ophthalmol 1981; 25:112–118.
27. Dellaporta A. Central serous retinopathy. Trans Am Ophthalmol Soc 1976; 74:144–153.
28. Lyons DE. Conservative management of central serous retinopathy. Trans Ophthalmol Soc UK 1977; 97:214–216.
29. Yannuzzi LA. Type A behavior and central serous chorioretinopathy. Trans Am Ophthalmol Soc 1986; 84:799–845.
30. Yannuzzi LA, Schatz H, Gitter KA. Central serous chorioretinopathy. In: The macula: a comprehensive text and atlas. Baltimore: Williams & Wilkins; 1979.
31. Masuda T. A study of chorioretinitis centralis. Chuo Ganka Iho 1915; 7:123–152.
32. Masuda T. Clinical studies of central serous chorioretinitis. Acta Soc Ophthalmol Jpn 1916; 20:1518–1552.
33. Masuda T. Clinical studies of central serous chorioretinitis. Acta Soc Ophthalmol Jpn 1917; 20:158–186, 478–508, 1049–1066, 1381–1399, 1518–1552.
34. Mitsui Y, Sakanashi R. Central angiospastic retinopathy. Am J Ophthalmol 1956; 41:105–114.
35. Bouzas EA, Scott MH, Mastorakos G et al. Central serous chorioretinopathy in endogenous hypercortisolism. Arch Ophthalmol 1993; 111:1229–1233.
36. Carvalho-Recchia CA, Yannuzzi LA, Negrao AS et al. Corticosteroids and central serous chorioretinopathy. Ophthalmology 2002; 109:1834–1837.
37. Thoelen AM, Bernasconi PP, Schmid C et al. Central serous chorioretinopathy associated with a carcinoma of the adrenal cortex. Retina 2000; 20:98–99.
38. Dollery CT, Henkind P, Kohner EM et al. Effect of raised intraocular pressure on the retinal and choroidal circulation. Invest Ophthalmol 1968; 7:191–198.
39. Hayreh SS. The choriocapillaris. Graefes Arch Clin Exp Ophthalmol 1974; 192:165–179.
40. Shimizu K, Ujiie K. Structure of ocular vessels. Tokyo: Igaku-Shoin; 1978:1–7, 50–92.
41. Yoneya S, Tso MOM. Angioarchitecture of the human choroid. Arch Ophthalmol 1987; 105:681–687.
42. Gaudric A, Coscas G, Bird AC. Choroidal ischemia. Am J Ophthalmol 1982; 94:489–498.
43. Morse PH. Elschnig's spots and hypertensive choroidopathy. Am J Ophthalmol 1968; 66:844–852.
44. Fastenberg DM, Fetkenhour CL, Choromokos E et al. Choroidal vascular changes in toxemia of pregnancy. Am J Ophthalmol 1980; 89:362–368.
45. Gitter KA, Houser BP, Sarin LK et al. Toxemia of pregnancy. an angiographic interpretation of fundus changes. Arch Ophthalmol 1968; 80:449–454.
46. Mabie WC, Ober RR. Fluorescein angiography in toxemia of pregnancy. Br J Ophthalmol 1980; 64:666–671.
47. Oliver M, Uchenik D. Bilateral exudative retinal detachment in eclampsia without hypertensive retinopathy. Am J Ophthalmol 1980; 90:792–796.
48. Jampol LM, Lahav M, Albert DM et al. Ocular clinical findings and basement membrane changes in Goodpasture's syndrome. Am J Ophthalmol 1975; 79:452–463.
49. Percival SPB. Ocular findings in thrombotic thrombocytopenic purpura (Moschcowitz's disease). Br J Ophthalmol 1970; 54:73–78.
50. Stefani FH, Brandt E, Pielsticker K. Periarteritis nodosa and thrombotic thrombocytopenic purpura with serous retinal detachment in siblings. Br J Ophthalmol 1978; 62:402–407.

51. Cogan DG. Ocular involvement in disseminated intravascular coagulopathy. Arch Ophthalmol 1975; 93:1–8.

52. Foulds WS. Do we need a retinal pigment epithelium (or choroid) for the maintenance of retinal apposition? Br J Ophthalmol 1985; 69:237–239.

52a. Foulds WS, Lee WR, Taylor WOG. Clinical and pathological aspects of choroidal ischaemia. Trans Ophthalmol Soc UK 1971; 91:325–343.

53. Amalric P. Le territoire chorioretinien de l'artère ciliaire longue postérieure. Etude clinique. Bull Soc Ophthalmol Fr 1963; 63:342–351.

54. Amalric P. Acute choroidal ischaemia. Trans Ophthalmol Soc UK 1971; 91:305–324.

55. Goldbaum MH, Galinos SO, Apple D et al. Acute choroidal ischemia as a complication of photocoagulation. Arch Ophthalmol 1976; 94:1025–1035.

56. Anderson DR, Davis EB. Retina and optic nerve after posterior ciliary artery occlusion: an experimental study in squirrel monkeys. Arch Ophthalmol 1974; 92:422–426.

57. Hayreh SS, Baines JAB. Occlusion of the posterior ciliary artery. II. Chorioretinal lesions. Br J Ophthalmol 1972; 56:736–753.

58. Ernest JT, Stern WH, Archer DB. Submacular choroidal circulation. Am J Ophthalmol 1976; 81:574–582.

59. Stern WH, Ernest JT. Microsphere occlusion of the choriocapillaris in rhesus monkeys. Am J Ophthalmol 1974; 78:438–448.

60. Deutman AF, Lion F. Choriocapillaris nonperfusion in acute multifocal placoid pigment epitheliopathy. Am J Ophthalmol 1977; 84:652–658.

61. Young NJA, Bird AC, Sehmi K. Pigment epithelial diseases with abnormal choroidal perfusion. Am J Ophthalmol 1980; 90:607–618.

62. Gass JDM, Jallow S. Idiopathic serous detachment of the choroid, ciliary body, and retina (uveal effusion syndrome). Ophthalmology 1982; 89: 1018–1032.

63. Schepens CL, Brockhurst RJ. Uveal effusion. 1. Clinical picture. Arch Ophthalmol 1963; 70:189–210.

63a. Calhoun FP Jr. The management of glaucoma in nanophthalmos. Trans Am Ophthalmol Soc 1975; 73:97–122.

64. Bok D. Retinal photoreceptor–pigment epithelium interactions. Invest Ophthalmol Vis Sci 1985; 26:1659–1694.

65. Brockhurst RJ. Nanophthalmos with uveal effusion: a new clinical study. Arch Ophthalmol 1975; 93:1289–1299.

66. Vine AV. Uveal effusion in Hunter's syndrome. Retina 1986; 6:57–60.

67. Brockhurst RJ. Vortex vein decompression for nanophthalmic uveal effusion. Arch Ophthalmol 1980; 98:1987–1990.

68. Stiebel-Kalish H, Setton A, Nimii Y et al. Cavernous sinus dural arteriovenous malformations: patterns of venous drainage are related to clinical signs and symptoms. Ophthalmology 2002; 109:1685–1691.

69. Gass JDM. Uveal effusion syndrome: a new hypothesis concerning pathogenesis and technique of surgical treatment. Trans Am Ophthalmol Soc 1983; 81:246–260.

70. Mashayekhi A, Shields CL. Circumscribed choroidal hemangioma. Curr Opin Ophthalmol 2003; 14:142–149.

71. Gass JDM. Pathogenesis of disciform detachment of the neuroepithelium. III. Senile disciform macular degeneration. Am J Ophthalmol 1967; 63:617–644.

72. Gass JDM. Pathogenesis of tears of the retinal pigment epithelium. Br J Ophthalmol 1984; 68:513–519.

73. Casswell AG, Kohen D, Bird AC. Retinal pigment epithelial detachments in the elderly: classification and outcome. Br J Ophthalmol 1985; 69: 397–403.

74. Chuang EL, Bird AC. Repair after tears of the retinal pigment epithelium. Eye 1988; 2:106.

75. Pagliarini S, Barondes MJ, Chisholm IH et al. Detection of subpigment epithelial neovascularization in cases of retinal pigment eithelial detachments: a review of the Moorfields treatment trial. Br J Ophthalmol 1992; 76:8–10.

75a. Moorfields Macular Study Group. Retinal pigment epithelial detachments in the elderly: a controlled trial of argon laser photocoagulation. Br J Ophthalmol 1982; 66:1–16.

75b. Chen J, Fitzke F, Pauliekhoff D et al. Functional loss in age-related Bruch's membrane change with choroidal perfusion defect. Invest Ophthalmol Vis Sci 1992; 33:334–340.

76. Tsuboi S. Measurement of the volume flow and hydraulic conductivity across the isolated dog retinal pigment epithelium. Invest Ophthalmol Vis Sci 1987; 28:1776–1782.

77. Moore DJ, Hussain AA, Marshall J. Age related variation in the hydraulic conductivity of Bruch's membrane. Invest Ophthal Vis Sci 1995; 36: 1290–1297.

78. Loffler KU, Lee WR. Basal linear deposit in the human macula. Graefes Arch Clin Exp Ophthalmol 1986; 224:493–501.

79. Pauleikhoff D, Harper CA, Marshall J et al. Aging changes in Bruch's membrane: a histochemical and morphological study. Ophthalmology 1990; 97:171–180.

80. Sheraidah G, Steinmetz R, Maguire J et al. Correlation between lipids extracted from Bruch's membrane and age. Ophthalmology 1993; 100:47–51.

81. Pauleikhoff D, Zuels S, Sheraidah G et al. Determinants of the fluorescence of drusen in Bruch's membrane. Ophthalmology 1992; 99:1548–1553.

82. Decker WL, Sanborn GE, Ridley M et al. Retinal pigment epithelial tears. Ophthalmology 1983; 90:507–512.

83. Hoskin A, Bird AC, Sehmi K. Tears of detached retinal pigment epithelium. Br J Ophthalmol 1981; 65:417–422.

84. Krishan NR, Chandra SR, Stevens TS. Diagnosis and pathogenesis of retinal pigment epithelial tears. Am J Ophthalmol 1985; 100:698–707.

85. Chuang EL, Bird AC. Bilaterality of tears of the retinal pigment epithelium. Br J Ophthalmol 1988; 72:918–920.

86. Schoeppner G, Chuang EL, Bird AC. Retinal pigment epithelial tears: risk to the second eye. Am J Ophthalmol 1989; 108:683–685.

87. Chuang EL, Bird AC. The pathogenesis of tears of the retinal pigment epithelium. Am J Ophthalmol 1988; 105:285–290.

88. Coffey AJH, Brownstein S. The prevalence of macular drusen in postmortem eyes. Am J Ophthalmol 1986; 102:164–171.

89. Barondes M, Pauleikhoff D, Chisholm IH et al. Bilaterality of drusen. Br J Ophthalmol 1990; 74:180–182.

90. Pauleikhoff D, Chen JC, Chisholm IH et al. Choroidal perfusion abnormalities in age related macular disease. Am J Ophthalmol 1990; 109: 211–217.

91. Korte GE, Repucci V, Henkind P. RPE destruction causes choriocapillary atrophy. Invest Ophthalmol Vis Sci 1984; 25:1135–1145.

92. Glaser BM, Campochiaro PA, Davis JL Jr et al. Retinal pigment epithelial cells release an inhibitor of neovascularization. Arch Ophthalmol 1985; 103:1870–1875.

93. Olver J, Pauleikhoff D, Bird AC. Morphometric analysis of age changes in the choriocapillaris. Invest Ophthalmol Vis Sci 1990; 31(Suppl):47.

94. Sunness JS, Massoff RW, Johnson MA et al. Diminished foveal sensitivity may predict the development of advanced age-related macular degeneration. Ophthalmology 1989; 96:375–380.

95. Slakter JS, Yannuzzi LA, Schneider U et al. Retinal choroidal anastomoses and occult choroidal neovascularization in age-related macular degeneration. Ophthalmology 2000; 107:742–753.

96. Weinberger D, Lichter H, Goldenberg-Cohen N et al. Retinal microangiopathies overlying pigment epithelial detachment in age-related macular degeneration. Retina 2002; 22:406–411.

97. Yannuzzi LA, Negrao S, Iida T et al. Retinal angiomatous proliferation in age-related macular degeneration. Retina 2001; 21:416–434.

98. Ahuja RM, Stanga PE, Vingerling JR et al. Polypoidal choroidal vasculopathy in exudative and haemorrhagic pigment epithelial detachments. Br J Ophthalmol 2000; 84:479–484.

99. Kwok A, Lai TY, Chan CW et al. Polypoidal choroidal vasculopathy in Chinese patients. Br J Ophthalmol 2002; 86:892–897.

100. Tateiwa H, Kuroiwa S, Gaun S et al. Polypoidal choroidal vasculopathy with large vascular network. Graefes Arch Clin Exp Ophthalmol 2002; 240:354–361.

101. Yannuzzi LA, Freund KB, Goldbaum M et al. Polypoidal choroidal vasculopathy masquerading as central serous chorioretinopathy. Ophthalmology 2000; 107:767–777.

Chapter

55

Steroids in Macular Disease

Carl H. Park
Glenn J. Jaffe

INTRODUCTION

The use of periocular and intravitreal corticosteroids to manage posterior segment disease is undergoing a minor renaissance. As the limitations and the complications of systemic corticosteroid therapy to treat ocular diseases became evident, much effort has been made to develop localized, safe, and efficacious ocular corticosteroid drug delivery methods.

Currently there are three important ocular steroid delivery modalities: (1) periocular or posterior sub-Tenon's injection; (2) intravitreal injection; (3) sustained drug delivery device systems. The first two delivery methods have a long history. The use of periocular depot corticosteroids to manage uveitis dates back to at least the 1960s.[1] In 1980, Tano, Machemer, McCuen, and others described the safety and efficacy of intravitreal triamcinolone to treat proliferative vitreoretinopathy in an animal model.[2–4] Over the last three to four years, there has been a significant increase in the use of intravitreal steroids to manage a variety of macular and retinal vascular diseases.[5] This rapid acceptance in light of the paucity of randomized controlled data may reflect the increasing frustration by clinicians with currently available treatment techniques. Although it is uncertain whether or not intraocular steroids will live up to its current popularity, it is likely that intraocular steroids will continue to have a role in the management of variety of macular diseases.

HISTORY AND BASIC SCIENCE OF CORTICOSTEROIDS

Corticosteroid use dates back to the early 1950s and the first rational use of prednisone and prednisolone for ocular diseases is attributed to Gordon in 1956.[6] Gordon described the use of both topical and systemic corticosteroids and for far ranging ocular diseases from episcleritis to sympathetic ophthalmia. It is of historical interest to note that in this paper, Gordon presented a case of a man with central serous retinopathy and 20/200 vision, who had been treated with 20 mg of Meticorten (hydrocortisone derivative) daily for three weeks with no improvement. He stated that the dose was increased to 40 mg daily with subsequent visual improvement to 20/30 by the third day.

All synthetic corticosteroids are derived from the basic sterol structure, modified to elicit different potencies as well as durations suitable for the clinical needs. In ophthalmology, the most commonly used local steroid agents are prednisolone, dexamethasone, triamcinolone, and betamethasone. Table 55-1 outlines the relative potency of different corticosteroids used in ophthalmology.

Corticosteroids have important immuno-suppressive activities. For example, systemic corticosteroids reduce helper T cell recruitment.[7,8] Neutrophil migration is also reduced following corticosteroid therapy, an effect that further blocks the immune response.[7] Cumulatively, these actions result in an anti-inflammatory effect at end organs, including the eye. There is a decreased hypersensitivity response, a decrease in phagocytic/ bactericidal activity, decreased cytokine/lymphokine production, and decreased vascular permeability.[8] Wilson et al.[9] demonstrated that a single injection of intravitreal triamcinolone acetonide (2 mg) can reduce the severity of blood–retinal barrier breakdown following pan retinal photocoagulation in a rabbit model. Sakamoto et al.[10] used triamcinolone acetonide as a surgical tool during pars plana vitrectomy for complex diabetic retinopathy and discovered that in the postoperative period, the blood–ocular barrier was more preserved compared to eyes that underwent routine vitrectomy without intraoperative triamcinolone acetonide.

Corticosteroids also have a significant anti-angiogenic capacity. Folkman and others first promulgated the angiostatic properties of corticosteroids and its derivatives.[11] The primary mechanism of action of angiostatic steroids appears to be in aiding the breakdown and blocking the formation of capillary endothelial basement membranes.[12]

Of the synthetic glucocorticosteroids, it is thought that triamcinolone and betamethasone have the most potent anti-angiogenic properties.[13] Triamcinolone acetonide appears to modulate the permeability and adhesion of human choroidal endothelial cells in culture. Penfold and associates[14] demonstrated that cytokine-induced expression of intercellular adhesion molecule-1 is down-regulated by triamcinolone acetonide. They also showed that interferon gamma-induction of vascular permeability was decreased by triamcinolone acetonide. Wang and colleagues[15] found that triamcinolone acetonide can prevent tube formation in bovine choroidal endothelial cells in a cell culture model. These investigators also demonstrated that matrix metalloproteinases were down regulated following incubation with triamcinolone suggesting that the active remodeling of the

Table 55-1 Relative steroid potency (adapted from Nussenblatt et al.[8])		
Steroid	Equivalent dosage (mg)	Relative potency
Hydrocortisone	20	1.0
Prednisolone	5	4.0
Methylprednisolone	4	5
Triamcinolone	4	5
Dexamethasone	0.75	26
Betamethasone	0.6	33

extracellular matrix necessary for neovascularization can be inhibited. Ciulla et al.[16] have shown that intravitreal triamcinolone acetonide completely inhibited laser-induced choroidal neovascularization in rats. These experiments provide rationale for using triamcinolone acetonide to treat choroidal neovascularization in exudative macular degeneration and other retinal vascular diseases.

The safety of intravitreal corticosteroids has been extensively studied in animal models. The initial interest in utilizing intravitreal steroid was aimed at the pharmacological management of proliferative vitreoretinopathy. McCuen et al.[4] injected 1 mg of triamcinolone acetonide in 21 rabbit eyes with the fellow eye serving as the control. The anterior and posterior segments, evaluated by slit lamp examination, tonometry, ophthalmoscopy, and electroretinography, did not differ between treated and control groups during the three months follow-up period. Kwak and D'Amico[17] evaluated the toxicity of dexamethasone sodium phosphate intravitreal injection at doses of 0.4 to 4.0 mg in the rabbit model. At the higher doses, on histopathology, there was increased disruption of Muller cells suggesting possible retinal toxicity at these doses. However, other animal studies have failed to demonstrate toxicity after up to 4.8 mg intravitreal injection of dexamethasone.[18] Shimada and Matsui[19] injected up to 80 mg of dexamethasone sodium phosphate (as well as equal doses of betamethasone sodium phosphate) in a rabbit model and found that doses higher than 10 mg produced localized retinal degeneration, degradation and vitreous inflammation. Hainsworth et al.[20] evaluated the safety of a sustained release preparation of dexamethasone (embedded in polymer pellet) in a rabbit model. The measured delivery rate was 1.5 μg/h. After implantation into the vitreous cavity there were no signs of retinal toxicity or functional abnormalities, as evaluated by histopathology and electroretinography, respectively.

There are data to suggest that human intravitreal steroid injection is in most part safe with minimal risk of acute drug related toxicity. Blankenship[21] evaluated the efficacy and toxicity of dexamethasone phosphate following pars plana vitrectomy for diabetic retinopathy. Twenty-seven eyes received a single intravitreal dose of 0.8 mg dexamethasone phosphate and thirty eyes that did not receive the injection served as the control

group. There were no clinical signs of toxicity in the treated group at six months. All outcome measures, including visual acuity, cataract formation, and post-vitrectomy membrane formations were equal between the two groups. Also the increased use of intravitreal triamcinolone acetonide use to treat various macular diseases has produced a literature body of "human safety trials." Although most studies have used 4 mg of triamcinolone acetonide for intravitreal injection, single doses up to 25 mg injected in to the human vitreous cavity, do not appear to cause significant toxicity.[22]

The pharmacokinetics of the various intravitreal steroid delivery modalities have been studied to gain insight to the possible duration of the therapeutic effect. There have been several animal studies and human investigations to examine the pharmacokinetics of intravitreal steroid clearance. Short acting corticosteroid formulations, such as dexamethasone sodium phosphate have a relatively short half-life measured in days.[17] Schindler and co-workers[23] evaluated to clearance rate for intravitreal triamcinolone acetonide injection in a rabbit model. They performed both ophthalmoscopy and colorimetric tests to determine the clearance of 0.5 mg triamcinolone acetonide injected into rabbit eyes that underwent no surgery, vitrectomy, or vitrectomy combined with lensectomy. They found that in eyes that had no surgery, the drug disappeared in 41 days compared to 16.8 days and 6.5 days for eyes that had vitrectomy and vitrectomy–lensectomy, respectively.

Scholes et al.[24] evaluated the clearance rate of 0.4 mg intravitreal triamcinolone acetonide also in a nonvitrectomized rabbit model. By high-performance liquid chromatography the elimination half-life was 1.6 days. This value is significantly shorter than that observed in studies described above. The peak triamcinolone concentration was 235 μg, which decreased to 66 μg at 13 days. No drug was detectable by 21 days in most of the eyes. Interestingly, by ophthalmoscopic examination white aggregates of presumed triamcinolone acetonide were visible up to 23 days, suggesting that the visible presence of the white aggregate may not correlate with therapeutic triamcinolone acetonide levels.

The pharmacokinetics of intravitreal triamcinolone acetonide have been studied in humans.[25] In this study, five patients received a single 4 mg triamcinolone acetonide intravitreal injection. The aqueous humor samples were obtained by anterior chamber tap at several time points up to 31 days. The peak aqueous humor concentration ranged from 2000 to 7000 ng/ml and the half-life of the drug was 76 to 635 hours. The mean elimination half-life for nonvitrectomized eyes was 18.6 days while the half-life for vitrectomized eyes was only 3.2 days. Given the calculated half-life, a single 4 mg intravitreal injection of triamcinolone acetonide could be expected to last approximately three months in a nonvitrectomized eye.

Sustained drug delivery devices have potential pharmacodynamic advantages. Depending on the device configuration, they can release a constant drug concentration over a prolonged time period, ideally over the disease duration. Fluocinolone acetonide is a synthetic corticosteroid, with an extremely low aqueous solubility. This low solubility allowed development of a sustained release device with a relatively small "footprint."[68] In a rabbit model, the fluocinolone acetonide implant (Control Delivery Systems, Watertown, Mass., USA) provided steady state drug levels ranging from 0.10 to 0.21 μg/ml over a one-year period. The predicted life span of the two mg device was estimated to be almost three years. Further studies are underway to evaluate its use in patients with refractory uveitis, age-related macular degeneration, diabetic macular edema, and macular edema associated with vein occlusion.

AGE-RELATED MACULAR DEGENERATION

The treatment of choroidal neovascularization associated with age-related macular degeneration has evolved from thermal photocoagulation expounded by the Macular Photocoagulation Studies to ocular photodynamic therapy with verteporfin.[26,27] As the limitations of laser treatments have become apparent, there has been great interest in developing pharmacological therapies for choroidal neovascularization. Various antiangiogenic factors, including rhuFab (Lucentis, Genentech, USA) and Pegaptanib sodium aptamer (Macugen, EyeTech Pharm, USA) are currently undergoing multicenter phase three clinical trials. Corticosteroids with antiangiogenic properties are also being investigated as possible treatment for neovascular age-related macular degeneration.

Penfold et al.[28] published a pilot study for the treatment of neovascular age-related macular degeneration with intravitreal triamcinolone acetonide. Their preliminary data evaluating 30 eyes treated with intravitreal triamcinolone injection demonstrated decreased leakage by fluorescein angiography and increased visual acuity. A small, randomized clinical trial was conducted to evaluate the safety and effectiveness of a single 4 mg intravitreal triamcinolone acetonide injection for neovascular age-related macular degeneration.[29] At both the three and six-month follow-up visits, the treated group had statistically significant better visual acuity than the control group. The angiographic appearance was also better in the treated group compared to the control group. Adverse events from the injection included intraocular pressure elevation seen in 25% of the patients and cataract progression in the treated group.

In a separate report, triamcinolone acetonide was injected into the vitreous cavity of 14 consecutive patients with recurrent choroidal neovascularization following extrafoveal thermal laser treatment.[30] Following intravitreal injection, the mean visual acuity remained stable; these results were comparable to the laser re-treatment group in the Macular Photocoagulation Study.[31]

Jonas et al.[32] performed an uncontrolled study of intravitreal triamcinolone acetonide to treat exudative age-related macular degeneration. Of 71 treated eyes, 68 had predominantly or totally occult choroidal neovascularization, as determined by fluorescein angiography. With a mean follow-up of 7 months, the visual acuity was found to increase from a preinjection mean of 0.16 to a maximum of 0.23 ($P < 0.001$). The maximal visual acuity was attained at one to three months postinjection. The average intraocular pressure increased from a baseline of 15.1 mmHg to 23.0 mmHg. There were no significant postoperative complications, such as endophthalmitis and retinal detachment.

Gillies and associates[33] conducted a randomized, double-masked, placebo-controlled trial of single-dose 4 mg triamcinolone acetonide intravitreal injection in patients with classic choroidal neovascularization associated with age-related macular degeneration. At 12 months the risk of severe visual loss (30 letters) was 35% for both the treated group and the placebo group. Although the visual acuity did not differ between the treated and control groups, at three months, the choroidal neovascular complex appeared to be smaller in the treated group. At 12 months, however, there was no difference in lesion size between the groups. The smaller lesion size at three months suggested an anti-angiogenic effect of intravitreal triamcinolone acetonide over the three months following injection, which may have diminished as the drug was cleared. It is not known whether repeated injections would provide a sustained benefit to stabilize visual acuity and lesion size. However, there was a statistically significant elevation in intraocular pressure in the treated group compared to the placebo group, which may be one of the factors (among others) that may limit a long-term reinjection protocol for the treatment of choroidal neovascularization.

Verteporfin ocular photodynamic therapy has been combined with intravitreal triamcinolone acetonide to treat choroidal neovascularization associated with age-related macular degeneration.[34] The rationale for this approach is to decrease the number of photodynamic treatments (as well as the cost associated with these multiple treatments) by combining the angiostatic properties of triamcinolone acetonide with the vascular occlusion induced by ocular photodynamic therapy. In a small pilot study of 26 eyes (13 eyes naïve to photodynamic therapy and 13 eyes previously treated with photodynamic therapy), the retreatment rate at three-month follow-up was 7.7% (two of 26 eyes). At the six-month follow-up visit, no eyes required retreatment. A multicenter, randomized trial is currently underway to compare verteporfin ocular photodynamic therapy alone to ocular photodynamic therapy with intravitreal triamcinolone acetonide for neovascular age-related macular degeneration. The main outcome measures include visual acuity improvement and the number of verteporfin treatments.

Anecortave acetate (Alcon Research, Ltd., Fort Worth, TX) is currently being investigated to treat subfoveal choroidal neovascularization associated with age-related macular degeneration.[35,36] Anecortave acetate is a novel steroid compound, which has been shown to have potent antiangiogenic properties with minimal glucocorticoid effects.[37] It is an effective antiangiogenic drug in corneal neovascularization, intraocular tumor, and retinopathy of prematurity animal models.[38–40] Anecortave acetate is injected through a proprietary cannula. It is introduced at the juxtascleral plane at the superotemporal quadrant and advanced to reach the posterior juxtascleral space (see Fig. 55-1). The twelve month results from a masked, randomized, placebo-controlled trial indicates that a 15 mg posterior juxtascleral anecortave acetate depot, injected at six month intervals, reduced severe vision loss (30 letters) compared to

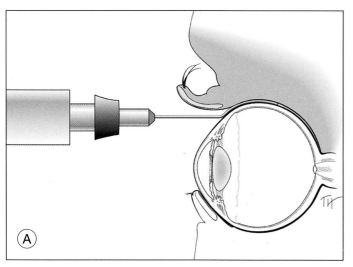
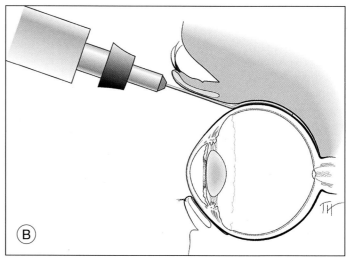

Fig. 55-1 Posterior juxtascleral administration of anecortave acetate. (A) Proprietary 56-degree posterior juxtascleral cannula is introduced through a small superotemporal quadrant incision 8 mm posterior to the limbus. (B) The cannula is "glided" along bare sclera until the full advancement is reached. The medicine is injected slowly with cotton swab pressure along the cannula to prevent reflux. (Courtesy Alcon Research, Ltd.)

the placebo group (0% vs. 23%, respectively).[36] Eighty percent of the enrolled eyes had predominantly classic lesions on fluorescein angiography. There were no significant safety concerns that were attributed to the injection. Notably, there were no reports of globe perforation. There were no serious adverse events reported during the follow-up period and the intraocular pressure levels remained unchanged. Interestingly, the 30 mg dose of anecortave acetate appeared to be less efficacious than the 15 mg dose. Further studies are currently underway to evaluate anecortave acetate treatment of neovascular age-related macular degeneration, including a study in which anecortave acetate is compared to verteporfin photodynamic therapy.

DIABETIC MACULAR EDEMA

Diabetic macular edema is the most frequent cause of visual loss in patients with nonproliferative diabetic retinopathy. The Early Treatment of Diabetic Retinopathy Study Research Group studies[41,42] found that the three-year risk of moderate visual loss (doubling of the visual angle) for patients with foveal or perifoveal macular edema was 24% for the control group and 12% for the laser-treated group. Only 2% of the treated eyes had a three or more line visual acuity improvement. Although laser can control the diabetic macular edema extent, it may be less safe when microaneurysms are near the foveal center. Furthermore, the efficacy may be limited by development of focal scotomas, by development of choroidal neovascularization, and by underlying macular ischemia.[42,43] Often patients have refractory macular edema despite several focal or grid laser treatments.

Martidis and co-workers[44] prospectively evaluated sixteen eyes with refractory diabetic macular edema (no response to at least two previous laser photocoagulation sessions) following intravitreal triamcinolone acetonide injection (4 mg) (see Fig. 55-2). The mean visual acuity improved by 2.4 Snellen lines

at one month post-injection. At three and six months follow-up, the visual acuity improvement was 2.4 and 1.3 Snellen lines, respectively. The mean central macular thickness as measured by optical coherence tomography decreased from 540 μm preinjection to 242 μm at one month. At three and six months, the macular thickness measured 224 μm and 335 μm, respectively. No significant complications were noted except for a temporary increase in intraocular pressure in five of 16 eyes at the one-month follow-up visit. The authors concluded that intravitreal triamcinolone was a promising form of therapy, especially since these study eyes had a long history of macular edema (average 32 months) and multiple failed laser photocoagulation treatments (2.6 sessions). Jonas and associates[45] also prospectively evaluated 26 eyes with diffuse macular edema treated with intravitreal triamcinolone acetonide injection (25 mg). In this study, visual acuity improved from a baseline of 0.12 LogMar units to a maximum of 0.19 LogMar units during the study follow-up period. Intraocular pressure also increased significantly from 16.9 to 17.7 mmHg and returned to normal by the end of the follow-up period.

At least two sustained corticosteroid drug delivery systems are currently undergoing clinical trials to treat diabetic macular edema. A nonbiodegradable intravitreal fluocinolone acetonide implant (Retisert™, Bausch & Lomb, Rochester, NY and Control Delivery Systems, Watertown, Mass.), designed to release over a three year period has been evaluated in a multicenter, randomized clinical trial for use in patients with refractory macular edema.[46] Eighty patients were randomized to receive either an implant (0.5 mg and 2.0 mg) or standard of care (macular laser or observation). At 12 months follow-up, 49% of the eyes treated with the 0.5 mg implant had resolution of their macular edema compared to 25% for the standard of care group ($P < 0.05$). The 0.5 mg implant group was more likely to show an improvement of 15 letters compared to standard of care group (20% vs. 7%) but the difference did not reach statistical significance.

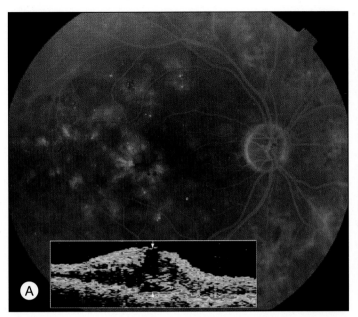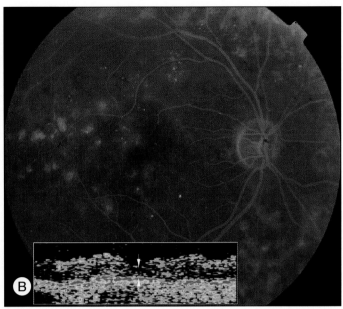

Fig. 55-2 Diabetic macular edema. (A) Right eye of a 56-year-old man with history of two previous focal lasers. Vision was 20/80. Fluorescein angiogram demonstrated focal microaneurysmal leakage and cystoid type macular edema. Horizontal optical coherence tomogram (inset) of the fovea demonstrated cystic intraretinal edema with a trace subretinal fluid. (B) Four months after intravitreal triamcinolone acetonide (4 mg) injection the vision has improved to 20/30. Angiogram demonstrates decreased leakage. Horizontal tomogram (inset) demonstrates restoration of the foveal contour. (Courtesy Adam Martidis, MD.)

More patients in the standard of care group had worsening diabetic retinopathy at twelve-months compared to the 0.5 mg implant group (30% vs. 5%). The incidence of serious ocular adverse events, which included increased intraocular pressure, vitreous hemorrhage, and cataract formation, was significantly higher in the implant group (59%) vs. the standard of care group (11%). The trial is expected to continue for an additional three years to monitor implant efficacy and safety. Another steroid drug delivery system undergoing investigation is the biodegradable dexamethasone posterior segment drug delivery system (Posurdex®, Allergan, Irvine, CA), which is being studied for patients with macular edema associated with diabetic retinopathy, vein occlusions, pseudophakia, and uveitis. In a phase 2 study, eyes that received the 700 μg dexamethasone implant had a statistically significant improvement in visual acuity and retinal thickness compared to the control group (Kupperman et al., American Academy of Ophthalmology 2003 Annual Meeting paper presentation). A phase 3 trial is currently ongoing.

RETINAL VASCULAR DISEASES

Retinal vein occlusion

A natural history study of perfused central retinal vein occlusion suggests that approximately 50% of eyes with an initial visual acuity of 20/50 or worse will have a visual acuity of 20/250 or worse at three years.[47] Cystoid macular edema is the most significant ocular morbidity that accounts for visual acuity loss in these patients. In the Central Vein Occlusion Study[48] 155 eyes with a visual acuity of 20/50 or worse and cystoid macular edema were randomly assigned to observation or mac-

ular grid pattern laser photocoagulation. The study demonstrated that macular grid pattern laser photocoagulation did not have a beneficial effect on visual acuity. There is clearly a need for new treatments to manage cystoid macular edema associated central retinal vein occlusion.

Greenberg and colleagues[49] were the first to report intravitreal triamcinolone acetonide to treat macular edema associated with central retinal vein occlusion. They reported a case of an 80-year-old woman who presented with a chronic central retinal vein occlusion in the right eye and an acute occlusion in the left. The left eye was injected with 4 mg of triamcinolone acetonide. The visual acuity improved from 20/400 to 20/30 at three months. The improvement in visual acuity was associated with macular edema resolution; the central macular thickness (measured by optical coherence tomography) decreased from 489 μm to 160 μm at three months. At six months, the edema returned with concurrent drop in vision to 20/400. Triamcinolone acetonide was reinjected and the visual acuity improved to 20/50. Subsequently, triamcinolone acetonide was injected into the right eye (with chronic central retina vein occlusion). The macular edema resolved in the right eye; however, there was no improvement in visual acuity, suggesting that the macular edema chronicity may have contributed to irreversible photoreceptor damage and vision loss.

There have been several other case reports of using intravitreal triamcinolone acetonide to treat macular edema associated with retinal vein occlusion.[50,51] Park and co-workers reported a case series of triamcinolone acetonide to treat macular edema in eyes with perfused central retinal vein occlusion and visual acuity of 20/50 or worse.[52] Following a single 4 mg intravitreal triamcinolone injection, the mean visual acuity improved from 58 ETDRS letters to 78 letters at last follow-up (see Fig. 55-3). Before treatment, all ten treated eyes had both angiographic and optical coherence tomographic evidence of macular edema. Following treatment, macular edema, as demonstrated by optical coherence tomography, improved in all eyes (see Fig. 55-3). The mean macular volume decreased from 4.2 mm^3 to 2.6 mm^3 at last follow-up. One eye required re-injection five months following initial therapy because of cystoid macular edema recurrence. Four of ten eyes required either initiation or escalation of glaucoma therapy secondary to increased intraocular pressure during the follow-up period. There were no other significant complications.

The Branch Vein Occlusion Study[53] supported the finding that grid type laser photocoagulation may reduce the risk of visual loss from macular edema. In this study, patients without macular ischemia, without foveal hemorrhages, and vision acuity better than 20/40 were specifically enrolled. There have been reports of using intravitreal triamcinolone either as a first line treatment or as a rescue treatment following macular grid laser for cystoid macular edema associated with branch vein occlusion. In a case series of 20 eyes with cystoid macular

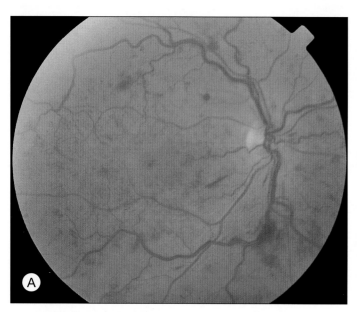

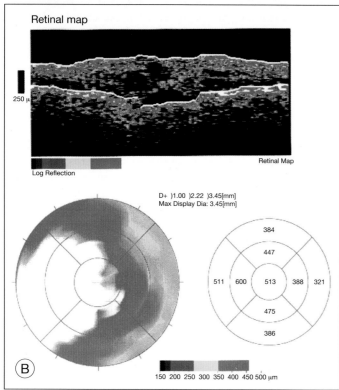

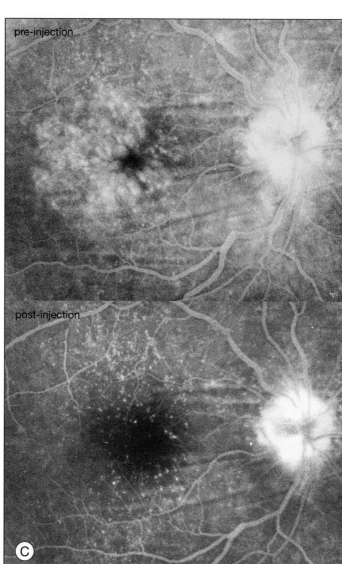

Fig. 55-3 (A) A 58-year-old man presented with a six-month history of central retinal vein occlusion. Vision was 20/60. Pre-injection fundus photograph demonstrated a congested optic nerve and diffuse intraretinal hemorrhages. There was marked cystoid macular edema. (B) Optical coherence tomogram demonstrated diffuse thickening of the neurosensory retina. The mean central retinal thickness was 513 micron with total macular volume of 4.07 mm^3. (C) Pre-injection and three months post-intravitreal triamcinolone acetonide injection fluorescein angiograms show resolution of the cystoid macular edema.

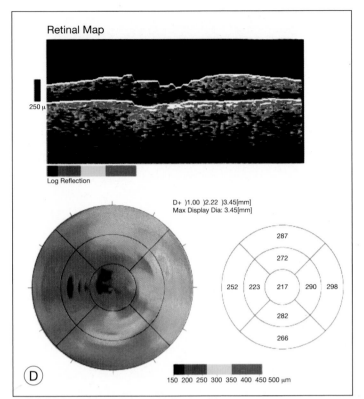

Retinal Map

250 µ

Log Reflection

D+)1.00)2.22)3.45[mm]
Max Display Dia: 3.45[mm]

287
272
252 223 217 290 298
282
266

150 200 250 300 350 400 450 500 µm

(D)

Fig. 55-3—cont'd (D) Six months post-injection the vision has improved to 20/20. OCT demonstrates restoration of the foveal contour. The mean central retinal thickness is 217 microns. The total macular volume is 2.51 mm³.

edema secondary to branch vein occlusion and no previous laser (baseline vision of 20/40 to 20/200), there was an average three Snellen lines of visual acuity improvement at six months (Martidis, Retina Congress 2002, San Francisco, CA). Macular edema, as determined by optical coherence tomography, resolved in nearly all eyes (see Fig. 55-4). Chen et al.[54] have reported a case of a patient with ischemic macular edema secondary to branch vein occlusion treated successfully with intravitreal triamcinolone acetonide injection. A randomized clinical trial is clearly needed to further define the safety and efficacy of intravitreal steroid injection in the management of patients with vein occlusions.

Idiopathic juxtafoveal telangiectasis and other retinal vascular diseases

Idiopathic juxtafoveal telangiectasis is a disease typically seen in middle-aged men who have unilateral, localized perifoveal capillary telangiectasis, usually on the temporal side.[55] Most commonly, patients have good vision and no treatment is necessary. There is also a bilateral form of idiopathic juxtafoveal telangiectasis seen in both males and females; these patients have more significant retinal telangiectasis accompanied by retinal pigment epithelium changes. There may be a systemic association of abnormal glucose metabolism in these patients.[56] The vision can be decreased, both acutely and chronically, with secondary changes of macular edema associated with the retinal

telangiectasis. Usually, laser therapy is contraindicated because of the close proximity of the retinal telangiectasis to the fovea and the risk of choroidal neovascularization. There has been a case published by Alldredge and Garretson[57] describing successful use of intravitreal triamcinolone to treat juxtafoveal telangiectasis. There also has been a report of using intravitreal triamcinolone acetonide to manage radiation-induced retinopathy.[58]

PSEUDOPHAKIC CYSTOID MACULAR EDEMA AND UVEITIC CYSTOID MACULAR EDEMA

Postoperative cystoid macular edema is seen in approximately 16 to 24% of patients following extracapsular cataract extraction.[59] Although most of these patients are asymptomatic, a small percentage may develop visually disabling, chronic macular edema that does not respond to topical steroid or nonsteroidal therapy.

Conway et al.[60] reported a retrospective review of eight eyes with refractory pseudophakic cystoid macular edema treated with 1 mg of intravitreal triamcinolone acetonide. Visual acuity and fluorescein angiographic leakage improved following triamcinolone acetonide injection. However, all eyes required relatively early re-injections for recurrent macular edema. Benhamou et al.[61] reported a prospective case series of three eyes undergoing 8 mg injection of intravitreal triamcinolone acetonide for refractory pseudophakic cystoid macular edema. They reported that one month after injection, there was a decrease in macular thickness as measured by optical coherence tomography with a corresponding improvement in visual acuity. However triamcinolone acetonide was re-injected in two of the three eyes, and by three months, macular edema had again recurred.

Refractory cystoid macular edema is one of the most important reasons for decreased visual acuity in patients with chronic uveitis.[62] Yoshikawa et al.[63] described a case series of 39 eyes treated with sub-Tenon's corticosteroids for uveitis-associated cystoid macular edema. Following the injection, visual acuity improved by two or more lines, and macular edema decreased, in 22 of 39 eyes. Helm and Holland[64] described a series of twenty consecutive eyes treated with posterior sub-Tenon's injection of triamcinolone acetonide. Visual acuity improvement was seen in 67% of the patients. There was a significant incidence of increased intraocular pressure (30%), which peaked at 14 weeks after injection. Intraocular pressure elevation following posterior sub-Tenon's injection can be seen in 13 to 44% of eyes, with higher incidence of pressure elevation in eyes with previous history of topical steroid response and eyes with uveitis.[65]

Antcliff et al.[66] have described the use of intravitreal injection of triamcinolone acetonide for treatment of uveitic cystoid macular edema. In a case series of six patients who were refractory to systemic and periocular steroids, 2 mg of triamcinolone acetonide was injected into the vitreous cavity. Optical coherence tomography of the fovea demonstrated a complete resolution of the cystoid macular edema in five of six patients within one week of injection. The mean visual acuity at one year was 0.27.

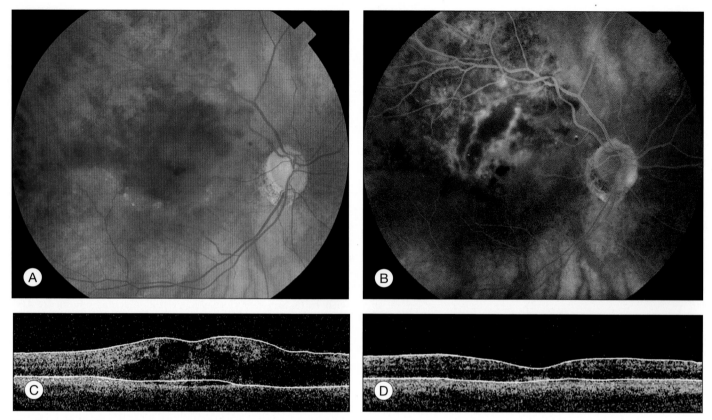

Fig. 55-4 (A) A 54-year-old woman presented with an eight-month history of branch retinal vein occlusion. Vision was 20/200. There was a superotemporal branch vein occlusion with significant intraretinal hemorrhage and edema. (B) Fluorescein angiogram demonstrated areas of nonperfusion as well as leakage. (C) Optical coherence tomogram demonstrated massive cystic intraretinal thickening. (D) One-month post-intravitreal triamcinolone acetonide injection, the vision has improved to 20/50. Tomogram demonstrates resolution of the foveal contour (Courtesy Adam Martidis, MD.)

A fluocinolone acetonide sustained drug delivery device has been used to treat severe uveitis refractory to conventional systemic immunosuppression and periocular steroid injections.[67] Fluocinolone acetonide is a synthetic corticosteroid with a low aqueous solubility.[68] The drug is encased in a polyvinyl acetate/silicone laminate, which is designed to be surgically implanted through the pars plana. In pharmacokinetic studies, the drug has been shown to maintain a constant vitreous level over at least one-year period.[68] In a pilot study, the fluocinolone acetonide sustained drug delivery device was implanted into seven eyes with refractory, severe uveitis.[67] All eyes demonstrated clinical evidence of decreased inflammation and four of seven eyes demonstrated at least three lines of visual acuity improvement. Four eyes developed increased intraocular pressure, which was controlled with topical therapy. Currently, further studies are underway to demonstrate the feasibility of using this implant in other refractory retinal vascular diseases including chronic diabetic maculopathy and retinal vein occlusions.

COMPLICATIONS OF PERIOCULAR AND INTRAVITREAL STEROID INJECTIONS

The complications of periocular and intravitreal steroid injections can include injection complications (globe perforation, retinal/choroidal vascular occlusion,[69] vitreous hemorrhage, retinal detachment), cataract progression, elevated intraocular pressure, and endophthalmitis. The most common complications seen following both periocular and intravitreal steroid injection is elevated intraocular pressure seen in approximately 10 to 50% of the patients. Periocular injection, if done correctly, to place the entire depot of steroid in the posterior space, probably has a lower risk of intraocular pressure elevation than the intravitreal injection of steroids. Jonas et al.[70] prospectively evaluated the intraocular pressure of 75 eyes undergoing 25 mg intravitreal injection of triamcinolone acetonide for various posterior segment diseases. The intraocular pressure increased from a baseline of 14.9 mmHg to a peak of 20.8 mmHg at six months (approximately 50% of patients lost to follow-up). They concluded that 50% of eyes that undergo 25 mg injection of intravitreal triamcinolone acetonide develop an intraocular pressure elevation; however, most eyes could be controlled with topical medications alone and the pressure normalized after six months. Bakri and Beer[71] published a retrospective series of 43 consecutive eyes undergoing 4 mg intravitreal triamcinolone injection for various pathologies. At 12 weeks, 49% of the eyes demonstrated an intraocular pressure elevation of greater than or equal to 5 mmHg. Twenty-eight percent of the eyes demonstrated a pressure rise of 10 mmHg or more. However, all patients responded well to topical glaucoma medications. Given that the cumulative data for periocular and intravitreal steroid therapy suggest a moderate to severe elevated intraocular pressure in a significant percentage eyes, the informed consent for steroid injection should include a careful discussion of the possibility of steroid-induced glaucoma and/or decompensation of an existing glaucoma.

Perhaps the most feared complication following intravitreal triamcinolone injection is infectious endophthalmitis. This is to be differentiated from the numerous reports of sterile intraocular inflammation seen after intravitreal triamcinolone injection. Because steroid is presumed to cause a local area of immunosuppression in the vitreous cavity, the risk of increased rate of endophthalmitis compared to other intravitreal injection drugs has been speculated. The endophthalmitis risk following triamcinolone acetonide injection should be judged against the risk of endophthalmitis following other pharmacological interventions requiring intravitreal injection. For comparison, Heinemann[72] reported one case of *Staphylococcus epidermis* endophthalmitis in 1372 total intravitreal injections (infection rate of 0.29%) for the treatment of cytomegalovirus retinitis.

Jonas et al.[22] have reported an interventional case series of 454 eyes that received a 25 mg injection of triamcinolone acetonide for variety of pathologies, including diabetic retinopathy, macular degeneration, uveitis, and vein occlusions. The preparatory steps for the injection were thorough, including 5% topical povidone-iodine scrub, local eye draping, and lid speculum placement. A 27-gauge sharp needle was used to enter the inferotemporal pars plana. Post-injection topical antibiotic ointment was applied. The supernatant was removed from the mixture prior to injection. At slitlamp evaluation on day one and one week, no patients demonstrated a true hypopyon or vitreitis. One patient had a pseudo-hypopyon, which was lavaged and found to contain triamcinolone acetonide crystals. Microbiological analysis was unremarkable. Given the case series number, the estimated risk of infectious endophthalmitis in this series was less than 0.2%

Moshfeghi et al.[73] reported a multicenter, interventional case series of acute endophthalmitis following intravitreal triamcinolone acetonide injection. The preparatory steps included a lid speculum, topical anesthesia, 10% povidone iodine scrub of conjunctiva, lids, and lashes. A single 4 mg dose of triamcinolone acetonide was obtained from either a single use or multi-use vial. The supernatant was not removed. The suspension was injected through the inferior or inferotemporal pars plana. The calculated rate of infectious endophthalmitis was 0.87% (eight of 922 injections). The median time to presentation was 7.5 days. Seven of eight eyes had pain at the time of presentation. Interestingly, there was a high proportion of endophthalmitis cases at two academic centers, and elimination of these two centers would have decreased the rate to 0.3% (two of 623 injections.). Seven of eight eyes had a final visual acuity outcome worse than their preinjection vision. Three eyes were no light perception.

There are also reports of noninfectious endophthalmitis after intravitreal triamcinolone acetonide injections. Nelson et al.[74] reported a case series of seven eyes that presented with blurred vision, hypopyon, and pain within two days of intravitreal triamcinolone injection. These patients were followed closely without intervention with rapid resolution of the hypopyon and discomfort within a few days. Similarly, Roth et al.[75] reported a case series of seven patients who presented within one or two days after injection with an inflammatory response, including hypopyon, anterior chamber reaction, and vitreitis. Six of the seven patients were treated for presumed infectious endophthalmitis. The cultures were negative for organisms and all eyes had rapid resolution of their inflammatory response in a few days with recovery to preinjection vision. This type of clinical course was thought to be atypical for a true infectious endophthalmitis. The seventh eye with presumed endophthalmitis was observed without treatment and the eye responded favorably in a few days with rapid resolution of the inflammation. Five of the seven eyes had previously had a vitrectomy suggesting that absence of vitreous bulk may predispose the eye to a more rapid anterior chamber displacement of the drug contributing to the inflammatory response. The authors felt that a hyperacute inflammatory response seen after triamcinolone acetonide could be considered to be noninfectious endophthalmitis and could be observed carefully without treatment. Sutter and Gillies[76] have reported a similar hyperacute inflammatory response in four patients following intravitreal triamcinolone acetonide injection, which resolved without specific treatment.

These reports appear to suggest that the clinical entity of noninfectious, pseudo-endophthalmitis does exist in the setting of intravitreal triamcinolone acetonide injection. The identity of the offending agent in these sterile inflammatory responses is uncertain. The commercial preparation of triamcinolone acetonide (Kenalog®) includes the preservative benzyl alcohol, which has been shown to cause systemic toxicity when used in intravenous medication.[77] However intradermal use of normal saline with benzyl alcohol for intravenous cannulation pain has been shown to be safe with no evidence of local toxicity.[78] Benzyl alcohol vehicle incubation of human retinal pigment epithelium cell culture does not appear to cause adverse cellular reaction or toxicity.[79]

Other commercial preparations of corticosteroids cause an intraocular toxic response. Hida et al.[80] have evaluated the intraocular toxicity of commercial corticosteroid preparations in a rabbit eye model. Two of the corticosteroid preparations, Celestone Soluspan® (betamethasone sodium phosphate) and Depo-Medrol® (methylprednisolone acetate), produced both retinal and lens damage within 24 hours. The preservative/carrier in these commercial preparations was benzalkonium chloride, myristyl gamma-picolinium chloride, and ethylenediaminetetraacetic acid (EDTA). Kenalog® (triamcinolone acetonide) and did not produce toxic effects in the rabbit model.

Some guidelines can be derived from the above literature review on endophthalmitis and pseudo-endophthalmitis following intravitreal triamcinolone acetonide injection. It makes sense to make the injection environment as sterile as possible, including proper povidone iodine preparation of the lids, lashes, and the conjunctiva. The use of a lid speculum is indicated especially if the physician feels that he or she cannot isolate the lashes during the injection. A single use vial of triamcinolone acetonide should be used (although this is not specifically supported in literature). The removal of the supernatant may reduce the risk of the sterile inflammatory response[22]; however, this must be balanced with potential risk of organism introduction during the steps of supernatant removal and reintroduction of a solvent. The hyperacute response seen within one or two days following triamcinolone acetonide injection may be a sterile intraocular inflammatory response to the drug.[74–76]

The presence or absence of pain at this hyperacute presentation does not seem to be a reliable marker for either an infectious or a noninfectious etiology. Close observation may be warranted (perhaps with addition of topical steroid therapy) for this hyperacute inflammatory response and a lack of significant improvement within 24 to 48 hours may indicate a possible infectious etiology. True infectious endophthalmitis following intravitreal triamcinolone acetonide infection typically presents within seven to fourteen days following injection. The presence or absence of pain is not a reliable indicator of an infectious or sterile endophthalmitis. Prompt intravitreal antibiotic treatment is indicated for this situation. Given these guidelines however, if any doubts exist regarding the potential infectious or noninfectious etiology of the endophthalmitis presentation, an intravitreal antibiotic injection may be warranted given the relative low morbidity associated with such injection. See Table 55-2 for a review of the various ocular steroid delivery modalities.

CONCLUSION

The current, cumulative review of literature for therapeutic use of steroid in macular diseases is lacking in that most studies are retrospective, nonrandomized, and of small numbers with a relatively short follow-up time. However, the literal explosion in the use of steroid therapy for macular diseases over the last three years (this currently being written in early 2004), especially in the use of intravitreal triamcinolone acetonide for diabetic macular edema and retinal vascular diseases, suggests that clinicians are finding value in its use for managing these often refractory, chronic diseases.

Currently, two randomized studies are underway evaluating the efficacy of intravitreal triamcinolone acetonide for the treatment of macular diseases. The Intravitreal Steroid Injection Studies (ISIS) trial is a multicenter, prospective trial evaluating the effectiveness of intravitreal triamcinolone acetonide for the treatment of macular edema secondary to diabetic retinopathy, vein occlusions, and pseudophakia. The National Eye Institute is currently sponsoring a study (protocol number 04-EI-0013) investigating the use of intravitreal triamcinolone acetonide for the treatment of choroidal neovascularization associated with age-related macular degeneration, diabetic macular edema, and cystoid macular edema associated with vein occlusions. The study was initiated in late 2003 and a three-year follow-up period is expected. The results of these two studies will go a long way to fully exploit the potential values and benefits of steroid therapy for macular diseases.

REFERENCES

1. Schlaegel TF Jr. Essential of uveitis. Boston: Little, Brown, 1969.
2. Tano Y, Sugita G, Abrams G et al. Inhibition of intraocular proliferation with intravitreal corticosteroids. Am J Ophthalmol 1980; 89:131–136.
3. Tano Y, Chandler D, Machemer R. Treatment of intraocular proliferation with intravitreal injection of triamcinolone acetonide. Am J Ophthalmol 1980; 90:810–816.
4. McCuen BW II, Bressler M, Tano Y et al. The lack of toxicity of intravitreal administered triamcinolone acetonide. Am J Ophthalmol 1981; 91:785–788.
5. American Society of Retina Specialists. PAT Survey, 2003.
6. Gordon DM. Prednisone and prednisolone in ocular disease. Am J Ophthalmol 1956; 41:593–600.
7. Fauci AS. Clinical aspects of immunosuppression: use of cytotoxic agents and corticosteroids. Immunology. Philadelphia: WB Saunders, 1978.
8. Nussenblatt RB, Whitcup SM, Palestine AG. Uveitis: fundamentals and clinical practice. St Louis: Mosby, 1996.
9. Wilson CA, Berkowitz BA, Sato Y et al. Treatment with intravitreal steroid reduces blood-retinal barrier breakdown due to retinal photocoagulation. Arch Ophthalmol 1992; 110:1155–1159.
10. Sakamoto T, Miyazaki M, Hisatomi T et al. Triamcinolone-assisted pars plana vitrectomy improves the surgical procedure and postoperative blood–ocular barrier breakdown. Graefes Arch Clin Exp Ophthalmol 2002; 240: 423–429.

Table 55-2 Summary of steroid delivery modalities

	Systemic steroid	Periocular steroid (TA)	Intravitreal steroid (TA)	Sustained drug delivery device (FA)
Intraocular concentration	Low	Medium	High	High
Duration of action	NA	1–2 months	2–4 months	6 months–3 years
Systemic complications	Yes	Possible	No	No
Ocular complications	Cataract	Cataract, globe perforation	Cataract, endophthalmitis, RD, hemorrhage	Cataract, surgical complications including RD, hemorrhage
Risk of intraocular pressure rise	Low	10–40%	20–50%	30–40%

NA, not applicable; TA, triamcinolone acetonide; FA, fluocinolone acetonide; RD, retinal detachment.

11. Crum R, Szabo S, Folkman J. A new class of steroids inhibits angiogenesis in presence of heparin or a heparin fragment. Science 1985; 230: 1375–1378.

12. Ingber DE, Madri JA, Folkman J. A possible mechanism for inhibition of angiogenesis by angiostatic steroids: induction of capillary basement membrane dissolution. Endocrinology 1986; 119:1768–1775.

13. Hasa Q, Tan ST, Xu B et al. Effects of five commonly used glucocorticoids in haemangioma in vitro. Clin Exp Pharmacol Physiol 2003; 30:140–144.

14. Penfold PL, Wen L, Madigan MC et al. Modulation of permeability and adhesion molecule expression by human choroidal endothelial cells. Invest Ophthalmol Vis Sci 2002; 43:3125–3130.

15. Wang YS, Friedrichs U, Eichler W et al. Inhibitory effects of triamcinolone acetonide on bFGF-induced migration and tube formation in choroidal microvascular endothelial cells. Graefes Arch Clin Exp Ophthalmol 2002; 240:42–48.

16. Ciulla TA, Criswell MH, Danis RP et al. Intravitreal triamcinolone acetonide inhibits choroidal neovascularization in a laser-treated rat model. Arch Ophthalmol 2001; 119:399–404.

17. Kwak HW, D'Amico DJ. Evaluation of the retinal toxicity and pharmacokinetics of dexamethasone after intravitreal injection. Arch Ophthalmol 1992; 110:259–266.

18. Nabih M, Peyman GA, Tawakol ME et al. Toxicity of high dose intravitreal dexamethasone. Int Ophthalmol 1991; 15:234–235.

19. Shimada H, Matsui M. Effects of intravitreal steroid injection on rabbit eye. Nippon Ganka Gakkai Zasshi 1989; 93:510–510.

20. Hainsworth DP, Pearson PA, Conklin JD et al. Sustained release intravitreal dexamethasone. J Ocul Pharmacol Ther 1996; 12:57–63.

21. Blakenship GW. Evaluation of a single intravitreal injection of dexamethasone phosphate in vitrectomy surgery for diabetic retinopathy complications. Graefes Arch Clin Exp Ophthalmol 1991; 229:62–65.

22. Jonas JB, Kreissig I, Degenring RF. Endophthalmitis after intravitreal injection of triamcinolone acetonide. Arch Ophthalmol 2003; 121:1663–1664.

23. Schindler RH, Chandler D, Thresher R et al. The clearance of intravitreal triamcinolone acetonide. Am J Ophthalmol 1982; 93:415–417.

24. Scholes GN, O'Brien WJ, Abrams GW et al. Clearance of triamcinolone from vitreous. Arch Ophthalmol 1985; 103:1567–1569.

25. Beer PM, Bakri SJ, Sing RJ et al. Intraocular concentration and pharmacokinetics of triamcinolone acetonide after a single intravitreal injection. Ophthalmology 2003; 110:681–686.

26. Macular Photocoagulation Study Group. Visual outcome after laser photocoagulation for subfoveal choroidal neovascularization secondary to age-related macular degeneration: the influence of initial lesion size and initial visual acuity. Arch Ophthalmol 1994; 112:480–488.

27. Treatment of Age-Related Macular Degeneration With Photodynamic Therapy (TAP) Study Group. Photodynamic therapy of subfoveal choroidal neovascularization in age-related macular degeneration with verteporfin: 1-year results of 2 randomized clinical trials. TAP Report. Arch Ophthalmol 1999; 117:1329–1345.

28. Penfold PL, Gyory JF, Hunyor AB et al. Exudative macular degeneration and intravitreal triamcinolone. A pilot study. Aust NZ J Ophthalmol 1995; 23:293–298.

29. Danis RP, Ciulla TA, Pratt LM et al. Intravitreal triamcinolone acetonide in exudative age-related macular degeneration. Retina 2000; 20:244–250.

30. Ranson NT, Danis RP, Ciulla TA et al. Intravitreal triamcinolone in subfoveal recurrence of choroidal neovascularization after laser treatment in macular degeneration. Br J Ophthalmol 2002; 86:527–529.

31. Macular Photocoagulation Study Group. Five-year follow-up of fellow eyes of patients with age-related macular degeneration and unilateral extrafoveal choroidal neovascularization. Arch Ophthalmol 1993; 111:1189–1199.

32. Jonas JB, Kreissig I, Hugger P et al. Intravitreal triamcinolone acetonide for exudative age related macular degeneration. Br J Ophthalmol 2003; 87: 462–468.

33. Gillies MC, Simpson JM, Luo W et al. A randomized clinical trial of a single dose intravitreal triamcinolone acetonide for neovascular age-related macular degeneration: one-year results. Arch Ophthalmol 2003; 121:667–673.

34. Spaide RF, Sorenson J, Maranan L. Combined photodynamic therapy with verteporfin and intravitreal triamcinolone acetonide for choroidal neovascularization. Ophthalmology 2003; 110:1517–1525.

35. Slakter JS. Anecortave Acetate Clinical Study Group. Anecortave acetate as monotherapy for treatment of subfoveal neovascularization in age-related macular degeneration: interim (month 6) analysis of clinical safety and efficacy. Retina 2003; 23:14–23.

36. Slakter JS. Anecortave Acetate Clinical Study Group. Anecortave acetate as monotherapy for treatment of subfoveal neovascularization in age-related macular degeneration: twelve-month clinical outcomes. Ophthalmology 2003; 110:2372–2383.

37. Crum R, Szabo S, Folkman J. A new class of steroids inhibits angiogenesis in presence of heparin or a heparin fragments. Science 1985; 230: 1375–1378.

38. BenEzra D, Griffin BW, Maftzir G et al. Topical formulations of novel angiostatic steroids inhibit corneal neovascularization. Invest Ophthalmol Vis Sci 1997; 38:1954–1962.

39. Clark AF, Mellon J, Li XY et al. Inhibition of intraocular tumor growth by topical application of angiostatic steroid anecortave acetate. Invest Ophthalmol Vis Sci 1999; 40:2158–2162.

40. Penn JS, Rajaratnam VS, Collier RJ et al. The effect of an angiostatic steroid on neovascularization in a rat model of retinopathy of prematurity. Invest Ophthalmol Vis Sci 2001; 42:283–290.

41. Early Treatment Diabetic Retinopathy Study Research Group. Treatment techniques and clinical guidelines for photocoagulation of diabetic macular edema. ETDRS report no 1. Arch Ophthalmol 1985; 103:1796–1806.

42. Early Treatment Diabetic Retinopathy Study Research Group. Treatment techniques and clinical guidelines for photocoagulation of diabetic macular edema. ETDRS report no 2. Ophthalmology 1987; 97:761–774.

43. Lewis H, Schachat AP, Haimann MH et al. Choroidal neovascularization after laser photocoagulation for diabetic macular edema. Ophthalmology 1990; 97:503–510.

44. Martidis A, Duker JS, Greenberg PB et al. Intravitreal triamcinolone for refractory diabetic macular edema. Ophthalmol 2002; 109:920–927.

45. Jonas JB, Kreissig I, Sofker A et al. Intravitreal injection of triamcinolone for diffuse diabetic macular edema. Arch Ophthalmol 2003; 121:57–61.

46. Control Delivery Systems Press Release. Analysis of 12-month data from diabetic macular edema clinical trial. Online. Available: http://www.control delivery.com/prmay72003.htm 7 May 2003.

47. The Central Vein Occlusion Study Group. Natural history and clinical management of central retinal vein occlusion. Arch Ophthalmol 1997; 115:486–491.

48. The Central Vein Occlusion Study Group. Evaluation of grid laser pattern photocoagulation for macular edema in central vein occlusion. Ophthalmology 1995; 102:1425–1433.

49. Greenberg PB, Martidis A, Rogers AH et al. Intravitreal triamcinolone acetonide for macular oedema due to central retinal vein occlusion. Br J Ophthalmol 2002; 86:247–248.

50. Jonas JB, Kreissig I, Degenring RF. Intravitreal triamcinolone acetonide as treatment of macular edema in central retinal vein occlusion. Graefes Arch Clin Exp Ophthalmol 2002; 240:782–783.

51. Ip MS, Kumar KS. Intravitreous triamcinolone acetonide as treatment for macular edema from central retinal vein occlusion. Arch Ophthalmol 2002; 120:1217–1219.

52. Park CH, Jaffe GJ, Fekrat S. Intravitreal triamcinolone acetonide in eyes with cystoid macular edema associated with central retinal vein occlusion. Am J Ophthalmol 2003; 136:419–425.

53. Branch Vein Occlusion Study Group. Argon laser photocoagulation for macular edema in branch vein occlusion. Am J Ophthalmol 1984; 98:271–282.

54. Chen SDM, Lochhead J, Patel CK et al. Intravitreal triamcinolone acetonide for ischaemic macular oedema caused by branch retinal vein occlusion. Br J Ophthalmol 2004; 88:154–155.

55. Gass JDM, Blodi BA. Idiopathic juxtafoveolar retinal telangiectasis: update of classification and follow-up study. Ophthalmology 1993; 100:1536–1546.

56. Millay RH, Klein ML, Handelman IL et al. Abnormal glucose metabolism and parafoveal telangiectasia. Am J Ophthalmol 1986; 102: 363–370.

57. Alldredge CD, Garretson BR. Intravitreal triamcinolone for the treatment of idiopathic juxtafoveal telangiectasis. Retina 2003; 23:113–116.

58. Sutter FK, Gillies MC. Intravitreal triamcinolone for radiation-induced macular edema. Arch Ophthalmol 2003; 121:1491–1493.

59. Wright PL, Wilkinson CP, Balyeat HD et al. Angiographic cystoid macular edema after posterior chamber lens implantation. Arch Ophthalmol 1988; 106:740–744.

60. Conway MD, Canakis C, Livir-Rallatos C et al. Intravitreal triamcinolone acetonide for refractory chronic pseudophakic cystoid macular edema. J Cataract Refract Surg 2003; 29:27–33.

61. Benhamou N, Massin P, Haouchine B et al. Intravitreal triamcinolone for refractory pseudophakic macular edema. Am J Ophthalmol 2003; 135: 246–249.

62. Rothova A, Suttorp van Schulten MSA, Treffers WF et al. Causes and frequency of blindness in patients with intraocular inflammatory diseases. Br J Ophthalmol 1996; 80:332–336.

63. Yoshikawa K, Kotake S, Ichiishi A et al. Posterior sub-Tenon injections of repository corticosteroids in uveitis patients with cystoid macular edema. Jpn J Ophthalmol 1995; 39:71–6.

64. Helm CJ, Holland GN. The effects of posterior subtenon injection of triamcinolone acetonide in patients with intermediate uveitis. Am J Ophthalmol 1995; 120:54–64.

65. Levin DS, Han DP, Dev S et al. Subtenon's depot corticosteroid injections in patients with a history of corticosteroid-induced intraocular pressure elevation. Am J Ophthalmol 2002; 133:196–202.

66. Antcliff RJ, Spalton DJ, Stanford MR et al. Intravitreal triamcinolone for uveitis cystoid macular edema: an optical coherence tomography study. Ophthalmology 2001; 108:765–772.
67. Jaffe GJ, Ben-nun J, Guo H et al. Fluocinolone acetonide sustained drug delivery device to treat severe uveitis. Ophthalmology 2000; 107:2024–2033.
68. Jaffe GJ, Yang CH, Guo H et al. Safety and pharmacokinetics of an intra-ocular fluocinolone acetonide sustained delivery device. Invest Ophthalmol Vis Sci 2000; 41:3569–3575.
69. Moshfeghi DM, Lowder CY, Roth DB et al. Retinal and choroidal vascular occlusion after posterior sub-tenon triamcinolone injection. Am J Ophthalmol 2002; 134:132–134.
70. Jonas JB, Kreissig I, Degenring R. Intraocular pressure after intravitreal injection of triamcinolone acetonide. Br J Ophthalmol 2003; 87:24–27.
71. Bakri SJ, Beer PM. The effect of intravitreal triamcinolone acetonide on intraocular pressure. Ophthalmic Surg Lasers Imaging 2003; 34:386–390.
72. Heinemann MH. *Staphylococcus epidermis* endophthalmitis complicating intravitreal antiviral therapy of cytomegalovirus retinitis: case report. Arch Ophthalmol 1989; 107:643–644.
73. Moshfeghi DM, Kaiser PK, Scott IU et al. Acute endophthalmitis following intravitreal triamcinolone acetonide injection. Am J Ophthalmol 2003; 136: 791–796.
74. Nelson ML, Tennant MT, Sivalingam A et al. Infectious and presumed non-infectious endophthalmitis after intravitreal triamcinolone acetonide injection. Retina 2003; 23:686–691.
75. Roth DB, Chieh J, Spirn MJ et al. Noninfectious endophthalmitis associated with intravitreal triamcinolone injection. Arch Ophthalmol 2003; 121: 1279–1282.
76. Sutter FK, Gillies MC. Pseudo-endophthalmitis after intravitreal injection of triamcinolone. Br J Ophthalmol 2003; 87:972–974.
77. Lopez-Herce J, Bonet C, Meana A et al. Benzyl alcohol poisoning following diazepam intravenous infusion. Ann Pharmacother 1995; 29:632.
78. McNelis KA. Intradermal bacteriostatic 0.9% sodium chloride containing the preservative benzyl alcohol compared with intradermal lidocaine hydrochloride 1% for attenuation of intravenous cannulation pain. AANA J 1998; 66:583–585.
79. Yeung CK, Chan KP, Chiang SW et al. The toxic and stress responses of cultured human retinal pigment epithelium (ARPE19) and human glial cells (SVG) in the presence of triamcinolone. Invest Ophthalmol Vis Sci 2003; 44:5293–5300.
80. Hida T, Chandler D, Arena JE et al. Experimental and clinical observations of the intraocular toxicity of commercial corticosteroid preparations. Am J Ophthalmol 1986; 101:190–195.

Chapter

56

Choroidal Neovascularization

Stephen J. Ryan
David R. Hinton
Toshinori Murata

Choroidal neovascularization (CNV) denotes the pathologic growth of new blood vessels from pre-existing choroidal vessels into the subretinal space. The newly formed vessels lie between the choroid and the retinal pigment epithelium (RPE) or between the native RPE and the neurosensory retina; thus, CNV is also referred to as subretinal neovascularization (SRN). A wide range of disorders that affect the RPE–Bruch's membrane–choriocapillaris complex result in the development of CNV (Table 56-1). The importance of CNV is that it is the determinant of the disciform process; the disc-shaped, subretinal, fibrovascular membrane ultimately progresses to cicatrization, and loss of macular function.

HISTORICAL REVIEW

The disciform process was first described by Pagenstecher & Genth[1,2] in 1875; the term *disciform* was coined and first used by Oeller[3] in 1903. In 1926, Junius & Kuhnt[4] provided the first comprehensive description of the disciform process and noted that the pathologic findings could extend beyond the macula. Their description was widely accepted and their names were an eponym for this condition for many years.[5–10] Verhoeff & Grossman[11] were the first to suggest that CNV represents a vascular ingrowth from the choroid. That the disciform process is the ultimate outcome of many disease processes was emphasized in a series of papers by Maumenee.[12–14]

Many of our current concepts regarding the pathogenesis of the disciform process can be attributed to the seminal monograph of Gass,[15] who recognized age-related (senile) macular degeneration (AMD) as the most common cause of disciform macular degeneration.[16–24] CNV is recognized as the cause of more than 80% of cases of significant visual loss in patients with AMD in the USA.[1,20,23–25] The evolution of the disciform process involves repeated episodes of serous and hemorrhagic detachments as a result of leakage from CNV, with eventual cicatrization and formation of a subretinal fibrovascular scar.

More than 40 other disease processes may exhibit similar manifestations and result in the disciform response (Table 56-1). Some of the processes most commonly associated with disciform lesions include presumed ocular histoplasmosis syndrome,[15,26–32] angioid streaks,[33–47] myopia,[48–54] blunt trauma,[55–61] laser therapy,[47,62–69] and a group of idiopathic processes[68,70–75] that affect young adults as discrete macular lesions without the diffuse changes of the RPE characteristic of the disciform process in AMD.

PATHOGENESIS OF CHOROIDAL NEOVASCULARIZATION ASSOCIATED WITH AGE-RELATED MACULAR DEGENERATION

The mechanisms involved in the pathogenesis of CNV and associated CNV membrane (CNVM) formation are being elucidated but are still not fully understood.[76–78] Aging and genetically determined changes in the RPE–Bruch's membrane–choriocapillaris complex are important in inducing CNV, and wound-healing responses are instrumental for their progression and resolution. The process of CNV formation in AMD can be divided into five steps.

Aging and senescence of retinal pigment epithelium

The incidence and progression of nearly every feature of AMD including CNV relates to age. The Beaver Dam Eye Study[79] showed that those individuals 75 years of age and older had significantly ($P < 0.01$) higher 5-year incidence of exudative macular degeneration than people between the ages of 43 and 54 (1.8% versus 0%). Lipofuscin accumulates with age in RPE as a byproduct of photoreceptor outer-segment digestion by lysosomes. A decrease in lysosomal activity of RPE accompanies aging,[80] and age-related progressive accumulation of lipofuscin results in disturbance of RPE function.[81] Cathepsin D is important for opsin proteolysis. Transgenic expression of an enzymatically inactive form of cathepsin D in mice results in accumulation of autofluorescent debris in RPE, formation of basal laminar and linear deposits, and progressive photoreceptor degeneration.[82] Successive passage of cultured RPE cells results in diminished production of pigment epithelium-derived growth factor (PEDF), suggesting that there could be an age-related decline in the production of this antiangiogenic growth factor.[83]

Senescence is generally defined as having occurred when cells are in an irreversible state of G(1) cell cycle arrest, and are refractory to growth factor stimulation. The presence of senescence-related beta-galactosidase activity in RPE of older monkey eyes has been documented.[84,85] The mRNA phenotype

Table 56-1 Conditions in which choroidal neovascularization may occur

Condition	References
Age-related macular degeneration	15,17,19,210–226
Angioid streaks	33–41,42–47
Anterior ischemic optic neuropathy	227
Bacterial endocarditis	228
Best disease	229–231
Birdshot retinochoroidopathy	232,233
Choroidal hemangioma	234
Choroidal nevi	235–239
Choroidal nonperfusion	240
Choroidal osteomas	53,241–249
Choroidal rupture	58,60,61,250,251
Choroideremia	252
Chronic retinal detachment	253
Coloboma of the retina	224
Diabetes mellitus	134
Drusen	15,17,19,20,23,72,210–212,215,218,219,221,223–226,254,255
Endogenous *Candida* endophthalmitis	256
Extrapapillary hamartomas of the retinal pigment epithelium	257,258
Fundus flavimaculatus	259
Idiopathic	68,73,74,260–262
Macular hole	263
Malignant melanoma	264
Membranoproliferative glomerulonephritis (type II)	265,266
Metallic intraocular foreign body	267
Morning-glory disc syndrome	268
Multiple evanescent white-dot syndrome (MEWDS)	260,269
Myopia	48–54
Neovascularization at ora serrata	210,253,270,271
Operating microscope burn	156
Optic glioma	272
Optic nerve head pits	273
Photocoagulation	62–69,274,275
Presumed ocular histoplasmosis syndrome	22,31,75,276–286
Punctate inner choroidopathy	287
Radiation retinopathy	288
Retinal cryoinjury	290

Table 56-1 Conditions in which choroidal neovascularization may occur—cont'd

Condition	References
Retinitis pigmentosa	290
Retinochoroidal coloboma	291
Rubella	292,293
Sarcoidosis	293,294
Serpiginous or geographic choroiditis	295–298
Subretinal fluid drainage	299,300
Tilted disc syndrome	301
Toxoplasma retinochoroiditis	237,302,303
Tuberculosis	304
Vogt–Koyanagi–Harada syndrome	305,306

of a human RPE cell line at replicative senescence has been examined; changes similar to those found in repairing wounds were demonstrated.[86]

Drusen, basal laminar/linear deposit formation

Hard drusen (nodular drusen) are localized, rounded, dome-shaped deposits lying between Bruch's membrane and uplifted RPE (Fig. 56-1). Soft drusen have an indistinct margin and more readily become confluent. Soft drusen, unlike hard drusen, appear to be an important associated and predisposing feature of CNV.[87,88] Several mechanisms for the formation of soft drusen have been proposed: (1) membranous accumulation of debris as part of a diffuse disturbance of the RPE (soft membranous drusen);[87] (2) softening of hard drusen;[87] and (3) cleavage in basal laminar/linear deposits that may occur with the formation of a localized detachment.[89] Histopathologic studies also reveal that basal laminar deposits, accumulating between the plasma and basement membrane of the RPE, and basal linear deposits, with a thickening of the inner collagenous zone of the Bruch's membrane (i.e., external to the basement membrane of the RPE), also have important associations with CNV.[89] Therefore, abnormal deposits that occur between the RPE layer and Bruch's membrane and that have a diffuse distribution pattern are predisposing features of CNV.

One possible hypothesis for the proangiogenic role of these deposits is shown in Figure 56-2. Deposits between the RPE layer and Bruch's membrane may block the diffusion of oxygen and nutrients from choriocapillaris to the RPE monolayer and photoreceptors.[90] It is speculated that localized cellular hypoxia results in overexpression of growth factors such as vascular endothelial growth factor (VEGF), which in turn, induce neovascularization from the choroidal vasculature. VEGF expression is enhanced by hypoxia in cultured RPE[91] and photoreceptor cells.[92] The deposits may also serve as a reservoir for sequestration of growth factors[93] and other angiogenic factors (e.g.,

advanced glycation end-products or AGEs[94]) that may affect the function of adjacent RPE and choroidal endothelial cells. The accumulation of AGEs in Bruch's membrane and basal laminar/lineal deposits has been reported in AMD tissue samples.[94]

Enzymatic and mechanical disruption of Bruch's membrane

In CNV, activated endothelial cells migrate through Bruch's membrane; this process occurs by degradation of an intact Bruch's membrane, or growth through an existing Bruch's membrane break. Clinicopathologic studies suggest that classic CNVMs are predominantly subretinal in location, whereas occult CNVMs are predominantly sub-RPE.[95] Bruch's membrane may be

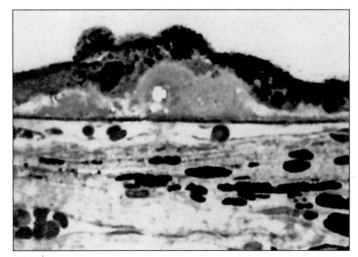

Fig. 56-1 Light microphotograph of typical drusen with dome-shaped granular nodule beneath the pigment epithelium (Richardson's stain, ×660). (Reproduced from Ishibashi T, Patterson R, Ohnishi Y et al. Formation of drusen in the human eye. Am J Ophthalmol 1986; 101: 342–353.)

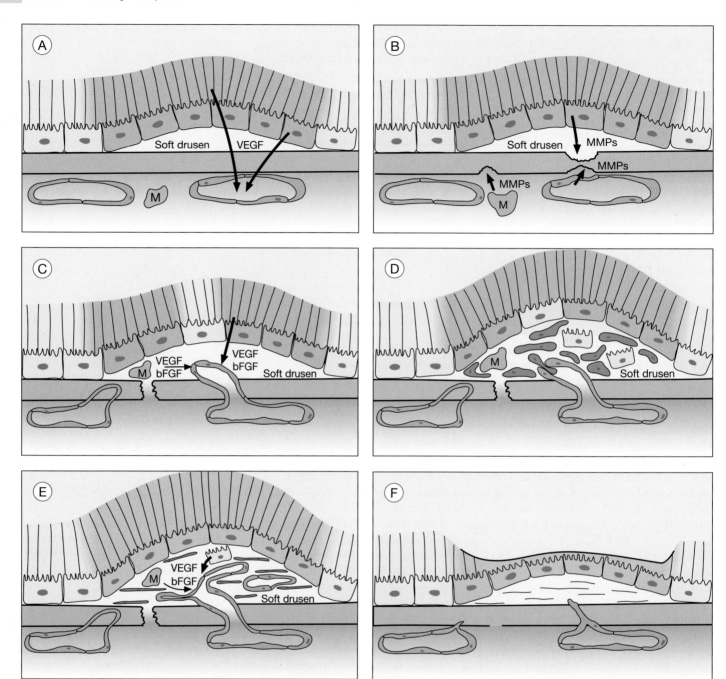

Fig. 56-2 Presumed pathologic stages required for the development and progression of choroidal neovascularization (CNV). A, Retinal cells (retinal pigment epithelium, photoreceptor cells) adjacent to soft drusen secrete vascular endothelial growth factor (VEGF) in response to hypoxia, inflammatory cytokines, or advanced glycosylation end-products. Macrophages (M) are attracted to the lesion in response to locally expressed chemokines (e.g., monocyte chemoattractant protein-1). B, Development of CNV requires the development of a break in Bruch's membrane. Proteolysis of Bruch's may occur by local secretion of matrix metalloproteinases (MMPs) by retinal pigment epithelium, choroidal endothelial cell sprouts, or macrophages. C, Activated choroidal endothelial sprouts grow through the break in Bruch's membrane in response to angiogenic growth factors (VEGF, basic fibroblast growth factor (bFGF)). Macrophages are recruited into the subretinal space. D, The newly formed vessels are fragile, often resulting in subretinal hemorrhage. Retinal pigment epithelium transdifferentiates and migrates from the monolayer into the stroma of the lesion. E, Organization of the cellular lesion continues in response to continued expression of angiogenic growth factors and hemorrhage. A disciform lesion is formed with damage to adjacent photoreceptor cells. F, Cellular, vascular membranes gradually change into inactive cicatricial membranes. This loss of cellularity is most likely due to apoptosis.

disrupted when the balance between proteolytic enzymes such as matrix metalloproteinases (MMPs) and their inhibitors, the tissue inhibitors of metalloproteinases (TIMPs), favors a proteolytic environment. RPE cells express MMP-1 (interstitial colla-genase),[96] MMP-2 (72 kDa gelatinase),[96,97] MMP-3 (stromolysin),[96] and MMP-9 (92 kDa gelatinase),[96] as well as TIMP-1,[97,98] TIMP-2,[98] and TIMP-3.[98] Thus, proteolysis of Bruch's membrane may potentially result from reduced expression of TIMPs, or increased expression of MMPs. MMPs also play an important role in degrading the extracellular matrix at the leading edge of neovascular fronds (Fig. 56-2B). Studies in transgenic mice support the contention that Bruch's membrane disruption is required for the development of CNV. Transgenic mice with an intact Bruch's membrane that overexpress VEGF in photoreceptors develop SRN; however, the subretinal vessels extend from retinal vessels rather than the choroidal vasculature.[99] In contrast, transgenic mice that overexpress VEGF in RPE cells show intrachoroidal CNV.[100] These findings support the notion that CNV requires both the expression of an angiogenic factor and a break in Bruch's membrane (by proteolysis, physical disruption, or pre-existing break).

Macrophages are an alternative source of enzymes such as MMPs that could cause focal disruption of Bruch's membrane.[101] Histopathologic studies reveal that macrophages accumulate near thinned segments of Bruch's membrane.[102] In AMD, the RPE shows increased expression of monocyte chemoattractant protein-1 (MCP-1); a factor critical for macrophage recruitment.[103] Macrophages in the choroid may subsequently degrade Bruch's membrane, thus forming a passage that can be used by activated choroidal endothelial cells to gain entrance to the sub-RPE space.

Choroidal neovascularization membrane formation

Green & Enger[89] reported a series of 760 eyes with AMD from 450 patients; 310 eyes (40.8%) demonstrated a disciform membrane. The mean diameter of these membranes was 3.73 mm, and the mean thickness was 0.27 mm. Preservation of photoreceptor cells was seen when the thickness of the disciform scars was 0.2 mm or less. Histologic studies of highly vascular CNVM show that they contain endothelial cell-lined channels, RPE cells, and macrophages within the extracellular matrix-rich stroma. The stromal RPE are immunoreactive for smooth-muscle actin, indicating a transdifferentiated phenotype. The transdifferentiated RPE often expresses VEGF, suggesting that these RPE have a proangiogenic role, and that VEGF is a mediator of AMD-related CNV.[104]

Choroidal angiogenesis is a multistep process that includes degradation of vascular basement membrane, proliferation and migration of choroidal endothelial cells, choroidal endothelial cell tube formation, and restoration of the vascular basement membrane.[105,106] CNV occurs when there is an imbalance between proangiogenic and antiangiogenic growth factors (Fig. 56-3). Angiogenic growth factors, such as VEGF, angiopoietins (Ang 1, Ang 2), connective tissue growth factor (CTGF),[107] and basic fibroblast growth factor (bFGF), released from RPE cells and/or other retinal cells, promote CNV (Fig. 56-2C). Choroidal angiogenesis is inhibited by antiangiogenic growth factors such as thrombospondin-1 and PEDF[108] and Fas-mediated killing of new vessels by Fas-ligand-positive RPE or leukocytes.[109]

Macrophages are an additional source of angiogenic growth factors that may promote the development of CNV. Depletion of macrophages diminishes the lesion size and severity in experimental laser-induced CNV.[110,111] Ccr-2 knockout mice, characterized by hampered macrophage recruitment, also show inhibition of laser-induced CNV.[112] Activated macrophages show increased expression of inflammatory cytokines such as tumor necrosis factor-alpha and interleukin-1-beta, which may promote angiogenesis by stimulating VEGF expression in RPE.[113]

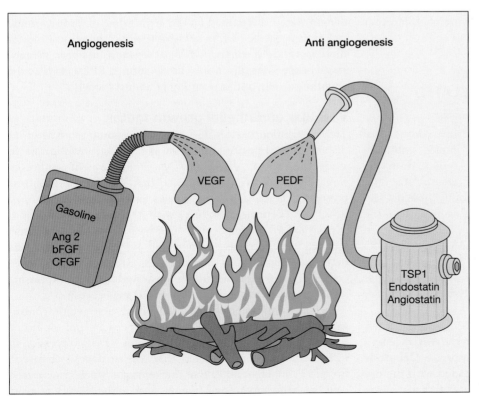

Fig. 56-3 The competing effects of growth factors on angiogenesis. When the angiogenic process is thought of as a "fire," this fire can be "fueled" by proangiogenic growth factors (e.g., vascular endothelial growth factor (VEGF), basic fibroblast growth factor (bFGF), angiopoietin-2 (Ang 2)), or "put out with water" by antiangiogenic growth factors (e.g., pigment epithelial-derived factor (PEDF), thrombospondin-1 (TSP-1), angiostatin).

The contribution of bone marrow-derived endothelial cells to CNV has been evaluated by inducing CNV in irradiated mice that have received bone marrow transplants from green fluorescent protein (GFP)-expressing mice. These studies show that GFP+ endothelial cells are incorporated into the laser-induced CNVM, suggesting that bone marrow-derived progenitor cells provide an additional source of endothelial cells in CNV.[114–116]

CNV lesions are leaky and often show evidence of hemorrhage. In fact, the evolution of the CNVM often involves repeated episodes of serous leakage and hemorrhage (Fig. 56-2D). In response to these changes, fibrovascular membrane formation occurs around the CNV, resulting in a disciform lesion (Fig. 56-2E). The presence of hemosiderin within the disciform CNVM suggests that fibrovascular organization of hemorrhage is important in its evolution. Over time, the newly formed vessels mature, perhaps in response to angiopoietin-1, and show reduced leakage that may result from the perivascular growth of RPE.

Cicatricial membrane formation

Cellular and highly vascularized membranes gradually evolve into paucicellular cicatricial membranes (Fig. 56-2F). The loss of cellularity is most likely due to apoptosis, or programmed cell death of stromal cells.[117] Surgically excised AMD-related CNVM contain apoptotic stromal RPE, endothelial cells, and macrophages. Apoptosis may be associated with a local decrease in the expression of angiogenic growth factors that promote survival of activated cells. Fas and Fas-ligand expression may also be involved in the induction of apoptosis in these cells.[118] Little is known about the mediators of collagenous scar formation in CNVM. Recent studies show that CTGF, a proangiogenic and profibrotic growth factor, is expressed in stromal RPE cells in surgically excised CNVM.[107] The development of a cicatricial disciform lesion promotes overlying photoreceptor cell loss.[119]

GENETIC ASPECTS OF CHOROIDAL NEOVASCULARIZATION IN AGE-RELATED MACULAR DEGENERATION

AMD is a multifactorial disease in which critical environmental factors (e.g., aging, smoking, oxidant stress) interact within an AMD-susceptible genetic phenotype that results from the contributions from multiple predisposing genes.[120] Several approaches are being employed in order to identify these disease-associated genes. One unbiased approach is based on the genome-wide evaluation of hundreds of thousands of common single nucleotide polymorphisms for their association with AMD in case-control studies. Another approach is to evaluate the contributions of mutations or polymorphisms in candidate genes such as those mediating monogenetic early-onset hereditary macular dystrophies.

Stargardt disease is an autosomal recessive juvenile macular dystrophy characterized by mutations within the *ABCR* gene, a rod-specific ATP-binding cassette (ABC) transporter. One study suggested that *ABCR* mutations were associated with the dry form of AMD;[121] however another study reported that there were no significant differences between the proportion of *ABCR* genetic variations in patients with and without AMD.[122]

Sorsby fundus dystrophy is an autosomal dominant disorder that manifests histologic changes similar to those of neovascular AMD. Mutations in the gene encoding TIMP-3, an inhibitor of proteolysis found within Bruch's membrane, are present in patients with Sorsby fundus dystrophy.[123,124] TIMP-3 dysfunction in Bruch's membrane may lead to membrane disruption and may facilitate CNV. Although a direct association between TIMP-3 mutations and neovascular AMD has not been found,[125,126] these studies highlight the importance of MMP/TIMP imbalance in the pathogenesis of CNV.

Best macular dystrophy is an autosomal dominant disorder characterized by egg-yolk macular lesions and accumulation of lipofuscin within and beneath the RPE. Degeneration of the RPE and overlying photoreceptors results in geographic atrophy and/or CNV. Best disease is a result of mutations within the *VMD2* gene that encodes the protein bestrophin.[127]

Malattia levantinese and Doyne honeycomb retinal dystrophy are autosomal dominant disorders associated with drusen formation. A single, nonconservative mutation in the epidermal growth factor-containing, fibrillin-like extracellular matrix protein (EFEMP1) gene has been identified in affected individuals. Although this change was not seen in control or AMD patients, EFEMP1 protein has been found to accumulate beneath RPE cells overlying drusen in AMD and may be linked to drusen formation.[128]

ANGIOGENIC FACTORS IN CHOROIDAL NEOVASCULARIZATION

Pathologic studies of surgically excised human CNVM have demonstrated alterations in the expression of proangiogenic and antiangiogenic factors in these tissues. The critical role of these factors in mediating CNV pathogenesis has been demonstrated experimentally in vitro using cultured RPE and choroidal endothelial cells, and in a variety of animal models.

Vascular endothelial growth factor

The recognition that VEGF was an important mediator of diabetic retinal neovascularization encouraged investigators to study the role of VEGF in CNV.[129] Subsequent studies of surgically excised CNVMs showed that VEGF expression was present in choroidal endothelial cells, macrophages, and stromal RPE.[104,130,131] Furthermore, eyes with AMD also showed VEGF expression in photoreceptors overlying CNVM.[119] In laser-induced CNV in monkeys, increased expression of VEGF was detected in infiltrating macrophages, RPE cells, and Müller cells.[132] In vitro experiments demonstrated that RPE expressing VEGF promote experimental choroidal angiogenesis.[133]

Increased expression of VEGF in CNVM suggested the controversial hypothesis that tissue hypoxia may be an etiologic factor for this disorder, since hypoxia stimulates VEGF expression in RPE.[134] It has been suggested that drusen deposits between Bruch's membrane and RPE or thickening of Bruch's membrane could mediate outer retinal hypoxia even in the absence of overt choriocapillaris damage. Clinical studies show that the most peripheral choroidal arterial segments are detected as hypofluorescent zones in early-phase indocyanine green angiograms. The demonstration of a comparatively reduced choroidal vascularity in some AMD eyes with CNV suggests that this may represent another cause of hypoxia in AMD.[135] Other potential inducers of VEGF expression include bFGF, transforming growth factor-β (TGF-β),[119] and AGEs.[136]

Advanced glycosolation end-products and choroidal neovascularization

AGEs, which are formed by nonenzymatic protein glycation, have been found to play an important role in both aging changes and neovascularization. AGEs have been localized in basal laminar/linear deposits or soft drusen in AMD.[94] In surgically excised CNVM, AGE deposition is spatially associated with RPE that express VEGF.[94] AGEs induce VEGF expression by RPE cells in vitro,[136] and growth of RPE on AGE leads to the upregulation of genes associated with RPE aging[137] and down-regulation of cathepsin D expression.[138] AGEs are also involved in lipofuscin formation in RPE cells.[139] Reactive oxygen intermediates are generated in parallel with AGEs either directly or through AGE–RAGE (receptor for AGEs) interaction.[140] Consistent with the ability of AGEs to induce VEGF expression in vitro,[136] AGEs can also induce angiogenesis in vivo.[141]

Basic fibroblast growth factor (bFGF, FGF-2)

The fibroblast growth factors (FGFs) are a family of heparin-binding proteins with key roles in neovascularization. Expression of bFGF (FGF-2), acidic FGF (aFGF, FGF-1), and FGF-5 has been demonstrated in the normal retina and RPE.[142] In surgically removed CNVM, bFGF expression is upregulated in RPE and choroidal endothelial cells.[104,130,131,143] Sustained release of bFGF from subretinal pellets induces CNV in rabbits.[144] However, targeted disruption of the FGF-2 gene does not prevent the development of laser-induced CNV in the mouse, suggesting that, at least in this model, bFGF is not required for CNV formation.[145] Co-localization of bFGF and VEGF in the same cells of CNVM was observed, suggesting that bFGF and VEGF may act together to accelerate CNV.[130] Although bFGF does not have a signal sequence typically required for cell secretion, sublethal injury could result in release of bFGF into the extracellular space. Low-intensity photocoagulation lesions that damage photoreceptors and RPE cells, but not Bruch's membrane, result in CNV in mice whose photoreceptors overexpress bFGF but not in wild-type mice.[146] These data suggest that bFGF overexpression in the retina could promote CNV in the setting of photoreceptor and RPE injury.

Angiopoietins

Angiopoietin-1 (Ang 1) is a largely endothelial-specific growth factor that acts through the tyrosine kinase receptor Tie2. Ang 1 promotes vascular integrity and has a critical role in vascular development, as its absence leads to embryonic lethality.[147] Angiopoietin-2 (Ang 2) is also a natural ligand for Tie2 and may act as a competitive inhibitor of Ang 1. Activation of Tie2 by

Ang 1 may be important in the maturation and reduction in leakiness of newly formed blood vessels[148] that have been stimulated to grow by VEGF. Ang 2 overexpression induced by hypoxia or VEGF is localized at the site of neovascularization in CNVMs or experimental retinal neovascularization. Overexpression of Ang 2 can promote angiogenesis, since it destabilizes existing vasculature by competing with the stabilizing effect of Ang 1.[149] Histologic studies have shown the expression of Ang 1 and Ang 2, as well as Tie2, in human CNVMs.[150]

Pigment epithelium-derived factor

PEDF is a glycoprotein that is abundantly produced by RPE cells and functions as a neurotrophic factor for photoreceptors. PEDF is strongly antiangiogenic in the eye and is one of the factors that may be responsible for the avascularity of vitreous body and cornea.[151] The fact that RPE cells produce both PEDF and VEGF suggests that they have a dual role (i.e., angiogenic and antiangiogenic) in CNV pathogenesis. In patients with CNV due to AMD, the vitreous concentration of PEDF is decreased when compared to vitreous samples from patients with other retinal disorders not involving neovascularization.[152] Systemic delivery of recombinant PEDF inhibited ischemia-induced retinopathy in mice,[153] and viral vector-mediated transfection of PEDF inhibited laser-induced CNV in mice.[154] The antiangiogenic activity of PEDF may stem from its ability to induce endothelial cell apoptosis.[153]

Other growth factors

Platelet-derived growth factor (PDGF) expression has been reported in the outer nuclear layer of the macula from patients with AMD.[119] RPE cells in CNVM are strongly immunoreactive for TGF-β, and it may act by modulating the effects of other growth factors such as bFGF and VEGF.[143] This hypothesis is supported by the fact that TGF-β and interleukin-1 induce VEGF expression in cultured choroidal fibroblasts.[155] CTGF is a proangiogenic and profibrotic growth factor that is expressed in stromal cells in human CNVM.[107] It also plays a role in mediating and modulating the effects of other growth factors; CTGF is upregulated in vitro by VEGF in choroidal endothelial cells and by TGF-β in RPE cells. However, the relative importance of these growth factors, in comparison with VEGF, has not been determined.

ANIMAL MODELS OF CHOROIDAL NEOVASCULARIZATION

Photocoagulation as a model for induction of choroidal neovascularization

There is no reproducible animal model of CNV in which CNV develops spontaneously over a short time period and demonstrates the constellation of clinical and pathologic changes typical of the human disorder. Two factors are necessary for the development of CNV in animal models: (1) disruption of Bruch's membrane; and (2) expression of angiogenic stimuli/growth factors. Intense photocoagulation provides both factors by creating a focal lesion at the RPE with extension to, and disruption of, Bruch's membrane. The RPE injury stimulates a wound-healing response with infiltration of leukocytes and increased expression of angiogenic growth factors and MMPs. The CNV that results may be thought of as a form of granulation tissue developing in response to the photocoagulation injury. Similarly, disciform CNVM can also be regarded as a kind of granulation tissue that is formed in response to subretinal hemorrhage or exudates from CNV. Consequently, the photocoagulation model of CNV is relevant for investigating the mechanisms of CNV progression.

Photocoagulation choroidal neovascularization model in primates

Clinical reports noted the occasional development of CNV after photocoagulation with xenon arc[62,65] and laser,[62,63,65,68] as well as after photic injury from an operating microscope burn.[156] Archer & Gardiner[157] noted CNV in animals after branch vein occlusion was induced by argon laser photocoagulation. In their model, about 25% of photocoagulation burns that disrupted Bruch's membrane resulted in the development of CNV. Ryan[158,159] showed that argon laser photocoagulation, if sufficiently intense, caused reproducible CNV in a high percentage of burns. The successful development of a reproducible primate model of CNV led to a number of studies in which the parameters of laser burns, topographic variation, development, natural history, ultrastructure, and clinicopathologic correlation of CNV were studied. The clinical relevance of the model was based on its pathologic features and the angiographic definition of leaking and pooling of fluorescein in the subretinal space.

Natural history of experimental, laser-induced choroidal neovascularization in primates

The natural history, parameters of laser application, and results from 50 treated monkey eyes have been described.[160] A total of 779 lesions (either parafoveal or in the nasal retina) that could be followed by fluorescein angiography were produced. Evidence of macular CNV and fluorescein leakage and pooling was found in 39% of burns in the macula (Fig. 56-4), but the same evidence was found in only 3% of retinal burns that were applied nasal to the optic disc and in less than 1% of peripheral retinal burns. The CNV typically developed within 3 weeks after the laser injury, continued to evolve for an average of 13 weeks (although with a wide range), and then involuted, ceasing to leak and pool fluorescein.

Origin of laser-induced choroidal neovascularization

Derivation of CNV from choroidal vessels was proved in primates by the use of intravascular casts of the choroid.[161] A choroidal origin of CNV had previously been described by Verhoeff & Grossman,[11] Behr,[6] Holloway & Verhoeff,[8] Klien,[162] Paul,[163] Braun,[164] Rintelen,[165] Sandoz,[166] and others. The vessels from which CNV develops were studied in the laser-induced primate model by scanning electron microscopy of plastic casts of the vasculature. Although the procedure[161,167] was technically difficult and prone to artifacts, it was possible to trace the

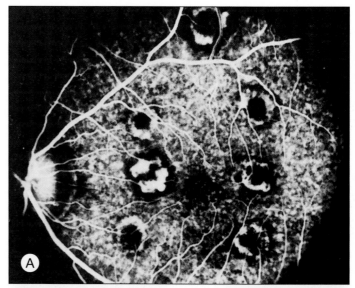

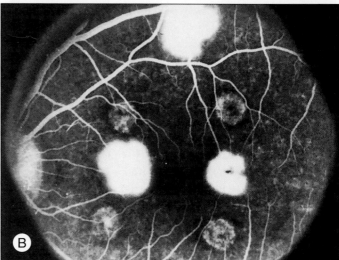

Fig. 56-4 Angiogram shows first clinical evidence of subretinal neovascularization 4 weeks after laser photocoagulation. Note that, in three of eight spots, neovascularization did develop. The leaking lasted for 17, 32, and 44 weeks. A, Early-phase fluorescein angiogram. Note beginning tufts of neovascularization at the edge of the laser burn. B, Late-phase angiogram demonstrates profuse leakage of fluorescein.

feeder vessels from arterioles to the new frond, which drained via the choriocapillaris. In late CNV, feeding vessels of the new frond continued to be derived from choroidal arterioles, but this frond drained via the choroidal venules rather than from the choriocapillaris (Figs 56-5 and 56-6). This preparation provided the opportunity to examine a number of adjacent lesions in three-dimensional detail.

Correlation of histology with fluorescein angiography

The topography of experimental CNV and the relation of CNV to serous detachment of the sensory retina were studied by serial reconstruction and light microscopic studies.[168] These data were correlated with the results of fluorescein angiographic

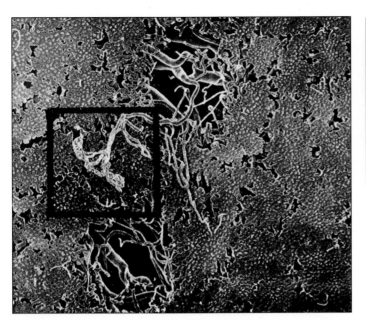

Fig. 56-5 Scanning electron photomicrograph of a vascular cast of a neovascular frond elicited in a monkey retina by laser photocoagulation. The frond was located by pooling and leakage of fluorescein. Choriocapillaris is perforated by two laser lesions through which choroidal vessels can be seen to give rise to the frond (×50). (Reproduced from Ohkuma H, Ryan SJ. Vascular casts of experimental subretinal neovascularization in monkeys: a preliminary report. Jpn J Ophthalmol 1982; 26:150–158.[161])

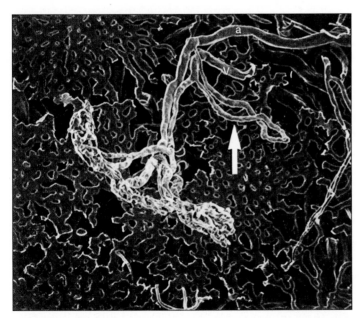

Fig. 56-6 Scanning electron photomicrograph at higher magnification of the neovascular frond shown in Figure 56-4. A simple neovascular loop is indicated by the arrow. The arterial supply (a) and venous drainage (v) of the frond are indicated (×195). (Reproduced from Ohkuma H, Ryan SJ. Vascular casts of experimental subretinal neovascularization in monkeys: a preliminary report. Jpn J Ophthalmol 1982; 26:150–158.[161])

examination. All laser lesions that demonstrated leakage and pooling of fluorescein (leaky lesions) contained subretinal vessels, with an overlying fluid-filled space (Fig. 56-7). The subretinal vessels extended beyond the area of demonstrable leakage,

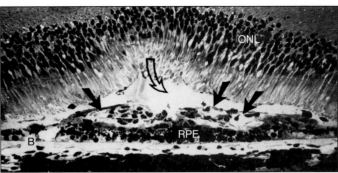

Fig. 56-7 The periphery of a laser lesion. The newly formed subretinal vessels (solid arrows) have proliferated on top of Bruch's membrane (B) and a layer of proliferating retinal pigment epithelial (RPE) cells. The subretinal tissue is separated from the sensory retina by a fluid-filled space (open arrow). ONL, Outer nuclear layer. (Periodic acid–Schiff; ×280.) (Reproduced from Miller H, Miller B, Ryan SJ. Correlation of choroidal subretinal neovascularization with fluorescein angiography. Am J Ophthalmol 1985; 99:263–271.)

whereas the fluid-filled space overlying the subretinal vessels correlated closely with the demonstrated area of leakage (Fig. 56-8). All leaky lesions gradually stopped leaking fluorescein (i.e., they underwent involution). The cessation of leakage was not accompanied by a reduction in the number of subretinal vessels but, rather, with disappearance of the overlying fluid. Furthermore, 80% of the lesions that never leaked fluorescein also contained subretinal vessels in a fibrovascular scar, but these lesions exhibited no overlying fluid. These findings suggest that subretinal vessels can only be detected by fluorescein angiography if they lie beneath a fluid-filled space; fluorescein angiography thus does not necessarily rule out the presence of CNV.

Ultrastructure of choroidal neovascularization

One characteristic of CNV is its tendency to leak and pool. Vessels of the normal choriocapillaris differ from retinal vessels in that they leak fluorescein freely, giving rise to the "choroidal flush" of the normal angiogram. It is considered that leakage of the choriocapillaris is due to the presence of their fenestrations. It was of interest to examine CNV, in its "leaky" stage and after involution, for the presence of fenestrations. Studies with step serial sections and electron microscopic examination revealed that CNV, whether active or involuted, is fenestrated.[168] Consequently, cessation of clinical leakage of fluorescein could not be attributed to loss of CNV fenestrations in involuted CNV.[168] As noted above, in CNV, there is an association between clinical leaking and the presence of an enlarged subretinal space. Because CNV involution was shown not to occur on the basis of loss of fenestrations from the new vessels, additional detailed studies of CNV were done. These suggested an alternative hypothesis.[169] When the first visible signs of leakage appeared on angiographic examination, newly formed vessels had spread into the subretinal space around the break in Bruch's membrane, fluid was accumulating in the subretinal space, and RPE cells were proliferating in a papillary pattern around the newly formed vessels (Fig. 56-9). The RPE proliferation began with the undamaged cells at the edges of the laser injury. With

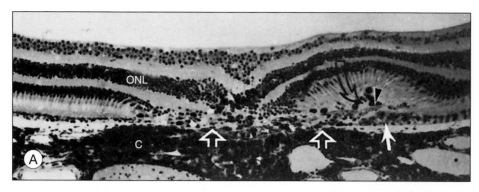

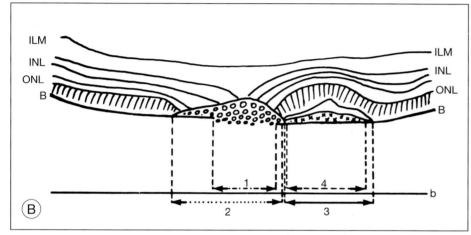

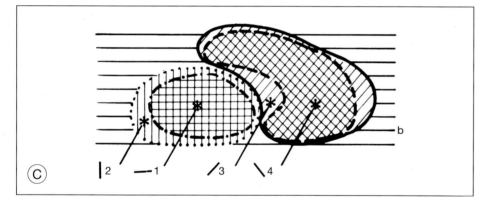

Fig. 56-8 A, The center and periphery of a laser lesion. The edges of the laser injury are defined by the break in Bruch's membrane (open arrows). Subretinal vessels (arrowhead) have proliferated from the edge of the laser injury toward the periphery, where they are found on top of proliferating cells (white solid arrow). Subretinal membrane is present on only one side of the laser injury and is separated from the sensory retina by a fluid-filled space (curved open arrow). Note that the fluid-filled space of this lesion correlates well with the amount of fluorescein leakage and pooling that the lesion demonstrates. C, Choroid; ONL, outer nuclear layer. (Periodic acid–Schiff; ×120.) B, Camera lucida drawing of A (×70). Subretinal neovascularization (SRN) is denoted by x; a fluid-filled space is overlying the neovascularization, and the chorioretinal scar tissue is denoted by o. ILM, Internal limiting membrane; INL, inner nuclear layer; ONL, outer nuclear layer. On a line (b) parallel to Bruch's membrane (B), the orthogonal projection of the following areas is shown: 1, the break in Bruch's membrane; 2, the chorioretinal scar tissue; 4, the neovascular subretinal membrane; and 3, its overlying fluid-filled space. C, Orthogonal serial reconstruction of the lesion. Each line on the reconstructed lesion represents a camera lucida drawing of a cross-section, that is, line b is of the upper drawing. The drawings were made every 40 μm. Areas 1 to 4 show the reconstructed orthogonal features noted in the middle drawing. The neovascular membrane with its overlying fluid is found on only one side of the laser injury. Note the resemblance between the reconstructed shape of the fluid-filled space overlying the SRN (area 4) and the distribution of fluorescein dye during angiography. (Reproduced from Miller H, Miller B, Ryan SJ. Correlation of choroidal subretinal neovascularization with fluorescein angiography. Am J Ophthalmol 1985; 99:263–271.)

further maturation, the RPE continued to envelope the subretinal vessels. This RPE proliferation was associated with the disappearance of fluid between the enveloped vessels and the sensory retina and the gradual cessation of fluorescein leakage and pooling during angiography. At the end of the involution process, when the neovascular membrane no longer demonstrated any leakage, the subretinal vessels were found to be tightly enveloped by RPE cells and no fluid separated them from the sensory retina (Fig. 56-10). These results suggest that involution of the neovascular membrane with maturation, as demonstrated by the cessation of visible fluorescein leakage, is associated with, and may well be the result of, growth of RPE such that they tightly envelop the newly formed vessels. The RPE may be involved in the resorption of the previously accumulated subretinal fluid, as well as in the prevention of its further accumulation in the subretinal space[170] (Fig. 56-11). Histologically, this is supported by a study by Gehrs et al.[171] that used transmission electron microscopy to examine sections of a subretinal choroidal vascular membrane from a patient with AMD. In cross-section, the disciform scar was divided by a thickened RPE cell layer. The choroidal side consisted of fibrovascular tissue with active neovascular buds and inflammatory cells, including macrophages, attached to the RPE basement membrane. The retinal side was fibrous and formed by metaplastic RPE cells and elements of fibrovascular ingrowth in the choroid.

The relevance of this model to the study of human CNV is supported by the similarities in histology and cell types found in established lesions, the identification of VEGF as a major angiogenic protein in these membranes,[132] and the similarity of angiographic features. The model has been used to establish the

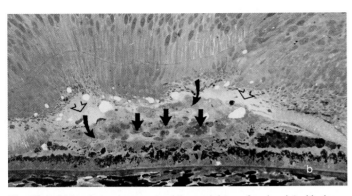

Fig. 56-9 Light photomicrograph of the periphery of an involuted lesion. Retinal pigment epithelial (RPE) cells (curved arrows) are enveloping subretinal vessels (straight black arrows). Note the fluid (open arrows) separating the enveloped subretinal vessels from the sensory retina (×970). b, Bruch's membrane. (Reproduced from Miller H, Miller B, Ryan SJ. The role of retinal pigment epithelium in the involution of subretinal neovascularization. Invest Ophthalmol Vis Sci 1986; 27:1644–1652.)

efficacy of steroids[172] and indometacin[173] in inhibiting CNV formation, thus providing support for the role of an inflammatory component in this model.

Photocoagulation choroidal neovascularization models in other animals

The primate laser model of CNV has been translated to rabbits,[174] rats,[175,176] and mice,[145] since experiments in these animals are much more practical and cost-effective. In rabbits, although photocoagulation does not cause clinically apparent CNV (i.e., associated with leaking and pooling of fluorescein), all photocoagulation lesions produced contained microscopic CNV. Laser-induced CNV in rodents is highly reproducible and is being widely used to evaluate compounds for their ability to inhibit choroidal angiogenesis. Murine laser-induced CNV models have also made it possible to investigate the effect of gene manipulation using knockout or transgenic mouse technology. Fluorescein angiography can be performed in both rat and mouse eyes (Fig. 56-12A). Exogenous gene (β-galactosidase gene) transfer to laser-induced CNVM is also possible (Fig. 56-12B). By

transducing antiangiogenic genes, this model could be useful for investigating the possibility of gene therapy to inhibit formation of the CNV in AMD. A variety of methods have been established to image the laser-induced CNV lesion histologically in exquisite detail (Fig. 56-13).

Choroidal neovascularization models without mechanical disruption of Bruch's membrane

While the photocoagulation model of CNV is relevant for investigating the mechanisms of CNV progression, it may not be appropriate for investigating the initiation of CNV. In the photocoagulation model, Bruch's membrane is mechanically disrupted before the initiation of CNV and the retina is extensively damaged. This extensive tissue damage does not exist in clinical CNV in AMD. Consequently, models of CNV without mechanical damage of Bruch's membrane and overlying retina are of great interest. Two models that induce true CNV without mechanical disruption of Bruch's membrane have been reported. One is a model of CNV (rabbits, rats, or monkeys) induced by implantation of subretinal gelatin microspheres inpregnated with bFGF or VEGF.[144,177] Microspheres are injected from the vitreous side to avoid Bruch's membrane damage using a micropipet. In rabbits, 83% of the eyes showed fluorescein leakage in 2 weeks. Histopathologic examination revealed microscopic CNV in all experimental eyes (Fig. 56-14), but not in the control eyes in which non-bFGF-impregnated microspheres were injected. A second, very recently reported model uses Ccr-2 or Ccl-2 knockout mice; MCP-1 (also known as Ccl-2) and its cognate C-C chemokine receptor-2 (Ccr-2) are critical for extravasation of monocytes. With prolonged aging of the Ccr-2 and Ccl-2 mice, prominent extracellular deposits (similar to drusen) were seen as well as spontaneous CNV.[78] Other transgenic models in which VEGF is overexpressed are relevant to this discussion; however, these models do not result in true CNV. Transgenic mice that overexpress VEGF in photoreceptors develop SRN; however, the subretinal vessels extend from retinal vessels rather than the choroidal vasculature.[99] In contrast, transgenic mice that overexpress VEGF in RPE cells show intrachoroidal CNV.[100]

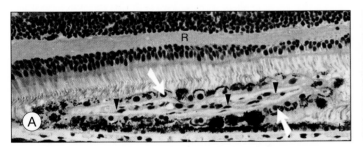

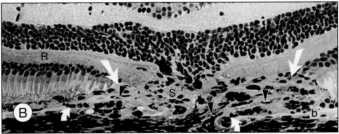

Fig. 56-10 Two representative serial sections of an involuted lesion that had leaked for 4 weeks. The eye was enucleated 8 months after involution was completed. A, Light photomicrograph of periphery of lesion. Retinal pigment epithelial (RPE) cells (white arrows) have formed a tight envelope around the subretinal vessel (arrowheads). Note papillary arrangement of RPE cells and absence of subretinal fluid. R, retina. B, Light photomicrograph 140 μm further into the center of the scar. RPE envelope (long white arrows) on each side seems to end at the edge of the break in Bruch's membrane (short white arrows). Subretinal vessels (arrowheads) are connected to choroidal vasculature through the center of the lesion, where a chorioretinal scar (S) is formed. b, Bruch's membrane. (Reproduced from Miller H, Miller B, Ryan SJ. The role of retinal pigment epithelium in the involution of subretinal neovascularization. Invest Ophthalmol Vis Sci 1986; 27:1644–1652.)

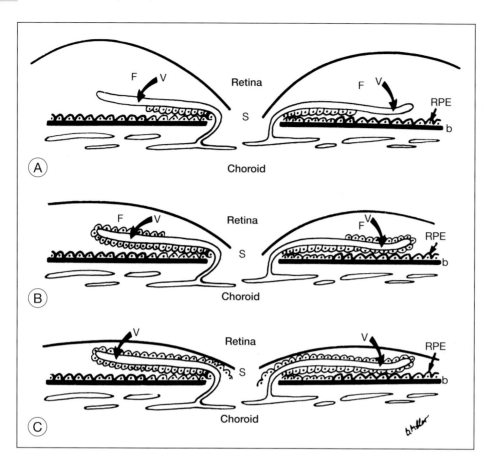

Fig. 56-11 Schematic drawings presenting progression of retinal pigment epithelium (RPE) proliferation around the newly formed subretinal vessels with maturation of the neovascular membrane. A, Early leakage stage. Newly formed subretinal vessels (V) have proliferated into the subretinal space. Fluid (F) leaks from vessels and accumulates in the subretinal space. RPE cells are proliferating in a papillary pattern around the newly formed subretinal vessels. B, Proliferation begins at the edges of the scar with the undamaged cells (heavy line). The finer line represents the newly formed RPE cells that partially envelop the subretinal vessels (V). Less fluid (F) is seen between the enveloped vessels and the sensory retina. C, Involuted stage. RPE cells have formed a tight envelope around the subretinal vessels (V). No fluid is present in the subretinal space. b, Bruch's membrane; S, chorioretinal scar. (Reproduced from Miller H, Miller B, Ryan SJ. The role of retinal pigment epithelium in the involution of subretinal neovascularization. Invest Ophthalmol Vis Sci 1986; 27:1644–1652.)

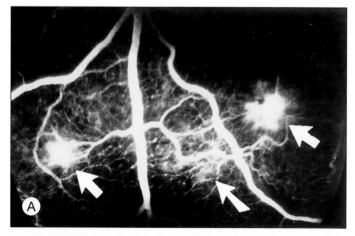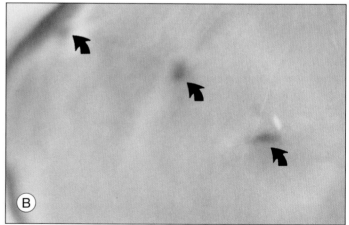

Fig. 56-12 A, Fluorescein leakage indicating choroidal neovascularization development (short arrows) is observed. The other lesion (long arrow) does not show leakage. B, Three photocoagulation lesions (arrows) show a blue reaction product, indicating successful retroviral vector-mediated β-galactosidase transduction and expression.

TARGETED MOLECULAR THERAPY

Specific inhibitors of vascular endothelial growth factor

Currently, many of the basic studies and clinical trials for CNV are focused on the inhibition of VEGF. Strategies that are being investigated include: (1) an oligonucleotide-inhibiting expression of VEGF; (2) a humanized antibody fragment (rhu-Fab V2, or ranibizumab) that neutralizes all isoforms of VEGF; and (3) a synthetic RNA aptamer that specifically binds VEGF and inhibits binding to its receptor.[178]

Steroids

The antiangiogenic activity of steroids is typically a result of broad suppression of inflammation. For example, a single intravitreal injection of triamcinolone acetonide in patients with classic CNV associated with AMD led to a significant

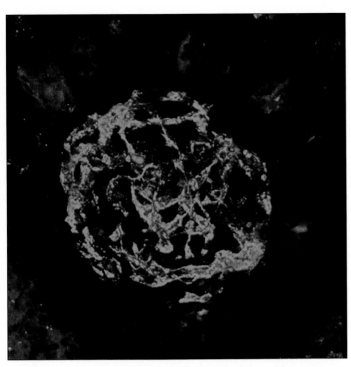

Fig. 56-13 Laser-induced choroidal neovascularization in the mouse. The animal was perfused with fluorescein isothiocyanate (FITC)-dextran 1 week after laser lesion. The retina was dissected from the well-defined lesion, and the FITC-filled neovascular choroidal vessels were identified using confocal microscopy. Z-section series was reconstructed, and a single projection of the image is presented. (Courtesy of Dr. Masanori Hangai and Dr. Naoko Yagi.)

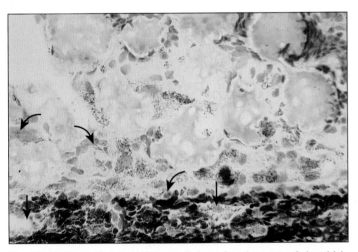

Fig. 56-14 The native choroidal vessels (arrow) and sprouts of choroidal neovascularization (curved arrows) are positive for von Willebrand factor, a marker for endothelial cells. The pale spheres represent microspheres.

reduction in lesion size at 3 months, although there was no apparent difference at 12 months.[179] Combined use of photodynamic therapy and triamcinolone injection has also been investigated. Angiostatic steroids have antiangiogenic activity independent of glucocorticoid action.[180] Anecortave acetate, the most widely studied drug of this class, possesses significant antiangiogenic activity.[181] Sub-Tenon injection of anecortave

acetate stabilized vision in patients with predominantly classic subfoveal CNV.[182]

Signal transduction therapy

Ligand binding to angiogenic growth factor receptors leads to activation of downstream intracellular signaling pathways and subsequent modulation of gene expression and cellular behavior. Targeting inhibition of distinct intracellular signaling pathways, or those common to several growth factor/cell surface receptors, may provide a strategy for therapy of CNV. Peroxisome proliferator-activated receptor-gamma ligands have been shown to have an inhibitory effect on mitogen-activated protein kinase signaling, and they inhibit laser photocoagulation-induced CNV in rats and primates.[183] A VEGF receptor-2 (KDR)-selective tyrosine kinase inhibitor also suppressed laser-induced CNV.[184] Similarly, inhibition of the protein kinase C pathway, currently under evaluation for inhibition of neovascularization in diabetic retinopathy,[185] may be valuable for treatment for CNV.[186]

Radiation therapy

Radiation therapy induces vascular damage leading to vascular occlusion and it may be useful for the therapy of subfoveal CNV. Trials are underway to determine optimal conditions to inhibit CNV formation with fewest side-effects (e.g., radiation retinopathy or cataract).[187]

Photodynamic therapy (PDT)

In PDT, a photosensitizing compound is intravenously injected, and the CNV lesion is irradiated by a sensitizing laser beam of a specific wavelength. Reactive oxygen species are generated that locally damage endothelial cells and result in occlusion of the neovascular channels. Damage to the overlying retina is significantly less than that caused by conventional laser photocoagulation.[188] Several randomized, placebo-controlled trials have demonstrated a functional benefit for PDT in AMD patients with classic subfoveal CNV.[189,190] Currently, PDT combined with another therapeutic modality (e.g., steroids[191] or macular translocation[192]) is being evaluated for its ability to improve the effectiveness of the therapy.

Transplantation of retinal pigment epithelium

During surgical excision of CNVM in AMD, the overlying and adjacent RPE cells are inevitably removed because of their intimate association with the neovascular membrane. Clinical observations and animal studies suggest that RPE removal leads to delayed atrophy of the subfoveal choriocapillaris[193,194] A rationale for RPE transplantation is that the replacement of dysfunctional RPE (removed at the time of submacular surgery) with healthy RPE will both improve RPE function and prevent secondary choriocapillaris atrophy. RPE transplantation could potentially be performed in high-risk AMD patients prior to initiation of CNV.

Gene therapy

The potential of gene therapy for the treatment of CNV is currently being explored in experimental studies that focus on appropriate vector development, selectivity, targeting, and safety, and the stability of transgene expression. Subretinal injection of viral vectors has been used to induce the overexpression of antiangiogenic factors. Delivered in such a manner, vectors expressing tissue inhibitor of metalloproteinases-2,[195] angiostatin,[196] soluble flt-1 receptor,[197] PEDF[198] inhibited the development of laser-induced CNVM. A phase I study of intravitreal injection of an adenoviral vectors encoding PEDF has been commenced in AMD patients with CNV.[199]

We have previously shown that the angiogenic potential of RPE and choroidal endothelial cells can be modulated in vitro by gene transfer.[200] We have shown that retrovirus-mediated TIMP-2 gene transfer into choroidal endothelial cells resulted in sustained expression of TIMP-2 protein, and that the ability of the transduced cells to migrate and form capillary-like tubes was markedly inhibited.[201] These data suggest the possibility that TIMP-2-transduced choroidal endothelial cells may lack the proteolytic ability to penetrate Bruch's membrane and that such treatment may inhibit the development of CNV in vivo. Similarly, RPE cells that have been modified to overexpress TIMP-3 also inhibit CNV.[202]

In most cases, a gene therapy approach for the treatment of CNV would require long-term expression of the therapeutic gene; thus retroviral or lentiviral vectors have been studied for the delivery of antiangiogenic genes to the subretinal space.[203-205] Successful transduction by retroviral vectors requires that target cells are proliferating. Laser photocoagulation initiates a local wound-healing response in which cell proliferation occurs. We have previously shown that retroviral vectors transduced the β-galactosidase (*β-gal*) gene exclusively into photocoagulation sites with relatively high transduction efficiency (Fig. 56.12B).[205,206] Potential candidate genes for delivery using this strategy would be TIMPs, PEDF, or VEGF antisense. Lentiviral vectors do not require cell division for gene transfer; recently, a novel lentiviral vector derived from the nonpathogenic simian immunodeficiency virus from African green monkeys (SIVagm) has been applied to experimental gene therapy for retinal degeneration.[203,204]

Another gene therapy approach for CNV would be the intraocular transplant of RPE cells transduced ex vivo with genes encoding antiangiogenic factors. RPE cells that have been transduced with *β-gal* gene and transplanted into the subretinal space of rabbit eyes remained viable and continued to express the β-gal protein for several months without apparent photoreceptor cell loss (Fig. 56-15).[195]

FAILED STRATEGIES FOR CHOROIDAL NEOVASCULARIZATION TREATMENT

Drugs that have been shown to inhibit angiogenesis in vitro, and CNV in animal models, may not be successful when brought to clinical trial. For example, a clinical trial of the antiangiogenic agent thalidomide for CNV was unsuccessful due to the high incidence of patient side-effects. Interferon-alfa-2a had been shown to be effective as an antiangiogenic agent for several systemic human disorders; however, a randomized, placebo-

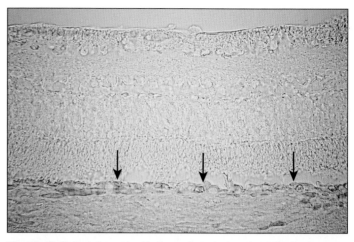

Fig. 56-15 Retinal pigment epithelium cells transduced with β-galactosidase gene (blue) that were transplanted into the subretinal space (arrows).

controlled, multicenter double-blind trial concluded that interferon-alfa-2a provided no benefit as a treatment for CNV secondary to AMD.[207] Although it had been reported that drusen in patients with AMD may resolve after macular laser photocoagulation,[208] enrollment in a clinical trial testing this therapy was halted when possible laser-induced CNV was noted in these patients.[209]

REFERENCES

1. Ryan SJ, Mittl RN, Maumenee AE. The disciform response: an historical perspective. Von Graefes Arch Klin Exp Ophthalmol 1980; 215:1–20.
2. Pagenstecher H, Genth C. Atlas der pathologischen Anatomie des Augenapfels. Wiesbaden, Germany: CW Kriedel; 1875.
3. Oeller J. Atlas seltener ophthalmoskopischer Befunde. Wiesbaden, Germany: JF Bergmann; 1903.
4. Junius P, Kuhnt H. Die scheibenformige Entartung der Netzhautmitte (Degeneratio maculae luteae disciformis). Berlin: Karger; 1926.
5. Behr C. Zur Anatomie der scheibenformigen Maculadegeneration. Klin Monatsbl Augenheilkd 1929; 83:109–110.
6. Behr C. Ein weiterer Beitrag zur Anatomie und zur Pathogenese der scheibenformigen Degeneration am hinteren Augenpol. Z Augenheilkd 1931; 75:216–237.
7. Brown EVL. Retroretinal tissue from the choroid in Kuhnt–Junius degeneration of the macula: anatomic study. Arch Ophthalmol 1940; 23:1157–1168.
8. Holloway TB, Verhoeff FH. Disc-like degeneration of the macula with microscopic report concerning a tumor-like mass in the macular region. Trans Am Ophthalmol Soc 1981; 91:177–183.
9. Khaler AR, O'Brien CS. Disciform degeneration of the macula. Arch Ophthalmol 1935; 13:937–959.
10. Pallares J. Degeneratio disciformis maculae luteae. Klin Monatsbl Augenheilkd 1931; 86:201–203.
11. Verhoeff FH, Grossman HP. Pathogenesis of disciform degeneration of the macula. Arch Ophthalmol 1937; 18:561–585.
12. Maumenee AE. Further advances in the study of the macula. Arch Ophthalmol 1967; 78:151–165.
13. Maumenee AE. Serous and hemorrhagic disciform detachment of the macula. Trans Pa Coast Otolaryngol Ophthalmol Soc 1959; 40:139–160.
14. Maumenee AE. Macular disease: clinical manifestations. Trans Am Acad Ophthalmol Otolaryngol 1965; 69:605–613.
15. Gass JDM. Pathogenesis of disciform detachment of the neuroepithelium. Am J Ophthalmol 1967; 63:573–711.
16. Friedman E, Smith TR, Kuwabara T. Senile choroidal vascular patterns and drusen. Arch Ophthalmol 1963; 69:220–230.
17. Green WR, Key SI. Senile macular degeneration: a histopathologic study. Trans Am Ophthalmol Soc 1977; 75:180–254.
18. Hogan MJ, Alvarado J. Studies on the human macula. IV. Aging changes in Bruch's membrane. Arch Ophthalmol 1967; 77:410–420.

19. Mazow ML, Ruiz RS. Eccentric disciform degeneration. Trans Am Acad Ophthalmol Otolaryngol 1973; 77:68–73.
20. Sarks SH. New vessel formation beneath the retinal pigment epithelium in senile eyes. Br J Ophthalmol 1973; 57:9519–9565.
21. Sarks SH. Ageing and degeneration in the macular region: a clinico-pathological study. Br J Ophthalmol 1976; 60:324–341.
22. Sheffer A, Green WR, Fine SL et al. Presumed ocular histoplasmosis syndrome. A clinicopathologic correlation of a treated case. Arch Ophthalmol 1980; 98:335–340.
23. Teeters VW, Bird AC. A clinical study of the vascularity of senile disciform macular degeneration. Am J Ophthalmol 1973; 75:53–65.
24. Teeters VW, Bird AC. The development of neovascularization of senile disciform macular degeneration. Am J Ophthalmol 1973; 76:1–18.
25. Hyman LG. Senile macular degeneration: an epidemiologic case control study (doctoral dissertation). Baltimore: The Johns Hopkins University; 1981.
26. Ryan SJ. De novo subretinal neovascularization in the histoplasmosis syndrome. Arch Ophthalmol 1976; 94:321–327.
27. Pau H. Die zentrale seröse Retinitis oder Chorioretinitis (Retinopathie oder Chorioretinopathie) und die zentral hämorrhagische Chorioretinitis (juvenile disciforme Makulaablösung: fokale hämorrhagische Choriodditis, presumed Histoplasmosis). Klin Monatsbl Augenheilkd 1979; 175:634–640.
28. Woods AC, Wahlen HE. The probable role of benign histoplasmosis in the etiology of granulomatous uveitis. Trans Am Ophthalmol Soc 1959; 57:318–343.
29. Fine SL, Owens SL, Haller JA et al. Choroidal neovascularization as a late complication of ocular toxoplasmosis. Am J Ophthalmol 1981; 91:318–322.
30. Kleiner RC, Ratner CM, Enger C et al. Subfoveal neovascularization in the ocular histoplasmosis syndrome. A natural history study. Retina 1988; 8:225–229.
31. Krill AE, Archer D. Choroidal neovascularization in multifocal (presumed histoplasmin) choroiditis. Arch Ophthalmol 1970; 84:595–604.
32. Maumenee AE, Ryan SJ. Photocoagulation of disciform macular lesions in the ocular histoplasmosis syndrome. Am J Ophthalmol 1973; 75:13–16.
33. Deutman AF, Kovacs B. Argon laser treatment in complications of angioid streaks. Am J Ophthalmol 1979; 88:12–17.
34. Dreyer R, Green WR. The pathology of angioid streaks: a study of twenty-one cases. Trans Pa Acad Ophthalmol Otolaryngol 1978; 31:158–167.
35. Erkkila H, Raitta C, Niemi KM. Ocular findings in four siblings with pseudoxanthoma elasticum. Acta Ophthalmol (Copenh) 1983; 61:589–599.
36. Esente S, Francais C, Soubrane G et al. Stries angioides et neovaisseaux sous-retiniens: étude retrospective des resultats de la photocoagulation au laser au krypton et au laser à argon vert. Bull Soc Ophtalmol Fr 1987; 87:293–296.
37. Francois J, De LJ, Cambie E et al. Neovascularization after argon laser photocoagulation of macular lesions. Am J Ophthalmol 1975; 79:206–210.
38. Gass JD, Clarkson JG. Angioid streaks and disciform macular detachment in Paget's disease (osteitis deformans). Am J Ophthalmol 1973; 75:576–586.
39. Moriarty BJ, Webb DK, Serjeant GR. Treatment of subretinal neovascularization associated with angioid streaks in sickle cell retinopathy. Case report. Arch Ophthalmol 1987; 105:1327–1328.
40. Shields JA, Federman JL, Tomer TL et al. Angioid streaks. I. Ophthalmoscopic variations and diagnostic problems. Br J Ophthalmol 1975; 59:257–266.
41. Singerman LJ, Hatem G. Laser treatment of choroidal neovascular membranes in angioid streaks. Retina 1981; 1:75–83.
42. Coscas G, Soubrane G. Photocoagulation des néovaisseaux sousrétiniens dans la dégénérescence masculaire sénile par laser à argon: résultats de l'étude randomisée de 60 cas. Bull Mem Soc Fr Ophtalmol 1983; 94:149–154.
43. Elwin H. Heredodegenerations and heredoconstitutional defects of the retina. Arch Ophthalmol 1955; 53:619–633.
44. Gifford SR, Cushman B. Certain retinopathies due to changes in the lamina vitrea. Arch Ophthalmol 1940; 23:60–75.
45. Goodman RM, Smith EW, Paton D et al. Pseudoxanthoma elasticum: a clinical and histopathological study. Medicine (Baltimore) 1963; 42:297–334.
46. Smith JL, Gass JDM, Justice JJ. Fluorescein fundus photography of angioid streaks. Br J Ophthalmol 1964; 48:517–521.
47. Clay GE, Baird JM. Angioid streaks of the choroids and pseudoxanthoma elasticum. South Med J 1910; 3:127–133.
48. Levy JH, Pollock HM, Curtin BJ. The Fuchs' spot: an ophthalmoscopic and fluorescein angiographic study. Ann Ophthalmol 1977; 9:1433–1443.
49. Klein RM, Curtin BJ. Lacquer crack lesions in pathologic myopia. Am J Ophthalmol 1975; 79:386–392.
50. Hotchkiss ML, Fine SL. Pathologic myopia and choroidal neovascularization. Am J Ophthalmol 1981; 91:177–183.
51. Hampton GR, Kohen D, Bird AC. Visual prognosis of disciform degeneration in myopia. Ophthalmology 1983; 90:923–926.
52. Fleury I, De LJ. Prognosis of the disciform response in high myopia. Bull Soc Belge Ophtalmol 1983; 206:91–102.
53. Avila MP, Weiter JJ, Jalkh AE et al. Natural history of choroidal neovascularization in degenerative myopia. Ophthalmology 1984; 91:1573–1581.
54. Green WR. Retina. In: Spencer WH, ed. Ophthalmic pathology: an atlas and textbook. Philadelphia: WB Saunders; 1985:913–924.
55. Doyne RW. Choroidal and retinal changes as the result of blows on the eyes. Trans Ophthalmol Soc UK 1889; 9:128.
56. Wallace W, Neame H. Retinitis proliferans: clinical report, with illustration of a case which developed after gunshot wound of orbit; pathological report, with notes of other cases and review. Trans Ophthalmol Soc UK 1923; 43:296–324.
57. Paton D, Goldberg MF. Management of ocular injuries. Philadelphia: WB Saunders; 1976.
58. Fuller B, Gitter KA. Traumatic choroidal rupture with late serous detachment of macula. Report of successful argon laser treatment. Arch Ophthalmol 1973; 89:354–355.
59. Goldberg MF. Choroidoretinal vascular anastomoses after blunt trauma to the eye. Am J Ophthalmol 1976; 82:892–895.
60. Hilton GF. Late serosanguineous detachment of the macula after traumatic choroidal rupture. Am J Ophthalmol 1975; 79:997–1000.
61. Smith RE, Kelley JS, Harbin TS. Late macular complications of choroidal ruptures. Am J Ophthalmol 1974; 77:650–658.
62. Francois J, De Laey JJ, Cambie E et al. Neovascularization after argon laser photocoagulation of macular lesions. Am J Ophthalmol 1975; 79:206–210.
63. Berger AR, Boniuk I. Bilateral subretinal neovascularization after focal argon laser photocoagulation for diabetic macular edema. Am J Ophthalmol 1989; 108:88–90.
64. Chandra SR, Bresnick GH, Davis MD et al. Choroidovitreal neovascular ingrowth after photocoagulation for proliferative diabetic retinopathy. Arch Ophthalmol 1980; 98:1593–1599.
65. Fine SL, Patz A, Orth DH et al. Subretinal neovascularization developing after prophylactic argon laser photocoagulation of atrophic macular scars. Am J Ophthalmol 1976; 82:352–357.
66. Galinos SO, Asdourian GK, Woolf MB et al. Choroido-vitreal neovascularization after argon laser photocoagulation. Arch Ophthalmol 1975; 93:524–530.
67. Goldbaum MH, Galinos SO, Apple D et al. Acute choroidal ischemia as a complication of photocoagulation. Arch Ophthalmol 1976; 94:1025–1035.
68. Schatz H, Yannuzzi LA, Gitter KA. Subretinal neovascularization following argon laser photocoagulation treatment for central serous chorioretinopathy: complication or misdiagnosis? Trans Am Acad Ophthalmol Otolaryngol 1977; 83:893–906.
69. Wallow I, Johns K, Barry P et al. Chorioretinal and choriovitreal neovascularization after photocoagulation for proliferative diabetic retinopathy. A clinicopathologic correlation. Ophthalmology 1985; 92:523–532.
70. Cleasby GW. Idiopathic focal subretinal neovascularization. Am J Ophthalmol 1976; 81:590–599.
71. Lepori JC, Raspiller A, Heymann V et al. Membrane neovasculaire choroidienne et maladie de Lobstein. Bull Soc Ophtalmol Fr 1984; 84:305–307.
72. Macular Photocoagulation Study Group. Argon laser photocoagulation for senile macular degeneration. Results of a randomized clinical trial. Arch Ophthalmol 1982; 100:912–918.
73. Meyer D, Harris WP, Fine SL et al. Clinicopathologic correlation of argon-laser photocoagulation of an idiopathic choroidal neovascular membrane in the macula. Retina 1984; 4:107–114.
74. Soubrane G, Koenig F, Coscas G. Choroidopathie maculaire hemorragique du sujet jeune. J Fr Ophtalmol 1983; 6:25–34.
75. Yassur Y, Gilad E, Ben SI. Treatment of macular subretinal neovascularization with the red-light krypton laser in presumed ocular histoplasmosis syndrome. Am J Ophthalmol 1981; 91:172–176.
76. Campochiaro PA, Soloway P, Ryan SJ et al. The pathogenesis of choroidal neovascularization in patients with age-related macular degeneration. Mol Vis 1999; 5:34.
77. Zarbin MA. Age-related macular degeneration: review of pathogenesis. Eur J Ophthalmol 1998; 8:199–206.
78. Ambati J, Anand A, Fernandez S et al. An animal model of age-related macular degeneration in senescent Ccl-2- or Ccr-2-deficient mice. Nat Med 2003; 9:1390–1397.
79. Klein R, Klein BE, Jensen SC et al. The five-year incidence and progression of age-related maculopathy: the Beaver Dam Eye Study [see comments]. Ophthalmology 1997; 104:7–21.
80. Wilcox DK. Vectorial accumulation of cathepsin D in retinal pigmented epithelium: effects of age. Invest Ophthalmol Vis Sci 1988; 29:1205–1212.
81. Kennedy CJ, Rakoczy PE, Constable IJ. Lipofuscin of the retinal pigment epithelium: a review. Eye 1995; 9:763–771.
82. Rakoczy PE, Zhang D, Robertson T et al. Progressive age-related changes similar to age-related macular degeneration in a transgenic mouse model. Am J Pathol 2002; 161:1515–1524.

83. Tombran-Tink J, Shivaram SM, Chader GJ et al. Expression, secretion, and age-related downregulation of pigment epithelium-derived factor, a serpin with neurotrophic activity. J Neurosci 1995; 15:4992–5003.

84. Hjelmeland LM, Cristofolo VJ, Funk W et al. Senescence of the retinal pigment epithelium. Mol Vis 1999; 5:33.

85. Okubo A, Rosa RH Jr, Bunce CV et al. The relationships of age changes in retinal pigment epithelium and Bruch's membrane. Invest Ophthalmol Vis Sci 1999; 40:443–449.

86. Matsunaga H, Handa JT, Gelfman CM et al. The mRNA phenotype of a human RPE cell line at replicative senescence. Mol Vis 1999; 5:39.

87. Sarks JP, Sarks SH, Killingsworth MC. Evolution of soft drusen in age-related macular degeneration. Eye 1994; 8:269–283.

88. Abdelsalam A, Del Priore L, Zarbin MA. Drusen in age-related macular degeneration: pathogenesis, natural course, and laser photocoagulation-induced regression. Surv Ophthalmol 1999; 44:1–29.

89. Green WR, Enger C. Age-related macular degeneration histopathologic studies. The 1992 Lorenz E. Zimmerman lecture. Ophthalmology 1993; 100:1519–1535.

90. Starita C, Hussain AA, Patmore A et al. Localization of the site of major resistance to fluid transport in Bruch's membrane. Invest Ophthalmol Vis Sci 1997; 38:762–767.

91. Punglia RS, Lu M, Hsu J et al. Regulation of vascular endothelial growth factor expression by insulin-like growth factor I. Diabetes 1997; 46:1619–1626.

92. Pe'er J, Shweiki D, Itin A et al. Hypoxia-induced expression of vascular endothelial growth factor by retinal cells is a common factor in neovascularizing ocular diseases [see comments]. Lab Invest 1995; 72:638–645.

93. Lutty GA, McLeod DS, Merges C et al. Localization of vascular endothelial growth factor in human retina and choroid. Arch Ophthalmol 1996; 114:971–977.

94. Ishibashi T, Murata T, Hangai M et al. Advanced glycation end products in age-related macular degeneration. Arch Ophthalmol 1998; 116:1629–1632.

95. Lafaut BA, Bartz-Schmidt KU, Vanden Broecke C et al. Clinicopathological correlation in exudative age related macular degeneration: histological differentiation between classic and occult choroidal neovascularisation. Br J Ophthalmol 2000; 84:239–243.

96. Alexander JP, Bradley JM, Gabourel JD et al. Expression of matrix metalloproteinases and inhibitor by human retinal pigment epithelium. Invest Ophthalmol Vis Sci 1990; 31:2520–2528.

97. Padgett LC, Lui GM, Werb Z et al. Matrix metalloproteinase-2 and tissue inhibitor of metalloproteinase-1 in the retinal pigment epithelium and interphotoreceptor matrix: vectorial secretion and regulation. Exp Eye Res 1997; 64:927–938.

98. Vranka JA, Johnson E, Zhu X et al. Discrete expression and distribution pattern of TIMP-3 in the human retina and choroid. Curr Eye Res 1997; 16:102–110.

99. Okamoto N, Tobe T, Hackett SF et al. Transgenic mice with increased expression of vascular endothelial growth factor in the retina: a new model of intraretinal and subretinal neovascularization. Am J Pathol 1997; 151:281–291.

100. Schwesinger C, Yee C, Rohan RM et al. Intrachoroidal neovascularization in transgenic mice overexpressing vascular endothelial growth factor in the retinal pigment epithelium. Am J Pathol 2001; 158:1161–1172.

101. Goetzl EJ, Banda MJ, Leppert D. Matrix metalloproteinases in immunity. J Immunol 1996; 156:1–4.

102. Killingsworth MC, Sarks JP, Sarks SH. Macrophages related to Bruch's membrane in age-related macular degeneration. Eye 1990; 4:613–621.

103. Grossniklaus HE, Ling JX, Wallace TM et al. Macrophage and retinal pigment epithelium expression of angiogenic cytokines in choroidal neovascularization. Mol Vis 2002; 8:119–126.

104. Lopez PF, Sippy BD, Lambert HM et al. Transdifferentiated retinal pigment epithelial cells are immunoreactive for vascular endothelial growth factor in surgically excised age-related macular degeneration-related choroidal neovascular membranes. Invest Ophthalmol Vis Sci 1996; 37:855–868.

105. Murata T, Ishibashi T, Inomata H et al. Media conditioned by coculture of pericytes and endothelial cells under a hypoxic state stimulate in vitro angiogenesis. Ophthalm Res 1994; 26:23–31.

106. Zetter BR. Angiogenesis and tumor metastasis. Annu Rev Med 1998; 49:407–424.

107. He S, Jin ML, Worpel V et al. Connective tissue growth factor and its role in the pathogenesis of choroidal neovascularization. Arch Ophthalmol 2003; 121:1283–1288.

108. Miyajima-Uchida H, Hayashi H, Beppu R et al. Production and accumulation of thrombospondin-1 in human retinal pigment epithelial cells. Invest Ophthalmol Vis Sci 2000; 41:561–567.

109. Kaplan HJ, Leibole MA, Tezel T et al. Fas ligand (CD95 ligand) controls angiogenesis beneath the retina. Nat Med 1999; 5:292–297.

110. Espinosa-Heidmann DG, Suner IJ, Hernandez EP et al. Macrophage depletion diminishes lesion size and severity in experimental choroidal neovascularization. Invest Ophthalmol Vis Sci 2003; 44:3586–3592.

111. Sakurai E, Anand A, Ambati BK et al. Macrophage depletion inhibits experimental choroidal neovascularization. Invest Ophthalmol Vis Sci 2003; 44:3578–3585.

112. Tsutsumi C, Sonoda KH, Egashira K et al. The critical role of ocular-infiltrating macrophages in the development of choroidal neovascularization. J Leukoc Biol 2003; 74:25–32.

113. Oh H, Takagi H, Takagi C et al. The potential angiogenic role of macrophages in the formation of choroidal neovascular membranes. Invest Ophthalmol Vis Sci 1999; 40:1891–1898.

114. Tomita M, Yamada H, Adachi Y et al. Choroidal neovascularization is provided by bone marrow cells. Stem Cells 2004; 22:21–26.

115. Espinosa-Heidmann DG, Caicedo A, Hernandez EP et al. Bone marrow-derived progenitor cells contribute to experimental choroidal neovascularization. Invest Ophthalmol Vis Sci 2003; 44:4914–4919.

116. Sengupta N, Caballero S, Mames RN et al. The role of adult bone marrow-derived stem cells in choroidal neovascularization. Invest Ophthalmol Vis Sci 2003; 44:4908–4913.

117. Wyllie AH. Glucocorticoid-induced thymocyte apoptosis is associated with endogenous endonuclease activation. Nature 1980; 284:555–556.

118. Hinton DR, He S, Lopez PF. Apoptosis in surgically excised choroidal neovascular membranes in age-related macular degeneration. Arch Ophthalmol 1998; 116:203–209.

119. Kliffen M, Sharma HS, Mooy CM et al. Increased expression of angiogenic growth factors in age-related maculopathy. Br J Ophthalmol 1997; 81:154–162.

120. Yates JR, Moore AT. Genetic susceptibility to age related macular degeneration. J Med Genet 2000; 37:83–87.

121. Allikmets R, Singh N, Sun H et al. A photoreceptor cell-specific ATP-binding transporter gene (ABCR) is mutated in recessive Stargardt macular dystrophy [see comments]. Nat Genet 1997; 15:236–246.

122. Webster AR, Heon E, Lotery AJ et al. An analysis of allelic variation in the ABCA4 gene. Invest Ophthalmol Vis Sci 2001; 42:1179–1189.

123. Weber BH, Vogt G, Pruett RC et al. Mutations in the tissue inhibitor of metalloproteinases-3 (TIMP3) in patients with Sorsby's fundus dystrophy. Nat Genet 1994; 8:352–356.

124. Fariss RN, Apte SS, Olsen BR et al. Tissue inhibitor of metalloproteinases-3 is a component of Bruch's membrane of the eye. Am J Pathol 1997; 150:323–328.

125. Felbor U, Doepner D, Schneider U et al. Evaluation of the gene encoding the tissue inhibitor of metalloproteinases-3 in various maculopathies. Invest Ophthalmol Vis Sci 1997; 38:1054–1059.

126. De La Paz MA, Pericak-Vance MA, Lennon F et al. Exclusion of TIMP3 as a candidate locus in age-related macular degeneration. Invest Ophthalmol Vis Sci 1997; 38:1060–1065.

127. Petrukhin K, Koisti MJ, Bakall B et al. Identification of the gene responsible for Best macular dystrophy. Nat Genet 1998; 19:241–247.

128. Marmorstein LY, Munier FL, Arsenijevic Y et al. Aberrant accumulation of EFEMP1 underlies drusen formation in Malattia Leventinese and age-related macular degeneration. Proc Natl Acad Sci USA 2002; 99:13067–13072.

129. Aiello LP, Avery RL, Arrigg PG et al. Vascular endothelial growth factor in ocular fluid of patients with diabetic retinopathy and other retinal disorders. N Engl J Med 1994; 331:1480–1487.

130. Frank RN, Amin RH, Eliott D et al. Basic fibroblast growth factor and vascular endothelial growth factor are present in epiretinal and choroidal neovascular membranes. Am J Ophthalmol 1996; 122:393–403.

131. Kvanta A, Algvere PV, Berglin L et al. Subfoveal fibrovascular membranes in age-related macular degeneration express vascular endothelial growth factor. Invest Ophthalmol Vis Sci 1996; 37:1929–1934.

132. Ishibashi T, Hata Y, Yoshikawa H et al. Expression of vascular endothelial growth factor in experimental choroidal neovascularization. Graefes Arch Clin Exp Ophthalmol 1997; 235:159–167.

133. Sakamoto T, Sakamoto H, Murphy TL et al. Vessel formation by choroidal endothelial cells in vitro is modulated by retinal pigment epithelial cells. Arch Ophthalmol 1995; 113:512–520.

134. Cao J, McLeod S, Merges CA et al. Choriocapillaris degeneration and related pathologic changes in human diabetic eyes. Arch Ophthalmol 1998; 116:589–597.

135. Ross RD, Barofsky JM, Cohen G et al. Presumed macular choroidal watershed vascular filling, choroidal neovascularization, and systemic vascular disease in patients with age-related macular degeneration. Am J Ophthalmol 1998; 125:71–80.

136. Lu M, Kuroki M, Amano S et al. Advanced glycation end products increase retinal vascular endothelial growth factor expression. J Clin Invest 1998; 101:1219–1224.

137. Honda S, Farboud B, Hjelmeland LM et al. Induction of an aging mRNA retinal pigment epithelial cell phenotype by matrix-containing advanced glycation end products in vitro. Invest Ophthalmol Vis Sci 2001; 42:2419–2425.

138. McFarlane S, McMullen CB, Henry DN. Advanced glycation end products (AGEs) modulate cathepsin D expression in retinal pigment epithelium (RPE): implications for age-related macular dysfunction. Invest Ophthalmol Vis Sci 2001; 42:S414.

139. Schutt F, Bergmann M, Holz FG et al. Proteins modified by malondialdehyde, 4-hydroxynonenal, or advanced glycation end products in lipofuscin of human retinal pigment epithelium. Invest Ophthalmol Vis Sci 2003; 44:3663–3668.

140. Yan SD, Schmidt AM, Anderson GM et al. Enhanced cellular oxidant stress by the interaction of advanced glycation end products with their receptors/binding proteins. J Biol Chem 1994; 269:9889–9897.

141. Okamoto T, Tanaka S, Stan AC et al. Advanced glycation end products induce angiogenesis in vivo. Microvasc Res 2002; 63:186–195.

142. Kitaoka T, Morse LS, Schneeberger S et al. Expression of FGF5 in choroidal neovascular membranes associated with ARMD. Curr Eye Res 1997; 16:396–399.

143. Amin R, Puklin JE, Frank RN. Growth factor localization in choroidal neovascular membranes of age-related macular degeneration. Invest Ophthalmol Vis Sci 1994; 35:3178–3188.

144. Kimura H, Sakamoto T, Hinton DR et al. A new model of subretinal neovascularization in the rabbit. Invest Ophthalmol Vis Sci 1995; 36:2110–2119.

145. Tobe T, Ortega S, Luna JD et al. Targeted disruption of the FGF2 gene does not prevent choroidal neovascularization in a murine model. Am J Pathol 1998; 153:1641–1646.

146. Yamada H, Yamada E, Kwak N et al. Cell injury unmasks a latent proangiogenic phenotype in mice with increased expression of FGF2 in the retina. J Cell Physiol 2000; 185:135–142.

147. Suri C, Jones PF, Patan S et al. Requisite role of angiopoietin-1, a ligand for the TIE2 receptor, during embryonic angiogenesis. Cell 1996; 87:1171–1180.

148. Thurston G, Suri C, Smith K et al. Leakage-resistant blood vessels in mice transgenically overexpressing angiopoietin-1. Science 1999; 286:2511–2514.

149. Oh H, Takagi H, Suzuma K et al. Hypoxia and vascular endothelial growth factor selectively up-regulate angiopoietin-2 in bovine microvascular endothelial cells. J Biol Chem 1999; 274:15732–15739.

150. Otani A, Takagi H, Oh H et al. Expressions of angiopoietins and Tie2 in human choroidal neovascular membranes. Invest Ophthalmol Vis Sci 1999; 40:1912–1920.

151. Dawson DW, Volpert OV, Gillis P et al. Pigment epithelium-derived factor: a potent inhibitor of angiogenesis. Science 1999; 285:245–248.

152. Holekamp NM, Bouck N, Volpert O. Pigment epithelium-derived factor is deficient in the vitreous of patients with choroidal neovascularization due to age-related macular degeneration. Am J Ophthalmol 2002; 134:220–227.

153. Stellmach V, Crawford SE, Zhou W et al. Prevention of ischemia-induced retinopathy by the natural ocular antiangiogenic agent pigment epithelium-derived factor. Proc Natl Acad Sci USA 2001; 98:2593–2597.

154. Mori K, Gehlbach P, Ando A et al. Regression of ocular neovascularization in response to increased expression of pigment epithelium-derived factor. Invest Ophthalmol Vis Sci 2002; 43:2428–2434.

155. Kvanta A. Expression and regulation of vascular endothelial growth factor in choroidal fibroblasts. Curr Eye Res 1995; 14:1015–1020.

156. Leonardy NJ, Dabbs CK, Sternberg PJ. Subretinal neovascularization after operating microscope burn. Am J Ophthalmol 1990; 109:224–225.

157. Archer DB, Gardiner TA. Morphologic fluorescein angiographic, and light microscopic features of experimental choroidal neovascularization. Am J Ophthalmol 1981; 91:297–311.

158. Ryan SJ. The development of an experimental model of subretinal neovascularization in disciform macular degeneration. Trans Am Ophthalmol Soc 1979; 77:707–745.

159. Ryan SJ. Subretinal neovascularization after argon laser photocoagulation. Von Graefes Arch Klin Exp Ophthalmol 1980; 215:29–42.

160. Ryan SJ. Subretinal neovascularization. Natural history of an experimental model. Arch Ophthalmol 1982; 100:1804–1809.

161. Ohkuma H, Ryan SJ. Vascular casts of experimental subretinal neovascularization in monkeys. Invest Ophthalmol Vis Sci 1983; 24:481–490.

162. Klien BA. Macular lesions of vascular origin. Am J Ophthalmol 1951; 34:1279–1289.

163. Paul L. Choroditis exsudative unter dem Bilde der scheibenförmigen Entartung der Netzhautmitte. Z Augenheilkd 1927; 63:295–723.

164. Braun R. Pathologisch-anatomischer Beitrag zur Frage der scheibenförmigen Entartung der Fundusmitte. Arch Augenheilkd 1937; 110:535–548.

165. Rintelen F. Zur Histologie des submakulären senilen Pseudotumors. Z Augenheilkd 1937; 92:306–321.

166. Sandoz YL. Beidseitiger histologischer Befund bei senilem Maculapseudotumor, der zu einer neuen Auffassung dieser Altersveränderung führt. Graefes Arch Exp Ophthalmol 1939; 140:725–747.

167. Ohkuma H, Ryan SJ. Vascular casts of experimental subretinal neovascularization in monkeys: a preliminary report. Jpn J Ophthalmol 1982; 26:150–158.

168. Miller H, Miller B, Ryan SJ. Correlation of choroidal subretinal neovascularization with fluorescein angiography. Am J Ophthalmol 1985; 99:263–271.

169. Miller H, Miller B, Ryan SJ. Newly-formed subretinal vessels. Fine structure and fluorescein leakage. Invest Ophthalmol Vis Sci 1986; 27:204–213.

170. Miller H, Miller B, Ryan SJ. The role of retinal pigment epithelium in the involution of subretinal neovascularization. Invest Ophthalmol Vis Sci 1986; 27:1644–1652.

171. Gehrs KM, Heriot WJ, de Juan E Jr. Transmission electron microscopic study of a subretinal choroidal neovascular membrane due to age-related macular degeneration. Arch Ophthalmol 1992; 110:833–837.

172. Ishibashi T, Miki K, Sorgente N et al. Effects of intravitreal administration of steroids on experimental subretinal neovascularization in the subhuman primate. Arch Ophthalmol 1985; 103:708–711.

173. Sakamoto T, Soriano D, Nassaralla J et al. Effect of intravitreal administration of indomethacin on experimental subretinal neovascularization in the subhuman primate. Arch Ophthalmol 1995; 113:222–226.

174. elDirini AA, Ogden TE, Ryan SJ. Subretinal endophotocoagulation. A new model of subretinal neovascularization in the rabbit. Retina 1991; 11:244–249.

175. Dobi ET, Puliafito CA, Destro M. A new model of experimental choroidal neovascularization in the rat. Arch Ophthalmol 1989; 107:264–269.

176. Frank RN, Das A, Weber ML. A model of subretinal neovascularization in the pigmented rat. Curr Eye Res 1989; 8:239–247.

177. Cui JZ, Kimura H, Spee C et al. Natural history of choroidal neovascularization induced by vascular endothelial growth factor in the primate. Graefes Arch Clin Exp Ophthalmol 2000; 238:326–333.

178. Eyetech SG. Anti-vascular endothelial growth factor therapy for subfoveal choroidal neovascularization secondary to age-related macular degeneration: phase II study results. Ophthalmology 2003; 110:979–986.

179. Gillies MC, Simpson JM, Luo W et al. A randomized clinical trial of a single dose of intravitreal triamcinolone acetonide for neovascular age-related macular degeneration: one-year results. Arch Ophthalmol 2003; 121:667–673.

180. Crum R, Szabo S, Folkman J. A new class of steroids inhibits angiogenesis in the presence of heparin or a heparin fragment. Science 1985; 230:1375–1378.

181. Penn JS, Rajaratnam VS, Collier RJ et al. The effect of an angiostatic steroid on neovascularization in a rat model of retinopathy of prematurity. Invest Ophthalmol Vis Sci 2001; 42:283–290.

182. Slakter JS. Anecortave acetate as monotherapy for treatment of subfoveal neovascularization in age-related macular degeneration: twelve-month clinical outcomes. Ophthalmology 2003; 110:2372–2383.

183. Murata T, He S, Hangai M et al. Peroxisome proliferator-activated receptor-gamma ligands inhibit choroidal neovascularization. Invest Ophthalmol Vis Sci 2000; 41:2309–2317.

184. Takeda A, Hata Y, Shiose S et al. Suppression of experimental choroidal neovascularization utilizing KDR selective receptor tyrosine kinase inhibitor. Graefes Arch Clin Exp Ophthalmol 2003; 241:765–772.

185. Aiello LP, Bursell SE, Clermont A et al. Vascular endothelial growth factor-induced retinal permeability is mediated by protein kinase C in vivo and suppressed by an orally effective beta-isoform-selective inhibitor. Diabetes 1997; 46:1473–1480.

186. Saishin Y, Silva RL, Callahan K et al. Periocular injection of microspheres containing PKC412 inhibits choroidal neovascularization in a porcine model. Invest Ophthalmol Vis Sci 2003; 44:4989–4993.

187. Bergink GJ, Hoyng CB, van der Maazen RWM et al. A randomized controlled clinical trial on the efficacy of radiation therapy in the control of subretinal choroidal neovascularization in age-related macular degeneration: radiation versus observation. Graefes Arch Clin Exp Ophthalmol 1998; 236:321–325.

188. Schmidt-Erfurth UJM, Bunse A, Laqua H et al. Photodynamic therapy of subfoveal choroidal neovascularization: clinical and angiographic examples. Graefes Arch Clin Exp Ophthalmol 1998; 236:365–374.

189. Blinder KJ, Bradley S, Bressler NM et al. Effect of lesion size, visual acuity, and lesion composition on visual acuity change with and without verteporfin therapy for choroidal neovascularization secondary to age-related macular degeneration: TAP and VIP report no. 1. Am J Ophthalmol 2003; 136:407–418.

190. Blumenkranz MS, Bressler NM, Bressler SB et al. Verteporfin therapy for subfoveal choroidal neovascularization in age-related macular degeneration: three-year results of an open-label extension of 2 randomized clinical trials – TAP report no. 5. Arch Ophthalmol 2002; 120:1307–1314.

191. Spaide RF, Sorenson J, Maranan L. Combined photodynamic therapy with verteporfin and intravitreal triamcinolone acetonide for choroidal neovascularization. Ophthalmology 2003; 110:1517–1525.

192. Stanga P, Hiscott P, Li K et al. Macular relocation after photodynamic therapy for recurrent choroidal neovascular membrane: visual results and histopathological findings. Br J Ophthalmol 2003; 87:975–976.

193. Akduman L, Del PL, Desai VN et al. Perfusion of the subfoveal choriocapillaris affects visual recovery after submacular surgery in presumed ocular histoplasmosis syndrome. Am J Ophthalmol 1997; 123:90–96.

194. Pollack JS, Del PL, Smith ME et al. Postoperative abnormalities of the choriocapillaris in exudative age-related macular degeneration. Br J Ophthalmol 1996; 80:314–318.

195. Murata T, Cui J, Taba KE et al. The possibility of gene therapy for the treatment of choroidal neovascularization. Ophthalmology 2000; 107:1364–1373.

196. Lai CC, Wu WC, Chen SL et al. Suppression of choroidal neovascularization by adeno-associated virus vector expressing angiostatin. Invest Ophthalmol Vis Sci 2001; 42:2401–2407.

197. Honda M, Sakamoto T, Ishibashi T et al. Experimental subretinal neovascularization is inhibited by adenovirus-mediated soluble VEGF/flt-1 receptor gene transfection: a role of VEGF and possible treatment for SRN in age-related macular degeneration. Gene Ther 2000; 7:978–985.

198. Mori K, Gehlbach P, Yamamoto S et al. AAV-mediated gene transfer of pigment epithelium-derived factor inhibits choroidal neovascularization. Invest Ophthalmol Vis Sci 2002; 43:1994–2000.

199. Rasmussen H, Chu KW, Campochiaro P et al. Clinical protocol. An open-label, phase I, single administration, dose-escalation study of ADGVPEDF.11D (ADPEDF) in neovascular age-related macular degeneration (AMD). Hum Gene Ther 2001; 12:2029–2032.

200. Sakamoto T, Spee C, Scuric Z et al. Ability of retroviral transduction to modify the angiogenic characteristics of RPE cells. Graefes Clin Exp Ophthalmol 1998; 236:220–229.

201. Murata T, Cui JZ, Taba KE et al. The possibility of gene therapy for the treatment of choroidal neovascularization. Ophthalmology 2000; 107:1364–1373.

202. Takahashi T, Nakamura T, Hayashi A et al. Inhibition of experimental choroidal neovascularization by overexpression of tissue inhibitor of metalloproteinases-3 in retinal pigment epithelium cells. Am J Ophthalmol 2000; 130:774–781.

203. Ikeda Y, Goto Y, Yonemitsu Y et al. Simian immunodeficiency virus-based lentivirus vector for retinal gene transfer: a preclinical safety study in adult rats. Gene Ther 2003; 10:1161–1169.

204. Miyazaki M, Ikeda Y, Yonemitsu Y et al. Simian lentiviral vector-mediated retinal gene transfer of pigment epithelium-derived factor protects retinal degeneration and electrical defect in Royal College of Surgeons' rats. Gene Ther 2003; 10:1503–1511.

205. Murata T, Hoffmann S, Ishibashi T et al. Retrovirus-mediated gene transfer targeted to retinal photocoagulation sites. Diabetologia 1998; 41:500–506.

206. Murata T, Hangai M, Ishibashi T et al. Retrovirus-mediated gene transfer to photocoagulation-induced choroidal neovascular membranes. Invest Ophthalmol Vis Sci 1998; 39:2474–2478.

207. Pharmacological Therapy for Macular Degeneration Study Group. Interferon alfa-2a is ineffective for patients with choroidal neovascularization secondary to age-related macular degeneration. Results of a prospective randomized placebo-controlled clinical trial. Arch Ophthalmol 1997; 115:865–872.

208. Ho AC. Laser treatment in eyes with drusen. Curr Opin Ophthalmol 1999; 10:204–208.

209. Owens SL, Bunce C, Brannon AJ et al. Prophylactic laser treatment appears to promote choroidal neovascularisation in high-risk ARM: results of an interim analysis. Eye 2003; 17:623–627.

210. Annesley WJ. Peripheral exudative hemorrhagic chorioretinopathy. Trans Am Ophthalmol Soc 1980; 78:321–364.

211. Blair CJ, Aaberg TM. Massive subretinal exudation associated with senile macular degeneration. Am J Ophthalmol 1971; 71:639–648.

212. Garner A. Pathology of macular degeneration in the elderly. Trans Ophthalmol Soc UK 1975; 95:54–61.

213. Gass JD. Drusen and disciform macular detachment and degeneration. Trans Am Ophthalmol Soc 1972; 70:409–436.

214. Gass JD. Drusen and disciform macular detachment and degeneration. Arch Ophthalmol 1973; 90:206–217.

215. Gass JD. Choroidal neovascular membranes – their visualization and treatment. Trans Am Acad Ophthalmol Otolaryngol 1973; 77:OP310–OP320.

216. Gass JDM. Pathogenesis of disciform detachment of the neuroepithelium. Am J Ophthalmol 1967; 63:573–711.

217. Gass JD, Jallow S, Davis B. Adult vitelliform macular detachment occurring in patients with basal laminar drusen. Am J Ophthalmol 1985; 99:445–459.

218. Gaynon MW, Boldrey EE, Strahlman ER et al. Retinal neovascularization and ocular toxoplasmosis. Am J Ophthalmol 1984; 98:585–589.

219. Gold D, Friedman A, Wise GN. Predisciform senile macular degeneration. Am J Ophthalmol 1973; 76:763–768.

220. Gospodarowicz D. Brain and pituitary-fibroblast growth factors. Hormonal Proteins Peptides 1984; 12:205–230.

221. Gragoudas ES, Chandra SR, Friedman E et al. Disciform degeneration of the macula. II. Pathogenesis. Arch Ophthalmol 1976; 94:755–757.

222. Green WR, McDonnell PJ, Yeo JH. Pathologic features of senile macular degeneration. Ophthalmology 1985; 92:615–627.

223. Gregor Z, Bird AC, Chisholm IH. Senile disciform macular degeneration in the second eye. Br J Ophthalmol 1977; 61:141–147.

224. Kenyon KR, Maumenee AE, Ryan SJ et al. Diffuse drusen and associated complications. Am J Ophthalmol 1985; 100:119–128.

225. Small ML, Green WR, Alpar JJ et al. Senile macular degeneration. A clinicopathologic correlation of two cases with neovascularization beneath the retinal pigment epithelium. Arch Ophthalmol 1976; 94:601–607.

226. Smiddy WE, Fine SL. Prognosis of patients with bilateral macular drusen. Ophthalmology 1984; 91:271–277.

227. Giuffre G, Brancato G. Subretinal neovascularization in anterior ischemic optic neuropathy. Graefes Arch Clin Exp Ophthalmol 1991; 229:19–23.

228. Munier F, Othenin GP. Subretinal neovascularization secondary to choroidal septic metastasis from acute bacterial endocarditis. Retina 1992; 12:108–112.

229. Turet P, Malthieu D, Douillet A. Pseudo-retinite pigmentaire rubeolique et membrane neo-vasculaire choroidienne. Bull Soc Ophtalmol Fr 1982; 82:595–597.

230. Frangieh GT, Green WR, Fine SL. A histopathologic study of Best's macular dystrophy. Arch Ophthalmol 1982; 100:1115–1121.

231. Benson WE, Kolker AE, Enoch JM et al. Best's vitelliform macular dystrophy. Am J Ophthalmol 1975; 79:59–66.

232. Brucker AJ, Deglin EA, Bene C et al. Subretinal choroidal neovascularization in birdshot retinochoroidopathy. Am J Ophthalmol 1985; 99:40–44.

233. Soubrane G, Coscas G, Binaghi M et al. Birdshot retinochoroidopathy and subretinal new vessels. Br J Ophthalmol 1983; 67:461–467.

234. Witschel H, Font RL. Hemangioma of the choroid. A clinicopathologic study of 71 cases and a review of the literature. Surv Ophthalmol 1976; 20:415–431.

235. Snip RC, Green WR, Jaegers KR. Choroidal nevus with subretinal pigment epithelial neovascular membrane and a positive P-32 test. Ophthalm Surg 1978; 9:35–42.

236. Waltman DD, Gitter KA, Yannuzzi LA et al. Choroidal neovascularization associated with choroidal nevi. Am J Ophthalmol 1978; 85:704–710.

237. Skorska I, Soubrane G, Coscas G. Choroidite toxoplasmique et neo-vaisseaux sous-retiniens. J Fr Ophtalmol 1984; 7:211–218.

238. Mines JA, Freilich DB, Friedman AH et al. Choroidal (subretinal) neovascularization secondary to choroidal nevus and successful treatment with argon laser photocoagulation. Case reports and review of literature. Ophthalmologica 1985; 190:210–218.

239. Gonder JR, Augsburger JJ, McCarthy EF et al. Juxtapapillary choroidal nevi. Trans Pa Acad Ophthalmol Otolaryngol 1982; 35:13–15.

240. Melrose MA, Magargal LE, Goldberg RE et al. Subretinal neovascular membranes associated with choroidal nonperfusion and retinal ischemia. Ann Ophthalmol 1987; 19:396–399.

241. Kelinske M, Weinstein GW. Bilateral choroidal osteomas. Am J Ophthalmol 1981; 92:676–680.

242. Kayazawa F, Shimamoto S. Choroidal osteoma: two cases in Japanese women. Ann Ophthalmol 1981; 13:1053–1056.

243. Joffe L, Shields JA, Fitzgerald JR. Osseous choristoma of the choroid. Arch Ophthalmol 1978; 96:1809–1812.

244. Grand MG, Burgess DB, Singerman LJ et al. Choroidal osteoma. Treatment of associated subretinal neovascular membranes. Retina 1984; 4:84–89.

245. Gass JD, Guerry RK, Jack RL et al. Choroidal osteoma. Arch Ophthalmol 1978; 96:428–435.

246. Gass JD. New observations concerning choroidal osteomas. Int Ophthalmol 1979; 1:71–84.

247. Coston TO, Wilkinson CP. Choroidal osteoma. Am J Ophthalmol 1978; 86:368–372.

248. Burke JFJ, Brockhurst RJ. Argon laser photocoagulation of subretinal neovascular membrane associated with osteoma of the choroid. Retina 1983; 3:304–307.

249. Baum MD, Pilkerton AR, Berler DK et al. Choroidal osteoma. Ann Ophthalmol 1979; 11:1849–1851.

250. Pearlstone AD. Delayed loss of central vision following multiple posterior segment trauma. Ann Ophthalmol 1980; 12:409–411.

251. Aguilar JP, Green WR. Choroidal rupture. A histopathologic study of 47 cases. Retina 1984; 4:269–275.

252. Robinson D, Tiedeman J. Choroideremia associated with a subretinal neovascular membrane. Case report. Retina 1987; 7:70–74.

253. Green WR. The uveal tract. In: Spencer WH, ed. Ophthalmic pathology: an atlas and textbook, Philadelphia: WB Saunders; 1985:1515–1520.

254. Sorenson JA, Yannuzzi LA, Shakin JL. Recurrent subretinal neovascularization. Ophthalmology 1985; 92:1059–1074.

255. Spitznas M, Bornfeld N. Development and ultrastructure of peripheral subretinal neovascularizations. Von Graefes Arch Klin Exp Ophthalmol 1978; 208:125–133.

256. Beebe WE, Kirkland C, Price J. A subretinal neovascular membrane as a complication of endogenous *Candida* endophthalmitis. Ann Ophthalmol 1987; 19:207–209.

257. Green WR. Retina. In: Spencer WH, ed. Ophthalmic pathology: an atlas and textbook. Philadelphia: WB Saunders; 1985:1239–1244.

258. Flood TP, Orth DH, Aaberg TM et al. Macular hamartomas of the retinal pigment epithelium and retina. Retina 1983; 3:164–170.

259. Klein R, Lewis RA, Meyers SM et al. Subretinal neovascularization associated with fundus flavimaculatus. Arch Ophthalmol 1978; 96:2054–2057.

260. Yannuzzi LA, Shakin JL, Fisher YL et al. Peripheral retinal detachments and retinal pigment epithelial atrophic tracts secondary to central serous pigment epitheliopathy. Ophthalmology 1984; 91:1554–1572.

261. Macular Photocoagulation Study Group. Argon laser photocoagulation for idiopathic neovascularization. Results of a randomized clinical trial. Arch Ophthalmol 1983; 101:1358–1361.

262. Cleasby GW, Fung WE, Fiore JJ. Photocoagulation of exudative senile maculopathy. Arch Ophthalmol 1971; 85:18–26.

263. Smith T, Magargal LE, Donoso LA et al. Choroidal neovascularization in an eye with a macular hole. Ann Ophthalmol 1989; 21:331–336.

264. Lubin JR, Gragoudas ES, Albert DM. Choroidal neovascularization associated with malignant melanoma: a case report. Acta Ophthalmol (Copenh) 1982; 60:412–418.

265. Wildi G. Zur Fundusentartung mit angioider Streifenbildung. Klin Monatsbl Augenheilkd 1925; 76:177–194.

266. Leys A, Michielsen B, Leys M et al. Subretinal neovascular membranes associated with chronic membranoproliferative glomerulonephritis type II. Graefes Arch Clin Exp Ophthalmol 1990; 228:499–504.

267. Trimble SN, Schatz H. Subretinal neovascularization following metallic intraocular foreign-body trauma. Arch Ophthalmol 1986; 104:515–519.

268. Sobol WM, Bratton AR, Rivers MB et al. Morning glory disk syndrome associated with subretinal neovascular membrane formation. Am J Ophthalmol 1990; 110:93–94.

269. Wyhinny GJ, Jackson JL, Jampol LM et al. Subretinal neovascularization following multiple evanescent white-dot syndrome. Arch Ophthalmol 1990; 108:1384–1385.

270. Silva VB, Brockhurst RJ. Hemorrhagic detachment of the peripheral retinal pigment epithelium. Arch Ophthalmol 1976; 94:1295–1300.

271. Bec P, Secheyron P, Arne JL et al. Le neovascularisation sous-retinienne peripherique et ses consequences pathologiques. J Fr Ophtalmol 1979; 2:329–336.

272. Shields JA, Shields CL, De PP, Milner RS. Choroidal neovascular membrane as a feature of optic nerve glioma. Retina 1997; 17:349–350.

273. Borodic GE, Gragoudas ES, Edward WO et al. Peripapillary subretinal neovascularization and serous macular detachment. Association with congenital optic nerve pits. Arch Ophthalmol 1984; 102:229–231.

274. Dizon-Moore RV, Jampol LM, Goldberg MF. Chorioretinal and choriovitreal neovascularization. Their presence after photocoagulation of proliferative sickle cell retinopathy. Arch Ophthalmol 1981; 99:842–849.

275. Benson WE, Townsend RE, Pheasant TR. Choriovitreal and subretinal proliferations: complications of photocoagulation. Ophthalmology 1979; 86:283–289.

276. Weingeist TA, Watzke RC. Ocular involvement by Histoplasma capsulatum. Int Ophthalmol Clin 1983; 23:33–47.

277. Watzke RC, Claussen RW. The long-term course of multifocal choroiditis (presumed ocular histoplasmosis). Am J Ophthalmol 1981; 91:750–760.

278. Stafford TJ, Anness SH, Fine BS. Subretinal neovascularization after experimental ocular histoplasmosis in a subhuman primate [letter]. Am J Ophthalmol 1986; 101:132–133.

279. Rosenberg PR, Zinn KM. Peripapillary subretinal neovascularization in presumed ocular histoplasmosis: a case report. Mt Sinai J Med 1980; 47:405–409.

280. Olk RJ, Burgess DB, McCormick PA. Subfoveal and juxtafoveal subretinal neovascularization in the presumed ocular histoplasmosis syndrome. Visual prognosis. Ophthalmology 1984; 91:1592–1602.

281. Meredith TA, Green WR, Key SN et al. Ocular histoplasmosis: clinico-pathologic correlation of 3 cases. Surv Ophthalmol 1977; 22:189–205.

282. Macular Photocoagulation Study Group. Argon laser photocoagulation for ocular histoplasmosis. Results of a randomized clinical trial. Arch Ophthalmol 1983; 101:1347–1357.

283. Klein ML, Fine SL, Knox DL et al. Follow-up study in eyes with choroidal neovascularization caused by presumed ocular histoplasmosis. Am J Ophthalmol 1977; 83:830–835.

284. Jester JV, Smith RE. Subretinal neovascularization after experimental ocular histoplasmosis in a subhuman primate. Am J Ophthalmol 1985; 100:252–258.

285. Irvine AR, Spencer WH, Hogan MJ et al. Presumed chronic ocular histoplasmosis syndrome: a clinical-pathologic case report. Trans Am Ophthalmol Soc 1977; 74:91–106.

286. Baskin MA, Jampol LM, Huamonte FU et al. Macular lesions in blacks with the presumed ocular histoplasmosis syndrome. Am J Ophthalmol 1980; 89:77–83.

287. Watzke RC, Packer AJ, Folk JC et al. Punctate inner choroidopathy. Am J Ophthalmol 1984; 98:572–584.

288. Boozalis GT, Schachat AP, Green WR. Subretinal neovascularization from the retina in radiation retinopathy. Retina 1987; 7:156–161.

289. Theodossiadis GP. Choroidal neovascularization after cryoapplication. Von Graefes Arch Klin Exp Ophthalmol 1981; 215:203–208.

290. Fogle JA, Welch RB, Green WR. Retinitis pigmentosa and exudative vasculopathy. Arch Ophthalmol 1978; 96:696–702.

291. Maberley AL, Gottner MJ, Antworth MV. Subretinal neovascularization associated with retinochoroidal colobomas. Can J Ophthalmol 1989; 24:172–174.

292. Frank KE, Purnell EW. Subretinal neovascularization following rubella retinopathy. Am J Ophthalmol 1978; 86:462–466.

293. Deutman AF, Grizzard WS. Rubella retinopathy and subretinal neovascularization. Am J Ophthalmol 1978; 85:82–87.

294. Gragoudas ES, Regan CD. Peripapillary subretinal neovascularization in presumed sarcoidosis. Arch Ophthalmol 1981; 99:1194–1197.

295. Mansour AM, Jampol LM, Packo KH et al. Macular serpiginous choroiditis. Retina 1988; 8:125–131.

296. Laatikainen L, Erkkila H. Subretinal and disc neovascularisation in serpiginous choroiditis. Br J Ophthalmol 1982; 66:326–331.

297. Jampol LM, Orth D, Daily MJ et al. Subretinal neovascularization with geographic (serpiginous) choroiditis. Am J Ophthalmol 1979; 88:683–689.

298. Blumenkranz MS, Gass JD, Clarkson JG. Atypical serpiginous choroiditis. Arch Ophthalmol 1982; 100:1773–1775.

299. Gottlieb F, Fammartino JJ, Stratford TP et al. Retinal angiomatous mass. A complication of retinal detachment surgery. Retina 1984; 4:152–157.

300. Goldbaum MH, Weidenthal DT, Krug S et al. Subretinal neovascularization as a complication of drainage of subretinal fluid. Retina 1983; 3:114–117.

301. Stur M. Congenital tilted disk syndrome associated with parafoveal subretinal neovascularization. Am J Ophthalmol 1988; 105:98–99.

302. Kennedy JE, Wise GN. Retinochoroidal vascular anastomosis in uveitis. Am J Ophthalmol 1971; 71:1221–1225.

303. Fine SL, Owens SL, Haller JA et al. Choroidal neovascularization as a late complication of ocular toxoplasmosis. Am J Ophthalmol 1981; 91:318–322.

304. Chung YM, Yeh TS, Sheu SJ et al. Macular subretinal neovascularization in choroidal tuberculosis. Ann Ophthalmol 1989; 21:225–229.

305. Ober RR, Smith RE, Ryan SJ. Subretinal neovascularization in the Vogt–Koyanagi–Harada syndrome. Int Ophthalmol 1983; 6:225–234.

306. Inomata H, Minei M, Taniguchi Y et al. Choroidal neovascularization in long-standing case of Vogt–Koyanagi–Harada disease. Jpn J Ophthalmol 1983; 27:9–26.

Chapter

57

Management of Intraocular Inflammation

Narsing A. Rao

Uveitis and other intraocular inflammations are major causes of blindness. In approximately 70% of cases, the etiologic basis and pathogenesis of these intraocular inflammations remain obscure, even after exhaustive clinical and laboratory investigations.[1] In the remaining 30% the intraocular inflammation is caused by trauma or by an infectious agent, most commonly *Toxoplasma gondii*. Most cases of nontraumatic and noninfectious uveitis are believed to represent autoimmunity to ocular tissue components. Regardless of their cause, however, those forms of uveitis that appear with signs of severe intraocular inflammation have a poor visual prognosis, primarily because of retinal and uveal tissue damage in the form of vascular leakage, cystoid macular edema, secondary glaucoma, cataract, and other alterations mediated by cytokines, proteolytic enzymes, and oxygen metabolites and free radicals.[2,3]

Clear experimental evidence demonstrates that retinal and retinal pigment epithelial (RPE) proteins, including choroidal melanin-associated proteins, can function as autoantigens and perpetuate uveitis. These antigen-induced uveitis models (Fig. 57-1) have allowed investigations of the cellular and molecular mechanisms involved in the development and perpetuation of uveitis in various laboratory animals.[4–7] Based on these experimental animal studies, it appears that the induction of uveitis may be initiated by an altered tolerance to retinal or RPE-choroidal proteins, probably triggered by an infectious agent.[8]

For the appropriate management of uveitis today, it is important to recognize and differentiate infectious from noninfectious autoimmune uveitis, as well as from those masquerade syndromes that may clinically simulate uveitis, such as retinoblastoma, leukemia, or juvenile xanthogranuloma in children and lymphoma or other necrotic malignancies in adults.[9]

Using the appropriate antimicrobial agents, with or without corticosteroids, makes the management of infectious uveitis fairly straightforward.[10] Noninfectious uveitis, on the other hand, necessitates further investigation before administration of antiinflammatory or immunosuppressive agents.[11] These cases require a clear understanding of the autoimmune processes that can lead to uveitis.

Many factors must be considered when deciding when and how to treat patients with noninfectious uveitis. The presence of inflammation alone is not always an indication for treatment. For example, a patient who has pars planitis with moderate vitreous cells but with no cystoid macular edema and a visual acuity of 20/25 does not require treatment. Likewise, a patient who has Fuchs' heterochromic iridocyclitis should not be given intensive topical corticosteroid treatment, since this will only hasten the development of cataract. On the other hand, a patient who has juvenile rheumatoid arthritis (JRA) and chronic flare alone does not require corticosteroid medications, but he or she may require chronic mydriatic therapy to prevent the synechiae. In all instances a risk–benefit analysis should be performed, and therapy should be instituted only when the benefits of such therapy outweigh the potential complications.

Once infectious processes and neoplastic possibilities are excluded, noninfectious uveitis should be classified as anterior, intermediate, posterior, or panuveitis on the basis of slit-lamp and ophthalmoscopic findings. For most cases of anterior uveitis, frequent topical corticosteroids combined with cycloplegic agents should be sufficient; in severe cases periocular injections or a short course of systemic corticosteroids may be necessary. For intermediate or posterior uveitis, periocular injections are the preferred route; however, systemic corticosteroids are used for bilateral cases or if the patient is intolerant of periocular injections.

Mydriatic or cycloplegic agents are used primarily to relieve the ciliary spasm and pain that often accompany iridocyclitis and to prevent the development of posterior synechiae. In general, the intermediate-acting agents, such as homatropine, are preferred in most cases of anterior uveitis. The stronger, longer-acting agents may be indicated to help break synechiae that have already formed, whereas shorter-acting agents may be preferred if there is a high likelihood of posterior synechiae formation (e.g., severe iritis with intense flare), since these agents tend to keep the pupil relatively mobile.

Nonsteroidal anti-inflammatory drugs (NSAIDs) exert their effects by interfering with prostaglandin synthesis. Although these drugs appear to have some role in the treatment of aphakic cystoid macular edema and certain types of scleritis, they have generally been found to be of little value in the treatment of most uveitis entities.

CORTICOSTEROIDS

Corticosteroids are the mainstay of antiinflammatory therapy for most types of uveitis because they effectively suppress the

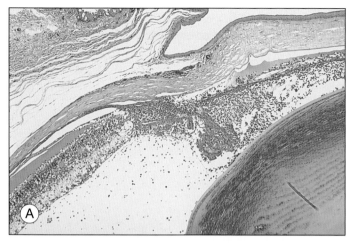

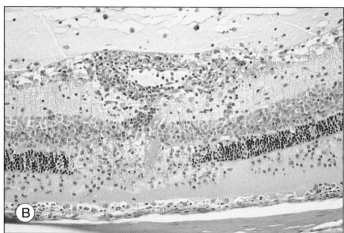

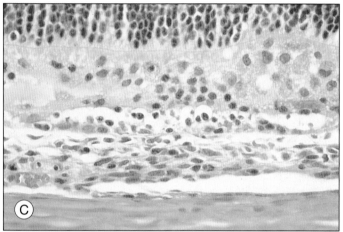

Fig. 57-1 Retinal soluble protein (S antigen)-induced uveoretinitis in Lewis rat. A, Note iridocyclitis and inflammation involving retina with serous detachment (hematoxylin & eosin; ×60). B, Note retinal vasculitis and foci of necrosis (hematoxylin & eosin; ×200). C, Higher magnification shows photoreceptor damage at the site of inflammatory cell infiltration. The choroid is thickened from the inflammatory cell infiltration (hematoxylin & eosin; ×320).

inflammatory response regardless of its cause. The anti-inflammatory effects are initiated when the corticosteroid molecule enters the target cell and combines with the appropriate receptor within the cytoplasm. This steroid–receptor complex is then transported to the cell nucleus, where it influences DNA transcription, resulting in changes in messenger RNA production, protein synthesis, and cell function.

Topical application of corticosteroid drops produces fewer side-effects than corticosteroids administered by periocular injection or oral therapy. These corticosteroid drops are used for most cases of anterior uveitis and can be given as frequently as every hour if necessary. Only in particularly severe cases of anterior uveitis may periocular or systemic corticosteroids be indicated. However, since topical corticosteroids do not penetrate the posterior segment well, topical application is not usually indicated in the treatment of intermediate or posterior uveitis. In these instances periocular injections should be given, if possible, particularly in unilateral cases. In general, the preferred method of delivery is by injection into the posterior sub-Tenon's space through one of the temporal quadrants. This can easily be accomplished by using only topical anesthesia, such as proparacaine or tetracaine. The periocular injection results in high concentrations of corticosteroids in both the anterior and posterior compartments of the eye.[12]

Systemic therapy is most often administered by the oral route. It is generally used for patients with bilateral uveitis or those with severe unilateral inflammation who are intolerant of or unresponsive to periocular injections. An initial oral dose of 1 mg/kg of prednisone per day is usually given; the dosage is then gradually tapered as the inflammation subsides. In selected cases with severe intraocular inflammation, some clinicians will begin with intravenous methylprednisolone at a dosage of 1 g/day for 3 days followed by the oral prednisone, 60 to 80 mg/day in an adult. Generally, the high-dose corticosteroids are continued for no longer than 1 month and if there is no response within 4 weeks an immunosuppressive agent is added. In patients with satisfactory anti-inflammatory response, the corticosteroids are gradually tapered and discontinued if possible. If the systemic corticosteroids lasts for more than 2 weeks, the corticosteroids should not be stopped abruptly at a high dose. Generally, they are tapered 10 mg/day every 1 to 2 weeks while the patient is on over 40 mg/day. Once the oral prednisone is reduced to 20 to 40 mg/day, the corticosteroids can be decreased by 5 mg/day every 1 to 2 weeks and subsequently decreased by 2.5 mg/day every 1 to 2 weeks. Once the dose has been reduced to between 10 and 20 mg/day, the dosage can be doubled and taken on alternate days to reduce the systemic side-effects of chronic corticosteroid use. However, some patients may have an exacerbation of symptoms on alternate-day therapy and may need to take daily doses until the medicine is tapered. When either topical or systemic corticosteroids are being used, it is generally preferred to begin with a higher or more frequent dose (e.g., one drop every 1 to 2 h or 60 to 80 mg of prednisone per day), tapering the medication as the inflammation subsides, rather than to start with a low dose and increase the dose to control the inflammation.

Regardless of the route of administration, steroid therapy can be associated with both ocular and systemic complications, including elevated intraocular pressure, predisposition to infections, posterior subcapsular cataract formation, gastric ulceration, hypertension, osteoporosis, diabetes, and mental changes such as euphoria or psychosis. Although the periocular route decreases the incidence and severity of these systemic effects, it does not completely eliminate the risk. In general, the development of these side-effects is related to the dose of medication and the duration of treatment. Patients need to be advised of the possible side-effects before beginning therapy, and they should be monitored (blood pressure, weight, glucose every 3 months, blood lipids annually, bone density within the first 3 months and annually thereafter) closely while receiving corticosteroids.

CYTOTOXIC AND IMMUNOSUPPRESSIVE AGENTS

Use of cytotoxic and immunosuppressive agents is reserved for severe, sight-threatening cases of uveitis that are poorly responsive to corticosteroids or for patients who develop intolerable side-effects from corticosteroids. In contrast to the more cytostatic effects of corticosteroids, cytotoxic agents (antimetabolites and alkylating agents) are believed to exert their beneficial effects in uveitis by killing the rapidly dividing lymphocyte clones that are responsible for the inflammation[13] (Table 57-1).

In general, the use of immunosuppressive agents is only indicated when certain conditions are met: (1) the intraocular inflammation is of a vision-threatening nature; (2) the disease process is reversible; and (3) there is no response to corticosteroid treatment, or such treatment is contraindicated because of a systemic problem.

In addition, several guidelines should be followed before initiation of therapy with any cytotoxic agent: (1) there should be an absence of infection; (2) the patient should have no hematologic contraindications to therapy; (3) there should be meticulous follow-up by an ophthalmologist or internist or a medical oncologist, if necessary; and (4) an objective evaluation of the disease process should be done.

The immunosuppressive/cytotoxic agents used in treatment of uveitis include methotrexate, azathioprine, mycophenolate mofetil, chlorambucil, and cyclophosphamide.[14] Azathioprine, methotrexate, and mycophenolate mofetil are examples of antimetabolites. Azathioprine can suppress both antibody production and cell-mediated function. The degree of T-cell immunosuppression by this agent is unclear, and it appears that much of its anti-inflammatory activity can be attributed to the inhibition of monocyte function. Methotrexate has an inhibitory activity against many enzymes in the metabolic pathway of folic acid. The long-term use of low-dose methotrexate therapy

Table 57-1 Some clinically useful cytotoxic and immunosuppressive agents in uveitis

Agent	Class	Mode of action	Dose	
			Initial	Maximum
Methotrexate	Antimetabolite	Inhibits dihydrofolate reductase	7.5 to 12.5 mg/week	25 mg/week PO, SC, or IM
Azathioprine	Antimetabolite	Inhibits nucleic acid synthesis in lymphocytes	1 mg/kg per day	2.5 to 4 mg/kg per day PO
Mycophenolate mofetil	Antimetabolite	Inhibits inosine monophosphate and lymphocyte proliferation	500 mg BID	1.5 g BID PO
Cyclophosphamide	Alkylating agent	Cross-links DNA; blocks cell division	2 mg/kg per day	3 mg/kg per day PO
Chlorambucil	Alkylating agent	Cross-links DNA; lymphotoxicity	0.1 mg/kg per day	0.2 mg/kg per day
Ciclosporin	T-cell inhibitor	Binds calcineurin, inhibits nuclear factor of activated T cell; early events in T-cell activation	2.5–5.0 mg/kg per day (divided dose)	10 mg/kg per day PO

PO, orally; SC, subcutaneously; IM, intramuscularly; BID, twice daily.

(≤ 25 mg once a week) inhibits the production of thymidylate, purines, and methionines and leads to the accumulation of adenosine, a potent anti-inflammatory substance. These actions inhibit cellular proliferation, decrease the formation of antibodies, and decrease the production of interleukins and eicosanoids.[15] Mycophenolate mofetil inhibits inosine monophosphate dehydrogenase and prevents lymphocyte proliferation and decreases recruitment of leukocytes to sites of inflammation. Azathioprine is usually given at a dose of 1 to 4 mg/kg per day (Table 57-1), whereas methotrexate can be given as a weekly oral or subcutaneous or intramuscular dose of 7.5 to 25 mg. Methotrexate may be an effective therapy for corticosteroid-resistant uveitis including intermediate uveitis, vitritis, scleritis, and sarcoid-associated uveitis.[12,16] Side-effects of methotrexate include hepatotoxicity, cytopenias, interstitial pneumonia, stomatitis, alopecia, and rash. This agent is contraindicated in pregnancy and patients should be advised to abstain from alcohol consumption. Monitoring of liver functions and complete blood count should be obtained every 4 to 8 weeks. Azathioprine can be used as a steroid-sparing agent in uveitis. Patients receiving standard doses of both azathioprine and allopurinol should be observed for possible life-threatening granulocytopenia caused by a marked increase in the azathioprine effect, which is increased about fivefold. Allergic phenomena that may occur with azathioprine include rash, fever, hepatitis, and gastrointestinal intolerance. Severe side-effects include bone marrow suppression and hepatotoxicity. Complete blood count and liver function tests should be performed every 4 to 6 weeks.

Mycophenolate mofetil is often used in combination with corticosteroids or in some cases in combination with ciclosporin.[17] Adverse effects of mycophenolate mofetil include myalgia, headache, nausea, and fatigue and patients should be monitored with complete blood count, blood chemistry, and liver functions.

Chlorambucil is an alkylating agent. At high doses it causes a suppressed maturation of bone marrow cells. At lower doses it exerts its effects on lymphopoiesis and then on granulopoiesis. The daily oral dosage varies from 0.1 to 0.2 mg/kg. Both leukopenia and thrombocytopenia may occur, and irreversible bone marrow suppression has been reported in some patients.

Cyclophosphamide is metabolized in the liver. Concomitant administration of phenobarbital, adrenocorticosteroids, or other agents that induce the hepatic mixed-oxidase system leads to more complete metabolism of cyclophosphamide. The metabolites accumulate in patients with renal insufficiency; therefore such patients should receive lower doses of cyclophosphamide. Cyclophosphamide may be administered either orally or intravenously; however, uveitis is usually managed by oral administration. Adverse events include bone marrow suppression, hemorrhagic cystitis, azoospermia, ovarian failure, alopecia, nausea, and vomiting. The patient should be advised to take adequate fluids to prevent the cystitis. Complete blood count and urine analysis should be performed at least every 4 weeks.

The side-effects and potential complications of any of the above cytotoxic agents are many and, at times, can be fatal. Leukopenia is more common than thrombocytopenia or significant anemia with azathioprine.

The most feared complication of these agents is the future development of malignancies, such as leukemia, lymphoma, or soft-tissue tumors, as well as teratogenesis (e.g., chromosomal damage or azoospermia), which makes their use in younger patients particularly troublesome. Whenever these agents are used, the patient should be fully advised of all potential complications, including the development of opportunistic bacterial, fungal, and viral infections. Because cytotoxic agents have such serious side-effects, their use in the treatment of uveitis is restricted to severe and chronic cases that do not respond to other therapy. Treatment should be discontinued either at the first sign of major toxicity or when it is clear that no benefit has been obtained with therapeutic levels of the drug.

When a combination of cytotoxic agents is administered, a synergistic effect can occur. This synergy takes place when methylprednisolone is used with cyclophosphamide, chlorambucil, or azathioprine. The synergistic effect is also noted when treatment includes either cyclophosphamide and methotrexate or cyclophosphamide with azathioprine and methylprednisolone.

The International Uveitis Study Group attempted to categorize the indications for immunosuppressive agents as "absolute" and "relative" (Table 57-2), except in the rare cases in which the agents might not be selected, such as in early pregnancy. Some uveitis entities do warrant the use of cytotoxic agents for suppression of the intraocular inflammation. These include Behçet's disease and rheumatoid necrotizing sclerouveitis. Although these intraocular inflammatory disorders may initially respond well to corticosteroids, the long-term prognosis and the morbidity associated with these entities are unacceptable. Initial treatment of these conditions with cytotoxic agents has been shown to improve the long-term prognosis and to lessen the visual morbidity. There is an absolute indication for the use of cytotoxic agents in patients with chronic Vogt–Koyanagi–Harada syndrome and patients with serpiginous choroidopathy.

Relative indications for the cytotoxic agents include those conditions for which corticosteroids are the initial agents of choice. If these agents fail to control the inflammation, then cytotoxic agents may be tried. The clinical entities in this category include intermediate uveitis (pars planitis), retinal vasculitis,

Table 57-2 Indications for cytotoxic and immunosuppressive agents in adults as recommended by the International Uveitis Study Group	
Indications	Uveitis entities
Absolute	Behçet's syndrome
	Rheumatoid sclerouveitis
	Chronic Vogt–Koyanagi–Harada syndrome
	Serpiginous choroidopathy
Relative	Intermediate uveitis (pars planitis)
	Retinal vasculitis
	Chronic cyclitis

and chronic iridocyclitis. With some of these conditions, however, particularly in children, it is not clear whether these cytotoxic agents should be used (e.g., a child with intermediate uveitis). Because of the long-term, serious side-effects of these agents, their use in children should generally be avoided. For pediatric patients the newer immunosuppressive agents, such as ciclosporin and related drugs, may be helpful. However, a recent multicenter, controlled clinical trial has shown that weekly low-dose methotrexate treatment (5 to 15 mg) with low-dose steroids and other anti-inflammatory agents is effective in cases of JRA, with minimal side-effects in the short term (6 months).[18] Similar results have been reported with JRA-associated uveitis.[12]

CICLOSPORIN A AND FK 506

Ciclosporin is a naturally occurring compound produced by soil fungi. It has a much more specific effect on immune function than that of either corticosteroids or cytotoxic agents. It inhibits T-cell activation and recruitment, most likely through its inhibition of interleukin-2 (IL-2) production, which is necessary for the activation of T lymphocytes. Ciclosporin binds to calcineurin and inhibits nuclear factor of activated T cells during early events in T-cell activation.[13]

Ciclosporin has been shown to be clinically effective in treating various types of uveitis, such as Behçet's disease and Vogt–Koyanagi–Harada syndrome.[19,20] Therapy is usually begun at a daily dose of 5 mg/kg; prednisone 20 to 40 mg may be added for a more potent anti-inflammatory effect. It should be noted that ciclosporin is not cytolytic (i.e., it does not kill the lymphocytes responsible for the inflammation); thus its beneficial effects often disappear when the medication is discontinued, making long-term treatment necessary in some patients.

The major side-effects of ciclosporin are nephrotoxicity and hypertension, which occur in up to 75% and 25% of patients, respectively. Renal impairment is often reversible if the dose is decreased, but irreversible tubular damage has occurred in patients undergoing prolonged therapy. Other side-effects include paresthesia, gastrointestinal upset, fatigue, hypertrichosis, gingival hyperplasia, elevated sedimentation rate, and a normochromic, normocytic anemia. Patients receiving ciclosporin should be closely followed up by an internist to monitor their renal function, blood pressure, and hematologic status. It is recommended that the dosage be reduced if the serum creatinine level increases by more than 20 to 30% above the pretreatment baseline value.

At present, the use of ciclosporin should only be considered in cases of severe bilateral posterior uveitis that is poorly responsive to more conventional therapy. Although ciclosporin is probably not carcinogenic, in contrast to the cytotoxic agents, its teratogenic effects are unknown. The use of ciclosporin in pregnancy should be avoided unless absolutely necessary, and it should only be used after consultation with the patient's obstetrician or internist or both.

Similar to ciclosporin, FK 506 is a potent immunosuppressive agent used in the management of severe uveitis.[21] This agent has been tried in a very limited number of patients with uveitis, and further studies are required to evaluate the indications and contraindications of its use and the use of other such potent immunosuppressive agents.

MONOCLONAL ANTIBODIES

In recent years monoclonal antibodies have been used in the treatment of uveitis. However, such treatment was used in select cases including uveitis associated with JRA and Behçets disease.[12] These biological agents include etanercept, infliximab, and daclizumab. Etanercept (Enbrel) is an anti-TNF (tumor necrosis factor) agent and its main effect is to block TNF receptor, thereby inhibiting the activity of TNF, which is a potent proinflammatory cytokine. Etanercept is administered 25 mg twice a week subcutaneously. Infliximab (Remicade) is a chimeric monoclonal antibody against the inflammatory TNF-α and this agent is administered initially at 0, 2, and 6 weeks, followed by maintenance intravenous injections every 8 weeks, 3 mg/kg. Daclizumab (Zenapax) is an anti-IL-2 receptor antibody and is known to inhibit IL-2.[13] All these agents can be associated with side-effects such as sepsis, autoantibodies, and infection.[12]

PARS PLANA VITRECTOMY

Pars plana vitrectomy may have a role in the treatment of uveitis. In some cases a core vitrectomy has altered the course of the disease. This beneficial effect was seen in some patients with intermediate uveitis and in others with chronic uveitis associated with vitreitis. Vitreous surgery is usually reserved for patients who fail to respond to systemic corticosteroids.[22,23]

REFERENCES

1. Henderly DE, Genstler AJ, Smith RE et al. Changing patterns of uveitis. Am J Ophthalmol 1987; 103:131–136.
2. Rao NA. Role of oxygen free radicals in retinal damage associated with experimental uveitis. Trans Am Ophthalmol Soc 1990; 88:797–850.
3. Rao NA, Romero JL, Fernandez MA et al. Role of free radicals in uveitis. Surv Ophthalmol 1987; 32:209–213.
4. Broekhuyse RM, Kuhlmann ED, Winkens HJ et al. Experimental autoimmune anterior uveitis (EAAU), a new form of experimental uveitis. I. Induction by a detergent-insoluble, intrinsic protein fraction of the retinal pigment epithelium. Exp Eye Res 1991; 52:465–474.
5. Hirose S, Kuwabara T, Nussenblatt RB et al. Uveitis induced in primates by interphotoreceptor retinoid-binding protein. Arch Ophthalmol 1986; 104:1698–1702.
6. Rao NA, Naidu YM, Bell R et al. Usage of T cell receptor beta-chain variable gene is highly restricted at the site of inflammation in murine autoimmune uveitis. J Immunol 1993; 150:5716–5721.
7. Rao NA, Wacker WB, Marag GE Jr. Experimental allergic uveitis: clinicopathologic features associated with varying doses of S antigen. Arch Ophthalmol 1979; 97:1954–1958.
8. Rao NA, Wong V. Aetiology of sympathetic ophthalmitis. Trans Ophthalmol Soc UK 1981; 101:357–360.
9. Read RW, Zamir E, Rao NA. Neoplastic masquerade syndromes. Surv Ophthalmol 2002; 47:81–124.
10. Holland GN. Ocular toxoplasmosis: a global reassessment. Part II: Disease manifestations and management. Am J Ophthalmol 2004; 137:1–17.
11. Ozdal PC, Ortac S, Taskintuna I et al. Longterm therapy with low dose cyclosporin A in ocular Behçet's disease. Doc Ophthalmol 2002; 105: 301–312.
12. Jabs DA, Rosenbaum JT, Foster SC et al. Guidelines for the use of immunosuppressive drugs in patients with ocular inflammatory disorders: recommendation of an expert panel. Am J Ophthalmol 2000; 130:492–513.

13. Nusssenblatt RB, Thompson DJ, Li Z et al. Humanized anti-interleukin-2 (IL-2) receptor alpha therapy: long-term results in uveitis patients and preliminary safety and activity data for establishing parameters for subcutaneous administration. J Autoimmun 2003; 21:283–293.

14. Hemady R, Tauber J, Foster CS. Immunosuppressive drugs in immune and inflammatory ocular disease. Surv Ophthalmol 1991; 35:369–385.

15. Egan U, Sandbom WJ. Methotrexate for inflammatory bowel disease: pharmacology and preliminary results. Mayo Clin Proc 1996; 71:69–80.

16. Shah SS, Lowder CY, Schmitt MA et al. Low-dose methotrexate therapy for ocular inflammatory disease. Ophthalmology 1992; 99:1419–1423.

17. Lau CH, Comer M, Lightman S. Longterm efficacy of mycophenolate mofetil in the control of severe intraocular inflammation. Clin Exp Ophthalmol 2003; 31:487–491.

18. Giannini EH, Brewer EJ, Kuzmina N et al. Methotrexate in resistant juvenile rheumatoid arthritis: results of the USA–USSR double-blind, placebo-controlled trial. The Pediatric Rheumatology Collaborative Study Group and the Cooperative Children's Study Group. N Engl J Med 1992; 326:1043–1049.

19. Nussenblatt RB, Palestine AG. Cyclosporine: immunology, pharmacology, and therapeutic uses. Surv Ophthalmol 1986; 31:159–169.

20. Ozyazgan Y, Yurdakul S, Yazici H et al. Low-dose cyclosporin A versus pulsed cyclophosphamide in Behçet's syndrome: a single masked trial. Br J Ophthalmol 1992; 76:241–243.

21. Mochizuki M, Masuda K, Sakane T et al. A multicenter clinical open trial of FK 506 in refractory uveitis, including Behçet's disease. Japanese FK 506 Study Group on Refractory Uveitis. Transplant Proc 1991; 23:3343–3346.

22. Dugel PU, Rao NA, Ozler S et al. Pars plana vitrectomy for intraocular inflammation-related cystoid macular edema unresponsive to corticosteroids: a preliminary study. Ophthalmology 1992; 99:1535–1541.

23. Scott RA, Haynes RJ, Orr GM et al. Vitreous surgery in the management of chronic endogenous posterior uveitis. Eye 2003; 17:221–227.

Chapter

58

Epidemiology of Age-Related Macular Degeneration

Johanna M. Seddon
Clara A. Chen

Age-related macular degeneration (AMD) is the leading cause of irreversible blindness.[1,2] The disease adversely affects quality of life and activities of daily living, causing many affected individuals to lose their independence in their retirement years. AMD is estimated to affect more than 8 million individuals in the USA;[3] the advanced form of the disease affects more than 1.75 million individuals.[4] The population over age 85 years is expected to increase by 107% by the year 2020,[5] so the prevalence of this disease will continue to rise dramatically.

The only proven treatment available for the dry or nonexudative forms of this disease, comprising 85% of cases, is an antioxidant/mineral supplement which can slow the progression of the disease by 25% over 5 years.[6] For the remaining 15% of cases, laser treatment and photodynamic therapy are the only therapies that have been demonstrated by randomized clinical trials to be of limited benefit for certain subgroups of these patients. Preventive measures are needed to reduce the burden of this disease. Smoking is the most consistently identified modifiable risk factor.[7–9] Obesity, sunlight exposure, and factors including antioxidants and dietary fat intake may also affect AMD incidence and progression.[10–20] Nonmodifiable risk factors include increasing age, gender, and family history of the disease. Although much progress has been made over the past decade, finding the causes and mechanisms of this condition remains a challenge.

CLASSIFICATION

Macular degenerative changes have typically been classified into two clinical forms, dry or wet, both of which can lead to visual loss. The wet form is also called exudative or neovascular. In the dry form visual loss is usually gradual. Ophthalmoscopy reveals yellow subretinal deposits called *drusen*, or retinal pigment epithelial (RPE) irregularities, including hyperpigmentation or hypopigmentary changes. Larger drusen may become confluent and evolve into drusenoid RPE detachments. These drusenoid RPE detachments often progress to geographic atrophy and less frequently to neovascular AMD. Geographic atrophy involving the center of the macula leads to visual loss. Each of these signs can be further subdivided according to the number and size of the lesions. In the wet (exudative) form, vision loss can appear to occur suddenly, when a choroidal neovascular membrane leaks fluid or blood into the subpigment epithelial or subretinal space.

Serous RPE detachments with or without coexisting choroidal neovascularization (CNV) are also classified as the wet form. Exudative serous RPE detachments often, but not always, advance to the neovascular stage. This phenotypic heterogeneity, or wide range of clinical findings, has led to the use of various definitions of AMD and also to some difficulties with comparisons among studies.

It is important for investigators to standardize definitions of a disease and its subtypes, to enhance comparability, and to promote collaborative efforts.[21] Toward this goal, an international classification and grading system for AMD was recommended, although it is not universally applied.[22] In this system early age-related maculopathy (ARM) is defined as the presence of drusen and RPE irregularities, and the terms *late ARM* and *AMD* are limited to the occurrence of geographic atrophy and neovascular disease, the forms most often associated with greater visual loss. The clinical manifestations can be subcategorized even further according to the specific type of early ARM and AMD, which, for example, can yield a four- or five-step grading system.[23–25] The Clinical Age-Related Maculopathy grading System (CARMS), which we have described,[23] has been used in several studies.[19,20,25,26] Alternative and more detailed systems have been used in some of the population-based studies described below.[27,28] New subcategories of AMD will evolve as genetic and epidemiologic studies provide further insight into the pathogenesis of this disease.

PREVALENCE

Population-based studies that have provided information on the prevalence of AMD within the USA include the National Health and Nutrition Examination Survey (NHANES),[29,30] the Framingham Eye Study (FES),[31] the Chesapeake Bay Watermen Study,[27] the Beaver Dam Eye Study (BDES),[32] the Baltimore Eye Survey,[33] and the Salisbury Eye Evaluation Project.[34] Population-based studies outside the USA include the Rotterdam Study in the Netherlands,[35] the Blue Mountains Eye Study (BMES) in Australia,[36] the Barbados Eye Study,[37] and a study in Italy.[38] Prevalence rates are quite variable for all types of AMD combined, because of differences in definitions of AMD, but are more consistent for "advanced AMD."

The BDES, sponsored by the US National Eye Institute, was a census of the population of Beaver Dam, Wisconsin.[32] This study found that the early forms are much more common than the late stages of ARM, and both types increase in frequency with increasing age. The prevalence of late ARM was 1.6% overall; exudative maculopathy was present in at least one eye in 1.2% of the population; and geographic atrophy was present in 0.6%. The prevalence of late ARM rose to 7.1% in persons who were 75 or older. The third NHANES, conducted from 1988 to 1991, sampled approximately 40 000 persons and used a complex multistage–area probability design.[39] The total prevalence of any AMD in the 1991 civilian noninstitutionalized population of the USA aged 40 years or older was 9.2% (8.5 million persons), and 417 000 persons were estimated to have the late stage of AMD.[30]

Total prevalence of AMD in the USA was also estimated in 2004 using pooled findings from seven large population-based studies both inside and outside the USA, and applying those prevalence rates to the US population.[4] This meta-analysis by the Eye Diseases Prevalence Group calculated the overall prevalence of neovascular AMD and/or geographic atrophy to be 1.47% of the US population aged 40 years or older. This is more than 1.75 million individuals affected with advanced AMD in the USA, with an estimated increase of 50% to 2.95 million by 2020. These numbers are lower than the NHANES predictions because they focus on advanced AMD and included studies conducted outside the USA.

Studies conducted outside the USA have found similar or lower rates of maculopathy compared to those conducted inside the USA. In the Rotterdam Study in the Netherlands, fundus photographs of 6251 participants aged 55 to 98 years were reviewed for drusen, pigmentary changes, and atrophic or neovascular AMD.[35] The prevalence of AMD was observed to be slightly lower in that study compared with the BDES in Wisconsin. In the BMES in Australia, the authors also found lower prevalence of all lesions related to AMD in each age stratum.[36] After adjusting for age, differences were significant for both soft drusen and retinal pigmentary abnormalities; they were lower but not significantly different for geographic atrophy and exudative disease. In a population-based study of 354 participants in rural southern Italy, the prevalence rates of ARM and AMD were also lower than those found in the USA.[38] Methodological differences between studies may exist, but the lower prevalence rates found in these countries may also reflect genetic or environmental differences compared with the US population.

INCIDENCE

Few studies have been done to evaluate the incidence of AMD. The FES used the age-specific prevalence data to estimate 5-year incidence rates of AMD, according to the definition of AMD in that study. These estimates were 2.5%, 6.7%, and 10.8% for individuals who were 65, 70, and 75 years of age, respectively.[40] The BDES determined the 5-year cumulative incidence of developing early and late AMD in a population of 3583 adults (age range 43 to 86 years).[41] Incidence of early AMD increased from 3.9% in individuals aged 43 to 54 years to 22.8% in persons 75 years of age and older. The overall 5-year incidence

of late AMD was 0.9%. Persons 75 years of age or older had a 5.4% incidence rate of late AMD. The Visual Impairment Project of Melbourne, Australia, described the 5-year incidence of early ARM lesions in a population of 3271 participants aged 40 years and older.[42] The overall 5-year incidence of AMD was 0.49%, and overall incidence of early ARM was 17.3% in this population. As with the BDES, incidence of AMD increased with age – up to 6.3% for people aged 80 years and older at baseline. The Barbados Eye Study described a 4-year incidence of early macular changes as 5.2% in a black population, with an extremely low incidence of exudative AMD.[43] The differences in prevalence and incidence rates by race/ethnicity are discussed below.

QUALITY OF LIFE

The psychologic and economic costs associated with AMD underscore the growing importance of this disease on the expanding older adult population. For this reason it is important to incorporate a functional component into studies of AMD. However, measures of visual function and quality of life have rarely been included in studies of AMD, even though patients with visual loss resulting from AMD often report AMD as their worst medical problem and have a diminished quality of life.[44–46] The severity of AMD is associated with poorer visual function,[46] and more recently instruments such as the National Eye Institute Visual Function Questionnaire have been used.[47] In one study of well-being, patients with AMD had lower scores than patients with chronic obstructive pulmonary disease and acquired immunodeficiency syndrome (AIDS); the lower quality of life in patients with AMD was related to greater emotional distress, worse self-reported general health, and greater difficulty carrying out daily activities. Not only is AMD associated with a higher rate of depression in the community-dwelling adult population when compared to the unaffected adult population,[48,49] but depression also exacerbates the effects of AMD.[50]

SOCIODEMOGRAPHIC RISK FACTORS

Age

All studies demonstrate that the prevalence, incidence, and progression of all forms of AMD rise steeply with increasing age. There was a 17-fold increased risk of AMD comparing the oldest to the youngest age group in the Framingham Study.[31] In the Watermen Study, the prevalence of moderate to advanced AMD doubled with each decade after age 60.[27] In the BDES, approximately 30% of individuals 75 years of age or older had early ARM; of the remainder, 23% developed early ARM within 5 years.[32,41] By age 75 years and older in that study, 7.1% had late ARM or AMD, compared with 0.1% in the age group 43 to 54 years and 0.6% among persons aged 55 to 64 years. Pooled data in a prevalence paper showed similar rates, with dramatic increases in rates for both men and women older than 80 years.[4]

Gender

Several studies[4,31,32,35] have shown no overall difference in the frequency of AMD between men and women, after controlling for age. However, in NHANES III, men, regardless of race and age, had a lower prevalence of AMD than women.[30] Incidence rates within the Beaver Dam population also suggest a gender difference. After adjusting for age, women aged 75 years or older had approximately twice the incidence of early ARM compared with men.[41] A study using reported incidence of exudative AMD in the USA among Medicare beneficiaries supported the Beaver Dam results.[51] In the BMES, there were consistent, though not significant, gender differences in prevalence for most lesions of ARM, with women having higher rates for AMD and soft, indistinct drusen, but not for retinal pigmentary abnormalities.[36] A case-control study in the Age-Related Eye Disease Study (AREDS) study also found women had a higher risk for intermediate drusen.[52] Residual confounding by age in the broad age category "75 and older" may partially explain the differences between studies. However, true gender differences may exist, and further research is needed to confirm and expand these findings.

Race/ethnicity

Ophthalmologists rarely observe visual loss caused by CNV among ethnic-minority groups. In the Baltimore Eye Survey, AMD accounted for 30% of bilateral blindness among whites and for 0% among blacks.[53] Data from a population-based study of blacks in Barbados, West Indies,[37,43] revealed that incidence of ARM and signs of ARM changes occurred commonly but at a lower frequency than in predominantly white populations in other studies. Hispanics also have a lower prevalence of advanced AMD than non-Hispanics. A prevalence study compared Hispanics in Colorado with non-Hispanic whites in Beaver Dam (odds ratio (OR), 0.07; 95% confidence interval (CI), 0.01 to 0.49).[54] Preliminary reports from the ongoing Los Angeles Latino Eye Study indicate Latinos have a relatively high rate of early AMD but not late AMD.[55] There have not been enough population-based data on ARM in Asians to draw meaningful conclusions. Studies in Canada[56] and Japan[56,57] noted a lower prevalence of ARM in people of Asian descent than Caucasians, although a comparison of individuals in two cities (one primarily Asian, the other Caucasian) showed no difference in the prevalence of ARM.[58]

Overall, the literature to date suggests that early ARM is common among blacks and Hispanics, although less common than among non-Hispanic whites, whereas late ARM or AMD is much less common in these groups compared with non-Hispanic whites. These observations provide support for a potential genetic component to this disease. Furthermore, differences in prevalence rates between non-Hispanic whites in different regions of the USA suggest that ethnicity is an important determinant of AMD.

Socioeconomic status

Although less education and lower income have been shown to be related to increased morbidity and mortality from a number of diseases,[59] this has not been convincingly demonstrated for AMD. The Eye Disease Case Control Study (EDCCS), a National Eye Institute-sponsored multicenter study, was designed to study risk factors for several types of maculopathy, including neovascular AMD.[60] Persons with higher levels of education had a slightly reduced risk of neovascular AMD, but the association

did not remain statistically significant after multivariate modeling.[60] Education was also inversely related to AMD in a case-control study within the AREDS population.[52] In the BDES, no association was found between education, income, employment status, or marital status and maculopathy.[61] Furthermore, no associations were noted in another case-controlled study[62] or in the FES,[31] although different definitions of macular degeneration were used in those reports, compared with the more recent studies.

OCULAR RISK FACTORS

Refractive error

Several case-control studies have shown an association between AMD and hyperopia.[52,60,62–64] The potential problem with some of these studies is the clinical setting in which they were conducted. Because ophthalmology practices tend to contain a disproportionate number of myopic patients, controls selected from such practices would tend to have a higher prevalence of myopia than that of the general population. Population-based data from the BMES, unlikely to have such potential bias, has also suggested a weak association between hyperopia and early ARM, but not late ARM.[65] The population-based Rotterdam Study also showed an association between hyperopia and both incident and prevalent ARM.[66] This association therefore might implicate structural and mechanical differences which render some eyes predisposed to maculopathy.[67]

Iris color

Higher levels of ocular melanin may be protective against light-induced oxidative damage to the retina, since melanin can act as a free radical scavenger and may have an antiangiogenesis function. To date, the literature is inconclusive about the relationship between iris color and AMD. Darker irides have been found to be protective in some studies[62,68–72] but not in others.[60,73–77] Differences between studies may be partly related to the use of different definitions of disease, different number and types of other factors evaluated simultaneously, and residual confounding by ethnicity in some studies.

Lens opacities, cataracts, and cataract surgery

Data regarding the relationship between cataracts and AMD are inconsistent. FES investigators found no relationship,[78] whereas data from the NHANES did support a relationship between AMD and lens opacities.[79] In the BDES, in which photographs of the lens and macula were graded, nuclear sclerosis was associated with increased odds of early ARM (OR, 1.96; 95% CI, 1.3 to 3.0) but not of late ARM. Neither cortical nor posterior subcapsular cataracts were related to ARM.[80] A case-control study of 1844 cases and 1844 controls indicated that lens opacities or cataract surgery were associated with an increased risk of AMD.[63]

Although AMD-affected individuals reported better visual function and quality of life after cataract surgery,[81] a history of cataract surgery may be associated with an increased risk for advanced AMD.[82] Investigators have postulated that this association might arise because the cataractous lens can block damaging ultraviolet light. Inflammatory changes after cataract surgery may also cause progression of early to late ARM. In the NHANES, aphakia was associated with a twofold increased risk of AMD (OR, 2.00; 95% CI, 1.44 to 2.78).[29] Another study evaluated 47 patients with bilateral, symmetric early AMD who underwent extracapsular cataract extraction with intraocular lens implantation in one eye.[83] Progression of AMD occurred more often in the surgical eyes compared with the fellow eyes. In the BDES, previous cataract surgery at baseline was associated with a statistically significant increased risk for progression of ARM (OR, 2.7) and for development of late ARM (OR, 2.8; 95% CI, 1.03 to 7.6).[74] The relationship between cataract surgery and ARM and AMD requires clarification and confirmation in other studies, since cataract surgery is such a common exposure among the older population at risk of AMD.

Cup-to-disc ratio

The EDCCS demonstrated that eyes with larger cup-to-disc ratios had a reduced risk of exudative AMD. This effect persisted even after multivariate modeling,[60] adjusting for known and potential confounding factors. Whether this finding, which is consistent with the association between AMD and hyperopic refractive error mentioned earlier, is meaningful in terms of the mechanisms associated with the development of AMD awaits further study.

BEHAVIORAL AND LIFESTYLE FACTORS

Smoking

The preponderance of epidemiologic evidence indicates a strong positive association between both wet and dry AMD and smoking. Two large prospective cohort studies have evaluated the relationship between smoking and wet AMD and dry AMD associated with visual loss.[7,8,84] In the Nurses' Health Study, women who currently smoked 25 or more cigarettes per day had a relative risk (RR) of 2.4 (95% CI, 1.4 to 4), and women who were past smokers had an RR of 2.0 (95% CI, 1.2 to 3.4) for AMD compared with women who never smoked.[7,8] There was a dose–response relationship between AMD and pack-years of smoking, and risk remained elevated for many years after smoking cessation. Results were consistent for various definitions of AMD, including wet AMD and dry AMD, with different levels of visual loss, and for different definitions of smoking. Among women, it was estimated that 29% of the AMD cases in that study could be attributable to smoking.[8] These results were supported by a study among men participating in the Physicians' Health Study.[84] Several other studies have also shown an increased risk for AMD among smokers.[52,60,85–87] Smoking is an important, independent, avoidable risk factor for AMD.

Mechanisms by which smoking may increase the risk of developing macular degeneration include its adverse effect on blood lipids by decreasing levels of high-density lipoprotein (HDL) and increasing platelet aggregability and fibrinogen, increasing oxidative stress and lipid peroxidation, and reducing plasma levels of antioxidants.[8] In animal models, nicotine has been shown to increase the size and severity of experimental CNV, suggesting that nonneuronal nicotinic receptors may also play a part in the effect of smoking on advanced AMD.[88]

Antioxidants, vitamins, and minerals

The role of antioxidant vitamins in the pathogenesis of AMD has received a great deal of attention. Antioxidants, which include vitamin C (ascorbic acid), vitamin E (alpha-tocopherol), and the carotenoids (including alpha-carotene, beta-carotene, cryptoxanthin, lutein, and zeaxanthin), may be relevant to AMD because of their physiologic functions and the location of some of these nutrients in the retina. Lutein and zeaxanthin, in particular, are associated with macular pigment.[89,90] Trace minerals such as zinc, selenium, copper, and manganese may also be involved in antioxidant functions of the retina.[91] Antioxidants could prevent oxidative damage to the retina, which could in turn prevent development of AMD.[17,92,93] Damage to retinal photoreceptor cells could be caused by photo-oxidation or by free radical-induced lipid peroxidation.[94,95] This could lead to impaired function of the RPE and eventually to degeneration involving the macula. The deposit of oxidized compounds in healthy tissue may result in cell death because they are indigestible by cellular enzymes.[93,96] Antioxidants may scavenge, decompose, or reduce the formation of harmful compounds.

Antioxidant and zinc supplementation has been shown to decrease the risk of AMD progression and vision loss in the AREDS.[6] This study included a double-blind clinical trial in 11 centers around the USA, randomly assigning 3640 participants to take daily oral supplements of antioxidants, zinc, antioxidants and zinc, or placebo. Both zinc alone and antioxidants and zinc together significantly reduced the odds of developing advanced AMD in participants with intermediate signs of AMD in at least one eye. The zinc supplement included zinc (80 mg) as zinc oxide and copper (2 mg) as cupric oxide; the antioxidant supplement included vitamin C (500 mg), vitamin E (400 IU), and beta-carotene (15 mg). If the AREDS formulation were used to treat the 8 million individuals in the USA who are at risk for developing advanced AMD, the AREDS study estimates that more than 300 000 would avoid advanced AMD and the associated vision loss during the next 5 years.[3] AREDS supplements are a cost-effective way of reducing visual loss due to the progression of AMD,[97] although the effect of dietary antioxidants on the incidence of early AMD has not yet been established.

Diets high in antioxidant-rich fruits and vegetables may be related to a lower risk of exudative AMD. The first study launched to evaluate diet and AMD, the Dietary Intake Study, ancillary to the EDCCS, showed an inverse association between exudative AMD and dietary intake of carotenoids from foods.[15] In that study, a diet rich in green leafy vegetables containing the carotenoids lutein and zeaxanthin was associated with a reduction in the risk of exudative AMD. A prospective double-masked study involving lutein and antioxidant supplementation in a group of 90 individuals showed that visual function was improved with 10 mg of lutein or a lutein/antioxidant formula.[98] In a British study of 380 men and women, lower plasma levels of zeaxanthin were also found to be associated with an increased risk of ARM.[99] A cross-sectional study using previously collected NHANES I data found a weak protective effect with increased consumption of fruits and vegetables rich in vitamin A (which are also rich in carotenoids).[100] A prospective follow-up study has shown that fruit intake is inversely associated with exudative AMD. Participants who consumed three or more servings of fresh fruit per day have an RR of 0.64 (95% CI, 0.44 to 0.93) compared to those who consumed less than 1.5 servings per day.[11]

Alcohol intake

Studies that have examined the relationship between AMD and alcohol consumption have yielded mixed results. In the EDCCS, no significant relationship between alcohol intake and exudative AMD was noted in univariate analyses,[60] but an inverse association could not be ruled out in multivariate analyses.[101] Another case-controlled study found a suggestion of a nonlinear trend with higher risk of AMD in persons who had five drinks or more per day and a lower risk in persons who had one or two drinks per day compared with nondrinkers.[102] In a case-controlled study using NHANES I data, moderate wine consumption was associated with a decreased risk of developing AMD, although the analysis did not control for the potential confounding effects of smoking.[103] In a large prospective study, no support was found for a protective association between moderate alcohol consumption and risk of AMD, although there was a suggestion of a modest increased risk of AMD in heavier drinkers.[104] The BDES found heavy drinkers were more likely to develop late AMD,[86] whereas the BMES found an increased risk of early ARM only in current spirits drinkers.[105] The evidence to date indicates that alcohol intake does not have a large effect on the development of AMD.

Obesity

There is an association between AMD and obesity.[19,106–109] In a prospective cohort study of 261 individuals with some sign of nonadvanced AMD in at least one eye,[19] individuals with a body mass index (BMI) between 25 and 29 had an RR of 2.32 (95% CI, 1.32 to 4.07) for progression of AMD when compared to those with a BMI of less than 25. Those with a BMI of at least 30 had an RR of 2.35 (95% CI, 1.27 to 4.34) compared to the lowest category (BMI < 25), after controlling for other factors. Similarly, the highest tertile of waist circumference had a twofold increased risk compared to the lowest tertile, and the highest tertile of waist-to-hip ratio had an RR of 1.84 compared to the lowest tertile. Thus, both overall and abdominal obesity were related to AMD progression. Vigorous physical activity three times a week reduced the risk of AMD progression by 25% compared to no physical activity. Obesity and physical activity are modifiable factors that may alter an individual's risk of AMD incidence and progression.

Sunlight exposure

The literature to date regarding the association between sunlight exposure and AMD is conflicting. Overall, the data do not support a strong association between ultraviolet radiation exposure and risk of AMD, although a small effect cannot be ruled out. In the BDES,[110] increased time spent outdoors in the summer was associated with a twofold increased risk of advanced AMD. The 5-year[111] and 10-year incidence[112] of early ARM in the BDES confirmed these associations, although the 10-year incidence study showed few significant associations between environmental light and incidence and progression of early ARM. The EDCCS[60] and the Pathologies Oculaires Liées a l'Age (POLA) study in France[113] showed no significant association between advanced AMD and sunlight exposure. Sensitivity to sunburn may also be a risk factor. Both an Australian case-control study[114] and the BMES noted an association between sun-sensitive skin and risk of neovascular AMD.[115] Conflicting results in these studies exemplify the difficulties encountered when studying this complex exposure. These include challenges in measuring acute and chronic lifetime exposure and the effect of potential confounding variables, such as sun sensitivity and sun avoidance behaviors. Furthermore, different populations with different stages of AMD and people with varying intensity of exposures have been evaluated.

Medications

The use of certain medications may be associated with ARM, although studies have yielded mixed results. Some studies have shown borderline statistically significant associations between increased risk of early ARM with use of antihypertensive medication, especially beta-blockers.[116] Other studies have shown a decreased rate of CNV among AMD patients taking aspirin[117] or cholesterol-lowering drugs such as statins.[117,118] However, the prospective Rotterdam Study did not find a relationship between cholesterol-lowering drugs and risk of ARM.[119] The use of statins, in particular, may be associated with decreased CNV because of their anti-inflammatory and antioxidant properties.[120] Increased levels of C-reactive protein in patients with AMD have implicated an inflammatory role in the pathophysiology of the disease,[121] and it may be the anti-inflammatory effects of statins that affect risk, rather than the medication's cholesterol-lowering effect. Other commonly prescribed medications may also be associated with ARM. For example, the BDES has shown an inverse relationship between ARM and antidepressants.[122]

The effects of hormone replacement therapy and ARM are discussed below, in the section on hormonal and reproductive factors.

CARDIOVASCULAR-RELATED FACTORS

Cardiovascular diseases

Some studies have suggested an association between AMD and clinical manifestations of cardiovascular disease (CVD).[123–126] The presence of atherosclerotic lesions, determined by ultrasound, was examined in relation to risk of macular degeneration in a large population-based study conducted in the Netherlands.[126] Results obtained from this cross-sectional study showed a 4.5-fold increased risk of late AMD (defined as geographic atrophy or neovascular macular degeneration, as determined by grading of fundus photographs) associated with plaques in the carotid bifurcation and a twofold increased risk associated with plaques in the common carotid artery. Lower-extremity arterial disease (as measured by the ratio of the systolic blood pressure (SBP) level of the ankle to the SBP of the arm) was also associated with a 2.5-times increased risk of AMD.

In addition, a case-control study found a relationship between AMD and a history of one or more CVDs.[62] The NHANES I study reported a positive association between AMD and cerebrovascular disease, but positive associations with other vascular diseases did not reach statistical significance.[100] A Finnish study reported a significant correlation between occurrence of AMD and the severity of retinal arteriosclerosis.[127] However, other studies found that individuals who reported a history of cerebrovascular disease did not have a significantly greater risk of AMD.[60,85,128] On the other hand, many CVD risk factors are associated with AMD.

Blood pressure and hypertension

The role of blood pressure in the etiologic complex of AMD remains unclear. There was a small and consistent statistically significant relationship between AMD and systemic hypertension in two cross-sectional population-based studies.[100,129] A case-control study found that individuals with AMD were significantly more likely to be taking antihypertensive medication.[130] Also, a significant relationship was found between AMD and diastolic blood pressure measured several years before the eye examination in the FES[131] and in a small Israeli study.[132] The BDES reported that SBP was associated with incidence of RPE depigmentation,[133] 10-year incidence of advanced AMD lesions and progression of ARM.[123] The study has also shown that arteriovenous nicking, a retinal vascular characteristic associated with hypertension, is associated with an increased incidence of ARM.[134] The Rotterdam Study also showed a relationship between elevated SBP and incidence of AMD.[125] In the Macular Photocoagulation Study, there was an increased incidence of exudative AMD associated with hypertension in the second eye of individuals with exudative AMD in one eye at baseline (RR, 1.7; 95% CI, 1.2 to 2.4).[135] In another case-control study, dry AMD was not associated with hypertension, but exudative AMD was significantly associated with both hypertension and antihypertensive medication use.[116]

On the other hand, cross-sectional[85,126,136] and case-controlled studies,[60] as well as one prospective study,[128] in which duration of hypertension was not taken into account did not show an increased risk of late AMD associated with current hypertension or systolic or diastolic blood pressure. However, in the EDCCS, a nonsignificant trend for an increased risk associated with higher SBP was evident.[60]

Taken together, the evidence suggests a possible mild to moderate association between elevated blood pressure and AMD. Assessment of this relationship could be enhanced by evaluating the duration of hypertension and its subsequent effects on onset and progression of maculopathy.

Cholesterol levels and dietary fat intake

There is some evidence linking cholesterol level to AMD, but not all results are consistent. The EDCCS reported a statistically significant fourfold increased risk of exudative AMD associated with the highest serum cholesterol level (>4.88 mmol/l) and a twofold increased risk in the middle-cholesterol-level group, compared with the lowest-cholesterol-level group, controlling for other factors.[60] A positive association was found between risk of AMD and increasing high-density lipoprotein–cholesterol (HDL-C) levels in both the population-based POLA study[107] and the Rotterdam Study.[137] The BDES found that early AMD was related to low total serum cholesterol levels in women and men older than 75. Furthermore, men with early AMD had higher HDL-C and lower total cholesterol-to-HDL-C ratios.[85,133] Slightly, but not significantly, increased risk of wet AMD was seen with increasing triglyceride level in the EDCCS.[60] This finding was not seen in the Rotterdam Study[126] or the BDES[85] (both of which had small numbers of exudative AMD cases and therefore limited power).

Dietary fat intake was associated with an elevated risk of exudative AMD in the Dietary Ancillary Study of EDCCS.[16,18] This association was primarily caused by vegetable fat rather than animal fat. For omega-3 fatty acid intake, an inverse association was found in the multivariate model.[16,18] Also reported are positive associations between risk of AMD and total fat,[10] vegetable, monounsaturated, and polyunsaturated fats and linoleic acid.[18] All of these relationships were confirmed in a prospective longitudinal study of AMD.[20] A high intake of fish and omega-3 fatty acids reduced the risk when linoleic acid intake was low.[18,20] Nuts have also been shown to decrease the risk of AMD progression.[20] In the BDES, individuals with greater saturated fat and cholesterol intake also had increased risk for early AMD.[13] However, no relationship was found between AMD and dietary fat intake in NHANES III.[138]

In summary, serum cholesterol levels may be related to exudative AMD, and the relationship with dietary fat is more consistent.[60] The possible association between AMD and dietary fat and cholesterol intake may indicate a relationship with atherosclerosis.[139]

Diabetes and hyperglycemia

Many studies have investigated the relationship between diabetes and/or hyperglycemia and AMD, and most have found no significant relationships. Only a few studies suggested a possible positive association.[30,140] Based on the scant literature to date, the association between hyperglycemia or diabetes and AMD, if any, is probably weak. One difficulty with these studies is the uncertainty of diagnosing AMD in the presence of diabetic retinopathy. Also, many studies of AMD exclude persons with diabetic retinopathy. This could result in attenuated relationships between AMD and diabetes in published studies.

HORMONAL AND REPRODUCTIVE FACTORS

There is evidence to support a small protective effect of hormone therapy on AMD,[60,141] but associations with pregnancies[60,115] or the menopause[115,142] are more mixed. The EDCCS showed a marked decrease in the risk of neovascular AMD among postmenopausal women who used estrogen therapy,[60] as did a cross-sectional study.[141] No relationship was found in the BDES between years of estrogen therapy and exudative AMD (OR, 0.9 (per 1 year of therapy); 95% CI, 0.8 to 1.1) or any of the less severe forms of AMD among women.[115] However, this study had limited power to detect a potential effect of estrogen therapy on late AMD. The POLA study did not show an association between AMD and hormone therapy, hysterectomy, or oophorectomy.[143] Some studies,[144] including the BMES,[142] reported no relationship between AMD and hormone replacement therapy or early menopause. However, the BMES did describe a small but significant decrease in risk of early ARM with increasing number of years between menarche and menopause. The evidence is sparse, but a protective effect of estrogen on AMD is possible and potentially important, and further research is warranted. Although the Women's Health Initiative has refuted the association between hormone therapy and decreased CVD,[145,146] the potential protective effect of hormone therapy on AMD may be due to inflammatory factors.

INFLAMMATORY FACTORS

Studies have suggested that inflammation plays a role in the pathogenesis of drusen and AMD.[121,124,147–149] Examination of tissue samples has shown that "cellular debris" from RPE cells becomes trapped in the RPE basal lamina and Bruch's membrane, potentially causing a chronic inflammatory response which may prompt drusen formation.[147] Drusen contain proteins that are associated with chronic and acute inflammatory responses[148] and other age-related diseases, including amyloid P component and complement proteins.[149] Inflammation is also associated with angiogenesis, and may play a role in the neovascularization seen in the advanced forms of AMD.

A study of 930 individuals has shown that serum levels of the systemic inflammatory marker, C-reactive protein, are significantly elevated in individuals with advanced AMD.[121] This study showed that, after adjusting for variables such as age, gender, BMI, and smoking, the odds ratio for AMD between the highest and lowest quartiles of C-reactive protein was 1.65 (95% CI, 1.07 to 2.55, P for trend = 0.02). In stratified analyses, the highest levels of C-reactive protein were associated with a twofold increased risk among both smokers and nonsmokers. These elevated levels suggest that reducing inflammation may slow the progression of AMD. Some studies raise the possibility that medications with anti-inflammatory properties, such as statins[117,118,120] and triamcinolone,[150] may be beneficial. C-reactive protein may be a good marker of risk or response to treatment.[121] Additional research regarding the potential association between the inflammatory pathway and AMD is underway.

GENETIC FACTORS

Genetic or familial factors play a role in the etiologic basis of AMD. The evidence includes studies demonstrating familial aggregation,[151–154] twin studies,[25,155–158] segregation and linkage analyses,[159,160] genome-wide scans,[26,161–164] and candidate gene studies.[165–174] The degree of heritability and the relative role of

genetic and environmental factors, however, is still unknown. This is currently under investigation.

Several difficulties are associated with evaluating the genetics of this disease. AMD occurs late in life, and usually only one generation in the appropriate age range is available for study. The parents are often deceased, and the children are too young to manifest the disease. The phenotype is heterogeneous, with potentially all stages of AMD represented within families. Furthermore, this disease is likely complex, involving multiple genes and environmental factors. These challenges can be partially addressed by applying genetic epidemiologic methods of analysis, involving affected and discordant siblings, and other affected relatives in addition to evaluating large families and twins.

Using these techniques, familial aggregation has been shown in AMD.[151–154] The risk of AMD among families of cases is 2.4 times higher than among families of controls; for exudative AMD, the risk among families of cases is 3.1 times higher.[153] In another study,[154] 20 of 81 siblings of affected patients had AMD compared with only one of 78 siblings of control subjects. In a case-control study, case subjects were twice as likely to report a family history of this disease.[61] Additional evidence for a genetic component was suggested by a segregation analysis involving the Beaver Dam population.[159] Complex analyses with assumptions suggested that 55% to 57% of the variability in AMD could be attributed to single gene segregation.

Several genome-wide scans have been published recently, in which several promising areas have appeared. The most replicated linkage signals have been at 1q25-31 and 10q26,[164] although linkage peaks have been found in chromosomal regions 2, 3, 4, 5, 6, 7, 8, 9, 11, 12, 14, 15, 16, 17, 19, 21, and X.[26,161–164,175,176] The identification of so many areas of interest is consistent with a complex oligogenic disease, and more studies are needed to pinpoint the genes in these regions that may contribute to the pathogenesis of AMD.

Candidate gene analyses and linkage analyses have identified several genes of interest. ABCR, an adenosine triphosphate-binding transporter protein, was one of the earliest genes reported to be associated with AMD.[166,172] Allelic variation of apolipoprotein E, which transports lipids and cholesterol in the nervous system, is related to CVD and some forms of retinal degenerations. Although two studies did not find an association or linkage between apolipoprotein E alleles and AMD,[171,177] others have found a protective association with the E4 allele and variable associations with the E2 allele.[167,169,174,178] Two studies have shown hemicentin-1[179] or variants very close to this locus are associated with AMD,[162] but others have not.[161,180] Hemicentin-1, also known as the fibulin 6 gene, is an extracellular member of the immunoglobulin superfamily. Another gene, fibulin 5, has come to light in a recent linkage association study that showed missense mutations in this gene to be associated with AMD.[180]

The recent increased interest in the genetic component of AMD underscores the need to determine more definitively the degree of heritability of various forms of this disease, the role of mutations in various genes, and the relative contributions of genetic, lifestyle, and environmental factors.

CONCLUSION

AMD is a multifactorial disease that affects a large segment of the population and research to date has yielded some preventive measures but few effective treatments. Several modifiable risk factors have been identified, including smoking, dietary intake of omega-3 and vegetables with lutein, and exercise, but population-based studies have shown mixed effects of sunlight exposure, medication use, and alcohol intake. Familial aggregation studies clearly suggest a genetic component to AMD, as well as an environmental one. The role of inflammation and genetics is being explored with increasing interest, as studies focus on the etiology of this disease.

REFERENCES

1. National Advisory Eye Council (US). Vision research: a national plan 1994–1998. NIH publication no. 93-3186. Bethesda, MD: US Department of Health and Human Services; 1993.
2. National Institute for Neurological Diseases and Blindness, Section on Blindness Statistics. Statistics on blindness in the model reporting area, 1969–1970. DHEW publication no. (NIH) 73-427. US Department of Health Education, and Welfare. Washington, DC: US Government Printing Office; 1973.
3. Age-Related Eye Disease Study Research Group. Potential public health impact of Age-Related Eye Disease Study results: AREDS report no. 11. Arch Ophthalmol 2003; 121:1621–1624.
4. Eye Diseases Prevalence Research Group. Prevalence of age-related macular degeneration in the United States. Arch Ophthalmol 2004; 122:564–572.
5. Thylefors B. A global initiative for the elimination of avoidable blindness. Am J Ophthalmol 1998; 125:90–93.
6. Age-Related Eye Disease Study Research Group. A randomized, placebo-controlled, clinical trial of high-dose supplementation with vitamins C and E, beta carotene, and zinc for age-related macular degeneration and vision loss: AREDS report no. 8. Arch Ophthalmol 2001; 119:1417–1436.
7. Seddon JM, Hankinson S, Speizer F et al. A prospective study of smoking and age-related macular degeneration. Am J Epidemiol 1995; 241:136 (abstract).
8. Seddon JM, Willett WC, Speizer FE et al. A prospective study of cigarette smoking and age-related macular degeneration in women. JAMA 1996; 276:1141–1146.
9. Tomany SC, Wang JJ, van Leeuwen R et al. Risk factors for incident age-related macular degeneration: pooled findings from three continents. Opthalmol 2004; 111:1280–1287.
10. Cho E, Hung S, Willett WC et al. Prospective study of dietary fat and the risk of age-related macular degeneration. Am J Clin Nutr 2001; 73:209–218.
11. Cho E, Seddon JM, Rosner B et al. Prospective study of intake of fruits, vegetables, vitamins, and carotenoids and risk of age-related maculopathy. Arch Ophthalmol 2004; 122:883–896.
12. Eye Disorders Case-Control Study Group. Antioxidant status and neovascular age-related macular degeneration. Arch Ophthalmol 1993; 111:104–109.
13. Mares-Perlman JA, Brady WE, Klein R. Dietary fat and age-related maculopathy. Arch Ophthalmol 1995; 113:743–748.
14. Mares-Perlman JA, Brady WE, Klein R et al. Serum antioxidants and age-related macular degeneration in a population-based case-control study. Arch Ophthalmol 1995; 113:1518–1523.
15. Seddon JM, Ajani UA, Sperduto RD et al. Dietary carotenoids, vitamins A, C, and E, and advanced age-related macular degeneration. JAMA 1994; 272:1413–1420.
16. Seddon JM, Ajani U, Sperduto R et al. Dietary fat intake and age-related macular degeneration. Invest Ophthalmol Vis Sci 1994; 25:2003.
17. Seddon JM, Hennekens CH. Vitamins, minerals, and macular degeneration. Arch Ophthalmol 1994; 112:176–179.
18. Seddon JM, Rosner B, Sperduto RD et al. Dietary fat and risk for advanced age-related macular degeneration. Arch Ophthalmol 2001; 119:1191–1199.
19. Seddon JM, Cote J, Davis N et al. Progression of age-related macular degeneration: association with body mass index, waist circumference, and waist–hip ratio. Arch Ophthalmol 2003; 21:785–792.
20. Seddon JM, Cote J, Rosner B. Progression of age-related macular degeneration: association with dietary fat, transunsaturated fat, nuts, and fish intake. Arch Ophthalmol 2003; 121:1728–1737.
21. Seddon JM, Gragoudas E, Egan K. Standardized data collection and coding in eye disease epidemiology: the uveal melanoma data system. Ophthalm Surg 1991; 22:127–136.
22. Bird AC, Bressler NM, Bressler SB et al. An international classification and grading system for age-related maculopathy and age-related macular degeneration. Surv Ophthalmol 1995; 39:367–374.
23. Afshari MA, Sharma S, Seddon JM. Evaluation of the clinical age-related maculopathy staging system (CARMS). Presented at the American Academy of Ophthalmology annual meeting, 2000.
24. Age-Related Eye Disease Study Research Group. The Age-Related Eye Disease Study (AREDS): design implications. AREDS report no. 1. Control Clin Trials 1999; 20:573–600.
25. Seddon JM, Samelson U, Page WF et al. Twin study of macular degeneration: methodology and application to genetic epidemiologic studies. Invest Ophthalmol Vis Sci 1996; 38:676.
26. Seddon JM, Santangelo SL, Book K et al. A genomewide scan for age-related macular degeneration provides evidence for linkage to several chromosomal regions. Am J Hum Genet 2003; 73:780–790.
27. Bressler NM, Bressler SB, West SK et al. The grading and prevalence of macular degeneration in Chesapeake Bay watermen. Arch Ophthalmol 1989; 107:847–852.
28. Klein R, Davis MD, Magli YL et al. The Wisconsin age-related maculopathy grading system. Ophthalmology 1991; 98:1128–1134.
29. Ganley J, Roberts J. Eye conditions and related need for medical care among persons 1–74 years of age, United States, 1971–72. Vital and health statistics, series 11, no. 228. DHHS publication no. (PHS) 83–1678. Washington, DC.
30. Klein R, Rowland ML, Harris MI. Racial/ethnic differences in age-related maculopathy: third national health and nutrition examination survey. Ophthalmology 1995; 102:371–381.
31. Leibowitz HM, Krueger DE, Maunder LR et al. The Framingham Eye Study monograph. Surv Ophthalmol 1980; 24:335–610.
32. Klein R, Klein BEK, Linton KLP. Prevalence of age-related maculopathy. Ophthalmology 1992; 99:933.
33. Friedman DS, Katz J, Bressler NM et al. Racial differences in the prevalence of age-related macular degeneration: the Baltimore Eye Survey. Ophthalmology 1999; 106:1049–1055.
34. West SK, Muñoz B, Rubin GS et al. Function and visual impairment in a population-based study of older adults. The SEE project. Salisbury Eye Evaluation. Invest Ophthalmol Vis Sci 1997; 38:72–82.
35. Vingerling JR, Dielemans I, Hofman A et al. The prevalence of age-related maculopathy in the Rotterdam Study. Ophthalmology 1995; 102:205–210.
36. Mitchell P, Smith W, Attebo K et al. Prevalence of age-related maculopathy in Australia: the Blue Mountains Eye Study. Ophthalmology 1995; 102:1450–1460.
37. Schachat AP, Hyman L, Leske C et al. Features of age-related macular degeneration in a black population. Arch Ophthalmol 1995; 113:728–735.
38. Pagliarim S, Moramarco A, Wormald RPL et al. Age-related macular disease in rural southern Italy. Arch Ophthalmol 1997; 115:616–622.
39. National Center for Health Statistics. Plan and operation of the NHANES III: United States 1988–1994. Vital Health Stat vol 1, 1994.
40. Podgor MJ, Leske MC, Ederer F. Incidence estimates for lens changes, macular changes, open-angle glaucoma and diabetic retinopathy. Am J Epidemiol 1983; 118:208–212.
41. Klein R, Klein BEK, Jensen SC et al. The five-year incidence and progression of age-related maculopathy. Ophthalmology 1997; 104:7–21.
42. Mukesh BN, Dimitrov PN, Leikin S et al. Five-year incidence of age-related maculopathy: The Visual Impairment Project. Ophthalmology 2004; 111:1176–1182.
43. Leske MC, Wu SY, Hyman L, et al. Barbados Eye Studies Group. Four-year incidence of macular changes in the Barbados Eye Studies. Ophthalmology 2004; 111:706–711.
44. Alexander MF, Maguire MG, Lietman TM et al. Assessment of visual function in patients with age-related macular degeneration and low visual acuity. Arch Ophthalmol 1988; 105:1543–1547.
45. Davis C, Lovie-Kitchin J, Thompson B. Psychosocial adjustment to age-related macular degeneration. J Vis Impair Blind 1995; 1:16–27.
46. Mangione CM, Gutierrez P, Lowe G et al. Influence of age-related maculopathy on visual functioning and health-related quality of life. Am J Ophthalmol 1999; 128:45–53.
47. Age-Related Eye Disease Study Research Group. National Eye Institute visual function questionnaire in the Age-Related Eye Disease Study (AREDS). AREDS report no. 10. Arch Ophthalmol 2003; 121:211–217.
48. Brody BL, Gamst AC, Williams RA et al. Depression, visual acuity, comorbidity, and disability associated with age-related macular degeneration. Ophthalmology 2001; 108:1893–1900; discussion 1900–1901.
49. Casten RJ, Rovner BW, Tasman W. Age-related macular degeneration and depression: a review of recent research. Curr Opin Ophthalmol 2004; 15:181–183.

50. Rovner BW, Casten RJ, Tasman WS. Effect of depression on vision function in age-related macular degeneration. Arch Ophthalmol 2002; 120:1041–1044.

51. Javitt JC, Zhou Z, Maguire MG et al. Incidence of exudative age-related macular degeneration among elderly Americans. Ophthalmology 2003; 110:1534–1539.

52. Age-Related Eye Disease Study Research Group. Risk factors associated with age-related macular degeneration. A case-control study in the Age-Related Eye Disease Study: AREDS report no. 3. Ophthalmology 2000; 107:2224–2232.

53. Sommer A, Tielsch JM, Katz J et al. Racial differences in the cause-specific prevalence of blindness in East Baltimore. N Engl J Med 1991; 325:1412–1417.

54. Cruickshanks KJ, Hamman RF, Klein R et al. The prevalence of age-related maculopathy by geographic region and ethnicity. Arch Ophthalmol 1997; 115:242–250.

55. Varma R, Fraser-Bell S, Tan S et al. Los Angeles Latino Eye Study Group. Prevalence of age-related macular degeneration in Latinos. Ophthalmology 2004; 111:1288–1297.

56. Oshima Y, Ishibashi T, Murata T et al. Prevalence of age related maculopathy in a representative Japanese population: the Hisayama study. Br J Ophthalmol 2001; 85:1153–1157.

57. Miyazaki M, Nakamura H, Kubo M et al. Risk factors for age related maculopathy in a Japanese population: the Hisayama study. Br J Ophthalmol 2003; 87:469–472.

58. Das BN, Thompson JR, Patel R et al. The prevalence of eye disease in Leicester: a comparison of adults of Asian and European descent. J R Soc Med 1994; 87:219–222.

59. Adler NE, Boyce WT, Chesney MA et al. Socioeconomic inequalities in health: no easy solution. JAMA 1993; 269:3140–3145.

60. Eye Disease Case-Control Study Group. Risk factors for neovascular age-related macular degeneration. Arch Ophthalmol 1992; 110:1701–1708.

61. Klein R, Klein BEK, Jensen SC et al. The relation of socioeconomic factors to age-related cataract, maculopathy and impaired vision. Ophthalmology 1994; 101:1969–1979.

62. Hyman LG, Lilienfeld AM, Ferris FL et al. Senile macular degeneration: a case-control study. Am J Epidemiol 1983; 118:213–227.

63. Chaine G, Hullo A, Sahel J et al. Case-control study of the risk factors for age related macular degeneration. France–DMLA study group. Br J Ophthalmol 1998; 82:996–1002.

64. Maltzman BA, Mulvihill MN, Greenbaum A. Senile macular degeneration and risk factors: a case-control study. Ann Ophthalmol 1979; 11:1197–1201.

65. Wang JJ, Mitchell P, Smith W. Refractive error and age-related maculopathy: the Blue Mountains Eye Study. Invest Ophthalmol Vis Sci 1998; 39:2167–2171.

66. Ikram MK, van Leeuwen R, Vingerling JR et al. Relationship between refraction and prevalent as well as incident age-related maculopathy: the Rotterdam Study. Invest Ophthalmol Vis Sci 2003; 44:3778–3782.

67. Friedman E, Ivry M, Ebert E et al. Increased scleral rigidity and age-related macular degeneration. Ophthalmology 1989; 96:104–108.

68. Frank RN, Puklin JE, Stock C et al. Race, iris color, and age-related macular degeneration. Trans Am Ophthalmol Soc 2000; 98:109–115.

69. Holz FG, Piguet B, Minassian DC et al. Decreasing stromal iris pigmentation as a risk factor for age-related macular degeneration. Am J Ophthalmol 1994; 117:19–23.

70. Mitchell P, Smith W, Wang JJ. Iris color, skin sun sensitivity, and age-related maculopathy. The Blue Mountains Eye Study. Ophthalmology 1998; 105:1359–1363.

71. Sandberg MA, Gaudio AR, Miller S et al. Iris pigmentation and extent of disease in patients with neovascular age-related macular degeneration. Invest Ophthalmol Vis Sci 1994; 35:2734–2740.

72. Weiter JJ, Delori FC, Wing GL et al. Relationship of senile macular degeneration to ocular pigmentation. Am J Ophthalmol 1985; 99:185–187.

73. Gibson JM, Shaw DE, Rosenthal AR. Senile cataract and senile macular degeneration: an investigation into possible risk factors. Trans Ophthalmol Soc UK 1986; 105:463–468.

74. Klein R, Klein BEK, Jensen SC et al. The relationship between ocular factors to the incidence and progression of age-related maculopathy. Arch Ophthalmol 1998; 116:506–513.

75. Tomany SC, Klein R, Klein BE et al. The relationship between iris color, hair color, and skin sun sensitivity and the 10-year incidence of age-related maculopathy: the Beaver Dam Eye Study. Ophthalmology 2003; 110:1576–1633.

76. Wang JJ, Jakobsen K, Smith W et al. Five-year incidence of age-related maculopathy in relation to iris, skin or hair colour, and skin sun sensitivity: the Blue Mountains Eye Study. Clin Exp Ophthalmol 2003; 31:317–321.

77. West SK, Rosenthal FS, Bressler NM et al. Exposure to sunlight and other risk factors for age-related macular degeneration. Arch Ophthalmol 1989; 107:875–879.

78. Sperduto R, Hiller R, Seigel D. Lens opacities and senile maculopathy. Arch Ophthalmol 1981; 99:1004–1008.

79. Liu IY, White L, LaCroix AZ. The association between age-related macular degeneration and lens opacities in the aged. Am J Public Health 1989; 79:765–769.

80. Klein R, Klein BE, Wang Q et al. Is age-related maculopathy associated with cataracts? Arch Ophthalmol 1994; 112:191–196.

81. Lundstrom M, Brege KG, Floren I et al. Cataract surgery and quality of life in patients with age related macular degeneration. Br J Ophthalmol 2002; 86:1330–1335.

82. Freeman EE, Munoz B, West SK et al. Is there an association between cataract surgery and age-related macular degeneration? Data from three population-based studies. Am J Ophthalmol 2003; 135:849–856.

83. Pollack A, Marcovich A, Bukelman A et al. Age-related macular degeneration after extracapsular cataract extraction with intraocular lens implantation. Ophthalmology 1996; 103:1546–1554.

84. Christen WG, Glyim RJ, Manson JE et al. A prospective study of cigarette smoking and risk of age-related macular degeneration in men. JAMA 1996; 276:1147–1151.

85. Klein R, Klein BEK, Franke T. The relationship of cardiovascular disease and its risk factors to age-related maculopathy. Ophthalmology 1993; 100:406–414.

86. Klein R, Klein BE, Tomany SC et al. Ten-year incidence of age-related maculopathy and smoking and drinking: the Beaver Dam Eye Study. Am J Epidemiol 2002; 156:589–598.

87. POLA Study Group. Smoking and age-related macular degeneration. The POLA study. Pathologies Oculaires Liées à l'Age. Arch Ophthalmol 1998; 116:1031–1035.

88. Suner IJ, Espinosa-Heidmann DG, Marin-Castano ME et al. Nicotine increases size and severity of experimental choroidal neovascularization. Invest Ophthalmol Vis Sci 2004; 45:311–317.

89. Bone RA, Landrum JT, Guerra LH et al. Lutein and zeaxanthin dietary supplements raise macular pigment density and serum concentrations of these carotenoids in humans. J Nutr 2003; 133:992–998.

90. Krinsky NI, Landrum JT, Bone RA. Biologic mechanisms of the protective role of lutein and zeaxanthin in the eye. Annu Rev Nutr 2003; 23:171–201.

91. Hung S, Seddon JM. The relationship between nutritional factors and age-related macular degeneration. In: Bendich A, Deckelbaum R, eds. Preventive medicine: the comprehensive guide for health professionals. Totowa, NJ: Humana Press; 1997.

92. Evereklioglu C, Er H, Doganay S et al. Nitric oxide and lipid peroxidation are increased and associated with decreased antioxidant enzyme activities in patients with age-related macular degeneration. Doc Ophthalmol 2003; 106:129–136.

93. Sperduto RD, Ferris FL, Kuriij N. Do we have a nutritional treatment for age-related cataract or macular degeneration? Arch Ophthalmol 1990; 108:1403–1405.

94. Anderson RE, Kretzer FL, Rapp LM. Free radicals and ocular disease. Adv Exp Med Biol 1994; 366:73–86.

95. Anderson RE, Rapp LM, Wiegand RD. Lipid peroxidation and retinal degeneration. Curr Eye Res 1984; 3:223–227.

96. Young RW. Pathophysiology of age-related macular degeneration. Surv Ophthalmol 1987; 31:291–306.

97. Hopley C, Salkeld G, Wang JJ et al. Cost utility of screening and treatment for early age related macular degeneration with zinc and antioxidants. Br J Ophthalmol 2004; 88:450–454.

98. Richer S, Stiles W, Statkute L et al. Double-masked, placebo-controlled, randomized trial of lutein and antioxidant supplementation in the intervention of atrophic age-related macular degeneration: the Veterans LAST study (Lutein Antioxidant Supplementation Trial). Optometry 2004; 75:216–230.

99. Gale CR, Hall NF, Phillips DI et al. Lutein and zeaxanthin status and risk of age-related macular degeneration. Invest Ophthalmol Vis Sci 2003; 44:2461–2465.

100. Goldberg J, Flowerdew G, Smith E et al: Factors associated with age-related macular degeneration: an analysis of data from the first National Health and Nutrition Examination Survey. Am J Epidemiol 1988; 128:700–710.

101. Ajani UA, Willett W, Miller D et al. Alcohol consumption and neovascular age-related macular degeneration. Am J Epidemiol 1993; 138:646 (abstract).

102. Vinding T, Appleyard M, Nyboe J et al. Risk factor analysis for atrophic and exudative age-related macular degeneration: an epidemiologic study of 1000 aged individuals. Acta Ophthalmol 1992; 70:66–72.

103. Obisesan TO, Hirsch R, Kosoko O et al. Moderate wine consumption is associated with decreased odds of developing age-related macular degeneration in NHANES-1. J Am Geriatr Soc 1998; 46:1–7.

104. Seddon JM, Cho E, Stampfer M et al. Prospective study of alcohol consumption and the risk of age-related macular degeneration. Invest Ophthalmol Vis Sci 1999; 40:568.

105. Smith W, Mitchell P. Alcohol intake and age-related maculopathy. Am J Ophthalmol 1996; 122:743–745.

106. Klein BE, Klein R, Lee KE et al. Measures of obesity and age-related eye diseases. Ophthalm Epidemiol 2001; 8:251–262.

107. POLA Study Group. Associations of cardiovascular disease and its risk factors with age-related macular degeneration: the POLA study. Ophthalm Epidemiol 2001; 8:237–249.

108. Schaumberg DA, Christen WG, Hankinson SE et al. Body mass index and the incidence of visually significant age-related maculopathy in men. Arch Ophthalmol 2001; 119:1259–1265.

109. Smith W, Mitchell P, Leeder SR et al. Plasma fibrinogen levels, other cardiovascular risk factors, and age-related maculopathy: the Blue Mountains Eye Study. Arch Ophthalmol 1998; 116:583–587.

110. Cruickshanks KJ, Klein R, Klein BEK. Sunlight and age-related macular degeneration: the Beaver Dam Eye Study. Arch Ophthalmol 1993; 111:514–518.

111. Cruickshanks KJ, Klein R, Klein BE et al. Sunlight and the 5-year incidence of early age-related maculopathy: the Beaver Dam Eye Study. Arch Ophthalmol 2001; 119:246–250.

112. Tomany SC, Cruickshanks KJ, Klein R et al. Sunlight and the 10-year incidence of age-related maculopathy: the Beaver Dam Eye Study. Arch Ophthalmol 2004; 122:750–757.

113. POLA Study Group. Light exposure and the risk of age-related macular degeneration: the Pathologies Oculaires Liées à l'Age (POLA) study. Arch Ophthalmol 2001; 119:1463–1468.

114. Darzins P, Mitchell P, Heller RF. Sun exposure and age-related macular degeneration: an Australian case-control study. Ophthalmology 1997; 104:770–776.

115. Klein BEK, Klein R, Jensen SC et al. Are sex hormones associated with age-related maculopathy in women? The Beaver Dam Eye Study. Trans Am Ophthalmol Soc 1994; 92:289–295.

116. Age-Related Macular Degeneration Risk Factors Study Group. Hypertension, cardiovascular disease, and age-related macular degeneration. Arch Ophthalmol 2000; 118:351–358.

117. Wilson HL, Schwartz DM, Bhatt HR et al. Statin and aspirin therapy are associated with decreased rates of choroidal neovascularization among patients with age-related macular degeneration. Am J Ophthalmol 2004; 137:615–624.

118. Hall NF, Gale CR, Syddall H et al. Risk of macular degeneration in users of statins: cross sectional study. Br Med J 2001; 323:375–376.

119. van Leeuwen R, Vingerling JR, Hofman A et al. Cholesterol lowering drugs and risk of age related maculopathy: prospective cohort study with cumulative exposure measurement. Br Med J 2003; 326:255–256.

120. Hall N, Martyn C. Could statins prevent age-related macular degeneration? Exp Opin Pharmacother 2002; 3:803–807.

121. Seddon JM, Gensler G, Milton RC et al. Association between C-reactive protein and age-related macular degeneration. JAMA 2004; 291:704–710.

122. Klein R, Klein BE, Jensen SC et al. Medication use and the 5-year incidence of early age-related maculopathy: the Beaver Dam Eye Study. Arch Ophthalmol 2001; 119:1354–1359.

123. Klein R, Klein BE, Tomany SC et al. The association of cardiovascular disease with the long-term incidence of age-related maculopathy: the Beaver Dam Eye Study. Ophthalmology 2003; 110:1273–1280.

124. Snow KK, Seddon JM. Do age-related macular degeneration and cardiovascular disease share common antecedents? Ophthalm Epidemiol 1999; 6:125–143.

125. van Leeuwen R, Ikram MK, Vingerling JR et al. Blood pressure, atherosclerosis, and the incidence of age-related maculopathy: the Rotterdam Study. Invest Ophthalmol Vis Sci 2003; 44:3771–3777.

126. Vingerling JR, Dielemans I, Bots ML et al. Age-related macular degeneration is associated with atherosclerosis: the Rotterdam Study. Am J Epidemiol 1995; 142:404–409.

127. Hirvela H, Luukinen H, Laara E et al. Risk factors of age-related maculopathy in a population 70 years of age or older. Ophthalmology 1996; 103:871–877.

128. Vinding T. Age-related macular degeneration: an epidemiological study of 1000 elderly individuals with reference to prevalence, funduscopic findings, visual impairment, and risk factors. Acta Ophthalmol Scand 1995; 21 (suppl.):1–32.

129. Sperduto RD, Hiller R. Systemic hypertension and age-related macular degeneration in the Framingham Eye Study. Arch Ophthalmol 1986; 104:216–226.

130. Delaney WV, Oates RIP. Senile macular degeneration: a preliminary study. Ann Ophthalmol 1982; 14:21–24.

131. Kahn HA, Leibowitz HM, Ganley JP et al. The Framingham Eye Study. II. Association of ophthalmic pathology with single variables previously measured in the Framingham Heart Study. Am J Epidemiol 1977; 106:33–41.

132. Vidaurri JS, Peter J, Halfon ST et al. Association between drusen and some of the risk factors for coronary artery disease. Ophthalmologica 1984; 188:243–247.

133. Klein R, Klein BEK, Jensen SC. The relation of cardiovascular disease and its risk factors to the 5-year incidence of age-related maculopathy: the Beaver Dam Eye Study. Ophthalmology 1997; 104:1804–1812.

134. Klein R, Klein BE, Tomany SC et al. The relation of retinal microvascular characteristics to age-related eye disease: the Beaver Dam eye study. Am J Ophthalmol 2004;137:435–444.

135. Macular Photocoagulation Study Group. Risk factors for choroidal neovascularization in the second eye of patients with juxtafoveal or subfoveal choroidal neovascularization secondary to age-related macular degeneration. Arch Ophthalmol 1997; 151:741–747.

136. Klein R, Klein BE, Marino EK et al. Early age-related maculopathy in the cardiovascular health study. Ophthalmology 2003; 110:25–33.

137. van Leeuwen R, Klaver CC, Vingerling JR et al. Cholesterol and age-related macular degeneration: is there a link? Am J Ophthalmol 2004; 137:750–752.

138. Heuberger RA, Mares-Perlman JA, Klein R et al. Relationship of dietary fat to age-related maculopathy in the Third National Health and Nutrition Examination Survey. Arch Ophthalmol 2001; 119:1833–1838.

139. Friedman E. Dietary fat and age-related maculopathy. Arch Ophthalmol 1996; 114:235–236.

140. Klein R, Klein BEK, Moss SE. Diabetes, hyperglycemia and age-related maculopathy: the Beaver Dam Eye Study. Ophthalmology 1992; 99:1527–1534.

141. Snow KK, Cote J, Yang W et al. Association between reproductive and hormonal factors and age-related maculopathy in postmenopausal women. Am J Ophthalmol 2002; 134:842–848.

142. Smith W, Mitchell P, Wang JJ. Gender oestrogen, hormone replacement and age-related macular degeneration: results from the Blue Mountains Eye Study. Aust NZ J Ophthalmol 1997; 25 (suppl.):13–15.

143. POLA Study Group. Sex steroids and age-related macular degeneration in older French women: the POLA study. Ann Epidemiol 2004; 14:202–208.

144. Abramov Y, Borik S, Yahalom C et al. The effect of hormone therapy on the risk for age-related maculopathy in postmenopausal women. Menopause 2004; 11:62–68.

145. Women's Health Initiative Investigators. Risks and benefits of estrogen plus progestin in healthy postmenopausal women: principal results from the Women's Health Initiative randomized controlled trial. JAMA 2002; 288:321–333.

146. Women's Health Initiative Investigators. Estrogen plus progestin and the risk of coronary heart disease. N Engl J Med 2003; 349:523–534.

147. Anderson DH, Mullins RF, Hageman GS et al. A role for local inflammation in the formation of drusen in the aging eye. Am J Ophthalmol 2002; 134:411–431.

148. Johnson LV, Leitner WP, Staples MK et al. Complement activation and inflammatory process in drusen formation and age related macular degeneration. Exp Eye Res 2001; 73:887–896.

149. Mullins RF, Russell SR, Anderson DH et al. Drusen associated with aging and age-related macular degeneration contain proteins common to extracellular deposits associated with atherosclerosis, elastosis, amyloidosis, and dense deposit disease. FASEB J 2000; 14:835–846.

150. Jonas JB, Kreissig I, Hugger P et al. Intra-vitreal triamcinolone acetonide for exudative age related macular degeneration. Br J Ophthalmol 2003; 87:462–468.

151. Klaver CC, Wolfs RC, Assink JJ et al. Genetic risk of age-related maculopathy: population-based familial aggregation study. Arch Ophthalmol 1998; 116:1646–1651.

152. Piguet B, Wells JA, Palmvang IB et al. Age-related Bruch's membrane change: a clinical study of the relative role of heredity and environment. Br J Ophthalmol 1993; 77:400–403.

153. Seddon JM, Ajani UA, Mitchell BD. Familial aggregation of age-related maculopathy. Am J Ophthalmol 1997; 123:199–206.

154. Silvestri G, Johnston PB, Hughes AE. Is genetic predisposition an important risk factor in age-related macular degeneration? Eye 1994; 8:564–568.

155. Grizzard SW, Arnett D, Haag SL. Twin study of age-related macular degeneration. Ophthalm Epidemiol 2003; 10:315–322.

156. Hammond CJ, Webster AR, Snieder H et al. Genetic influence on early age-related maculopathy: a twin study. Ophthalmology 2002; 109:730–736.

157. Klein ML, Mauldin WM, Stoumbos VD. Heredity and age-related macular degeneration: observations in monozygotic twins. Arch Ophthalmol 1994; 112:932–937.

158. Meyers SM, Greene T, Gutman FA. A twin study of age-related macular degeneration. Am J Ophthalmol 1995; 120:757–766.

159. Heiba IM, Elston RIC, Klein BEK et al. Sibling correlations and segregation analysis of age-related maculopathy: the Beaver Dam Eye Study. Genet Epidemiol 1994; 11:51–67.

160. Kenealy SJ, Schmidt S, Agarwal A et al. Linkage analysis for age-related macular degeneration supports a gene on chromosome 10q26. Mol Vis 2004; 10:57–61.

161. Abecasis GR, Yashar BM, Zhao Y et al. Age-related macular degeneration: a high-resolution genome scan for susceptibility loci in a population enriched for late-stage disease. Am J Hum Genet 2004; 74:482–494.

162. Iyengar SK, Song D, Klein BE et al. Dissection of genomewide-scan data in extended families reveals a major locus and oligogenic susceptibility for age-related macular degeneration. Am J Hum Genet 2004; 74:20–39.

163. Schick JH, Iyengar SK, Klein BE et al. A whole-genome screen of a quantitative trait of age-related maculopathy in sibships from the Beaver Dam Eye Study. Am J Hum Genet 2003; 72:1412–1424.

164. Weeks DE, Conley YP, Tsai HJ et al. Age-related maculopathy: a genomewide scan with continued evidence of susceptibility loci within the 1q31, 10q26, and 17q25 regions. Am J Hum Genet 2004; 75.

165. Allikmets R, Seddon JM, Bernstein PS et al. Evaluation of the Best disease gene in patients with age-related macular degeneration and other maculopathies. Hum Genet 1999; 104:449–453.

166. Allikmets R, Singh N, Sun H et al. A photoreceptor cell-specific ATh-binding transporter gene (ABCR) is mutated in recessive Stargardt macular dystrophy. Nat Genet 1997; 124:331–343.

167. Baird PN, Guida E, Chu DT et al. The epsilon2 and epsilon4 alleles of the apolipoprotein gene are associated with age-related macular degeneration. Invest Ophthalmol Vis Sci 2004; 45:1311–1315.

168. De La Paz MA, Pericak-Vance MA, Lennon F et al. Exclusion of TIMP3 as a candidate locus in age-related macular degeneration. Invest Ophthalmol Vis Sci 1997; 38:1060–1065.

169. Schmidt S, Klaver C, Saunders A et al. A pooled case-control study of the apolipoprotein E (APOE) gene in age-related maculopathy. Ophthalm Genet 2002; 23:209–223.

170. Seddon JM, Afshari MA, Sharma S et al. Assessment of mutations in the Best macular dystrophy (VMD2) gene in patients with adult-onset foveomacular vitelliform dystrophy, age-related maculopathy, and bull's-eye maculopathy. Ophthalmology 2001; 108:2060–2067.

171. Seddon JM, De La Paz M, Clements K et al. No association between apolipoprotein E and advanced age-related macular degeneration. Am J Hum Genet 1996; 559:388.

172. Sun H, Nathans J. Stargardt's ABCR is localized to the disc membrane of retinal rod outer segments. Nat Genet 1997; 17:15–16.

173. Weber BHF, Vogt G, Pruett RC et al. Mutations in the tissue inhibitor of metalloproteinases-3 (TIMP3) in patients with Sorsby's fundus dystrophy. Nat Genet 1994; 8:352–356.

174. Zareparsi S, Reddick AC, Branham KE et al. Association of apolipoprotein E alleles with susceptibility to age-related macular degeneration in a large cohort from a single center. Invest Ophthalmol Vis Sci 2004; 45:1306–1310.

175. Weeks DE, Conley YP, Mah TS et al. A full genome scan for age-related maculopathy. Hum Mol Genet 2000; 9:1329–1349.

176. Weeks DE, Conley YP, Tsai HJ et al. Age-related maculopathy: a genomewide scan with continued evidence of susceptibility loci within the 1q31 and 17q25 regions. Am J Ophthalmol 2001; 132:682–692.

177. Pang CP, Baum L, Chan WM et al. The apolipoprotein E epsilon4 allele is unlikely to be a major risk factor of age-related macular degeneration in Chinese. Ophthalmologica 2000; 214:289–291.

178. Souied EH, Benlian P, Amouyel P et al. The E4 allele of the apolipoprotein E gene as a potential protective factor for exudative age-related macular degeneration. Am J Ophthalmol 1998; 125:353–359.

179. Schultz DW, Klein ML, Humpert AJ et al. Analysis of the ARMD1 locus: evidence that a mutation in HEMICENTIN-1 is associated with age-related macular degeneration in a large family. Hum Mol Genet 2003; 12:3315–3323.

180. Stone EM, Braun TA, Russell SR et al. Missense variations in the fibulin 5 gene and age-related macular degeneration. N Engl J Med 2004; 351:346–353.

Age Changes in Bruch's Membrane and Related Structures

Robyn Guymer
Alan C. Bird

Research into age-related macular disease (AMD) is assuming increasing importance because of the high prevalence of this disease in Western society and its reported increasing prevalence in Eastern Asia.[1–7] Visual loss occurs as a consequence of choroidal neovascularization, detachment of the retinal pigment epithelium (RPE), or geographic atrophy, which occur as a response to age-related changes at the level of Bruch's membrane. These changes in Bruch's membrane are associated with the accumulation of material that is thought to be derived from the RPE. This chapter examines the nature, causes, and consequences of this accumulation.

RETINAL PIGMENT EPITHELIUM

The RPE is metabolically highly active with specialized functions to sustain the photoreceptor cells and, in particular, outer segment renewal. Unlike other phagocytes, the RPE cells remain in situ for a lifetime, and loss of RPE cells with age results in an increasing metabolic demand on each cell.[8] These cells are believed to discharge cytoplasmic material into the inner portion of Bruch's membrane to achieve cytoplasmic renewal, a mechanism common to all metabolically active but nondividing cells.[9–13]

Throughout life the RPE cells phagocytose and degrade the shed tips of rod outer segments. It has been calculated that each rat RPE cell is in contact with about 300 rods, and each day 25% of these rods shed 100 discs, so an RPE cell engulfs about 7500 discs per day, or 1 million discs per year.[14] The RPE has a highly developed catalytic lysosomal system to handle this load.[15] Engulfed rod outer segments are contained in a phagocytic vacuole (phagosome), and a primary lysosome fuses with the vacuole to deliver degradative enzymes, forming a secondary lysosome, or phagolysosome. The undigested end products within the phagolysosome, called *residual bodies*, contain the fluorescent granules.[8,16–25] Residual bodies may fuse with melanophores, forming melanolipofuscin.[16,17,26] The residual bodies are all acidified, indicating that lysosomal vesicles are constantly fusing with the long-term phagosomes, a conclusion supported by the observation by Feeney[17] that all phagosomes showed degradative enzyme activity. Residual bodies therefore would be expected to have a finite half-life, a conclusion supported by the observation that lipofuscin slowly disappears with loss of photoreceptor cells.[27] Some of the products resulting from degradation of the contents of these various intracytoplasmic vesicles are recycled, and it is assumed that the remainder are extruded through the basal surface of the RPE into Bruch's membrane and diffuse into the choroidal circulation.

Age changes

RPE changes with age are characterized by the accumulation of residual bodies that contain lipofuscin. These are similar to the "age pigment" found in other organs, including the brain.[28] In vitro studies report that very few fluorescent granules are present in young individuals, and those present are in secondary lysosomes with no typical lipofuscin granules. With increasing age, the number of fluorescent granules increases; by age 16 years they are prominent in the basilar portions of posterior pole RPE. Wing et al.[29] reported a biphasic increase, but a subsequent study showed a quadratic relationship between accumulation of residual bodies and autofluorescence with age.[30] The periphery always has less lipofuscin than the posterior pole.

With the use of a confocal scanning laser ophthalmoscope (CSLO), it is now possible to measure and image auto-fluorescence of the fundus in vivo.[27,31–33] The optical characteristics and distribution of fluorescence seen with the CSLO imply that it is derived from lipofuscin in the pigment epithelium. Early in vivo measurements confirm that it increases with age. The RPE residual body content also increases with age, and the relationship is also best approximated by a quadratic model.[30] At age 40 years residual bodies occupy approximately 8% of cytoplasmic volume of the RPE, increasing to 19% by age 80.[17,34] The quadratic model of accumulation of material in the RPE can be explained if loss of central photoreceptors occurs in late life, if intracellular accumulation is related to metabolic activity, and if the material had a finite half-life.[30,35] There is evidence to support these three concepts. It is likely that the quantity of residual bodies formed reflects photoreceptor outer segment renewal,[36] and the photoreceptor population in the posterior pole decreases after the sixth decade of life.[37,38] Although it does not necessarily follow that outer segment turnover would decrease as a consequence, this is likely the case. The presence of enzyme activity in long-term phagosomes has led to the conclusion that they are constantly being degraded.[17] A direct relationship has been shown between RPE autofluorescence and residual body content, which is best approximated by linear regression.

However, the relationship between the two is not precise ($R^2 = 0.26$).[30] The observed large variation between specimens should not be surprising, since there are many fluorophores,[39] only a small proportion of the material in residual bodies fluoresces, and this proportion may be influenced by factors such as diet.[40]

It may be that the failure of the RPE to manage the metabolic load leads to lipofuscin accumulation and possibly disease. It is not known if accumulation of lipofuscin-containing residual bodies leads to RPE functional compromise. After the seventh decade the RPE basement membrane becomes thickened, and the number and complexity of basal convolutions of the RPE lessen. These changes have been interpreted as indicating RPE cellular stress, and their presence correlates closely with the risk of choroidal neovascularization.[41–43]

BRUCH'S MEMBRANE

Bruch's membrane is crucial because of its strategic location. It is interposed between the RPE and metabolically active photoreceptors and their major source of nutrition, the choriocapillaris. In addition to acting as a support element and an attachment site for the RPE, Bruch's membrane provides a semipermeable filtration barrier through which major metabolic exchange takes place. Nutrients pass from the choriocapillaris to the photoreceptors and the RPE, and cellular breakdown products travel in the opposite direction.[44]

Bruch's membrane can be divided ultrastructurally into five layers: (1) the basement membrane of the RPE, which forms the innermost layer; (2) an inner collagenous zone (ICZ); (3) an elastic zone; (4) an outer zone of collagen (OCZ); and (5) an outermost basement membrane elaborated by the endothelial cells of the choriocapillaris.[45] The interfiber matrix of Bruch's membrane is composed largely of heparan sulfate and chondroitin/dermatan sulfate, and it has been suggested that the chondroitin sulfate side chains provide an electrolytic barrier to diffusion. Heparan sulfate appears to be concentrated in the basement membrane portion adjacent to the RPE, and chondroitin/dermatan sulfate is located predominantly within the collagenous layers and along the basal laminar of the choriocapillaris.[46]

Diffusion through Bruch's membrane depends on local concentration of salts, glucose, and pH. Maximum diffusion occurs at the membrane's isoelectric point of pH 5. At physiologic pH, there is a negative charge, and this may result in impedance to the passage of negatively charged macromolecules.[46–49] Any alteration in the structure or composition of Bruch's membrane might influence its diffusion properties and ultimately the function of the RPE and outer retina.

Age changes

Bruch's membrane has long been known to change in thickness, ultrastructure, and histochemistry with age.[42,50] These changes occur in both the posterior pole and the periphery but are generally greater at the posterior pole.[51–53] Alteration in the extracellular matrix and the biophysical properties of Bruch's membrane would lead to altered nutrition and consequent abnormal functioning of the RPE and photoreceptors. It has

been suggested that these changes in Bruch's membrane have a major influence on the development and subsequent outcome of disease.[54]

Changes in collagen, elastin, and glycosaminoglycan components

As Bruch's membrane ages, a highly significant, almost linear, decline occurs in the solubility of collagen from nearly 100% in the first decade of life to 40% to 50% in the ninth decade in both the macula and the periphery.[55] This decrease in solubility is thought to be the result of an increase in cross-linking of collagen fibers, although the nature of the cross-links is not yet known. Nonenzymatic glycosylation of collagen, as occurs in other aging tissue, has yet to be shown in Bruch's membrane.[55] This increase in cross-linking would have an effect on permeability and may change the nature of the extracellular matrix. In addition, it would result in decreased susceptibility of Bruch's membrane collagen to the enzymatic action of the RPE collagenolytic enzymes, resulting in less effective turnover of collagen. With age there is also a significant decrease in the proportion of hydroxyproline and an increase in tyrosine, methionine, and phenylalanine in the macular region of Bruch's membrane but not in the periphery. The increase in these amino acids, low in collagen, indicates deposition of noncollagenous proteinaceous material and may reflect debris accumulation.[55]

Deposition of long-space material also occurs in Bruch's membrane, and its significance to disease has been the subject of great debate.[56] It is widely believed to be derived from collagen and has been termed *fibrous*, or *long-space*, *collagen* (LSC). One study appeared to show localization of type VI collagen to LSC, but subsequent studies have failed to confirm that type VI or any other collagen is present in LSC. Some have stated that there is no justification for considering the long spacing structures as collagen derivatives,[56,57] and they make a distinction between LSC and fibrous-banded material, which has a shorter periodicity and lacks the fine structure of LSC. LSC is found between the OCZ and the basal lamina of the choriocapillaris, whereas the fibrous-banded material is found in both the OCZ and the ICZ. LSC is described as material running in a parallel fashion and varying in periodicity from 100 to 140 nm. This material may be more widespread than appreciated, since bundles of fibers cut in cross-section appear amorphous rather than showing the characteristic banding (personal observation). The variation in periodicity can be explained if the cross-banded structures are planar in configuration and are formed as a result of polymerization rather than by a mechanism of twisting of bundled fibers, as seen in native collagen. With such a planar configuration, the obliquity of section would influence the apparent periodicity.[58]

Most attention has been devoted to LSC located between the plasma membrane and the basement membrane of the RPE, where it makes up part of the basal laminar deposits (BLD) and is implicated in the pathogenesis of AMD. LSC in Bruch's membrane has been presumed to be produced by the RPE cells and has generally been regarded as a sign of cellular distress.[34,59] A close relationship between LSC and the basement membrane of the choriocapillaris is also well described.[9,34,58,60] It is thought by some to be derived from RPE, and it has been argued that the LSC in the outer collagenous layer could be explained by diffusion of precursors of LSC from the RPE before polymerization occurs. However, the finding of LSC in the OCZ in the majority of young eyes suggests otherwise.[34,61] The concept of choroidal endothelial cell origin of the LSC in the young is implied by the finding of focal deposits of LSC at the site of cell processes protruding into Bruch's membrane, where there is focal thickening of the basement membrane.[61] These observations suggest that LSC is a normal feature in young eyes that may be the result of constant collagen turnover. Vascular endothelial cells produce enzymes that degrade collagen, and it has been proposed that under normal conditions there is constant formation and degradation of collagen, particularly if the formation of cellular intrusions is a dynamic process occurring in response to the changing environment. The apparent shift of LSC production from the choriocapillaris and outer choroid in the young to the pigment epithelium and inner choroid in older adults may be relevant to the pathogenesis of AMD.

The nature of the putative association between LCS and basement membrane is uncertain. The main components of basement membrane are type IV collagen, heparan sulfate proteoglycans, and laminin, with the distribution of the six type IV collagen chains in Bruch's membrane being recently described.[62] Fibronectin, an extracellular matrix protein involved in adhesion, is also found in basement membranes. By contrast, LSC exhibits only weak labeling for basement membrane components. Moreover, LSC contains carbohydrates not found in laminin and type IV collagen.[63] It has been suggested that LSC may form by direct polymerization of basement membrane material and that antigenicity is lost in the polymer.[64-66] Type VI collagen is known to have a tendency to form aggregates similar to LCS in vitro as a result of extensive disulfide bonding, and it is characteristically refractory to proteolytic enzymes.[67-69] Type VI collagen has been identified in relationship to the choriocapillaris by immunogold labeling, although this appeared to be on the scleral aspect of the capillaries. It is suggested that type VI collagen links the cell surface with extracellular fibrous structures and therefore may have a role in cell adhesion. The elastic tissue elements in Bruch's membrane, which form a continuous meshwork of intersecting elastic fibers, also change with age. The fiber number increases, and the immature elastic elements (oxytalan) mature from an anterior to posterior direction.[70] Calcification also occurs, rendering Bruch's membrane brittle.[65]

Change in lipid composition of Bruch's membrane

Progressive accumulation of lipids in Bruch's membrane with age has been shown by examination of cryosections of donor eyes.[71,72] Differences have been found in the specific types of lipids present among individuals. Some eyes stain for neutral lipids alone, some stain predominantly for phospholipids, whereas others stained equally for both neutral lipids and phospholipids.[71] To add support to these findings, lipids extracted from Bruch's membrane by lipid solvents have been analyzed using thin layer and gas chromatography, and the compounds have been identified by mass spectroscopy.[73,74] Little or no lipid was extracted

from donors younger than 50. For those older than 50, the quantity of lipid in Bruch's membrane increased exponentially. The ratio of phospholipids to neutral fats varied from one subject to another and did not correlate well with the total quantity of lipid extracted. The lipids consisted of phospholipids, triglycerides, fatty acids, and free cholesterol.[73] Generally, the amount of phospholipid was greater than the neutral lipids, but this was reversed in eyes from older donors.[74] Higher quantities of lipid were consistently extracted from the macular than from the periphery, and the magnitude of the difference increased with age.[73] If the extracellular deposits of lipid were derived from blood, cholesterol and cholesterol esters would have constituted the major fraction of the total lipids, and more than 90% of phospholipid would be phosphatidylcholine. Very little cholesterol ester was found, and no more than 50% of the phospholipid was phosphatidylcholine. This is in keeping with the abnormal material being cellular in origin rather than being derived from plasma, and in these respects it differs from other extracellular lipid deposits, such as atheroma and arcus senilis.[73-75] Conversely others find similarities that may link Bruch's membrane changes with those involved in atherogenesis.[76]

Deposition of extraneous material

The initial age-related change in Bruch's membrane, as seen by electron microscopy, is the accumulation of vesicles and granular and filamentous material.[45,77] These deposits are seen initially in the ICZ but with time occupy both collagenous zones.[52,78] The terms *basal linear deposits* and *diffuse drusen* have been used to describe such deposits, which cause diffuse thickening of the inner aspect of Bruch's membrane external to the basement membrane of the RPE. Sparsely scattered granules and fibrillary material have been documented as early as 10 years of age in the ICZ.[74] By middle age this material can be found in both collagenous zones and is present more commonly than not. Killingsworth[79] described the various deposits as coated membrane-bound (CMB) bodies, and their fragments have been called coated vesicle-like (CVL) bodies, fibrous-banded material, and focal areas of mineralization. CMB bodies have a uniform electron-dense coat covering their single membrane and contain fine granular material, electron-lucent droplets, dense particles, and $70 \mu m$ CVL bodies. CMB bodies are thought to be the main source of coated-membrane fragments, fine granular material, unbound droplets, and CVL bodies, which are released once the CMB body ruptures. CMB bodies make up the bulk of age-related deposits within the ICZ and the OCZ. These deposits increase with age, with proportionally more material in the OCZ than in the ICZ.[71,79]

Focal deposits of similar material may occur as discrete mounds between the basement membrane of the RPE and the inner collagenous layer; they are responsible for the clinical appearance of drusen. Drusen are the clinical hallmark of age-related maculopathy (ARM) and are seen ophthalmoscopically as pale deposits at the level of Bruch's membrane. Drusen are composed of polymorphous material of vesicular, granular, and filamentous appearance. Historically they have been divided into hard and soft drusen, according to the nature of their margins. Hard drusen are defined as $<63\ \mu m$; they are discrete, having distinct margins, and are formed of dense hyaline material that is continuous with the inner collagenous layer of Bruch's membrane. Their presence alone is thought not to signify increased risk of visual loss and has therefore been removed as a criterion for the diagnosis of ARM.[80] Soft drusen have indistinct edges, tend to be large, and may be confluent. Soft drusen are thought to form from clusters of small, hard drusen (soft clusters) or in late life from focal accentuation of the membranous debris within Bruch's membrane (soft membranous drusen).[42,81–83] Irregular pigmentation at the level of the RPE is commonly seen in subjects with drusen and is classified as part of ARM.

CHORIOCAPILLARIS

Choroidal blood flow is very high, achieving high oxygen tension in the outer retina, which is necessary to maintain the photoreceptor dark current in the dark-adapted state.[84] The capillary bed is sinusoidal, and the endothelial cells are fenestrated. Material from the RPE is believed to diffuse through Bruch's membrane and be cleared by the choriocapillaris. The mechanism of clearance of debris is not known, although many believe that this occurs by passive diffusion. Nutrients required by the RPE and photoreceptors travel in opposite directions.

Processes from choroidal capillary endothelial cells have been observed to protrude through the basement membrane of the endothelial cell into Bruch's membrane, although their functional significance is uncertain.[61] They have been observed in several species and are seen in normal human eyes of all ages.[85–89] Many have regarded these processes as evidence of nascent angiogenesis,[90–93] but there is increasing evidence to suggest that these are a feature of the normal choriocapillaris.[61,89,94] This phenomenon is common to other fenestrated thin-walled capillaries, and the primary function of these cellular protrusions into Bruch's membrane, together with the endothelial cytoskeleton, may be to stabilize the cell physically.[95–97] Arising from a network of cytoplasmic channels around the cell, they could have a widespread influence on cell form. This concept of a structural role is supported by the finding of actin filaments within the processes and the thickening of basement membrane around the base of the structure, which could serve to spread the physical load on the cell membrane.[61,94]

Age changes

With age, the cross-sectional area of choriocapillaris is reduced and the normal sinusoidal capillaries are replaced by a tubular system.[53,98,99] These changes are accompanied by widening of the intercapillary pillars. In ten decades the density of the choriocapillaris decreases by 45%, and its diameter decreases by 34%, whereas the thickness of Bruch's membrane increases by 135%.[53,99] There is a wide variation in the range of values of choriocapillaris density with increasing age, and the presence of AMD may mask the effect.[100] These changes could account for the perfusion defect seen on fluorescein angiography in Sorsby's fundus dystrophy and some cases of AMD.[101–103] It is of interest that a weak linear association has been noted between the number

of cellular processes from the endothelial cells of the choriocapillaris protruding into Bruch's membrane and the thickness of Bruch's membrane.[61] It is not possible to determine if thickening of Bruch's membrane precedes choriocapillaris changes in AMD, and therefore a causal relationship between the two has not yet been proved. An initial abnormality in the choriocapillaris could lead to a reduction in clearance of waste material from Bruch's membrane into the choroidal circulation. Alternatively, the diffuse deposits in Bruch's membrane may induce secondary changes in the capillaries by acting as a barrier to diffusion between the RPE and choroid. There is good evidence that diffusible agents from the RPE regulate the choriocapillaris morphology, so the interposition of a diffusion barrier between the two structures may alter the accessibility of these molecules to the capillaries, resulting in the vessels reverting to the more common tubular arrangement of capillary beds.[79,104,105] This concept has been illustrated by the expression at high levels of TIMP-3 in Bruch's membrane[106] and the demonstration that TIMP-3 influences endothelial function.[107]

INTERRELATIONSHIP BETWEEN AGING IN BRUCH'S MEMBRANE AND THE RETINAL PIGMENT EPITHELIUM

Despite the universal acceptance that the material in Bruch's membrane is derived from RPE, little information exists about the exact relationship between the accumulation of debris in both structures. This has been investigated recently.[30] A direct relationship was found between Bruch's membrane thickness and changes in the RPE cells, which is best described by a linear regression model. However, considerable variation exists between specimens of donors of similar age, with increasing variation in older age groups. The variation between specimens from donors of the same age may reflect sampling, but more likely it is due to the multiplicity of genetic and environmental factors influencing the aging processes.

The possibility that age-related changes in the different tissues may occur independently cannot be denied. However, it seems likely that at least some aspects of aging in these tissues are causally related. If the level of RPE residual body content and autofluorescence reflects metabolic activity, so might the discharge of waste material into Bruch's membrane. The linear relationship between Bruch's membrane thickness and RPE autofluorescence is likely to reflect this functional relationship. Logically the thickness of Bruch's membrane would be influenced by the rate of deposition of material into it and the rate of clearance. The linear relationship between Bruch's membrane thickness and RPE change is likely to reflect this functional relationship. The relationship between autofluorescence and Bruch's membrane thickness was closer ($R^2 = 0.37$) than that between Bruch's membrane thickness and residual body content ($R^2 = 0.18$).[30] This gives some support to the suggestion that the influence of fluorescence, rather than volume occupied by the residual bodies on RPE function, is critical to the disease process.[31,108] This belief was based on the proposal that free radicals emitted by the fluorescent material may influence the composition of lipids in the RPE that would in turn make them less amenable to enzymatic degradation.

In the recently proposed inflammatory hypothesis of drusen biogenesis it is proposed that the debris derived from the compromised RPE cells is the critical seeding event for drusen formation. The cellular debris constitutes a chronic inflammatory stimulus that becomes the target of encapsulation by a variety of inflammatory mediators.[109]

ACCUMULATION OF MATERIAL IN BRUCH'S MEMBRANE

Origin of material

The debris deposited into Bruch's membrane is believed to be derived from the RPE. The failure of the debris to traverse Bruch's membrane into the choriocapillaris is thought to result in its accumulation in Bruch's membrane.[9,45,49,78,110,111] There is no consensus regarding the actual mechanism of deposition. Whether the material is shed as parcels of cytoplasm from the basal surface of the RPE as a result of budding RPE cells, with degradation and fragmentation of the budded portion, or whether it arises from RPE cell death is in dispute.[10,110] One of the original theories of Donders[112] was that RPE cells were directly converted to drusen, but the lack of structures resembling outer segments, phagosomes, or lipofuscin granules is thought by some to make this unlikely.[110] There is also no consensus about the origin of CMB bodies, and similar theories abound. Hogan[45] proposed that they represented RPE residual bodies and partially digested phagosomes. Others thought that they originated from shed aliquots of cytoplasm by RPE that disposed of old or damaged membrane and organelles to account for the membrane-bound material.[9,12,13] Killingsworth[79] suggested that the CMB bodies represent RPE-derived plasma membrane-bound vesicles released through "pinching off" from the basal plasma membrane. These bodies are found in Bruch's membrane from eyes of donors of any age, suggesting that the budding off process is a normal phenomenon of RPE. The CMB bodies are thought to move unimpeded through the inner layers of Bruch's membrane and become lodged in the OCZ, explaining their higher concentration there. Alternatively, the membranes and vesicles may form in situ from discharged lipids or may even develop postmortem.

It has been considered unlikely that the material in Bruch's membrane is derived directly from photoreceptor outer segment breakdown or phagosomes, since neither rhodopsin epitopes nor phagosomal enzyme activity has been shown in Bruch's membrane deposits using monoclonal antibodies.[113] However, the presence of docosahexaenoic acid, which is found in quantity only in the outer segments, implies that material derived from the rod outer segment contributes toward the debris. It is generally considered that the debris in Bruch's membrane reflects RPE metabolic activity in general rather than being directly derived from outer segment material.

Cause of accumulation

The nature of the material deposited by the RPE, the diffusion characteristics of Bruch's membrane, and the ability of the choriocapillaris to clear the debris may all contribute to the kinetics of clearance. The material to be cleared may be abnormal as a consequence of incomplete degradation,[114] possibly because of failure of degradative enzymes. It has been demonstrated that, in the presence of antisense cathepsin D and cathepsin S, RPE cells in culture rapidly accumulate cytoplasmic inclusions when fed rod outer segments.[115] This is presumed to result from the reduced ability to degrade the contents of phagosomes. The evidence concerning the level of enzyme activity in RPE in humans is mixed,[18,116] but most studies imply that total activity increases with age. In addition, there is experimental evidence that increasing phagosomal load in cultured RPE cells results in a rise in degradative enzyme activity.[19,116] The finding that all residual bodies have enzyme activity suggests a possible competition for newly produced lysosomes, leading to a decrease in those available to newly formed phagosomes. Thus, even if total enzyme activity is increased, there may still be a relative deficiency, with resultant defective breakdown of newly ingested photoreceptor outer segment material within the RPE. The unsaturated fatty acids from the photoreceptor outer segments are liable to free radical damage, particularly in the high oxygen tension of RPE and outer segments.[29] It is postulated that the substrate for degradation may be altered by peroxidation, resulting in compounds that cross-link biologic molecules, causing them to be less susceptible to degradation by lysosomal enzymes.[117] The ability of highly active free radical scavenging systems in the outer retina to counteract this may alter with age.[118]

An additional major contributing factor may be structural alteration of Bruch's membrane. As Bruch's membrane ages, changes in the extracellular matrix may alter its permeability and impede normal filtration, and there is good evidence to support this.[46,47,49,55,60] Finally, reduction of the cross-sectional area of choriocapillaris in older adults may reduce the rate of clearance from Bruch's membrane. Why a small number of laser lesions, as used in clinical prophylactic studies in eyes with multiple drusen, causes drusen to disappear is unexplained.[119]

DETERMINANTS OF CHANGE IN BRUCH'S MEMBRANE

The factors that determine risk of developing AMD have yet to be well defined, but clinical studies imply that both genetic and environmental factors are involved. It is generally considered that genetic susceptibility becomes evident in the presence of appropriate environmental pressures.

Genetic factors

The greater concordance between siblings than between spouses in the prevalence and qualitative attributes of age change in Bruch's membrane demonstrates the importance of genetic factors to the pathogenesis of disease.[120-122] A twin study supports this conclusion.[123] It is possible that genetic sequence changes determine the risk of AMD by influencing a variety of functions such as: the turnover rates of outer segments,[124] the rates of lysosomal degradation, the efficiency in discharging material by the RPE, or the diffusional characteristics of Bruch's membrane. To date the one gene that has been associated with AMD in several studies is the Apolipoprotein E (APOE) gene which is involved in cholesterol transport and its presence in both drusen and the RPE suggest that it may be involved in lipid homeostasis in these tissues.[109,125–127]

AMD is likely to be a complex polygenic disorder dependent on the presence of one or several mutant genes or allelic variants. Thus many genes may contribute to the risk of AMD. The phenotypic expression of AMD varies widely[41] and differs in various communities. This is illustrated by observations in Japan, where a high proportion of second eyes of subjects with unilateral visual loss have no ophthalmoscopically visible age change (Uyama, personal communication, 1998), whereas in Western populations virtually all such eyes will have drusen. This might be explained if the prevalence of those genes influencing disease differed in various communities. In Greenland the phenotype of AMD is different from that in Western communities with more widespread atrophy, which progresses rapidly and results in worse visual acuity than usually seen in the Western counterpart.[128,129] This might be explained by a founder effect in a relatively isolated population.

Environmental factors

The relative lack of concordance of drusen between spouses[121] was thought to imply that either environment is not important in the pathogenesis of disease or that the variation in environment in the communities under study was insufficient to show an effect. Persuasive evidence of environmental influence comes from Japan and Greenland. In Japan AMD was reputedly rare 20 years ago, but it is now recognized as a common cause of blind registration in urban communities.[1–3] The prevalence of visual loss from macular disease among older adult Inuit in Greenland is the highest of any community in the world, including genetically similar communities, suggesting the possibility of a local environmental effect.[128,129] AMD has been shown to be rare in South African blacks, which could arguably be explained on a genetic basis.[130] However, this would not explain a low prevalence found in a preliminary survey of rural Southern Italy when compared with other European communities,[131] given that Europe is fairly genetically homogeneous.[132]

The search for major environmental influences on AMD has met with some success, but the evidence is mixed. Smoking has most consistently been associated with increased risk,[133,134] but, surprisingly, not all studies have demonstrated this.[135] Higher serum levels of combined antioxidants have been found by some to decrease the risk of neovascular AMD,[136] and recently a major study (AREDS) showed that there may be some benefit, for a small subpopulation of AMD subjects, in taking large quantities of multiple vitamins and zinc, although widespread supplementation is not advocated by all.[137–139] However other studies have not shown high oral intake of vitamins A, C, and E to be protective[140,141] and carries potential risk.[142] Zinc deficiency may play a role because it is a coenzyme in the lysosomal degradative processes within the RPE. One study appeared to show a beneficial effect of dietary supplementation,[143] but a subsequent controlled trial did not show any therapeutic benefit,[144] and an epidemiologic study gave only weak support to this concept.[145] Light has also been implicated,[146] and there has been particular interest in the potential protective influence of lutein and zeaxanthin,[147] which constitute the major luteal pigments. High intake of lutein in green vegetables and high levels of macular density may be associated with low prevalence of AMD.[140,148] Although there may be an association between these factors and AMD, none has been shown to alter the odds ratio sufficiently to account for observed differences in prevalence between various communities. The suspicion is that the most important factors have not been identified to date.

RELEVANCE OF AGE CHANGE TO DISEASE

Both drusen and end-stage disciform lesions were described in the nineteenth century,[112,149] and yet a causal relationship between the two conditions was not recognized until well into the twentieth century.[150–153] Drusen vary widely in their appearance and location from one patient to another, although there is remarkable symmetry between the two eyes of an individual with respect to drusen size, density, and fluorescence on angiography.[152,154,155] There is good evidence that the type of deposit may influence the outcome of the disease.[156]

Drusen, even small subclinical drusen, have recently been shown to cause overlying changes in photoreceptors.[157] However it is the diffuse, rather than focal, deposits that might logically be expected to have the greater influence on the outcome of disease. However, although well documented histologically, these diffuse deposits have received little attention by clinicians until recently, since no recognizable clinical correlate of their presence existed. As a result of studies on patients with Sorsby's fundus dystrophy, an angiographic correlate of diffuse Bruch's membrane thickening has been proposed. In this autosomal dominant condition, a continuous layer of abnormal material up to 30 μm thick is deposited between the inner collagenous layer of Bruch's membrane and the basement membrane of the RPE.[158] On fluorescein angiography there is prolonged, patchy choroidal filling with normal fluorescence not apparent until the venous phase of the retinal circulation.[103,159] As a result of this observation, fluorescein angiograms of patients with ARM degeneration were examined, and approximately one quarter had an angiographic appearance consistent with prolonged choroidal filling.[73] It was suggested that this may be a useful clinical sign of diffuse thickening of Bruch's membrane in ARM.

Metabolic exchange

Thickening of Bruch's membrane may alter its biophysical properties, particularly if it contains neutral lipids, and consequently impede diffusion between the RPE and choroid. This concept is supported by studies on the hydraulic conductivity of Bruch's membrane with age. Fisher[160] reported that hydraulic conductivity of Bruch's membrane decreased with age and predicted from extrapolation of his data that by the age of 130 years there would be no flow of water through Bruch's membrane. More recently, an exponential decrease in hydraulic conductivity with increasing age has been shown, with changes being more marked in the macula than in the periphery.[161] An association between age-related loss of conductivity and the profile of lipid extracted from Bruch's membrane was shown.[161] The major contributor to the decrease in conductivity appears to be in the inner half of Bruch's membrane.[162]

Normal photoreceptor function depends on free diffusion through Bruch's membrane from the choriocapillaris to the RPE[44,163] which would not occur through a hydrophobic layer of debris. The magnitude of change would depend on the thickness, matrix components and chemical composition of the material within Bruch's membrane and would be particularly marked in the presence of a large quantity of neutral lipids.[164] Scotopic dysfunction with scotopic threshold elevation of up to several log units and slow dark adaptation have been documented in subjects with symptoms of poor vision in the dark, dark-adapted central scotomas, and fading vision in bright light. These are common complaints of subjects with good vision but age-related change at the level of Bruch's membrane.[165,166] This abnormality was found consistently in eyes with abnormal choroidal filling patterns on fluorescein angiography.[167] The deficit is similar to that seen in vitamin A deficiency. It has been shown that the functional deficits in Sorsby's fundus dystrophy can be reversed by vitamin A supplementation,[168] indicating that retinal dysfunction reflects lack of vitamin A rather than a global defect in metabolic supply. The improvement was lost within 4 weeks of discontinuing supplementation. Thus loss of sensitivity, slow dark adaptation, and delayed choroidal perfusion on angiography may all be consequent on diffuse deposits within Bruch's membrane sufficient to compromise the metabolic exchange between choroid and retina.

Age-related macular degeneration

The lesions identified as causing loss of central vision in AMD are growth of new blood vessels from the choroid through Bruch's membrane toward the retina, detachment of the RPE, and geographic atrophy of the outer retina and choriocapillaris.[151] At what stage the universal deposition of material with age becomes abnormal and predisposes to disease is not clear. The prevalence of all types of drusen within the older adult Western population has been estimated at between 10% and 80%, depending on definitions and methods used for detection.[155,169,170] The risk of visual loss in subjects with drusen has been estimated in several studies. A large and recent study to quantify this risk is the Age-Related Eye Disease Study (AREDS) which concluded that eyes with mild AMD (multiple small drusen, nonextensive intermediate drusen) had a lower rate of progression to late AMD in 5 years (1.3%), compared to eyes with more severe AMD (at least one large druse, extensive intermediate drusen, or noncentral geographic atrophy) (18%).[137] The risk continues to increase with larger and more drusen. The clinical study of drusen has revealed a relationship between the characteristics of the drusen seen clinically and the form of lesion causing visual impairment, implying that the chemical composition and the quantity of the deposits may play a role in determining the form of complication and the magnitude of risk of visual loss. It has been hypothesized that hyperfluorescent drusen are hydrophilic, allowing free diffusion of water-soluble sodium fluorescein into the deposits, whereas hypofluorescent drusen imply hydrophobic drusen.[54] It is concluded that the former are rich in polar compounds and the latter are rich in neutral fats. This hypothesis was supported by in vitro staining, since the specimens with deposits containing little neutral lipids bound sodium fluorescein, whereas those with high levels did not.[171] The presence of serum fibronectin in the latter but not in the former provides further support to the concept. The proposal that the form of Bruch's membrane deposits determines the nature of the retinal disease suggests that the two eyes of a patient should behave similarly if the deposits in both eyes are similar. This observation is not new.[149] Symmetry of drusen has been shown with respect to their quantity, distribution, and chemical composition. In one study the fluorescence of drusen on fluorescein angiography had the greatest symmetry between eyes. This implies that the chemical composition and therefore the biophysical properties of the drusen were similar in the two eyes of an individual.[154] Several authors have reported that greater numbers and confluence of soft drusen and focal hyperpigmentation at the level of the RPE are associated with greater-than-average risk of visual loss.[51,172–175] In a hospital population there is an overall risk of 12% to 15% per year of developing a disciform lesion in the other eye if the first has an end-stage lesion, but this risk is even higher if the second eye has high-risk drusen characteristics.[137,150] Those with unilateral tears of the RPE have been reported to have an 80% risk of a similar lesion occurring in the other eye over 3 years.[176]

Pigment epithelial detachments

Large confluent hypofluorescent, hydrophobic soft drusen predispose to pigment epithelial detachments (PED).[41,171,177] It was initially postulated that detachments of the RPE were induced by passage of fluid through Bruch's membrane from the choriocapillaris, the physical attachment of RPE to Bruch's membrane having been disturbed by progressive accumulation of debris on the inner surface of Bruch's membrane.[151] However, this explanation requires either high hydrostatic pressure in the choroid compared with the subretinal space or flow induced by an osmotic pressure gradient from the choroid into the sub-RPE space. The little evidence that exists does not support the proposal that the hydrostatic pressure in choroid is higher than in the outer retina[178] or that there is high concentration of large polar molecules in the sub-RPE space. Choroidal blood vessels growing through Bruch's membrane might provide an alternative source of sub-RPE fluid.[179] However, neovascularization is not universal in PEDs,[180] implying that neovascularization is not always the initiating event in the pathogenesis of the lesion. An alternative concept was proposed in 1986 in which it was suggested that the sub-RPE fluid is derived from the RPE rather than from the choroid.[54] It is widely accepted that fluid moves from the retina into Bruch's membrane as a result of active movement of ions by the RPE cells. If Bruch's membrane became hydrophobic, resistance to water flow could cause fluid to collect between the RPE and Bruch's membrane. The concept that hydrophobicity of Bruch's membrane may be important to disease is illustrated by observations on the relationship of the characteristics of drusen and the lesion, subsequently causing visual loss. It has been shown that eyes with hypofluorescent drusen are at risk of developing a PED, whereas those with hyperfluorescent drusen are at risk of choroidal neovascularization.[171,176,177,180]

Geographic atrophy

From the preceding discussion it would follow that it may not only be water movement that is affected by reduction of diffusion through Bruch's membrane, but that there may be global reduction of metabolic exchange between the RPE and the choriocapillaris. Impairment of metabolic exchange between the choroid and RPE could compromise photoreceptor function and eventually lead to cell death. This would initially lead to loss of retinal sensitivity seen in ARM and subsequently to the loss of photoreceptors seen in geographic atrophy.[167,181] This concept is supported by the observation that patients with prolonged choroidal perfusion on angiogram, thought to indicate diffuse thickening of Bruch's membrane, are at three times greater risk of losing two lines of vision because of geographic atrophy than are those without this clinical sign.[102]

Choroidal neovascularization

At present, the changes in Bruch's membrane that predispose to neovascularization are unclear. Inward growth of choroidal new vessels through Bruch's membrane is the common endpoint in several retinal diseases, leading to disciform scarring and visual loss. Drusen that are hyperfluorescent and presumed to be hydrophilic appear to predispose to choroidal neovascularization, but the precise reason why this occurs has not been defined.[71,166,172,182] It is likely that blood vessel growth is suppressed by the metabolic environment of Bruch's membrane, which may be influenced by diffusible agents produced by the RPE.[183,184] New vessel formation is thought to occur as a consequence of an imbalance in the stimulating and inhibiting influences of growth factors, and any disruption to their diffusion through Bruch's membrane to choroid could alter this balance.[185,186]

Cells invading Bruch's membrane may alter it and may release angiogenic factors. The number of macrophages increases at the outer surface of Bruch's membrane in AMD.[183] They are thought by some to be the factor common to all diseases involving neovascularization.[187] Macrophages promote growth of endothelial cells, pericytes, and fibroblasts, and macrophage-derived prostaglandins, especially prostaglandin E, may be a strong stimulus to neovascularization.[188] Activated macrophages secrete enzymes such as collagenases and elastases and may erode Bruch's membrane by a combination of mechanical disruption, phagocytosis, and extracellular release of enzymes.[81] This erosion involves first the OCZ then the ICZ, with the elastic layer being more resistant. This cellular response with increasing age is not seen until Bruch's membrane has membranous debris present beneath the RPE basement membrane and seems to occur preferentially beneath hard drusen. This may be related to the fact that the RPE is often anchored over hard drusen while it becomes separated from Bruch's membrane by membranous soft deposits, so any diffusible factors from the RPE

exert maximal effect where it remains attached.[81,183] Other cells, such as monocytes, lymphocytes, fibroblasts, and mast cells, may also play a role in damage and the formation of breaks in Bruch's membrane. However, preexisting breaks are not necessary for new vessels to invade.[92,189]

Endothelial cell processes have also been found to penetrate Bruch's membrane as a normal phenomenon.[61] Human endothelial budding through the capillary basement membrane is the initial step in neovascularization in other tissues and is thought to be activated by endothelial membrane-associated metallaproteinases, which digest types IV and V collagen found in basement membranes.[190] Endothelial cells also produce two proteases, plasminogen activator and latent collagenases, that facilitate connective tissue invasion.[92] The disruption of the basement membrane locally is believed to facilitate outgrowth of capillary sprouts.[190] The mechanisms that initiate and modulate the normal rate of basement membrane dissolution and protrusion formation and the conversion of this phenomenon to neovascularization are unknown. The response of the choriocapillaris to its environment has been amply demonstrated in vitro and in vivo.[86,106,185,191] Local control mechanisms must exist to prevent one phenomenon from translating into the other, and these may be altered in pathologic conditions.[190] The process thereafter is likely to be determined by the relative concentrations of various growth factors and the nature of the collagen and interfiber matrix of Bruch's membrane. Some have suggested that the basement membrane may bind factors, thereby modulating their immediate effect.[185] In this regard it is interesting that local increases in thickness of the endothelial basement membrane around the endothelial cell processes protruding into Bruch's membrane, at least in the young, have been noted.[61] There is ample evidence that various factors with the potential to modify cell behavior exist in Bruch's membrane and that Bruch's membrane changes with age.[17,34,42,65] These considerations imply that choroidal neovascularization as part of ARM may occur as a distortion of a normal mechanism rather than representing a process unique to the aging eye.[192] If choroidal neovascularization in ARM is a distortion of this process, its up-regulation, such as may occur following laser photocoagulation, would be associated with potential neovascular complications.[193]

REFERENCES

1. Kubo N, Ohno Y, Yanagawa H et al. Annual estimated number of patients with senile disciform macular degeneration in Japan. Research committee on chorioretinal degenerations. Tokyo: The Ministry of Health and Welfare of Japan, 1989.
2. Kubo N, Ohno Y, Yuzawa M et al. Report on nationwide clinico-epidemiological survey of senile disciform macular degeneration in Japan. Research committee on chorioretinal degenerations. Tokyo: The Ministry of Health and Welfare of Japan, 1990.
3. Maruo T, Ikebukuro N, Kawanabe K et al. Changes in causes of visual handicaps in Tokyo. Jpn J Ophthalmol 1991; 35:268–272.
4. Bird AC. Towards an Understanding of age-related macular disease, The Bowman Lecture. Eye 2003; 17:457–466.
5. Evans J. Causes of blindness and partial sight in England and Wales 1990-1991. Studies on medical and population subjects, no 57, London, 1995, Her Majesty's Stationery Office.
6. Evans J, Wormald R. Is the incidence of registrable are-related macular degeneration increasing? Br J Ophthalmol 1996; 80:9–14.

7. Kahn HA, Moorhead HB. Statistics on Blindness in the Model Reporting Areas 1969-70, Washington, DC, US Department of Health, Education and Welfare Publication, US Government Printing Office.

8. Dorey CK, Wum G, Ebenstein D et al. Cell loss in the ageing retina: relationship to lipofuscin accumulation and macular degeneration. Invest Ophthalmol Vis Sci 1989; 30:1691–1692.

9. Feeney-Burns L, Ellersieck M. Age-related changes in the ultrastructure of Bruch's membrane. Am J Ophthalmol 1985; 100:686–697.

10. Ishibashi T, Patterson R, Ohnishi Y et al. Formation of drusen in the human eye. Am J Ophthalmol 1986; 101:342–353.

11. Ishibashi T, Sorgente N, Patterson R et al. Pathogenesis of drusen in the primate. Invest Ophthalmol Vis Sci 1986; 27:184–193.

12. Reme C. Autophagy in visual cells and pigment epithelium. Invest Ophthalmol Vis Sci 1977; 16:807–814.

13. Rungger-Branche E, Englert U, Leuenberger PM. Exocytic clearing of degraded membrane material from pigment epithelial cells in frog retina. Invest Ophthalmol Vis Sci 1988; 28:2026–2037.

14. Bok D, Young RW. Phagocytic properties of the RPE. In: Zinn KM, Marmor MF, eds. The retinal pigment epithelium. Cambridge, Mass: Harvard University Press, 1979, p 148–174.

15. Feeney L. The phagolysosomal system of the pigment epithelium: a key to retinal disease. Invest Ophthalmol Vis Sci 1973; 12:635–638.

16. Boulton ME, Docchio F, Dayhaw-Braker P et al. Age-related changes in the morphology, absorption and fluorescence of melanosomes and lipofuscin granules of the retinal pigment epithelium. Vision Res 1990; 30:1291–1305.

17. Feeney L. Lipofuscin and melanin of human retinal pigment epithelium: fluorescence, enzyme cytochemical, and ultrastructural studies. Invest Ophthalmol Vis Sci 1978; 17:583–600.

18. Wyszynski RE, Brunar WE, Cano DB et al. A donor age-dependent change in the activity of alpha-mannosidase in human cultured RPE cells. Invest Ophthalmol Vis Sci 1989; 30:2341–2347.

19. Boulton ME. Ageing of the retinal pigment epithelium. In: Osborne NN, Chader GJ, eds. Progress in retinal research, vol 11. Oxford: Pergamon, 1991.

20. Boulton ME, Cabral L, Marshall J et al. Light and ageing as cofactors in retinal pigment epithelial disease. In Zingirian M, Piccolino FC, eds. Retinal pigment epithelium, Amsterdam, 1989, Kugler and Ghedini.

21. Boulton ME, McKechnie NM, Breda J et al. The formation of autofluorescent granules in cultured human RPE. Invest Ophthalmol Vis Sci 1989; 30:83.

22. Deguchi J, Yammamoto A, Yoshimori T et al. Acidification of phagosomes and degradation of rod outer segments in rat retinal pigment epithelium. Invest Ophthalmol Vis Sci 1994; 35:568–579.

23. Feeney-Burns L, Eldred GE. The fate of the phagosome: conversion to "age-pigment" and impact in human retinal pigment epithelium. Trans Ophthalmol Soc UK 1984; 103:414–421.

26. Weale RA. Do years or quanta age the retina? Photochem Photobiol 1989; 50:429–438.

27. von Rückmann A, Fitzke FW, Bird AC. Distribution of fundus autofluorescence with a scanning laser ophthalmoscope. Br J Ophthalmol 1995; 119:543.

28. Taudold RD. Studies on chemical nature of lipofuscin (age pigment) isolated from normal human brain. Lipids 1975; 10:383–390.

29. Wing GL, Blanchard GC, Weiter JL. The topographical and age relationship of lipofuscin concentration in the retinal pigment epithelium. Invest Ophthalmol Vis Sci 1978; 17:601–607.

30. Okubo A, Rosa RH, Fan JT et al. RPE residual body content, autofluorescence and aging. Invest Ophthalmol Vis Sci 1996; 37(suppl):380.

31. Docchio F, Boulton M, Cubeddu R et al. Age-related changes in the fluorescence of melanin and lipofuscin granules of the retinal pigment epithelium: a time-resolved fluorescence spectroscopy study. Photochem Photobiol 1991; 54:247–253.

32. von Rückmann A, Fitzke FW, Bird AC. In vivo fundus autofluorescence in age-related macular degeneration. Invest Ophthalmol Vis Sci 1997; 38:478–486.

33. Woon WH, Fitzke FW, Chester GH et al. The scanning laser ophthalmoscope: basic principles and applications. J Ophthalmol Photog 1990; 12:17.

34. van de Schaft TL, Bruijn WC, Mooy CM et al. Is basal laminar drusen unique for age-related macular degeneration? Arch Ophthalmol 1991; 109:420–425.

35. Delori FC, Arend O, Staurenghi G et al. Lipofuscin and drusen fluorescein aging and age-related macular degeneration. Invest Ophthalmol Vis Sci 1995; 36:718–729.

36. Yuodelis C, Hendrickson A. A qualitative and quantitative analysis of the human fovea during development. Vision Res 1986; 26:847–856.

37. Curcio CA, Millican CL, Allen KA et al. Aging of the human photoreceptor mosaic: evidence for selective vulnerability of rods in central retina. Invest Ophthalmol Vis Sci 1993; 34:3278–3296.

38. Keunen JEE, van Norren D, van Meel GJ. Density of foveal cone pigment at older age. Invest Ophthalmol Vis Sci 1987; 28:985–991.

39. Eldred GE, Katz ML. Fluorophores of the human retinal pigment epithelium: separation and spectral characterization. Exp Eye Res 1988; 47:71–86.

40. Katz ML, Norberg M. Influence of dietary vitamin A on autofluorescence of leupeptin-induced inclusions in the retinal pigment epithelium. Exp Eye Res 1992; 54:239–246.

41. Green WR, Enger C. Age-related macular degeneration histopathological studies. Ophthalmology 1993; 100:1519–1535.

42. Sarks SH. Ageing and degeneration in the macular region: a clinico-pathological study. Br J Ophthalmol 1976; 60:324–341.

43. van de Schaft TL, Bruijn WC, Mooy CM et al. Basal laminar deposit in the aging peripheral human retina. Graefes Arch Clin Exp Ophthalmol 1993; 231:470–475.

44. Bok D. Retinal photoreceptor-pigment epithelium interactions. Invest Ophthalmol Vis Sci 1985; 26:1659–1694.

45. Hogan MJ. Role of the retinal pigment epithelium in macular disease. Trans Am Acad Otolaryngol Ophthalmol 1972;76:64.

46. Hewitt TA, Nakazawa K, Newsome DA. Analysis of newly synthesized Bruch's membrane proteoglycans. Invest Ophthalmol Vis Sci 1989; 30:478–486.

47. Hewitt TA, Newsome DA. Altered synthesis of Bruch's membrane proteoglycans associated with dominant retinitis pigmentosa. Curr Eye Res 1985; 4:169–174.

48. Lyda W, Eriksen N, Krishna N. Studies of Bruch's membrane: flow and permeability studies in a Bruch's membrane-choroid preparation. Am J Ophthalmol 1957; 44:362–396.

49. Marshall J. The ageing retina: physiology or pathology. Eye 1987; 1:282.

50. Hogan MJ, Alvarado J. Studies on the human macula. IV. Aging changes in Bruch's membrane. Arch Ophthalmol 1967; 77:410–420.

51. Holz FG, Sheraidah G, Pauleikhoff D et al. Analysis of lipid deposits extracted from human macular and peripheral Bruch's membrane. Arch Ophthalmol 1994; 112:402–406.

52. Newsome DA, Huh W, Green WR. Bruch's membrane age-related changes vary by region. Curr Eye Res 1987; 6:1211–1221.

53. Ramrattan RS, van der Schaft TL, Mooy CM et al. Morphometric analysis of Bruch's membrane, the choriocapillaris, the choroid in aging. Invest Ophthalmol Vis Sci 1994; 35:2857–2864.

54. Bird AC, Marshall J. Retinal pigment epithelial detachments in the elderly. Trans Ophthalmol Soc UK 1986; 105:674–682.

55. Karwatowski WSS, Jeffries TE, Duance VC et al. Preparation of Bruch's membrane and analysis of the age-related changes in the structural collagens. Br J Ophthalmol 1995; 79:944–952.

56. Marshall GE, Konstas AGP, Lee WR. Collagens in ocular tissues. Br J Ophthalmol 1993; 77:515–524.

57. Lutjen-Drecoll E, Rittig M, Rauterberg J et al. Immunomicroscopical study of type VI collagen in the trabecular meshwork of normal and glaucomatous eyes. Exp Eye Res 1989; 48:139–147.

58. Sun CN, White HJ. Extracellular cross-striated banded structures in human connective tissue. Tissue Cell 1975; 7:419–432.

59. Sarks S. New vessel formation beneath the retinal pigment epithelium in senile eyes. Br J Ophthalmol 1973; 57:951–961.

60. Marshall GE, Konstas AGP, Reid GG et al. Collagens in the aged human macula. Graefes Arch Clin Exp Ophthalmol 1994; 232:133–140.

61. Guymer RH, Bird AC, Hageman GS. Cytoarchitecture of choroidal capillary endothelial cells. Invest Ophthalmol Vis Sci 2004; 45:1660–1666.

62. Chen L, Miyamura N, Ninomiya Y et al. Distribution of the collagen IV isoforms in human Bruch's membrane. Br J Ophthalmol 2003; 87:212–215.

63. Kliffen M, Mooy CM, Luider TM et al. Analysis of carbohydrate structures in basal laminar deposit in aging human maculae. Invest Ophthalmol Vis Sci 1994; 35:2901–2905.

64. Kajikawa K, Nakanishi I, Yamamura T. The effect of collagenase on the formation of fibrous long-spacing collagen aggregates. Lab Invest 1980; 43:410–417.

65. Loffler KU, Lee WR. Basal linear deposit in the human macula. Graefes Arch Clin Exp Ophthalmol 1986; 224:493–501.

66. van der Schaft TL, Mooy CM, de Bruijn WC et al. Immunohistochemical light and electron microscopy of basal laminar deposit. Graefes Arch Clin Exp Ophthalmol 1994; 232:40–46.

67. Bruns RR. Beaded filaments and long spacing fibrils: relation to type VI collagen. J Ultrastruct Res 1984; 89:136–145.

68. Bruns RR, Press W, Engvall E et al. Type VI collagen in extracellular 100-nm periodic filaments and fibrils: identification by immunoelectron microscopy. J Cell Biol 1986; 103:393–404.

69. Hirano K, Kobayashi M, Kobayashi K et al. Experimental formation of 100 nm periodic fibrils in the mouse corneal stroma and trabecular meshwork. Invest Ophthalmol Vis Sci 1989; 30:869–874.

70. Alexander RA, Garner A. Elastic and precursor fibres in the normal human eye. Exp Eye Res 1983; 36:305–315.

71. Pauleikhoff D, Harper CA, Marshall J et al. Aging changes in Bruch's membrane: a histochemical and morphological study. Ophthalmology 1990; 97:171–178.

72. Ruberti J, Curcio CA, Millican L et al. Quick-freeze/deep etch visualization of age-related lipid accumulation in Bruch's membrane. Invest Ophthalmol Vis Sci 2003; 44: 1753–1759.

73. Holz FG, Piguet B, Minasian DC et al. Decreasing stromal iris pigmentation as a risk factor for age-related macular degeneration. Am J Ophthalmol 1994; 117:19–25.

74. Sheraidah G, Steinmetz R, Maguire J et al. Correlation between lipids extracted from Bruch's membrane and age. Ophthalmology 1993; 100:47–51.

75. Bazan HE, Bazan NG, Feeney-Burns L et al. Lipids in human lipofuscin-enriched subcellular fractions of two age populations. Invest Ophthalmol Vis Sci 1990; 31:1433–1443.

76. Malek G, Li CM, Guidry C et al. Apolipoprotein B in cholesterol containing drusen and basal deposits of human eyes with related maculopathy. Am J Pathol 2003; 162:413–425.

77. Marshall GE, Konstas AGP, Reid GG et al. Type IV collagen and laminin in Bruch's membrane and basal linear deposit in the human macula. Br J Ophthalmol 1992; 76:607–614.

78. Grindle CFJ, Marshall J. Aging changes in Bruch's membrane and their functional implications. Trans Ophthalmol Soc UK 1978; 98:172–175.

79. Killingsworth MC. Age-related components of Bruch's membrane in the human eye. Graefes Arch Clin Arch Exp Ophthalmol 1987; 225:406–412.

80. The International ARM Epidemiological Study Group: An international classification and grading system for age-related macular maculopathy and age-related macular degeneration. Surv Ophthalmol 1995; 39:367–374.

81. Garner A, Sarks S, Sarks JP. Degenerative and related disorders of the retina and choroid. In: Garner A, Klintworth GK, eds. Pathobiology of ocular disease, 2nd edn. New York: Marcel Dekker,1994.

82. Sarks JP, Sarks SH, Killingsworth MC. Evolution of soft drusen in age-related macular degeneration. Eye 1994; 8:268–283.

83. Sarks SH. Drusen and their relationship to senile macular degeneration. Aust J Ophthalmol 1980; 8:117–130.

84. Steinberg RH. Monitoring communications between photoreceptors, pigment epithelial cells: effects of "mild" systemic hypoxia. Invest Ophthalmol Vis Sci 1987; 28:1888–1904.

85. Garron LK. The ultrastructure of the retinal pigment epithelium with observations on the choriocapillaris and Bruch's membrane. Trans Am Ophthalmol Soc 1963; 61:545.

86. Korte GE, Chase J. Additional evidence for remodeling of normal choriocapillaris. Exp Eye Res 1989; 49:299–303.

87. Leeson TS, Leeson CR. Choriocapillaris and lamina elastica (vitrea) of the rat eye. Br J Ophthalmol 1967; 51:599–616.

88. Matsusaka T. Undescribed endothelial processes of the choriocapillaris extending to the retinal pigment epithelium in chick. Br J Ophthalmol 1968; 52:887–892.

89. Yamamoto T, Yamashita H. Pseudopodia of choriocapillary endothelium. Jpn J Ophthalmol 1989; 33:327–336.

90. Ausprunk DH, Folkman J. Migration and proliferation of endothelial cells in preformed and newly formed blood vessels during tumour angiogenesis. Microvasc Res 1997; 14:53–65.

91. Folkman J. Angiogenesis: initiation and control. Ann NY Acad Sci 1982; 401:212–227.

92. Heriot WJ, Henkind P, Bellhorn RW et al. Choroidal neovascularization can digest Bruch's membrane. Ophthalmology 1984; 91:1603–1608.

93. Killingsworth MC. Angiogenesis in early choroidal neovascularization secondary to age-related macular degeneration. Graefes Arch Clin Exp Ophthalmol 1995; 233:313–323.

94. Yamamoto T, Yamashita H. Pseudopodia of choriocapillary endothelium in ocular tissues. Jpn J Ophthalmol 1990; 34:181–187.

95. Hageman GS, Kelly DE. Cytoskeletal support and anchorage of the choriocapillaris. Invest Ophthalmol Vis Sci 1983; 24(suppl):141.

96. Michel CC. Renal medullary microcirculation: architecture and exchange. Microcirculation 1995; 2:125–139.

97. Takahashi-Iwanaga H. The three-dimensional cytoarchitecture of the interstitial tissue in the rat kidney. Cell Tissue Res 1991; 264:269–281.

98. Olver J, Pauleikhoff D, Bird A. Morphometric analysis of age changes in the choriocapillaris. Invest Ophthalmol Vis Sci 1990; 31(suppl):47.

99. Sarks SH. Changes in the region of the choriocapillaris in aging and degeneration. Twenty-Third Concilium Ophthalmology, Kyoto, 1978.

100. Spraul CW, Lang GE, Grossniklaus HE. Morphometric analysis of the choroid, Bruch's membrane, retinal pigment epithelium in eyes with age-related macular degeneration. Invest Ophthalmol Vis Sci 1996; 37:2724.

101. Pauleikhoff D, Chen JC, Chisholm IH et al. Choroidal perfusion abnormalities in age-related macular disease. Am J Ophthalmol 1990; 109:211.

102. Piguet BP, Palmvang IP, Chisholm IH et al. Evolution of age-related macular disease with choroidal perfusion abnormality. Am J Ophthalmol 1992; 113:657.

103. Polkinghorne PJ, Capon MR, Berninger TA et al. Sorsby's fundus dystrophy: a clinical study. Ophthalmology 1989; 96:1763–1768.

104. Henkind P, Gartner S. The relationship between retinal pigment epithelium and the choriocapillaris. Trans Ophthalmol Soc UK 1983; 103:444–447.

105. Korte GE, Repucci V, Henkind P. RPE destruction causes choriocapillary atrophy. Invest Ophthalmol Vis Sci 1984; 25:1135–1145.

106. Vranka JA, Johnson E, Zhu X et al. Discrete expression and distribution pattern of TIMP-3 in the human retina and choroid. Curr Eye Res 1997; 16:102–110.

107. Anand-Apte B, Pepper MS, Voest E et al. Inhibition of angiogenesis by tissue inhibitor of metalloproteinase-3. Invest Ophthalmol Vis Sci 1997; 38:817–823.

108. Rozanowska M, Jarvis-Evans J, Korytowski W et al. Blue light-induced reactivity of retinal age pigment: in vitro generation of oxygen-reactive species. J Biol Chem 1995; 27:18825–18830.

109. Anderson DH, Mullins RF, Hageman GS et al. A role for local inflammation in the formation of drusen in the ageing eye. Am J Opthal 2002; 134:411–431.

110. Burns RP, Feeney-Burns L. Clinico-morphologic correlations of drusen and Bruch's membrane. Trans Am Ophthalmol Soc 1980; 78:206–225.

112. Donders FC. Beitrage zur pathologischen Anatomie des Aüges. Albrecht von Graefes Archiv Ophthalmol 1855; 2:106.

113. Feeney-Burns L, Gao CL, Tidwell M. Lysosomal enzyme cytochemistry of human RPE, Bruch's membrane, and drusen. Invest Ophthalmol Vis Sci 1987; 28:1138–1147.

114. Katz ML. Incomplete proteolysis may contribute to lipofuscin accumulation in the retinal pigment epithelium. Adv Exp Med Biol 1989; 266:109.

115. Rakoczy PE, Mann K, Cavaney DM et al. Detection and possible functions of a cysteine protease involved in digestion of rod outer segments by retinal pigment epithelial cells. Invest Ophthalmol Vis Sci 1994; 35:4100.

116. Boulton ME, Moriarty P, Unger W et al. Modulation of lysosomal enzyme content in cultured human RPE. Invest Ophthalmol Vis Sci 1991; 32 (suppl):1056.

117. Crabb J, Miyagi M, Gu X et al. Drusen proteome analysis: an approach to the etiology of age related macular degeneration. PNAS 2002; 99:14682–14687.

118. Penn JS, Anderson RE. Effect of light history on rod outer-segment membrane composition in the rat. Exp Eye Res 1987; 44:767–778.

119. Guymer RH, Gross-Jendroska M, Owens SL et al. Laser treatment in subjects with high risk clinical features of AMD. Arch Ophthalmol 1997; 155:595–603.

120. Heiba IM, Elston RC, Klein BEK et al. Sibling correlations and segregation analysis of age-related maculopathy: the Beaver Dam Eye Study. Genet Epidemiol 1994; 11:51.

121. Piguet B, Wells JA, Palmvang IB et al. Age-related Bruch's membrane change: a clinical study of the relative role of heredity and environment. Br J Ophthalmol 1993; 77:400–403.

122. Silvestri G, Johnston PB, Hughes AE. Is genetic predisposition an important risk factor in age-related macular disease? Eye 1994; 8:564–568.

123. Klein ML, Mauldin WM, Stoumbos VD. Heredity and age-related macular degeneration: observations in monozygotic twins. Arch Ophthalmol 1994; 112:932–937.

124. Bird AC. Retinal photoreceptor dystrophies. Am J Ophthalmol 1995; 119:543–552.

125. Baird P, Guida E, Cain M et al. Association studies of the apolipoprotein (APOE) gene and age-related macular degeneration. Invest Ophthalmol Vis Sci 2004; 45:1311–1315.

126. Klaver CCW, Kliffen M, Vasn Duijn CM et al. Genetic association of apolipoprotein E with age-related macular degeneration. Am J Hum Genet 1998; 63:200–206.

127. Souied EH, Benlian P, Amouyel P et al. The epsilon 4 allele of the apolipoprotein E gene as a potential protective factor for exudative age-related macular degeneration. Am J Ophthalmol 1998; 125:353–359.

128. Rosenberg T. Prevalence and causes of blindness in Greenland. Arch Med Res 1987; 46:13–17.

129. Rosenberg T. Prevalence of blindness caused by senile macular degeneration in Greenland. Arch Med Res 1987; 46:64–70.

130. Gregor Z, Joffe L. Senile macular changes in the black African. Br J Ophthalmol 1978; 62:547.

131. Pagliarini S, Moramarco A, Wormald RPL et al. Age-related macular disease in Southern Italy. Arch Ophthalmol 1997; 115: 616–622.

132. Cavalli-Sforza LL, Menozzi P, Liazza A. The history and geography of human genes. Princeton, NJ: Princeton University Press, 1994.

133. Klein R, Klein BEK, Linton KLP et al. The Beaver Dam Eye Study: the relation of age-related maculopathy to smoking. Am J Epidemiol 1993; 37:190–200.

134. Smith W, Mitchell P, Leeder SR. Smoking and age-related maculopathy: the Blue Mountains Eye Study. Arch Ophthalmol 1996; 114:1518–1523.

135. Hirvela H, Luukinen H, Laara E et al. Risk factors of age-related maculopathy in a population 70 years of age or older. Ophthalmology 1966; 103:871.

136. The Eye Disease Case Control Study Group. Antioxidant status and neo-vascular age-related macular degeneration. Arch Ophthalmol 1993; 111:104–109.

137. Age-related Eye Disease Study Research Group (AREDS report no 8). A randomized, placebo-controlled, clinical trial of high dose supplementation with vitamin C and E, beta-carotene, and zinc for age-related macular degeneration and vision loss. Arch Ophthalmol 2001; 119:1417–1436.

138. Lim L, Guymer RH. AMD: to supplement or not? Clinical Exp Ophth 2004; 32:341–343.

139. Seigel D. AREDS investigators distort findings (Letter). Arch Ophthalmol 2002; 120:100–101.

140. Seddon JM, Ajani UA, Sperduto RD et al. Dietary carotenoids, vitamins A, C, E and advanced age-related macular degeneration. JAMA 1994; 272:1413–1420.

141. Sperduto RD, Ferris FL, Kurinij N. Do we have a nutritional treatment for age-related cataract or macular degeneration? Arch Ophthalmol 1990; 108:1403.

142. Peterson K. Natural cancer prevention trial halted. Science 1996; 271:441.

143. Newsome DA, Swartz M, Leone NC et al. Oral zinc in macular degeneration. Arch Ophthalmol 1988; 106:192–198.

144. Stur M, Tittl M, Reitner A et al. Oral zinc and the second eye in age-related macular degeneration. Invest Ophthalmol Vis Sci 1996; 37:1225–1235.

145. Mares-Peerlman JA, Klein R, Klein BEK et al. Association of zinc and antioxidant nutrients with age-related maculopathy. Arch Ophthalmol 1966; 114:991.

146. West SK, Rosenthal FS, Bressler NM et al. Exposure to sunlight and other risk factors for age-related macular degeneration. Arch Ophthalmol 1989; 107:875–879.

147. Hammond BR, Wooten BR, Snoddely DM. Cigarette smoking and retinal carotenoids: implications for age-related macular degeneration. Vision Res 1996; 36:3003–3009.

148. Hammond BR, Wooten BR, Snoddely DM. Preservation of visual sensitivity of older subjects: association with macular pigment density. Invest Ophthalmol Vis Sci 1998; 39:397–406.

149. Hutchinson J, Tay W. Symmetrical central chorio-retinal disease occurring in senile persons. Roy Lond Ophthalmol Hosp Rep 1875; 83:275.

150. Gass JDM. Drusen and disciform macular detachment and degeneration. Trans Am Ophthalmol Soc 1972; 70:409–436.

151. Gass JDM. Pathogenesis of disciform detachment of the neuroepithelium. III. Senile disciform macular degeneration. Am J Ophthalmol 1976; 63:617.

152. Gifford SR, Cushman B. Certain retinopathies due to changes in the lamina vitrea. Arch Ophthalmol 1940; 23:6.

153. Verhoeff FH, Grossman HP. Pathogenesis of disciform degeneration of the macula. Arch Ophthalmol 1938; 19:561.

154. Barondes M, Pauleikhoff D, Chisholm IH et al. Bilaterality of drusen. Br J Ophthalmol 1990; 74:180–182.

155. Coffrey AJH, Brownstein S. The prevalence of macular drusen in post-mortem eyes. Am J Ophthalmol 1986; 102:164–171.

156. Bird AC. Bruch's membrane changes with age. Br J Ophthalmol 1992; 76:160.

157. Johnson PT, Lewis G, Talaga K et al. Invest Ophth Vis Sci 2003; 44:4484–4488.

158. Capon MRC, Marshall J, Kraft JI et al. Sorsby's fundus dystrophy: a light and electron microscopic study. Ophthalmology 1989; 96:1769–1777.

159. Hoskin A, Sehmi K, Bird AC. Sorsby's pseudo-inflammatory macular dystrophy. Br J Ophthalmol 1981; 65:859–865.

160. Fisher RF. The influence of age on some ocular basement membranes. Eye 1987; 1:184–189.

161. Moore DJ, Hussain AA, Marshall J. Age-related variation in the hydraulic conductivity of Bruch's membrane. Invest Ophthalmol Vis Sci 1995; 36:1290–1297.

162. Starita C, Hussain AA, Patmore A et al. Localization of the site of major resistance to fluid transport in Bruch's membrane. Invest Ophthalmol Vis Sci 1997; 38:762–767.

163. Bok D, Heller J. Transport of retinol from the blood to the retina: an autoradiographic study of the pigment epithelial cell surface receptor for plasma retinol-binding protein. Exp Eye Res 1976; 22:395–402.

164. Hillenkamp J, Hussain AA, Jackson TL et al. The influence of path length and matrix components on aging: characteristics of transport between the choroid and the outer retina. Invest Ophth Vis Sci 2004; 45:1493–1498.

165. Steinmetz RL, Haimovici R, Jubb C et al. Symptomatic abnormalities of dark adaptation in patients with age-related Bruch's membrane change. Br J Ophthalmol 1993; 77:549–554.

166. Steinmetz RL, Polkinghorne PC, Fitzke FW et al. Abnormal dark adaptation and rhodopsin kinetics in Sorsby's fundus dystrophy. Invest Ophthalmol Vis Sci 1992; 33:1633–1636.

167. Chen JC, Fitzke FW, Pauleikhoff D et al. Functional loss in age-related Bruch's membrane change with choroidal perfusion defect. Invest Ophthalmol Vis Sci 1992; 33:334–340.

168. Jacobson SG, Cideciyan AV, Regunath G et al. Night blindness in a TIMP3-associated Sorsby's fundus dystrophy is reversed by vitamin A. Nat Genet 1995; 11:27–32.

169. Gibson JM, Rosenthal AR, Lavery J. A study of prevalence of eye disease in the elderly in an English community. Trans Ophthalmol Soc UK 1985; 104:196–203.

170. Leibowitz H, Krueger DE, Maunder LR et al. The Framingham Eye Study monograph: an ophthalmological and epidemiological study of cataract, glaucoma, diabetic retinopathy, macular degeneration and visual acuity in a general population of 2631 adults, 1973–75. Surv Ophthalmol 1984; 25 (suppl):335.

171. Pauleikhoff D, Zuels S, Sheraidah G et al. Correlation between biochemical composition and fluorescein binding of deposits in Bruch's membrane. Ophthalmology 1993; 99:1548–1553.

172. Bressler SB, Maguire MG, Bressler NM et al. Relationship of drusen and abnormalities of the retinal pigment epithelium to the prognosis of neo-vascular macular degeneration. Arch Ophthalmol 1990; 108:1442–1447.

173. Bressler NM, Bressler SB, Seddon TM et al. Drusen characteristics in patients with exudative versus non-exudative age-related macular degeneration. Retina 1988; 8:109–114.

174. Boulton ME. Ageing of the retinal pigment epithelium. In Osborne NN, Chader GJ, eds. Progress in retinal research, vol 11. Oxford: Pergamon, 1991.

175. Smiddy WE, Fine SL. Prognosis of patients with bilateral macular drusen. Ophthalmology 1984; 91:271–277.

176. Schoeppner G, Chuang EL, Bird AC. The risk of fellow eye visual loss with unilateral retinal pigment epithelial tears. Am J Ophthalmol 1989; 108:683–685.

177. Chuang EL, Bird AC. The pathogenesis of tears of the retinal pigment epithelium. Am J Ophthalmol 1988; 105:285–290.

178. Foulds WS. Clinical significance of transscleral fluid transfer. Trans Ophthalmol Soc UK 1976; 96:290.

179. Gass JDM. Pathogenesis of tears of the retinal pigment epithelium. Br J Ophthalmol 1984; 68:513–519.

180. Barondes MJ, Pagliarini S, Chisholm IH et al. Controlled trial of laser photocoagulation of pigment epithelial detachments in the elderly: a four-year review. Br J Ophthalmol 1992; 76:5–7.

181. Bird AC. Pathogenesis of retinal pigment epithelial detachment in the elderly: the relevance of Bruch's membrane change. Eye 1991; 5:1–12.

182. Gregor Z, Bird AC, Chisholm IH. Senile disciform macular degeneration in the second eye. Br J Ophthalmol 1977; 61:141–147.

183. Killingsworth MC, Sarks JP, Sarks SH. Macrophages related to Bruch's membrane in age-related macular degeneration. Eye 1990; 4:613–621.

184. Penfold PL, Killingsworth MC, Sarks SH. Senile macular degeneration: the involvement of giant cells in atrophy of the retinal pigment epithelium. Invest Ophthalmol Vis Sci 1986; 27:364–371.

185. Glaser BM. Extracellular modulating factors and the control of intraocular neovascularization. Arch Ophthalmol 1988; 106:603–610.

186. Glaser BM, Campochiaro PA, Davis JL et al. Retinal pigment epithelial cells release an inhibitor to neovascularization. Arch Ophthalmol 1985; 103:1870–1875.

187. Ben Ezra D. Neovasculogenic ability of prostaglandins, growth factors and synthetic chemoattractants. Am J Ophthalmol 1978; 86:455–461.

188. Polverin PJ, Cotran RS, Gimbrone MA et al. Activated macrophages induce vascular proliferation. Nature 1977; 269:804.

189. Penfold P, Killingsworth M, Sarks S. An ultrastructural study of the role of leukocytes and fibroblasts in the breakdown of Bruch's membrane. Aust J Ophthalmol 1984; 12:23–31.

190. Kalebic T, Garbisa S, Glaser B et al. Basement membrane collagen degradation by migrating endothelial cells. Science 1983; 221:281–283.

191. Korte GE, Burns MS, Bellhorn RW. Epithelium–capillary interactions in the eye: the retinal pigment epithelium and the choriocapillaris. Int Rev Cytol 1989; 114:221–248.

192. Guymer RH, Hageman GS, Bird AC. Influences of laser photocoagulation on choroidal capillary cytoarchitecture. Br J Ophthalmol 2001; 85:40–46.

193. Owens SA, Bunce C, Brannon AJ et al. The Drusen Laser Study Group. Prophylactic laser treatment appears to promote choroidal neovascularization in high-risk ARM: results of an interim analysis. Eye 2003; 176:623–627.

Age-Related Macular Degeneration: Nonneovascular Early AMD, Intermediate AMD, and Geographic Atrophy

Susan B. Bressler
Neil M. Bressler
Shirley H. Sarks
John P. Sarks

Age-related macular degeneration (AMD) is not only the leading cause of legal blindness in patients aged 65 or over,[1] but it is also now the commonest overall cause of blindness in the western world. It is estimated that in the USA over 8 million people have some stage of AMD,[2,3] with hundreds of thousands of people aged 75 and over developing some stage of AMD over any 5-year period.[4] The incidence continues to rise as a result of the increasing percentage of elderly persons and the improved management of other eye diseases.[3] The prevalence of AMD has also increased steadily in the UK, accounting for approximately 50% of registered blindness in England and Wales that cannot be explained by the increasing age of the population alone.[5] In addition, macular degeneration is the commonest reason that patients with lesser handicaps attend low-vision clinics.

The advanced forms of AMD associated with visual acuity loss are divided into a nonneovascular atrophic (dry) type, and neovascular (wet) type. In atrophic AMD, gradual disappearance of the retinal pigment epithelium (RPE) results in one or more patches of atrophy that slowly enlarge and coalesce. Affected areas have no visual function, since loss of the RPE is associated with fallout of photoreceptors. Gass[6] applied the term "geographic atrophy of the retinal pigment epithelium" to this picture, which is the natural end-result of AMD in the absence of clinical evidence of choroidal neovascularization (CNV). This chapter is devoted to the clinical and pathologic features leading to this picture, as well as their management.

Senile macular degeneration was first reported as a clinical entity in 1885 by Otto Haab,[7] who described a variety of pigmentary and atrophic changes in the macular region, causing progressive impairment of central vision in patients over the age of 50. Subsequent observers referred to the different fundus manifestations of the disease as separate entities, resulting in a variety of descriptive eponyms. However, a review of dominantly inherited drusen[8] found that only Doyne's honeycomb familial choroiditis and Malattia levantinese were disorders that could be distinguished from each other by clinical criteria, and these entities are considered to be a separate category. A major step toward a better understanding of the disease was taken when Gass[9] clarified that drusen, senile macular degeneration, and senile disciform macular degeneration represented a single disease.

In the 1990s it had been proposed that the features should be termed either early or late *age-related maculopathy* (ARM),[10,11] to suggest that early ARM was not necessarily a pathologic state, with the term *age-related macular degeneration* (AMD) being reserved for late ARM and encompassing geographic atrophy and neovascular AMD. Since many epidemiologic studies are based on the International Epidemiological Age-related Maculopathy Study Group[10] description, it is described here. However, more recent descriptions of AMD from the Age-Related Eye Disease Study Group[12] have provided longitudinal information to understand features associated with an increased risk of developing advanced forms of AMD and are used in the description of the clinical management of AMD that follows.

In the International Epidemiological Age-related Maculopathy Study Group definitions used in many epidemiologic studies, early ARM was defined as a degenerative disorder in individuals ≥ 50 years of age, characterized by the presence of any of the following lesions:

- Soft (large, ≥ 63 μm) drusen. When occurring alone, soft, indistinct drusen are considered more likely to indicate AMD than soft, distinct drusen,[4,13,14] and drusen over 125 μm are more significant than smaller drusen.[15,16]
- Areas of hyperpigmentation associated with drusen but excluding pigment surrounding hard drusen.
- Areas of depigmentation or hypopigmentation associated with drusen. These areas, which commonly occur as drusen fade, are most often more sharply demarcated than drusen, but without exposure of the underlying choroidal vessels.
- *Visual acuity* is not used to define AMD because advanced changes may be present without affecting central fixation.

This definition of early ARM excluded small, hard drusen alone, pigment changes alone, and even pigment changes surrounding small, hard drusen for two reasons: (1) hard drusen become an almost constant finding in the fifth decade; and (2) a number of diverse processes can cause pigment abnormalities that may not be possible to distinguish from early ARM, so the inclusion of soft drusen limits the definition more specifically.[13] However, eyes with numerous small, hard drusen or eyes with pigment abnormalities in the absence of obvious drusen can also progress to AMD. Currently, prevalence studies have not existed long enough to confirm the significance of hard drusen or to determine how many drusen should be regarded as abnormal for the age of the patient.

Grading systems have been devised to permit comparison of severity over time of the size, number, and extent of drusen.[10,17–19] Grids are prepared on a transparent sheet and laid over one of a pair of stereoscopic color fundus transparencies. Because of the 3× magnification of the 30-degree fundus camera, 4.7 mm on the grid corresponds to 1500 μm, the diameter of the optic disc in the average fundus. Figure 60-1 illustrates a simplified form of the Wisconsin Age-Related Maculopathy Grading System.[19] The diameter of the circles are respectively 1000 μm, 3000 μm, and 6000 μm. The central and middle circles combined define the inner macula, which is two disc diameters across. The outer circle defines the macula itself. Figure 60-2 illustrates smaller standard circles, which are used to grade the size and area of specified lesions.[10]

These grading systems are applied to color transparencies and are intended primarily for epidemiologic studies and clinical trials. However, fluorescein angiography often provides additional insight into the natural history of the disease, as do pathologic studies,[20–24] which have demonstrated aging and degeneration to be a continuum based on diffuse morphologic changes at the level of the RPE under the macula, as distinct from focal abnormalities such as drusen. These diffuse changes comprise two sub-RPE or basal deposits separated by the RPE basement membrane. On the internal aspect lies a layer of abnormal basement membrane material, referred to as the *basal laminar deposit* (BLD); on the external aspect of the basement membrane is a

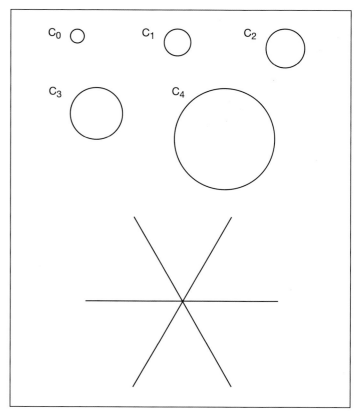

Fig. 60-2 Standard circles C_0, C_1, C_2, C_3, and C_4 that are used to grade the size of specified lesions. They are reduced on a transparent sheet to range from 1/24 to 1/3 disc diameter, thereby representing 63 μm, 125 μm, 175 μm, 250 μm, and 500 μm. Circle C_0 is used to differentiate small from large drusen, and circle C_2 indicates the minimum area on which to base a definition of geographic atrophy. The diagonal lines facilitate locating the central point and estimating size of lesions. (Reproduced from Bird AC, Bressler NB, Bressler SB et al. An international classification and grading system for age-related maculopathy and age-related macular degeneration. Surv Ophthalmol 1995; 39:367–374.[10])

layer of membranous debris, referred to as the *basal linear deposit*.[21] This latter deposit may build up into a type of soft drusen specific for AMD. However, although significant diffuse changes correlate with a decline in visual acuity,[22] they are difficult to see in the fundus, making a histologic definition of AMD based on basal laminar and basal linear deposits unworkable in a clinical setting. A study of donor postmortem eyes[25] suggests that objective markers for the presence of AMD might be the presence of at least one druse larger than 125 μm or an area of pigment-clumping 500 μm in diameter.

AGING

One of the difficulties in establishing the pathologic changes in AMD is separating the effects of age from those of disease. Aging is a fundamental biologic phenomenon that occurs even in the absence of disease, each cell having a genetically programmed lifespan. Tissues that do not undergo mitotic division to replace this cell fallout, such as the central nervous system and the retina, have a high incidence of aging

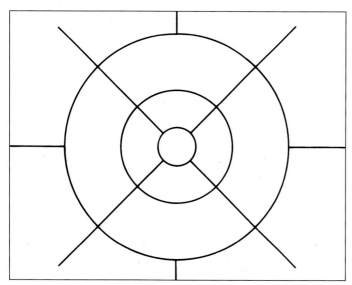

Fig. 60-1 Standard grid for classification of age-related macular degeneration. For a 30-degree fundus camera the diameters of the central, middle, and outer circles are 1000 μm, 3000 μm, and 6000 μm, respectively. These circles represent the central, inner, and outer subfields. The diagonal lines help to center the grid on the macula. (Reproduced from Klein R, Davis MD, Magli YL et al. The Wisconsin age-related maculopathy grading system. Ophthalmology 1991; 98:1128–1134.[19])

manifestations, particularly after 75 years of age. This age-related deterioration indicates a reduced anatomic reserve capacity in older subjects.

The aging eye – clinical findings

The normal aged fundus usually demonstrates loss of the foveal and foveolar reflexes. This may be due to fallout of cells from the inner retinal layers, shallowing of the walls of the foveal pit, and enlargement of the capillary-free zone.[26] A few small, hard drusen are almost always present.[11,13,15,17]

Irregularity of retinal pigmentation gives rise to a fine granularity, and the fundus commonly demonstrates a tigroid background. This senile tigroid fundus (see Fig. 60-5) is increasingly apparent with advancing age but remains compatible with normal vision. It is unrelated to skin pigmentation and differs from the tigroid fundus in youth in that the choroidal vessels become visible under the macula. There is commonly also a peripapillary halo of atrophy in which the exposed vessels may be sheathed and the intervascular spaces appear pale. Studies using blue-field stimulation[27] and scanning laser Doppler flowmetry[28] have shown a decrease in blood flow in the retinal macular capillaries of older individuals, and a lower number of perifoveal arterioles and venules have also been reported.[29] These findings are consistent with enlargement of the capillary-free zone[26] and loss of ganglion cells.[30]

Many aspects of visual function, not just visual acuity, show a decline with age, including dark adaptation, stereopsis, contrast sensitivity, sensitivity to glare, and visual field tests.[31,32] Color perception and foveal cone pigment densities show a decline.[33] The limits of normal aging are therefore difficult to define in terms of visual performance.

The aging eye – morphologic changes

The evolution of the aging process is easier to appreciate by studying morphologic changes. The RPE, Bruch's membrane, and choriocapillaris must function efficiently to serve as the nutritional complex for the photoreceptors. In a normal eye (Fig. 60-3A), the complement of photoreceptors is normal, the RPE forms a regular layer, Bruch's membrane is not unduly thickened, and the choroid consists of the usual three layers of vessels. Each of these tissues has at one time been regarded as primarily at fault in macular degeneration. Therefore it is first necessary to consider the changes developing in these structures during life (Fig. 65-3B).

Photoreceptors

The cone density at the foveal center does not appear to alter significantly during the first eight decades.[30,34,35] A significant loss beyond the ninth decade has been reported, but it is not invariable.[36]

In the rods the outer segments become convoluted, possibly as an expression of impaired phagocytosis.[37] This may lead to the accumulation of outer-segment material at the apical surface of the RPE.[36] Fallout of rods can also be demonstrated, with the fastest rate occurring between the second and fourth decades. Cells in the ganglion cell layer show a similar rate of

decrease, so the rod and ganglion cell layer densities maintain a constant ratio.[30] Rod photoreceptors and cells in the ganglion cell layer therefore appear to be more vulnerable than cones to loss during aging. In fact, this may be the initial subclinical stage of AMD because the spatial population of parafoveal rods decreases by 30% during adulthood, and AMD often commences in a similar parafoveal distribution.[34,38]

Retinal pigment epithelium

Each pigment epithelial cell must continue to engulf spent photoreceptor discs on a diurnal basis for life, the rods being digested by day and the cones by night,[39] and any undigested residual bodies remain as lipofuscin.[40] The RPE must also remove material from other retinal pigment cells or photoreceptors that may be eliminated, a burden that increases sharply once degeneration of these tissues commences. Finally, being a non-dividing tissue, autophagy alone could lead to the accumulation of lipofuscin in the same way that it builds up in the neurons of the central nervous system, which have no photoreceptors to phagocytose. The RPE is therefore particularly vulnerable to cell encumbrance.

Damage to molecules may occur in the photoreceptor outer segments as a result of free radical chain reactions initiated by radiation or oxygen metabolism. After phagocytosis, the lysosomal enzymes may fail to "recognize" these abnormal molecules, with a consequent failure of molecular degradation[41] and accumulation of lipofuscin. Free radicals also damage the cells' own molecules, and there is evidence that enzymatic inactivation occurs, particularly cathepsin D, which is the main lysosomal protease responsible for rod outer-segment digestion.[42] There is also an increase of complex granules of melanolysosomes and melanolipofuscin, which are thought to be melanin granules undergoing repair or degradation.

The accumulation of lipofuscin in the RPE, which can be demonstrated as early as the second decade of life,[43] reduces the cytoplasmic space. As the cell volume available to the organelles diminishes, the capacity to deal with photoreceptors is reduced. The issue of whether lipofuscin accumulation has significant deleterious effects on the RPE, and consequently on overall retinal function, continues to be of great interest.[44,45] Since lipofuscin is the predominant fluorophore responsible for fundus auto-fluorescence, the in vivo imaging and mapping of retinal autofluorescence using the confocal scanning laser ophthalmoscope[46] or fundus spectrophotometer[47] may prove helpful in estimating the risk for progression to AMD.

A certain loss of RPE cells occurs with age, particularly in the periphery. For the fovea this decrease in cell density has been estimated to be about 0.3% per year.[48] The ratio of photoreceptors to RPE cells remains the same,[30,36] the average cone-to-RPE ratio at the center of fovea being approximately 24:1. Photoreceptors and RPE cells therefore show a parallel loss during aging. However, the most notable changes in the RPE develop at the base of the cells, where there is loss of basal infoldings and deposition of patches of abnormal basement membrane material (Fig. 60-3B). (This BLD is described under Onset and progress of age-related macular degeneration, below.)

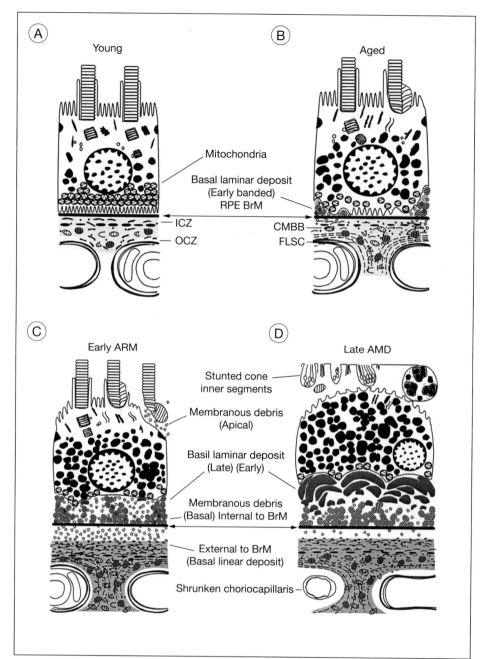

Fig. 60-3 Diagram depicting the ultrastructural features of aging and the evolution of age-related macular degeneration (AMD) in the retinal pigment epithelium (RPE) and Bruch's membrane (BrM). Bruch's membrane is defined as an inner and outer collagenous zone (ICZ and OCZ) separated by an elastic layer but excluding the basement membranes of the RPE and choriocapillaris, instead of as a five-layered structure. The principal distinguishing feature of each stage is the quantity and type of basal laminar deposit (BLD) present at the base of the RPE. A, Young. The BLD is absent. Mitochondria lie at the base of the cell. The pigment granules comprise elliptical melanin granules in the apical part of the cell and the incompletely degraded products of phagolysosomal digestion, or lipofuscin, toward the base. B, Aged. Patches of the early, or striated, type of BLD appear on the inner aspect of the RPE basement membrane, where the basal infoldings of the cells are reduced. Also, fewer apical microvilli are present, and elongated rod outer segments attest to impaired phagocytosis. Progressive accumulation of lipofuscin causes the RPE cells to enlarge. Coated membrane-bound bodies (CMBB) accumulate in Bruch's membrane and, together with an increase in fibrous long-spacing collagen (FLSC), cause thickening of the OCZ. C, Early age-related macular degeneration (AMD). The early type of BLD now forms a continuous layer. Membranous debris in the form of coiled lipid membranes is found: (1) at the apex of the RPE, where there is more distortion of outer segments; (2) at the base of the RPE interspersed among the strands of BLD, where it may form basal mounds; (3) as a layer between the RPE basement membrane and the ICZ (basal linear deposit), where it may build up into soft drusen; and (4) within the collagenous zones. CMBB and FLSC accumulating in Bruch's membrane can be seen in the intercapillary pillars extending to the level of the outer surface of the choroidal capillaries. D, Late age-related macular degeneration. A thick layer of late BLD is present, predominantly of the amorphous type. Being a later development, the amorphous layer lies on the internal aspect of the early type and appears to be formed in waves as the base of the RPE retracts. The retinal pigment cells are engorged with lipofuscin and become rounder, with loss of both apical microvilli and basal infoldings. Cell fallout occurs, and necrotic portions of cells containing membrane-bound granules are liberated into the subretinal space. The photoreceptor outer segments disappear, leaving stunted cone inner segments. The membranous debris disappears, resulting in "empty spaces" between the strands of early BLD internal to the basement membrane and the regression of any soft drusen present external to the basement membrane. The choroidal capillaries undergo disuse atrophy.

Bruch's membrane

Although anatomists regard Bruch's membrane as a five-layered structure, pathologic processes are more readily understood if one uses the definition proposed by Gass[49] that excludes the basement membranes of the RPE and choriocapillaris. Bruch's membrane can then be thought of as a sheet-like condensation of the innermost portion of the choroidal stroma that consists of an inner and outer collagenous zone separated by the elastic layer. In this way the location of drusen, RPE detachments, and sub-RPE neovascular membranes can be described more accurately than by using the all-embracing term "within Bruch's membrane." Also, thickening of Bruch's membrane then refers to the collagenous layers alone, which focuses on a possible etiologic role for Bruch's membrane in AMD, rather than on the actual manifestations of the disease mentioned above.

A linear relationship exists between the thickness of Bruch's membrane and age, the membrane increasing in thickness from 2 μm in the first decade of life to 4.7 μm by the 10th decade.[50] The debris that accumulates within the collagenous and elastic layers, which coincides with the buildup of lipofuscin in the RPE and is similarly first detected early in life on electron microscopy, takes three main forms:

1. A general increase in collagen. The 64-nm banded fibers found in increasing numbers in the collagenous layers with age are believed to be fibrillar type I collagen.[51] Clumps of fibrous long-spacing collagen with band periodicity of about 120 nm are found primarily in the outer collagenous layer or embedded in the basement membrane of the choriocapillaris.[52,53] Fibrous long-spacing collagen is thought to be a combination of collagen and proteoglycans or glycoprotein and may be formed by depolymerization of native collagen fibrils.[52] Other components that have been identified include collagen types III, IV, and V, fibronectin, chondroitin sulfate, dermatan sulfate, and proteoglycans.[51,54] A significant linear decline in solubility of Bruch's membrane collagen occurs with age and may be due to increase in crosslinking.[51]

2. Rounded, coated membrane-bound bodies (Fig. 60-4). Since these are found as early as the second decade,[55] it has been suggested that this material may result from the shedding of unwanted basal cytoplasm through the basement membrane of the RPE.[56] The actual separation of the bodies from the cells appears to have been demonstrated,[57] but it is such a rare finding that their derivation remains uncertain. These membrane-bound bodies then rupture, spilling their content of coated vesicles and granular material into Bruch's membrane and, together with fragments of the coated membrane wall, the resulting debris accounts for most of the thickening of Bruch's membrane with age.[58] However, most of the debris is found in the outer collagenous zone and even on the outer side of the choroidal capillaries, suggesting that it may also be derived from the choroid.[53]

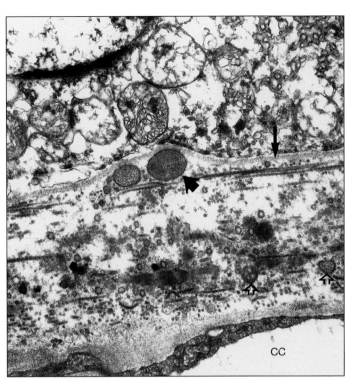

Fig. 60-4 Electron micrograph shows accumulation of debris in Bruch's membrane. The patient was 62 years of age and had 20/20 vision; however, this process can be detected as early as the second decade. Coated membrane-bound bodies (short arrow) are apparently trapped between the basement membrane of the retinal pigment epithelium (RPE) and the inner collagenous zone (entrapment sites). Others lie in the outer collagenous layer (open arrows). Some have ruptured, releasing vesicular and granular material and fragments of the coated membrane. Bruch's membrane is normally defined as a five-layered structure, but it may be more appropriate not to regard the basement membrane of the RPE (long arrow) or of the choriocapillaris (CC) as part of the membrane (×11 800). (Courtesy of MC Killingsworth.)

3. Mineralized deposits affect primarily the elastic lamina. The degeneration of elastin may be initiated by actinic damage.[23] The corresponding histologic findings in Bruch's membrane, which become evident in the fifth decade, comprise thickening, hyalinization, and patchy basophilia.[22,24] This diffuse deposition in the collagenous zones also extends down the intercapillary pillars and can be correlated with an increase in the lipid content of Bruch's membrane after the fourth decade.[59-61] The lipids consist largely of phospholipids, triglycerides, fatty acids, and free cholesterol. There is little cholesterol ester, which would have been expected to predominate if the lipids had been derived from the blood stream, suggesting that the source of the material is the RPE.[59] However, the specific inclusions seen with electron microscopy cannot be correlated with any particular type of lipid.[62]

Peroxidized lipids have recently been identified in Bruch's membrane, the total amount increasing exponentially with age. The peroxidized lipids identified were derived from long-chain polyunsaturated fatty acids, particularly docosahexaenoic acid and linolenic acid, which are polyunsaturated fatty acids found in photoreceptor outer segments. Lipid peroxides have recently been shown to induce neovascularization by inducing expression of a cascade of angiogenic cytokines.[63]

Changes in hydraulic conductivity

Hydraulic conductivity is the measurement of the bulk flow of fluid through a test membrane in response to applied pressure. Bruch's membrane would be expected to show increasing resistance to flow with age because it exhibits a linear increase in thickness[50] and a significant accumulation of lipid after the fourth decade.[61,62,64] However, studies undertaken on Bruch's membrane have shown that the decrease in hydraulic conductivity is exponential, being greatest in the first four decades of life[65,66]; it is unclear why this occurs before age 40. It has therefore been suggested that remodeling of collagen occurs as a result of increased cross-linkage, and this may cause an increase in rigidity of the membrane and reduced pore size, with entrapment of passing protein molecules.[67] After age 40 the increasing lipid content would be expected to have an increasing effect on hydraulic conductivity, while in the 60s a further reduction would result from the diffuse deposits that appear beneath the RPE.

The excimer laser has been used to remove progressively ultrathin shavings of Bruch's membrane to determine in which layer the major barrier to the flow of water lies. This demonstrated that the greatest resistance throughout life resides within the inner collagenous zone.[66] Serial ultrathin sections cut parallel to the plane of Bruch's membrane to estimate the porosity at sequential levels confirmed that the inner collagenous zone presented the lowest porosity. Calculations based on the pore radii and length further confirmed that the inner collagenous zone also had the lowest flow rate. However, ultrastructural studies would appear to indicate that it is mainly the outer collagenous zone that increases in thickness with age, with the inner collagenous zone remaining constant.[58] Clearly, further studies are required, as only a limited number of younger eyes have been examined.

The debris that accumulates in Bruch's membrane is probably the result, rather than the cause, of degeneration of the RPE. Nevertheless, the associated reduction in permeability may in turn further compromise the RPE.

Choroid

A decrease in choroidal blood flow with age can be demonstrated by laser Doppler flowmetry and is mainly due to a decrease in choroidal blood volume rather than in velocity of flow.[68] This is consistent with histologic changes in aged eyes. Comparing normal maculas in the first and 10th decades, the density of the choroidal capillaries (combined length of capillary lumina per unit length) decreased in a linear fashion by 45%, and the anteroposterior diameter by 34%.[50]

The middle layer of medium-sized vessels decreases with age, resulting in a progressive decrease in thickness of the choroid from 200 μm at birth to 80 μm by the age of 90 years.[50]

The resulting thinning of the choroid throws the remaining larger vessels into greater prominence, accounting for the senile tigroid fundus. This clinical appearance has generally been attributed to unmasking of the choroidal vessels by attenuation and loss of pigment from the retinal pigment cells. However, senile choroidal atrophy appears to contribute more significantly to the increased visibility of the vessels.

ONSET AND PROGRESS OF AGE-RELATED MACULAR DEGENERATION

Clinical features in the absence of drusen

The lipofuscin-laden RPE cells that fall out with age are phagocytosed by their neighbors. The fundi usually retain a normal appearance during this process, but in older eyes the number of cells shed may be sufficient to become visible in the fundus as a diffuse mottling of small pigment clumps or as a microreticular pattern of small lines, more obvious on fluorescein angiography. The progress of AMD is thus closely related to the degree of pigmentary disturbance evident in the fundus, and this may occur in the absence of typical drusen.

The patient illustrated in Figures 60-5 and 60-6 shows this evolution to geographic atrophy over 17 years. The first change detected was the presence of scattered, small drusen-like dots, 25 to 50 μm in size (Fig. 60-5B). A ring of small pigment clumps then developed around fixation (Fig. 60-5D), but vision remained 20/20, demonstrating the difficulty of determining when, on the basis of visual acuity alone, pigment changes become pathologic. This is due to the fact that fixation is often spared for many years. Hyperpigmentation is accompanied by hypopigmentation, with geographic atrophy (Fig. 60-6) then spreading into the area of attenuated RPE (incipient atrophy).

Morphologic changes (Fig. 60-3C)

The morphologic alterations considered thus far in the photoreceptors, RPE, Bruch's membrane, and choroid are progressive throughout life. However, by the seventh decade other changes have appeared at the base of the RPE that have no counterpart in earlier life. These comprise the deposition of basement membrane-like material and shedding of membranous debris. Although these changes first develop in a patchy distribution while the fundus and vision are still normal, their diffuse occurrence is the principal feature of AMD.[22,69,70]

Basal laminar deposit – early form

The BLD lies beneath the RPE, between the plasma membrane and the basement membrane, in contrast to typical drusen, which lie external to the basement membrane. It can be demonstrated consistently by the seventh decade,[22] but has been found even in the fifth decade.[24] It first appears in a patchy distribution over thickened or basophilic segments of Bruch's membrane, over intercapillary pillars, or over small drusen, suggesting a potential response to altered filtration at these sites. It can be quantified histologically[24] as class 1 (small, solitary patches), class 2 (a thin continuous layer), and class 3 (a thick layer, at least half the height of the RPE).

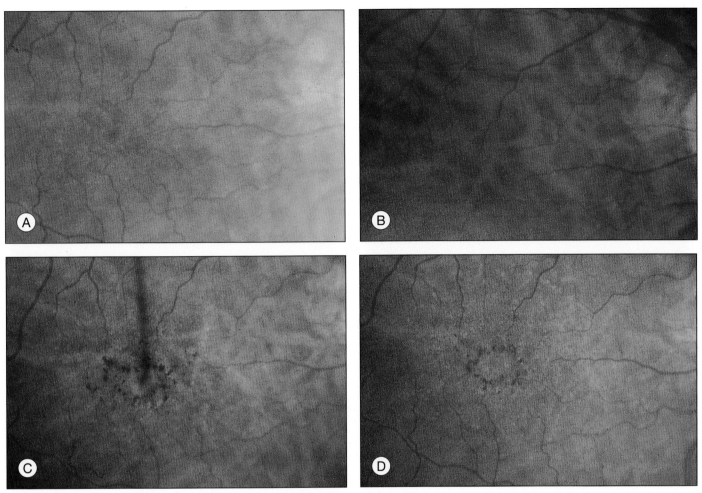

Fig. 60-5 Evolution of age-related macular degeneration, apparently unrelated to drusen, developing into geographic atrophy over 16 years. A, At age 68, the patient has a normal left fundus with senile tigroid pattern (vision 20/15). B, At age 73, small drusen-like dots are present, ≤ 63 µm in size (vision 20/20). C, At age 77, a ring of pigment clumps is developing around the center of the fovea. D, At age 79, the pigment clumping around fixation has increased; vision is still 20/20. The choroidal vascular pattern is more prominent. (Reproduced from Sarks JP, Sarks SH, Killingsworth M. Evolution of geographic atrophy of the retinal pigment epithelium. Eye 1988; 2:552–577.[79])

Histologically the deposit exists in two different forms, early and late, according to the stage of degeneration. The early BLD is a pale-staining eosinophilic material that stains blue with picro-Mallory and shows faint anteroposterior striations (Fig. 60-7). On electron microscopy the BLD consists of three phenotypes: fibrillar, amorphous, and polymerized. The fibrillar phenotype appears to be the earliest manifestation and may only be detected by electron microscopy as irregular nodules lying on the original basement membrane. The polymerized form resembles the fibrous long-spacing collagen seen in Bruch's membrane and is also found in the cornea, trabecular meshwork, and other tissues in the body.[53] It projects internally from the original RPE basement membrane[71] (Fig. 60-8) and accounts for the striations, or bush-like appearance, seen histologically.

The similarity of the BLD to basement membrane and its proximity to rough endoplasmic reticulum at the base of the cells suggest it is a secretory product of the RPE.[71] It reacts with antibodies against type IV collagen, heparan sulfate proteoglycans, and laminin,[54,72] but the BLD is biochemically distinct from the RPE basement membrane, and a faulty, degradative process rather than enhanced synthesis may account for its accumulation in aged maculas.[54]

Membranous debris

Coiled membrane fragments continuous with the plasma membrane of the RPE appear together with the BLD, but they are not found unless BLD is also present[23] (Fig. 60-8). This material has the bilayered structure of phospholipids and is not to be confused with the coated membrane-bound bodies described earlier in Bruch's membrane. Whereas by light microscopy the BLD was regarded as the hallmark of macular degeneration, by electron microscopy it is this membranous debris that correlates more closely with the degree of degeneration. These membranes are found in three locations, as described in the following paragraphs.

Internal to the retinal pigment epithelium basement membrane The coils appear to be extruded from the base of

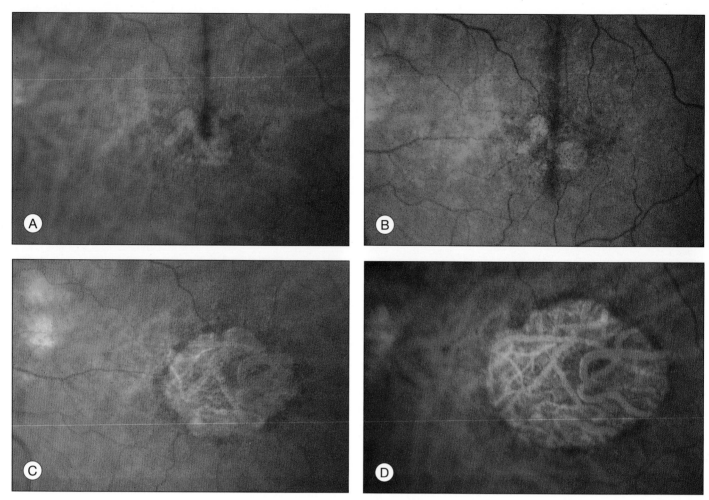

Fig. 60-6 Same patient as in Figure 60-5. A and B (red-free), At age 81, patient fixing between two small areas of atrophy that have developed. Pigment clumping and drusen-like dots are spreading outward. This surrounding incipient atrophy corresponds to the area of geographic atrophy that developed subsequently (D); vision is still 20/30. C, At age 82, atrophy involves fixation, and dots have faded. Vision has dropped to 20/200. D, At age 84, area of atrophy has almost doubled; vision is 20/400. Choroidal atrophy causes exposed vessels to appear white. Patient died at age 85. Pathology of this eye is shown in Figure 60-8. (Reproduced from Sarks JP, Sarks SH, Killingsworth M. Evolution of geographic atrophy of the retinal pigment epithelium. Eye 1988; 2:552–577.[79])

the cells, which have lost their infoldings, although they may alternatively result from a free-energy process in which lipid molecules are deposited by the RPE into Bruch's membrane and coalesce. The membranes form layers and then basal mounds internal to the RPE basement membrane (Fig. 60-3C and Fig. 60-9), which may account for the drusen-like dots noted clinically (Fig. 60-5B). The membranes are not demonstrated in conventional histologic sections, since the mounds manifest only as small, unstained spaces within the BLD (Fig. 60-10). As the mounds enlarge and fuse, the RPE shows more derangement and cell fallout.

External to the RPE basement membrane (basal *linear* deposit[21]).* Membranes appear to pass through the basement membrane to form a layer between the basement membrane and the inner collagenous layer of Bruch's membrane (Fig. 60-8). In this location the debris may build up into the soft drusen specific for AMD[77] (see Fig. 60-26). The debris also appears to disturb the normal attachment of the RPE to Bruch's mem-

brane, creating a cleavage plane, and it is in this plane that RPE detachments due to blood and serous fluid lie and into which early choroidal new vessels grow. The membranes even appear to percolate into the collagenous zones of Bruch's membrane.

---

*A uniform terminology for the diffuse deposits is gaining acceptance. The original observations by light microscopy distinguished only one deposit. This was referred to as the *basal linear deposit* and it proved a useful histologic marker for the stage of the disease.[22] Subsequent electron microscopic studies showed that this deposit lies internal to the RPE basement membrane, so the name was changed to *basal laminar deposit*, but another layer could also be demonstrated lying external to the basement membrane. Green & Enger[21] suggested retaining the term *basal laminar deposit* for the material internal to the basement membrane, but resurrecting *basal linear deposit* for the diffuse layer of vesicular and granular material on the external aspect. Unfortunately the acronym *BLD* could then be applied to either deposit, so recently the term *basement membrane deposit* (BMD) has been proposed for the basal laminar deposit.[74] Until the terminology and the abbreviations become standardized, this chapter will continue to apply the abbreviation *BLD* for the basal laminar deposit and use the terms *membranous debris*, or the unabbreviated *basal linear deposit*, when referring to the material external to the basement membrane. These definitions replace older terms such as *diffuse thickening of the inner aspect of Bruch's membrane* and *diffuse drusen*.[20,75,76]

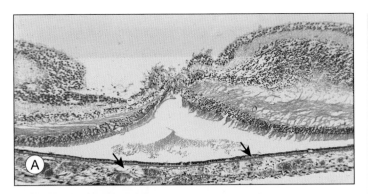

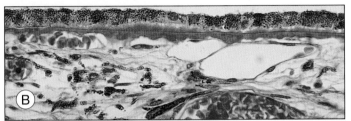

Fig. 60-7 A, Section through the macula of a 79-year-old man. Fundus appeared normal, and vision was 20/30. Early form of basal laminar deposit (BLD) is seen as continuous, blue-staining layer beneath the retinal pigment epithelium. Unstained spaces (right arrow) would correspond to membranous debris on electron microscopy. Arrow at left indicates area magnified in B (×75). B, BLD is most developed over a thicker segment of Bruch's membrane. Hyalinization of Bruch's membrane extends down intercapillary pillars (picro-Mallory stain; ×500). (Reproduced from Sarks SH. Aging and degeneration in the macular region: a clinico-pathological study. Br J Ophthalmol 1976; 60:324–341.[22])

At the apex of the retinal pigment epithelium   Morphologically similar membranous debris is also found over the apex of the RPE, lying in the subretinal space and presumably representing outer-segment material that has not been phagocytosed (see Fig. 60-12).

Membranous debris is therefore seen in three different locations: (1) in the subretinal space; (2) between the RPE and its basement membrane; and (3) external to the basement membrane, but it is always dependent on the presence of outer segments.

Basal laminar deposit – late form (diffuse thickening of the internal aspect of Bruch's membrane – see footnote)   With progressive degeneration of the RPE, another form of basal laminar material appears. On light microscopy it forms a thick, hyalinized layer that stains red with picro-Mallory, similar to hyalinized Bruch's membrane, and that is more periodic acid–Schiff-positive than the earlier, banded form. Being a later development, it forms a distinct layer on the internal surface of the earlier form (Fig. 60-3D) and may approximate the thickness of the normal RPE, occasionally displaying nodular elevations on its internal surface75 (Fig. 60-11).

On electron microscopy, the later form of the BLD has a flocculent appearance and consists mainly of amorphous material. It may be uplifted with the attenuated RPE over the

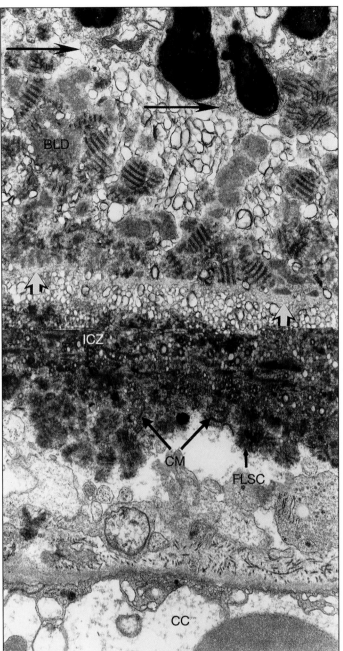

Fig. 60-8 Electron micrograph illustrating changes developing between retinal pigment epithelium and choriocapillaris (CC) in age-related maculopathy corresponding to Figure 60-3C. Horizontal black arrows indicate the basal plasma membrane of the RPE. Early-type basal laminar deposit (BLD) projects inward from the RPE basement membrane (white arrows) and comprises mainly banded material resembling fibrous long-spacing collagen. Coiled membranes with a bilayered structure of lipids lie among the clumps of BLD and appear to pass through the basement membrane to lie between it and the inner collagenous zone (ICZ), as well as filtering into the membrane itself. Identifiable structures within Bruch's membrane include fragments of coated membrane (CM) and fibrous long-spacing collagen (FLSC) (×11 780). (Reproduced from Killingsworth MC, Sarks JP, Sarks SH. Macrophages related to Bruch's membrane in age-related macular degeneration. Eye 1990; 4:613–621.[83])

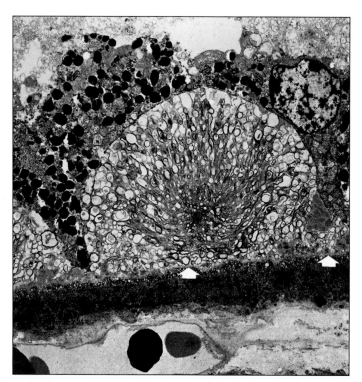

Fig. 60-9 Basal mound lying internal to RPE basement membrane. Electron micrograph shows build-up of coiled membranous debris separating the grossly abnormal RPE from its basement membrane. These collections are referred to as "basal mounds" and may account for the drusen-like dots noted clinically. Only a very thin layer of membranous debris lies external to the basement membrane (arrows), so there are no soft drusen (×1680). (Courtesy of MC Killingsworth.)

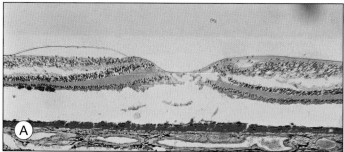
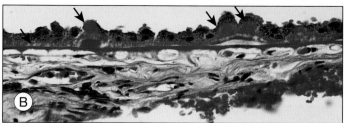

Fig. 60-11 A, Incipient atrophy, showing an unusually thick layer of late basal laminar deposit (BLD), which has also been referred to as diffuse thickening of the inner aspect of Bruch's membrane. This material is hyalinized and periodic acid–Schiff-positive; on electron microscopy it would have a corresponding amorphous appearance. The retinal pigment epithelium forms a very attenuated layer over the surface and seems about to disappear (periodic acid–Schiff; ×45). B, Parafoveal area from the same eye shows the different deposits. The two forms of the BLD are seen: the blue-staining, early form (long arrow) and, on its inner surface, nodular collections of the late hyalinized form (short arrows), also referred to as "basal laminar drusen." External to the BLD lie two typical drusen; beneath the short arrow at left is a small hard druse; beneath the two short arrows at right is a soft druse (picro-Mallory stain; ×500). (Reproduced from Sarks SH. Aging and degeneration in the macular region: a clinico-pathological study. Br J Ophthalmol 1976; 60:324–341.[22])

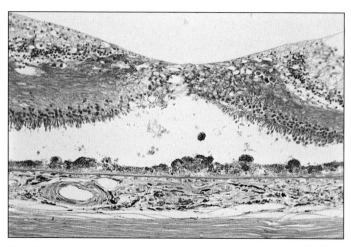

Fig. 60-10 Section through the macula of an 83-year-old man in whom pigment changes were evident clinically. Stretches of attenuated, hypopigmented retinal pigment epithelium (RPE) alternate with clumps from which hyperpigmented cells are shed into the subretinal space. Basal laminar deposit is thicker and comprises both early and late forms. Small, unstained patches beneath the RPE would correspond to mounds of membranous debris on electron microscopy (×525). (Reproduced from Sarks SH. Aging and degeneration in the macular region: a clinico-pathological study. Br J Ophthalmol 1976; 60:324–341.[22])

membranous mounds and appears to be formed in waves according to the level of the base of the cell at the time (Fig. 60-12). It indicates the altered metabolism of a severely stressed RPE and occurs typically over regressing drusen (see Fig. 60-30).

Clinically the BLD has not yet been identified in the fundus with any certainty, but the presence of the late form can be inferred by the presence of significant pigment changes and, since there is an associated reduction of the choriocapillary bed, by noting delayed choroidal perfusion on the fluorescein angiogram.

Retinal pigment epithelium and photoreceptors Lipofuscin and complex melanolipofuscin granules continue to accumulate in the retinal pigment cells, which enlarge and lose their regular shape. The external or basal surface of the cell shows loss of the basal infoldings (with a consequent reduction in surface area) and becomes increasingly separated from its basement membrane by thickening of the BLD and more membranous debris. Occasional cells undergo lipoidal degeneration.[78] Finally the hyperpigmented cells resulting from this phagocytic overload round off, so only a few stubby apical microvilli remain, and they lose their ability to phagocytose. Lipofuscin is packed into large degenerate retinal pigment cells or membrane-bound bodies and shed (Fig. 60-3D).

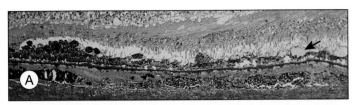

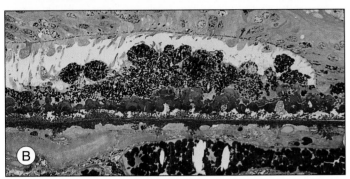

Fig. 60-12 Same eye as in Figures 60-5 and 60-6. Section passes through the temporal margin of the area of geographic atrophy. A, Photoreceptors become fewer and outer segments wider and stunted as they approach the edge. Vacuolated appearance under the retinal pigment epithelium (RPE) is due to disappearance of membranous debris. Collections of membranous debris can be seen on the internal (apical) surface of RPE (arrow), possibly due to failure of phagocytosis (×150). B, Hyperpigmented edge noted clinically corresponds to a double layer of RPE, the inner layer representing necrotic hyperpigmented cells in the process of being eliminated. Late amorphous form of basal laminar deposit (BLD) lies internal to striated form and has a multilaminar appearance, suggesting formation in successive waves according to the level of RPE (see Fig. 60-3D). Photoreceptors disappear, and external limiting membrane terminates on BLD (methylene blue and basic fuscin; ×500). (Reproduced from Sarks JP, Sarks SH, Killingsworth M. Evolution of geographic atrophy of the retinal pigment epithelium. Eye 1988; 2:552–577.[79])

The corresponding pigment abnormalities in the fundus may be classified[10] as increased pigmentation (or hyperpigmentation) and depigmentation (or hypopigmentation). Focal hyperpigmentation correlates histologically with localized areas of RPE cell hypertrophy, which may be accompanied by clumps of hyperpigmented cells in the sub-RPE space, in the subretinal space, and in the outer nuclear layer (see Fig. 60-10). Focal hypopigmentation correlates with attenuated depigmented RPE cells around the hyperpigmented cells.[75]

The sequence of events leading to pigment disturbance and, ultimately, atrophy seems to be the same irrespective of the cause. When a retinal pigment cell dies, the products are phagocytosed by its neighbors. These cells in turn become filled with lipofuscin and round off, losing their ability to phagocytose. As the cells are discarded, the nearby cells migrate and increase in surface area in an attempt to maintain the integrity of the blood–retinal barrier. This results in thinned, hypopigmented cells adjacent to focal hyperpigmentation. Finally, these cells can no longer stretch to fill the gap and atrophy results. Hyperpigmentation therefore precedes hypopigmentation, and this in turn is the prelude to the development of patches of atrophy.[79]

Another instance where pigment figures precede atrophy occurs over long-standing drusenoid pigment epithelial detachments (PEDs). However, atrophy is likely to occur only after the cell population is already depleted, and, in younger patients with focal hyperpigmentation related to drusen or in patients with pattern dystrophies of the RPE, patches of attenuated RPE may be present for many years without progressing to atrophy. Focal hyperpigmentation lying at or close to fixation is not uncommon after middle age and is believed to be part of the spectrum of adult vitelliform degeneration,[80] so it is not considered a stage of AMD.

Progressive derangement of the RPE is accompanied by dropout of photoreceptors, with a reduction in the number of nuclei in the outer nuclear layer. The inner segments tend to become shorter and more bulbous. The outer segments may terminate in collections of membranes over the apical surface of the RPE (Fig. 60-12).

Bruch's membrane and choroid Hyalinization and densification of Bruch's membrane extend down the intercapillary pillars and may even surround the choriocapillaris. The choroidal capillaries, already separated by widening of the intercapillary pillars, become further narrowed by retraction away from Bruch's membrane, and this is accompanied by a loss of fenestrations. Patent capillaries now begin to occupy less space than the intercapillary distances under the macula, in keeping with the reduced requirements of the attenuated RPE.

Macrophages, giant cells, fibroblasts, and occasional lymphocytes are found in relation to the outer surface of Bruch's membrane in the space formerly occupied by the choroidal capillaries.[81] Segments of the membrane begin to thin, and cell processes are occasionally observed splitting off and even enveloping small fragments of the membrane.[71] The choroidal capillaries in the vicinity may show signs of activation, and new vessels still confined entirely to the choroid have been identified.[82] This chronic, low-grade inflammatory reaction, which possibly develops in response to the membranous debris liberated by degenerating RPE, is often found in the choroid near breaks in Bruch's membrane,[83] and it appears to be a link in the chain of events leading to CNV.

DRUSEN

Clinical grading

Despite their apparently very significant role in the evolution of AMD, diffuse deposits detected on histopathology are difficult to study clinically, and hence prognostic significance is ascribed to the clinical presence of drusen, which are readily visible as yellowish deposits lying deep to the retina, representing accumulation of the materials described above. Drusen vary in size and shape and occasionally have a crystalline appearance resulting from calcification (the term *drusen* is also applied to a crust of crystals lining a rock cavity). The crystalline appearance is usually within or adjacent to areas of atrophy of the RPE. While it was previously recognized that patients with large (63 μm), soft, or confluent drusen are predisposed to develop advanced stages of AMD,[18,84] recent information from Age-Related Eye Disease Study (AREDS) has suggested the following description of nonneovascular AMD with respect to features within 3000 μm of the center of the macula (Fig. 60-1). The terminology is relevant to the management of nonneovascular AMD.

An eye is considered to have *no AMD* if there are no drusen or only a few small drusen (< 63 μm) in the absence of any other stage of AMD. An eye is considered to have the *early stage of AMD* if there are few (approximately < 20) medium-size drusen (63 to 124 μm) or pigment abnormalities (increased pigmentation or depigmentation and no other stage of AMD. The *intermediate stage of AMD* is usually the presence of at least one large drusen (at least 125 μm, approximately the width of a retinal vein as it crosses the optic nerve), but can also be numerous medium-size drusen (approximately 20 or more when the drusen boundaries are indistinct or amorphous or soft; and approximately 65 or more when the drusen boundaries are distinct or sharp or hard) or the presence of geographic atrophy that does not extend under the center of the macula. The *advanced stage of AMD* is geographic atrophy extending under the center of the macula or signs of CNV.

Grading in scientific studies

While the grading of drusen described above is relevant to management and relatively easy to apply in clinical practice, a means of more specific grading of drusen for scientific studies is desirable, ideally without requiring fluorescein angiography. The system proposed by the International Epidemiology Study Group,[10] which is based on stereoscopic color fundus photographs, grades for the predominant drusen type, the most severe drusen type, drusen numbers, largest drusen size, area involved by drusen, drusen confluence, and drusen disappearance (see Figs 60-1 and 60-2).

Drusen type

Drusen are broadly divided into hard and soft, with a number of subtypes. Soft drusen are generally larger and have a soft appearance. They have an obvious thickness and tend to become confluent, so they show greater variation in size and shape.

Drusen size

Clinically, drusen size can be related to the width of a major vein at the disc edge (approximately 125 μm). Small drusen are those less than 0.5 vein width (63 μm), and these are considered to be hard.[11,17] Drusen $\geq$ 125 μm (Fig. 60-2, circle C$_1$) are large, and these are considered to be soft unless they are in the process of regression. Drusen between 63 μm and 125 μm may be either hard or soft.

Extent of fundus involvement

This may be assessed by noting drusen numbers, the area of fundus involved,[19] and the density of drusen,[85] that is, whether discrete, touching, or confluent.

Drusen distribution

Most significance attaches to drusen in the inner macula,[86,87] which is defined as the area within a circle 3000 μm, or two disc diameters, across (see Fig. 60-1). This includes the fovea, which measures 1500 μm, or one disc diameter, but the central circle on the grid measures only 1000 μm in diameter, as this is more useful when only a few drusen are present in the center of the fovea. Moreover, the area between the smaller, central circle and the inner circle of 3000 μm diameter includes the foveal perimeter, where the greatest number of rods reside (which in cases of AMD show selective loss over the foveal cones[38]) and where soft drusen, pigmentary changes, and focal areas of geographic atrophy often begin. Different patterns of drusen distribution have been recorded,[14] the largest areas covered by drusen and the prevalence of soft, indistinct drusen being greater in the superior and temporal quadrants.

Imaging of drusen
Fluorescence of drusen

On fluorescein angiography, soft drusen fill more slowly and are not as brightly fluorescent as hard drusen, but they remain fluorescent for a longer period. Fluorescence may be graded[88] as: (1) equal to choroidal fluorescence; (2) slightly brighter than choroidal fluorescence; or (3) brightly fluorescent (during the dye transit and 3 min after the dye entry).

On indocyanine green angiography, hard drusen become hyperfluorescent 2 to 3 min after dye administration, and this persists through the middle and late phases. Soft drusen are either hypofluorescent throughout the angiogram or remain undetectable.[89]

Drusen color

Color is recorded as yellow, pale, or white, the last characterizing regressing drusen, which are best seen using red-free light.

Drusen symmetry[88,14,16,24]

Comparisons of the distribution, number, and type of drusen between the two eyes of a patient tend to show a remarkable symmetry, which often leads to similar behavior in both eyes. The drusen most frequently bilateral were reticular drusen and soft, indistinct drusen.[16]

On autofluorescence,[64] large drusen may or may not be appear apparent. However, areas of developing atrophy may be more apparent on autofluorescnce.[64]

Pathologic considerations

Drusen are deposits of extracellular material, lying typically between the basement membrane of the retinal pigment cells and the inner collagenous zone of Bruch's membrane (Fig. 60-13). Papillary drusen that develop beneath long-standing retinal detachments, diffuse thickening of the inner aspect of Bruch's membrane (see footnote), and cuticular drusen,[21,53] also called *basal laminar drusen*,[90] describe material internal to the basement membrane and appear to be similar to the late, amorphous form of BLD (Fig. 60-11). Basal laminar drusen are attributed to internal nodularity of the RPE basement membrane and can

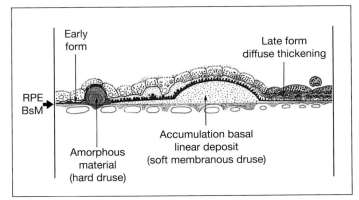

Fig. 60-13 Diagram showing the relationship to the retinal pigment epithelium (RPE) basement membrane (BsM) of the deposits accumulating under the RPE during the evolution of age-related macular degeneration. The basal laminar deposit (BLD) lies internal to the BsM, and typical drusen lie external. The BLD exists in an early striated form (shown in blue) and late amorphous form (shown in brown). Membrane coils are found both internal to BsM, as mounds at the base of the RPE, and external to the BsM, as the BLD, where it may form soft, membranous drusen. Hard drusen consist predominantly of amorphous material.

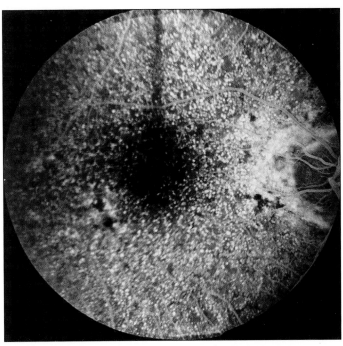

Fig. 60-14 Scattered, small, hard drusen in generalized distribution. Fluorescein angiogram of the right eye of a 59-year-old man. The whole posterior pole is studded with drusen, mostly of the discrete, small, hard variety, in the region of 25 to 75 µm. A few larger drusen, up to 150 µm across, have resulted from the fusion of several smaller drusen, and small reticular pigment figures are developing in relation to these larger drusen. Vision was still 20/20. The drusen were not obvious on ophthalmoscopy because most were only 30 µm tall. The patient died 6 months later. The pathology is shown in Figure 60-15. (Reproduced from Sarks JP, Sarks SH, Killingsworth MC. Evolution of soft drusen in age-related macular degeneration. Eye 1994; 8:269–283.[77])

produce a starry-sky appearance on fluorescein angiography, which can be impossible to distinguish clinically from myriads of small, hard drusen (Fig. 60-14). However, the condition can usually be recognized when a myriad of small drusen have a somewhat translucent appearance with retroillumination in an individual in their 40s or 50s, sometimes with a vitelliform detachment of yellowish material. (The latter will progressively accumulate fluorescein but should not be confused with progressive fluorescein leakage from CNV.) *Basal laminar drusen* is also applied to a dominantly inherited dystrophy of small, radially arranged drusen (Malattia levantinese). These have been confirmed pathologically to consist of basement membrane material.[91,92] Another type of small, yellow lesion resembling drusen, but which is nonfluorescent, has been found to be due to lipoidal degeneration of individual retinal pigment cells.[78] The present discussion is therefore confined to typical drusen external to the basement membrane.

The clinical classification of drusen mentioned above is based on ophthalmoscopic appearance, but fluorescein angiography and histopathologic examination add further information and suggest two main paths of development. Small, hard drusen with a hyalinized structure are the predominant type in younger persons, and some larger soft drusen show evidence of their derivation from clusters of these small drusen.[77] A clinicopathologic correlation study of 353 normal and aged eyes without AMD showed that, in the absence of the diffuse deposits, all the drusen were of the hyalinized variety.[93] Other drusen, however, develop de novo in the seventh decade, when the diffuse layer of membranous debris (basal linear deposit) appears, and these latter are specific for AMD. To these may be added a third presumed mechanism, the addition of proteinaceous fluid in those drusen ≥ 250 µm that resemble serous PEDs. Other authors have identified five distinct morphologic classes of drusen at the ultrastructural level. No attempt was made to correlate

these classes of drusen to clinical phenotypes described in the literature. However, class 1 corresponds to hard drusen and class 2 to soft drusen with the same composition as the basal linear deposit.[94] Therefore, until the complete life cycle of drusen can be recognized clinically, a classification of drusen must remain part clinical and part morphologic.

Clinicopathologic classification
1. Small, hard (hyalinized) drusen
2. Soft (pseudosoft), cluster-derived drusen
3. True soft drusen, which have three morphologic subtypes:
   a. Granular
   b. Fluid, including drusenoid PEDs
   c. Membranous (accumulation of basal linear deposit)
4. Reticular drusen (pseudodrusen)
5. Regressing (fading) drusen.

Small, hard (hyalinized, nodular[75]) drusen
Clinical features
Small, hard drusen are not visible in the fundus until they measure 30 to 50 µm, the width of two to three retinal pigment cells. They are difficult to see in fair fundi but can be seen more clearly in red-free light. They are readily demonstrated on fluo-

rescein angiography, even when as small as 25 μm, fluorescing brightly in the mid venous phase and fading soon after the background choroidal fluorescence (Fig. 60-14).

Small, hard drusen may first be noted in the central area, 1000 μm in diameter,[14] but when numerous they are most common on the temporal side of the fovea. They tend to occur in clusters, and histopathologic specimens show that, where hard drusen can be demonstrated clinically, there are often numerous intervening drusen too small to be seen (see Fig. 60-16). Another common pattern consists of a wide band outside the vascular arcades and passing on the nasal side of the disc, with sparing of the inner macula. Toward the equator they assume a linear arrangement in relation to a polygonal pattern of hyperpigmented lines, giving rise to the picture of reticular (honeycomb) degeneration of the pigment epithelium.

Formation

Small, hard drusen histologically are globular deposits of hyalinized material with staining properties similar to hyalinized Bruch's membrane and have an amorphous appearance on electron microscopy. They have been identified at the macula in 83% of postmortem eyes.[95]

Certain preceding changes in Bruch's membrane may determine their formation.[93] In eyes with only a few drusen, small hyalinized plaques of densification in Bruch's membrane are observed, sometimes with extensions into the outer collagenous zone and even on to its choroidal surface. Another early change, seen only by electron microscopy, appears as coated membrane-bound bodies, both ruptured and intact (see Fig. 60-4), similar to those found within the outer collagenous zone. However, here they appear "trapped" between the elevated RPE basement membrane and the inner collagenous zone. It has been proposed that they develop by the shedding of unwanted basal cytoplasm through the basement membrane of the RPE[56] by a process likened to apoptosis (from the Greek: "a falling off, as the petals of a flower"), but the process of evagination and pinching-off of cytoplasm from the base of the RPE is so difficult to find that it has not been established to be a mechanism by which drusen form, and the term *entrapment sites*[93] seems preferable to *shedding sites*. These entrapment sites are found at all ages and have also been detected in primate eyes, probably indicating a normal aging phenomenon.

In eyes with many small, hard drusen the preceding thickenings in Bruch's membrane are more extensive, appearing as a row of microdrusen, or rounded elevations 2 μm in diameter, and composed of very dense amorphous material[77] (Fig. 60-15). Hyalinized drusen form over these changes and as they grow they become hemispherical or almost globular. When small, hard drusen grow larger than about 63 μm, the amorphous contents become less compact and paler-staining, a process that begins in the lower part of the druse. Single hard drusen rarely exceed 125 μm, and further enlargement is the result of the fusion of several drusen. As the RPE over the drusen degenerates, the contents become increasingly dispersed (Fig. 60-15) or, especially in older patients, coarsely granular (Fig. 60-16). When the drusen finally fade, the basement membrane of the overlying

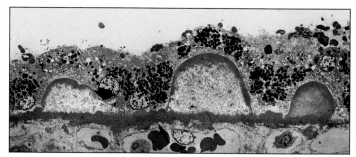

Fig. 60-15 Electron micrograph of small, hard drusen present in the eye shown in Figure 60-14. Druse at far right demonstrates greater electron density around the margin than in the center. Larger druse in middle shows dispersion of contents except for a peripheral shell of amorphous material, with the outline of the druse remaining sharp. Druse at left is similar but has lost rim of amorphous material on one side (arrowhead), and this edge is spreading out on Bruch's membrane. Note that the inner surface of Bruch's membrane is raised into a row of small, rounded, electron-dense elevations, or microdrusen (arrow), which also lie beneath the larger druse. Similar extensions occur on the choroidal side of the membrane (near arrow). Despite the presence of numerous drusen, there was no basal laminar deposit or membranous debris in this eye (the patient was only 62 years of age) (×7315). (Reproduced from Sarks JP, Sarks SH, Killingsworth MC. Evolution of soft drusen in age-related macular degeneration. Eye 1994; 8:269–283.[77])

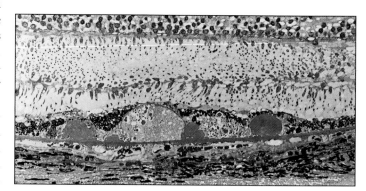

Fig. 60-16 Electron micrograph shows a parafoveal cluster of small, hard drusen measuring 250 μm in diameter, the drusen touching and fusing. Larger drusen inside the cluster are breaking down into globules of hyaline material, leaving small, hyalinized drusen around the perimeter. The smallest drusen would not be seen clinically, but they can be assumed to be present around the larger, visible drusen. Retinal pigment epithelium over the larger drusen is thinned. Fundus had shown only a few drusen clusters. Vision was 20/20 2 years before death at age 81; lens opacities and dementia precluded further documentation. The cluster would appear as a single deposit, and fluorescein angiography (not performed) would be expected to demonstrate brightly staining, small drusen around a more homogeneous center (methylene blue and basic fuchsin; ×290).

RPE becomes infolded and collapses on to Bruch's membrane, usually leaving a small patch of clinical hypopigmentation.

Significance

Population-based studies[11,13,15,17,96] all reported that one or more drusen were found commonly – in 95.5% of the population aged over 43 years[11] to 98.8% of those over 49 years[13] – with small, hard drusen less than 63 μm being the most frequent type in all age groups. Pathologic studies[21,97] support the conclusion that the presence of a few small, hard drusen is not a risk factor for AMD. However, several studies[4,96] have found that if a threshold of small, hard drusen is exceeded, the eye is more likely to develop larger drusen. Although, in 5-year studies, advanced AMD did not develop in eyes with only small, hard drusen at baseline, regardless of the area involved,[4] longer follow-up will likely reveal complications if numerous drusen are present or if a cluster occurs at fixation. These patients are generally younger, so even if the course is slow, geographic atrophy or, more rarely, CNV, may in time affect vision[98] and may be considered to have a hard drusen maculopathy (Fig. 60-17). It is also interesting that drusen with an appearance, distribution, and course similar to small, hard drusen develop in patients with membranoproliferative glomerulonephritis type II.[99] The number of these drusen was related to the duration of the disease and was independent of the age of the patient.

Soft (pseudosoft) cluster-derived drusen

Initially the small, hard drusen in a cluster may remain discrete, or even may be touching, but individual drusen can still be distinguished on ophthalmoscopy. As the drusen become so closely packed together, the cluster appears as a single larger

deposit that clinically appears soft, but the small drusen can usually still be made out in red-free light or on fluorescein angiography (Fig. 60-18). These fused drusen are up to 250 μm, depending on the number of drusen in the cluster. If sufficiently elevated, they may tent up the retina and cause a reddish halo around the base, which is a favorable sign because it reflects the hard, abruptly elevated margins and the integrity of the surrounding retina (Fig. 60-19). On fluorescein angiography they remain brightly fluorescent, although staining is not uniform. These clusters of fused, small, hard drusen occur in middle age, and the prognosis is generally good, with the drusen slowly regressing over many years and leaving a focal patch of atrophy (Fig. 60-19). It is of interest that this cycle may be completed in younger persons before the BLD and membranous debris characteristic of AMD have developed. Hard drusen therefore appear to occur independently of the intermediate or advanced stage of AMD.

True soft drusen

These soft drusen are not visibly derived from small, hard drusen. At least three separate processes may contribute to their formation, but since all may be present in the same druse, they often cannot be distinguished from one another clinically.

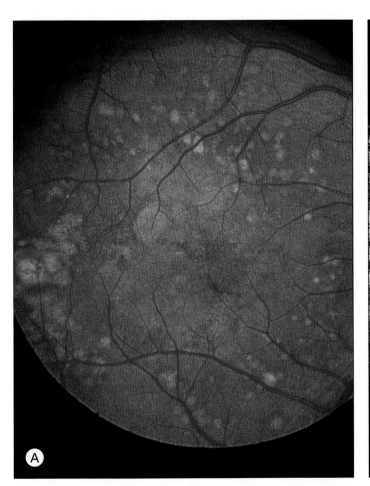

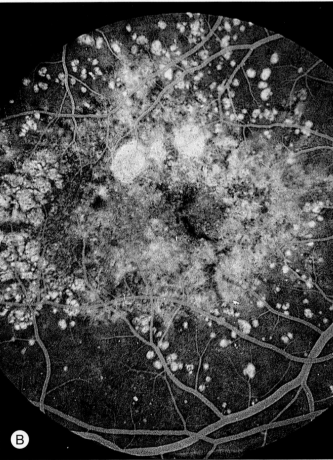

Fig. 60-17 Example of geographic atrophy developing in a 47-year-old man due to excessive numbers of drusen (A). Fluorescein angiogram (B) revealed numerous, mostly small, hard drusen, although many aggregated into clusters. Drusen are fading centrally in an area of incipient atrophy of the retinal pigment epithelium, which appears as a pinker area of the fundus, showing diffuse hyperfluorescence. Geographic atrophy commences as rounded, more circumscribed, brighter window defects within the incipient atrophy. Vision was still 20/15.

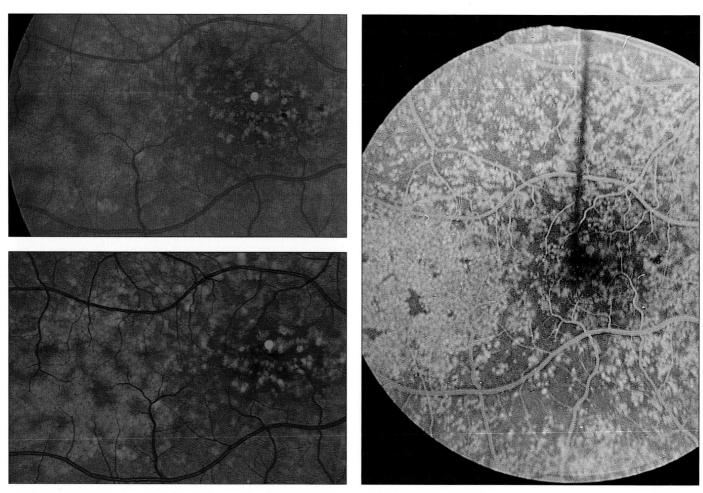

Fig. 60-18 Soft, cluster-derived drusen (pseudosoft drusen). Right fundus of a 50-year-old man with 20/20 vision (top left). Groups of mainly small, hard drusen associated with hyperpigmentation are seen at the fovea. Large, soft, confluent drusen appear to be located temporal to the fovea, but in red-free light (bottom left), and particularly on fluorescein angiography (right), the soft drusen can be seen to consist of closely packed clusters of small, hard drusen.

Moreover, the contents of soft drusen are easily lost during histopathologic processing, so not all the constituents will have been identified. In the following discussion, true soft drusen are subdivided according to their apparent pathogenesis.

Granular soft drusen (synonyms: serogranular drusen, semisolid drusen,[100] localized detachment of the basal linear deposit[21])

Clinically, most of these drusen are about 250 μm and have a yellow, solid appearance, their confluence resulting in crescentic or sinuous shapes (Fig. 60-20). Histologically, they have a coarsely granular structure, consisting of membrane-bound globules of amorphous material, small membrane fragments, and other cellular debris. The presence of microdrusen and the proximity of some of these drusen to hyalinized drusen (Fig. 60-16) suggest that the granular contents represent, in part, cluster-derived drusen in which the original hard drusen have broken down (Fig. 60-21). A thin layer of this granular material would appear to resemble the soft drusen described by Green & Enger[21] (see Fig. 60-8), as localized detachment of the RPE and basal linear deposit, in an eye with diffuse basal linear deposit.

Not all these drusen can be seen to be derived from the breakdown of hard drusen, but when this does occur the drusen in the center of the cluster seem to be affected first (Fig. 60-16), and small, hard drusen may remain identifiable around the perimeter of the cluster. The detection of this heterogeneous composition, either on fluorescein angiography or in histologic sections, led to the designation *semisolid*.[100] Calcified particles may also be found and, as these deposits are commonly observed around an area of atrophy, they appear to be in the early stages of regression.

Soft, fluid (serous) drusen and drusenoid pigment epithelial detachments

Soft, confluent drusen larger than 500 μm, and even some over 250 μm, may have pooled serous fluid if the lipoidal debris in Bruch's membrane has created a hydrophobic barrier[101] and interfered with the retinal pigment epithelial pump. This may be important in causing hard drusen to become soft and in fostering the enlargement and confluence of drusen.[49] As a result some larger drusen appear to have a fluid consistency, even appearing blister-like and being translucent on retroillumination.

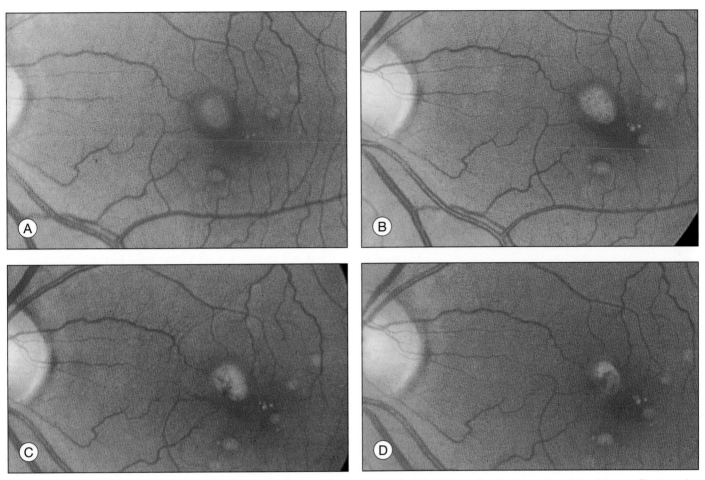

Fig. 60-19 Patient illustrating large pseudosoft druse with halo around base, apparently derived from a fused cluster of small, hard drusen. Photographs trace the regression of the druse over 9 years. The druse was located just above fixation, and vision remained unaffected. A, At age 48, druse is surrounded by a red halo. B, At age 52, the druse appears whiter, and pigment stippling is present over the surface. C, At age 54, the halo fades as the druse becomes shallower. D, At age 57, hyperpigmentation is preceding the formation of a patch of atrophy. The atrophy remains localized in younger persons in whom the retinal pigment epithelium between the drusen is normal. (Reproduced from Sarks SH. Drusen patterns predisposing to geographic atrophy of the retinal pigment epithelium. Aust J Ophthalmol 1982; 10:91–97.[98])

Further confluence leads to larger soft drusen that resemble serous PEDs (Fig. 60-22), often retaining a scalloped outline representing the original drusen. This subset of serous PEDs was characterized as the "drusen form"[102] when they were noted to have different ophthalmoscopic and angiographic features, as well as a better prognosis. The term *drusen* or *drusenoid*[75] *RPE detachments* may arbitrarily be applied to drusen over 500 μm but may be better reserved for those 1000 μm in greatest length, the central circle of the Wisconsin grid,[4] and involving the foveal center. However, they generally remain less than one disc diameter in size. This evolution occurs at times on a background of small, hard drusen; Figure 60-22 shows how the small drusen become incorporated into the larger fluid deposits. In the outer macula the brightly fluorescent small drusen remain discrete. In the inner macula they form clusters in which the individual drusen become progressively more difficult to distinguish. These now fill more slowly on the fluorescein angiogram but often show a few brightly fluorescent highlights around the edge of the deposits. Those drusen clusters closest to the fovea can

become completely homogeneous on fluorescein angiography, without highlights, and they take on a fluid appearance. Hyperpigmentation gradually develops over the surface, often in the form of a radiating pigment figure. On fluorescein angiography the drusenoid PEDs show faint late fluorescence similar to the filling of the surrounding fluid drusen. The overlying hyperpigmentation appears as a hypofluorescent figure separating the hyperfluorescent lobules.

Drusenoid PEDs are consistent with good vision, although large ones can cause mild distortion. However, as overlying hyperpigmentation and hypopigmentation develop, the contents appear whiter and more inspissated, and visual acuity begins to decline. Once heavy clumping has appeared, the drusenoid PED generally begins to collapse within a couple of years, and a rapidly evolving atrophy is then a more common outcome (Fig. 60-23) than CNV.[79,102–104]

Occasionally a drusenoid PED develops into an avascular PED (Fig. 60-23), becoming more elevated with a rounded outline. Fluorescein angiography then demonstrates rapid, bright, and

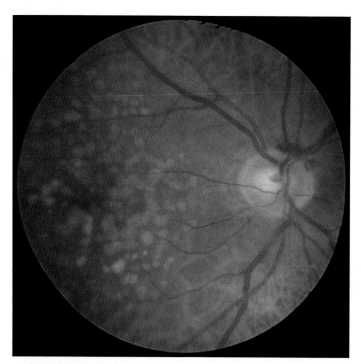

Fig. 60-20 Soft drusen of granular structure. Numerous soft, yellow drusen of solid appearance in the right eye of a 72-year-old man. Confluence of soft drusen results in a sinuous pattern. Patient died 3 years later, and corresponding histopathology (see Fig. 60-19) demonstrated a granular structure derived from broken down small, hard drusen. (Reproduced from Sarks SH. Drusen and their relationship to senile macular degeneration. Aust J Ophthalmol 1980; 8:117–130.[100])

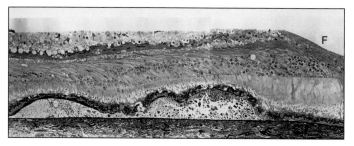

Fig. 60-21 Semithin section through edge of fovea (F) of eye shown in Figure 60-20 demonstrates confluence of three soft drusen. Drusen have a granular structure, comprising variably sized globules of amorphous material, some membrane-bound. This material appeared to be derived from the breakdown of small hard drusen, several of which were still present around the edge of these drusen. Note that, as the contents break down, drusen tend to lose sharp margins and nodular surface elevations present in fused clusters (see Figs 60-12 and 60-13). The fellow eye demonstrated similar drusen, but many were regressing (methylene blue and basic fuchsin; ×115). (Reproduced from Sarks JP, Sarks SH, Killingsworth MC. Evolution of soft drusen in age-related macular degeneration. Eye 1994; 8:269–283.[77])

even fluorescence, unlike the slow and faint staining observed in the typical drusenoid PED.[49]

Disappearance of drusen following prophylactic laser photocoagulation Although longitudinal studies have shown that drusen may come and go, another indication of the fluid

nature of drusenoid PEDs is the rapidity with which they clear away after application of laser photocoagulation. Drusenoid PEDs occur most commonly within the fovea and can be flattened over several months by the application of gentle laser burns around their margin, possibly because laser alters the lipids in Bruch's membrane, favoring the egress of fluid. Laser burns have been shown to cause a focal reduction in age-related lipid deposits in Bruch's membrane in the long term, but a cellular mechanism may also be invoked, since laser induces an inflammation with occasional cellular intrusions into the membrane.[105,106]

Based on these findings, a number of trials of prophylactic laser treatment of drusen have therefore been undertaken.[107,108,108a–108e] An increased short-term incidence of CNV was reported in patients with neovascular AMD in the fellow eye but not in patients with bilateral drusen.[107] Whether the treatment prevents visual acuity loss by lowering the incidence of CNV or delaying the development of geographic atrophy in these eyes still remains to be determined.[108,109b]

Soft (membranous) drusen (localized accumulation of the basal linear deposit[21])

Soft membranous drusen often appear paler and shallower than the yellow granular drusen (Fig. 60-24). They are usually smaller than 250 μm, most commonly 63 to 175 μm (0.5 to 1.5 vein widths). On fluorescein angiography they fluoresce later and less brightly than small, hard drusen. Small, distinct drusen of this type are commonly associated with reticular pseudodrusen (see Fig. 60-28). These drusen are specific for the intermediate stage or advanced stage of AMD. Since they represent focal accentuations of a continuous layer of debris, their margins are usually indistinct and they readily become confluent. Therefore they are most developed in the inner macula where this deposit occurs, and they do not form before the seventh decade. Histologically these drusen are pale-staining and faintly periodic acid–Schiff-positive, with a finely granular or ground-glass appearance; they even may appear optically empty. However, on electron microscopy they contain tightly packed membrane coils (Figs 60-25 and 60-26). A small amount of amorphous material may be present within the coils, so their contents have also been described as vesicular and granular electron-dense, lipid-rich material.[21,75] This membranous debris is morphologically similar to that which forms basal mounds internal to the RPE basement membrane, and continuity between the mounds and drusen through the basement membrane can at times be observed (Fig. 60-26). Similar material has also been found in autosomal dominant drusen.[52]

Membranous drusen have a high risk of CNV and are often found in advance of neovascular membranes in pathologic specimens, unlike granular drusen, which more often occur around areas of atrophy. They are significant because they are not simply a focal pathology but are part of a diffuse layer of debris external to the basement membrane that opens a cleavage plane for the spread of the new vessels. The BLD over these drusen is usually the early type because membranous material declines as late BLD appears. Although these soft drusen develop de

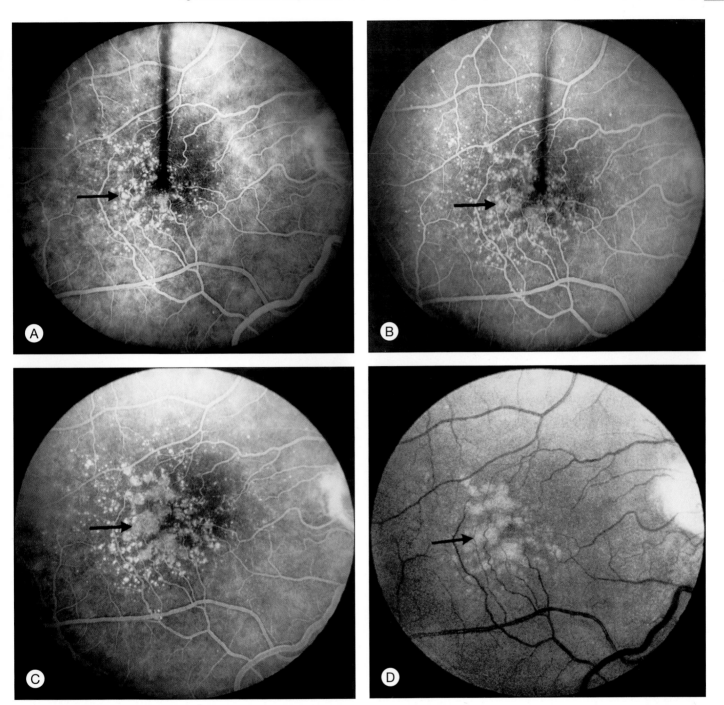

Fig. 60-22 Patient showing evolution of clusters of small, hard drusen into larger, soft, confluent drusen (arrows), presumably due to the addition of serous fluid. Fluorescein angiograms of the right eye of a man at age 55 (A), 58 (B), and 61 (C). The drusen farthest from the fovea remain discrete. In the inner macula they form clusters in which the individual drusen are more difficult to distinguish owing to confluence and breakdown. The more central clusters have become completely homogeneous on fluorescein angiography. D, Red-free photograph at age 61 shows corresponding clinical picture. Homogenized clusters have a soft, yellow appearance. Visual acuity remained 20/20, although the patient had been aware of some deterioration, the other eye being amblyopic.

novo, small, hard drusen are commonly also present and then become incorporated into the membranous drusen; their amorphous contents break down (Fig. 60-27).

This debris coincides with a macrophage response in the choroid, and segments of thinning of Bruch's membrane may be found, with signs of activation in the adjacent choroidal capil-laries.[82] This occurs preferentially beneath hard drusen, possibly because the RPE remains anchored to these for a time, while becoming increasingly separated from Bruch's membrane elsewhere by the membranous debris. An ischemic stimulus induced in the outer retina by this separation may cause the RPE to release diffusible angiogenic factors that would reach

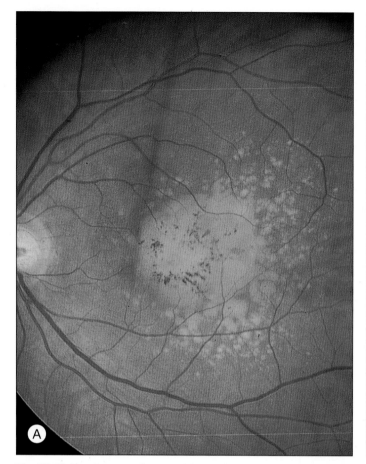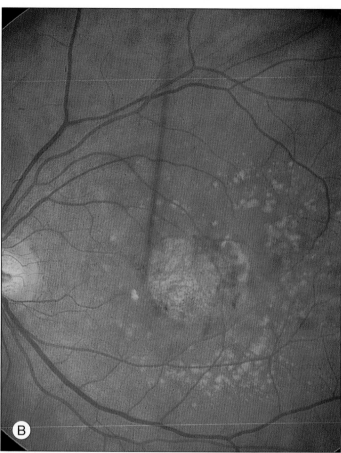

Fig. 60-23 Development of geographic atrophy after collapse of a pigment epithelial detachment (PED). A, Left eye of a 65-year-old woman with a PED that had been observed to develop from the confluence of soft, fluid drusen. It subsequently developed into an avascular, true PED that demonstrated bright hyperfluorescence. Hyperpigmentation developed over the surface (vision 20/50). B, Three years later the PED had collapsed, leaving an area of geographic atrophy abutting on fixation (vision 20/100).

the choroid in greatest concentration where the RPE remains attached to Bruch's membrane (Fig. 60-27).

Reticular pseudodrusen,[110] reticular drusen[13,19]

These drusen are characterized by a yellowish interlacing network about 250 μm in diameter[19] and first appear in the superior outer macula (Fig. 60-28). The network slowly extends into other quadrants and also peripherally, the transition with normal retina being marked by a scalloped line breaking up into islands. The picture resembles soft confluent drusen, but it is flat, appears to lie deep to drusen, and shows none of the signs drusen demonstrate when they are regressing. The pattern does not fluoresce on fluorescein angiography, being best observed in red-free light or the helium neon light of the scanning laser ophthalmoscope. The histologic counterpart remains uncertain, but it has not been confirmed to be due to drusen, so the term *pseudodrusen*[111] remains more appropriate. It has been suggested that the pattern results from fibrous replacement of the middle layer of the choroid,[110] especially since it may be associated clinically with delayed choroidal perfusion on fluorescein angiography. This picture carries a very high risk of the development of CNV.

Regressing (fading) drusen (localized detachment of the basal laminar deposit within an area of retinal pigment epithelium and photoreceptor atrophy[21])

All drusen types may in time disappear,[4,15,96,112] but this does not signify a return to a more normal state, since areas of drusen may be replaced by more severe manifestations. A proportion of eyes show changes in the appearance of the macula that might be considered "improved," but whether this is associated with a decreased risk of the advanced stage of AMD remains to be seen.[113] It is doubtful that the RPE remains unaffected, and fluorescein angiography generally shows increased transmission of fluorescence where drusen have faded.

Drusen commence to regress when the overlying RPE fails, often assuming a whiter and harder appearance (see Fig. 60-19). It has been suggested that the drusen have reverted to a previous type,[4] but hardening of the drusen in this situation is caused by inspissation of the contents and is associated with more advanced degeneration of the RPE, with hyperpigmentation and hypopigmentation often developing over the surface. Later the margins become irregular and foci of calcification may appear, especially after the age of 60 years. Ultimately the drusen fade,

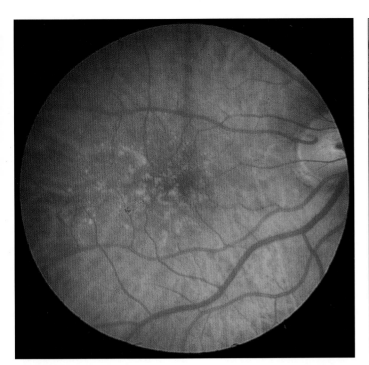

Fig. 60-24 Soft, indistinct drusen composed of membranous debris. The right eye of a 71-year-old man shows small, hard drusen and medium-sized soft drusen of smudgy appearance. This eye developed a hemorrhagic disciform lesion shortly before the patient died at age 75. The left eye had similar drusen and also proved to contain an early active neovascular membrane. The morphology of the drusen in the left eye is illustrated in Figures 60-25 to 60-27. (Reproduced from Sarks JP, Sarks SH, Killingsworth MC. Evolution of soft drusen in age-related macular degeneration. Eye 1994; 8:269–283.[77])

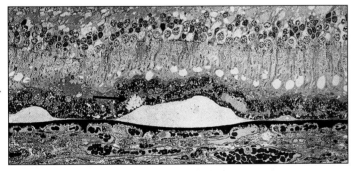

Fig. 60-25 Semithin section showing medium-sized soft drusen from the left eye of the patient illustrated in Figure 60-24. Since these deposits are focal accentuations of a continuous layer of debris, their margins are ill defined and they readily become confluent. It is into this plane that choroidal new vessels grow; a neovascular membrane was present nearby. Drusen appear empty or very finely granular at this magnification. The arrow points to a small basal mound of similar appearance, lying above the druse. Higher magnification is shown in Figure 60-26 (methylene blue and basic fuchsin; ×240). (Reproduced from Sarks JP, Sarks SH, Killingsworth MC. Evolution of soft drusen in age-related macular degeneration. Eye 1994; 8:269–283.[77])

leaving multifocal patches of RPE atrophy that reflect their original distribution and often sparing fixation (Fig. 60-29). Glistening calcium deposits may remain in these atrophic areas for many years.

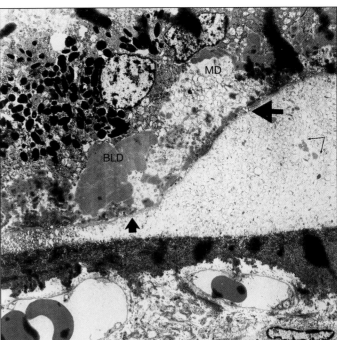

Fig. 60-26 Electron micrograph corresponding to the area indicated in Figure 60-25 shows formation of a soft druse made up of coiled lipid membranes lying external to the basement membrane of the retinal pigment epithelium (RPE) (arrows). The membranes appear first at the base of the RPE, where they may form basal mounds (MD). At the site of the right-hand arrow, some membranes can be seen within the basement membrane of the RPE and appear to be entering the soft druse from the basal mound. Some of the coils appear empty, and others contain amorphous material (double arrow). These drusen are specific for age-related macular degeneration, since they are only found after membranous debris develops. BLD, Basal laminar deposit (×2210). (Reproduced from Sarks JP, Sarks SH, Killingsworth MC. Evolution of soft drusen in age-related macular degeneration. Eye 1994; 8:269–283.[77])

Histopathologically, both RPE and photoreceptors over regressing drusen disappear, leaving a thick layer of late-type amorphous BLD over the apex (Fig. 60-30). Regressing drusen therefore not only have a reduced input of membranous debris due to loss of overlying RPE, but also show evidence of its removal by macrophages. Material not removed becomes invaded by glial cells or collagen fibers or undergoes dystrophic calcification. Regression of soft drusen therefore closes the cleavage plane created by membranous debris and, if CNV occurs, it remains localized (Fig. 60-30).

Outcome of drusen

The cumulative incidence of advanced AMD in individuals with bilateral drusen has been reported in several prospective studies. Among patients attending an ophthalmology clinic in England the 3-year cumulative incidence of the advanced stage of AMD were respectively, 23.5% and 18%,[104] one significant risk factor being the degree of confluence of drusen within 1600 μm of the center of the fovea. In the Beaver Dam study of persons with signs of what was characterized as "early ARM" in both eyes at baseline, the respective figures at 5 years were 11% and 7.1% in this study.[4] In patients who have developed CNV in the first

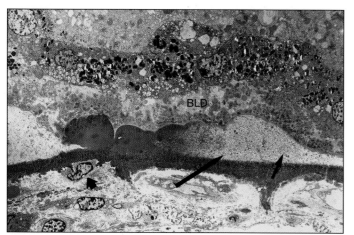

Fig. 60-27 Electron micrograph of the same eye in Figures 60-24 to 60-26 shows a cluster of subclinical, small, hard drusen apparently becoming eroded by membranous debris and breaking down into small membrane-bound particles (central arrow). At right (shorter arrow), druse consists of more characteristic membranous debris. This scenario suggests that small, hard drusen become incorporated into soft drusen once membranous debris develops. Early-type basal laminar deposit (BLD) lies over drusen. Note that the BLD and retinal pigment epithelium remain anchored at the site of hard drusen but are separated from Bruch's membrane on either side by soft drusen. This may permit a retinal stimulus to evoke the maximum cellular response in the choroid directly beneath these drusen. Small arrow at left points to macrophage-type cell adjacent to outer surface of Bruch's membrane, where retina remains attached (×1260). (Courtesy of MC Killingsworth.)

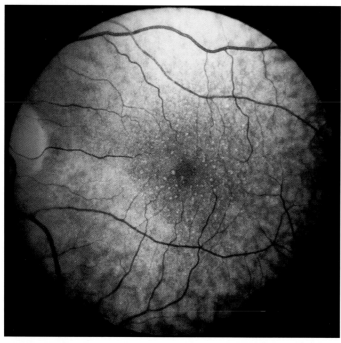

Fig. 60-28 Reticular pseudodrusen, a yellowish, lobular pattern in the outer macular region, in a 65-year-old woman with a disciform scar in the other eye. Pseudodrusen are not visible on fluorescein angiography and are best observed with red-free light. Delayed choroidal perfusion was present, and the appearance presumably results from choroidal ischemia. Vision was 20/30, and small, soft, distinct drusen are scattered over the fovea. This picture suggests a very high risk of choroidal neovascularization.

eye, the presence of five or more drusen, or one or more large drusen, were two factors associated independently with an increased risk of developing CNV within 5 years.[87] Another prospective study followed 101 patients with unilateral neovascular AMD and drusen only in the fellow eye for up to 9 years. Yearly incidence rates for the development of CNV or geographic atrophy in the fellow were between 5% and 14%. The risk of CNV peaked at 4 years and decreased thereafter. Longer follow-up was associated with a slightly increased incidence of geographic atrophy. The risk of CNV in patients with AMD was heralded by an increase in the number, size, and confluence of drusen (in decreasing order of significance). This risk eventually declines and is followed by later increased risk of geographic atrophy.[114] Most recently, the Age-Related Eye Disease Study Group[2,12] reported that the risk of progressing to the advanced stage of AMD within 5 years was extremely low for individuals with the early stage of AMD, approximately 6% for individuals with the intermediate stage in only one eye, approximately 25% for individuals with the intermediate stage in both eyes, and approximately 43% for individuals who already have the advanced stage in only one eye (Fig. 60-31). Another way of approximating the risk of progressing to the advanced stage adds up the presence of large drusen (one risk factor for each eye) and pigmentary abnormalities (one risk factor for each eye) and totaling the risk factors (or if counting the advanced stage in one eye to be equivalent to two risk factors for that eye).[115]

This risk is also reflected in pathologic specimens, in which active subretinal new vessels are more likely to be associated with soft membranous-type drusen, over which the BLD is of the early type. Cells of the macrophage series were found to be related to thinned segments of Bruch's membrane[83] (see Fig. 60-27) and are believed to precede the ingrowth of new vessels into the subretinal space.

Histochemistry

Drusen contain neutral fats and phospholipids,[116] as well as glycoconjugates containing specific carbohydrate residues. The latter were found in all classes of drusen, suggesting that both hard and soft drusen may have a similar origin.[117] Many hard and soft drusen contain specific cores with a carbohydrate-rich composition confined to distinct domains. These cores are positioned centrally within the drusen and are typically juxtapositioned to Bruch's membrane. Some researchers have suggested that they may represent an early nucleation site around which other drusen-associated molecules including lipid are subsequently deposited.[83,118,119]

Other distinct components common to all phenotypes of hard and soft drusen include apolipoprotein E, immunoglobulins, factor X, amyloid P component, complement C5 and C5b-9 terminal complexes, fibrinogen, and thrombospondin.[117] Vitronectin is a major constituent of both hard and soft drusen, and vitronectin mRNA is expressed locally in the RPE, suggesting that vitronectin may participate in the pathogenesis of AMD.[120] A number of these drusen-associated constituents are participants in humoral and cellular immunity, including a number of acute-phase reactants, plasma proteins that rapidly

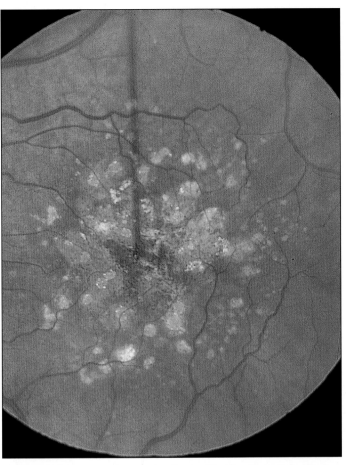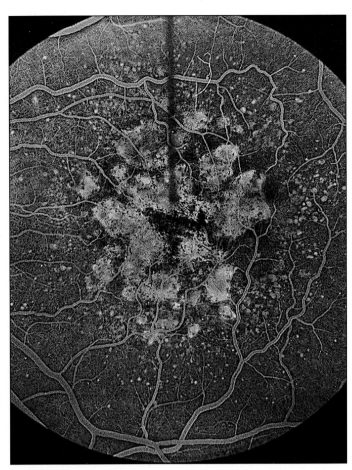

Fig. 60-29 Regressing drusen, showing multifocal pattern of atrophy, in a patient 69 years of age. The separate patches of atrophy have spread into the surrounding retina, and many have coalesced to produce the geographic pattern. The drusen within these areas have disappeared, and only calcified particles remain. Vision was 20/40, and although still capable of fixing on the small central island of retina, the patient was unable to read along a line.

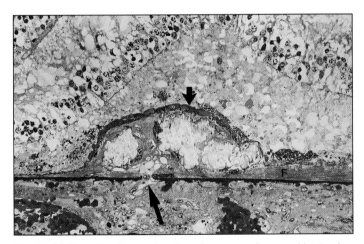

Fig. 60-30 Example of regressing druse in an area of geographic atrophy. The druse is covered by late, amorphous basal laminar deposit (short arrow) and has dystrophic calcification. A clinically unsuspected small vessel passes through a gap in Bruch's membrane beneath the druse (long arrow), but the surrounding atrophy has inhibited its further spread. A layer of fibrous tissue (F) lies on Bruch's membrane, with fibroblasts replacing macrophages as new vessels become less active (methylene blue and basic fuchsin; ×240). (Reproduced from Sarks JP, Sarks SH, Killingsworth M. Evolution of geographic atrophy of the retinal pigment epithelium. Eye 1988; 2:552–577.[79])

elevate in response to inflammatory stimuli. They are also common components of abnormal deposits associated with other diseases such as amyloidosis and atherosclerosis.[118]

The membranous debris appears to bleb from the surface of the RPE and pass through the RPE basement membrane to form soft drusen specific for intermediate or advanced stage of AMD. Ultrastructurally, this material resembles the extracellular lipid found in developing atheromatous plaque.[69,70] The debris probably arises indirectly at least from peroxidized lipid[63] derived from the photoreceptor outer segments, since membranous debris disappears with loss of photoreceptors.

The outer segments of the photoreceptors are rich in polyunsaturated fatty acids and subject to light and oxygen damage, promoting free radical production. This, combined with environmental factors (e.g., smoking) and inherited risk factors, may promote RPE damage and membrane production.

INCIPIENT ATROPHY (NONGEOGRAPHIC ATROPHY[17])

Incipient atrophy is the stage immediately preceding geographic atrophy and is a useful means of predicting its rate and direction of spread. Although not as sharply defined as actual geographic

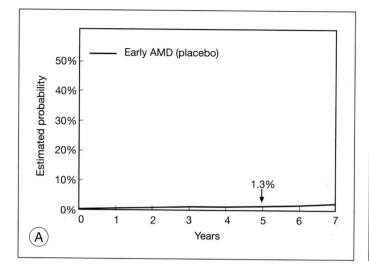

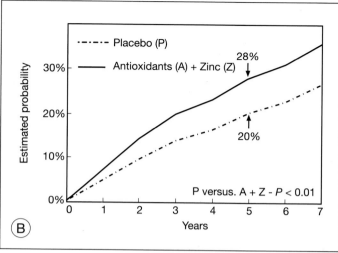

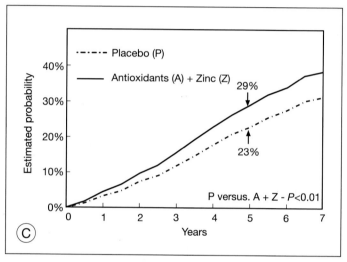

Fig. 60-31 Results of the Age-Related Eye Disease Study (AREDS) trial. Risk of progressing to advanced age-related macular degeneration (AMD) within 5 years for patients with (A) early AMD, (B) intermediate or monocular advanced AMD. The effect of treatment with antioxidants and zinc is also shown in (B). (C) Effect of antioxidants and zinc on vision loss in patients with intermediate or monocular advanced AMD within 5 years.

atrophy, areas of RPE thinning or depigmentation (incipient atrophy) can nevertheless be recognized. The affected retina appears pinker than the normal fundus background, and any drusen present appear whiter and harder before fading. Fluorescein angiography demonstrates diffuse hyperfluorescence, not as bright as an area of geographic atrophy (see Fig. 60-17), which is commonly associated with a reticular pattern of hyperpigmentation (Fig. 60-32). The areas may be more easily delineated on autofluorsecence.

Pathology

It has been shown that the character of the material liberated by the RPE reflects the stage of degeneration. The debris made up of coiled membranes (basal linear deposit) appears when the cells are also elaborating the early form of BLD. As degeneration develops, there is initially a marked increase in the quantity of both these diffuse deposits. However, with more advanced fallout of photoreceptors, the amount of membranous debris produced declines, and both the basal mounds internal to the basement membrane and the soft drusen fade, and the BLD is now the late amorphous type. Multinucleated giant cells and mononuclear inflammatory cells are observed lying on Bruch's

membrane at the margin of areas of geographic atrophy and may play a role in clearing the debris from necrotic cells at this site.[121] Therefore, as the late type of BLD increases, the quantity of membranous debris is reduced, which is particularly noticeable at the edge of an area of atrophy (see Fig. 60-12).

CHOROIDAL PERFUSION IN AGE-RELATED MACULAR DEGENERATION

The retina has the highest oxygen uptake in the body, most of which is provided by the choroid, but as AMD advances, the cross-sectional area of the choriocapillary bed progressively decreases. Histologic measurements made in eyes with (1) continuous BLD, (2) geographic atrophy, and (3) disciform scarring showed that the choriocapillary density, defined as the combined length of patent capillary lumina parallel to Bruch's membrane, was respectively 63%, 54%, and 43% of normal. The corresponding figures for the choriocapillary diameter measured perpendicular to Bruch's membrane were 81%, 73%, and 75% of normal.[50] In one study choriocapillary density was increased,[122,123] possibly representing an initial intrachoroidal neovascular response, but in long-standing atrophy the capillaries disappear. Not surprisingly, therefore, until recently the most popularly held belief has been that most cases of AMD are caused by ischemia. The macula is the watershed zone where branches of the short posterior ciliary arteries meet, and an area where multiple watershed zones meet is an area of poor vascularity and therefore most vulnerable to ischemic disorders.[124] Moreover, the distribution of diffuse deposits beneath the RPE is often closely related to regions of choroidal capillary dropout.[125]

Relationship to age-related macular degeneration

As a result of studies on Sorsby's fundus dystrophy, it has been suggested that delayed choroidal perfusion may indicate diffuse thickening of Bruch's membrane. In this autosomal dominant condition a continuous layer of abnormal material up to 30 μm thick is deposited internal to the inner collagenous zone,[97] and this material has a similar morphology to the late form of BLD. Similar angiographic characteristics have been found in patients with the intermediate and advanced stages of AMD and interpreted as a clinical sign for diffuse aging changes in Bruch's membrane,[126] especially in eyes with soft drusen.[127] A prolonged choroidal filling time, as evidenced by patchy and slow filling of the choroid in the early phase of fluorescein angiography, was found in 40% of eyes with AMD, and this was corroborated by indocyanine green angiography, by means of which a distinct area of reduced fluorescence of the choriocapillaris was noted in the middle phase in 44% of eyes.[128] A prolonged choroidal filling phase may therefore be a marker for loss of the choriocapillaris and the presence of diffuse deposits.

It was first reasoned,[129] and then confirmed,[130] that the RPE modulates the choroidal vasculature by secreting a diffusible growth factor. Since in the intermediate stage of AMD there is a continuous layer of debris internal to Bruch's membrane that may present a barrier to metabolic exchange between the RPE and the choriocapillaris, and since the RPE cells are degenerate, less growth factor would be expected to reach the choriocapillaris. This may be the reason why the choriocapillaris is initially slow to fill, then loses its endothelial fenestrations and ultimately atrophies. Hence the narrowing of the choriocapillaris, rather than causing the disease, may represent a disuse atrophy secondary to degeneration of the RPE. The alternative view, that impaired choroidal perfusion is responsible for dysfunction of the RPE, is supported by the use of color Doppler imaging, which demonstrated increased pulsatility and decreased velocity in the short posterior ciliary arteries. This suggested greater scleral rigidity in AMD, which increases the resistance of the choroid to the flow of blood.[131]

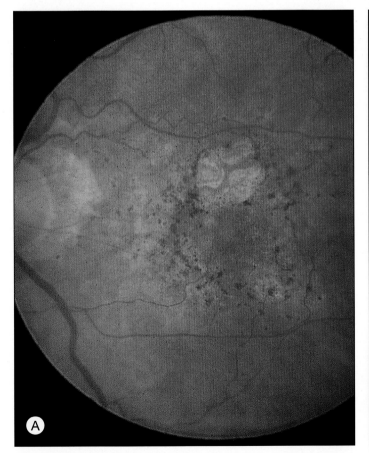

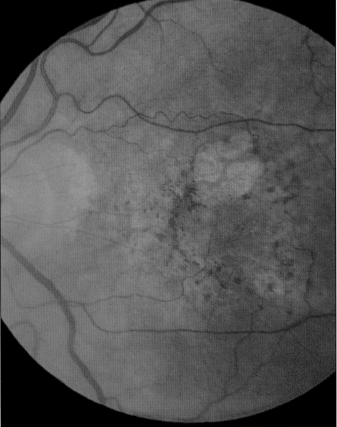

Fig. 60-32 An eye illustrating the spread of geographic atrophy unrelated to drusen. A, At age 68, atrophy was developing in relation to a ring of incipient atrophy, showing reticular pigmentation, located around the perimeter of the fovea.

Continued

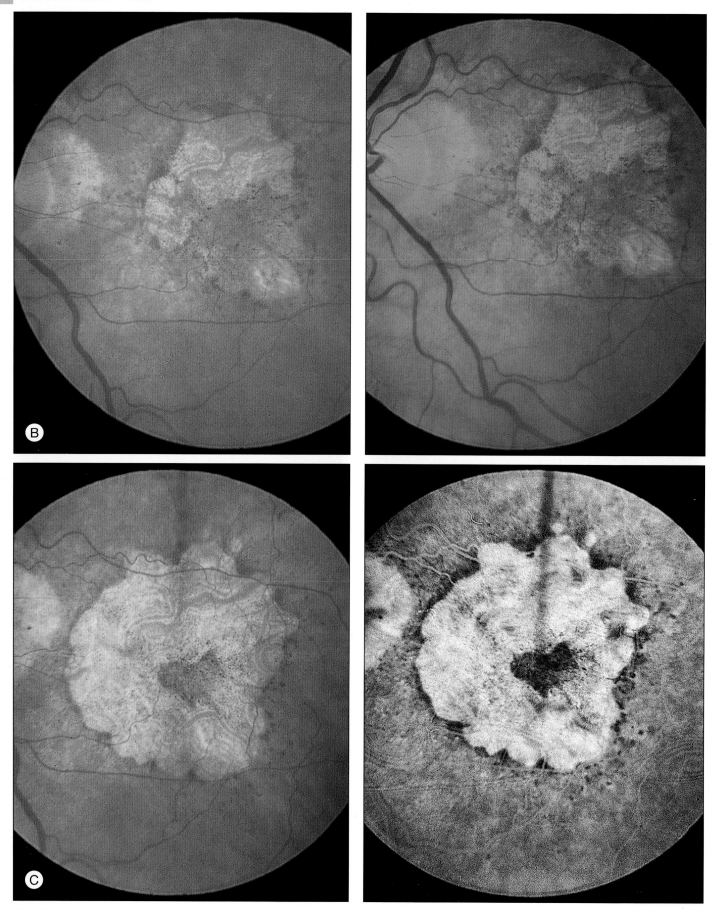

Fig. 60-32—cont'd B, One year later atrophy was progressing around the ring, but vision was still 20/30. C, At age 73, encirclement of the central island was complete. Atrophy occupied 75% of the fovea. Vision was 20/80.

Functional effects

In patients with AMD and delayed choroidal perfusion on fluorescein angiography, discrete areas of scotopic threshold elevation can be recorded that correspond to regions of choroidal perfusion abnormality.[132] It is interesting that these patients reported easy fatigability when doing close work,[132] the need for increased light intensity to read, fading of vision and slow recovery of vision after exposure to bright light,[132,133] and a central scotoma noticeable in the dark.[133] Patients may be reluctant to drive into tunnels. Delayed choroidal perfusion has also been linked to a prolonged foveal cone electroretinogram implicit time.[134] Since the diffuse deposits, especially the late amorphous BLD, are associated with some loss of RPE and photoreceptors, these deposits may account for the functional disturbances, as well as the perfusion abnormality.[133]

Prognostic value

Eyes with prolonged choroidal filling have been found to be at greater risk of visual loss, compared with eyes with normal choroidal filling. Whereas the proportion of eyes that develop CNV is the same in the two groups, the difference is caused by a higher incidence of geographic atrophy in the eyes with prolonged choroidal filling.[135] In eyes with drusen, a reduced retinal sensitivity may similarly predict the development of advanced AMD, especially drusen PEDs,[136] which are usually followed by geographic atrophy.

A prolonged choroidal filling phase was also found to be associated with more evidence of atrophy of the RPE in the fellow eye[128] and, together with reduced foveal sensitivity, may therefore be a predictor that geographic atrophy will develop. Areas of incipient atrophy around a region of geographic atrophy, a region where the late form of the BLD is maximally developed with an associated fallout of RPE and photoreceptors, would also be expected to have reduced retinal sensitivity under dark-adapted conditions, so in addition it may be possible to predict the rate and spread of geographic atrophy.[137]

GEOGRAPHIC ATROPHY

Geographic atrophy is the end-result of the atrophic form of AMD and is currently defined[10] as any sharply delineated round or oval area of hypopigmentation or depigmentation or apparent absence of the RPE, in which choroidal vessels are more visible than in surrounding areas and which must be at least 175 μm in diameter (see Fig. 60-2, circle C_2). However, since such a small area could result from regression of a single druse, other dimensions proposed have been wider, varying from 200 μm,[138] to 500 μm,[139] to 700 μm,[17] to 1 mm.[79] If a larger size is chosen, it has greater prognostic significance, especially if the atrophy has already entered the fovea, because CNV is then less likely to develop or, if it should occur, is more likely to be muted. It should be noted that for epidemiologic purposes an eye that shows any evidence of CNV is classified as neovascular AMD, even if atrophy predominates.

Evolution

Drusen-unrelated atrophy

This is an extension of AMD considered thus far. Stippling and small drusen often coexist, but atrophy is not seen to commence in relation to individual drusen. Instead, the atrophy often commences around the perimeter of the fovea in a band of microreticular hyperpigmentation[79,138] (Fig. 60-32), although this is not always the case (see Figs 60-5 and 60-6).

Spread continues into retina affected by incipient atrophy and is more rapid when the ring of pigment clumps is pronounced. It tends to expand in a horseshoe-like fashion around the central fovea or develops simultaneously in several areas around the foveal perimeter.[79,138-141] The nasal or temporal side of the ring is usually the last part to close, completing the bull's-eye that may spare fixation for several years.

The spread of geographic atrophy is therefore different from that of choroidal neovascular membranes, which, although they also often commence outside the rod-free area, have a propensity to spread toward fixation. The reason atrophy tends to skirt fixation may be determined by the manner in which lipofuscin accumulates at the posterior pole. This parallels the distribution of rods in the human retina and reflects the greater vulnerability to fallout of rods than cones.[34] In the central rod-free area the lipofuscin content in the pigment epithelium is lower;[142] a sharp increase occurs on the foveal slope.[35] This sparing of the central fovea is also attributable to the distribution of macular pigment. In humans this consists of two major carotenoids, lutein and zeaxanthin, which are thought to function as antioxidants and as blue-light filters, to protect the macula from phototoxic damage.[142,143]

Drusen-related atrophy

Most cases of geographic atrophy occur in eyes with prominent drusen and develop as the drusen regress.[6] Degeneration of the RPE is usually more advanced over drusen, and the pattern of atrophy therefore initially reflects the distribution of the drusen. In younger patients such foci of atrophy remain discrete for many years (see Fig. 60-19), but when AMD affects the intervening RPE, the patches enlarge and coalesce in an irregular manner (Fig. 60-29).

This pattern of evolution similarly tends to be more advanced around the perimeter of the fovea and spreads into the center. Ultimately the only evidence that atrophy evolved in a multifocal distribution in relation to drusen may be some scattered calcified deposits and a few small outlying islands of atrophy. In those younger patients with widespread drusen, there is an initial diffuse pigmentary disturbance, within which focal patches of atrophy then develop (see Fig. 60-17).

Following pigment epithelial detachments Geographic atrophy may follow collapse of an RPE detachment (see Fig. 60-23), especially those drusenoid RPE detachments formed by the confluence of large soft confluent drusen.[102] Vision remains satisfactory only as long as the RPE detachment is intact. Ultimately the RPE over a long-standing detachment fails, leading to loss of vision, flattening of the detachment, and a rapidly developing area of atrophy. If an RPE detachment is complicated by a rip, the resulting retraction of the pigment epithelium can also resemble an area of geographic atrophy.

Pathology

The changes causing an area of atrophy to spread are best studied at the junctional zone (see Fig. 60-12), where in vivo studies have demonstrated increased lipofuscin-induced autofluorescence.[64] Here the lipofuscin content of the RPE is maximal, presumably the result not only of autophagy and outer-segment phagocytosis, but also of engulfment of discarded RPE and their photoreceptor cells. The few surviving photoreceptors comprise grossly abnormal cones with widened inner segments and absent outer segments, with no evidence of phagocytosis. The photoreceptors and the RPE then disappear together.

The heaping-up of necrotic RPE cells as they are shed into the subretinal space accounts for the hyperpigmented edge commonly noted clinically around an area of atrophy. These pigment-laden cells have been referred to as *macrophages*, but certain features point to their pigment epithelial origin. Some have a few distorted apical villi or remain associated with basal laminar material; they may contain abundant smooth endoplasmic reticulum, and they occasionally demonstrate cell junctions with the underlying pigment epithelial cells. However, although the RPE seems capable of phagocytosing the debris released as a result of the normal cell deletion that occurs with age, an excessive amount of debris may attract macrophages and giant cells.

Within the area of atrophy itself there is absence of photoreceptors, RPE, and choriocapillaris; the loss of RPE precedes the loss of the choroidal capillaries. An occasional surviving whorl of persisting photoreceptors may be observed converging on a group of degenerating pigment cells, but only if there are some surviving choroidal capillaries. The outer nuclear layer disappears, causing the outer plexiform layer to rest directly on the BLD. The outer plexiform layer is thinned and vacuolated, but the inner nuclear layer is less affected.

Once there is loss of RPE and photoreceptors, the membranous material (basal linear deposit) disappears, but the BLD, particularly the late amorphous form, can be traced throughout the area of atrophy for a long time. Obliteration of the choriocapillaris is followed by erosion of the intercapillary pillars of Bruch's membrane, and in long-standing cases the membrane becomes thinner. Fibroblasts and macrophage processes are found in contact with the outer surface of the membrane, commonly splitting off fragments or even passing through small breaks.

Choroidal atrophy

In long-standing geographic atrophy, there are fewer large choroidal vessels,[122] and the exposed choroidal arteries may display white sheathing of their walls or even appear bloodless. This picture was formerly called *senile choroidal sclerosis*, but on histologic examination the white fibrotic appearance does not result from sclerosis; the majority of arteries show only fibrous replacement of the media without thickening of the walls and with retention of wide lumina.

The appearance is instead an expression of choroidal atrophy;[22] loss of the choriocapillaris and the middle layer of vessels throws the remaining larger vessels into greater prominence. The white sheathing is due to the disproportionate thickening of the vessel walls by becoming flattened in the thinned choroid, but in many cases it also reflects a reduced blood column.

Since choroidal atrophy is a normal aging change, the white sheathing of the exposed choroidal arteries develops much more rapidly in patients over 80 years of age. In many patients with senile tigroid fundi and good vision, even the unexposed choroidal vessels assume this whiter appearance (see Fig. 60-5).

Clinical significance of geographic atrophy

Two case studies[9,144] found that geographic atrophy accounts for only 12% to 21% of eyes with severe visual loss due to AMD. However, visual acuity does not relate closely to functional handicap, since a large area of atrophy may spare fixation but still cause the patient difficulty with reading a line of print. The reading rate is slowed not only by the paracentral scotomata, but also because eyes with geographic atrophy demonstrate abnormal foveal dark-adapted sensitivity, reduced visual acuity in dim illumination, and reduced contrast sensitivity.[139] Magnifying aids rarely help these reading difficulties because the image will be enlarged on to nonfunctioning retina.

In one study central fixation was not completely lost until atrophy occupied more than 80% of the fovea, and this occurred about 5 years earlier in drusen-related atrophy as compared with drusen-unrelated atrophy.[79] Even when fixation is affected, vision may vary depending on the patient's ability to find a surviving island of retina within the atrophic area, or the least affected portion of retina outside the area.[145–147] There seems to be a preference to fix with the scotoma to the right,[141] favoring the ability to see the beginning of a line rather than the end. Visual retraining may enable a patient to use the closest viable area of retina.

Prognosis

Once geographic atrophy has commenced, the factors that influence the rate and direction of further spread are the number, distribution, and regression of drusen and the extent of incipient atrophy. When this extends into the central fovea, visual acuity can be expected to drop more rapidly (see Fig. 60-6). In general, the percentage of foveal involvement increases rapidly at first, slowing once all the area of incipient atrophy has become involved.

Prognostication therefore requires each case to be assessed individually, but in one study the average interval from onset of geographic atrophy to legal blindness was about 9 years.[140] In another study an interval of just over 5 years elapsed from the time atrophy first encroached into the fovea until vision fell to 20/200; fixation was lost earlier in the drusen-related group.[79] In a third study the average rate of expansion in one direction was 139 μm per year (the width of a major retinal vein at the edge of the disc is about 125 μm), and 8% of affected eyes had significant visual loss (from 20/50 or better to 20/100 or worse) per year.[138] In another series in which visual acuity was 20/50 or better at baseline, 50% of eyes lost three or more lines of acuity, and 25% lost six or more lines of acuity at 2-year follow-up.[139] Areas of atrophy continue to enlarge over time, even if large at baseline. The combination of reduced visual acuity with enlargement of atrophy, occurring bilaterally in most patients, can lead to significant impairment of visual acuity.[146]

Geographic atrophy and choroidal neovascularization

Histologic studies have shown that eyes with geographic atrophy may also contain small areas of CNV and that CNV is more frequently bilateral than clinical impressions suggest.[21,22] Eyes with this CNV are more likely to have soft drusen of granular composition, often showing foci of calcification or other signs of regression. The BLD over these drusen is of the late type and is associated with more advanced degeneration of the RPE, whereas the cells adjacent to Bruch's membrane are more often fibroblasts than macrophages. A neovascular response is therefore more likely to occur at an earlier stage, while the RPE is still viable; the vessels then spread in the plane created by the layer of membranous debris beneath the RPE basement membrane. Although they may be found close to an area of atrophy, they do not appear to grow into the area in which there is no such debris.

Geographic atrophy also tends to be a bilateral disease. In one series of over 200 patients with geographic atrophy, the fellow eye was affected in over 50% of cases, and there was a tendency to symmetry between the two eyes, the area of atrophy being only about 20% smaller in the fellow eye.[79] In about 25% of cases the fellow eye had developed an earlier disciform process, and these are the patients who are most at risk of developing CNV in the second eye despite the presence of geographic atrophy, although the neovascular response will usually remain limited. In one study 152 patients with geographic atrophy and no CNV in at least one eye were examined annually. For patients with CNV in the fellow eye, 18% developed CNV in the study eye by 2 years and 34% by 4 years. In contrast, for patients with bilateral geographic atrophy, the risk for developing CNV was relatively low – 2% by 2 years and 11% by 4 years.[146] As geographic atrophy enlarges in the first eye, the risk of subsequently developing clinically obvious CNV decreases in both eyes.[79,139,148]

Intermediate stage of age-related macular degeneration and cataract

In this aged population, the question of cataract extraction commonly arises, requiring an estimation of the postoperative visual acuity and of how long it may be expected to last. A preoperative fluorescein angiogram can map out any sharply demarcated areas of atrophy, but unsteady fixation and indistinct landmarks can make it difficult to tell where the center of the fovea lies.[79] However, in one series of cases with mainly the intermediate stage of AMD noted preoperatively, two-thirds of patients believed the operation had been worthwhile, based largely on an improvement in visual acuity.[149] The Beaver Dam study showed that its study participants who had previously

undergone cataract surgery were found to be more likely to demonstrate progression of the disease at 5 years than phakic eyes.[60] This may have reflected easier visualization of the fundus after surgery, but damage due to photic injury or inflammation was also hypothesized. More recent information from AREDS, with a matched-pair analysis or a Cox regression analysis, could not show an increased risk of developing CNV following cataract surgery. A definitive increased risk of developing geographic atrophy extending under the center of the macula could also not be found. Therefore, the best evidence at this time does not suggest that cataract surgery increases the risk that AMD will progress. Ophthalmologists should be cognizant of the possibility that advanced AMD (especially geographic atrophy in a blonde fundus or CNV with minimal subretinal fluid, hemorrhage, lipid, or scarring) might not be readily apparent through a cataract. However, pre-existing advanced AMD might be a cause of vision loss mistakenly attributed to the cataract before surgery and a cause of continued vision loss after cataract surgery. Furthermore, the patient may presume that loss of vision following cataract surgery, which is really due to progression of AMD unrelated to cataract surgery, was due to progression of AMD caused by the cataract surgery because of the temporal relationship of loss of vision soon after cataract surgery. Careful examination for the advanced stage of AMD before cataract surgery in any individual at risk for AMD, therefore, is important. Other clues for the ophthalmologist that may assist in this evaluation include having a high level of suspicion that the advanced stage of AMD exists in the fellow eye of an individual with the advanced stage in the first eye, noting senile reticular pigmentary degeneration at the equator (since it has been associated with AMD in the posterior pole,[150] seeing pigmentary abnormalities in the macula (which may be associated with less visible atrophy or CNV), or glistening from calcification (which is usually associated with geographic atrophy).

Age-related macular degeneration and age

Reference has already been made to the physiologic visual decline with age. If AMD is present in addition, these subjective tests, such as the time for visual recovery after exposure to a glare source,[32] become increasingly abnormal. The incidence and progression of AMD are closely related to age. Over a 5-year period,[4] compared to persons 43 to 54 years, persons 75 years of age and over were more than 10 times as likely to develop earlier stages of AMD and more than 40 times as likely to develop drusen 250 μm in diameter. The 5-year incidence of soft indistinct drusen, increased retinal pigment, and depigmentation was strongly associated with age, the most marked increase being found in people 75 and over.[4,96,112] This accelerated deterioration in older persons coincides with the accumulation of the diffuse deposits and makes prognostication in younger persons difficult.

Management of nonneovascular AMD

The management of nonneovascular AMD (Fig. 60-33) begins with the recognition that most people with the intermediate stage of AMD, while at risk of progressing to the advanced stage

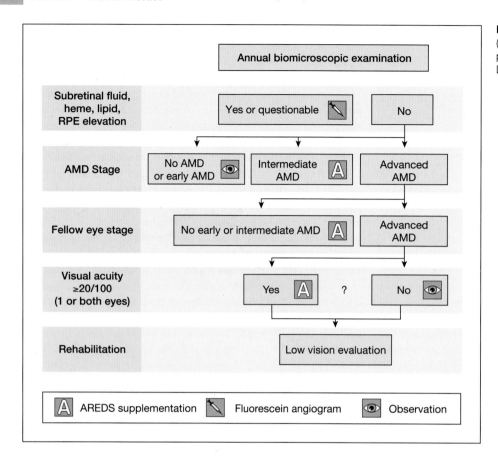

Fig. 60-33 Age-related macular degeneration (AMD) management algorithm. RPE, retinal pigment epithelium; AREDS, Age-Related Eye Disease Study.

of AMD, have no symptoms. Since, in the USA alone, it is estimated that approximately 8 million of the 60 million people aged 55 or older have the intermediate stage of AMD,[3,12] usually without symptoms, annual ophthalmologic examination of all people in this age group should include an evaluation of the retina to determine the stage of AMD, if any. If subretinal fluid, hemorrhage, lipid, or elevation of the RPE to suggest the presence of neovascular AMD is noted, then fluorescein angiography is indicated to determine the management, as outlined in Chapter 61.

If none of these features of neovascular AMD is noted, then the stage of AMD in each eye should be determined. If there is no AMD or only the early stage of AMD in either eye, then no management for AMD is indicated at that time. Specifically, AREDS could find no evidence that taking a dietary supplement of antioxidants as was used in AREDS reduced the risk of progression to advanced AMD or to the intermediate stage of AMD, even when the individual had a family history for AMD.

If the intermediate stage of AMD is noted in at least one eye, then the individual should consider taking a dietary supplement such as that used in AREDS, provided the individual's physicians know of no contraindication to taking this formulation of antioxidants (daily dose of 500 mg vitamin C, 400 international units of vitamin E, and 15 mg beta carotene) and zinc (daily dose of 80 mg zinc oxide with 2 mg cupric oxide added to try to reduce the risk of a copper-deficiency anemia). Individuals with the intermediate stage of AMD in at least one eye, or the

advanced stage of AMD in one eye but not the fellow eye, who were assigned to this formulation had a decreased risk of progression to advanced AMD (Fig. 60-31B) and a decreased risk of vision loss from advanced AMD (Fig. 60-31C) through at least 5 years. The risks of such a regimen are small (Tables 60-1 and 60-2) but should be reviewed with the patient in order to weigh the risks and benefits. Cigarette smokers should be warned that higher doses of beta-carotene in other randomized trials resulted in a definite, although small, increased risk of developing lung cancer.[151] Individuals should also realize that

Table 60-1 Safety – antioxidants		
Condition	No antioxidants (%)	Antioxidants (%)
Hospitalization for mild/ moderate symptoms	10.1	7.4
Hospitalization for infections	0.8	1.6
Circulatory	0.8	0.3
Skin, subcutaneous tissue	1.0	2.2
Change in skin color	6.0	8.3
Chest pain	23.1	20.2

Table 60-2 Safety – zinc oxide

Condition	No zinc (%)	Zinc (%)
Hospitalization for mild/ moderate symptoms	7.8	9.7
Hospitalization for genitourinary	4.9	7.5
Hospitalization for genitourinary problems in men	4.4	8.6
Circulatory	0.3	0.9
Anemia	10.2	13.2
Difficulty swallowing pills	15.3	17.8

benefits of other formulations, such as those containing lutein, have not been proven in randomized clinical trials. Also, the risks of other formulations are unknown, but individuals should be reminded that micronutrients, such as beta-carotene, have been shown to be harmful, so the safety of other micronutrient formulations may be unknown. In addition, individuals with no AMD or the early stage of AMD should recognize that there is no evidence from randomized clinical trials at this time to

suggest that dietary supplements such as those used in AREDS can reduce the risk of progression to the intermediate stage of AMD, even in individuals in whom a family member has the intermediate or advanced stage of AMD.

As seen in the algorithm (Fig. 60-33), if the advanced stage of AMD is noted in one eye, the physician should then determine if the fellow eye has either no or early or an intermediate stage of AMD. Then a dietary supplement such as that used in AREDS should be considered, as explained above. If the advanced stage of AMD is noted in one eye, and the fellow eye has the advanced stage, the physician should consider a dietary supplement such as that used in AREDS if the visual acuity is relatively good in at least one eye. This consideration is based on data from AREDS which showed that when an individual had the advanced stage of AMD at baseline in one eye (in which the fellow eye did not have the advanced stage at baseline), taking a dietary supplement was associated with a decreased risk of vision loss in the eye with the advanced stage at baseline when the baseline visual acuity in the eye with advanced AMD was 20/100 or better, but not when the acuity was 20/200 or better (Table 60-3).

Data from AREDS[2] have shown that if all 8 million people with the intermediate stage of AMD in the USA took a dietary supplement such as that used in AREDS, approximately 300 000 individuals would avoid the development of advanced AMD in at least one eye over 5 years. Nevertheless, an additional 1 million

Table 60-3 Effect of treatment on risk of moderate vision loss from baseline in eyes with neovascular age-related macular degeneration at baseline

A. Baseline visual acuity 20/100 or better (n = 260)*

	Odds ratio	99% CI	P-value
Antioxidant versus no antioxidant	0.54	0.30–0.95	0.005
Zinc versus no zinc	0.99	0.56–1.74	0.96
Antioxidant versus placebo	0.35	0.15–0.81	0.001
Zinc versus placebo	0.65	0.28–1.50	0.18
Antioxidant + zinc versus placebo	0.53	0.23–1.24	0.05

CI, confidence interval.
*206 participants with moderate vision loss.

B. Baseline visual acuity 20/200 or better (n = 352)*

	Odds ratio	99% CI	P-value
Antioxidant versus no antioxidant	0.66	0.40–1.07	0.03
Zinc versus no zinc	1.10	0.67–1.79	0.62
Antioxidant versus placebo	0.56	0.27–1.13	0.03
Zinc versus placebo	0.93	0.46–1.89	0.79
Antioxidant + zinc versus placebo	0.72	0.36–1.46	0.24

CI, confidence interval.

people will still develop the advanced stage, of whom approximately two-thirds will develop the neovascular stage, for which treatment might be considered to reduce the risk of vision loss. Therefore, individuals with the intermediate stage are also told to return for the following reasons: (1) to evaluate periodically to receive further updates on AMD management; (2) to identify any asymptomatic neovascular AMD for which further treatment or closer follow-up might be indicated; (3) to review the need and methods for periodic monitoring to increase the chance that the individual will identify progression to the neovascular stage when the neovascular lesion is small, before significant visual acuity has been lost, when treatment has been shown to be more likely to be most effective; and (4) to be aware of an ophthalmologist to contact promptly who treats neovascular AMD should progression be suspected. Although an Amsler grid has not been shown to be very sensitive at detecting neovascular AMD,[152–155] many physicians recommend its use to individuals with the intermediate stage of AMD. More recently, a perimetry device, the Preferential Hyperacuity Perimeter (PreView PHP, Carl Zeiss Meditec, Dublin, CA) was shown to identify recent-onset neovascular AMD (often small lesions with relatively good levels of visual acuity when treatment will likely be most effective) among individuals with either the intermediate stage of AMD or recent-onset neovascular AMD with both a high sensitivity (82%) and high specificity (88%), making it likely that individuals identified as having progressed to neovascular AMD by the PHP will indeed have progressed.[156] Based on this information, individuals with the intermediate stage of AMD should consider periodic monitoring with the PHP to assist in the identification of recent-onset neovascular AMD. Since such monitoring will not identify all neovascular lesions, periodic examinations for asymptomatic progression are still indicated.

Finally, as noted in the algorithm (Fig. 60-33), if the advanced stage is noted in one or both eyes, then rehabilitation with a low-vision service should be considered to determine what services or devices might help the individual cope with the visual loss from the advanced stage of AMD. It is hopeful that future research will elucidate further the causes, treatments, and prevention of drusen, atrophy, and CNV, as well as additional ways to rehabilitate the individual who has lost vision from the advanced stage of AMD.

REFERENCES

1. Ferris FL III. Senile macular degeneration: review of epidemiologic features. Am J Epidemiol 1983; 118:132–151.
2. The Age-Related Eye Disease Study Research Group. Potential public health impact of AREDS results: AREDS report no. 11. Arch Ophthalmol 2003; 121:1621–1624.
3. The Eye Diseases Prevalence Research Group. Prevalence of age-related macular degeneration in the United States. Arch Ophthalmol 2004; 122:567–572.
4. Klein R, Klein BEK, Jensen SC et al. The five-year incidence and progression of age-related maculopathy. Ophthalmology 1997; 104:7–21.
5. Evans J, Wormold R. Is the incidence of registrable age-related macular degeneration increasing? Br J Ophthalmol 1996; 80:9–14.
6. Gass JDM. Drusen and disciform macular detachment and degeneration. Arch Ophthalmol 1973; 90:206–217.
7. Haab O. Erkrankungen der Macula Lutea, Centralblat Augenheilkd 1885; 9:384–391. (Cited by Duke-Elder S. System of ophthalmology, vol. 9. London: Kimpton; 1966.)
8. Piguet B, Haimovici R, Bird AC. Dominantly inherited drusen represent more than one disorder: a historical review. Eye 1995; 9:34–41.
9. Gass JDM. Pathogenesis of disciform detachment of the neuroepithelium (parts I and III). Am J Ophthalmol 1967; 63:573–711.
10. Bird AC, Bressler NB, Bressler SB et al. An international classification and grading system for age-related maculopathy and age-related macular degeneration. Surv Ophthalmol 1995; 39:367–374.
11. Klein R, Klein BEK, Linton KLP. Prevalence of age-related maculopathy: the Beaver Dam Eye Study. Ophthalmology 1992; 99:933–943.
12. The Age-Related Eye Disease Study Research Group. A randomized, placebo-controlled, clinical trial of high-dose supplementation with vitamins C and E, beta carotene, and zinc for age-related macular degeneration and vision loss: AREDS report no. 8. Arch Ophthalmol 2001; 119:1417–1436.
13. Mitchell P, Smith W, Attebo K et al. Prevalence of age-related maculopathy in Australia. Ophthalmology 1995; 102:1450–1460.
14. Wang Q, Chappell RJ, Klein R et al. Patterns of age-related maculopathy in the macular area, the Beaver Dam Eye Study. Invest Ophthalmol Vis Sci 1996; 37:2234–2242.
15. Vingerling JR, Dielemans I, Hofman A et al. The prevalence of age-related maculopathy in the Rotterdam study. Ophthalmology 1995; 102:205–210.
16. Wang JJ, Mitchell P, Smith W et al. Bilateral involvement by age-related maculopathy lesions in a population, the Blue Mountains Eye Study. Br J Ophthalmol 1998; 82:743–747.
17. Bressler NM, Bressler SB, West SK et al. The grading and prevalence of macular degeneration in Chesapeake Bay watermen. Arch Ophthalmol 1989; 107:847–852.
18. Gregor Z, Bird AC, Chisholm IH. Senile disciform macular degeneration in the second eye. Br J Ophthalmol 1977; 61:141–147.
19. Klein R, Davis MD, Magli YL et al. The Wisconsin age-related maculopathy grading system. Ophthalmology 1991; 98:1128–1134.
20. Green WR, McDonnell PJ, Yeo JH. Pathologic features of senile macular degeneration. Ophthalmology 1985; 92:615–627.
21. Green WR, Enger C. Age-related macular degeneration histopathologic studies: the 1992 Lorenz E. Zimmerman lecture. Ophthalmology 1993; 100:1519–1535.
22. Sarks SH. Aging and degeneration in the macular region: a clinico-pathological study. Br J Ophthalmol 1976; 60:324–341.
23. Spraul CW, Grossniklaus HE. Characteristics of drusen and Bruch's membrane in postmortem eyes with age-related macular degeneration. Arch Ophthalmol 1997; 115:267–273.
24. van der Schaft TL, Mooy CM, de Bruijn WC et al. Histologic features of the early stages of age-related macular degeneration. A statistical analysis. Ophthalmology 1992; 99:278–286.
25. Curcio CA, Medeiros NE, Millican CL. The Alabama age-related macular degeneration grading system for donor eyes. Invest Ophthalmol Vis Sci 1998; 39:1085–1096.
26. Laatikainen L, Karinkari J. Capillary-free area of the fovea with advancing age. Invest Ophthalmol Vis Sci 1977; 161:1154–1157.
27. Grunwald JE, Piltz J, Patel N et al. Effect of aging on retinal macular microcirculation: a blue-field simulation study. Invest Ophthalmol Vis Sci 1994; 34:3609–3613.
28. Groh MJM, Michelson G, Langhans MJ et al. Influence of age on retinal and optic nerve head blood circulation. Ophthalmology 1996; 103:529–534.
29. Ibrahim YWM, Bots ML, Mulder PGH et al. Number of perifoveal vessels in aging, hypertension, and atherosclerosis: the Rotterdam Study. Invest Ophthalmol Vis Sci 1998; 39:1049–1053.
30. Gao H, Hollyfield JG. Aging of the human retina: differential loss of neurons and retinal pigment epithelial cells. Invest Ophthalmol Vis Sci 1992; 33:1–17.
31. Rubin GS, West SK, Munoz B et al. A comprehensive assessment of visual impairment in a population of older Americans, the SEE study. Invest Ophthalmol Vis Sci 1977; 38:557–568.
32. Sandberg MA, Gaudio AR. Slow photostress recovery and disease severity in age-related macular degeneration. Retina 1995; 15:407–412.
33. Liem AT, Keunen JE, van Norren D. Clinical applications of fundus reflection densitometry. Surv Ophthalmol 1996; 41:37–50.
34. Curcio CA, Millican CL, Allen KA et al. Aging of the human photoreceptor mosaic: evidence for selective vulnerability of rods in central retina. Invest Ophthalmol Vis Sci 1993; 34:3278–3296.
35. Dorey CK, Wu G, Ebenstein D et al. Cell loss in the aging retina: relationship to lipofuscin accumulation and macular degeneration. Invest Ophthalmol Vis Sci 1989; 30:1691–1699.
36. Feeney-Burns L, Burns RP, Gao C. Age-related macular changes in humans over 90 years old. Am J Ophthalmol 1990; 109:265–278.
37. Marshall J, Grindle J, Ansell PL et al. Convolution in human rods: an ageing process. Br J Ophthalmol 1979; 63:181–187.
38. Curcio CA, Medeiros NE, Millican CL. Photoreceptor loss in age-related macular degeneration. Invest Ophthalmol Vis Sci 1996; 37:1236–1249.
39. Young RW. The Bowman Lecture, 1982. Biological renewal: applications to the eye. Trans Ophthalmol Soc UK 1982; 102:42–75.

40. Feeney-Burns L, Berman ER, Rothman H. Lipofuscin of human retinal pigment epithelium. Am J Ophthalmol 1980; 90:783–791.

41. Young RW. Pathophysiology of age-related macular degeneration. Surv Ophthalmol 1987; 31:291–306.

42. Rakoczy PE, Baines M, Kennedy C et al. Correlation between autofluorescent debris accumulation and the presence of partially processed forms of cathepsin D in cultured retinal pigment epithelial cells challenged with rod outer segments. Exp Eye Res 1996; 63:159–167.

43. Feeney-Burns L, Hilderbrand ES, Eldridge S. Aging human RPE: morphometric analysis of macular, equatorial, and peripheral cells. Invest Ophthalmol Vis Sci 1984; 25:195–200.

44. Beatty S, Boulton M, Henson D et al. Macular pigment and age-related macular degeneration. Br J Ophthalmol 1999; 83:867–877.

45. Kennedy CJ, Rakoczy PE, Constable IJ. Lipofuscin of the retinal pigment epithelium: a review. Eye 1995; 9:763–771.

46. von Ruckmann A, Fitzke FW, Bird AC. In vivo fundus autofluorescence in macular dystrophies. Arch Ophthalmol 1997; 115:609–615.

47. Delori FC, Dorey CK, Staurenghi G et al. In vivo fluorescence of the ocular fundus exhibits retinal pigment epithelium lipofuscin characteristics. Invest Ophthalmol Vis Sci 1995; 36:718–729.

48. Panda-Jonas S, Jonas JB, Jakobczyk-Zmija M. Retinal pigment epithelial cell count, distribution, and correlations in normal human eyes. Am J Ophthalmol 1996; 121:181–189.

49. Gass JDM. Stereoscopic atlas of macular diseases: diagnosis and treatment, 4th edn. St Louis: Mosby; 1997.

50. Ramrattan RS, van der Schaft TL, Mooy CM et al. Morphometric analysis of Bruch's membrane, the choriocapillaris, and the choroid in aging. Invest Ophthalmol Vis Sci 1994; 35:2857–2864.

51. Karwatowski WSS, Jeffries TE, Duance VC et al. Preparation of Bruch's membrane and analysis of the age-related changes in the structural collagens. Br J Ophthalmol 1995; 79:944–952.

52. Holz FG, Owens SL, Marks J et al. Ultrastructural findings in autosomal dominant drusen. Arch Ophthalmol 1997; 115:788–792.

53. van der Schaft TL, de Bruijn WC, Mooy CM et al. Is basal laminar deposit unique for age-related macular degeneration? Arch Ophthalmol 1991; 109:420–425.

54. Marshall GE, Konstas AGP, Reid GG et al. Type IV collagen and laminin in Bruch's membrane and basal linear deposit in the human macula. Br J Ophthalmol 1992; 76:607–614.

55. Feeney-Burns L, Ellersieck MR. Age-related changes in the ultrastructure of Bruch's membrane. Am J Ophthalmol 1985; 100:686–697.

56. Burns RP, Feeney-Burns L. Clinico-morphologic correlations of drusen of Bruch's membrane. Trans Am Ophthalmol Soc 1980; 78:206–225.

57. Ishibashi T, Sorgente N, Patterson R et al. Aging changes in Bruch's membrane of monkeys: an electron microscopic study. Ophthalmologica 1986; 192:179–190.

58. Killingsworth MC. Age-related components of Bruch's membrane in the human eye. Graefes Arch Clin Exp Ophthalmol 1987; 225:406–412.

59. Holz FG, Sheraidah G, Pauleikhoff D et al. Analysis of lipid deposits extracted from human macular and peripheral Bruch's membrane. Arch Ophthalmol 1994; 112:402–406.

60. Klein R, Klein BEK, Jensen SC et al. The relationship of ocular factors to the incidence and progression of age-related maculopathy. Arch Ophthalmol 1998; 116:506–513.

61. Sheraidah G, Steinmetz R, Maguire J et al. Correlation between lipids extracted from Bruch's membrane and age. Ophthalmology 1993; 100:47–52.

62. Pauleikhoff D, Harper CA, Marshall J et al. Aging changes in Bruch's membrane: a histochemical and morphologic study. Ophthalmology 1990; 97:171–178.

63. Spaide RF, Ho-Spaide WC, Browne R et al. Characterization of peroxidized lipids in Bruch's membrane. Retina 1999; 19:141–147.

64. Holz FG, Bellmann C, Margaritidis M et al. Patterns of increased in vivo fundus autofluorescence in the junctional zone of geographic atrophy associated with age-related macular degeneration. Graefes Arch Clin Exp Ophthalmol 1999; 237:145–152.

65. Moore DJ, Hussain AA, Marshall J. Age-related variation in the hydraulic conductivity of Bruch's membrane. Invest Ophthalmol Vis Sci 1995; 36:1290–1297.

66. Starita C, Hussain AA, Patmore A et al. Localization of the site of major resistance to fluid transport in Bruch's membrane. Invest Ophthalmol Vis Sci 1997; 38:762–767.

67. Marshall J, Hussain AA, Starita C et al. (eds) The retinal pigment epithelium: function and disease. New York: Oxford University Press; 1998.

68. Grunwald JE, Hariprasad SM, Dupont J. Effect of aging on foveolar choroidal circulation. Arch Ophthalmol 1998; 116:150–154.

69. Curcio CA, Millican CL. Basal linear deposit and large drusen are specific for early age-related maculopathy. Arch Ophthalmol 1999; 117:329–339.

70. Zarbin MA. Age-related macular degeneration: review of pathogenesis. Eur J Ophthalmol 1998; 8:199–206.

71. Löffler KU, Lee WR. Basal linear deposit in the human macula. Graefes Arch Clin Exp Ophthalmol 1986; 224:493–501.

72. van der Schaft TL, Mooy CM, de Bruijn WC et al. Immunohistochemical light and electron microscopy of basal laminar deposit. Graefes Arch Clin Exp Ophthalmol 1994; 232:40–46.

73. Hirata A, Feeney-Burns L. Autoradiographic studies of aged primate macular retinal pigment epithelium. Invest Ophthalmol Vis Sci 1992; 33:2079–2090.

74. Löffler KU, Lee WR. Terminology of sub-RPE deposits: do we all speak the same language? Br J Ophthalmol 1998; 82:1104–1105.

75. Bressler NM, Silva JC, Bressler SB et al. Clinicopathologic correlation of drusen and retinal pigment epithelial abnormalities in age-related macular degeneration. Retina 1994; 14:130–142.

76. Green WR, Key SN III. Senile macular degeneration: a histopathologic study. Trans Am Ophthalmol Soc 1997; 75:180–254.

77. Sarks JP, Sarks SH, Killingsworth MC. Evolution of soft drusen in age-related macular degeneration. Eye 1994; 8:269–283.

78. El Baba F, Green WR, Fleischmann J et al. Clinicopathologic correlation of lipidization and detachment of the retinal pigment epithelium. Am J Ophthalmol 1986; 101:576–583.

79. Sarks JP, Sarks SH, Killingsworth M. Evolution of geographic atrophy of the retinal pigment epithelium. Eye 1988; 2:552–577.

80. Greaves AH, Sarks JP, Sarks SH. Adult vitelliform macular degeneration: a clinical spectrum. Aust NZ J Ophthalmol 1990; 18:171–178.

81. Penfold PL, Killingsworth MC, Sarks SH. Senile macular degeneration: the involvement of immunocompetent cells. Graefes Arch Clin Exp Ophthalmol 1985; 223:69–76.

82. Sarks JP, Sarks SH, Killingsworth MC. Morphology of early choroidal neovascularisation in age-related macular degeneration. Eye 1997; 11:515–522.

83. Killingsworth MC, Sarks JP, Sarks SH. Macrophages related to Bruch's membrane in age-related macular degeneration. Eye 1990; 4:613–621.

84. Bressler NM, Bressler SB, Seddon JM et al. Drusen characteristics in patients with exudative versus nonexudative age-related macular degeneration. Retina 1988; 8:108–114.

85. Chuang MD, Bird AC. The pathogenesis of tears of the retinal pigment epithelium. Am J Ophthalmol 1988; 105:285–290.

86. Eye Disease Case-Control Study Group. Risk factors for neovascular age-related macular degeneration. Arch Ophthalmol 1992; 110:1701–1708.

87. Macular Photocoagulation Study Group. Risk factors for choroidal neovascularization in the second eye of patients with juxtafoveal or subfoveal choroidal neovascularization secondary to age-related macular degeneration. Arch Ophthalmol 1997; 115:741–747.

88. Barondes M, Pauleikhoff D, Chisholm IC et al. Bilaterality of drusen. Br J Ophthalmol 1990; 74:180–182.

89. Arnold JJ, Quaranta M, Soubrane G et al. Indocyanine green angiography of drusen. Am J Ophthalmol 1997; 124:344–356.

90. Gass JDM, Jallow S, Davis B. Adult vitelliform macular detachment occurring in patients with basal laminar drusen. Am J Ophthalmol 1985; 99:445–459.

91. Dusek J, Streicher T, Schmidt K. Hereditäre Drusen der Bruchschen Membran II Untersuchung von Semidtünnschnitten und elektronenmikroskopischen Ergebnissen. Klin Monatsbl Augenheilkd 1982; 181:79–83.

92. Streicher T, Schmidt K, Dusek J. Hereditäre Drusen der Bruchschen Membran. I. Klinische und lichtmikroskopische Beobachtungen. Klin Monatsbl Augenheilkd 1982; 181:27–31.

93. Sarks SH, Arnold JJ, Killinsworth MC et al. Early drusen formation in the normal and aging eye and their relationship to age-related maculopathy: a clinicopathological study. Br J Ophthalmol 1999; 83:358–368.

94. Hageman GS, Mullins RF. Molecular composition of drusen as related to substructural phenotype. Mol Vis 1999; 5:28–37.

95. Coffey AJH, Brownstein S. The prevalence of macular drusen in postmortem eyes. Am J Ophthalmol 1986; 102:164–171.

96. Bressler NM, Munoz B, Maguire MG et al. Five-year incidence and disappearance of drusen and retinal pigment epithelial abnormalities, Chesapeake Bay Watermen study. Arch Ophthalmol 1995; 113:301–308.

97. Capon MRC, Marshall J, Krafft JI et al. Sorsby's fundus dystrophy: a light and electron microscopic study. Ophthalmology 1989; 96:1769–1777.

98. Sarks SH. Drusen patterns predisposing to geographic atrophy of the retinal pigment epithelium. Aust J Ophthalmol 1982; 10:91–97.

99. Leys A, Vanrenterghem Y, Van Damme B et al. Fundus changes in membranoproliferative glomerulonephritis type II: a fluorescein angiographic study of 23 patients. Graefes Arch Clin Exp Ophthalmol 1991; 229:406–410.

100. Sarks SH. Drusen and their relationship to senile macular degeneration. Aust J Ophthalmol 1980; 8:117–130.

101. Bird AC. Pathogenesis of retinal pigment epithelial detachment in the elderly: the relevance of Bruch's membrane change, Doyne lecture. Eye 1991; 5:1–12.

102. Casswell AG, Kohen D, Bird AC. Retinal pigment epithelial detachments in the elderly: classification and outcome. Br J Ophthalmol 1985; 69:397–403.

103. Hartnett ME, Weiter JJ, Garsd A et al. Classification of retinal pigment epithelial detachments associated with drusen. Graefes Arch Clin Exp Ophthalmol 1992; 230:11–19.

104. Holz FG, Wolfensberger TJ, Piguet B et al. Bilateral macular drusen in age-related macular degeneration: prognosis and risk factors. Ophthalmology 1994; 101:1522–1528.

105. Duvall J, Tso MOM. Cellular mechanisms of resolution of drusen after laser photocoagulation: an experimental study. Arch Ophthalmol 1985; 103:694–703.

106. Ruskovic D, Ulbig MW, Mueller AJ et al. Cellular response to hard drusen and lipid deposits in human Bruch's membrane following diode laser photocoagulation. Invest Ophthalmol Vis Sci 1998; 39 (suppl.):369.

107. The Choroidal Neovascularization Prevention Trial Research Group. Laser treatment in eyes with large drusen: short-term effects seen in a pilot randomized clinical trial, Ophthalmology 1998; 105:11–23.

108. The Complications of Age-Related Macular Degeneration Prevention Trial Study Group. The Complications of Age-Related Macular Degeneration Prevention Trial (CAPT): rationale, design, methodology. Clin Trials 2004; 1:91–107.

108a. Figueroa MS, Regueras A, Bertrand J et al. Laser photocoagulation for macular soft drusen: updated results. Retina 1997; 17:378–384.

108b. Ho AC, Maguire MG, Yoken J et al. Laser-induced drusen reduction improves visual function at 1 year. Ophthalmology 1999; 106:1367–1374.

108c. Klein R, Klein BEK, Jensen SC. The relation of cardiovascular disease and its risk factors to the 5-year incidence of age-related maculopathy, Beaver Dam Eye Study. Ophthalmology 1997; 104:1804–1812.

108d. Little HL, Showman JM, Brown BW et al. A pilot randomized controlled study on the effect of laser photocoagulation of confluent soft macular drusen. Ophthalmology 1997; 104:623–631.

108e. Owen SL, Guymer R, Gross-Jendroska M et al. Fluorescein angiographic abnormalities after prophylactic macular photocoagulation for high-risk age-related maculopathy. Am J Ophthalmol 1999; 127:681–687.

109. Olk RJ, Friberg TR, Stickney KL et al. Therapeutic benefits of infrared (810-nm) diode laser macular grid photocoagulation in prophylactic treatment of nonexudative age-related macular degeneration: two-year results of a randomized pilot study. Ophthalmology 1999; 106:2082–2090.

110. Arnold JJ, Sarks SH, Killingsworth MC et al. Reticular pseudodrusen: a risk factor in age-related maculopathy. Retina 1995; 15:183–191.

111. Mimoun G, Soubrane G, Coscas G. Macular drusen. J Fr Ophtalmol 1990; 13:511–530.

112. Dickinson AJ, Sparrow JM, Duke AM et al. Prevalence of age-related maculopathy at two points in time in an elderly British population. Eye 1997; 11:301–314.

113. Maguire MG. More pieces for the age-related macular degeneration puzzle. Ophthalmology 1997; 104:5–6.

114. Sarraf D, Gin T, Yu F et al. Long-term drusen study. Retina 1999; 19:513–519.

115. The Age-Related Eye Disease Study Research Group. Report no. 16. Ocular risk factors for development of neovascular age-related macular degeneration in the fellow eyes of patients with unilateral neovascular AMD. AREDS Report No. 20. Arch Ophthalmol 2005; in press.

116. Pauleikhoff D, Zuels S, Sheraidah GS et al. Correlation between biochemical composition and fluorescein binding of deposits in Bruch's membrane. Ophthalmology 1992; 99:1548–1553.

117. Mullins RF, Johnson LV, Anderson DH et al. Characterization of drusen-associated glycoconjugates. Ophthalmology 1998; 104:288–298.

118. Hageman GS. Pathogenesis and treatment of age-related macular degeneration. Paper presented at the Twenty-eighth Anniversary Meeting, The Wilmer Ophthalmological Institute at Johns Hopkins, June 4–6, 1998.

119. Mullins RF, Hageman GS. Human ocular drusen possess novel core domains with a distinct carbohydrate composition. J Histochem Cytochem 1999; 47:1533–1539.

120. Hageman GS, Mullins RF, Russell SR et al. Vitronectin is a constituent of ocular drusen and the vitronectin gene is expressed in human retinal pigmented epithelial cells. FASEB J 1999; 13:477–484.

121. Penfold PL, Killingsworth MC, Sarks SH. Senile macular degeneration: the involvement of giant cells in atrophy of the retinal pigment epithelium. Invest Ophthalmol Vis Sci 1986; 27:364–371.

122. Spraul CW, Lang GE, Grossniklaus HE. Morphometric analysis of the choroid, Bruch's membrane, and retinal pigment epithelium in eyes with age-related macular degeneration. Invest Ophthalmol Vis Sci 1996; 37:2724–2735.

123. Spraul CW, Lang GE, Grossniklaus HE et al. Histologic and morphometric analysis of the choroid, Bruch's membrane, and retinal pigment epithelium in postmortem eyes with age-related macular degeneration and histologic examination of surgically excised choroidal neovascular membranes. Surv Ophthalmol 1999; 44 (suppl. 1):10–32.

124. Hayreh SS. In vivo choroidal circulation and its watershed zones. Eye 1990; 4:273–289.

125. McLeod DS, Lutty GA. High-resolution histologic analysis of the human choroidal vasculature. Invest Ophthalmol Vis Sci 1994; 35:3799–3811.

126. Pauleikhoff D, Chen JC, Chisholm IH et al. Choroidal perfusion abnormality with age-related Bruch's membrane change. Ophthalmology 1990; 109:211–217.

127. Staurenghi G, Bottoni F, Lonati C et al. Drusen and choroidal filling defects: a cross-sectional survey. Ophthalmologica 1992; 205:178–186.

128. Pauleikhoff D, Spital M, Radermacher M et al. Regression of the choriocapillaris in age-related macular degeneration. Invest Ophthalmol Vis Sci 1997; 38 (suppl.):967.

129. Henkind P, Gartner S. The relationship between retinal pigment epithelium and the choriocapillaris. Trans Ophthalmol Soc UK 1983; 103:444–447.

130. Glaser BM. Extracellular modulating factors and the control of intraocular neovascularization. Arch Ophthalmol 1988; 106:603–607.

131. Friedman E, Krupsky S, Lane AM et al. Ocular blood flow velocity in age-related macular degeneration. Ophthalmology 1995; 102:640–646.

132. Chen JC, Fitzke FW, Pauleikhoff D et al. Functional loss in age-related Bruch's membrane change with choroidal perfusion defect. Invest Ophthalmol Vis Sci 1992; 33:334–340.

133. Steinmetz RL, Haimovici R, Jubb C et al. Symptomatic abnormalities of dark adaptation in patients with age-related Bruch's membrane change. Br J Ophthalmol 1993; 77:549–554.

134. Remulla JFC, Gaudio AR, Miller S et al. Foveal electroretinograms and choroidal perfusion characteristics in fellow eyes of patients with unilateral neovascular age-related macular degeneration. Br J Ophthalmol 1995; 79:558–561.

135. Piguet B, Palmvang TB, Chisholm IH et al. Evolution of age-related macular degeneration with choroidal perfusion abnormality. Am J Ophthalmol 1992; 113:657–663.

136. Sunness JS, Massof RW, Johnson MA et al. Diminished foveal sensitivity may predict the development of advanced age-related macular degeneration. Ophthalmology 1989; 96:375–381.

137. Sunness JS, Johnson MA, Massof RW et al. Retinal sensitivity over drusen and nondrusen areas: a study using fundus perimetry. Arch Ophthalmol 1988; 106:1081–1084.

138. Schatz H, McDonald HR. Atrophic macular degeneration: rate of spread of geographic atrophy and visual loss. Ophthalmology 1989; 96:1541–1551.

139. Sunness JS, Rubin GS, Applegate CA et al. Visual function abnormalities and prognosis in eyes with age-related geographic atrophy of the macula and good visual acuity. Ophthalmology 1997; 104:1677–1691.

140. Maguire P, Vine AK. Geographic atrophy of the retinal pigment epithelium. Am J Ophthalmol 1986; 102:621–625.

141. Sunness JS, Applegate CA, Haselwood D et al. Fixation patterns and reading rates in eyes with central scotomas from advanced atrophic age-related macular degeneration and Stargardt's disease. Ophthalmology 1996; 103:1458–1466.

142. Weiter JJ, Delori F, Dorey CK. Central sparing in annular macular degeneration. Am J Ophthalmol 1988; 106:286–292.

143. Snodderly DM. Evidence for protection against age-related macular degeneration by carotenoids and antioxidant vitamins. Am J Clin Nutr 1995; 62 (suppl.):1448–1461.

144. Hyman LG, Lilienfeld AM, Ferris FL III et al. Senile macular degeneration: a case-control study. Am J Epidemiol 1983; 118:213–227.

145. Harris MJ, Robins D, Dieter JM Jr et al. Eccentric visual acuity in patients with macular disease. Ophthalmology 1985; 92:1550–1553.

146. Sunness JS, Gonzalez-Baron J, Applegate CA et al. Enlargement of atrophy and visual acuity loss in the geographic atrophy form of age-related macular degeneration. Ophthalmology 1999; 106:1768–1779.

147. Weiter JJ, Wing GL, Trempe CL et al. Visual acuity related to retinal distance from the fovea in macular disease. Ann Ophthalmol 1984; 16:174–176.

148. Sunness JS, Gonzalez-Baron J, Bressler NM et al. The development of choroidal neovascularization in eyes with geographic atrophy form of age-related macular degeneration. Ophthalmology 1999; 106:910–919.

149. Shuttleworth GN, Luhishi EA, Harrad RA. Do patients with age-related maculopathy and cataract benefit from cataract surgery? Br J Ophthalmol 1998; 82:611–616.

150. Lewis H, Straatsma BR, Foos RY et al. The prevalence of macular drusen in postmortem eyes. Am J Ophthalmol 1986; 102:801–803.

151. Alpha-tocopherol Beta Carotene Study. NEJM The Alpha-Tocopherol, Beta Carotene Cancer Prevention Study Group. The effect of vitamin E and beta carotene on the incidence of lung cancer and other cancers in male smokers. N Engl J Med 1994; 330:1029–1035.

152. Fine AM, Elman MJ, Ebert JE et al. Earliest symptoms caused by neovascular membranes in the macula. Arch Ophthalmol 1986; 104:513–514.

153. Achard OA, Safran AB, Duret FC, Ragama E. Role of the completion phenomenon in the evaluation of Amsler grid results. Am J Ophthalmol 1995; 120:322–329.

154. Schuchard RA. Validity and interpretation of Amsler grid report. Arch Ophthalmol 1993; 111:776–780.

155. Goldstein M, Loewenstein A, Barak A et al. Results of a multicenter clinical trial to evaluate the preferential hyperacuity perimeter for detection of age-related macular degeneration. Retina 2005; 25:296–303.

156. Preferential Hyperacuity Perimetry (PHP) Research Group. Preferential Hyperacuity Perimeter (PreView PHP™) for detecting choroidal neovascularization study. Ophthalmology 2005; in press.

Neovascular (Exudative) Age-Related Macular Degeneration

Neil M. Bressler
Susan B. Bressler
Stuart L. Fine

EPIDEMIOLOGY

Age-related macular degeneration (AMD) is the major cause of severe visual loss in older adults.[1] Most AMD patients have macular drusen or retinal pigment epithelial abnormalities or both.[2] However, approximately 10% of AMD patients manifest the neovascular form of the disease.[3] Neovascular AMD includes choroidal neovascularization (CNV) and associated manifestations such as retinal pigment epithelial detachment (PED), retinal pigment epithelial tears, fibrovascular disciform scarring, and vitreous hemorrhage.[2] The vast majority of people with severe vision loss (20/200 or worse in either eye) from AMD have the neovascular form.[3]

RISK FACTORS

The prevalence of AMD-associated vision loss in at least one eye increases with age. For example, AMD was the leading cause of blindness in white (prevalence, 2.7 per 1000; 95% confidence interval [CI], 1.2 to 5.4) but not black subjects randomly selected to participate in the Baltimore Eye Survey. In this study, AMD resulting in blindness affected 3% of all white subjects 80 years of age or older.[4]

AMD may be a multifactorial syndrome with different causative factors damaging the macula and resulting in common clinical manifestations that are recognized clinically as AMD. Risk factors implicated in clinical and laboratory studies include drusen, visible (but not ultraviolet) injury, micronutrient deficiency as measured in blood serum levels or by dietary history, cigarette smoking, family history (genetic predisposition[5]), and cardiovascular risk factors (including systemic hypertension).[6,7] More detailed information regarding the epidemiology of AMD is reviewed in Chapter 58.

CLINICAL (INCLUDING BIOMICROSCOPIC) PRESENTATION

Overview

Blurred vision and distortion, especially distorted near vision, are the symptoms most patients with CNV notice first.[2,8] Patients may also complain of decreased vision, micropsia, metamorphopsia, or a scotoma; however, many times they volunteer no symptoms or report only vague visual complaints.[8] Symptoms generally arise from subretinal fluid, intraretinal fluid, blood, or destruction of photoreceptors and the retinal pigment epithelium (RPE) by fibrous or fibrovascular tissue.[9–12] In some cases, areas of distortion or scotoma can be mapped out on an Amsler grid. Visual acuity, although frequently decreased, may not always be affected. Functional vision generally declines in accordance with Snellen visual acuity. Thus patients with poor Snellen acuity generally report decreased ability to perform functional tasks (e.g., face recognition, telling time) with the affected eye.[38]

In some patients with AMD, CNV may appear as a gray-green elevation of tissue deep to the retina with overlying detachment of the neurosensory retina (Fig. 61-1). The gray-green color may arise from hyperplastic RPE in response to the CNV,[13] as has typically been seen in patients, usually younger individuals, with ocular histoplasmosis syndrome (OHS), pathologic myopia, and other conditions complicated by CNV. This gray-green appearance is not always present in older individuals with AMD. Often, the presence of blood or lipid or a sensory retinal detachment in an elderly patient with vision loss indicates the presence of CNV. The CNV capillary network may become more apparent when the overlying RPE has atrophied. Occasionally, a shallow neurosensory detachment may be the only presenting sign of underlying CNV. Elevated RPE, also termed a *pigment epithelial detachment* (PED), even without overlying subretinal fluid, may also suggest the presence of CNV to be identified subsequently by a fluorescein angiogram. RPE folds beneath a shallow RPE elevation usually indicate the presence of CNV.[14] These subtle clinical findings can easily be missed without careful stereoscopic slit-lamp biomicroscopic examination, facilitated with a contact lens.

Retinal pigment epithelial detachments

Retinal PEDs appear clinically as sharply demarcated, dome-shaped elevations of the RPE (Fig. 61-2). They usually transilluminate if they are filled with serous fluid only. Often, there is accompanying RPE atrophy and "pigment figure" formation. Pigment figures, a reticulated pattern of increased pigmentation extending radially over the PED, indicate chronicity of disease and probably have no prognostic significance. Although an overlying sensory retinal detachment may be a clue to the presence of CNV beneath a PED,[15] sometimes a shallow

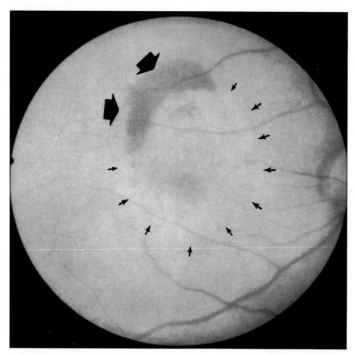

Fig. 61-1 Fundus photograph of choroidal neovascularization. Note area of hemorrhage (large arrows), as well as neurosensory retinal detachment (small arrows). (Reproduced from Elman MJ. Age-related macular degeneration. Int Ophthalmol Clin 1986; 26:117–144.)

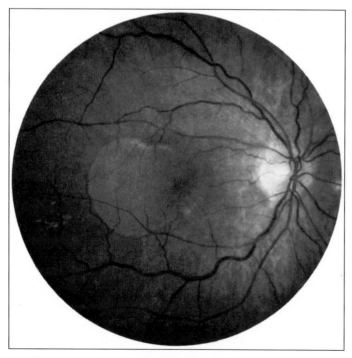

Fig. 61-2 Fundus photograph in which a round, sharply demarcated mound indicates the detached retinal pigment epithelium. (Reproduced from Bressler NM, Bressler SB, Fine SL. Age-related macular degeneration. Surv Ophthalmol 1988; 32:375–413.[2])

neurosensory detachment may occur as a result of breakdown of the physiologic RPE pump or from disruption of the tight junctions between adjacent RPE cells in the absence of CNV. Unlike a PED, the borders of a neurosensory detachment are not sharply demarcated. The presence of a PED may or may not be a feature of CNV. The fluorescein angiographic pattern (see subsequent discussion) can differentiate a drusenoid PED,[16] which does not have CNV, from a fibrovascular PED, which is a form of occult CNV,[17] as well as from a serous PED, which may or may not overlie an area with CNV.[17] Several clinical signs suggest the presence of CNV underlying an area of PED identified biomicroscopically, including overlying sensory retinal detachment and lipid, blood, and chorioretinal folds radiating from the PED.[2] Blood within or surrounding a PED implies the presence of CNV (Fig. 61-3). When confined to the sub-RPE space, the blood may appear as a discretely elevated, green or dark red mound. The hemorrhage can dissect through the RPE into the subsensory retinal space or into the retina. Rarely, blood may pass through the retina into the vitreous cavity, causing extensive vitreous hemorrhage. The Submacular Surgery Trials (SST) Research Group suggested that this event was more likely in predominantly hemorrhagic lesions that were large (>12 disc areas) or associated with very poor visual acuity (worse than 20/1280 Snellen equivalent).[18]

Breakthrough vitreous hemorrhage

In most cases of neovascular AMD, the peripheral visual field remains unaffected. However, if bleeding breaks through the retina into the vitreous cavity, patients may complain of severe and sudden visual loss involving the peripheral visual field, as well as the central field. This may be accompanied by pain believed to result from stretching of the nerve fibers within the choroid.[19]

Massive subretinal hemorrhage

Massive subretinal hemorrhage is an unusual complication of neovascular AMD. If – extremely rarely – total hemorrhagic retinal detachment occurs, secondary angle-closure glaucoma may develop. These patients may report sudden visual loss followed by pain.[20] Anticoagulation therapy may contribute to massive subretinal hemorrhage. In a report by el Baba et al.,[21] 19% of AMD patients with massive subretinal hemorrhage were taking sodium warfarin or aspirin. Although sodium warfarin therapy may have contributed to the massive subretinal hemorrhage, the antiplatelet therapy was likely a chance association because several Macular Photocoagulation Study (MPS) reports did not observe any increased risk of hemorrhage associated with the use of aspirin.[22–24] Furthermore, comparing baseline characteristics in study participants with predominantly choroidal neovascular lesions in the SST Group N Trial[25] with participants with predominantly hemorrhagic lesions,[18] no difference in use of aspirin was detected. Thus, patients with AMD who need to follow a regimen of aspirin therapy should continue to do so without unnecessary fear of any evidence to suggest they will increase their risk of vitreous hemorrhage.

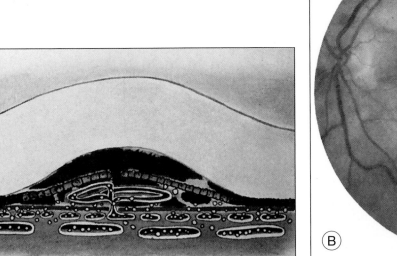
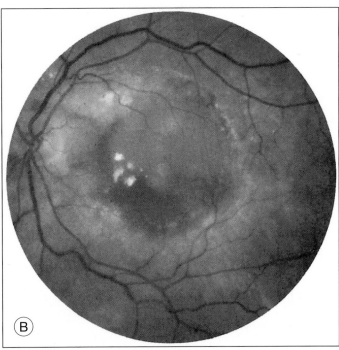

Fig. 61-3 Hemorrhagic retinal pigment epithelial detachment (PED). A, Sketch of hemorrhagic detachment in which the blood has also dissected underneath the sensory retina. B, Fundus photograph of hemorrhagic PED. (Reproduced from Bressler NM, Bressler SB, Fine SL. Age-related macular degeneration. Surv Ophthalmol 1988; 32:375–413.[2])

Retinal pigment epithelial tears

RPE dehiscence or tears have been described as a complication associated with CNV, often in an eye with a serous or fibrovascular PED, and secondary to or unassociated with laser photocoagulation.[26-30] Gass[31] suggested that CNV underlying a detached RPE can contribute to RPE tear formation. Tears occur at the junction of attached and detached RPE, perhaps when the PED can no longer resist the stretching forces from the fluid in the sub-RPE space emanating from the underlying occult CNV (Fig. 61-4) or from the contractile forces of the underlying fibrovascular tissue that may be intimately associated or entwined with the overlying RPE. When the RPE tears, the free edge of the RPE retracts and rolls toward the mound of fibrovascular tissue. Acutely, a serous detachment of the sensory retina may be caused by the leaking of fluid from the exposed choriocapillaris.[16] This is rarely seen after a few days following the tear.

Disciform scars

Histologically, CNV is usually accompanied by fibrous tissue, even when no fibrous tissue is readily apparent on initial presentation to an ophthalmologist.[9,33,34] This fibrous tissue may be accompanied by CNV (fibrovascular tissue) or not (fibroglial tissue).[9] The fibrous tissue complex may be beneath the RPE (usually proliferating within the inner aspect of an abnormally thickened Bruch's membrane), termed *type I* by Gass, or between the RPE and the photoreceptors, termed *type II* by Gass.[31] While some people speculate that these types differentiate classic CNV from occult CNV,[35,36] there is little evidence to support that these histologic types are always differentiated by histopathologic correlation.[37] Often, over time, the plane of the RPE is destroyed by the fibrovascular or fibroglial tissue, so the location of the CNV with respect to the RPE can no longer be identified readily. When the fibrous tissue becomes apparent clinically, the CNV and fibrous tissue complex may be termed a *disciform scar*.

Clinically, disciform lesions may vary in color, although typically they appear white to yellow. Hyperpigmented areas may be present depending on the degree of RPE hyperplasia within the scar tissue. Disciform fibrovascular scars may continue to grow, with neovascularization recurring along the edge, invading previously unaffected areas (Fig. 61-5). Varying degrees of subretinal hemorrhage and lipid may overlie or surround the scar. Occasionally, fibrovascular scars may precipitate massive transudation of fluid, mimicking a retinal detachment. The scars may be accompanied by massive lipid, as might be seen in retinal telangiectasis from Coats disease, and hence are sometimes called a "senile Coats response" in AMD. Disciform scars occasionally masquerade as choroidal tumors when much pigment is seen.[31] Not infrequently, anastomoses are observed between the retina and the fibrovascular tissue.[12] As a rule, most fibrovascular scars involve the fovea and cause severe visual loss. However, surviving islands of intact photoreceptor cells noted histologically may explain the better visual performance than would be predicted from the morphologic appearance alone in some scars. Reading vision, rarely better than 20/200, becomes severely compromised in most cases with extensive scars.

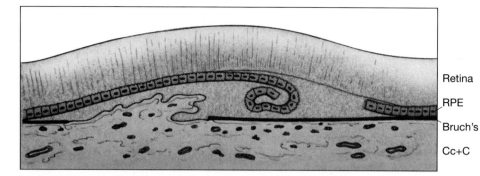

Fig. 61-4 Sketch of tear or rip of the retinal pigment epithelium (RPE), showing contracted RPE tear. Cc + C, choriocapillaris and choroid. (Reproduced from Bressler NM, Bressler SB, Fine SL. Age-related macular degeneration. Surv Ophthalmol 1988; 32:375–413.[2])

Retina

RPE

Bruch's

Cc+C

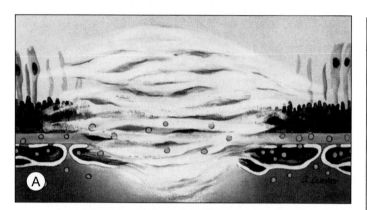

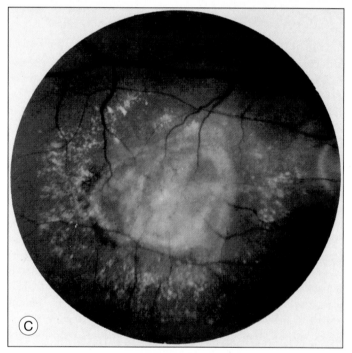

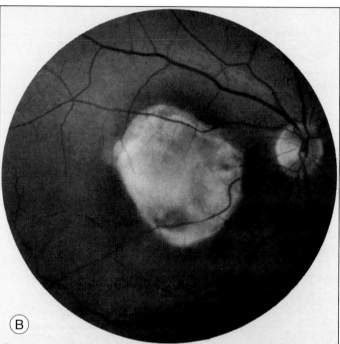

Fig. 61-5 Disciform scar. A, Sketch demonstrating that most of the sensory retina, pigment epithelium, and inner choroid has been replaced by a fibrovascular scar. B, Fundus photograph of a disciform scar after choroidal neovascularization. C, Fundus photograph of a disciform scar in which continued subretinal fluid and lipid from persistent choroidal neovascularization at the periphery of the fibrous tissue can be seen. (Reproduced from Bressler NM, Bressler SB, Fine SL. Age-related macular degeneration. Surv Ophthalmol 1988; 32:375–413.[2])

FLUORESCEIN ANGIOGRAPHIC FEATURES

Overview

Whenever one suspects CNV for which treatment might be indicated, stereoscopic fluorescein angiography should be performed promptly. Fluorescein angiography frequently allows one to determine the pattern (classic or occult), boundaries (well defined or poorly defined), composition (e.g., predominantly CNV, predominantly classic CNV, predominantly CNV with a minimally classic composition, predominantly CNV with an occult with no classic composition, predominantly hemorrhagic) and location of the neovascular lesions with respect to the geometric center of the foveal avascular zone (FAZ). High-quality stereoscopic fluorescein angiograms, together with meticulous contact lens examination, facilitate detecting obvious and subtle features of CNV on angiography.[17,38,39] It should be noted that the descriptive terms below refer to patterns of fluorescence on fluorescein angiography that have been shown to be reliable and reproducible in multicenter clinical trials,[17,40,41] and in practice, and are not related to terms based on other imaging such as indocyanine green angiography, ocular coherence tomography, histopathology, or immunohistochemistry.

Classic choroidal neovascularization

The fluorescein angiographic appearance of classic CNV consists of a discrete, well-demarcated focal area of hyperfluorescence that can be discerned in the early phases of the angiogram, sometimes before dye has completely filled the retinal vessels during choroidal filling.[17,40,41] Although fluorescein can occasionally be observed within the actual capillary network of CNV in the early phase of the angiogram (Fig. 61-6A), the ability to visualize the appearance of actual new vessels is not needed to diagnose classic CNV and is not a specific feature of classic versus occult CNV.[17,40-42] Since both classic and occult patterns of CNV contain new vessels histologically, early-phase angiography may be able to demonstrate these vessels in either pattern. As the angiogram is evaluated within the area of classic CNV, hyperfluorescence increases in intensity and extends beyond the boundaries of the hyperfluorescent area identified in earlier phases of the angiogram through mid- and late-phase frames. Fluorescein may also pool in subsensory retinal fluid overlying the classic CNV (Fig. 61-6B), best seen when visualizing early- and late-phase frames of classic CNV on stereoscopic images. This presentation of classic CNV is in contrast to the appearance of an area of RPE atrophy on fluorescein angiography. RPE atrophy, like classic CNV, is hyperfluorescent during the early phase of the angiogram (Fig. 61-7A). The increased fluorescence through the atrophic patch results from increased transmission of fluorescein through an overlying RPE with a reduced amount of pigment that normally obscures the choroidal blush (sometimes termed a window, or transmission, defect). Unlike the increase in extent and intensity of hyperfluorescence due to leakage from the fluorescence of classic CNV, RPE atrophy does not show leakage of fluorescein at its boundaries through the mid- and late-phase frames. The fluorescence fades after several minutes (Fig. 61-7B), without leakage of fluorescein beyond the boundaries of hyperfluorescence defined in the early stages. Two other lesions in AMD that may show an area of discrete hyperfluorescence in the early phase of the angiogram include a serous PED and a rip or tear of the RPE (angiographic features that differentiate these abnormalities from classic CNV are discussed later). Neither one of these latter abnormalities should show fluorescein leakage in later phases of the angiogram at the boundary of the hyperfluorescence noted in earlier phases.

Occult choroidal neovascularization

Occult CNV refers to two hyperfluorescent patterns on fluorescein angiography.[17,40,41] The first pattern, termed a *fibrovascular pigment epithelial detachment* (FVPED), is best appreciated with stereoscopic views, usually at approximately 1 to 2 min after dye injection. It appears as an irregular elevation of the RPE, often stippled with hyperfluorescent dots (Fig. 61-8). The boundaries may or may not show leakage in the late-phase frames as fluorescein collects within the fibrous tissue or pools in the subretinal space overlying the FVPED. The exact boundaries of a FVPED can usually be determined most accurately only when fluorescence sharply outlines the elevated RPE. The amount of elevation depends on the quality of the stereoscopic photographs and the thickness of the fibrovascular tissue. Stereoscopic pairs of fluorescein angiogram frames can sometimes facilitate identification of the boundaries of the elevated RPE, although

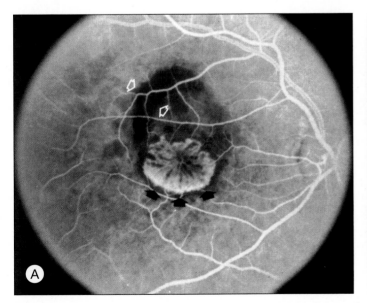
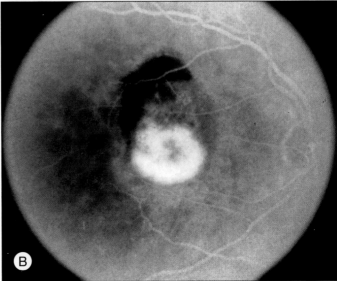

Fig. 61-6 A, Early transit phase of fluorescein angiogram showing fine net of vessels corresponding to part of choroidal neovascular lesion (black arrows). B, Late phase of the fluorescein angiogram, demonstrating an increase in the degree and size of fluorescence. In both A and B, there is blocked fluorescence resulting from overlying hemorrhage (white arrows). (Reproduced from Elman MJ. Age-related macular degeneration. Int Ophthalmol Clin 1986; 26:117–144.)

not always, as the elevation can slope gradually down to the normal level of the RPE. The second pattern, late leakage of an undetermined source (Fig. 61-9), refers to late choroidal-based leakage in which there is no clearly identifiable classic CNV or FVPED in the early or mid phase of the angiogram to account for an area of leakage in the late phase. Often, this pattern of occult CNV can appear as speckled hyperfluorescence with pooling of dye in the subretinal space overlying the speckles. Usually, the boundaries of this type of CNV cannot be determined precisely, and a lesion with this component should not be considered for photocoagulation treatment if it contributes to poorly demarcated boundaries of the lesion.

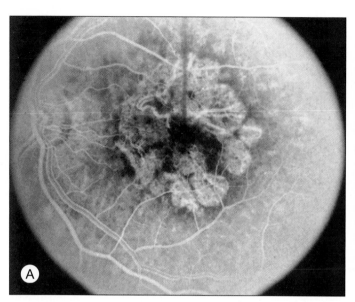

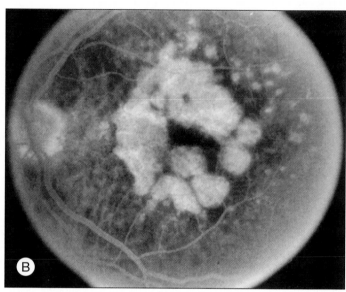

Fig. 61-7 A, Transit phase of fluorescein angiogram, showing hyperfluorescence corresponding to atrophic zones of the retinal pigment epithelium (transmission, or window, defect) and easily visualized choroidal vessels (too large to be vessels of choroidal neovascularization). B, Hypofluorescence does not increase in size and fades with the later phases of the angiogram. This is in contrast to the pattern seen in choroidal neovascularization (Fig. 61-5). (Reproduced from Elman MJ. Age-related macular degeneration. Int Ophthalmol Clin 1986; 26:117–144.)

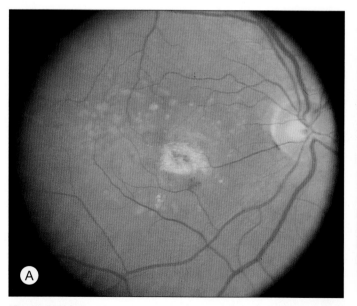

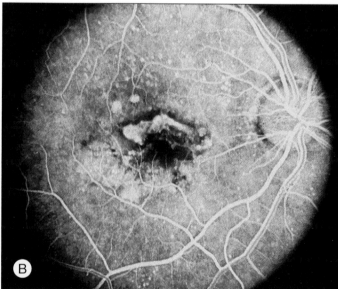

Fig. 61-8 Classic and occult choroidal neovascularization (CNV) with well-demarcated borders. A, Color photograph shows scar from prior photocoagulation surrounded by several clues to suggest recurrent CNV, including subretinal hemorrhage, subretinal lipid, irregular elevation of retinal pigment epithelium (RPE) below the area of prior laser treatment, and overlying subretinal fluid. B, Early phase of fluorescein angiogram shows area of classic CNV, scar from prior laser treatment, and irregular elevation of RPE with stippled hyperfluorescence representing fibrovascular pigment epithelial detachment (PED) inferior and temporal to the scar.

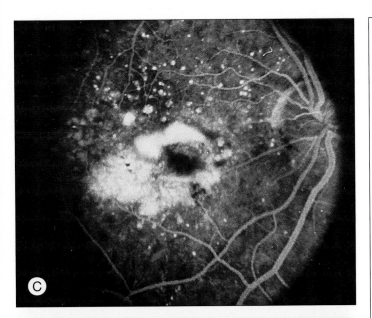

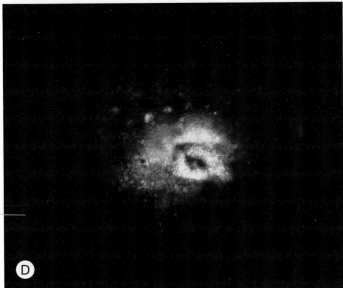

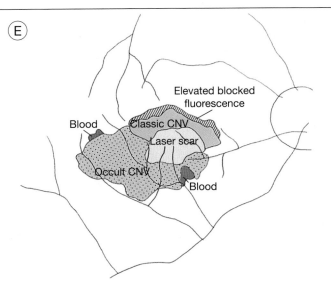

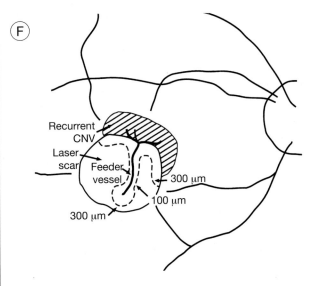

Angiographic eligibility criteria

Lesion must include some classic CNV.
    Eyes that did not undergo previous photocoagulation must have CNV underlying fovea; eyes that did undergo previous photocoagulation must have recurrent CNV underlying fovea or extension of original treatment to extrafoveal or juxtafoveal CNV must underlie fovea, with recurrent CNV <150 μm from foveal center.

Entire subfoveal CNV lesion must have well-demarcated boundaries.
    Eyes that did not undergo previous photocoagulation must have lesions ≤3.5 standard disc areas; eyes that did undergo previous photocoagulation must have lesion ≤6 standard disc areas (considering previous treatment scar, recurrent neovascular lesion, and area of additional treatment), and some area of uninvolved retina within 1500 μm of foveal center must remain untreated if treatment of neovascular lesion was applied according to protocol.

Ratio of CNV to other lesion components, ≥1.0.

Fig. 61-8—cont'd C, Stereoscopic photograph of the same eye 1 min after fluorescein injection. Note fluorescein leakage already apparent from classic CNV and increased intensity of stippled hyperfluorescence corresponding to fibrovascular PED. The boundaries of the fibrovascular PED remain well demarcated. D, Angiogram taken 10 min after fluorescein injection shows persistence of fluorescein staining and leakage within a sensory retinal detachment overlying the lesion. It is difficult to determine the precise demarcation of fluorescence outlining the elevated RPE from these photographs alone. Although a fairly well-demarcated border can be seen in C, the intensity of fluorescence at the boundary of elevated RPE is quite irregular in these late-phase photographs, with some areas fading relative to fluorescence of remaining areas of elevated RPE (D). E and F, Composite drawings using multiple stereoscopic photographs from angiogram show interpretation of the boundaries of the lesion. At each clock-hour, the boundary of the lesion is clearly demarcated; the lesion included classic CNV, which occupies the foveal center, and met all the angiographic eligibility criteria listed in the accompanying box. (Reproduced from Macular Photocoagulation Study Group. Subfoveal neovascular lesions in age-related macular degeneration: guidelines for evaluation and treatment in the Macular Photocoagulation Study. Arch Ophthalmol 1991; 109:1242–1257.[17])

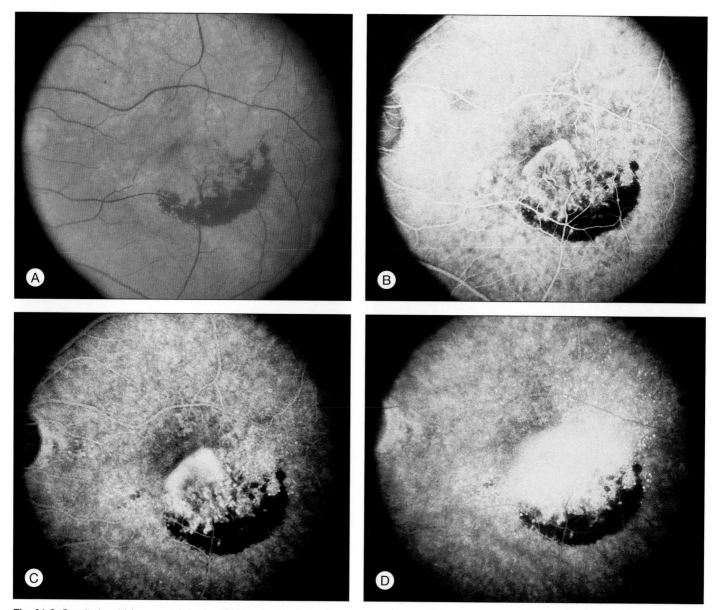

Fig. 61-9 Occult choroidal neovascularization (CNV) with poorly demarcated boundaries accompanied by classic CNV. A, Subretinal fluid and hemorrhage in eye with drusen. B, Early phase of fluorescein angiogram shows both feeder vessels to classic CNV and fibrovascular pigment epithelial detachment (PED). Blocked fluorescence due to thick blood obscures inferior boundary of occult CNV. C, Mid-phase stereoscopic photographs of angiogram show leakage from classic CNV. D, Late phase of angiogram shows other areas of late leakage of undetermined source with no discernible, discrete, well-demarcated area of hyperfluorescence from classic CNV or fibrovascular PED detectable in early or mid-phase frames of angiogram that might be considered a source of late leakage. (Reproduced from Macular Photocoagulation Study Group. Subfoveal neovascular lesions in age-related macular degeneration: guidelines for evaluation and treatment in the Macular Photocoagulation Study. Arch Ophthalmol 1991; 109:1242–1257.[17])

Other terms relevant to interpreting fluorescein angiography of choroidal neovascularization

The terms *lesion component* versus *lesion* are important to differentiate in the discussion of fluorescein interpretation and treatment of CNV.[17,40,41] Lesion component is classic or occult CNV or any of four angiographic features that could obscure the boundaries of classic or occult CNV. These four features include: (1) blood that is visible on color fundus photographs and thick enough to obscure the normal choroidal fluorescence; (2) hypofluorescence due to hyperplastic pigment or fibrous tissue, or blood not visible on color fundus photographs; (3) a serous detachment of the RPE (Fig. 61-10); and (4) scar from CNV which either stains or blocks fluorescence (depending on the extent of RPE within the scar). The first two of these four features block the angiographic view of the choroid, making it impossible to determine whether CNV is located in the area of this component. The bright, reasonably uniform, early hyperfluorescence associated with a serous detachment of the RPE (described later) may obscure hyperfluorescence from classic or occult CNV and therefore interfere with the ability to judge whether CNV extends under the area of the serous detachment. The term *lesion*, in contrast, refers to the entire complex of lesion components.

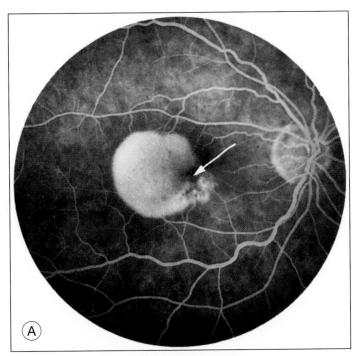
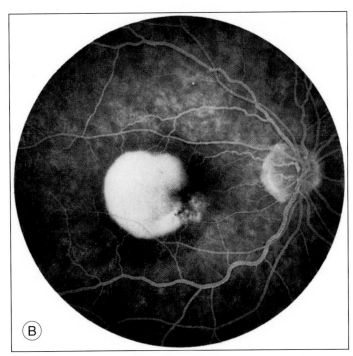

Fig. 61-10 Fluorescein angiogram of serous retinal pigment epithelial detachment. A, Early transit phase of a fluorescein angiogram demonstrates uniform fluorescence under the dome of the detachment. Note the deformation of the otherwise round detachment by a notch of the hyperfluorescence (arrow). B, Later phase of the fluorescein angiogram demonstrates persistent hyperfluorescence that does not extend beyond the margins of the hyperfluorescence seen in the early transit phase. (Reproduced from Bressler NM, Bressler SB, Fine SL. Age-related macular degeneration. Surv Ophthalmol 1988; 32:375–413.[2])

The terms *well-defined* (synonymous with *well-demarcated*) and *poorly defined* (synonymous with *poorly demarcated* or *ill-defined*) refer to a description of the boundaries of the entire lesion (not of individual lesion components). In a well-defined lesion, the entire boundary for 360 degrees is well demarcated (for example, Figs 61-8, 61-11, and 61-12). If the entire boundary is not well demarcated for 360 degrees, then the lesion is poorly defined (for example, Fig. 61-9). Thus the terms *well-defined* and *classic* should not be used interchangeably, nor should *poorly defined* and *occult*. *Well-defined* and *poorly defined* describe lesion boundaries (for a lesion that may be composed of classic CNV, or occult CNV, or both). Classic and occult CNV refer to patterns of fluorescence. In addition, the term *poorly defined* should not be used to describe situations in which blood blocks the ability to see fluorescence from CNV,[17,40,41] even though earlier publications had alluded to descriptions incorporating this possibility.[43]

The term *predominantly CNV* indicates that at least 50% of the lesion is composed of either classic CNV or occult CNV, or both, while the term *predominantly hemorrhagic* indicates that at least 50% of the lesion is composed of hemorrhage.[40,41] These terms are critical in the management of AMD (Fig. 61-13), since treatments for CNV with laser photocoagulation, photodynamic therapy (PDT), surgery, and intravitreal drugs have only been tested in lesions that are predominantly CNV or predominantly hemorrhagic. After determining whether a lesion's composition is predominantly CNV, it should be determined whether the lesion is predominantly classic, rather than minimally classic or

occult with no classic. If predominantly classic, then treatment could be considered with or without evidence of presumed recent disease progression (defined as evidence of blood associated with CNV, or definite visual acuity loss within 3 months, or definite growth of the lesion within 3 months). If minimally classic or occult with no classic, then treatment should only be considered with evidence of presumed recent disease progression, and usually only in relatively small lesions.

Retinal pigment epithelium detachments in age-related macular degeneration

Various changes in an eye with AMD may result in elevation or detachment of the RPE, as seen on stereoscopic biomicroscopic or angiographic evaluation. The term *RPE detachment* or *retinal pigment epithelial detachment (retinal PED)* secondary to AMD in the ophthalmic literature remains confusing because various RPE detachments may have quite different compositions, fluorescein angiographic appearances, prognoses, and management. Fortunately, these various RPE detachments can usually be differentiated on the basis of fluorescein angiographic patterns of fluorescence. The patterns include the following: (1) fibrovascular PEDs,[17] which are a subset of occult CNV (see Figs 61-8 and 61-9); (2) serous detachments of the RPE[44] (see Fig. 61-10); (3) hemorrhagic detachments of the RPE, in which blood from a choroidal neovascular lesion is noted beneath or exterior to the RPE (see Fig. 61-3); and (4) drusenoid RPE detachments,[8] in which large areas of confluent, soft drusen are noted. Potentially it is difficult to differentiate between fibrovascular

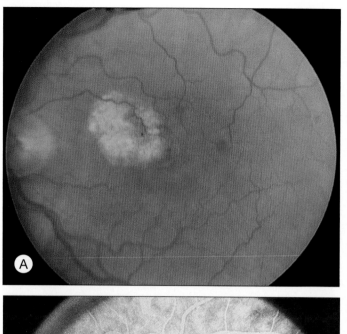

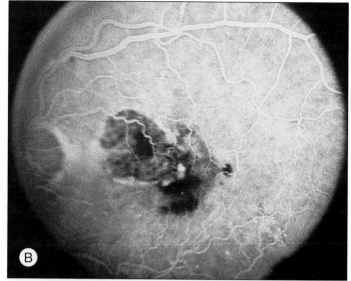

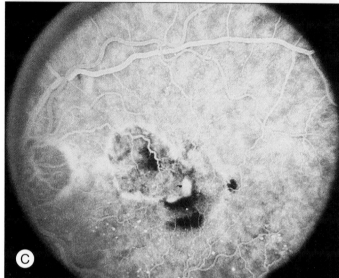

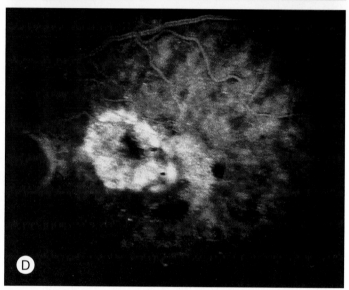

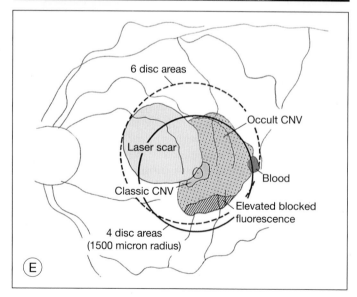

Fig. 61-11 Classic and occult choroidal neovascularization (CNV) and elevated blocked fluorescence (EBF) with well-demarcated borders. A, Recurrent subfoveal CNV. Note small area of hemorrhage temporal to recurrence. B, Early phase of fluorescein angiogram shows sharp demarcation of hyperfluorescence of classic CNV. C, Mid-phase photograph of angiogram with fluorescein leakage from classic CNV and sharply demarcated hyperfluorescence of elevated retinal pigment epithelium due to fibrovascular pigment epithelial detachment and indicative of occult CNV (curved arrows). Elevated blocked fluorescence still obscures choroidal fluorescence and possibly the inferior boundary of CNV. D, Late phase of angiogram demonstrates fluorescein leakage from both classic and occult neovascularization. Note hardly discernible EBF. E, Composite drawing using multiple stereoscopic photographs of angiogram shows interpretation of boundaries of lesion. Since each lesion component (classic CNV, occult CNV, blood, and EBF) has well-demarcated boundaries, boundaries of entire lesion are considered well demarcated. Furthermore, lesion meets size criteria for recurrent CNV cases that benefited from laser photocoagulation because the recurrent neovascular lesion, previous laser treatment scar, and area of additional treatment to be applied will not exceed six standard disc areas and, if recurrence is treated according to Macular Photocoagulation Study protocol (with treatment extending 100 μm beyond boundaries of recurrence), some area of retina will remain untreated within 1500 μm of foveal center. However, this lesion would also benefit from photodynamic therapy with verteporfin. (Reproduced from Macular Photocoagulation Study Group. Subfoveal neovascular lesions in age-related macular degeneration: guidelines for evaluation and treatment in the Macular Photocoagulation Study. Arch Ophthalmol 1991; 109:1242–1257.[17])

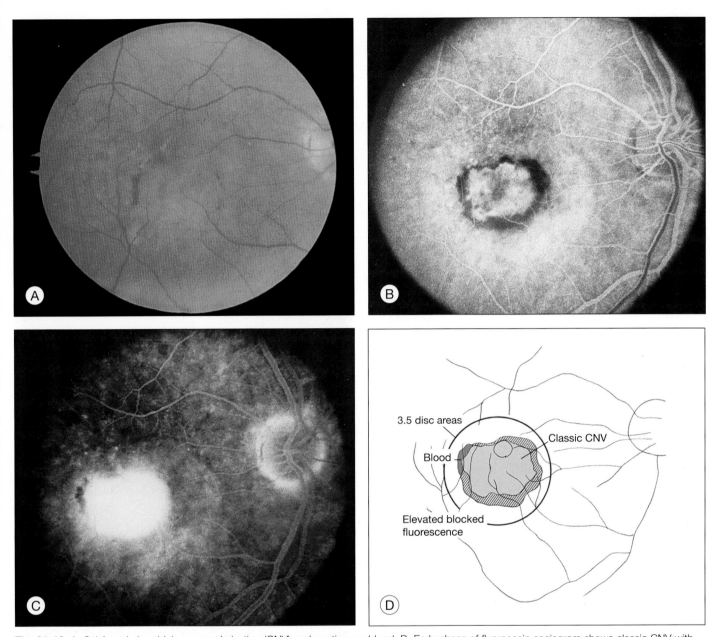

Fig. 61-12 A, Subfoveal choroidal neovascularization (CNV) and contiguous blood. B, Early phase of fluorescein angiogram shows classic CNV with blocked fluorescence corresponding to contiguous blood that obscures boundaries of CNV along temporal border. Remaining blocked fluorescein surrounding CNV (elevated when viewed stereoscopically) was probably due to the fibrous component of CNV. C, Late phase of fluorescein angiogram demonstrates that borders of CNV, blood, and elevated blocked fluorescence (green, red, and blue, respectively, in D) were derived from viewing the entire stereoscopic fluorescein angiogram taken according to study protocol. D, Drawing demonstrates that combined areas of blood and elevated blocked fluorescence that obscured borders of CNV did not exceed area of visible CNV. Total lesion size, including CNV, blood, and elevated blocked fluorescence, was less than 3.5 disc areas (circle) and would meet criteria for lesions that would benefit from laser photocoagulation or photodynamic therapy with verteporfin. (Reproduced from Macular Photocoagulation Study Group. Subfoveal neovascular lesions in age-related macular degeneration: guidelines for evaluation and treatment in the Macular Photocoagulation Study. Arch Ophthalmol 1991; 109:1242–1257.[17])

PEDs and serous PEDs. Using descriptions from the MPS Group, fibrovascular PEDs (as a subset of occult CNV) have been distinguished from a typical serous detachment of the RPE, in that the former do not have uniform, bright hyperfluorescence in the early phase. Instead, they show a stippled fluorescence along the surface of the RPE by the middle phase of the angiogram and may show pooling of dye in the overlying subsensory retinal space in the late phase (see Fig. 61-8). Serous PEDs show uniform, bright hyperfluorescence in the early phase, with a smooth contour to the RPE by the middle phase, and little, if any, leakage at the borders of the PED by the late phase (see Fig. 61-10). The fluorescent pattern of a serous PED obscures the ability to determine whether classic or occult CNV exists within or beneath the area of the serous PED. In contrast, a fibrovascular PED is an area of occult CNV.

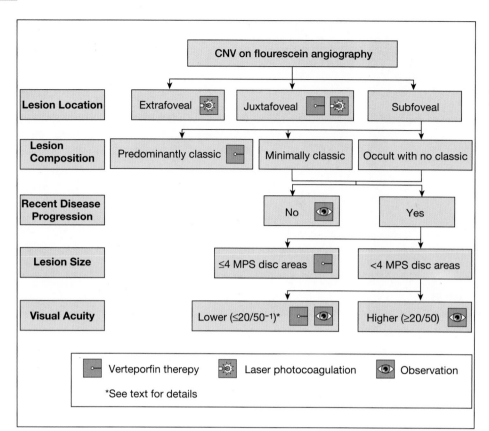

Fig. 61-13 Algorithm for verteporfin therapy or laser photocoagulation or observation for symptomatic patients with age-related macular degeneration, pathologic myopia, or other causes of choroidal neovascularization (CNV) in which the natural course is likely worse without treatment. MPS, Macular Photocoagulation Study.

A hemorrhagic detachment of the RPE will block choroidal fluorescence because of the mound-like collection of blood beneath the RPE (see Fig. 61-3). Occasionally a hemorrhagic detachment of the RPE may be mistaken for a choroidal melanoma, but usually hemorrhagic detachments of the RPE do not demonstrate low internal reflectivity, as is seen characteristically in choroidal melanomas.

One other feature of AMD that appears as an elevated or detached RPE is a drusenoid RPE detachment,[16] which represents extensive areas of large, confluent drusen. Drusenoid RPE detachments can be distinguished from serous detachments of the RPE in that drusenoid RPE detachments fluoresce faintly during the transit and do not progress to bright hyperfluorescence in the late phase of the angiogram. In contrast, serous detachments of the RPE fluoresce brightly in the early-transit phase and remain brightly hyperfluorescent in the late phase. In addition, serous detachments will usually have a smoother, sharper boundary compared with drusenoid RPE detachments. Drusenoid RPE detachments can be distinguished from fibrovascular PEDs in occult CNV by noting that fibrovascular PEDs show areas of stippled hyperfluorescence with persistence of staining or leakage within a sensory retinal detachment overlying the area in the late phase of the angiogram. RPE detachments due to large, soft, confluent drusen are usually smaller, shallower, and more irregular in outline than are fibrovascular PEDs. In addition, the drusenoid RPE detachments often have reticulated pigment clumping overlying the large, soft, confluent drusen, a scalloped border, and have less fluorescence in late-phase frames as compared with earlier-phase frames.

Other angiographic features
Fading choroidal neovascularization

CNV may occasionally be recognized in the early- or middle-transit phase of the angiogram with fading in the late phase, so little fluorescein staining or leakage can be discerned in the late phase within an area that was presumed to harbor CNV on the basis of its early-phase features[17] (Fig. 61-14). A vascular pattern of the fibrovascular tissue can occasionally be discerned in early-phase frames.[42] Most ophthalmologists are reluctant to treat areas of CNV that fade. These areas are usually not associated with overlying subretinal fluid (in conjunction with the lack of fluorescein leakage on angiography), so one can only presume that this region may proceed to disciform scarring. Perhaps these areas represent CNV histologically, but without evidence of subretinal fluid or late leakage, one cannot be certain that this pattern definitively represents CNV, and treatment of this area may damage retina unnecessarily.

Feeder vessels

These vessels may be identified as choroidal vessels apparent during the transit phase of the angiogram and connected unequivocally to leaking choroidal capillaries[17] (see Fig. 61-8). Although feeder vessels have been described as extending from a laser-treated area to recurrent CNV across the perimeter of

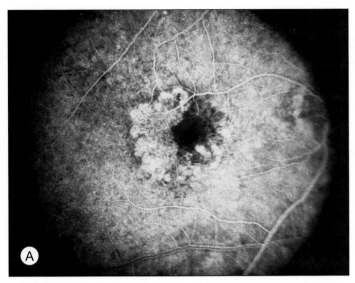

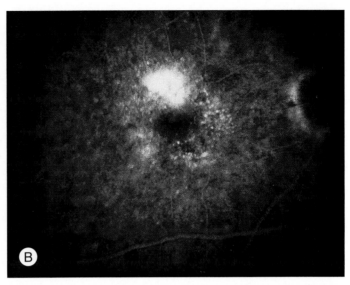

Fig. 61-14 Fading fluorescence of occult choroidal neovascularization (CNV) contiguous with classic CNV. A, Early phase of angiogram shows classic CNV with contiguous areas of slightly elevated hyperfluorescent retinal pigment epithelium (RPE) with a vascular pattern, presumably a fibrovascular pigment epithelial detachment, and other less well-demarcated areas of hyperfluorescence nasal to the fovea. B, Later phase of angiogram shows fluorescein leakage from classic CNV. However, areas of elevated hyperfluorescent RPE on early phase of angiogram (left) begin to fade, and vascular pattern is no longer apparent. Faded area is not considered a lesion component because hyperfluorescence does not meet minimal leakage/staining standard for occult CNV. Before 1988, most Macular Photocoagulation Study (MPS) investigators would have treated the area of classic CNV with late leakage. By current MPS interpretations, treatment of the area of classic CNV might still be contemplated, but investigators would be concerned about untreated areas of presumed occult CNV that fade in the late phase of the angiogram. (Reproduced from Macular Photocoagulation Study Group. Subfoveal neovascular lesions in age-related macular degeneration: guidelines for evaluation and treatment in the Macular Photocoagulation Study. Arch Ophthalmol 1991; 109:1242–1257.[17])

the laser-treated areas, feeder vessels may also be seen in untreated eyes (see Fig. 61-9). In the latter situation, peripheral, untreated areas of CNV may be connected by feeder vessels to more central areas of CNV that are evolving toward natural scar formation.

Retinal lesion anastomosis ("retinal angiomatous proliferans" or "chorioretinal anastomosis")

Retinal vessels can anastomose with CNV from AMD.[45] The vessels can be seen dividing at right angles from the surface of the retina to the neovascular lesion (as may be seen with idiopathic parafoveal telangiectasis).

Loculated fluid

This fluid consists of a well-demarcated area of hyperfluorescence that appears to represent pooling of fluorescein in a compartmentalized space anterior to the choroidal neovascular leakage, usually seen in the late phase of the angiogram.[46] Although the loculated fluid may conform to a pattern of typical cystoid macular edema, it can also pool within an area deep to the sensory retina in a shape that does not bear any resemblance to cystoid macular edema.

Retinal pigment epithelial tears

RPE tears have a characteristic fluorescein angiographic appearance.[47] The denuded RPE displays marked early hyperfluorescence. Later, staining of the choroid and sclera may be observed, but fluorescein generally does not leak from the denuded area. The folded pigment epithelial mound blocks fluorescence; However, this area may leak later during the angiogram, presumably from underlying CNV. Tears may occur following development of a serous PED in the absence of CNV. In addition, tears may occur following development of CNV, sometimes accompanied by large areas of hemorrhage. Tears in any of these situations may occur without any antecedent treatment or may occur soon after laser photocoagulation or PDT.

Disciform scars

Fibrovascular scars frequently hyperfluoresce from both fluorescein leakage and staining. One may also notice chorioretinal anastomoses or, more precisely, retinal anastomoses into fibrovascular tissue. These vessels have also been called retinal angiomatous proliferans (RAP)[45] or chorioretinal anastomoses or retinal lesion anastomoses. Some descriptions of these vessels have suggested that they can develop *prior to* the development of CNV (as is seen in the subretinal neovascularization that can develop in an individual with idiopathic parafoveal telangiectasis). However, there is no evidence that these vessels develop in the absence of CNV from AMD on histopathology. Furthermore, most cases show evidence of CNV in the presence of these anastomoses of retinal vessels with the neovascular lesion, and those cases that do not show obvious CNV often have difficult angiograms to interpret to state with certainty that CNV is not present. The area of anastomosis, when noted before development of extensive visible scar tissue, often shows a bright area of fluorescence in the early phase, occasionally accompanied by a small area of intraretinal hemorrhage. While some reports have suggested that the natural history of lesions with these anastomoses is worse than the natural history without these anastomoses, there is no strong evidence to support this impression at this time.

PATHOGENESIS

Choroidal neovascularization

Histopathology

CNV appears as a neovascular sprout growing under or through the RPE through breaks in Bruch's membrane[12] (Figs 61-15 and 61-16). Usually this occurs in association with evidence of fibroblasts, myofibroblasts, lymphocytes, and macrophages.[48] Various growth factors are suspected to be involved in the development of this CNV, such as vascular endothelial growth factor (VEGF).[49] However, while drugs designed to interfere with VEGF have been shown to reduce the risk of vision loss,[50,51] vision loss still occurred in many treated cases, and it is not yet clear how much these drugs produce an antiangiogenic effect or an antipermeability effect. Following penetration of the inner aspect of Bruch's membrane, the new vessels proliferate laterally between the RPE and Bruch's membrane.[12] As these neovascular twigs mature, they develop a more organized vascular system stemming from a trunk of feeder vessels off the choroid, as well as proliferation of fibrous tissue. The endothelial cells in the arborizing neovascular tufts lack the barrier function of more mature endothelial cells. Hence these new vessels can leak fluid (and fluorescein) in the neurosensory, subsensory, and RPE layers of the retina. Proteins and lipids may accompany this process and precipitate in any layer of the retina. In addition, the fragile vessels are prone to hemorrhage. Occasionally, blood may extend through all the layers of the retina, breaking through into the vitreous cavity. Ultimately, a fibrovascular scar results, usually causing disruption and death of the overlying sensory retinal tissue accompanied by severe visual loss.

Associated factors

The stimulus for vascular ingrowth of choroidal vessels remains unknown, but several theories have been advanced. Soft drusen

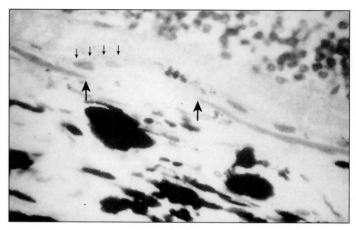

Fig. 61-15 Photomicrograph of choroidal neovascularization (outlined by small arrows) beneath the retinal pigment epithelium growing through a break in Bruch's membrane (large arrows). (Reproduced from Elman MJ. Age-related macular degeneration. Int Ophthalmol Clin 1986; 26:117–144.)

have been associated histopathologically with CNV. The soft drusen represent focal accumulation of membranous debris (ultrastructurally termed *basal linear deposits*) accumulated as a diffuse, shallow layer between the RPE basement membrane and the inner aspect of Bruch's membrane.[10–12,52–57] This material should not be confused with *basal laminar deposit*, which is material that collects between the RPE plasma membrane and the basement membrane of the RPE and accumulates with age but may not lead to vision loss from CNV or geographic atrophy and therefore may not be part of AMD.[52,53] The term should also not be confused with *basal laminar drusen*, also called *cuticular drusen*. (Basal laminar, or cuticular, drusen usually present in midlife with a myriad of small, translucent drusen that appear like a starry sky on a fluorescein angiogram and may be associated with vitelliform macular detachments: see below.[2,58]) Some investigators believe that soft drusen represent extracellular matrix material produced by the RPE.[52,59] Deposition of this material may suggest a widespread RPE abnormality.[18] The diffusely thickened area is weakly attached, allowing the development of

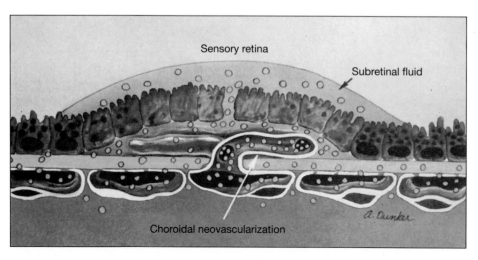

Fig. 61-16 Sketch of choroidal neovascularization showing ingrowth of vessels from the choriocapillaris, through a break in Bruch's membrane, into the subretinal pigment epithelial space. (Reproduced from Bressler NM, Bressler SB, Fine SL. Age-related macular degeneration. Surv Ophthalmol 1988; 32:375–413.[2])

Sensory retina

Subretinal fluid

Choroidal neovascularization

localized detachments seen clinically as soft drusen. These localized detachments can coalesce into larger drusenoid or serous RPE detachments.[11] Alternatively, drusen may act as an indirect angiogenic factor by attracting macrophages from the choroid.[48]

Breaks in Bruch's membrane permit ingrowth of new vessels from the choriocapillaris. However, these breaks can also be seen without ingrowth of choroidal new vessels. Some investigators have suggested that endothelial cells of growing CNV may actually produce the break in Bruch's membrane rather than grow through pre-existing breaks in Bruch's membrane.[60] An inflammatory component seen in association with AMD may play a role in the development of CNV.[61] Eyes with AMD show an increased prevalence of lymphocytes, fibroblasts, and macrophages within Bruch's membrane as compared with control eyes without AMD. However, these findings are not specific to eyes with neovascular AMD.[61,62] The presence of macrophages and lymphocytes near breaks in Bruch's membrane suggests that leukocytes may be involved in the induction of CNV growth and the release of collagenases from endothelial cells. It is postulated that leukocytes may initially stimulate neovascular proliferation, promote the release of factors leading to breakdown of Bruch's membrane, and even affect (with pericytes) the dilation of new vessels.[63] Whether these inflammatory cells act as mediators of the degenerative changes seen in Bruch's membrane or directly stimulate new vessel growth remains unknown. Finally, as mentioned above, other angiogenic factors, such as VEGF or a platelet-derived growth factor (PDGF),[49,51,64] may contribute to the ingrowth of new vessels from the choroid through Bruch's membrane into the sub-RPE space. Growth factors leading to neovascular formation may arise from an imbalance between stimulating and inhibiting chemical modulators. The RPE has been implicated as the source of these factors, but RPE cells may also act indirectly through the attraction of macrophages.[65]

DIFFERENTIAL DIAGNOSIS

Choroidal neovascularization

CNV may arise in association with a number of conditions other than AMD, such as OHS, pathologic myopia, angioid streaks (especially when associated with pseudoxanthoma elasticum), choroidal ruptures, and idiopathic causes. Whether AMD is present when CNV arises in patients older than 50 without drusen is controversial.

CNV may masquerade as central serous chorioretinopathy. Although the classic case of central serous chorioretinopathy shows a "smokestack" configuration on fluorescein angiography, the more common presentation is a dot of hyperfluorescence that merely increases in size and intensity of fluorescence, much like a small area of CNV. One must strongly consider CNV in patients aged 50 and older who have typical central serous chorioretinopathy. In these cases the increased age contrasts to the third to fifth decades, when central serous chorioretinopathy is most commonly seen. Presentation of central serous chorioretinopathy in an elderly patient with drusen can be difficult to distinguish and should alert one to the possibility of CNV, necessitating careful follow-up. If CNV is indeed present, growth of the area of hyperfluorescence might be detected while treatment may still be beneficial.

Basal laminar, or cuticular, drusen may be complicated by foveal detachments of vitelliform material in one or both eyes that may mimic neovascular AMD. Contact lens examination with transillumination of the fundus in these cases reveals an appearance similar to that of pigskin, with a myriad of small drusen. Angiographically, literally hundreds of bright spots appear very early during the angiogram, an appearance that has been described as a "starry sky." These patients are usually asymptomatic until they accumulate vitelliform lesions in the fovea. The ensuing foveal detachment by this material, which can be unilateral or bilateral, simulates the foveal detachment that occurs with subfoveal CNV. The hyperfluorescence usually progressively fills the area of vitelliform material, rather than showing one area of bright fluorescence early that leaks late in classic CNV. Unlike subfoveal CNV, which most often progresses to a disciform scar with visual acuity of 20/200 or worse, eyes with a foveal detachment secondary to cuticular drusen resolve without scarring. The retina then may or may not have an area of RPE atrophy about one to two disc areas in size. Foveal acuity with atrophy is more often in the range of 20/80 to 20/125, in contrast to the more severe visual loss that accompanies true subfoveal CNV. Patients with cuticular drusen can still develop typical drusen associated with AMD or CNV.

Pattern dystrophies of the RPE may also have vitelliform detachments in which the angiographic pattern can mimic CNV. When one identifies any condition with a vitelliform detachment, it is critical to determine if the late-phase bright fluorescence is progressive fluorescein staining of the vitelliform material or leakage of fluorescein from CNV. The former would not benefit from laser photocoagulation, whereas the latter might. As discussed earlier, usually the fluorescence from a vitelliform detachment shows one or more areas of hyperfluorescence in the early phase of the angiogram with progressive hyperfluorescence of the entire area of yellow vitelliform material by the late phase. In contrast, a diffuse area of hyperfluorescence in the late phase that corresponds to classic CNV (rather than the stippled fluorescence of occult CNV) should show an area of bright hyperfluorescence in the early phase that is only slightly smaller than the area of hyperfluorescent leakage in the late phase.

Vitreous hemorrhage

If a new patient has vitreous hemorrhage in one eye and signs of AMD in the other eye, other causes of vitreous hemorrhage must first be ruled out. Common causes of vitreous hemorrhage include retinal tear formation and retinal vascular diseases such as diabetic retinopathy or branch vein occlusion. Ultrasonography usually differentiates breakthrough vitreous hemorrhage secondary to neovascular AMD or retinal vascular causes from that caused by a tumor (Fig. 61-17).

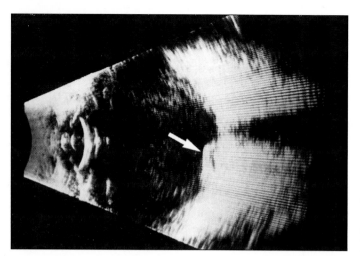

Fig. 61-17 Ultrasound image of a vitreous hemorrhage associated with neovascular age-related macular degeneration in which a relatively flat and broad-based posterior pole lesion (arrow) with a fairly homogeneous pattern and with no choroidal excavation is seen. (Reproduced from Bressler NM, Bressler SB, Fine SL. Age-related macular degeneration. Surv Ophthalmol 1988; 32:375–413.[2])

NATURAL HISTORY

Most prospective natural history data of CNV comes from control (untreated) groups of individuals participating in randomized clinical trials. As such, *the natural-history information is specific to the eligibility criteria of those trials and is not necessarily reflective of the natural history of the universe of choroidal neovascular lesions in the population*, and precludes precise comparisons of natural histories from one study to another. With this caveat in mind, the natural history from these trials is reviewed to provide some evidence regarding the outcome of these lesions without treatment.

Well-defined extrafoveal and juxtafoveal choroidal neovascularization

Patients assigned to observation in the MPS trials provide natural-history information on cases that met criteria for these studies. When lesions have well-defined boundaries, the CNV lesion can be classified according to the location of the most posterior boundary of the lesion with respect to the center of the FAZ on the fluorescein angiogram. CNV lesions located more than 200 μm from the FAZ center are termed *extrafoveal*; those between 1 and 199 μm from the center are *juxtafoveal*; CNV lesions extending under the center of the FAZ are termed *subfoveal*. In contrast to other pathologic conditions predisposing to CNV (e.g., OHS and pathologic myopia) in eyes with AMD, CNV presents more frequently under the FAZ center. In addition, subfoveal CNV from AMD tends to be larger on initial presentation than when seen in other conditions.[66] In a retrospective review of fluorescein angiograms of AMD ordered at a community hospital over a 9.5-year period, only 8% (19/244) of the CNV lesions were extrafoveal.[67] Other retrospective reports not derived solely from a retinal referral practice have suggested that most patients with CNV from AMD present to an ophthalmologist with subfoveal CNV with poorly demar-

cated boundaries.[66,68] However, there is no information from population-based studies to describe precisely how many choroidal neovascular lesions are subfoveal versus not subfoveal, and for those that are not subfoveal, how many are well-demarcated on laser photocoagulation. Furthermore, there are no studies to determine how many cases that are subfoveal are predominantly classic, and if not predominantly classic, how many have presumed recent disease progression after developing.

In the MPS, 62% of untreated eyes with well-defined, extrafoveal CNV (posterior boundary of lesion located at least 200 μm from the FAZ center) lost six or more lines of visual acuity by 3 years of follow-up.[69] By 5 years, this percentage was similar at 64%.[70] Furthermore, in nearly 75% of the untreated eyes, the CNV extended under the FAZ center.[71] For juxtafoveal lesions, 49% of untreated eyes had lost six or more lines of visual acuity by 3 years of follow-up.[24]

Subfoveal choroidal neovascularization

For subfoveal lesions, the MPS reported that 48% of untreated eyes with well-defined subfoveal CNV that was predominantly CNV and included a component of classic CNV in which the entire lesion was no greater than 3.5 MPS disc areas lost six or more lines of vision from baseline by 48 months.[22,72] Similar outcomes were noted for untreated eyes with recurrent subfoveal CNV with similar features as for new subfoveal lesions except the total size of the lesion plus any area of prior treatment was to be no greater than six MPS disc areas.[23,72] A broader group of subfoveal lesions in the Treatment of Age-related macular degeneration with Photodynamic therapy (TAP) investigation described the natural history in subfoveal lesions that were predominantly CNV with evidence of classic CNV and a lesion size no greater than nine disc areas in which 62% lost three or more lines at 2 years after entry, including 30% losing six or more lines of visual acuity.[73] With increasing size of predominantly classic lesions on presentation, the average visual acuity is more likely to be worse by 2 years.[74]

A variety of studies have shown that cases of predominantly CNV with a composition that is occult CNV with no classic CNV or minimally classic CNV have a more heterogeneous outcome.[43,74–79] Most of this information is from series in clinical trials with presumed recent disease progression. Some cases may remain stable for years without visual loss, whereas other cases may develop severe visual loss at a rate similar to the deterioration noted for cases of classic CNV only. Furthermore, increasing size of minimally classic or occult with no classic lesions is not associated with a worse natural history outcome.[74]

Up to 50% of the cases with no classic CNV may develop classic CNV within a year of presentation.[43,75,76,80] Cases that develop some classic CNV may be more likely to have severe visual acuity loss.[75,76,80] Results from several clinical trials suggest that the natural history of lesions with classic CNV but no occult CNV is worse than the natural history of lesions with classic and occult CNV or occult CNV with no classic CNV.[76,78,81] It is likely that the natural history of lesions with classic and occult CNV may lie somewhere between the natural course of lesions with classic CNV only and occult CNV only.[76]

Natural course of large subfoveal subretinal hemorrhage in age-related macular degeneration

Some eyes with subfoveal subretinal hemorrhage associated with AMD have poor outcomes.[82–84] However, the visual acuity of other eyes does not deteriorate or may improve spontaneously.[82,84] Such findings underscore the importance of evaluating the role of therapeutic interventions for these cases, such as surgery[85,86] to remove subretinal hemorrhage and associated CNV, in randomized clinical trials.[87] The SST Group B Trial of relatively large, predominantly hemorrhagic subfoveal lesions demonstrated that 41% of untreated eyes remained stable or improved, although 36% had severe visual acuity loss after enrollment into the trial. Furthermore, this trial suggested that 18% of large subfoveal subretinal hemorrhages will progress to a vitreous hemorrhage as blood dissects from the subretinal space through the retina and into the vitreous.[25]

Retinal pigment epithelial tears

Patients with RPE tears involving the foveal center may initially maintain good vision but usually develop severe visual loss. However, cases with RPE tears through the fovea and preservation of good visual acuity have been reported.[32] Unfortunately, there is a substantial risk of AMD-related visual loss in the fellow eye. Schoeppner and associates[88] reported a cumulative risk of visual loss in the fellow eye of patients who had an RPE tear in the eye as 37% at 1 year, 59% at 2 years, and 80% at 3 years of follow-up. Visual loss usually arose from development of a PED, RPE tear, or CNV.

LASER PHOTOCOAGULATION TREATMENT

Laser treatment of well-defined choroidal neovascular lesions

Laser photocoagulation has only been shown to be beneficial for well-defined lesions. If the entire boundary of the lesion is not well defined, then the treating ophthalmologist cannot determine where to apply laser photocoagulation with certainty in order to cover the lesion in its entirety; undertreatment or overtreatment will likely occur. Failure to cover the entire lesion increases the likelihood of recurrent CNV[89–91] and, for extrafoveal and juxtafoveal lesions, of additional visual acuity loss.[89,91,92] Overtreatment will likely destroy retinal tissue (and corresponding function) that was not overlying CNV unnecessarily.[91] Therefore cases that were evaluated in clinical trials for which treatment results are available are limited to well-defined lesions. For extrafoveal and juxtafoveal lesions, results were evaluated on well-defined lesions before any differentiation of angiographic patterns (classic or occult) was recognized. For subfoveal lesions, results were evaluated on relatively small, well-defined lesions that were to include a component of classic CNV.

Results of laser photocoagulation treatment
Extrafoveal choroidal neovascularization
Initial MPS trials in patients with AMD evaluated well-defined, extrafoveal CNV lesions in which the entire complex was located at least 200 μm from the center of the FAZ in eyes with a baseline visual acuity of 20/100 or better.[69–71] Classic and occult CNV were not differentiated at this time. CNV was defined angiographically as leakage at the level of the outer retina. This initial study, sometimes referred to as the "argon" study, was designed to test laser photocoagulation in a group of eyes thought to have the best prognosis for maintaining vision with or without treatment. Patients were enrolled between 1979 and 1982. In 1982 the MPS group reported that argon blue-green or green laser photocoagulation treatment, applied with the intent to have an intensity to whiten the retina and cover the entire extent of the extrafoveal CNV and contiguous blood, reduced the risk of additional severe visual acuity loss when compared with the natural course of the disease[71] (Fig. 61-18).

The benefits of argon laser photocoagulation were greatest during the first posttreatment year. The treatment benefit persisted over 5 years of follow-up; at that time 64% of untreated eyes versus 46% of treated eyes progressed to severe visual loss[70] (see Fig. 61-18). The relative risk of losing six or more lines of visual acuity from the baseline level among untreated eyes compared to treated eyes was 1.5 from 6 months to 5 years after enrollment.[70] After 5 years, laser-treated eyes lost a mean of 5.2 lines of visual acuity, whereas untreated eyes lost a mean of 7.1 lines.[70] By the end of the 5-year follow-up, recurrent CNV had been observed in 54% of the laser-treated eyes.[70] Recurrence of CNV was responsible for most of the deterioration seen in the treatment group, occurring with greatest frequency within the first 2 years after the initial photocoagulation.[92] Thus prompt argon laser photocoagulation treatment of extrafoveal CNV lesions in AMD reduces the likelihood of severe visual loss when compared with the natural course of the disease. Two other randomized, prospective clinical trials in the UK[93] and France[94] reached similar conclusions.

Juxtafoveal choroidal neovascularization

In 1981, after the introduction of the krypton laser and over 1 year before the results of the argon trial were announced, the MPS Group initiated a trial to determine whether krypton laser photocoagulation would prevent visual acuity loss in AMD eyes with potentially treatable CNV lesions not eligible for the argon trial but not requiring treatment to extend under the center of the FAZ. The krypton red laser was used because investigators thought it would allow treatment within the FAZ with theoretically less risk of damaging the fovea owing to the lack of uptake by foveal xanthophyll. In addition, krypton laser photocoagulation theoretically might facilitate sparing of the inner retina from damage, especially in the treatment of large peripapillary lesions.[95] Eligible lesions included cases with CNV that extended 1 to 199 μm from the FAZ center (but not under the center) or CNV 200 μm or farther from the FAZ center with blood or blocked fluorescence or both extending within 200 μm from the FAZ center (Figs 61-19 and 61-20). This MPS trial, sometimes called the "krypton" study, differed from the argon study in the type and location of CNV lesions, qualifying visual acuity at baseline (20/400 or better best corrected), the wavelength used (krypton red versus argon blue-green or green), and in the

Medical Retina

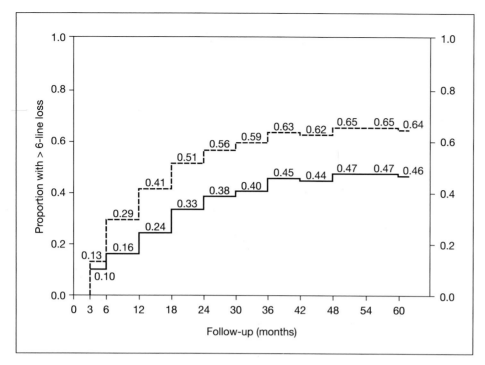

Fig. 61-18 Proportion of eyes at each follow-up examination with decrease in visual acuity of six or more lines from baseline in the Senile Macular Degeneration Study of extrafoveal lesions. Dashed line indicates eyes assigned randomly at entry to no treatment; solid line indicates eyes assigned at entry to laser treatment. (Reproduced from Macular Photocoagulation Study Group. Subfoveal neovascular lesions in age-related macular degeneration: guidelines for evaluation and treatment in the Macular Photocoagulation Study. Arch Ophthalmol 1991; 109:1242–1257.[17])

treatment protocol. In contrast to the argon study, treatment over all the blood associated with the CNV lesion was not required, and photocoagulation was permitted up to the center of the FAZ. Specifically, treatment on the foveal side of the CNV was to cover the CNV and then extend up to 100 μm into any blood (or up to the foveal center, whichever came first).

At 3 years after randomization, 86 (49%) of 174 treated eyes compared to 98 (58%) of 169 untreated eyes had lost six or more lines of visual acuity.[24] The average visual acuity at that time point was 20/200 in the treated eyes and 20/250 in the untreated eyes. Most of the visual loss in treated and untreated eyes occurred within the first 3 to 9 months after randomization. As compared to no treatment, krypton laser photocoagulation reduced the risk of severe visual loss by approximately 10%. Laser treatment showed its greatest benefit in patients without any evidence of systemic hypertension, but showed reduced or no benefit in patients with highly elevated blood pressure or those treated with antihypertensive medication. However, treatment should still be considered in patients who are not normotensive because of the lack of a consistent similar finding in other MPS trials in AMD.[22,23] The relative risk of losing six or more lines of visual acuity from baseline to any examination from 6 months through 5 years after enrollment was 1.2.[24]; 25% of the treated eyes compared to 15% of the untreated eyes maintained their baseline level of visual acuity. In addition, more than twice as many treated patients as untreated patients retained visual acuity of 20/40 or better.[24]

In the extrafoveal and juxtafoveal trials, persistence and recurrence of CNV after initial treatment with laser photocoagulation were the major contributors to visual loss. Persistent CNV, defined as leakage detected during the first 6 weeks after laser treatment, was higher in the krypton study; 32% of eyes

had persistent neovascularization[3] compared to only 10% in the argon study.[92] Recurrent CNV is defined as leakage detected for the first time 6 weeks or more after laser treatment. In both studies, the overall recurrence rate (including persistence and recurrence) was almost 50% by the 2-year follow-up.[89,92]

In the krypton study, the persistence rate in eyes having 10% or more of the foveal side of the neovascular lesion not covered by treatment was twice as high as in the eyes with more extensive treatment coverage.[91] It is apparently more difficult to photocoagulate within the avascular zone; 41% of CNV lesions in the krypton study were not completely covered on the foveal side with laser treatment, even though the treating ophthalmologists attempted to cover the entire area of neovascularization. Reluctance to treat within the avascular zone and reduced visibility of retinal landmarks probably contribute to this difficulty.

Covering the entire lesion with adequate intensity of treatment also reduces the risk of persistent CNV and associated visual loss.[89] Posttreatment photographs that demonstrated adequate intensity of the entire treatment also identified a case with a reduced risk of persistent CNV.[89]

Most ophthalmologists managing juxtafoveal CNV choose to try PDT with verteporfin in cases where the treating ophthalmologist believes that applying adequate photocoagulation would likely extend under the center of the FAZ (see section on photodynamic therapy, below).

Subfoveal choroidal neovascularization

In 1986 the MPS Group initiated two additional randomized clinical trials to evaluate laser treatment in eyes with subfoveal CNV.[22,23] One trial evaluated the effect on vision of laser treatment (argon green or krypton red, assigned randomly) compared to observation in previously untreated AMD eyes (also termed

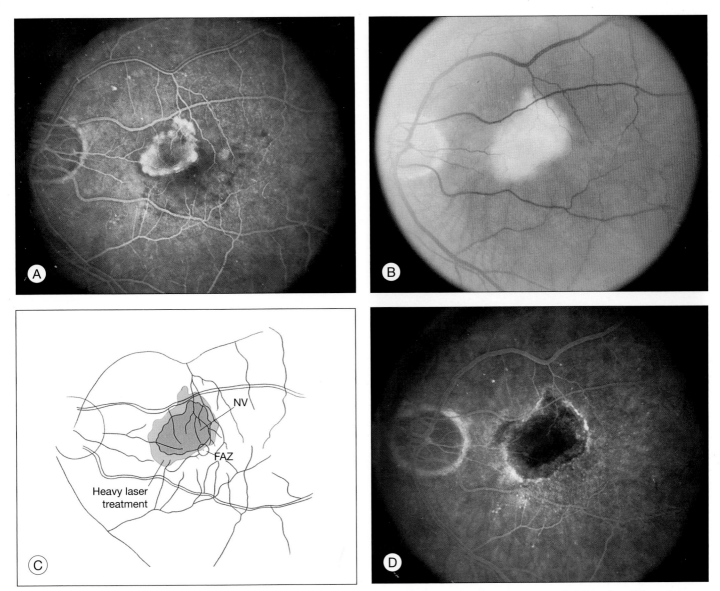

Fig. 61-19 Juxtafoveal choroidal neovascularization (CNV) lesion. A, Early-phase fluorescein angiogram shows classic CNV less than 200 μm from center of foveal avascular zone (FAZ). B, Photograph taken 24 h after treatment shows photocoagulation burn of adequate intensity. C, Composite drawing made from early-phase angiogram (A) and posttreatment photograph (B) demonstrates complete coverage of neovascularization (NV) by heavy treatment. D, Early-phase fluorescein angiogram 6 weeks after treatment shows no persistence (no fluorescein leakage at periphery of treated area). (Reproduced from Macular Photocoagulation Study Group. Subfoveal neovascular lesions in age-related macular degeneration: guidelines for evaluation and treatment in the Macular Photocoagulation Study. Arch Ophthalmol 1991; 109:1242–1257.[17])

"new" lesions) with a CNV lesion that had a component of classic CNV in which the entire lesion was well demarcated and in which CNV (classic or occult) extended directly beneath the geometric center of the FAZ. The neovascular lesions could be no larger than 3.5 MPS disc areas. Total area of treatment (extending 100 μm beyond all borders of the lesion) could not exceed four disc areas (see Fig. 61-12). Baseline best-corrected vision was no better than 20/40 and no worse than 20/320.

In 1991 the MPS group reported that laser treatment of new subfoveal neovascular lesions meeting the eligibility criteria outlined above was better than observation alone in preventing large losses of acuity, provided the patient and the ophthalmologist were prepared for the possibility of a substantial decrease in visual acuity (three lines, on average) immediately after treatment.[22] At 3 months after randomization, visual acuity dropped by six or more lines in 37 (20%) of 184 laser-treated eyes compared to only 19 (11%) of 178 untreated eyes. However, untreated eyes continued to lose vision, whereas laser-treated eyes remained relatively stable after any initial laser-related drop in vision. By 24 months, visual acuity had still decreased by six or more lines in 23 (20%) of 114 laser-treated eyes compared to 41 (37%) of 112 untreated eyes. The average visual acuity decreased three lines from baseline in treated eyes versus four lines in untreated eyes. Of note, approximately 30% of treated eyes compared to approximately 60% of untreated eyes were 20/400 or worse by the 48-month follow-up examination.

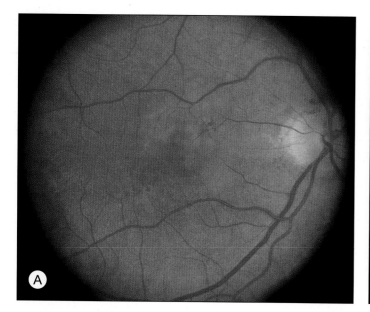

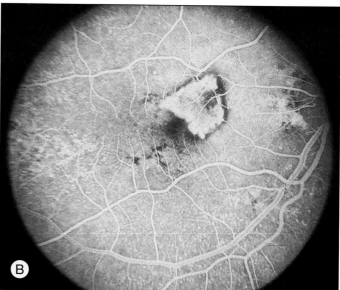

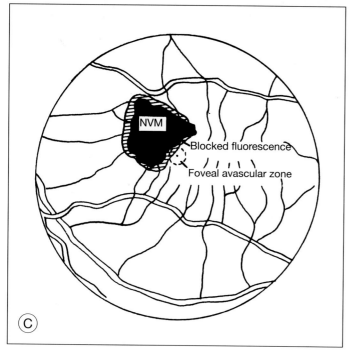

Fig. 61-20 Juxtafoveal choroidal neovascularization lesion. A, Fluorescein angiogram shows choroidal neovascularization (CNV) in which the posterior edge of the CNV is more than 200 μm from the foveal center and is associated with blocked fluorescence on the posterior edge of the lesion within 200 μm of the foveal center. B, Red-free photograph of same eye demonstrating that, except for a small amount of blood superonasal to the neovascular lesion, the blocked fluorescence is not due to subretinal blood visible on photograph. C, Drawing of CNV or neovascular membrane (NVM) in which blocked fluorescence is represented by hatched area surrounding the neovascular lesion. (Reproduced from Macular Photocoagulation Study Group. Subfoveal neovascular lesions in age-related macular degeneration: guidelines for evaluation and treatment in the Macular Photocoagulation Study. Arch Ophthalmol 1991; 109:1242–1257.[17])

In addition, laser-treated eyes were more likely to be able to read large text at 40 words or more per minute, a rate judged necessary to maintain comprehension of what is read. Furthermore, laser-treated eyes maintained baseline contrast sensitivity, whereas untreated eyes worsened. Patients with better contrast sensitivity appear better able to perform functional tasks than patients with poorer contrast thresholds at similar visual acuities.[96] These treatment benefits were maintained with additional follow-up information provided in 1993.[72] The benefits of treatment varied significantly with the lesion size and initial visual acuity at baseline.[97] Eyes with smaller lesions and relatively poorer visual acuity seemed to benefit most from treatment. Larger lesions with relatively good visual acuity had no obvious treatment benefit, and larger lesions with relatively poor visual acuity had only a small treatment benefit. These findings, although based on subgroup analysis with relatively small numbers, suggest that extrapolating these results to lesions larger than what were enrolled in this trial (> 3.5 MPS disc areas) would not be prudent.

Because of the high rate of persistence and recurrence in the argon and krypton trials and their association with poorer visual outcome, a companion study to the trial on "new" lesions was started to evaluate laser treatment versus observation of subfoveal recurrent CNV developing along the perimeter of a laser-treated area after earlier treatment of an extrafoveal or juxtafoveal CNV lesion. In the recurrent subfoveal study, eligibility criteria were similar to the new subfoveal study except the total area treated (previous area of laser treatment plus new laser treatment to recurrent CNV) was not to exceed six MPS disc areas. Additionally, some area within four MPS disc areas centered on the fovea had to be left untreated (see Figs 61-8 and 61-11). Again, baseline best-corrected visual acuity was no better than 20/40 and no worse than 20/320. The risk of severe visual loss was greater in untreated eyes than treated eyes.[23] The mean visual acuity of laser-treated eyes by 3 years was 20/250, one line better than untreated eyes. However, more than twice as many treated eyes as untreated eyes had visual acuity better than 20/200 at the 3-year examinations, and fewer than half as many treated eyes as untreated eyes had visual acuity of 20/400 or worse. Thus treatment is recommended for recurrent subfoveal lesions that meet the criteria used in this trial. Subgroup analyses of the recurrent trial also showed that treatment was beneficial regardless of the initial visual acuity, in contrast to similar subgroup analyses for new (no prior laser) subfoveal lesions.

With the advent of PDT, shown to reduce the risk of moderate and severe visual acuity loss for lesions that were shown to benefit from laser photocoagulation (see below), most ophthalmologists treating such lesions use PDT instead of laser photocoagulation for several reasons. First, PDT applies to a larger range of lesion sizes; second, it does not require that lesion boundaries be well demarcated; and third, it is less likely to cause immediate loss of vision. While few cases of neovascular AMD are treated with laser photocoagulation, the treatment approach is reviewed as it applies to well-demarcated extrafoveal lesions and some well-demarcated juxtafoveal lesions.

Preparation for laser photocoagulation treatment

Before photocoagulation treatment, patients with a potentially treatable CNV lesion should be informed that laser treatment will create a permanent blank area, or blind spot, corresponding to the area of retina to be treated. The postoperative vision will correlate with the extent of central retina destroyed with laser photocoagulation treatment. Whereas patients with binocular macular vision and a treated lesion away from the center of the FAZ frequently remain unaware of this treatment scotoma unless they cover the untreated fellow eye, patients with a central scotoma in the fellow eye are usually immediately aware of the laser-induced scotoma in the treated eye. Because laser treatment may cause hemorrhage or increase sensory retinal detachment during the immediate postoperative period, all patients, especially those with juxtafoveal or extrafoveal lesions, should be warned that they may experience increased distortion and decreased vision after treatment and that this may persist for several weeks. In addition, the ophthalmologist must emphasize that laser treatment is not a cure for AMD; rather, laser photocoagulation treatment is designed to obliterate the neovascular complex and thereby reduce the risk of additional severe visual loss in the future. Furthermore, the treating ophthalmologist must recall that, even under the best conditions in the MPS, many of the treated eyes progressed to severe visual loss despite careful protocol treatment by ophthalmologists experienced in the laser management of CNV and despite meticulous follow-up.

Following the treatment protocol established by the MPS (discussed below), a recent fluorescein angiogram (if possible, less than 72 to 96 h old) should be used to guide the ophthalmologist during treatment. Because the CNV may grow, a fluorescein angiogram older than a few days may no longer depict the extent of CNV accurately. A suitable frame from the angiogram is displayed near the laser console top. The angiogram thus displayed permits rapid and accurate orientation of critical retinal vascular and CNV landmarks.

Drawing the CNV lesion and its relationship to the FAZ, made before treatment from selected frames of the fluorescein angiogram using a digital image or a microfilm reader, can assist in planning and later in assessing the laser treatment (Fig. 61-21). Alternatively, a drawing may be obtained by projecting the angiogram on a piece of paper mounted on the wall or by using an acetate sheet placed on a slide viewer screen. Whatever the method, the CNV lesion's perimeter, the FAZ, and the key landmarks around the CNV lesions, such as retinal vessels and subretinal blood, can be drawn to familiarize the ophthalmologist with the planned extent of treatment.[98]

Retrobulbar anesthesia was required in the MPS argon and krypton studies; it was recommended but optional in the subfoveal trials. Although the risks of retrobulbar anesthesia include retrobulbar hemorrhage, globe perforation, and optic nerve damage, the akinesia and anesthesia of the globe were thought to facilitate treatment in many cases. Because of the advantages of reduced patient discomfort and ocular motility, retrobulbar or peribulbar anesthesia may be useful in laser photocoagulation of CNV if needed to insure coverage of the entire lesion with adequately intense laser treatment. With a cooperative patient, an ophthalmologist with adequate experience in the treatment of CNV may elect to treat without retrobulbar or peribulbar anesthesia.

Macular Photocoagulation Study photocoagulation techniques

Using a 200-μm spot size and duration of at least 0.2 s, a test burn is placed along the lesion's perimeter to determine the necessary power setting. This burn is placed away from the foveal edge in juxtafoveal and extrafoveal lesions and recommended along an inferior border of the lesion in subfoveal CNV. The foveal edge of the CNV is treated next in juxtafoveal and extrafoveal lesions, using overlapping 200-μm laser burns with a duration of 0.2 to 0.5 s. After the foveal edge is treated, the rest of the lesion is outlined with laser burns. Ideally, one should start at the inferior edge of a lesion and work superiorly in case intraoperative bleeding occurs and tracks inferiorly, obscuring retinal landmarks; this area will have been treated. To obliterate the CNV, the burns should be sufficiently intense to produce retinal whitening. Finally, the center of the CNV is obliterated (Fig. 61-22).

To increase the chances of a successful result, one should be thoroughly familiar with the eligibility criteria and different treatment protocols used in the MPS trials. To ensure adequate treatment, the MPS protocol required that the entire CNV lesion be covered by a uniformly intense area of whitening extending 100 μm beyond the angiographically visible lesion for extrafoveal and subfoveal cases. In the krypton study, treat-ment on the foveal side of the lesion had to cover the CNV completely and extend up to 100 μm into areas of blood on the foveal side (with less extension, as needed, to avoid having treatment extend under the center of the FAZ). Treatment was to extend 100 μm beyond the boundaries of the lesion on the

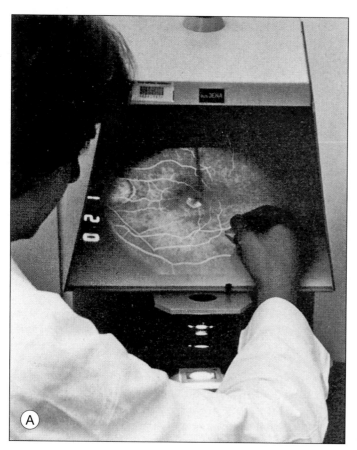

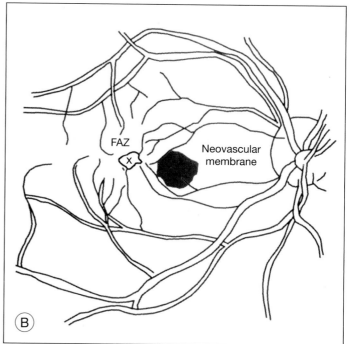

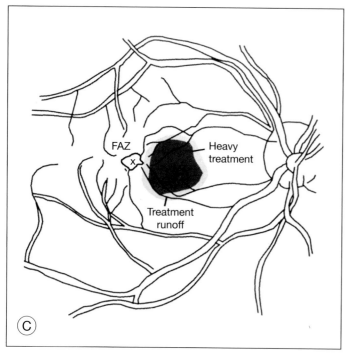

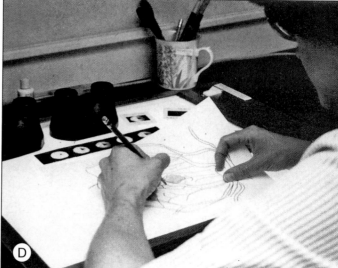

Fig. 61-21 Evaluation of choroidal neovascularization treatment. A, Angiogram is projected on a suitable apparatus. B, This allows the lesion, key landmarks around the lesion, such as subretinal blood and retinal vessels, and the foveal center, to be drawn. FAZ, foveal avascular zone. C, A posttreatment photograph is projected. The area of heavy treatment and the same landmark vessels can be outlined on a separate piece of paper. D, The treatment drawing (see Fig. 61-17) is placed under the pretreatment drawing (B) on a light box.

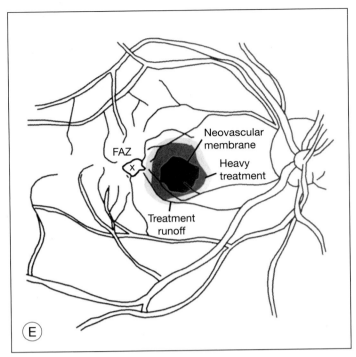

Fig. 61-21—cont'd E, The area of heavy treatment can then be traced on the pretreatment drawing to determine whether the treatment has covered the lesion entirely. (Reproduced from Bressler NM, Bressler SB, Fine SL. Age-related macular degeneration. Surv Ophthalmol 1988; 32:375–413.[2])

There is probably little hesitancy in extending treatment slightly beyond the borders of the lesion in an effort to ensure adequate coverage when the lesion is far away from the foveal center. Slight extension of treatment should have little effect on the visual acuity, since the treatment in these situations will not affect central foveal photoreceptors.

Conversely, when one is treating a juxtafoveal lesion, even the most experienced ophthalmologist may be reluctant to treat the foveal perimeter of the CNV too extensively. Excessive treatment in this situation could easily contribute to visual loss. However, failure to cover the CNV in its entirety could lead to increased persistence within 6 weeks of treatment, as noted earlier.[89–91]

Rarely, choroidal hemorrhage occurs as a treatment complication. Generally, choroidal hemorrhage stops spontaneously. If not, it can usually be controlled by applying pressure to the globe with the contact lens while treating the area of hemorrhage with repetitive laser spots, employing a larger spot size and longer duration than might have been used for CNV treatment. Long burns (0.5 to 1.0 s) and large spot sizes (200 μm or larger) decrease the chances of additional choroidal hemorrhage.

Wavelength selection for photocoagulation

When the MPS was begun in 1978, the argon blue-green laser was the wavelength most commercially available to investigators. This laser is no longer recommended for treatment within the macular region because macular xanthophyll pigment directly absorbs the blue light of the argon blue-green laser, thereby inducing thermal damage to the inner retina. In addition, the risk of inducing internal limiting membrane wrinkling, although rarely of clinical significance, is probably greatest with the argon blue-green laser. Subsequent trials in the MPS for juxtafoveal lesions employed the krypton red laser because of its theoretical advantage of penetrating through xanthophyll and passing through thin layers of red hemorrhage, allowing the uptake of the laser to be concentrated within the RPE and melanocytes of the

nonfoveal side. For recurrent lesions, additional photocoagulation 300 μm into the area of previous laser treatment at the interface with recurrent neovascularization was required. Feeder vessels were to be covered with laser treatment extending 100 μm beyond it on both sides and 300 μm beyond the base.[17,23]

If CNV is not very close to the foveal center, it is usually not difficult for an ophthalmologist experienced in treating CNV to extend laser treatment over the entire extent of the lesion.

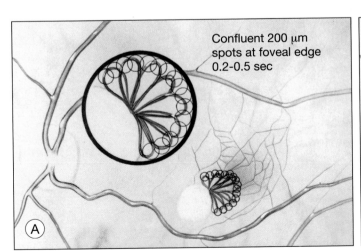

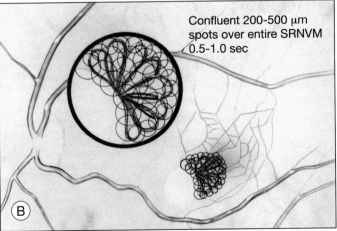

Fig. 61-22 Macular Photocoagulation Study (MPS) treatment protocol for photocoagulation of choroidal neovascularization. A, An initial burn (200 μm, 0.2 to 0.5 s) is placed along the perimeter of the lesion away from the fovea to determine the necessary power setting. Starting with the foveal side, the entire lesion is outlined with overlapping burns. B, Finally, the entire lesion or subretinal neovascular membrane (SRNVM) is treated with overlapping burns of sufficient intensity (200 to 500 μm, 0.5 to 1.0 s) to produce adequate intensity. (Reproduced from Elman MJ. Age-related macular degeneration. Int Ophthalmol Clin 1986; 26:117–144.)

inner choroid. When the MPS trials for subfoveal lesions were designed, eyes randomized to the treatment group were further randomized to either the argon green or the krypton red wavelength for treatment. None of the findings from the subfoveal trials suggests a reason to favor either the argon green or the krypton red wavelength.[99] If there was any theoretical advantage to using one wavelength over another for treatment of CNV, one might have expected to have detected a difference within the MPS subfoveal trials. Although these trials did not have sufficient power to demonstrate a small or moderate difference between the two wavelengths, a large difference has been ruled out by these studies.[99] Recurrence and persistence rates were also similar between the two laser wavelengths.[99] The recurrence and persistence rates were similar to those observed when the krypton red laser alone was used to treat neovascular lesions in the MPS trial of juxtafoveal neovascularization. Thus no visible wavelength appears to have a significant advantage over other wavelengths. Small differences in convenience of achieving the end-point of a uniform white burn might be seen with red or yellow wavelengths when penetrating through the increased yellow color of the lens nucleus in the older age group afflicted with CNV secondary to AMD, but any significant difference of clinical importance has not been shown.

Special circumstances relevant to laser photocoagulation

When treating CNV that lies under a major retinal vessel, the laser burns should straddle the retinal vessel to reduce the possibility of causing hemorrhage or damaging the vessel by thermal vasculitis. No evidence has suggested that this technique compromised the effectiveness of treatment.

When treating CNV that is contiguous with the optic nerve, it should be kept in mind that laser treatment directly over the optic nerve can cause thermal necrosis of disc tissue and nerve fiber bundle defects. Therefore one should consider refraining from treatment within 100 to 200 μm of the optic nerve. Similarly, when treating a peripapillary area of CNV, one may want to consider treatment only when at least 1½ clock-hours of papillomacular bundle on the temporal side of the disc is uninvolved with CNV so that at least 1½ clock-hours of papillomacular bundle can be spared of treatment, as was done in several of the MPS trials. Treatment to nasal or peripapillary lesions that met criteria for MPS trials will likely not lead to severe visual loss from damage to the nerve fiber layer that serves the central macula if the treatment guidelines outlined previously are followed.[100] In these situations, the MPS group reported that severe visual acuity loss was noted after treatment only when recurrent CNV extended through the center of the fovea.[100] This finding suggests that, in the absence of subfoveal recurrence, severe visual loss only from nerve fiber layer damage after this treatment approach must be a rare complication.

As previously discussed, certain subgroups in the various trials had different treatment benefits, which should be considered when determining whether treatment would be beneficial for a particular patient. This subgroup analysis should probably not completely sway the decision to recommend or deny treatment. Rather, the subgroup analysis data should serve as a guideline when deciding whether treatment should be recommended to a particular individual. For instance, in the krypton trial of juxtafoveal lesions, patients who were normotensive had a marked treatment benefit. Patients who had evidence of hypertension, either by elevated systolic or diastolic blood pressure or by the use of antihypertensive medication, had no treatment benefit. Although similar trends were noted in the argon trial for patients with CNV secondary to the OHS,[101] similar trends were not noted in the argon trial of CNV secondary to AMD[70] or in the subfoveal trials in AMD.[22,23] Therefore, although the data in the juxtafoveal trial failed to detect a treatment benefit for a subgroup of hypertensive patients, lack of corroboration of this finding in other prospective trials on CNV secondary to AMD cautions one from withholding treatments in patients who are hypertensive.

In the subfoveal trial for new lesions, subgroup analysis showed that the greatest treatment benefit was noted in lesions that were less than two MPS disc areas in size.[97] The impact of the initial size and visual acuity on the treatment benefit suggested that treatment was not likely to be beneficial for lesions greater than two MPS disc areas in size when the visual acuity was better than 20/200. In general, the relative risks and benefits of PDT with verteporfin need to be considered for these lesions (see below).

Drusenoid RPE detachments should not be included as a component to be treated in conjunction with subfoveal CNV. Most lesions that include serous RPE detachments were not evaluated in treatment trials in which the serous RPE detachment and not the subfoveal CNV was the major component of the lesion.

On rare occasions, an area of extrafoveal CNV is contiguous to a serous detachment of the RPE in which the serous detachment extends under the center of the FAZ. There have been case reports in which only the extrafoveal CNV in these lesions is treated, resulting in prompt flattening of the RPE detachment with improvement of vision in selected cases.[102] Nevertheless, with follow-up, many of these eyes have acquired recurrent CNV with extensive scarring and visual loss. In these situations, one should consider the possibility that the extrafoveal CNV is associated with a subfoveal fibrovascular PED – a pattern of occult CNV in which treatment of the extrafoveal CNV alone has not been shown to be of any benefit.

Occult choroidal neovascularization and laser photocoagulation

When the original studies demonstrating the benefit of laser photocoagulation for lesions not involving the fovea (juxtafoveal or extrafoveal lesions) were initiated, a distinction was not made between occult and classic CNV. A subsequent reanalysis of all fluorescein angiograms from the juxtafoveal AMD MPS trial strengthened the conclusion that treatment of lesions that involved classic CNV with no occult CNV was beneficial as compared with observation when treatment covered the entire lesion.[76] The risk of severe visual loss after photocoagulation treatment of classic CNV but not occult CNV in lesions that had both classic and occult components was essentially equivalent to no treatment. There were too few eyes with occult CNV only (i.e., occult CNV without evidence of classic CNV) with variable coverage of the lesion to draw conclusions about the benefit of treatment compared with observation in this subgroup. However, 41% of the eyes with occult CNV only that were not treated lost significant vision by 1 year after study entry, usually following the development of classic CNV, confirming the variable and sometimes poor outcome of subfoveal occult CNV without classic CNV.[76]

When a lesion with occult CNV only that does not extend into the foveal center and has well-demarcated boundaries presents in a symptomatic patient, it is probably reasonable to consider photocoagulation. This treatment may decrease the likelihood that the CNV will extend into the center of the fovea. However, since some of these lesions may remain stable for years, close follow-up to monitor for vision loss, lesion growth, or the development of classic CNV should be considered.

Posttreatment care following laser photocoagulation

A 35-mm black-and-white Polaroid transparency (Polaroid Polapan 35-mm film, CT 135-36) or video image of the treated eye obtained immediately after treatment allows the treating ophthalmologist to evaluate treatment adequacy within minutes of photocoagulation. Compared with the pretreatment angiogram, these images provide rapid feedback, while the patient is still in the office, as to whether the entire lesion has been completely covered by treatment. A drawing from the posttreatment transparency, outlining the area of heavy treatment, can be compared with the pretreatment drawing of the CNV (see Fig. 61-21). To facilitate the alignment of the two drawings, the same landmarks drawn from the pretreatment fluorescein angiogram should be retraced or identified by using image software that can match points (e.g., vessel crossings) from pretreatment and posttreatment images. The posttreatment and pretreatment drawings are then superimposed and the landmark vessels aligned. With this technique, the area of heavy treatment can be traced on to the original pretreatment drawing to determine, in an unbiased fashion, whether treatment has indeed covered the CNV lesion completely. In this way, an additional touch-up treatment may be considered before retrobulbar anesthesia has worn off or without need to recall the patient soon after leaving the office. This technique may be of value in preventing persistent or recurrent CNV from inadequate coverage or intensity. Because persistence and recurrence have an adverse effect on visual outcome, any measures that can reduce the likelihood of persistence or recurrence should have a positive effect on visual acuity treatment.

Whenever employing retrobulbar anesthesia, a light-pressure dressing should be applied after treatment to protect the eye from exposure keratitis and discomfort from diplopia. The patch can be removed several hours later. Beginning with the first postoperative day, patients should be instructed to monitor the size of the resulting scotoma and surrounding distortion by observing distance and near vision. An evaluation for new distortion surrounding the scotoma on an Amsler grid may also be beneficial. Any increase in the scotoma size or in the surrounding distortion on the first posttreatment day should prompt a call to the treating ophthalmologist. Early evaluation is usually appropriate. Such a change from baseline may indicate persistent or recurrent leakage.

Evaluations following laser photocoagulation

A follow-up evaluation that includes best-corrected vision, biomicroscopy of the fundus, and fluorescein angiography is obtained 2 to 3 weeks after treatment. Follow-up earlier than 2 weeks is often difficult to evaluate because swelling and leakage from the treatment itself may obscure persistent or recurrent CNV. At follow-up, an angiogram should be scrutinized for the presence of leakage at the periphery of the laser-treated area to identify the presence of persistent or recurrent CNV. Simultaneous projection of the fluorescein angiogram during biomicroscopy may help differentiate areas of atrophy, which stain, from areas of recurrent leakage with subretinal fluid. If no residual or recurrent CNV is noted at this time, a similar evaluation is repeated 2 to 4 weeks later because the risk of recurrent CNV is so high within the first 6 weeks to 12 months after treatment. By 6 weeks after treatment, a patient should be encouraged to monitor the central vision of the treated eye daily for clarity of distance and near vision, as well as for any distortion, blurry vision, or increase in scotoma. These latter symptoms might indicate leakage from persistent or recurrent CNV and are an indication for prompt examination. The ophthalmologist's office staff should also be aware that these patients may need prompt re-evaluation if such symptoms develop and not necessarily schedule such patients for the "next available opening" 2 or 3 weeks later. Furthermore, although the risk of recurrent CNV after treatment in eyes with AMD is high, results showing the benefits of treating selected cases of recurrent subfoveal CNV make follow-up warranted for identifying these recurrences before they become too large.

Clinical examination probably cannot replace fluorescein angiography in detecting all recurrent CNV after laser treatment. In one prospective evaluation in which recurrent CNV was not suspected on biomicroscopy within approximately 1 year after laser photocoagulation to CNV, definite or questionable recurrent CNV was identified on the fluorescein angiogram 12% of the time.[39] Most of these recurrent cases that were not identified on biomicroscopy alone were treated promptly after review of the fluorescein angiogram. This study also showed that questionable recurrences that showed focal staining along the edge of the laser lesion and speckled hyperfluorescence were the patterns that were most likely to progress to definite recurrence.[38]

Since many recurrences occur within 3 to 6 months after treatment, an evaluation, including fluorescein angiography, is again repeated at 3 to 4 and 6 to 8 months after treatment. Subsequent evaluations, probably with angiography, at 9 to 12 months after treatment appear to be indicated for CNV secondary to AMD that has been treated because many recurrences develop between 6 and 12 months after treatment. After 2 years, recurrences are unusual; follow-up every 6 to 12 months without angiography (unless signs or symptoms suggest a recurrence) is probably sufficient.

Recurrent CNV is also frequently seen in eyes that have previously undergone *foveal* photocoagulation,[90] although this situation occurs very infrequently at this time now that laser photocoagulation of subfoveal lesions is rarely employed with the advent of PDT.

Predicting recurrences following laser photocoagulation

It may be possible to reduce the risk of persistent CNV after treatment by ensuring that a uniform white laser treatment covers the extent of the CNV in its entirety. However, in the MPS trials for extrafoveal and juxtafoveal lesions secondary to AMD, recurrence was also likely if the fellow eye already had CNV or disciform scarring at the time of treatment of the study eye. If no CNV or scarring is present in the fellow eye at the time of treatment of the first eye, studies have suggested that the presence of large drusen in the macula of the fellow eye is associated with an increased risk of developing recurrent CNV in the first eye. Other factors that might increase the rate of recurrence include cigarette smoking, hypertension, and CNV that is very lightly pigmented.[89,90,92] This last finding may be a reflection of the difficulty in obtaining a uniform white confluent treatment in CNV that is very lightly pigmented; the inability to obtain a uniform white treatment burn is associated with an increased risk of persistent CNV after treatment.

Complications of laser photocoagulation

Immediate complications from treatment of CNV are uncommon. Rates of choroidal hemorrhage, which can occur when attempting to achieve a white burn, may be minimized by avoiding a spot size less than 200 μm and an exposure time shorter than 0.2 s. Macular pucker, observed with some frequency after argon blue-green laser treatment, is rarely clinically significant and is far less common when employing argon green or krypton red wavelengths.[67] Rates of inadvertent treatment of the foveola in extrafoveal or juxtafoveal lesions, the most serious treatment complication, can be minimized by concurrent comparison of vascular landmarks in the patient's fundus to landmarks seen on the fluorescein angiogram projection. Before treatment, the ophthalmologist must be confident that he or she has identified the center of the FAZ accurately. Drawing the landmarks of the pretreatment angiogram before commencing laser treatment increases the clinician's familiarity with a given patient's critical vascular landmarks. In addition, the use of retrobulbar or peribulbar anesthesia probably minimizes the likelihood of unplanned foveal photocoagulation resulting from sudden eye movement during treatment.

Delayed perfusion of choroidal vessels, thought to result from vascular spasm, has been reported following the use of the krypton red laser.[103] In most cases, normal choroidal perfusion returns rapidly without any permanent visual sequelae. The krypton red laser has also been implicated in RPE tears arising from treatment of CNV.[30] However, RPE tears may be observed spontaneously and after treatment of CNV using any wavelength, particularly in patients with associated RPE detachments, either serous or fibrovascular.

Visual acuity might decline several years after treatment with late remodeling and enlargement of the area of RPE disturbance. These areas have been reported by Morgan & Schatz[115] to increase in size by 50 to 100 μm over serial follow-up. In their series, 4 (3%) of 174 eyes lost vision when the area of disturbance extended into the fovea. The peripheral zone of atrophy in a laser-treated area may correspond with the runoff or spread of the laser burn during the treatment. "Runoff" refers to the border of less-intense whitening surrounding the area of heavy treatment; it probably represents less severe damage to the RPE, retina, and choroid. When runoff extends through the foveal center, vision may actually decrease several lines 1 year or more after treatment, unrelated to recurrence (Fig. 61-23). Rice et al.[104] correlated the degree of late RPE atrophy with "runoff," or "spread," seen immediately after treatment. However, whenever visual acuity declines after prior stabilization, one must scrutinize the eye intensely, both ophthalmoscopically and angiographically, for evidence of CNV recurrence.

PHOTODYNAMIC THERAPY

Until 1999, no treatment other than laser photocoagulation had been shown to reduce the risk of vision loss in patients with CNV from AMD in large-scale, randomized clinical trials. The TAP Study Group[73,105] reported that PDT with verteporfin (Visudyne) can reduce the risk of moderate and severe visual acuity loss for at least 2 years in patients who present with subfoveal lesions in AMD with a predominantly classic lesion composition (in which the area of classic CNV is at least 50% of the area of the lesion). The results were even greater in the absence of occult CNV.[81] The therapy also reduced the risk of contrast sensitivity loss at a level likely to be beneficial for a patient's visual function.[106] For occult with no classic lesions, the Verteporfin In Photodynamic therapy (VIP) Trial in AMD showed that PDT could reduce the risk of moderate and severe visual acuity loss by 2 years after randomization compared with a sham treatment.[79] While the primary outcome for the VIP trial, avoiding at least 15 letters (or three lines) of visual acuity loss at 1 year after randomization, was not statistically significantly different between the PDT and control group, the totality of the vision results (including avoiding three lines of loss at 2 years, avoiding six lines of loss at 1 and 2 years, mean visual acuity loss at 1 and 2 years, percentage 20/200 or worse) support considering this therapy for selected occult with no classic lesions. Specifically, occult with no classic lesions for which therapy was shown to reduce the risk of vision loss included lesions with recent disease progression (having blood associated with CNV, or definite loss of visual acuity within the past 3 months, or growth of the lesion on fluorescein angiography). Furthermore, therapy appeared to be beneficial for relatively small occult with no classic lesions or larger lesions with relatively poorer levels of visual acuity. While minimally classic

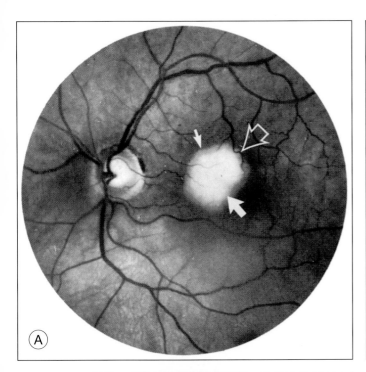

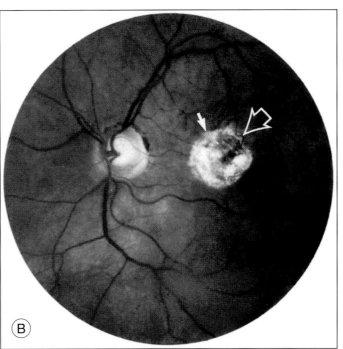

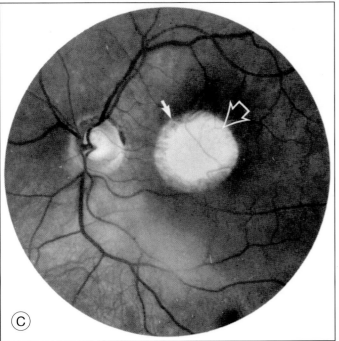

Fig. 61-23 Atrophy of the retinal pigment epithelium after laser photocoagulation of choroidal neovascularization. A, One day after treatment, an area of runoff, or spread, is seen as milder whitening (small arrow) surrounding the intense coagulation (large solid arrow). B, One year after treatment, the extent of retinal pigment epithelial atrophy (small arrow) appears to correlate with the extent of runoff seen immediately after treatment. Note the position of the atrophy relative to retinal vessel (open arrow). C, Three years after treatment, the retinal pigment epithelial atrophy (small arrow) appears to extend beyond the original area of runoff (note same retinal vessel). (Reproduced from Bressler NM, Bressler SB, Fine SL. Age-related macular degeneration. Surv Ophthalmol 1988; 32:375–413.[2])

lesions evaluated within a subgroup of classic-containing lesions in the TAP investigation showed no benefit of therapy, subsequent retrospective analyses of relatively small minimally classic lesions[79] and a small randomized clinical trial of relatively smaller minimally classic lesions,[107] showed a treatment benefit.

PDT involves the use of an intravenously injected photosensitizing drug combined with a low-intensity laser light to cause damage of choroidal neovascular tissue through a photochemical reaction by the light-activated drug that appears to result in direct cellular injury, including damage to vascular endothelial cells and vessel thrombosis.[108,109] An important advantage of this therapy is the potentially selective destruction of the CNV tissue. Retinal and choroidal tissue surrounding the CNV may be minimally disturbed, thus maintaining function of surrounding and overlying sensory retina, RPE, and choroid. Three multicenter, randomized clinical trials using benzoporphyrin-derivative monoacid verteporfin as the photosensitizing agent are currently under way to evaluate the effectiveness of this therapy, with additional trials evaluating other drugs, which have yet to show benefit in randomized clinical trials. When complexed with low-density lipoprotein (LDL) and injected intravenously, verteporfin may be taken up selectively by rapidly proliferating endothelial cells that have an increased number of LDL receptors active in their plasma membranes. Infrared laser light of low power (to avoid thermal damage) is used to irradiate the neovascular complex after verteporfin injection. Although the treatment can result in cessation of fluorescein dye leakage from CNV without significant visual loss at 1 and 4 weeks after treatment, fluorescein leakage from CNV is often apparent by 12 weeks after treatment,[108] with fewer and fewer treated cases showing fluorescein leakage with each subsequent follow-up after treatment is given.

Results of photodynamic therapy treatment and overall management approach to choroidal neovascularization in age-related macular degeneration

Outcomes of PDT compared with no treatment are summarized in Tables 61-1 through 61-4. Based on these results and the findings from the MPS regarding laser photocoagulation, a current approach to management of subfoveal CNV in AMD in which the CNV is the predominant component (that is, the area of any classic CNV plus any occult CNV is at least 50% of the area of the lesion) is summarized in Figure 61-13. For lesions that are predominantly scar or predominantly a serous PED, it is unknown if any treatment is beneficial, For lesions that are predominantly hemorrhagic (area of blood at least 50% of the area of the lesion), submacular surgery might be considered to reduce the risk of additional severe visual acuity loss if the lesion is not very large (< 16 disc areas) and visual acuity is better than 20/200 as measured in the SST.[18]

Preparation for photodynamic therapy

Before PDT, patients with a potentially treatable CNV lesion should be informed that PDT will not likely improve vision, although it does not reduce the chance of improving vision compared with no treatment, and it does reduce the risk of additional moderate and severe visual acuity loss. Further, patients should understand that most individuals lose some vision after PDT, usually within the first 12 months, and that there is a small risk of acute severe visual acuity decrease (loss of at least

Table 61-1 Evidence supporting benefits of verteporfin therapy at month 12[83,134] and month 24[82,83] examination in the Treatment of Age-related macular degeneration with Photodynamic therapy (TAP) investigation

Visual acuity loss (lines)	Visit (months)	Verteporfin n (%)	Placebo n (%)	P
Total patient population (verteporfin n = 402; placebo n = 207)				
≥ 3	12	156 (39)	111 (54)	<0.001
	24	189 (47)	129 (62)	<0.001
≥ 6	12	59 (15)	49 (24)	<0.006
	24	73 (18)	62 (30)	<0.001
Patients with predominantly classic CNV* (verteporfin n = 159; placebo n = 83)				
≥ 3	12	52 (33)	50 (60)	<0.001
	24	65 (41)	57 (69)	<0.001
≥ 6	12	19 (12)	28 (34)	<0.001
	24	24 (15)	30 (36)	<0.001
Patients with predominantly classic CNV with no occult CNV (verteporfin n = 90; placebo n = 44)				
≥ 3	12	21 (23)	32 (73)	<0.001
≥ 6	12	9 (10)	18 (41)	<0.001
Patients with predominantly classic CNV with occult CNV (verteporfin n = 69; placebo n = 40)				
≥ 6	12	10 (14)	10 (25)	0.17
	24	12 (17)	14 (36)	0.03
Patients with minimally classic CNV† (verteporfin n = 202; placebo n = 104)				
≥ 3	12	89 (44)	47 (45)	0.85
	24	106 (52)	58 (56)	0.584
≥ 6	12	34 (17)	17 (16)	0.62
	24	40 (20)	28 (27)	0.24

*In an exploratory analysis of patients with predominantly classic choroidal neovascularization (CNV), prior laser photocoagulation was not found to have a statistically significant effect on the treatment benefits of verteporfin therapy. At the month-24 examination, 10 (40%) of the 25 verteporfin-treated patients who had received prior laser photocoagulation had lost at least 15 letters of visual acuity compared with 5 (71%) of the 7 patients who received placebo (P = 0.21). The percentage of eyes that lost at least 30 letters of visual acuity at the month-24 examinations was also lower in verteporfin-treated patients in the subgroup that had received prior laser photocoagulation. Two verteporfin-treated patients (8%) had lost at least 30 letters of visual acuity at the month-24 examination compared with 3 patients (43%) who received placebo (P = 0.06).[83]
†In a retrospective analysis of patients with minimally classic subfoveal CNV due to age-related macular degeneration, in the subgroup with small lesions (≤ 4 Macular Photocoagulation Study (MPS) disc areas) and lower levels of visual acuity (< 65 letters, approximately worse than 20/50 Snellen equivalent), 42% of 57 verteporfin-treated patients lost at least 15 letters of visual acuity at the 12-month examination, compared with 63% of 27 patients given placebo. These benefits were sustained at the month-24 examination (also see Figs 61-2 and 61-3).[98]

Table 61-2 Evidence regarding outcomes of verteporfin therapy at month-12 and month-24 examinations in the Verteporfin In Photodynamic therapy (VIP) trial

Visual acuity change*	Visit (months)	Verteporfin n (%)	Placebo n (%)	P[†]
Patients with AMD with occult CNV with no classic CNV[‡67] (verteporfin n = 166; placebo n = 92)				
≥ 3 line loss	12	85 (51%)	51 (55%)	0.515
	24	91 (55%)	63 (68%)	0.032
≥ 6 line loss	12	37 (22%)	30 (33%)	0.07
	24	48 (29%)	43 (47%)	0.004
Patients with AMD with occult CNV with no classic CNV presenting either with smaller lesions or lower levels of visual acuity[67] (verteporfin n = 123; placebo n = 64)				
≥ 3 line loss	24	60 (49%)	48 (75%)	<0.001
≥ 6 line loss	24	26 (21%)	31 (48%)	<0.001
Patients with AMD with occult CNV with no classic CNV presenting with both larger lesions and higher levels of visual acuity[67] (verteporfin n = 43; placebo n = 27)				
≥ 3 line loss	24	31 (72%)	14 (52%)	0.09[§]
≥ 6 line loss	24	22 (51%)	11 (41%)	0.40[§]
Patients with pathologic myopia[16,84] (verteporfin n = 81; placebo n = 39)				
< 1.5 line loss	12	58 (72%)	17 (44%)	<0.01
	24	52 (64%)	19 (49%)	0.106
≥ 1.0 line gain	12	26 (32%)	6 (15%)	<0.01
	24	32 (40%)	5 (13%)	0.003

AMD, age-related macular degeneration; CNV, choroidal neovascularization.
*Values are approximate; there are five letters per line.
[†]Test for treatment effect within subgroups.
[‡]At the month-24 examination in the VIP trial, in the subgroup of patients presenting with occult CNV with no classic CNV, 5 of the 10 verteporfin-treated patients (50%) who had evidence of prior laser photocoagulation lost at least 15 letters of visual acuity compared with both of the patients (100%) given placebo (P = 0.19). Two verteporfin-treated patients (20%) had lost at least 30 letters of visual acuity by the month-24 examination compared with both (100%) of the placebo-treated patients (P = 0.03).[67]
[§]The placebo-treated group had the better outcome.

Table 61-3 Contrast sensitivity change at month-12[134] and month-24[82] examination in the Treatment of Age-related macular degeneration with Photodynamic therapy (TAP) investigation and at month-24 examination in the Verteporfin In Photodynamic therapy (VIP) trial

Visit (months)	Contrast sensitivity letters lost		P
	Verteporfin (letters)	Placebo (letters)	
TAP investigation: total patient population* (verteporfin n = 402; placebo n = 207)			
12	1.3	4.5	<0.001
24	1.3	5.2	<0.001
VIP trial: patients with occult CNV with no classic CNV (verteporfin n = 166; placebo n = 92)			
12	3.6	4.4	0.164
24	3.7	6.1	0.004

* In an exploratory analysis of patients with predominantly classic choroidal neovascularization (CNV) with occult CNV, the mean change in contrast sensitivity score from baseline was almost 0 at the month-24 examination in verteporfin-treated eyes compared with a decrease of approximately six letters (approximately two segments of contrast) in eyes receiving placebo.[83]

four lines of visual acuity compared with pretreatment levels within 7 days of treatment). Such events can occur from sudden hemorrhages (sometimes associated with tears or rips of the RPE), or choroidal perfusion abnormalities (sometimes associated with extensive subretinal fluid accumulation).[81]

Following the treatment protocol established by the TAP investigation and VIP trial, a recent fluorescein angiogram (if possible, less than 2 weeks old) should be used to guide the ophthalmologist during treatment. Because the CNV may grow or bleed, the treating ophthalmologist should confirm with careful biomicroscopic examination on the day of treatment that the lesion has not changed on that day if different from the day of the fluorescein angiogram. A suitable frame from the fluorescein angiogram can be displayed near the laser console

Table 61-4 Selected subgroup analyses in the Treatment of Age-related macular degeneration with Photodynamic therapy (TAP) investigation[82,83] and Verteporfin In Photodynamic therapy (VIP) trial[67] at month-24 examination

Characteristic	No. of eyes		Loss of ≥ 15 letters		P*
	Verteporfin	Placebo	Verteporfin n (%)	Placebo n (%)	
TAP investigation: total patient population (verteporfin n = 402; placebo n = 207)					
Greatest linear dimension (diameter of MPS disc area circle)					
≤ 3	107	46	41 (38.3)	23 (50.0)	0.219
> 3 to ≤ 6	152	97	68 (44.7)	66 (68.0)	
> 6 to ≤ 9	109	52	65 (59.6)	32 (61.5)	
> 9	25	8	14 (56.0)	6 (75.0)	
Initial visual acuity score in study eye (letters)					
73–54	203	101	114 (56.2)	66 (65.3)	0.158
53–34	199	106	75 (37.7)	63 (59.4)	
Age (years)					
<75	194	87	79 (40.7)	51 (58.6)	0.533
≥ 75	208	120	110 (52.9)	78 (65.0)	
Systemic hypertension					
Definite[†]	170	77	80 (47.1)	52 (67.5)	0.327
Others	232	130	109 (47.0)	77 (59.2)	
TAP investigation: patients with predominantly classic CNV (verteporfin n = 159; placebo n = 83)					
Evidence of prior laser photocoagulation					
Yes	25	7	10 (40)	5 (71)	0.85
No	134	76	55 (41)	52 (68)	
Phakic at enrolment					
Yes	124	62	51 (41)	41 (66)	0.44
No	35	21	14 (40)	16 (76)	
Micronutrient use					
Yes	80	45	33 (41)	33 (73)	0.44
No	79	38	32 (41)	24 (63)	
VIP trial: patients with occult CNV with no classic CNV (verteporfin n = 166; placebo n = 92)					
Lesion size (MPS disc areas)					
≤ 4	80	39	36 (45.0)	28 (71.8)	0.04
> 4	84	52	55 (65.5)	34 (65.4)	
Initial number of letters read (approximate Snellen equivalent visual acuity) in study eye					
≥ 65 (≥20/50)	87	51	58 (66.7)	32 (62.7)	0.004
< 65 (≤20/50⁻¹)	79	41	33 (41.8)	31 (75.6)	
Age (years)					
< 75	74	40	39 (52.7)	22 (55.0)	0.09
≥ 75	92	52	52 (56.5)	41 (78.8)	
Systemic hypertension					
Definite[†]	80	43	38 (47.5)	28 (65.1)	0.61
Others	86	49	53 (61.6)	35 (71.4)	

MPS, Macular Photocoagulation Study; CNV, choroidal neovascularization.
*Test of interaction between subgroups using a single logistic regression model that includes treatment.
[†]Definite hypertension was defined as systolic blood pressure of 160 mmHg or higher or of 140 to 159 mmHg with a history of hypertension or use of antihypertension medications or diastolic blood pressure of 95 mmHg or higher or of 90 to 94 mmHg with a history of hypertension or use of antihypertension medications.

top. Once the area of the entire lesion is determined, one can determine the greatest linear dimension (GLD) of the lesion. If the GLD is determined from a film angiogram, the ophthalmologist should divide that dimension by the magnification factor of the camera used to obtain the angiogram to get the GLD on the retina. The spot size to be used to activate the verteporfin should be approximately 1 mm greater than the GLD of the lesion on the retina. The ophthalmologist then enters the magnification of the lens to be used for applying laser light to activate verteporfin on the laser console *before* entering the spot size to be applied to the retina. Then the ophthalmologist should enter the spot size to be applied to the retina (that is, the GLD of the

lesion on the retina, plus 1 mm). The ophthalmologist should confirm that the laser is set to a standard fluence rate shown to be beneficial (50 J/cm²), which should indicate 83 s at 600 mW/cm².

The patient should also be warned of potential side-effects, including photosensitivity reactions, which are usually transient and mild, occurring in 2% of treated eyes. Verteporfin-treated patients should avoid significant light exposure for up to 2 days, when almost all photosensitivity reactions were reported in clinical trials (although the Food and Drug Administration recommended avoiding significant light exposure for up to 5 days). The physician or nurse overseeing the infusion of verteporfin over 10 min should watch for extravasations which might not cause pain during the extravasation but which can cause significant pain or edema at the injection site or, rarely, skin damage if exposed to sunlight. The patient should also understand that any extravasations should be covered from sunlight until the drug is believed to have been completely resorbed. Transient visual disturbance (20% of the time) and infusion-related back pain (2% of the time), not noted to be of any lasting significance, may also be seen.

Ophthalmologists should identify potentially treatable cases as soon as possible to preserve as much vision as possible. Treating ophthalmologists will need to identify the entire lesion and be able to distinguish between classic and occult CNV in order to determine if the lesion is predominantly classic CNV. Posttreatment follow-up will require identification of fluorescein leakage following previous PDT to judge when and where retreatment should be applied.

Follow-up after photodynamic therapy

Follow-up after PDT is summarized in Figure 61-24. Any decreased vision within 5 weeks after treatment may need prompt evaluation. If a change in the biomicroscopic examination is noted compared with the pretreatment appearance, fluorescein angiography may be indicated to try to understand why decreased vision has occurred, for example, due to growth of the lesion, additional fluid accumulation associated with classic CNV, bleeding, choroidal perfusion abnormalities, tears of the RPE, or other causes. Additional treatment for growth of the lesion earlier than 5 to 6 weeks has not been studied extensively, so that additional treatment at this time is probably not warranted, even if growth of the lesion or persistent fluorescein leakage with visual acuity loss is noted. If decreased vision is noted prior to 10 to 12 weeks after treatment and growth of the lesion is noted or persistent fluorescein leakage is noted on angiography, an additional course of PDT might be considered since no harm was shown when therapy was given as often as every 6 weeks.[110] However, retreatment as early as 6 weeks was not shown to result in significantly different outcomes from retreatment as early as 12 weeks, so that one could wait until 12 weeks before considering retreatment. Even if no change in vision is noted by 12 weeks after treatment, re-examination should occur at that time. If no fluorescein leakage from CNV is noted at that time, then no additional treatment is needed, although re-examination in another 6 to 12 weeks is warranted to see if leakage develops subsequently. If fluorescein leakage is noted, then treatment should be applied using the GLD on the area of leakage and any contiguous blood plus 1 mm when determining the spot size. This follow-up approach should be repeated indefinitely until treatment either seems futile (because the lesion is so large and the visual acuity is so decreased that reducing the risk of visual acuity loss would not likely impact on the patient's quality of life or visual function) or the

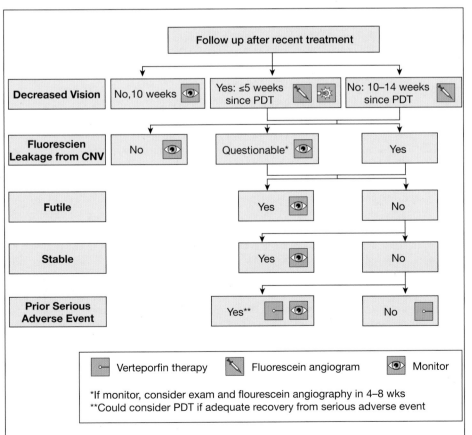

Fig. 61-24 Algorithm for monitoring, obtaining fluorescein angiography, or considering verteporfin therapy during follow-up of patients who have received a course of photodynamic therapy (PDT) with verteporfin. "Futile" indicates that a relatively large lesion is associated with a particularly low level of visual acuity such that additional treatment is judged unlikely to prevent further deterioration, and hence unlikely to have a positive impact on the patient's quality of life. "Stable" indicates that best-corrected visual acuity is stable or improved, the biomicroscopic and fluorescein angiographic appearance of the lesion is unchanged or improved with respect to the preceding pretreatment examination, including, a flat, scar-like appearance to the lesion, minimal or no subretinal fluid, and minimal fluorescein leakage from choroidal neovascularization without progression of fluorescein leakage beyond the boundaries of the area treated at the previous visit.

situation has stabilized (because there is minimal leakage associated with a relatively flat scar and no change in visual acuity, biomicroscopic appearance, or fluorescein angiographic appearance for at least 6 months). Usually, patients will need two to three treatments in the first year, and possibly one to two treatments in the second year after initiating PDT when following this schedule.

SUBMACULAR SURGERY

Recent studies have shown that visual acuity outcomes with submacular surgery are no different compared with observation for subfoveal CNV in patients with AMD in which a majority of the lesion is CNV and there is evidence of classic CNV.[25] However, for lesions which are predominantly hemorrhagic (at least 50% of the lesion is blood), submacular surgery can reduce the risk of additional severe visual acuity loss compared with observation, although many patients undergoing surgery lost at least two lines of visual acuity.[18] Specifically, 21% of patients undergoing removal of hemorrhage lost six or more lines of visual acuity compared with 36% assigned to observation. Almost half of the patients who were phakic at the time of undergoing submacular surgery had cataract surgery by 2 years. Furthermore, there was a relatively high risk of rhegmatogenous retinal detachment, especially when the lesion was > 16 disc areas or the visual acuity was very poor after enrollment. For this reason, submacular surgery for predominantly hemorrhagic lesions could be considered for lesions that were no greater than 16 disc areas if identified before visual acuity was very poor. More details on the findings of the trials investigating surgery for CNV in patients with AMD is included in the surgery volume of the book, in Chapter 150.

EARLY IDENTIFICATION OF CHOROIDAL NEOVASCULARIZATION

It has become critically important to identify, while potentially still at a treatable stage, those eyes at high risk for visual loss. Unfortunately, the likelihood of finding a case that will benefit from treatment appears to be time-dependent. Fluorescein angiographic studies have suggested growth of CNV lesions at an average rate of 10 μm to 18 μm per day.[111,112] Grey and colleagues[113] reported that patients with acute visual loss from AMD are more likely to have extrafoveal CNV if they are examined within the first month after the onset of symptoms.

Clearly, identifying lesions before they had extended under the foveal center, when laser photocoagulation can be considered, is worthwhile. Furthermore, identifying lesions while they are relatively small can result in better levels of final visual acuity when applying PDT (Figs 61-25 and 61-26). Finally, predominantly hemorrhagic lesions may benefit from intervention if identified while relatively small and before a large amount of visual acuity loss has occurred. Thus, a key approach in the management of AMD is to identify lesions promptly, recognizing new signs or symptoms of CNV so that treatment can more likely be applied when therapy is most likely to be beneficial.

PREVENTION OF CHOROIDAL NEOVASCULARIZATION

Two studies sponsored by the National Eye Institute of the US National Institutes of Health are evaluating treatments designed to prevent complications of AMD that lead to visual loss, including CNV. These studies include the Age-Related Eye Disease Study (AREDS) and the Complications of Age-Related Macular Degeneration Prevention Trial (CAPT). AREDS is evaluating whether micronutrients or zinc can prevent the development of complications of AMD, including CNV. CAPT is evaluating whether light laser photocoagulation, which has been associated with a decreased visualization of drusen,[114] can prevent the development of complications of AMD associated with visual loss, including CNV and geographic atrophy. Only cases with bilateral drusen without CNV or significant geographic atrophy in either eye are being enrolled. Previous studies[114] suggested that such treatment in the fellow eye of a patient who already developed CNV in the first eye could increase the risk of developing CNV in the treated eye, although without significant visual acuity loss recorded to date.[115] Another industry-sponsored study is evaluating whether light diode laser treatment can reduce the risk of developing vision loss from CNV.

RISK OF FELLOW-EYE INVOLVEMENT

When one eye has developed CNV, it is important to monitor the other eye for CNV, especially since substantial loss of vision in the first eye is highly likely.[116] Development of CNV in the second eye can be devastating, since patients may have functioned quite well with good vision in their remaining eye but would be abruptly confronted for the first time with severe lifestyle impairment with development of CNV in both eyes. Often, they may not have planned for this eventuality despite proper counseling at the time of the first eye involvement. It is therefore paramount to discover and treat CNV as soon as possible to maximize the possibility of detecting treatable lesions. Because patients may only be aware of symptoms when the fovea has become involved, it would be useful to stratify risk based on fundus appearance and perhaps employ more aggressive monitoring strategies in those deemed at high risk.

The investigators of the MPS Group have studied the eyes of 670 patients enrolled in the trials of laser therapy for extrafoveal, juxtafoveal, and subfoveal CNV to identify fundus characteristics that might be predictive of CNV development in the uninvolved fellow eyes.[117–119] Follow-up ranged from 3 to 5 years and revealed an overall incidence of 35%, which is consistent with previously reported figures. Application of life table estimation methods to this data yielded cumulative incidence rates of 10%, 28%, and 42% at 1, 3, and 5 years respectively. Three characteristics of the central macula and one systemic factor were associated independently with increased risk of developing CNV: the presence of five or more drusen, one or more large drusen, focal hyperpigmentation, and systemic hypertension. A substantial difference in prognosis was seen depending on the number of risk factors present. Estimated 5-year incidence rates ranged from 7% for the subgroup with no risk factors to

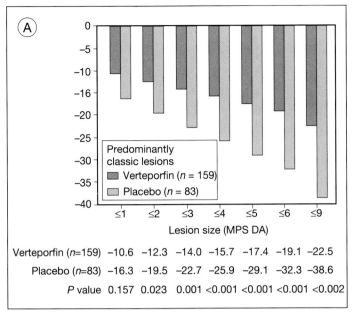

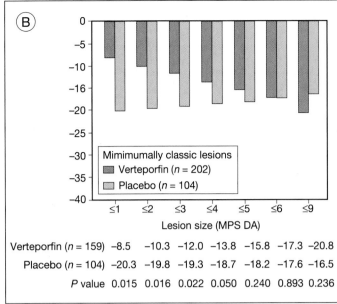

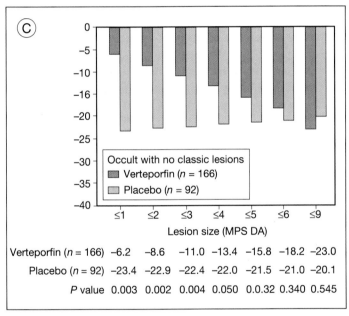

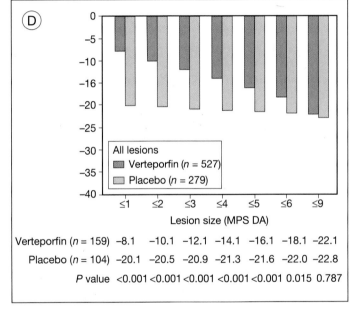

Fig. 61-25 Model-adjusted means of visual acuity change between baseline and month-24 examination for treated and untreated lesions by baseline lesion size based on multiple linear regression analysis in (A) patients with predominantly classic choroidal neovascularization (CNV), (B) patients with minimally classic CNV, (C) patients with occult with no classic CNV, and (D) all patients regardless of lesion composition at baseline. MPS DA, Macular Photocoagulation Study disc area. Reprinted with permission from Elsevier Inc. (Treatment of Age-related Macular Degeneration with Photodynamic Therapy (TAP) Study Group. Effect of lesion size, visual acuity, and lesion composition on visual acuity change from baseline with and without verteporfin therapy in choroidal neovascularization secondary to age-related macular degeneration: TAP and VIP report no 1. Am J Ophthalmol 2003; 136:407–418).

87% for the subgroup with all four risk factors. Similarly, in AREDS, subjects enrolled with advanced AMD (either neovascular AMD or central atrophy of the RPE) in one eye only at study entry had a 43% chance of developing advanced AMD in the fellow eye by 5 years.[120] The type of CNV present in the affected eye, classic versus occult, appeared to have no effect on the rate of CNV development in the fellow eye. It must be stressed that these figures do not apply to patients with nonneovascular abnormalities only in both eyes. They are, however, very important in counseling the AMD patient who has just experienced the initial development of CNV in one eye with respect to prognosis and frequency of follow-up to try to protect the vision in the other eye.

ADDITIONAL THERAPIES

Submacular surgery

Although there is no strong evidence to support benefits of submacular surgery,[25,87,105,121] except for reducing the risk of additional severe visual acuity loss in selected cases of predominantly hemorrhagic lesions, alternative surgical approaches under investigation for managing CNV and its neovascular complications

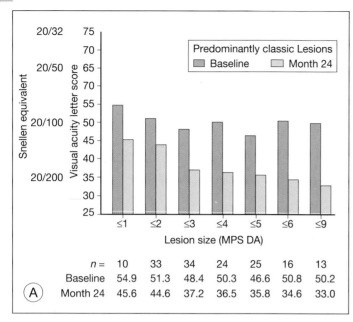

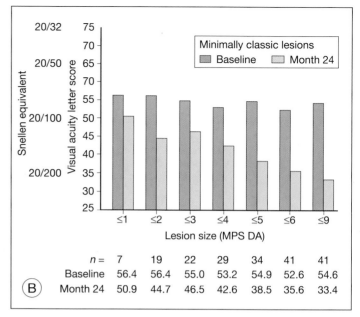

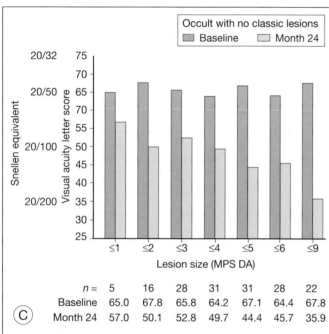

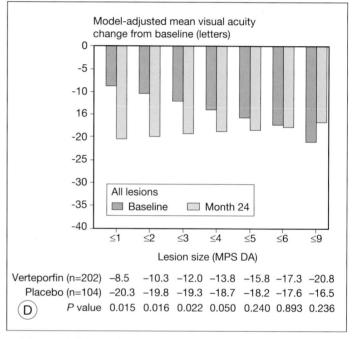

Fig. 61-26 Mean visual acuity among verteporfin-treated lesions at baseline and the month-24 examination for each lesion size category in (A) predominantly classic lesions, (B) minimally classic lesions, (C) occult with no classic lesions at baseline, and (D) all lesions. Reprinted with permission from Elsevier Inc. (Treatment of Age-related Macular Degeneration with Photodynamic Therapy (TAP) Study Group. Effect of lesion size, visual acuity, and lesion composition on visual acuity change from baseline with and without verteporfin therapy in choroidal neovascularization secondary to age-related macular degeneration: TAP and VIP report no 1. Am J Ophthalmol 2003; 136:407–418).

include macular translocation and mechanical displacement of relatively large submacular hemorrhages using intraocular gas injection. Macular translocation can be accomplished by vitrectomy combined with retinotomy or by vitrectomy combined with external sclerochoroidal foreshortening.[122] After translocation has been accomplished and the CNV lesion is no longer subfoveal, laser photocoagulation is applied with sparing of the foveal center from photocoagulation. These techniques might be shown to have applications for relatively small subfoveal lesions in which laser treatment or PDT with verteporfin is not

as beneficial. The American Academy of Ophthalmology published an *Ophthalmic Procedure Preliminary Assessment* of this technique,[123] highlighting the need for large-scale case series and randomized trials before widespread acceptance of this approach should be considered.

When AMD-related CNV is associated with a large submacular hemorrhage, intraocular injection of gas and face-down positioning may allow for mechanical displacement of the blood and at least temporary recovery of visual acuity.[124] The improvement may not have long-term benefit if the underlying neovascular lesion and its accompanying destruction of the retina, not the blood, determines the ultimate visual outcome. More experience is needed to evaluate the safety and benefit of these surgical approaches.

Indocyanine green angiography

Indocyanine green is a dye that is more highly protein-bound than sodium fluorescein and that fluoresces in the near-infrared wavelength. These properties were suggested to be useful in the evaluation and management of CNV. Many cases are ineligible for laser photocoagulation because the borders of the CNV are not well defined. In other cases, if the CNV fluorescence is blocked by the hemorrhage, then the blocked zone might be harboring CNV and should be included in the area under consideration for treatment. If the area of blocked fluorescence from blood on fluorescein angiography is very large, then treatment must be withheld and the lesion monitored to see if criteria for which treatment might be considered are met. The wavelength at which indocyanine green fluoresces allows it to penetrate blood better than that of sodium fluorescein. If CNV tissue adequately takes up this dye, then it is theoretically possible for CNV borders to be better visualized through blood that is thick enough to block fluorescein but not indocyanine green dye fluorescence.

Three basic patterns of fluorescence have been reported in indocyanine green angiography of CNV judged to be occult on fluorescein angiography: a small, focal "hot spot" (a bright area of fluorescence more than one disc area that usually shows by the mid-phase of the angiogram), a plaque (a well-demarcated area of fluorescence more than one disc area in size that emerges relatively late in the angiogram), and ill-defined fluorescence.[125,126] Because the hot spot is small and may be extrafoveal in location, attention is drawn to it as a possible treatment site. Pilot studies utilizing photocoagulation of this site have reported improvement or stabilization of visual acuity, as well as resolution of "exudative features."[125-128] However, similar outcomes have been observed in eyes with occult CNV that have not received any treatment.[76,129] For example, a reanalysis of data used in the MPS juxtafoveal trial suggested that eyes with occult only CNV may have a more favorable natural course than eyes with classic CNV only. It is possible that the outcome of treating hot spots is no better than that of the natural course of these lesions. As described previously, eyes with both classic and occult CNV did not benefit from photocoagulation of the classic component alone. Treatment of the entire neovascular complex appears to be necessary. Treatment of a "hot spot" alone, identified on indocyanine green and associated with a larger area judged to be occult CNV on fluorescein angiography, may be similar to the unsuccessful strategy of treating just the classic CNV in an eye with both classic and occult CNV on fluorescein angiography. Until carefully designed, randomized clinical trials are conducted that show that indocyanine green-guided laser therapy of AMD-related CNV results in a better visual outcome than no treatment, one cannot know for sure if this particular intervention is beneficial.[129]

Radiation therapy

The use of radiation therapy for CNV in AMD is based on the possibility that radiation can damage rapidly proliferating neovascular tissue. Studies have been inconsistent in documenting a benefit to this approach.[130-132]

Pharmacologic therapy with angiogenesis inhibitors

Recombinant interferon-alpha-2a administered systemically is a weak inhibitor of angiogenesis that is commercially available. However, when tested in a randomized clinical trial, the treatment was found to be of no benefit, and possibly harmful, compared to placebo treatment.[133] This outcome, which confirmed the variable course of untreated subfoveal CNV in AMD, especially within the first year after presentation, underscores the need for randomized clinical trials in any evaluation of pharmacologic or other therapies for CNV in AMD.

Pegaptanib sodium, a modified oligonucleotide that binds to an isoform of vascular endothelial growth factor (VEGF), has been studied in two recent phase II/III multicenter trials involving 1186 patients randomized 1:1:1:1 to sham, or 0.3 mg, 1 mg, or 3 mg of pegaptanib intraocular injections. Injections were given every 6 weeks. The trials enrolled patients with subfoveal CNV due to AMD with lesions smaller than 12 disc areas, of which at least 50% of the lesion had to be CNV (i.e., the lesion was *predominantly* CNV). In addition, there could not be atrophy or fibrosis in the center of the macula. Individuals with minimally classic or occult with no classic lesion compositions required evidence of recent disease progression.[133a]

For the primary endpoint of the proportion of patients losing less than 3 lines of visual acuity by week 54, a combined analysis found an absolute difference of 15% in favor of treatment (70% vs 55%; $P < 0.001$) for the 294 patients receiving pegaptanib 0.3 mg. No dose response was seen in the pegaptanib studies; pegaptanib at 1.0 mg or 3.0 mg was less effective than at 0.3 mg for all outcomes.

The percentage of patients losing less than 3 lines of visual acuity was not reported for the different lesion compositions. As prognosis varies according to lesion characteristics at baseline it will be important to examine the efficacy for the different lesion subtypes. Furthermore, although there was a possible trend for the treatment effect to be greater for smaller lesions, it is unknown if the therapy reduces the risk of vision loss for all small or large lesions, or those that are predominantly classic, or minimally classic, or occult with no classic. Natural history data from the verteporfin trials suggest that *both* lesion size *and* lesion composition need to be considered when deciding if a therapy is beneficial for CNV in AMD. Also, for predominantly classic lesions treated with pegaptanib injections, the results should be interpreted with the recognition that these patients could also receive PDT. PDT almost never was added to patients who had at baseline a minimally classic or occult with no classic lesion in VISION.

Although the incidence of endophthalmitis was low when expressed on a per-injection basis, the need to administer treatment at 6-week intervals increases this risk. During the 12 months of the studies, 1.3% of pegaptanib recipients had endophthalmitis; of these, few (8%) lost 6 or more lines of visual acuity. The optimal duration of pegaptanib therapy has yet to be established. In the phase II/III clinical trials treatment through 1 year followed by re-randomization for a further year was investigated with a different endpoint, namely first time to loss of at least 15 letters, with some patients initially assigned to sham able to receive pegaptanib. Further long-term data are expected to be published regarding long-term efficacy and safety. Just as this book was being printed, favorable results about another anti-VEGF agent, ranibizumab, have been announced via press release but results of the large phase 3 trials are not yet published. The parent molecule of ranibizumab, bevacizumab, which is larger and must be administered systemically, showed favorable results in a pilot study.[133b]

PATIENT EDUCATION AND REHABILITATION

Patient education is an extremely important part of the management of patients with AMD. All patients over the age of 50 who have drusen should be made aware of the importance of regular central visual acuity testing in each eye to facilitate early detection of CNV. Although the Amsler grid is often recommended, it is not particularly sensitive or specific; frequently, changes in near or distance vision herald underlying neovascularization not detected by the patient on an Amsler grid.[8] Therefore patients experiencing any change in vision in eyes at risk for neovascularization should be encouraged to contact their ophthalmologist promptly. Although patients should be counseled about the risk of severe central visual loss, they should also be reassured that AMD almost never leads to total blindness. Patients at risk should be informed that, in its more severe neovascular form, central visual tasks can be severely and permanently impaired. In light of the therapeutic implications of prompt laser photocoagulation or PDT, the importance of quickly reporting new visual symptoms must be stressed to all patients. At the same time, they should be reassured that no harm will come by continuing to read or perform routine visual tasks. On the contrary, patients should be encouraged to continue reading and to pursue vigorously any visual activity that they enjoy.

Treatment does not end in the physician's office when the diagnosis is established or when laser treatment or PDT is applied. Visual rehabilitation forms an integral part of patient care in AMD. Patients with central visual impairment should be evaluated and educated in the use of visual aids such as magnifiers. Magnification and improved contrast sensitivity through bright illumination are particularly helpful. To arrive at the best magnifying aid, one starts with a complete low visual evaluation. In addition, the patient should be counseled on available low-vision materials such as large-print newspapers, magazines, and books. Large-print materials permit many people who are unable to read normal print to continue reading for a considerable period of time. Newspapers such as the *New York Times* and periodicals such as *Reader's Digest* and *Newsweek* are currently published in large-print editions. The local library can assist with the selection of magazines and books available in large print. The Library of Congress in Washington, DC, maintains a list of books and magazines available on loan without cost on virtually every subject. The combination of bright illumination, powerful magnification, and large type allows all but the most severely impaired patients to continue reading, albeit on a more limited scale. Reading skills frequently need to be relearned in a painstakingly slow process. Nevertheless the ability to continue reading, even on a limited basis, may provide tremendous psychologic support to these patients. Some patients with AMD may find the use of a closed-circuit television viewer helpful for reading. This machine uses a projection device to magnify one or several words on to a television screen. Unfortunately, this instrument is large and fairly expensive; thus it is generally purchased by people with sufficient economic means who use it primarily in one location such as at work or at home. For those patients who are unable to take advantage of large-print materials or who cannot use magnification devices, talking books or tapes are available. These may be borrowed through local libraries or from the Library of Congress. Audiotapes of popular books are also sold at many bookstores.

Patients with severe visual loss require early referral to an appropriate agency for low vision so that they can take advantage of community support services. Information can be obtained from the Directory of Agencies serving the visually handicapped in the USA through the American Foundation for the Blind. The American Foundation for the Blind also provides information regarding other aids such as talking books and clocks and watches that audibly tell time.

Because AMD can place severe restrictions on many activities such as driving and rapid reading of small print, visual rehabilitation efforts are directed toward preserving the patient's independence as much as possible. Toward this end, social service consultations are invaluable. In addition, in-house evaluations by agencies designed to assist the visually impaired are useful in helping with activities of daily living. Simple recommendations, such as using brightly colored utensils on a white or black background in the kitchen, as well as suggestions on improving existing lighting, can be of tremendous benefit. Similar ideas aimed at increasing contrast may improve the quality of life for these patients. Patients often become frustrated because of their inability to perform certain fine visual tasks, such as reading and sewing. Unable to recognize faces from across the room, patients with visual loss from AMD may feel isolated and withdraw from social contact. In the absence of any external tell-tale signs of blindness, friends and relatives may attribute the lack of recognition to a sudden "snobbishness" rather than to visual impairment. Patient and family alike should be educated about these problems. In particular, patients should be encouraged to become more outgoing, which in turn fosters recognition of others through speech rather than vision. Discussion of the patient's problems by the physician often helps to relieve patients of much of their burdens.

Ophthalmologists must recognize that elderly patients can have difficulty coping with the new onset of severe visual loss. Patients may resist efforts to use magnifying devices for a variety of reasons, including denial and secondary gain. Often tremulousness interferes with the patient's ability to use certain aids. All these conditions may increase the tendency to depression or anxiety that many patients with visual loss have, including patients with AMD. In addition to caring for the eye, the ophthalmologist should serve as the patient's advocate, marshaling his or her resources for the patient's benefit. This includes compassionate support, educating the patient and family, and making appropriate referrals to maintain the patient's quality of life. With complete care of the patient, many individuals at risk for, or suffering severe visual loss from, AMD can continue to enjoy fulfilling lives.

REFERENCES

1. Eye Diseases Prevalence Research Group. Prevalence of age-related macular denegeration in the United States. Arch Ophthalmol 2004; 122:564–572.
2. Bressler NM, Bressler SB, Fine SL. Age-related macular degeneration. Surv Ophthalmol 1988; 32:375–413.
3. Ferris FL III, Fine SL, Hyman LA. Age-related macular degeneration and blindness due to neovascular maculopathy. Arch Ophthalmol 1984; 102:1640–1642.
4. Sommer A, Tielsch JM, Katz J et al. Racial differences in the cause-specific prevalence of blindness in east Baltimore. N Engl J Med 1991; 325:1412–1417.
5. Schultz DW, Klein M, Humpert AJ et al. Analysis of the ARMDI locus: evidence that a mutation in HEMICENTIN-1 is associated with age-related macular degeneration in a large family. Hum Mol Genet 2003; 12:3315–3323.
6. Hyman L, Schachat AP, He Q et al. Hypertension, cardiovascular disease, and age-related macular degeneration. Age-Related Macular Degeneration Risk Factors Study Group. Arch Ophthalmol 2000; 118:351–358.
7. Loewenstein A, Bressler NM, Bressler SB. Epidemiology of RPE disease. In: Marmor MF, Wolfensberger TJ, eds. Retinal pigment epithelium: current aspects of function and disease. New York: Oxford University Press; 1999.
8. Fine AM, Elman MJ, Ebert JE et al. Earliest symptoms caused by neovascular membranes in the macula. Arch Ophthalmol 1986; 104:513–514.
9. Bressler SB, Silva JC, Bressler NM et al. Clinicopathologic correlation of occult choroidal neovascularization in age-related macular degeneration. Arch Ophthalmol 1992; 110:827–832.
10. Green WR, Key SN. Senile macular degeneration: a histopathologic study. Trans Am Ophthalmol Soc 1977; 75:180–254.
11. Green WR, McDonnell PH, Yeo JH. Pathologic features of senile macular degeneration. Ophthalmology 1985; 92:615–627.
12. Green WR, Enger C. Age-related macular degeneration histopathologic studies. The 1992 Lorenz E. Zimmerman lecture. Ophthalmology 1993; 100:1519–1535.
13. Doyle WJ, Davidorf FH, Makley TA et al. Histopathology of an active lesion of ocular histoplasmosis. Ophthalm Forum 1984; 2:105–111.
14. Schatz H, McDonald HR, Johnson RN. Retinal pigment epithelial folds associated with retinal pigment epithelial detachment in macular degeneration. Ophthalmology 1990; 97:658–665.
15. Elman MJ, Fine SL, Murphy RP et al. The natural history of serous retinal pigment epithelium detachments in patients with age-related macular degeneration. Ophthalmology 1986; 93:224–230.
16. Bird AC, Marshal J. Retinal pigment epithelial detachment in the elderly. Trans Ophthalmol Soc UK 1986; 105:674–682.
17. Macular Photocoagulation Study Group. Subfoveal neovascular lesions in age-related macular degeneration: guidelines for evaluation and treatment in the Macular Photocoagulation Study. Arch Ophthalmol 1991; 109:1242–1257.
18. Submacular Surgery Trials (SST) Research Group. Surgery for hemorrhagic choroidal lesions of age-related macular degeneration: ophthalmic findings. SST report no. 13. Ophthalmology 2004; 111:1993–2006.
19. Taylor HR, West S, Munoz B et al. The long-term effects of visible light on the eye. Arch Ophthalmol 1992; 110:99–104.
20. Wood WJ, Smith TR. Senile disciform macular degeneration complicated by massive hemorrhagic retinal detachment and angle closure glaucoma. Retina 1983; 3:296–303.
21. el Baba F, Jarrett WH II, Harbin IS et al. Massive hemorrhage complicating age-related macular degeneration. Ophthalmology 1986; 93:1281–1592.
22. Macular Photocoagulation Study Group. Laser photocoagulation of subfoveal neovascular lesions in age-related macular degeneration: results of a randomized clinical trial. Arch Ophthalmol 1991; 109:1220–1231.
23. Macular Photocoagulation Study Group. Subfoveal neocular lesions in age-related macular degeneration: results of a randomized clinical trial. Arch Ophthalmol 1991; 109:1232–1241.
24. Macular Photocoagulation Study Group. Laser photocoagulation of juxtafoveal choroidal neovascularization: 5-year results from randomized clinical trials. Arch Ophthalmol 1994; 111:500–509.
25. Submacular Surgery Trials (SST) Research Group. Surgery for subfoveal choroidal neovascularization of age-related macular degeneration: ophthalmic findings. SST report no. 11. Ophthalmology 2004; 111:1967–1980.
26. Cantrill HL, Ramsay RC, Knoblock WH. Rips in the pigment epithelium. Arch Ophthalmol 1983; 101:1074–1079.
27. Decker WL, Sanborn GF, Ridley M et al. Retinal pigment epithelial tears. Ophthalmology 1983; 90:507–512.
28. Green SN, Yarian D. Acute tears of the retinal pigment epithelium. Retina 1983; 3:16–20.
29. Hoskin A, Bird AC, Sehow K. Tears of detached retinal pigment epithelium. Br J Ophthalmol 1981; 65:417–422.
30. Yeo JH, Marcus S, Murphy RP. Retinal pigment epithelial tears: patterns and prognosis. Ophthalmology 1988; 95:813.
31. Gass JDM. Stereoscopic atlas of macular disease and treatment, 4th edn. St Louis: Mosby; 1997.
32. Bressler NM, Finkelstein D, Sunness JS et al. Retinal pigment epithelial tears through the fovea with preservation of good visual acuity. Arch Ophthalmol 1990; 108:1694–1697.
33. Grossniklaus HE, Green WR, for the Submacular Surgery Trials Research Group. Histopathologic and ultrastructural findings of surgically-excised choroidal neovascularization. Arch Ophthalmol 1998; 116:745–749.
34. Submacular Surgery Trials Research Group. Histopathological and ultrastructural features of surgically-excised subfoveal choroidal neovascularization and associated tissue. SST report no. 6. Arch Ophthalmol 2005; 122: in press.
35. Grossniklaus HE, Green WR. Choroidal neovascularization. Am J Ophthalmol 2004; 137:496–503.
36. Lafaut BA, Bartz-Schmidt KU, Vanden Broecke C et al. Clinicopathologic correlation in exudative age related macular degeneration: histological differentiation between classic and occult choroidal neovascularization. Br J Ophthlamol 2000; 84:239–243.
37. Comparison of two-dimensional reconstructions of surgically-excised subfoveal choroidal neovascularization with fluorescein angiographic features: SST report no. 15. Ophthalmology 2005; 112: in press.
38. Dyer DS, Brant AM, Schachat AP et al. Questionable recurrent choroidal neovascularization: angiographic features and outcome. Am J Ophthalmol 1995; 120:497–505.
39. Sykes SO, Bressler NM, Maguire MG et al. Detecting recurrent choroidal neovascularization: comparison of clinical examination with and without fluorescein angiography. Arch Ophthalmol 1994; 111:1561–1566.
40. Treatment of Age-Related Macular Degeneration with Photodynamic Therapy (TAP) and Verteporfin In Photodynamic Therapy Study Groups. Photodynamic therapy of subfoveal choroidal neovascularization with verteporfin: fluorescein angiographic guidelines for evaluation and treatment – TAP and VIP report no. 2. Arch Ophthalmol 2003; 121:1253–1268.
41. Submacular Surgery Trials (SST) Research Group. Guidelines for interpreting retinal photographs in the Submacular Surgery Trials (SST). SST Report No. 8. Retina 2005; 25:253–268.
42. Koenig F, Soubrane G, Coscas G. Angiographic aspects of senile macular degeneration: spontaneous course. J Fr Ophtalmol 1984; 7:93–98.
43. Frost L, Bressler NM, Bressler SB et al. Natural course of poorly defined choroidal neovascularization associated with age-related macular degeneration. Invest Ophthalmol 1988; 29 (suppl.):120.
44. Hyman L, Lilienfeld AM, Ferris FL III et al. Senile macular degeneration: a case-control study. Am J Epidemiol 1983; 118:213–227.
45. Yannuzzi LA, Negrao S, Iida T et al. Retinal angiomatous proliferation in age-related macular degeneration. Retina 2001; 21:416–434.
46. Bressler NM, Bressler SB, Alexander J et al. Loculated fluid: a previously undescribed angiographic finding in macular degeneration. Arch Ophthalmol 1991; 109:211–215.
47. Chuang EL, Bird AC. The pathogenesis of tears of the retinal pigment epithelium. Am J Ophthalmol 1988; 105:285–290.
48. Killingsworth MC, Sarks JP, Sarks SH. Macrophages related to Bruch's membrane in age-related macular degeneration. Eye 1990; 4:613–621.
49. Ambati J, Ambati BK, Yoo SH et al. Age-Related Macular Degeneration: Etiology, Pathogenesis, and Therapeutic Strategies. Survey of Ophthalmol 2003; 48:257–293.
50. Gragoudas ES, Adamis AP, Cunningham Jr. ET al, for the VEGF Inhibition Study in Ocular Neovascularization Clinical Trial Group. Pegaptanib for neovascular age-related macular degeneration. N Engl J Med 2004; 351:2805–2816.

51. Preliminary Phase III Data Show Lucentis Maintained Or Improved Vision In Nearly 95 Percent Of Patients With Wet Age-Related Macular Degeneration, http://www.gene.com/gene/news/press-releases/. Date accessed, June 2005.

52. Bressler NM, Silva JC, Bressler SB et al. Clinicopathologic correlation of drusen and retinal pigment epithelial abnormalities in age-related macular degeneration. Retina 1994; 14:130–142.

53. Curcio CA, Millican CL. Basal linear deposit and large drusen are specific for early age-related macular degeneration. Arch Ophthalmol 1999; 117:329–339.

54. Sarks SH. Aging and degeneration in the macular region: a clinicopathological study. Br J Ophthalmol 1976; 60:324–341.

55. Sarks SH. Drusen and their relationship to senile macular degeneration. Aust J Ophthalmol 1980; 8:117–130.

56. Sarks SH, Penfold PL, Killingsworth MC et al. Patterns in macular degeneration. In: Ryan SJ, Dawson AK, Little HL, eds. Retinal diseases. Orlando: Grune & Stratton; 1985.

57. Sarks SH, Van Driel D, Maxwell L et al. Softening of drusen and subretinal neovascularization. Trans Ophthalmol Soc UK 1980; 100:414–422.

58. Kenyon KR, Maumenee AE, Ryan SJ et al. Diffuse drusen and associated complications. Am J Ophthalmol 1985; 100:119–128.

59. Eagle RC. Mechanisms of maculopathy. Ophthalmology 1984; 91:613–625.

60. Heriot WJ, Henkind P, Bellhorn RW et al. Choroidal neovascularization can digest Bruch's membrane: a prior break is not essential. Ophthalmology 1984; 91:1603–1608.

61. Loffler KU, Lee WR. Basal linear deposit in the human macula. Graefes Arch Clin Exp Ophthalmol 1986; 224:493–501.

62. Penfold PL, Killingsworth MC, Sarks SH. Senile macular degeneration: the involvement of immunocompetent cells. Graefes Arch Clin Exp Ophthalmol 1985; 223:69–76.

63. Penfold PL, Provis JM, Billson FA. Age-related macular degeneration: ultrastructural studies of the relationship of leukocytes to angiogenesis. Graefes Arch Clin Exp Ophthalmol 1987; 225:70–76.

64. Campochiaro PA, Hackett SF, Vinores SA et al. Platelet-derived growth factor is an autocrine growth stimulator in retinal pigmented epithelial cells. J Cell Sci 1994; 107:2459–2469.

65. Glaser BM. Extracellular modulating factors and the control of intraocular neovascularization. Arch Ophthalmol 1988; 106:603–607.

66. Bressler NM, Bressler SB, Gragoudas ES. Clinical characteristics of choroidal neovascular membranes. Arch Ophthalmol 1987; 105:209–213.

67. Berkow JW. Subretinal neovascularization in senile macular degeneration. Am J Ophthalmol 1984; 97:143–147.

68. Moisseiev J, Alhalel A, Masuri R et al. The impact of the Macular Photocoagulation Study results on the treatment of exudative age-related macular degeneration. Arch Ophthalmol 1995; 113:185–189.

69. Macular Photocoagulation Study Group. Argon laser photocoagulation for neovascular maculopathy: 3-year results from randomized clinical trials. Arch Ophthalmol 1986; 104:694–701.

70. Macular Photocoagulation Study Group: Argon laser photocoagulation for neovascular maculopathy after 5 years: results from randomized clinical trials. Arch Ophthalmol 1991; 109:1109–1114.

71. Macular Photocoagulation Study Group. Argon laser photocoagulation for senile macular degeneration: results of a randomized clinical trial. Arch Ophthalmol 1982; 100:912–918.

72. Macular Photocoagulation Study Group. Laser photocoagulation of subfoveal neovascular lesions of age-related macular degeneration: updated findings from two clinical trials. Arch Ophthalmol 1993; 111:1200–1209.

73. Treatment of Age-Related Macular Degeneration with Photodynamic Therapy (TAP) Study Group. Photodynamic therapy of subfoveal choroidal neovascularization in age-related macular degeneration with verteporfin: Two year results of 2 randomized clinical trials – TAP report no. 2. Arch Ophthalmol 2001; 119:198–207.

74. Treatment of Age-Related Macular Degeneration with Photodynamic Therapy (TAP) Study Group. Effect of lesion size, visual acuity, and lesion composition on visual acuity change from baseline with and without verteporfin therapy in choroidal neovascularization secondary to age-related macular degeneration: TAP and VIP report no. 1. Am J Ophthalmol 2003; 136:407–418.

75. Bressler NM, Maguire MG, Murphy PL et al. Macular scatter ("grid") laser treatment of poorly demarcated subfoveal choroidal neovascularization in age-related macular degeneration: results of a randomized pilot trial. Arch Ophthalmol 1996; 114:1456–1464.

76. Macular Photocoagulation Study Group. Occult choroidal neovascularization: influence on visual outcome in patients with age-related macular degeneration. Arch Ophthalmol 1996; 114:400–412.

77. Soubrane G, Coscas G, Francais C et al. Occult subretinal new vessels in age-related macular degeneration: natural history and early laser treatment. Ophthalmology 1990; 97:649–657.

78. Tani PM, Buettner H, Robertson DM. Massive vitreous hemorrhage and senile macular choroidal degeneration. Am J Ophthalmol 1980; 90:525–533.

79. Verteporfin in Photodynamic Therapy (VIP) Study Group. Photodynamic therapy of subfoveal choroidal neovascularization in age-related macular degeneration with verteporfin: Two year results of a randomized clinical trial including lesions with occult but no classic neovascularization – VIP report no. 2. Am J Ophthalmol 2001; 131:541–560.

80. Treatment of Age-Related Macular Degeneration with Photodynamic Therapy (TAP) Study Group. Natural history of minimally classic subfoveal choroidal neovascular lesions in the Treatment of Age-related macular degeneration with Photodynamic therapy (TAP) Investigation: Outcomes potentially relevant to management – TAP Report no. 6. Arch Ophthalmol 2004; 122:325–329.

81. Treatment of Age-Related Macular Degeneration with Photodynamic Therapy (TAP) Study Group. Verteporfin therapy of subfoveal choroidal neovascularization in patients with age-related macular degeneration: additional information regarding baseline lesion composition's impact on vision outcomes – TAP Report No. 3. Arch Ophthalmol 2002; 120:1443–1454.

82. Avery RL, Fekrat S, Hawkins BS et al. Natural history of subfoveal subretinal hemorrhage in age-related macular degeneration. Retina 1996; 16:183–189.

83. Bennett SR, Folk JC, Blodi CF et al. Factors prognostic of visual outcome in patients with subretinal hemorrhage. Am J Ophthalmol 1990; 109:33–37.

84. Berrocal MH, Lewis ML, Flynn HW Jr. Variations in the clinical course of submacular hemorrhage. Am J Ophthalmol 1996; 122:486–493.

85. Hanscom TA, Diddie KP. Early surgical drainage of macular subretinal hemorrhage. Arch Ophthalmol 1987; 105:1722–1723.

86. Lewis H, Jaffe GJ, Blumenkranz MS. Management of submacular hemorrhage with vitreoretinal surgery and subretinal injection of tissue plasminogen activator. Invest Ophthalmol Vis Sci 1992; 33:898.

87. Bressler NM. Submacular surgery: are randomized trials necessary? Arch Ophthalmol 1995; 113:1557–1560.

88. Schoeppner G, Chuang EL, Bird AC. The risk of fellow eye visual loss with unilateral retinal pigment epithelial tears. Am J Ophthalmol 1989; 108:683–685.

89. Macular Photocoagulation Study Group. Persistent and recurrent neovascularization after krypton laser photocoagulation for neovascular lesions of age-related macular degeneration. Arch Ophthalmol 1990; 108:825–833.

90. Macular Photocoagulation Study Group. Persistent and recurrent choroidal neovascularization after laser photocoagulation for subfoveal choroidal neovascularization of age-related macular degeneration. Arch Ophthalmol 1994; 112:489–499.

91. Macular Photocoagulation Study Group. The influence of treatment coverage on the visual acuity of eyes treated with krypton laser for juxtafoveal choroidal neovascularization. Arch Ophthalmol 1995; 113:190–194.

92. Macular Photocoagulation Study Group. Recurrent choroidal neovascularization after argon laser photocoagulation for neovascular maculopathy. Arch Ophthalmol 1986; 104:503–512.

93. Moorfields Macular Study Group. Treatment of senile disciform macular degeneration: a single, blind, randomized trial by argon laser photocoagulation. Br J Ophthalmol 1982; 66:745–753.

94. Coscas G, Soubrane G. Photocoagulation des neovaisseaux sous retiniens dans le degénérescence maculaire senile par laser à argon: resultats de l'etude randomisée de 60 cas. Bull Mem Soc Fr Ophthalmol 1982; 94:149–154.

95. Guyer DR, Fine SL, Murphy RP et al. Clinicopathologic correlation of krypton and argon laser photocoagulation in a patient with a subfoveal choroidal neovascular membrane. Retina 1986; 6:157–163.

96. Rubin GA, Bandeen-Roche K, Prasada-Rao P et al. Visual impairment and disability in older adults. Optom Vis Sci 1994; 71:750–760.

97. Macular Photocoagulation Study Group. Visual outcome after laser photocoagulation for subfoveal choroidal neovascularization secondary to age-related macular degeneration: the influence of initial lesion size and initial visual acuity. Arch Ophthalmol 1994; 112:480–488.

98. Chamberlin JA, Bressler NM, Bressler SB et al. The use of fundus photographs and fluorescein angiograms in the identification and treatment of choroidal neovascularization in the Macular Photocoagulation Study. Ophthalmology 1989; 96:1526–1533.

99. Macular Photocoagulation Study Group. Evaluation of green versus red laser for photocoagulation of subfoveal choroidal neovascularization in the Macular Photocoagulation Study. Arch Ophthalmol 1994; 112:1176–1184.

100. Macular Photocoagulation Study Group. Laser photocoagulation for neovascular lesions nasal to the fovea associated with ocular histoplasmosis or idiopathic causes. Arch Ophthalmol 1995; 113:56–61.

101. Macular Photocoagulation Study Group. Argon laser photocoagulation for ocular histoplasmosis syndrome: results of a randomized clinical trial. Arch Ophthalmol 1983; 101:1347–1357.

102. Maguire JI, Benson WE, Brown GC. Treatment of foveal pigment epithelial detachments with contiguous extrafoveal choroidal neovascular membranes. Am J Ophthalmol 1990; 109:523–529.

Chapter 61

Neovascular (Exudative) Age-Related Macular Degeneration   1113

103. Cohen SMZ, Fine SL, Murphy RP et al. Transient delay in choroidal filling after krypton red laser photocoagulation for choroidal neovascular membranes. Retina 1983; 3:284–290.

104. Rice TA, Murphy RP, Fine SL et al. Stability of size of argon laser photo-coagulation scars in ocular histoplasmosis. In: Fine SL, Owens SL, eds. Management of retinal vascular and macular disorders. Baltimore: Williams & Wilkins; 1983.

105. Treatment of Age-Related Macular Degeneration with Photodynamic Therapy (TAP) Study Group. Verteporfin (Visudyne) therapy of subfoveal choroidal neovascularization in age-related macular degeneration: 1-year results of two randomized clinical trials, TAP report no 1. Arch Ophthalmol 1999; 117:1329–1345.

106. Rubin GS, Bressler NM. Treatment of Age-related Macular Degeneration with Photodynamic Therapy (TAP) Study Group. Effects of verteporfin therapy on contrast sensitivity; results from the Treatment of Age-related Macular Degeneration with Photodynamic therapy (TAP) Investigation: TAP Report No. 4. Retina 2002; 22:536–544.

107. Visudyne® In Minimally Classic Choroidal Neovascularization Study Group. Verteporfin therapy of subfoveal minimally classic choroidal neovascularization in age-related macular degeneration: 2-Year Results of a Randomized Clinical Trial. Arch Ophthalmol 2005; 123:448–457.

108. Miller JW, Schmidt-Erfurth U, Sickenberg M et al. Photodynamic therapy for choroidal neovascularization due to age-related macular degeneration with verteporfin: results of a single treatment in a phase I and II study. Arch Ophthalmol 1999; 117:1161–1173.

109. Schmidt-Erfurth U, Miller JW, Sickenberg M et al. Photodynamic therapy of choroidal neovascularization due to age-related macular degeneration with verteporfin: results of retreatments in a phase I and II study. Arch Ophthalmol 1999; 117:1177–1187.

110. Verteporfin Early Retreatment Study Group. Verteporfin Early Retreatment (VER) Trial Study Group. Verteporfin therapy of choroidal neovascularization due to age-related macular degeneration at early treatment intervals compared to standard treatment intervals: 2-year results of the Verteporfin Early Retreatment (VER) Trial. Ophthalmology 2005; submitted for publication.

111. Klein ML, Jorizzo PA, Watzke RC. Growth features of choroidal neovascular membranes in age-related macular degeneration. Ophthalmology 1989; 96:1416–1419.

112. Vander JF, Morgan CM, Schatz H. Growth rate of subretinal neovascularization in age-related macular degeneration. Ophthalmology 1989; 96:1422–1426.

113. Grey RHB, Bird AC, Chisholm IH. Senile disciform macular degeneration: features indicating suitability for photocoagulation. Br J Ophthalmol 1986; 104:702–705.

114. Choroidal Neovascularization Prevention Trial Research Group. Laser treatment in eyes with large drusen. Ophthalmology 1998; 105:11–23.

115. Choroidal Neovascularization Prevention Trial Research Group. Choroidal neovascularization prevention trial research. Ophthalmology 1998; 105:1364–1372.

116. Thomas MS, Grand MG, Williams DF et al. Surgical management of subfoveal choroidal neovascularization. Ophthalmology 1992; 99:952–966.

117. Bressler SB, Maguire MG, Bressler NM et al. Relationship of drusen and abnormalities of the retinal pigment epithelium to the prognosis of neovascular macular degeneration. The Macular Photocoagulation Study Group. Arch Ophthalmol 1990; 108:1442–1447.

118. Macular Photocoagulation Study Group. Five-year follow-up of fellow eyes of patients with age-related macular degeneration and unilateral extrafoveal choroidal neovascularization. Arch Ophthalmol 1993; 111:1189–1199.

119. Macular Photocoagulation Study Group. Risk factors for choroidal neovascularization in the second eye of patients with juxtafoveal or subfoveal choroidal neovascularization secondary to age-related macular degeneration. Arch Ophthalmol 1997; 115:741–747.

120. The Age-Related Eye Disease Study Research Group. A randomized, placebo-controlled, clinical trial of high-dose supplementation with vitamins C and E, beta carotene, and zinc for age-related macular degeneration and vision loss: AREDS report no. 8. Arch Ophthalmol 2001; 119:1417–1436.

121. Berger AS, Kaplan HJ. Clinical experience with the surgical removal of subfoveal neovascular membranes. Ophthalmology 1992; 99:969–976.

122. deJuan E Jr, Loewenstein A, Bressler NM et al. Translocation of the retina for management of subfoveal choroidal neovascularization. II. A preliminary report in humans. Am J Ophthalmol 1998; 125:635–646.

123. American Academy of Ophthalmology. Macular translocation. Ophthalmic procedure preliminary assessment. Ophthalmology 2000; 107:1015–1018.

124. Hassan AS, Johnson MW, Regillo CD et al. Management of submacular hemorrhage with intravitreal tPA injection and pneumatic displacement. Invest Ophthalmol Vis Sci 1998; 39 (suppl.):227.

125. Regillo CD, Benson WE, Maguire JI et al. Indocyanine green angiography and occult neovascularization. Ophthalmology 1994; 101:280–288.

126. Yannuzzi LA, Slakter JS, Sorenson JA et al. Digital indocyanine green videoangiography and choroidal neovascularization. Retina 1992; 12:191–223.

127. Guyer DR, Yannuzzi LA, Ladas I et al. Indocyanine green-guided laser photocoagulation of focal spots at the edge of plaques of choroidal neovascularization. Arch Ophthalmol 1996; 114:693–697.

128. Regillo CD, Blade KA, Custis PH et al. Evaluating persistent and recurrent choroidal neovascularization: the role of indocyanine green angiography. Ophthalmology 1998; 105:1821–1826.

129. Bressler NM, Bressler SB. Indocyanine green angiography: can it help preserve the vision of our patients? Arch Ophthalmol 1996; 114:747–749.

130. Bergink GJ, Hoyng CB, van der Maazen RW et al. A randomized controlled clinical trial on the efficacy of radiation therapy in the control of subfoveal choroidal neovascularization in age-related macular degeneration: radiation versus observation. Graefes Arch Clin Exp Ophthalmol 1998; 236:321–325.

131. Holz FG, Unnebrink K, Engenhart-Cabillic R et al. Results of a prospective, randomized, controlled, double-blind multicenter trial on external beam radiation therapy for subfoveal choroidal neovascularization secondary to ARMD (RAD-study). Invest Ophthalmol Vis Sci 1999; 40 (suppl.):2115.

132. Spaide RF, Guyer DR, McCormick B et al. External beam radiation therapy for choroidal neovascularization. Ophthalmology 1998; 105:24–30.

133. Pharmacological Therapy for Macular Degeneration Study Group. Interferon alfa-2a is ineffective for patients with choroidal neovascularization secondary to age-related macular degeneration: results of a prospective, randomized, placebo-controlled clinical trial. Arch Ophthalmol 1997; 115:865–782.

133a. Gragoudas ES, Adamis AP, Cunningham ET Jr, et al. VEGF, Inhibition Study in Ocular Neovascularization Clinical Trial Group. Pegaptanib for neovascular age-related macular degeneration. N Engl J Med 2004; 351:2805–16.

133b. Michels S, Rosenfeld PJ, Puliafito CA et al. Systemic bevacizumab (Avastin) therapy for neovascular age-related macular degeneration twelve-week results of an uncontrolled open-label clinical study. Ophthalmology 2005; 112:1035–1047.

134. Alexander MF, Maguire MG, Lietman TM et al. Assessment of visual function in patients with age-related macular degeneration and low visual acuity. Arch Ophthalmol 1988; 106:1543–1547.

Chapter

62

Choroidal Neovascular Membrane in Degenerative Myopia

Gisele Soubrane
Gabriel J. Coscas

Degenerative myopia is one of the leading causes of blindness in the world. Macular degeneration is a major complication of the posterior staphyloma – the hallmark of degenerative myopia. In addition, breaks in Bruch's membrane (lacquer cracks) may herald a decrease in central vision, especially when associated with hemorrhages. The occurrence of hemorrhaging can also be related to the submacular invasion by choroidal neovascular membrane: central visual function may be affected by serous or hemorrhagic detachments of the retina, or by both. Macular degeneration commonly occurs during the productive years of young adulthood and may progress to central atrophy of the retinal pigment epithelium (RPE), with or without previous detachments. A major advance in the management of choroidal neovascularization (CNV) in myopia has been obtained by photodynamic therapy (PDT) with verteporfin. Surgical techniques have been suggested as alternative methods.

EPIDEMIOLOGY

Simple, congenital, and degenerative myopia are generally considered to be distinct conditions. Simple myopia is a normal chance variation in the refractive error; congenital myopia tends to be stationary and nonprogressive; degenerative myopia (> –6 D), however, is characterized by increased axial length (> 26 mm), with progressive choroidal degeneration in the posterior pole.[1]

Myopia is the seventh greatest cause of registered blindness in adults in Europe[2] and in the USA.[3] The prevalence of myopia in developed countries is reported to be between 11% and 36%.[3–5] Prevalence shows a marked change with age, the peak being at 20 years,[2,5] but decreases with increasing age.[6] The frequency of degenerative myopia has been reported to range from 27% to 33.2% of the myopic population,[7–9] which corresponds to rates of 1.7% to 2.1% for the general population.[8]

The overall prevalence of myopia, including degenerative myopia, demonstrates substantial differences among races and ethnic groups.[5,10] For example, the prevalence of degenerative myopia varies from 0.2% in Egypt, to 9.6% in Spain,[11] and to 18% in Japan.[12] In the USA, approximately 2.1% of 17-year-olds exhibit more than 5 D of myopia.

Prevalence of myopia was found to increase in the youngest birth cohorts.[6,13] Lower prevalence rates were found for males than for females;[14] also, women are thought to be more likely to develop higher degrees of myopia as well as the subsequent degenerative changes. Numerous reports show a positive association between myopia and educational level,[15] near working habits,[4,16] and higher socioeconomic classes.[17]

PATHOGENESIS

The pathogenesis of the degenerative changes in and about the macula of the myopic eye is not clearly understood, although the lesions are thought to be due to either biomechanical abnormalities or heredodegenerative factors.[18,19]

In the biomechanical concept, the chorioretinal lesions are viewed as a consequence of excessive axial elongation.[11,14] It is believed that progressive distention of the posterior pole stretches the ocular coats, as evidenced by the straightening of the temporal retinal vessels, the appearance of a supertractional crescent, and thinning of the retina and choroid.[7,20,21] Crescent formation and chorioretinal atrophy have been directly related to increased axial length.[22] Although the pathophysiology of staphyloma formation is unknown, it has been suggested that the abnormal sclera has a low mechanical resistance and gradually stretches or creeps in response to forces such as intraocular pressure or extraocular muscle tension.[11] Fuchs' spot and lacquer cracks, which occur in eyes with increased axial length, cannot however be directly correlated with axial length.

The heredodegenerative theory considers the chorioretinal changes as a genetically determined abiotrophic process[23] that is associated with, but independent of, the anatomic changes on the scleral wall. There is some evidence that pathologic myopia is autosomal dominant. A number of studies have reported a greater similarity in refractive error, and in various ocular measurements that contribute to refractive status in monozygotic twins[24] as well as between siblings.[6] Genetic studies are in progress in myopic families based on linkage.[6] However the relative importance of genetic and environmental factors remains unclear.

HISTOPATHOLOGY

The abnormal histologic changes found in the posterior pole of eyes with degenerative myopia are characteristic.

Sclera

The sclera is thinned, with localized ectasia of the posterior pole, or staphyloma which was observed in 35.4% of 308 myopic eyes.[25] The architectural changes in the longitudinal fibers consist of thinning of the collagen bundles, reduced diameter of collagen fibrils, loss of striations, and diminished scleral lamellae.[26] The modification of elastic tissue remains controversial. Ultramicroscopic alterations seen in myopic sclera indicate a derangement of the diameter, number, and organization of its fibrils surrounded by an abundant extracellular matrix.[11]

Choroid and retinal pigment epithelium

The degenerative changes initially involve the choriocapillaris, Bruch's membrane, and the RPE.[25] Changes affecting the choroid are essentially degenerative and atrophic (see Figs 62-2A, 62-6C, and 62-8D). The choroid is thin, with a lack of vessels in some areas and a loss of choroidal melanocytes.[27] Ultramicroscopic alterations include a pronounced thinning of the choriocapillaris.[28] The RPE cells appear flatter and larger than usual,[29] prior to their degeneration. In some sections, pigment epithelial and visual cells are completely replaced by Mueller cells.[30] Bruch's membrane undergoes a variety of changes, including thinning, splitting, and rupturing.

Degenerative myopia causes thinning of the sensory retina associated with choroidal atrophy. Myopic retinal degeneration was found in 11.4% in a retrospective histopathologic study.[25] A distinct thinning of the macular area appears to be due at least partially to loss of the ganglion cell layer.

ANIMAL MODELS

To investigate the structural abnormalities of degenerative myopia, various experimental models have been developed by altering the visual input in young animals (chick, cat, monkey, and tree shrew[31]). Form-deprivation myopia causes elongation of the posterior segment by blurring the image on the retina in young animals by various means (suture of the eyelids,[32] dome or arch occluders to obstruct the entire visual field or lateral field respectively).[33] Continuous illumination,[34] dark-rearing, forced near vision,[35] and reduction in the level of visual contrast result in an increased axial length, with a shallow anterior chamber.[33] The results of these experiments suggest that axial myopia is produced by excessive accommodation during eye growth,[29] which would explain the significantly enlarged nasotemporal equatorial diameter. After the use of continuous illumination,[36] lid sutures,[32] and dome devices, retinal thickening is considered as an inflammatory response.[22] In addition, regulatory changes in scleral metabolism can result in a change in the eye size.[16] Although no animal model faithfully reproduces human pathologic myopia, prolonged retinal exposure in monkeys to formless images caused myopia with choroidal attenuation and peripapillary scleral crescent on fundus examination.[37]

FEATURES OF THE MYOPIC FUNDUS

Myopic conus

The myopic disc is typically tilted and oblique, with the temporal side flattened (Figs 62-1A, 62-3D, and 62-6E). The nasal side frequently has a raised edge, sometimes called supertraction. In addition, the temporal side is often surrounded by a concentric area of depigmentation, the so-called myopic conus or temporal crescent. The myopic crescent usually appears as a white, sharply defined area where the inner surface of the sclera is seen distinctly (Figs 62-1A and 62-3C). The choroidal layer usually extends closer to the temporal edge of the disc than does the pigment epithelium. This dragging may be caused by a mechanical factor secondary to progressive enlargement of the globe. Some temporal crescents are pigmented, while some show vascular changes as a result from the presence of choroidal vessels and choroidal pigmentation. The crescent may appear nasally or even inferiorly. The crescent surrounds the entire disc in 10% of cases; in some cases it extends into the macular region.

Staphylomas

Posterior staphyloma is pathognomonic of degenerative myopia. Its frequence is clinically underestimated (10%) compared to histopathology (35%).[25] A localized ectasia involves the sclera, the choroid, and the pigment epithelium. Posterior-pole staphyloma is present early in life and increases gradually with age.[38] Its prevalence increases with axial length as well as with myopic refraction.[39] Chorioretinal atrophy and conus formation are correlated with the increasing staphyloma depth.

The depth and size of a posterior staphyloma are best appreciated with stereopsis and B-scan or optical coherence tomography (OCT) examination. In contrast to fluorescein angiography, indocyanine green (ICG) angiography may disclose the borders of the staphyloma as a circular brilliant reflex and allow the visualization of extraocular vessels[40] (Fig 62-2G). Localizations of the staphyloma are various, including nasal, macula-centered, disc-centered, and tiered staphylomas.[1] Staphyloma underlying the macula is commonly associated with decreased vision,[41] whereas in other locations in the posterior pole, central vision may not be affected. Rarely, a serous retinal detachment overlies the crest of the staphyloma and is due to deep leaking of the central serous chorioretinopathy type.[42]

Retinal pigment epithelium and choroid disturbances

The thinning of the pigment epithelium and choroid, referred to as "tigroid" or "tesselated" fundus, allows easy visibility of the larger choroidal vessels. This thinning is often inferior to the disc and localized in the lower fundus (Figs 62-2A, 62-3A, and 62-6A). Blach[7] found that the electro-oculogram, which reflects the overall function of the RPE, was diminished in the majority of high myopes (< –0.6 D), but was not useful in differentiating children who will or will not develop myopic degeneration. Standard electroretinograms may show a decrease in amplitude.[43]

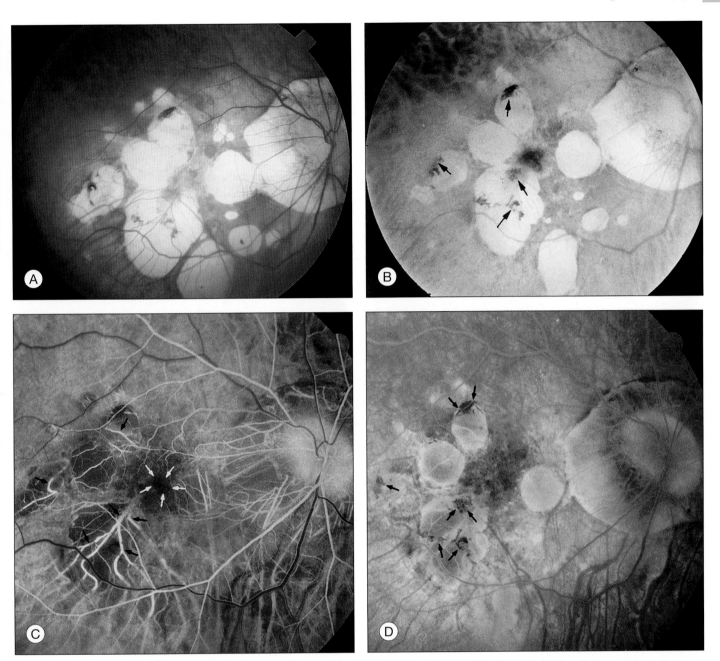

Fig. 62-1 Areas of focal atrophy. A, Color photograph: numerous areas of atrophy of the pigment epithelium and choriocapillaris extend into the macular region, sparing the fovea. A circular myopic crescent is visible. B, In a photograph taken in red light, pigmentary clumping (arrows) is seen within the atrophic areas. The pigment epithelium is irregular in the macular area. C, On fluorescein angiography, the large choroidal vessels (black arrows) crossing the punched-out areas fill early with dye. The large choroidal vessels are also visible in the myopic crescent. The atrophic areas are hypofluorescent secondary to choriocapillaris atrophy. The foveal avascular zone is visible (white arrows). D, On late-frame fluorescein angiography, the atrophic patches stain with the dye; pigment clumping is visible (arrows).

Marked thinning of the choroid and pigment epithelium reduces blood flow in the choroid. Consequently, light from the sclera is reflected, frequently causing decreased contrast during fluorescein angiography obscuring the exact limits of the foveal avascular zone. Since the macular retina is also thinned, the luteal pigment may be barely visible. Therefore, the direction of the macular arterioles may be the only useful landmark to locate the fovea (Fig. 62-8A).

Choroidal vessels

The large choroidal vessels are usually visible across the posterior pole (Figs. 62-3C and 62-6F). The choroidal arteries have a hook-like entrance into the globe, and the choroidal veins appear worm-like even on fluorescein angiography. On ICG angiography, the scarcity of the entire choroidal vasculature is obvious (Fig 62-5D). The choroidal arteries are reduced in number and in caliber in the macular region whereas the veins are only attenuated in the area of the staphyloma. Areas of remaining choriocapillaris show as irregular gray hyperfluorescent zones.[44] Moreover, in degenerative myopia the arrangement of the major choroidal veins is abnormal. Large veins flow together to form vortex-like confluence of choroidal veins crossing the macular area

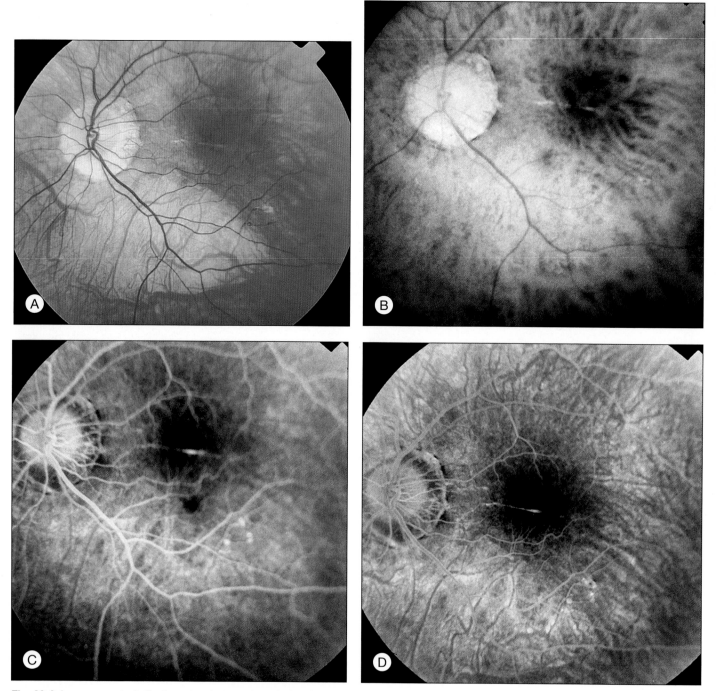

Fig. 62-2 Lacquer crack. A, On the color photograph, an isolated macular lacquer crack shows as a depigmented, irregular line. The area inferior to the disc is very depigmented. B, On the red-light photograph, discrete pigment clumping extends along the foveal part of the lacquer crack as well as along the myopic temporal crescent. C, On the venous phase of fluorescein angiography, the hyperfluorescence of the lacquer crack is more striking in its temporal portion. D, On a late frame, its hyperfluorescence is more even. The rupture is extending along the lower part of the foveal avascular zone.

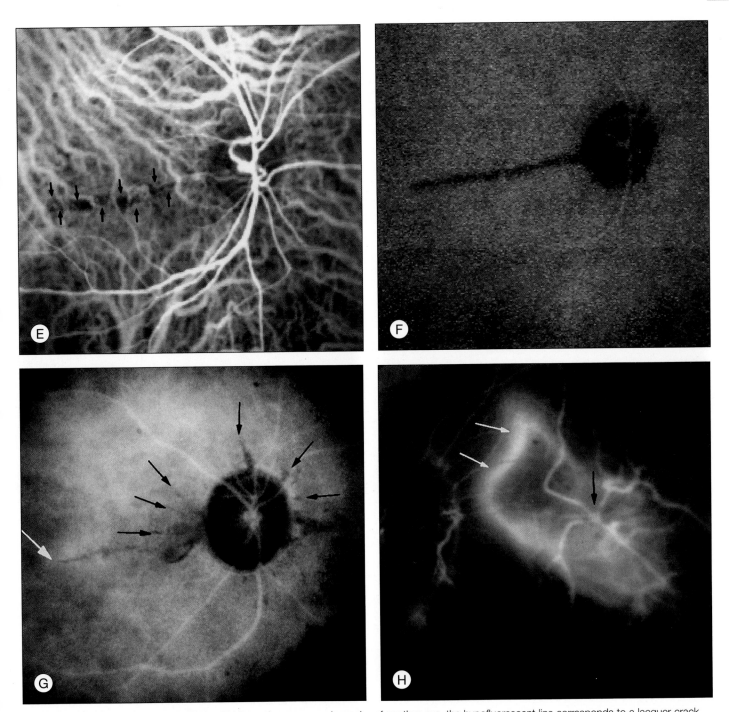

Fig. 62-2—cont'd E, On the early frame of indocyanine green angiography of another eye, the hypofluorescent line corresponds to a lacquer crack (arrows). The filling of the choroidal veins is already completed and some are visible within the crack. F, On the late frame of indocyanine green angiography, the lacquer crack is evident as a dark line extending from the optic nerve to the temporal macular area. G, In another eye, on a late frame of indocyanine green angiography, multiple small lacquer cracks (black arrows) are radiating from the optic disc in addition to a faint macular Bruch's membrane rupture (white arrow). H, On this very early phase of indocyanine green angiography, extraocular vessels (white arrows) are visible as the sclera is transparent to infrared light. The site of a choroidal artery penetration (black arrow) can be identified as well as its major branches.

(Figs 62-3C and 62-6F) or surrounding the optic disc, suggesting a hereditary component.

Atrophic areas

Areas of focal atrophy may be round or irregularly shaped, small or extensive, isolated or multiple, and yellowish-white (Fig. 62-1A). Their sharp margins are sometimes underlined by a pigmented line. A variable amount of pigment clumping may exist within these areas (Fig. 62-1B). With progressive atrophy, yellowish or whitish choroidal vessels appear in the atrophic zone and are sheathed on ophthalmoscopic examination. The term *choroidal sclerosis* was previously used to describe this

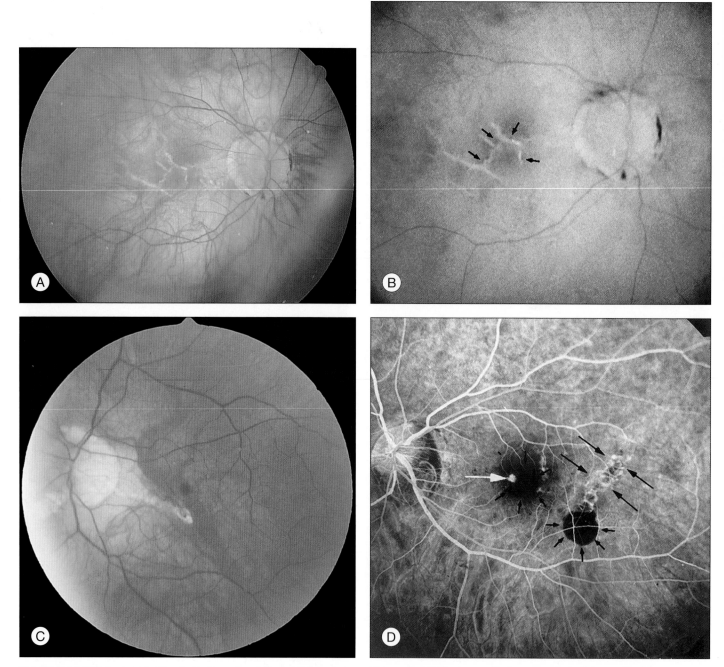

Fig. 62-3 Multiple lacquer cracks. A, On the color photograph there is branching and crisscrossing on the linear cracks in the macular area. The pigment epithelium and the choriocapillaris of the entire posterior pole are atrophic. The myopic crescent is limited. B, Bruch's membrane ruptures are particularly evident on the red-light photograph. Some pigment clumping is visible at the border of the cracks (arrows). C, In another eye, a large lacquer crack extends from the temporal myopic crescent toward the macula. Note next to the lacquer crack that major choroidal vessels flow into a large vortex-like vein. D, A large temporal lacquer crack (black arrows) presents at its inferior extremity a round subretinal hemorrhage (small black arrows). In addition, fluorescein angiography allows identification of choroid neovascularization (white arrow).

pattern. However, these vessels fill with fluorescein and ICG, and appear to be so because of the changes in the overlying RPE cells.

On fluorescein angiography, the atrophic areas are hypofluorescent and crossed by large choroidal vessels that fill early (Fig. 62-1C). The overlying retinal vessels appear normal. During recirculation the atrophic areas, on which the pigmentary clumping contrasts, show progressive staining (Fig. 62-1D). The extent of the patches of staining remains identical, as there is no leakage of dye.

On ICG angiography, these areas are hypofluorescent, traversed only by rare choroidal vessels. In the late phases, these dark patches contrast on the otherwise uniformly gray choroidal background.[40]

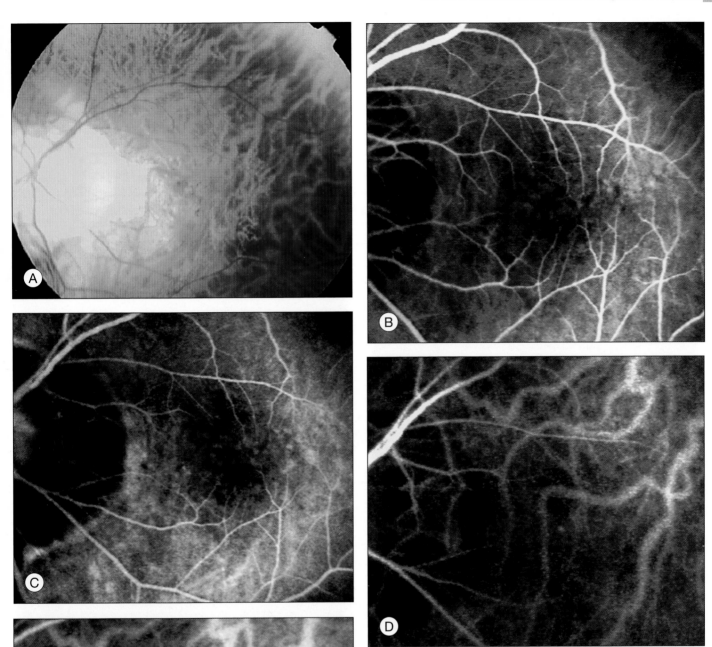

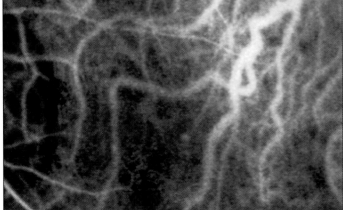

Fig. 62-4 Myopic pseudoretinoschisis. A, Color photograph, peripapillar and interpapillar area of moderate chorioretinal atrophy. B, C, On fluorescein angiography, the macular area does not show evidence of significant changes and no intraretinal cystoid accumulation of dye. D, E, On early and late frames of indocyanine green angiography, there is relative rarefaction of choroidal vessels without obvious changes.

Continued

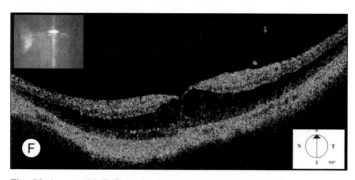

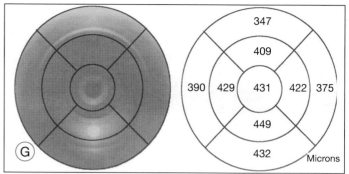

Fig. 62-4—cont'd F. On optical coherence tomography, there is accentuated increase of sensory retinal thickness in the macular area and relative conservation of the foveal depression. Note the accentuated accumulation of fluid in the outer retinal layers with very large cystoid spaces, quite confluent and simulating a retinoschisis.

With time, all of these areas demonstrate a strong tendency to coalesce into larger lesions, which assume rather irregular shapes. When the lesions extend into the fovea, central vision can be markedly decreased. The whole posterior pole may finally become atrophic.

Lacquer cracks

Ruptures of Bruch's elastic lamina are typical features of degenerative myopia. Progressive posterior segment elongation, uveal and scleral thinning, and RPE degeneration are thought to create a predisposition to crack formation. Located in the posterior pole within the staphylomata area, lacquer cracks are clinically noted in 4.2% of eyes with an axial length superior to 26.5 mm[21] and are found histopathologically in 0.6%.[8] Regardless of the extent of the rupture, visual acuity may be altered.[45]

Lacquer cracks are linear or stellate. The lines are fine, irregular in caliber, yellowish-white, horizontally oriented, single (Figs 62-2A and 62-3C) or multiple (Figs 62-3A and 62-3B), often branching with crisscrossing. They are located in the deepest layers of the retina. On their borders a fine pigmentary mottling (Fig. 62-3B) is often noted. When the lacquer cracks are large, choroidal vessels may traverse the lesion posteriorly. There is no irregularity or distortion of the neurosensory retina or retinal vessels overlying the lacquer cracks; the inner layers of the retina are undisturbed as well.

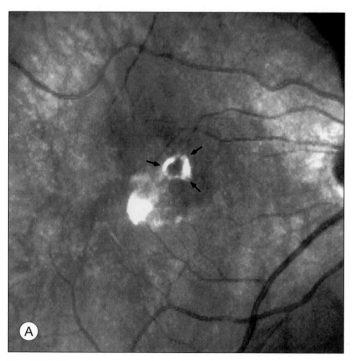

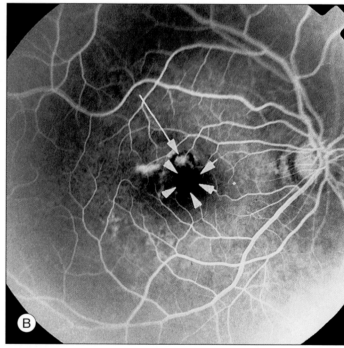

Fig. 62-5 Choroidal new vessels. A, On the red-free photograph this fundus exhibits a temporal transparent pigment epithelium and an atrophic choriocapillaris. There is a dark lesion (arrows) visible in the macular area. B, On fluorescein angiography, the hyperfluorescence of the neovascular network (white arrow) spares the foveal avascular zone (arrowheads). A temporal lacquer crack is visible.

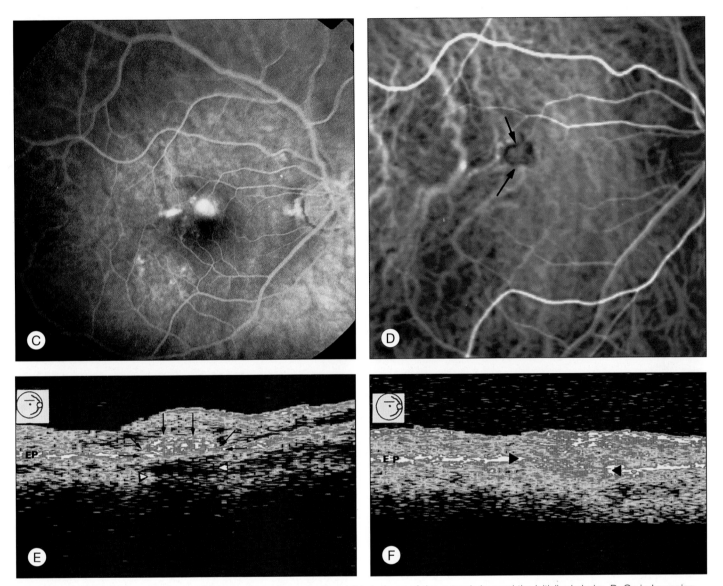

Fig. 62-5—cont'd C, On a late frame of fluorescein angiography, the visible leakage of dye extends beyond the initially dark rim. D, On indocyanine green angiography (2 min, 33), the new vessels (arrows) are in exactly the same location and underlined by a dark rim as on fluorescein angiography. However, its form differs by a superior extension. E, On optical coherence tomography, the new vessels (arrows) are located within and anterior to the pigment epithelium (EP), Bruch's membrane, and choriocapillaris complex and induce an underlying shadow (in between arrowheads) (horizontal section). F, Postlaser treatment optical coherence tomography shows the hyperechogenicity of the entire retina in the photocoagulated area (horizontal section). Note the rupture in Bruch's membrane (in between arrowheads).

The pattern of myopic lacquer crack formation was studied in 20 eyes (refractive error from −6.37 D to −27.00 D) using a graphic composition technique and computer analysis of digitized color, monochromatic, and fluorescein angiographic photographs.[46] Seventeen percent of the cracks were connected with the temporal crescent, which was noticed in all eyes. When cracks are numerous, a reticular or fishnet pattern predominates.

Fluorescein angiography helps to detect lacquer cracks that may be subtle and missed or incompletely identified on routine examination. In the early phase, the crack is an irregular and discretely hyperfluorescent line produced by abnormal transmission from a partially atrophic choriocapillaris (Figs 62-2C and 62-3D). The fluorescence increases moderately during transit. In the late phase, the linear lesion is only faintly hyperfluorescent, probably as a consequence of some scleral or scar-tissue staining (Fig. 62-2D). The hyperfluorescence does not extend into the width of the crack. No intraretinal or subretinal leakage of dye has been noted in uncomplicated lacquer cracks. On late ICG angiography frames, lacquer cracks appear as well-delineated hypofluorescent lines more numerous and longer than on fluorescein angiography (Figs 62-2E and 62-2F). Furthermore, unexpected fine lacquer cracks radiating from the optic disc are only detectable on ICG angiography[40] (Fig. 62-2G).

The natural history of lacquer cracks is variable. With time, the number and the dimension of Bruch's membrane ruptures increase (Fig. 62-3D). Focal areas of chorioretinal atrophy develop at the peripheral end and gradually enlarge until they cover the full extent of the lacquer crack. It was shown that patchy atrophy begins with a tiny hypofluorescent area of choroidal filling delay on fluorescein angiography.[30] Lacquer cracks carry a guarded prognosis for the retention of central vision because of their association with focal degenerative lesions and subretinal neovascularization along their course.

The occurrence or extension of a lacquer crack can be associated with a macular hemorrhage (Fig. 62-3D). These occur in the absence of choroidal neovascular membrane (CNV) and have different features. A sudden positive scotoma, sometimes with metamorphopsia, occurs, usually in the teenage years. The subretinal hemorrhage is focal, dense, round, deep, and often centered on the fovea. There is no retinal detachment. The hemorrhage may totally obscure the associated lacquer crack, even on

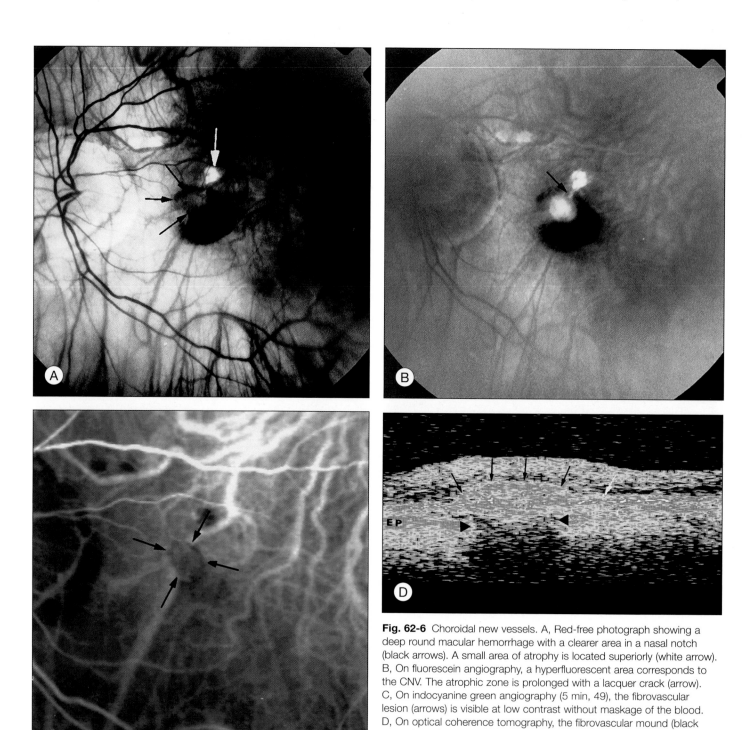

Fig. 62-6 Choroidal new vessels. A, Red-free photograph showing a deep round macular hemorrhage with a clearer area in a nasal notch (black arrows). A small area of atrophy is located superiorly (white arrow). B, On fluorescein angiography, a hyperfluorescent area corresponds to the CNV. The atrophic zone is prolonged with a lacquer crack (arrow). C, On indocyanine green angiography (5 min, 49), the fibrovascular lesion (arrows) is visible at low contrast without maskage of the blood. D, On optical coherence tomography, the fibrovascular mound (black arrows) produces an external shadowing (in between arrowheads). Note the reflectivity of the deep retinal blood (white arrow).

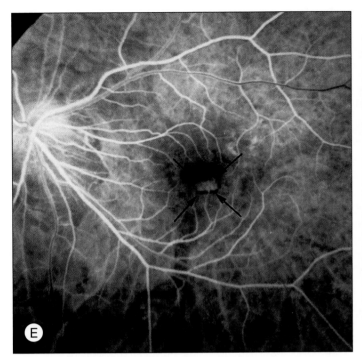
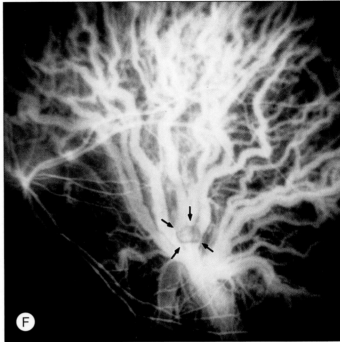

Fig. 62-6—cont'd E, In another patient, the mid-phase of fluorescein angiography shows a hyperfluorescent zone located at the margin of the avascular zone, outlined by a thin hypofluorescent ring (arrows). F, The late indocyanine green picture of the same eyes shows a strikingly huge choroidal venous confluent on which the neovascular membrane is barely visible (arrows).

fluorescein angiography. ICG angiography may detect the lacquer crack underlying the hemorrhage. Macular hemorrhages have been associated with lacquer cracks in 96% of cases, mostly along the lacquer crack itself and rarely in its immediate vicinity.[47,48] Hemorrhages resolve but may recur in the same or in another location. The most plausible explanation for the origin of hemorrhagic lesions relates to the intimate anatomic relationship between Bruch's membrane and the choriocapillaris. The prognosis for the retention of central vision in nearly all cases is good after the hemorrhage resolves.[7,45,47,49,50]

The lack of leakage of fluorescein from the choriocapillaris through the rupture in Bruch's membrane suggests that the defect is closed by an avascular barrier, such as scar tissue. Lacquer cracks have been ascribed to either a degenerative process of Bruch's membrane or sclerosis of the choroidal vessels. The filling of the choroidal vessels posterior to the lacquer cracks with fluorescein indicates that the latter hypothesis is improbable. Moreover, their association with fresh hemorrhaging would argue against that concept. The most generally accepted explanation for lacquer crack formation is that they are mechanical tears in Bruch's membrane that also involve the choriocapillaris and RPE. Their development or expansion after laser photocoagulation has been documented.[51]

Treatment of degenerative myopia

Equatorial scleral resection using homologous donor sclera was developed to reduce the volume of myopic eye in an attempt to ameliorate chorioretinal degeneration.[52] It was claimed[20] that myopia increased in none of the eyes operated on and that visual acuity increased in one-third of the cases. The dangers of this approach limit the acceptance of this procedure. Surgical reinforcement of the posterior pole has been performed since 1957[53] to arrest staphyloma progression. A number of materials have been employed, including donor sclera, autologous fascia lata, dura mater, silicone rubber, dacron mesh, and polytetrafluoroethylene in experimental animal models and in humans.[54,55] Long-term follow-up shows continued axial elongation.[19] Furthermore, no surgical technique has protected affected eyes from the occurrence of a Fuchs' spot (which occurred in six of the 10 eyes followed for more than 4 years). Although prevention of posterior staphyloma or of irreversible damage would be ideal, the value of surgical techniques must be demonstrated by a long-term investigation with careful monitoring and controls before general recommendation can be made. A retrospective multicenter study in children suggested that reduced quality of the retinal image during infancy and early childhood triggers an elongation of the posterior chamber at the eye.[56] A recent retrospective study of 214 children followed for a median period of 3.5 years supports the view that atropine is associated with decreased progression of myopia and that the beneficial effect remains after treatment discontinuation.[56] Other prospective studies suggested that this pharmacological treatment should be evaluated in children who are at high risk of degenerative myopia (Asiatic children with a family history of degenerative myopia and performing long hours of work).

NEOVASCULARIZATION

Since Foerster's[57] and Fuchs' original description,[58] common usage considers Foerster–Fuchs' spot as any dark spot in the posterior pole of patients with high myopia. It is generally accepted that the pigmented lesion described by Fuchs and the hemorrhagic lesions reported by Foerster represent different stages of the process of the development of CNV in myopia. Fuchs believed the dark macular spot to be related to proliferation of RPE rather than to hemorrhage. Saltzmann[59] noted that the cells of the pigment epithelium were increased in size and number surrounding a previously described hyaline material. Saltzmann has called attention to breaks in the lamina vitrea and Lloyd[23] to stretching of the choriocapillaris as being possible factors. Fuchs' spot represents subretinal or intraretinal migration of RPE accompanying CNV.[25] Hyperplasia of the RPE completely surrounds each individual choroidal vessel.

With the advent of fluorescein angiography, neovascularization extending from the choroid into the subpigment epithelial space has been identified as preceding the development of the Fuchs' spot.[60–62] Gass[62] has indicated that an acute hemorrhagic detachment ensures the development of new vessels. Subsequently, the subepithelial hemorrhage organizes and may combine with the proliferation of pigment epithelium, resulting in a dark Fuchs' spot in the macula.

Choroidal new vessels

Myopia is globally the second most common cause of choroidal new vessels and the first in young adults.[24] CNVs are generally believed to affect 5%[1] to 10%[60] of myopes with an axial length of 26.5 mm or more or with more than 5 D of myopia. Hotchkiss & Fine[46] reported that 40.7% of high myopic patients in their study demonstrated CNV. Histopathologic evidence of CNV and Fuchs' spot were respectively found in 5.2% and 3.2% of 308 high myopic eyes.[25]

The bilateral involvement of CNV or Fuchs' spot was estimated to be 12% by Hotchkiss & Fine,[46] 18% by Curtin,[1] 24% by Fuchs,[58] 28% by Campos,[60] and 41% by Fried and colleagues.[61] The observations of Fried et al. were made within a period of days to 8 years (mean time, 2.4 years).

The ingrowth of choroidal new vessels induces a sudden painless reduction in vision, usually associated with metamorphopsia. The neovascular lesion presents biomicroscopically as a light-gray round or elliptic macular lesion (Fig. 62-5A), which is usually small. The lesion is limited and located next to the fovea. A grayish circle may partially outline the lesion (Figs 62-7A and 62-8C). The retinal detachment is shallow and best detectable by stereopsis and OCT. Hemorrhages are not extensive and are primarily located in the deep neuroretina (Fig. 62-6D). Hard exudates are rare. The exudative detachment must be clearly differentiated from a localized serous detachment caused by a tiny macular hole and/or a retinal schisis evidenced by OCT (Fig. 62-4 A to F).

Fluorescein angiography relates the macular lesion to the ingrowth of a choroidal neovascular membrane. This ingrowth is the turning point of the natural history of macular lesions in myopic patients. In young myopes, a small neovascular tuft exhibits early hyperfluorescence in the juxtafoveal region (Figs 62-5B,

62-6E and 62-7A). On late frames, the leakage of dye suggests the presence of new vessels (Figs 62-5C and 62-6B). Although the leakage does not increase significantly throughout the transit (Fig. 62-5C), it is evidenced by the vanishing of the peripheral hypofluorescent rim of pigmentation. In fact, blood flow in the choroidal vessels is delayed in degenerative myopia, and the diffusely thinned choriocapillaris shows severe circulatory disturbances[1,41,63] with loss of choroidal stroma and the obliteration of some of the vessels. Since new vessels originate from the choroid, the hemodynamic characteristics must depend on those of the choroid. In elderly patients, CNV is larger and exhibits more leakage, resulting in the extension of dye beyond the boundaries of the neovascular net that was delineated in the early dye transit (Figs 62-7B and 62-7C). This increase in exudation may be due to associated age-related degenerative changes. The modification of the new vessels' behavior on the late phases of angiography with increasing age of the patient explains the description by some authors of two types of CNV.[47] Most studies include elderly patients (up to 96 years),[47,60,61,64,65] which might confuse neovascularization due to degenerative myopia in elderly eyes with age-related macular degeneration in myopic eyes. Therefore, only patients younger than 50 years can be considered to have pure myopic choroidal new-vessel ingrowth.

During the choroidal arterial and venous phase ICG angiography may detect a focal hyperfluorescent area (Figs 62-5D and 62-6C) that fades with dye washout, especially in its center. In the late phases, the focal area may stain and remain mildly hyperfluorescent in advanced lesions (Fig. 62-6F). In some cases, the intensity of the CNV is similar to that of the choroidal background but remains detectable because of the presence of a surrounding dark rim[40] (Fig. 62-6F). On OCT, the CNV extend within the RPE, Bruch's membrane, and choriocapillaris complex but protruding in front of it. Fluid accumulation within the neurosensory retina is moderate in degenerative myopia (Figs 62-5E and 62-6D).

An association between the development of posterior staphyloma and CNV was observed. Up to a point (staphyloma ≤ 2 mm on B-scan), the incidence of neovascularization may increase with increasing chorioretinal damage. However, as the depth of the staphyloma increases, the number of CNV decreases.[39] This decrease in neovascularization suggests that development of CNV requires relative preservation of the choriocapillaris, as occurs in eyes with less advanced stages of posterior staphyloma formation.

A break in Bruch's membrane or an atrophic area may precede the development of CNV.[62] Several clinical studies have suggested a relationship between lacquer cracks and the development of CNV.[7,41] The incidence of lacquer cracks was found to be higher in eyes with CNV than in eyes without detectable new vessel growth,[46] reaching 82% of eyes with CNV in one study.[47] This prevalence is probably even higher, because lacquer cracks may be incorporated into areas of choroidal atrophy.[21] On biomicroscopic examination, the lacquer crack exhibits a grayish zone, usually in the portion next to the fovea, with an overlying serous detachment. Fluorescein angiography shows the choroidal new vessels to arise from the lacquer crack directly or to be contiguous with it (Fig. 62-7A). The late

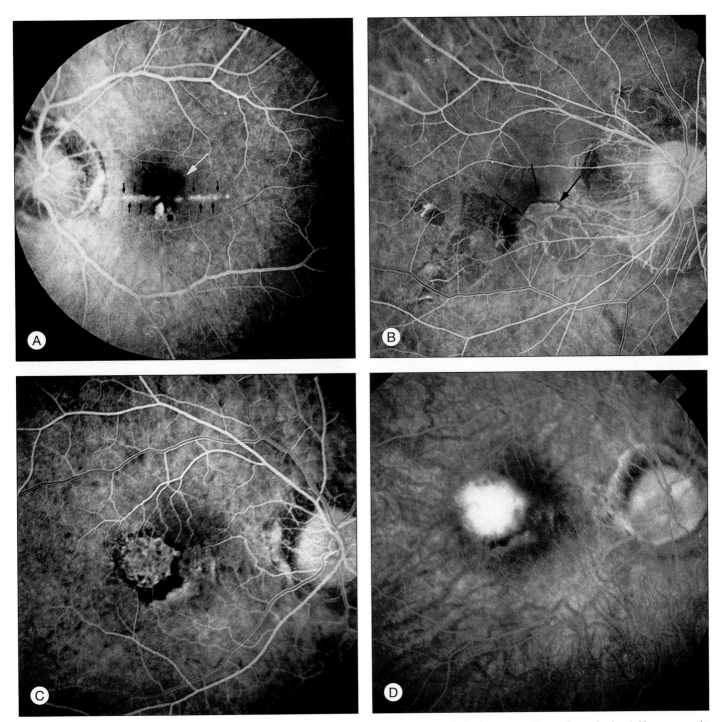

Fig. 62-7 Choroidal new vessels. A, A neovascular lesion at the margin of the avascular zone is hyperfluorescent as well as a horizontal lacquer crack (black arrows), to which the neovascular network is probably related. Note the artifact visible in high myopic eyes (white arrow), identifiable as a black area which appears in the same location of each photograph and can be misinterpreted as the foveal avascular zone. B, A choroidal neovascular membrane (arrows) is proliferating from the border of an atrophic area. C, Elderly myopic patient presenting with extensive lacy choroidal neovascularization in the early phase of fluorescein angiography. D, On the late phase, the important leakage of dye is a special feature of elderly myopics, suggesting some age-related modification.

leakage of dye confirms the diagnosis. When the new vessels arise from atrophic patches, the diagnosis may be quite difficult (Fig. 62-7B). The small and minimally leaking CNV are not always easily distinguishable from the mild hyperfluorescence of lacquer cracks and focal atrophy. Moreover, subretinal hemorrhages may partly or totally obscure all CNV features. ICG angiography allows the differentiation of the late hypofluorescence of lacquer cracks and RPE atrophy from the early hyperfluorescence of CNV.[40] However, in 43% of eyes, CNV develops in the absence of clinically visible lacquer cracks, although they have been detected microscopically.[45] No prospective study has focused on the relation between new vessels and lacquer cracks or atrophic areas on the basis of fluorescein and ICG angiography.

The neovascular tissue is frequently subfoveal at the time of presentation. Hampton et al.[27] found 58% of neovascularization directly involving the foveal zone on initial examination, while another study reported the incidence to be 74%.[66] Nearly all of the remaining membranes are located within 100 to 300 μm of the fovea, which restricts the number of eyes that are eventually amenable to photocoagulation. This foveal location is a major feature and clinically characteristic of new vessel growth in degenerative myopia.

Natural history

The picture of choroidal new vessels varies with the age of the lesion. The early picture is that of a dark-brown spot in the center of the macula, which is due to collected blood. Recurrent hemorrhaging may occur (Figs 62-8A and 62-8B) As the pigmented lesion degenerates, it evolves into a yellowish-gray, round or oval, and slightly elevated lesion, the Foerster–Fuchs' scar. There is usually some degree of visual improvement after the acute stage passes. This can best be attributed to the absorption of the transudate and hemorrhage, together with the establishment of an eccentric point of fixation.

As time passes, chorioretinal atrophy develops around the Foerster–Fuchs' spot and enlarges gradually (Figs 62-8C and 62-8D); the only evidence of the previous existence of CNV may be a certain amount of clumped pigment in a flat macular area. Some lesions appear to contain widespread fibrosis and atrophy in addition to macular hyperpigmentation. In histology, the fibrous tissue contains melanin, waste products secondary to hemosiderin degradation, and xanthophyll.

The visual prognosis in cases of choroidal new vessels in degenerative myopia remains controversial. All studies agree that a rapid decrease in central vision occurs after the onset of the disease. In a retrospective study, Hampton et al.[27] have shown a short neovascular growth phase with early visual loss directly related to the distance of the neovascular tissue from the foveola. Fried et al.[61] noted stabilization of visual acuity after the acute phase in 63% of patients studied (206 eyes). However, CNV was not detected by fluorescein angiography in 36% of patients, thus eyes without CNV may have been included in the study. Even so, the authors concluded that the visual prognosis was relatively benign, especially for near vision, although 50% of the new vessels grew into the foveola in a 5-year follow-up period. Hotchkiss & Fine[46] have documented choroidal new vessels in 23 patients and have demonstrated a worse prognosis, since visual acuity deteriorated in approximately 51% of the study eyes and 48% progressed to 20/200 or worse; 22% of eyes in the study underwent laser photocoagulation. After 2 years of follow-up,[27] the general prognosis is poor in that 43% of patients lost two or more lines of vision, and 60% had 20/200 visual acuity or worse. Thirty-five percent of the potentially treatable eyes when first seen became untreatable. A recent retrospective study of 50 consecutive eyes in which CNV spared the fovea at presentation demonstrated that after 5 years the center of the fovea

was involved, resulting in a visual acuity of 20/160,[19,67] and of less than 20/200 in another study after a follow-up of more than 10 years.[12] Furthermore, Curtin[38] found a 34% prevalence of legal blindness at long-term follow-up as a result of the enlargement of chorioretinal atrophy (Fig. 62-8D) around the Foerster–Fuchs' spot, causing decentration of fixation and subsequently extension of the central scotoma. Therefore, the presence of Fuchs' spot indicates a guarded prognosis for visual acuity.

Laser photocoagulation

Laser photocoagulation of choroidal new vessels may be considered when the membrane reduces or threatens to reduce central vision, as shown in the study of Fried et al.[61] (Figs 62-3D, 62-5B, and 62-9A). Photocoagulation could thus be applied in juxtafoveal lesions. In another study,[47] 16 eyes received argon green laser photocoagulation for typical myopic CNV; this completely closed the membrane in all eyes, as documented by fluorescein angiography. Immediately after treatment, or 1 year later, six eyes had visual acuities the same or better than the acuities at pretreatment. By the end of the follow-up period (21 to 52 months), however, visual acuities had deteriorated in all eyes. In another study, three wavelengths of the dye laser have been successful in 100 out of 133 consecutive eye patients.[68] Follow-up reached 60 months for 47 eyes. Visual acuity remained stable (0.36 at baseline; 0.33 at 5 years). Recurrences occurred in 58% of the treated eyes.

A randomized controlled trial[66] was designed to assess if krypton red laser photocoagulation was useful in preventing visual loss in myopic eyes with evidence of choroidal neovascular membranes, outside the fovea. Only patients younger than 55 years were included in this study. The visual symptoms had to be related to an angiographically visible choroidal neovascular network that was 100 to 1000 μm from the center of the foveal avascular zone. The main difficulty in the treatment was related to the precise localization of the foveola in relation to the neovascular network. When xanthophyll pigment was enhanced on blue-light frames, or the foveal avascular zone was visible on early frames of fluorescein angiography (Figs 62-5B and 62-7A), the foveola was quite readily located. However, these landmarks were not discernible in some myopic eyes (Fig. 62-9A), so these eyes were excluded. At 2 years, results of this study were statistically significant with respect to the outcome of distance vision ($P < 0.01$) and of reading vision ($P < 0.001$). Fourteen (40%) of the 35 treated eyes, compared with five (13%) of the 35 observed eyes, experienced an increase in visual acuity of approximately two lines; 14 (40%) patients in the treated group, compared with 27 (77%) in the observed group, had decreased visual acuity of this level. After 5 years of follow-up, the difference between the treated and the observed eyes was no more statistically significant. Treated eyes lost central vision, by subfoveal recurrences and even more by expansion of the treatment scar (92%). However, 26% of the treated eyes in comparison with 8% of the observed eyes maintained a visual acuity better than 20/100. Similar results were obtained in a retrospective study.[19]

Recurrences were observed in 31.4% of cases. However, in only three of 11 cases did the recurrent neovascular membrane

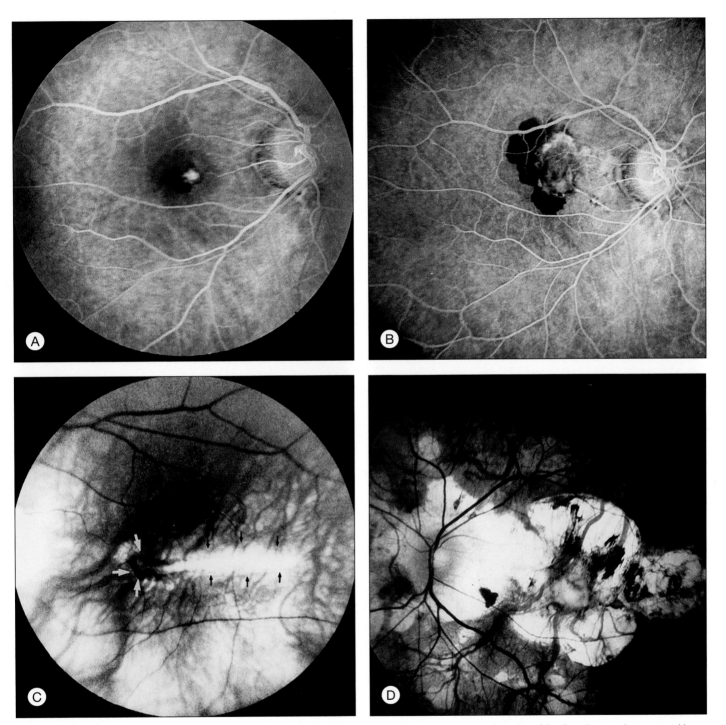

Fig. 62-8 Natural history of choroidal new vessels. A, A hyperfluorescent network extends into the nasal portion of the foveal avascular zone and is underlined with a deep hemorrhage. The myopic crescent is limited and the retinal vessels straightened. B, Three months later, the neovascular network has extended and a large subretinal hemorrhage has occurred. C, In another eye, the choroidal membrane (white arrows) is outlined by a dark rim and is originating from a large temporal lacquer crack (black arrows). D, Two years later the neovascular membrane has progressed to a fibrous lesion surrounded by a large atrophic area involving the entire posterior pole.

involve the center of the foveal avascular zone, thereby precluding further photocoagulation. Two-thirds of recurrences occurred during the first year of follow-up, and in half of these eyes, on the foveal side of photocoagulation scar. This high recurrence rate (up to 72%) indicates that close follow-up is needed for the early detection and treatment of recurrent CNV.

The increase in size of the atrophic scar following laser therapy[47,64,66,69] may induce central visual loss when the foveal area is affected (Fig. 62-9 B to D). Both the photocoagulation scars and the spontaneous atrophic scars may enlarge progressively.[69] This spontaneous enlargement should be considered when a decision is made to photocoagulate new vessels for

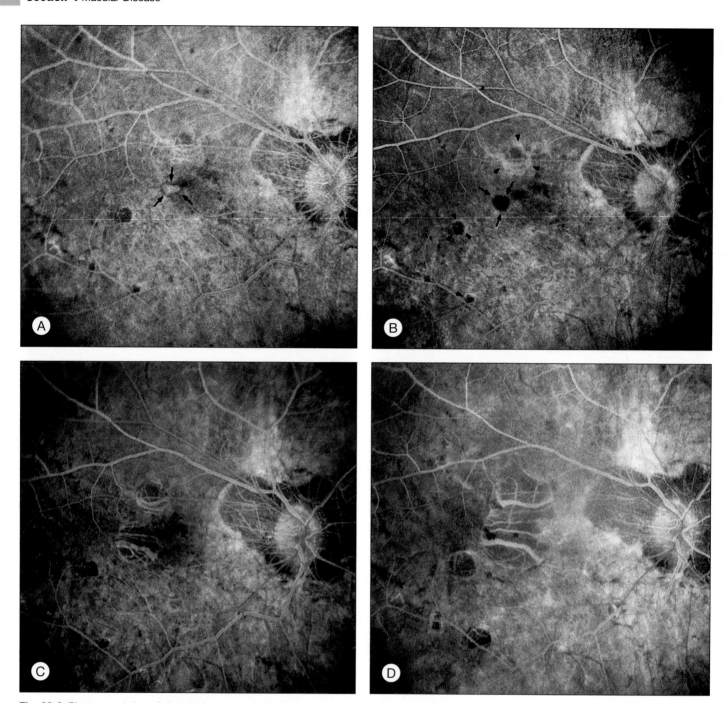

Fig. 62-9 Photocoagulation of choroidal new vessels. A, Before treatment, a discrete hyperfluorescent membrane is seen in the temporal part of the fovea (black arrows). Since the membrane is located in a zone reached by the retinal vessels, the choroidal neovascular membrane is outside the foveal avascular zone. B, Two weeks after krypton laser photocoagulation, the treatment scar (arrows) is hypofluorescent with well-defined borders. Note spontaneous atrophic areas in the posterior pole (arrowheads). C, One year after treatment the photocoagulation area as well as the spontaneous atrophic area have extended. D, Five years later, two scars have merged, resulting in a large macular atrophy. The spontaneous atrophic patches at a greater distance have also extended.

degenerative myopia. Progressive enlargement of the atrophic photocoagulation scar was seen with various wavelengths.

Photodynamic therapy

PDT has been evaluated for subfoveal CNV, which is the most prominent location in degenerative myopia.[70] The Verteporfin In Photodynamic therapy (VIP) trial, a randomized, multinational, double-masked, placebo-controlled clinical trial of PDT with verteporfin (Visudyne) included eyes with subfoveal CNV secondary to pathologic myopia.[71] At follow-up examinations every 3 months, retreatment was indicated if leakage from CNV was observed on fluorescein angiography. At the 12-month examination, only 28% ($n = 23$) of the 81 eyes given PDT lost eight or more letters of visual acuity, compared with 56% ($n = 22$) of the 39 eyes given placebo ($P < 0.01$). Moderate vision loss (> 15 letter loss of visual acuity) occurred in fewer PDT-treated eyes than placebo (14% versus 33%, $P = 0.01$). However, the 24-months data showed no statistical significance in benefit on visual acuity for either the percentage of eyes losing at least eight letters (verteporfin 36%, placebo 51%, $P = 0.11$) or the percentage losing at least 15 letters (verteporfin 21%, placebo 28%, $P = 0.38$).[72] Conversely, an increase in visual acuity of at least five letters was more likely to occur in eyes in the verteporfin group than in eyes in the placebo group (40% versus 13%). At 36 months, 19 (32%) and 17 (29%) eyes of 59 patients enrolled in the VIP extension had lost at least eight letters and at least 15 letters respectively, whereas 23 eyes (39%) had gained more than one line of visual acuity compared with baseline. PDT was well tolerated with few clinical relevant adverse events.

Thus, the results of the VIP trial indicate that eyes receiving PDT with verteporfin have vision benefits sustained through month 36.[73]

Surgical approaches

The goal of surgical options was in order to restore (versus stabilize) vision.[74] The first results of surgical removal of subfoveal CNV in high myopia were controversial.[75] Improvement in vision of two lines or more occurred in 45% of 65 operated eyes reviewed retrospectively, with final visual acuity of 20/200 or better in 66% (follow-up from 6 to 48 months). This study emphasized that the postoperative (RPE) defect was 4.6 times larger than the original membrane.[76] However surgical removal did not achieve any significant improvement of best-corrected visual acuity in a recent study of 22 eyes.[59] The recurrence rate was relatively high, ranging from 18% to 57%.[23] The imprecision of the removal may have increased atrophy and prevented regrowth of the RPE and choriocapillary.[25] A choriocapillaris perfusion defect was related to the pathway of CNV extraction.[77]

The introduction of macular translocation offers a surgical alternative.[78] Two surgical techniques have been performed, either limited macular translocation by scleral shortening or macular translocation involving a 360-degree retinotomy. Limited macular translocation, developed in the 1990s, allows the fovea to be moved away from the neovascular lesion after artificial retinal detachment without performing retinotomy.[79] In one prospective study, eight of nine eyes improved two lines or more in visual acuity, including three eyes improving by at least six lines.[80] In a Japanese prospective study, visual acuity improved by two lines or more in five out of 17 eyes (29%), was unchanged in seven eyes (41%), and worsened in five eyes.[12] The shift in the fixation point was in average 0.5 disc diameter in the first study and 0.75 disc diameter in the second study, resulting in amenability of CNVs to possible laser photocoagulation. The recurrence rate was of 11% after 4 to 9 months' follow-up[80] to 25% after 6 to 68 months' follow-up.[12] Retinal translocation by 360-degree retinotomy comprises the deliberate detachment of the entire retina from the RPE, followed by a peripheral 360-degree retinotomy.[78] The retina is then rotated around the optic nerve head

to reposition the fovea superiorly at distance from the CNV area. A two-line or more vision acuity improvement was obtained in 18 out of 28 eyes (64%), a visual acuity stabilization in four eyes, and visual acuity decrease in six eyes. The foveal displacement varied from 550 to 6090 μm (mean 2970 μm).[81] However, scanning laser ophthalmoscope fundus perimetry showed that the surgically disturbed area previously occupied by CNV can remain functional 6 months postoperatively.[27]

Macular translocation seems to offer an alternative therapy for subfoveal CNVs with the possibility of improvement in visual acuity. OCT discloses the sub-RPE position of the membrane and thus could be a reliable tool for selection of cases for surgery, as suggested by Gass.[74] A comparison of a large series of operated eyes with a natural history of subfoveal CNV is necessary before considering those invasive approaches.

SUMMARY

Eyes with degenerative myopia, lacquer cracks, and atrophic areas portend a poor prognosis. These eyes are at risk of developing choroidal new vessels, which further worsens the visual prognosis. Moreover, these new vessels are difficult to manage: first, their location in relation to the foveola is usually difficult to pinpoint; second, the CNV penetrates Bruch's membrane very close to the fovea; and third, the atrophic photocoagulation or surgical scar may extend to the foveola.

However, randomized trials have demonstrated a statistically significant beneficial effect on visual outcome following krypton laser photocoagulation of extrafoveal subretinal new vessels at 2 years (but no more at 5 years) and following PTD with verteporfin of subfoveal choroidal new vessels at 3 years. A number of alternative pharmacological therapeutic approaches could be tested and might provide new treatment for the management of subfoveal CNV of degenerative myopia in the near future at 3 years.

REFERENCES

1. Curtin BJ. The pathogenesis of congenital myopia: a study of 66 cases. Arch Ophthalmol 1963; 69:166–173.
2. Ghafour IM, Allan D, Foulds WS. Common causes of blindness and visual handicap in the west of Scotland. Br J Ophthalmol 1983; 67:209–213.
3. Sperduto RD, Seigel D, Roberts J et al. Prevalence of myopia in the United States. Arch Ophthalmol 1983; 101:405–407.
4. Leibowitz HM, Krueger DE, Maunder LR et al. The Framingham Eye Study monograph. VIII. Visual acuity. Surv Ophthalmol 1980; 24:472–479.
5. Sorsby A, Sheridan M, Leary GA et al. Vision, visual acuity and ocular refraction of young men. Br Med J 1960; 1:1394–1398.
6. The Framingham Offspring Eye Study Group. Familial aggregation and prevalence of myopia in the Framingham Offspring Eye Study. Arch Ophthalmol 1996; 114:326–332.
7. Blach RK. Degenerative myopia. In: Krill AE, Archer DB, eds. Hereditary retinal and choroidal diseases, vol. 2. Clinical characteristics. Hagerstown, MD: Harper & Row; 1977:911–937.
8. Guttmann E. Klinische-statistische Beitrage zur Aetiologie der hochgradigen Kurzsichtigkeit. Graefes Arch Clin Exp Ophthalmol 1902; 54:268–299.
9. Hertel E. Uber Myopie: Klinisch-statistische Mitteilungen. Graefes Arch Clin Exp Ophthalmol 1903; 56:326–386.
10. Hyams SW, Pokotilo E, Shkurko G. Prevalence of refractive errors in adults over 40: a survey of 8102 eyes. Br J Ophthalmol 1977; 61: 428–432.
11. Curtin BJ. "The myopias": basic science and clinical management. Philadelphia: Harper & Row; 1985.

12. Tano Y. Pathologic myopia: where are we now? Am J Ophthalmol 2002; 134:645–660.

13. Wang Q, Klein BEK, Klein R et al. Refractive status in the Beaver Dam Eye Study. Invest Ophthalmol Vis Sci 1994; 5:4344–4347.

14. Stromberg E. Uber Refraktion und Achsenlange des menschlichen Auges. Acta Ophthalmol 1936; 14:281–293.

15. Wong L, Coggon D, Cruddas M et al. Education, reading, and familial tendency as risk factors for myopia in Hong Kong fishermen. J Epidemiol Commun Health 1993; 47:50–53.

16. McBrien NA, Adams DW. A longitudinal investigation of adult-onset and adult-progression of myopia in an occupational group. Invest Ophthalmol Vis Sci 1997; 38:321–333.

17. Rosner M, Belkin M. Intelligence, education and myopia in males. Arch Ophthalmol 1987; 105:1508–1511.

18. Curtin BJ. Physiologic vs pathologic myopia: genetics vs environment. Ophthalmology 1979; 86:681–691.

19. Secretan M, Soubrane G, Kuhn D et al. Long-term follow-up of choroidal neovascularization in pathologic myopia: natural history compared to laser treatment. Eur J Ophthalmol 1997; 7: 307–316.

20. Balacco-Gabrieli C. Aetiopathogenesis of degenerative myopia: a hypothesis. Ophthalmologica 1982; 185:199–204.

21. Curtin BJ, Karlin DB. Axial length measurements and fundus changes of the myopic eye. Am J Ophthalmol 1971; 71:42–53.

22. Hayes BP, Fitzke FW, Hodos W et al. A morphological analysis of experimental myopia in young chickens. Invest Ophthalmol Vis Sci 1986; 27:981–991.

23. Lloyd RI. Clinical studies of the myopic macula. Trans Am Ophthalmol Soc 1953; 51:273–284.

24. Angi MR, Clementi M, Sardei C et al. Heritability of myopic refractive errors in identical and fraternal twins. Grafes Arch Clin Exp Ophthalmol 1993; 231:580–585.

25. Grossniklaus HE, Green WR. Pathologic findings in pathologic myopia. Retina 1992; 12: 127–133.

26. Curtin BJ, Iwamoto T, Renaldo DP. Normal and staphylomatous sclera of high myopia: an electron microscopic study. Arch Ophthalmol 1979; 97:912–915.

27. Hampton GR, Kohen D, Bird AC. Visual prognosis of disciform degeneration in myopia. Ophthalmology 1983; 90:923–926.

28. Okabe S, Nobuhiko M, Okamoto S et al. Electron microscopic studies on retinochoroidal atrophy in the human eye. Acta Med Okayama 1982; 36:11–21.

29. Greene PR. Mechanical considerations in myopia: relative effects of accommodation, convergence intraocular pressure and the extraocular muscles. Am J Optom Physiol Opt 1980; 57:902–914.

30. Ohno-Matsui K, Tokoro T. The progression of lacquer cracks in pathologic myopia. Retina 1996; 16:29–37.

31. McBrien NA, Lawlor P, Gentle A. Scleral remodeling during the development of and recovery from axial myopia in the tree shrew. Invest Ophthalmol Vis Sci 2000; 41:3713–3719.

32. Tucker GS, Yinon U. Refractive error, gross morphometry and light microscopy of eyes from chickens following lid suture (abstract). Neuroscience 1983; 9:376–380.

33. Yinon U. Myopia induction in animals following alteration of the visual input during development: a review. Curr Eye Res 1984; 3:677–690.

34. Wallman J, Turkel J, Trachtman J. Extreme myopia produced by modest change in early visual experience. Science 1978; 201: 1249–1254.

35. Young FA, Leary GA. Visual optical characteristics of caged and semifree ranging monkeys. Am J Phys Antrop 1973; 38:377–382.

36. Lauber JK, Boyd JE, Boyd TAS. Intraocular pressure and aqueous outflow facility in light-induced avian buphthalmos. Exp Eye Res 1970; 9:181–187.

37. Raviola E, Wiesel TN. An animal model of myopia. N Engl J Med 1985; 312:1609.

38. Curtin BJ. The posterior staphyloma of pathologic myopia. Trans Am Ophthalmol Soc 1977; 75:67–86.

39. Steidl SM, Pruett RC. Macular complications associated with posterior staphyloma. Am J Ophthalmol 1997; 123:181–187.

40. Quaranta M, Arnold J, Coscas G. Indocyanine green angiographic features of pathologic myopia. Am J Ophthalmol 1996; 122:663–671.

41. Noble KG, Carr RE. Pathologic myopia. Ophthalmology 1982; 89:1099–1100.

42. Leys AM, Cohen SY. Subretinal leakage in myopic eyes with a posterior staphyloma or tilted disk syndrome. Retina 2002; 22: 659–665.

43. Yoshii M, Yanashima K, Nagasaka E et al. Nonlinear component of the electroretinogram recorded from posterior pole of normal and highly myopic human eyes. Ophthalm Res 2002; 34: 393–399.

44. Soubrane G, Arnold J, Quaranta M. Atteintes dégénératives de l'épithélium pigmentaire. In: Soubrane G, ed. Les affections acquises de l'épithélium pigmentaire. Marseille: Fuery-Lamy, 1995;169–204.

45. Klein RM, Curtin BJ. Lacquer crack lesions in pathologic myopia. Am J Ophthalmol 1975; 79:386–392.

46. Hotchkiss ML, Fine SL. Pathologic myopia and choroidal neovascularization. Am J Ophthalmol 1981; 91:177–183.

47. Avila MP, Weiter JJ, Jalkh AE et al. Natural history of choroidal neovascularization in degenerative myopia. Ophthalmology 1984; 91:1573–1581.

48. Milch FA, Yannuzi LA, Rudick AJ. Pathologic myopia and subretinal hemorrhages. Ophthalmology 1987; 94 (suppl.): 117.

49. D'Hoine G, Turut P, Francois P et al. L'atteinte maculaire des myopes. Bull Soc Ophtalmol Fr 1974; 74:821–826.

50. Pruett RC, Weiter JJ, Goldstein RB. Myopic cracks, angioid streaks, and traumatic tears in Bruch's membrane. Am J Ophthalmol 1987; 103:537–543.

51. Johnson DA, Yannuzzi LA, Shakin JL et al. Lacquer cracks following laser treatment of choroidal neovascularization in pathologic myopia. Retina 1998; 18:118–124.

52. Blegvad O. Die Prognose der excessiven Myopie. Acta Ophthalmol 1987; 5:49.

53. Borley WE, Snyder AA. Surgical treatment of high myopia: the combined lamellar scleral resection with scleral reinforcement using donor eye. Trans Am Acad Ophthalmol Otolaryngol 1958; 62:791–802.

54. Malbran J. Una nueva orientacion quinigica contra la myopia. Arch Soc Oftal Hisp Am 1954; 14:1167–1169.

55. Vancea P. New concept in the treatment of progressive myopia. Ann Ophthalmol 1971; 3:1105–1108.

56. Kennedy RH, Dyer JA, Kennedy MA et al. Reducing the progression of myopia with atropine: a long term cohort study of Olmsted County students. Binocul Vis Strabismus Q 2000; 15: 281–304.

57. Foerster R. Ophthalmologische Beitrage. Berlin: Enslin; 1862:55.

58. Fuchs E. Der centrale schwarze Fleck bei Myopie. Z Augenheilkd 1901; 5:171–178.

59. Saltzmann M. The choroidal changes in high myopia. Arch Ophthalmol 1902; 31:41–42.

60. Campos R. La tache de Fuchs. In: Problemes actuels d'ophtalmologie. Basel: Karger; 1957:364–363.

61. Fried M, Siebert A, Meyer-Schwickerath G et al. Natural history of Fuch's spot: a long-term follow-up study. Doc Ophthalmol Proc Ser 1981; 28:215–221.

62. Gass JDM. Pathogenesis of disciform detachment of the neuroepithelium. VI. Disciform detachment secondary to heredodegenerative, neoplastic and traumatic lesions of the choroids. Am J Ophthalmol 1967; 63:689–711.

63. Avetisov ES, Savitskaya NF. Some features of ocular microcirculation in myopia. Ann Ophthalmol 1977; 9:1261–1264.

64. Jalkh AE, Weiter JJ, Trempe CL et al. Choroidal neovascularization in degenerative myopia: role of laser photocoagulation. Ophthalm Surg 1987; 18:721–725.

65. Levy JH, Pollock HM, Curtin BJ. The Fuchs' spot: an ophthalmoscopic and fluorescein angiographic study. Ann Ophthalmol 1977; 9:1433–1443.

66. Soubrane G, Pison J, Bornert P et al. Neo-vaisseaux sous-rétiniens de la myopie dégénérative: résultats de la photocoagulation. Bull Soc Ophtalmol Fr 1986; 86:269–272.

67. Tabandeh H, Flynn HW Jr, Scott IU et al. Visual acuity outcomes of patients 50 years of age and older with high myopia and untreated choroidal neovascularization. Ophthalmology 1999; 106:2063–2067.

68. Pece A, Brancato R, Avanza P et al. Laser photocoagulation of choroidal neovascularization in pathologic myopia: long-term results. Int Ophthalmol 1995; 18:339–344.

69. Brancato R, Pece A, Avanza P et al. Photocoagulation scar expansion after laser therapy for choroidal neovascularization in degenerative myopia. Retina 1990; 10:239–243.

70. Sickenberg M, Schmidt-Erfurth U, Miller JW et al. Preliminary results of photodynamic therapy for choroidal neovascularization in pathologic myopia, ocular histoplasmosis syndrome and idiopathic causes within a phase I/II study. Invest Ophthalmol Vis Sci 1997; 38 (suppl).

71. Verteporfin in Photodynamic Therapy Study Group. Verteporfin therapy of subfoveal choroidal neovascularization in age-related macular degeneration: two-year results of a randomized clinical trial including lesions with occult with no classic choroidal neovascularization – Verteporfin in Photodynamic Therapy report 2. Am J Ophthalmol 2001; 131:541–560.

72. Verteporfin in Photodynamic Therapy (VIP) Study Group. Verteporfin therapy of subfoveal choroidal neovascularization in pathologic myopia with verteporfin: two-year results of a randomized clinical trial VIP report no. 3. Ophthalmology 2003; 110:667–673.

73. Verteporfin in Photodynamic therapy (VIP) Trial Study Group. Verteporfin therapy for subfoveal choroidal neovascularization in pathologic myopia: three-year results – VIP report no. 5. Ophthalmology (submitted).

74. Gass JDM. Biomicroscopic and histopathologic considerations regarding the feasibility of surgical excision of subfoveal neovascular membranes. Am J Ophthalmol 1994; 118:285–298.

75. Thomas MA, Dickinson JD, Melberg NS et al. Visual results after surgical removal of subfoveal choroidal neovascular membranes. Ophthalmology 1994; 101:1384–1396.

76. Uemura A, Thomas MA. Subretinal surgery for choroidal neovascularization in patients with high myopia. Arch Ophthalmol 2000; 118:334–360.

77. Hamelin N, Glacet-Bernard A, Brindeau C et al. Surgical treatment of subfoveal neovascularization in myopia: macular translocation versus surgical removal. Am J Ophthalmol 2002; 133:530–536.

78. Machemer R, Steinhorst UH. Retinal separation, retinotomy, and macular relocation: II. A surgical approach for age-related maculopathy? Graefes Arch Clin Exp Ophthalmol 1993; 231:635–641.

79. de Juan E Jr. Retinal translocation: rationale and results. Ophthalmologica 2001; 215:10–19.

80. Glacet-Bernard A, Simon P, Hamelin N et al. Translocation of the macula for management of subfoveal choroidal neovascularization: comparison of results in age-related macular degeneration and degenerative myopia. Am J Ophthalmol 2001; 131:78–89.

81. Abdel-Meguid A, Lappas A, Hartmann K et al. One year follow up of macular translocation with 360 degree retinotomy in patients with age-related macular degeneration. Br J Ophthalmol 2003; 87:615–621.

Chapter

63

Central Serous Chorioretinopathy

Christina M. Klais
Michael D. Ober
Antonio P. Ciardella
Lawrence A. Yannuzzi

In 1866, von Graefe first described a disease of the macula characterized by recurrent serous macular detachment and named it *recurrent central retinitis*.[1] Almost 100 years later, in 1955, Bennet applied the term *central serous retinopathy*.[2] At the same time, Maumenee observed using fluorescein angioscopy that the detachment of the macula resulted from a leak at the level of the retinal pigment epithelium (RPE).[3] In 1967, Gass provided the classic description of the pathogenesis and clinical features of the condition which he called *idiopathic central serous choroidopathy*.[4–6] Since the disease appears to involve both the choroid and the retina, the currently accepted name is *central serous chorioretinopathy* (CSC).

CSC is characterized by accumulation of transparent fluid at the posterior pole of the fundus. There are two main types of CSC.[7] The more common type, typical or classic CSC, is seen in younger patients and causes an acute localized detachment of the retina with mild to moderate loss of visual acuity associated with one or a few focal leaks seen during fluorescein angiography (Fig. 63-1). The second presentation of CSC has widespread alteration of pigmentation of the RPE related to chronic presence of shallow subretinal fluid. This variant has been termed diffuse retinal pigment epitheliopathy, decompensated RPE, or chronic CSC (Fig. 63-2).[8] This type is common in patients with CSC associated with chronic corticosteroid usage.[9] There is a third less common form of CSC which causes bullous retinal detachments usually located inferiorly. This variant is often associated with shifting fluid and appears to be more frequently observed after organ transplantation, in patients using corticosteroids, and in patients of Asian descent.

PATHOGENESIS

The pathophysiology of CSC is still not completely understood. Fluorescein angiography demonstrates one or multiple focal sites of leakage resulting in detachment of the RPE and/or neurosensory retina in cases of active CSC (Fig. 63-3). With the cessation of these leaks, the detachment regresses. This suggests that the fluorescein findings represent fluid emanating from the choroid which escapes into the subretinal space through a defect in the tight junctions between cells of the RPE.[10] Ordinarily, the balance of the tissue osmotic and hydrostatic pressures causes fluid flow from the retina toward the choroid. In experimental studies,

destruction or injury of the RPE speeds the resorption of subretinal defect.[11,12] These results suggests that a simple defect of integrity of the RPE alone could not explain the findings seen in CSC.[13]

One theory suggested that affected RPE cells lose their normal polarity and pump fluid from the choroid towards the retina, causing a neurosensory detachment.[14] This theory is unable to explain why the cells pumped in the wrong direction or how pigment epithelial detachments (PEDs) form, since pigment epithelial cells pumping in the wrong direction should drive the pigment epithelium towards Bruch's membrane, and not away from it. It is also difficult to accept that a single isolated disturbance of a few RPE cells may overwhelm the physiologic RPE pump of the neighboring normal RPE. Furthermore, theories on the pathogenesis of CSC must address the formation of protein, particularly fibrin, in the subretinal space (Fig. 63-4). Fibrinogen, a monomeric precursor of fibrin, is ordinarily restricted to the intravascular space because of its molecular weight of 345 kDa.

Clinical findings of CSC and abnormalities of choroidal circulation in patients with CSC obtained by indocyanine green (ICG) angiography have led to new theoretical considerations.[15,16] ICG angiogram reveals multifocal areas with choroidal vascular hyperpermeability in patients with CSC.[17] Excessive tissue hydrostatic pressure within the choroid from vascular hyperpermeability may lead to mechanical disruption of the RPE barrier, damage of RPE cells, and abnormal egress of fluid under the retina. Functional loss of contiguous RPE cells may allow the fluid to accumulate in the subretinal space, causing neurosensory detachment. It has been shown that leaks at the level of the RPE seen on fluorescein angiography were contiguous with areas of choroidal vascular hyperpermeability in ICG angiography.[17] On the other hand, most areas of choroidal hyperpermeability were not associated with actual fluorescein leaks. Focal areas of ICG hyperfluorescence are also often noted in clinically unaffected fellow eyes (Fig. 63-5).[7] These areas of hyperpermeability without leaks may not be clinically silent; increased tissue hydrostatic pressure within the choroid could affect the ability of the overlying RPE to pump fluid from the retina to the choroid. This would potentially limit the absorption of subretinal fluid and contribute to size, shape, and chronicity of the overlying neurosensory detachment. In patients with CSC, segments with late choroidal hyperpermeability also show a delay in filling which

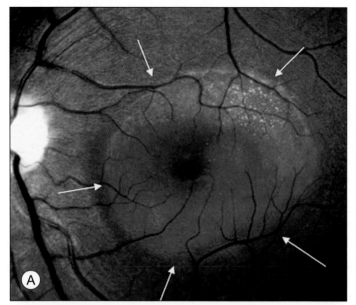

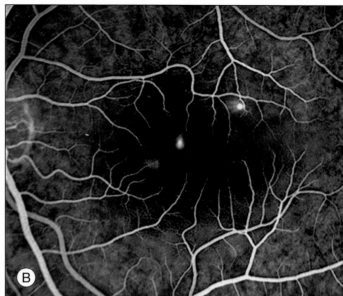

Fig. 63-1 This 34-year-old Caucasian male presented with complaints of blurred vision in the left eye for 1 week. A, Red-free photograph of the left eye shows serous neurosensory macular detachment (white arrows). B and C, Fluorescein angiography demonstrates pinpoint areas of hyperfluorescence in the central macula leading to the characteristic smokestack configuration in the late phase.

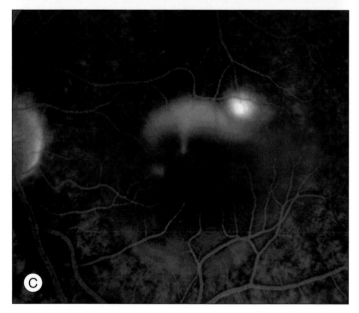

has been attributed to decreased arterial perfusion or decreased venous outflow.[18] This may create a pressure overload and cause choroidal vascular hyperpermeability.[14]

Clinically, patients with CSC have frequently had a preceding stressful event[19] and are more likely to have type A personalities.[21,22] CSC has also been associated with increased cortisol levels, thus implying higher incidence in patients with Cushing's disease.[22–24] Particularly severe CSC can occur in patients who have had organ transplants and are being treated with medications to prevent rejections, such as corticosteroids.[10,25,26] Furthermore, CSC is more common in women during pregnancy, a state with increased level of free circulating endogenous cortisol.[27–29] Another study identified hypertension and the use of corticosteroids as important risk factors for patients with CSC.[30] Also increased levels of catecholamines have been associated with CSC.[30,31] In

animal studies, clinical findings of CSC have been produced by repeated injections of norepinephrine (noradrenaline) and corticosteroids.[32–34]

Although the role played by corticosteroids and catecholamines in CSC is not well understood, the effects of endogenous circulating adrenergic effectors and sympathetic innervation combine to produce vasoconstriction and alteration of blood flow in the choroidal vascular beds. Corticosteroids also reduce the production of nitric oxide, an autoregulatory vasodilator, which controls local blood flow.[35] Increased corticosteroid levels may also cause increased capillary fragility and hyperpermeability, which, in turn, may lead to decompensation of the choroidal circulation and leakage of fluid into the subretinal space.[36,37] Furthermore, the anti-inflammatory properties of steroids may cause delayed healing of the RPE defect. By suppressing synthesis

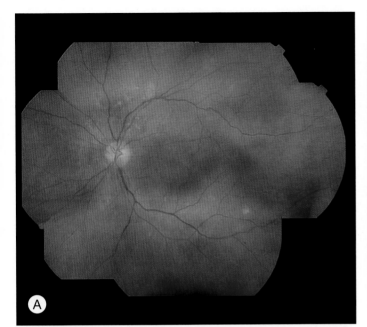

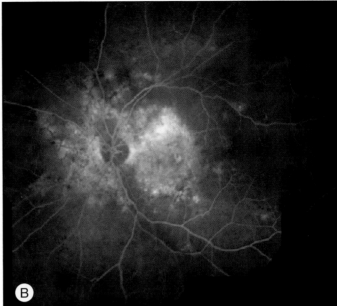

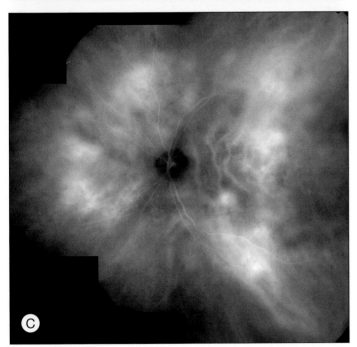

Fig. 63-2 A, The color photograph composite of an 87-year-old male with a history of long-standing central serous chorioretinopathy (CSC) in the left eye and visual acuity of 20/100 shows diffuse pigmentary changes in the posterior pole. B, Fluorescein angiogram composite reveals diffuse decompensation of the retinal pigment epithelium. C, Mid-phase indocyanine green (ICG) angiography illustrates multiple patchy areas of hyperfluorescence in the left eye. Note that the areas of hyperfluorescence on ICG do not correspond to the areas of leakage shown on fluorescein angiography.

of extracellular matrix components and inhibiting fibroblastic activity, corticosteroids may also directly damage RPE cells or their tight junctions, delaying the reparative process in the damaged cells.[38–40] Experimental animal models have demonstrated that increased levels of corticosteroids and catecholamines disturb the autoregulation of choriocapillaris blood flow.[32,33,41] Steroids also directly affect ion transport and thus may reverse the polarity of RPE cells, resulting in secretion of ions into the subretinal space. This would in turn change the osmotic pressure gradient to favor fluid flow from the choroid to the retina, resulting in a neurosensory detachment.[42–44]

We hypothesize that a protracted disturbance in the microcirculation of the choriocapillaris leads to leakage of fluid into the sub-RPE space (Fig. 63-1). Initially, the RPE cells are able to maintain their integrity and pump fluid in the retinal–choroidal direction; however, prolonged stress ultimately causes pump failure and loss of function. A combination of choroidal hyperpermeability and impaired RPE function leads to pooling of fluid in the sub-RPE space with eventual leakage through the RPE into the subretinal space. Spontaneous healing and resorption of fluid may occur during the healing process. However, the perpetuating microcirculatory disturbance leads to new damage and recurrence of

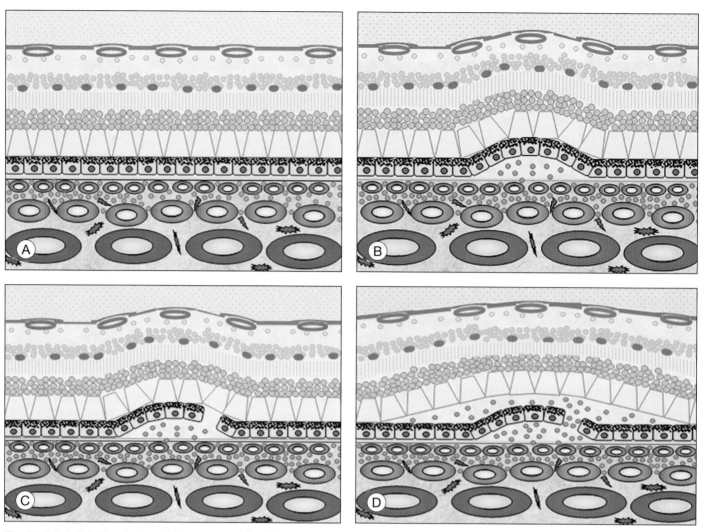

Fig. 63-3 A, Initially there is choroidal hyperpermeability with congestion of the choriocapillaris along with exudation of protein and fluid. B, Retinal pigment epithelium (RPE) pump decompensation occurs over time with the formation of a pigment epithelial detachment. C, Eventually, RPE defect develops, leading to leakage into the subretinal space. D, This leads to elevation of the neurosensory retina and a neurosensory retinal detachment.

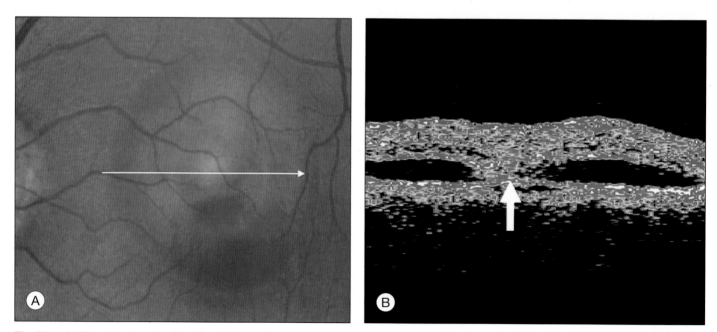

Fig. 63-4 A, Clinical photograph of a patient with macular neurosensory detachment and subfoveal fibrinous exudation. White arrow corresponds to the line of the optical coherence tomography (OCT) scan. B, OCT confirms the presence of a serous neurosensory detachment. The fibrinous exudation appears as a subretinal deposit (white arrow).

the process. This theory provides an explanation for some of the clinical characteristics of CSC: diffuse choroidal hyperpermeability in areas that appear clinically normal, recurrence of the disease, progressive damage of the RPE layer, and multifocal pinpoint areas of leakage in more severe or chronic cases. Further clinical and experimental studies are needed to provide evidence for the pathophysiology of CSC.

CLINICAL FEATURES

Demographics

Greater understanding of the clinical manifestations of CSC has considerably changed our knowledge of its demographics.

In the past, CSC has been considered predominantly a disease of males between 30 and 50 years of age. No case of CSC has been reported in patients under the age of 20 years, with the exception of a 7-year-old girl who might have had a posterior scleritis.[45] The overall incidence in men versus women in numerous reports was approximately 8 or 9 to 1, but the incidence in women was noted to double between the ages of 31 and 40, as compared with ages 21 to 30.[46] Very little is known about age-specific prevalence and clinical findings of CSC in older adults. Neurosensory macular detachment in an adult over 50 years of age, in fact, suggests the presence of choroidal neovascularization (CNV) secondary to age-related macular degeneration (AMD), the most common cause of blindness in older adults.[47] In 1996,

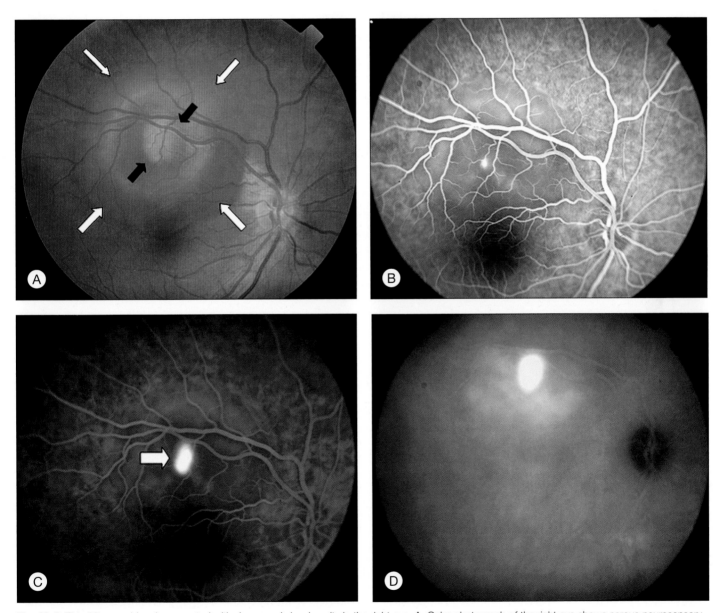

Fig. 63-5 This 36-year-old male presented with decreased visual acuity in the right eye. A, Color photograph of the right eye shows serous neurosensory detachment (white arrows) in the superior area of the macula with ring-like yellowish subretinal nodular deposits consistent with fibrin surrounding the localized pigment epithelial detachment (PED) (black arrows). B, Early-phase fluorescein angiogram reveals localized area of hyperfluorescence. C, Late-phase fluorescein angiogram demonstrates hyperfluorescence due to pooling beneath the serous PED (white arrow). D, Late-phase indocyanine green angiogram shows an area of hyperfluorescence corresponding to the serous PED and staining of the subretinal fibrin deposits.

Continued

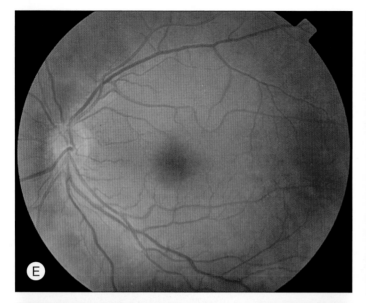

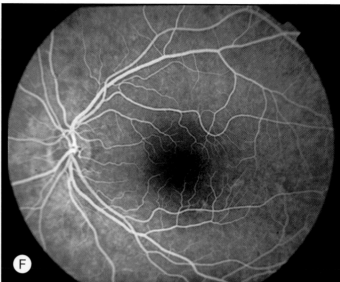

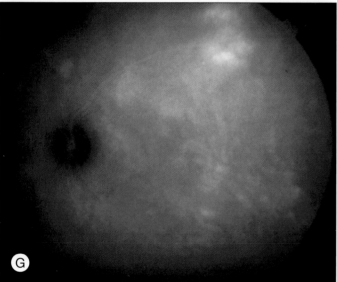

Fig. 63-5—cont'd E and F, The fellow eye appears normal both clinically and on fluorescein angiography. G, Late-phase indocyanine green angiogram reveals multiple areas of hyperfluorescence consistent with diffuse choroidal vascular hyperpermeability and bilateral disease.

Spaide et al. reported a study conducted on 130 older patients with neurosensory macular detachment.[48] More than half the subjects were 50 years of age or older, and 57 were diagnosed with CSC after they turned 50. The male-to-female ratio was 2.6 to 1 with no differences among the age groups. Another study found the same male-to-female ratio in 230 consecutive patients with CSC.[30] On the basis of such results, we can consider CSC a disease that, although typical of young adult males, is more frequent among females and older adults than was traditionally thought.

Predisposing conditions

It has been speculated that psychological factors may play a causative role in CSC.[21,49,50] Patients with CSC show significantly higher values on the hypochondria and hysteria scale[51] and are more likely to use psychopharmacological medications.[30] Most CSC cases are diagnosed in patients with no refractive error or mild

hyperopia.[21,52] There may be racial predisposition, with higher incidence among Caucasians, Hispanics, and possibly Asians, and extremely low occurrence in African Americans.[7,53–55] The more severe form of CSC occurs more frequently in individuals from South Asia and those of Latin descent.[56]

Symptoms

Many patients first notice a minor blurring of vision followed by various degrees of metamorphopsia, micropsia, dyschromatopsia, hypermetropization, and central scotoma, as well as loss of contrast sensitivity and increasing hyperopia. In some patients the onset of symptoms is preceded or accompanied by migraine-like headaches.[6]

The anterior displacement of the retinal plane may account for hypermetropization, and irregularities in the shape of the retinal plane may result in metamorphopsia. The cause of micropsia is not completely understood, but it may be due to the hyper-metropization[57] or a result of increased distance between photoreceptors in the detached retinal area.[58] There was no correlation between dyschromatopsia and the anatomic derangements, such as size and form of the detachment, obtained with optical coherence tomography (OCT).[59]

Typically, the area of metamorphopsia is reproducible on Amsler grid testing. Visual acuity in the acute stages ranges from 20/20 to 20/200.[60,61] Vision can usually be improved with a small hyperopic correction.

EXAMINATION/CLINICAL FINDINGS

Neurosensory retina

The biomicroscopic examination with a fundus contact lens reveals a detachment of the neurosensory retina which appears as a well-delineated transparent blister at the posterior pole. The normal foveal light reflex is usually absent and replaced by a halo of light reflex delimiting the elevated area. The detached neurosensory retina is usually transparent and of normal thickness. Sometimes a yellowish discoloration of the fovea is visible caused by increased visibility of retinal xanthophyll. It is not uncommon for patients with CSC to have multiple yellowish-white dot-like deposits covering the posterior surface of the detached retina.[7,10,27,62]

Retinal pigment epithelium

Careful scanning with the OCT reveals serous PED under the neurosensory elevation more often than previously recognized (Fig. 63-6). Sometimes there are two or more PEDs which are usually located superior to the neurosensory detachment since gravity forces the fluid inferiorly. The PED has a round or oval shape. A pink halo surrounding the PED is caused by shallow separation of the retina at the edge of the PED. Long-standing and recurrent PEDs may present with pigment migration or atrophy. Although the subretinal fluid is usually transparent, allowing clear visualization of the underlying RPE and choroidal details, it may become cloudy and grayish.[7,56] Histopathologic studies have demonstrated the presence of subretinal and sub-pigment epithelial fibrin.[10] With increasing concentrations, fibrin molecules polymerize to form oval yellow or gray membranes, causing the subretinal fluid progressively to opacify. A PED can often be found adjacent to fibrin accumulation.

In most cases the fibrin deposits dissolve; rarely do they stimulate subretinal fibrosis and fibrotic scar formation, leading to permanent visual loss. Subretinal neovascularization and RPE tears complicate the situation.[62,63] Conditions predisposing to subretinal fibrin exudation include large and multiple PEDs, chronic and recurrent disease, pregnancy, systemic administration of corticosteroids, organ transplant, diabetes, and male gender.[26,64] Subretinal lipid may also occur, particularly in patients with chronic CSC.[7,65]

Peripheral retinal detachments and RPE atrophic tracts

Peripheral dependent bullous neurosensory detachments have been described in patients with CSC.[25,66–69] Yannuzzi et al. first characterized the presence of such detachments and offered a pathophysiologic explanation for their development.[65] Presumably, particularly severe and/or prolonged leakage of fluid into the

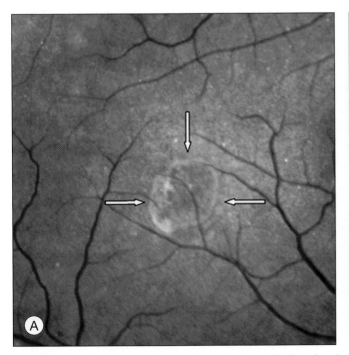

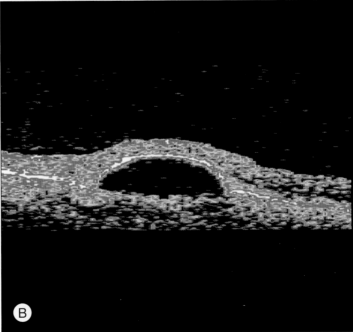

Fig. 63-6 Optical coherence tomography of pigment epithelium detachment (white arrows in the red-free photograph) in a patient with central serous chorioretinopathy confirms the presence of localized elevation consistent with serous pigment epithelial detachment.

subretinal space occurs at the posterior pole in these patients. The subretinal fluid gravitates inferiorly to form a neurosensory detachment in a flask, teardrop, dumbbell, or hourglass pattern (Fig. 63-7). Sometimes the tract of subretinal fluid connecting the macular detachment with the bullous neurosensory detachment in the inferior hemisphere is very shallow and therefore difficult to assess. The RPE under the chronic retinal detachment develops atrophic changes that appear as atrophic RPE tracts connecting the posterior pole with the dependent detachment (Fig. 63-8). The retina undergoes changes, including pigment migration, capillary dilation (telangiectasia) proximally, and capillary non-perfusion (ischemia) distally in the area of the detached retina. The RPE changes consist of both atrophy and perivascular pigment deposits or occasionally bone spicules. Gass first described this pseudoretinitis pigmentosa-like atypical CSC presentation.[70] Other complications of chronic CSC include cystoid retinal changes in the areas of chronic detachment, cystoid macular edema (Fig. 63-9), subretinal lipid deposition, choriocapillaris atrophy, and CNV.[71,72] Iida et al. also reported intraretinal cystoid spaces without intraretinal leakage, or cystoid macular degeneration in patients with chronic CSC.[73] In these cases the reduced visual acuity remains after resolution of subretinal fluid.

CENTRAL SEROUS CHORIORETINOPATHY AND SYSTEMIC DISEASE

By definition CSC is an idiopathic disease; however, particularly severe forms of CSC have been associated with pregnancy (Fig. 63-10),[27–31] end-stage renal disease,[25,68,74] organ transplantation,[26,75] systemic lupus erythematosus,[76] increased endogenous cortisol production,[23] endogenous mineralocorticoid dysfunction,[77] use of inhaled nasal corticosteroids,[78] systemic corticosteroid treatment,[24,26,79] and epidural corticoid injection.[80] In addition, a severe variant of CSC appears to be more frequent in patients of Hispanic or Asian ancestry, associated with frequent recurrences, permanent central vision loss, and significant superior visual field loss.

In our experience, patients with end-stage renal disease under systemic corticosteroid treatment tend to develop a severe bilateral form of CSC complicated by giant tears of the RPE and permanent loss of vision. Serous retinal and RPE detachments resembling CSC have also been described in patients with paraproteinemia who are on steroid therapy.[81] In addition, CSC has been described in patients using methylenedioxymethamfetamine (ecstasy).[82]

A number of systemic diseases characterized by ischemia of the choroid may present with PEDs and bullous neurosensory detachment resembling CSC. These include systemic lupus erythematosus,[76] polyarteritis nodosa,[83] Goodpasture's syndrome,[84] Wegener' granulomatosis,[85] accelerated hypertension,[86,87] toxemia of pregnancy,[88–90] disseminated intravascular coagulopathy (DIC),[91] and thrombotic thrombocytopenic purpura (TTP).[92] Ischemia of the choriocapillaris may be the final common pathway to serous retinal detachments in these diseases with different pathogenesis and systemic manifestations. Ischemia may be caused by vasospasm (e.g., malignant hypertension, toxemia during pregnancy), by intravascular clots (e.g., DIC, TTP), or by intravascular precipitation of circulating immunocomplexes (e.g., lupus erythematosus, and other collagen vascular diseases). Choriocapillaris ischemia may ultimately lead to the damage of the RPE and subretinal fluid exudation.

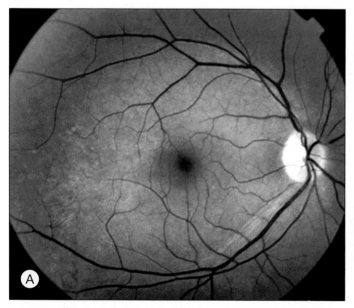 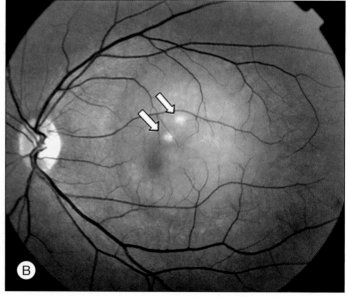

Fig. 63-7 A 41-year-old male with the diagnosis of central serous chorioretinopathy in both eyes for 10 years presented complaining of sudden decrease of vision in the left eye. A, Red-free photograph of the right eye reveals pigmentary changes temporal to the fovea. B, Red-free photograph of the left eye shows a well-circumscribed neurosensory detachment of the macula with two areas of focal pigment epithelial detachment (PED) (arrows).

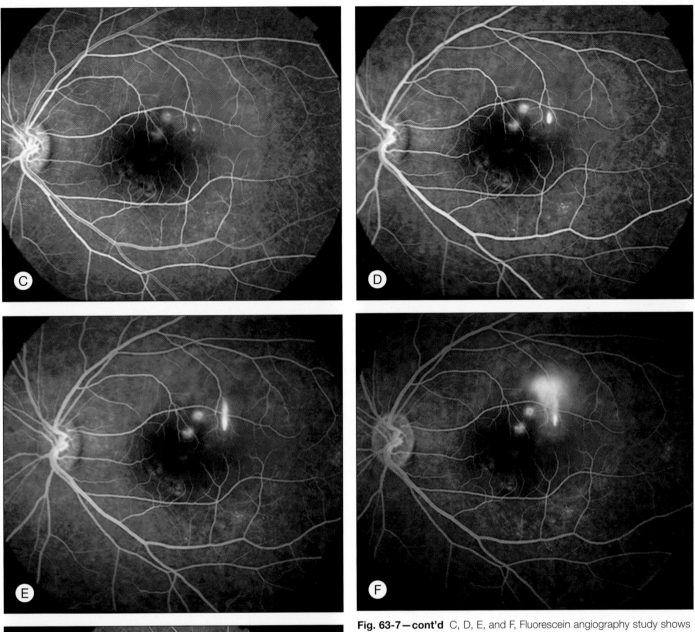

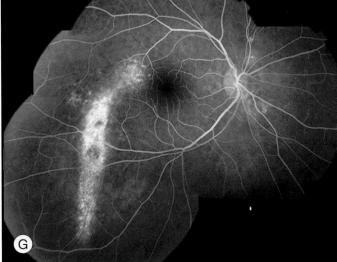

Fig. 63-7—cont'd C, D, E, and F, Fluorescein angiography study shows two localized areas of PED and typical "smokestack" appearance of the dye leaking under the detached retina. Note the dye expanding in an umbrella-like fashion once it reaches the upper limit of the detachment. G, Mid-phase fluorescein angiography study of the fellow eye shows window defect hyperfluorescence corresponding to the atrophic retinal pigment epithelial tract extending inferiorly.

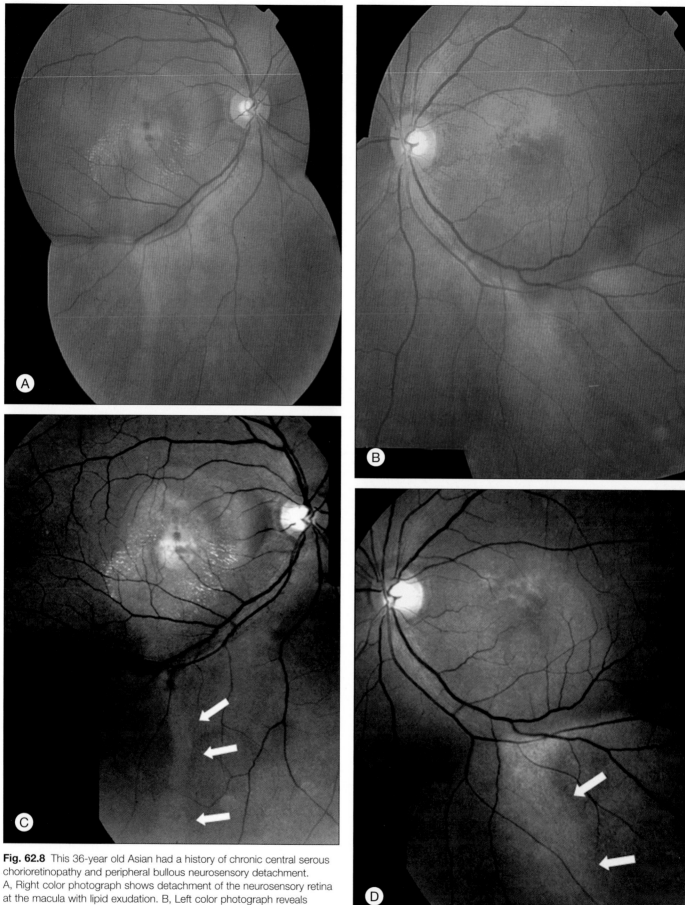

Fig. 62.8 This 36-year old Asian had a history of chronic central serous chorioretinopathy and peripheral bullous neurosensory detachment.
A, Right color photograph shows detachment of the neurosensory retina at the macula with lipid exudation. B, Left color photograph reveals changes in the retinal pigment epithelium (RPE) at the posterior pole.
C, Right red-free photograph confirms neurosensory detachment, lipid exudation, and an atrophic RPE tract (arrows). D, There is also an atrophic RPE tract (arrows) in the fellow eye.

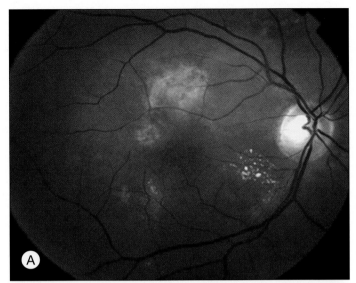

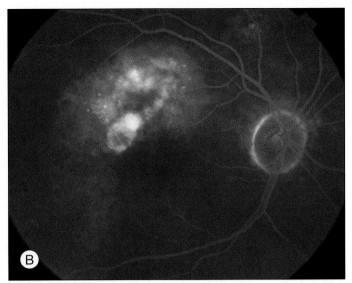

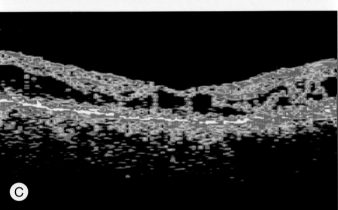

Fig. 63-9 A, This 46-year-old male patient has chronic central serous chorioretinopathy (CSC) with decreased visual acuity in his right eye. Red-free photograph shows changes in the retinal pigment epithelium (RPE) at the posterior pole. Note that areas above the optic disc are also involved. B, Fluorescence angiogram reveals diffuse RPE decompensation which is typical for this form of CSC. C, Optical coherence tomography shows multiple cystic retinal spaces in the foveal area consistent with cystoid macular degeneration.

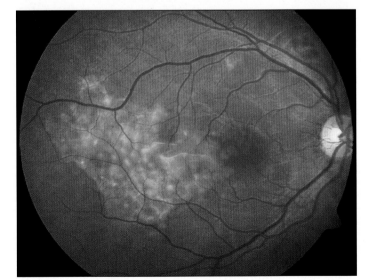

Fig. 63-10 This is a clinical photograph of the right eye of a 26-year-old female who developed bilateral bullous neurosensory detachments during childbirth complicated by preeclampsia. After resolution of the neurosensory detachment in the right eye there was a triangular-shaped area of subretinal fibrinous exudation consistent with occlusion of a short posterior ciliary artery.

IMAGING TECHNIQUES

Fluorescein angiography

The typical angiographic finding in fluorescein angiography is the presence of one or several hyperfluorescent leaks in the level of the RPE (Fig. 63-11).[93] In the majority of the cases, the dye spreads symmetrically to all sides, slowly and evenly staining the subretinal detachment. Even though the initial diffusion of the dye occurs rather quickly, it often does not reach the borders of the detachment by the late phases of the angiogram. Fluorescein does not stain the retina beyond the edges of the detachment. In approximately 10% of cases, the dye rises within the neurosensory detachment in a "smokestack" pattern and expands laterally in a mushroom-like or umbrella-like fashion at the upper limit of the detachment. This pattern is believed to be related to an increased concentration of protein within the subretinal fluid.[94] There are usually one or two leakage points; however, there may be as many as seven or more.[93] In rare cases, there may be no definite leakage point, but rather an area of diffuse hyperfluorescence. Other times, a mechanical defect at the margin of the PED may be apparent as a puncture, or "blow-out." Large PEDs with multiple fracture sites at their margins have also been

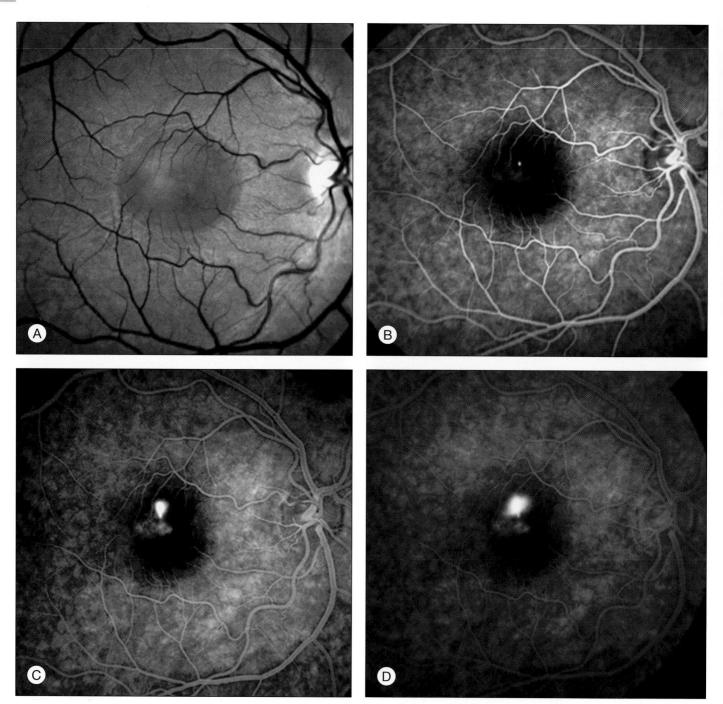

Fig. 63-11 A, Red-free photograph of a 28-year-old male with decreased vision reveals a large neurosensory detachment at the macula. B, Early fluorescein angiogram shows a small pinpoint leak which progresses in the mid (C) and late (D) phase of the study into a typical smokestack.

described.[95] Although exudates usually extend into or beyond the fovea, the leakage point is found in the foveal area in less than 10%. It is most frequently located in a 1-mm-wide ring-like zone immediately adjacent to the fovea: incidence rapidly decreases beyond this area.[14,96] The leakage points are most commonly found in the superonasal quadrant of the posterior pole, followed in decreasing frequency by the inferonasal quadrant, the superotemporal quadrant, and the inferotemporal quadrant.[97] There are no anatomical differences in the neurosensory retina,

RPE, Bruch's membrane, or choriocapillaris that may account for this phenomenon; however, the absence of rod cells in the fovea resulting in weaker adhesion between the neurosensory retina and the RPE may explain both the predominance of leakage points and the tendency for extension of the exudate in this area.[96] In almost one-third of cases, the leakage point is found within the papillomacular bundle and the incidence above the horizontal raphe is almost twice that of those below this line.[98]

If the leakage point is not visualized under the retinal detachment, the most likely location is the superior portion of the affected area. In some cases, the leaking point cannot be found because the area has healed. Patients with CSC may also have window defects in areas uninvolved by subretinal fluid during fluorescein angiography.[99] These window defects occur over areas of choroidal vascular hyperpermeability observed during ICG angiography. In chronic CSC, atrophic RPE tracts appear as mottled hyperfluorescence.

Indocyanine green angiography

The application of ICG angiography to study CSC has expanded our knowledge of the disease.[7,17,18,100–103] A consistent finding in reports about CSC is hyperpermeability of the choroid during ICG angiography.[18,48,104,105] These areas are best seen in the mid-phase of the angiogram and appear localized in the inner choroid (Fig. 63-12). As the liver removes ICG from circulation, the dye that has leaked into the choroid appears to disperse, particularly into the deeper layers of the choroid. This produces a characteristic appearance of hyperfluorescent patches in the choroid with negative staining or silhouetting of the larger choroidal vessels in the later phases of the ICG angiogram.[7] The areas of hyperfluorescence appear to enlarge centrifugally during the later stages of ICG angiography (Fig. 63-13), radiating from the loci of hyperpermeability.[101] These areas of hyperfluorescence are found not only in correspondence with the leaking point seen on fluorescein angiography, but also in areas that appear clinically normal as well as unaffected fellow eyes. These multifocal hyperpermeable areas noted on wide-angle ICG angiography are presumed to be occult PEDs and extend far beyond the posterior pole, emphasizing that CSC may be more diffuse and widespread than previously believed (Fig. 63-14).[103] Many areas of choroidal vascular hyperpermeability may be seen during ICG angiography in patients with CSC but do not appear to be associated with active leaks.[7] Choroidal vascular hyperpermeability is a unifying feature of all types of CSC,

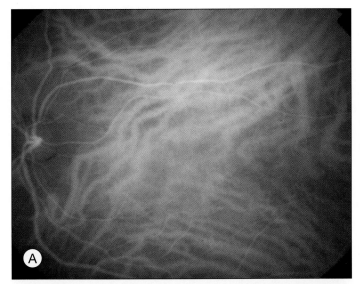

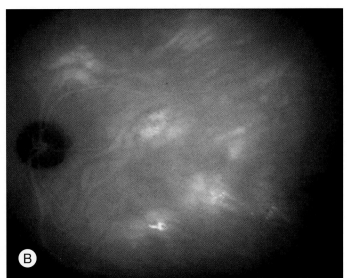

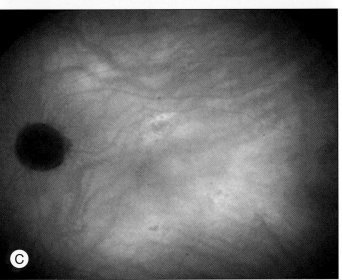

Fig. 63-12 A, The early indocyanine green angiogram of a 28-year-old male with central serous chorioretinopathy shows no pathology. B, Hyperpermeability of the choroid is better observed during the mid-phase of the study when compared to the late phase (C).

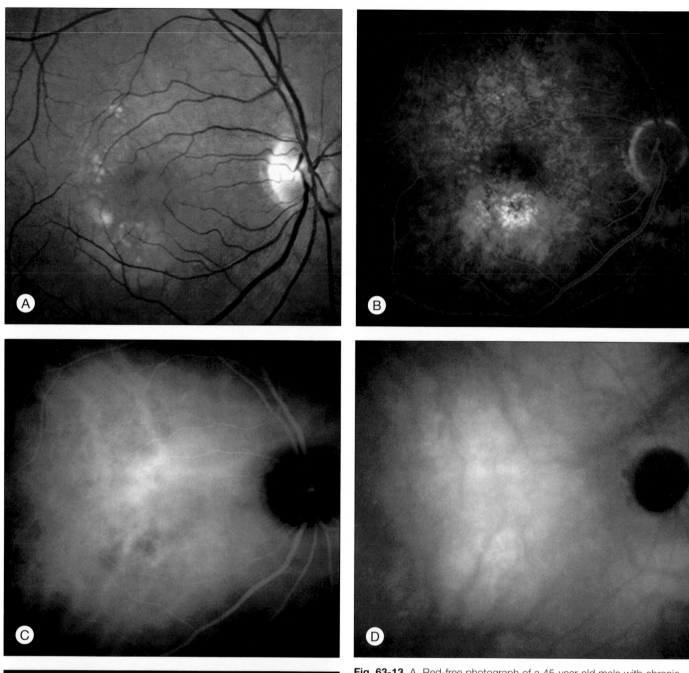

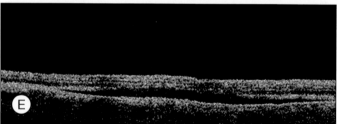

Fig. 63-13 A, Red-free photograph of a 45-year-old male with chronic central serous chorioretinopathy shows diffuse retinal pigment epithelial (RPE) changes at the posterior pole and a shallow detachment of the neurosensory retina. B, Fluorescence angiogram demonstrates RPE decompensation. C, Early indocyanine green angiogram shows hyperfluorescent areas at the posterior pole which appear to enlarge during the late phase (D). E, Optical coherence tomography reveals a shallow neurosensory detachment.

independent of the age, subtype, or relationship to corticosteroid treatment or past organ transplantation.[7,105] Several investigators have noted areas of slow filling during ICG angiography in CSC patients.[18,104] The choroidal veins in patients with CSC may also appear to be engorged. The speed and variation in filling of the choroid are not well known in normal patients, making interpretation of these findings in CSC difficult. It is possible that the flow through and pressure within the choriocapillaris is altered by inappropriate alteration of choroidal arteries, choroidal veins, or both.[15]

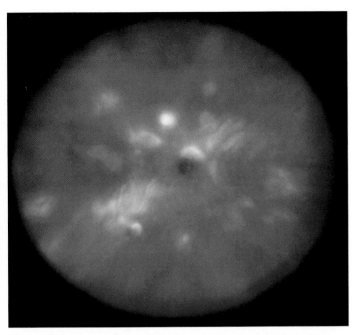

Fig. 63-14 The wide-angle indocyanine green angiogram of a patient with central serous chorioretinopathy shows multiple hyperfluorescent areas including the retina far beyond the posterior pole.

Optical coherence tomography

OCT is an effective method for quantifying serous detachments of the retina and the RPE (Fig. 63-15).[106,107] Longitudinal measurements can track the resolution of subretinal fluid and provide an objective measure of the clinical course, thus reducing the need for angiograms.[108]

Natural history

Neurosensory detachment in CSC generally resolves spontaneously within 3 months, with most recovering baseline visual acuity. After healing, a pigment epithelial scar can be observed; this occupies an area considerably larger than the original leakage point and is characterized by the accumulation of dot-like areas of hyperfluorescence and hypofluorescence with no signs of dye leakage. Recurrences develop in about one-third to one-half of all cases after the first episode and 10% have three or more recurrences.[5,6,109] In almost half of the patients the recurrence occurs within 1 year of the primary episode while others develop up to 10 years later. A single episode may also be followed by a chronic, slowly progressing disturbance of the RPE at the posterior pole. Some cases may suffer a persistent and progressive macular detachment with visual loss. A small percentage of patients develop CNV, perifoveal RPE atrophy, or cystic macular degeneration with severe and irreversible loss of visual acuity. The clinical course is also variable in patients with larger PEDs, multiple recurrences, subretinal fibrin deposits, multifocal leaks, dependent neurosensory detachments, and atrophic RPE tracts, but they seem to be at greater risk for visual impairment.

Differential diagnosis

Although the clinical diagnosis of CSC is usually confirmed by fluorescence angiography and OCT, several entities should be considered in the differential diagnosis (Fig. 63-16).

INFECTIOUS AND INFLAMMATORY DISORDERS

Any infectious and inflammatory disorder involving the posterior pole that causes serous macular detachment, such as presumed

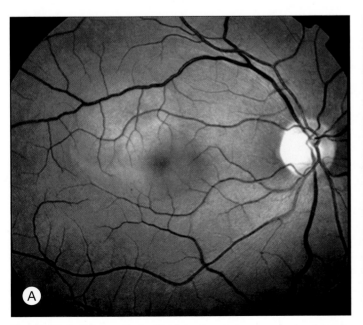

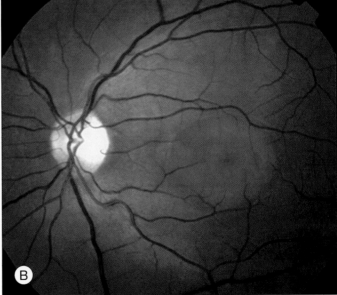

Fig. 63-15 A, B, In a patient with bilateral central serous chorioretinopathy and bilateral vision deterioration, red-free photographs reveal bilateral subretinal fluid within the macula.

Continued

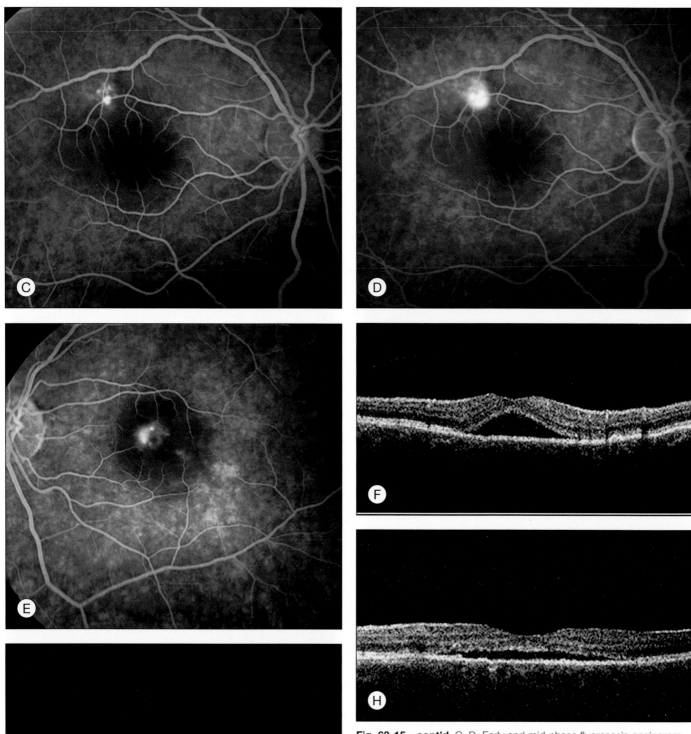

Fig. 63-15—cont'd C, D, Early and mid-phase fluorescein angiogram of the right eye identifies a hyperfluorescent area in the temporal superior macula. E, There is also a hyperfluorescent area at the macula of the fellow eye. Vertical (F) and horizontal (G) optical coherence tomography of the right macula shows subretinal fluid including the subfoveal area. H, There is a shallow detachment of the neurosensory retina at the foveal optical coherence tomography of the fellow eye.

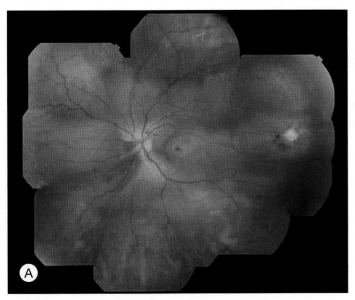
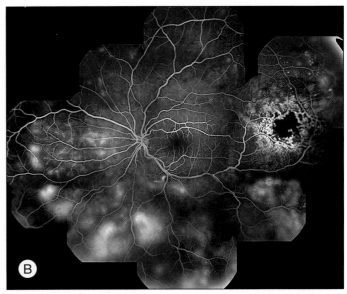

Fig. 63-16 A 14-year-old female noticed a sudden decrease of left vision to 20/400. A, Composite fundus photograph of the left eye demonstrates a neurosensory macular detachment simulating central serous chorioretinopathy. There is a localized area of retinal capillary telangiectasia in the temporal periphery. The intraretinal yellowish material is consistent with dehemoglobinized blood. There are also intraretinal exudates scattered throughout the fundus. B, Composite fluorescein angiography study of the same eye reveals diffuse retinal capillary telangiectasia and intraretinal leakage. The dilated retinal telangiectatic vessels are actively leaking, leading to neurosensory macular detachment. The patient was diagnosed with Coats disease.

ocular histoplasmosis syndrome (POHS), is considered in the differential diagnosis of CSC. POHS can be easily differentiated from CSC by the concomitant presence of peripheral "punched-out" chorioretinal lesions, peripapillary atrophy, and arcuate striae in the mid-periphery. Idiopathic CNV also presents with serous macular detachment in young, otherwise healthy subjects. The presence of CNV, subretinal hemorrhages, unilateral involvement, and the lack of spontaneous resolution of the maculopathy help to distinguish it from CSC.

Infiltrative or inflammatory disorders of the choroid, such as Harada's disease, may also present with serous macular detachment. The presence of vitritis, optic disc hyperemia, associated systemic manifestations, disturbances of the internal limiting membrane, and prompt response to anti-inflammatory therapy are helpful in differentiating Harada's disease from CSC. Posterior scleritis can also present with exudative neurosensory detachment of the macula; it can be distinguished from CSC by the presence of scleral thickening, vitreous cells, and pain with ocular movements. The diagnosis can be confirmed with ultrasound examination which reveals nodular scleral thickening and an echolucent area at the posterior pole behind the echo of the sclera (T-sign). Sympathetic ophthalmia may also present with serous macular detachment, and associated intraocular inflammation, yellowish cellular detachments of the RPE (Dalen–Fuchs nodules), and a history of trauma to the fellow eye. In addition, idiopathic uveal effusion syndrome and benign reactive lymphoid hyperplasia of the choroid may present with exudative neurosensory detachment in otherwise healthy subjects.

Tumors

Choroidal melanoma, choroidal hemangioma, choroidal metastasis, choroidal osteoma, and leukemic choroidal infiltrates can present with exudative macular detachment. Although clinical examination of the fundus is usually sufficient to recognize the choroidal tumor, some cases, especially choroidal hemangioma, can be confused with a large PED and associated neurosensory detachment. In these cases ultrasound examination and angiography may be helpful in determining the correct diagnosis.

Vascular disorders

Collagen-vascular diseases such as systemic lupus erythematosus, polyarteritis nodosa, scleroderma, dermatomyositis, and relapsing polychondritis may develop serous detachment of the macula caused by fibrinoid necrosis of the choroidal vessels. Furthermore, in such disease the prolonged systemic use of corticosteroids may be complicated by CSC. Malignant hypertension, toxemia of pregnancy, and DIC can present with a neurosensory detachment secondary to acute multifocal occlusion of choroidal arteries and choriocapillaris as well as necrosis of the overlying RPE (Elschnig's spots).

Optic nerve pit with serous macular detachment

The macular elevation that communicates with an optic nerve pit is often a schisis-like separation of the internal layers of the retina. The outer-layer detachment starts in the macula without apparent communication with the pit, and it can be distinguished because it is relatively opaque. The inner-layer separation is transparent and communicates with the pit. On fluorescein angiography, there may be neither pinpoint leakage nor filling of the macular detachment, as seen in CSC. OCT may also be helpful in the presence of a macular detachment associated with an optic pit to image the schisis-like separation of the retinal layers at the posterior pole.

Age-related macular degeneration

The differentiation between AMD and CSC is necessary when CSC is present in adults over 50 years of age. CSC in older patients may present with more diffuse RPE damage, multifocal areas of leakage, and subretinal deposits of fibrin and lipids. Furthermore, chronic CSC may be complicated by secondary CNV. Although fluorescein angiography is helpful in distinguishing between the two conditions, when there is a well-defined CNV in AMD and a well-defined pinpoint leakage in CSC, it is much less helpful in the presence of diffuse, ill-defined hyperfluores-

cence, which may be caused either by an ill-defined CNV or by a diffuse "ooze" of the RPE. In these cases ICG angiography may be helpful. In fact, ICG angiograms typically reveal multifocal, early hyperfluorescence that fades in the late phase in CSC, and late hyperfluorescence corresponding to the CNV in AMD.[17]

Polypoidal choroidal vasculopathy

Polypoidal choroidal vasculopathy is presumed to be a variant of occult CNV.[110] The typical clinical presentation of this entity poses little challenge; however, an isolated macular variant of polypoidal choroidal vasculopathy may have clinical and fluorescein angiographic characteristics resembling CSC (Fig. 63-17). These atypical cases of polypoidal choroidal vasculopathy involve small-caliber vascular abnormalities and may present exclusively with a neurosensory detachment of the neurosensory retina (Fig. 63-18).

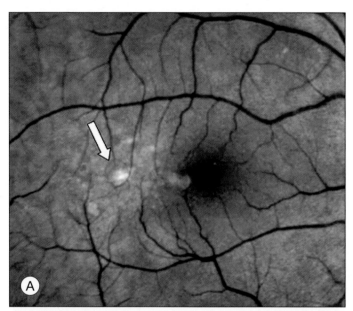

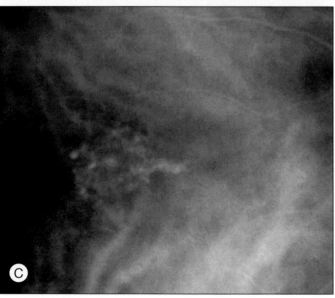

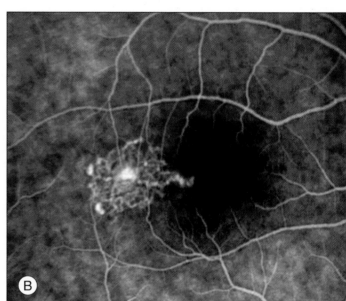

Fig. 63-17 This 56-year-old Caucasian male had three transient episodes of vision disturbance diagnosed as central serous chorioretinopathy. A, Red-free photograph reveals a flat macula overlying multiple, nummular elevations suggestive of small serous pigment epithelial detachments. At the center of the lesion there is a patch of fibrous metaplasia (white arrow). B, Fluorescein angiogram reveals a net of inner choroidal vessels terminating in aneurysmal or polypoidal lesions. C, Late indocyanine green angiogram confirms the presence of a polypoidal vascular abnormality.

The polyoidal lesions may resemble small PEDs clinically and by fluorescein angiography. These cases masquerade as CSC.[111] ICG angiography is important in differentiating these two disorders. In polypoidal choroidal vasculopathy, ICG angiogram reveals a small-caliber vascular network terminating in multiple, polypoidal lesions.[112]

Treatment

In most cases CSC resolves spontaneously within a few months and visual acuity returns to 20/25 or better.[2,46,113] Only 5% of all CSC cases experience severe, permanent visual loss.[5] A beneficial effect of photocoagulation has been shown in several studies (Figs 63-19 and 63-20).[109,114-117] Photocoagulation typically shortens the course of the disease, accelerating the resorption of fluid; however, it has no effect on final visual acuity. Some authors have reported that treatment of CSC with laser coagulation reduces the recurrence rate,[116] whereas other investigators have observed no difference.[109,118,119]

Because CSC is usually a self-limiting disease and there are possible complications associated with laser treatment,

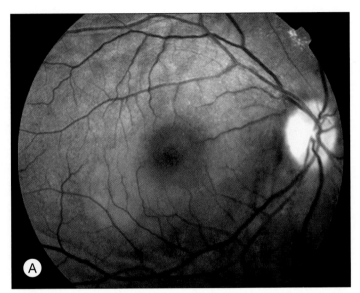
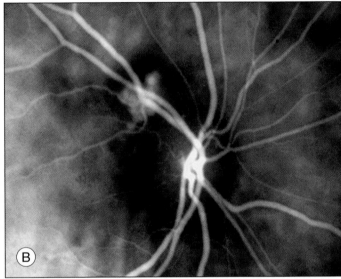

Fig. 63-18 A, This clinical photograph shows a 62-year-old female who had a neurosensory retinal detachment in the central macula and was diagnosed with central serous chorioretinopathy. B, Indocyanine green angiogram reveals the presence of a polypoidal choroidal vascular abnormality in the superior temporal juxtapapillary region.

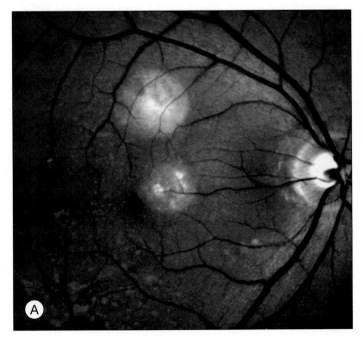
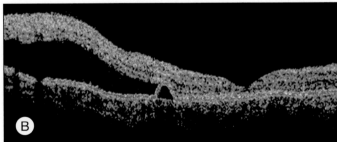

Fig. 63-19 This 34-year-old male was diagnosed with recurrent central serous chorioretinopathy. A, The red-free photograph reveals retinal pigment epithelium (RPE) changes in the papillomacular bundle caused by a previous episode. There is an acute neurosensory detachment of the retina inferior to the temporal superior arcade. B, Vertical optical coherence tomography (OCT) confirms subretinal fluid and in addition shows a small RPE detachment.

Continued

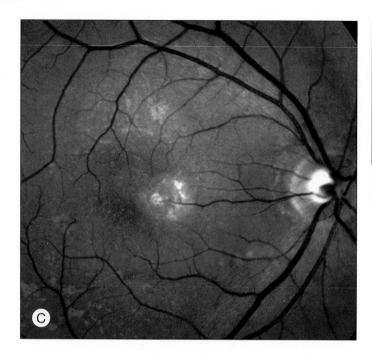

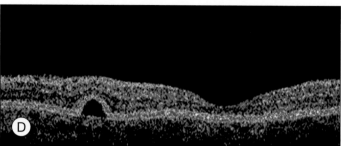

Fig. 63-19—cont'd C, Two weeks after focal laser treatment there is complete resolution of the subretinal fluid but vertical OCT reveals the remaining RPE detachment (D).

particularly when applied very close to the fovea, a recommendation for photocoagulation can only be based on clinical judgment. As a general rule, we recommend observing a new-onset acute serous macular detachment for the first 3 months, unless the patient has special occupational considerations that require rapid improvement of visual acuity or in the case of monocular patients. If the macular detachment has not resolved after the first 3 months and the leakage point is remote from the center of the fovea, it is reasonable to treat a symptomatic patient. If the leakage point is within $500\,\mu m$ from the center of the fovea, it is reasonable to observe for 6 months before treatment. Other indications for laser treatment are

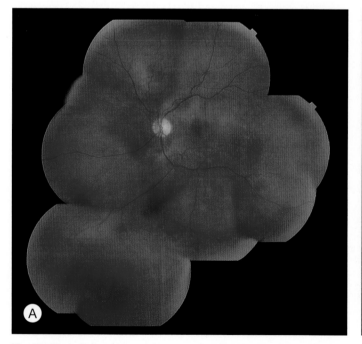

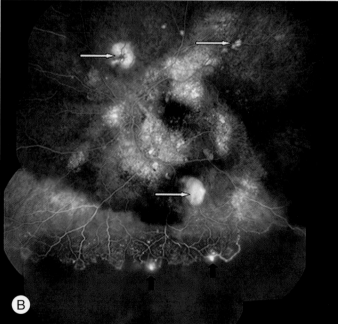

Fig. 63-20 A, Color photograph composite of a 47-year-old female with an 18-year history of bilateral central serous chorioretinopathy (CSC) shows bullous dependent detachment of the neurosensory retina inferiorly. B, Fluorescein angiogram composite reveals diffuse decompensation of the retinal pigment epithelium, multiple scattered pigment epithelial detachments (white arrows), and obliteration of the retinal capillaries in the region of the detachment. Note the presence of early neovascularization at the junction between perfused and nonperfused retina (black arrows).

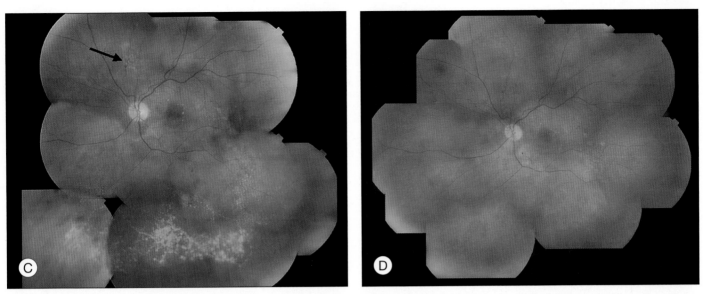

Fig. 63-20—cont'd C, Color photograph composite of the same eye 2 months after the laser treatment of the site of leakage (black arrow) reveals partial resolution of the detachment and lipid precipitation. D, Clinical photograph composite 16 months after the laser treatment in the area of the leakage shows complete resolution of the detachment.

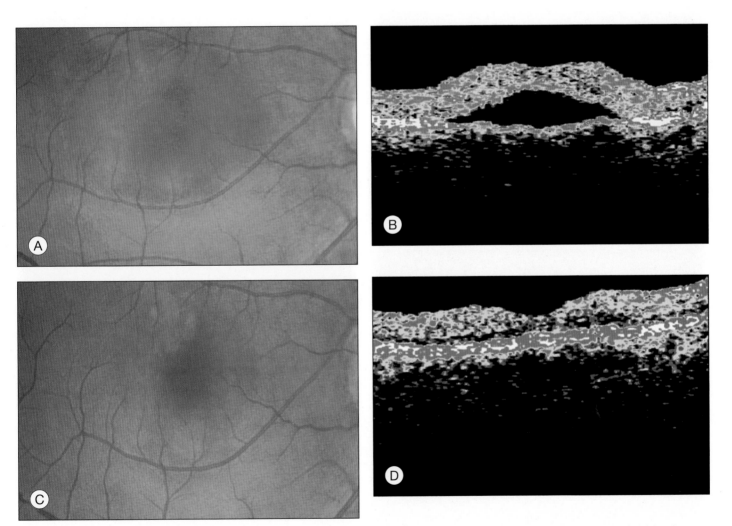

Fig. 63-21 A, This color photograph of a patient with acute decrease in vision shows a large detachment of the neurosensory retina involving the fovea. B, Subretinal fluid is shown on the optical coherence tomography (OCT). C, Four weeks after focal laser treatment visual acuity increased to 20/20 and there was no retinal thickening noted on the color photograph. D, OCT confirmed the complete resolution of subretinal fluid.

primary detachment with visual decline in a patient who has experienced permanent visual loss from an untreated macular detachment in the fellow eye and recurrent macular detachment in the eye of a patient who has experienced permanent visual loss from the initial episode. Furthermore, laser treatment is indicated in particularly severe forms of CSC that are known to have a poor prognosis if left untreated. These include cases complicated by multiple serous detachments of the RPE and bullous sensory retinal detachment, dependent neurosensory detachment, epithelial tracts, diffuse RPE decompensation, subretinal deposits of fibrin and lipids, and those forms of CSC associated with secondary CNV.

After laser photocoagulation of the leakage point anatomic

resolution of the macular detachment generally occurs in about 2 weeks in uncomplicated cases, but it may require up to 6 weeks in long-standing detachments with turbid subretinal fluid (Fig. 63-21). Complete visual recovery usually requires twice that time.

Recently, ICG angiographic-guided photodynamic therapy for treatment of chronic CSC has shown promising results, especially in cases with diffuse decompensation of RPE (Fig. 63-22).[120–124] Even after long-standing macular detachments of years' duration, a complete resolution of the fluid was observed in the majority of patients (Fig. 63-23). The rationale behind such a therapeutic approach is to cause a reduction of the blood flow in the hyperpermeable choriocapillaris (Fig. 63-24).

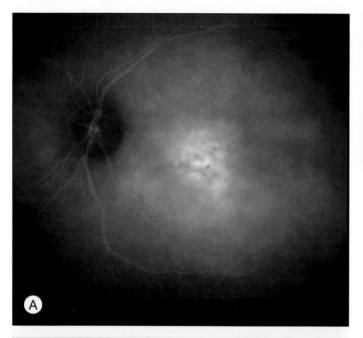

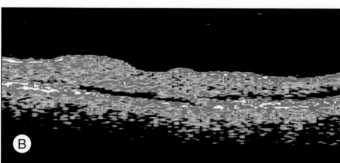

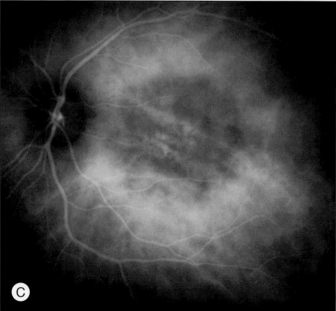

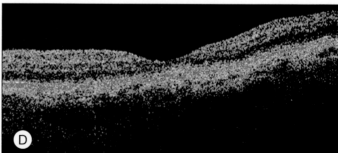

Fig. 63-22 This 42-year-old male had decreased visual acuity due to a chronic form of central serous chorioretinopathy. A, Mid-phase indocyanine green (ICG) angiogram shows a large area of hyperfluorescence in the macula. B, Optical coherence tomography (OCT) reveals a shallow detachment of the neurosensory retina. C, Photodynamic therapy with verteporfin was performed and the patient noticed a slight increase in vision. There was a circular hypofluorescence at the macula in the ICG angiogram 3 weeks later. D, OCT confirms the complete resolution of fluid. There are some hyperreflective changes in the retinal pigment epithelial layer due to a long-standing history of subretinal fluid.

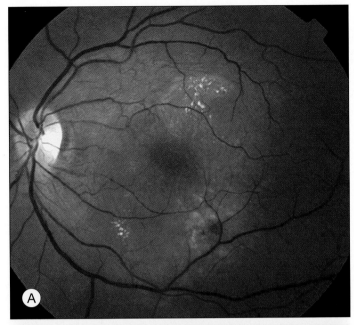

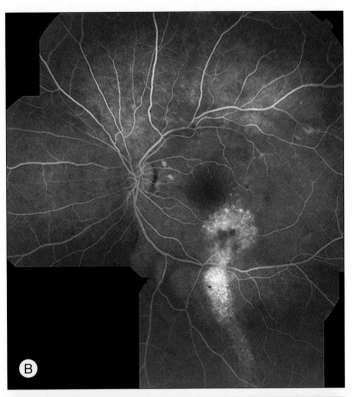

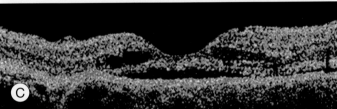

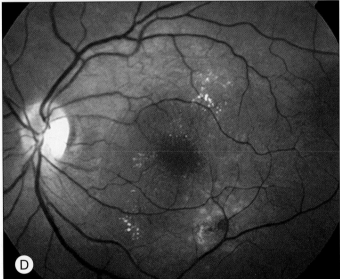

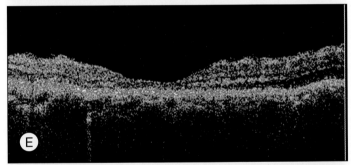

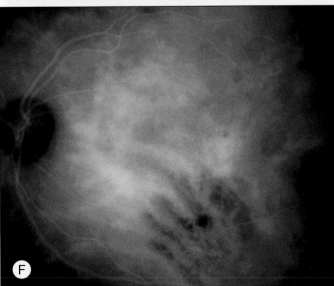

Fig. 63-23 A, Red-free photograph of a 52-year-old male with a chronic form of central serous chorioretinopathy reveals diffuse retinal pigment epithelium (RPE) changes at the posterior pole accompanied by subretinal fluid. B, Composite of fluorescein angiogram shows areas of RPE decompensation at the posterior pole and the mid peripheral retina. Note the atrophic RPE tract expanding inferiorly from the hyperfluorescent macular area. C, Cystoid macular degeneration, as seen on this optical coherence tomography (OCT), causes the decrease in visual acuity. D, Photodynamic therapy was performed leading to resolution of subretinal fluid. E, OCT confirms the resolution of subretinal fluid as well as the absence of the retinal cystic spaces. Note the foveal atrophy which might be caused by long-standing chronic disease and the cystoid degeneration. F, Mid-phase indocyanine green angiogram shows circular hypofluorescence in the area the laser was applied.

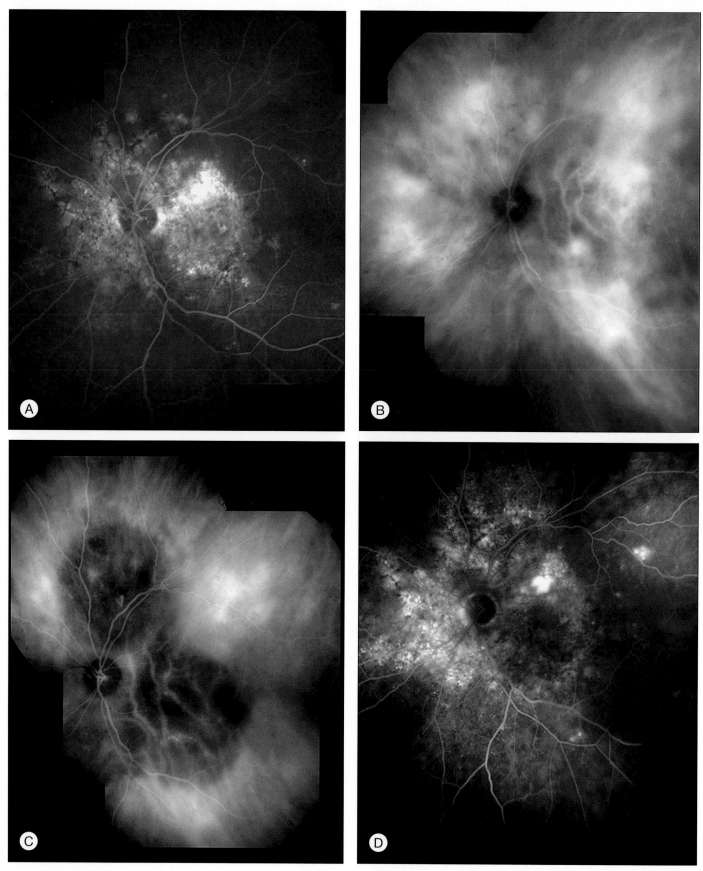

Fig. 63-24 A, Composite of the fluorescein angiogram of a patient with chronic central serous chorioretinopathy reveals diffuse retinal pigment epithelium decompensation also outside the arcades. B, Composite of the indocyanine green (ICG) angiogram shows multiple hyperfluorescent areas which do not always correspond to hyperfluorescent regions on fluorescein angiography. C, Photodynamic therapy was performed on two different areas resulting in two circular hypofluorescent regions at the macula and superior to the optic disc, as noted on the ICG angiogram 4 weeks after treatment. D, At the same time the fluorescein angiogram reveals a reduction in hyperfluorescence in the treated areas. Note the two temporal hyperfluorescent areas which are still leaking.

Although rare, there are some recognized complications of laser treatment of CSC, the worst of which is inadvertent photocoagulation of the fovea. The patient should always be informed that a persistent scotoma, corresponding to the site of laser photocoagulation, may occur after the treatment. Secondary CNV may be induced by laser treatment, especially when excessive intensity is used.[109,125,126] In some instances this complication may be induced by the treatment, but sub-retinal neovascular membranes may also occur in untreated eyes.[109,125,127] In addition, an often underestimated complication is the slow but progressive enlargement of the area of RPE atrophy caused by the laser treatment. When the treatment site is close to the center of the fovea, the enlargement of the RPE scar, with time, may eventually involve the fovea and cause delayed irreversible visual loss. When possible, the laser treatment of a leaking point in CSC should be avoided within the foveal avascular zone.

REFERENCES

1. von Graefe A. Central recurrent retinitis. Graefes Arch Clin Exp Ophthalmol 1866; 12:211–215.
2. Bennet G. Central serous retinopathy. Br J Ophthalmol 1955; 39:605–618.
3. Maumenee AE. Symposium: Macular disease, clinical manifestations. Trans Pacific Coast Oto-Ophthalm Soc 1959; 40:139–160.
4. Gass JDM. Stereoscopic atlas of macular diseases, 4th edn. St. Louis: CV Mosby; 1997:49–70.
5. Gass JDM. Pathogenesis of disciform detachment of the neuro-epithelium. I. General concepts and classification. Am J Ophthalmol 1967; 63:573–585.
6. Gass JDM. Pathogenesis of disciform detachment of the neuro-epithelium. II. Idiopathic central serous choroidopathy. Am J Ophthalmol 1967; 63:587–615.
7. Spaide RF, Campeas H, Haas L et al. Central serous chorioretinopathy in younger and older adults. Ophthalmology 1996; 103:2070–2079.
8. Jalkh AE, Jabbour N, Avila MP et al. Retinal pigment epithelial decompensation. I. Clinical features and natural course. Ophthalmology 1984; 91:1544–1548.
9. Polak BC, Baarsma GS, Snyers B. Diffuse retinal pigment epitheliopathy complicating systemic corticosteroid treatment. Br J Ophthalmol 1995; 79:922–925.
10. de Venecia G. Fluorescein angiographic smoke stack. Verhoeff Society Meeting, Washington, DC, April 24–25, 1982. [Quoted from Gass JDM. Stereoscopic atlas of macular diseases. St. Louis: CV Mosby; 1987:56–57.]
11. Negi A, Marmor MF. The resorption of subretinal fluid after diffuse damage of the retinal pigment epithelium. Invest Ophthalmol Vis Sci 1983; 24:1475–1479.
12. Negi A, Marmor MF. Experimental serous retinal detachment and focal pigment epithelium damage. Arch Ophthalmol 1984; 102:445–449.
13. Marmor MF. New hypotheses on the pathogenesis and treatment of serous retinal detachment. Graefes Arch Clin Exp Ophthalmol 1988; 226:548–552.
14. Spitznas M. Pathogenesis of central serous retinopathy: a new working hypothesis. Graefes Arch Clin Exp Ophthalmol 1986; 224:321–324.
15. Spaide RF, Goldbaum M, Wong DWK et al. Serous detachment of the retina. Retina 2003; 23:820–846.
16. Ciardella AP, Borodoker N, Costa DLL et al. The expanding clinical spectrum of central serous chorioretinopathy. Comp Ophthalmol Update 2003; 4:71–84.
17. Guyer DR, Yannuzzi LA, Slakter JS et al. Digital indocyanine green video-angiography of central serous chorioretinopathy. Arch Ophthalmol 1994; 112:1057–1062.
18. Prunte C, Flammer J. Choroidal capillary and venous congestion in central serous chorioretinopathy. Am J Ophthalmol 1996; 121:26–34.
19. Gelber GS, Schatz H. Loss of vision due to central serous chorioretinopathy following psychological stress. Am J Psychiatry 1987; 144:46–50.
20. Yannuzzi LA. Type-A behavior and central serous chorioretinopathy. Retina 1987; 7:111–130.
21. Horniker E. Ueber eine Form von zentraler Retinitis auf angio-neurotischer Grundlage (Retinitis centralis angio-neurotica). Graefes Arch Clin Exp Ophthalmol 1929; 123:286–360.
22. Garg SP, Dada T, Talwar D et al. Endogenous cortisol profile in patients with central serous chorioretinopathy. Br J Ophthalmol 1997; 81:962–964.
23. Bouzas EA, Scott MH, Mastorakos G et al. Central serous chorioretinopathy in endogenous hypercortisolism. Arch Ophthalmol 1993; 111:1929–1932.
24. Haimovici R, Koh S, Gagnon DR et al. Risk factors for central serous chorioretinopathy: a case-control study. Ophthalmology 2004, 111:244–249.
25. Gass JDM, Little HL. Bilateral bullous exudative retinal detachment complicating idiopathic central serous chorioretinopathy during systemic corticosteroid therapy. Ophthalmology 1995, 102:737–747.
26. Friberg TR, Eller AW. Serous retinal detachment resembling central serous chorioretinopathy following organ transplantation. Graefes Arch Clin Exp Ophthalmol 1990; 288:305–309.
27. Gass JDM. Central serous chorioretinopathy and white subretinal exudation during pregnancy. Arch Ophthalmol 1991; 109:677–681.
28. Fastenburg DM, Ober RR. Central serous choroidopathy in pregnancy. Arch Ophthalmol 1983; 101:1055–1058.
29. Quillen DA, Gass JDM, Brod R et al. Central serous chorioretinopathy in women. Ophthalmology 1996; 103:72–79.
30. Tittl K, Spaide RF, Wong D et al. Systemic and ocular findings in central serous chorioretinopathy. Am J Ophthalmol 1999; 128:63–68.
31. Yoshioka H, Sugita T, Nagayoski K. Fluorescein angiography findings in experimental retinopathy produced by intravenous adrenaline injection. Folia Ophthalmol Jpn 1970; 21:648–652.
32. Yoshioka H, Katsume Y. Experimental central serous chorioretinopathy. III: ultrstructural findings. Jpn J Ophthalmol 1982; 26:397–409.
33. Yoshioka H, Katsume Y, Akune H. Experimental central serous chorioretinopathy in monkey eyes fluorescein angiographic findings. Ophthalmologica 1982; 185:168–178.
34. Miki T, Sunada I, Higaki T. Studies on chorioretinitis induced in rabbits by stress (repeated administration of epinephrine). Acta Soc Ophthalmol Jpn 1972; 75:1037–1045.
35. Warren JB, Loi RK, Coughlan ML. Involvement of nitric oxide in the delayed vasodilator response to ultraviolet light irradiation of rat skin in vivo. Br J Pharmacol 1993; 109:802–806.
36. Chrousos GP, Gold PW. The concepts of stress and stress system disorders. Overview of physical and behavioral homeostatsis. JAMA 1992; 267:1244–1252.
37. Gill GN. Adrenal gland. In: West JB, ed. Best and Taylor's physiological basis of medical practice. Baltimore, MD: Williams & Wilkins, 1990:820–830.
38. Smith TJ. Dexamethasone regulation of glycosaminoglycan synthesis in cultured human skin fibroblast. Similar effects of glucocorticoid and thyroid hormones. J Clin Invest 1984; 74:2157–2163.
39. Ehrlich HP, Traver H, Hunt TK. Effects of vitamin A upon inflammation and collagen synthesis. Ann Surg 1973; 177:222–227.
40. Pratt WB, Aronow L. The effect of glucosteroids on protein and nucleic acid synthesis in mouse fibroblasts growing in vitro. J Biol Chem 1966; 241:5244–5250.
41. Yasuzumi T, Miki T, Sugimoto K. Electromicroscopic studies of epinephrine choroiditis in rabbits. I. Pigment epithelium and Bruchs mmbrane in the healed stage. Nippon Ganka Gakkai Zasshi 1974; 78:588–598.
42. Basti CP. Regulation of cation transport by low doses of glucocorticoids. J Clin Invest 1987; 80:848–856.
43. Sandle GI, McGlone F. Acute effects of dexamethasone on cation transport in colonic epithelium. Gut 1987; 28:701–706.
44. Smith OB, Benos DJ. Epithelial Na+ channels. Ann Rev Physiol 1991; 53:509–530.
45. Fine SL, Owens SL. Central serous chorioretinopathy in a 7-year old girl. Am J Ophthalmol 1980; 90:871–873.
46. Klein ML, van Buskirk EM, Friedman E et al. Experience with non-treatment of central serous choroidopathy. Arch Ophthalmol 1974; 91:247–250.
47. Leibowitz HM, Kreuger DE, Maunder LR et al. The Framingham Eye Study monograph: an ophthalmological and epidemiological study of cataract, glaucoma, diabetic retinopathy, macular degeneration, and visual acuity in a general population of 2631 adults. Surv Ophthalmol 1980; 24:335–610.
48. Spaide RF, Hall L, Haas A et al. Indocyanine green videoangiography of older patients with central serous chorioretinopathy. Retina 1996; 16:203–213.
49. Cordes FC. A type of foveo-macular retinitis observed in the US Navy. Am J Ophthalmol 1944; 27:803–816.
50. Harrington DO. The autonomic nervous system in ocular diseases. Am J Ophthalmol 1946; 29:1405–1425.
51. Werry H, Arends C. Untersuchung zur Objektivierung von Persoenlichkeitsmerkmalen bei Patienten mit Retinopathia centralis serosa. Klin Monatsbl Augenheilkd 1978; 172:363–370.
52. Yannuzzi LA, Gitter KA, Schatz H. Central serous chorioretinopathy. In: Yannuzzi LA, Gitter KA, Schatz H, eds. The macula: a comprehensive text and atlas. Baltimore, MD: Williams & Wilkins; 1979:145–165.
53. Fukunaga K. Central chorioretinopathy with disharmony of the autonomic nervous system. Acta Soc Ophthalmol Jpn 1969; 73:1468–1477.

54. Guyer DR, Gragoudas ES. Central serous chorioretinopathy. In: Albert DM, Jakobiec FA, eds. Principles and practice of ophthalmology, vol. 2. Philadelphia, PA: WB Saunders, 1994:818–825.

55. Desai UR, Alhalel AA, Campen TJ et al. Central serous chorioretinopathy in African Americans. J Natl Med Assoc 2003; 95:553–559.

56. Gass JDM. In: Stereoscopic atlas of macular diseases: diagnosis and treatment, 4th edn. St. Louis: Mosby; 1997:52–70.

57. Jaeger WA, Nover A. Stoerungen des Lichtsinns und Farbsinns bei Chorioretinitis centralis serosa. Graefes Arch Clin Exp Ophthalmol 1951; 52:11–120.

58. Frisén L, Frisén M: Micropsia and visual acuity in macular edema. A study of neuroretinal basis of visual acuity. Graefes Arch Clin Exp Ophthalmol 1979; 210:69–77.

59. Bek T, Kandi M. Quantitative anomaloscopy and optical coherence tomography scanning in central serous chorioretinopathy. Acta Ophthalmol Scand 2000; 78:632–637.

60. Klien BA. Retinal lesions associated with uveal disease, part 1. Am J Ophthalmol 1956; 42:831–847.

61. Peyman GA, Bok D. Peroxidase diffusion in the normal and laser-coagulated primate retina. Invest Ophthalmol Vis Sci 1972, 11:35–45.

62. Ie D, Yannuzzi LA, Spaide RF et al. Subretinal exudative deposits in central serous chorioretinopathy. Br J Ophthalmol 1993; 77:349–353.

63. Schatz H, McDonald HR, Johnson RN et al. Subretinal fibrosis in central serous chorioretinopathy. Ophthalmology 1995; 102:1077–1088.

64. Hooymans JM. Fibrotic scar formation in central serous chorioretinopathy developed during systemic treatment with corticosteroids. Graefes Arch Clin Exp Ophthalmol 1998; 236:876–879.

65. Yannuzzi LA, Shakin JL, Fisher YL et al. Peripheral retinal detachments and retinal pigment epithelial atrophic tracts secondary to central serous pigment epitheliopathy. Ophthalmology 1984; 91:1554–1572.

66. Cohen D, Gaudric A, Coscas G et al. Epitheliopathie retinienne diffuse et chorioretinopathie sereuse centrale. J Fr Ophtalmol 1983; 6:339–349.

67. Zweng HC, Little HL, Vassiliadis A. Argon laser photocoagulation. St Louis: Mosby; 1977.

68. Gass JDM. Bullous retinal detachment: an unusual manifestation of idiopathic central serous choroidopathy. Am J Ophthalmol 1973;75:810–821.

69. Nadel AJ, Turan MI, Coles RS. Central serous retinopathy: a generalized disease of the pigment epithelium. Mod Probl Ophthalmol 1979; 20:76–88.

70. Gass JDM. Photocoagulation treatment of idiopathic central serous choroidopathy. Trans Am Acad Ophthalmol Otolaryngol 1977; 83:456–463.

71. Schatz H, D'Oesterloh M, McDonald RH et al. Development of retinal vascular leakage and cystoid macular edema secondary to central serous chorioretinopathy. Br J Ophthalmol 1993; 77:744–746.

72. Weiler W, Foerester MH, Wessing A. Exudative retinal detachment, pigment epithelium tear, and subretinal exudate in a case of central serous chorioretinopathy. Klin Monatsbl Augenheilkd 1991; 199:450–453.

73. Iida T, Yannuzzi LA, Spaide RF et al. Cystoid macular degeneration in chronic central serous chorioretinopathy. Retina 2003; 23:1–7.

74. Hilton AF, Harrison JD, Lamb AM et al. Ocular complications in haemodialysis and renal transplant patients. Aust NZ J Ophthalmol 1982; 10:247–253.

75. Gass JDM, Slamovits TL, Fuller DG et al. Posterior chorioretinopathy and retinal detachment after organ transplantation. Arch Ophthalmol 1992;110:1717–1722.

76. Eckstein MB, Spalton DJ, Holder G. Visual loss from central serous retinopathy in systemic lupus erythematosus. Br J Ophthalmol 1993; 77:607–609.

77. Haimovici R, Rumelt S, Melby J. Endocrine abnormalities in patients with central serous chorioretinopathy. Ophthalmology 2003; 110:698–703.

78. Haimovici R, Gragoudas ES, Duker JS et al. Central serous chorioretinopathy associated with inhaled or intranasal coricosteroids. Ophthalmology 1997; 104:1653–1660.

79. Wakakura M, Ishikawa S. Central serous chorioretinopathy complicating systemic corticosteroid treatment. Br J Ophthalmol 1984; 68:329–331.

80. Iida T, Spaide RF, Negrao SG et al. Central serous chorioretinopathy after epidural corticosteroid injection. Am J Ophthalmol 2001; 132:423–425.

81. Cohen SM, Kokame GT, Gass JDM. Paraproteinemias associated with serous detachments of the retinal pigment epithelium and neurosensory retina. Retina 1996; 16:467–473.

82. Hassan L, Carvalho C, Yannuzzi LA et al. Central serous chorioretinopathy in a patient using methylenedioxymethamphetamine (MDMA) or ecstasy. Retina 2001; 21:559–561.

83. Googe JM, Brady SE, Argyle JC et al. Choroiditis in infantile periarteritis nodosa. Arch Ophthalmol 1985; 103:81–83.

84. Jampol LM, Lahav M, Albert DM et al. Ocular clinical findings and basement membrane changes in Goodpasture's syndrome. Am J Ophthalmol 1975; 79:452–463.

85. Kihyoun JL, Kalina RE, Klein ML. Choroidal involvement in systemic necrotizing vasculitis. Arch Ophthalmol 1987; 105:939–942.

86. Stropes LL, Luft FC. Hypertensive crisis with bilateral bullous retinal detachment. JAMA 1977; 238:1948–1949.

87. Venecia G, Jampol LM. The eye in accelerated hypertension. II. Localized serous detachments of the retina in patients. Arch Ophthalmol 1984; 102:68–73.

88. Gass JDM, Pautler SE. Toxemia of pregnancy pigment epitheliopathy masquerading as heredomacular dystrophy. Trans Am Ophthalmol Soc 1985; 83:114–130.

89. Gitter KA, Houser BP, Sarin LK et al. Toxemia of pregnancy: an angiographic interpretation of fundus changes. Arch Ophthalmol 1968; 80:449–454.

90. Menchini U, Lanzetta P, Virgili G et al. Retinal pigment epithelium tear following toxemia of pregnancy. Eur J Ophthalmol 1995; 5:139–141.

91. Cogan DG. Ocular involvement in disseminated intravascular coagulopathy. Arch Ophthalmol 1975;93:1–8.

92. Spraul CW, Lang CE, Lang GK. Central serous chorioretinopathy in systemic therapy with corticosteroids. Ophthalmology 1997; 94:392–396.

93. Spitznas M, Huke J. Number, shape, and topography of leakage points in acute type I central serous chorioretinopathy. Br J Ophthalmol 1993; 77:349–353.

94. Shimizu K, Tobari I. Central serous retinopathy dynamics of subretinal fluid. Mod Probl Ophthalmol 1971; 9:152–157.

95. Goldstein BG, Pavan PR. "Blow outs" in the retinal pigment epithelium. Br J Ophthalmol 1987; 71:676–681.

96. Spitznas M, Hogan MJ. Outer segments of photoreceptors and the retinal pigment epithelium: interrelationship in the human eye. Arch Ophthalmol 1970; 84:810–819.

97. Wessing A. Grundsaetzliches zum diagnostischen Fortschritt durch die Fluoreszenzangiographie. Berl Dtsch Ophthalmol Ges 1973; 73:566–568.

98. Wessing A, Meyer-Schwickerath G. Lichtchirurgische Behandlung und sonstige chirurgische Massnahmen. Berl Dtsch Ophthalmol Ges 1971; 73:585–593.

99. Levine R, Brucker AJ, Robinson F. Long-term follow-up of idiopathic central serous chorioretinopathy by fluorescein angiography. Ophthalmology 1989; 96:854–859.

100. Hayashi K, Hasegawa Y, Tokoro T. Indocyanine green angiography of central serous chorioretinopathy. Int Ophthalmol 1986; 9:37–41.

101. Piccolino FC, Borgia L. Central serous chorioretinopathy and indocyanine green angiography. Retina 1994; 14:231–242.

102. Giovannini A, Scasellati-Sforzolini B, D'Altobrando E. Choroidal findings in the course of idiopathic serous pigment epithelium detachment detected by indocyanine green videoangiography. Retina 1997; 17:286–293.

103. Spaide RF, Orlock D, Herrmann-Delemazure B et al. Wide-angle indocyanine green angiography. Retina 1998; 18:44–49.

104. Iida T, Kishi S, Hagimura N et al. Persistent and bilateral choroidal vascular abnormalities in central serous chorioretinopathy. Retina 1999; 19:508–512.

105. Iida T, Spaide RF, Haas A et al. Leopard-spot pattern of yellowish subretinal deposits in central serous chorioretinopathy. Arch Ophthalmol 2002; 120:37–42.

106. Huang D, Swanson EA, Lin CP et al. Optical coherence tomography. Science 1991; 254:1178–1181.

107. Hee MR, Puliafito CA, Wong C et al. Optical coherence tomography of central serous chorioretinopathy. Am J Ophthalmol 1995; 120: 65–74.

108. Iida T, Hagimura N, Sato T et al. Evaluation of central serous chorioretinopathy with optical coherence tomography. Am J Ophthalmol 2000; 129:16–20.

109. Ficker L, Vafadis G, While A et al. Long-term follow-up of a prospective trial of argon laser photocoagulation in the treatment of central serous retinopathy. Br J Ophthalmol 1988; 72:829–834.

110. Yannuzzi LA, Ciardella A, Spaide RF et al. The expanding spectrum of idiopathic polypoidal choroidal vasculopathy. Arch Ophthalmol 1997; 115:478–485.

111. Yannuzzi LA, Freund KB, Goldbaum M et al. Polypoidal choroidal vasculopathy masquerading as central serous chorioretinopathy. Ophthalmology 2000; 107:767–777.

112. Spaide RF, Yannuzzi LA, Slakter JS et al. Indocyanine green videoangiography of idiopathic polypoidal choroidal vasculopathy. Retina 1995; 15:100–110.

113. Watzke RC, Burton TC, Leaverton PA. Ruby laser photocoagulation therapy of central serous retinopathy. Trans Am Acad Ophthalmol Otolaryngol 1974; 78:205–211.

114. Wessing A. Changing concepts of central serous retinopathy and its treatment. Trans Am Acad Ophthalmol Otolaryngol 1973; 77:275–280.

115. L'Esperance FA. Argon and ruby laser photocoagulation of disciform macular disease. Trans Am Acad Ophthalmol Otolaryngol 1971; 75:609–628.

116. Yap EY, Robertson DM. The long-term outcome of central serous chorioretinopathy. Arch Ophthalmol 1996; 114:689–692.

117. Yannuzzi LA, Slakter JS, Kaufman SR et al. Laser treatment of diffuse retinal pigment epitheliopathy. Eur J Ophthalmol 1992; 2:103–114.

118. Brancato R, Scialdone A, Pece A et al. Eight-year follow-up of central serous chorioretinopathy with and without laser treatment. Graefes Arch Clin Exp Ophthalmol 1987; 225:166–168.

119. Castro-Correia J, Coutinho MF, Rosas V. Long-term follow-up of central serous chorioretinopathy in 150 patients. Doc Ophthalmol 1992; 81:379–386.

120. Yannuzzi LA, Slakter JS, Gross NE et al. Indocyanine green angiography-guided photodynamic therapy for treatment of chronic central serous chorioretinopathy. Retina 2003; 23:288–298.

121. Chan WM, Lam DS, Lai TY, et al. Treatment of choroidal neovascularization in central serous chorioretinopathy by photodynamic therapy with verteporfin. Am J Ophthalmol 2003; 136:836–845.

122. Cardillo Piccolino F, Eandi CM, Ventre L et al. Photodynamic therapy for chronic central serous chorioretinopathy. Retina 2003; 23:752–763.

123. Taban M, Boyer DS, Thomas EL et al. Chronic central serous chorioretinopathy: photodynamic therapy. Am J Ophthalmol 2004; 137:1073–1080.

124. Canakis C, Livir-Rallatos C, Panayiotis Z et al. Ocular photodynamic therapy for serous macular detachment in the diffuse retinal pigment epitheliopathy variant of idiopathic central serous chorioretinopathy. Am J Ophthalmol 2003; 136:750–752.

125. Faurschou S, Rosenberg T, Nielsen N. Central serous retinopathy and presenile disciform macular degeneration. Acta Ophthalmol 1977; 55:515–524.

126. Schatz H, Yannuzzi LA, Gitter KA. Subretinal neovascularization following argon laser photocoagulation treatment for central serous chorioretinopathy: complication or misdiagnosis? Trans Am Acad Ophthalmol Otolaryngol 1977; 83:893–906.

127. Ergun E, Tittl M, Stur M. Photodynamic therapy with verteporfin in subfoveal choroidal neovascularization secondary to central serous chorioretinopathy. Arch Ophthalmol 2004; 122: 37–41.

Chapter

64

Macular Dystrophies

August F. Deutman
Carel B. Hoyng
Janneke J.C. van Lith-Verhoeven

As recently as 1967 it was claimed that the many different clinical pictures described as hereditary macular dystrophies probably represent phenotypical manifestations of a fundamentally single dystrophic process and not a number of autonomous lesions.[1] Leber and particularly Behr stated long ago that all the numerous types of hereditary dystrophies of the central retina constitute a single clinical entity with more than one mode of inheritance.[2,3] This monistic view was espoused by many investigators. However, since then the literature clearly indicates the existence of several foveal dystrophies determined by different genes.[4,5]

Stargardt was the first to suggest an adequate and clear classification of the dystrophies of the retina and to separate progressive macular dystrophy with dementia from that without.[6] Furthermore, he distinguished different entities among the central tapetoretinal dystrophies. In his classic work *Genetics and Ophthalmology*, Waardenburg was critical of Behr's monistic view and pointed out that the field was still too imperfectly explored to permit a well-reasoned and workable classification.[7] He devised several classifications, indicating that there are many different dystrophies of the posterior pole of the eye. Waardenburg noted the peculiarity of a number of investigations, concluding on the one hand that the many macular dystrophies are homogenetically determined, while on the other hand accepting a polygenic theory in the classification of various corneal dystrophies. The anatomy and function of the human retina are determined by several hundreds of the 100 000 genes of the human genome. Until now several genes causing macular dystrophies have been located. The finding of the causative gene in some of these macular dystrophies suggests that the primary defect is located elsewhere than was supposed by the clinical investigations. For example, in butterfly dystrophy the clinical picture suggests that the pigment epithelium is the causative structure. However, in several families the *peripherin/RDS* gene, encoding for a rim protein of the photoreceptors, was found as the causative gene in this disease. For the general clinical ophthalmologist the morphological classification seems to be the most appropriate one in order to understand and predict the clinical course. Once all genes involved in macular dystrophies and its functions are known, a genetic classification might be more appealing.

However, the scarcity of knowledge about the histologic and ultrastructural changes involved does not make it easy to construct a morphologic classification. Nearly all eyes obtained for histologic study come from patients of advanced age. Consequently, these eyes show senile and often postmortem autolytic changes. Nevertheless, electrophysiologic examinations, photographic studies, and fluorescein angiographic examinations are helpful in determining what tissues seem to be primarily involved.

In this chapter the classification described is limited to dystrophies in which affection of the posterior pole of the eye plays a predominant role. In cases in which histologic data are not available, the classification is based on retinal function and photographic test results. The retinal function tests necessary for such a classification are visual acuity, color vision, dark adaptation, photopic and scotopic electroretinography (ERG), electrooculography (EOG), and visual fields. The photographic tests most helpful for this classification are fluorescein angiography and photography with monochromatic light and preferably with different types of films.[8]

Based on observations obtained through these modalities, the following tentative classification can be proposed:

1. Nerve fiber layer
   a. X-linked juvenile retinoschisis
2. Photoreceptors and retinal pigment epithelium (RPE)
   a. Cone (-rod) dystrophy
   b. Stargardt's disease (atrophic macular dystrophy with fundus flavimaculatus)
   c. Pericentral retinitis pigmentosa
   d. Progressive atrophic macular dystrophy
3. Retinal pigment epithelium
   a. Vitelliform dystrophy
   b. Fundus flavimaculatus
   c. Butterfly-shaped pigment dystrophy, or pattern dystrophy
   d. Reticular dystrophy
   e. Dominant cystoid macular dystrophy (DCMD)
   f. Familial grouped pigmentations
   g. Benign concentric annular macular dystrophy
   h. Dominant drusen
4. Bruch's membrane
   a. Pseudoinflammatory dystrophy
   b. Angioid streaks
   c. Age-related macular dystrophy
   d. Myopic macular degeneration

5. Choroid
   a. Central areolar choroidal dystrophy.

There are nevertheless still a few dystrophies that might be separate entities because they do not fit easily into the entities just mentioned. These include:

1. Polymorphic macular dystrophy with an autosomal dominant inheritance pattern as identified by Lefler et al.[9] Macular lesions vary from scattered drusen and pigment dispersion to confluent drusen and ultimately choroidal atrophy. ERG and EOG results are normal, as are those of dark adaptometry and color vision testing.
2. Dominant pigment epithelial dystrophy of Noble et al.[10] Myopia, nystagmus, and mild retinal pigment epithelial dystrophy develop with changes in the ERG results.
3. Fenestrated sheen macular dystrophy. In five patients from three generations, macular changes consisting of a yellowish refractile sheen and red fenestration within the sensory retina at the macula were reported. The prognosis for maintenance of good central vision is excellent.[11–13]

Degeneration is a pathologic anatomic concept covering certain conditions or processes that involve cell death. The underlying mechanisms are diverse, and no hereditary origin need be involved. Like Waardenburg, Blodi, Braley, and others, we prefer the designation *dystrophy* for hereditary disorders that lead to early and premature cell changes and cell death and for which no clearly demonstrable cause has been determined.[8,14,15] These affections become manifest at a certain age as a result of a genetically determined enzymatic and metabolic malfunction. Therefore, because this chapter deals with inherited disorders, the term *dystrophy* will be used when the macular degeneration appears to be caused directly by an inherited lack or deficiency of enzymes or other biochemical compounds. Furthermore, diffuse choroidoretinal disorders in which the macula may be involved are not discussed here. These include retinopathia pigmentosa (retinitis pigmentosa), diffuse choroidal dystrophy (choroideremia),

Leber's congenital amaurosis, and Goldmann–Favre disease. Nevertheless, it is worthwhile to mention here the tapetal reflex with inverse Mizuo phenomenon in carriers of X-linked retinopathia pigmentosa[16] and the cystoid macular changes in Goldmann–Favre disease. The phakomatoses, which have an autosomal dominant inheritance, may occasionally also give rise to macular changes.

Tortuosity of the small retinal vessels may cause hemorrhages in the macular area, and because this disease is inherited in an autosomal dominant fashion, the hemorrhages may mimic an apparently dominantly inherited macular dystrophy. The same accounts for crater-like holes in the optic disc, giving rise to a central serous detachment of the retina (Fig. 64-1). This condition has also been seen in pedigrees showing an autosomal dominant pattern of transmission.[17]

Macular colobomata (Fig. 64-2) may also be inherited in an autosomal dominant pattern; however, because there is no dystrophy involved, we do not discuss this entity.[5]

A type of foveal dysplasia was described as "progressive bifocal chorioretinal abiotrophy."[18] In these cases there is a connatal white atrophic focus at the site of the fovea. In the early years of life, an atrophic focus develops at a site nasal to the disc, and finally a progressive chorioretinal dystrophy occurs, without total loss of vision. The mode of transmission is dominant. Hypoplasia of the fovea is seen in a variety of hereditary anomalies, such as aniridia, achromatopsia, X-linked hemeralopia, ocular and general complete and incomplete albinism, and microphthalmia.

NERVE FIBER LAYER

X-linked juvenile retinoschisis

X-linked juvenile retinoschisis belongs to the still poorly defined group of vitreoretinal dystrophies. It was initially considered to be a relatively rare abnormality. However, recently it has become apparent that it is fairly common.[5] Although no evidence exists for genetic heterogeneity, there is wide phenotypic variation.[19]

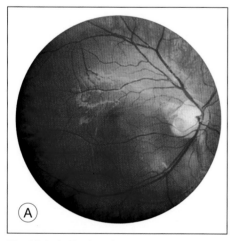 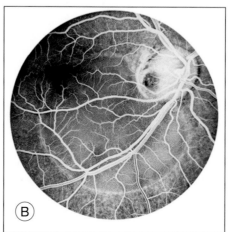 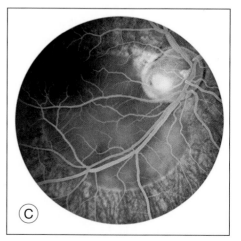

Fig. 64-1 A, Fundus of a patient with optic pit and central serous retinopathy. B and C, Note the leakage of fluorescein, which seems to originate in the optic pit.

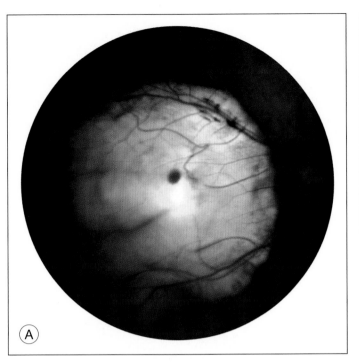 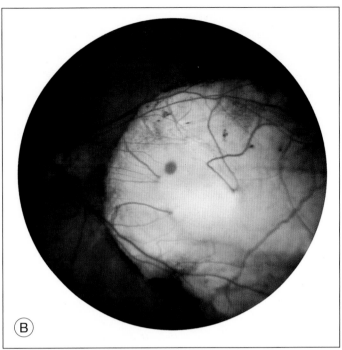

Fig. 64-2 Macular colobomata, also called macular dysplasia, in both eyes of an infant.

We have seen 100 patients with this condition. Because in many cases the only or most prominent abnormality consists of macular changes, the condition has often been diagnosed falsely as "juvenile macular degeneration," or Stargardt's disease. Since Haas's exact description, many articles, under a variety of titles, have been devoted to this subject: "congenital vascular veils in the vitreous" and "congenital cystic retinal detachment" are examples.[20] Owing to its X-linked inheritance pattern, this disease occurs virtually exclusively in males. Furthermore, because it is congenital, it will be seen first in boys.

Symptoms
The macular abnormality appears to have been present since birth in virtually all cases. The reasons why patients with this condition visit an ophthalmologist, are poor vision and sometimes vitreous hemorrhage, due to rupture of one of the vessels in the vitreous veils. Strabismus and nystagmus occur more frequently in this condition than in a control group.

Ophthalmoscopic features and evolution
Foveal retinoschisis is the characteristic sign of X-linked juvenile retinoschisis, and it appears to be present in all patients. In approximately 50% of patients the foveal retinoschisis is the only abnormality present on ophthalmoscopic examination. It consists of an optically empty zone delimited by two retinal layers, of which the more superficial one is very thin. This layer shows a typical radiate plication, formed by small folds in the internal limiting membrane and resulting from the presence of a cystoid structure in the foveal center (Fig. 64-3). Round microcysts are often seen in the perifoveal area (see Fig. 64-3). Narrow-beam ophthalmoscopic examination and red-free light

facilitate the identification of this peculiar pathognomonic structure.

Other ophthalmoscopic findings are silver-gray, glistening spotty areas, grayish white arborescent and dendritiform structures (Fig. 64-4), perivascular silver-gray cuffs, true retinoschisis in the retinal periphery, mostly in the lower temporal quadrant, veils in the vitreous, with or without retinal vessels enclosed, a pseudopapillitis picture, pigmentations and grayish white spots suggestive of scars of chorioretinitis, and posterior and also anterior vitreous detachment, with syneresis of the vitreous. True retinal detachment is rare. Nasal dragging of the retinal vessels has been described.[21] There is usually a slow progression of disease. Bilateral congenital retinal detachment has been seen in a few cases.[22,23]

Fluorescein angiography
In many cases the fluorescein angiographic picture of the macula is normal. In some cases there is evidence of pigment epithelial atrophy at the site of the macula[24] (see Fig. 64-3). In more severe cases there may be more or less diffuse or blotchy pigment epithelial atrophy and even choroidal atrophy in certain areas. Flow in the retinal vessels appears to be delayed in most cases. This implies a decreased flow in the retinal vasculature, which correlates very well with ERG findings. In some cases the fluorescein angiogram shows leakage of the retinal vessels.

Optical coherence tomography
Optical coherence tomography (OCT) can be a valuable diagnostic tool in the diagnosis of X-linked retinoschisis. OCT findings demonstrate a wide hyporeflective space with vertical palisades that split the neurosensory retina into a thin outer layer and a thicker inner retinal layer.[25]

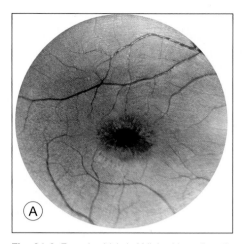
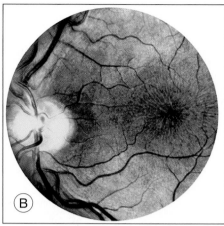
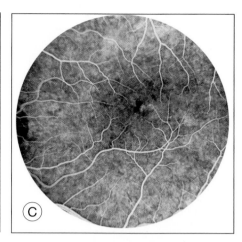

Fig. 64-3 Foveal schisis in X-linked juvenile retinoschisis. A and B, The pathognomonic macular abnormality of the condition. C, Fluorescein angiogram shows only mild pigment epithelial atrophy.

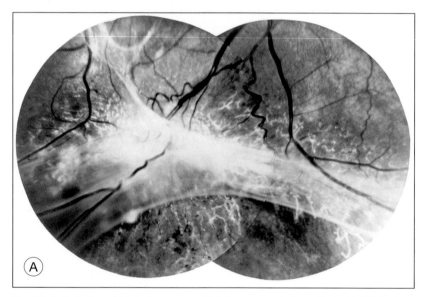
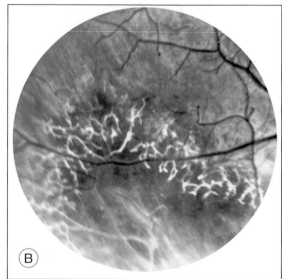

Fig. 64-4 A, Retinoschisis in the temporal inferior quadrant of a patient with X-linked juvenile retinoschisis. B, Note the denuding of the retina inferiorly and the dendritiform structures, probably caused by closure of capillaries.

Retinal function tests

Visual acuity   Visual acuity is often in the range of 0.2 to 0.4. However, vision may be 1.0 or 0.1 or even lower, depending on the stage of the process or the manifestation of the disorder. Refraction tends to be hyperopic and astigmatic in most cases, although emmetropia and slight myopia have been seen as well, although rarely.

Visual fields   Visual fields nearly always show a relative central scotoma. Reduction of the peripheral visual field is frequently encountered, primarily in the upper nasal quadrant of the visual field. The defects correspond largely to the ophthalmoscopically visible areas of retinoschisis.

Color vision   As in most other macular diseases, color vision is often affected.[26] An aberration is indicated by a mild, red-green dyschromatopsia with Hardy–Rand–Rittler pseudoisochro-matic plates and a wider-than-normal Rayleigh equation on the anomaloscope (i.e. more red than normally is required in this equation). The Farnsworth–Munsell 100-hue test shows mostly a tritan axis and not so many errors (fewer than 400) as, for example, in the cone dystrophies (generally more than 500).

Dark adaptation   Dark adaptation is normal or minimally affected. If affected, it is rarely decreased more than 1 log unit. Both the cone and rod portions are generally slightly subnormal.

Electroretinography   Invariably, the electroretinogram shows disturbed b-waves, but the a-waves are usually normal. Damage at the level of the bipolar cell layer is indicated. This type of ERG corresponds completely with the slow retinal circulation demonstrated on fluorescein angiogram. On the other hand, it may be due to the Müller's cell disturbance that has been seen in histologic specimens.[27,28] Dowling suggested that at least a considerable part of the b-wave arises from these Müller's cells.[29] Photopic and scotopic ERGs are approximately equally affected. In long-standing cases, often only ERG a-wave remnants are present, and, finally, the ERG virtually ceases to be recordable or cannot be recorded at all.

Electro-oculography   The electro-oculogram is normal in young patients or in patients with only macular involvement. In advanced cases, however, the EOG tends to become subnormal, and in extensively affected persons the EOG may be subnormal at a relatively young age. These findings indicate a normally functioning RPE in mild cases. Therefore pigment epithelial changes in this condition appear to be secondary rather than primary.

Histology and pathogenesis

Yanoff et al. were the first to conduct a histologic investigation of a well-documented case of X-linked juvenile retinoschisis.[28] Manschot also had occasion to examine the eyes of a 60-year-old man who had been a member of the family investigated by Jager.[27,30] Both examinations showed a splitting of the retina in the nerve fiber layer and not in deeper retinal layers, as is seen in senile retinoschisis. Yanoff et al. thought that the superficial retinoschisis is probably due to an inherited defect in the innermost portion of the cytoplasm of Müller cells, causing the internal limiting membrane and attached parts of Müller's cells to split away from the rest of the retina.[28] Manschot suggested that the inherited defect may also be located in the retinal nerve fibers, because he found severe atrophy of nerve fibers centrally as well as peripherally.[27] In our opinion, this nerve fiber and optic atrophy are probably secondary to defects in Müller's cells.

Condon et al. studied two eyes postmortem and one surgically enucleated eye from two related men with congenital hereditary retinoschisis.[31] Ultrastructural examination of this material showed numerous extracellular filaments, measuring approximately 11 nm in diameter. Similar filaments were found in the vitreous. These authors believe that the intraretinal filaments are produced by defective Müller cells and that their extracellular accumulation may lead to degeneration of these cells and subsequent schisis formation.

Mode of inheritance

The mode of inheritance is clearly X-linked and recessive; male patients transmit this pathologic gene to all their apparently normal daughters, whereas their sons are entirely normal. The daughters, indistinguishable from normal subjects, produce sons who are affected in 50% of the cases and daughters who, in 50% of cases, carry the gene like their mothers. It is regrettable that carriers cannot be detected with objective function tests. Lewis et al. described foveal retinoschisis in three daughters of normal (determined ophthalmoscopically) parents with a non-consanguineous marriage.[32] Autosomal recessive inheritance might therefore be possible in rare cases.[33]

Genetics

The gene for X-linked retinoschisis (*XLSRS1* gene) has been localized to the short arm of the X chromosome. Several muta-

tions in this gene have already been found in families with X-linked retinoschisis.[34] Because of the X-linked transmission retinoschisis seems to be caused by loss-of-function mutations only. Mutations occur nonrandomly: exons 4 to 6, encoding the discoidin domain, contain most, mainly missense mutations. A polyclonal antibody against a peptide from a unique region within retinoschisin was created.[35] Using in situ hybridization and immunohistochemistry, they showed that the gene is expressed only in the photoreceptor layer, but the protein product is present both in the photoreceptors and within the inner portions of the retina. So the expression is limited to photoreceptors but the protein must be secreted into the inner retina.

Differential diagnosis

The differential diagnosis encompasses an entity such as the autosomal recessive Goldmann–Favre disease, in which there is an extensive vitreoretinal dystrophy with bone corpuscle pigmentations and severe night blindness. The macula in this disease may show abnormalities that strikingly resemble those of the macula in X-linked retinoschisis. However, it is much coarser in the Goldmann–Favre type of dystrophy. Other diseases that might make differential diagnosis necessary are the other types of macular dystrophy described in this chapter, as well as idiopathic peripheral vasculopathy (Eales' disease), retinal periphlebitis, chorioretinitis, Wagner's vitreoretinal dystrophy, ablatio falciformis, inferior dialysis of the young, senile retinoschisis, autosomal juvenile retinoschisis, and sickle cell ocular disease. Choroidal folds (Fig. 64-5) and folds in the internal limiting membrane, due to vitreoretinal traction, give rise to an ophthalmoscopic picture that slightly resembles foveal retinoschisis; therefore they need to be differentiated. Fluorescein angiographic studies may be helpful in the diagnosis of these different nosologic entities and definitely in the differentiation from DCMD.

PHOTORECEPTORS AND RETINAL PIGMENT EPITHELIUM

Cone dystrophy

There are several known types of cone dysfunction, stationary as well as progressive. Goodman et al.[36] distinguished the following so-called cone dysfunction syndromes:

1. Congenital color vision defects without amblyopia: deuteranopia and protanopia – X-linked recessive transmission; tritanopia – probably autosomal dominant transmission.
2. Complete color blindness without amblyopia: cone monochromatism – mode of transmission remains to be established.
3. Congenital incomplete color blindness with subnormal visual acuity: incomplete achromatopsia – X-linked recessive and possibly also autosomal recessive transmission.
4. Congenital complete color blindness with subnormal visual acuity: complete achromatopsia with amblyopia; rod monochromatism – autosomal recessive transmission.
5. Progressive cone degenerations.

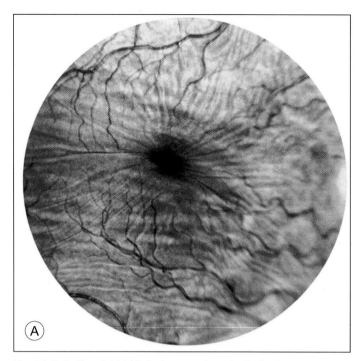 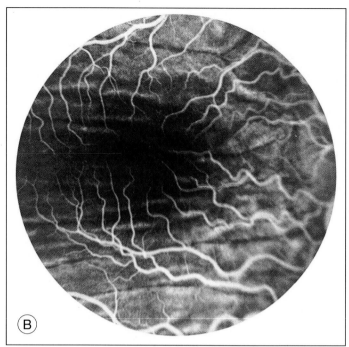

Fig. 64-5 A, Choroidal folds in the posterior pole. B, On fluorescein angiography the characteristic dark lines are visible.

6. Generalized cone–rod deficiencies in which symptoms relating to the cone dysfunctions predominate.
7. Generalized cone–rod deficiencies in which rod disorders predominate: retinitis pigmentosa is a good example of this category.

Herein, the inherited cone dysfunctions are dealt with exclusively. The noncongenital cone dysfunctions will be called *cone dystrophy* whenever they appear to be inherited, which usually is the case, or *cone degeneration* when the origin is obscure.

After a study of a large pedigree in Chicago, it became clear that it is not possible to differentiate sharply between progressive cone degeneration and "generalized cone–rod deficiencies in which symptoms relating to the cone dysfunction predominate," because both categories occurred in one and the same pedigree.[37] There is often a gradual transition from group 5 to group 6 during life. Depending on the genetic defect, there is pure cone dysfunction in several cases, while in some other cases additional rod dysfunction may develop. It also appeared that many pedigrees described so far as "dominantly inherited macular degeneration" are in reality nothing else than autosomal dominant cone dystrophies.[5,37]

All these pedigrees have been compiled, and cone dystrophy was established as a unique hereditary retinal disease.[37] Autosomal dominantly inherited cone dystrophies show great variability in severity and rate of progression from family to family and sometimes within the same family. However, there are enough similar features in the various pedigrees to conclude that this entity is unique.[37] Aside from the autosomal dominant cases, there are many sporadic cases of acquired cone dysfunction, as well as cases in which an autosomal recessive mode of inheritance is sug-gested.[38] In most cases, cone involvement appears to be diffuse; in some cases, however, there is evidence only of central cone involvement.[38,39] Pronounced acquired diffuse cone disease is evidenced by predominant involvement of the photopic ERG. Cone disease of the macula is shown by decreased visual acuity and very poor color discrimination.

Some reports have been devoted to the characteristic functional changes in cone degenerations.[39,40] Ophthalmoscopic changes, however, have hardly been mentioned. It appears that several characteristic fundus pictures are seen in combination with cone dystrophy. All the functional and ophthalmoscopic abnormalities of cone dystrophy have been compiled in a report by Krill et al.[38]

Symptoms

Visual loss is the predominant symptom, and photophobia is almost invariably present. Color vision problems arise early in this condition, in contrast to other macular diseases, in which they occur in later stages. Acquired nystagmus may be observed. Patients see better at dusk and prefer to wear dark glasses. Symptoms are exactly the reverse of those in retinopathia pigmentosa.

Ophthalmoscopic features and evolution

Visual loss typically precedes definite macular changes on ophthalmoscopic examination. As in Stargardt's disease, the fluorescein angiogram may reveal hyperfluorescence, indicating changes in the RPE in these early stages (Fig. 64-6).

Generally, four types of macular lesions are seen:

1. The most common type has a bull's-eye appearance and consists of a sharply defined, doughnut-like zone of atrophic pigment epithelium surrounding a central homogeneous darker

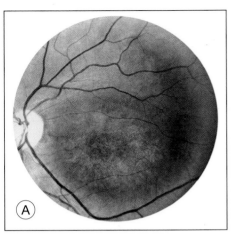
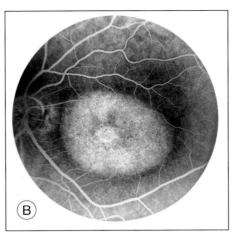
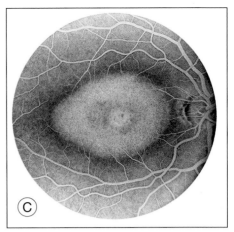

Fig. 64-6 Bull's-eye macula typical of cone dystrophy. In this case there is also an olivopontocerebellar atrophy.

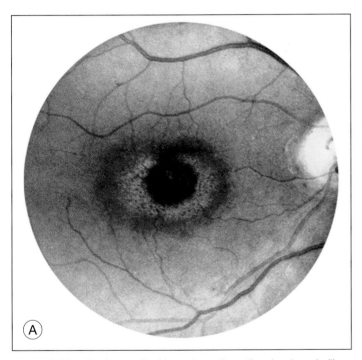
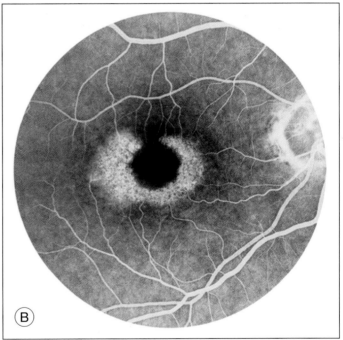

Fig. 64-7 Macular changes in chloroquine retinopathy, showing a bull's-eye macular pattern with perifoveal pigmentary atrophy.

area (see Fig. 64-6). This pattern is reminiscent of that seen in the macula of patients with chloroquine retinopathy (Fig. 64-7).

2. Pigment stippling and diffuse, round pigment clumps in the posterior pole is another, less frequent form of cone dystrophy. There is rather diffuse atrophy of the posterior pole in this variety, which is mostly seen in recessive pedigrees. Bone corpuscles may appear in the midperiphery, and they often appear as pigmented cuffs along the veins (Fig. 64-8).

3. Atrophy of the choriocapillaris and larger choroidal vessels is seen in a few patients at an early age. In general, though, it seems to occur rarely in this condition.

4. Ophthalmoscopic changes such as those seen in Stargardt's disease and fundus flavimaculatus are seen in a few patients. However, in contrast to the majority of patients with flavimaculatus, there are definite signs of acquired cone dysfunction. This category appears to be a specific one, which ophthalmoscopically links fundus flavimaculatus with atrophic macular dystrophy (Stargardt's disease), but functionally includes it in the cone dystrophy group.

In all groups, optic atrophy is a common finding. Initially, there is temporal pallor, but later the discs may become waxy, in a manner similar to that seen in retinitis pigmentosa. Also, vessels may become attenuated, and bone corpuscles and spider-like pigmentations may appear in the perimacular area and also in the midperiphery and far periphery of the retina (Fig. 64-9). A tapetal reflex was noted in some of our patients.

Fluorescein angiography

The type of ophthalmoscopic change determines what kind of fluorescein angiographic findings are observed, because cone

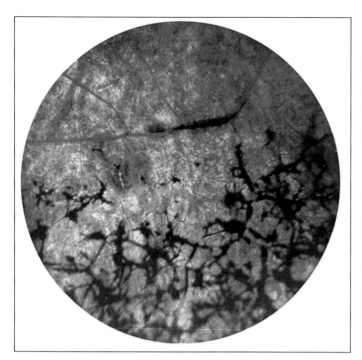

Fig. 64-8 Bone corpuscles in the fundus of a patient with an advanced form of cone (-rod) dystrophy.

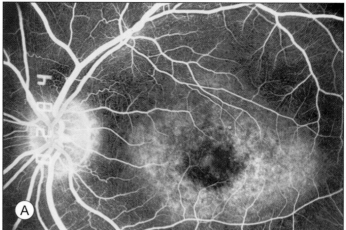

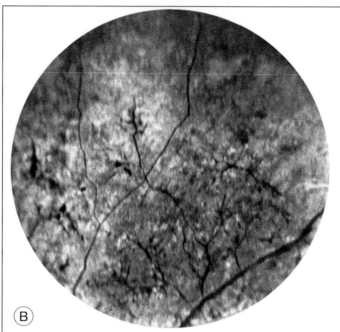

Fig. 64-9 Patient with cone dystrophy, showing perimacular pigment epithelial atrophy and peripheral pigmentary changes.

dystrophy is, at least ophthalmoscopically, a polymorphous condition. In group 1 (bull's-eye appearance), there is a horizontal ovoid zone of hyperfluorescence surrounding a nonfluorescent center (see Fig. 64-6). In the second group there is diffuse hyperfluorescence in a large part of the posterior pole. Often, there are sharp boundaries between the hyperfluorescent and the nonfluorescent areas (see Fig. 64-9). In the third group, fluorescein angiographic findings are like those in central choroidal atrophy. In the fourth group the picture resembles that of Stargardt's disease and fundus flavimaculatus. In late stages, with obvious cone–rod involvement, the fluorescence picture is similar to that in retinitis pigmentosa.

Retinal function tests

Visual acuity   Vision usually deteriorates gradually, but it can deteriorate rapidly to 0.1; later, in more severe cases, it drops to counting fingers. In advanced cases, acuity may go down as far as hand movements.

Visual fields   Generally, visual fields are normal, except for central scotomata. In cases with the typical bull's-eye appearance, there is often relative central sparing; in such cases a small central island is surrounded by a dense paracentral circular scotoma. In more severe cases, partial ring and large paracentral scotomata may be seen. These are usually cases in which rod dysfunction is also present. In late stages there may be some constriction of the fields.

Color vision   On the Hardy–Rand–Rittler (HRR) series, errors are made on both red-green and blue-yellow plates, with many errors also made on the Ishihara plates. There are almost always more than 500 errors, and often more than 600, on the Farnsworth–Munsell 100-hue test. Sometimes, the error distribution is along a deutan axis. This test appeared to be very sensitive in detecting cone abnormalities. Very wide or wider-than-normal equations are often found on the Nagel anomaloscope. These equations are often shifted toward the red end of the instrument. A typical feature in severe cases is the finding that red-green mixtures close to pure red may be very dim, whereas red-green mixtures close to green may be very bright.[37] We may conclude that there is severe color blindness, often resembling the features of congenital achromatopsia.

Dark adaptation   The cone portion of the dark adaptation curve usually shows abnormalities consisting of an elevated cone plateau, a cone plateau of shorter-than-normal duration, or a completely absent cone plateau, with a rapid fall to the final threshold. The final thresholds are usually either normal or only mildly elevated. A marked elevation similar to that seen in retinopathia pigmentosa is only rarely found in severe cases with extensive rod involvement.[37]

Electroretinography   The single-flash photopic ERG is generally very low or unrecordable, whereas photopic flicker ERG is either absent or gives minimal responses. Fusion frequencies are generally much lower than in normal persons (40 cps instead of 80 cps). The scotopic ERG is often normal in early or mild cases with involvement limited to the cones. Subnormal scotopic records are often found in more severe cases or in cases of longer standing. A completely extinguished photopic and scotopic ERG is found in the most severe cases, which are often long standing.[37]

Electro-oculography   In mild cases the EOG may be normal, but in more severe cases the EOG is definitely affected. Acquired fixation nystagmus may be first noted on the EOG record.[37]

Histology and pathogenesis
Histologic examinations are rarely made in cone dystrophy. In the pedigree described by Vail and Shoch,[41] the affected persons probably suffered from cone dystrophy. The eyes of one of these patients, a 78-year-old woman, were submitted for histologic examination, which showed that the outer nuclear layer of rods and cones had disappeared completely, whereas the RPE showed pronounced pigment changes. There was atrophy of the temporal disc.

In this condition the dystrophy appears to be primary. Distinct subjective and objective abnormalities of cone function are already found when ophthalmoscopic changes are still absent or very subtle. However, the RPE rapidly becomes involved, and then a tapetoretinal dystrophy occurs with predominant central changes.

The hypothesis of enzymatic or structural disorder in the cones themselves seems attractive. This may account for the early atrophy of the papillomacular nerve fibers and, consequently, for the early temporal pallor of the disc that usually is seen in this condition.

Mode of inheritance
The mode of inheritance is in many cases autosomal dominant. However, a number of cases appear to be sporadic, and instances of autosomal recessive heredity have been seen as well.[38] In several pedigrees a sex-linked inheritance pattern could be demonstrated.

Genetics
So far, adCOD has been found to be associated with mutations in the *guanylate cyclase activator 1A* (*GUCA1A*) gene on chromosome 6p21.1, and with as yet unidentified genes on chromosomes 6q25-26 and 17p13-p12.[42-45] The locus in one of the X-linked families was identified at chromosome Xq27[46] In three families with autosomal recessive cone dystrophy, mutations in the RPGR gene at chromosome Xp11.4 were found.[47]

Differential diagnosis
In addition to the other macular dystrophies, the hereditary optic atrophies must be taken into account in the differential diagnosis. Fluorescein angiography, ERG, and color vision tests are important methods of examination to facilitate diagnosis in early stages.

Stargardt's disease: atrophic macular dystrophy with flecks (fundus flavimaculatus)
Much confusion still exists about the use of the terms *juvenile macular degeneration* and *Stargardt's disease*. Many authors refer to any juvenile macular dystrophy as Stargardt's disease. However, distinctly different types of macular dystrophy have been shown to exist among the so-called juvenile macular degenerations.[4,5] X-linked juvenile retinoschisis, cone dystrophy, and vitelliform dystrophy, together with atrophic macular dystrophy with flecks (Stargardt's disease), are by far the most common entities in the group of juvenile macular dystrophies.[4,48,49] If the term *Stargardt's disease* is to be used correctly, it should be reserved for patients who show an atrophic macular area surrounded by some or many yellowish, ill-defined flecks. It was Stargardt who described this condition for the first time in a clear and comprehensive manner.[50] However, not all patients described by Stargardt had an atrophic macular dystrophy with flecks (later called *fundus flavimaculatus* with atrophic macular degeneration). Family S, for example, described in 1913, suffered from what we now know to be a cone (–rod) dystrophy.[51] The siblings mentioned in that report suffered from poor vision, poor color vision, photophobia, and day blindness. It now appears that the cases described by Stargardt do not all fall into the same category. Therefore the term *Stargardt's disease* can give rise to confusion.

Our reason for restricting the use of Stargardt's disease to atrophic macular dystrophy with flecks (fundus flavimaculatus with atrophic macular dystrophy)[49] is that the first and all of Stargardt's publications on this subject,[6,50,52,53] except his 1913 article,[6] dealt with this condition. The disease "fundus flavimaculatus with atrophic macular degeneration"[54] appears to be nothing other than what had been described earlier by Stargardt and many others.[55,56] It is still open to discussion whether it is correct to use the term *Stargardt's disease* for atrophic macular dystrophy without flecks and without obvious cone dysfunction (which differentiates it from the diagnosis of cone dystrophy). In such a condition, flecks may develop later. This section on Stargardt's disease will deal with atrophic macular dystrophy with flecks (fundus flavimaculatus with atrophic macular dystrophy). However, it is clear that it would be equally appropriate to discuss this topic in the section on fundus flavimaculatus. Meanwhile Stargardt's disease, as well as fundus flavimaculatus, seem to be caused by the same gene (*ABCR* gene) on the short arm of chromosome 1. This, however, does not mean that these diseases are necessarily one entity. For example, some types of cone–rod dystrophy and retinitis pigmentosa are also caused by mutations in the ABCR gene.[19,57,58]

Symptoms
The patients usually report between the ages of 6 and 20 years with bilateral gradual diminution of vision, but stating that visual

acuity had previously been entirely normal. The ophthalmologist often cannot find distinct foveal changes in initial cases, and patients are suspected of being neurasthenic or hysterical. The bilateral symmetric diminution of visual acuity, however, should alarm the physician. Often, several children in the same family are affected, and consanguinity of the parents is not infrequently found.

Ophthalmoscopic features and evolution

In the initial stage there are either no ophthalmoscopic changes or virtually none. Fluorescein angiographic examination may be helpful in showing a pigment epithelial defect centrally, often surrounded by a horizontally ovoid zone of faint hyperfluorescent flecks (Fig. 64-10). Disc, vessels, midperiphery, and periphery are normal at this stage. The first ophthalmoscopic sign is disappearance of the foveolar reflex. Changes in the pigment epithelium become visible in the form of grayish-yellowish spots. The fovea may show a granulated appearance and may give an impression of being covered by varnish or snail slime (Fig. 64-11). As in Stargardt's original cases, one frequently observes yellowish, ill-defined perifoveal flecks, which are localized beneath the vessels and are situated in the RPE (Fig. 64-12). Sometimes, a few of these perifoveal flecks may be the first signs present.

Finally, a horizontal oval of atrophic pigment epithelium appears, which usually measures 2.0 disc diameters in width and 1.5 disc diameters in height (Fig. 64-13). The appearance of this atrophic glistening area has been described as "beaten-bronze atrophy." A broad ring of flecks usually surrounds this area (see Fig. 64-13). As the beaten-bronze atrophic area extends, new flecks occur. They extend as far as the midperiphery but without arising in the periphery (Fig. 64-14). Discs and vessels generally remain normal. In long-standing cases the flecks may become less yellow, and pigmentations may occur in the form of black dots surrounded by whitish halos. The midperiphery eventually may have a pepper-and-salt appearance, and the central focus of atrophy may extend into the deeper layers of the posterior pole. Extensive atrophy of the choriocapillaris – and larger choroidal vessels – may be found in these long-standing cases. Rosehr[59] described two of Stargardt's patients 50 years after the original examination, and he found essentially normal discs, retinal peripheries, and vessels, whereas the posterior pole showed extensive choroidal atrophy, with blotchy pigment deposits.

Fluorescein angiography and photography

Fluorescein angiography in early cases shows a central ovoid zone of hyperfluorescence, mostly surrounded even in the early stages by some hyperfluorescent flecks (see Fig. 64-10). In these cases there is often "choroidal silence" because of an increased filtering action of the RPE. Retinal capillaries are then more clearly visible than normal.

As the disease progresses, more flecks appear, until the entire posterior pole may show a blotchy pattern of hyperfluorescence (see Fig. 64-13). Often no hyperfluorescence occurs at the site of the flecks, probably because the yellow acid mucopolysaccharide stored in the pigment epithelial cells, together with the still relatively intact cells, blocks the choroidal fluorescence. The hyperfluorescent flecks may ultimately show confluence because of widespread retinal pigment epithelial atrophy. Leakage of fluorescein never occurs. In late stages, central choroidal atrophy is visible (Fig. 64-15).

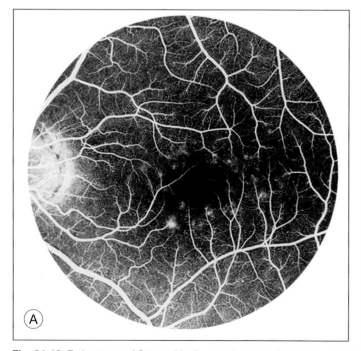

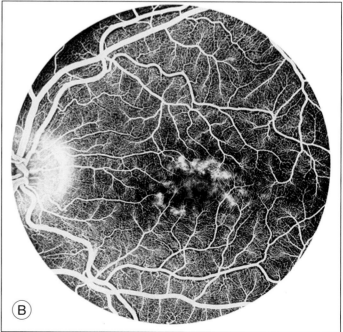

Fig. 64-10 Early stages of Stargardt's disease shown on fluorescein angiography. Note "choroidal silence" and striking visibility of the retinal capillaries. Some hyperfluorescent spots indicate pigment epithelial atrophy.

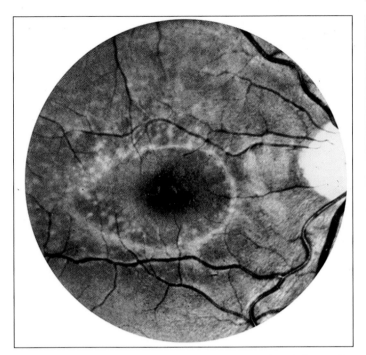

Fig. 64-11 Characteristic macular appearance in relatively early Stargardt's disease.

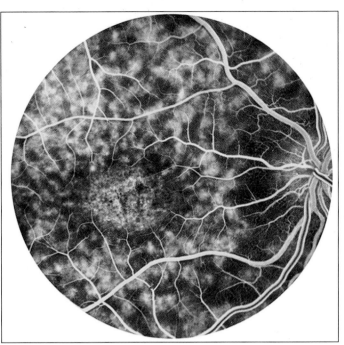

Fig. 64-13 Advanced stage of Stargardt's disease (atrophic macular dystrophy with fundus flavimaculatus). There is a central area of beaten-bronze atrophy surrounded by many yellowish flecks, showing defective retinal pigment epithelium on fluorescein angiography.

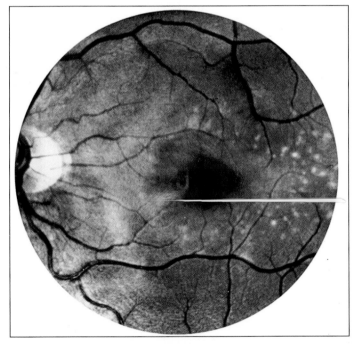

Fig. 64-12 Snail-slime appearance of the macula with yellowish flecks temporal to the fovea. Typical appearance of early Stargardt's disease.

Retinal function tests

Visual acuity   Visual acuity gradually decreases to 0.1. Generally, the diminution is symmetric. In some patients, however, we found a striking asymmetry in acuity (0.1 and 0.9) even though the ophthalmoscopic pattern in both eyes did not show clear differences. In cases of longer standing, acuity may decrease to counting fingers.

Visual fields   Generally the visual fields retain the normal peripheral boundaries, whereas the midperipheral areas have normal or slightly diminished sensitivity. At first, relative central scotomata are found; later, absolute central scotomata are found.

Color vision   As in most other macular diseases, color vision is affected. The HRR test shows a mild red-green dyschromatopsia. The Nagel anomaloscope shows a wider-than-normal Rayleigh equation, requiring more red than normal.[5,49,50] The Farnsworth 100-hue test shows mostly a tritan axis and generally fewer than 400 errors. In later stages there may be an acquired achromatopsia. Functionally, therefore, Stargardt's disease may ultimately be a *central cone dystrophy* in which the photopic ERG is still normal, which distinguishes it from a genuine diffuse cone dystrophy.

If severely defective color vision is found early, as in congenital achromatopsia, we make the diagnosis of cone dystrophy.[38] This diagnosis was made in a few patients with atrophic macular dystrophy with flecks and with functional abnormalities typical of cone dystrophy.

Dark adaptation   Dark adaptation is normal or slightly delayed. Gross abnormalities have never been found.

Electroretinography   Generally, the implicit time and amplitudes of the photopic and scotopic ERG are normal. However, a slight delay in attaining the otherwise normal maximum b-wave is not infrequently seen. In cases of longer standing, however, in which pigmentations are often seen in the midperiphery, the ERG amplitudes may decrease.[5] Unrecordable ERGs, as in retinopathia pigmentosa, have never been seen.

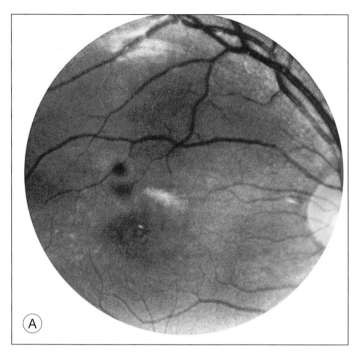

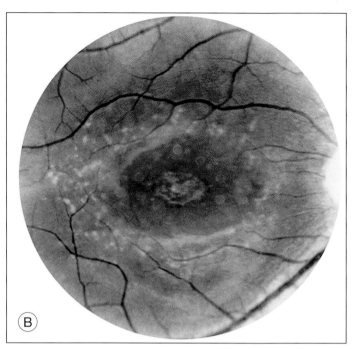

Fig. 64-14 Follow-up of Stargardt's disease over a period of 6 years, showing an increase in the number of flecks.

Electro-oculography   The EOG tends to be subnormal in most patients. This indicates a diffuse disturbance of the function of the RPE.[5]

Histology and pathogenesis

Histologic studies are scarce. Blodi summarized the histologic findings reported as follows[14]:

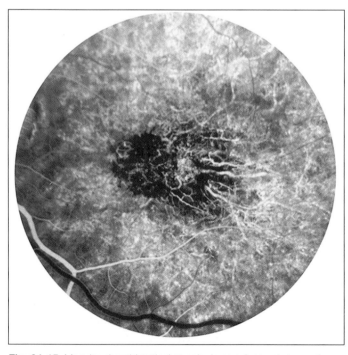

Fig. 64-15 Macular choroidoretinal atrophy in an advanced stage of Stargardt's disease.

The hallmark is a complete disappearance of the visual elements in the macular area. The macular cones are gone and so are the cones and rods in the perimacular area. The pigment epithelium has also disappeared in this area and only a few degenerated nuclei are visible between Bruch's membrane and the external limiting membrane.

Klien and Krill[60] presented an extensive histologic study of a patient who showed flecks such as those seen in Stargardt's disease. There was an accumulation of a pathologic substance in circumscribed areas, largely within the inner half of the pigment epithelial cells. Neuroepithelium, Bruch's membrane, and choroid were normal. The pathologic substance in the apex of the pigment epithelial cells was identified as an acid mucopolysaccharide.

This condition appears to start centrally in the photoreceptors, because severely affected acuity is often seen in patients in whom the ophthalmoscopic findings are almost normal. The involvement in the paramacular and perimacular areas, however, appears to arise mainly in the pigment epithelium. This is supported by the histologic studies of Klien and Krill[60] and by the subnormal EOG findings. The differences between the macular and perimacular changes are difficult to understand. A primary dystrophy of the RPE remains an attractive hypothesis, although the macular part of this condition appears to start in or close to the photoreceptors. A more recent histopathologic study suggests that the defects in the photoreceptors are secondary to a retinal pigment epithelial abnormality.[61] Re-examination of an (autopsy) eye of an infant of 16 months, who had developed Stargardt's disease at the age of 9 months, revealed increased autofluorescence, increased reactivity to periodic acid–Schiff staining, and a displacement of melanin granules toward the apex of retinal epithelial cells.[62]

Mode of inheritance

The mode of inheritance is mostly autosomal recessive. A few pedigrees with atrophic macular dystrophy and flecks suggest autosomal dominant inheritance.[63-65] However, Stargardt's original patients, and nearly all other patients, show autosomal recessive inheritance. Often, several siblings are affected, and the parents are frequently consanguineous.

Genetics

In recessive Stargardt's disease the affected gene is the ATP-binding transporter gene (*ABCA4 gene*) located on the short arm of chromosome one.[57] Different kinds of mutations in this gene may lead to different phenotypes of Stargardt's disease, fundus flavimaculatus, or even cone–rod dystrophy and retinitis pigmentosa. Heterozygous mutations in the *ABCR* gene also may play a role in the development of age-related macular degeneration.[57,58] The autosomal dominant pedigrees have been mapped to chromosomes 4p (STGD4) and 6q14 (STGD3).[66,67] At locus 6q14, the causative gene is the *elongation of very long chain fatty acids-4 gene* (*ELOVL4*).[68,69]

Differential diagnosis

The other disorders that are presented in this chapter must be considered in the differential diagnosis. Furthermore, incipient Spielmeyer–Vogt (Batten–Mayou) disease and hereditary optic nerve atrophy may present problems in differential diagnosis. It is important to remember that Spielmeyer–Vogt manifests a severely affected ERG and that optic nerve atrophies may have completely unrecordable visually evoked cortical responses in the presence of a normal ERG.

Pericentral (and central) retinitis pigmentosa

The term *pericentral retinitis pigmentosa* is used here in the sense of Duke-Elder[1]: "A dystrophy in which the pigmentary disturbances, either as spiderlike clumps or scattered black dots, take the form of an island round the macula." The picture lies between the true macular lesions and the classic equatorial lesions. A pigmented zone occurs immediately around the macula, and patients often may have good central vision.[5]

There is one diagnostic restriction, however. An observation indicated that in cone dystrophies pigment clumps often occur in the posterior pole of the eye and narrow vessels and waxy discs also may occur.[38] These cases often have been called *inverse* or *central retinitis pigmentosa* because of the fundus picture. Such cases, with obvious cone disease, have been discussed in the section on cone dystrophy. Other cases, with pericentral retinitis pigmentosa, show symptoms and signs that are more or less similar to those seen in classic retinitis pigmentosa. In some cases it may be difficult or even impossible to distinguish between pericentral retinitis pigmentosa and cone–rod dystrophies, and the diagnosis depends on the classification that is used. For example, the classification made by Szlyk et al.[70] is so broad that some cases of pericentral retinitis pigmentosa could well be fitted into some subtypes of this classification.

Symptoms

In the early stages, patients are asymptomatic. Night blindness is a common early complaint. Later, visual acuity may diminish considerably.

Ophthalmoscopic features and evolution

The first signs are bone corpuscles along the vessels in the perimacular region (Fig. 64-16). The macula itself does not show these spiderlike pigmentations. Choroidal atrophy is also frequently seen in these patients. Later, the pigmentations and atrophy may spread centrally as well as peripherally, and sometimes only a peripheral sector becomes involved. Vessels tend to become attenuated, and discs may become waxy and pale. Ultimately, blindness may ensue.

Fluorescein angiography

The pericentral parts of the fundus show atrophic pigment epithelium and black, spiderlike pigmentations in front of a fluorescent choroid. Hyperfluorescence is present, particularly pericentrally, and patches of choroidal atrophy are frequently seen. Sometimes, fluorescent abnormalities extend farther than the ophthalmoscopic eyeground changes. Extensive abnormalities of the retinal vasculature are generally found in cases of longer standing.

Retinal function tests

Visual acuity   Vision is initially normal. After a certain amount of time the macula may become affected, and vision may decrease considerably, even so far as to counting fingers.

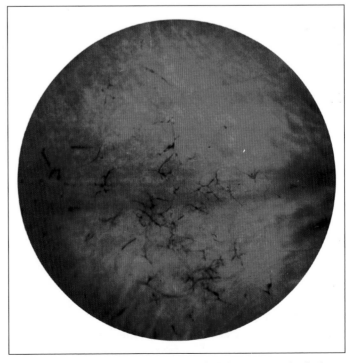

Fig. 64-16 Pericentral retinitis pigmentosa with bone corpuscles in the perifoveal area.

Visual fields   Visual fields are usually abnormal only in the area corresponding to the involved pericentral retinal sector. An absolute field defect is often seen in advanced stages, but in others it is relative and elicited only with smaller targets. Occasionally, field defects extend beyond the area of ophthalmoscopic involvement.

Color vision   Although initially normal, color vision diminishes when visual acuity decreases. Generally, color vision defects are comparable to those seen in other macular diseases. There is no predominant loss of color vision in this condition, as, for instance, in the cone dystrophies or in chloroquine retinopathy.[26,37]

Dark adaptation   Dark adaptation may be close to normal initially, when the fundus as a whole is tested. Perimetric dark adaptation data usually indicate a more widespread disease than ophthalmoscopy suggests. In advanced stages the extent of functional involvement on threshold evaluation is often much greater than predicted from ophthalmoscopic evaluation.

Electroretinography   The ERG almost always shows subnormal results, but with the scotopic ERG more affected than the photopic ERG. If the photopic ERG appears to be predominantly affected, the diagnosis is cone dystrophy, which usually shows rod involvement as well in advanced cases, as previously indicated. The degree of involvement varies considerably from one person to another, but usually the ERG is not so diminished or is not extinguished so early as in the classic type of retinitis pigmentosa.

Electro-oculography   The EOG mainly shows subnormal test results. Generally, it is affected soon and often more severely than the ERG. In mild cases the EOG may be close to normal or even normal.

Histology and pathogenesis

A primary dystrophic process at the site of the photoreceptors and pigment epithelium has to be accepted in this condition. There is no known reason why in most cases there are diffuse pathologic findings, whereas in others there is only localized (sector, pericentral) involvement. Histologic examinations will presumably reveal the same abnormalities as are seen in the classic type of retinitis pigmentosa. It has been demonstrated that the pigment epithelium of the dystrophic rat shows an inability to remove its rod outer segment material. Normal phagocytic removal of old outer segments was never seen.[71]

Mode of inheritance

Most data from the literature and from clinical experience point to an autosomal recessive mode of inheritance. It is not rare to see sporadic cases, and in such cases it becomes impossible to conclude anything definite about the inheritance pattern.

Differential diagnosis

Classic retinitis pigmentosa and sector retinitis pigmentosa closely resemble this condition.[72] The distribution of the lesions, however, is definitely different. Pigmented paravenous retinal degeneration is still a rather unclear entity and potentially is caused by an old inflammation. This condition may be reminiscent of sector retinitis pigmentosa in particular. Occasionally, in Stargardt's disease, gross pigment deposits may be present in the atrophic macular area. Scars of an old chorioretinitis and choroidal dystrophies occasionally may need differentiation, although generally there will be no problem in differential diagnosis. And as mentioned before, cone dystrophy may demonstrate spiderlike pigmentations all over the posterior pole. In such cases, retinal functional studies are of considerable value in providing a reliable diagnosis.

Progressive atrophic macular dystrophy

Apart from Stargardt's disease (atrophic macular dystrophy with flecks [fundus flavimaculatus]), X-linked juvenile retinoschisis, cone dystrophy, and vitelliform dystrophy, there is a small group of patients in whom an atrophic macular dystrophy occurs without flecks and without obvious cone dysfunction. In my (A.F.D.) thesis,[5] if there was evidence of autosomal recessive heredity, I presented these patients in the chapter on Stargardt's disease. Possibly, they deserve a specific place as "Stargardt without flecks." However, in patients who show atrophic macular dystrophy, flecks may develop later in life; in this event, the patients would undoubtedly fit into the Stargardt category.

The dominant cases were presented in the same report as dominant progressive dystrophy of the fovea.[5] We know that many of these so-called dominant macular degenerations are really cone dystrophies. However, there are a few pedigrees in the literature in which no definite cone dysfunction was present; I (A.F.D.) have examined a similar pedigree. These pedigrees, then, belong to this subdivision.

Symptoms

Loss of visual acuity is the only initial complaint.

Ophthalmoscopic features and evolution

An atrophic macular lesion develops gradually, and, in my experience, often starts in the second or third decade of life. Usually, this lesion is sharply defined and looks similar to the beaten-bronze atrophy seen in Stargardt's disease (Fig. 64-17). I (A.F.D.) have never witnessed an evolution beyond atrophy of the RPE. Discs, vessels, and retina outside the macula are normal. There are no flecks.

Fluorescein angiography

Fluorescein angiographic studies show a round or horizontal ovoid zone of hyperfluorescence, indicating atrophic pigment epithelium.

Retinal function tests

Visual acuity   Visual acuity drops gradually to 0.1 or even lower.

Visual fields   Visual fields are normal except for central scotomata.

Color vision   As in other macular diseases, color vision is affected, but by no means so severely as in cone dystrophy.

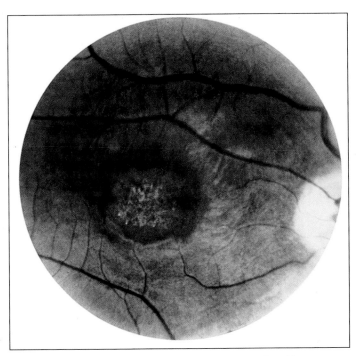

Fig. 64-17 Advanced case of atrophic macular dystrophy without any flecks.

Dark adaptation　　Dark adaptation is normal.

Electroretinography　　The ERG is normal. In contrast to cone dystrophy, photopic responses are normal.

Electro-oculography　　There are not many data available. In a few cases I (A.F.D.) examined, there were subnormal values. However, the EOG is usually normal.

Histology and pathogenesis

No histologic examinations are known to us. Atrophy of photoreceptors and retinal pigment epithelium at the macula is probable in such cases. A primary dystrophic process at the macula, probably due to enzyme defects, is a possibility. Retinal pigment epithelium and photoreceptors appear to be affected more or less simultaneously.

Mode of inheritance

Autosomal dominant pedigrees have been published. However, there are cases in which autosomal recessive heredity is likely. Sporadic cases have been seen as well.

Differential diagnosis

A large number of pathologic macular processes may at first glance mimic this dystrophy. Apart from the other dystrophies described here, choroidoretinal scars, vitreomacular traction, and solar retinopathy should be distinguished. In instances of unclear macular changes, optic atrophy is an important differential diagnosis. In such cases, fluorescein angiography and a combination of diffuse electroretinography and visual evoked responses (VERs) may definitely establish the diagnosis.

RETINAL PIGMENT EPITHELIUM

Vitelliform dystrophy

Vitelliform dystrophy of the fovea is a clearly separate entity among the inherited macular dystrophies. Many different terms have been used to describe this condition, which was first reported by Adams.[73] The first pedigree was presented by Best, and consequently the condition, until recently, was often called *Best's disease*.[74] The following designations have also been used: *vitelline dystrophy* and *vitelliruptive degeneration*,[75,76] Zanen and Rausin[77]

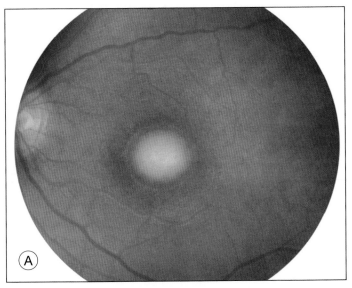

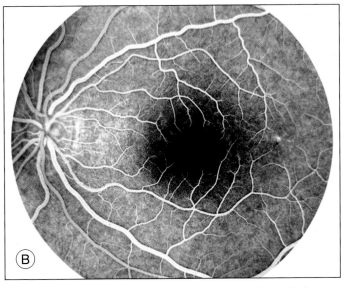

Fig. 64-18 Pathognomonic picture of vitelliform dystrophy (Best, A), showing hypofluorescence at the site of the intact macular disc (egg yolk-like lesion, B).

introduced the term *vitelliform*. Vitelliform dystrophy has been seen all over the world, and, in the relatively short time of 4 years, we have seen well over 100 cases in the Netherlands. Occasionally, Stargardt's name has been attached to cases of vitelliform dystrophy.[78] However, as far as we know, Stargardt, in contrast to Behr,[79] never described cases of vitelliform dystrophy.

Symptoms

The typical vitelliform structures usually are found during routine ophthalmoscopy. Visual acuity often is only minimally affected. However, severely diminished acuity may occur, particularly in older age groups. Sometimes, the decrease in vision is so rapid that an inflammatory process is suspected. Usually, however, gradual diminution in visual acuity occurs over a period of years. No symptoms, other than a decrease in visual acuity, are predominant. In one of our patients the rise of vitelliform discs occurred together with light flashes; in two other patients retinal detachment complicated the picture. Refraction is generally hyperopic and often is combined with astigmatism.

Ophthalmoscopic features and evolution

Vitelliform dystrophy is usually a bilateral abnormality, although unilateral changes frequently have been described, both in young people and in adults. The classic vitelliform structure is an egg-yellow, sometimes orange, round, slightly elevated structure surrounded by a somewhat darker border (Fig. 64-18). The retinal vessels take an undisturbed course past the edge of this macular disc, which may measure from 0.5 to 3.0 disc diameters. There is an unmistakable resemblance to the intact yolk of a fried egg or to a canned peach half. Very often this classic structure is not

seen at the time of examination, and sometimes it never occurs. One occasionally may see multiple vitelliform structures in the posterior pole[5,80] (Fig. 64-19). The ophthalmoscopic findings range from an exceedingly small, round, yellow dot at the fovea to a condition resembling the scar of a toxoplasmosis retinochoroiditis. The vitelliform stage is usually seen in patients between 3 and 15 years old. However, we observed typical vitelliform discs in both eyes of a 44-year-old man, whereas 1 year previously both maculae had been normal at ophthalmoscopic examination.

The evolution of vitelliform dystrophy can be summarized in a strictly schematic way as follows:

Normal fovea (but already pathologic EOG)
Previtelliform stage
Vitelliform stage
Scrambled-egg stage
Cyst stage
Pseudohypopyon stage
Round chorioretinal atrophy stage.

The previtelliform stage may show a small, round, yellowish dot at the site of the foveola or a tiny honeycomb structure centrally (Fig. 64-20). In the vitelliform stage the disc may disappear completely, leaving a macula that is ophthalmoscopically almost normal. This has been observed several times.[5] After this, a new disc may arise. Also, the yellowish material in the disc may disintegrate, leaving a scrambled-egg appearance (Fig. 64-21).

Sometimes the disc appears to rupture at a certain spot. This also results in a scrambled-egg appearance, which is often seen together with a decrease in visual acuity. The contents of the

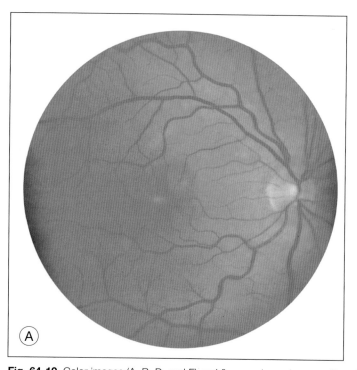

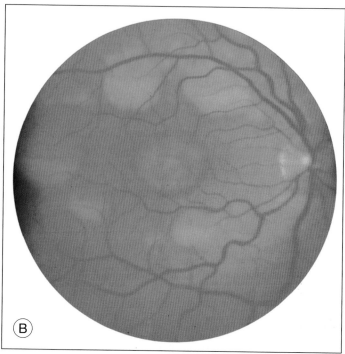

Fig. 64-19 Color images (A, B, D, and E) and fluorescein angiograms (C and F) of a patient who originally had one vitelliform lesion but gradually developed more lesions.

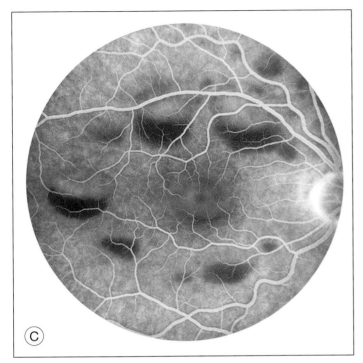

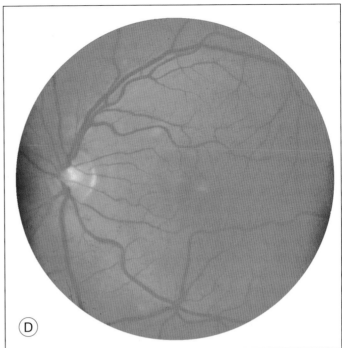

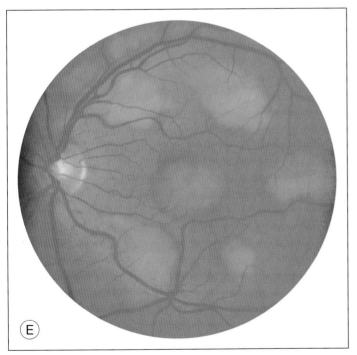

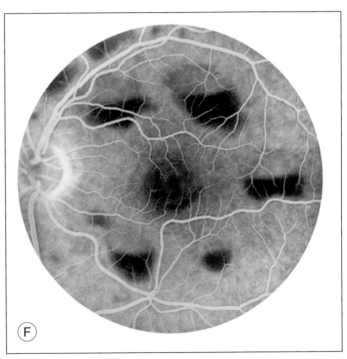

Fig. 64-19—cont'd

disc may disintegrate or become subject to syneresis, giving rise to a cyst with a fluid level. Because of the striking resemblance to a hypopyon, this stage is sometimes called a pseudohypopyon stage.

Subretinal neovascularization may occur, after which visual acuity drops considerably. Ultimately, round areas of chorioretinal atrophy are seen at the site of the macula, whereas other times marked pigmentations resulting from proliferation of pigment epithelium are observed.

Fluorescein angiography

The fluorescein angiogram shows hypofluorescence at the site of the macula in the intact disc stage. The yellowish material does not transmit the choroidal fluorescence (see Fig. 64-18). As soon as the disc disintegrates, areas of hyperfluorescence, indicating atrophic pigment epithelium, become visible, and ultimately one may see a hyperfluorescent circle at the macula. In cases of longer standing the choriocapillaris may disappear, and the larger choroidal vessels are rendered visible.

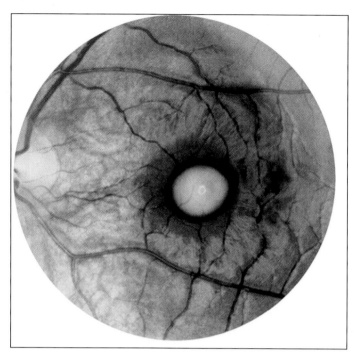

Fig. 64-20 Small, shining vitelliform lesion surrounded by wrinkling of the internal limiting membrane.

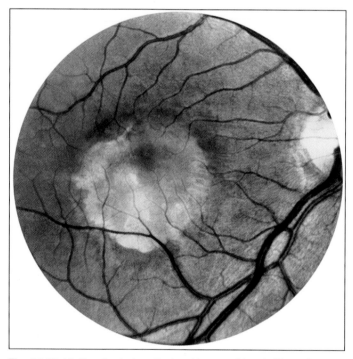

Fig. 64-21 Vitelliruptive lesion after breaking up of the vitelliform disc.

Retinal function tests

Visual acuity Vision is initially normal or only slightly subnormal, even in the presence of a fully developed vitelliform disc. In many patients, vision may be only slightly affected, even until old age. In quite a few patients, however (even in youth), visual acuity may diminish considerably, even as low as counting fingers.

Loss of vision is rarely symmetric, and it is virtually impossible to predict the acuity from ophthalmoscopic results. Hemorrhage in the vitelliform structure or rupture or disintegration of the disc may cause a sudden and considerable decrease in visual acuity. Quite often in these patients, this decrease appears to be reversible to some unpredictable extent.

Visual fields Visual fields are normal except for the central visual fields, which may be normal but often show some decrease in sensitivity. Scotomata occur, initially for red and later for green, followed by relative scotomata for white light. In serious cases an absolute central scotoma can occur.

Color vision As in most macular diseases, color vision is affected.[5,26] This means a mild red–green dyschromatopsia with the HRR test and a wider-than-normal Rayleigh equation on the anomaloscope, requiring more red than normal in this equation. The Farnsworth–Munsell 100-hue test mainly shows a tritan axis and not so many errors (fewer than 400) as, for instance, in the cone dystrophies (usually over 500 errors).

Dark adaptation Dark adaptation is generally completely normal.

Electroretinography The ERG is completely normal. Scotopic and photopic a- and b-waves have normal amplitudes and implicit times. The oscillatory potentials appear to be normal as well.[5]

Electro-oculography The EOG is almost always definitely subnormal in this condition and therefore is a very important diagnostic tool in the differential diagnosis. The EOG light–dark ratio is rarely higher than 1.5. Carriers, who are ophthalmoscopically normal, also have a definitely subnormal EOG.[80] Thus the EOG enables us to determine who is a carrier and who is not. Our understanding of this disease is much increased by this feature, which also may be of importance in genetic counseling.

Histology and pathogenesis

Histologic examinations have shown a predominant atrophy of the RPE. Andersen and Barkman[5] demonstrated a spotty thinning and degeneration of the RPE with few or no melanin granules in the macular area of a patient who died at the age of 59 years. The inner retinal layer, which was artificially detached from the pigment epithelium, showed a severe defect of the sensory cells, which were lacking in the same area as the degeneration of the RPE. Choriocapillaris and Bruch's membrane were fairly well preserved. McFarland[81] examined another eye with vitelliform dystrophy from an 87-year-old man (the histologic specimen was assessed by Klien). His finding agreed with those of the previous examiners. No histologic examination has been made so far in an eye with an intact vitelliform disc, and consequently no histochemical examination of the yellowish material has been carried out. The vitelliform disc is probably located in the superficial half of the cells of the pigment epithelium.[5]

Binocular slit-lamp examination of the fundus, fluorescein angiography, and photography with monochromatic light and with films with different absorption characteristics all favor a localization in the RPE.[5,76] Retinal function tests, such as visual acuity, ERG, and EOG, all indicate the primary disturbance to be located in or close to the pigment epithelium. Because histologic studies also show that the main changes occur at the site of the RPE, we may accept a primary disturbance of the pigment epithelial cells in this condition. An inborn error of metabolism or a membrane disturbance could be a possible mechanism of this pathologic condition. Many of the characteristics of fundus flavimaculatus are seen in vitelliform dystrophy. Fluorescein angiographic and retinal function patterns are almost identical in these conditions. Because fundus flavimaculatus lesions appeared to originate in the apex of the pigment epithelial cells, it is a fair proposition to accept a similar pathogenesis in vitelliform dystrophy.[60]

Weingeist et al.[82] reported an abnormal accumulation of lipofuscin granules. Lipopigment appeared to accumulate within the RPE, within macrophages in the subretinal space, and within the choroid. Frangieh et al.[83] found flattened retinal pigment epithelial cells, with displacement of the nuclei toward the apex and diffuse deposition of abnormal lipofuscin and pleomorphic melanolipofuscin granules.

Mode of inheritance

The mode of inheritance in vitelliform dystrophy is unquestionably that of an irregular autosomal dominant. The penetrance is diminished, and the expression is highly variable. In many pedigrees the ophthalmoscopic changes show a regular autosomal dominant pattern, and in almost all pedigrees a regular autosomal dominant inheritance pattern can be demonstrated for the EOG abnormalities.[80] Men and women appear to be equally affected, and roughly 50% of the children of affected persons or carriers are affected as well. Whenever one finds a "sporadic" case, one must perform EOGs in the parents or in other relatives. In many cases one of the parents and some of the ophthalmoscopically normal relatives will show a definitely subnormal EOG, thus indicating that they are carriers.[80]

Genetics

VMD maps to chromosome 11q13 and the causative gene is VMD2, encoding bestrophin.[84-88] This protein has been localized to the basolateral plasma-membrane of RPE cells and is important in the formation of oligomeric chloride channels.[89,90] Abnormal chloride conductance, caused by mutations in the VMD2 gene, might disturb the fluid transport across the RPE which could result in accumulation of debris between RPE and photoreceptors and between RPE and Bruch's membrane, and alter the EOGs of individuals with VMD.[90,91] Linkage of the disease locus to the same region of chromosome 11 has been significantly excluded in a German family, thereby providing evidence of locus heterogeneity in this clinically unique condition.[92]

Differential diagnosis

Some fundus pictures resemble vitelliform dystrophy closely. Instances of central serous choroidopathy, serous detachment of the RPE, toxoplasmotic retinochoroiditis, macular colobomata, solar retinopathy, and old foveal hemorrhages may occasionally require an exact differential diagnosis (Fig. 64-22).

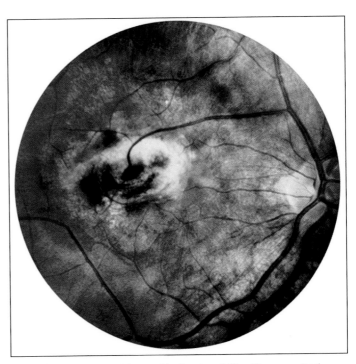

Fig. 64-22 Scar of toxoplasmosis retinochoroiditis with an acquired retinochoroidal anastomosis.

Juvenile disciform and senile disciform macular degeneration are generally easily differentiated on the basis of their subretinal choroidal neovascularization. In Europe we have occasionally seen the picture of juvenile disciform macular degeneration, but without a positive histoplasmin skin test. Other mechanisms probably give rise to multifocal choroiditis (presumed histoplasmotic choroiditis). (In Europe there frequently are no "histo spots" in the retinal midperiphery and periphery, whereas the peripapillary atrophy also is often absent.) Multiple vitelliform structures, particularly when they are small, may be reminiscent of some of the flecked retina diseases, such as dominant drusen or fundus flavimaculatus, or of some kind of systemic inflammatory process. In general, however, the clinical picture will be distinct enough to facilitate diagnosis. If necessary, an EOG can assist in making the diagnosis. In our opinion, the adult-onset foveomacular pigment epithelial dystrophy of Vine and Schatz[93] is a polymorphous type of Best's vitelliform dystrophy.

Fundus flavimaculatus

The term *fundus flavimaculatus* was introduced in ophthalmology by Franceschetti[54] to describe a fundus picture, noted by him since 1953, that was characterized by the presence of ill-defined, yellowish spots in the deeper retinal layers of the posterior pole of the eye. Previously this abnormality often had been diagnosed as chorioretinitis disseminata or retinitis punctata albescens, but unlike these two conditions the retinal abnormality had a stationary course and a fairly good prognosis.[54] Retinal function tests, such as dark adaptation, ERG, and EOG, appeared to show far fewer pathologic changes than in retinopathia pigmentosa.

Many patients previously described also had shown these flecks. Franceschetti and Francois[54] mentioned in this context publications on Stargardt's disease, drusen and retinitis punctata albescens by several other authors. From this it is clear that the entity fundus flavimaculatus was no newly discovered disease. The term merely grouped together all conditions showing fuzzy, yellowish flecks in the posterior pole of the eye. Great confusion has occurred because of this new nomenclature, primarily because Stargardt's disease in the strict sense is atrophic macular dystrophy with fundus flavimaculatus[6,50,52,53] or fundus flavimaculatus with macular dystrophy. In my (A.F.D.) thesis[5] I therefore classified as fundus flavimaculatus the forms with typical fundus flavimaculatus lesions only (but without macular involvement) or the forms with late involvement of the macula caused by invading flecks. Fundus flavimaculatus is still a rather heterogeneous category with many different appearances and occasionally with different retinal function patterns.

It may be disturbing not to group Stargardt's disease and fundus flavimaculatus together in the classification presented, because in many cases these terms are interchangeable. Because the term *Stargardt's disease* has found a place in the literature for more than 50 years, using this designation is justifiable. However, it is important to clarify the meaning of this term adequately whenever it is used. There can be no objection if Stargardt's disease is classified as one of the various types of fundus flavimaculatus.

Grossly, we can differentiate the following categories on an ophthalmoscopic basis:

- Pure fundus flavimaculatus: no, or late, macular involvement and occurring mainly in adults.
- Atrophic macular dystrophy with fundus flavimaculatus (Stargardt's disease): occurring mainly in juveniles.

Usually, fundus flavimaculatus has a very distinct retinal functional pattern, characterized by a subnormal EOG together with a normal or near-normal ERG and dark adaptation.[60] However, some patients with these flecks show a severe cone dysfunction. Furthermore, it is confusing that patients with a cone dystrophy may sometimes have a few tiny yellowish flecks in the perifoveal area. We have also noted the presence of typical fundus flavimaculatus flecks in patients with an otherwise classic retinopathia pigmentosa. Thus typical fundus flavimaculatus and fundus flavimaculatus with predominant cone involvement can be distinguished best by functional tests.

Although fundus flavimaculatus is nearly always inherited in an autosomal recessive pattern, some pedigrees have been seen with dominant transmission.[89] Some of these dominant cases may show a progressive deterioration of peripheral retinal function, as well as an atrophic macular degeneration.

These examples indicate that it is very difficult to delineate sharply the entity of fundus flavimaculatus.

Symptoms

Fundus flavimaculatus may be found at a very early age in combination with atrophic macular dystrophy. In our experience, the types without macular dystrophy occur mainly in adulthood. Normal visual acuity is present in these patients if the fovea is not invaded by flecks. If there is foveal involvement, visual acuity may decrease rapidly to counting fingers. This is generally the symptom that brings the patient to the ophthalmologist.

Ophthalmoscopic features and evolution

The posterior poles of both eyes show a virtually symmetric fundus picture consisting of yellowish spots below the level of the retinal vessels. They are often ill-defined and shaped like a crescent, shark fin, fishtail, or fish; linear and circular forms may also be present (Fig. 64-23). Often there is confluence of these flecks, which are never seen peripheral to the equator but are always central to it. The flecks frequently form garlands surrounding the foveal area. Old flecks may disappear, and new ones may arise. In advanced cases the flecks become less conspicuous; pigmentations occur, particularly close to the equator, and often there are pigment dots surrounded by lighter halo-like areas. Often, the flecks are arranged in a reticular pattern, as is seen in reticular dystrophy of the RPE.

There may be an atrophic macular lesion of beaten-bronze atrophy, such as that described by Stargardt.[50] In that event the condition may be called Stargardt's disease. In these cases it is striking to note the great differences between the affection of the macular and nonmacular areas. Sometimes, the macula is completely normal; later, flecks may invade the macular area, eventually also giving rise to an atrophic appearance (Fig. 64-24). Ultimately, the central retinal area may show severe choroidoretinal atrophy and coarse pigmentations. However, discs, vessels, and the far periphery always remain normal.

Fluorescein angiography

More defects are visible in the pigment epithelium with fluorescein angiographic examination than with normal ophthalmoscopic methods, and many spots prove to be confluent. Flecks of recent origin do not show hyperfluorescence, probably because the pigment epithelial cells are still intact and contain a yellowish

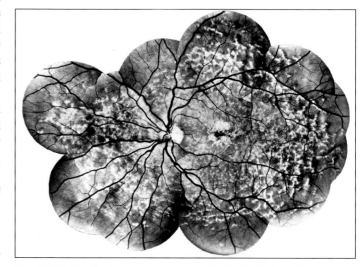

Fig. 64-23 Fundus flavimaculatus in a patient in his forties with late macular involvement.

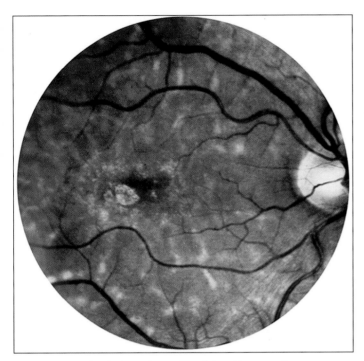

Fig. 64-24 Fundus flavimaculatus with mild and late macular involvement.

a deutan axis. Then, the Nagel anomaloscope often shows wide equations, frequently shifted toward the red end of the instrument. Typical findings in these patients are that red-green mixtures close to pure red appear to be very dim, whereas red-green mixtures close to green appear to be bright.

Dark adaptation Adaptation to dark is mostly normal or only slightly disturbed. A delayed dark adaptation with ultimately normal cone and rod thresholds is often found.[5,60]

Electroretinography The ERG is normal or only slightly subnormal in most cases. A slight delay in attaining an otherwise normal maximum b-wave amplitude is typical for this condition.[60] In this respect, fundus flavimaculatus clearly differs from the diffuse tapetoretinal dystrophies, in which the ERG is often unrecordable. In certain patients with a cone dysfunction syndrome, the photopic ERG appears to be severely affected, whereas the scotopic ERG is normal or only slightly affected.

Electro-oculography The light-peak-dark-trough ratio is subnormal in virtually all patients. Of all retinal function tests, the EOG is the test that is affected most consistently,[5,60] indicating a widespread functional disturbance of the RPE. This view is strengthened to a substantial degree by the histologic studies of Klien and Krill,[60] which showed that the flecks are found exclusively in the RPE.

Histology and pathogenesis

Only one histologic study has been conducted so far in a patient with fundus flavimaculatus.[60] A pathologic substance appeared to accumulate in circumscribed areas, largely within the inner half of the cells of the pigment epithelium. The substance was identified as an acid mucopolysaccharide. Recent flecks proved to be contained in still fully intact pigment epithelial cells. Unlike drusen, in which the base of the cell is predominantly involved, fundus flavimaculatus involves the apex. Electron microscopic studies of the same eye were disappointing because of marked autolytic changes that did not make a detailed analysis rewarding.[94] Condensation of melanin granules, variation in size of the cells, and displacement of the nucleus involved were the most important findings. The pathogenesis appears to be a primary fault in the metabolism of the RPE, which gives rise to the accumulation of the acid mucopolysaccharide. This appears to be mainly hyaluronic acid in the cells of the RPE.[94]

It is difficult to understand why the atrophic macular lesion seen in the Stargardt type of fundus flavimaculatus shows such a completely different appearance when compared with the perimacular flecked areas.

substance at the surface.[60] On the other hand, areas that show no flecks may show hyperfluorescence, resulting from pigment epithelial atrophy. No leakage of fluorescein is seen.

Retinal function tests

Visual acuity Visual acuity may be normal in patients with pure fundus flavimaculatus with macular involvement. When the macula is affected, as in Stargardt's disease, vision decreases gradually to 0.1 or to counting fingers. If flecks invade the otherwise normal macula, visual acuity may be anywhere from 1.0 to 0.1. As in all retinal diseases, and particularly in this disease, visual acuity depends on the variable amount of macular involvement.

Visual fields Fields are generally normal. If the macula is involved, relative or even absolute central scotomata may occur.

Color vision Color vision often is affected, as in any other macular disease. This means mild red-green dyschromatopsia with the HRR test and a wider-than-normal Rayleigh equation on the anomaloscope, requiring more red than normal in this equation. The Farnsworth–Munsell 100-hue test shows mostly a tritan axis and not very many errors (fewer than 400). Occasionally, there may be an acquired achromatopsia. There appears to be a separate group of patients with fundus flavimaculatus who show predominant cone involvement in functional examinations.[38] In these patients the HRR test shows rather severe errors on both red-green and blue-yellow plates, while the Farnsworth–Munsell 100-hue test demonstrates many errors (over 500 or even 600), with the error distribution often along

Mode of inheritance

The mode of inheritance appears to be autosomal recessive in far more than 90% of patients. In those showing autosomal dominant inheritance,[37] the disorder seemed to have a more severe and more polymorphous appearance than in the autosomal recessive type. Sporadic cases are often seen; here, the mode of transmission cannot be determined.

Genetics

In several cases the ABCA4 gene, located on the short arm of chromosome 1, seems to be the affected gene.[95] Other retinal dystrophies, like cone–rod dystrophy and retinitis pigmentosa, are also caused by mutations in this gene.[58]

Differential diagnosis

Differential diagnosis has to be made with other conditions showing a flecked retina, such as drusen, fundus albipunctatus, multiple vitelliform lesions, and neck retina of Kandori.[5] If there is an atrophic beaten-bronze macula that is uninvolved by flecks, the terms *Stargardt's disease* and *atrophic macular dystrophy with fundus flavimaculatus* are interchangeable. The peau d'orange appearance of the fundus in pseudoxanthoma elasticum is also different from fundus flavimaculatus (see Fig. 64-36). Once in a while, yellowish-whitish flecks are seen in disseminated choroiditis and in retinopathia pigmentosa. In general, however, the differential diagnosis will not present many difficulties, although there will always remain sporadic cases that are difficult or impossible to classify.

Patterned pigment dystrophy of the fovea

In 1970, four brothers and the son of one of them were found to have black, pigmented, butterfly-shaped structures in their maculae.[96] Before 1970, another instance of a dystrophy showing even a slight resemblance to this condition has not appeared in the literature.

Symptoms

Patients may have a decrease in visual acuity. Metamorphopsia also may be present. However, it appears that most cases will be found in the course of routine ophthalmoscopic examination in patients with no obvious complaints, because normal acuity has been seen in the presence of these structures.

Ophthalmoscopic features and evolution

A virtually symmetric, bilateral pigmentation, which may be polymorphous but in most cases is butterfly shaped, is seen in the deeper layers of the central retina (Fig. 64-25). Binocular slit-lamp examination reveals that the pigmented deposits are localized in or near the RPE. The retinal vessels continue their course undisturbed across the pigment butterfly. The pigmentations seem to consist of closely packed pigment granules that have migrated from the perifoveal area to the center.

At examination with red-free light, the pigmentation is less clearly visible, indicating localization deep in the retina. The superficial retinal layers are normal, as are the foveolar and foveal reflexes. Discs and retinal vessels are also normal, and the choroid, too, appears to be normal. In two of the five patients originally evaluated, there were unmistakable peripheral changes in the form of small bone corpuscles, and there were also drusen-like structures.

The course of this condition is very slowly progressive. The oldest of the patients still had normal visual acuity at age 43 years. The pigment deposits barely tend to involve the layers anterior and posterior to the pigment epithelium.

In some families, patients may have lesions that are suggestive of Best's vitelliform macular dystrophy. In those rare pedigrees it may be difficult to make a sharp distinction between pattern and vitelliform dystrophy.[97,98]

Fluorescein angiography

The black, pigmented, butterfly-shaped structures stand out, clearly outlined by the choroidal fluorescence, as if held in front of a light box (Fig. 64-26). Some hyperfluorescence usually surrounds the pigmented structure, which of course shows no fluorescence at all. These findings are indicative of localization of the pigmented, butterfly-shaped structures in the pigment epithelium.

Retinal function tests

Visual acuity   Visual acuity is virtually normal or only very slightly diminished. The lowest vision recorded so far is 0.8. More serious loss of acuity, however, might occur in old age.

Visual fields   Except for a slightly diminished central sensitivity, visual fields are normal.

Color vision   Color vision is normal. It may be only minimally affected, as in most other mild macular degenerations. We found essentially normal color vision in our patients who had virtually normal visual acuity.

Dark adaptation   Dark adaptation is normal.

Electroretinography   The ERG shows normal findings. Photopic and scotopic ERG a- and b-waves, as well as the oscillatory potentials, are all within normal limits. Also, the local foveal ERG appeared to be normal in one of our patients.[5]

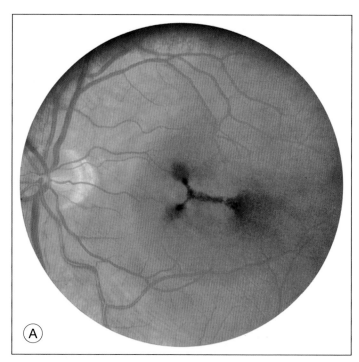

Fig. 64-25 A, Color image of a butterfly-shaped pigment dystrophy of the macula.

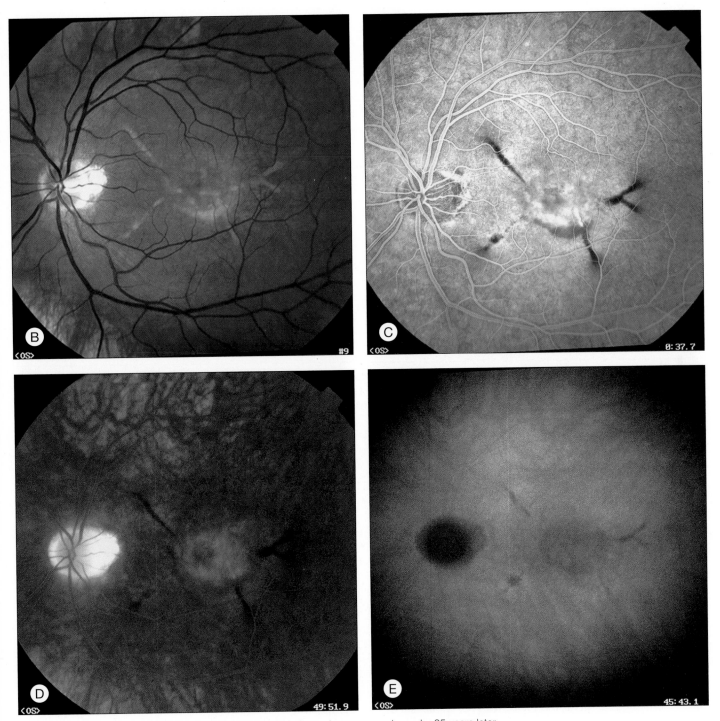

Fig. 64-25—cont'd B to E, Fluorescein angiography and indocyanine green angiography 25 years later.

Electro-oculography EOGs showed markedly subnormal results in four of the five patients originally tested. A patient seen at the University of Chicago also had a definitely subnormal EOG light-rise-dark-trough ratio. Some of the EOGs closely resembled the low EOGs found in vitelliform dystrophy.

The finding of virtually normal visual acuity, accompanied by normal color vision, normal visual fields, normal dark adaptation, and normal ERG, indicates intactness of the photoreceptors and the innermost retinal layers. The finding of a disturbed EOG almost certainly indicates a diffuse disturbance in the function of the pigment epithelium. Because ophthalmoscopic, fluorescein angiographic, and photographic studies show that the pigment epithelium is the site of the pigment changes and that layers outside the pigment epithelium appear to be unaffected, there is strong evidence that the EOG light–dark ratio is an index of the function of the pigment epithelium.

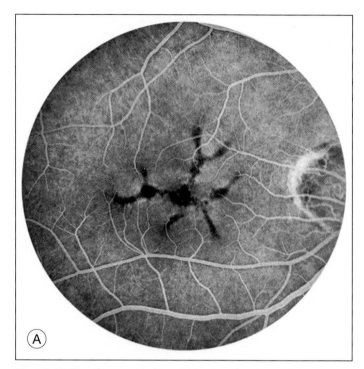

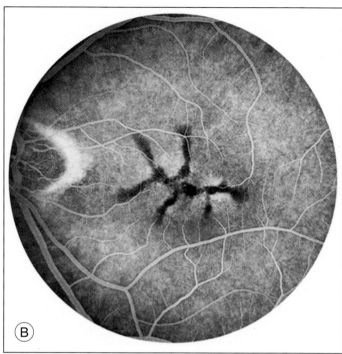

Fig. 64-26 Hypofluorescent pigmented pattern in autosomal dominant butterfly (pattern) dystrophy.

Histology and pathogenesis

Microscopic examination of one eye of a patient with butterfly shaped macular dystrophy, revealed an area of total loss of the RPE and photoreceptor cell layer with intact choriocapillaris and lipofuscin-containing cells in the subretinal space. Outside the area of RPE atrophy, the RPE was greatly distended by lipofuscin.[99] Ophthalmoscopy, retinal function tests, and fluorescein angiography all indicate a primary dysfunction of the RPE.

Mode of inheritance

This dystrophy has an autosomal dominant transmission.

Genetics

Several mutations in the human *peripherin/RDS* gene have been found to be associated with butterfly-shaped pattern dystrophy.[100,101] In the original family with butterfly shaped macular dystrophy, the *peripherin/RDS* gene as well as 44 loci involved in retinal dystrophies could be excluded.[102] A novel locus at chromosome 5q21.2-q33.2 was identified (yet unpublished).

Differential diagnosis

The other pigment dystrophies and other macular dystrophies described in this chapter must be differentiated from this condition. Furthermore, rubella retinopathy, fundus pulverulentus, pigmented paravenous chorioretinal degeneration, drug-induced degenerations, primary and secondary retinopathia pigmentosa, and angioid streaks are among the entities that occasionally may show some resemblance to butterfly-shaped pigment dystrophy.[16,103] In general, however, differential diagnosis will offer little difficulty because of the specific changes of butterfly-shaped pigment dystrophy.

One exception is the macular pattern in myotonic dystrophy of Steinert–Curschmann. In these patients the macular changes resemble pattern dystrophy almost completely[104] (Fig. 64-27).

Reticular dystrophy of the retinal pigment epithelium (Sjögren's disease)

An exceedingly rare, peculiar affection of the retinal pigment epithelium was observed by H. Sjögren in five children from a Swedish family.[105] In view of the reticular character of the retinal pigmentations found in these children, he named this condition *dystrophia reticularis laminae pigmentosae retinae*. The fovea in these children showed accumulations of dark pigment, surrounded by a finely meshed network of polygonally arranged pigment granules with densification at the sites of the knots of the network. To our knowledge, only several pedigrees have been reported so far.[105–109]

Symptoms

Generally, visual acuity is unaffected or is only minimally affected in advanced stages. Routine ophthalmoscopic examinations may disclose this striking abnormality in patients who have no specific complaints.

Ophthalmoscopic features and evolution

In the initial stages, pigment granules accumulate at the site of the fovea. A network gradually forms around the central accumulation and extends toward the periphery, until finally it closely resembles a knotted fishnet.

In more advanced cases the shape of the network becomes irregular, and its appearance is bleached. In later stages the

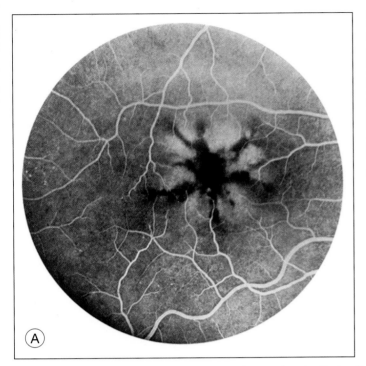

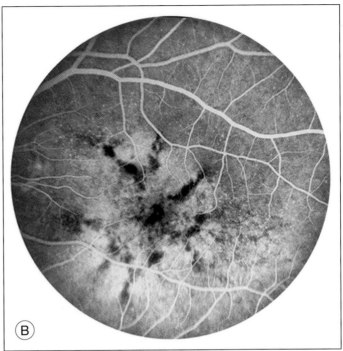

Fig. 64-27 Patterned hypofluorescent structures in maculae of patients with myotonic dystrophy.

pigment disappears gradually. The meshes of the net, which are arranged around a dark pigment spot at the fovea, are less than 1 disc diameter in size and of irregular shape (Fig. 64-28).

Binocular slit-lamp examination of the retina shows that the pigmentations are localized below the neuroepithelium and very likely in the pigment epithelium. Ophthalmoscopic study in red-free light discloses a barely discernible network. This, too, indicates that the pigmentations are not localized in the superficial retinal layers. Foveal reflexes are normal, as are discs and vessels. The reticulum extends approximately 4 to 5 disc diameters from the macula in all directions. The midperiphery and periphery are not affected. The reticulum probably appears in infancy and may be fully developed at age 15 years. In older persons the pigmentations may disappear, and in these cases the initial characteristics may disappear.

Fluorescein angiography

The network stands out, as if held in front of a light box, as soon as the choroid is filled by fluorescein (see Fig. 64-28). There is no fluorescence at the site of the pigment and hyperfluorescence within the meshes of the reticulum. No leakage of fluorescein is observed, and the vessels are normal. This fluorescein pattern suggests an intracellular pigment epithelial localization of the network.

Retinal function tests

Visual fields   Visual fields are normal.

Color vision   Color vision is normal.

Dark adaptation   Adaptation to dark is normal.

Electroretinography   The ERG shows normal findings.

Electro-oculography   EOG gives values at the lower limit of normal.[5,107,108]

Histology and pathogenesis

No histologic studies are available. It would seem that this condition is a primary dystrophy of the cells of the pigment epithelium, which, for the most part, leaves these cells functionally intact. It is interesting that the pigment granules form such a mosaic-like pattern in the pigment epithelial cells. In fundus flavimaculatus, drusen, and angioid streaks, as well as in older patients, there may also be a peculiar arrangement of polygonal shapes.[5] It might well be that each mesh of the reticulum constitutes a functional or anatomic unit.

Mode of inheritance

Both autosomal recessive and dominant mode of transmission have been described.[5,107,108]

Differential diagnosis

The differential diagnosis is not difficult. In elderly persons, reticular pigment changes frequently are found in the midperiphery and far periphery of the retina. This is often the case in patients who also have drusen. Patients with fundus flavimaculatus, angioid streaks, and dominant drusen may also show reticular patterns. Dystrophia macroreticularis laminae pigmentosae retinae[110] shares a few characteristics with reticular dystrophy and also butterfly-shaped dystrophy and therefore is reminiscent of these conditions (Fig. 64-29).

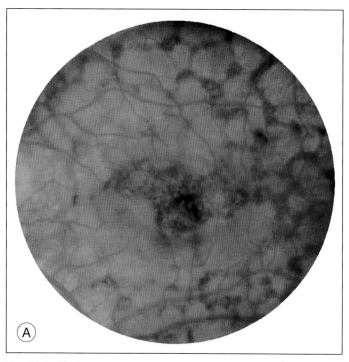

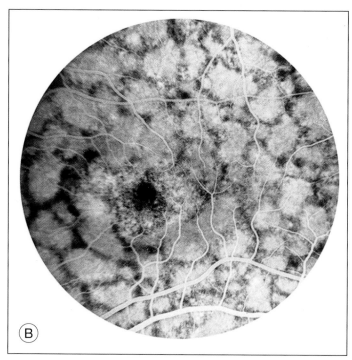

Fig. 64-28 Reticular dystrophy of the retinal pigment epithelium (A) and its characteristic fluorescein angiogram (B).

Dominant cystoid macular dystrophy

In the Institute of Ophthalmology in Nijmegen, we have seen at least 71 patients with dominantly inherited cystoid macular edema. A useful term for this entity appears to be *dominant cystoid macular dystrophy (DCMD)*.[111,112] In this dystrophy there is an early onset of cystoid macular edema that ultimately results

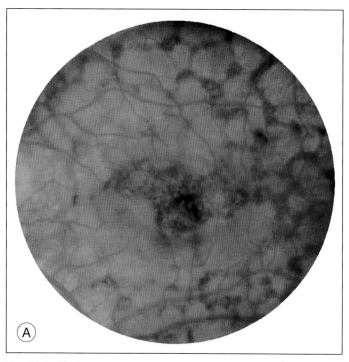

Fig. 64-29 Patient with "macroreticular" dystrophy of the retinal pigment epithelium.

in macular atrophy and sometimes pericentral pigmentary deposits.

Symptoms
Young patients usually have somewhat decreased visual acuity, and affected parents usually have a much lower visual acuity. Visual acuity decreases gradually with age.

Ophthalmoscopic features and evolution
The maculae show the typical pattern of cystoid macular edema in younger affected persons. Later, macular atrophy is seen, but the vessels and discs remain normal. There may be pigmentary changes in the midperiphery and far retinal periphery (Fig. 64-30).

Fluorescein angiography
Fluorescein angiography shows the characteristic features of leaking perimacular capillaries in young patients (Fig. 64-31). The capillaries throughout the posterior pole may be leaky. Later, hyperfluorescence resulting from defective retinal pigment epithelium may be seen.

Retinal function tests
An ERG is usually normal, whereas the EOG tends to be subnormal in most cases. The EOG tends to become more subnormal with increasing age. Color vision will show both blue-yellow and red-green defects.[113]

Histology and pathogenesis
So far there has been no histologic specimen available. Retinal function suggests a primary affection of retinal pigment epithelium, with secondary breakdown of the inner and outer blood–retinal barrier.

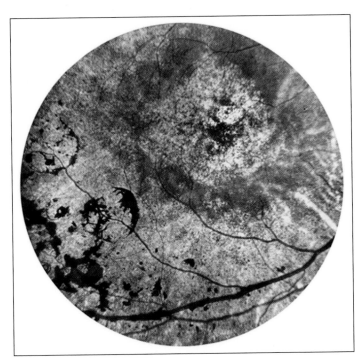

Fig. 64-30 Pigmentary changes in the posterior pole of the eye and atrophic macula in advanced stage of dominant cystoid macular dystrophy (DCMD).

Genetics

In the large family with dominant cystoid macular edema, linkage was detected within an area on the short arm of chromosome 7.[114] The gene has not yet been identified.

Differential diagnosis

Differential diagnosis must be made with X-linked juvenile retinoschisis, dominantly inherited retinitis pigmentosa with cystoid macular edema, and other types of retinitis pigmentosa. Rarely, differentiation has to be made from mild cases of epimacular fibrosis or cellophane retinopathy.

Cystoid macular edema as a postoperative complication will be readily distinguished. Furthermore, patients with uveitis, diabetes, vein obstruction, or other such factors have to be separated. Idiopathic parafoveal telangiectasia is another separate entity that needs differentiation.

Grouped pigmentations of the foveal area

It may be inappropriate to deal with grouped pigmentations in this chapter because it has been shown repeatedly that no obvious hereditary factors are involved in this condition.[5] Possible hereditary components have been mentioned only by Forgacs and Bozin,[114,115] who described two sisters with grouped pigmentations in the foveal area. However, these patients did not show the classic picture of grouped pigmentations. Perhaps a better term can be found for the fundus picture in this condition if additional, similar cases are found.

Classic grouped pigmentations of the fundus are rarely found in the posterior pole.[115,116] They are often unilateral, but may be bilateral.

Symptoms

In classic cases no symptoms are present, and routine ophthalmoscopic examination reveals the diagnosis. However, Forgacs and Bozin[115] reported that one of their patients showed some visual loss and that the other showed some metamorphopsia.

Ophthalmoscopic features and evolution

The patients in whom the condition was possibly inherited showed small, round pigmentations, always surrounded by a light halo. These pigmentations were localized in the fovea or its immediate surroundings. Loewenstein and Steel[117] also described such foveal pigmentations surrounded by a light halo in a sporadic case.

Classic grouped pigmentations of the retina, however, are found mostly in the retinal periphery and have no halos. They are often seen in a triangular area, the apex of which points to the center of the retina. Their size ranges from 0.1 to 1.0 disc diameter, and their shape often is irregular. They are also ill defined and can vary considerably in number. They are reminiscent of bear tracks or footprints in the snow.

Fluorescein angiography

The fluorescein angiogram shows no fluorescence at the site of the pigmentations and no pathologic fluorescence elsewhere. The fluorescein pattern therefore is similar to that in butterfly-shaped pigment dystrophy and in reticular dystrophy of the RPE.

Retinal function tests

Visual acuity   Acuity is generally normal. In one of the siblings described,[115] there was some decrease in acuity.

Visual fields   Visual fields are completely normal.

Color vision   Color vision is normal.

Dark adaptation   Dark adaptation is normal.

Electroretinography   The ERG is normal. In one of the supposed hereditary cases, it appeared to be slightly subnormal.[115]

Electro-oculography   The EOG is normal in the classic bear-track, grouped pigmentations. EOG studies were not performed in the presumably hereditary cases.

Histology and pathogenesis

Classic grouped pigmentations show accumulation of pigment and pigment epithelium cells at the site of the pigmentations, with absence of the photoreceptors. The cases of Forgacs and Bozin[115] probably represent a primary dystrophy of the pigment epithelium.

Mode of inheritance

It is well established now that classic grouped pigmentations of the retina are not inherited. It seems likely that the Swiss sisters described[115] suffered from an autosomally (recessive?) inherited condition, which, at this time, probably requires a

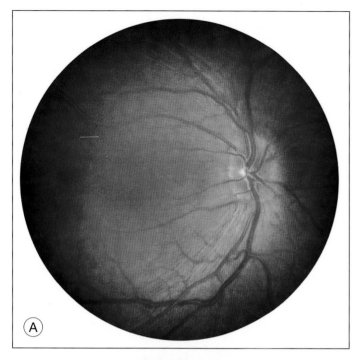

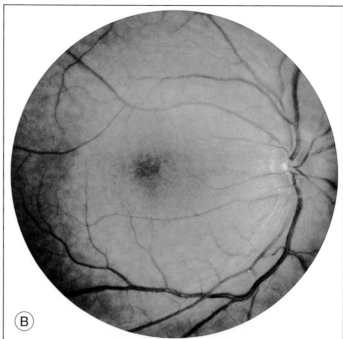

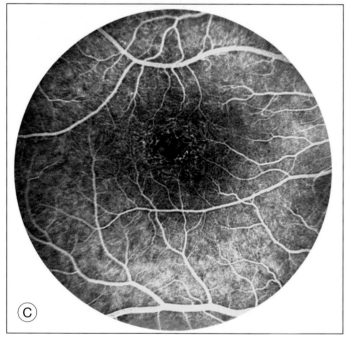

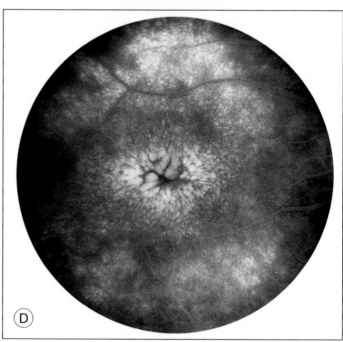

Fig. 64-31 Conventional color picture (A) and red-free color picture (B) of DCMD. Early (C) and late phases (D) of angiograms of DCMD.

separate nosologic place among the numerous different retinal diseases.

Differential diagnosis

All other pigment dystrophies described in this chapter need to be differentiated from grouped pigmentations of the foveal area. Furthermore, other pigment changes, such as in the choroideremia-carrier state, melanosis bulbi, acute pigment epithelitis,[118] rubella retinopathy, and other post-inflammatory reactions, have to be differentiated.

Benign concentric annular macular dystrophy

Among the autosomal dominant macular dystrophies, we have found a dystrophy with a ringlike depigmentation around the fovea associated with unusually good visual acuity, even in the oldest patients affected (Fig. 64-32). Despite the presence of a so-called bull's-eye macular degeneration, there was no history of chloroquine ingestion. There were no signs or symptoms typical of a cone dystrophy in these patients.[119]

Ten years later we performed a follow-up examination.[120] Some patients complained of deterioration of visual acuity, night vision,

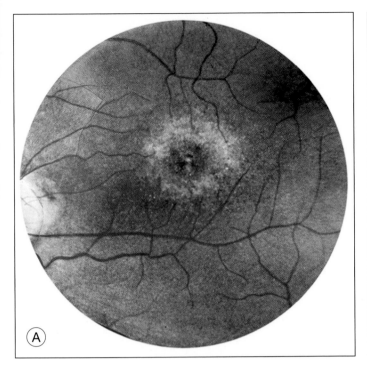

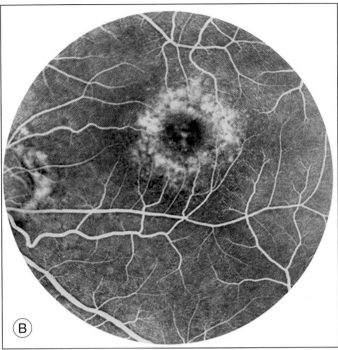

Fig. 64-32 Macular area and fluorescein angiogram in patient with benign concentric annular macular dystrophy.

and color vision. The macular dystrophy had progressed, and the fundus periphery was more involved. In two patients there were bone corpuscle-like pigmentations. Electrophysiologic examination showed increased photoreceptor dysfunction, with equal involvement of the rod and cone system. The patients had an acquired type III blue-yellow defect with pseudoprotanomaly. The dystrophy appeared to have developed into a more diffuse but mild pigmentary retinopathy, with functional characteristics of a relatively benign cone–rod dystrophy.

Mode of inheritance
The original family has an autosomal dominant mode of transmission. Several other patients have been reported with clinical features similar to this initial stage of BCAMD including a three generation family, and six isolated patients.[121–124]

Genetics
The original family was linked to a novel locus at chromosome 6p12.3-q16.[125]

Dominant drusen
Dominant drusen of the retina are found on the vitreal side of Bruch's membrane. They are secreted by the RPE.[5,126]

It is usually possible to separate hereditary drusen from degenerative drusen. There is no clear justification for separating familial drusen into four different categories, as is often done. The following terms have been used for these categories in this respect: *Hutchinson–Tay choroiditis, Holthouse–Batten* superficial chorioretinitis, Doyne's honeycomb dystrophy, and *Malattia levantinese.* All these "hyaline" dystrophies are nothing other than dominantly inherited drusen, also called *familial,* or *dominant, drusen.*[5,126]

Symptoms
Initially, there are no symptoms at all, and drusen may be found during routine ophthalmoscopy. Later, decrease in visual acuity is the predominant reason for the patient's visit to the ophthalmologist. Metamorphopsia is also a frequent complaint.

Ophthalmoscopic features and evolution
Usually in patients between age 20 and 30 years, but sometimes earlier, a few round, brownish yellow, later whitish, structures appear in the deep retinal layers of the posterior pole (Fig. 64-33). In middle age the posterior pole is usually already covered by many round, sharply defined white dots, which may be arranged in a mosaic or honeycomb pattern (Fig. 64-34). Often, there is striking symmetry in both eyes. Usually, the closer to the fovea, the larger are the drusen (Fig. 64-35). The flecks are rounded, whiter, and more sharply delineated than in fundus flavimaculatus. Later, these spots show confluence, particularly close to the center, and the retina shows an atrophic pigment epithelium. Then, pigmentations may occur, and atrophy of the choriocapillaris and of the larger choroidal vessels ensues. Occasionally, drusen may disappear and leave atrophic areas. Generally, these drusen also extend nasally to the disc. Optic discs, vessels, and retinal peripheries remain normal. In advanced stages, oval-shaped or almost rectangular white plaques surrounding the disc are characteristic findings in this dystrophy.

Fluorescein angiography
During the arterial phase, the fluorescein angiogram reveals multiple, round, sharply defined fluorescent spots, the contours of which correspond partly to the lesions observed at normal ophthalmoscopy (Fig. 64-35). Fluorescein angiography also often

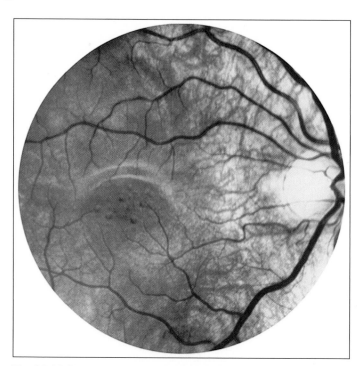

Fig. 64-33 Dominant drusen in a 12-year-old boy.

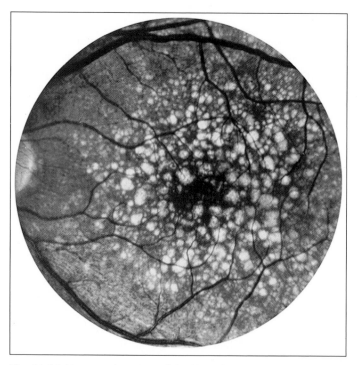

Fig. 64-34 Honeycomb pattern of dominant drusen of the retinal pigment epithelium.

discloses several areas of atrophic pigment epithelium, which are not clearly visible at normal ophthalmoscopy (see Fig. 64-35). Sometimes, drusen, particularly large ones, do not show hyperfluorescence. This is probably the case when the hyaline bodies consist of a large mass. This mass, then, may block the choroidal fluorescence, whereas small drusen usually transmit the choroidal

fluorescence. No leakage of fluorescein is seen. Discs, vessels, and retinal periphery are normal.

Retinal function tests

Visual acuity Visual acuity is initially normal; vision may decrease gradually. It often takes more than 10 or even 20 years before drusen inflict the first damage on the photoreceptors. Diminution of acuity is rarely seen before age 40 years. The photoreceptors remain unharmed for a long time because the pigment epithelium secretes the degenerative products to its choroidal side (unlike fundus flavimaculatus).

Visual fields Fields retain their normal peripheral boundaries. In more advanced cases, central scotomata occur.

Color vision Color vision is affected, as in most other macular diseases. (As long as vision is normal, however, color vision is also normal.) This means a mild red-green dyschromatopsia with the HRR test and a wider-than-normal Rayleigh equation on the anomaloscope, requiring more red than normal in this equation. The Farnsworth–Munsell 100-hue test mainly shows a tritan axis and not so many errors (fewer than 400) as, for instance, in the cone dystrophies (mostly more than 500 errors).

Dark adaptation Dark adaptation is usually normal. In more advanced cases there may be some delay, although normal cone and rod thresholds are ultimately found.

Electroretinography ERG usually gives normal results. A delay in attaining an otherwise normal maximum b-wave amplitude has been seen in more severe cases.

Electro-oculography The EOG is normal in the initial stages, but ultimately becomes subnormal to a degree that depends on the extent of the retinal involvement. The EOG is generally less severely affected than in fundus flavimaculatus.[5] We found that the EOG becomes subnormal before dark adaptation abnormalities develop and the ERG becomes abnormal. This suggests an important correlation between the light-rise-dark-trough ratio of the EOG and the integrity of the RPE. In other primary disorders of the pigment epithelium, such as fundus flavimaculatus (and probably vitelliform dystrophy as well), a pathologic EOG is similarly often found in combination with normal dark adaptation and ERG.

Histology and pathogenesis

This dystrophy appears to be an inborn error of metabolism, localized in the RPE. Coats[127] postulated a pathogenesis of drusen on the basis of transformation or deposition. Both types of drusen occur together, and both result in large hyaline structures on Bruch's membrane, with destruction of adjacent cells of the pigment epithelium. Wolter[128] found two different developmental types of drusen: (1) those developing by accumulation of hyaline substance within slowly degenerating cells of the pigment epithelium; and (2) those developing by extracellular deposition of hyaline substance between the pigment epithelium and Bruch's membrane.

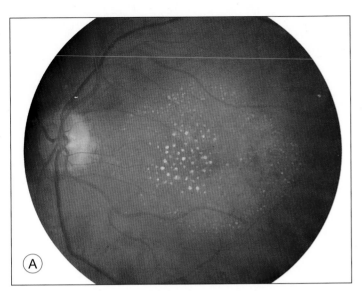
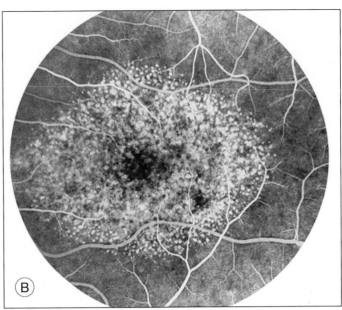

Fig. 64-35 Conventional photograph (A) and fluorescein angiogram (B) from a patient with dominant drusen of the macula. There is a large area of defective retinal pigment epithelium centrally.

Histologic examination discloses round accumulations of hyaline in the pigment epithelium. These hyaline bodies are connected with the inner layer of Bruch's membrane.[128–130] Choroid and neuroepithelium are normal in the initial stages, but in the advanced stages these structures may show marked atrophy. The eosinophilic hyaline bodies have a stratified structure. Histochemical examination reveals that these structures are made up of carbohydrate compounds, proteins, and minute quantities of nucleoproteins.[131] Farkas et al.[132] found that drusen were composed of at least two major constituents: mucopolysaccharide, identified as sialomucins, and a lipid, characterized as a cerebroside.

With the help of ultrastructural and histochemical studies, it was found that degenerating retinal pigment epithelial cells are converted into an amorphous material that eventually fills the inner collagenous zone of Bruch's membrane, forming drusen.[133] Discontinuities in the elastic layer of Bruch's membrane permit accumulation of drusen material within the inner choroid. Large numbers of lysosomes are present in degenerating pigment epithelial cells and drusen material. Therefore, it was suggested by these investigators[133] that drusen formation is due to uncontrolled activity of lysosomal enzymes, causing cytolysis of the RPE.

Mode of inheritance

The mode of transmission is doubtless autosomal dominant, with variable expressivity. Pearce[134] studied a large pedigree and concluded that there is a regular autosomal dominant inheritance pattern.

Genetics

In most families with dominant drusen, a single mutation Arg345Trp (R345W) has been found in the *EFEMP1* gene at 2p16-p21.[135–138] *EFEMP1* encodes the EGF-containing, fibulin-like extracellular matrix protein-1. In a few other dominant drusen families that map to 2p16-p21, no mutations were found in the *EFEMP1* gene, suggesting an *EFEMP1* promoter sequence mutation or a second dominant drusen gene at this locus.[139] The defect underlying dominant drusen was also located in one family at 6q14,[140,141] and a *peripherin/RDS* mutation is associated with CACD and dominant drusen in three families.[142]

Differential diagnosis

Degenerative drusen are the primary consideration in the differential diagnosis. These are frequently seen in the fellow eye of a patient with senile disciform macular degeneration (Kuhnt–Junius). A great variety of other conditions also may demonstrate these degenerative drusen. Of these conditions, hyalinosis cutis et mucosae (Urbach–Wiethe syndrome)[143] should be mentioned particularly. Other "flecked retina syndromes" have to be distinguished, including fundus flavimaculatus, fundus albipunctatus, "fleck retina with congenital hemeralopia," and multiple vitelliform lesions. The fundus in angioid streaks may also show a typical finely mottled, yellowish flecked pattern (peau d'orange) (see Fig. 64-36), which is definitely different from drusen. In other conditions, whitish flecks may also be present, as in disseminated choroiditis and retinopathia pigmentosa. In general, however, there will be no diagnostic problems in these patients.

BRUCH'S MEMBRANE

Pseudoinflammatory macular dystrophy (Sorsby)

In 1949, Sorsby and co-workers[144] reported five pedigrees with fundus changes reminiscent of an inflammatory process of the

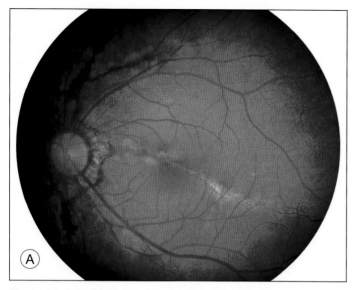

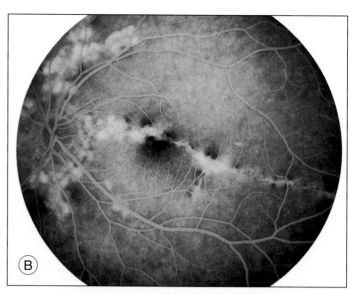

Fig. 64-36 Color image (A) and fluorescein angiogram (B) of angioid streaks and peau d'orange with defective retinal pigment epithelium at the side of the streaks.

posterior pole of the eye. Symmetric, bilateral fundus changes were seen, and acute visual loss occurred. This dystrophy was inherited as an autosomal dominant disease.

The lesions may look very similar to those found in central areolar choroidal dystrophy, which also may be inherited as an autosomal dominant disease. Differential diagnosis from disciform macular degeneration or from real inflammatory processes may be very difficult.[145] Several families from all over the world have been described. In some families the ancestors originate in the United Kingdom and a founder effect is suggested.[144,146,147]

Symptoms
This condition usually becomes manifest at about age 40 years, and visual acuity diminishes within a few months to very low levels.

Ophthalmoscopic features and evolution
The first changes consist of edema, hemorrhages, and exudates in the central retina of both eyes. Next, cicatrization occurs, with a varying degree of pigment proliferation. Marked atrophy of the pigment epithelium develops after some time; the choroidal vessels are exposed and become visible. Over the course of several years the process extends to the periphery, and differentiation from diffuse choroidal dystrophy becomes difficult. Almost complete blindness ultimately results.

Fluorescein angiography
Extensive defects of the pigment epithelium and pigmentations were disclosed.[148,149] The results of this method of examination are largely dependent on the stage the dystrophy has reached. If there is edema, there probably will be leakage of fluorescein. In later stages, atrophy of the choriocapillaris and some of the larger choroidal vessels will certainly be seen.

Retinal function tests
Visual acuity   Visual acuity diminishes rapidly, and, as indicated previously, almost complete blindness may ultimately result.

Visual fields   A central scotoma soon occurs and increases progressively in size and intensity, until a large part of the central visual field is finally involved.

Color vision   It appears that color vision is affected, as in most other macular diseases.[150,151]

Dark adaptation   Dark adaptation is generally unaffected. In advanced stages it may be slightly delayed.[151]

Electroretinography   The ERG is normal initially but becomes subnormal in advanced stages, when a sizable part of the retina is involved.

Electro-oculography   No distinct reports are available on the EOG in Sorsby's pseudoinflammatory dystrophy. We assume that the EOG will be normal initially but will become subnormal in advanced stages.

Histology and pathogenesis
Ashton and Sorsby[152] made a histologic examination of the eyes of two patients (70 and 71 years old) with Sorsby's pseudo-inflammatory dystrophy. A significant objection to this work is that, precisely in these patients' families, dominant transmission was not demonstrable. The following histologic changes were found:

1. Sclerosis and atrophy of the choroid, with fibrous mural degeneration of the remaining vessels.
2. Numerous ruptures of Bruch's membrane in the posterior fundus, with degeneration of the elastic layer in the same area.

3. Newly formed subretinal vascular tissue, originating from the choroid and related to the dehiscences in Bruch's membrane.
4. Disturbance of the pigment epithelium.
5. Destruction of the outer layers of the retina with glial replacement.

Babel[153] examined the eyes of a 52-year-old man with a 12-year history of diminishing vision, whose condition had been diagnosed as Sorsby's pseudoinflammatory dystrophy. The choriocapillaris of the right eye had largely disappeared. The corresponding pigment epithelium was atrophic but also showed areas of proliferation. The neuroepithelium and outer retinal layers also showed atrophy. The large choroidal vessels were either fibrotic or hyalinized. Bruch's membrane was greatly changed, showing irregular rarefactions and deposits of fine granulations. Circumscribed exudates were found between the more or less marked pigment epithelium changes and the external limiting membrane, and small localized hemorrhages were visible in the inner retinal layers. The left eye showed a less completely affected choriocapillaris, and its neuroepithelium showed unmistakable degenerative changes.

Histopathologic studies thus disclosed changes of the type usually found in disciform macular degeneration and angioid streaks. The principal common lesion in these three conditions is degeneration and rupture of Bruch's membrane, followed by formation of subretinal vessels, hemorrhages, and tissue.

The findings indicate that in Sorsby's pseudoinflammatory dystrophy, the fundamental pathologic condition seems to be a primary dystrophic change of Bruch's membrane, followed by secondary organization of subretinal hemorrhages and exudates originating in the choriocapillaris and passing through the ruptures in Bruch's membrane. Nevertheless, the physiochemical changes that lead to involvement of the elastic tissue of Bruch's membrane are still obscure, and the possibility remains that this involvement results from pathologic alteration of the choroid or the choriocapillaris proper. Histologic examination in early stages of this dystrophy may lead to a solution to this problem.

For the time being, it seems best to follow Ashton and Sorsby's suggestion and assume that pseudoinflammatory dystrophy is primarily caused by genetically determined defects in Bruch's membrane, thus indicating a histopathologic relationship of this condition to angioid streaks and disciform macular degeneration.[152]

Mode of transmission
The mode of transmission of this condition is always autosomal dominant. Sorsby et al.[144] reported on four families, including a family with 16 patients in four generations, a family with 10 patients in two generations, a family with 25 patients in four generations, and a family with 16 patients in three generations. Burn[154] described 11 cases in three generations.

Genetics
Mutations in the tissue inhibitor of metalloproteinase-3 gene (*TIMP3*) have been found to be the cause of this disease. As yet, no other retinal dystrophy has been found to be caused by mutations in this gene.[155,156]

Differential diagnosis
Differential diagnosis of Sorsby's pseudoinflammatory dystrophy encompasses the other dystrophies of the central retina and choroid discussed in this chapter, none of which shows really marked similarities to the entity Sorsby described. Vitelliform dystrophy of the fovea can show exudative changes and must therefore be borne in mind in the differential diagnosis. Edema, hemorrhages, exudates, drusen, gross pigment changes, and subsequent generalized chorioretinal atrophy are more reminiscent of the complications of angioid streaks or of disciform macular degeneration, and choroiditis disseminata can also show similarities to this condition. The entities thus defined are not accompanied by angioid streaks, and disciform macular degeneration usually is confined to the retinal center, not affecting the retinal midperiphery. Also, disciform macular degeneration rarely occurs in patients under the age of 55 years and has no dominant transmission. In chorioretinitis disseminata, an infectious cause can often be found, and hereditary factors are not at all involved. In the terminal stages, an extensive choroidal atrophy may call for differentiation from one of the forms of choroidal atrophy, choroideremia, gyrate atrophy, or chorioretinal atrophy associated with high myopia.

Angioid streaks
Angioid streaks are found in several different conditions, among them pseudoxanthoma elasticum (Grönblad–Strandberg syndrome), osteitis deformans (Paget's disease), sickle cell anemia, senile elastosis of the skin, hypertensive cardiovascular disorders, and, rarely, fibrodysplasia hyperelastica (Ehlers–Danlos syndrome). By far the commonest cause of angioid streaks is pseudoxanthoma elasticum, in which the streaks may already be seen in young adults. In Paget's disease they are late developments, and in sickle cell disease the diagnosis has probably been made before angioid streaks are noted. Senile elastosis with angioid streaks is considered rare. An interesting monograph was presented on this subject by Paton.[157]

Angioid streaks may lead to a disciform type of macular degeneration, and this is why we include this condition here.

Symptoms
Loss of visual acuity and metamorphopsia occur when there is leakage of fluid through Bruch's membrane at the posterior pole of the eye.

Ophthalmoscopic features and evolution
Angioid streaks are grayish or dark reddish lines that surround the optic disc and extend from there radially (Fig. 64-36A). They lie deeper than the retinal vessels and have a crackline appearance. A characteristic speckled appearance of the fundus in patients with pseudoxanthoma elasticum has frequently been seen. This fundus mottling is most distinct in the area temporal to the macula, and it may antedate the appearance of angioid streaks or hemorrhagic disciform macular degeneration. Sometimes, a macular degeneration arises before real angioid streaks are present (see Fig. 64-36). Angioid streaks are rarely noted in children; they develop in the second or third decade. Extensive

hemorrhaging may occur, but spontaneous resolution has been seen (see Fig. 64-36A). Ultimately, disciform degeneration and hypertrophic scars are frequently seen. Drusen of the optic disc are also often seen in patients with angioid streaks.

Laser treatment may be beneficial in treating subretinal neovascularization in this disorder.[158,159]

Fluorescein angiography

Fluorescence of most of the streaks occurs in the arterial phase, and this persists after the dye has disappeared from the retinal veins. These findings indicate atrophic pigment epithelium at the site of the hyperfluorescent angioid streaks. Leakage of fluorescein occasionally is noted in some of the cracks (Fig. 64-36B).

Retinal function tests

Visual acuity   Visual acuity is normal as long as there is no leakage of fluid from the choroid through Bruch's membrane and the RPE.

Visual fields   Visual fields are normal. Centrally decreased sensitivity occurs when the macula is damaged as a result of leaking fluid.

Color vision   Color vision is affected only if visual loss occurs; then, loss of color vision is like that in other macular diseases.[26]

Dark adaptation   Dark adaptation is normal.

Electroretinography   The ERG is normal.

Electro-oculography   The EOG is normal. Only in advanced cases have we seen subnormal results.

Histology and pathogenesis

Angioid streaks probably represent visible cracks in Bruch's membrane. Klien[160] proposed a dual mechanism as a cause of these cracks: (1) a primary abnormality of the fibers of Bruch's membrane; and (2) an increased availability of metal salts or a tendency for their pathologic deposition, resulting in secondary brittleness of the membranes. Adelung[161] demonstrated that the lines of force within the eye resulting from the pull of intrinsic and extrinsic ocular muscles on the relatively fixed site of the optic nerve have the same configuration as the peripapillary interlacement and radial extensions of angioid streaks. Such forces acting on Bruch's membrane, in which residual strength of matrix fibers is diminished or in which deposition of metabolic salts such as calcium or iron has rendered the membrane brittle, undoubtedly account for the configuration of the breaks.

As in all the other dystrophies, the fundamental biochemical alterations of pseudoxanthoma elasticum and angioid streaks are yet to be identified. In patients with pseudoxanthoma elasticum, fibroblasts with metachromatic granules have been reported in tissue culture studies of these cells.[162] The significance of these findings is still undetermined.

Studies with the high-resolution electron microscope indicate that the lesion of pseudoxanthoma elasticum has no identifiable normal elastic units; instead, there is an abundant granulofila-mentous material related to an abnormal elastica.[163] Huang et al.,[163] who carried out these studies, concluded that there is an abnormal elastogenesis in pseudoxanthoma elasticum, and they suggest the term *elastodysplasia calcificans* as a substitute for the old terms *elastorrhexis* and *elastotic degenerations*.

Mode of inheritance

The mode of inheritance depends on the underlying condition. Pseudoxanthoma elasticum is autosomal recessive, although some authors suggest the possibility of an autosomal dominant form as well. Sickle cell disease, Paget's disease, and Ehlers–Danlos syndrome, however, are autosomal dominant.

Genetics

In linkage studies both autosomal recessive and dominant variants of pseudoxanthoma elasticum have been mapped to chromosome 16.[164] Mutations in *ABCC6* (formerly *MRP6*) are associated with PXE.[165]

Differential diagnosis

In general, differential diagnosis will not pose any problems. Disciform macular degeneration, both juvenile and senile, occasionally has to be differentiated. Pseudoangioid streaks in high myopia also may look slightly like real angioid streaks. The pigment lines in reticular dystrophy of the RPE are definitely different, but may at first glance be misinterpreted.

Age-related macular dystrophies

It appears that there are age-related macular degenerations with a hereditary character. Behr[79] and Waardenburg[166] were among the first to emphasize the occurrence of hereditary senile macular degenerations. Other pedigrees were reported by several authors, among which Baillart,[167] Francois and Deweer.[168,169] These pedigrees had several affected siblings. A few pedigrees have been reported in which an autosomal dominant senile macular dystrophy may have been present.[166,168,169] We have seen a few pedigrees in which more than one sibling suffered from an exudative disciform macular degeneration (Kuhnt–Junius type).

Because parents have died, and children are still too young to demonstrate macular changes, it seems to be difficult to find out whether real senile macular dystrophies are present in more than one generation. In some of the well-established macular dystrophies described in this chapter, patients may be seen at a relatively old age, which may suggest that the condition is a senile hereditary macular dystrophy. In general, we reject a classification of macular dystrophies based on the age at which the disease manifests itself because it is impossible to work with such a classification.[5] Therefore we do not like to present this category of senile macular dystrophies because there might be different entities among them. On the other hand, we are convinced that certain macular dystrophies of a hereditary character appear at age 60 years or later. The ones we have seen belonged to the category of the exudative disciform macular degenerations (Kuhnt–Junius). Generally, retinal function test results in these patients are normal or close to normal.

With Klien, we believe that senile macular degeneration is neither a clinical, histopathologic, nor genetic entity.[170] It comprises end stages of true hereditary diseases and secondary degenerations of the percipient retinal elements. These secondary degenerations are due to diffuse and pronounced thickening and degeneration of the intercapillary connective tissue and to damage to Bruch's membrane. In none of these secondary degenerations can genetic influences in a wider sense be ruled out completely. Among the "true" hereditary macular diseases, there does not seem to be an entity that appears only and consistently in old age.

Genetics
Genome-wide association studies using families with at least two siblings affected by ARMD reveal susceptibility loci at 1q31 and 17q25.[109] Only a single family with monogenic ARMD has been described so far. A genome scan mapped the underlying defect in this family to chromosome 1q25-q31 (ARMD1), and it was suggested HEMICENTIN-1 is the causative gene.[171]

High myopia
Hereditary factors are frequently involved in high myopia. Because this condition often leads to extensive macular changes, it is worthwhile to present the most common fundus abnormalities in this disease.

Symptoms
The refractive error dominates the clinical picture. Sudden visual loss may occur as a result of macular hemorrhage at the site of the fovea when Bruch's membrane decompensates (Fuchs' fleck). Gradual visual loss and metamorphopsia may result from breaks in Bruch's membrane.

Ophthalmoscopic features and evolution
Initially there are, in the main, no distinct ophthalmoscopic changes except for a myopic crescent. A generally blond fundus renders the choroidal vessels visible. Peripapillary chorioretinal atrophy (Fig. 64-37) occurs early, and pigmentary changes in the macula may be seen. Then, owing to cracks in Bruch's membrane, pseudoangioid streaks (lacquer cracks) (Fig. 64-38) occur and may lead to macular hemorrhage (Fuchs' fleck) (Fig. 64-39). Pseudoholes of the macula may result from vitreoretinal traction. Ultimately, large areas of chorioretinal atrophy may be found in the posterior pole of the eye. The retinal periphery often shows pigmentary changes and may show areas of lattice-like and snail-track degeneration. Holes are not infrequently found in the periphery of these retinas; retinal detachment is therefore often seen. However, in a few of these patients, the retinal hole appears to be at the site of the macula.

Fluorescein angiography
The ophthalmoscopic abnormality determines what kind of fluorescence abnormalities are seen. At the site of the pseudoangioid streaks, there is mostly hyperfluorescence, which is due to pigment epithelial atrophy. Leakage of fluorescein may be noted occasionally in these lacquer crack areas, particularly if there is a Fuchs' fleck. In the areas of chorioretinal atrophy, there is sometimes hardly any fluorescence at all, owing to the disappearance of pigment epithelium, choriocapillaris, and a large part of the choroidal vasculature.

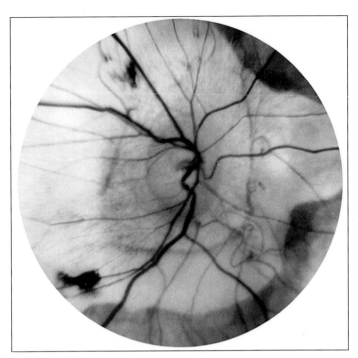

Fig. 64-37 Extensive peripapillary choroidoretinal atrophy in high myopia.

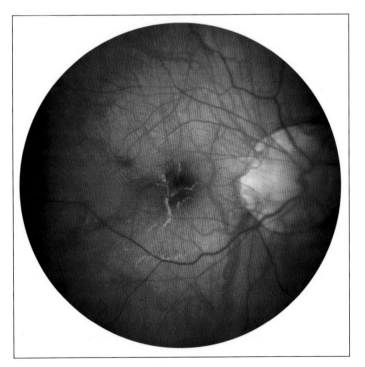

Fig. 64-38 Lacquer cracks in high myopia.

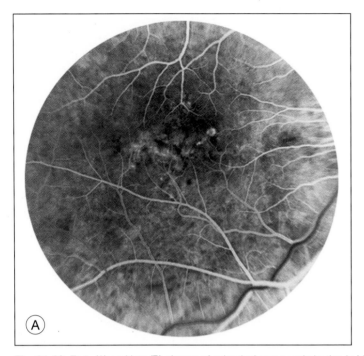
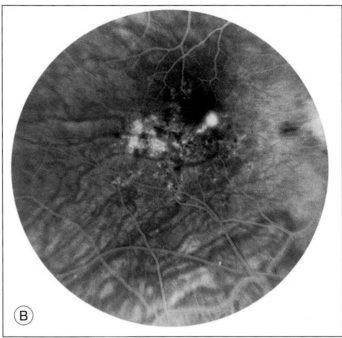

Fig. 64-39 Early (A) and late (B) phases of subretinal neovascularization in high myopia.

Retinal function tests

Visual acuity   Visual acuity may be normal for a long time. Sudden loss may occur when there is hemorrhaging at the macula. Visual loss may also be gradual, because of pigmentary changes and lacquer cracks in Bruch's membrane. Ultimately there is severe visual loss as a result of extensive chorioretinal atrophy.

Visual fields   The fields are usually not constricted. Relative and absolute central scotomata may occur following chorioretinal changes. Retinal detachment, of course, may lead to gross field defects.

Color vision   Color vision is affected, as in other macular diseases.

Dark adaptation   Dark adaptation is normal or slightly delayed in long-standing cases.

Electroretinography   The ERG initially is normal but frequently is mildly subnormal in advanced stages of myopic chorioretinal atrophy.

Electro-oculography   The EOG may be subnormal, indicating early involvement of the RPE.[172]

Histology and pathogenesis

Atrophic changes are found in the sclera, around the disc, in the choroid, in Bruch's membrane and the retina in the central area, and in the peripheral parts of the retina. The atrophic thinning of the sclera is confined to its posterior half, where it may be very attenuated. Atrophic choroidal changes are also mainly in the central area of the fundus, with gradual disappearance of the small vessels. Lacunae appear, making irregular areas of atrophy

around the disc and at the macula. The fundus changes appear to be primary in nature and are not just due to the mechanical effects of stretching. Clinically, the retinal changes are secondary to changes in the choroid. Genetic factors play a prominent part, possibly by means of primary changes in the RPE.

Mode of inheritance

Some pedigrees have been described in which autosomal dominant inheritance is established. However, there are pedigrees in which autosomal recessive inheritance is clearly indicated.[7]

Differential diagnosis

Some of the choroidal dystrophies and angioid streaks must be differentiated from high myopia. Central areolar choroidal dystrophy, choroideremia, and the congenital but progressive bifocal chorioretinal atrophy have certain features similar to those seen in high myopia.[18]

CHOROIDAL PROBLEMS

Central areolar choroidal dystrophy

Central choroidal, or, preferably, central choroidoretinal, dystrophies are a category of disorders that are still difficult to classify, owing to the scarcity of distinct pedigrees. Some autosomal dominant pedigrees have been described with central areolar choroidal dystrophy.[173–175] In a few pedigrees presented, there was indication of autosomal recessive inheritance.[5,176] The faulty term *choroidal sclerosis* has often been applied to these cases. Since the histologic studies of Ashton[177] and others,[178] it has been clear that in the end stage there is no sclerosis of the choroidal vessels, but there is atrophy of the neuroepithelium, pigment epithelium, and part of the choroid.

Sporadic cases are often found, and then it is very difficult or impossible to know whether the condition is an inherited dystrophy, a degenerative condition, or even an inflammatory disease.

In recent years an attempt was made to classify central choroidal dystrophy into two altogether different groups[176]: (1) *central choriocapillaris dystrophy*, in which the larger choroidal vessels remain unaffected; and (2) *central total choroidal vascular dystrophy*. Although at least two different groups of central choroidoretinal dystrophies appear to exist, more information has to be gathered in order to conclude definitely that two such groups exist.

We have seen patients in whom only the choriocapillaris appeared to be absent and in whom the atrophy did not extend to deeper choroidal layers even after years of observation. On the other hand, we have seen patients in whom almost the full thickness of the choroid disappeared rapidly in a few months' time. On clinical evaluation it may be difficult to decide if only the choriocapillaris is gone and if the intermediate and larger choroidal vessels are intact.

A complete total choroidal dystrophy is rarely seen; some choroidal vessels nearly always remain. The fluorescein angiogram always demonstrates many more deep choroidal vessels to be patent than routine ophthalmoscopy suggests. Also, some cases appear to be somewhere between choriocapillaris atrophy and full-thickness choroidal atrophy. In the patients in whom only the superficial choroidal layers are affected, there is often a horizontal oval, slightly areolar zone of atrophy. These cases are rather often clearly inherited. The patients in whom most of the choroidal thickness is affected often show a serpiginous geographic configuration, and these cases are almost always sporadic.

In our experience and that of others, there are no edematous reactions in the choriocapillaris variety, although they are often seen in the full-thickness choroidal dystrophy. Because of these reactions, some investigators[92,131] think that the latter type may be due to an inflammatory process, and they have designated this condition as *serpiginous*, or *geographic choroiditis*.[179,180] We saw one such patient, who also had bouts of iritis without any obvious cause. However, in other patients we never saw any sign of inflammation.

It is confusing that Sorsby and Crick[175] report that edematous-exudative reactions may be the earliest changes in central areolar choroidal dystrophy, since their pedigree appears to fit best into the choriocapillaris dystrophy category. This makes differential diagnosis with Sorsby's pseudoinflammatory dystrophy and "total" choroidal vascular dystrophy much more complicated.

Because there is not yet enough known to be certain about definitely different categories in central areolar choroidal dystrophy, and because there are no large differences in retinal function, the varieties are presented together here. Intermediate cases, which are not clearly superficial or almost complete choroidal dystrophies, justify such a presentation. Some pedigrees have been presented[22] in which affected children were seen with nonspecific macular changes.[181] We think that these pedigrees do not fit into this group.

In some of the so-called juvenile macular degenerations (atrophic macular dystrophy with flecks [Stargardt], cone dystrophy), a picture of distinct central choroidal atrophy may eventually develop. In early cases of cone dystrophy, this has also been noted.[37]

Central areolar choroidal dystrophy (CACD) rarely occurs before age 30 years and develops mainly after the age of 40 years. Mild ophthalmoscopic changes possibly may occur at earlier ages.

Symptoms

Patients have a history of experiencing gradual visual loss in one or both eyes. Sparing of the fovea may occur, and in this event visual loss may be absent or only unilateral.

Ophthalmoscopic features and evolution

Early macular changes in choriocapillaris dystrophy are characterized by pigment stippling and mottling, indicating pigment epithelial dystrophy (Fig. 64-40A). Later, around the age of 40, the atrophy of the pigment epithelium affects the whole macular area, sometimes leaving the fovea intact. In the following years, patches of atrophy of the choriocapillaris start to develop. Often this atrophy has a horseshoe shape around the fovea. This explains why visual acuity may be satisfactory to the age of 60. Then, the fovea starts to be affected, and visual acuity may drop dramatically within several years to the level of finger counting.[182]

Fluorescein angiography

Fluorescein angiographic study in early cases shows hyperfluorescence, due to pigment epithelial atrophy, whereas in cases of longer standing the choriocapillaris and, consequently, the diffuse background fluorescence disappear. The intermediate and large choroidal vessels are beautifully outlined by fluorescein in these cases. In late stages of the subtotal CACD, there are always many more vessels visible on the fluorescein angiogram than from normal ophthalmoscopic examination. At the margins of the lesions, hyperfluorescence resulting from leakage of dye is visible from intact choriocapillaris (see Fig. 64-40F).

Visual functions

Visual acuity Vision is often severely affected, as far down as 0.1 or counting fingers. In patients in whom there is macular sparing, acuity may be, and may remain, 1.0, despite extensive paramacular chorioretinal atrophy (see Fig. 64-40, C to H).

Visual fields Fields are normal in the periphery. Central or paracentral scotomata, or both, are always present.

Color vision Color vision is moderately affected, as in most other macular diseases.[5,26]

Dark adaptation Adaptation to dark is often normal. In some patients there may be slightly pathologic dark adaptation curves.

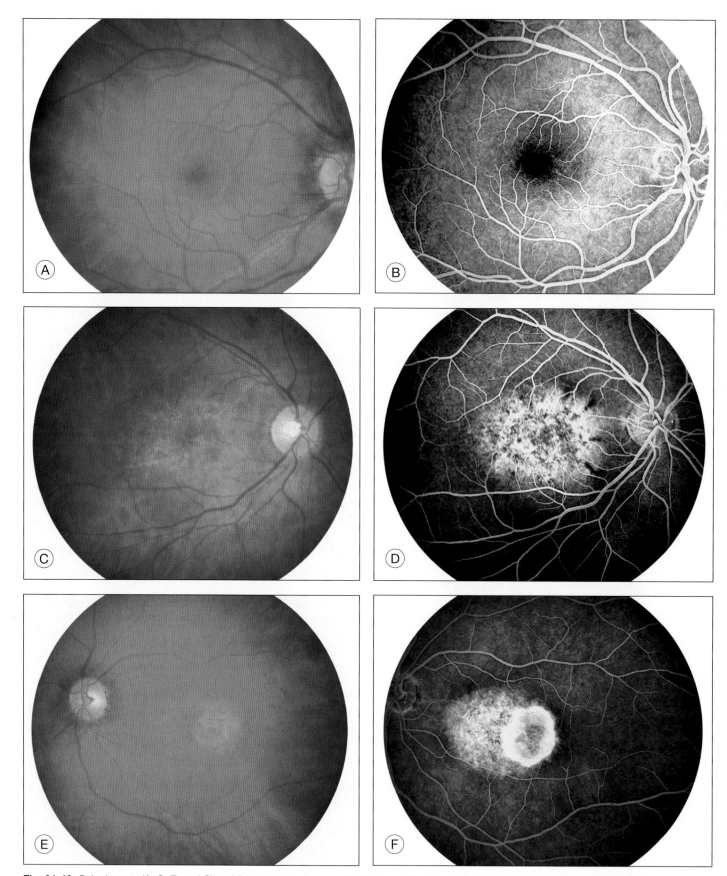

Fig. 64-40 Color images (A, C, E, and G) and fluorescein angiograms (B, D, F, and H) of four stages of central areolar choroidal dystrophy.

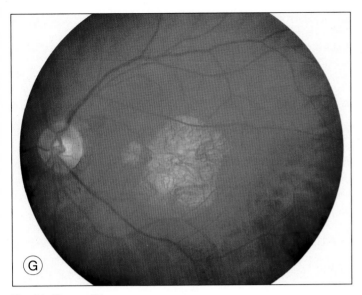

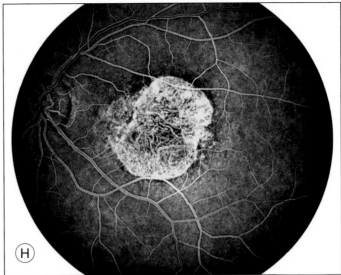

Fig. 64-40—cont'd

Electroretinography   The ERG is normal in many patients. However, subnormal values have been obtained, particularly in patients with central choriocapillaris dystrophy, pale discs, and attenuated vessels. In subtotal CACD the ERG is usually normal.

Electro-oculography   The EOG is normal in many patients. However, subnormal values are occasionally obtained.

Histology and pathogenesis

Ashton[177] had occasion to make a histologic examination of the eyes of a 56-year-old woman from a family described by Sorsby and Crick.[175] His findings were as follows:

1. A well-demarcated avascular zone, extending from the submacular region to the disc, was present in the posterior choroid.
2. Histologically, this avascular zone was found to be atrophic and fibrosed. No arteriosclerotic changes were found in the affected area or elsewhere in the choroid. Dissection of the posterior ciliary arteries failed to reveal constriction or occlusion.
3. The outer layers of the retina, together with the pigment epithelium, had disappeared without glial replacement in an area corresponding exactly to the underlying choroidal atrophy.
4. Bruch's membrane was little affected by the failure of the choroidal blood supply.

Babel[153] examined the eyes of a 64-year-old man with CACD and found numerous drusen surrounding the atrophic area from which choriocapillaris, pigment epithelium, and neuroepithelium had disappeared. Bruch's membrane showed secondary irregularities, ruptures, and a lamellar structure. Babel ascribed the clinical features of vascular sclerosis to the sharp contrast between the remaining choroidal vessels and the atrophic area.

Klien described the histologic features of CACD in the eye of a 71-year-old man in whose family there was no history of eye disease[170]:

The macular area showed grossly an area 2.0 by 2.0 disc diameters in size, of pigmentary and choroidal atrophy, beginning near the temporal edge of the disc. Histologically this lesion represented a rather well-defined macular defect of the neuroepithelium, pigment epithelium and choriocapillaris. These three structures had normal appearance up to the edges of the defect where they ceased rather abruptly. In the peripheral portion of the atrophic area a few scattered lumens of capillaries were still visible, while in the central portion all of these and the medium-sized vessels had disappeared, leaving only a few arteries surrounded by fibrosed stroma. No breaks were found in Bruch's membrane. The histopathologic findings in this eye resemble closely those described by Ashton in central areolar choroidal atrophy.

However, it is our impression that in long-standing dystrophies of the first retinal neuron the choroid also becomes atrophic. Howard and Wolf[183] carried out a histopathologic study in one case. They found atrophy and loss of the choriocapillaris, beginning near the equator and becoming more pronounced at the posterior pole. There were degenerative changes in Bruch's membrane and RPE. A selective loss of the outer retinal elements was particularly marked posteriorly.

The pathogenesis of CACD is probably to be found in primary dystrophy of the choroidal vessels, although primary tapetochoroidal dystrophy or primary dystrophy of the pigment epithelium with secondary choroidal involvement cannot be ruled out. Sclerosis of the choroidal vessels as a causative factor is unlikely in view of the histologic absence of sclerotic vessels. However, considering the early stages of this condition, in which only slight pigment changes of the macula are seen with already markedly diminished vision,[173,181] the question arises whether or not this condition involves a primary tapetoretinal lesion, as does progressive foveal dystrophy.

Mode of inheritance

There are reports of families with autosomal dominant transmission of CACD,[173,175,181] as well as of families in which an autosomal recessive pattern seems to prevail.[174,175]

Genetics

In the patients we examined, we were able to demonstrate autosomal dominant inheritance in seven pedigrees.[184] In these pedigrees we found that this dystrophy was caused by a mutation in the peripherin/RDS gene, located on the short arm of chromosome 6.[185] The defect in a CACD family from Northern Ireland has been linked to chromosome 17p13, but the gene has not yet been identified.[186,187]

Differential diagnosis

Differential diagnosis may be difficult, particularly if we deal with sporadic cases. We merely mention the following conditions that may be considered:

Pseudoinflammatory dystrophy (Sorsby)
Choroideremia
Myopia gravior
Macular coloboma
Angioid streaks
Diffuse, generalized choroidal dystrophy (gyrate atrophy)
Peripapillary and circinate choroidal dystrophy
End stages of Stargardt's disease

Cone dystrophy
Progressive bifocal chorioretinal atrophy[18]
Multifocal placoid pigment epitheliopathy[188]
Serpiginous choroiditis (Fig. 64-41).

ACUTE MACULAR NEURORETINOPATHY

Acute macular neuroretinitis causes a sudden decrease in visual acuity or paracentral scotomata. The ophthalmoscopic lesions consist of darkish, brown-red, wedge-shaped dots in the macula, pointing to the foveola. These dots are located mostly on the nasal side of the macula and have been seen by us in five women and one man (Figs 64-42 and 64-43).

Neuroretinitis occurs in young adults and may be unilateral or bilateral. Biomicroscopic examination shows that the lesions are located in the superficial layers of the retina. The retinal vessels, pigment epithelium, and optic disc show no distinct pathologic features. The fluorescein angiogram shows no abnormalities or only questionably dilated perimacular capillaries without leakage. Static perimetric analysis delineates dense paracentral scotomata. Recovery is very slow, and the affection may last longer than 1 or 2 years. Ophthalmoscopic, fluorescein angiographic, and perimetric analyses exclude an affection of the pigment epithelium, the nerve fiber layer, or the optic disc.

The affection appears to be localized superficially in the retina and is therefore called *acute macular neuroretinopathy*.[189–191]

ACUTE PIGMENT EPITHELIITIS

Acute retinal pigment epitheliitis is an eye affection in which the patient experiences, rather acutely, a considerable loss of

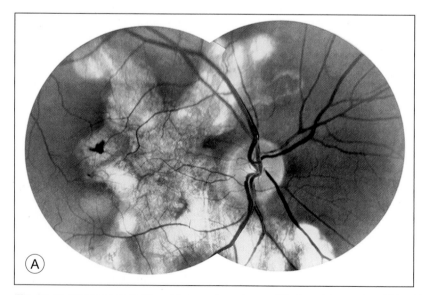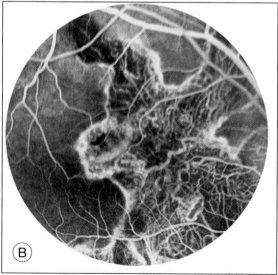

Fig. 64-41 Red-free image (A) and fluorescein angiogram (B) of serpiginous choroiditis with helicoid extensions in the posterior pole. There is extensive atrophy of the retinal pigment epithelium and choriocapillaris in the posterior pole.

visual acuity in one or both eyes and in which particularly subtle changes are perceptible in the pigment epithelium.

The ophthalmoscopic abnormalities consist of one or several clusters of dark spots, each surrounded by a small halo resulting from defects in the macular pigment epithelium. No leakage of fluorescein, as in central serous choroidopathy, is present.

The complaints of the patient, a young adult, disappear after 7 to 11 weeks, and visual acuity returns to normal values.

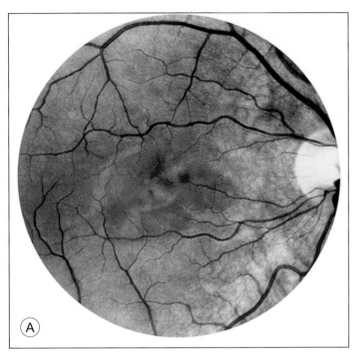
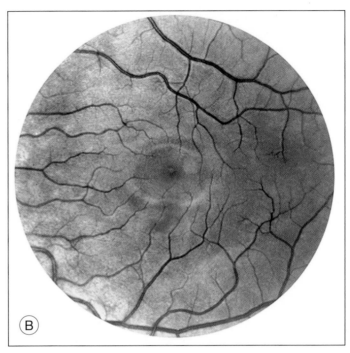

Fig. 64-42 Characteristic macular changes in acute macular neuroretinopathy.

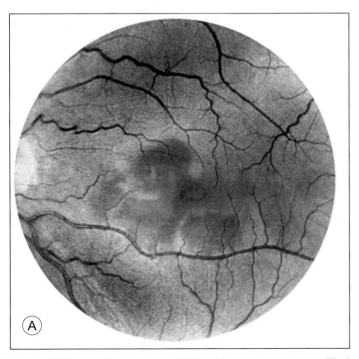
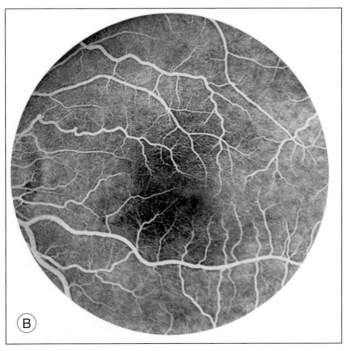

Fig. 64-43 Conventional photograph (A) and fluorescein angiogram (B) of acute macular neuroretinopathy.

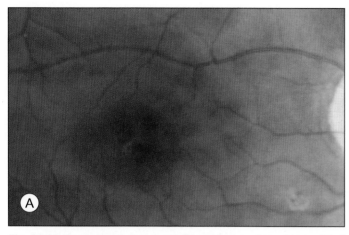 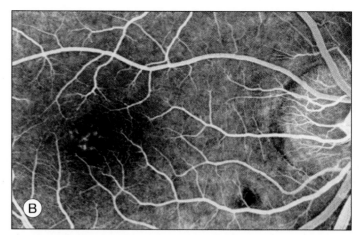

Fig. 64-44 Conventional photograph (A) and fluorescein angiogram (B) of acute retinal pigment epitheliitis.

The pigmentary changes usually remain visible. No other ocular or general disturbances are found. The EOG appears to be affected in the early stages of the disease. The acute occurrence of the affection and the self-limiting course suggest a viral inflammation of the pigment epithelium[37,48] (Figs 64-44 and 64-45).

MOLECULAR GENETICS OF MACULAR DYSTROPHIES

More genetic localizations and the genes causing macular dystrophies have been discovered in the past few years. At the time we wrote this chapter the localizations and genes presented in Table 64-1 were known.

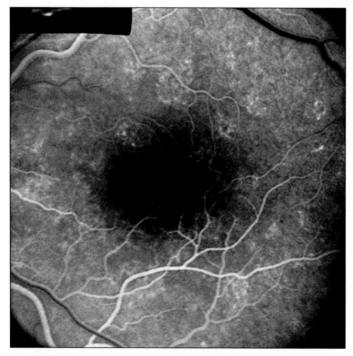

Fig. 64-45 Fluorescein angiogram of acute retinal pigment epitheliitis, showing spots of mild pigment epithelial atrophy around the fovea.

SUMMARY

The long-accepted view that many different manifestations of hereditary foveal dystrophies are all expressions of the same basic dystrophic process is untenable. There are many different, distinguishable entities among the hereditary macular dystrophies. In the future it is likely that more "splitting" will present new entities with individual, distinct properties.

This may be illustrated by our recent discovery of a pedigree with exceptional ophthalmoscopic and retinal functional findings. Because this dystrophy cannot be fitted into one of the existing dystrophy categories, this might possibly be a "new" dystrophy. A mother and her two children (girl and boy), who had hardly any complaints, demonstrated typical bull's-eye lesions in their maculae, slightly attenuated vessels, and pigment mottling in the peripheries. Visual acuity and color vision were normal, or close to normal, and visual fields demonstrated some loss of central sensitivity and normal peripheries. ERG resulted in scotopic and photopic values that were 50% of normal, and the EOGs were subnormal. Dark adaptation was slightly delayed and elevated. This appears to be a dominant, benign bull's-eye dystrophy, definitely different from cone dystrophy and other similar conditions.

To investigate foveal dystrophies properly it is necessary to perform detailed retinal function tests (visual acuity, visual fields, color vision, dark adaptation, ERG, EOG, and fluorescein angiography).

Histochemical and biochemical research, it is hoped, will yield more information on the pathologic changes underlying this interesting group of conditions. As long as no truly effective therapies are available, it is important to correct refractive errors, assure most patients that total blindness will not ensue, and refrain from unnecessary therapy.

ACKNOWLEDGMENT

We would like to thank Mr A.L. Aandekerk FOPS, for his kind help with the photographic part of this chapter.

Table 64-1 Chromosomal localization and genes typically associated with macular dystrophies

Chromosome	Locus	Gene	Diagnosis	Reference
1p21-p22	STGD1	ABCA4	Stargardt disease, fundus flavimaculatus, cone–rod dystrophy; age-related macular degeneration	Allikmets[57,192] Lewis[193]
1q25-q31	ARMD	HEMICENTIN-1	Age-related macular degeneration	Klein[194] Schultz[171]
1q12-q24	CORD8	–	Recessive cone–rod dystrophy	Khaliq[182]
2p16	DHRD MTLV	EFEMP1	Doyne honeycomb retinal dystrophy (dominant drusen)	Edwards[195] Kermani[196] Stone[138]
3p13-p12	ADCA2	SCA7	Progressive macular dystrophy and cerebellar atrophy	Del-Favero[197]
4p	STGD 4	–	Dominant Stargardt-like macular dystrophy	Kniazeva[66]
4p16.3-p15.2	MCDR2	–	Bull's-eye macular dystrophy	Michaelides[198]
5p15.33-p13.1	MCDR3	–	Macular dystrophy	Michaelides[199]
6p21.2	RDS	Peripherin/RDS	(Adult vitelliform) macular dystrophy, dominant central areolar choroidal dystrophy	Arikawa[200] Felbor[201] Hoyng[185]
6p21.1	COD3	GUCA1A	Dominant cone dystrophy	Payne[43] Sokal[202]
6p12.3-q16	BCAMD	–	Benign concentric annular macular dystrophy	Van Lith-Verhoeven[125]
6q13	CORD7	RIM1	Dominant cone–rod dystrophy	Kelsell[203] Johnson[204]
6q14-q16.2	MCDR1 PBCRA	–	North Carolina macular dystrophy, progressive bifocal choroidal dystrophy	Small[205] Kelsell[206]
6q25-q26	RCD1	–	Dominant retinal cone dystrophy	Online Mendelian
6q14.1	STGD3 DD	ELOVL4	Dominant Stargardt-like disease	Griesinger[207] Zhang[69]
7p21-p15	CYMD	–	Dominant cystoid macular edema	Kremer[114]
8p11	CORD9	–	Recessive cone–rod dystrophy	Danciger[208]
11q13	VMD2	Bestrophin	Dominant macular dystrophy, Best type	Petrukhin[86] Marquardt[209]
11q23.3	CTRP5	C1QTNF5	Dominant MD, late onset	Hayward[210]
12q13.2	RDH1	RDH5	Recessive fundus albipunctatus; recessive cone dystrophy	Yamamoto[211]
16p13.11	PXE	ABCC6	Recessive and dominant pseudoxanthoma elasticum	Bergen[165]
17p	CACD	–	Dominant central areolar choroidal dystrophy	Hughes[186]
17p13.2	–	AIPL1	Dominant cone–rod dystrophy	Sohocki[212]
17p13.1	CORD6	GUCY2D	Dominant cone–rod dystrophy	Kelsell[213,214]
17q11.2	–	UNC119	Dominant cone–rod dystrophy	Kobayashi[215]
19q13.3	CORD2	CRX	Dominant cone–rod dystrophy	Freund[216]
22q12.1-q13.2	SFD	TIMP3	Dominant Sorsby's fundus dystrophy	Weber[155,156]
Xp22.13	XLRS1	RS1	Retinoschisis	Sauer[217]
Xp11.4-q13.1	COD4	–	X-linked progressive cone–rod dystrophy	Jalkanen[218]
Xp11.4	–	RPGR	X-linked cone dystrophy, X-linked atrophic MD	Ayyagari[73]
Xq27	COD2	–	X-linked progressive cone dystrophy	Bergen[46]

REFERENCES

1. Duke-Elder S, ed. System of ophthalmology, vol 10: Diseases of the retina. St Louis: Mosby, 1967.
2. Behr C. Die Heredodegeneration der Makula. Klin Monatsbl Augenheilkd 1920; 65:465.
3. Leber T. Die Krankheiten der Netzhaut. In: Graefe–Saemisch–Hess Handbuch des gesamten Augenheilkunde, 2nd edn, vol 7. Leipzig: Engelmann, 1915–1916.
4. Deutman AF. Hereditary dystrophies of the central retina and choroid. In: Winkelman JE, Crone RA, eds. Perspectives in ophthalmology, vol 2. Amsterdam: Excerpta Medica, 1970.
5. Deutman AF. The hereditary dystrophies of the posterior pole of the eye. Assen, Netherlands: Van Gorcum, 1971.
6. Stargardt K. Ueber familiare Degeneration in der Maculagegend des Auges, mit und ohne psychische Storungen. Arch Psychiatr Nervenkr 1917; 58:852.
7. Waardenburg PJ. Genetics and ophthalmology, vol 2. Assen, Netherlands: Van Gorcum, 1963.
8. Craandijk A, AandeKerk AL. Retinal photography using panchromatic and orthochromatic films. Br J Ophthalmol 1969; 53:568–573.
9. Lefler WH, Wadsworth JA, Sidbury JB Jr. Hereditary macular degeneration and amino-aciduria. Am J Ophthalmol 1971; 1:224–230.
10. Noble KG, Carr RE, Siegel IM. Pigment epithelial dystrophy. Am J Ophthalmol 1977; 83:751–757.
11. Daily MJ, Mets MB. Fenestrated sheen macular dystrophy. Arch Ophthalmol 1984; 102:855–856.
12. O'Donnell FE Jr, Welch RB. Fenestrated sheen macular dystrophy. A new autosomal dominant maculopathy. Arch Ophthalmol 1979; 97:1292–1296.
13. Slagsvold JE. Fenestrated sheen macular dystrophy. A new autosomal dominant maculopathy. Acta Ophthalmol. (Copenh) 1981; 59:683–688.
14. Blodi F. The pathology of central tapeto-retinal dystrophy (hereditary macular degenerations). Trans Am Acad Ophthalmol Otolaryngol 1966; 70:1047.
15. Braley AE. Dystrophy of the macula. Am J Ophthalmol 1966; 61:1–24.
16. Ricci, A: Case of tapetal reflex with inverse Mizuo phenomenon. Bull Soc Ophtalmol Fr 1968; 68:459–461.
17. Babel J, Farpour H. The genetic origin of colobomatous fossae of the optic nerve. J Genet Hum. 1967; 16:187–198.
18. Douglas AA, Waheed I, Wyse CT. Progressive bifocal chorio-retinal atrophy. A rare familial disease of the eyes. Br J Ophthalmol 1968; 52:742–751.

19. George ND, Yates JR, Moore AT. Clinical features in affected males with X-linked retinoschisis. Arch Ophthalmol 1996; 114:274–280.
20. Haas J. Ueber das Zusammenvorkommen von Veranderungen der Retina und Chorioidea. Arch Augenheilkd 1898; 37:343.
21. Tasman W, Greven C, Moreno R. Nasal retinal dragging in X-linked retinoschisis. Graefes Arch Clin Exp Ophthalmol 1991; 229:319–322.
22. Chew E, Pinckers A. Bilateral retinal detachment in X-linked juvenile retinoschisis. Ophthalmic Paediatr Genet 1983; 2:89.
23. Laatikainen L, Tarkkanen A, Saksela T. Hereditary X-linked retinoschisis and bilateral congenital retinal detachment. Retina 1987; 7:24–27.
24. Krause U, Vainio-Mattila B, Eriksson A et al. Fluorescein angiographic studies on X-chromosomal retinoschisis. Acta Ophthalmol (Copenh) 1970; 48:794–807.
25. Eriksson U, Larsson E, Holmstrom G. Optical coherence tomography in the diagnosis of juvenile X-linked retinoschisis. Acta Ophthalmol Scand 2004; 82:218–223.
26. Krill AE, Fishman GA. Acquired color vision defects. Trans Am Acad Ophthalmol Otolaryngol 1971; 75:1095–1111.
27. Manschot WA. Hereditary diseases with retinal detachment. Ned Tijdschr Geneeskd 1969; 113:2260–2261.
28. Yanoff M, Kertesz RE, Zimmerman LE. Histopathology of juvenile retinoschisis. Arch Ophthalmol 1968; 79:49–53.
29. Dowling JE. Organization of vertebrate retinas. Invest Ophthalmol 1970; 9:655–680.
30. Jager G. A hereditary affection of the retina. Ophthalmologica 1953; 125:470.
31. Condon GP, Brownstein S, Wang NS et al. Congenital hereditary (juvenile X-linked) retinoschisis. Histopathologic and ultrastructural findings in three eyes. Arch Ophthalmol 1986; 104:576–583.
32. Lewis RA, Lee GB, Martonyi CL et al. Familial foveal retinoschisis. Arch Ophthalmol 1977; 95:1190–1196.
33. Forsius E, Erikson A, Damsten M et al. Recessive central retinoschisis. Doc Ophthalmol Proc Ser 1978; 17:245.
34. Sauer CG, Gehrig A, Warneke-Wittstock R et al. Positional cloning of the gene associated with X-linked juvenile retinoschisis. Nat Genet 1997; 17:164–170.
35. Grayson C, Reid SN, Ellis JA et al. Retinoschisin, the X-linked retinoschisis protein, is a secreted photoreceptor protein, and is expressed and released by Weri-Rb1 cells. Hum Mol Genet 2000; 9:1873–1879.
36. Goodman G, Ripps H, Siegel I. Cone dysfunction syndromes. Arch Ophthalmol 1963; 70:214.
37. Krill AE, Deutman AF. Dominant macular degenerations. The cone dystrophies. Am J Ophthalmol 1972; 73:352–369.
38. Krill AE, Deutman AF, Fishman M. The cone degenerations. Doc Ophthalmol 1973; 35:1–80.
39. Siegel IM, Smith BF. Acquired cone dysfunction. Arch Ophthalmol 1967; 77:8–13.
40. Berson EL, Gouras P, Gunkel RD. Progressive cone degeneration, dominantly inherited. Arch Ophthalmol 1968; 80:77–83.
41. Vail D, Shoch D. Hereditary degeneration of the macula. II. Follow-up report and histopathologic study. Trans Am Ophthalmol Soc 1965; 63:51–63.
42. Balciuniene J, Johansson K, Sandgren O et al. A gene for autosomal dominant progressive cone dystrophy (CORD5) maps to chromosome 17p12-p13. Genomics 1995; 30:281–286.
43. Payne AM, Downes SM, Bessant DA et al. A mutation in guanylate cyclase activator 1A (GUCA1A) in an autosomal dominant cone dystrophy pedigree mapping to a new locus on chromosome 6p21.1. Hum Mol Genet 1998; 7:273–277.
44. Small KW, Syrquin M, Mullen L et al. Mapping of autosomal dominant cone degeneration to chromosome 17p. Am J Ophthalmol 1996; 121:13–18.
45. Tranebjaerg L, Sjo O, Warburg M. Retinal cone dysfunction and mental retardation associated with a de novo balanced translocation 1;6(q44;q27). Ophthalmic Paediatr Genet 1986; 7:167–173.
46. Bergen AA, Pinckers AJ. Localization of a novel X-linked progressive cone dystrophy gene to Xq27: evidence for genetic heterogeneity. Am J Hum Genet 1997; 60:1468–1473.
47. Demirci FY, Rigatti BW, Wen G et al. X-linked cone–rod dystrophy (locus COD1): identification of mutations in RPGR exon ORF15. Am J Hum Genet 2002; 70:1049–1053.
48. Deutman AF. Acute retinal pigment epitheliitis. Am J Ophthalmol 1974; 78:571–578.
49. Krill AE, Deutman AF. The various categories of juvenile macular degeneration. Trans Am Ophthalmol Soc 1972; 70:220–245.
50. Stargardt K. Ueber familiare Degeneration in der Maculagegend des Auges. Graefes Arch Clin Exp Ophthalmol 1909; 71:534.
51. Stargardt K. Ueber familiare Degeneration in der Maculagegend des Auges. Graefes Arch Clin Exp Ophthalmol 1913; 30:95.
52. Stargardt K. Zur kasuistik der "familiaren, progressiven degeneration in der makulagegend des auges." Z Augenheilk 1916; 35:249.
53. Stargardt K. Ein fall von familiarer progressiver Makuladegeneration-degeneration. Klin Monatsbl Augenheilkd 1925; 75:246.
54. Franceschetti A, Francois J. Fundus flavimaculatus. Arch Ophthalmol Rev Gen Ophtalmol 1965; 25:505–530.
55. Agatston II. Retinitis albescens with macular involvement. Am J Ophthalmol 1949; 32:275.
56. Friemann W. Heredodegeneration der Makula mit Hyperkinesen. Klin Monatsbl Augenheilkd 1955; 126:460–469.
57. Allikmets R, Singh N, Sun H et al. A photoreceptor cell-specific ATP-binding transporter gene (ABCR) is mutated in recessive Stargardt macular dystrophy. Nat Genet 1997; 15:236–246.
58. Cremers FP, van de Pol DJ, van Driel M et al. Autosomal recessive retinitis pigmentosa and cone–rod dystrophy caused by splice site mutations in the Stargardt's disease gene ABCR. Hum Mol Genet 1998; 7:355–362.
59. Rosher K. Ueber den weiteren verlauf der von Stargardt und Behr beschriebenen familiaren degeneration der Makula. Klin Monatsbl Augenheilkd 1954; 124:171.
60. Klien BA, Krill AE. Fundus flavimaculatus. Clinical, functional and histopathologic observations. Am J Ophthalmol 1967; 64:3–23.
61. Eagle RC Jr, Lucier AC, Bernardino VB Jr et al. Retinal pigment epithelial abnormalities in fundus flavimaculatus: a light and electron microscopic study. Ophthalmology 1980; 87:1189–1200.
62. Steinmetz RL, Garner A, Maguire JI et al. Histopathology of incipient fundus flavimaculatus. Ophthalmology 1991; 98:953–956.
63. Cibis GW, Morey M, Harris DJ. Dominantly inherited macular dystrophy with flecks (Stargardt). Arch Ophthalmol 1980; 98:1785–1789.
64. Lopez PF, Maumenee IH de la CZ, Green WR. Autosomal-dominant fundus flavimaculatus. Clinicopathologic correlation. Ophthalmology 1990; 97:798–809.
65. Mansour AM. Long-term follow-up of dominant macular dystrophy with flecks (Stargardt). Ophthalmologica 1992; 205:138–143.
66. Kniazeva M, Chiang MF, Morgan B et al. A new locus for autosomal dominant Stargardt-like disease maps to chromosome 4. Am J Hum Genet 1999; 64:1394–1399.
67. Stone EM, Brain E, Kimura AE et al. Clinical features of a Stargardt-like dominant progressive macular dystrophy with genetic linkage to chromosome 6q. Arch Ophthalmol 1994; 112:765–772.
68. Bernstein PS, Tammur J, Singh N et al. Diverse macular dystrophy phenotype caused by a novel complex mutation in the ELOVL4 gene. Invest Ophthalmol Vis Sci 2001; 42:3331–3336.
69. Zhang K, Kniazeva M, Han M et al. A 5-bp deletion in ELOVL4 is associated with two related forms of autosomal dominant macular dystrophy. Nat Genet 2001; 27:89–93.
70. Szlyk JP, Fishman GA, Alexander KR et al. Clinical subtypes of cone–rod dystrophy. Arch Ophthalmol 1993; 111:781–788.
71. Herron WL Jr, Riegel BW, Rubin ML. Outer segment production and removal in the degenerating retina of the dystrophic rat. Invest Ophthalmol 1971; 10:54–63.
72. Krill AE, Archer D, Martin D. Sector retinitis pigmentosa. Am J Ophthalmol 1970; 69:977–987.
73. Ayyagari R, Demirci FY, Liu J et al. X-linked recessive atrophic macular degeneration from RPGR mutation. Genomics 2002; 80:166–171.
74. Best F. Ueber eine hereditaere Makulaaffection. Beitraege zur Vererbungslehre. Zschr Augenheilk 1905; 13:199–212.
75. Braley AE, Spivey BE. Hereditary vitelline macular degeneration. A clinical and functional evaluation of a new pedigree with variable expressivity and dominant inheritance. Arch Ophthalmol 1964; 72:743–762.
76. Krill AE, Morse PA, Potts AM et al. Hereditary vitelliruptive macular degeneration. Am J Ophthalmol 1966; 61:1405–1415.
77. Zanen J, Rausin G. Kyste vitelliforme congenital de la macula. Bull Soc Belge Ophtalmol 1950; 96:544.
78. Berard P. In: Discussion. Bonnet JL et al. Bull Soc Ophtalmol Fr 1966; 66:977.
79. Behr C. Die Anatomie der "senilen Macula" (der senilen Form der makularen Heredodegeneration). Klin Monatsbl Augenheilkd 1921; 67:551.
80. Deutman AF. Electro-oculography in families with vitelliform dystrophy of the fovea. Detection of the carrier state. Arch Ophthalmol 1969; 81:305–316.
81. McFarland CB. Heredodegeneration of the macula lutea; a study of the clinical and pathologic aspects. Am Arch Opthalmol 1955; 53:224–228.
83. Frangieh GT, Green WR, Fine SL. A histopathologic study of Best's macular dystrophy. Arch Ophthalmol 1982; 100:1115–1121.
83. Weingeist TA, Kobrin JL, Watzke RC. Histopathology of Best's macular dystrophy. Arch Ophthalmol 1982; 100:1108–1114.
84. Graff C, Forsman K, Larsson C et al. Fine mapping of Best's macular dystrophy localizes the gene in close proximity to but distinct from the D11S480/ROM1 loci. Genomics 1994; 24:425–434.
85. Nichols BE, Bascom R, Litt M et al. Refining the locus for Best vitelliform macular dystrophy and mutation analysis of the candidate gene ROM1. Am J Hum Genet 1994; 54:95–103.

86. Petrukhin K, Koisti MJ, Bakall B et al. Identification of the gene responsible for Best macular dystrophy. Nat Genet 1998; 19:241–247.

87. Stone EM, Nichols BE, Streb LM et al. Genetic linkage of vitelliform macular degeneration (Best's disease) to chromosome 11q13. Nat Genet 1992; 1:2 46–250.

88. Weber BH, Walker D, Muller B et al. Best's vitelliform dystrophy (VMD2) maps between D11S903 and PYGM: no evidence for locus heterogeneity. Genomics 1994; 20:267–274.

89. Marmorstein AD, Marmorstein LY, Rayborn M et al. Bestrophin, the product of the Best vitelliform macular dystrophy gene (VMD2), localizes to the basolateral plasma membrane of the retinal pigment epithelium. Proc Natl Acad Sci USA 2000; 97:12758–12763.

90. Sun H, Tsunenari T, Yau KW et al. The vitelliform macular dystrophy protein defines a new family of chloride channels. Proc Natl Acad Sci USA 2002; 99:4008–4013.

91. Pianta MJ, Aleman TS, Cideciyan AV et al. In vivo micropathology of Best macular dystrophy with optical coherence tomography. Exp Eye Res 2003; 76:203–211.

92. Mansergh FC, Kenna PF, Rudolph G et al. Evidence for genetic heterogeneity in Best's vitelliform macular dystrophy. J Med Genet 1995; 32:855–858.

93. Vine AK, Schatz H. Adult-onset foveomacular pigment epithelial dystrophy. Am J Ophthalmol 1980; 89:680–691.

94. Newell FW, Krill AE, Farkas TG. Drusen and fundus flavimaculatus: clinical, functional, and histologic characteristics. Trans Am Acad Ophthalmol Otolaryngol 1972; 76:88–100.

95. Gerber S, Rozet J, Bonneau D et al. A gene for late-onset fundus flavimaculatus with macular dystrophy maps to chromosome 1p13. Am J Hum Genet 1995; 56:396–399.

96. Deutman AF, van Blommestein JD, Henkes HE et al. Butterfly-shaped pigment dystrophy of the fovea. Arch Ophthalmol 1970; 83:558–569.

97. Gutman I, Walsh JB, Henkind P. Vitelliform macular dystrophy and butterfly-shaped epithelial dystrophy: a continuum? Br J Ophthalmol 1982; 66:163–173.

98. Lodato G, Giuffre G. Unusual associations of pattern dystrophies. J Fr Ophtalmol 1985; 8:147–154.

99. Zhang K, Garibaldi DC, Li Y et al. Butterfly-shaped pattern dystrophy: a genetic, clinical, and histopathological report. Arch Ophthalmol 2002; 120:485–490.

100. Nichols BE, Drack AV, Vandenburgh K et al. A 2 base pair deletion in the RDS gene associated with butterfly-shaped pigment dystrophy of the fovea. Hum Mol Genet 1993; 2:1347.

101. Nichols BE, Sheffield VC, Vandenburgh K et al. Butterfly-shaped pigment dystrophy of the fovea caused by a point mutation in codon 167 of the RDS gene. Nat Genet 1993; 3:202–207.

102. Lith-Verhoeven JJC, Cremers FPM, van den Helm B et al. Genetic heterogeneity of butterfly-shaped pigment dystrophy of the fovea. Mol Vis 2003; 9:138–143.

103. Amalric P, Schum U. Pigmented, paravenous retinal and choroidal atrophy. Klin Monatsbl Augenheilkd 1968; 153:763–775.

104. Chew E, Deutman A, Cruysberg J. Macular changes in myotonic dystrophy. In: Ryan SJ, Dawson AK, Little HL, eds. Retinal diseases. Orlando, Fla: Grune & Stratton, 1985.

105. Sjögren H. Dystrophia reticularis laminae pigmentosae retinae: an earlier not described hereditary eye disease. Acta Ophthalmol (Copenh) 1950; 28:279.

106. Benedikt O, Werner W. Retikulare Pigmentdystrophie der Netz-haut. Klin Monatsbl Augenheilkd 1971; 159:794.

107. Deutman AF, Rumke AM. Reticular dystrophy of the retinal pigment epithelium. Dystrophia reticularis laminae pigmentosa retinae of H. Sjogren. Arch Ophthalmol 1969; 82:4–9.

108. Kingham JD, Fenzl RE, Willerson D et al. Reticular dystrophy of the retinal pigment epithelium. A clinical and electrophysiologic study of three generations. Arch Ophthalmol 1978; 96:1177–1184.

109. Weeks DE, Conley YP, Tsai HJ et al. Age-related maculopathy: an expanded genome-wide scan with evidence of susceptibility loci within the 1q31 and 17q25 regions. Am J Ophthalmol 2001; 132:682–692.

110. Mesker RP, Oosterhuis JA, Delleman JW. A retinal lesion resembling Sjögren's dystrophia reticularis laminae pigmentosae retinae. In: Winkelman JE, Crone RA, eds. Perspectives in ophthalmology, vol 2. Amsterdam: Excerpta Medica, 1970.

111. Deutman AF, Pinckers A, Aandekerk AL. Dominantly inherited cystoid macular edema. Am J Ophthalmol 1976; 82:540–548.

112. Notting JG, Pinckers JL. Dominant cystoid macular dystrophy. Am J Ophthalmol 1977; 83:234–241.

113. Pinckers A, Deutman AF, Notting JG. Retinal functions in dominant cystoid macular dystrophy (DCMD). Acta Ophthalmol (Copenh) 1976; 54:579–590.

114. Kremer, H, Pinckers, A, van den Helm, B et al. Localization of the gene for dominant cystoid macular dystrophy on chromosome 7p. Hum Mol Genet 1994; 3:299–302.

115. Forgacs J, Bozin I. Familial manifestations of grouped pigmentation in macular region. Ophthalmologica 1966; 152:364–368.

116. Perera C. Congenital grouped pigmentation of the retina: report of a case. Arch Ophthalmol 1939; 21:108.

117. Loewenstein A, Steel J. Special case of melanosis fundi: bilateral congenital group pigmentation of the central area. Br J Ophthalmol 1941; 25:417.

118. Krill AE, Deutman AF. Acute retinal pigment epitheliitus. Am J Ophthalmol 1972; 74:193–205.

119. Deutman AF. Benign concentric annular macular dystrophy. Am J Ophthalmol 1974; 78:384–396.

120. van den Biesen PR, Deutman AF, Pinckers AJ. Evolution of benign concentric annular macular dystrophy. Am J Ophthalmol 1985; 100:73–78.

121. Coppeto J, Ayazi S. Annular macular dystrophy. Am J Ophthalmol 1982; 93:279–284.

122. Miyake Y, Shiroyama N, Horiguchi M et al. Bull's-eye maculopathy and negative electroretinogram. Retina 1989; 9:210–215.

123. Sadowski B, Rohrbach JM, Partsch M et al. Benign concentric annular macular dystrophy. Klin Monatsbl Augenheilkd 1994; 205:173–175.

124. Singh AJ. Concentric annular macular dystrophy. Eye 2001; 15:340–342.

125. Lith-Verhoeven JJC, Hoyng CB, van den Helm B et al. The benign concentric annular macular dystrophy locus maps to 6p12.3-q16. Invest Ophthalmol Vis Sci 2004; 45:30–35.

126. Deutman AF, Jansen LM. Dominantly inherited drusen of Bruch's membrane. Br J Ophthalmol 1970; 54:373–382.

127. Coats G. The structure of the membrane of Bruch, and its relation to the formation of colloid excrescences. R Lond Ophthalmol Hosp Rep 1904; 16:164.

128. Wolter J. Die Histogenese der Drusen im Pigmentepithel der Netzhaut des menschlichen Auges. Klin Monatsbl Augenheilkd 1957; 130:86.

129. Forni S, Babel J. Clinical and histological study of the disease of Leventina. Disease belonging to the group of hyaline degenerescences of the posterior pole. Ophthalmologica 1962; 143:313–322.

130. Wolter J. Hyaline bodies of ganglion-cell origin in the human retina. Arch Ophthalmol 1959; 61:127.

131. Seitz R. The drusen of the retina. Ber Zusammenkunft Dtsch Ophthalmol Ges 1968; 68:373–376.

132. Farkas TG, Sylvester V, Archer D et al. The histochemistry of drusen. Am J Ophthalmol 1971; 71:1206–1215.

133. Farkas TG, Sylvester V, Archer D. The ultrastructure of drusen. Am J Ophthalmol 1971; 71:1196–1205.

134. Pearce W. Genetic aspects of Doyne's honeycomb degeneration of the retina. Ann Hum Genet 1967; 31:173.

135. Gregory CY, Evans K, Wijesuriya SD et al. The gene responsible for autosomal dominant Doyne's honeycomb retinal dystrophy (DHRD) maps to chromosome 2p16. Hum Mol Genet 1996; 5:1055–1059.

136. Heon E, Piguet B, Munier F et al. Linkage of autosomal dominant radial drusen (malattia leventinese) to chromosome 2p16-21. Arch Ophthalmol 1996; 114:193–198.

137. Matsumoto M, Traboulsi EI. Dominant radial drusen and Arg345Trp EFEMP1 mutation. Am J Ophthalmol 2001; 131:810–812.

138. Stone EM, Lotery AJ, Munier FL et al. A single EFEMP1 mutation associated with both Malattia Leventinese and Doyne honeycomb retinal dystrophy. Nat Genet 1999; 22:199–202.

139. Tarttelin EE, Gregory-Evans CY, Bird AC et al. Molecular genetic heterogeneity in autosomal dominant drusen. J Med Genet 2001; 38:381–384.

140. Kniazeva M, Traboulsi EI, Yu Z et al. A new locus for dominant drusen and macular degeneration maps to chromosome 6q14. Am J Ophthalmol 2000; 130:197–202.

141. Stefko ST, Zhang K, Gorin MB et al. Clinical spectrum of chromosome 6-linked autosomal dominant drusen and macular degeneration. Am J Ophthalmol 2000; 130:203–208.

142. Klevering BJ, van Driel M, van Hogerwou AJ et al. Central areolar choroidal dystrophy associated with dominantly inherited drusen. Br J Ophthalmol 2002; 86:91–96.

143. Francois J, Bacskulin J, Follmann P. Ocular manifestations of the Urbach–Wiethe syndrome. Hyalitis of the skin and the mucosa. Ophthalmologica 1968; 155:433–448.

144. Sorsby A, Mason M, Gardener N. A fundus dystrophy with unusual features. Br J Ophthalmol 1949; 33:67.

145. Hoskin A, Sehmi K, Bird AC. Sorsby's pseudoinflammatory macular dystrophy. Br J Ophthalmol 1981; 65:859–865.

146. Peters AL, Greenberg J. Sorsby's fundus dystrophy. A South African family with a point mutation on the tissue inhibitor of metalloproteinases-3 gene on chromosome 22. Retina 1995; 15:480–485.

147. Wijesuriya SD, Evans K, Jay MR et al. Sorsby's fundus dystrophy in the British Isles: demonstration of a striking founder effect by microsatellite-generated haplotypes. Genome Res 1996; 6: 92–101.

148. Lip PL, Good PA, Gibson JM. Sorsby's fundus dystrophy: a case report of 24 years follow-up with electrodiagnostic tests and indocyanine green angiography. Eye 1999; 13:16–25.

149. Rosen ES, Leighton D. Fluorescein photography of generalized dominant fundus dystrophy. Br J Ophthalmol 1968; 52:828–832.

150. Cox J. Colour vision defects acquired in diseases of the eye. Br J Physiol Opt 1960; 17:195–216.

151. Franceschetti A, Francois J, Bable J. Les heredo-degenerescences chorioretiniennes: degenerescences tapeto-retiniennes. Paris: Masson, 1963.

152. Ashton N, Sorsby A. Fundus dystrophy with unusual features: a histological study. Br J Ophthalmol 1951; 35:751.

153. Babel J. Le role de la choriocapillaire dans lens affections degeneratives du pole posterieur. Bull Mem Soc Fr Ophtalmol 1958; 71:389.

154. Burn R. Further cases of a fundus dystrophy with unusual features. Br J Ophthalmol 1950; 34:393.

155. Weber BH, Vogt G, Pruett RC et al. Mutations in the tissue inhibitor of metalloproteinases-3 (TIMP3) in patients with Sorsby's fundus dystrophy. Nat Genet 1994; 8:352–356.

156. Weber BH, Vogt G, Wolz W et al. Sorsby's fundus dystrophy is genetically linked to chromosome 22q13-qter. Nat Genet 1994; 7:158–161.

157. Paton D. The relation of angioid streaks to systemic disease. Springfield, Ill: Charles C Thomas, 1972.

158. Deutman AF, Kovacs B. Argon laser treatment in complications of angioid streaks. Am J Ophthalmol 1979; 88:12–17.

159. Gelisken O, Hendrikse F, Deutman AF. A long-term follow-up study of laser coagulation of neovascular membranes in angioid streaks. Am J Ophthalmol 1988; 105:299–303.

160. Klien B. Angioid streaks: a clinical and histopathologic study. Am J Ophthalmol 1947; 30:955.

161. Adelung J. Zur Genese der angioid streaks (Knapp). Klin Monatsbl Augenheilkd 1951; 119:241.

162. Cartwright E, Danks DM, Jack I. Metachromatic fibroblasts in pseudoxanthoma elasticum and Marfan's syndrome. Lancet 1969; 1:533–534.

163. Huang SN, Steele HD, Kumar G et al. Ultrastructural changes of elastic fibers in pseudoxanthoma elasticum. A study of histogenesis. Arch Pathol 1967; 83:108–113.

164. Struk B, Neldner KH, Rao VS et al. Mapping of both autosomal recessive and dominant variants of pseudoxanthoma elasticum to chromosome 16p13.1. Hum Mol Genet 1997; 6:1823–1828.

165. Bergen AA, Plomp AS, Schuurman EJ et al. Mutations in ABCC6 cause pseudoxanthoma elasticum. Nat Genet 2000; 25:228–231.

166. Waardenburg P. Ueber familiarer-erbliche Falle von seniler Maculadegeneration. Genetica 1936; 18:38.

167. Bailliart P. Degenerescence maculaire senile. In: Bailliart P, Coutela CH, Redslob E et al., eds. Traite d'ophthalmologie, vol 5. Paris: Masson, 1939.

168. Francois J. Heredity of senile macular degeneration. Arch Ophtalmol Rev Gen Ophtalmol 1969; 29:899–902.

169. Francois J, Deweer JP. Hereditary senile degenerescence of the macula. Ann Ocul (Paris) 1952; 185:136–154.

170. Klien BA. Some aspects of classification and differential diagnoses of senile macular degeneration. Am J Ophthalmol 1964; 58:927–939.

171. Schultz DW, Klein ML, Humpert AJ et al. Analysis of the ARMD1 locus: evidence that a mutation in HEMICENTIN-1 is associated with age-related macular degeneration in a large family. Hum Mol Genet 2003; 12:3315–3323.

172. Arden G, Fojas M. Electrophysiological abnormalities in pigmentary degenerations of the retina. Arch Ophthalmol 1962; 68:369.

173. Sandvig K. Familial, central, areolar, choroidal atrophy of autosomal dominant inheritance. Acta Ophthalmol (Copenh) 1955; 33:71–78.

174. Sandvig K. Central, areolar choroidal atrophy: a report on four cases. Acta Ophthalmol (Copenh) 1959; 37:325–329.

175. Sorsby, A and Crick, R: Central areolar choroidal sclerosis. Br J Ophthalmol 1953; 37:129.

176. Krill AE, Archer D. Classification of the choroidal atrophies. Am J Ophthalmol 1971; 72:562–585.

177. Ashton N. Central areolar choroidal sclerosis: a histopathological study. Br J Ophthalmol 1953; 37:140.

178. Ferry AP, Llovera I, Shafer DM. Central areolar choroidal dystrophy. Arch Ophthalmol 1972; 88:39–43.

179. Maumenee AE. Clinical entities in "uveitis." An approach to the study of intraocular inflammation. Am J Ophthalmol 1970; 69:1–27.

180. Schlaegel TF Jr. Essentials of uveitis. Symposium on differential diagnostic problems of posterior uveitis. Boston: Little, Brown, 1969.

181. Carr RE. Central areolar choroidal dystrophy Arch Ophthalmol 1965; 73:32–35.

182. Khaliq S, Hameed A, Ismail M et al. Novel locus for autosomal recessive cone–rod dystrophy CORD8 mapping to chromosome 1q12-Q24. Invest Ophthalmol Vis Sci 2000; 41:3709–3712.

183. Howard GM, Wolf E. Central choroidal sclerosis. A clinical and pathological study. Trans Am Acad Ophthalmol Otolaryngol 1964; 68:647–660.

184. Hoyng CB, Deutman AF. The development of central areolar choroidal dystrophy. Graefes Arch Clin Exp Ophthalmol 1996; 234:87–93.

185. Hoyng CB, Huetink P, Testers L et al. Autosomal dominant central areolar choroidal dystrophy caused by a mutation in codon 142 in the peripherin/RDS gene. Am J Ophthalmol 1996; 121:623–629.

186. Hughes AE, Lotery AJ, Silvestri G. Fine localisation of the gene for central areolar choroidal dystrophy on chromosome 17p. J Med Genet 1998; 35:763–772.

187. Lotery AJ, Ennis KT, Silvestri G et al. Localisation of a gene for central areolar choroidal dystrophy to chromosome 17p. Hum Mol Genet 1996; 5:705–708.

188. Gass, JD: Acute posterior multifocal placoid pigment epitheliopathy. Arch Ophthalmol 1968; 80:177–185.

189. Bos PJ, Deutman AF. Acute macular neuroretinopathy. Am J Ophthalmol 1975; 80:573–584.

190. Priluck IA, Buettner H, Robertson DM. Acute macular neuroretinopathy. Am J Ophthalmol 1978; 86:775–778.

191. Rush JA. Acute macular neuroretinopathy. Am J Ophthalmol 1977; 83:490–494.

192. Allikmets R, Shroyer NF, Singh N et al. Mutation of the Stargardt disease gene (ABCR) in age-related macular degeneration. Science 1997; 277:1805–1807.

193. Lewis RA, Shroyer NF, Singh N et al. Genotype/phenotype analysis of a photoreceptor-specific ATP-binding cassette transporter gene, ABCR, in Stargardt disease. Am J Hum Genet 1999; 64:422–434.

194. Klein ML, Schultz DW, Edwards A et al. Age-related macular degeneration. Clinical features in a large family and linkage to chromosome 1q. Arch Ophthalmol 1998; 116:1082–1088.

195. Edwards AO, Klein ML, Berselli CB et al. Malattia leventinese: refinement of the genetic locus and phenotypic variability in autosomal dominant macular drusen. Am J Ophthalmol 1998; 126:417–424.

196. Kermani S, Gregory K, Tarttelin EE et al. Refined genetic and physical positioning of the gene for Doyne honeycomb retinal dystrophy (DHRD). Hum Genet 1999; 104:77–82.

197. Del Favero J, Krols L, Michalik A et al. Molecular genetic analysis of autosomal dominant cerebellar ataxia with retinal degeneration (ADCA type II) caused by CAG triplet repeat expansion. Hum Mol Genet 1998; 7:177–186.

198. Michaelides M, Johnson S, Poulson A et al. An autosomal dominant bull's-eye macular dystrophy (MCDR2) that maps to the short arm of chromosome 4. Invest Ophthalmol Vis Sci 2003; 44:1657–1662.

199. Michaelides M, Johnson S, Tekriwal AK et al. An early-onset autosomal dominant macular dystrophy (MCDR3) resembling North Carolina macular dystrophy maps to chromosome 5. Invest Ophthalmol Vis Sci 2003; 44:2178–2183.

200. Arikawa K, Molday LL, Molday RS et al. Localization of peripherin/rds in the disk membranes of cone and rod photoreceptors: relationship to disk membrane morphogenesis and retinal degeneration. J Cell Biol 1992; 116:659–667.

201. Felbor U, Schilling H, Weber BH. Adult vitelliform macular dystrophy is frequently associated with mutations in the peripherin/RDS gene. Hum Mutat 1997; 10:301–309.

202. Sokal I, Li N, Surguncheva I et al. GCAP1 (Y99C) mutant is constitutively active in autosomal dominant cone dystrophy. Mol Cell 1998; 2:129–133.

203. Kelsell RE, Gregory-Evans GK, Gregory-Evans CY et al. Localization of a gene (CORD7) for a dominant cone–rod dystrophy to chromosome 6q. Am J Hum Genet 1998; 63:274–279.

204. Johnson S, Halford S, Morris AG et al. Genomic organisation and alternative splicing of human RIM1, a gene implicated in autosomal dominant cone–rod dystrophy (CORD7). Genomics 2003; 81:304–314.

205. Small KW, Weber JL, Roses A et al. North Carolina macular dystrophy is assigned to chromosome 6. Genomics 1992; 13:681–685.

206. Kelsell RE, Godley BF, Evans K et al. Localization of the gene for progressive bifocal chorioretinal atrophy (PBCRA) to chromosome 6q. Hum Mol Genet 1995; 4:1653–1656.

207. Griesinger IB, Sieving PA, Ayyagari R. Autosomal dominant macular atrophy at 6q14 excludes CORD7 and MCDR1/PBCRA loci. Invest Ophthalmol Vis Sci 2000; 41:248–255.

208. Danciger M, Hendrickson J, Lyon J et al. CORD9 a new locus for arCRD: mapping to 8p11, estimation of frequency, evaluation of a candidate gene. Invest Ophthalmol Vis Sci 2001; 42:2458–2465.

209. Marquardt A, Stohr H, Passmore LA et al. Mutations in a novel gene, VMD2, encoding a protein of unknown properties cause juvenile-onset vitelliform macular dystrophy (Best's disease). Hum Mol Genet 1998; 7:1517–1525.

210. Hayward C, Shu X, Cideciyan AV et al. Mutation in a short-chain collagen gene, CTRP5, results in extracellular deposit formation in late-onset retinal degeneration: a genetic model for age-related macular degeneration. Hum Mol Genet 2003; 12:2657–2667.

211. Yamamoto H, Simon A, Eriksson U et al. Mutations in the gene encoding 11-cis retinol dehydrogenase cause delayed dark adaptation and fundus albipunctatus. Nat Genet 1999; 22:188–191.

212. Sohocki MM, Perrault I, Leroy BP et al. Prevalence of AIPL1 mutations in inherited retinal degenerative disease. Mol Genet Metab 2000; 70:142–150.

213. Kelsell RE, Evans K, Gregory CY et al. Localisation of a gene for dominant cone–rod dystrophy (CORD6) to chromosome 17p. Hum Mol Genet 1997; 6:597–600.

214. Kelsell RE, Gregory-Evans K, Payne AM et al. Mutations in the retinal guanylate cyclase (RETGC-1) gene in dominant cone–rod dystrophy. Hum Mol Genet 1998; 7:1179–1184.

215. Kobayashi A, Higashide T, Hamasaki D et al. HRG4 (UNC119) mutation found in cone–rod dystrophy causes retinal degeneration in a transgenic model. Invest Ophthalmol Vis Sci 2000; 41:3268–3277.

216. Freund CL, Gregory-Evans CY, Furukawa T et al. Cone–rod dystrophy due to mutations in a novel photoreceptor-specific homeobox gene (CRX) essential for maintenance of the photoreceptor. Cell 1997; 91:543–553.

217. Sauer CG, Gehrig A, Warneke-Wittstock R et al. Positional cloning of the gene associated with X-linked juvenile retinoschisis. Nat Genet 1997; 17:164–170.

218. Jalkanen R, Demirci FY, Tyynismaa H. et al. A new genetic locus for X linked progressive cone–rod dystrophy. J Med Genet 2003; 40:418–423.

Chapter

65

Pharmacotherapy of Age-Related Macular Degeneration

Mark S. Blumenkranz
Darius M. Moshfeghi

INTRODUCTION

Age-related macular degeneration (ARMD) is a spectrum of related diseases that have in common the progressive decline of vision as a consequence of dysfunction of the central retina and its underlying supporting elements, principally the retinal pigment epithelium and choroid in older adults.[1] Although the disease is seen in all racial and ethnic groups, it is more commonly encountered in females and light-skinned individuals and typically presents after the 7th decade.[2-5] The disease has been traditionally classified into early and late stages.[1]

The early stages consist of alterations in the coloration of the macular pigment epithelium, both hypo and hyperpigmentation, and the presence of drusen of greater than 125 microns in diameter. Although patients with the early form of the disease may have modest visual symptoms including microscotomata, reduced contrast sensitivity, metamorphosia and nyctalopia, most patients have reasonably good Snellen visual acuity, typically 20/40 or better. The early phases have been variously referred to as atrophic, nonexudative, pre-angiogenic, or dry ARMD (Fig. 65-1).

In contrast, exudative or neovascular ARMD is typically a later onset phenomenon, occurring in eyes with high-risk characteristics including the presence of extensive soft drusen, Bruch's membrane thickening, and focal hyperpigmentation. This phase of the disease is characteristically accompanied by rapid loss of vision over a period of 6 to 12 months and the development of a central discform fibrotic scar. Without intervention, the visual acuity generally decreases to the range 20/200 or worse, 12 months following the onset of this phase.[3,4] Conventional forms of treatment including thermal laser photocoagulation and surgery have limited benefit for this condition, particularly when it presents with involvement of center of the fovea.[6-10]

Relevant to the purpose of this chapter, it is important to understand that the mechanisms of vision loss in age-related macular degeneration differ according to the stage, and even within stages may be amenable to different points of attack. Because the exudative form of the disease accounts for a disproportionate degree of the legal blindness associated with ARMD, much of the effort expended to date, has been on the development of drugs, which address this form, or drugs which may reduce the likelihood of progression from the nonexudative to the exudative form.[2,4] Importantly, there appear to be at least two separate and distinct mechanisms by which vision loss occurs in the exudative form:

1. Proliferation of new capillaries is accompanied by secondary fibrosis and disorganization of the pigment epithelium and outer retina, a somewhat gradual process.
2. Secondary alterations in both retinal capillary and pigment epithelial permeability lead to the accumulation of serous or serosanguineous fluid beneath the pigment epithelium, neurosensory retina, or within the retina itself, and are associated with more acute visual dysfunction.

Similarly, with increased understanding of the mechanisms underlying drusen formation, pigment epithelial senescence, and loss of photoreceptors and choriocapillaris, it is also now possible to address therapeutically, visual dysfunction arising from the atrophic form of the disease (Fig. 65-2).

EPIDEMIOLOGY

The need for pharmacologic forms of therapy is especially urgent considering the magnitude of the unmet need.[11] Based upon US Census Data and population based studies of ARMD, it is estimated that there are more than 7 million individuals with drusen measuring 125 microns or larger who are at substantial risk for developing the advanced forms of age-related macular degeneration.[11] In the US population aged 40 and older, it is estimated that 1.4–7% of this population, or in excess of 1.75 million persons, already have the advanced forms of the disease including either choroidal neovascularization and/or geographic atrophy.[12] The prevalence of the condition increases dramatically with age, with estimates of more than 15% of Caucasian women aged 80 or over having the advanced form of the disease currently, and as many as 3 million persons having the advanced forms by the year 2020.[12] Once choroidal neovascularization has developed in one eye, the fellow eye is thought to be at increased risk, with annual incidence rates ranging from approximately 5 to 14%. Consequently the risk of legal blindness constituting 20/200 or worse vision in the better eye, in the fellow eye of patients with unilateral vision, loss from choroidal neovascularization is thought to be approximately 12% over five years.[2]

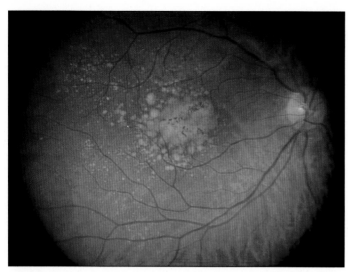

Fig. 65-1 Color fundus photograph of right eye patient with early age-related macular degeneration. Note the extensive drusen throughout the posterior pole, some of which appear calcific and others large and soft. The patient has not yet progressed to the stage of either geographic atrophy, or choroidal neovascularization.

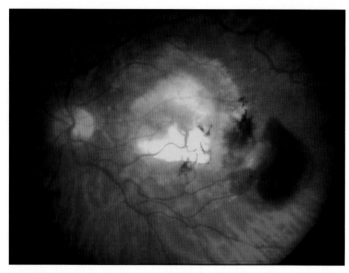

Fig. 65-2 Color photograph of the left eye of another patient with the severe form of late exudative age-related macular degeneration. Note the extensive scarring beneath the sensory retina, hemorrhage and lipid exudation.

ETIOLOGIC FACTORS

A variety of factors are thought to play a role in the development of age-related macular degeneration including genetic susceptibility and a host of potentially modifiable environmental factors, including comorbidities, diet, medications and light exposure.[13]

Genetic susceptibility

Multiple sources suggest that genetic susceptibility plays some role in this disease with first-degree relatives of patients with exudative AMD three times more likely than controls to develop the disease. Twin studies suggest concordance in 37% of monozy-

gotic twins vs. 19% of dizygotic twins, and sibling analyses suggest approximately 56% of the variability in AMD can be attributed to single gene segregation.[2,14] High-resolution genome scans for susceptibility loci in populations enriched for either choroidal neovascularization, or geographic atrophy or both suggest susceptibility loci on chromosomes 1q31, 5p, 9q, and 17q25. Subanalysis of patients exclusively with CNV provided additional evidence of susceptibility loci on chromosome 2p(10cM), and 22q(25cM).[2,15–17] An ARG to TRP mutation in EFEMP1, which codes for an elastin-related protein, fibulin 3, is thought to cause the abnormal accumulation of extensive drusen in malattia leventinese, an inherited macular degenerative disease with phenotypic characteristics closely correlated with advanced nonexudative ARMD.[18,19] Deposits of wild-type EFEMP1 accumulate within RPE cells and between the retinal pigment epithelium and drusen in eyes with ARMD and drusen, but not in regions where there is no apparent pathology.[20] Missense variations in the gene for a related structural protein involved in elastin and collagen cell adhesion, fibulin 5, are also more commonly found in patients with advanced AMD than in the general population to a statistically significant degree, although still relatively uncommon, representing approximately 1.7% of patients with AMD.[21] The gene for tissue inhibitor for metalloproteinase 3 (TIMP-3) which is a binding partner of EFEMP1, and like EFEMP1, acts to inhibit the stimulatory effects of VEGF on vascular cells, is coded for in the carboxy terminal end of chromosome 22, which was independently associated with neovascular ARMD in genome scans mentioned previously.[22,20] Multiple distinct alleles in exon 5 of the gene encoding tissue inhibitor metalloproteinase 3 TIMP-3, have been causally linked to an autosomal dominant form of neovascular macular degeneration Sorsby's fundus dystrophy (SFD) with strong phenotypic similarities to exudative ARMD,[23,24] although it is not thought to account for the majority of patients with exudative ARMD.[25] TIMP-3 is also found in increasing quantities and associated with thickening of Bruch's membrane during aging, including within drusen and the pigment epithelium.[18,26,27] The increased frequency of genome alterations coding for these two proteins (TIMP-3 and fibulin), which are important in the regulation of the extracellular matrix, particularly Bruch's membrane, provides support for the hypothesis proposed by Blumenkranz that generalized increased susceptibility of elastic fibers to photic degeneration is an important risk factor for choroidal neovascularization.[3] If disregulation of regulatory proteins including members of the TIMP and fibulin classes either through mutations in the genome, or post-transcriptional events are important in the pathologic thickening of Bruch's membrane and development of drusen that precede the advanced forms of ARMD, then pharmacologic therapies which address these families of proteins either directly through gene therapy, or by other conventional means, may prove to be valuable.

Apolipoprotein E-4 allele has been associated with a 50 to 70% reduction in the risk of exudative AMD while the E-2 allele has been associated with a 50% increase risk. These findings have been further corroborated by the presence of immuno-reactive apolipoprotein E in drusen and the basal laminar deposits in patients with AMD.[2,28] Correlations have been drawn between the lipoidal accumulation seen within drusen, and the known genetically determined relationship between apolipoprotein alleles and the neurofibulary tangles associated with Alzheimer's disease, another slowly degenerative process associated with aging. Potentially, drugs targeting this pathway may be useful in slowing the rate of drusen formation and the secondary complications associated with them.

Recently new evidence suggests that single nucleotide polymorphisms (SNPs) in the regulation of the complement activation locus (RCA) of chromosome 1q31.3 increase the risk of ARMD. The RCA locus spans 338 kb of genomic DNA that contain the gene encoding complement factor H (CFH). Mutations centered over a tyr402his protein polymorphism incearse the risk of ARMD between 2.7 and 7.4 fold and appear to account for between 43% and 50% of the attributable risk of ARMD. CFH which binds to C-Reactive Protein (CRP) and heparin consists of 20 repetitive units of 60 amino acids called short consensus repeats (SCR) and is responsible for downregulating activation of the complement system, including c5b-9. This molecule is thought to be important in immune mediated damage to Bruch's membrane and an important pathogenetic component of drusen.[29,30]

Early onset retinal degeneration characterized by the accumulation of lipofuscin within the pigment epithelium, and autofluorescence, using specialized photographic filters, has shed light on both the pathophysiology of RPE apoptosis and potential therapeutic avenues.[31] Stargardt's macular degeneration, an autosomal recessive condition manifesting in childhood, is causally linked to mutations in the ABCR gene.[32] While initial reports also suggested that ABCR might be a dominant susceptibility locus for AMD being found in 3.4% of cases and only 0.95% of controls, subsequent investigators have been unable to confirm this apparent increased frequency.[16,33] Nonetheless, the fact that increased amounts of lipofuscin are present in both Stargardt's disease, and in the earlier stages of the nonexudative forms of ARMD, later characterized by geographic atrophy, suggests that pharmacologic therapeutics insights might be gained from understanding the common pathways phenotypically expressed by these two different entities. Biochemical studies on the lipofuscin found in both Stargardt's disease and ARMD confirm that the principal component is N retinylidene-N-retinylethanolamine (A2E), which accumulates in cells of the retinal pigment epithelium and results in RPE apoptosis, photoreceptor death and vision loss.[30,34] This process is thought to be initiated by light activation of rhodopsin in the course of normal visual transduction as the first reactant in A2E biosynthesis. Isotretinoin (Accutane) which slows the synthesis of 11-cis retinaldehyde and regeneration of rhodopsin, was able to slow the accumulation of lipofuscin in ABCR knock-out mice and also aged wild-type mice.[34] This suggests that compounds with mechanisms of action similar to isotretinoin, which is structurally related to vitamin A, may represent another therapeutic avenue for the slowing or prevention of ARMD, independent of the effects of other agents acting primarily on the extracellular matrix.[31-34] Aside from providing targets of opportunity for correction of mutations in the genome as a method of treatment for age-related macular degeneration,

genetic studies provide the opportunity to target known protein products of altered genes for pharmacologic intervention, and the ability to create more relevant animal models that permit testing of agents with differing mechanisms of action.

ENVIRONMENTAL FACTORS

Diet

The principal environmental factors thought to be associated with age-related macular degeneration include diet, history of smoking, light exposure and use of supplemental medications. To the extent that coexisting morbidities such as hypertension or hypercholesterolemia can be considered environmental factors, they are also thought to play a potentially important role. Prospective dietary studies have indicated conflicting results with regard to the role of the dietary fat in age-related macular degeneration. While some studies have suggested that increased intake of saturated fats, particularly linoleic acid may increase the risk, other studies have had conflicting results. In the third National Health and Nutrition examination survey (NHANES), after adjustment for age, race, eye color and lifestyle, the odds ratio for early ARMD was 1.4 among persons in high vs. low quintiles of total fat intake, but 0.7 for late ARMD, calling into question the consistency of the observation.[36] A large case-control study suggested that higher dietary intake of carotenoids was associated with a lower risk of AMD with the highest quintile having a 43% reduction compared with those in the lowest quintile and the specific carotenoids lutein and zeaxanthine most strongly correlated. In that study no reduction could be found with the use of oral vitamin A, vitamin E or vitamin C.[37] Subsequent studies suggest that the use of foods, particularly fruits rich in antioxidants and carotenoids, when consumed at the level of three servings or more per day result in a pooled multivariate reduced relative risk of 0.64 compared with persons who consumed less than 1.5 servings per day.[2] Although the patients in two other studies, the Nurses Health Studies (NHS) and the Men in Health Profession Follow-up Study did not derive benefit from the use of either vegetables, antioxidants or carotenoids compared with fruits, subsequent prospective studies demonstrated benefit from comparable regimens in patients with more advanced forms of established ARMD.[22,38-40]

Smoking

Most studies have consistently implicated smoking as a statistically significant risk factor for the development of late-stage ARMD.[2,41] In a meta-analysis of three pooled studies from the United States, The Netherlands and Australia, smoking was one of only two significant associations identified with incident AMD along with total serum cholesterol. Current smoking was associated with an increased incidence of geographic atrophy and late AMD with an odds ratio relative to nonsmokers of 2.83 and 2.35 respectively.[41]

Light exposure

Although there is a considerable body of compelling experimental data to suggest that increased retinal irradiance is positively correlated with an increased likelihood of advanced age-related macular degeneration, the epidemiological evidence supporting this hypothesis is modest.[3,42,43] In the Beaver Dam eye study, participants exposed to summer sun for more than five hours a day during selected periods of time were at increased risk for increased retinal pigment (relative ratio 3.17) and early ARM (relative risk 2.14) after ten years of follow-up compared with those exposed to less than two hours per day.[43] Persons who experienced more than ten severe sunburns during youth were more likely than those who experienced one or no burns to develop drusen with greater than 250 micron diameter size or larger as well.[43] A similar increased susceptibility to sunburning and glare, but not actual hours of sun exposure, were found in an Australian cohort.[42]

The underlying rationale for the hypothesis that increased light stress predisposes to ARM rests on the role of oxidative stress inherent with photo bleaching of the photoreceptors and to a lesser extent pigment epithelium. In particular, reactive oxygen intermediates (ROI) including hydrogen peroxide, singlet oxygen, and other short-lived species, which arise as the byproducts of cellular metabolism are known to have a toxic effect on cellular membranes.[38] Experimental studies have confirmed the deleterious effect of chronic light and in particular blue and ultraviolet light on the retinal pigment epithelium in part through the creation of A2E oxiranes, a major component of lipofuscin. This effect is magnified in experimental animals and presumably humans with defects either in the *ABCR* gene, or in the regulatory gene product protein associated with *ABCR*.[34] Although ROIs can be of therapeutic importance following irradiance with major photodynamic agents such as verteporforin,[44-46] it is felt that the cumulative effects of chronic low levels of these species result in profound damage to the retina and pigment epithelium through lipid peroxidation, mitochondrial DNA damage and induction of apoptosis.[2,38] The presence of natural antioxidants derived from dietary sources including lutein, zeaxanthin, lycopene, and ascorbate are thought to mitigate the effects of photo-oxidation by quenching free radicals and other intermediate species.[38] It has been hypothesized that this represents one, but not the only mechanism of action, of the antioxidants in the AREDS study.[47] Additionally it is known that photoaging of skin following solar irradiation is mediated by the induction of matrix metalloproteinase and that the effect can be ameliorated by the use of inhibitory molecules such as blocking antibodies or presumably naturally incurring inhibitors such as the TIMP class.[48] It is possible that one of the beneficial effects of zinc may relate to its requirements as a cofactor for the matrix metalloproteinases. Additional studies using a variety of naturally occurring antioxidants and related agents such as green tea polyphenols suggest that this and similar classes of compounds may also be capable of preventing light-induced matrix metalloproteinase damage.[49]

Use of medications

Meta-analyses of pooled prospective studies suggest that certain medications may be associated with an increased or decreased risk of age-related macular degeneration.[50] Antihypertensive medications, particularly beta-blockers, are associated with modest increased risk, whereas hormone replacement therapy in women, and tricyclic antidepressants, confer some relative protection.[50] These observations may be able to be further exploited in the development of new classes of drugs in addition to avoiding potentially harmful drug interactions.

SYSTEMIC RISK FACTORS

In addition to smoking and possibly hyperlipidemia, hypertension is thought by some to be an independent risk factor for the development of ARMD. The mechanism by which this occurs is unknown, but it may relate to deleterious effects hypertension has on the choroidal vasculature, confounded by the use of antihypertensives, or other mechanisms. This has been confirmed in several different risk factor studies, and it appears also to be an independent risk factor for recurrence of choroidal neovascularization following successful photocoagulation of extra foveal lesions[7-9,13]

One new and intriguing observation is the potential association between levels of ocular inflammation or systemic inflammatory disease and age-related macular degeneration. It has long been known that there is a relationship between VEGF and inflammation.[2,51] Inflammatory foci and white cells, principally monocytes, are commonly seen in the choroid in autopsy specimens of patients with choroidal neovascularization. Macrophages as well as pigment epithelial cells express angiogenic cytokines and are found in choroidal neovascular membranes removed from patients surgically.[52-56] Aside from the well-known association between choroidal neovascularization and presumed ocular histoplasmosis syndrome and multifocal choroiditis, it has also been more recently postulated that other markers for chronic inflammation including serologic exposure to *Chlamydia pneumonia* infection and elevated C-reactive protein levels may also be associated with a greater likelihood of advanced ARMD in addition to elevated white blood count seen in one case-control study.[3,57,58] Some investigators have hypothesized that inflammation associated either with free radical formation resulting from reactive oxygen intermediates, or generation of epoxides, and other intermediate compounds related to the genesis of A2E oxiranes, may stimulate inflammation that further increases both apoptosis and angiogenic signals[38,30] (Fig. 65-3). To the extent that inflammation does have a causative effect on the development of ARMD, therapy aimed at reducing inflammation either through immunomodulation or stabilization of intracellular organelles such as lysosomes and resultant proteolysis, may be successful pharmacologic strategies. In animal models, intravitreal triamcinolone has been shown to inhibit preretinal and choroidal neovascularization induced by laser injury.[59] There is increasing evidence of the linkage between VEGF, inflammation, and intracellular adhesion molecule 1 (ICAM-1) (Fig. 65-3). It is known that inhibition of ICAM-1 prevents both leukostasis and vascular leakage in streptozotocin-induced diabetic retinopathy.[60,61] Triamcinolone acetonide modulates permeability and intracellular adhesion and ICAM-1 expression in cell culture, and it has further been shown that upregulation

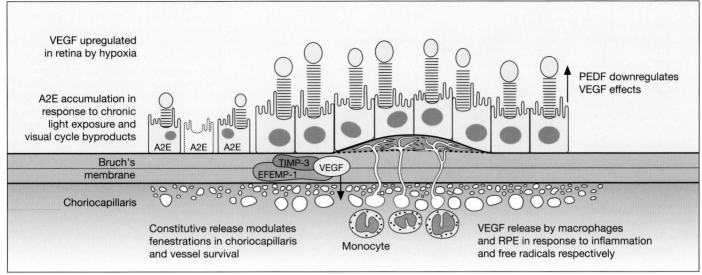

Fig. 65-3 Schematic diagram of pathogenic mechanisms associated with atrophic and exudative age-related macular degeneration. Normal constitutive release of VEGF, which is responsible for maintenance of fenestrations and other desirable permeability effects on the normal choriocapillaris through basal lateral secretion in an outward direction, appears to be effectively counterbalanced by the apical secretion of cytokines inhibitory for angiogenesis, including pigment epithelial derived (PEDF). This results in the relative avascularity of the outer retina as seen in the diagram on the right. In response to chronic light exposure and oxidation of phospholipids associated with the visual cycle, A2E and other oxidative byproducts accumulate in the retinal pigment epithelium, accounting for the characteristic autofluorescence seen on fundus photography. They also result in senescence of the pigment epithelium and apoptotic death associated with secondary atrophic effects on the overlying photoreceptors and underlying choriocapillaris, seen on the left in the diagram. The accumulation of increased lipoproteins as well as other glycoproteins including TIMP-3 and EFEMP-1 contribute to the thickening of Bruch's membrane, characteristically seen in patients with more advanced forms of the disease (seen centrally). Low-grade inflammation, chemoattraction of monocytes, and proangiogenic signals both from the pigment epithelium and inflammatory cells lead to vascular ingrowth from the choroid through defects in calcific and fragmented Bruch's membrane.

of ICAM-1 and invasion by CD18 positive leukocytes follows laser injury and proceeds neovascularization.[62,63] Comparable laser injury in ICAM-1 knock-out mice demonstrated considerable reduction in neovascularization, confirming the likely participation of this class of molecules in VEGF-mediated angiogenesis. Other therapies that target CD18-positive leukocytes or ICAM-1 are likely to be beneficial in reducing the angiogenic stimulus associated with inflammation and aging.

Definition and steps in angiogenesis

Angiogenesis refers to the creation of new blood vessels from existing blood vessels, and therefore is contrasted from the process of vasculogenesis seen characteristically in utero in which vessels are created de novo. The angiogenesis cascade has been characterized as occurring in multiple sequenced steps (adapted from The Angiogenesis Foundation, http://www.angio.org/understanding/understanding.html):

1. Release of angiogenic growth factors by diseased tissue.
2. Binding of the angiogenic growth factors to adjacent existing vascular endothelial cells (EC).
3. Activation of EC to produce molecules, including enzymes.
4. Dissolution of the surrounding basement membrane by activated enzymes.
5. Proliferation and migration of EC.
6. Adhesion molecules (integrins) help to serve as framework for advancing EC.

7. Further dissolution of tissue and remodeling with matrix metalloproteinases.
8. Formation of vascular tubes by EC.
9. Formation of blood vessel loops from EC tubes.
10. Stabilization of new blood vessels by smooth muscle cells and pericytes. Antiangiogenic therapies currently under investigation are thought to inhibit angiogenesis at various different steps in this process (Fig. 65-4).

THE PATHOPHYSIOLOGY OF EXUDATIVE ARMD: THE CRUCIAL ROLE OF CYTOKINES

VEGF and other positive and negative modulators of angiogenesis

Regardless of the inciting stimulus involved in the development of pathologic neovascularization, it is now well established that vascular endothelial growth factor (VEGF) plays a principal role including not only the neovascular forms of age-related macular degeneration, but also diabetic retinopathy, iris neovascularization, and retinopathy of prematurity. Additionally other cytokines may play an important role as well, including FGF, PEDF, the integrins, angiopoietins, and matrix metalloproteinase inhibitors.[2,23,65–68]

VEGF undoubtedly represents the putative factor X first postulated by Michaelson associated with pathologic neovascularization.[2] First described as a vasopermeability factor associated with tumors, the molecule has since been cloned and well-characterized.[69,70] VEGF has two important characteristics relevant

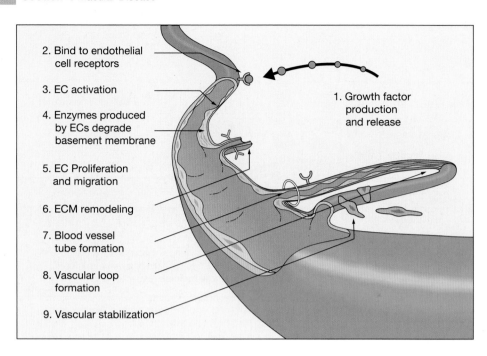

2. Bind to endothelial
   cell receptors

3. EC activation

4. Enzymes produced
   by ECs degrade
   basement membrane

5. EC Proliferation
   and migration

6. ECM remodeling

7. Blood vessel
   tube formation

8. Vascular loop
   formation

9. Vascular stabilization

1. Growth factor
   production
   and release

Fig. 65-4 The cascade of events associated with angiogenesis are schematically diagrammed, including the release of angiogenic factors, binding by endothelial receptors, followed by endothelial cell activation, proliferation and directed migration. With remodeling of the extracellular matrix, vascular tubes and loops form, associated eventually with the histologic appearance of neovascularization. From The Angiogenesis Foundation. http://www.angio.org/understanding/understanding.html

to its role in the pathogenesis of the neovascular forms of age-related macular degeneration: (1) induction of angiogenesis through endothelial proliferation, migration and new capillary formation; and (2) enhancement of vascular permeability.

Vascular permeability

VEGF produces important increases in hydraulic conductivity of isolated microvessels that are mediated by increased calcium influx and likely changes in levels of nitric oxide caused by induction of nitric oxide synthetase (NOS). While VEGF is both necessary and sufficient when administered exogenously to induce both these effects in vitro and in vivo, it is also well-known that a number of other growth factors participate in this process. Some represent steps in a cascade initiated by VEGF while others act upstream.[71,72] The chemical structure of VEGF is that of a heparin binding homodimeric glycoprotein of 45 kilodaltons (Fig. 65-5).[69] VEGF has significant homology to platelet-derived growth factor (PDGF). The human *VEGF* gene is organized into eight exons separated by seven introns and is localized in chromosome 6p21.3. Although there is only a single gene for VEGF-A, alternate post-translational exon splicing results in the generation of between four and six different isoforms having 121, 145, 165, 183, 189, and 206, amino acids respectively after signal sequence cleavage[69,68] (Fig. 65-6). While VEGF 165 is thought to be predominantly responsible for pathologic neovascularization, other isoforms are also thought to be important.[69,51] VEGF 189 and VEGF 206 are highly basic and bind to heparin with high affinity, remaining almost completely sequestered in the extracellular matrix. In contrast VEGF 121 is an acidic polypeptide that fails to bind heparin and is principally found freely diffusible. VEGF 165 exists in both soluble and bound forms[69] (Figs 65-6 and 65-7).

While the participation of VEGF in pathologic neovascularization in the eye is well understood, as well as the role of the

VEGF and its various isoforms in embryogenesis during development of the ocular vasculature, its regulatory function in the retinal pigment epithelium and in the retina remains somewhat poorly understood. It probably plays a role as a vascular survival factor for the choriocapillaris as well as for the maintenance of fenestrations in the choriocapillaris through directed secretion from the basal portion of the pigment epithelium. In contrast another regulatory cytokine secreted by the pigment epithe-

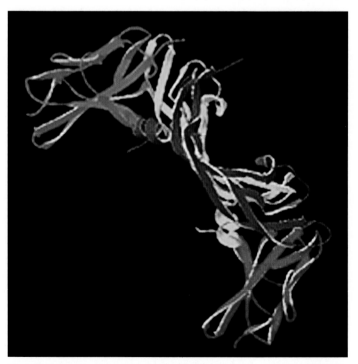

Fig. 65-5 Structural formula of vascular endothelial growth factor (VEGF), demonstrating the characteristic folding pattern of the pathologic isoform VEGF 165 in a computerized rendering.

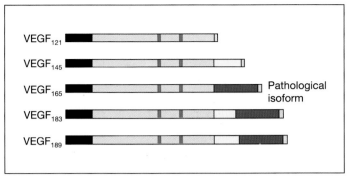

VEGF_{121}

VEGF_{145}

VEGF_{165}   Pathological isoform

VEGF_{183}

VEGF_{189}

Fig. 65-6 Multiple isoforms of VEGF exist in nature and appear to participate to a differential degree in the normal events of vasculogenesis, as well as the pathologic events of angiogenesis occurring in response to local stimuli. Although there is only a single gene for VEGF, alternate splicing as well as post-transcriptional modification by plasminogen in the extracellular matrix accounts for a variety of isoforms that determine the relative balance between normal vascular homeostasis and pathologic neovascularization (see also Fig. 65-7). The shorter amino acid length isoforms VEGF 121 and 145 are principally found in soluble form, whereas the longer spliced lengths 183, 189, and 206 are principally tissue fixed and bound by heparin. VEGF 165 is thought to stimulate pathologic neovascularization and exists both in soluble and tissue fixed configurations.

lium in an apical direction, pigment epithelial-derived factor (PEDF) has an inhibitory effect relative to VEGF and may serve to counteract some of the effects of VEGF release in the normal retina[64,73] (Figs 65-3 and 65-7).

VEGF receptors

VEGF exerts its effects on cells through two highly related receptor tyrosine kinases (RTKs) VEGFR-1 and VEGFR-2.[69] VEGFR-1, also termed FLT-1 (FMS-like tyrosine kinase), was described first, but its role remains open to debate. Like VEGF, VEGFR-1 is upregulated by a hypoxia-inducing factor dependent mechanism (HIF). The receptor undergoes weak tyrosine autophosphorylation in response to VEGF. It is thought not to be primarily a mitogenic stimulus but rather a "decoy" receptor, which downregulates the activity of VEGF by sequestering and rendering the factor less available to VEGFR-2 (Figs 65-7 and 65-8). This receptor may be most important during embryogenesis rather than during pathologic neovascularization as well as in hematopoietic bone marrow-derived cells and neural signaling.[69,74]

VEGFR-2 (KDR in humans or FLK-1 in mice)

VEGFR-2 binds VEGF with lower affinity relative to VEGFR-1, but is felt to be the major mediator of the mitogenic, angiogenic, and permeability enhancing effects of VEGF. The binding site for VEGF on VEGFR-2 has been mapped to the second and third IgG-like domains and it undergoes dimerization and strong ligand depend tyrosine phosphorylation resulting in a mitogenic chemotactic and prosurvival signal. It appears to have at least two separate tyrosine phosphorylation sites. VEGFR-2 is thought to be critical as a survival factor with apoptosis occurring in its absence (Fig. 65-8).

In addition to VEGFR-1 and -2, there appear to be several other receptors on tumors and endothelial cells that bind VEGF principally neuropilin (NRP1 and NRP2). The precise function of these binding sites is unknown, but they may induce neuronal guidance and are thought to be specific for VEGF 165 but not VEGF 121. NRP1 may also present VEGF 165 to the VEGFR-2 in such a manner that it enhances the effectiveness of the VEGFR-2-mediated signal. NRP2 may be linked to lymphatic vessel development.[69]

A large body of evidence exists to support the critical and probably rate limiting role of VEGF in neovascular forms of age-related macular degeneration. High messenger RNA levels and increased VEGF receptor levels are observed in areas of choroidal neovascularization in primates as well as in the extracted neovascular membranes of patients removed at surgery and following autopsy.[2,54] Additionally there are strong indications that elevated levels of VEGF are the proximal cause for the hyperpermeability seen not only in diabetic macular edema, but in patients with subsensory and intraretinal fluid associated with choroidal neovascularization as well. The permeability changes resulting from VEGFR-2 are thought to be mediated to a large extent by an endothelial nitric oxide synthetase-based generation of increased nitric oxide levels, and associated changes in calcium flux (Fig. 65-8). These alterations are able to be reversed either by direct blockade of VEGF, the receptor, or NOS using a knock-out model.[2,70,71] Inactivation of soluble VEGF by monoclonal antibodies directed against it, or inhibition of ICAM also appear to be effective as well. In addition to either the indirect inhibition of VEGF effects through modulation of ICAM, or indirect effects on nitric oxide phosphorylase, nitric oxide synthetase, or protein kinase C, another modulator of permeability, there are several other methods by which VEGF effects can be blocked in the eye and elsewhere. These include the use of a class of compounds termed aptamers, which are chemically synthesized single strand nucleic acids, either RNA or DNA, that bind to target molecules with high selectivity and affinity leaving nontargeted protein functions intact[75,76] (see subsequent section).

Other methods of direct inhibition of VEGF include inhibition of its tyrosine kinase receptors (VEGFR-1 and -2), either by systemic administration or gene transfer. Several laboratories have described the use of small interfering RNA (siRNAs) in effectively downregulating gene regulation[77] (see subsequent section).

Although all the above VEGF inhibitors share in common an attempt to mitigate the proliferative and permeability effects of VEGF on normal and neovascular tissue, there are likely to be differences in both efficacy and safety related to the choice of agents for several reasons. It remains unclear, and a point of some debate, as to the relative desirability and safety of complete blockade of all major VEGF isoforms compared with exclusively VEGF 165. At present there are no definitive data to suggest the superiority of one versus the other, although with the availability of complete phase 3 trial data with both sodium pegaptanib, which has now been completed, and Rhufab which is still under way at the time of writing, some clarity should be

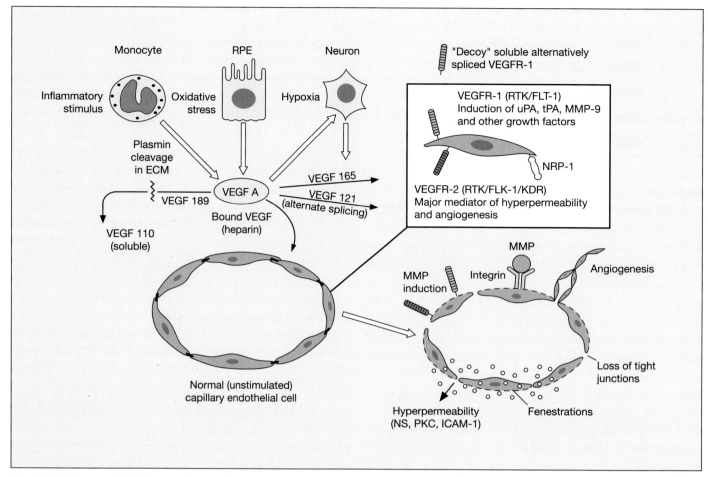

Fig. 65-7 Pathways of VEGF expression and effects on vascular cells are demonstrated schematically. A variety of cells contribute to VEGF release, including monocytes, retinal pigment epithelial cells and neurons responding to inflammation, oxidative stress and hypoxia respectively. These and other cell types produce predominantly VEGF-A which is expressed in various isoforms through transcriptional and post-translational steps. VEGF 165 and VEGF 121 are the predominant forms, with VEGF 189 being cleaved in the extracellular matrix to VEGF 110, a soluble form by activated plasmin. Each of these molecules, but principally VEGF 165, bind to endothelial cells through specific receptors VEGFR-1 and VEGFR-2. A sequence of events is set in motion through subsequent intracellular messaging systems as well as extracellular events that result in the loss of tight junctions between individual endothelial cells, the formation of fenestrations within endothelial cells and calcium-mediated permeability channels resulting in loss of the normal inner and outer blood–retinal barriers. Additionally matrix metalloproteinase activation occurs through its interaction with integrin receptors alpha v beta 3 and alpha v beta 5, which are found on the surface of endothelial cells exclusively following induction of the cell through activation with the VEGFR-1.

achievable, even if it is to conclude that the two act to bind soluble VEGF in the extracellular space and are comparable. From a theoretical standpoint, since VEGF 165 is the principal isoform involved in pathologic neovascularization, it has been argued that leaving the other three principal isoforms intact (121 which is principally diffusible in soluble form, and 189 and 206 which are principally matrix-bound through high-affinity heparin binding sites), avoids the possibility of inter-ference with normal homeostatic mechanisms associated with constitutive VEGF expression. There is some experimental evidence to suggest that blockage of VEGF 164 in the mouse (equivalent to VEGF 165 in man) is as effective as nonselective antibody-mediated VEGF blockage in preventing pathologic neovascularization in the hypoxia-induced model, while not interfering with normal physiologic development of retinal vasculature.[51,78] Additionally, VEGF 164 was found to be more potent in stimulating ICAM expression in endothelial cells and inducing chemotaxis of monocytes through its interaction with VEGFR-1 than VEGF 121. On the other hand, the effects of soluble 121 as well as matrix-bound 189 and 206 VEGF iso-forms may prove to be important in patients who may benefit from a broader blockade. These results should be answered by the human clinical trials currently underway.

Other cytokine regulators of angiogenesis

Although VEGF appears to have been clearly established as the rate-limiting step in the control of angiogenesis, it is thought that a number of other cytokines, both soluble and tissue-fixed, may play an important regulatory role as well. This is particu-larly true in the case of age-related macular degeneration where VEGF is, in all likelihood, the rate-limiting step rather than the initiating step. In contrast, in other forms of ocular neovas-

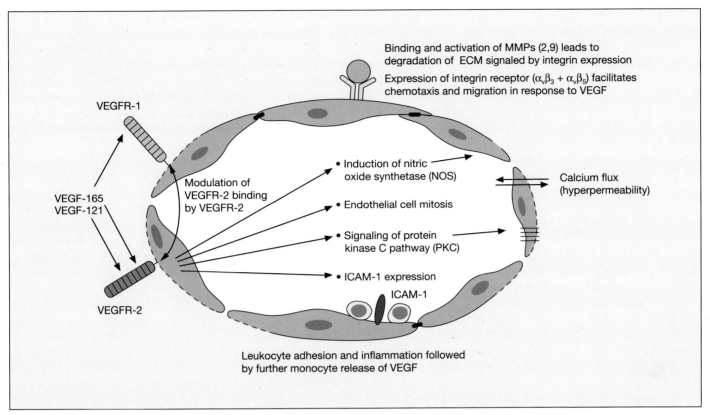

Fig. 65-8 Intracellular signaling including induction of nitric oxide synthetase (NOS), protein kinase C activation (PKC) and expression of ICAM-1 leading to leukocyte adherence and further changes in permeability mediated by calcium flux and protein kinase C.

cularization, particularly those associated solely with ischemia or hypoxia, VEGF may be both necessary and sufficient for all the manifestations of the disease. In age-related macular degeneration, as detailed in an earlier section, it is likely that key signaling steps occur prior to the upregulation of VEGF either initiated by, or facilitated by, cytokines, which act under normal constitutive conditions to counterbalance constitutive VEGF effects, and in pathologic circumstances may either counteract or serve to amplify the process.

Cytokines may be generally divided into two classes, those that upregulate VEGF or VEGF associated effects, and those that act in an inhibitory capacity. In some instances, the same compounds may perform both functions depending upon the other extracellular signals present in the milieu as well as post-transcriptional or post-translational events, including cleavage by proteases, or binding by soluble receptors such as the family of tyrosine kinases.[2] Accordingly, any of this class of normally occurring compounds can be considered either in their native form, through splice or cleavage products, or chemical substitution to be potential therapeutic compounds in the treatment of pathologic neovascularization. Stimulatory cytokines in addition to vascular endothelial growth factor include basic and acidic fibroblast growth factor, the angiopoietins, transforming growth factor, and platelet-derived growth factor.[65,66] Naturally occurring inhibitory factors include interferon alpha, thrombospondin 1, angiostatin, endostatin, hemopexin-like domain of matrix metalloproteinase 2 (PEX), and pigment epithelial-

derived factor (PEDF).[2,64,79,80-86] Additionally it is likely there are many other naturally occurring compounds, as yet not recognized or well-characterized biochemically. The relative balance between naturally occurring stimulatory and inhibitory factors is thought to contribute to the tight control of ocular vascular homeostasis, and may explain the differential ability of normal vascular as well as neovascular tissue to respond exquisitely both spatially and temporally to various stimuli.

NATURALLY OCCURRING UPREGULATORS OF ANGIOGENESIS

Fibroblast growth factor

Basic fibroblast growth factor (FGF2) has been found to be elevated in excised choroidal neovascular membranes from patients undergoing surgery for ARMD, and is capable when implanted within the eye or adjacent to the retina of inducing pathologic neovascularization.[65,66] Laser models of choroidal neovascularization are accompanied by upregulation of FGF2-associated mRNA, which precedes the development of histologically identifiable new vessels. However, while FGF2 is sufficient when inserted exogenously in creating choroidal neovascularization, it is not necessary in that *FGF2* gene knock-out animals are also capable of developing laser-induced choroidal neovascularization, indicating that alternative pathways exist. FGF upregulation of angiogenesis is thought to be in part mediated by adhesion-mediated signals including expression of the cell membrane-associated integrins. In experimental models of neovascularization, including the corneal micropocket assay and chorioallantoic membrane (CAM) induced by fibroblast growth factor, neovascularization depends on the expression of alpha v beta 3 integrin, and can be blocked by selective monoclonal antibodies to this molecule. In contrast, experimental neovascularization upregulated by VEGF was blocked by a separate and distinct monoclonal antibody to another integrin, alpha v beta 5, and had no effect on the FGF-mediated pathway. Both, however, were blocked by a cyclic peptide antagonist (RGDfv) suggesting the differential expression of separate integrin-based pathways to VEGF and FGF, by a potential common inhibitory pathway within the intracellular signaling process.[2,65,66] Although the alpha v beta 3 and alpha v beta 5 integrins appear to differentially represent the stimulatory effects of FGF2 and VEGF respectively in laboratory studies, there is conflicting evidence as to whether these pathways are distinct with regard to the separate disease processes of age-related macular degeneration and diabetic retinopathy respectively. As a result, therapeutic approaches to integrin inhibition directed at downstream events such as intracellular signaling probably represent a more logical point of attack than targeted inhibition of the individual receptors through monoclonal antibodies or related mechanisms.

Angiopoietins, which are also highly specific for endothelial cells, perform a variety of other regulatory activities related to supporting cells and the extracellular matrix. A laboratory study suggests that two different isoforms. Angiopoietin 1 and angiopoietin 2 appear to have differential and counteracting effects on the vasculature. Angiopoietin 2, which is upregulated by both hypoxia and VEGF, binds to an endothelial cell receptor TIE2 and augments neovascularization incited by VEGF, but does not stimulate endothelial cells or proliferation in vitro.[2] ANG1 appears to play a maturation role, is associated with nonleaky behavior and may have potential therapeutic benefit through its inhibition of ICAM-1 and other inflammatory-associated pathways.[2]

Intracellular adhesion molecule 1 (ICAM-1) is a peptide known to mediate leukocyte adhesion and transmigration and is thought to be important in the pathogenesis of a variety of disorders characterized by abnormal vascular permeability including age-related macular degeneration, as well as diabetic retinopathy. ICAM-1 is constitutively expressed on retinal pigment epithelial and choroidal vascular endothelial cell surfaces and mediates leukocyte adhesion and extravasation from retinal and choroidal capillaries in response to inflammation as well as VEGF stimulation through its effects on adherens and occludens junctions. Because leukocytes both possess receptors for and migrate in response to VEGF, VEGF-stimulated leukostasis and expression of ICAM-1 leukocyte adhesion can be blocked by specific inhibitors of ICAM-1. Antibody-based neutralization of ICAM-1 and CD-18 have been shown to prevent both leukocyte adhesion and retinal endothelial cell injury and death. In addition to specific inhibitors of ICAM-1, other anti-inflammatory molecules including triamcinolone acetonide have been shown to negatively modulate the hyper-

permeability associated with increased expression of ICAM-1 in cultured cells, suggesting a mechanism by which the beneficial effects of triamcinolone on retinal and choroidal vascular hyperpermeability might be explained.[62,63]

Expression of matrix metalloproteinases and their associated RNA, particularly MMP-2 and MMP-9, have been associated with pathologic neovascularization. Both matrix metalloproteinases, which are bound to the integrin receptors alpha v beta 3 and alpha v beta 5 on endothelial cells, are activated by VEGF and other regulatory cytokines and act to digest the extracellular matrix and thereby facilitate the spreading and chemotaxis of actively proliferating endothelial cells as they aggregate to form new capillaries.[2] Matrix metalloproteinases (MMPs) appear to be modulated and principally downregulated by naturally occurring tissue inhibitors of metalloproteinases (TIMPs) of which TIMP-1, TIMP-2 and TIMP-4 are thought to be soluble, and TIMP-3 principally extracellular matrix bound. TIMP-3 is thought to play an important and possibly critical role in the natural modulation of matrix metalloproteinase regulation in Bruch's membrane, and is found in increased amounts in drusen and thickened basement membranes associated with age-related macular degeneration.[27,87] Mutations in exon-5 of the TIMP-3 molecule are associated with Sorby's fundus dystrophy, and an experimental model that either delivers increased amounts of TIMP-3 or induces overexpression of TIMP-3 by gene therapy demonstrate potent antiangiogenic effects for this molecule.[88,89] MMP-2 appears to localize to a greater extent in surgical specimens at sites of new vessel proliferation, whereas MMP-9 expression appears greatest at the margins, suggesting possible synergy in addition to MMP-7.[2] Despite the likely involvement of MMPs in pathologic neovascularization, a recent trial of a synthetic MMP-2 and MMP-9 inhibitor, which was effective in experimental models of neovascularization in animals, failed to show a therapeutic benefit in humans (personal communication, Pfizer/Agouron 2002). In addition to these well-characterized molecules, it is also thought that a variety of other factors may play a contributing, if less important, role including tumor necrosis factor alpha (TNF-alpha), transforming growth factor beta (TGF-beta) which have both inhibitory and inhibitory effects paradoxically, and other inflammatory cell mediated molecules. Monocyte chemoattractant protein (MCP) a cytokine involved with macrophage recruitment is prominently expressed in surgically excised choroidal neovascular membranes and probably plays an important up regulatory function. It has been implicated as a possible critical regulatory cytokine in the genesis of drusen and CNV in experimental animal models.[90]

Naturally occurring downregulators

A variety of naturally occurring cytokines are known to have a downregulatory effect on angiogenesis and VEGF-mediated effect on cells.

Pigment epithelial-derived factor, which is secreted by the pigment epithelium in vivo as well as in cell culture, has been shown to be biochemically identical to the product of the wild-type of retinoblastoma tumor suppressor gene (RB) and is thought to induce differentiation of retinoblastoma cells, inhibit microglial growth, and other important regulatory functions in addition to its effects on angiogenesis.[42]

Another interesting class of regulatory cytokines, which appear to have an inhibitory effect on angiogenesis relate to the class of aminoacyl-tRNA synthetases, which are associated with the first step of protein synthesis. Tryptophanyl-tRNA synthetase (TrpRS, a homolog of TyrRS) has no effect in its native form on angiogenesis or angiogenesis signaling. In contrast, an alternatively spliced fragment reported to be stimulated by interferon alpha lacking a portion of the NH_2 terminal fragment, has potent antiangiogenic effects, both in vitro and in vivo.[91]

Interferon alpha is a naturally occurring cytokine expressed in response to a variety of stimuli. Based on its known ability to inhibit certain vascular tumors of childhood as well as experimental ocular neovascularization in a primate model, it was tested in a large multicenter randomized clinical trial and ultimately shown not to be of benefit in patients with neovascular forms of AMD[81,92] (see subsequent section).

Thrombospondin 1 has been described as both an up and downregulator of VEGF. Under specified conditions TSP-1, which is produced by platelets and monocytes, enhances simulated VEGF release and is dependent upon binding to alpha v beta 5 and alpha v beta 1 integrins. In separate studies, TSP-1 has also been noted to inhibit endothelial cell proliferation, migration, and angiogenesis. VEGF and TSP-1 appear to participate in a feedback loop and its potential role as a therapeutic agent remains uncertain.[2] Angiostatin is a 38 kilodalton internal fragment of plasminogen that encompasses the first four cringles of the molecule. It shows inhibitory effects on vascular endothelial proliferation in vitro and in vivo, particularly within tumors.[86,93] Endostatin, a cleavage product of collagen XVIII is structurally related to and shares homology with angiostatin, and inhibits tumor-associated angiogenesis.[85] Each of these classes is further described in the following section as they relate to preclinical or clinical studies.

AGENTS CURRENTLY IN USE OR UNDER INVESTIGATION

Antioxidants, vitamins and cofactors

The rationale for the use of antioxidants, multivitamins and other cofactors is based upon several lines of evidence including the essential role of vitamin A in the visual transduction cycle, the known and predicted effects of oxidative stress resulting in reactive oxygen intermediates, and the requirement of certain critical metal ions including zinc in the functioning of critical proteases and other naturally occurring defense mechanisms against oxidative injury. Prior to the release of the data from the AREDS study, there remained some controversy as to whether or not antioxidant multivitamin therapy was efficacious or not, with some studies suggesting a protective effect, and others not.[39,40,94]

The AREDS trial was a large well-designed multicenter randomized clinical trial, which evaluated the effect of high-dose vitamin C and E, beta-carotene, and zinc supplements on AMD progression and visual acuity.[47] A total 4757 persons were enrolled and stratified into one of four categories of increasing severity of disease. Due to the low rate of progression of category 1 consisting of drusen area of less than five small drusen of 63 microns or less, statistical analysis was only performed on the remaining 3640 patients with categories 2, 3, 4. Only the latter two (categories 3 and 4) were ultimately found to be at more than a trivial risk for progression. Patients in category 2 with at least one intermediate size druse, but not extensive drusen, had only a 1.3% probability of progression to advanced AMD by year 5 and no meaningful inference could be drawn regarding their risk with or without intervention. Patients in category 3 had either extensive intermediate drusen, large drusen or noncentral geographic atrophy, and patients in category 4 had visual acuity of less than 20/32 due to AMD in one eye related either to geographic atrophy involving the center of the macula or choroidal neovascularization in the fellow eye, but not the study eye, which had visual acuity 20/32 or better. The average follow-up of the 3640 enrolled study participants aged 55 to 80 was 6.3 years, and by comparison with placebo, patients treated with antioxidants plus zinc demonstrated a statistically significant odds reduction for the development of advanced AMD (odds ratio 0.72, 99% confidence interval, 0.52–0.98. The odds ratio for zinc alone and antioxidants alone were 0.75 and 0.8 respectively, and the odds reduction estimates increased when only patients with category 3 or category 4 drusen were included reducing to 0.66, 0.71 and 0.76 for antioxidants plus zinc, zinc alone and antioxidants alone respectively. These data are further reflected in Fig. 65-9.

Based upon these findings, and extrapolation of the US population at risk, it has been estimated that of the 8 million persons in the United States aged 55 or more with ARMD, if those at highest risk including categories 3 and 4 were to receive therapy with the formulation employed in the AREDS trial, as many as 300 000 of the 1.3 million at highest risk for advancement might avoid progression to the severe forms of the disease.[95] Additionally, based upon recent epidemiologic data, exclusion of beta-carotene is recommended for persons with a current history of smoking, or a long smoking history based upon a theoretical increased risk of lung cancer.

Intriguing data also exist with regard to the use of other naturally occurring and synthetic analogs of beta-carotene. Conflicting evidence exists with regard to the potential benefit of vitamin A supplementation in patients with advanced forms of retinitis pigmentosa. Additionally at least one study suggests that patients with symptomatic nyctalopia associated with Sorsby's fundus dystrophy, which in turn is known to be associated with mutations in TIMP-3, can be benefited visually and electrophysiologically by supraphysiologic doses of vitamin A (50 000 IU per day).[96]

Unlike Sorsby's fundus dystrophy, which in addition to producing nyctalopia, also results in choroidal neovascularization, Stargardt's disease, which has onset at an earlier stage results in pigment epithelial abnormalities and geographic atrophy, and as previously described, is thought to occur as a result of a homozygous mutation in the ABCR gene resulting in accumulation of

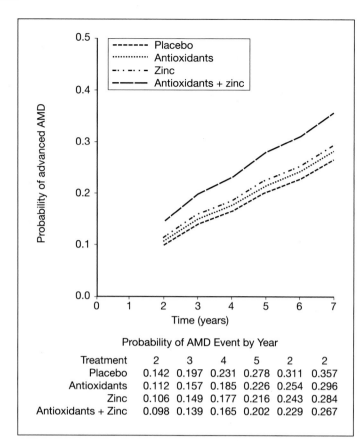

Probability of AMD Event by Year

Treatment	2	3	4	5	2	2
Placebo	0.142	0.197	0.231	0.278	0.311	0.357
Antioxidants	0.112	0.157	0.185	0.226	0.254	0.296
Zinc	0.106	0.149	0.177	0.216	0.243	0.284
Antioxidants + Zinc	0.098	0.139	0.165	0.202	0.229	0.267

Fig. 65-9 Repeated-measures estimates of the probability of loss in the visual acuity score of at least 15 letters in at least one study eye of participants within categories 3 and 4. From AREDS Research Group. Arch Ophthalmol 2001; 19:1417.

large amounts of a major fluorophore of lipofuscin A2E.[34] This molecule, which is thought to represent the end-stage of visible and particularly blue light-induced reactive oxidative intermediates (ROI) associated with the visual cycle transduction, is amenable to treatment in animal models with isotretinoin (Accutane), a congener of vitamin A, an inhibitor of rhodopsin regeneration at supraphysiologic concentrations.[33] It has been proposed that by using Accutane, or other related molecules, that it might be possible to favorably affect the progressive accumulation of lipofuscin and eventual geographic atrophy seen in patients with the conventional advanced forms of atrophic age-related macular degeneration, that are recognized in most patients with this disease who do not suffer from a mutation in the ABCR. It is also conceivable that some of the beneficial effects related to compounds used in the AREDS trial may have been from influences of the supplementation of beta-carotene, a potential precursor of 11 cis-retinal.

A variety of other compounds from naturally occurring sources, with antioxidant or related capabilities, may also be of benefit in pharmacologic treatment of some less advanced forms of ARMD.[38] Genistein, a naturally occurring product found within soy beans, has antioxidant properties, and is also thought to be a tyrosine kinase inhibitor. It has been shown to normalize retinal vascular permeability in an experimental model of diabetes

mellitus when administered orally to rats made diabetic by streptozotocin injection.[97,98] The macular carotenoids thought to be the principal contributors to macular yellow include lutein and zeaxanthin. One study suggested that a high dietary intake of these carotenoids protected against AMD, adjusting for other risk factors with a 43% reduction in risk for AMD compared when the upper quartile of use was compared with the lowest quartile.[37] Other prospective studies have not yet confirmed this phenomenon although in yet other studies, measurement of serum concentrations appeared to indicate that elevated levels of these compounds were associated with reduced risk. The critical dependence of the naturally occurring antioxidant enzymes, superoxide dismutase, catalase, and glutathione peroxidase like the matrix metalloproteinases, particularly copper, zinc and manganese, provides yet another potential mechanism by which AREDS supplementation of both copper and zinc, as well as the naturally occurring antioxidants vitamin E and vitamin C might have a beneficial effect on the progression of ARMD.[38] At present no definitive recommendations can be made regarding the supplemental use of either zeaxanthine, lutein or other naturally occurring carotenoids such as lycopene, in the absence of unequivocal prospective trial data, although future studies evaluating some of these compounds and omega free fatty acids are planned (personal communication, Emily Chew MD).

Steroids and other immunomodulators
Steroids

Steroids have long known to be associated with neovascularization reduction by mechanisms that were not clearly understood. Folkman and colleagues were the first to suggest that the anti-angiogenic effects of steroids could be separated into two categories: (1) those related to anti-inflammatory effects paralleling convention glucocorticoid and mineralocorticoid activity; and (2) a separate structural configuration of the pregnan nucleus conferring distinct antiangiogenic capability.[79,80] This antiangiogenic effect was shown to be potentiated by heparin, short-chain fragments of heparin, and other related molecules such as cyclodextrin, and was associated with the alpha hydroxyl group on the C-ring as well as 17 and 21 hydroxyl groups on the D-ring. The relative potencies for antiangiogenic glucocorticoid and mineral corticoid effects of various naturally occurring and synthetic steroids are given in Fig. 65-10.[99]

Conventional steroid therapy
Preclinical studies There is increasing experimental and clinical evidence to connect the processes of inflammation and neovascularization. It is known that vascular endothelial growth factor-induced retinal vascular permeability is mediated by intracellular adhesion molecule 1 (I-CAM-1). The inhibition of I-CAM-1 bioactivity with a neutralizing antibody inhibits the permeability associated with leukostasis, and suggests that anti-inflammatory molecules such as steroids including triamcinolone may exert their salutary effects on the blood–retinal barrier breakdown seen in diabetes and possibly ARMD by this mechanism. These same effects are seen in both animals exposed to VEGF stimulation in which I-CAM-1 inflammation is thought

	Anti-angiogenic	Gluco-corticoid	Mineralo-corticoid
Hydrocortisone	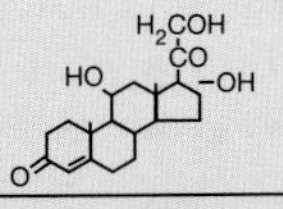 361	11	11
11α-Epihydrocortisol	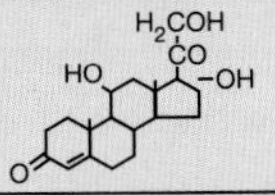 102	0	0
Cortexolone	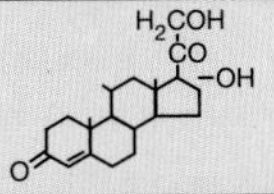 86	0*	0*
17α-Hydroxyprogesterone	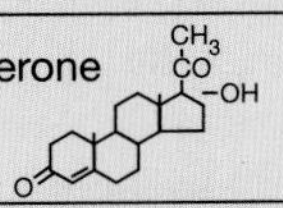 397	0*	0*
Corticosterone	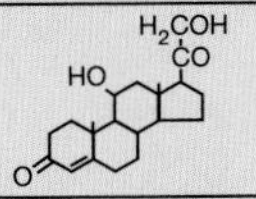 86	0.3	1.6
Desoxycorticosterone	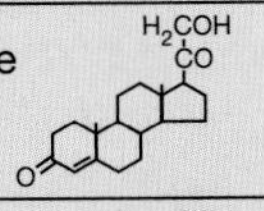 62	0	10
Progesterone	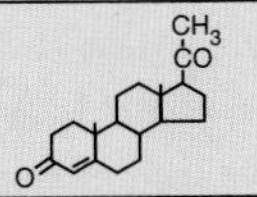 0	0	0
Testosterone	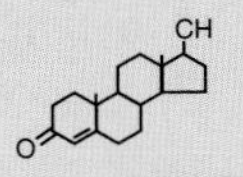 25	0	0
Estrone	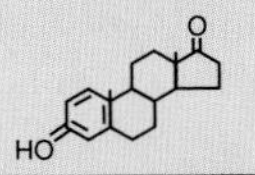 13	0	0
Pregnenolone	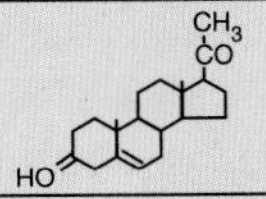 0	0	0
Tetrahydro S	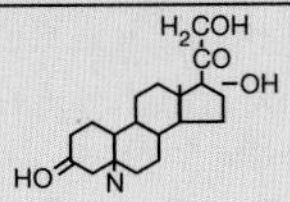 704	0	0

Fig. 65-10 A table of relative antiangiogenic potencies of normally occurring steroids related to their antiangiogenic moieties. Traditional leukocorticoid and mineralocorticoid activities are shown for comparison at right. The antiangiogenic index was determined by the percentage of avascular CAMs at the most active dose. From Crum et al. Nature 1985; 320:1375.

to play a critical role, and in experimental models induced by streptozotocin rather than exogenous VEGF administration.[51,61] Tissue specimens indicate that macrophages and other cell types express a variety of proinflammatory cytokines that may additionally contribute to this phenomenon.[54] In vitro studies with triamcinolone acetonide and a cultured epithelial cell line (ECV304) suggest that when epithelial cells are exposed to either naturally occurring stimulators of I-CAM expression such as interferon gamma or tumor necrosis factor, that triamcinolone acetonide significantly decreases permeability associated with this effect through normalization of transepithelial resistance to both fluid flow and normalization of junctional morphology.[62]

Clinical studies Clinical studies employing conventional steroids alone have shown relatively unimpressive effects on the natural history of age-related macular degeneration. In one study, intravitreal triamcinolone was used to treat eyes with recurrent subfoveal choroidal neovascularization rather than subfoveal laser, but vision showed no significant improvement over baseline. This was interpreted by the authors as a relative stabilization of vision loss over time in a small series of 14 patients.[100] The results were not as impressive as animal models of choroidal neovascularization. When triamcinolone acetonide was administered coincident with the neovascular stimulus, potent inhibition of fibrovascular proliferation was seen.[59] In one randomized clinical trial, a single dose of 4 mg of intravitreal triamcinolone was administered to 73 eyes in the treatment group receiving laser and matched to 70 eyes in the control group with a follow-up of one year.[53] Although the change in size of the neovascular membrane was significantly less in eyes receiving triamcinolone than those receiving placebo three and 12 months after treatment, there was no significant difference in the visual acuity between the two groups, although eyes receiving treatment were at a higher risk of elevated intraocular pressure (41%) than those without treatment (4%).[101]

Although the results using intravitreal triamcinolone alone have been generally interpreted as disappointing, there has been considerable enthusiasm for potential beneficial effects associated with the use of intravitreal triamcinolone combined with conventional photodynamic therapy (PDT) using Visudyne for subfoveal choroidal neovascularization.[102] Although there are limited clinical data available, in one uncontrolled clinical trial, 26 patients undergoing PDT received intravitreal triamcinolone acetonide. Of 13 patients being treated for the first time with both modalities sequentially on the same day, there was an apparent improvement in visual acuity of 1.9 lines at three months following treatment (30.8%) and only two patients (15.4%) required retreatment at three months compared with less than 10% of patients achieving visual improvement following PDT alone, the large majority requiring retreatment at three months similar to the TAP and VIP trials. The treatment benefit appeared to be less notable in patients who had already received at least one session of PDT.[102] Subsequent studies as well as our own experience[103] have confirmed this apparent beneficial effect and better controlled prospective randomized clinical trials are now under way to test further this potential beneficial interaction (personal communication, Richard Spaide 2004).

Angiostatic steroids Based upon the initial observations of a specific antiangiogenic capacity of steroids, further research has been performed further delineating the structure activity relationship for this behavior by minimizing glucocorticoid and mineralocorticoid side effects. The synergistic effect of angiostatic steroids and heparin and related compounds have been further confirmed, and a mechanism proposed in which naturally occurring compounds such as the metabolite tetrahydrocortisol alters basement membrane turnover in growing capillary blood vessels, such that the extracellular matrix is less hospitable to the budding tubes and primitive lumina seen in angiogenesis. Two important and relatively under-appreciated phenomena were discovered in conjunction with this class of angiostatic steroids: (1) a bimodal effect occurs for inhibition with actual stimulation of angiogenic response recurring at concentrations above the preferred angiostatic effect; (2) the specific angiogenic effect of specially modified steroids is strongly synergized by interaction with co-administered heparin and heparin-related compounds.[18] As an example, hydrocortisone 21 phosphate at a concentration of 60 micrograms per 10 microliters and in the presence of heparin 50 micrograms per 10 microliters, reproducibly resulted in avascular zones in 49 to 50% of chorioallantoic membranes. In contrast at even slightly higher concentrations of 70 to 200 micrograms there was reduced inhibition of angiogenesis and the appearance of an angiogenic reaction on the CAM which was further increased in the absence of heparin, but not observed with steroids that lacked glucocorticoid activity. Even moderately antiangiogenic steroids when administered in the

absence of heparin in this study failed to inhibit angiogenesis nor did heparin when administered alone, with the potentiation effect of the heparin on angiostatic steroids in the range of ten-fold or greater.[104] It was found that heparin could be substituted by a synthetic pentasaccharide with little loss in synergy, and furthermore that this synergy of coadministration could also be substituted by the use of a sulfated cyclodextrin. The combination of tetrahydrocortisol-S, a purely angiostatic corticosteroid paired with beta-cyclodextrin tetradecasulfate, or 6-alpha fluoro-17,21dihydroxy-16-beta-methyl-pregna-4,9,11 diene,3,20-dione results in a marked reduction in induced corneal neovascularization in animal models.[104] However, the inhibition of angiogenesis, as measured by eyes with normal vascularization in the CAM assay, with a conventional (nonangiostatic steroid) such as hydrocortisone was still approximately twice as great as that seen with the angiostatic steroid tetrahydrocortisol-S. Hydrocortisone cyclodextrin suppressed virtually all inflammation and cellular infiltrates compared with the angiostatic compounds which only partially reduced inflammation.[104] The reduced anti-inflammatory capability of angiostatic steroids may in part explain the failure of anecortave to enhance outcomes with Visudyne compared with triamcinolone. It is thought that therapeutic effects of photodynamic therapy which are mediated largely by the creation of free radicals and single oxygen damage to neovascular tissue may also be associated with a proangiogenic inflammatory response, including VEGF and I-CAM-1-mediated upregulation.

Subsequent to the work of Folkman, further enhancement in the chemical synthesis of specific antiangiogenic steroids have occurred, including the identification of a candidate molecule AL-3789 (Anecortave) in animal models including the CAM assay, which demonstrates the ability of anecortave to inhibit neovascularization with minimal glucocorticoid and anti-inflammatory effects[105,106] (Fig. 65-11). These results have been further confirmed in animal models of corneal neovascularization and in rat models of retinopathy prematurity in which significant benefit has been demonstrated.[107] One of the mechanisms of action is thought to

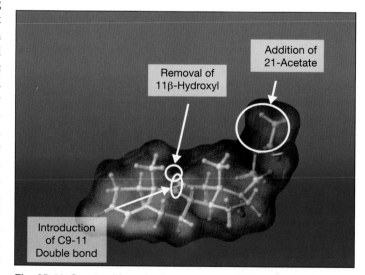

Fig. 65-11 Structural formula of anecortave acetate. Courtesy of Jason Slakter/Alcon.

be upregulation of naturally occurring plasminogen activator inhibitor 1 (PAI-1) in the extracellular matrix. The drug has shown a favorable safety and efficacy profile in preclinical studies and has recently completed phase 2 study in humans administered as a juxtascleral injection described below.[10,108] (Fig. 65-12).

In addition to anecortave and a related compound, AL-4940, additional work has been performed on another class of compounds, the estratropones.[109] 2-Methoxyestradiol, which is a mammalian metabolite of estradiol, is the prototype of this class of agents and is thought to exert its antiangiogenic effects through interaction at the colchicine scene binding site on the tubulin monomer. Further investigation of the structure activity relationship of this molecule and related molecules has elucidated a class of compounds possessing an A-ring tropone system with the ketofunction at either the C-2, C-3 or C-4 position of the steroid nucleus. Preclinical animal studies have been performed indicating 2-methoxyestradiol (2ME-2) can be placed within a silicone-based reservoir and implanted within the eye of a rabbit safely for extended delivery producing 2ME-2 vitreous levels within a therapeutic range for inhibition of endothelial cell proliferation.[110] A trial employing 2ME-2 (Panzem™) has been proposed for the eye and currently additional phase 1 and phase 2 trials are under way for malignancies thought to be sensitive to antiangiogenic effects (Entremed 2003).

Human trial with an angiostatic steroid (anecortave)

Rationale A clinical trial was performed in which the route of administration of anecortave acetate was by posterior juxtascleral injection under topical anesthesia using a custom 56-degree cannula. The goal was to place the anecortave acetate in a juxtascleral position immediately posterior to the macula. In an initial safety and efficacy trial in humans, it was determined that a single 15 mg posterior juxtascleral administration of anecortave acetate was safe and resulted in improved visual acuity outcomes when compared to the 30 mg, 3 mg, and placebo groups in the treatment of subfoveal choroidal neovascularization due to AMD. The study design was masked, randomized, and placebo-controlled. A total of 128 eyes of 128 patients were initially enrolled.[90] CNV-specific entry criteria included diagnosis of AMD, subfoveal location, size less than 12 Macular Photocoagulation Study (MPS) disc areas, angiographic evidence of the CNV occupying at least 50% of the total lesion size, with at least 50% of the CNV being classic or at least 0.75 MPS disc areas of classic CNV. Visual acuity in the experimental eye was between 20/40 and 20/320, and greater than 20/800 in the fellow eye. Patients were randomized 1:1:1:1 to one of three doses of anecortave acetate or placebo (anecortave acetate suspension). Following administration of the anecortave acetate, patients were examined on day 1 or 2, week 2, week 6, month 3, and at 6 months. At the 6-month evaluation, retreatment was left to the discretion of a masked examining ophthalmologist, based upon whether they felt the patient would benefit from further treatment. An identical follow-up plan ensued for patients who were retreated. Patients who did not receive retreatment were exited from the study. Digital fluorescein angiography was performed at week 2, week 6, month 3, retreatment, and exit. The main outcome measure was the mean change from baseline in logMar visual acuity. At the 12-month follow-up, 76 patients (59.4%) were available for evaluation. The 15 mg dose of anecortave acetate was superior to a statistically significant degree to placebo in mean change from baseline logMar visual acuity at the 12-month evaluation ($P = 0.0131$). Additionally, for the 15 mg anecortave acetate group, 79% vs. 53% of placebo-treated eyes demonstrated stabilization of visual acuity (change of <15 logMar letters, $P = 0.0323$) and 3% of 15 mg anecortave acetate vs. 23% of placebo-treated eyes had severe visual acuity loss (change of 30 logMar letters, $P = 0.0224$). Subgroup analysis demonstrated that among patients with predominantly classic subfoveal CNV, anecortave acetate (15 mg) treated patients demonstrated less change from baseline visual acuity than placebo at the month 6, 6.5, 7.5, 9, and 12 evaluations ($P < 0.0102$), with 84% of anecortave acetate (15 mg) eyes and 50% of placebo eyes demonstrating stabilization of visual acuity ($P = 0.0100$). There were no safety concerns identified related to the administration of anecortave acetate report through the month 12 evaluation. Adverse events were described as "typically mild and transient," with only one resulting in the interruption of patient participation in the study (mild visual acuity decrease that lasted following discontinuation of therapy). The two most common adverse events were cataractous lens change and visual acuity decreases of 20 logMar letters, and were evenly distributed among the four groups. Evaluation of the patients receiving anecortave acetate versus patients receiving placebo revealed only two differences: in early adverse events; mild vision abnormalities (15% for anecortave acetate, 0% for placebo) and ocular foreign body sensation (7% for anecortave acetate, 0% for placebo). This study is ongoing (Fig. 65-12).[108,111]

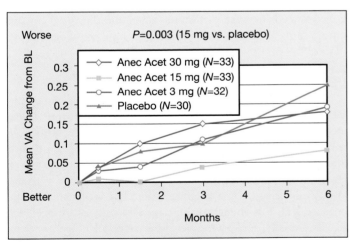

Fig. 65-12 The effects of anecortave on logMar visual acuity are summarized 6 months following treatment. There is a significant difference between treatment with anecortave acetate 15 mg and placebo with intermediate effects seen for anecortave acetate 30 mg. These results persist through one year of follow-up. The lack of a traditional escalating dose–response curve suggests that there are factors including a nonlinear dose–response effect, or the previously described paradoxical bimodal effect of increasing angiostatic steroids causing increased angiogenesis at higher doses compared with lower doses. From Acetate Clinical Study Group, Retina 2003; 23:18.

Cox-2 inhibitors

In addition to conventional steroids and angiostatic steroids as well as nontraditional methods of I-CAM-1 inhibition, Cox-2 inhibitors have been proposed as potential therapeutic approaches to neovascularization.[112] In preclinical animal models, Cox-2 inhibitors have been shown to be effective inhibitors of angiogenesis and have also decreased retinal vascular endothelial growth factor expression and vascular leakage in the streptozotocin-induced diabetic rat. Celecoxib nearly normalized VEGF mRNA expression and leakage in diabetic animals and was found to reach the retina after oral administration.[60] These studies have been further confirmed on VEGF-induced retinal vascular leakage and suggest that this approach may be applicable to the treatment of diabetic retinopathy and retinopathy of prematurity, and perhaps by extension to other ocular vascular diseases including age-related macular degeneration.[113] Clinical trials are currently under way to evaluate these effects in diabetic retinopathy (personal communication, Fredrick Ferris 2004).

I-CAM inhibitors

I-CAM inhibition through the use of conventional steroids with glucocorticoid and mineralocorticoid activity, including triamcinolone, is covered in the preceding sections.[62] A well-characterized I-CAM-1 neutralizing monoclonal antibody (aAmAb) is available as a laboratory investigational tool. At the present time the author is not aware of any human trial employing a humanized version of this monoclonal antibody. Similarly, monocyte lineage cells which are known to secrete cytokines resulting in increased expression of I-CAM-1 are able to be inhibited experimentally with clodronate encapsulated in liposomes and may represent another therapeutic avenue.[63]

Alpha interferon

The initial postulation of a potential inhibitory effect of interferon alpha 2A was based upon the known ability of this naturally occurring cytokine with anti-inflammatory properties to induce regression of childhood hemangiomas.[81] While pilot studies on this compound were equivocal,[114] a definitive large multicenter prospective randomized clinical trial unequivocally demonstrated no efficacy of subcutaneous interferon given in dosages of either 1.5, 3.0 or 6.0 m international units.[92] A total of 281 patients were prospectively randomized at one of 35 ophthalmic centers worldwide to one of three dosages or placebo and were slightly more likely to lose three lines of vision at 12 months than placebo (50% vs. 38% for the three treatment groups pooled). As a result no further studies have been performed with this modality and it is currently not recommended as a therapeutic approach to choroidal neovascularization, although therapy continues for other indications.

Rapamycin

Rapamycin (sirolimus) is a macrocyclic, naturally occurring lactone that was initially isolated from the species *Streptomyces hygroscopicus* and given its name from the region of Rapa Nui on Easter Island during the course of a search for novel antifungal agents. Rapamycin is structurally related to the immuno-suppressive agent FK506 (tacrolimus), which has been used extensively for the prevention of organ transplant rejection. Rapamycin requires direct interaction with at least two intracellular proteins to exert its action of arresting cell phase progression. FK binding protein (FKBP12) forms a rapamycin FK complex, which in turns binds to and inhibits the activity of the mammalian target of rapamycin (mTOR) through which it exerts its intracellular effects. Other FKBPs have been identified and interact with heat shock proteins. When bound to mTor, phosphorylation does not occur, and the cells' ability to mitose is blocked in addition to other effects involving protein kinase C delta, and I IL-2 dependent functions that control the progression of T cells into the S phase.[115]

Rapamycin inhibits primary metastatic tumor growth by inhibition of angiogenesis through direct inhibition of vascular endothelial growth factors as well as endothelial cell responses to VEGF.[116] It is also known that in autosomal dominant tuberous sclerosis, mutations in either the *TSC-1* or *TSC-2* gene cause loss of negative regulation of mTor activity resulting in increased endogenous secretion of vascular endothelial growth factor (VEGF) by fibroblasts. Treatment with rapamycin in vitro reduces the production of VEGF by TSC-1 and TSC-2 null fibroblasts back to normal levels associated with reduction in serum VEGF levels in knockout mice with tuberous sclerosis.[76] Additionally rapamycin through its intrinsic immunomodulatory effects may reduce macrophage chemotaxis and activation with concomitant reduction in release of VEGF and other angiogenic cytokines.

In experimental models, rapamycin has been shown to inhibit the development of ocular neovascularization in rats in response to subretinal matrigel placement orally at a dose of 2.5 mg per kilograms per day, or as in intraocular injection. Inhibition was also seen in a murine model of retinopathy of prematurity and laser-induced neovascularization when administered by an intraperitoneal route in doses of 2 mg to 4 mg per kilograms per day.[117,118]

VEGF inhibitors

A variety of methods are now available to directly inhibit the VEGF 165 molecule as well as its various other isoforms. These include the use of oligonucleotides with chain-specific sequences corresponding to the VEGF protein, monoclonal antibodies directed at one or more isoforms, and molecules directed at one or more of the VEGF receptors including native decoys, tyrosine kinase inhibitors, fusion proteins, and TIE2 receptors. Finally, because VEGF is thought to initiate a cascade of intracellular signals initially, and subsequently extracellular events, it is possible to inhibit VEGF effects either through prevention of secretion of the molecule, direct inhibition of the molecule in the extracellular space, blockade of the receptors, or through interruption in the downstream intracellular signaling pathways leading to both intra and extracellular events.[119]

Direct VEFG inhibitors – oligonucleotides

Aptamers (pegaptanib sodium [Macugen]) Aptamers are short nucleic acid sequences of specified strand shape and length, which result in a high degree of specificity and affinity for target polypeptides.[120] Unlike antibodies, aptamers are single strands of nucleic acid complementary to the polypeptide target, either RNA or DNA, which are chemically synthesized through a process termed systematic evolution of ligands by exponential enrichment (Selex).[76,121] In the case of pegaptanib, a large library of RNA sequences ranging from 10^{14} to 10^{15} sequences are incubated with the target molecule, VEGF isoform 165; the unbound sequence is washed away, the target uncoupled from the candidate strands and the process repeated between eight and 15 times resulting in increased specificity of the aptamer for the polypeptide for VEGF 165. After modification of the complementary backbone of the oligonucleotide to increase resistance to endonuclease degradation, and the attachment of a polyethylene moiety (PEG) to extend the half-life, the molecule is capable of selectively binding only VEGF 165, and not the other isoforms or other receptors. It provides sustained inhibition for in excess of 20 days in vitro, corresponding to a desired intraocular concentration in excess of the minimal inhibitory concentration necessary to inhibit VEGF 165 for a period of approximately 6 weeks.[122] Unlike proteins, aptamers are not thought to elicit an immune response nor to result in systemic inhibition of VEGF following intravitreal injection in the doses employed. The molecule is a 28-base ribonucleic acid covalently linked to two branched 20 kD polyethylene glycol moieties, and is illustrated in Fig. 65-13.[121]

Extensive preclinical studies suggested the efficacy of the molecule as a potent inhibitor of VEGF 165-related effects encompassing both permeability, and proliferation and migration of capillary endothelial cells and new vessels. In an assay of cutaneous vascular permeability (Miles Assay), pegaptanib almost completely inhibited VEGF 165-induced leakage of Evans blue dye from the vasculature of the guinea pig following intravitreal VEGF injection. In a corneal angiogenesis assay, pegaptanib resulted in approximately 65% inhibition of VEGF 165-dependent angiogenesis compared with PBS control, and in a retinopathy of prematurity study in the mouse, pegaptanib reduced retinal neovascularization relative to untreated control eyes by approximately 80% at two different doses with no untoward toxicity identified.[121] The estimated terminal half-life of the drug was found to range from 83 to 94 hours in rabbits and rhesus monkeys respectively, and 4 weeks following administration of the drug

in the vitreous humor was found to be greater than the quantity required for inhibition of VEGF, consistent with first order elimination kinetics. Selected blockade of VEGF 164 in mice, equivalent to VEGF 165 in humans, appeared to inhibit pathologic neovascularization, but did not cause a significant reduction in normal vasculogenesis. It was also not associated with regression of normal vasculature, which was seen in eyes with nonselective VEGF inhibition resulting in regression on normal vessels in the adult mouse trachea.[51,121]

In a phase 1a clinical evaluation of sodium pegaptanib, no toxicity was encountered in a single ascending dose study of intravitreal injections in 15 patients with subfoveal choroidal neovascularization.[121] In a phase 2 study, 21 patients were treated with intravitreal injection of pegaptanib in doses of 3 mg per injection in a volume of 100 microliters on three occasions at 28 day intervals.[123] The results, which were not statistically significant, suggested an improved outcome relative to control although the lack of randomization prohibited definitive conclusion. The clinical results with the combination of pegaptanib and Visudyne also appeared promising, although the sample size was too small to draw definitive conclusions.

Based upon the results of the phase 1 and phase 2 data, two randomized prospective double masked multicenter dose-ranging phase 2/3 clinical trials with broad entry criteria were conducted in humans in the United States and in Europe concurrently.[124] Patients received one of three doses of sodium pegaptanib (0.3 mg, 1 mg or 3 mg) vs. a sham injection, each of which was administered every 6 weeks for 48 weeks with a primary endpoint being the number and percentage of patients losing less than 15 letters of visual acuity. Additional efficacy endpoints included proportion of patients maintaining or gaining 0, 5, 10, or 15 letters, those losing more than 30 letters, mean changes in visual acuity at 6 week intervals from baseline to week 44, and the proportion of patients having visual acuity of 20/200 or worse constituting legal blindness at week 54.

A total of 1186 patients were randomized to one of the three treatments arms in a ratio of 1:1:1:1. With 0.3 mg pegaptanib, 70% of patients lost less than 15 letters of best-corrected visual acuity vs. 55% of controls ($P < 0.001$) for the pooled aggregate data. The risk of severe visual loss, greater than or equal to 30 letters, was reduced from 33% to 10% ($P < 0.001$), and compared with sham patients, more patients receiving 0.3 mg of pegaptanib maintained or gained visual acuity (33% vs. 23%) ($P < 0.003$). Visual acuity results were evident as early as 6 weeks following the first injection, and the treatment benefit appeared to cross all angiographic subtypes and lesion sizes. Beneficial effects were also seen for additional doses including 1 mg and 3 mg, with the results for all three doses compared with sham as well interdose comparisons presented in Table 65-1. Serious adverse events were encountered infrequently and were exclusively related to the intravitreal injection procedure rather than the drug itself. The most common serious side effect was endophthalmitis, occurring in 0.16% of eyes per injection, or 1.3% of patients overall. This complication was successfully managed in the large majority of patients and only one patient of 1186 was thought to have had severe loss of vision as a result of this

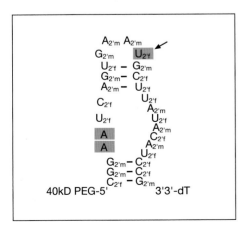

Fig. 65-13 Chemical structure of sodium pegaptanib.

Table 65-1 Results of phase 2/phase 3 clinical trial with pegaptanib. Primary endpoints (<15 letters of vision loss) and additional endpoints

Primary endpoint: patients losing <15 Letters of Visual Acuity (intention-to-treat population, $N = 1186$).*

Time point	Pegaptanib			Sham (N = 296)
	0.3 mg (N = 294)	1 mg (N = 300)	3 mg (N = 296)	
Week 12	256 (87)	259 (86)	251 (85)	237 (80)
Week 24	242 (82)	239 (80)	224 (76)	190 (64)
Week 36	220 (75)	229 (76)	222 (75)	175 (59)
Week 54	206 (70)	213 (71)	193 (65)	164 (55)

Comparisons with sham				**Interdose comparisons**		
Time point	0.3 mg vs. sham	1 mg vs. sham	3 mg vs. sham	0.3 mg vs. 1 mg	0.3 mg vs. 3 mg	1 mg vs. 3 mg
Week 12	0.012	0.049	0.13	0.99	0.54	0.75
Week 24	<0.001	<0.001	0.003	0.39	0.058	0.26
Week 36	<0.001	<0.001	<0.001	0.90	0.85	0.63
Week 54	<0.001	<0.001	0.031	0.86	0.29	0.13

Additional efficacy endpoints (intention-to-treat population, $N = 1186$).*

Endpoints	Pegaptanib			Sham (N = 296)
	0.3 mg (N = 294)	1 mg (N = 300)	3 mg (N = 296)	
Maintain/gaining ≥0 letters	98 (33)	110 (37)	93 (31)	67 (23)
P value vs. sham	0.003	<0.001	0.021	
Gaining ≥5 letters	64 (22)	69 (23)	49 (17)	36 (12)
P value vs. sham	0.004	0.002	0.12	
Gaining ≥10 letters	33 (11)	43 (14)	31 (10)	17 (6)
P value vs. sham	0.024	0.001	0.028	
Gaining ≥15 letters	18 (6)	20 (7)	13 (4)	6 (2)
P value vs. sham	0.040	0.024	0.16	
Losing ≥30 letters	28 (10)	24 (8)	40 (14)	65 (22)
P value vs. sham	<0.001	<0.001	0.014	
Visual acuity 20/200 or worse (legal blindness in study eye)	111 (38)	128 (43)	129 (44)	165 (56)
P value vs. sham	<0.001	<0.001	0.001	

*For missing data, the last observation carried forward method was used. Data are numbers of patients (%) unless otherwise noted. P values from the Cochran–Mantel–Haenszel test.
From Gragoudas ES, Adamis AP, Cunningham ET Jr et al. Pegaptanib for neovascular age-related macular degeneration. N Engl J Med 2004; 391:2805–2816.

complication. Five of 7545 intravitreous injections resulted in traumatic injury to the lens for a percent per injection rate of 0.07%. A similar number of patients sustained a retinal detachment of whom none were thought to have permanent loss as a result of this complication (Table 65-2).[125]

Small interfering RNA (siRNA) RNA interference is the process of sequence specific post-transcriptional gene silencing in animals and plants, which is initiated by double-stranded RNA (dsRNA) that is homologous in sequence to the silent gene. Con-fronted with double-stranded RNA, eukaryotic cells respond by destroying their own messenger RNA (mRNA) that shares these sequences with the double-strand.[126] The process appears to be mediated by 21 and 22 nucleotide, small interfering RNAs (siRNAs), that are generated by ribonuclease 3 cleavage from longer dsRNAs.[75] siRNA differs from an aptamer in being double rather than single-stranded RNA and results in the inhibition of synthesis of VEGF through the destruction of VEGF-specific RNA rather than through the binding of free VEGF 165 by pegaptanib.

Table 65-2 Injection-related serious adverse events in patients treated with pegaptanib (N = 892)

Condition	Occurrence of event			Occurrence of severe visual acuity loss*	
	Number of patients	Percent patients	Percent per injection	Number of patients	Percent patients
Endophthalmitis	12†	1.3	0.16	1	0.1
Traumatic lens injury	5	0.6	0.07	1	0.1
Retinal detachment	5	0.6	0.07	0‡	0

A total of 7545 intravitreous injections of pegaptanib were administered.
*Severe visual acuity loss is defined as a loss of ≥30 letters.
†Three quarters of the endophthalmitis patients remained in the trial, ¾ were associated with protocol violations.
‡ Post-event vision not available in one patient.
From Gragoudas ES, Adamis AP, Cunningham ET Jr et al. Pegaptanib for neovascular age-related macular degeneration. N Engl J Med 2004; 391:2805–2816.

siRNA specific for human vascular endothelial growth factor (VEGF), and an enhanced green fluorescent protein (EGFP) were designed and tested as active molecule and negative control in both in vitro cell lines chemically induced to simulate hypoxia as well as in a laser-induced model of choroidal neovascularization in mice. siRNA was delivered by co-injection with recombinant viruses carrying small hVEGF cDNA to induce expression of the appropriate siRNA in the subretinal space. Production of siRNA was confirmed by the expression of EGFP in the subretinal space with positive controls, and as evidence of VEGF transgene expression, which resulted in significant inhibition of choroidal neovascularization compared with negative controls after laser photocoagulation.[126] Conventionally injected siRNA at dosages of 70, 150 or 350 micrograms in a 0.05 ml volume with a vehicle serving as a negative control was also successful in reducing choroidal neovascularization in a primate model following standardized laser injury between 15 and 36 days after treatment in conjunction with reduced permeability, angiographically and reduced lesion sizes measured by planimetric methods in a masked fashion[77] (Fig. 65-14). Presently studies are under way to test the safety and efficacy of this molecule in humans (personal communication, Michael Tolentino, Acuity Pharmaceuticals).

Monoclonal antibodies

Bevacizumab is a mouse-derived monoclonal antibody to VEGF produced by humanization of the mouse epitopes that was designed to neutralize the effects of all isoforms of VEGF in clinical disease. Preclinical studies in animal models of various tumor cell lines as well as different forms of ocular neovascularization indicated that the fully sized antibody had excellent efficacy against the primary permeability and proliferative effects of VEGF isoforms. It was found to be effective in slowing tumor growth through its effects on angiogenesis.[69] Following extensive clinical testing, bevacizumab was shown to increase duration and survival, response rate, and duration of response compared with conventional therapy consisting of irinotecan fluorouracil and leukovorin for metastatic colorectal cancer.[127] However, because of the relatively large molecular weight of a fully sized IgG molecule of approximately 150 000 daltons, the compound was found not to be able to cross the retina following intravitreal injection and therefore was probably unable to exert a potential effect against VEGF in the subretinal space or beneath the pigment epithelium. As a result parallel efforts to assess its efficacy in human ocular neovascularization were not pursued initially. Subsequently, using pepsin cleavage techniques, it was possible to create rhuFab VEGF (recombinant humanized fragment of antibody) representing the Fab portion (antigen-binding portion) of the anti-VEGF monoclonal antibody, that consisted of two parts. The first was a nonbinding human sequence making it less antigenic in primates as well as a high affinity binding epitope derived from the mouse serving to bind the antigen. Its molecular weight of 48 000 made it a significantly smaller molecule than the full-length monoclonal antibody with a molecular weight 148 000, thus rendering

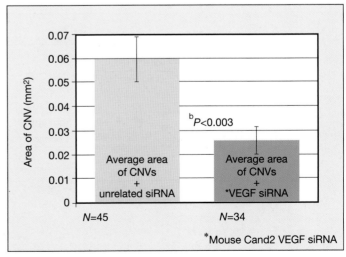

Fig. 65-14 Effects of siRNA treatment in murine model of choroidal neovascularization. From Reich et al. Mol Vis 2003; 9:210–216.

it capable of penetrating the internal limiting membrane of the retina and crossing the subretinal space in order to inhibit VEGF in that region. This molecule termed rhuFab is demonstrated in Fig. 65-15 with the active portion representing one of the two arms of the Fab fragment contrasted with the full size molecule on the left and its relative conformational shape seen on the right (Fig. 65-15).

Ranibizumab (rhuFab): primate and human studies

Ranibizumab (rhuFAB VEGF, Lucentis), the antigen-binding portion of the monoclonal antibody directed against VEGF was tested in a phase I/II preclinical cross-over study. The phase I/II cross-over study consisted of cynomolgus monkeys receiving intravitreal injections of ranibizumab in one eye and vehicle in the other eye at 2-week intervals. Beginning at day 21, laser photo-coagulation was performed in each eye to induce CNV develop-ment. Eyes receiving vehicle alone were crossed over 21 days after laser photocoagulation to receive ranibizumab intravitreal injections at day 42 and day 56. Fluorescein angiography, fundus photography, and clinical examination were performed. All eyes developed an anterior chamber inflammatory response within the first 24 hours after intravitreal injection of ranibizumab that was self-limited, resolving within one week. Subsequent injections were associated with recurrent, yet blunted, inflammatory responses. Control eyes demonstrated no inflammatory response until the point of cross-over. At that time, they too demonstrated an inflammatory response. Eyes receiving intravitreal ranibizumab were less likely to develop grade 4 leakage on angiography following induction of CNV when compared to control eyes ($P < 0.001$). In the cross-over study eyes, the number of eyes with grade 4 leakage was reduced at the 1, 2, and 3-week follow-up when compared to the same eyes prior to the cross-over time point ($P = 0.001$).[128]

The rhuFAB V2 fragment was evaluated for tolerance at doses of 300 mg following 4-monthly intravitreal injections in a phase Ib/II study and noted to have no adverse effects in 30 human subjects. A follow-up study compared rhuFAB V2 (0.3 mg or

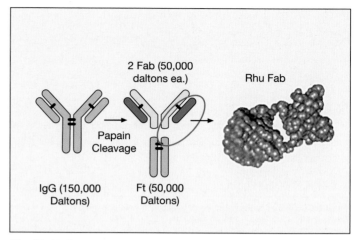

Fig. 65-15 Structural formal of recombinant fragment of human monoclonal antibody directed against VEGF (rhuFAB). Courtesy of William Greene MD, Genentech.

0.5 mg) to "usual care" (4:1 rhuFAB V2: "usual care"). Patients receiving the 0.3 mg dose had an improvement of 8.5 ± 3.3 letters on the ETDRS chart, compared to a loss of 3.0 ± 5.6 letters in the "usual care" group. Following cross-over, the "usual care" group received intravitreal rhuFAB V2 and improved to a gain of 7.3 ± 6.6 letters at day 210.[29,129]

These results are summarized in Fig. 65-16, demonstrating a net gain of approximately nine letters for patients receiving either doses of 300 μg or 500 μg of rhuFab V2 as contrasted with a decline of approximately five letters at 112 weeks for patients receiving usual care.[29,130] Two large prospective masked controlled trials are currently under way (Anchor and Marina) comparing the efficacy of rhuFab (Lucentis®), as an intravitreal injection compared with a sham injection in patients with pre-dominantly classic choroidal neovascularization as well as occult forms of choroidal neovascularization. The entry criteria and efficacy endpoints are generally comparable to those employed

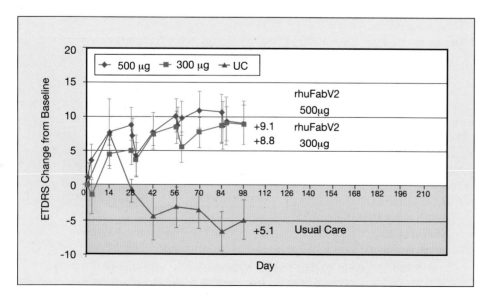

Fig. 65-16 Results of Phase I/II rhuFAB trial in humans. Courtesy of Jeffrey Heier MD.[29,129]

in the TAP and VIP studies, as well as the VISION Trials with pegaptanib (Macugen). Therefore a relative comparison of these forms of therapy against one another for primary disease should be possible, although at the time of writing the data have not yet been released.

VEGF receptor (VEGFR) inhibitors

A variety of techniques are available to utilize the receptors normally bound to the cell surface, principally tyrosine kinases to act as competitive inhibitors of VEGF either in their native state soluble in the extracellular matrix as may be occasionally seen as a normal decoy situation with VEGFR-1, or through specialized chemical modifications (Fig. 65-7).

VEGF-TRAP (R1R2) is a fusion protein which combines ligand binding elements taken from the extracellular domains of VEGF receptors 1 and 2 fused to the Fc portion of IgG. This is used as a means of blocking the normal VEGF signaling pathway by inhibiting binding of VEGF to its normal receptors rather than to the decoy soluble receptors. Potent anti-VEGF effects can be achieved.[131,132] These include the inhibition of tumor growth and vascularization in response to VEGF-TRAP administration and the suppression of choroidal neovascularization using a similar molecule after laser-induced rupture of Bruch's membrane in mice by the intravitreal injection of VEGF-TRAP. These molecules are now being tested in preliminary clinical trials (Regeneron Pharmaceuticals). A selective small molecule kinase inhibitor of vascular endothelial growth factor VEGFR2 with activity against both VEGF-induced angiogenesis and vascular permeability (SU10944) has demonstrated a dose–response effect in reducing corneal neovascularization following oral administration doses of approximately 30 mg per kilogram with maximum inhibition of 95% at 300 mg per kilogram as well as in the Miles Permeability Assay.[133] Other similar approaches have included the administration of Tie-2, an endothelial specific receptor tyrosine kinase, that when administered through adenovirus-mediated gene delivery inhibited experimental retinal and choroidal neovascularization by as much as 47% as well as fluorescein leakage by a comparable degree.[134] The Tie-2 receptor is thought to be an endothelial specific receptor tyrosine kinase that is phosphorylated and activated upon binding of angiopoietin-1.[2] In addition to adenovirus vector-mediated expression of soluble Tie-2, the soluble Fl-1 receptor has been utilized as another alternate ligand for VEGF following adeno-associated virus secretion by intraocular injection.[135] Delivery of the vector into the anterior chamber results in transgene expression in the iris pigment epithelium and vascular endothelium, and reduces the development of corneal neovascularization in the treated rats by 36% compared with cauterized control groups as well as in suppressing choroidal neovascularization following subretinal delivery utilizing a different vector.[136]

Intracellular signaling blockers

Nitric oxide synthetase inhibitors (NOS)
Nitric oxide synthetase and its product nitric oxide are thought to play a critical role in VEGF-induced angiogenesis and vascular permeability. It is believed that its effects are mediated through its activation

of VEGFR2 (KDR) and through stimulation of a KDR-C-SRC complex which triggers calcium release through the second messenger pathway. As a result, NOS, which is calcium-dependent and constitutively expressed in vascular endothelial cells is almost immediately activated. There appears to be at least three isoforms of NOS: neuronal NOS (nNOS), inducible NOS (iNOS), and endothelial (eNOS).[71] It is known that inhibition of in vivo NO production results in reduced angiogenesis and vascular permeability induced by VEGF. eNOS stimulation through the KDR-C-SRC complex appears to be the most important of the three isoforms and it is regulated by protein kinase Akt. iNOS is found to be expressed in avascular tissue in proliferative retinopathy in vivo. It is responsible for retinal neuronal cell death by apoptosis.[72] NOS suppression either by the inhibitor N-nitro-l-arginine (l-NNA) or through knockout with a homozygous targeted disruption of the gene for endothelial NOS (eNOS) resulted in approximately 43% reduction in oxygen-induced retinal vaso-obliteration.[137] A similar blockade of NOS resulted in neovascularization, although depending upon the type of NOS blocked, differential results were noted. In ischemia-induced retinal neovascularization, nitric oxide produced by eNOS is stimulatory, but nitric oxide produced in other retinal cells by iNOS and/or nNOS is inhibitory.[138] At the present time NOS inhibitors and other related forms of therapy do not occupy an important role in the mitigation of VEGF-associated hyperpermeability in neovascularization in patients, but may become important in the future.

TrpRS inhibitors
Another class of compounds that appear to play an important role in intracellular signaling following VEGF stimulation are the human aminoacyl-t-RNA synthetases. These molecules, which catalyze the first step of protein synthesis by aminoacylation of transfer RNA appear to have novel cytokine functions in addition to their role in protein synthesis. The catalytic core domain of tryptophanyl-tRNA synthetase (TrpRS) is a close homolog of the catalytic domain of tyrosine RS (TyRS).[91] In normal human cells the TrpRS exists as two forms. The major form is a full-length protein, which is stimulated by interferon gamma and has no cytokine activity. The other is truncated TrpRS (miniTrpRS) in which most of the extra NH_2 terminal domain is deleted through alternate splicing of the mRNA. In addition to its production by alternative splicing, shorter fragment lengths of TrpRS can also be created by PMN elastase cleavage of full human length TrpSR into two forms of miniTrpRS, both of which show cytokine-related activity. In contrast neither full-length TrpRS nor miniTrpRS induced migration of endothelial cells.[139] When cells were induced with VEGF 165 and then treated with TrpRS, migration was inhibited by the miniTrp fraction, but not the full-length fraction. VEGF 165-induced angiogenesis in CAMs was inhibited by miniTrpRS, but not full-length TrpRS, as was neovascularization induced in a murine matrigel model. Following digestion with leukocyte elastase, of the two shortened products found, both of which underwent truncation at the NH terminal end, the smaller of the two, T2-TrpRS in which the entire NH_2 terminal domain had been deleted, appeared to be the most potent antiangiogenesis agent with dose-dependent angiostatic activity. The molecule appeared to be bound within the retina

to endothelial cells.[91] The efficacy of this molecule appears to be not as an intrinsic inhibitor, but as a downregulator of stimulation induced by VEGF suggesting it represents a portion of the downstream signal cascade following VEGF stimulation, along with NOS, and expression of surface integrins.[140] A recombinant form of the human T2-TrpRS13 now being tested for potential efficacy in human models of choroidal neovascularization (personal communication, Martin Friedlander, Angiosyn).

PKC inhibitors Protein kinase C isoforms, particularly beta isoform, are thought to play an important regulatory role in intracellular signaling following VEGF stimulation of endothelial and other cells through phosphorylation mechanisms.[141] Most of the work detailing the interaction between VEGF effects on vascular permeability and PKC beta has been performed in experimental diabetic retinopathy and in preliminary human trials. The beta isoform of PKC (protein kinase C) has been implicated in both the early and late stage manifestations of diabetic retinopathy with studies suggesting that orally administered ly333531, a beta isoform specific PKC inhibitor may be effective in reducing retinopathy progression proliferation and leakage.[141,142] Protein kinases transfer terminal high-energy phosphate groups of ATP to the target site on proteins, triggering enzyme cell membrane receptors and ion transport channels.[143] A recent large multicenter randomized trial evaluating the use of a specific protein kinase C beta isoform inhibitor, ly333531, showed improved vision and trends towards improvement in the severity of retinopathy and macular edema, although not to a statistically significant degree for the group as a whole. New trials are underway to attempt to show benefit for this class of compound and diabetic retinopathy (personal communication, Lloyd Aiello 2004, Eli Lilly). An alternative protein kinase C inhibitor PKC412, that blocks several isoforms of protein kinase C was administered via a periocular injection within microspheres containing either 25% or 50% drug. Ten to 20 days following laser rupture and injection, CNV at Bruch's membrane rupture sites were smaller in eyes receiving drug than those receiving control microspheres without drugs. Additionally, 20 days following periocular injection, high levels of the inhibitor were measured in the choroid vitreous and retina for eyes with 50% loading and to a lesser extent with 25% loading.[144]

Naturally occurring inhibitory polypeptides and inducible cleavage products

While the protein miniTrpRC might also be considered in this category, a broader category is reserved for those agents, which are thought to be naturally secreted into the extracellular space rather than acting as intracellular signals and include normal inducible homeostatic regulators. An example is PEDF, which is thought to modulate neuronal differentiation in the outer retina following apical secretion by the pigment epithelium in addition to its downregulation of VEGF effects on endothelial cells. Although TrpRS seems to function principally as an intracellular messenger in the cascade associated with VEGF-stimulation of VEGFR 1 and 2, it may also be secreted into the extracellular space and thus fulfill the above criteria. In addition to these compounds, there are pathologically expressed circulating molecules that are formed as a result of cleavage by specific proteases from larger pre-existing polypeptides that have intrinsic antiangiogenic potency. These also include angiostatin and endostatin, in addition to PEDF.[137]

PEDF

Pigment epithelial derived factor (PEDF) was first purified in the conditioned media of human retinal pigment epithelial cells that induced neuronal differentiation as well as inhibiting microglial growth. The protein shares sequence and structural homology with the serum proteinase inhibitor family (Serpen). One of its most striking abilities is the capacity to inhibit endothelial cell migration in a dose-dependent manner with a greater degree of potency than either angiostatin, thrombospondin-1 or endostatin. A variety of potentially attractive therapeutic avenues are possible with endostatin, which is naturally secreted by retinal pigment epithelial cells, but not iris pigment epithelial cells.[64] It has been possible to use adenovirus vector-mediated gene transfer of cDNA constructs to iris pigment epithelium (IPE) resulting in autologous IPE cells gaining the capacity to support the choriocapillaris and outer retina in vivo.[145] Iris pigment epithelial cells which overexpressed in PEDF were capable of rescuing photoreceptors in RCS rats, reducing laser-induced CNV and partially reversing the effects of ischemic retinopathy in various animal models.[83] This has led to the initiation of an open label phase 1 single administration dose escalation study of ADGVEPVF.11D (ADPEVF) in patients with choroidal neovascularization (oxyiGENE). The results of the study are not known and await further testing and analysis.[146]

Pathologically expressed circulating molecules

Angiostatin Angiostatin is an internal proteolytic fragment of a known protein, plasminogen, expressed in association with tumor growth in the serum such that it inhibits primary metastatic tumor growth by blocking tumor angiogenesis. Angiostatin does not appear to have a specific gene locus resulting in transcription, but rather represents a cryptic fragment produced in response to pathologic rather than physiologic conditions, such as primary tumor growth. The molecule has a molecular weight of 38 kilodaltons and inhibits endothelial cell proliferation in vitro and angiogenesis in vivo.[93] It appears that tumor cells do not themselves express angiostatin or other fragments of plasminogen. Rather gelatinase A also known as matrix metalloproteinase-2, which is produced by rapidly growing tumor cells such as experimental Lewis lung carcinoma, performs the proteolysis of plasminogen.[86] When administered systemically, angiostatin can regress a wide variety of malignant tumors through its inhibitory effects on angiogenesis. Adenovirus-associated vectors causing overexpression of angiostatin in a murine model of choroidal neovascularization were effective in causing regression. Expression of the angiostatin gene in choroidoretinal tissue for up to 150 days was possible as was reduction in the average size of CNV lesions in treated eyes as compared with control eyes. There were no significant adverse events reported in the animal model using target gene therapy.[82,136]

Endostatin   Another compound from this class, endostatin, is thought to represent a proteolytic fragment of 20 kD created by digestion of the C terminal fragment of collagen XVIII.[85] Endostatin inhibits both endothelial cell proliferation in vitro and angiogenesis and tumor growth in vivo and is capable of being delivered by a variety of methods including sustained delivery or adenovirus vector.[84] Zinc binding of endostatin is thought to be essential for its antiangiogenic activity and metal chelating agents can induce internal degradation of endostatin with associated loss of activity.[147] Full-length human type 18 collagen CDNAs that encode 1516 or 336 residue alpha chains exhibit homology with endostatin. Incorporated with adenoviral vectors and administered intravenously, it can be demonstrated that endostatin levels tend to rise with concomitant reduction in CNV size in experimental models.[84] The zinc requirement for endostatin may be one component of the apparent beneficial effect of zinc in the AREDs trial along with other effects on matrix metalloproteinases and dismutases.[148]

Extracellular matrix modulators

A variety of targets exist outside the cell in the extracellular matrix for therapeutic intervention. Some such as the alpha v beta 3 and alpha v beta 5 integrins are expressed on the cell surface in response to VEGF stimulation and participate in the adhesion of other regulatory molecules as well as interaction with metalloproteinases responsible for degradation of the extracellular matrix, facilitating migration and sprouting of new vessels.[149] Additionally others such as the naturally occurring tissue inhibitors of metalloproteinase (TIMP) or other synthetic metalloproteinase inhibitors may actually precede the VEGF activation step and represent both early and late targets for intervention.

Integrin antagonists

Examination of tissues from eyes with pathologic neovascularization indicate that at least two cytokine-dependent pathways of angiogenesis exist and both may be important in pathologic neovascularization. In in vivo models including both corneal and chorioallantoic membrane angiogenesis induced by basic fibroblast growth factor or tumor necrosis factor alpha, the cell surface expressed integrin alpha v beta 3 predominates, whereas in models initiated by vascular endothelial growth factor (VEGF) transforming growth factor alpha (TgF-alpha), or phorbol ester the pathway is characterized by dependence on and expression of the related cytokine alpha v beta 5.[65,66] These findings are further confirmed by several lines of evidence that have therapeutic implications, including the fact that inhibition of protein kinase C, an intracellular messenger discussed earlier, using a specific inhibitor calphostin C blocked angiogenesis induced by VEGF and TGF alpha, but had only a small effect on basic fibroblast growth factor or TNF alpha-mediated angiogenesis. This suggests the specificity of the two pathways: (1) dependent on alpha v beta 3 and relatively independent of PKC; (2) the second potentiated by alpha v beta 5, but dependent upon both VEGF stimulation and PKC activation.[65,66]

Therapeutically several alternative methods for the inhibition of alpha v beta 3 and alpha v beta 5 expression exists. In immunohistochemical examination of tissues removed from eyes with pathologic neovascularization, it appears that for the purposes of inhibiting choroidal rather than retinal neovascularization, selective inhibition of the alpha v beta 3 pathway may be preferred. When neovascular membranes removed from patients with choroidal neovascularization secondary to age-related macular degeneration were examined, only the expression of alpha v beta 3 was observed whereas both alpha v beta 3 and alpha v beta 5 were present on vascular cells and tissues from patients with proliferative diabetic retinopathy.

A cyclic peptide antagonist of alpha v beta 3 and alpha v beta 5 was capable of dramatically reducing retinal vessel blood growth contrasted with a control peptide in a neonatal mouse model of retinopathy of prematurity. The cyclic peptide cyclo RGDv was composed of a sequence of arg-gly-aspartic acid-phenylalanine-valene. Other molecules including XJ735 and the alpha v beta 3 antagonist, $XKOO_2$, a combined antagonist of alpha v beta 3 and alpha v beta 5, also inhibit retinal neovascularization in a murine model.[150] Cyclic RGDfV peptide was found to represent an antagonist of vitronectin receptor type integrins by other groups.[2]

Another approach rather than specific receptor binding with polypeptide molecules is the use of selective monoclonal antibodies directed against cell surface integrins. Specific mouse monoclonal antibodies to integrins alpha v beta 3 (LM609) and alpha v beta 5 (P1F6) have been prepared, and in addition to demonstrating the presence of expressed integrins on vascular cell surfaces, have also been used therapeutically to inhibit neovascularization. Antibodies directed against alpha v beta 3 appeared to selectively block bVGF-induced angiogenesis whereas antibodies directed against antibeta 1 and alpha v beta 5 had dramatically less effect and appeared to spare pre-existing preformed vessels.[65,66] Other approaches have included the conjugation of mitomycin C dextran to a monoclonal anti-integrin alpha v beta 3 antibody, which was more effective than the use of a mouse monoclonal alone in a rat model of laser-induced choroidal neovascularization.[151] It is anticipated that these confirmatory preclinical studies will soon lead to early stage human trials of both polypeptide antagonists and also monoclonal antagonists of alpha v beta 3, alpha v beta 5 integrins, and other classes of integrins.

MMP inhibitors

The naturally occurring class of tissue inhibitors of metalloproteinase (TIMP), particularly TIMP-3 are thought to be critically important in the homeostasis of the extracellular matrix and thereby to factors contributing to the development of choroidal neovascularization. Large quantities of TIMP-3 have been found with increasing age in Bruch's membrane where it is thought to be a normal structural component and particularly in areas where there is pathologic thickening of Bruch's membrane.[23,27,87] The COOH terminal end of TIMP-3, unlike TIMP-1, TIMP-2 and TIMP-4 which are soluble, is exclusively membrane-bound and the NH terminal end appears to inhibit MMPs 2 and 9, which are known to be expressed in choroidal new vessel membranes removed from patients with subfoveal choroidal neovascularization.[88] TIMP-3 naturally inhibits VEGF and is capable of reducing angiogenesis in vitro and in vivo, including CAM assays and also when overexpressed by selective gene therapy in rat eyes undergoing laser photocoagulation for the induction of choroidal neovascularization.[88,89] Although mutations in TIMP-3 are not thought to account for the vast majority of patients with genetically determined choroidal neovascularization based upon linkage analysis,[25] it is well-known that point mutations in the carboxy terminal-end of exon-5 of the *TIMP* gene in chromosome 22 are causal for Sorsby's fundus dystrophy, an early onset form of choroidal neovascularization associated with extensive thickening of Bruch's membrane, drusen formation, and many of the other cardinal features of the exudative form of age-related macular degeneration.[4,96] Thus pharmacologic therapies directed at replacement or modification of TIMP-3 and potentially other related compounds may have utility as a pharmacologic strategy not only for regulation of the extracellular matrix in response to late VEGF stimulation, but potentially earlier in regulating the homeostatic mechanisms which lead to Bruch's membrane thickening and the other inducible factors for choroidal neovascularization preceding VEGF activation (Fig. 65-17).[131]

Matrix metalloproteinase inhibitors (MMPI) have been tested for their ability to inhibit pathologic ocular neovascularization. AG3340, a synthetic MMP2,9 inhibitor was shown to significantly inhibit neovascularization in a mouse model of retinopathy of prematurity leading to a human phase 2/3 trial.[152] However, the study was unable to confirm any inhibitory effect of the small molecular weight binding inhibitor of MMP-2 MMP-9 in any dose tested either with regards to lesion size, or final visual acuity and

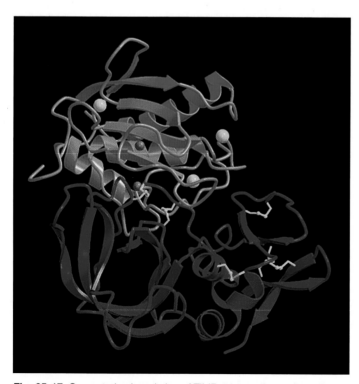

Fig. 65-17 Computerized rendering of TIMP-1 interacting as its active NH site with MMP-3 catalytic domain. From Gornis et al. Nature 1997; 389:77–81.

efforts were halted (personal communication, Agouran/Pfizer Pharmaceuticals 2002). Other MMP inhibitors continue to be tested in preclinical studies.

Other molecules

A variety of molecules with varying mechanisms of action are undergoing preliminary evaluation. Combrestatin A-4, a naturally occurring agent from tree bark that binds tubulin and causes necrosis and shrinkage of tumors by inhibition of the blood supply is capable of suppressing experimental choroidal neovascularization in response to photocoagulation.[130,153] Preliminary trials are under way in humans to test its efficacy and early stage neovascularization AMD (Oxigene 2003).

Squalamine

Squalamine is an anti-angiogenic amino sterol derived from shark fin which inhibits iris neovascularization when administered by intravenous injection, although it is ineffective when administered by intravitreal injection.[154,155] Squalamine also induces regression of experimental retinopathy of prematurity in a mouse model[156] and has been tested in a phase 1 study of choroidal neovascularization in patients with no safety concerns expressed leading to the announcement of additional studies in humans (Genera 2004).

Photodynamic therapy

Pharmacology of photodynamic sensitizers   Photodynamic therapy actually represents the combination of a pharmacologic therapy and a laser-based therapy in a two-step process capable of successfully treating subfoveal choroidal neovascularization. Photosensitizers have biophysical properties well-suited to the thrombotic closure of abnormal neovascularization while preserving normal physiologic vessels. Most agents possess strong absorption properties in the far-red spectral region (660 to 780 nanometers) where light has the greatest penetration through blood and tissue. Photosensitizers also selectively bind to abnormal neovascularization through its expression of increased numbers of lipoprotein receptors contrasted with normal mature vessels, thus achieving the desirable feature of selectivity. Most photosensitizing molecules, including Visudyne which has been approved for human use, as well as a number of agents under clinical evaluation are structurally related to porphyrins (Fig. 65-18). Porphyrins are fused tetrapyrrolic macromolecules found in nature as pigments such as protoporphyrin IX, the nonprotein portion of hemoglobin. Benzoporphyrin derivative monoacid verteporfin (Visudyne) consists of two isomers that differ in the location of the carboxylic acid and methyl ester on the lower pyrrole rings of the chlorine macrocycle. Because Visudyne is hydrophobic, it requires formulation within liposomes, which in addition to improving penetration into cells and delivery by an intravenous route, also may actually further enhance its selectivity. Visudyne is activated with a monochromatic laser light in the range of approximately 689–691 nanometers at a power setting of 600 milliwatts per cm[2] and produces selective closure of abnormal choroidal neovascularization while minimizing damage to adjacent normal choroid as well as the overlying pigment

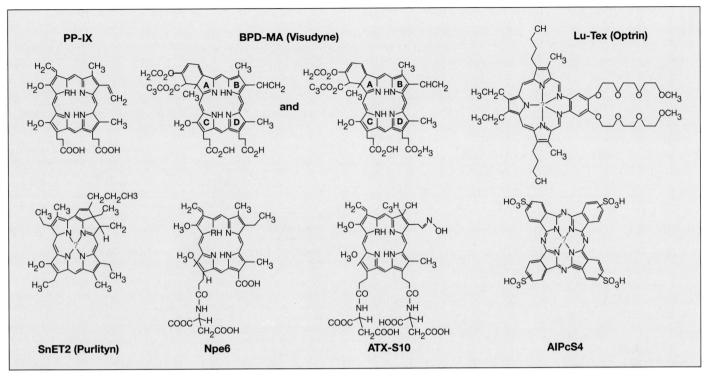

Fig. 65-18 Structural formulae of photodynamic therapy agents either approved (Visudyne) or under investigation for use in humans. From Woodburn et al. Retina 2002; 22:391–405.

epithelium and neurosensory retina. The molecule is well-tolerated following intravenous administration and cutaneous light sensitivity is kept to a minimum compared with other molecules which either have longer periods of photosensitization, or less favorable therapeutic indices.

Other molecules undergoing evaluation although not yet approved for use in humans include tin-ethyl-etiopurpurin (Purlytin), monotexafin lutetium (Optrin, Lu-tex), Npe6, and ATX-S10. Their chemical formulas are listed in Fig. 65-18. Purlytin was subjected to a large multicenter phase 2/phase 3 clinical trial, which demonstrated a trend towards efficacy in selected subgroups, although it failed to meet the pre-approved regulatory efficacy endpoint. Concerns also exist regarding its larger potential for longer term photosensitization than Visudyne. Currently the drug is undergoing further regulatory review.

Lu-tex underwent a phase 1 dose escalation trial in humans, which demonstrated its ability to achieve photodynamic closure. However it is associated with a greater degree of surrounding choroidal damage than Visudyne, and is also associated with peripheral paresthesias and occasional periocular pain in selected patients. NPE6 and ATX-10 are currently the subject of continuing preclinical studies and at the time of writing no human trials are under way.[157]

Visudyne Verteporfin photodynamic therapy (PDT) was the first photosensitizer approved for the treatment of exudative AMD. The technique involves infusion of 6 mg/m² verteporfin over a 10 minute period followed by laser irradiation using a 689 nm diode laser (light dose: 50 J/cm²; power density: 600 mW/cm²;

duration: 83 seconds) 15 minutes after the start of the infusion. Verteporfin demonstrated safety and efficacy in selectively localizing to choroidal neovascular membranes in preclinical trials in nonhuman primates. The mechanism of action is postulated to occur by activation of verteporfin to a triplet state following laser irradiation, resulting in the creation of singlet and reactive oxygen species that induces endothelial cellular damage and, ultimately, occlusion of the neovascular membranes through activation of the clotting cascade. This vascular occlusion was demonstrated in nonhuman primates both angiographically and histologically.[158–162] Several histopathologic studies in humans have subsequently demonstrated that while vascular occlusion does occur following verteporfin PDT, this effect is transient, usually disappearing by 1 month after treatment.[55] Flower and others have proposed that Sattler layer vessels are temporarily damaged following verteporfin PDT, resulting in the typical hypofluorescent spot seen on angiography, and accounting for the high recurrence rate after therapy.[111,158] Unfortunately the generation of free radicals necessary for the photothrombotic effect, may also serve as a proangiogenic stimulus, possibly accounting for the apparent benefit associated with concomitant administration of steroids.

Verteporfin PDT was demonstrated to be safe and effective for treatment of CNV due to AMD in phase 1 and 2 testing.[163,164] The Treatment of Age-related Macular Degeneration with Photodynamic Therapy (TAP) Study demonstrated that patients with CNV due to AMD demonstrated a beneficial effect following verteporfin PDT. The greatest benefit was seen among the subset of patients with predominantly classic subfoveal CNV due to AMD, with 67% of verteporfin-treated eyes vs. 39% of placebo-treated eyes prevented from progressing to moderate visual loss, namely, loss of <15 letters on the Early Treatment Diabetic Retinopathy Study (ETDRS) scale or approximately three lines of vision ($P < 0.001$). Lesions that were less than 50% classic did not demonstrate a treatment benefit. These results were valid through the 2-year follow-up.[165,166] Further discussion of the role of verteporfin in AMD is covered in Chapter 60. Presently, verteporfin PDT is approved for the treatment of AMD lesions which are predominantly classic subfoveal CNV or for occult or minimally classic subfoveal CNV less than four disc diameters in size.[124,167,168]

SUMMARY

A variety of molecules, specifically targeted to different pathologic pathways in AMD, have been identified for their therapeutic potential. Research is actively being pursued in preclinical models both in academic laboratories and in the pharmaceutical industry, including multiple early stage clinical trials. It is anticipated that molecules with activity at various stages of the disease, and especially including those multiple stages relating to RPE function, the visual transduction cycle, metalloproteinase homeostasis, and VEGF inhibition, will find prominent roles either alone or in combination such as photodynamic therapy and combined laser and drug surgical therapies.

REFERENCES

1. Bird AC, Bressler NM, Bressler SB et al. The International ARM Epidemiological Study Group. An international classification and grading system for age-related maculopathy and age-related macular degeneration. Surv Ophthalmol 1995; 39:367–374.
2. Ambati J, Ambati BK, Yoo SH et al. Age-related macular degeneration: etiology, pathogenesis, and therapeutic strategies. Surv Ophthalmol 2003; 48:257–293.
3. Blumenkranz MS, Russell SR, Robey MD et al. Risk factors in age-related maculopathy complicated by choroidal neovascularization. Ophthalmology 1986; 93:552–558.
4. Ferris FL 3rd, Fine SL, Hyman L. Age-related macular degeneration and blindness due to neovascular maculopathy. Arch Ophthalmol 1984; 102:1640–1642.
5. Ferris FL 3rd. Senile macular degeneration: review of epidemiologic features. Am J Epidemiol 1983; 118:132–151.
6. Bressler NM, Hawkins BS, Sternberg P Jr et al. Are the submacular surgery trials still relevant in an era of photodynamic therapy? Ophthalmology 2001; 108:435–436.
7. Macular Photocoagulation Study Group. Argon laser photocoagulation for senile macular degeneration: results of a randomized clinical trial. Arch Ophthalmol 1982; 100:912–918.
8. Macular Photocoagulation Study Group. Argon laser photocoagulation for neovascular maculopathy: three-year results from randomized clinical trials. Arch Ophthalmol 1986; 104:694–701.
9. Macular Photocoagulation Study Group. Laser photocoagulation of subfoveal neovascular lesions of age-related macular degeneration: updated findings from two clinical trials. Arch Ophthalmol 1993; 111:1200–1209.
10. Slakter JS, Yannuzzi L, Sorenson J et al. A pilot study of indocyanine given videoangiography guided laser photocoagulation of occult choroidal neovascularization in age-related macular degeneration. Arch Ophthalmol 1994; 112:465–472.
11. Klein BE, Klein R. Cataracts and macular degeneration in older Americans. Arch Ophthalmol 1982; 100: 571–573.
12. Friedman DS, O'Colmain BJ, Munoz B et al. Prevalence of age-related macular degeneration in the United States. Arch Ophthalmol 2004 ; 122:564–572.
13. Leibowitz H, Krueger DE, Maunder LR et al. The Framingham Eye Study monograph: an ophthalmological and epidemiological study of cataract,

14. Flower RW. Experimental studies of indocyanine green dye-enhanced photocoagulation of choroidal neovascularization feeder vessels. Am J Ophthalmol 2000; 129:510–512.
15. Abecasis GR, Yashar BM, Zhao Y et al. Age-related macular degeneration: a high-resolution genome scan for susceptibility loci in a population enriched for late-stage disease. Am J Hum Genet 2004; 74:482–494.
16. Allikmets R. Further evidence for an association of ABCR alleles with age-related macular degeneration. The International ABCR Screening Consortium. Am J Hum Genet 2000; 67:487–491.
17. Weeks DE, Conley YP, Tsai HJ et al. Age-related maculopathy: an expanded genome-wide scan with evidence of susceptibility loci within the 1q31 and 17q25 regions. Am J Ophthalmol 2001; 132:682–692.
18. Marmorstein LY, Munier FL, Arsenijevic Y et al. Aberrant accumulation of EFEMP1 underlies drusen formation in malattia leventinese and age-related macular degeneration. Proc Natl Acad Sci USA 2002; 99:13067–13072.
19. Stone EM, Lotery AJ, Munier FL et al. A single EFEMP1 mutation associated with both Malattia Leventinese and Doyne honeycomb retinal dystrophy. Nat Genet 1999; 22:199–202.
20. Klenotic PA, Munier FL, Marmorstein LY et al. Tissue inhibitor of metalloproteinases-3 (TIMP-3) is a binding partner of epithelial growth factor-containing fibulin-like extracellular matrix protein 1 EFEMP1). Implications for macular degeneration. J Biol Chem 2004; 279:30469–30473.
21. Stone EM, Braun TA, Russell SR et al. Missense variations in the fibulin 5 gene and age-related macular degeneration. N Engl J Med 2004; 351:346–353.
22. Albig AR, Schlemann WP. Fibulin-5 antagonizes vascular endothelial growth factor (VEGF) signaling and angiogenic sprouting by endothelial cells. DNA Cell Biol 2004; 23:367–379.
23. Fariss RN, Apte SS, Olsen BR et al. Tissue inhibitor of metalloproteinase-3 is a component of Bruch's membrane of the eye. Am J Pathol 1997; 150:323–328.
24. Felbor U, Stohr H, Amann T et al. A second independent Tyr168Cys mutation in the tissue inhibitor of metalloproteinases-3 (TIMP3) in Sorsby's fundus dystrophy. J Med Genet 1996; 33:233–236.
25. De La Paz MA, Pericak-Vance MA, Lennon F et al. Exclusion of TIMP3 as a candidate locus in age-related macular degeneration. Invest Ophthalmol Vis Sci 1997; 38:1060–1065.
26. Chong NH, Alexander RA, Gin T et al. TIMP-3, collagen, and elastin immunohistochemistry and histopathology of Sorsby's fundus dystrophy. Invest Ophthalmol Vis Sci 200; 41:898–902.
27. Kamei M, Hollyfield JG. TIMP-3 in Bruch's membrane: changes during aging and in age-related macular degeneration. Invest Ophthalmol Vis Sci 1999; 40:2367–2375.
28. Baird PN, Guida E, Chu DT et al. The epsilon2 and epsilon4 alleles of the apolipoprotein gene are associated with age-related macular degeneration. Invest Ophthalmol Vis Sci 2004 ; 45:1311–1315.
29. Klein RJ, Zeiss C, Chew EY et al. Complement Factor H Polymorphism in Age Related Macular Degeneration. Science 2005; Mar 10 Epub
30. Edwards AO, Ritte Iii R, Abel KJ et al. Complement Fator H Polymorphism in Age Related Macular Degeneration Science 2005 March 10 Epub
31. Mata NL, Weng J, Travis GH. Biosynthesis of a major lipofuscin fluorophore in mice and humans with ABCR-mediated retinal and macular degeneration. Proc Natl Acad Sci USA 2000; 97:7154–7159.
32. Zhang K, Garibaldi DC, Kniazeva M et al. A novel mutation in the ABCR gene in four patients with autosomal recessive Stargardt disease. Am J Ophthalmol 1999; 128:720–724.
33. Bernstein PS, Leppert M, Singh N, Dean M et al. Genotype–phenotype analysis of ABCR variants in macular degeneration probands and siblings. Invest Ophthalmol Vis Sci 2002; 43:466–473.
34. Radu RA, Mata NL, Nusinowitz S et al. Treatment with isotretinoin inhibits lipofuscin accumulation in a mouse model of recessive Stargardt's macular degeneration. Proc Natl Acad Sci USA 2003; 100:4245–4344.
35. Thomson DA, Gal A. Vitamin A metabolism in the retinal pigment epithelium: genes, mutations, and diseases. Prog Retin Eye Res 2003; 22:683–703.
36. Heuberger RA, Mares-Perlman JA, Klein R et al. Relationship of dietary fat to age-related maculopathy in the Third National Health and Nutrition Examination Surgery. Arch Ophthalmol 2002; 119:1833–1838.
37. Seddon JM, Ai UA, Sperduto RD et al. Dietary carotenoids, vitamins A, C, and E, and advanced age-related macular degeneration. Eye Disease Case-Control Study Group. JAMA 1994; 272:1455–1456.
38. Beatty S, Koh HH, Phil M et al. The role of oxidative stress in the pathogenesis of age-related macular degeneration. Surv Ophthalmol 2000; 45:115–133.
39. Cho E, Stampfer MJ, Seddon JM et al. Prospective study of zinc intake and the risk of age-related macular degeneration. Ann Epidemiol 2001; 11:328–336.

glaucoma, diabetic retinopathy, macular degeneration, and visual acuity in a general population of 2631 adults, 1973–1975. Surv Ophthalmol 1980; 24 (suppl):335–610.

40. Cho E, Seddon JM, Rosner B et al. Prospective study of intake of fruits, vegetables, vitamins, and carotenoids and risk of age-related maculopathy. Arch Ophthalmol 2004; 122:883–892.

41. Tomany SC, Wang JJ, Van Leeuwen R et al. Risk factors for incident age-related macular degeneration: pooled findings from 3 continents. Ophthalmology 2004; 111:1280–1287.

42. Darzins P, Mitchell P, Heller RF. Sun exposure and age-related macular degeneration. An Australian case-control study. Ophthalmology 1997; 104:770–776.

43. Tomany SC, Cruickshank KJ, Klein R et al. Sunlight and the 10-year incidence of age-related maculopathy: the Beaver Dam Eye Study. Arch Ophthalmol 2004; 122:750–757.

44. Schmidt-Erfurth U, Hasan T. Mechanisms of action of photodynamic therapy with verteporfin for the treatment of age-related macular degeneration. Surv Ophthalmol 2000; 45:195–214.

45. Schmidt-Erfurth U, Michels S, Barbazetto I et al. Photodynamic effects on choroidal neovascularization and physiological choroid. Invest Ophthalmol Vis Sci 2002; 43:830–841.

46. Sickenberg M, Schmidt-Erfurth U, Miller JW et al. A preliminary study of photodynamic therapy using verteporfin for choroidal neovascularization in pathologic myopia, ocular histoplasmosis syndrome, angioid streaks, and idiopathic causes. Arch Ophthalmol 2000; 118:327–336.

47. AREDS Study Group. A randomized, placebo-controlled, clinical trial of high-dose supplementation with vitamins C and E, beta carotene, and zinc for age-related macular degeneration and vision loss: AREDS report no. 8. Arch Ophthalmol 2001; 119:1417–1436.

48. Brennan M, Bhatti H, Nerusu KC et al. Matrix metalloproteinase-1 is the major collagenolytic enzyme responsible for collagen damage in UV-irradiated human skin. Photochem Photobiol 2003; 78:43–48.

49. Vayalil PK, Mittal A, Hara Y et al. Green tea polyphenols prevent ultraviolet light-induced oxidative damage and matrix metalloproteinases expression in mouse skin. J Invest Dermatol 2004; 122:1480–1487.

50. van Leeuwen R, Tomany SC, Wang JJ et al. Is medication use associated with the incidence of early age-related maculopathy? Pooled findings from 3 continents. Ophthalmology 2004; 111:1169–1175.

51. Ishida S, Usui T, Yamashiro K et al. VEGF165-mediated inflammation is required for pathological, but not physiological, ischemia-induced retinal neovascularization. J Exp Med 2003; 198:483–489.

52. Arroyo JG, Michaud N, Jakobiec FA. Choroidal neovascular membranes treated with photodynamic therapy. Arch Ophthalmol 2003; 121:898–903.

53. Ghazi NG, Jabbour NM, de la Cruz ZC et al. Clinicopathologic studies of age-related macular degeneration with classic subfoveal choroidal neovascularization treated with photodynamic therapy. Retina 2001; 21:478–486.

54. Grossniklaus HE, Ling JX, Wallace TM et al. Macrophage and retinal pigment epithelium expression of angiogenic cytokines in choroidal neovascularization. Mol Vis 2002; 21:119–126.

55. Moshfeghi DM, Kaiser PK, Grossniklaus HE et al. Clinicopathologic study after submacular removal of choroidal neovascular membranes treated with verteporfin ocular photodynamic therapy. Am J Ophthalmol 2003; 135:343–350.

56. Schnurrbusch UEK, Welt K, Horn L-C et al. Histological findings of surgically excised choroidal neovascular membranes after photodynamic therapy. Br J Ophthalmol 2001; 85:1086–1091.

57. Kalayoglu MV, Galvan C, Mahdi OS et al. Serological association between Chlamydia pneumoniae infection and age related macular degeneration. Arch Ophthalmol 2003; 121:478–482.

58. Seddon JM, Gensler G, Milton RC et al. Association between C-reactive protein and age-related macular degeneration. JAMA 2004; 292:43.

59. Ciulla TA, Criswell MH, Danis RP et al. Intravitreal triamcinolone acetonide inhibits choroidal neovascularization in a laser-treated rat model. Arch Ophthalmol 2001; 119:399–404.

60. Ayalasoaa SP, Kompella UB. Celecoxib, a selective cyclooxygenase-2 inhibitor, inhibits retinal vascular endothelial growth factor expression and vascular leakage in a streptozotocin-induced diabetic rate model. Eur J Pharmacol 2003; 458:283–289.

61. Miyamoto K, Khosrof S, Bursell SE et al. Prevention of leukostasis and vascular leakage in streptozotocin-induced diabetic retinopathy via intercellular adhesion molecule-1 inhibition. Proc Natl Acad Sci USA 1999; 96:10836–10841.

62. Penfold PL, Wen MC, Madigan MC et al. Triamcinolone acetonide modulates permeability and intercellular adhesion molecule-1 (ICAM-1) expression of the ECV304 cell line: Implications for macular degeneration. Clin Exp Immunol 2000; 121:458–465.

63. Sakurai E, Taguchi H, Anand A et al. Target disruption of the CD18 or ICAM-1 gene inhibits choroidal neovascularization. Invest Ophthalmol Vis Sci 2003; 44:2743–2749.

64. Dawson DW, Volpert OV, Gillis P et al. Pigment epithelium-derived factor: a potent inhibitor of angiogenesis. Science 1999; 285:245–248.

65. Friedlander M, Theesfeld CL, Sugita M et al. Involvement of integrins alpha v beta 3 and alpha v beta 5 in ocular neovascular diseases. Proc Natl Acad Sci USA 1996; 93:9764–9769.

66. Friedlander M, Brooks PC, Shaffer RW et al. Definition of two angiogenic pathways by distinct alpha v integrins. Science 1995; 270:1500–1502.

67. Miller JW. Vascular endothelial growth factor and ocular neovascularization. Am J Path 1997; 151:13–23.

68. Robinson C, Stringer S. The splice variants of vascular endothelial growth factor (VEGF) and their receptors. J Cell Sci 2001; 114:853–865.

69. Ferrara N. Vascular endothelial growth factor: basic science and clinical progress. Endocr Rev 2004; 25:581–611.

70. Senger DR, Galli SJ, Dvorak AM et al. Tumor cells secrete a vascular permeability factor that promotes accumulation of ascites fluid. Science 1983; 219:983–985.

71. Fukumura D, Gohongi T, Kadambi A et al. Predominant role of endothelial nitric oxide synthase in vascular endothelial growth factor-induced angiogenesis and vascular permeability. PNAS 2001; 98:2604–2609.

72. Sennlaub F, Courtois Y, Goureau O. Inducible nitric oxide synthase mediates retinal apoptosis in ischemic proliferative retinopathy. J Neurosci 2002; 22:3987–3993.

73. Blaauwgeers HG, Holtkamp GM, Rutten H et al. Polarized vascular endothelial growth factor secretion by human retinal pigment epithelium and localization of vascular endothelial growth factor receptors on the inner choriocapillaris. Evidence for a trophic paracrine relation. Am J Pathol 1999; 155:421–428.

74. Mayerhofer M, Valent P, Sperr WR et al. BCR/ABL induces expression of vascular endothelial growth factor and its transcriptional activator, hypoxia inducible factor-1alpha, through a pathway involving phosphoinositide 3-kinase and the mammalian target of rapamycin. Blood 2002; 100:3767–3775.

75. El Bashir S, Harborth, Lenkel W et al. Duplexes of 21 nucleotide RNAs mediate RNA interference in cultured mammalian cells. Nature 2001; 411:494.

76. El-Hashemite N, Walker V, Zhang H et al. Loss of Tsc1 or Tsc2 induces vascular endothelial growth factor production through mammalian target of rapamycin. Cancer Res 2003; 63:5173–5177.

77. Tolentino MJ, Brucker AJ, Fosnot J et al. Intravitreal injection of vascular endothelial growth factor small interfering RNA inhibits growth and leakage in a nonhuman primate, laser-induced model of choroidal neovascularization. Retina 2004; 24:132–138.

78. Usui T, Ishida S, Yamashiro K et al. VEGF164(165) is the pathological isoform: differential leukocyte and endothelial responses through VEGFR1 and VEGFR2. Invest Ophthalmol Vis Sci 2004; 45:368–374.

79. Folkman J, Ingber DE. Angiostatic steroids. Method of discovery and mechanism of action. Ann Surg 1987 ; 206:374–383.

80. Folkman J, Weisz BV, Joullie MM et al. Control of angiogenesis with synthetic heparin substitutes. Science 1989 Mar; 243:1490–1493.

81. Fung WE. Interferon alpha 2a for treatment of age-related macular degeneration. Am J Ophthalmol 1991; 112:349–350.

82. Lai CC, Wu WC, Chen SL, Xiao X et al. Suppression of choroidal neovascularization by adeno-associated virus vector expressing angiostatin. Invest Ophthalmol Vis Sci 2001; 42:2401–2407.

83. Mori K, Duh E, Gehlbach P et al. Pigment epithelium-derived factor inhibits retinal and choroidal neovascularization. J Cell Physiol 2001; 188:253–263.

84. Mori K, Ando A, Gehlbach P et al. Inhibition of choroidal neovascularization by intravenous injection of adenoviral vectors expressing secretable endostatin. Am J Pathol 2001; 159:313–320.

85. O'Reilly MS, Boehm T, Shing Y et al. Endostatin: an endogenous inhibitor of angiogenesis and tumor growth. Cell 1997; 88:277–285.

86. O'Reilly MS, Wiederschain D, Stetler-Stevenson WG et al. Regulation of angiostatin production by matrix metalloproteinase-2 in a model of concomitant resistant. J Biol Chem 1999; 274:29568–29571.

87. Crabb JW, Miyagi M, Gu Z et al. Drusen proteome analysis: an approach to the etiology of age-related macular degeneration. PNAS 2002; 99:14682–14687.

88. Anand-Apte B, Pepper MS, Voest E et al. Inhibition of angiogenesis by tissue inhibitor of metalloproteinase-3. Invest Ophthalmol Vis Sci 1997; 38:817–823.

89. Takahashi T, Nakamura T, Hayashi A et al. Inhibition of experimental choroidal vascularization by overexpression of tissue inhibitor of metalloproteinases-3 in retinal pigment epithelium cells. Am J Ophthalmol 2000; 130:774–781.

90. Ambati J, Anand A, Fernandez S, Sakurai E et al. An animal model of age-related macular degeneration in senescent Ccl-2 or Ccr-2-defiicient mice. Nat Med 2003; 9:1390–1397.

91. Otani A, Slike BM, Dorrell MI et al. A fragment of human TrpRS as a potent antagonist of ocular angiogenesis. Proc Natl Acad Sci USA 2002; 99:178–183. Epub 2002 02.

92. Pharmacological Therapy for Macular Degeneration Study Group. Interferon alfa-2A is ineffective for patients with choroidal neovascularization secondary to age-related macular degeneration. Results of a prospective randomized placebo-controlled clinical trial. Arch Ophthalmol 1997; 115:865–872.

93. Cao Y, Xue L. Angiostatin. Semin Thromb Hemost 2004; 30:83–93.

94. Newsome DA, Swartz M, Leone NC et al. Oral zinc in macular degeneration. Arth Ophthalmol 1988; 106:192–198.

95. Bressler NM, Bressler SB, Congdon NG et al., Age-related Eye Disease Study Research Group. Potential public health impact of Age-related Eye Disease Study results: AREDS report no. 11. Arch Ophthalmol 2003; 121:1621–1624.

96. Jacobson SG, Ciiyan AV, Regunath G et al. Night blindness in Sorsby's fundus dystrophy reversed by vitamin A. Nat Genet 1995; 11:27–32.

97. Luke E, Krott R, Luke M et al. Effects of protein tyrosine kinase inhibitor genistein on retinal function in superfused vertebrate retina. J Ocul Pharmacol Therap 2001; 17:151–158.

98. Nakajima M, Cooney MJ, Tu AH et al. Normalization of retinal vascular permeability in experimental diabetes with genistein. Invest Ophthalmol Vis Sci 2001; 42:2110–2114.

99. Crum R, Szabo S, Folkman J. A new class of steroids inhibits angiogenesis in the presence of heparin or a heparin fragment. Science 1985; 20:1375–1378.

100. Ranson NT, Danis RP, Ciulla TA et al. Intravitreal triamcinolone in subfoveal recurrence of choroidal neovascularization after laser treatment in macular degeneration. Br J Ophthalmol 2002; 86:527–529.

101. Gillies MC, Simpson JM, Luo W et al. A randomized clinical trial of a single dose of intravitreal triamcinolone acetonide for neovascular age-related macular degeneration: one-year results. Arch Ophthalmol 2003; 121:667–673.

102. Spaide RF, Sorenson J, Maranan L. Combined photodynamic therapy with verteporfin and intravitreal triamcinolone acetonide for choroidal neovascularization. Ophthalmology 2003; 110:1517–1525.

103. Bilbao KV, Kreidl KO, Blumenkranz MS. Angiographic improvement in a patient with subfoveal choroidal neovascularization following Verteporfin photodynamic therapy with adjuvant intravitreal triamcinolone acetonide. Am J Ophthalmol 2004 (accepted for publication with revisions).

104. Li WW, Casey R, Gonzalez EM et al. Angiostatic steroids potentiated by sulfated cyclodextrins inhibit corneal neovascularization. Invest Ophthalmol Vis Sci 1991; 32:2898–2905.

105. Clark AF, Mellon J, Li XY et al. Inhibition of intraocular tumor growth by topical application of the angiostatic steroid anecortave acetate. Invest Ophthalmol Vis Sci 1999; 40:2158–2162.

106. McNatt LG, Weimer L, Yanni J et al. Angiostatic activity of steroids in the chick embryo CAM and rabbit cornea models of neovascularization. J Ocul Pharmacol Ther 1999; 15:413–423.

107. Penn JS, Rajaratnam VS, Collier RJ et al. The effect of an angiostatic steroid on neovascularization in a rat model of retinopathy of prematurity. Invest Ophthalmol Vis Sci 2001; 42:283–290.

108. D'Amico DJ, Goldberg MF, Hudson H et al. Anecortave Acetate Clinical Study Group. Anecortave acetate as monotherapy for the treatment of subfoveal lesions in patients with exudative age-related macular degeneration (AMD): interim (month 6) analysis of clinical safety and efficacy. Retina 2003; 23:14–23.

109. Miller TA, Bulman AL, Thompson CE et al. Synthesis and structure profiles of A-homoestranes, and estratropones. J Med Chem 1997; 40:3836–3841.

110. Robinson MR, Baffi J, Yuan P et al. Safety and pharmacokinetics of intra-vitreal 2-methoxyestradiol implants in normal rabbit and pharmacodynamics in a rat model of choroidal neovascularization. Exp Eye Res 2002; 74:309–317.

111. Slakter JS. Anecortave Acetate Clinical Study Group. Anecortave acetate as monotherapy for treatment of subfoveal neovascularization in age-related macular degeneration: twelve-month clinical outcomes. Ophthalmology 2003; 110:2372–2383; discussion 2384–2385.

112. Masferrer JL, Koki A, Seibert K. COX-2 inhibitors. A new class of anti-angiogenic agents. Ann NY Acad Sci 1999; 889:84–86.

113. Castro MR, Lutz D, Edelman JL. Effect of COX inhibitors on VEGF-induced retinal vascular leakage and experimental corneal and choroidal neovascularization. Exp Eye Res 2004; 79:275–285.

114. Poliner LS, Tornambe PE, Michelson PE et al. Interferon alpha-2a for subfoveal neovascularization in age-related macular degeneration. Ophthalmology 1993; 100:1417–1424.

115. Napoli K, Taylor P. Beach to bedside: history of the development of sirolimus therapeutic drug monitoring 2001; 23:559–586.

116. Guba M, von Breittenbuch P, Steinbauer MG et al. Rapamycin inhibits primary and metastatic tumor growth by antiangiogenesis: involvement of vascular endothelial growth factor. Nat Med 2002; 8:128–135.

117. Kuroki A, Dejenka N, Fosnot TJ et al. Rapamycin inhibits retinal and choroidal neovascularization in mice. Invest Ophthalmol Vis Sci Suppl 2003.

118. Wen R, Wang Z, Song Y et al. Rapamycin inhibits choroidal neovascularization. Invest Ophthalmol Vis Sci 2003; Suppl Program #3928.

119. Campochiaro P. Ocular neovascularization and excessive vascular permeability. Expert opinion. Biol Ther 2004; 9:1395–1402.

120. Jellinek D, Green LS, Bell C et al. Inhibition of receptor binding by high-affinity RNA ligands to vascular endothelial growth factor. Biochemistry 1994; 33:10450–10456.

121. Eyetech Study Group. Anti-vascular endothelial growth factor therapy for subfoveal choroidal neovascularization secondary to age-related macular degeneration: phase II study results. Ophthalmology 2003; 110:979–986.

122. Puliafito CA, Duker JS, Blumenkranz MS et al. Targeting VEGF in vascular diseases. Dulany Foundation Webcast, 2004.

123. Eyetech Study Group. Preclinical and phase 1A clinical evaluation of an anti-VEGF pegylated aptamer (EYE001) for the treatment of exudative age-related macular degeneration. Retina 2002; 22:143–152.

124. Verteporfin in Photodynamic Therapy Study Group. Verteporfin therapy of subfoveal choroidal neovascularization in age-related macular degeneration: two-year results of a randomized clinical trial including lesions with occult with no classic choroidal neovascularization – verteporfin in photodynamic therapy report 2. Am J Ophthalmol 2001; 131:541–560.

125. Gragoudas ES, Adamis AP, Cunningham ET Jr et al. Pegaptanib for neovascular age-related macular degeneration. N Engl J Med 2004; 391:2805–2816.

126. Reich SJ, Fosnot J, Kuroki A et al. Small interfering RNA (siRNA) targeting VEGF effectively inhibits ocular neovascularization in a mouse model. Mol Vis 2003; 9:210–216.

127. Hurwitz H, Fehrenbacher L, Novotny W et al. Bevacizumab plus irinotecan, fluorouracil, and leucovorin for metastatic colorectal cancer. N Engl J Med 2004; 350:2335–2342.

128. Krzystolik MG, Afshari MA, Adamis AP et al. Prevention of experimental choroidal neovascularization with intravitreal anti-vascular endothelial growth factor antibody fragment. Arch Ophthalmol 2002; 120:338–346.

129. Heier JS et al. ARVO. Invest Ophthalmol Vis Sci 2003;44: E-Abstract 972.

130. Hageman GS, Luthert PJ, Chong NHV et al. An integrated hypothesis that considers drusen as biomarkers of immune-mediated processes at the RPE-Bruch's membrane interface in aging and age-related macular degeneration. Prog Retinal Eye Res 2001; 20:705–732.

131. Gornis F, Maskos K, Betz M et al. Mechanism of inhibition of the human MMP stromelysin-1 by TIMP-1. Nature 1997; 389:77–81.

132. Saishin S, Saishin Y, Takahashi K et al. VEGF-TRAP (RIR2) suppresses choroidal neovascularization and VEGF-induced breakdown of the blood retinal barrier. J Cell Physiol 2003; 195:241–248.

133. Patel N, Sun L, Moshinsky D et al. A selective and oral small molecule inhibitor of vascular epithelial growth factor receptor (VEGFR)-2 and VEGFR-1 inhibits neovascularization and vascular permeability. J Pharmacol Exp Ther 2003; 306:838–845.

134. Hangai M, Moon YS, Kitaya N et al. Systemically expressed soluble Tie2 inhibits intraocular neovascularization. Human Gene Therapy 2001; 12:1311–1321.

135. Honda M, Sakamoto T, Ishibashi T et al. Experimental subretinal neovascularization is inhibited by adenovirus-mediated soluble VEGF/flt-1 receptor gene transfection: a role of VEGF and possible treatment for SRN in age-related macular degeneration. Gene Therapy 2000; 7:978–985.

136. Lai YKY, Shen WY, Brankov M et al. Potential long-term inhibition of ocular neovascularization by recombinant adeno-associated virus-mediated secretion gene therapy. Gene Therapy 2002; 9:804–813.

137. Brooks SE, Gu Z, Samuel S et al. Reduced severity of oxygen-induced retinopathy in eNOS-deficient mice. Invest Ophthalmol Vis Sci 2001; 42:222–228.

138. Ando A, Yang A, Nambu H et al. Blockade of nitric-oxide synthase reduces choroidal neovascularization. Mol Pharmacol 2002; 62:539–544.

139. Otani A, Slike B, Dorrell M et al. A fragment of human Trp RS as a potent antagonist of ocular angiogenesis. PNAS 2002; 99:178–183.

140. Wakasugi K, Slike BM, Hood J et al. A human aminoacyl-tRNA synthetase as a regulator of angiogenesis. Proc Natl Acad Sci USA 2002; 99:173–177.

141. Aiello LP. The potential role of PKC beta in diabetic retinopathy and macular edema. Surv Ophthalmol 2002; 47 Suppl 2:S263–269.

142. Aiello L, Cahil M, Cavallerand J. Growth factors and protein kinase C inhibitors as novel therapies for medical management of diabetic retinopathy. Eye 2004; 18:117–125.

143. Frank RN. Potential news medical therapies for diabetic retinopathy: protein kinase C inhibitors. Am J Ophthalmol 2002; 133:693–698.

144. Saishin Y, Silva RL, Saishin Y et al. Periocular injection of microspheres containing PKC412 inhibits choroidal neovascularization in a porcine model. Invest Ophthalmol Vis Sci 2003; 44:4989–4993.

145. Semkova I, Kreppel F, Welsandt G et al. Autologous transplantation of genetically modified iris pigment epithelial cells: a promising concept for the treatment of age-related macular degeneration and other disorders of the eye. PNAS 2002; 99:19090–19095.

146. Rasmussen H, Chu KW, Campochiaro P et al. Clinical protocol. An open-label, phase 1, single administration, dose-escalation study of ADGVPEDF.11D (ADPEDF) in neovascular age-related macular degeneration (AMD). Hum Gene Ther 2001; 12:2029–2032.

147. Boehm T, O'Reilly MS, Keough K et al. Zinc-binding of endostatin is essential for its antiangiogenic activity. Biochem Biophys Res Commun 1998; 252:190–194.

148. Mori K, Ando A, Gehlbach P et al. Inhibition of choroidal neovascularization by intravenous injection of adeiral vectors expressing secretable endostatin. Am J Path 2001; 159:313–320.

149. Brooks PC, Clark RA, Cheresh DA. Requirement of vascular integrin alpha v beta 3 for angiogenesis. Science 1994; 264:569–571.

150. Luna J, Tobe T, Mousa SA et al. Antagonists of integrin alpha v beta 3 inhibit retinal neovascularization in a murine model. Lab Invest 1996; 75:563–573.

151. Kamitzuru H, Kimura H, Yasukawa T et al. Monoclonal antibody-mediated drug targeting to choroidal neovascularization in the rat. Invest Ophthalmol Vis Sci 2001; 42:2664–2672.

152. Garcia C, Bartsch D, Riverio M et al. Efficacy of drinomastat (AG3340), a MMP inhibitor in treatment of retinal neovascularization. Curr Eye Res 2002; 24:33–38.

153. Nambu H, Nambu R, Melia M. Combretastatin A-4 phosphate suppresses development and induces regression of choroidal neovascularization. Invest Ophthalmol Vis Sci 2003; 44:3650–3655.

154. Genaidy M, Kazi AA, Peyman GA et al. Effect of squalamine on iris neovascularization in monkeys. Retina 2002; 22:772–778.

155. Jones SR, Kinney WA, Zhang X et al. The synthesis and characterization of analogs of the antimicrobial compound squalamine: 6 beta-hydroxy-3-aminosterols synthesized from hyodeoxycholic acid. Steroids 1996; 61:565–571.

156. Higgins RD, Yan Y, Geng Y et al. Regression of retinopathy by squalamine is a mouse model. Pediatr Res 2004; 56:144–149.

157. Woodburn K, Engelman C, Blumenkranz MS. Photodynamic therapy for choroidal neovascularization. A review. Retina 2002; 22:391–405.

158. Flower RW, von Kerczek C, Zhu L et al. Theoretical investigation of the role of choriocapillaris blood flow in treatment of subfoveal choroidal neovascularization associated with age-related macular degeneration. Am J Ophthalmol 2001; 132:85–93.

159. Husain D, Miller JW, Michaud N et al. Intravenous infusion of liposomal benzoporphyrin derivative for photodynamic therapy of experimental choroidal neovascularization. Arch Ophthalmol 1996; 114:978–985.

160. Husain D, Kramer M, Kenny AG et al. Effects of photodynamic therapy using verteporfin on experimental choroidal neovascularization and normal retina and choroid up to 7 weeks after treatment. Invest Ophthalmol Vis Sci. 1999; 40:2322–2331.

161. Kramer M, Miller JW, Michaud N et al. Liposomal benzoporphyrin derivative verteporfin photodynamic therapy. Selective treatment of choroidal neovascularization in monkeys. Ophthalmology 1996; 103:427–438.

162. Miller JW, Walsh AW, Kramer M et al. Photodynamic therapy of experimental choroidal neovascularization using lipoprotein-delivered benzoporphyrin. Arch Ophthalmol 1995; 113:810–818.

163. Miller JW, Schmidt-Erfurth U, Sickenberg M et al. Photodynamic therapy with verteporfin for choroidal neovascularization caused by age-related macular degeneration: results of a single treatment in a phase 1 and 2 study. Arch Ophthalmol 1999; 117:1161–1173.

164. Schmidt-Erfurth U, Miller JW, Sickenberg M et al. Photodynamic therapy with verteporfin for choroidal neovascularization caused by age-related macular degeneration: results of retreatments in a phase 1 and 2 study. Arch Ophthalmol 1999; 117:1177–1187.

165. Treatment of Age-related Macular Degeneration with Photodynamic Therapy (TAP) Study Group. Photodynamic therapy of subfoveal choroidal neovascularization in age-related macular degeneration with verteporfin. One-year results of 2 randomized clinical trials – TAP Report 1. Arch Ophthalmol 1999; 117:1329–1345.

166. Treatment of Age-related Macular Degeneration with Photodynamic Therapy (TAP) Study Group. Photodynamic therapy of subfoveal choroidal neovascularization in age-related macular degeneration with verteporfin. Two-year results of 2 randomized clinical trials – TAP Report 2. Arch Ophthalmol 2001; 119:198–207.

167. Blinder KJ, Bradley S, Bressler NM et al. Effect of lesion size, visual acuity, and lesion composition on visual acuity change with and without verteporfin therapy for choroidal neovascularization secondary to age-related macular degeneration: TAP and VIP report no 1. Am J Ophthalmol 2003; 136:407–418.

168. Verteporfin in Photodynamic Therapy Study Group. Photodynamic therapy of subfoveal choroidal neovascularization in pathologic myopia with verteporfin. 1-year results of a randomized clinical trial – VIP report no. 1. Ophthalmology 2001; 108:841–852.

Chapter

66

Etiologic Mechanisms in Diabetic Retinopathy

Robert N. Frank

This chapter considers the hypothetical mechanisms of the development of diabetic retinopathy. Clinical manifestations of the disease, and concepts of treatment, are discussed elsewhere in this volume.

EPIDEMIOLOGY

Studies of the epidemiology of a disease are important for establishing hypotheses of its pathogenesis. Who is most at risk? What factors modify that risk? For diabetic retinopathy, the major risk factor is, of course, the presence of diabetes mellitus. Although there have been some claims of "diabetic retinopathy" without diabetes,[1,2] following publication of the results of the Diabetes Control and Complications Trial (DCCT),[3] this concept has been abandoned. The major point at issue in this dispute is that the genetic loci that are responsible for the development of diabetic retinopathy and other complications of diabetes are distinct from those loci that determine diabetes itself and (in the original hypothesis) do not require the presence of chronic hyperglycemia. The alternative hypothesis, that the complications of diabetes are direct consequences of long-term hyperglycemia, was decisively confirmed by the results of the DCCT, a randomized, controlled clinical trial involving 27 clinical centers in the USA and Canada[3] that will be discussed in detail below. Although the DCCT, and the more recent UK Prospective Diabetes Study (UKPDS),[4,5] conclusively demonstrated the importance of hyperglycemia in the development of retinopathy and other complications of diabetes, they did not eliminate the possible ancillary role of genetic factors. The current status of investigations on the genetic susceptibility to diabetic retinopathy will also be considered later in this chapter.

Duration of diabetes and the development of diabetic retinopathy

Several large studies[6-8] in which retinal photographs and fluorescein angiograms were evaluated by observers who were masked to the subjects' identities in order to eliminate bias have clearly demonstrated that retinopathy in young people with type 1 (insulin-dependent) diabetes does not occur for at least 3 to 5 years after the onset of the systemic disease (Fig. 66-1). Similar results have been obtained[9] for persons with type 2 (noninsulin-dependent) diabetes (Fig. 66-2), but in such cases

the time of onset and therefore the duration have been more difficult to determine precisely, so that patients with newly diagnosed type 2 diabetes occasionally present with retinopathy as the initial sign of their diabetes, or are found to have retinopathy soon after the diagnosis of their systemic disease.

The time course of development of specific lesions of diabetic retinopathy has been studied with similar photographic methods. Such studies[7] have shown that the prevalence of minimal retinopathy in individuals with type 1 diabetes approaches 100% after 20 years. However, the prevalence of proliferative retinopathy is not greater than about 50% in subjects with type 1 diabetes after a duration of 15 years or longer (Fig. 66-1), and is much less in persons with type 2 diabetes of similar duration[9] (Fig. 66-2). There are at least two possible explanations for this observation. First, proliferative disease may be the result of prolonged, very high average blood glucose levels, which are more likely to occur in persons with type 1 diabetes than in those with type 2. Second, proliferative retinopathy may result from a certain metabolic state of the retina that is more likely to be present in young persons with type 1 diabetes than in (the usually) older people with type 2 disease.

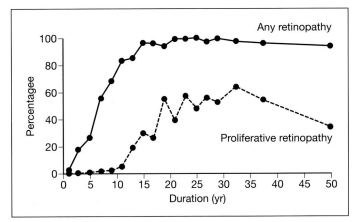

Fig. 66-1 Frequency of diabetic retinopathy in subjects with type 1 diabetes (as a percentage of the total number of diabetic subjects affected) as a function of duration of diabetes in years. (Redrawn from Klein R, Klein BE, Moss SE et al. The Wisconsin Epidemiologic Study of Diabetic Retinopathy. III. Prevalence and risk of diabetic retinopathy when age at diagnosis is 30 or more years. Arch Ophthalmol 1984; 102:527–532.[7] Copyright © 1984 American Medical Association.)

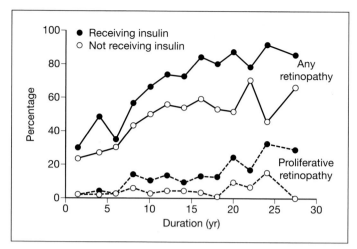

Fig. 66-2 Frequency of diabetic retinopathy in subjects with type 2 diabetes (as a percentage of the total number of diabetic subjects affected) as a function of the duration of diabetes in years. (Redrawn from Klein R, Klein BE, Moss SE et al. The Wisconsin Epidemiologic Study of Diabetic Retinopathy. II. Prevalence and risk of diabetic retinopathy when age at diagnosis is less than 30 years. Arch Ophthalmol 1984; 102:520–526.[7] Copyright 1984, American Medical Association.)

In addition to proliferative retinopathy, the other major vision-threatening form of diabetic retinopathy is macular edema. Macular edema has generally been assumed to be more common in older people with type 2 diabetes than in those with type 1 and, as such, is related to the age of the person affected. Aiello et al.[10] reported just this result, and they also noted that when young persons with type 1 diabetes had macular edema, they usually also had proliferative retinopathy. Klein et al.,[11] in the extensive population-based Wisconsin Epidemiologic Study of Diabetic Retinopathy (WESDR), found that the prevalence of macular edema as a function of duration of diabetes was virtually identical in persons with type 1 and type 2 diabetes. In a more recent follow-up of this study, they reported the 10-year incidence of macular edema in diabetic subjects to be 20.1% in type 1 diabetics, 25.4% in type 2 diabetics who required insulin, and 13.9% in type 2 diabetics not requiring insulin.[12] There is an impression among clinicians that the incidence, and hence likely the prevalence, of diabetic retinopathy may be decreasing in recent years because of the increased emphasis on maintenance of more nearly normal blood glucose levels in diabetic individuals. However, a 14-year follow-up of the WESDR, reported in 1998, found that the 20-year cumulative incidence of any retinopathy in persons with type 1 diabetes was 97%, compared to a nearly 100% prevalence reported from this group in 1984.[13] The same study reported that the cumulative incidence of proliferative retinopathy over 15 years in persons with type 1 diabetes was only 37% as assessed in 1998, as compared to a 50% prevalence reported in 1984. Of course, cumulative incidence over an interval and prevalence at one point in time are not the same measures, but, except for deaths or complete regression of disease in the study population, the former should approach the latter if the follow-up is long enough. The similarity of these 1984 and 1998 figures from the same population suggests that there has been no substantial reduction in the occurrence of diabetic retinopathy, or of its more severe forms, in recent years.

Systemic factors that may affect diabetic retinopathy

In addition to duration and type of diabetes, numerous other factors have been described as influencing the development and progression of diabetic retinopathy. One of these is puberty. Knowles et al.[14] were the first to suggest that the onset of puberty might be important. We,[6] as well as several other investigators,[8,15–17] have provided evidence on this point, based on studies involving photographic, and sometimes fluorescein angiographic, documentation and evaluation by masked observers. The mechanism by which puberty might exert its effect on the development of retinopathy is unknown, but several studies suggest a role for hormonal factors related to growth in the pathogenesis of proliferative retinopathy in young people. Daneman et al.[18] described five young patients with Mauriac syndrome, a rare form of extremely brittle type 1 diabetes, fatty liver, and delayed growth and puberty. When the blood glucose levels in these patients were brought under tight control, they experienced an increased rate of somatic growth, the onset of puberty, and the rapid development of proliferative retinopathy. Chantelau et al.[19] reported that patients with Mauriac syndrome before the onset of proliferative retinopathy had substantially increased serum levels of insulin-like growth factor 1 (IGF-1), a polypeptide that closely resembles the A chain of insulin and that is produced largely in the liver under the influence of growth hormone (somatotropin) secreted by the pituitary gland. Merimee et al.[20] reported that persons with type 1 diabetes and proliferative diabetic retinopathy had much higher serum levels of IGF-1. Meyer-Schwickerath et al.[21] found elevated levels of IGF-1 and IGF-2, as well as some of their specific binding proteins, in the vitreous of diabetic patients undergoing vitrectomy for complications of proliferative retinopathy, in comparison with controls. This confirmed an earlier report of increased levels of IGF-1 in the vitreous of diabetics with proliferative retinopathy who underwent vitrectomy.[22] The IGFs have several effects on cells, but one of the most important seems to be to enhance mitogenesis. Thus, elevated levels of IGFs may enhance the development of proliferative diabetic retinopathy, in particular, the rapidly progressive, or florid,[23] retinopathy that is occasionally seen in young people late in adolescence or in young adulthood. Rabbits injected intravitreally with IGF-1 develop dilation of the epiretinal vessels of their "visual streak," together with microaneurysms and actual neovascularization.[24] Although this finding indicates that IGF-1 can cause vascular abnormalities, including neovascularization, the experimental arrangement in which these vessels were produced was somewhat artificial (injection of the putative angiogenic agent directly into the vitreous in concentrations that may not be physiologic). Also, the rabbit does not have true retinal vessels like those of humans, and its retinal metabolism is based primarily on glycolysis rather than on oxygen-requiring pathways of glucose metabolism. Chantelau and

Kohner[25] have argued that the worsening of retinopathy that occurs in 5 to 10% of cases of type 1 diabetes following rapid improvement of glycemic control[3,26–29] is due to an increase in serum IGF. The reduction in IGF levels after destruction of the pituitary gland may also account for the remission of proliferative retinopathy that has been reported after pituitary ablation occurring spontaneously,[30] or after intervention by surgery[31] or radiation.[32] Subcutaneously injected IGF-1, given as a supplement to insulin, has been suggested as a way to improve glycemic control and thereby limit the complications of diabetes. In a clinical study that explored this point, patients with type 1 diabetes were placed on a 3-month regimen of high-dose or low-dose injections of recombinant human IGF-1 or placebo.[33] Over the course of this study, several patients on the high-dose regimen developed dilated, elevated vessels arising from the optic nerve head with fluorescein leakage (Fig. 66-3). No treatment was administered to the patient whose right optic nerve head is shown in Fig. 66-3, and the appearance of her optic nerves reverted to normal 2 months after discontinuing the IGF-1. Although this appearance strongly resembles optic disc neovascularization, it differs in some important respects. The patient shown in Fig. 66-3 had no other evidence of diabetic retinopathy, and the fluorescein angiogram showed no capillary nonperfusion. This is probably an example of diabetic

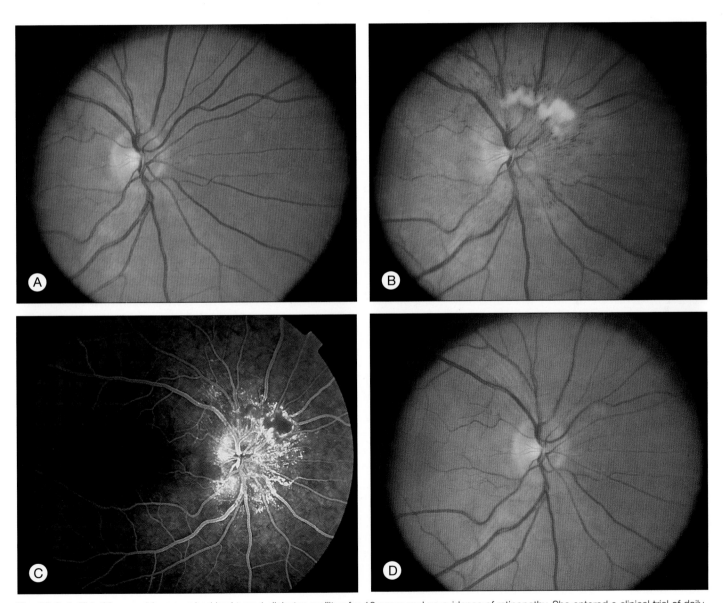

Fig. 66-3 A, This 28-year-old woman had had type 1 diabetes mellitus for 10 years and no evidence of retinopathy. She entered a clinical trial of daily insulin-like growth factor-1 (IGF-1) injections to improve blood glucose control, using a high-dose regimen. This baseline photograph shows a normal-appearing optic nerve head. B, After 3 months of treatment with IGF-1, the optic nerve head is swollen, with dilated vessels, small flame-shaped hemorrhages, and cottonwool spots. The left optic nerve showed a similar but less severe appearance. The remainder of the retinal examination remained entirely normal. C, A fluorescein angiogram taken on the same day as the photograph shown in Fig. 66-3B shows profuse dye leakage from the vessels on the right optic nerve head. D, Two months after discontinuing the IGF-1 injections, and with no further treatment, the right optic nerve has returned to a normal appearance.

papillopathy, a form of optic neuropathy that is occasionally seen in young people with type 1 diabetes but that is apparently unrelated to glycemic control or any other known features of diabetes.[34] The apparent correlation with exogenous IGF-1 administration in this study is therefore of interest.

In an experimental animal study, Smith and co-workers[35] demonstrated that growth hormone and IGF-1 are important permissive factors for the development of retinal neovascularization but are most likely not directly causal. Neonatal mice placed in hyperoxic environments develop peripheral retinal ischemia followed by neovascularization, analogous to retinopathy of prematurity in human infants. In the study of Smith et al., transgenic mice that express a growth hormone antagonist had a marked reduction in retinal neovascularization following neonatal hyperoxic exposure, by comparison with control animals, while transgenic mice with increased growth hormone levels did not demonstrate increased retinal new vessel formation by comparison with controls. Treatment of normal mice with an agent that prevents the release of growth hormone also reduced neovascularization following neonatal hyperoxia, but treatment of these animals with exogenous growth hormone or with IGF-1 restored the neovascular response. None of these animals had reduced expression of vascular endothelial growth factor (VEGF) or its receptors, which at present are considered to be the major mediators of retinal neovascularization.

Among systemic disorders that may affect the course of diabetic retinopathy, hypertension has been the subject of the most investigation. Several reports[5,36–38] have indicated that progression of both background and proliferative diabetic retinopathy is directly related to levels of systemic systolic and diastolic blood pressure. However, only a few of these reports[5,36–38] took care to clarify whether the hypertension was primary (and thus more likely to be a causal factor in progression of the retinopathy) or secondary to advancing diabetic nephropathy and thus likely simply to be an associated event, indicating individuals who might be at greater risk for several microvascular complications of diabetes. A more definitive approach to the role of hypertension in the development and progression of diabetic retinopathy was carried out in the UKPDS, which randomly allocated 1148 patients with type 2 diabetes and hypertension to "tight" blood pressure control (blood pressure < 150/85 mmHg) or "less tight" control (blood pressure <180/105 mmHg) with either atenolol, a beta-adrenergic blocker, or with captopril, an angiotensin convertase inhibitor.[5] After 9 years' follow-up and a mean blood pressure reduction in the tight control group to 144/82 mmHg and 154/87 in the less tight group, there was a 34% reduction in risk of deterioration of retinopathy by two steps on an arbitrary, photographic scale in the tight control group ($P = 0.0004$), and a 47% reduction in risk of a three-line deterioration in visual acuity in this group ($P = 0.004$). These results therefore clearly establish that increased blood pressure as well as increased blood sugar levels present an increased risk for the development and progression of diabetic retinopathy.

The effects of pregnancy on diabetic retinopathy have been controversial. Some authors claim that it accelerates the course of the disease, while others believe that it has no effect. Klein et al.[39] have provided the best evidence that pregnancy does promote the progression of diabetic retinopathy. They compared pregnant women with diabetes to nonpregnant women of comparable age and duration of diabetes. When the data were adjusted for various risk factors, these authors found that current pregnancy was significantly associated with progression of retinopathy ($P < 0.005$; adjusted odds ratio, 2.3).

The effect of "control" of blood glucose

As I have indicated previously, the major controversy in all discussions of the pathogenesis of diabetic retinopathy has been the role of hyperglycemia in the development of this disorder. For many years, the question could not be investigated properly in humans, because of the difficulty in documenting blood glucose levels in diabetic subjects many times each day over a period of several years. With the development of home blood glucose monitoring to make possible the rapid, simple, and accurate determination of blood glucose levels by patients at home or at their work, and the use of total glycosylated hemoglobin (or the closely related hemoglobin A_{1c}) measurements to determine average blood glucose levels over the past 6 to 12 weeks, it is possible to evaluate levels of blood glucose "control" in patients unequivocally. In addition, the increasing use of multiple daily injections of mixed ultrashort- or short-, and intermediate- or long-acting insulins, or of semiautomated insulin pumps that inject a continuous baseline dose of insulin, and that can be programmed to inject larger, bolus doses at mealtimes, has permitted patients to receive their daily insulin in a more nearly physiologic temporal profile.

In consequence of these developments, as well as the use of standardized techniques for performing retinal photography and the use of a standardized protocol and observers masked to the identity of the patient for evaluating the photographs, it has become possible to conduct randomized, controlled, clinical trials of the efficacy of "tight" blood glucose management by comparison with "standard" management in preventing the development, or slowing the progression, of diabetic retinopathy. The first of these were three relatively small-scale trials, none of which had a duration longer than 2 years,[26–29] and which studied young (less than 30 years of age at the outset of the study) persons with type 1 diabetes. None of these investigations demonstrated a beneficial effect of tight blood glucose control over these short time intervals. One surprising result of these studies was that the retinopathy in about 10% of the subjects who entered the studies with pre-existing nonproliferative retinopathy and who were assigned to the tight control group actually worsened over the first year of the follow-up, as compared with subjects in the standard control group. The worsening consisted primarily of an increased number of cotton-wool spots. In the one study that reported 2 years of follow-up, the two treatment groups had become essentially equal in their levels of retinopathy by the end of the second year.[29] The DCCT, a much larger randomized, controlled clinical trial, was completed and its major results published in 1993.[3] This study, which involved over 1400 patients with type 1 diabetes of less than 10 years' duration and less than 30 years of age at the beginning of the study, resolved definitively the role of hyperglycemia in the development of the late complications of type 1 diabetes mellitus. Patients were randomly allocated to "tight control" and "standard control" groups that were further (nonrandomly) divided into primary prevention and secondary intervention groups. The primary group patients had no evidence of diabetic retinopathy at the outset of the study, either on examination by an ophthalmologist who had been certified to participate or by standardized, stereoscopic retinal photography that was evaluated at a centralized facility. The secondary group patients had retinopathy that ranged from early background retinopathy through mild preproliferative changes. At the conclusion of the study, all patients had been followed for 5 to 10 years. Over the first 2 years of follow-up, there were no differences in the severity of retinopathy between the strict and standard control patients in either the primary or secondary groups. In fact, just as in the smaller, earlier trials, approximately 10% of the strict control patients in the secondary group showed "early worsening" of their retinopathy compared to patients on the standard control regimen. However, after 2 to 2½ years of follow-up, the strict control patients in both the primary and secondary intervention groups showed decreased progression of their retinopathy that was statistically highly significant by comparison with patients on the standard control regimen. "Progression" in this study was considered to be a change in retinopathy, as judged by evaluation of the standard photographs, of at least three steps on a defined grading scale. This three-step change was believed to represent a worsening of retinopathy that virtually every ophthalmologist would consider to represent a clinically important deterioration. Further, the significant differences between the treatment groups were present whether the three-step change was observed at only one visit, or was sustained, i.e., was present at two or more successive visits.

Although less impressive than the retinopathy results, studies of the progression of diabetic nephropathy (as judged primarily by 24-hour urinary microalbumin excretion) and of diabetic neuropathy (judged by clinical evaluation and by motor nerve conduction studies) also showed substantial, though not statistically highly significant, differences in favor of the patients on the "strict" control regimen.

A similar result was reported in 1998 for patients with type 2 diabetes in the UKPDS, a large controlled clinical trial in the UK.[4] In this study, over 3800 patients with newly diagnosed type 2 diabetes were randomly assigned either to dietary control alone, or to insulin, or to one of three different sulfonylureas to obtain the best possible blood glucose control. Patients were followed for at least 10 years and three different aggregate (i.e., combinations of several individual) endpoints were assessed, as well as some single endpoints. The drug therapy regimens in subjects with type 2 diabetes in the UKPDS achieved a reduction in glycemia to a mean hemoglobin A_{1c} level of 7.0% by comparison with 7.9% in the diet alone (control) group. Although statistically significant, this was a smaller reduction than was achieved in patients with type 1 diabetes in the

DCCT (mean hemoglobin A_{1c} 7.5% in the tight control group versus 9.5% in the standard control group). Better glycemic control with insulin or sulfonylureas (all modalities of pharmacologic therapy produced similar reductions in blood glucose levels in the UKPDS) yielded a 25% ($P = 0.0099$) reduction in risk for all microvascular endpoints combined, but the most prominent reduction was a decreased risk of retinal photocoagulation. Thus, at this time, the importance of hyperglycemia in the development of retinopathy and other complications of all forms of diabetes is no longer open to question.

Genetic and other factors

Although several investigators have suggested that genetic or environmental (e.g., the effect of dietary composition) factors may alter the prevalence of diabetes mellitus among people of differing racial or national groups, no such racial, national, or ethnic differences have been reported with respect to the development of diabetic retinopathy.

Several studies have explored the relationship between human leukocyte antigen (HLA) antigens, expressed on cell surfaces (and customarily tested with leukocytes withdrawn by venepuncture), and the presence, or severity, of diabetic retinopathy. Rand et al.[40] used case–control design and found a strong association (relative risk, 3.74) between proliferative retinopathy and the presence of HLA-DR phenotypes 4/0, 3/0, and X/X (neither 3 nor 4). Subjects who had HLA-DR phenotypes 3/4, 3/X, and 4/X had no increased risk of proliferative retinopathy as compared with "control" diabetic subjects, matched for age, sex, and diabetes duration, but without retinopathy. This question was also investigated in a group of 425 subjects with insulin-dependent diabetes who were randomly selected from a much larger population-based study.[41] After adjustments were made for duration of diabetes, glycemic control, hypertension, and nephropathy, these authors also found a significantly increased risk of proliferative diabetic retinopathy in subjects with the HLA DR4+ DR3 phenotype. No other HLA phenotype, or any of a variety of other genetic markers studied, conferred such increased risk. Previous studies indicating an increased, or decreased, risk of diabetic retinopathy, or of retinopathy of varying degrees of severity, in the presence of different HLA-A, HLA-B, or HLA-C group phenotypes may have been confounded by linkage disequilibrium. In this phenomenon, the major HLA antigen (in this case, in the D group) associated with the disease in question is frequently found closely linked, genetically, to an HLA antigen in another group (A, B, or C). Thus, if the investigation does not examine D-group antigens, an apparent association with an HLA antigen in another group will be found and reported as the primary association until later study discloses an even more highly statistically significant association with another antigen that was not initially studied but that is frequently in genetic linkage to the first.

More recent studies have investigated other aspects of the genetics of diabetic retinopathy. Of particular note is a report from the DCCT research group,[42] which examined familial clustering of severe diabetic retinopathy (Early Treatment Diabetic

Retinopathy Study (ETDRS) score > 47, i.e., severe preproliferative disease) among families of DCCT subjects with multiple diabetic members. Significant associations were found when the correlation of retinopathy severity among family members was investigated in several different ways. However, a less strong familial clustering of diabetic nephropathy was found, which is surprising because evidence from other studies has demonstrated considerable familial clustering of diabetic nephropathy, a complication of diabetes that is now considered to have a strong genetic component.[43–46] With increased sophistication in molecular biology, a number of investigators have examined several genetic loci for abnormalities that might be related to a hereditary susceptibility to complications of diabetes. Although these studies are not definitive, one of these claimed that a mutation in the aldose reductase gene conferred increased susceptibility to early-onset diabetic retinopathy in patients with type 2 diabetes.[47]

There appears to be considerable value in further investigation of genetic factors related to the pathogenesis of the more severe forms of diabetic retinopathy: advanced preproliferative and proliferative retinopathy and macular edema. Nearly all individuals with type 1 diabetes, and most with type 2 disease, will demonstrate some of the lesions of early retinopathy if they have their diabetes long enough, but only 50% or less will develop proliferative disease.[7,9] Like clinically evident diabetic nephropathy, which similarly affects fewer than 50% of all diabetic subjects regardless of the duration of their diabetes, this suggests that factors, quite possibly genetic, in addition to chronic hyperglycemia must be involved in the development of these severe forms of retinopathy.

Ocular factors

Becker[48] reported in 1967 that glaucoma reduced the prevalence and severity of diabetic retinopathy in affected eyes. Other studies have reported similar results. This has never been confirmed in a methodologically precise epidemiologic study, although Becker's claim seems to me to be correct based on my own clinical observations (Fig. 66-4). This is an important point that should be evaluated in a proper case–control study. If it is true, the explanation is unclear. If the effect is observable only in true glaucoma and not in ocular hypertension, in which the intraocular pressure is chronically elevated without damage to the retinal ganglion cell or optic nerve fiber layers, then it may be related in some way to loss of metabolic activity in the retina with degeneration of ganglion cells. If the effect is related simply to elevated intraocular pressure, the explanation for this observation would be less obvious.

It has also been reported that myopia reduces the prevalence and severity of diabetic retinopathy.[49] This effect of myopia on the prevalence of proliferative diabetic retinopathy has been confirmed by Rand et al.,[40] who found an interesting interaction between myopia of greater than 2 D and HLA-D-group antigens. Fewer subjects in their "case" group with proliferative retinopathy had myopia of this degree than did subjects in the control group, who had diabetes of 15 years' or more duration and minimal or no retinopathy. Subjects with 2 D or more of myopia and HLA-D group phenotypes 3/0, 4/0, or X/X had a relative risk for proliferative disease of 1.0 as compared with the control group (i.e., their risk was no different from that of the controls), while the overall risk for all subjects, regardless of refractive error, with these HLA-D group phenotypes was 3.74 (see above).

The initial observations leading to the development of panretinal photocoagulation (or scatter) treatment for proliferative diabetic retinopathy were made by Aiello and colleagues,[50] to the effect that eyes with a great deal of retinochoroidal scarring from trauma, inflammatory disease, etc. had markedly reduced prevalence and severity of diabetic retinopathy. The effect is unexplained, but the most widespread current hypothesis is that it results from decreased retinal metabolism – in particular,

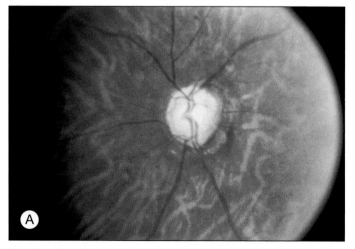
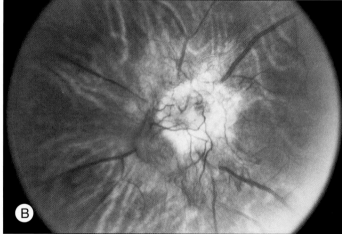

Fig. 66-4 This 64-year-old man presented with asymmetric, chronic open-angle glaucoma and markedly asymmetric diabetic retinopathy. Intraocular pressure in the right eye was 32 mmHg, visual acuity was 20/80, and there was a glaucomatous visual field defect and pronounced glaucomatous cupping of the optic nerve head. In the left eye, the pressure was 16 mmHg, visual acuity was 20/20, and there was only physiologic cupping. The patient had had diabetes mellitus for 15 years. A, Photograph of the right optic nerve head shows extensive cupping of the optic nerve, though without nasal displacement of the vessels. B, Photograph of the left optic nerve shows extensive neovascularization.

a decreased need for oxygen, with a resultant diminished production of a vasoproliferative (angiogenic) factor.[51–53] The immediate practical application of this observation was the attempt, through extensive photocoagulation of the mid peripheral retina (panretinal or scatter photocoagulation), to produce the same effect iatrogenically, a technique that significantly reduces the rate of progression to severe visual loss in proliferative diabetic retinopathy.[54]

Retinopathy in different forms of diabetes

There is no evidence that retinopathy differs in different forms of diabetes. Proliferative retinopathy is more prevalent at any given duration of the systemic disease in type 1 than in type 2 diabetes,[7,9] but, as noted earlier, it is not clear whether this is due to different metabolic factors in the two types of diabetes, to differences in the ages of the patients (type 1 patients are, on average, much younger), or to the higher mean blood glucose levels in type 1 patients. Macular edema probably occurs with equal prevalence as a function of disease duration in both type 1 and type 2 diabetes.[11] Type 2 diabetes is more common after the age of 30[7,9] (although "type 2 diabetes of youth" is becoming increasingly frequently recognized[55]) but, despite the apparently mild metabolic defect, proliferative retinopathy can occur as well in this form of the disease (Fig. 66-5). Similarly, vision-threatening retinopathy can occur in patients with "secondary" diabetes – that which occurs, for example, following pancreatitis, hemochromatosis, or acromegaly. The patient whose retinal photographs are shown in Fig. 66-6 A and B had acromegaly secondary to a pituitary adenoma and also developed background diabetic retinopathy with macular edema. Since the acromegaly had been treated and the patient had normal levels

of circulating growth hormone, the retinopathy may have been related to diabetes secondary to the acromegaly, or to a type 2 diabetes that would have developed regardless of the presence of acromegaly.

METHODS OF RESEARCH IN DIABETIC RETINOPATHY

Epidemiologic studies

The results of a number of epidemiologic investigations have been summarized above. In the evaluation of these and other studies, it is important to understand the methodologies employed. Sometimes investigators have employed an inappropriate method, or have used the appropriate method incorrectly. Even when the proper methodology has been used appropriately, it is important to understand its limitations. Although complete discussion of these problems is beyond the scope of this chapter, I would like here to summarize several of the epidemiologic methods used.

Studies of the *prevalence* of diabetic retinopathy (i.e., the number of cases that are present at a single point in time in the general population), or of the prevalence of visual disability or blindness resulting from diabetic retinopathy, have been, at best, inaccurate. The reason is, that many such studies[56] were performed by tabulating the numbers of cases of blindness resulting from diabetic retinopathy reported, on a voluntary basis, to governmental agencies and expressing these as a fraction of the total population. Such prevalence data will be flawed, since it is entirely possible that many blind people will not report to the agencies. Less likely, because a variety of examiners have certified the causes of blindness, it is possible that the reported diagnoses will be in error in at least some cases.

A better method of determining the prevalence of diabetic retinopathy in a population is the *population-based* study. In such a study, one chooses at random a predetermined fraction of the entire population of a given geographic region and determines the prevalence of the disease by performing a standardized examination on those individuals.[57] The WESDR,[7,9,11–13] an excellent example of such a population-based study, was designed to evaluate the prevalence of various levels of severity of diabetic retinopathy in a population of diabetic people in a 10-county area of southern Wisconsin. By surveying the primary care physicians in this geographic area, the investigators obtained a listing of all people with diabetes in the area. They then randomly selected about one-tenth of these persons for further evaluation.

The WESDR should be compared with two preceding studies[6,8] that reported very similar results regarding the prevalence of retinopathy in persons with type 1 diabetes in much smaller populations, drawn from diabetes clinics at university medical centers. The diabetic persons who participated in these studies were chosen by their attendance at a particular clinic. Because these individuals were not chosen at random, but rather were selected, they might possess "special" (even if unrecognized by the investigators) characteristics that distinguish them from the general population of type 1 diabetic persons. The

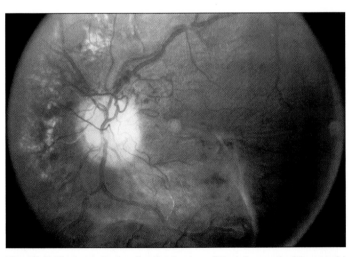

Fig. 66-5 Photograph showing the fundus of the left eye of a 32-year-old woman who had had diabetes mellitus since the age of 12 but had never required insulin. At the time of this photograph, she was being maintained on dietary management and sulfonylurea medication. She therefore has the diagnosis of "type 2 diabetes of youth." As the photograph demonstrates, she has developed substantial proliferative diabetic retinopathy with extensive optic nerve head neovascularization and fibroglial proliferation producing traction on the macula. The right eye had been lost because of proliferative diabetic retinopathy with neovascular glaucoma.

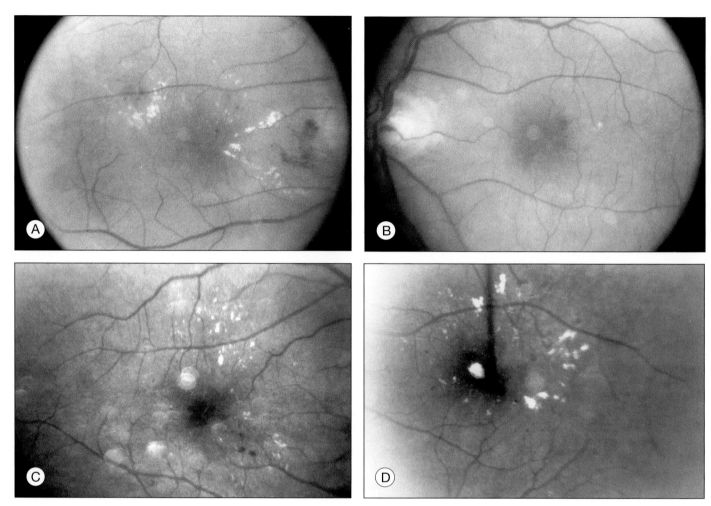

Fig. 66-6 A, Photograph of the macular region of the right eye of an 84-year-old man who had developed acromegaly 12 years previously. Treatment with bromocriptine has maintained serum growth hormone levels in the normal range. Subsequent to his development of acromegaly, he was found to have type 2 diabetes mellitus, and he developed background diabetic retinopathy with macular edema, for which he received focal argon laser photocoagulation. Subsequently, he developed a central retinal vein occlusion in his right eye, for which he received panretinal argon laser photocoagulation. Nevertheless, neovascular glaucoma ensued, requiring cyclocryotherapy and medical therapy to manage the intraocular pressure and maintain at least some visual acuity. B, The left eye of the same patient shows a few microaneurysms and minimal lipid deposition. C, Photograph of the right eye of a 52-year-old man with acromegaly and type 2 diabetes mellitus. Bromocriptine treatment brought serum growth hormone levels to the normal range. Background diabetic retinopathy and macular edema are present. D, The left macular region of the same patient, also showing background diabetic retinopathy with macular edema.

similarity of the results of these two studies (within the 95% confidence limits for each) to the results of the population-based Wisconsin study is strong evidence that such selection factors were not present.

To study whether a particular factor, present in certain people, may be causally related to the development of a disease, one can examine whether the antecedent presence of that factor predisposes to the future development of the disease – i.e., a *prospective* study – or whether a statistically significant relationship between the presumed causal factor and the disease existed in cases examined in the past – i.e., a *retrospective* study. Prospective studies are nearly always preferable, since, if proper methodology is used, it is much easier to isolate presumed causal factors and eliminate confounding interactions. However, because of the difficulties of designing such studies, and the much greater time and expense involved, prospective studies

have been conducted much less frequently than have retrospective ones.

A particular type of retrospective study that has merit is the *case–control* study.[40] In such a study, a population of persons with a given characteristic (in this example, type 1 diabetes of at least 15 years' documented duration) is separated into two groups: cases, persons who have, or have had, proliferative retinopathy, and controls, who have little or no retinopathy.. Various characteristics that differ between the two groups are sought, since these may be causally related to the development of diabetic retinopathy. However, in such retrospective investigations, these factors may simply be associated with the retinopathy and are not causally linked.

A particularly desirable, but difficult and expensive, type of prospective investigation is the *randomized, controlled clinical trial*. In this type of study, subjects who fulfill the characteristics previously determined as qualifying them for entry, and who volunteer for the study by completing appropriate informed-consent procedures, are randomly allocated to treatment or control groups. If the study group is sufficiently large, the random allocation statistically ensures that the many possible individual variables will be distributed equally in the treatment and control groups, so that treatment or nontreatment (or treatment by one of two or more different methods) is the only significant difference between the groups. If the groups are sufficiently large and the follow-up sufficiently long, it should be possible to determine if one or more of the treatments being studied is truly beneficial, by producing a statistically significant reduction in the chosen endpoint (e.g., progression to blindness from proliferative diabetic retinopathy[54]). If the treatment to be chosen has only local effects on the eye, e.g., photocoagulation therapy, then the randomization procedure may involve individual eyes of the same patient, provided that the patient has binocular, relatively symmetric disease.[54,58] This is advantageous because systemic factors that may vary among patients (e.g., individual variations in the blood glucose level) cancel out when each patient is his or her own control. However, despite their advantages, care must still be exercised in the design and conduct of randomized, controlled clinical trials, since inadvertent failure in various aspects of the design of these studies can leave their results open to great controversy.[59]

Techniques to study retinal blood flow

Fluorescein angiography, now in use for almost 40 years, is discussed in Chapter 51. Vitreous fluorophotometry[60–62] was designed to measure the passage of the small molecule sodium fluorescein (molecular weight 327) across the various components of the blood–retinal barrier. Unlike fluorescein angiography, vitreous fluorophotometry does not give a graphic picture of retinal or choroidal blood flow. In this technique, fluorescein dye is injected intravenously. Approximately 1 h later, the vitreous cavity is scanned by a fluorometer, usually attached to a slit lamp. The fluorometer scans small volumes of the vitreous cavity and converts the fluorescence measurements to concentrations, so that one can plot concentration of fluorescein as a function of location within the vitreous, and also (if measurements are performed at different intervals after the injection) as a function of time. A dramatic result that has been reported with this technique is that, in humans and in animals with diabetes mellitus of very brief onset and no retinopathy detectable either by clinical examination or by fluorescein angiography, increased concentrations of fluorescein dye can be detected in the vitreous, close to the retinal surface, in diabetic patients as compared with nondiabetic controls or with diabetic patients or animals whose blood glucose levels are normalized.[63–65] This suggests that one of the earliest functional lesions in the eyes of diabetic persons is a breakdown of the blood–retinal barrier. However, not all investigators have been able to reproduce these fluorophotometric results.[66,67] Because of the inconsistent results obtained by different investigators who have used vitreous fluorophotometry, this technique has lost favor.

Several other techniques permit quantitative evaluation of flow within the retinal vessels. Laser Doppler velocimetry[68–73] uses an argon laser beam, aimed perpendicular to the direction of blood flow in major retinal vessels (usually the major quadrantic arteries and veins near the margins of the optic nerve head), to measure flow in these vessels by means of the Doppler effect. In one study, when blood glucose levels in a group of 12 subjects with noninsulin-dependent diabetes were decreased acutely with insulin from more than 300 mg/dl to 80 to 120 mg/dl, retinal blood flow decreased by an average of 15% ($P < 0.001$).[71] When a group of patients with insulin-dependent diabetes were rendered normoglycemic by means of multiple daily insulin injections, 16 of 20 eyes that demonstrated an initial reduction in retinal blood flow by laser Doppler velocimetry 5 days after institution of the strict control regimen showed no progression of retinopathy after 6 months of follow-up. However, 6 of 8 eyes that showed an increase in retinal blood flow after 5 days of normoglycemia demonstrated retinopathy progression at 6 months.[68] Laser Doppler studies performed on subjects with background or proliferative diabetic retinopathy showed a significant reduction in maximum blood flow velocity in major retinal veins compared to measurements made in normals.[72] Because of venous dilation in the diabetic retinal circulation, however, the calculated volume flow in the eyes of diabetic subjects with retinopathy was not significantly different from that in normals. Following panretinal photocoagulation, the calculated volume flow in the eyes of diabetic subjects decreased significantly below that of normals. Eyes that showed regression of neovascularization after such laser treatment also demonstrated a significantly larger posttreatment recovery of the vascular regulatory response (i.e., vasoconstriction and reduction of flow) to hyperoxia than did those eyes whose proliferative retinopathy did not regress after panretinal laser treatment.[69]

Comparable results were obtained when patients with type 1 diabetes but no retinopathy were studied by video fluorescein angiography to quantitate retinal blood flow.[74] Diabetic subjects without retinopathy had reduced retinal blood flow compared to age-matched controls. However, when blood glucose was increased to fixed levels that were maintained for 1 h using the "glucose clamp" technique, blood flow in the diabetic subjects increased. Measurement of retinal blood flow in diabetic subjects must, therefore, consider not only the diabetic state, but also the acute blood glucose level.

This group of investigators used the same technique to study retinal blood flow in normal and diabetic rats.[75] They also found reduced retinal blood flow in the diabetic rats which could be corrected by intravitreal injection of a blocker of one of the receptors (the so-called ET_A receptor) for the powerful polypeptide vasopressor hormone, endothelin-1 (ET-1) or by a blocker of endothelin-converting enzyme. There is evidence that ET-1 is strongly upregulated in the retinas of diabetic rats.[76] An inhibitor of angiotensin-converting enzyme, however, had no effect. Levels of messenger RNA for preproendothelin-1 were approximately doubled in the retinas and brains of diabetic rats by comparison with normals, and intravitreal injection of

ET-1 into normal rats caused a decrease in retinal blood flow comparable to that observed in diabetic animals.

The blue-field entoptic phenomenon is a method of studying blood flow in the perifoveal capillary network.[77,78] The subject looks with one eye at a bright, uniform field of blue light and can then observe a pulsatile pattern of moving particles. Since the number of particles greatly increases in subjects with a marked leukocytosis and decreases in those with leukopenia, and since the pattern of moving particles resembles the anatomic distribution of perifoveal capillaries, this pattern is evidently produced by leukocytes flowing through these capillaries. Using computer simulation of the flow, which the subject can compare with that which he/she observes within his/her own eyes, and which can be adjusted to match precisely his/her own entoptic images, the method can provide a semiquantitative measure of flow in the perifoveal capillaries.

An experimental study in animals by Ernest et al.[79] deals with the important circulatory phenomenon of autoregulation. ("Autoregulation" refers to the ability of the retinal vessels to adjust blood flow locally, which they must do, since they have no sympathetic innervation, in response to appropriate stimuli, e.g., breathing hyperoxic or hypercarbic gas mixtures.) These investigators studied a group of four normal dogs and a group of four dogs that were made diabetic with alloxan and maintained in "poor" blood glucose control for 8 months. At the end of this time, the investigators measured preretinal oxygen tension in all animals, using a microelectrode inserted into the vitreous, under conditions of hyperglycemia following a rapid intravenous glucose infusion and during breathing of 100% oxygen. The average preretinal oxygen tension was higher in both the diabetic and in the normal animals when they were made acutely hyperglycemic. This result (which should be compared with the measurements of retinal blood flow in humans during glucose clamp conditions[74]) suggests that hyperglycemia per se impairs retinal vascular autoregulation. In addition, the diabetic animals had somewhat higher preretinal oxygen tensions while breathing 100% oxygen, suggesting that diabetes produces a further impairment of autoregulation. These authors therefore proposed that when "tight" blood glucose control is suddenly imposed on a person with chronic diabetes, the impaired retinal vascular autoregulation caused by the prolonged diabetic state may cause a sudden decrease in the retinal oxygen supply, producing areas of retinal infarction. This may result in the "early worsening" of retinopathy that has been observed in some cases clinically.[3,25–27]

In another study,[78] diabetic subjects used the blue-field entoptic technique to evaluate changes in autoregulation of the macular capillary circulation before and after panretinal laser treatment for proliferative diabetic retinopathy. Eyes in which the retinopathy regressed following laser treatment demonstrated improved vascular autoregulation, tested by measuring perifoveal capillary flow with the blue-field technique, or large-vessel flow with laser Doppler velocimetry, while the subjects were breathing hyperoxic or hypercarbic gas mixtures. These results are interesting but puzzling. Eyes with proliferative retinopathy have substantial anatomic abnormality. As judged from the extensive areas of nonperfusion usually demonstrable

in them by fluorescein angiography, these eyes have evidently suffered extensive retinal capillary cell loss. If retinal vascular autoregulation is governed by contractile cells (presumably pericytes) in the microcirculation, it is difficult to understand how these cells could regenerate following laser treatment. Alternatively, even in the presence of extensive cellular loss, the effect could have been mediated by cells that never actually degenerated, but simply diminished their functional capacity and then recovered following metabolic changes after photocoagulation. Another explanation, consistent with the laser Doppler results (which deal with the large vessels in the retinal circulation and not the capillaries), is that the variations in macular capillary flow measured in these experiments are actually governed by changes in the caliber of the retinal arterioles regulated by the arterial smooth-muscle cells rather than by the pericytes of the capillaries.

Finally, a new method that has been developed and tested in animals, and in preliminary fashion in humans, is the measurement of retinal oxygenation noninvasively, using magnetic resonance imaging.[80–82] The method does not measure the retinal Po_2 directly, but rather the change in Po_2 when the animal is switched from breathing room air to either 100% O_2 or to carbogen (95% O_2, 5% CO_2). Since the method measures this "ΔPo_2" at the inner retinal surface, the contribution of the choroidal circulation is minimal. Although certain assumptions are required, it is likely that the ΔPo_2 correlates with the Po_2 at the inner retinal surface. If further studies confirm its efficacy in humans, this method should have considerable value for assessing the role of retinal oxygenation in the development of proliferative diabetic retinopathy (see below) and other retinal vasoproliferative diseases.

Animal models in the study of diabetic retinopathy

Studies of the pathogenesis and treatment of human disease can be facilitated by the development of models of the disease in animals. There have been numerous attempts to reproduce the lesions of diabetic retinopathy in animals. Although several authors have claimed positive results, there are only a few animal models in which one or more of the lesions of diabetic retinopathy have been produced with unquestioned validity. Foremost among these are dogs, with spontaneous[83] or induced[84,85] diabetes of 3 to 5 years' duration. These animals develop loss of capillary pericytes and ultimately also of endothelial cells with nonfunctional, acellular capillaries; capillary basement membrane thickening; and microaneurysm formation. Early intraretinal neovascularization has also been observed. However, more advanced lesions, including retinal edema (dogs do not have a macula, so true macular edema cannot develop) and neovascularization into the vitreous, have not been reported.

Because of the ease of working with them, there have been many attempts to develop diabetic retinopathy in rodents, including mice and, in particular, rats. Claims to have produced lesions such as microaneurysms[86] and pericyte dropout[86] in rats with experimental diabetes of less than 1 year have not been validated by Engerman et al.[84] or Tilton et al.,[87] or in my own experiments (unpublished). However, rats with diabetes[88] or galactosemia[89,90] develop retinal capillary basement membrane thickening, a lesion that has been widely observed in many microvascular systems in the body in human and animal diabetes.[91–93] In addition, rats that have been galactosemic for 18 months or more develop pericyte loss and, eventually, capillary acellularity,[88,94–97] and some rats that have been fed a 30 to 50% galactose diet for up to 24 months develop a halo of dilated, hypercellular vessels surrounding the optic nerve.[88,94–97] Whether these represent intraretinal neovascularization or simply dilated pre-existing vascular channels is uncertain. Of particular interest is a report that pericyte and endothelial cell nuclei in short-term diabetic or galactosemic rats, and in retinal capillaries from donor eyes of humans with diabetes, undergo apoptosis as demonstrated by appropriate nuclear labeling techniques.[98] It is unknown what stimulus is induced by prolonged hyperglycemia, or galactosemia, that causes programmed death of retinal capillary cells to a greater extent than capillary cells elsewhere in the body.

Because of the similarity of their retinal anatomy to that of humans, one might expect that nonhuman primates with diabetes of sufficient duration would be good models for human diabetic retinopathy. However, studies of rhesus monkeys with diabetes for as long as 10 years have revealed occasional microaneurysms but no other lesions.[84,99]

Doubtless a major reason for the difficulty in producing lesions of diabetic retinopathy in animals with diabetes is the factor of disease duration. In diabetic dogs a minimum disease duration of 3 to 5 years is necessary for the development of the earliest lesions of retinopathy,[85] and this is identical to the duration required for retinopathy to develop in humans with type 1 diabetes.[6–8] Rats and mice normally have a lifespan of under 3 years, and after the onset of diabetes it is difficult to maintain these animals for much more than 1 year. Several investigators have reported the development of lesions resembling diabetic retinopathy in rats fed a 50% galactose diet for 28 months.[94–96] These lesions include pericyte "ghosts," acellular capillaries, and vascular dilation and tortuosity. Whether microaneurysms occur in galactosemic rats is controversial.[94–99] The use of a high-galactose diet to produce a model of diabetic retinopathy originated from the hypothesis that the enzyme sequence known as the "sorbitol pathway" is responsible for the earliest lesions of diabetic retinopathy. Since galactose, along with glucose, is a substrate for this pathway, its use in producing models of retinopathy is a good test of the hypothesis. Previously, Engerman & Kern,[100] as well as Kador and associates,[101,102] have produced a diabetic-like retinopathy in dogs fed a 50% galactose diet for 3 to 4 years. Kern & Engerman have also reported a diabetic-like retinopathy in mice fed a 30% galactose diet for 21 to 26 months.[103] They reported that, unlike galactosemic rats, galactosemic mice developed true microaneurysms. These findings raise two important questions. First, why might mice, dogs, and humans develop microaneurysms after chronic diabetes, or galactosemia, and rats do not? Second, how might the presence of retinopathy in chronically galactosemic mice be relevant to the hypothesis that the "sorbitol pathway" is an important causal mechanism for diabetic retinopathy? Both of these questions will be considered in more detail in later sections of this chapter.

Species- and organ-specific variations in anatomy and in metabolic pathways may be important considerations in the development of microvascular lesions in the retina or other organs. Pericyte dropout and microaneurysm formation have not been found either in the brains of diabetic human subjects,[104] or in those of diabetic or galactosemic dogs,[105] even though these lesions are common in the retina and were present in the retinas of the same human or animal subjects in whose cerebral cortexes they could not be found. It might be argued that in these studies, retinas were examined by the trypsin digest procedure in which the entire, intact retinal vasculature can be spread on a microscope slide and examined in detail. This cannot be done with cerebral cortical vasculature, which must be examined histologically following homogenization and sieving through a nylon mesh that retains only vascular fragments. Capillaries that have lost cells or are otherwise abnormal may be sufficiently fragile that they are broken into smaller pieces by this technique and are lost in the sieving process. Although the retina is derived embryologically from the brain, and both retina and brain have a microvasculature featuring thick endothelial cell cytoplasm and tight junctions between endothelial cells that produce a blood–tissue barrier to many molecules, pericyte coverage of the endothelial cell tube of capillaries of the retina is substantially greater in the two species that have been studied (rat and monkey) than it is in the brains of these species.[106,107] The same is probably true in humans, where the data from retina closely resemble data from the retinas of monkeys, but it has not been possible to obtain retinal and brain tissue from the same human donors adequate to perform these morphometric studies. Although galactosemic rats develop a diabetic-like retinopathy, rats have a much smaller ratio of pericytes to endothelial cells in their retinal microcirculations than do humans.[87,106,108] Comparisons of the retinal and cerebral pericyte:endothelial cell ratios in retinas and brains of rats with those of dogs, mice, and humans have not been carried out, but would be of interest because dogs, humans, and (at least according to one group of investigators) mice develop true capillary microaneurysms with long-term diabetes (dogs and humans) and galactosemia (dogs and mice), while rats do not.

Two useful animal models of neovascularization exist, both in nondiabetic animals. The first, originally described by Ashton[51] and by Patz,[109] is produced by exposing neonatal kittens or puppies to an atmosphere high in oxygen for just a few days just after birth. This produces at least a peripheral, or in more severe cases a generalized,[110] vasoconstriction, followed by the development of retinal new vessels. These vessels are transient, however, and regress spontaneously after a few weeks. This model was initially developed to simulate retinopathy of prematurity, following exposure of premature human infants to a high-oxygen atmosphere. The development of the new vessels, according to the hypothesis that has been favored for a number of years,[53] presumably resulted from production by the hypoxic retina cells (*hypoxic* because of the profound vasoconstriction that followed the *hyperoxia*) of an "angiogenesis factor."[111,112]

More recently, hyperoxygenation during the neonatal period has been applied to mice and rats, producing a model of peripheral retinal neovascularization similar to that of retinopathy of prematurity in human infants (Fig. 66-7), that has been exploited for studies of the production, and inhibition, of angiogenesis factors.[35,113,114]

A second model of intraretinal and subretinal (beneath the neural retina, but arising from the retinal and not the choroidal circulation) neovascularization has recently been described, using transgenic mice that overexpress the gene for VEGF.[115] This model is additional evidence that VEGF is capable of producing retinal neovascularization, although in a quite artificial situation that may not be relevant to neovascularizing ocular diseases in humans. The new vessels in these transgenic mice extend from the retinal circulation to beneath the photoreceptor layer of the neural retina but do not enter the RPE. The reason for this outward growth, rather than inward into the vitreous, is that the promoter used to carry the VEGF gene into the retina is the rhodopsin gene, which is localized to the photoreceptor cells.

Cell culture studies

The intact human, or experimental animal, is a complex organism, in which the study of the intricate metabolic pathways that ultimately lead to diabetic retinopathy may be difficult.

Since the mid-1970s, techniques have been developed to isolate and grow in culture the component cells of both large and small blood vessels, including those from the retina. In 1975, our laboratory described the culture of retinal microvascular pericytes from bovine and monkey eyes.[116] Subsequently we[117] and others[118–120] described the culture of retinal microvascular endothelial cells. More recent evidence indicates that glial cells of the retina and optic nerve may also be important in the development, at least in the later stages of diabetic retinopathy, of neovascularization and, perhaps, macular edema. Methods are available for retinal glial cell culture.[121] These techniques add an extra tool for research in diabetic retinopathy, but one that must be used with caution. One can use cell culture studies to investigate certain biochemical processes, but with great caution that the processes being studied have not been greatly modified in culture from those that occur in vivo. The same can be said for the investigation of physiologic function, e.g., phagocytosis, cell contraction, or cell motility. Diabetic retinopathy requires years to develop in the intact human or experimental animal. It has not yet been possible to maintain cultures of retinal cells for that duration, and there is no way of ascertaining that alterations produced in cells by exposure to high glucose or galactose over a short time in culture are truly related to the development of the anatomic and functional lesions of diabetic retinopathy over a very long time in the intact retina. Finally, although capillary tube-like structures composed of micro- and macrovascular endothelial cells have been produced under certain conditions in culture,[122–124] these may not be truly analogous

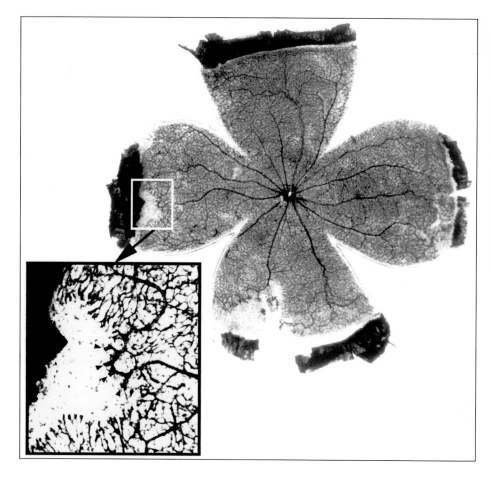

Fig. 66-7 Flat mount of the retinal vessels from an eye of a neonatal albino rat that had been exposed with its mother to an atmosphere in which the oxygen level was varied in stepwise fashion between 50% and 10% every 24 h over the first 14 days after birth. The animal was then returned to room air for the next 6 days and then euthanized, the eyes enucleated, and the retinal vessels visualized using a histochemical technique that demonstrates ADPase activity. The inset demonstrates a tuft of new vessels (arrowheads) in the peripheral retinal vasculature, similar to those that develop in human infants with retinopathy of prematurity. Magnifications: main figure, ×15; inset, ×75. (Courtesy of Bruce Berkowitz, Ph.D., Department of Anatomy and Cell Biology, Wayne State University School of Medicine.)

either to normal vessels or to abnormal new vessels in the intact retina.

Despite these caveats, there are several results using cultured retinal microvascular cells that appear to be relevant to the physiology of the intact retinal microcirculation. These include the elegant studies of D'Amore and associates,[125,126] in which microvascular endothelial cells were co-cultured with a variety of other cell types that had been growth-arrested with an antibiotic and were then plated together with endothelial cells in different proportions. Most of the cells used for the co-cultures, including bovine RPE cells, human skin fibroblasts, mouse 3T3 fibroblasts, and Madin-Darby canine kidney cells, greatly stimulated endothelial cell proliferation. By contrast, pericytes and vascular smooth-muscle cells dramatically inhibited endothelial cell proliferation, even when the pericytes or smooth-muscle cells were added in ratios as low as 1:10 with the endothelial cells.[125] For the co-culture to be effective in retarding endothelial cell proliferation, pericyte or smooth-muscle cell processes had to make contact with the endothelial cells. Transfer of "conditioned media" from pericyte or smooth-muscle cell cultures was ineffective in producing growth inhibition. In studying the mechanism of the inhibition, these authors found that it was produced by the release, and activation, of transforming growth factor β (TGF-β).[126] Pericytes or smooth-muscle cells alone produce this polypeptide in an inactive form. The co-cultured cells, in physical contact with one another, both produce and activate TGF-β. This finding suggests that one function of pericytes in the retina is to inhibit the proliferation of endothelial cells. Thus, the loss of pericytes that occurs early in the course of diabetic retinopathy may facilitate the later development of microaneurysms (clusters of newly formed endothelial cells) and of frank neovascularization. In fact, just this result has been reported in an experiment using mice with a targeted disruption ("knockout") of the gene for the B-chain of platelet-derived growth factor (PDGF-B).[127] This genetic defect is lethal, but histopathologic examination of the fetal PDGF-B-deficient animals shows an absence of capillary pericytes – whose antenatal development is evidently controlled by this growth factor – and the frequent appearance of microaneurysms throughout the microcirculation of the retina and brain.

Pericytes are considered to be contractile cells, regulating flow through the capillaries analogous to the function of the smooth-muscle cells of the larger vessels. Cultured pericytes are immunocytochemically positive for smooth-muscle actin,[128] and in culture they contract either spontaneously[129] or in response to a variety of agents.[130–132] Thus, loss of pericytes from the retinal microcirculation may produce alterations in retinal blood flow. However, direct evidence for pericyte contraction in the circulation of the intact retina has never been obtained. Tilton et al.[133] performed a morphometric study of capillaries in rats following infusion of various vasoconstrictor agents and found evidence of contraction of pericytes in skeletal muscle capillaries but not in those of cardiac muscle. We conducted a similar study in the retinal vessels of rats following intravitreal infusion of ET-1, an extremely powerful vasoconstrictor.[134] Although we found evidence of contraction of arteriolar smooth muscle, we could not demonstrate contraction of retinal capillary pericytes.

Anatomic lesions and the pathogenesis of diabetic retinopathy
Capillary basement membrane thickening

This well-known lesion of diabetes has usually been measured by electron microscopic morphometry. Additional basement membrane abnormalities of diabetes include "Swiss cheese-like" vacuolization and deposition of fibrillar collagen in the midst of the usual homogeneous pattern of basement membrane collagen when viewed by electron microscopy. The biochemical events that bring about these changes are not known, nor is it clear what, if any, alteration of physiologic function occurs because of the anatomic abnormalities of the basement membrane. In regard to the biochemical events that may cause the basement membrane changes, several studies implicate the sorbitol pathway in this process.[88–90,135,136] Nondiabetic rats fed for prolonged periods on diets rich in galactose develop thickened retinal capillary basement membranes, together with Swiss-cheese vacuolization and fibrillar collagen deposition (Fig. 66-8), whereas animals on a control diet, or on a high-galactose diet together with sorbinil, an aldose reductase inhibitor, do not develop the basement membrane abnormalities. Robison et al.[89,136] have shown that basement membrane thickening can be prevented in galactosemic animals by using various structurally different aldose reductase inhibitors. It is not clear how the action of the enzymes of the sorbitol pathway, aldose reductase and sorbitol dehydrogenase, can affect the structure of basement membranes. Against the possibility that the basement membrane thickening in the retinal capillaries of diabetic humans and animals, and of galactosemic animals, is a direct result of sorbitol pathway activity is the observation that, in the renal glomeruli of diabetic[92] and galactosemic[137] rats, basement membrane thickening that is structurally and immunochemically similar to that which occurs in the retina is not prevented by aldose reductase inhibitors. Thus basement membrane thickening may be a nonspecific, secondary response to a primary biochemical lesion in one of the types of cells that borders the basement membrane. In some cases, as in the retinal microcirculation, this primary lesion may involve the sorbitol pathway. In other cases, as in the renal glomerulus, it apparently does not.

Other biochemical mechanisms may also play a role in basement membrane thickening in the diabetic human or in diabetic or galactosemic animals. Basement membrane collagen is extensively glycated, and this glycation may be either qualitatively or quantitatively altered by enzymatic[138] or nonenzymatic[139] processes. Although type IV collagen is the major collagenous component of the basement membrane, other collagen types, as well as noncollagen macromolecules such as laminin,[140] entactin, heparan sulfate proteoglycan (HSPG),[141,142] and various basement membrane-bound growth factors are also present.[141] The structure of the basement membrane appears to be altered by variation in the relative amounts as well as the chemical composition of these substances.

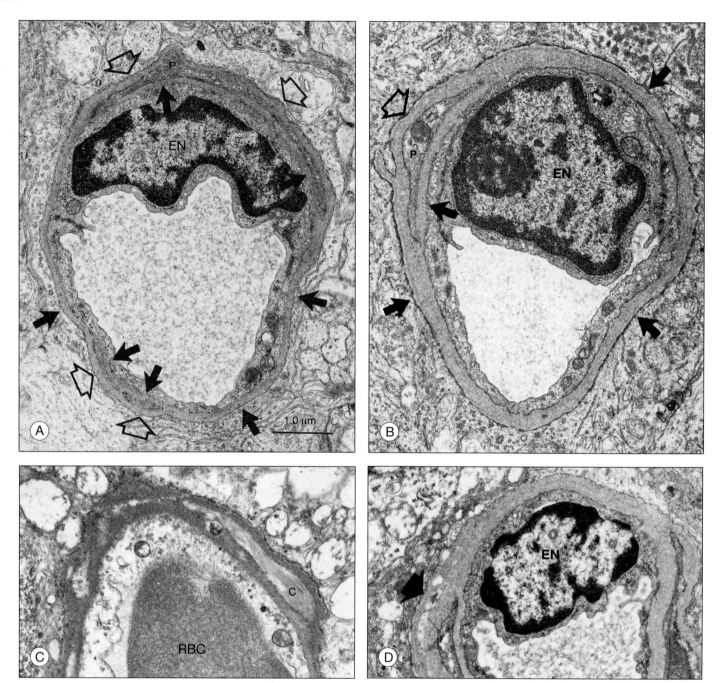

Fig. 66-8 A, Retinal capillary from a Wistar-Kyoto rat, aged 15 months, that had been maintained on a normal diet. The basement membrane surrounding the endothelial cells (closed arrows) is of normal thickness. Open arrows indicate basement membrane surrounding pericyte processes, whose thickness was not measured in the experimental protocol. An endothelial cell nucleus (EN) and a pericyte process (P) are indicated. B, Uniform thickening of the basement membrane surrounding the retinal capillary in a 17-month spontaneously hypertensive rat that had received a diet containing 30% by weight galactose for 15 months. C, A portion of a retinal capillary from a Wistar-Kyoto rat that had been fed the 30% galactose diet for 15 months. There is extensive, focal endothelial basement membrane thickening. Fibrillar collagen (C) is found within the basement membrane. An erythrocyte (RBC) is present in the capillary lumen. D, A retinal capillary from a Wistar-Kyoto rat that had received the high-galactose diet for 21 months. Note the diffuse basement membrane thickening and Swiss-cheese vacuolization of the basement membrane (arrow). (Reproduced with permission from Frank RN, Keirn RJ, Kennedy A et al. Galactose-induced retinal capillary basement membrane thickening: prevention by sorbinil. Invest Ophthalmol Vis Sci 1983; 24:1519–1524,[90] by permission of the Association for Research in Vision and Ophthalmology.)

On the basis of experiments performed on mice implanted with a tumor that produces copious amounts of basement membrane material, and then made diabetic, it has been proposed that an important biochemical lesion of basement membranes in diabetes is a marked decrease in the production of the heparan sulfate proteoglycan, with a resultant secondary overproduction of basement membrane collagen.[143] However, this result could not be repeated by another group of investigators.[144]

Shimomura & Spiro[145] and Spiro & Spiro[146] have reported decreased HSPG in kidney glomeruli from humans with diabetes. Quantitative electron microscopic immunocytochemical studies show that the increased retinal and renal capillary basement membrane thickness in galactosemic rats is accompanied by an increase in the relative concentrations of type IV collagen and laminin, while the relative concentration of HSPG core protein did not change.[135,137] While not identical to the findings of Rohrbach et al.[143] and Shimomura & Spiro[145] in different tissues, these results are comparable in that they show an increased ratio of other basement membrane macromolecules relative to HSPG. All of these changes in galactosemic rat retinal microvascular basement membranes were prevented by administration of sorbinil.

A second immunocytochemical finding in the galactosemic retinal capillary basement membranes was that regions of fibrillar collagen in these membranes (which were not found in the control animals or in those receiving sorbinil along with the high-galactose diet) stained immunocytochemically positive for type III collagen, a molecule not normally found in basement membranes in vivo[135] (Fig. 66-9). However, type III collagen is produced by retinal microvascular pericytes and endothelial cells in culture,[147] indicating that these cells possess the gene for this collagen, but that its production is normally suppressed in intact tissues of living animals.

What are the functions of basement membranes? How might these be affected by alterations in their structure? One obvious function of basement membranes is to serve as a "skeleton," giving structural rigidity to organs like blood vessels. This is unlikely to be altered by the basement membrane thickening of diabetes. Basement membranes may also serve as filtration

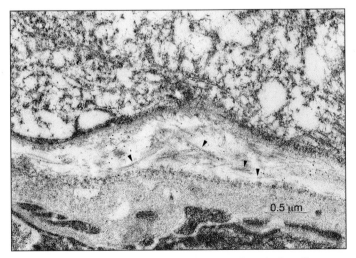

Fig. 66-9 A portion of the basement membrane of a retinal capillary from a galactose-fed rat showing focal thickening and deposition of thin striated fibrils (arrowheads) near the outer border of the basement membrane. Immunogold staining with collagen type III antibody shows strong labeling of these fibrils. (Reprinted from Das A, Frank RN, Zhang NL et al. Increases in collagen type IV and laminin in galactose-induced retinal capillary basement membrane thickening – prevention by an aldose reductase inhibitor. Exp Eye Res 1990; 50:269–280,[135] with permission from Elsevier.)

barriers for molecules of various sizes and electrical charges. Farquhar[148] originally proposed this for the renal glomerular basement membrane. Perhaps alterations in the amount or degree of sulfation, or in the anatomic distribution of the highly negatively charged heparan sulfate proteoglycan molecules within basement membranes, can affect their permeability properties to various ions.[149] Studies of the molecular filtration properties of the glomerular basement membrane[148] and of Bruch's membrane at the base of the RPE[150] indicate that the normal size cutoff is somewhat below serum albumin, whose molecular weight is 68 000. Alterations in this property might affect the function of the blood–retinal barrier, which breaks down in diabetic retinopathy, quite possibly very early in the diabetic state. Yet this breakdown would not appear to be caused by alterations in permeability of the blood–retinal barrier to molecules the size of serum albumin, since fluorescein (molecular weight 327) is only weakly bound to albumin and other serum proteins[151] and therefore much of the "leakage" seen in vitreous fluorophotometry and fluorescein angiography is likely due to the passage of free fluorescein.

A third function of basement membranes is to regulate cell proliferation and differentiation.[152–155] Several different cell types, when cultured in vitro, assume a more highly differentiated morphology when they are grown on collagenous substrates.[122,123,156,157] In a model of retinovitreal neovascularization that we have described in spontaneously hypertensive rats with dystrophic retinas,[158] the proliferating vessels grow through the retina accompanied by a sheath of RPE cells. When the vessels and RPE cells reach the inner limiting membrane of the retina, the RPE cells spread out in a monolayer against the inner limiting membrane, while the vessels burst through the membrane into the vitreous. This demonstrates, first, that basement membranes (such as the inner limiting membrane of the retina) can serve as a barrier to vasoproliferation, and therefore that newly forming vessels must be able to break throughout basement membranes, perhaps by elaborating appropriate enzymes.[159] The role of proteolytic enzymes that degrade basement membrane components is thought to be important in blood vessel growth, whether in normal development, in tissue repair, or in the pathologic neovascularization of disease, and the activation and inhibition of such enzymes in tissues (such as the retina) where neovascularization occurs has been the subject of considerable study.[160] The RPE cells, which do not make such enzymes, remain behind. For these cells, the basement membrane serves as a guide to differentiation, since the monolayer of RPE cells lined up along the inner limiting membrane of the retina develops a polarization exactly the opposite of that which they have in their normal anatomic location against Bruch's membrane.[158]

A fourth function of basement membranes is their ability to bind various growth factors. In particular, the fibroblast growth factors (FGFs) are potent mitogens that are especially active toward vascular endothelial cells, and are found in many tissues throughout the body. The binding of basic FGF (bFGF, now designated FGF-2)[161,162] as well as acidic fibroblast growth factor (aFGF, now designated FGF-1)[163] to basement membrane HSPG is well documented. Other growth factors are also found in basement membranes.[141] Since the retina is rich in these growth factors, their sequestration by HSPG residues may serve to restrain neovascularization. If the relative or actual quantity of HSPG is reduced in retinal microvascular basement membranes, then the ability of the basement membranes to prevent neovascularization may also be decreased.

Loss of microvascular intramural pericytes

This lesion, the classic histologic finding of early diabetic retinopathy in the human retina, was first described by Cogan, Kuwabara, and colleagues[164,165] when they examined flat mounts of the retinal vasculature of diabetic human subjects that had been prepared using an enzymatic digest method that they had developed.[166] Their findings have now been confirmed by many investigators.[4,167,168] In digest preparations from the retinal vessels of diabetic humans or dogs, one can easily recognize pericyte dropout by the observation of empty, balloonlike spaces bulging from the side of the capillary wall (Fig. 66-10A). In these species, normal pericyte nuclei appear as regularly spaced, darkly staining bulges in the wall of the capillary, like "bumps on a log" (Fig. 66-10B). They are not so easily recognized by light microscopic examination of digest preparations from other species, e.g., rats and mice, in which many pericyte nuclei do not bulge out from the wall of the vessel and, by light

microscopy, are difficult to distinguish from the nuclei of endothelial cells[45] (Fig. 66-10C).

The mechanism by which pericytes are specifically lost early in diabetic retinopathy is unknown. Akagi et al.[169] have proposed that it may be related to the action of the sorbitol pathway, since they find aldose reductase specifically in retinal capillary pericytes but not in endothelial cells in human specimens, using an immunohistochemical technique. This result would seem to provide a satisfactory explanation for the specific loss of pericytes, not only in the retinal microcirculation but also elsewhere in the body,[170] in diabetes. However, it has not been reported by other investigators. Two other groups have failed to find any aldose reductase immunoreactivity in retinal microvessels in rats and dogs,[171,172] while, conversely, we[173] have found biochemical evidence for aldose reductase activity both in cultured bovine retinal microvascular pericytes and in retinal microvascular endothelial cells. However, we have also found aldose reductase activity in cultured monkey retinal pericytes,[174] yet these animals develop only the most minimal early lesions of diabetic retinopathy after 10 years of diabetes. Since PDGF-B has now been described as essential for pericyte development in fetal life,[127] it is possible that much lower concentrations of this molecule are required as a "maintenance factor" for the viability of these cells postnatally. Alterations of PDGF-B

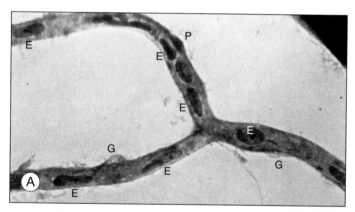

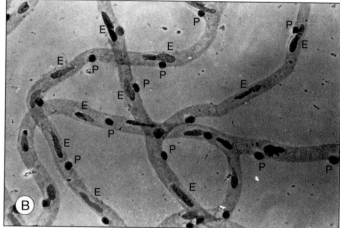

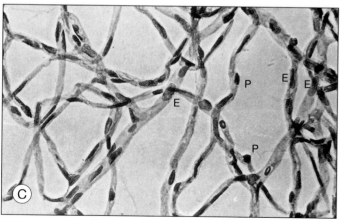

Fig. 66-10 A, Pericyte ghosts (G) in a trypsin digest preparation from a 42-year-old woman with background diabetic retinopathy who died of a dissecting aneurysm of the aorta. The ghost represents the vacant space in the capillary basement membrane, formerly occupied by an intramural pericyte nucleus that has degenerated. Normal pericyte (P) and endothelial cell (E) nuclei are also shown. The preparation was stained with periodic acid–Schiff (PAS) reagent and hematoxylin. Magnification ×575. B, A trypsin digest preparation from the retina of a nondiabetic, 55-year-old man who died of a myocardial infarction. Note the regular array of pericyte (P) and endothelial cell (E) nuclei. The preparation was stained with PAS reagent and hematoxylin. Magnification ×450. C, A trypsin digest preparation from the retina of a normal, adult male Sprague-Dawley rat, aged 12 months. Obvious pericyte (P) and endothelial cell (E) nuclei can be seen, but the type of cell represented by many other nuclei in this preparation cannot be distinguished unequivocally. Although the magnification is identical to that of the human digest preparation of B, the capillaries appear to be of smaller caliber. The preparation was stained with PAS and hematoxylin. Magnification ×450.

secretion or function produced by prolonged hyperglycemia or galactosemia may selectively affect pericyte viability, leading to their loss by apoptosis.[98]

Microaneurysms

Pericyte loss is detectable only in histologic preparations. The earliest clinically observable lesion of diabetic retinopathy is the microaneurysm,[175] which appears as a tiny, red dot by ophthalmoscopic examination, and as a hyperfluorescent dot by fluorescein angiography (Fig. 66-11). By light microscopy, in retinal vascular digest preparations, microaneurysms appear as grapelike or spindle-shaped dilations of retinal capillaries[164]. They may be hypercellular or acellular.

Retinal capillary microaneurysms may represent focal regions of endothelial cell proliferation, where the antiproliferative effect of pericytes has been lost.[125–127] This may explain the development of cellular microaneurysms, but not acellular ones. Perhaps all microaneurysms are initially cellular, but some become acellular as a result of extensive apoptosis[98] involving endothelial cell as well as pericyte nuclei.

A second explanation for microaneurysm formation is that they may arise from weak points in the capillary wall following the loss of pericytes. Since there is now strong anatomic,[128–130] biochemical,[176] and functional[129–132] evidence that pericytes are contractile elements in the capillary wall, much like the smooth-muscle cells of larger vessels, the tonus exerted by the myofibrils in the pericytes may counteract the transmural pressures produced by the flowing blood, and when this tonus is lost, the microvessel wall may dilate focally, producing a microaneurysm. However, one objection to the reasoning used in this discussion is that retinal capillary microaneurysms may be observed in other diseases in which pericyte loss has not been observed.[177,178]

Capillary acellularity

A more advanced microvascular lesion of diabetic retinopathy (and one that is not unique to this disease) is the complete loss of all cellular elements from the retinal microvessels. Clinicopathologic correlations between fluorescein angiograms that were performed shortly before an eye was enucleated for therapeutic purposes (or the patient died and had the eye removed at autopsy) and retinal vascular digest preparations that were performed on the enucleated specimens have demonstrated that acellular capillaries are nonfunctional, since they appear as dark spaces on the angiogram.[179,180] The sequence of events that leads to the total loss of cells in a capillary network in diabetes, or in other retinal vascular diseases, or in experimental diabetes or galactosemia in laboratory animals, is unknown. Since capillary acellularity appears in many diseases of the retinal blood vessels, a variety of etiologic mechanisms may produce this lesion.

Breakdown of the blood–retinal barrier

Breakdown of the blood–retinal barrier may occur early in the course of diabetes, before retinopathy is observed clinically, and it is certainly present when retinopathy is clinically evident. What are the anatomic, and biochemical, correlates of this functional abnormality?

One possible cause of blood–retinal barrier breakdown is opening of the tight junctions (zonulae occludentes) between adjacent microvascular endothelial cell processes.[18,181] Seen at high magnification with the electron microscope, such junctions normally have a pentalaminar structure, with two outer and one central electron-dense layers sandwiching two electron-lucent layers, as though the plasma membranes of the adjoining endothelial cell processes had fused. With appropriate magnification, it can be seen that electron-dense "tracers," such as

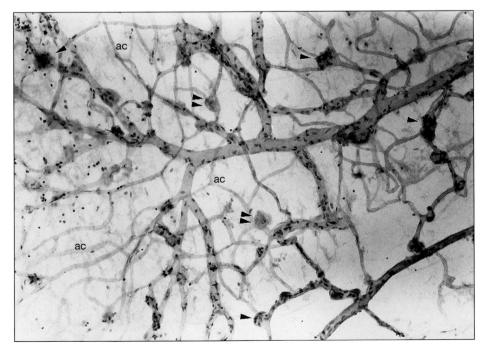

Fig. 66-11 A high-power field from a trypsin digest preparation of a human subject who died with long-standing diabetes. Multiple hypercellular (single arrowheads) and acellular (double arrowheads) microaneurysms are visible, as well as acellular capillaries (ac). Periodic acid–Schiff stain. Magnification ×250. (Reproduced with permission from Amin RH, Frank RN, Kennedy A et al. Vascular endothelial growth factor is present in glial cells of the retina and optic nerve of human subjects with nonproliferative diabetic retinopathy. Invest Ophthalmol Vis Sci 1997; 38:36–47,[259] by permission of the Association for Research in Vision and Ophthalmology.)

lanthanum chloride or horseradish peroxidase, cannot pass through tight junctions, but when the junctions are opened,[181] they become permeable to such tracers. Several proteins are closely involved with tight junction formation and function. The most widely studied of these are known as ZO-1 (for zonula occludens) and occludin. Gardner and associates[182] have reported that the expression of ZO-1 in cultured retinal microvascular endothelial cells is reduced by histamine in a dose-dependent fashion. Culture in astrocyte-conditioned medium (though with the astrocytes not present) increased ZO-1 expression, but high glucose reduced this expression.[183] Fluorescein leakage into the vitreous was reduced in experimentally diabetic rats and in diabetic humans by treatment with antihistamines.[184,185] These experiments suggest a role for normally functioning glial cells and normoglycemia in maintaining the integrity of the retinal vasculature, which forms the inner blood–retinal barrier. Further experiments by these investigators showed reduced expression and anatomic distribution of occludin in experimental diabetes.[186] They also showed that intravitreal injection of the polypeptide growth factor VEGF in rats increased production of the free radical nitric oxide (NO) and increased phosphorylation of ZO-1 and occludin.[187,188] All of these modifications may be critical for the breakdown of the blood–retinal barrier in diabetes, and the role of VEGF in facilitating this breakdown.

Another vascular endothelial cell abnormality that may contribute to breakdown of the blood–retinal barrier is fenestration of the endothelial cell cytoplasm. Fenestrae, which are gaps in the continuity of the endothelial cell cytoplasm, usually bridged by a thin, unilaminar membrane, are thought to explain the porousness of the thin endothelium of the normal choriocapillaris.[189] Fenestrae are normally absent from the thick endothelium of the retinal capillaries, but they have been observed in specimens from human and animal subjects with retinal neovascularization (Fig. 66-12) in which the blood–retinal barrier has broken down.[91,158,181,190]

A third possible anatomic explanation for blood–retinal barrier breakdown is an increase in transport by endocytic vesicles. Essner and colleagues[191,192] have observed this electron micro-

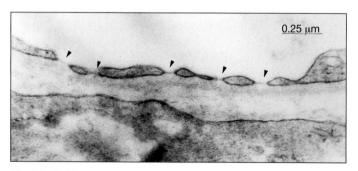

Fig. 66-12 Electron micrograph of endothelial fenestrae (arrowheads) in a neovascular tuft from a 59-year-old man with proliferative diabetic retinopathy. The eyes were obtained at autopsy following death from a cerebrovascular accident. (Modified from Wallow IHL, Geldner PS. Endothelial fenestrae in proliferative diabetic retinopathy. Invest Ophthalmol Vis Sci 1980; 19:1176–1183, by permission of Dr. Ingolf Wallow and the Association for Research in Vision and Ophthalmology.)

scopically, using horseradish peroxidase as a "tracer" in abnormal vessels penetrating the outer layers of the neural retina in animals with retinal dystrophies. However, this mechanism has not yet been reported from human or experimental animal subjects with diabetes.

Neovascularization

The anatomic features of retinovitreal neovascularization and some of the current theories regarding its pathogenesis have been presented above. Some years ago, a controversy existed as to the origins of the new vessels within the retinal circulation: Did certain dilated and tortuous loops of fine, intraretinal vessels represent pre-existing vessels that simply became dilated "shunts" through areas of nonperfusion, or were these truly intraretinal neovascularization? The debate was initially resolved by avoiding the issue, through the use of the noncommittal term "intraretinal microvascular abnormalities."[193] Subsequent clinicopathologic studies, in eyes in which such vessels were recognized ophthalmoscopically and fluorescein angiographically prior to enucleation, and which were then found to be early, intraretinal new vessels in the enucleated specimen, appear to have settled the controversy.[179,194]

BIOCHEMICAL MECHANISMS IN THE PATHOGENESIS OF DIABETIC RETINOPATHY

It is now undisputed that prolonged hyperglycemia is the major etiologic agent in all of the microvascular complications of diabetes, including diabetic retinopathy. The cellular mechanisms through which hyperglycemia acts currently remain unclear. Among mechanisms that have been proposed are:

1. Prolonged hyperglycemia may alter the expression of one or more genes, leading to increased (or decreased) amounts of certain gene products that can alter cellular functions leading to the lesions of diabetic retinopathy. Similar alterations of gene expression may occur in the presence of a chronic elevation of other hexoses, which would explain the similarity of at least some of the lesions in experimentally galactosemic animals to those in humans with diabetes.

2. Several types of sugars can bind nonenzymatically to proteins, leading to glycated products with very long cellular lifetimes.[139] Glycated proteins can then undergo a series of additional reactions, leading to inter- and intrachain crosslinking with considerable alteration of protein function.[139,195] Because such "advanced glycation endproducts" may be particularly long-lived, and because they may have important pathophysiologic functions, they are a plausible causal mechanism for the complications of diabetes.[86,139]

3. The chronic hyperglycemia of diabetes may produce accelerated oxidative stress in cells, leading to the formation of an excess of "toxic endproducts of oxidation" including peroxides, superoxides, nitric oxide, and oxygen free radicals.[196–198] Although these molecules are short-lived,

their production may be persistently elevated due to chronic changes in appropriate metabolic pathways, perhaps because of alterations in gene expression or increased production and longevity of advanced glycation endproducts. In that sense, this mechanism may simply be a variation of the two preceding ones, but its importance lies in the possibility of a simple therapeutic modality, treatment with antioxidants.[199,200]

There has been considerable recent interest in the possibility that diabetic retinopathy has characteristics of an inflammatory disease. These characteristics are not the classic "rubor, tumor, calor, and dolor," nor do they involve copious infiltration of inflammatory cells into the retinas of diabetic animals or human patients. The resemblance to inflammation derives from observations of increased leukocyte activation in the retinas of diabetic rats, with elaboration of increased amounts of inflammatory cytokines and adhesion molecules that enhance the adhesion of leukocytes to retinal capillary walls, thus increasing capillary stasis and occlusion and leading to the hypoxia that characterizes diabetic retinopathy.[201–203] Observations that intravitreal corticosteroid injections reduce diabetic macular edema, often with improvement of visual acuity, may be consistent with an anti-inflammatory effect of the steroid.[204] Although the ETDRS found that aspirin at a dose of 650 mg/day had no beneficial effect on diabetic retinopathy,[205] Kern et al. found that a higher dose (per unit body weight) in diabetic rats did retard the development of the lesions of retinopathy.[206] In light of all of these findings, further trials of anti-inflammatory agents for the prevention or treatment of diabetic retinopathy in humans are warranted.

An important observation from the DCCT was that the benefits of "tight" blood glucose control for the prevention of diabetic retinopathy, as well as nephropathy and neuropathy, did not become evident until more than 2 years after the institution of the intensive control regimen.[3] Similar observations were made by Engerman & Kern in long-term diabetic[207] and galactosemic[208] dogs. In these studies, dogs were rendered diabetic or placed on a diet containing 30% galactose without the induction of diabetes. In the study with diabetic dogs, the animals were assigned to one of three experimental groups. In the first group, blood glucose levels were tightly controlled for 5 years. In the second group, blood glucose levels were poorly controlled for the entire 5-year period. In the third group, the dogs were poorly controlled for the initial 2½ years, and then strict blood glucose control was maintained for the final 2½ years of the experiment. After the first 2½ years, one eye of each animal was enucleated and examined by light microscopy following preparation by the trypsin-digest technique. No retinopathy was observed in any of the eyes examined at this time. At the end of 5 years, all of the animals were killed, and the remaining eyes were examined histologically following trypsin digestion of the retinas. Little or no retinopathy was observed in the animals maintained in good control for 5 years, but substantial retinopathy was observed in those dogs that were either poorly controlled for all 5 years or were poorly controlled only for the first

2½ years, even though no retinopathy had been observed after this period.[207] The study with galactosemic dogs was conducted similarly, save that removal of the galactose diet and replacement by a normal diet after 2½ years[208] was substituted for the institution of "tight" blood glucose control in the study with diabetic animals. In similar fashion, no retinopathy was observed in the galactosemic animals after 2½ years on the galactose diet, while the dogs that had remained on this diet for the full 5 years of the study as well as those that were returned to the normal diet after 2½ years demonstrated the development of diabetic-like retinopathy. These important results in diabetic humans and diabetic and galactosemic dogs suggest that the metabolic changes that occur during the initial period of chronic hyperhexosemia set the stage for the eventual anatomic abnormalities, even though these lesions themselves do not appear for several more years. Any mechanism proposed to explain the biochemical basis for the development of diabetic retinopathy must account for these observations. Of the mechanisms discussed above, alterations of gene expression by chronic hyperglycemia (or galactosemia) seem most plausible because they are most likely to persist for the requisite duration of several years. Using a technique called "differential display," Aiello et al.[209] demonstrated the upregulation of several mRNA species in bovine retinal pericytes cultured in high-glucose medium in comparison with pericytes cultured in normal medium. While the gene products produced by these mRNAs, and their functions, were not described, these experiments show that the mechanism of altered gene expression by elevated glucose levels does occur and may be biologically important.

The sorbitol pathway

Of enzymatic mechanisms that have been proposed to cause retinopathy and other complications of diabetes, and which might be subject to regulation of their gene expression by chronic hyperhexosemia, the sorbitol pathway has been the most prominent. This is the name given to the sequence of reactions involving the enzymes aldose reductase and sorbitol dehydrogenase, which occur in many cells.[210,211] Using the reduced form of triphosphopyridine nucleotide (NADPH) as cofactor, aldose reductase reduces many aldose sugars to their respective sugar alcohols. Many of these, but not all (and specifically not galactitol, the sugar alcohol of galactose), may then be oxidized to their respective ketosugars by sorbitol dehydrogenase. In particular, glucose is reduced to sorbitol, which in turn is oxidized to fructose. However, since the latter reaction occurs slowly in many cells, sorbitol may build to high and possibly toxic concentrations in certain cells (in particular, those of the ocular lens epithelium of certain species), because intracellular sorbitol does not easily traverse cell membranes to the extracellular fluid. Among aldose sugars, glucose is a relatively poor substrate for aldose reductase (glucose has a very high binding constant, or K_m, for this enzyme). Therefore, aldose reductase is not operative in this pathway unless the glucose level is high, as in uncontrolled hyperglycemia, at which time the usual pathways for glucose metabolism are saturated. Because galactitol is not a substrate for sorbitol dehydrogenase, its intracellular level builds even more rapidly than does sorbitol in susceptible cells, which is why galactose is often used as a "model" for the presumed effects of the sorbitol pathway in producing the complications of diabetes. For this reason, reports of diabetic-like vascular basement membrane changes in galactosemic animals[89,90] have been considered important clues to the pathogenesis of retinopathy and, perhaps, other complications of diabetes. An especially important study was that of Engerman & Kern,[100] who reported pericyte dropout, microaneurysms, and capillary acellularity in nondiabetic dogs fed for more than 3 years on a diet enriched in galactose (Fig. 66-13). In this initial study, the animals were not given aldose reductase inhibitors to determine if these prevented the lesions.

This experiment was also performed by Kador et al.[101,102] and by Robison et al.,[96,136] who reported that the development of diabetic-like retinopathy is greatly retarded in dogs and rats fed high-galactose diets together with aldose reductase inhibitors, although most animals do develop it to some degree. However, this result has proved highly controversial.[212–214] Engerman[215] was unable to find any reduction in the rate of development or severity of retinopathy in galactosemic dogs also fed the aldose reductase inhibitor sorbinil. To the argument that they did not use the inhibitor in sufficiently high or frequent doses to maintain a constant, severe reduction in sugar alcohol formation, Kern & Engerman[216] have demonstrated that blood and tissue levels of galactitol in dogs receiving their experimental dose of sorbinil are extremely low, indicating almost complete inhibition of aldose reductase. These authors also described retinal microangiopathy in galactosemic rats, which they could not inhibit when rats were fed the galactose diet together with sorbinil.[95] We[94] have found that rats fed a 50% galactose diet for 2 years and concurrently dosed with a potent aldose reductase inhibitor (WAY-509, which was also used by Robison et al.[96]) developed much less retinopathy than galactosemic animals that did not receive the inhibitor. We argued[94] that one differ-

ence between our results in galactosemic rats and those of Kern & Engerman may have been the much more substantial enzyme inhibition produced by the inhibitor we used, which reduced retinal galactitol levels in these animals by at least 90%, substantially greater than the reduction reported by these investigators using sorbinil.[95] Dosing with the inhibitor after the animals had been on the diet for 1 year did not prevent the retinopathy.

An argument against a role for aldose reductase in the development of diabetic retinopathy was suggested by Kern & Engerman,[103] who found that mice given a 30% galactose diet for 2 years developed a diabetic-like retinopathy that included microaneurysms, lesions that both they[95] and we[94] could not find in long-term galactosemic rats. Unlike rats, mice do not develop cataracts after long-term diabetes or galactosemia. Cataracts were the first lesions to be described as consequences of the sorbitol pathway in diabetic and galactosemic animals,[212] and the etiologic relationship of this biochemical mechanism to cataracts in certain species of experimental animals, including rats, is unequivocal. By contrast with the rat enzyme, aldose reductase in mice has markedly decreased activity. However, when transgenic mice that expressed an active form of the enzyme in their lenses were made diabetic, cataracts appeared.[217] Given the relative inactivity of the wild-type mouse aldose reductase, this result and that reported by Kern & Engerman imply that the sorbitol pathway is unlikely to be the major causal factor for diabetic, or galactosemic, retinopathy. However, the lens in species that develop diabetic and galactosemic cataracts is notable for its relatively high concentration of sorbitol pathway enzymes by comparison with the enzymes of the classic pathways of glucose metabolism. Also, these cataracts are clearly produced by high levels of sugar alcohols which have osmotic effects. If the lesions of the complications of diabetes in other organs result from sorbitol pathway activity, much lower concentrations of sugar alcohols may be sufficient, and an extremely active enzyme may not be necessary.

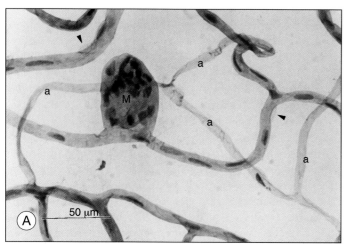

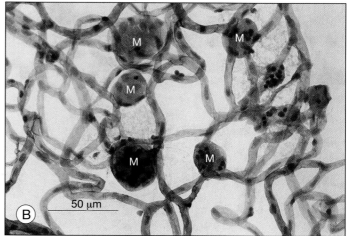

Fig. 66-13 A and B, Acellular capillaries and capillary microaneurysms in a trypsin-digest preparation from the retina of a nondiabetic dog that had been fed a diet containing 30% by weight galactose for 40 months. Many microaneurysms (M) and acellular capillaries (a) are evident. Pericyte ghosts (arrowheads) are also evident. The preparation was stained with periodic acid–Schiff reagent and hematoxylin. (Copyright © 1984 American Diabetes Association. From Diabetes, vol 33, 1984:97–100. Reprinted with permission from The American Diabetes Association.)

There have been two clinical trials of aldose reductase inhibitors in human diabetic retinopathy. In the first of these,[189] a total of 406 subjects were followed for at least 30 months, approximately half being randomized to 250 mg/day sorbinil and the remainder randomized to placebo; 125 subjects received drug or placebo for 48 months, the longest duration of follow-up in the study. Patients entered the study with type 1 (insulin-dependent) diabetes and no, or very minimal, retinopathy, entry criteria similar to those in the DCCT. The Sorbinil-Retinopathy Trial found no evidence that sorbinil, at this dose and duration, prevented the development or retarded the progression of diabetic retinopathy when retinopathy was evaluated by masked observers in accord with the protocol used in the ETDRS and DCCT studies. However, there was a slight reduction in the mean number of microaneurysms counted in the macular photographic fields of subjects who received sorbinil, by comparison with those who received placebo. The second trial of an aldose reductase inhibitor for diabetic retinopathy in humans evaluated tolrestat, a drug with somewhat greater inhibitory efficacy and a better safety profile than sorbinil. This study involved many more subjects than the Sorbinil-Retinopathy Trial and included subjects with both type 1 and type 2 diabetes, and subjects without prior retinopathy (prevention study) and with mild pre-existing retinopathy (intervention study). The duration of treatment was also longer, being approximately 4 to 5 years. Results of this study have not been published, but were reported by the sponsor both to investigators and to study subjects as negative. Although these results appear discouraging for the sorbitol pathway hypothesis of diabetic retinopathy, they may not definitively refute this hypothesis. The Sorbinil-Retinopathy Trial was of relatively short duration – only some 3 years, and the dose of the drug administered was reduced because of toxicity. Although the Tolrestat Study was longer, even this might not have been long enough in view of the duration required to demonstrate a significant treatment effect in subjects with similar degrees of retinopathy in the DCCT. Additionally, the degree of aldose reductase inhibition by this drug in the human retina following daily oral administration is not known, but in view of the very substantial inhibition we found necessary to prevent retinopathy in rats, and the fact that we could not reduce the retinopathy in animals given the inhibitor after 1 year of galactosemia (i.e., as an intervention, not as a prevention),[94] a much longer duration of study with a much more powerful aldose reductase inhibitor may be necessary to determine if this class of drugs has value in the treatment of diabetic retinopathy.

Nonenzymatic glycation

Hammes et al. reported that, when rats made diabetic with streptozotocin were dosed for 75 weeks with aminoguanidine, there was a substantial reduction of acellular retinal capillaries and retinal capillary microaneurysms by comparison with diabetic rats that did not receive aminoguanidine.[86] Aminoguanidine has been studied as an inhibitor of the formation of advanced glycation endproducts,[195] although it also inhibits inducible NO synthase, another action that is possibly relevant to the development of complications of diabetes. In my opinion, the photomicro-

graphs of retinal capillary lesions presented by these authors as examples of "diabetic" retinopathy[86] are unconvincing. Galactose also attaches nonenzymatically to proteins and forms advanced glycation endproducts similar to those produced by glucose. However, when we dosed galactosemic rats with aminoguanidine either from the outset of the galactose diet or after 1 year, we found no reduction in the retinopathy by comparison with that in animals receiving the galactose diet alone.[94] However, Kern & Engerman[206] reported that aminoguanidine substantially inhibited retinopathy over a 5-year follow-up in diabetic dogs. When they performed similar studies over a shorter term in diabetic and galactosemic rats, they found that aminoguanidine prevented capillary cell apoptosis over 6 to 8 months and retinopathy after 18 months in the diabetic animals, but (consistent with our findings) not in the galactosemic ones.[206] The mechanism for these different results remains unclear. The hypothesis that diabetic retinopathy and, perhaps, other complications of diabetes are related to nonenzymatic glycation remains challenging, but convincing evidence in its favor is still lacking. Aminoguanidine was used in a clinical trial for diabetic nephropathy, which was halted by its sponsor for undisclosed reasons. This agent is unlikely to be used in further studies on diabetic retinopathy in humans, but if they are safe, other agents that can block the formation of advanced glycation endproducts may be worth testing in humans.

Diacylglycerol and protein kinase C

Xia and associates proposed a mechanism by which hyperglycemia and galactosemia can stimulate a biochemical pathway possibly leading to the complications of diabetes, but without involvement of aldose reductase.[218,219] Both diabetes and galactosemia can produce within a few months a substantial elevation of diacylglycerol (DAG) within cells of the retina and of the aorta in dogs. This elevation is not prevented by sorbinil so it is unlikely to be due to activity of the sorbitol pathway. In turn, elevated DAG leads to increased activity of the ubiquitous enzyme protein kinase C (PKC). Elevated DAG levels and PKC activity in the retinas of diabetic rats correlate with decreased retinal blood flow as measured by fluorescein video angiography.[220] These alterations in flow (as well as renal abnormalities, including increased albumin excretion and glomerular filtration rate) could be corrected with a specific inhibitor of the β-isoform of PKC.[220] This isoform of PKC is also specifically activated by VEGF following binding of the growth factor to its cell membrane receptors, and PKC-β has therefore been implicated as an important mediator of the effects of VEGF in retinal neovascularization and in blood–retinal barrier breakdown leading to macular edema.[221] One concern about this hypothesis is that increases in DAG levels and PKC activity occur in the brains as well as in the retinas of diabetic rats,[220] while the lesions of diabetic retinopathy appear in the retinal vessels, but not the cerebral vessels, of diabetic humans[104] and dogs[105] (whether the same is true of rats has not yet been reported). A second and more important difficulty is that two initial randomized, controlled clinical trials of a PKC-β inhibitor, LY333531 (ruboxistaurin) for preventing the progression of preproliferative to proliferative diabetic retinopathy, and for preventing the progression of diabetic macular edema, both showed no significant benefit. Results of one of these trials have been presented in abstract form.[222]

Staurosporin (PKC412) is an inhibitor of several isoforms of PKC. It also blocks VEGF receptors 1 and 2, the PDGF receptor, and stem cell factor receptor. A relatively brief (3-month) randomized, controlled clinical trial in human subjects with diabetic macular edema showed that this molecule, administered orally, reduced macular edema fairly substantially, as measured by optical coherence tomography, compared to placebo, and also produced a very modest (less than one line) average improvement of visual acuity.[223] This drug does, however, have some toxicities.

Finally, it is possible that diabetic retinopathy is a multifactorial disease in which several pathways contribute to its pathogenesis. Such a possibility may explain why clinical trials of agents that principally block single mechanisms have been unsuccessful. Hammes et al.[224] have described an experiment in which benfotiamine, which blocks the hexosamine pathway, the increased formation of advanced glycation endproducts, the DAG–PAC pathway, and the upregulation of the transcription factor NF-kappa B, prevents the development of retinopathy in diabetic Wistar rats. Further studies of this drug are warranted.

Insulin receptors and glucose transporters

In certain types of cells, such as adipocytes and skeletal muscle cells, insulin is required to transport glucose from the extracellular fluid across the plasma membrane into the cytoplasm. This action requires a specific receptor for insulin on the plasma membrane. Although it has been commonly stated that the microvascular complications of diabetes do not occur in tissues in which insulin is required for the transport of glucose into cells, insulin receptors have been reported on the pericytes and endothelial cells of the retinal microvessels.[225] However, there is no evidence that the retinal microvascular insulin receptors are required for glucose transport, although insulin does enhance glycogen synthesis from radiolabeled glucose in retinal microvascular pericytes and endothelial cells and aortic smooth-muscle cells, but not in aortic endothelial cells.[225] Insulin in physiologic concentrations (as low as 10 ng/ml) stimulated [³H]-thymidine incorporation into retinal microvascular pericytes and endothelial cells and aortic smooth-muscle cells but not aortic endothelial cells.[225] It is noteworthy that, in these experiments, such low concentrations of insulin produced an effect, because unphysiologically high (e.g., 1 mg/ml) concentrations of insulin will stimulate proliferation of many types of cultured cells. However, since microvascular endothelial cells and pericytes do not normally proliferate in the mature retina,[112,,226] the importance of these results for normal retinal vascular physiology is unclear. Additionally, these results indicate that there are metabolic differences between microvascular endothelial cells and the endothelial cells of larger vessels, so that translation of results from one type of vascular endothelial cell to another must be done with great caution.

There are at least five different types of facilitated cell membrane glucose transporters, designated GLUT1, GLUT2, GLUT3, GLUT4, and GLUT5, that appear to be most important for the intracellular transport of glucose in tissues like the retina that do not require insulin. Of these, GLUT1 appears to be the most prevalent in the retina,[227–229] occurring in microvascular and macrovascular endothelial cells and on RPE cells, as well as in the Müller cells. GLUT2 localization has been reported by immunocytochemistry at the apical ends of the Müller cells of the rat retina, facing the interphotoreceptor matrix,[230] while GLUT3 has been reported by similar techniques to be localized to the plexiform layers of the rat[231] and human[229] retina. An initial report using light microscopic immunocytochemistry in human eyes[227] also reported GLUT1 in the nerve fiber layer of the retina and in photoreceptor cell bodies, but GLUT1 was absent from retinal neovascular proliferations in the eyes of diabetic subjects. Subsequently, these investigators used quantitative immunogold electron microscopic immunocytochemistry to examine GLUT1 localization in the eyes of two nondiabetic subjects and three diabetic subjects with little or no retinopathy.[228] In approximately half of the retinal microvessels from the diabetic subjects there was no quantitative difference in GLUT1 immunoreactivity by comparison with microvessels from the two normal individuals. However, in the other half of the retinal microvessels studied from diabetic individuals, these investigators reported an increase of GLUT1 immunoreactivity of about 18-fold over normal on the luminal plasma membranes. If these findings can be confirmed in a much larger number of eyes, such upregulation could be a mechanism that initiates glucose-mediated cellular damage by permitting a much greater influx of glucose into cells.

Whether galactose also enters cells by one or more of these facilitated glucose transporters has not been directly tested. However, the fact that rats fed a 50% galactose diet – which also contains the normal amount of glucose – double their food intake by comparison with normal rats, but nevertheless gain weight at only 60–70% of the rate of the normal animals,[94] suggests that the excessive amount of galactose competes with glucose for the transport sites, thereby limiting the entry of glucose into cells and diminishing glucose-requiring cellular energy metabolism. However, galactose can participate in other cellular pathways along with glucose, including protein glycation/advanced glycation endproduct formation and synthesis of DAG to activate PKC.[218] Whether glucose or galactose can upregulate the mRNAs governing synthesis of any of the GLUT proteins in a fashion such that this upregulation persists long after cessation of the hyperglycemic or galactosemic state has not yet been explored.

VEGF and other growth factors

In 1948, Isaac Michaelson proposed the hypothesis that a soluble, diffusible "factor X" that is produced in the retina stimulates retinal neovascularization.[111] It was not until the mid-1970s that the first soluble "growth factors" were discovered. With substantial further progress in this field, Michaelson's original hypothesis appears to be true, save that the story is more complicated than he could have anticipated over 50 years ago. The peptide growth factors that were initially considered most likely to stimulate retinal neovascularization were the FGFs,[232] a family of acidic and basic peptides, originally isolated from brain[233] as well as other tissues,[232,234] and which promote proliferation of a variety of cell types, in particular vascular endothelium. The most prominent of these have been acidic FGF or aFGF, now also designated FGF-1, and basic FGF or bFGF, now frequently designated FGF-2. A retinal-derived growth factor, first reported several years ago from aqueous extracts of bovine retina,[235] promotes proliferation of vascular endothelial cells. Subsequent investigations indicated that this extract contains a mixture of, among other things, aFGF and bFGF.[236,237] These two growth factors have several unique properties. They are strongly bound by heparin,[232] so that extracellularly they are highly associated with the heparan sulfate proteoglycan of basement membranes.[161–163] However, both aFGF and bFGF peptides lack a signal sequence, which means that they cannot normally be secreted from the cells in which they are synthesized.[238,239] Nevertheless, these growth factors can be found by immunocytochemistry in extracellular locations in ocular tissues from human subjects with retinal or choroidal neovascular diseases.[240–242] It is possible that only extracellular bFGF can exert a mitogenic effect by binding to specific receptors on the outer surface of cell plasma membranes.[243,244] Additionally, however, bFGF may serve as an autocrine growth factor, perhaps stimulating proliferation of the cells in which it is produced.[245] Basic FGF has been reported in vitreous specimens from human subjects undergoing vitrectomy for proliferative diabetic retinopathy, with levels higher than in subjects undergoing vitrectomy for nonneovascular diseases.[246] However, immunocytochemical studies of neovascular membranes in humans with proliferative diabetic retinopathy did not consistently demonstrate bFGF positivity,[242] and studies using polymerase chain reaction (PCR) technology to detect evidence of growth factor biosynthesis in such surgically excised membranes consistently showed the presence of VEGF mRNA, but not that for aFGF, bFGF, or other growth factors.[247] On the other hand, our own immunocytochemical studies of retinal and choroidal neovascular membranes including membranes from patients with proliferative diabetic retinopathy[241] show frequent co-localization of bFGF and VEGF within microvascular endothelial cells of these membranes, and bFGF and VEGF are synergistic, at least in vitro, in stimulating proliferation and in vitro angiogenesis of microvascular endothelial cells.[124] The most widespread current view is that aFGF and in particular bFGF may be ancillary factors in promoting retinal neovascularization in diabetic retinopathy and other retinal neovascular diseases, but they are not the molecules principally responsible for this process.

The most extensively investigated angiogenic factor at the present time with reference to retinal and choroidal neovascularizing diseases is VEGF. Unlike the FGFs, which constitute a family of similar molecules all derived from different genes, there is only one gene for VEGF but alternative splicing accounts for four different forms, ranging from 121 to 206 amino acids in size.[248] VEGF was first discovered as a molecule that increased the permeability of vessels, hence, its alternative name "vascular permeability factor." For this reason, VEGF has also been postulated to have a major role in diabetic macular edema.[249] VEGF expression is increased in tissues by a variety of factors, but of particular interest for proliferative diabetic retinopathy is its substantial upregulation by hypoxia.[250–252] VEGF levels in the vitreous of patients undergoing vitrectomy for proliferative diabetic retinopathy are substantially increased by comparison with individuals undergoing such surgery for nonvasoproliferative disease,[253,254] and where samples can be obtained both from the aqueous and from the vitreous, those obtained from vitreous have higher levels of the growth factor, suggesting a posterior site of secretion.[253] When vitreous samples can be obtained a second time following laser-induced regression of the neovascularization, they are reduced.[253] In a model of transient iris neovascularization produced in monkeys by laser photocoagulation to the major retinal veins, creating the equivalent of a central retinal vein occlusion, VEGF expression by the retina (as evaluated by in situ hybridization) increases during the period of neovascularization and diminishes thereafter.[255] In this model, and in retinal neovascularization in the neonatal mouse subjected to hyperoxia (analogous to human retinopathy of prematurity), various maneuvers designed to prevent VEGF synthesis or to block its action substantially retard the neovascularization. These include intravitreal injection of anti-VEGF antibodies[256] or of a soluble chimeric molecule consisting of a VEGF receptor linked to an immunoglobulin,[113] and the intravitreal infusion of an "antisense" strand of the VEGF DNA sequence to block the synthesis of the growth factor.[257] Two additional intriguing findings are, first, that VEGF cannot be demonstrated, at least with the sensitivity of light microscopic immunocytochemistry, in the retinas of nondiabetic human subjects obtained postmortem, but it is evident in the retinas of individuals with diabetes even when little or no retinopathy is present in these eyes when studied by other light microscopic techniques.[258,259] Second, VEGF is prominent by immunocytochemistry in retinal glial cells (including in particular the Müller cells), and also in the glial cells of the optic nerve of eyes from humans with diabetes[259] and in eyes from long-term galactosemic rats (Fig. 66-14).[94] While these findings indicate only the localization of VEGF protein and not necessarily where it is synthesized, the likelihood that the predominant site of synthesis of this molecule is in nonvascular cells of the retina and optic nerve implies that the initial metabolic abnormality that eventually results in the vascular lesions of diabetic retinopathy does not occur in the cells of the retinal vasculature.

Synthesis of the FGFs appears to be possible in several types of cells in the retina,[260–262] but the normal (as opposed to the pathological) function of these molecules is unclear. Perhaps they are principally active in fetal life where they may assist in the development of the vascular system,[260] or, when synthesized at very low levels, they may have a maintenance function for cell viability and differentiation. VEGF, however, appears clearly to be critical for the fetal development of the vascular system throughout the body since a targeted disruption of the VEGF gene in mice is lethal, and the nonviable fetuses fail to develop a vasculature.[263,264]

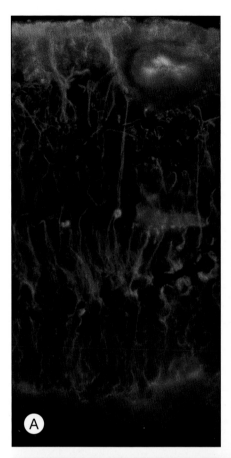

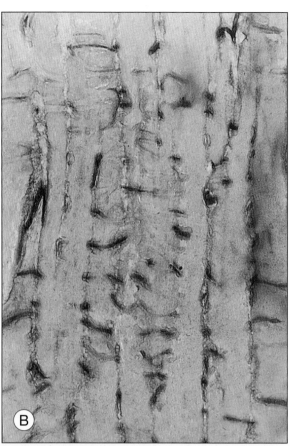

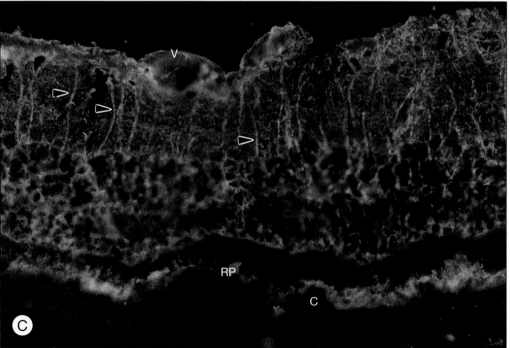

Fig. 66-14 A, Immunostaining for vascular endothelial growth factor (VEGF) using a fluorescein isothiocyanate (FITC)-labeled second antibody of a retinal section from a 60-year-old woman with diabetes. Note the elongated processes that immunostain and extend through all retinal layers except for the photoreceptor layer. There is also positive immunostain in the endothelial layer of a large retinal arteriole. The neurosensory retina has been detached artefactually. Other sections from this retina demonstrated a similar staining pattern of the long processes using antibodies to glial fibrillary acidic protein (GFAP) and to vimentin, and a similar staining pattern of the vascular endothelium using an antibody to factor VIII, suggesting that the staining processes are Müller cells and vascular endothelial cells, respectively. Magnification ×200. B, Immunostain for VEGF of a portion of the optic nerve from one eye of a 70-year-old woman with diabetes. The second antibody in this preparation was conjugated with biotin and the slide was then incubated with an avidin-conjugated color reagent to produce a colored reaction product that was visible by light microscopy. A similar staining pattern was obtained using antibodies to GFAP, indicating that the processes that stained for VEGF are glial cells. Magnification ×250. (Parts A and B reprinted from Amin RH, Frank RN, Kennedy A et al. Vascular endothelial growth factor is present in glial cells of the retina and optic nerve of human subjects with nonproliferative diabetic retinopathy. Invest Ophthalmol Vis Sci 1997; 38:36–47.[259] Copyright 1997, Association for Research in Vision and Ophthalmology.) C, Immunostaining for VEGF in a rat that received a diet containing 50% by weight galactose for 24 months. RP, retinal pigment epithelium; C, choriocapillaris; V, larger retinal vessel. Arrowheads indicate elongated staining processes that appear to be Müller cells, based on their morphologic characteristics and on their staining properties with antibodies to GFAP and to vimentin (original magnification ×950). (Part C reproduced from Frank RN, Amin R, Kennedy A et al. An aldose reductase inhibitor and aminoguanidine prevent vascular endothelial growth factor expression in rats with long-term galactosemia. Arch Ophthalmol 1997; 115:136–147.[94] Copyright © (1997) American Medical Association. All rights reserved.)

If VEGF is the principal retinal angiogenic factor, the "factor X" of Michaelson,[111] then several approaches might be attempted to devise a medical therapy for retinal vasoproliferation. These include anti-VEGF antibodies or "antisense" DNA technology, or the use of small molecules to block the effects of VEGF after it is bound to its cell membrane receptors. An apparently important postreceptoral event in this cascade is the activation of the β-isoform of PKC.[219] Specific inhibition of this isoform of PKC appears to prevent various vascular abnormalities in diabetic rats[220] and in pigs with retinal neovascularization produced by laser-induced retinal vein occlusion.[265] However, as previously noted, a clinical trial of a selective PKC-β inhibitor for the prevention of proliferative diabetic retinopathy and macular edema has thus far been unsuccessful.[222]

Other approaches to blockade of the action of VEGF, which to date have been used primarily as experimental treatments for the neovascular form of age-related macular degeneration, include an aptamer (a modified sequence of nucleotide bases) that binds to the VEGF peptide when injected intravitreally and blocks its action;[266] a VEGF-blocking antibody fragment;[267] specific blockers of VEGF receptors on cell membranes;[268] and an angiostatic, steroid-like molecule (anecortave acetate) that has been tested in humans for its efficacy in treating neovascular age-related macular degeneration.[269] Anecortave acetate has also shown efficacy for treating retinal neovascularization in hyperoxygenated, neonatal rats.[114]

Pigment epithelial-derived factor (PEDF) is a relatively recently described polypeptide factor that may have considerable importance for regulating vascular growth in the retina, and also for promoting neural differentiation.[270] It is a member of the serine protease inhibitor (serpin) family. Although there is evidence that PEDF is secreted by retinal ganglion cells, and other cells throughout the eye, its major site of secretion is the RPE.[271] A preliminary report, which has not yet appeared in other than abstract form, indicates that PEDF is secreted largely from the apical plasma membrane.[272] (VEGF, which is also produced copiously by RPE cells, is largely secreted from the basal plasma membrane of the RPE.[273]) The outer layers of the neural retina, adjacent to the apical surface of the RPE, are normally avascular, which is consistent with the finding that PEDF appears to inhibit neovascularization.[274,275] There is evidence that, in neovascular eye diseases, VEGF expression increases while PEDF expression decreases.[276] A clinical trial using gene therapy technology is testing the efficacy of upregulating PEDF expression in the retina and RPE of patients with neovascular age-related macular degeneration (similar methods could be used in proliferative diabetic retinopathy) by injecting intravitreally a nonreplicating adenovirus containing the gene for human PEDF.[277] This, and other approaches described in this chapter, illustrate the advanced technologies that are being brought to bear on the continuing problem of diabetic retinopathy.

ACKNOWLEDGMENTS

The studies from my laboratory reported here were supported in part by grants RO1 EY-01857 and RO1 EY-02566 from the National Eye Institute, National Institutes of Health, by research grants from the Juvenile Diabetes Foundation International, New York, by a postdoctoral fellowship to Dr. Arup Das from the Juvenile Diabetes Foundation International, and by a departmental unrestricted grant and an individual Senior Investigator Award from Research to Prevent Blindness, New York.

REFERENCES

1. Linner E, Svanborg A, Zelander T. Retinal and renal lesions of diabetic type, without obvious disturbances in glucose metabolism, in a patient with family history of diabetes. Am J Med 1965; 39:298–304.
2. Hutton WL, Snyder WB, Vaiser A et al. Retinal microangiopathy without associated glucose intolerance. Trans Am Acad Ophthalmol Otolaryngol 1972; 76:968–980.
3. DCCT Research Group. The effect of intensive treatment of diabetes in the development and progression of long-term complications in insulin-dependent diabetes. N Engl J Med 1993; 329:977–986.
4. UK Prospective Diabetes Study (UKPDS) Group. Intensive blood-glucose control with sulphonylureas or insulin compared with conventional treatment and risk of complications in patients with type 2 diabetes (UKPDS 33). Lancet 1998; 352:837–853.
5. UK Prospective Diabetes Study Group. Tight blood pressure control and risk of macrovascular and microvascular complications in type 2 diabetes. UKPDS 38. Br Med J 1998; 317:703–713.
6. Frank RN, Hoffman WH, Podgor MJ et al. Retinopathy in juvenile-onset type 1 diabetes of short duration. Diabetes 1982; 31:874–882.
7. Klein R, Klein BEK, Moss SE et al. The Wisconsin Epidemiologic Study of Diabetic Retinopathy. II. Prevalence and risk of diabetic retinopathy when age at diagnosis is less than 30 years. Arch Ophthalmol 1984; 102:520–526.
8. Palmberg P, Smith M, Waltman S et al. The natural history of retinopathy in insulin dependent juvenile-onset diabetes, Ophthalmology 1981; 88:613–618.
9. Klein R, Klein BEK, Moss SE et al. The Wisconsin Epidemiologic Study of Diabetic Retinopathy. III. Prevalence and risk of diabetic retinopathy when age at diagnosis is 30 or more years. Arch Ophthalmol 1984; 102:527–532.
10. Aiello LM, Rand LI, Briones JC et al. Diabetic retinopathy in Joslin Clinic patients with adult-onset diabetes. Ophthalmology 1981; 88:619–623.
11. Klein R, Klein BEK, Moss SE et al. The Wisconsin Epidemiologic Study of Diabetic Retinopathy. IV. Diabetic macular edema. Ophthalmology 1984; 91:1464–1474.
12. Klein R, Klein BE, Moss SE et al. The Wisconsin Epidemiologic Study of Diabetic Retinopathy. XV. The long-term incidence of macular edema. Ophthalmology 1995; 102:7–16.
13. Klein R, Klein BE, Moss SE et al. The Wisconsin Epidemiologic Study of Diabetic Retinopathy: XVII. The 14-year incidence and progression of diabetic retinopathy and associated risk factors in type 1 diabetes. Ophthalmology 1998; 105:1801–1815.
14. Knowles HC Jr, Guest GM, Lampe J et al. The course of juvenile diabetes treated with unmeasured diet. Diabetes 1965; 14:239–273.
15. Klein BEK, Moss SE, Klein R. Is menarche associated with diabetic retinopathy? Diabetes Care 1990; 13:1034–1038.
16. Klein R, Klein BEK, Moss SE et al. Retinopathy in young-onset diabetic patients. Diabetes Care 1985; 8:311–315.
17. Murphy RP, Nanda M, Plotnick L et al. The relationship of puberty to diabetic retinopathy. Arch Ophthalmol 1990; 108:215–218.
18. Daneman D, Drash AL, Lobes LA et al. Progressive retinopathy with improved control in diabetic dwarfism (Mauriac's syndrome). Diabetes Care 1981; 4:360–365.
19. Chantelau E, Eggert H, Seppel T et al. Elevation of serum IGF-1 precedes proliferative diabetic retinopathy in Mauriac's syndrome (letter to the editor). Br J Ophthalmol 1997; 81:169–170.
20. Merimee TJ, Zapf J, Froesch ER. Insulin-like growth factors: studies in diabetes with and without retinopathy. N Engl Med 1983; 309:527–530.
21. Meyer Schwickerath R, Pfeiffer A, Blum WF et al. Vitreous levels of the insulin-like growth factors I and II, and the insulin-like growth factor binding proteins 2 and 3, increase in neovascular eye disease: studies in nondiabetic and diabetic subjects. J Clin Invest 1993; 92:2620–2625.
22. Grant M, Russell B, Fitzgerald C et al. Insulin-like growth factors in vitreous: studies in control and diabetic subjects with neovascularization. Diabetes 1986; 35:416–420.
23. Kohner EM, Hamilton AM, Joplin GF et al. Florid diabetic retinopathy and its response to treatment by photocoagulation or pituitary ablation. Diabetes 1976; 25:104–110.

24. Grant MB, Mames RN, Fitzgerald C et al. Insulin-like growth factor-1 acts as an angiogenic agent in rabbit cornea and retina: comparative studies with basic fibroblast growth factor. Diabetologia 1995; 36:282–291.

25. Chantelau E, Kohner EM. Why some cases of retinopathy worsen when diabetic control improves. Br Med J 1997; 315:1105–1106.

26. Dahl-Jorgensen K, Brinchmann-Hansen O, Hanssen KF et al. Rapid tightening of blood glucose control leads to transient deterioration of retinopathy in insulin dependent diabetes mellitus: the Oslo study. Br Med J 1985; 290:811–815.

27. Lauritzen T, Larsen HW, Frost-Larsen K et al. Effect of 1 year of near-normal blood glucose levels on retinopathy in insulin-dependent diabetics. Lancet 1983; 1:200–204.

28. Kroc Collaborative Study Group. Blood glucose control and the evolution of diabetic retinopathy and albuminuria. N Engl J Med 1984; 311:365–372.

29. Lauritzen T, Frost-Larsen K, Larsen HW et al. Two-year experience with continuous subcutaneous insulin infusion in relation to retinopathy and neuropathy. Diabetes 1985; 34 (Suppl. 3):74–79.

30. Poulsen JE. The Houssay phenomenon in man: recovery from retinopathy in a case of diabetes with Simmonds' disease. Diabetes 1953; 2:7–12.

31. Lundbaek K, Malmros R, Andersen HC et al. Hypophysectomy for diabetic angiopathy: a controlled clinical trial. In: Goldberg MF, and Fine SL, eds: Symposium on the treatment of diabetic retinopathy. US Public Health Service publication no. 1890. Washington, DC: US Government Printing Office; 1968:291–311.

32. Oakley NW, Jopkin GF, Kohner EM et al. The treatment of diabetic retinopathy by pituitary implantation of radioactive yttrium. In: Goldberg MF, Fine SL, eds. Symposium on the treatment of diabetic retinopathy. US Public Health Service publication no. 1890. Washington, DC: US Government Printing Office; 1968:317–329.

33. Thrailkill KM, Quattrin T, Baker L et al. Cotherapy with recombinant human insulin-like growth factor I and insulin improves glycemic control in type 1 diabetes. RhIGF-I in IDDM Study Group. Diabetes Care 1999; 22:585–592.

34. Purvin VA, Yee RD. Neuro-ophthalmic disorders in diabetes mellitus. In: Feman SS, ed. Ocular problems in diabetes mellitus. Boston: Blackwell Scientific Publications; 1992:151–178.

35. Smith LEH, Kopchick JJ, Chen W et al.. Essential role of growth hormone in ischemia-induced retinal neovascularization. Science 1997; 276: 1706–1709.

36. Knowler WC, Bennett PH, Ballintine EJ. Increased incidence of retinopathy in diabetics with elevated blood pressure: a six-year follow-up study in Pima Indians. N Engl J Med 1980; 302:645–650.

37. Kornerup T. Studies in diabetic retinopathy: an investigation of 1000 cases of diabetes. Acta Med Scand 1955; 153:81–101.

38. Klein R, Klein BEK, Moss SE et al. Is blood pressure a predictor of the incidence or progression of diabetic retinopathy? Arch Intern Med 1989; 149:2427–2431.

39. Klein BEK, Moss SE, Klein R. Effect of pregnancy on progression of diabetic retinopathy. Diabetes Care 1990; 13:34–40.

40. Rand LI, Krolewski AS, Aiello LM et al. Multiple factors in the prediction of risk of proliferative diabetic retinopathy. N Engl J Med 1985; 313: 1433–1438.

41. Cruickshanks KJ, Vadheim CM, Moss SE et al. Genetic marker associations with proliferative retinopathy in persons diagnosed with diabetes before 30 yr of age. Diabetes 1992; 41:879–885.

42. DCCT Research Group. Clustering of long-term complications in families with diabetes in the diabetes control and complications trial. Diabetes 1997; 46:1829–1839.

43. Krolewski AS, Canessa M, Warram JH et al. Predisposition to hypertension and susceptibility to renal disease in insulin-dependent diabetes mellitus. N Engl J Med 1988; 318:140–145.

44. Krolewski AS, Doria A, Magre J et al. Molecular genetic approaches to the identification of genes involved in the development of nephropathy in insulin-dependent diabetes mellitus. J Am Soc Nephrol 1992; 3 (Suppl. 4):S9–S17.

45. Pettitt DJ, Saad MF, Bennett PH et al. Familial predisposition to renal disease in two generations of Pima Indians with type 2 (noninsulin-dependent) diabetes mellitus. Diabetologia 1990; 33:438–443.

46. Seaquist ER, Goetz FC, Rich S et al. Familial clustering of diabetic kidney disease: evidence for genetic susceptibility to diabetic nephropathy. N Engl J Med 1989; 320:1161–1165.

47. Ko BC, Lam KS, Wat NM et al. An (A-C)n dinucleotide repeat polymorphic marker at the 5' end of the aldose reductase gene is associated with early-onset diabetic retinopathy in NIDDM patients. Diabetes 1995; 44:727–732.

48. Becker B. Diabetes and glaucoma. In: Kimura SJ, Caygill WM, eds. Vascular complications of diabetes mellitus. St Louis: Mosby-Year Book; 1967:43–48.

49. Jain IS, Luthra CL, Das T. Diabetic retinopathy and its relation to errors of refraction. Arch Ophthalmol 1967; 77:59–60.

50. Aiello LM, Beetham WP, Balodimos MC et al. Ruby laser photocoagulation in treatment of diabetic proliferating retinopathy: preliminary report. In: Goldberg MF, Fine SL, eds. Symposium on the treatment of diabetic retinopathy. US Public Health Service publication no. 1890. Washington, DC: US Government Printing Office; 1968:437–464.

51. Ashton N. Oxygen and the growth and development of retinal vessels: in vivo and in vitro studies. In: Kimura SJ, Caygill WM, eds. Vascular complications of diabetes mellitus. St Louis: Mosby-Year Book; 1967:3–32.

52. Patz A. Studies on retinal neovascularization. Invest Ophthalmol Vis Sci 1980; 19:1133–1138.

53. Weiter JJ, Zuckerman R. The influence of the photoreceptor–RPE complex on the inner retina: an explanation for the beneficial effects of photocoagulation. Ophthalmology 1980; 87:1133–1139.

54. Diabetic Retinopathy Study Research Group. Photocoagulation treatment of proliferative diabetic retinopathy: clinical application of Diabetic Retinopathy Study (DRS) findings. DRS report number 8. Ophthalmology 1981; 88:583–600.

55. Tattersall RB, Fajans SS. A difference between the inheritance of classical juvenile-onset and maturity-onset type diabetes of young people. Diabetes 1975; 24:44–53.

56. Kahn HA, Moorhead HB. Statistics on blindness in the model reporting area, 1969–1970. US Department of Health, Education, and Welfare publication no. (NIH) 73–427. Washington, DC: US Government Printing Office; 1973.

57. Furcht LT. Critical factors controlling angiogenesis: cell products, cell matrix, and growth factors. Lab Invest 1986; 55:505–509.

58. Early Treatment Diabetic Retinopathy Study Research Group. Photocoagulation for diabetic macular edema, Early Treatment Diabetic Retinopathy Study report no. 1. Arch Ophthalmol 1985; 103:1796–1806.

59. Seltzer HS. A summary of criticisms of the findings and conclusions of the University Group Diabetes Program (UGDP). Diabetes 1972; 21:976–979.

60. Cunha-Vaz JG, Maurice DM. The active transport of fluorescein by the retinal vessels and the retina. J Physiol (Lond) 1967; 191:467–486.

61. Maurice DM. A new objective fluorophotometer. Exp Eye Res 1963; 2:33–38.

62. Waltman SR, Kaufman HE. A new objective slit lamp fluorophotometer. Invest Ophthalmol 1970; 9:247–249.

63. Cuhna-Vaz JG, Fonseca JR, Abreu JF et al. A follow-up study by vitreous fluorophotometry of early retinal involvement in diabetes. Am J Ophthalmol 1978; 86:467–473.

64. Krupin T, Waltman SR, Scharp DW et al. Ocular fluorophotometry in streptozotocin diabetes mellitus in the rat: effect of pancreatic islet isografts. Invest Ophthalmol Vis Sci 1979; 18:1185–1190.

65. Waltman SR, Santiago J, Krupin T et al. Vitreous fluorophotometry and blood-sugar control in diabetics. Lancet 1979; 2:1068.

66. Klein R, Wallow IH, Ernest JT. Fluorophotometry. III. Streptozotocin-treated rats and rats with pancreatectomy. Arch Ophthalmol 1980; 98:2235–2237.

67. Prager TC, Chu HH, Garcia CA et al. The use of vitreous fluorophotometry to distinguish between diabetics with and without observable retinopathy: effect of vitreous abnormalities on the measurement. Invest Ophthalmol Vis Sci 1983; 24:57–65.

68. Grunwald JE, Brucker AJ, Braunstein SN et al. Strict metabolic control and retinal blood flow in diabetes mellitus. Br J Ophthalmol 1994; 78:598–604.

69. Grunwald JE, Brucker AJ, Petrig BL et al. Retinal blood flow regulation and the clinical response to panretinal photocoagulation in proliferative diabetic retinopathy. Ophthalmology 1989; 96:1518–1522.

70. Grunwald JE, Riva CE, Brucker AJ et al. Altered retinal vascular response to 100% oxygen breathing in diabetes mellitus. Ophthalmology 1984; 91: 1447–1452.

71. Grunwald JE, Riva CE, Martin DB et al. Effect of an insulin-induced decrease in blood glucose on the human diabetic retinal circulation. Ophthalmology 1987; 94:1614–1620.

72. Grunwald JE, Riva CE, Sinclair SH et al. Laser Doppler velocimetry study of retinal circulation in diabetes mellitus. Arch Ophthalmol 1986; 104:991–996.

73. Riva CE, Feke GT. Laser Doppler velocimetry in the measurement of retinal blood flow. In: Goldman L, ed. The biomedical laser technology and clinical applications. New York: Springer-Verlag; 1981:135–161.

74. Bursell SE, Clermont AC, Kinsley BT et al. Retinal blood flow changes in patients with insulin-dependent diabetes mellitus and no diabetic retinopathy. Invest Ophthalmol Vis Sci 1996; 37:886–897.

75. Shiba T, Inoguchi T, Sportsman JR et al. Correlation of diacylglycerol level and protein kinase C activity in rat retina to retinal circulation. Am J Physiol 1993; 265:783–793.

76. Chakravarthy U, Hayes RG, Stitt AW et al. Endothelin expression in ocular tissues of diabetic and insulin-treated rats. Invest Ophthalmol Vis Sci 1997; 38:2144–2151.

77. Loebl M, Riva CE. Macular circulation and the flying corpuscles phenomenon. Ophthalmology 1978; 85:911–917.

78. Sinclair SH, Grunwald JE, Riva CE et al. Retinal vascular autoregulation in diabetes mellitus. Ophthalmology 1982; 89:748–750.

79. Ernest JT, Goldstick TK, Engerman RL. Hyperglycemia impairs retinal oxygen autoregulation in normal and diabetic dogs. Invest Ophthalmol Vis Sci 1983; 24:985–989.

80. Berkowitz BA. Adult and newborn rat inner retinal oxygenation during carbogen and 100% oxygen breathing. Comparison using magnetic resonance imaging delta pO_2 mapping. Invest Ophthalmol Vis Sci 1996; 37:2089–2098.

81. Berkowitz BA, McDonald C, Ito Y et al. Measuring the human retinal oxygenation response to a hyperoxic challenge using MRI: eliminating blinking artifacts and demonstrating proof of concept. Magn Reson Med 2001; 46:412–416.

82. Berkowitz BA, Wilson CA. Quantitative mapping of ocular oxygenation using magnetic resonance imaging. Magn Reson Med 1995; 33:579–581.

83. Patz A, Maumenee AE. Studies on diabetic retinopathy. I. Retinopathy in a dog with spontaneous diabetes mellitus. Am J Ophthalmol 1962; 54:532–541.

84. Engerman R, Finkelstein D, Aguirre G et al. Ocular complications. Diabetes 1982; 31 (Suppl. 1):82–88.

85. Engerman RL, Davis MD, Bloodworth JMB Jr. Retinopathy in experimental diabetes: its relevance to diabetic retinopathy in man. In: Rodriguez RR, Vallance-Owen JR, eds. Diabetes. Amsterdam: Excerpta Medica; 1971.

86. Hammes H-P, Martin S, Federlin K et al. Aminoguianidine treatment inhibits the development of experimental diabetic retinopathy. Proc Natl Acad Sci USA 1991; 88:11555–11558.

87. Tilton RG, LaRose LS, Kilo C et al. Absence of degenerative changes in retinal and uveal capillary pericytes in diabetic rats. Invest Ophthalmol Vis Sci 1986; 27:716–721.

88. Robison WG Jr, Laver NM, Lou MF. The role of aldose reductase in diabetic retinopathy: Prevention and intervention studies. In: Osborne NN, Chader GJ, eds. Progress in retinal and eye research, vol. 14. Oxford: Pergamon Press; 1995:593–640.

89. Robison WG Jr, Kador PF, Kinoshita JH. Retinal capillaries: basement membrane thickening by galactosemia prevented with aldose reductase inhibitor. Science 1983; 221:1177–1179.

90. Frank RN, Keirn RJ, Kennedy A et al. Galactose-induced retinal capillary basement membrane thickening: prevention by sorbinil. Invest Ophthalmol Vis Sci 1983; 24:1519–1524.

91. Kimura T, Chen C-H, Patz A. Ultrastructure of intravitreal proliferative tissue in human and puppy eyes. In: Shimizu K, ed. XXIII concilium ophthalmologicum. Tokyo: Igaku Shoin; 1979:1553–1556.

92. Tilton RG, Pugliese G, Williamson JR. Diabetes-induced glomerular changes in rats are not prevented by sorbinil. Diabetes 1989; 38 (Suppl. 2):94.

93. Engerman RL, Colquhoun PJ. Epithelial and mesothelial basement membranes in diabetic patients and dogs. Diabetologia 1982; 23:521–524.

94. Frank RN, Amin R, Kennedy A et al. An aldose reductase inhibitor and aminoguanidine prevent vascular endothelial growth factor expression in rats with long-term galactosemia. Arch Ophthalmol 1997; 115:136–147.

95. Kern TS, Engerman RL. Galactose-induced retinal microangiopathy in rats. Invest Ophthalmol Vis Sci 1995; 36:490–496.

96. Robison WG Jr, Laver NM, Jacot JL et al. Diabetic-like retinopathy ameliorated with the aldose reductase inhibitor WAY-121,509. Invest Ophthalmol Vis Sci 1996; 37:1149–1156.

97. Robison WG Jr, McCaleb ML, Feld LG et al. Degenerated intramural pericytes ('ghost cells') in the retinal capillaries of diabetic rats. Curr Eye Res 1991; 10:339–350.

98. Mizutani M, Kern TS, Lorenzi M. Accelerated death of retinal microvascular cells in human and experimental diabetic retinopathy. J Clin Invest 1996; 97:2883–2890.

99. Bloodworth JM Jr, Engerman RL, Anderson PJ. Microangiopathy in the experimentally diabetic animal. Adv Metab Disord 1973; 2 (Suppl.):245–250.

100. Engerman RL, Kern TS. Experimental galactosemia produces diabetic-like retinopathy. Diabetes 1984; 33:97–100.

101. Kador PF, Akagi Y, Takahashi Y et al. Prevention of retinal vessel changes associated with diabetic retinopathy in galactose-fed dogs by aldose reductase inhibitors. Arch Ophthalmol 1990; 108:1301–1309.

102. Kador PF, Akagi Y, Terubayashi H et al. Prevention of pericyte ghost formation in retinal capillaries of galactose-fed dogs by aldose reductase inhibitors. Arch Ophthalmol 1988; 106:1099–1102.

103. Kern TS, Engerman RL. A mouse model of diabetic retinopathy. Arch Ophthalmol 1996; 114:986–990.

104. DeOliveira F. Pericytes in diabetic retinopathy. Br J Ophthalmol 1966; 50:134–143.

105. Kern TS, Engerman RL. Capillary lesions develop in retina rather than cerebral cortex in diabetes and experimental galactosemia. Arch Ophthalmol 1996; 114:306–310.

106. Frank RN, Dutta SD, Mancini MA. Pericyte coverage is greater in the retinal than in the cerebral capillaries of the rat. Invest Ophthalmol Vis Sci 1987; 28:1086–1091.

107. Frank RN, Turczyn TJ, Das A. Pericyte coverage of retinal and cerebral capillaries. Invest Ophthalmol Vis Sci 1990; 31:999–1007.

108. Tilton RG, Miller EJ, Kilo C et al. Pericyte form and distribution in rat retinal and uveal capillaries. Invest Ophthalmol Vis Sci 1985; 26:68–73.

109. Patz A. The role of oxygen in retrolental fibroplasias. Trans Am Ophthalmol Soc 1968; 66:940–985.

110. Kremer I, Kissun R, Nissenkorn I et al. Oxygen-induced retinopathy in newborn kittens: a model for ischemic vasoproliferative retinopathy. Invest Ophthalmol Vis Sci 1987; 28:126–130.

111. Michaelson IC. The mode of development of the vascular system of the retina, with some observations on its significance for certain retinal diseases. Trans Ophthalmol Soc UK 1948; 68:137–180.

112. Wise GN, Dollery CT, Henkind P. The retinal circulation. New York: Harper & Row; 1971:34–54, 290–324.

113. Aiello LP, Pierce EA, Foley ED et al. Suppression of retinal neovascularization in vivo by inhibition of vascular endothelial growth factor (VEGF) using soluble VEGF-receptor chimeric proteins. Proc Natl Acad Sci USA 1995; 92:10457–10461.

114. Penn JS, Rajaratnam VS, Collier RJ et al. The effect of an angiostatic steroid on neovascularization in a rat model of retinopathy of prematurity. Invest Ophthalmol Vis Sci 2001; 42:283–290.

115. Okamoto N, Tobe T, Hackett SF et al. Transgenic mice with increased expression of vascular endothelial growth factor in the retina: a new model of intraretinal and subretinal neovascularization. Am J Pathol 1997; 151:13–23.

116. Buzney SM, Frank RN, Robison WG Jr. Retinal capillaries: proliferation of mural cells in vitro. Science 1975; 190:985–986.

117. Frank RN, Kinsey VE, Frank KW et al. In vitro proliferation of endothelial cells from kitten retinal capillaries. Invest Ophthalmol Vis Sci 1979; 18:1195–1200.

118. Bowman PD, Betz AL, Goldstein GW. Primary culture of microvascular endothelial cells from bovine retina: selective growth using fibronectin coated substrate and plasma derived serum. In Vitro 1982; 118:626–632.

119. Buzney SM, Massicotte SJ. Retinal vessels: proliferation of endothelium in vitro. Invest Ophthalmol Vis Sci 1979; 18:1191–1195.

120. Gitlin JD, D'Amore PA. Culture of retinal capillary cells using selective growth media. Microvasc Res 1983; 26:74–80.

121. Puro DG. Calcium channels of human retinal glial cells. In: Harahashi T, ed. Methods of neuroscience. Orlando, FL: Academic Press; 1994:68–81.

122. Madri JA, Williams SK. Capillary endothelial cell cultures: phenotypic modulation by matrix components. J Cell Biol 1983; 97:153–165.

123. Montesano R, Orci L, Vassalli P. In vitro rapid organization of endothelial cells into capillary-like networks is promoted by collagen matrices. J Cell Biol 1983; 97:1648–1652.

124. Goto F, Goto K, Weindel K et al. Synergistic effects of vascular endothelial growth factor and basic fibroblast growth factor on the proliferation and cord formation of bovine capillary endothelial cells within collagen gels. Lab Invest 1993; 69:508–517.

125. Orlidge A, D'Amore PA. Inhibition of capillary endothelial cell growth by pericytes and smooth muscle cells. J Cell Biol 1987; 105:1455–1462.

126. Antonelli-Orlidge A, Saunders KB, Smith SR et al. An activated form of transforming growth factor β is produced by cocultures of endothelial cells and pericytes. Proc Natl Acad Sci USA 1989; 86:4544–4548.

127. Lindahl P, Johansson BR, Levéen P et al. Pericyte loss and microaneurysm formation in PDGF-B-deficient mice. Science 1997; 277:242–245.

128. Herman IM, D'Amore PA. Microvascular pericytes contain muscle and nonmuscle actins. J Cell Biol 1985; 101:43–52.

129. Kelley C, D'Amore P, Hechtman HB et al. Microvascular pericyte contractility in vitro: comparison with other cells of the vascular wall. J Cell Biol 1987; 104:483–490.

130. Das A, Frank RN, Weber ML et al. ATP causes retinal pericytes to contract in vitro. Exp Eye Res 1988; 46:349–362.

131. Kelley C, D'Amore PA, Hechtman HB et al. Vasoactive hormones and cAMP affect pericyte contraction and stress fibres in vitro. J Muscle Res Cell Motil 1988; 9:184–194.

132. Chakravarthy U, Gardiner TA, Anderson P et al. The effect of endothelin 1 on the retinal microvascular pericyte. Microvasc Res 1992; 43:241–254.

133. Tilton RG, Kilo C, Williamson JR et al. Differences in pericyte contractile function in rat cardiac and skeletal muscle microvasculatures. Microvasc Res 1979; 18:336–352.

134. Butryn RK, Ruan H, Hull CM et al. Vasoactive agonists do not change the caliber of retinal capillaries of the rat. Microvasc Res 1995; 50:80–93.

135. Das A, Frank RN, Zhang NL et al. Increases in collagen type IV and laminin in galactose-induced retinal capillary basement membrane thickening – prevention by an aldose reductase inhibitor. Exp Eye Res 1990; 50:269–280.

136. Robison WG Jr, Kador PF, Akagi Y et al. Prevention of basement membrane thickening in retinal capillaries by a novel inhibitor of aldose reductase, tolrestat. Diabetes 1986; 35:295–299.

137. Das A, Frank RN, Zhang NL. Sorbinil does not prevent galactose-induced glomerular capillary basement membrane thickening. Diabetologia 1990; 33:515–521.

138. Nishio Y, Warren CE, Buczek-Thomas JA et al. Identification and characterization of a gene regulating enzymatic glycosylation which is induced by diabetes and hyperglycemia specifically in rat cardiac tissue. J Clin Invest 1995; 96:1759–1767.

139. Brownlee M, Cerami A. The biochemistry of the complications of diabetes mellitus. Annu Rev Biochem 1981; 50:385–432.

140. Timpl R, Rohde H, Robey PG et al. Laminin: a glycoprotein from basement membranes. J Biol Chem 1979; 254:9933–9937.

141. Grant DS, Kleinman HK. Regulation of capillary formation by laminin and other components of the extracellular matrix. In: Goldberg ID, Rosen EM, eds. Regulation of angiogenesis. Basel, Switzerland: Birkhäuser Verlag; 1997:317–333.

142. Kennedy A, Frank RN, Mancini MA. In vitro production of glycosaminoglycans by retinal microvessel cells and lens epithelium. Invest Ophthalmol Vis Sci 1986; 27:746–754.

143. Rohrbach DH, Wagner CW, Star VL et al. Reduced synthesis of basement membrane heparan sulfate proteoglycan in streptozotocin-induced diabetic mice. J Biol Chem 1983; 258:11672–11677.

144. Pihlajaniemi T, Myllyla R, Kivirikko KI et al. Effects of streptozotocin diabetes, glucose, and insulin on the metabolism of type IV collagen and proteoglycan in murine basement membrane-forming EHS tumor tissue. J Biol Chem 1982; 257:14914–14920.

145. Shimomura H, Spiro RG. Studies on macromacular components of human glomerular basement membrane and alterations in diabetes: decreased levels of heparan sulfate proteoglycan and laminin. Diabetes 1987; 36:374–381.

146. Spiro RG, Spiro MJ. Effect of diabetes on the biosynthesis of the renal glomerular basement membrane. Diabetes 1971; 20:641–648.

147. Kennedy A, Frank RN, Mancini MA et al. Collagens of the retinal microvascular basement membrane and of retinal microvascular cells in vitro. Exp Eye Res 1986; 42:177–199.

148. Farquhar MG. The glomerular basement membrane – a selective macromolecular filter. In: Hay ED, ed. Cell biology of the extracellular matrix. New York: Plenum Press; 1982:335–378.

149. Farquhar MG, Courtoy PJ, Lenkin MC et al. Current knowledge of the functional architecture of the glomerular basement membrane. In: Kuehn K, Schoene HH, Timpl R, eds. New trends in basement membrane research. New York: Raven Press; 1982:9–30.

150. Pino RM, Essner E. Permeability of rat choriocapillaris to hemeproteins: restriction of tracers by a fenestrated endothelium. J Histochem Cytochem 1981; 29:281–290.

151. Li W, Rockey JH. Fluorescein binding to normal human serum proteins demonstrated by equilibrium dialysis. Arch Ophthalmol 1982; 100:484–487.

152. Form DM, Pratt BM, Madri JA. Endothelial cell proliferation during angiogenesis: in vitro modulation by basement membrane components. Lab Invest 1986; 55:521–530.

153. Ingber DE, Folkman J. How does extracellular matrix control capillary morphogenesis? Cell 1989; 58:803–805.

154. Orlidge A, D'Amore PA. Cell specific effects of glycosaminoglycans on the attachment and proliferation of vascular wall components. Microvasc Res 1986; 31:41–53.

155. Trelstad RL. Glycosaminoglycans: mortar, matrix, mentor. Lab Invest 1985; 53:1–4.

156. Hall HG, Farson DA, Chin S et al. Extracellular matrix and morphogenesis: collagen overlay induces lumen formation by epithelial cell lines. In: Hawkes S, Wang JL, eds. Extracellular matrix. New York: Academic Press; 1982:233–238.

157. Kleinman HK, Klebe RJ, Martin GR. Role of collagenous matrices in the adhesion and growth of cells. J Cell Biol 1981; 88:473–485.

158. Frank RN, Mancini MA. Presumed retinovitreal neovascularization in dystrophic retinas of spontaneously hypertensive rats. Invest Ophthalmol Vis Sci 1986; 27:346–355.

159. Kalebic T, Garbisa S, Glaser B et al. Basement membrane collagen: degradation by migrating endothelial cells. Science 1983; 221:281–283.

160. van Hinsbergh VWM, Koolwijk P, Hanemaaijer R. Role of fibrin and plasminogen activators in repair-associated angiogenesis: in vitro studies with human endothelial cells. In: Goldberg ID, Rosen EM, eds. Regulation of angiogenesis. Basel, Switzerland: Birkhäuser Verlag; 1997:391–411.

161. Folkman J, Klagsbrun M, Sasse J et al. A heparin-binding angiogenic protein – basic fibroblast growth factor – is stored within basement membrane. Am J Pathol 1988; 130:393–400.

162. Vigny M, Ollier-Hartmann MP, Lavigne M et al. Specific binding of basic fibroblast growth factor to basement membrane-like structures and to purified heparan sulfate proteoglycan of the EHS tumor. J Cell Physiol 1988; 137:321–328.

163. Sakaguchi K, Yanagishita M, Takeuchi Y et al. Identification of heparan sulfate proteoglycan as a high affinity receptor for acidic fibroblast growth factor (aFGF) in a parathyroid cell line. J Biol Chem 1991; 266:7270–7278.

164. Cogan DG, Toussaint D, Kuwabara T. Retinal vascular patterns. IV. Diabetic retinopathy. Arch Ophthalmol 1961; 66:366–378.

165. Kuwabara T, Cogan DG. Retinal vascular patterns. VI. Mural cells of the retinal capillaries. Arch Ophthalmol 1963; 69:492–502.

166. Kuwabara T, Cogan DG. Studies of retinal vascular patterns. I. Normal architecture. Arch Ophthalmol 1960; 64:904–911.

167. Speiser P, Gittelsohn AM, Patz A. Studies on diabetic retinopathy. III. Influence of diabetes on intramural pericytes. Arch Ophthalmol 1968; 80:332–337.

168. Yanoff M. Diabetic retinopathy. N Engl J Med 1966; 274:1344–1349.

169. Akagi Y, Kador PF, Kuwabara T et al. Aldose reductase localization in human retinal mural cells. Invest Ophthalmol Vis Sci 1983; 24:1516–1519.

170. Tilton RG, Hoffmann PL, Kilo C et al. Pericyte degeneration and basement membrane thickening in skeletal muscle capillaries of human diabetics. Diabetes 1981; 30:326–334.

171. Kern TS, Engerman RL. Distribution of aldose reductase in ocular tissues. Exp Eye Res 1981; 33:175–182.

172. Ludvigson MA, Sorensen RL. Immunohistochemical localization of aldose reductase. II. Rat eye and kidney. Diabetes 1980; 29:450–459.

173. Kennedy A, Frank RN, Varma SD. Aldose reductase activity in retinal and cerebral microvessels and cultured vascular cells. Invest Ophthalmol Vis Sci 1983; 24:1250–1258.

174. Buzney SM, Frank RN, Varma SD et al. Aldose reductase in retinal mural cells. Invest Ophthalmol Vis Sci 1977; 16:392–396.

175. Friedenwald JS. Diabetic retinopathy. Am J Ophthalmol 1950; 33:1187–1199.

176. Joyce NC, DeCamilli P, Boyles J. Pericytes, like vascular smooth muscle cells, are immunocytochemically positive for cyclic GMP-dependent protein kinase. Microvasc Res 1984; 28:206–219.

177. Ashton N, Kok D'A, Foulds WS. Ocular pathology in macroglobulinaemia. J Pathol Bacteriol 1963; 86:453–461.

178. Duke JR, Wilkinson CP, Sigelman S. Retinal microaneurysms in leukaemia. Br J Ophthalmol 1968; 52:368–374.

179. DeVenecia G, Davis MD. Histology and fluorescein angiography of microaneurysms in diabetes mellitus. Invest Ophthalmol 1967; 6:555.

180. Kohner EM, Henkind P. Correlation of fluorescein angiogram and retinal digest in diabetic retinopathy. Am J Ophthalmol 1970; 69:403–414.

181. Wallow IHL, Engerman RL. Permeability and patency of retinal blood vessels in experimental diabetes. Invest Ophthalmol Vis Sci 1977; 16:447–461.

182. Gardner TW, Lesher T, Khin S et al. Histamine reduces ZO-1 tight-junction protein expression in cultured retinal microvascular endothelial cells. Biochem J 1996; 320:717–721.

183. Gardner TW. Histamine, ZO-1 and increased blood–retinal barrier permeability in diabetic retinopathy. Trans Am Ophthalmol Soc 1995; 93:583–621.

184. Enea NA, Hollis TM, Kern JA et al. Histamine H_1 receptors mediate increased blood–retinal barrier permeability in experimental diabetes. Arch Ophthalmol 1989; 107:270–274.

185. Gardner TW, Eller AW, Friberg TR et al. Antihistamines reduce blood–retinal barrier permeability in type I (insulin-dependent) diabetic patients with nonproliferative retinopathy. A pilot study. Retina 1995; 15:134–140.

186. Barber AJ, Antonelli DA, Gardner TW. Altered expression of retinal occludin and glial fibrillary acid protein in experimental diabetes. The Penn State Retinal Research Group. Invest Ophthalmol Vis Sci 2000; 41:3561–3568.

187. Antonetti DA, Barber AJ, Hollinger LA et al. Vascular endothelial growth factor induces rapid phosphorylation of tight junction proteins occludin and zonula occludens-1. A potential mechanism for vascular permeability in diabetic retinopathy and tumors. J Biol Chem 1999; 274:23463–23467.

188. Lakshminarayan S, Antonetti DA, Gardner TW et al. Effect of VEGF on retinal microvascular endothelial hydraulic conductivity: the role of NO. Invest Ophthalmol Vis Sci 2000; 41:4256–4261.

189. Sorbinil Retinopathy Trial Research Group. A randomized trial of sorbinil, an aldose reductase inhibitor, in diabetic retinopathy. Arch Ophthalmol 1990; 108:1234–1244.

190. Wallow IHL, Geldner PS. Endothelial fenestrae in proliferative diabetic retinopathy. Invest Ophthalmol Vis Sci 1980; 19:1176–1183.

191. Essner E. Role of vesicular transport in breakdown of the blood–retinal barrier. Lab Invest 1987; 56:457–460.

192. Essner E, Pino RM, Griewski RA. Breakdown of blood retinal barrier in RCS rats with inherited retinal degeneration. Lab Invest 1980; 43:418–426.

193. Davis MD, Norton EWD, Myers FL. The Airlie classification of diabetic retinopathy. In: Goldberg MF, Fine SL, eds. Symposium on the treatment of diabetic retinopathy. US Public Health Service publication no. 1890. Washington, DC: US Government Printing Office; 1968:7–22.

194. DeVenecia G, Davis M, Engerman R. Clinicopathologic correlations in diabetic retinopathy. I. Histology and fluorescein angiography of microaneurysms. Arch Ophthalmol 1976; 94:1766–1773.

195. Brownlee M, Vlassara H, Kooney A et al. Aminoguanidine prevents diabetes-induced arterial wall protein cross-linking. Science 1986; 232:1629–1632.

196. Tesfamariam B. Free radicals in diabetic endothelial cell dysfunction. Free Radic Biol Med 1994; 16:383–391.

197. Kuroki M, Voest EE, Amano S et al. Reactive oxygen intermediates increase vascular endothelial growth factor expression in vitro and in vivo. J Clin Invest 1996; 98:1667–1675.

198. Du Y, Smith MA, Miller CM et al. Diabetes-induced nitrative stress in the retina, and correction by aminoguanidine. J Neurochem 2002; 80:771–779.

199. Kunisaki M, Bursell SE, Clermont AC et al. Vitamin E prevents diabetes-induced abnormal retinal blood flow via the diacylglycerol–protein kinase C pathway. Am J Physiol 1995; 269 (2 Pt 1):E239–E246.

200. Kowluru RA, Tang J, Kern TS. Abnormalities of retinal metabolism in diabetes and experimental galactosemia. VII. Effect of long-term administration of antioxidants on the development of retinopathy. Diabetes 2001; 50:1938–1942.

201. Joussen AM, Murata T, Tsujikawa A et al. Leukocyte-mediated endothelial cell injury and death in the diabetic retina. Am J Pathol 2001; 158:147–152.

202. Joussen AM, Poulaki V, Mitsiades N et al. Nonsteroidal anti-inflammatory drugs prevent early diabetic retinopathy via TNF-alpha suppression. FASEB J 2002; 16:438–440.

203. Adamis AP. Is diabetic retinopathy an inflammatory disease? Br J Ophthalmol. 2002; 86:363–365.

204. Martidis A, Duker JS, Greenberg PB et al. Intravitreal triamcinolone for refractory diabetic macular edema. Ophthalmology 2002; 109:920–927.

205. Early Treatment Diabetic Retinopathy Study Research Group. Effects of aspirin treatment on diabetic retinopathy. ETDRS report number 8. Ophthalmology 1991; 98 (Suppl.):757–765.

206. Kern TS, Engerman RL. Pharmacological inhibition of diabetic retinopathy: aminoguanidine and aspirin. Diabetes 2001; 50:1636–1642.

207. Engerman RL, Kern TS. Progression of incipient diabetic retinopathy during good glycemic control. Diabetes 1987; 36:808–812.

208. Engerman RL, Kern TS. Retinopathy in galactosemic dogs continues to progress after cessation of galactosemia. Arch Ophthalmol 1994; 113:355–358.

209. Aiello LP, Robinson GS, Lin YW et al. Identification of multiple genes in bovine retinal pericytes altered by exposure to elevated levels of glucose by using mRNA differential display. Proc Natl Acad Sci USA 1004; 91:6231–6235.

210. Gabbay KH. The sorbitol pathway and the complications of diabetes. N Engl J Med 1973; 288:831–836.

211. Kinoshita JH. Cataracts in galactosemia. Invest Ophthalmol 1965; 4:786–799.

212. Robison WG Jr. Aldose reductase inhibition and retinopathy (letter to the editor). Diabetes 1994; 43:337–338.

213. Engerman RL, Kern TS. Response to Robison (letter to the editor). Diabetes 1994; 43:338–339.

214. Frank RN. Perspectives in diabetes. The aldose reductase controversy. Diabetes 1994; 43:169–172.

215. Engerman RL. Pathogenesis of diabetic retinopathy. Diabetes 1989; 38:1203–1206.

216. Kern TS, Engerman RL. Retinal polyol and myo-inositol in galactosemic dogs given an aldose reductase inhibitor. Invest Ophthalmol Vis Sci 1991; 32:3175–3177.

217. Lee AY, Chung SK, Chung SS. Demonstration that polyol accumulation is responsible for diabetic cataract by the use of transgenic mice expressing the aldose reductase gene in the lens. Proc Natl Acad Sci USA 1995; 92:2780–2784.

218. Xia P, Inoguchi T, Kern T et al. Characterization of the mechanism for the chronic activation of diacylglycerol-protein kinase C pathway in diabetes and hypergalactosemia. Diabetes 1994; 43:1122–1129.

219. Xia P, Aiello LP, Ishii H et al. Characterization of vascular endothelial growth factor's effect on the activation of protein kinase C, its isoforms, and endothelial cell growth. J Clin Invest 1996; 98:2018–2026.

220. Ishii H, Jirousek MR, Koya D et al. Amelioration of vascular dysfunctions in diabetic rats by an oral PKC beta inhibitor. Science 1996; 272:728–731.

221. Aiello LP, Bursell SE, Clermont A et al. Vascular endothelial growth factor-induced retinal permeability is mediated by protein kinase C in vivo and suppressed by an orally effective beta-isoform-selective inhibitor. Diabetes 1997; 46:1473–1480.

222. Milton R, Aiello L, Davis M et al. Initial results of the protein kinase C β inhibitor diabetic retinopathy study (PKC-DRS). Diabetes 2003; 52 (Suppl. 1):A-127 (abstract no. 544-P).

223. Campochiaro PA and the C99-PKC 412-003 Study Group. Reduction of diabetic macular edema by oral administration of the kinase inhibitor PKC 412. Invest Ophthalmol Vis Sci 2004; 45:922–931.

224. Hammes HP, Du X, Edelstein D et al. Benfotiamine blocks three major pathways of hyperglycemic damage and prevents experimental diabetic retinopathy. Nat Med 2003; 9:294–299.

225. King GL, Buzney SM, Kahn CR et al. Differential responsiveness to insulin of endothelial and support cells from micro- and macrovessels. J Clin Invest 1983; 71:974–979.

226. Engerman RL, Pfaffenbach D, Davis MD. Cell turnover of capillaries. Lab Invest 1967; 17:738–743.

227. Kumagai AK, Glasgow BJ, Pardridge WM. GLUT1 glucose transporter expression in the diabetic and nondiabetic human eye. Invest Ophthalmol Vis Sci 1994; 35:2887–2894.

228. Kumagai AK, Vinores SA, Pardridge WM. Pathological upregulation of inner blood–retinal barrier GLUT1 glucose transporter expression in diabetes mellitus. Brain Res 1996; 706:313–317.

229. Mantych GJ, Hageman GS, Devaskar SU. Characterization of glucose transporter isoforms in the adult and developing human eye. Endocrinology 1993; 133:600–607.

230. Watanabe T, Mio Y, Hoshino FB et al. GLUT2 expression in the rat retina: localization at the apical ends of Müller cells. Brain Res 1994; 65:128–134.

231. Watanabe T, Matsushima S, Okazaki M et al. Localization and ontogeny of GLUT3 expression in the rat retina. Dev Brain Res 1996; 94:60–66.

232. Burgess WH, Maciag T. The heparin-binding (fibroblast) growth factor family of proteins. Annu Rev Biochem 1989; 58:575–606.

233. Gospodarowicz D. Purification of a fibroblast growth factor from bovine pituitary. J Biol Chem 1975; 250:2515–2520.

234. Neufeld G, Gospodarowicz D. Basic and acidic fibroblast growth factors interact with the same cell surface receptors. J Biol Chem 1986; 261:5631–5637.

235. Glaser BM, D'Amore PA, Michels RG et al. Demonstration of vasoproliferative activity from mammalian retina. J Cell Biol 1980; 84:298–304.

236. Baird A, Esch F, Gospodarowicz D. Retina- and eye-derived endothelial cell growth factors: partial molecular characterization and identity with acidic and basic fibroblast growth factors. Biochemistry 1985; 24:7855–7860.

237. Schreiber AB, Kenney J, Kowalski JR et al. A unique family of endothelial cell polypeptide mitogens: the antigenic and receptor cross-reactivity of bovine endothelial cell growth factor, brain-derived acidic fibroblast growth factor, and eye-derived growth factor-II. J Cell Biol 1985; 101:1623–1626.

238. Abraham JA, Mergia A, Whang JL et al. Nucleotide sequence of a bovine clone encoding the angiogenic protein, basic fibroblast growth factor. Science 1986; 233:541–545.

239. Vlodavsky I, Fridman R, Sullivan R et al. Aortic endothelial cells synthesize basic fibroblast growth factor which remains cell associated and platelet-derived growth factor-like protein which is secreted. J Cell Physiol 1987; 13:402–408.

240. Amin R, Puklin JE, Frank RN. Growth factor localization in choroidal neovascular membranes of age-related macular degeneration. Invest Ophthalmol Vis Sci 1994; 35:3178–3188.

241. Frank RN, Amin RH, Eliott D et al. Basic fibroblast growth factor and vascular endothelial growth factor are present in epiretinal and choroidal neovascular membranes. Am J Ophthalmol 1996; 122:393–403.

242. Hanneken A, de Juan E Jr, Lutty GA et al. Altered distribution of basic fibroblast growth factor in diabetic retinopathy. Arch Ophthalmol 1991; 109:1005–1011.

243. Folkman J, Klagsbrun M. Angiogenic factors. Science 1987; 235:442–447.

244. Glaser BM. Extracellular modulating factors and the control of intraocular neovascularization. Arch Ophthalmol 1988; 106:603–607.

245. Schweigerer L, Neufeld G, Friedman J et al. Capillary endothelial cells express basic fibroblast growth factor, a mitogen that promotes their own growth. Nature 1987; 325:257–259.

246. Sivalingam A, Kenney J, Brown GC et al. Basic fibroblast growth factor levels in the vitreous of patients with proliferative diabetic retinopathy. Arch Ophthalmol 1990; 108:869–872.

247. Malecaze F, Clamens S, Simorre-Pinatel V et al. Detection of vascular endothelial growth factor messenger RNA and vascular endothelial growth factor-like activity in proliferative diabetic retinopathy. Arch Ophthalmol 1994; 112:1476–1482.

248. Brown LF, Detmar M, Claffey K et al. Vascular permeability factor/vascular endothelial growth factor: a multifunctional angiogenic cytokine. In: Goldberg ID, Rosen EM, eds. Regulation of angiogenesis. Basel: Birkhäuser Verlag; 1997:233–269.

249. Mathews MK, Merges C, McLeod DS et al. Vascular endothelial growth factor and vascular permeability changes in human diabetic retinopathy. Invest Ophthalmol Vis Sci 1997; 38:2729–2741.

250. Shweiki D, Itin A, Soffer D et al. Vascular endothelial growth factor induced by hypoxia may mediate hypoxia-initiated angiogenesis. Nature 1992; 359:843–845.

251. Aiello LP, Northrup JM, Keyt BA et al. Hypoxic regulation of vascular endothelial growth factor in retinal cells. Arch Ophthalmol 1995; 113:1538–1544.

252. Pe'er J, Shweiki D, Itin A et al. Hypoxia-induced expression of vascular endothelial growth factor (VEGF) by retinal cells is a common factor in neovascularization. Lab Invest 1995; 72:638–645.

253. Aiello LP, Avery RL, Arrigg PG et al. Vascular endothelial growth factor in ocular fluid of patients with diabetic retinopathy and other retinal disorders. N Engl J Med 1994; 331:1480–1487.

254. Adamis AP, Miller JW, Bernal M-T et al. Increased vascular endothelial growth factor levels in the vitreous of eyes with proliferative diabetic retinopathy. Am J Ophthalmol 1994; 118:445–450.

255. Miller JW, Adamis AP, Shima DT et al. Vascular endothelial growth factor/vascular permeability factor is temporally and spatially correlated with ocular angiogenesis in a primate model. Am J Pathol 1994; 145:574–584.

256. Adamis AP, Shima DT, Tolentino MJ et al. Inhibition of vascular endothelial growth factor prevents retinal ischemia-associated iris neovascularization in a nonhuman primate. Arch Ophthalmol 1996; 114:66–71.

257. Robinson GS, Pierce EA, Rook SL et al. Oligodeoxynucleotides inhibit retinal neovascularization in a murine model of proliferative retinopathy. Proc Natl Acad Sci USA 1996; 93:4851–4856.

258. Lutty GA, McLeod DS, Merges C et al. Localization of vascular endothelial growth factor in human retina and choroid. Arch Ophthalmol 1996; 114: 971–977.

259. Amin RH, Frank RN, Kennedy A et al. Vascular endothelial growth factor is present in glial cells of the retina and optic nerve of human subjects with nonproliferative diabetic retinopathy. Invest Ophthalmol Vis Sci 1997; 38:36–47.

260. Hanneken A, Lutty GA, McLeod DS et al. Localization of basic fibroblast growth factor to the developing capillaries of the bovine retina. J Cell Physiol 1989; 138:115–120.

261. Noji S, Matsuo T, Koyama E et al. Expression pattern of acidic and basic fibroblast growth factor genes in adult rat eyes. Biochem Biophys Res Commun 1990; 168:343–349.

262. Schweigere L, Malerstein B, Neufeld G et al. Basic fibroblast growth factor is synthesized in cultured retinal pigment epithelial cells. Biochem Biophys Res Commun 1987; 143:934–940.

263. Carmeliet P, Ferreira V, Breier G et al. Abnormal blood vessel development and lethality in embryos lacking a single VEGF allele. Nature 1996; 380: 435–439.

264. Ferrara N, Carver-Moore K, Chen H et al. Heterozygous embryonic lethality induced by targeted inactivation of the VEGF gene. Nature 1996; 380: 439–442.

265. Danis RP, Bingaman DP, Jrousek M et al. Inhibition of intraocular neo-vascularization due to retinal ischemia in pigs by PKCβ inhibition with LY333531. Invest Ophthalmol Vis Sci 1998; 39:171–179.

266. Eyetech Study Group. Anti-vascular endothelial growth factor therapy for subfoveal choroidal neovascularization secondary to age-related macular degeneration: phase II study results. Ophthalmology 2003; 110:979–986.

267. Ferrara N. Role of vascular endothelial growth factor in physiologic and pathologic angiogenesis: therapeutic implications. Semin Oncol 2002; 29 (Suppl. 16):10–14.

268. Rosen LS. Clinical experience with angiogenesis signaling inhibitors: focus on vascular endothelial growth factor (VEGF) blockers. Cancer Control 2002; 9 (Suppl. 2):36–44.

269. Slakter JS and the Anecortave Acetate Clinical Study Group. Anecortave acetate as monotherapy for treatment of subfoveal neovascularization in age-related macular degeneration: 12-month clinical outcomes. Ophthalmology 2003; 110:2372–2383.

270. Steele FR, Chader GJ, Johnson LV et al. Pigment epithelium-derived factor: neurotrophic activity and identification as a member of the serine protease inhibitor gene family. Proc Natl Acad Sci USA 1993; 90:1526–1530.

271. Ogata N, Wada M, Otsuji T et al. Expression of pigment epithelium-derived factor in normal adult rat eye and experimental choroidal neovascularization. Invest Ophthalmol Vis Sci 2002; 43:1168–1175.

272. Becerra SP, Wu YQ, Montuenga L et al. Pigment epithelium-derived factor (PEDF) in the monkey eye: apical secretion from the retinal pigment epithelium. Invest Ophthalmol Vis Sci 2001; 42:S772.

273. Blaauwgeers HG, Holtkamp GM, Rutten H et al. Polarized vascular endothelial growth factor secretion by human retinal pigment epithelium and localization of vascular endothelial growth factor receptors on the inner choriocapillaris. Evidence for a trophic paracrine relation. Am J Pathol 1999; 155:421–428.

274. Dawson DW, Volpert OV, Gillis P et al. Pigment epithelium-derived factor: a potent inhibitor of angiogenesis. Science 1999; 285:245–248.

275. Stellmach V, Crawford SE, Zhou W et al. Prevention of ischemia-induced retinopathy by the natural ocular antiangiogenic agent pigment epithelium-derived factor. Proc Natl Acad Sci USA 2001; 98:2593–2597.

276. Gao G, Li Y, Zhang D et al. Unbalanced expression of VEGF and PEDF in ischemia-induced retinal neovascularization. FEBS Lett 2001; 489: 270–276.

277. Rasmussen H, Chu KW, Campochiaro P et al. Clinical protocol. An open-label, phase I, single administration, dose-escalation study of $AD_{GV}PEDF.11D$ (ADPEDF) in neovascular age-related macular degeneration (AMD). Hum Gene Ther 2001; 12:2029–2032.

Chapter

67

Nonproliferative Diabetic Retinopathy

Emily Y. Chew
Frederick L. Ferris III

Diabetic retinopathy is a leading cause of new cases of blindness in people aged 20 to 74 years in the USA. The classification of diabetic retinopathy is generally based on the severity of intraretinal microvascular changes and the presence or absence of retinal neovascularization. The retinopathy is classified as nonproliferative diabetic retinopathy (NPDR) when there are only intraretinal microvascular changes. This early stage of retinopathy precedes the proliferative phase, in which new vessels or fibrous tissues, or both, form on the retina. The fundus abnormalities of nonproliferative retinopathy are microaneurysms and intraretinal abnormalities that result from altered retinal vascular permeability and eventual retinal vessel closure. The retinal vessel closure leads to nonperfusion, seen clinically as increasing hemorrhages, venous abnormalities, and intraretinal microvascular abnormalities. Nonperfusion of the retina is associated with the development of proliferative retinopathy in diabetes and other retinal vascular disorders. This chapter focuses on the natural course and treatment of NPDR; Chapter 67 discusses the diagnosis and treatment of proliferative diabetic retinopathy (PDR).

NATURAL COURSE OF NONPROLIFERATIVE DIABETIC RETINOPATHY

The pathologic processes associated with the progression of diabetic retinopathy include the formation of retinal capillary microaneurysms, the development of vascular permeability, and eventual vascular occlusion, or capillary closure.

Microaneurysms

The retinal capillary microaneurysm is usually the first visible sign of diabetic retinopathy. Microaneurysms, identified clinically by ophthalmoscopy as deep-red dots varying from 15 μm to 60 μm in diameter, are most common in the posterior pole. Although microaneurysms can be associated with other retinal vascular diseases, particularly those associated with vascular occlusion such as branch and central vein occlusions, they are the hallmark of NPDR.

Histologically, microaneurysms are hypercellular saccular outpouchings of the capillary wall, as demonstrated by trypsin digest retinal mounts.[1] Experimental models of diabetic retinopathy in dogs and rats and studies of human autopsy eyes indicate that the initial step of diabetic retinopathy is the loss of intramural capillary pericytes with subsequent microaneurysm formation and capillary closure leading to the development of acellular capillaries (Fig. 67-1). Another early morphologic finding in diabetic retinopathy is the thickening of the basement membrane of the retinal capillaries. The importance of this thickening in the pathogenesis of diabetic retinopathy is unknown.[2–4]

The mechanism for the formation of microaneurysms is also unknown. Possible mechanisms include release of a vasoproliferative factor with endothelial cell proliferation, weakness of the capillary wall (from loss of pericytes), abnormalities of the adjacent retina, and increased intraluminal pressure.[5–7]

Microaneurysms may be difficult to differentiate from punctate hemorrhages seen in diabetic retinopathy. However, on the early frames of a fluorescein angiogram, microaneurysms are easily distinguished from intraretinal hemorrhages because they exhibit bright hyperfluorescence against the darker choroidal background, whereas retinal hemorrhages block fluorescence (Fig. 67-2). Microaneurysms may show little change over many years, but the lumens can occlude, as demonstrated by hyperfluorescence on fluorescein angiography, and after recanalization the microaneurysms can disappear.[8] It is typical for individual microaneurysms to appear and disappear with time.

Fluorescein angiography is not clinically indicated for either detection or documentation of microaneurysms. Without the other components of diabetic retinopathy, microaneurysms alone have no apparent clinical significance. However, an increase in the number of microaneurysms in the retina is associated with progression of retinopathy.[9–11] When the number of microaneurysms increases, there is an increased likelihood that the other microvascular changes of diabetic retinopathy may also be present.

Vascular permeability

With the increasing formation of microaneurysms, excessive vascular permeability of the retinal capillaries can occur, resulting in the development of retinal edema, usually in the macular area. Macular edema is defined as retinal thickening from accumulation of fluid within one disc diameter of the macula.[12,13] Fluorescein angiography can be used to identify excessive permeability, but fluorescein leakage alone does not necessarily indicate the presence of macular edema. Macular edema is best detected with slit-lamp biomicroscopy or stereoscopic fundus photography. Macular edema is often accompanied by retinal hard exudates.

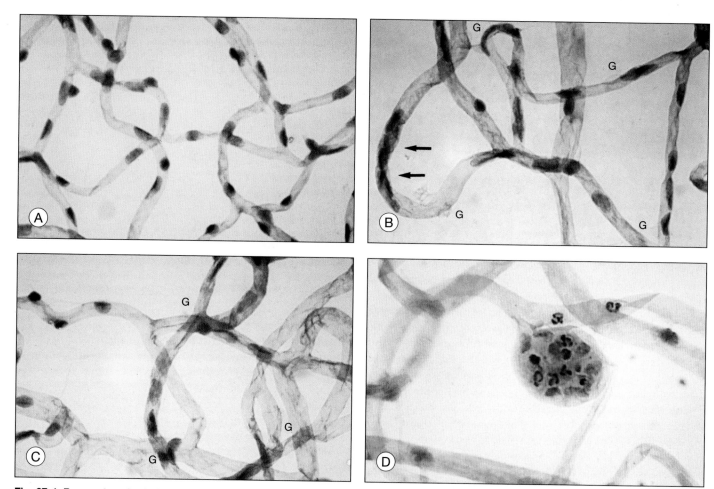

Fig. 67-1 Progression of retinal capillary changes in retinal vessel preparations from galactose-fed dog, isolated by trypsin digestion, mounted on gelatin-coated slides, and stained with periodic acid–Schiff–hematoxylin. A, Capillaries with normal distribution of pericyte and endothelial cells from a control dog fed with normal chow (original magnification ×825). B, Retinal vessels of a dog fed a galactose diet for 24 months illustrates the first visible change with the presence of pericyte ghosts (G) in the retinal vessels and the apparent proliferation of endothelial cells, as indicated by the arrows (original magnification ×825). C, Retinal changes from a dog fed galactose for 24 months shows acellular vessels as well as ghost pericytes (G) (original magnification ×925). D, The formation of a microaneurysm in a dog fed galactose for 27 months (original magnification ×570). (Courtesy of Dr. Peter Kador.)

These hard exudates are lipid deposits that presumably accumulate in association with lipoprotein leakage caused by breakdown of endothelial tight junctions in microaneurysms or retinal capillaries. Clinically, hard exudates are well-defined, yellowish-white intraretinal deposits, generally seen in the posterior pole, that are usually at the border of edematous and nonedematous retinas.

Edema fluid may come and go within the retina without visual consequence, but lipid deposits, especially when under the center of the macula, are associated with retinal damage and permanent visual loss.[14,15] The extent of these lipid deposits in the retina is associated with the degree to which serum lipids are elevated.[16,17]

More recently, optical coherence tomography (OCT) has been introduced in clinical studies of diabetic macular edema to provide high-resolution (e.g., 10 μm) imaging of the vitreoretinal interface, retina, and subretinal space.[18] OCT may be useful for quantifying retinal thickness and for identifying vitreomacular traction in selected patients with diabetic macular edema due to a taut posterior hyaloid face.[19,20]

Capillary closure

One of the most serious consequences of diabetic retinopathy is the obliteration of the retinal capillaries. When patches of acellular capillaries, seen early in the course of diabetic retinopathy, increase and become confluent, the terminal arterioles that supply these capillaries often become occluded. Adjacent to these areas of nonperfused retina, clusters of microaneurysms and tortuous, hypercellular vessels often develop. It is difficult to determine whether these vessels are dilated pre-existing capillaries or neovascularization within the retina. These vessels have been referred to as *intraretinal microvascular abnormalities* (IRMAs) clinically to include both possibilities.

As capillary closure becomes extensive, it is common to see many intraretinal hemorrhages or dilated segments of retinal veins (venous beading), or both (Fig. 67-3). The severity of IRMA (Fig. 67-3), intraretinal hemorrhages, and venous beading is directly associated with increasing nonperfusion and resulting ischemia (Fig. 67-4). This ischemia has a major pathogenic role in the development of retinal neovascularization. Endothelial

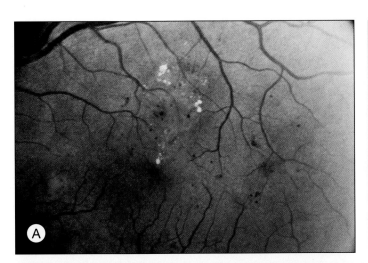

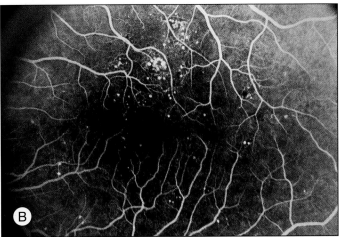

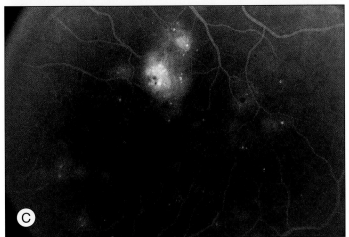

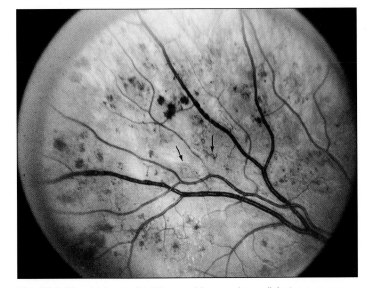

Fig. 67-2 The left eye of a 61-year-old man whose diabetes was diagnosed at age 55 years. A, A small zone of retinal thickening is located above the center of the macula, partially surrounded by hard exudates (thickening only discernible on stereoscopic examination, but suggested here by slight blurring of the retinal pigment epithelium pattern). There are scattered microaneurysms and punctate hemorrhages. B, Early-phase fluorescein angiogram demonstrates many microaneurysms (white dots) and very few hemorrhages (seen as a hypofluorescent spot). C, Late-phase fluorescein angiogram demonstrates fluorescein leakage, mainly from the two most prominent clumps of microaneurysms visible in B. The center of the macula was not involved, and visual acuity was 20/15.

Fig. 67-3 The right eye of a 25-year-old-man whose diabetes was diagnosed at age 12 years. Very severe nonproliferative diabetic retinopathy is present, characterized by extensive retinal hemorrhages, venous beading, and intraretinal microvascular abnormalities (IRMAs). Arrows indicate vessels at the borderline between IRMA and preretinal new vessels.

proliferation occurs following ischemia with subsequent preretinal new vessel proliferation.

CLASSIFICATION OF NONPROLIFERATIVE RETINOPATHY

Diabetic retinopathy is broadly categorized as nonproliferative (NPDR) or proliferative (PDR) (Table 67-1). In the nonproliferative stage, retinopathy is further categorized into four levels of severity: mild, moderate, severe, and very severe. The extent of IRMA, venous abnormalities, and the retinal hemorrhages are the factors that determine the level of severity of nonproliferative disease. Depending on the extent and severity of these lesions, an eye is classified as having moderate or severe NPDR.[21] In the mild to moderate nonproliferative categories (formerly termed *background retinopathy*), there are relatively few intraretinal hemorrhages and microaneurysms (H/MA) and only minimal venous changes or IRMA. The severe nonproliferative stage (formerly termed *preproliferative retinopathy*) represents increasing ischemia and is clinically detected by evaluating the four mid peripheral retinal quadrants using the so-called "4-2-1" rule.[22] Patients with any one of the following features are considered

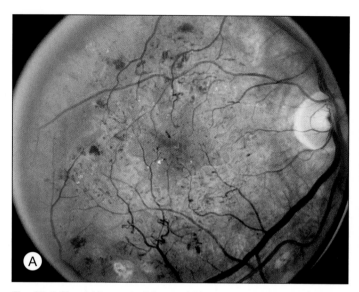 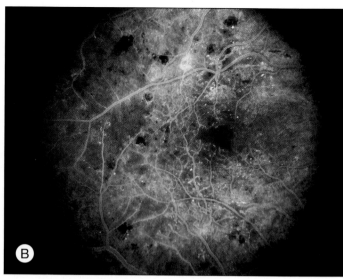

Fig. 67-4 The right eye of a 23-year-old man whose diabetes was diagnosed at age 9 years. A, Scattered retinal hemorrhages and microaneurysms are present in the posterior pole but not in the superior temporal part of the photograph, where the retina appears "featureless." B, Fluorescein angiogram shows capillary drop-out and pruned-off arteriolar side branches in "featureless" area. Foveal avascular zone is enlarged. Early new vessels were present on the disc and elsewhere.

Table 67-1 Classification of severity of diabetic retinopathy	
Severity	Lesions present
Nonproliferative	
No retinopathy	No retinal lesions
Microaneurysms only	No lesions other than microaneurysms
Mild NPDR, venous loops, or both	Microaneurysms plus retinal hemorrhage, hard exudate
Moderate NPDR	Mild NPDR plus cottonwool spots and/or IRMA
Severe NPDR	Presence of one of the following features: microaneurysms plus venous beading and/or H/MA ≥ Standard photograph 2A in four quadrants, or marked venous beading in two or more quadrants, or moderate IRMA (standard photograph 8A in one or more quadrants)
Very severe NPDR	Two or more of the above features described in severe NPDR
Proliferative	
PDR without HRC	New vessels and/or fibrous proliferations; or preretinal and/or vitreous hemorrhage
PDR with HRC	NVD ≥ standard photograph 10A; or less extensive NVD, if vitreous or preretinal hemorrhage is present; or NVE ≥ half disc area, if vitreous or preretinal hemorrhage is present
Advanced PDR	Extensive vitreous hemorrhage precluding grading, retinal detachment involving the macula, or phthisis bulbi or enucleation secondary to a complication of diabetic retinopathy

NPDR, Nonproliferative diabetic retinopathy; IRMA, intraretinal microvascular abnormalities; H/MA, hemorrhages and/or microaneurysms; PDR, proliferative diabetic retinopathy; HRC, high-risk characteristics; NVD, new vessels on or within one disc diameter of the optic disc, or in the vitreous cavity anterior to this area; NVE, new vessels elsewhere.

to have severe NPDR: (1) severe intraretinal hemorrhages and microaneurysms in all *four* quadrants (≥ standard photograph 2A, Fig. 67-5); (2) venous beading in *two* or more quadrants; or (3) moderate IRMA in at least *one* quadrant (≥ standard photograph 8A, Fig. 67-6). If any two of these features are present, the retinopathy level is considered to be very severe nonproliferative.

MACULAR EDEMA

Macular edema is the most frequent cause of visual impairment in patients with NPDR. However, the breakdown of endothelial tight junctions and loss of the blood–retinal barrier can be asso-

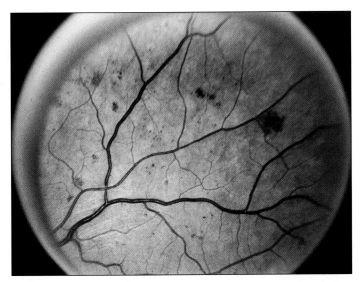

Fig. 67-5 Standard photograph 2A. Using the "4-2-1" rule, the presence of hemorrhages and microaneurysms in at least four mid peripheral fields, equaling or exceeding this standard photograph, would qualify as severe nonproliferative diabetic retinopathy.

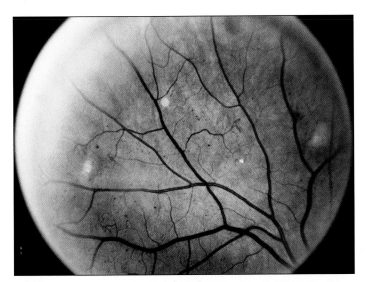

Fig. 67-6 Standard photograph 8A. Intraretinal microvascular abnormalities equaling or exceeding this standard photograph 8A in one or more quadrants would qualify as severe nonproliferative diabetic retinopathy.

ciated with both NPDR and PDR. This excessive vascular permeability, resulting in the leakage of fluid and plasma constituents, such as lipoproteins into the retina, leads to thickening of the retina. This macular edema is best detected by stereoscopic examination techniques (Fig. 67-2). When thickening involves or threatens the center of the fovea, there is a higher risk of visual loss. In the Early Treatment Diabetic Retinopathy Study (ETDRS), the 3-year risk of moderate visual loss (a doubling of the initial visual angle or a decrease of three lines or more on a logarithmic visual acuity chart) was 32%.

The ETDRS investigators classified macular edema by its severity. It was defined as clinically significant macular edema (CSME) if any of the following features were present: (1) thickening of the retina at or within 500 μm of the center of the macula; (2) hard exudates at or within 500 μm of the center of the macula, if associated with thickening of the adjacent retina (not residual hard exudates remaining after the disappearance of retinal thickening); or (3) a zone or zones of retinal thickening one disc area or larger, any part of which is within one disc diameter of the center of the macula.[23]

SIMPLIFIED CLASSIFICATION OF DIABETIC RETINOPATHY

In an attempt to improve communication between the ophthalmologists and the primary care physicians caring for patients with diabetes and between clinicians worldwide, a recent international classification of diabetic retinopathy and macular edema was developed. This classification is based on the data collected in the clinical trials and epidemiologic studies of diabetic retinopathy and it simplifies the ETDRS classification of diabetic retinopathy for clinical use (Box 67-1).[24]

With the introduction of this new simplified scale, it is hoped that these systems will be valuable in improving both screening of individuals with diabetes and communication and discussion among individuals caring for these patients.

EPIDEMIOLOGY OF DIABETES AND DIABETIC RETINOPATHY

The Centers for Disease Control estimate that 18.2 million American have diabetes and 5.2 million don't know they have it.[25] Type 2 diabetes accounts for up to 95% of all diabetes cases, affecting 8% of the population aged 20 and older. Among the population 60 years and older, 18.6% are affected with diabetes. The prevalence of type 2 diabetes has tripled in the last 30 years, much of it due to an increase in obesity.

More recent analyses utilized eight population-based studies to estimate the prevalence of diabetic retinopathy and of vision-threatening retinopathy, defined as PDR, severe NPDR, and/or macular edema.[26] Within each age stratum, the prevalence of diabetic retinopathy was estimated in the US population, by multiplying the prevalence rates found in the National Health Interview Survey[27] and the 2000 US population census. Among the estimated 10.2 million individuals in the USA older than 40 years of age and with known diabetes, the prevalence rates of

---

Box 67-1 Diabetic retinopathy disease severity scale

Proposed disease severity level
Findings observable upon dilated ophthalmoscopy
No apparent retinopathy
No abnormalities

Mild nonproliferative diabetic retinopathy
Microaneurysms only

Moderate nonproliferative diabetic retinopathy
More than just microaneurysms but less than severe nonproliferative diabetic retinopathy

Severe nonproliferative diabetic retinopathy
Any of the following:
- More than 20 intraretinal hemorrhages in each of four quadrants
- Definite venous beading in more than two quadrants
- Prominent intraretinal microvascular abnormalities in more than one quadrant and no signs of proliferative retinopathy

Proliferative diabetic retinopathy
One or more of the following:
- Neovascularization
- Vitreous/preretinal hemorrhage

Diabetic macular edema disease severity scale
Proposed disease severity level
Findings observable upon dilated ophthalmoscopy
Diabetic macular edema apparently absent
No apparent retinal thickening or hard exudates in posterior pole
Diabetic macular edema apparently present
Some apparent retinal thickening or hard exudates in posterior pole
If diabetic macular edema is present, it can be categorized as follows:
Proposed disease severity level
Findings observable upon dilated ophthalmoscopy*
Diabetic macular edema present

- **Mild diabetic macular edema**
Some retinal thickening or hard exudates in posterior pole but distant from the center of the macula

- **Moderate diabetic macular edema**
Retinal thickening or hard exudates approaching the center of the macula but not involving the center

- **Severe diabetic macular edema**
Retinal thickening or hard exudates involving the center of the macula

*Hard exudates are a sign of current or previous macular edema. Diabetic macular edema is defined as retinal thickening and this requires a three-dimensional assessment that is best performed by a dilated examination using slit-lamp biomicroscopy and/or stereofundus photography.

diabetic retinopathy and vision-threatening diabetic retinopathy were 40.3% and 82%, respectively. This translates to 4.1 million adults over the age of 40 years having diabetic retinopathy; one in every 12 known persons with diabetes has severe vision-threatening diabetic retinopathy.

Data from population-based studies such as the Wisconsin Epidemiologic Study of Diabetic Retinopathy (WESDR) provide valuable information regarding both the prevalence and the risk factors associated with the development of diabetic retinopathy. In the younger-onset group, which consists of patients whose age at diagnosis of diabetes was less than 30 years and who were taking insulin at the time of the examination (presumably those with type 1 diabetes), retinopathy, either proliferative or non-proliferative, was seen in 13% of patients with less than a 5-year duration of diabetes and in 90% of patients with a duration of 10 to 15 years.[28] PDR, the most vision-threatening form of the disease, is present in approximately 25% of patients with type 1 diabetes and a 15-year duration of the disease.

For patients with an onset of diabetes at 30 years of age or older (those with type 2 diabetes) and a duration of diabetes less than 5 years, 40% of those taking insulin and 24% of those not taking insulin have retinopathy.[29] These rates increase to 84% and 53%, respectively, with an increased diabetes duration of 15 to 19 years. PDR develops in 2% of patients with type 2 diabetes and a duration less than 5 years and 25% of patients with a duration of 25 or more years of diabetes.

The prevalence of diabetic macular edema did not vary as much by diabetes type. The prevalence of diabetic macular edema is approximately 18% to 20% in patients with either type 1 or type 2 (insulin-taking) diabetes.

RISK FACTORS FOR PROGRESSION OF RETINOPATHY

Severity of retinopathy

As retinopathy progresses from the mild to moderate to severe and then very severe stages, the risk of developing PDR or visual loss also increases. In the ETDRS, eyes with very severe NPDR or mild to moderate PDR, or both, had a 60-fold increased risk of developing high-risk PDR after 1 year of follow-up, compared with eyes with mild NPDR (48.5% versus 0.8%). After 5 years of follow-up, there was still a fivefold increased risk (74.4% versus 14.3%).[17]

The importance of retinopathy severity in predicting progression of retinopathy was also evaluated in the population-based WESDR.[30] In 708 insulin-dependent patients younger than 30 years of age at time of diagnosis of diabetes, the odds ratio for 4-year progression to PDR was 2.1 for each step increase in baseline retinopathy severity on an 11-step scale. For patients with bilateral moderate NPDR, the 4-year risk of progression to PDR was increased by 40-fold when compared with patients who had microaneurysms in only one eye.

Glycemic control

The relationship of glucose control and the chronic complications of diabetes has been extensively studied in observational studies. These studies all demonstrated that increased severity of diabetic retinopathy is associated with poorer glucose control. Randomized, controlled clinical trials of glycemic control were designed to address the causal role of glucose control in diabetic complications. In the Diabetes Control and Complications Trial (DCCT), 1441 patients with type 1 diabetes were randomly assigned to either conventional or intensive insulin treatment and followed for a period of 4 to 9 years.[31-35] The DCCT demonstrated that intensive insulin treatment is associated with a decreased risk of either the development or progression of diabetic retinopathy in patients with type 1 diabetes. In patients without any visible retinopathy when enrolled in the DCCT, the 3-year risk of developing retinopathy was reduced by 75% in the intensive insulin treatment group compared with the standard treatment group. However, even in the intensively treated group, retinopathy could not be completely prevented over the 9-year course of the study.

The benefit of the strict control was also evident in patients with existing retinopathy (50% reduction in the rate of progression of retinopathy compared with controls). At 6- and 12-month visits, a small adverse effect of intensive treatment on retinopathy progression was seen, similar to that described in other trials of glucose control. However, in eyes with little or no retinopathy at the time of initiating intensive glucose control, this early worsening of retinopathy is unlikely to threaten vision. When the DCCT results were stratified by hemoglobin A_1C (HbA$_1$C) levels, there was a 35% to 40% reduction in the risk of retinopathy progression for every 10% decrease in HbA$_1$C (e.g., from 8% to 7.2%). This represented a fivefold increase in the risk for patients with HbA$_1$C of about 10% versus those with 7%. Furthermore, there was a statistically significant reduction in both diabetic neuropathy and nephropathy with intensive blood glucose control in the DCCT. When the randomized controlled clinical trial was completed, the study participants were informed of the results and they were further enrolled into the follow-up phase of the study, known as the Epidemiology of Diabetes Intervention and Complications (EDIC) study.[36] With an additional 7 more years of follow-up when the HbA$_1$Cs in both treatment groups were not statistically significant (8.1% versus 8.2%, $P = 0.09$), the rate of progression of retinopathy remained statistically significantly less in those treated with the intensive therapy than in the conventional therapy. The intensive glycemic control over a period of 6.5 years conferred benefits well beyond the period of treatment. These data have resulted in recommendations for achieving intense control with HbA$_1$C level below 7% as soon as the diagnosis of diabetes is made.

The effect of glycemic control on the incidence and progression of diabetic retinopathy is similar in patients with type 2 diabetes, as assessed in observational studies and randomized studies conducted in Japan and the UK.[37-40] Findings in a study of Japanese patients with type 2 diabetes have shown that multiple insulin-injection treatment reduced the onset of retinopathy from 32% to 8% and reduced a two-step progression retinopathy from 44% to 19%, compared with people receiving conventional insulin treatments over 6 years.[38] In the UK Prospective Diabetes Study (UKPDS), the largest and longest study of patients with type 2 diabetes, there was a 25% reduction in the risk of the "any diabetes-related microvascular end point," including the need for retinal photocoagulation in the intensive treatment group compared to the conventional treatment group. After 6 years of follow-up, a smaller proportion of patients in the intensive treatment group than in the conventional group had a two-step progression (worsening) in diabetic retinopathy ($P < 0.01$). Epidemiologic analysis of the UKPDS data showed a continuous relationship between the risk of microvascular complications and glycemia, so for every percentage point decrease in HbA$_1$C (e.g., 9% to 8%), there was a 35% reduction in the risk of microvascular complications.

The results of both the DCCT and UKPDS show that, although intensive therapy of glucose does not prevent retinopathy completely, it reduces the risk of the development and progression of diabetic retinopathy. This may be translated clinically to both preservation of vision and reduction in therapy such as laser photocoagulation.

Hypertension

The findings of observational studies assessing the importance of blood pressure in the progression of NPDR are inconsistent. However, in the UKPDS a randomized comparison of more intensive blood pressure control versus less intensive blood pressure control in persons with type 2 diabetes demonstrated that intensive blood pressure control was associated with a decreased risk of retinopathy progression. Of the 1148 hypertensive patients in the UKPDS, 758 were allocated to tight control of blood pressure and 390 to less tight control with a median follow-up of 8.4 years.[41] Tight blood pressure control resulted in a 37% reduction in microvascular diseases, predominantly reduced risk of retinal photocoagulation, when compared to less tight control. A previously published study of blood pressure medication in diabetic retinopathy suggested that there might be a specific benefit of angiotensin-converting enzyme (ACE) inhibition and blood pressure reduction, even in normotensive persons, on the progression of diabetic retinopathy.[42] The UKPDS included a randomized comparison of beta-blockers and ACE inhibitors in the tight blood pressure control arm of that study. Benefits from tight blood pressure control were present in both the beta-blocker and ACE inhibitor treatment groups, with no statistically significant difference between them. This suggests that the treatment effect is more likely to be secondary to blood pressure reduction than to a specific effect of ACE inhibitors.

Elevated serum lipid levels

The WESDR, a population-based study, and the ETDRS found that elevated levels of serum cholesterol were associated with increased severity of retinal hard exudate.[16,17] Independent of the accompanying macular edema, the severity of retinal hard exudate at baseline was associated with decreased visual acuity in the ETDRS. The severity of retinal hard exudate was also a significant risk factor for moderate visual loss (15 letters or more loss) during the course of the study. In addition, the strongest risk factor for the development of subretinal fibrosis in ETDRS patients with diabetic macular edema was the presence of severe hard exudate.[43]

More recently, the DCCT investigators also evaluated the association of severity of retinopathy and retinal hard exudates with serum lipids.[44] The lipoproteins in the total cholesterol were further characterized by nuclear magnetic resonance lipoprotein subclass profile (NMR-LSP), apoA1, apoB, lipoprotein (a), and susceptibility of low-density lipoprotein to oxidation. They found that the severity of retinopathy was associated with increasing triglycerides and inversely associated with high-density lipoprotein cholesterol. The NMR-LSP results showed an increasing severity of retinopathy with small and medium very-low-density lipoprotein and inversely with very-low-density lipoprotein size. These data support the potential role for dyslipoproteinemia in the pathogenesis of diabetic retinopathy.

Elevated serum triglyceride levels were also associated with a greater risk of developing high-risk PDR in the ETDRS patients.[117] In a study in Pittsburgh, elevated triglycerides, as well as elevated low-density lipoprotein cholesterol, were found to be associated with PDR.[45] Although these are all observational findings, the data are compelling to recommend lowering elevated serum lipids in patients with diabetic retinopathy to reduce the risk of visual loss. In addition to reducing the risk of cardiovascular disease, reducing the risk of visual loss should be another motivating factor for patients to lower elevated serum lipids.

Pregnancy and diabetic retinopathy

Diabetic retinopathy may be accelerated during pregnancy because of the pregnancy itself or the changes in metabolic control.[46–48] In fact, both the pregnancy and changes in metabolic control may play important roles in accelerating the progression of diabetic retinopathy.[49] Ideally, patients who are planning to become pregnant should have their eyes examined before they attempt to conceive and should make every attempt to lower their blood glucose levels to as near normal as possible for the health of the fetus, as well as their own health. During the first trimester, another eye examination should be performed; subsequent follow-up will depend on the findings at the time of this examination. Pregnant women with less than severe NPDR should be examined every 3 months, whereas those with more severe stages should be seen every 1 to 3 months, as recommended by the American Academy of Ophthalmology *Preferred Practice Pattern*.[50]

Other systemic risk factors

Diabetic nephropathy, as measured by albuminuria, proteinuria, or renal failure, is found to be a risk factor associated with progression of retinopathy in some, but not all, studies.[51–53] Anemia has also been reported to be associated with progression of diabetic retinopathy in two small case series and two epidemiologic studies.[51,54–56] There was a progressive increase in the risk of development of high-risk PDR with decreasing hematocrit in an adjusted multivariate model in the ETDRS. This may add substantially to the evidence supporting the importance of anemia as a risk factor for diabetic retinopathy. History of diabetic neuropathy and cardiovascular autonomic neuropathy have also been suggested to be associated with increased risk of progression of retinopathy.[51,57,58]

MANAGEMENT OF NONPROLIFERATIVE DIABETIC RETINOPATHY

The treatment recommendations of diabetic retinopathy are based on the results of two major randomized clinical trials of laser photocoagulation, the Diabetic Retinopathy Study (DRS), and the ETDRS. The treatment of NPDR depends on the severity of retinopathy and the presence or absence of CSME, which may be present at any stage of NPDR.

Photocoagulation

The DRS enrolled patients with severe nonproliferative or PDR and visual acuity of 20/100 or better. The DRS results demonstrated a 50% reduction in severe visual loss (visual acuity of 5/200 or worse at two or more consecutively completed follow-up visits scheduled at 4-month intervals) in eyes that had received photocoagulation (scatter and focal photocoagulation) compared with eyes that did not receive photocoagulation. DRS reports also identify retinopathy features associated with a particularly high risk of severe visual loss.[59–62] These high-risk characteristics, which can be summarized as either neovascularization accompanied by vitreous hemorrhage or obvious neovascularization on or near the optic disc, even in the absence of vitreous hemorrhage, are described in further detail in Chapter 67.

Patients in the DRS had severe NPDR or PDR and were randomly assigned to either immediate photocoagulation or to no photocoagulation, regardless of retinopathy progression. Although that study identified a high-risk group of patients, it could not assess the appropriate timing of scatter photocoagulation. However, the ETDRS was designed to address this clinical question, as well as to evaluate the effects of laser photocoagulation for diabetic macular edema.[50] To be eligible for the ETDRS, patients had to have diabetic retinopathy in both eyes with less than high-risk proliferative retinopathy (allowing for mild, moderate, and severe NPDR and early PDR) with or without macular edema. One eye of each patient was randomly assigned to early photocoagulation using one of several strategies, and the fellow eye was assigned to deferral of photocoagulation.[63]

Scatter photocoagulation for nonproliferative diabetic retinopathy

The comparison of early photocoagulation versus deferral in the ETDRS revealed a small reduction in the incidence of severe visual loss in the early-treated eyes (Fig. 67-7), but 5-year rates were low in both the early treatment and deferral groups (2.6% and 3.7%, respectively).[64] For eyes with only mild to moderate NPDR, rates of severe visual loss were even lower, and any reductions in visual loss from early photocoagulation did not seem sufficient to compensate for the unwanted side-effects of scatter photocoagulation. As the retinopathy advances to the severe or very severe nonproliferative or early proliferative stage, the risk-to-benefit ratio becomes more favorable, and it is reasonable to consider initiating scatter photocoagulation before the development of high-risk PDR. Analyses of ETDRS data have suggested that early scatter treatment is particularly effective in reducing severe visual loss in patients with type 2 diabetes.[65] These data provide an additional reason to recommend early scatter photocoagulation in older patients with very severe NPDR or early PDR.

If patients with either type 1 or 2 diabetes present with both CSME and very severe NPDR or early PDR, the treatment of the macular edema should be considered first, if possible. Data from the ETDRS demonstrated the potential adverse effect of initial scatter photocoagulation in such patients.

Scatter photocoagulation for proliferative retinopathy

The technique of scatter photocoagulation for PDR is detailed in Chapter 67. This same technique is used for some eyes that are approaching high-risk PDR, for example, eyes with severe NPDR or early PDR. A standard "full" scatter panretinal photocoagulation should be applied (1200 to 1600 moderate intensity burns of approximately 500 μm in diameter).

Focal photocoagulation for diabetic macular edema

The ETDRS results also provide clinically important information to guide the treatment of diabetic macular edema.[23,63,66,67] In the ETDRS, eyes with mild or moderate NPDR and macular edema were randomly assigned to early focal/grid photocoagulation or no photocoagulation unless high-risk PDR developed. The main outcome variable was a decrease of three lines on a logarithmic visual acuity chart. This three-line decrease ($\geq$ 15-letter decrease) represents a doubling of the initial visual angle, for example, a change from 20/20 to 20/40 or from 20/100 to 20/200. After 3 years of follow-up, 24% of the control group experienced such a visual loss compared with 12% of the treated eyes. Focal/grid photocoagulation reduced the risk of moderate visual acuity loss for all eyes with diabetic macular edema and mild to moderate NPDR by about 50%. The group of untreated eyes with macular edema at highest risk for visual loss was the group with edema involving the center of the macula (Fig. 67-8). Prompt photocoagulation is indicated for these eyes, but treatment should be deferred for eyes with edema that is more remote

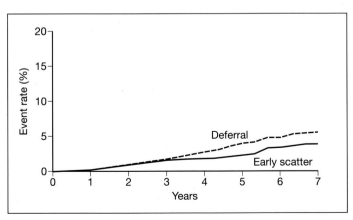

Fig. 67-7 Results of the Early Treatment Diabetic Retinopathy Study. Cumulative rates of severe loss (visual acuity <5/200 on two consecutive visits scheduled 4 months apart) in deferral eyes randomized to no treatment (dashed line) and to early scatter photocoagulation (solid line). At 5 years the rates were low in both the early treatment and deferral groups (2.6% and 3.7%, respectively).

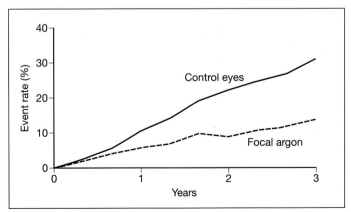

Fig. 67-8 Results of the Early Treatment Diabetic Retinopathy Study. Comparison of percentages of eyes that experienced visual loss of three or more lines (moderate visual loss) to eyes with clinically significant macular edema with center involvement. The control eyes were randomized to deferral of photocoagulation (solid line), and the treated eyes were assigned to immediate focal photocoagulation for macular edema (dashed line). There was more than a 50% reduction in the rates of moderate visual loss in the eyes treated with focal photocoagulation.

from the macular center. Also, if a large plaque of hard exudate is threatening the center, prompt treatment may be advised.

The effect of focal laser photocoagulation for diabetic macular edema was evaluated in eyes with a broad range of baseline edema severity, visual acuity levels, and various baseline fluorescein angiographic characteristics in the ETDRS.[68] Although these analyses were performed in eyes with mild to moderate NPDR only, the most important factor to consider in deciding whether to treat macular edema remains involvement of the center of the fovea.

Patients can notice the scotomas related to the focal laser burns, although there was limited documentation of this using the visual fields as measured in the ETDRS. For eyes with leakage arising close to the center of the macula, it may be preferable to observe closely rather than treat early because of increased risk of damage from direct treatment and possible subsequent migration of treatment scars. Careful follow-up with intervention when retinal thickening or lipid deposits threaten or involve

the center of the macula can reduce the risk of visual loss and limit the number of patients needing treatment.

The ETDRS used two types of treatment for diabetic macular edema: focal and grid. Focal refers to the direct treatment of all leaking microaneurysms in the edematous retina between 500 and 3000 μm from the center of the macula. Individual microaneurysms are treated with a spot size of 50 to 100 μm and an exposure time of 0.1 s. The power is set initially quite low and slowly increased to obtain either whitening or darkening of the microaneurysm with minimal power (Fig. 67-9). The grid treatment is primarily used for areas of diffuse leakage with no identifiable focal areas of leakage. The grid is composed of light intensity burns, 50 to rarely 200 μm in diameter, producing a grid of equally spaced burns more than one burn-width apart. One of the reported adverse effects of focal laser photocoagulation is the development of choroidal neovascularization and subsequent subretinal fibrosis.[69,70] However, in the ETDRS, only nine of 109 eyes with subretinal fibrosis associated with diabetic

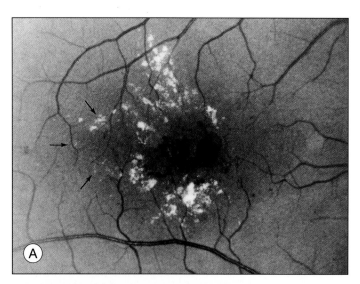

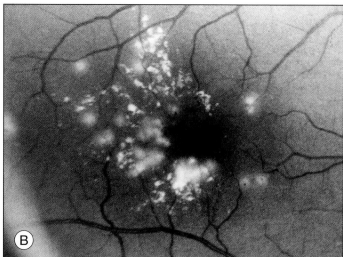

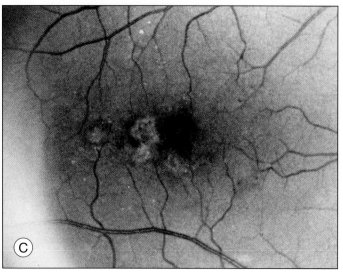

Fig. 67-9 The right eye of a 48-year-old man whose diabetes was diagnosed at age 21 years. A, Within the C-shaped ring of hard exudates, marked retinal thickening (edema) involving the center of the macula is present, although not visible in this nonstereoscopic photograph. Adjacent to this area temporally, there is a second zone of milder thickening within a smaller, more subtle hard exudate ring (arrows). Several microaneurysms are visible within the thickened areas. Best-corrected visual acuity was 20/30. B, Focal argon laser photocoagulation burns of moderate to strong intensity are visible immediately after treatment. C, Eight months after treatment, edema and hard exudates have absorbed. Treatment scars are visible. Visual acuity was 20/20.

macular edema could be directly attributed to focal photo-coagulation. The strongest risk factor for the development of subretinal fibrosis was the presence of severe hard exudate deposition in the retina, which is associated with elevated serum lipid levels.[43]

Other treatment of diabetic macular edema

Photocoagulation treatment for diabetic macular edema results in laser scars that tend to increase with time. The likelihood of experiencing vision improvement is low in these patients. In the ETDRS, about 17% of those treated with focal/grid laser photocoagulation will have a three-line improvement in 5 years compared to the 5% of those assigned to no laser treatment. More recently, patients with refractory macular edema – edema that has not responded to laser photocoagulation – are treated with intravitreal injections of triamcinolone acetonide.[71–73] These studies have small sample size with relatively short follow-up. Some have shown a mild improvement in visual acuity initially following treatment but longer-term evaluation is needed. In addition, the main adverse side-effects of raised intraocular pressure and increasing cataract formation have not been fully investigated. There are currently studies underway to assess this treatment. In addition, pharmacological agents that target vascular endothelial growth factor are also tested in early phases of controlled clinical trials for their role in the treatment of one of the major causes of vision loss in patients with diabetic retinopathy.

The use of OCT has played an important role in the design of these pharmacological studies in diabetic macular edema. With the completion of these trials, the data from the OCT may provide evidence to support the use of OCT as an important secondary endpoint.

A study comparing the detection of diabetic foveal edema with contact lens biomicroscopy or OCT suggested that mild diabetic macular edema may be more readily detected by OCT.[74] The biomicroscopic evaluation of the macula remains the standard technique for detecting macular edema in clinical practice, although fluorescein angiography and OCT are complementary studies that may help guide treatment decisions.

Medical therapy

Aspirin and antiplatelet treatments   Three randomized controlled clinical trials of antiplatelet treatments have been performed in patients with diabetic retinopathy. None has demonstrated a clinically beneficial effect of treatment. The Dipyridamole Aspirin Microangiopathy of Diabetes study[75] and the Ticlopidine Microangiopathy of Diabetes Study[76] enrolled 475 and 435 patients, respectively. These two studies found similar results with little difference in change in retinopathy severity as judged by visual acuity measurements or ophthalmoscopy. A difference was observed in counts of microaneurysms on fluorescein angiograms, with the increase greater in the placebo group and less in the aspirin group, the aspirin plus dipyridamole group, and the ticlopidine group. These small differences were of borderline statistical significance and uncertain clinical importance.

In the ETDRS, all patients were randomly assigned to 650 mg aspirin per day or a placebo, and one eye of each patient was randomly assigned to immediate photocoagulation, whereas the fellow eye was assigned to deferral of photocoagulation, that is, careful follow-up and prompt scatter photocoagulation if high-risk retinopathy developed. The eyes assigned to deferral of laser photocoagulation were assessed for the effects of aspirin on the progression of diabetic retinopathy.[77–81] Aspirin use did not affect the progression of retinopathy, nor did it affect the risk of visual loss.[67] Perhaps surprisingly, aspirin use did not increase the risk of vitreous hemorrhage in patients with proliferative retinopathy.[82,83] Aspirin use was associated with a 17% reduction in morbidity and mortality from cardiovascular disease.[84] Therefore aspirin should be considered for individuals with diabetes, not because of any effect on their diabetic retinopathy, but because of the benefits of aspirin that have been demonstrated for individuals who are at increased risk of cardiovascular disease. The presence of PDR should not be considered a contraindication to aspirin use.

Aldose reductase inhibitors   A medical approach for preventing the development of retinopathy that has been hypothesized for decades involves blocking the effects of the enzyme aldose reductase.[85] This enzyme facilitates the conversion of glucose to sorbitol. Animal experiments suggest that an aldose reductase inhibitor could slow the development of diabetic retinopathy.[86–90] Unfortunately, clinical trials in patients with diabetes have not yet demonstrated any slowing of the progression of retinopathy. The Sorbinil Retinopathy Trial enrolled 497 insulin-dependent diabetes mellitus patients with little or no retinopathy. After 3 to 4 years of follow-up, progression of diabetic retinopathy and neuropathy were apparently unaffected by administration of the drug Sorbinil.[91,92] However, interest continues in developing more potent inhibitors which will perhaps slow the progression of diabetic retinopathy or neuropathy.

Other medical treatments

A variety of other medical approaches to reducing the secondary complications of diabetes are currently under evaluation. Drugs with antiangiogenic activity, such as inhibitors of vascular endothelial growth factor and growth hormone antagonists, are in early clinical trials, as are inhibitors of advanced glycated end products.[93–96] Prevention will inevitably be more effective than treatment, and methods to prevent the development of diabetes and improved techniques for blood glucose control are also being tested.

SUMMARY

Based on the results of controlled clinical trials that have accumulated over the past several decades, we now have highly beneficial methods for the treatment of diabetic retinopathy. However, diabetic retinopathy remains the leading cause of visual loss in the USA among working-age Americans. This is unfortunate because, when properly treated, the 5-year risk of blindness for patients with PDR is reduced by 90% and the risk of visual loss from macular edema is reduced by 50%.[64] Unfortunately, only

50% of patients with diabetes receive regular dilated eye examinations, and many patients go blind without treatment,[97–99] despite the fact that the value of screening eye examinations has been well documented.[549] Many professional groups, including the American Diabetes Association, the American College of Physicians, the American Academy of Ophthalmology, and the American Optometric Association, have provided guidelines for their members as to when eye examinations should be performed (Table 67-2). The follow-up of patients with diabetic retinopathy depends on the status of the retinopathy (Table 67-3). It is hoped that heightened emphasis on identifying patients who are at risk and the use of new screening methods will reduce the number of patients who do not have regular eye examinations. Improved patient education programs, such as the National Eye Health Education Program, can motivate patients to take better care of themselves.[100–102] Access to the educational materials and facilities that will enable patients to improve the control of their diabetes will lead to fewer secondary complications. Prevention is cost-effective.[103,104] The record of carefully developing new treatments for diabetic retinopathy is a good one. With continued careful research, we can further reduce the risk of blindness from diabetic retinopathy.

ACKNOWLEDGMENT

The authors would like to thank Dr. Matthew D. Davis and the staff of the Fundus Reading Center at the University of Wisconsin for providing the fundus photographs.

REFERENCES

1. Kuwabara T, Cogan DG. Retinal vascular patterns. I. Normal architecture. Arch Ophthalmol 1960; 64:904–911.
2. Bloodworth JMB. Fine structure of retina in human and canine diabetes mellitus. In: Kimuara SJ, Caygill WM, eds. Vascular complications of diabetes mellitus. St Louis: Mosby; 1967.
3. Engerman RL. Pathogenesis of diabetic retinopathy. Diabetes 1989; 38:1203–1206.
4. Frank RN. On the pathogenesis of diabetic retinopathy – a 1990 update. Ophthalmology 1991; 98:586–593.
5. Cogan DG, Toussaint D, Kuwabara T. Retinal vascular patterns. IV. Diabetic retinopathy, Arch Ophthalmol 1961; 66:366–378.
6. Frank RN. Etiologic mechanisms in diabetic retinopathy. In: Ryan SJ, Schachat AP, Murphy RP et al., eds. Retina, vol. 2. Medical retina. St Louis: Mosby; 1989.
7. Wise GN. Retinal neovascularization. Trans Am Ophthalmol Soc 1956; 54:729–826.
8. De Venecia G, Davis M, Engerman R. Clinicopathologic correlations in diabetic retinopathy. I. Histology and fluorescein angiography of microaneurysms. Arch Ophthalmol 1976; 94:1766–1773.
9. Klein R, Meuer SM, Moss SE et al. The relationship of retinal microaneurysm counts to the 4-year progression of diabetic retinopathy. Arch Ophthalmol 1989; 107:1780–1785.
10. Klein R, Meuer SM, Moss SE et al. Retinal micro-aneurysm counts and 10-year progression of diabetic retinopathy. Arch Ophthalmol 1995; 113:1386–1391.
11. Kohner EM, Sleightholm M, and The Kroc Collaborative Study Group. Does microaneurysm count reflect severity of early diabetic retinopathy? Ophthalmology 1986; 93:586–589.
12. Ferris FL III, Patz A. Macular edema: a complication of diabetic retinopathy. Surv Ophthalmol 1984; 28 (suppl):452–461.
13. Patz A, Schatz H, Berkow JW et al. Macular edema – an overlooked complication of diabetic retinopathy. Trans Am Acad Ophthalmol Otolaryngol 1977; 77:34–42.
14. King RC. Exudative diabetic retinopathy. Br J Ophthalmol 1963; 47:666–672.
15. Sigurdsson R, Begg I. Organized macular plaques in exudative diabetic maculopathy. Br J Ophthalmol 1980; 64:392–397.
16. Chew EY, Klein ML, Ferris FL III et al. Association of elevated serum lipid levels with retinal hard exudate in diabetic retinopathy. Arch Ophthalmol 1996; 114:1079–1084.

Table 67-2 Eye examination schedule		
Time of onset of diabetes mellitus	Recommended time for first examination	Routine minimum follow-up
Less than 30 years of age	5 years after onset	Annually
Age 30 and older	At time of diagnosis	Annually
Before pregnancy	Before or soon after conception	At least every 3 months

Table 67-3 Recommended follow-up schedule	
Status of retinopathy	Follow-up (months)
No retinopathy or microaneurysms only	12
Mild/moderate NPDR without macular edema	6–12
Mild/moderate NPDR with macular edema that is not clinically significant	4–6
Mild/moderate NPDR with clinically significant macular edema	3–4
Severe/very severe NPDR	3–4

NPDR, Nonproliferative diabetic retinopathy.

17. Klein BEK, Moss SE, Klein R et al. The Wisconsin Epidemiologic Study of Diabetic Retinopathy. XIII. Relationship of serum cholesterol to retinopathy and hard exudates. Ophthalmology 1991; 98:1261–1265.

18. Strom C, Sander B, Larsen N et al. Diabetic macular edema assessed with optical coherence tomography and stereo fundus photography. Invest Ophthalmol Vis Sci 2002; 43:241–245.

19. Kaiser PK, Rieman CD, Sears JE et al. Macular traction detachment and diabetic macular edema associated with poster hyaloidal traction. Am J Ophthalmol 2001; 131:44–49.

20. Massin P, Graham D, Erginay A et al. Optical coherence tomography for evaluating diabetic macular edema before and after vitrectomy. Am J Ophthalmol 2003; 135:169–177.

21. Early Treatment Diabetic Retinopathy Study Research Group. Fundus photographic risk factors for progression of diabetic retinopathy. ETDRS report no 12. Ophthalmology 1991; 98:823–833.

22. Murphy RP. Management of diabetic retinopathy. Am Fam Phys 1995; 51:785–796.

23. Early Treatment Diabetic Retinopathy Study Research Group. Photocoagulation for diabetic macular edema. ETDRS report no 1. Arch Ophthalmol 1985; 103:1796–1806.

24. Wilkinson CP, Ferris FL, Klein RE et al. Proposed internation clinical diabetic retinopathy and diabetic macular edema disease severity scales. Ophthalmology 2003; 110:1677–1682.

25. Centers for Disease Control (www.cdc.gov/diabetes/news/docs/dpp.htm).

26. The Eye Disease Prevalence Research Group. The prevalence of diabetic retinopathy among adults in the United States. Arch Ophthalmol 2004; 122:552–563.

27. Harris M, Flega KM, Cowie CC et al. Prevalence of diabetes, impaired fasting glucose and impaired glucose tolerance in US adults: the Third National Health and Nutrition Examination Survey, 1988–1994. Diabetes Care 1998; 21:518–524.

28. Klein R, Klein BEK, Moss SE et al. The Wisconsin Epidemiologic Study of Diabetic Retinopathy. II. Prevalence and risk of diabetic retinopathy when age at diagnosis is less than 30 years. Arch Ophthalmol 1984; 102:520–526.

29. Klein R, Klein BEK, Moss SE et al. The Wisconsin Epidemiologic Study of Diabetic Retinopathy. III. Prevalence and risk of diabetic retinopathy when age at diagnosis is 30 or more years. Arch Ophthalmol 1984; 102:527–532.

30. Klein R, Klein BEK, Moss SE et al. Is blood pressure a predictor of the incidence or progression of diabetic retinopathy? Arch Intern Med 1989; 149:2427–2432.

31. Diabetes Control and Complications Trial Research Group. The effect of intensive treatment of diabetes on the development and progression of long-term complications in insulin-dependent diabetes mellitus. N Engl J Med 1993; 329:977–986.

32. Diabetes Control and Complications Trial Research Group. The effect of intensive diabetes treatment on the progression of diabetic retinopathy in insulin-dependent diabetes mellitus. Arch Ophthalmol 1995; 113:36–51.

33. Diabetes Control and Complications Trial Research Group. The relationship of glycemic exposures (HbA$_1$C) to the risk of development and progression of retinopathy in the Diabetes Control and Complications Trial. Diabetes 1995; 44:968–983.

34. Diabetes Control and Complications Trial Research Group. Perspectives in diabetes: the absence of a glycemic threshold for the development of long-term complications: the perspective of the Diabetes Control and Complications Trial. Diabetes 1996; 45:1289–1298.

35. Reichard P, Nilsson BY, Rosenqvist U. The effect of long-term intensified insulin treatment on the development of microvascular complications of diabetes mellitus. N Engl J Med 1993; 329:304–309.

36. The Diabetes Control and Complications Trial/Epidemiology of Diabetes Intervention and Complications Study Research Group. Effects of intensive therapy on the microvascular complications of type 1 diabetes mellitus. JAMA 2002; 287:2563–2569.

37. Klein R, Klein B, Moss S. Relation of glycemic control to diabetic microvascular complications in diabetes mellitus. Ann Intern Med 1996; 124:90–96.

38. Ohkubo Y, Hideke K, Eiichi A et al. Intensive insulin therapy prevents the progression of diabetic microvascular complications in Japanese patients with non-insulin-dependent diabetes mellitus: a randomized prospective 6-year study. Diabetes Res Clin Pract 1995; 28:103–117.

39. UK Prospective Diabetes Study Group. Effect of intensive blood-glucose control with metformin on complications in overweight patients with type 2 diabetes (UKPDS 34). Lancet 1988; 352:854–865.

40. UK Prospective Diabetes Study Group. Intensive blood-glucose control with sulphonylureas or insulin compared with conventional treatment and risk of complications in patients with type 2 diabetes (UKPDS 33). Lancet 1988; 352:837–853.

41. UK Prospective Diabetes Study Group. Tight blood pressure control and risk of macrovascular and microvascular complications in type 2 diabetes (UKPDS 38). Br Med J 1998; 317:703–713.

42. Chaturvedi N, Sjolie AK, Stephen JM et al. Effect of lisinopril on progression of retinopathy in normotensive people with type 1 diabetes. Lancet 1998; 351:28–31.

43. Fong DS, Segal PP, Myers F et al. Subretinal fibrosis in diabetic macular edema. ETDRS report no 23. Arch Ophthalmol 1997; 115:873–877.

44. Lyons TJ, Jenkins AJ, Zhen D et al. Diabetic retinopathy and serum lipoprotein subclasses in the DCCT/EDIC cohort. Invest Ophthalm Vis Sci 2004; 45:910–918.

45. Kostraba JN, Klein R, Dorman JS et al. The epidemiology of diabetes complications study. IV. Correlates of diabetic background and proliferative retinopathy, Am J Epidemiol 1991; 133:381–391.

46. Chew EY, Mills JL, Metzger BE et al. Metabolic control and progression of retinopathy. The Diabetes in Early Pregnancy Study. National Institute of Child Health and Human Development Diabetes in Early Pregnancy Study. Diabetes Care 1995; 18:631–637.

47. Klein BEK, Moss SE, Klein R. Effect of pregnancy on progression of diabetic retinopathy. Diabetes Care 1990; 13:34–40.

48. Phelps RL, Sakol P, Metzger BE et al. Changes in diabetic retinopathy during pregnancy: correlations with regulation of hyperglycemia. Arch Ophthalmol 1986; 104:1806–1810.

49. The Diabetes Control and Complications Trial Research Group. Effect of pregnancy on the microvascular complications. Diabetes Care 2000; 23:1084–1091.

50. American Academy of Ophthalmology. Preferred practice pattern. Diabetic retinopathy no. 110020. San Francisco: AAO; 1998.

51. Davis MD, Fisher MR, Gangnon RE et al. Risk factors for high-risk proliferative diabetic retinopathy and severe visual loss. ETDRS report no. 18, Invest Ophthalmol Vis Sci 1998; 39:233–252.

52. Janka HU, Warram JH, Rand LI et al. Risk factors for progression of background retinopathy in long-standing IDDM. Diabetes 1989; 38:460–464.

53. Rand LI, Prud'homme GJ, Ederer F et al. Factors influencing the development of visual loss in advanced diabetic retinopathy. DRS report no. 10. Invest Ophthalmol Vis Sci 1985; 26:983–991.

54. Berman DH, Friedman EA. Partial absorption of hard exudates in patients with diabetic end-stage renal disease and severe anemia after treatment with erythropoietin. Retina 1994; 14:1–5.

55. Qiao Q, Keinanen-Kiukaanniemi S, Laara E. The relationship between hemoglobin levels and diabetic retinopathy. J Clin Epidemiol 1997; 50:153–158.

56. Shorb SR. Anemia and diabetic retinopathy. Am J Ophthalmol 1985; 100:434–436.

57. Krolewski AS, Barzilay J, Warram JH et al. Risk of early-onset proliferative diabetic retinopathy in IDDM is closely related to cardiovascular autonomic neuropathy. Diabetes 1992; 41:430–437.

58. Tesfaye S, Stevens LK, Stephenson JM et al. Prevalence of diabetic peripheral neuropathy and its relation to glycaemic control and potential risk factors: The EURODIAB IDDM complications study. Diabetologia 1996; 39:1377–1384.

59. Diabetic Retinopathy Study Research Group. Photocoagulation treatment of proliferative diabetic retinopathy. DRS report no 2. Ophthalmology 1978; 85:82–105.

60. Diabetic Retinopathy Study Research Group. Four risk factors for severe visual loss in diabetic retinopathy. DRS report no 3. Arch Ophthalmol 1979; 97:654–655.

61. Diabetic Retinopathy Study Research Group. Clinical application of Diabetic Retinopathy Study (DRS) findings, DRS report no 8, Ophthalmology 88:583–600, 1981.

62. Diabetic Retinopathy Study Research Group. Photocoagulation treatment of proliferative diabetic retinopathy: relationship of adverse treatment effects to retinopathy severity. Dev Ophthalmol 1981; 2:248–261.

63. Early Treatment Diabetic Retinopathy Study Research Group. Techniques for scatter and local photocoagulation treatment of diabetic retinopathy. ETDRS report no. 3. Int Ophthalmol Clin 1987; 27:254–264.

64. Early Treatment Diabetic Retinopathy Study Research Group. Early photocoagulation for diabetic retinopathy. ETDRS report no. 9. Ophthalmology 1991; 98 (suppl):767–785.

65. Ferris F. Early photocoagulation in patients with either type I or type II diabetes. Trans Am Ophthalmol Soc 1996; 94:505–537.

66. Early Treatment Diabetic Retinopathy Study Research Group. Photocoagulation for diabetic macular edema. ETDRS report no. 4. Int Ophthalmol Clin 1987; 27:265–272.

67. Early Treatment Diabetic Retinopathy Study Research Group. Treatment techniques and clinical guidelines for photocoagulation of diabetic macular edema. ETDRS report no. 2. Ophthalmology 1987; 94:761–774.

68. Early Treatment Diabetic Retinopathy Study Research Group. Photocoagulation for diabetic macular edema: relationship of treatment effect to fluorescein angiographic and other retinal characteristics at baseline. ETDRS report no. 19. Arch Ophthalmol 1995; 113:1144–1155.

69. Han DP, Miller WF, Burton TC. Submacular fibrosis after photocoagulation for diabetic macular edema. Am J Ophthalmol 1992; 113:513–521.

70. Lewis H, Schachat AP, Haimann MH et al. Choroidal neovascularization after laser photocoagulation for diabetic macular edema. Ophthalmology 1990; 97:503–511.

71. Martidis A, Duker JS, Greenberg PB et al. Intravitreal triamcinolone for refractory diabetic macular edema. Ophthalmology 2002; 109:920–927.

72. Jonas JB, Kreissing I, Sofker A et al. Intravitreal injection of triamcinolone for diffuse macular edema. Arch Ophthalmol 2003; 121:57–61.

73. Massin P, Audren F, Haouchine B et al. Intravitreal triamcinolone acetonide for diabetic diffuse macular edema. Ophthalmology 2004; 111:218–225.

74. Brown JC, Soloman S, Bressler SB et al. Detection of diabetic foveal edema. Contact lens biomicroscopy compared with optical coherence tomography. Arch Ophthalmol 2004; 122:330–335.

75. Dipyridamole Aspirin Microangiopathy of Diabetes Study Group. Effect of aspirin alone and aspirin plus dipyridamole in early diabetic retinopathy: a multicenter, randomized, controlled clinical trial. Diabetes 1989; 38:491–498.

76. Ticlopidine Microangiography of Diabetes Study Group. Ticlopidine treatment reduces the progression of nonproliferative diabetic retinopathy. Arch Ophthalmol 1990; 108:1577–1583.

77. Carroll WW, Geeraets WJ. Diabetic retinopathy and salicylates. Ann Ophthalmol 1972; 4:1019–1046.

78. Kuwabara T, Cogan DG. Retinal vascular patterns. VI. Mural cells of retinal capillaries. Arch Ophthalmol 1963; 69:492–502.

79. Powell EDU, Field RA. Diabetic retinopathy and rheumatoid arthritis. Lancet 1964; 2:17–18.

80. Regnault F. Role des plaguettes dans la pathogenie de la retinopathie diabetique. Sem Hop Paris 1972; 48:893–902.

81. Sagel J, Colwell JA, Crook L et al. Increased platelet aggregation in early diabetes mellitus. Ann Intern Med 1975; 82:733–738.

82. Chew EY, Klein ML, Murphy RP et al. Effects of aspirin on vitreous/pre-retinal hemorrhage in patients with diabetes mellitus. ETDRS report no. 20. Arch Ophthalmol 1995; 113:52–55.

83. Early Treatment Diabetic Retinopathy Study Research Group. Effects of aspirin treatment on diabetic retinopathy. ETDRS report no. 8. Ophthalmology 1991; 98:757–765.

84. Early Treatment Diabetic Retinopathy Study Research Group. Aspirin effects on mortality and morbidity in patients with diabetes mellitus. ETDRS report no. 14. JAMA 1992; 268:1292–1300.

85. Frank RN. Perspectives in diabetes: the aldose reductase controversy. Diabetes 1994; 43:169–172.

86. Engerman RL, Kern TS. Experimental galactosemia produces diabetic-like retinopathy. Diabetes 1984; 33:97–100.

87. Kador PF, Akagi Y, Takahashi Y et al. Prevention of retinal vessel changes associated with diabetic retinopathy in galactose-fed dogs by aldose reductase inhibitors. Arch Ophthalmol 1990; 108:1301–1309.

88. Kador PF, Akagi Y, Takahashi Y et al. Prevention of pericyte ghost formation in retinal capillaries of galactose-fed dogs by aldose reductase inhibitors. Arch Ophthalmol 1988; 106:1099–1102.

89. Robison WG Jr, Laver NM, Jacot JL et al. Diabetic-like retinopathy ameliorated with the aldose reductase inhibitor WAY-121,509. Invest Ophthalmol Vis Sci 1996; 37:1149–1156.

90. Robison WG Jr, Nagata M, Laver N et al. Diabetic-like retinopathy in rats prevented with an aldose reductase inhibitor. Invest Ophthalmol Vis Sci 1989; 30:2285–2292.

91. Sorbinil Retinopathy Trial Research Group. A randomized trial of sorbinil, an aldose reductase inhibitor, in diabetic retinopathy. Arch Ophthalmol 1990; 108:1234–1244.

92. Sorbinil Retinopathy Trial Research Group. The sorbinil retinopathy trial: neuropathy results. Neurology 1993; 43:1141–1149.

93. Aiello LP, Pierce EA, Foley ED et al. Suppression of retinal neovascularization in vivo by inhibition of vascular endothelial growth factor (VEGF) using soluble VGEF-receptor dimeric proteins. Proc Nat Acad Sci USA 1995; 92:10457–10461.

94. Brownlee M, Cerami A, Vlassara H. Advanced glycosylation end products in tissue and the biochemical basis of diabetic complications. N Engl J Med 1986; 318:1315–1321.

95. Brownlee M, Vlassara H, Kooney A et al. Aminoguanidine prevents diabetes-induced arterial wall protein cross-linking. Science 1986; 232:1629–1632.

96. Smith LE, Kopchick JJ, Chen W et al. Essential role of growth hormone in ischemia-induced retinal neovascularization. Science 1997; 276:1706–1709.

97. Moss S, Klein R, Klein B. Factors associated with having eye examinations in persons with diabetes. Arch Fam Med 1995; 4:529–534.

98. Sprafka J, Fritsc T, Baker R et al. Prevalence of undiagnosed eye disease in high-risk diabetic individuals. Arch Intern Med 1990; 150:857–861.

99. Will J, German R, Schuman E et al. Patient adherence to guidelines for diabetes eye care: results from the diabetic eye disease follow-up study. Am J Public Health 1994; 84:1669–1671.

100. Klein R. Eye-care delivery for people with diabetes (commentary). Diabetes Care 1994; 17:614–615.

101. Klein R. Barriers to prevention of vision loss caused by diabetic retinopathy (editorial). Arch Ophthalmol 1997; 115:1073–1075.

102. Kupfer C. The challenge of transferring research results into patient care. Ophthalmology 1989; 96:737–738.

103. Ackerman SJ. Benefits of preventive programs in eye care are visible on the bottom line. Diabetes Care 1992; 15:580–581.

104. Diabetes Control and Complications Trial Research Group. Lifetime benefits and costs of intensive therapy as practiced in the diabetes control and complications trial. JAMA 1996; 276:1409–1415.

Chapter

68

Proliferative Diabetic Retinopathy

Matthew D. Davis
Barbara A. Blodi

Proliferation of vascular endothelial cells within the retina is considered an essential part of the pathogenesis of lesions such as intraretinal microvascular abnormalities (IRMAs) and venous beading or reduplication commonly seen in the severe stage of nonproliferative diabetic retinopathy (NPDR).[1–6] However, the presence of these lesions alone is not sufficient to meet the conventional definition of proliferative diabetic retinopathy (PDR), which requires *the presence of newly formed blood vessels or fibrous tissue, or both, arising from the retina or optic disc and extending along the inner surface of the retina or disc or into the vitreous cavity.* This section begins with a brief discussion of the circumstances under which preretinal new vessels appear and continues with their early clinical recognition. This is followed by a detailed description of the natural course of PDR, emphasizing four fundamental processes: (1) the cycle of proliferation and regression typical of new vessels; (2) proliferation of fibrous tissue accompanying new vessels; (3) formation of adhesions between the fibrovascular proliferations and the posterior vitreous surface; and (4) contraction of the posterior vitreous surface and associated proliferations. Other sections of this chapter consider the relationships of PDR to duration and type of diabetes, glycemic control, and other factors. Finally, the treatment of PDR is reviewed, with emphasis on findings of clinical trials and guidelines for management when the response to initial photocoagulation is disappointing.

ORIGIN AND EARLY RECOGNITION OF PRERETINAL NEW VESSELS

For many years most observers have agreed that the most plausible pathogenetic explanation for endothelial proliferation and new-vessel formation in the retina is ischemia of its inner layers secondary to closure of parts of the retinal capillary bed.[2,7–10] The ischemic retina is postulated to produce a new vessel-stimulating factor, capable of acting locally and diffusing through the vitreous to other areas of the retina, to the optic disc, and into the anterior chamber (where it is thought to be the cause of neovascularization on the iris and in the chamber angle).[8,10–12] Recent research has provided several candidates for the role of the postulated retinal angiogenesis factor, the most promising of which is vascular endothelial growth factor (VEGF), discussed in Chapter 65.

The background of intraretinal lesions against which preretinal new vessels arise is variable. The risk of PDR is greatest in eyes with severe NPDR (preproliferative retinopathy), characterized by the presence of soft exudates (cottonwool patches), IRMAs (a term chosen so as to be neutral about whether these abnormal vessels represent intraretinal new vessels or dilated pre-existing vessels), venous beading, and extensive retinal hemorrhages or microaneurysms (Fig. 68-1). In the Diabetic Retinopathy Study (DRS) *severe NPDR* was defined as the presence of at least three of the above four characteristics, each generally involving at least two quadrants of the fundus. About 50% of such eyes assigned to the untreated control group had developed PDR within 15 months.[13] Additional information concerning relationships between severity of NPDR and risk of PDR is included in the section on indications for photocoagulation, below.

The lesions characterizing severe NPDR are related to retinal capillary closure, and their frequent presence in eyes that are about to develop preretinal new vessels is one important observation linking these processes. Further evidence has been provided by the beautiful fluorescein angiographic montages of Shimizu et al.,[9] who found that the extent of capillary closure seen on angiography increased as the severity of new vessels increased on the following four-step scale: (1) none; (2) new vessels involving the retina but sparing the disc; (3) new vessels involving the disc; and (4) neovascularization of the anterior chamber angle with neovascular glaucoma. Muraoka & Shimizu[6] have provided serial fluorescein angiographic observations supporting the view that some lesions designated as IRMAs or reduplication of small venules are in fact intraretinal new vessels revascularizing areas of capillary loss.

Although there is little doubt that the presence of severe NPDR is predictive of subsequent neovascularization, the characteristic intraretinal lesions are not always present when preretinal new vessels are first recognized. A possible explanation for this is the relatively transient nature of some of these lesions. Soft exudates usually disappear within 6 to 12 months. Blot hemorrhages and IRMA tend to disappear after extensive capillary closure, when the number of small vascular branches decreases and some small arterioles become white threads, producing a picture aptly described as *featureless retina* (Fig. 68-2B). However, in some eyes intraretinal lesions are mild, and signs of extensive capillary closure are absent when new vessels are first recognized. It seems likely that at least some of these eyes have not previously had severe NPDR.

Although new vessels may arise anywhere in the retina, they are most frequently seen posteriorly, within about 45 degrees of

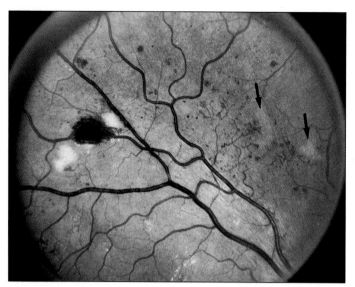

Fig. 68-1 Severe nonproliferative diabetic retinopathy (NPDR). On the left are two prominent soft exudates with a large blot hemorrhage between them. Venous beading is present where the superior branch of the superotemporal vein passes by the upper exudate. On the right are two faint soft exudates (arrows) and many intraretinal microvascular abnormalities. (Courtesy of Early Treatment Diabetic Retinopathy Study Research Group.)

the optic disc. They are particularly common on the disc itself (Davis[14]: 69% of 155 eyes with PDR; Taylor & Dobree[15]: 73% of 86 eyes). In the DRS, among 1377 control-group eyes with new vessels present in baseline photographs, 15% had new vessels only on or within 1 disc diameter (DD) of the disc or in the vitreous cavity anterior to this area (new vessels on disc, or NVDs); 40% had new vessels only outside this zone (new vessels elsewhere, or NVEs); and 45% had new vessels in both zones.[16]

NVDs begin as fine loops or networks of vessels lying on the surface of the disc or bridging across the physiologic cup. They are usually easily identified, but in their earliest stages they may be overlooked with the low magnification of binocular indirect ophthalmoscopy. They also may be difficult to distinguish from normal vessels in nonstereoscopic photographs or with monocular direct ophthalmoscopy. The most satisfactory examining methods are those that provide a magnified stereoscopic view, either biomicroscopy with contact or precorneal lens or stereoscopic 30-degree photography. If any doubt remains, it can usually be resolved by fluorescein angiography, which demonstrates the profuse leakiness characteristic of preretinal new vessels (Fig. 68-2).

Detection of early NVEs requires, first, that these vessels be found and, second, that they be differentiated from IRMAs. The ideal search for new vessels combines binocular indirect ophthalmoscopy of the entire retina with a biomicroscopic or direct ophthalmoscopic examination of the area within 5 or 6 DD of the disc and of any suspicious lesions outside this area noted during indirect ophthalmoscopy. A brief fundus diagram made during the indirect ophthalmoscopic examination is very helpful. It is also beneficial to add four colors to the six conventionally used in fundus diagrams: (1) purple, for new vessels on the surface of the retina or disc; (2) orange, for elevated new vessels; (3) pale green,

for fibrous proliferations; and (4) pink, for red hemorrhage in the vitreous (with red retained for retinal or preretinal hemorrhage and dark green used for white blood in the vitreous).[17] When the media are clear, fundus photographs may obviate the need for a fundus diagram (but not for the binocular indirect ophthalmoscopic examination). When new vessels or fibrous proliferations are extensive, wide-angle (45-degree or, preferably, 60-degree) photographs have the advantage of providing in one or two fields an integrated view of all or most of these lesions. However, a well-dilated pupil is necessary, particularly for stereophotographs, and subtle lesions are easily overlooked. For detection of early NVEs, stereophotographs with a 30-degree camera are superior, particularly if taken by an experienced photographer with the outstanding optical system of the original Zeiss fundus camera. In most patients an adequate stereoscopic effect can be obtained in all the seven standard fields of the modified Airlie House classification[18] (Fig. 68-3) with pupillary dilation of 4 or 5 mm, although maximal dilation should always be the aim. Photographers should routinely scan the fundus for definite or questionable NVEs outside the standard fields, particularly between and above fields 4 and 6, between and below fields 5 and 7, and temporal to fields 4 and 5. Subsequent follow-up visits are greatly facilitated by a set of 30-degree stereophotographs from the baseline examination.

When new vessels are not discovered by any of these techniques but are strongly suspected because of recent vitreous hemorrhage, examination of the more peripheral retina with biomicroscopy and the Goldmann three-mirror lens may be helpful. In this situation some observers also recommend fluorescein angioscopy using the binocular indirect ophthalmoscope with a dark-blue filter over the light source. In our experience this is rarely necessary. The possibility that the vitreous hemorrhage may come from a peripheral retinal tear, unrelated to diabetic retinopathy, should be kept in mind, and a careful examination of the peripheral fundus with scleral depression should be performed.

More difficult than finding NVEs may be distinguishing between NVEs and IRMAs. This is particularly true if IRMAs are extensive and NVEs do not yet show any of their unique features: formation of wheel-like networks, extension across both arterial and venous branches of the underlying retinal vascular network, and accompanying fibrous proliferations (see later discussion). Biomicroscopy with a flat, front-surfaced contact lens provides the best opportunity to recognize these features and to appreciate the slightly more superficial location characteristic of preretinal new vessels. It is desirable to begin this examination with a broad, low-intensity illuminating beam placed between the microscope objectives. This provides an overall view with easy orientation to other fundus features, good magnification, and excellent stereopsis. Subsequently, a narrow, bright illuminating beam can be placed at an angle to the viewing axis to assess vitreoretinal relationships and subtle changes in retinal thickness. For maximal image clarity it is important that the front surface of the contact lens be almost perpendicular to the viewing axis. In borderline cases fluorescein angiography can distinguish between the profuse leakiness of preretinal new vessels and IRMAs. However, this is usually unnecessary, since the true nature of such borderline lesions soon becomes clear with careful follow-up.

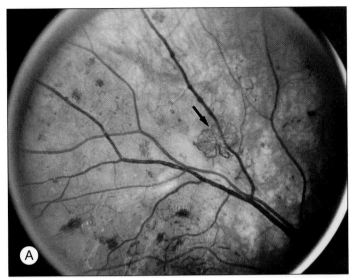

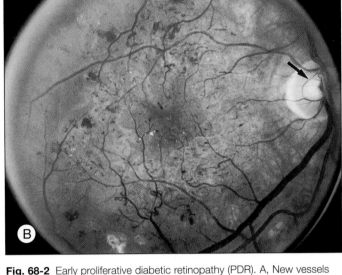

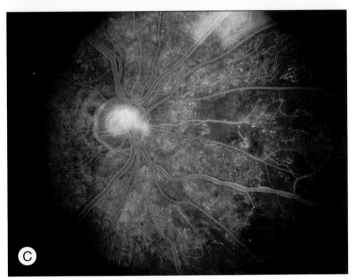

Fig. 68-2 Early proliferative diabetic retinopathy (PDR). A, New vessels form a small wheel-like network (arrow) in the superotemporal quadrant of an eye with venous beading, soft exudates, intraretinal microvascular abnormalities (IRMAs), and blot hemorrhages. B, Posterior pole of the same eye, showing IRMAs and retinal hemorrhages centrally and a featureless retina near the left edge of the figure. With stereoscopic examination, the vascular loop on the disc (arrow) could be seen to bridge the physiologic cup and was clearly a new vessel. C, In the late-stage angiogram, new vessels on the disc are no longer filled with fluorescent blood; they stand out in contrast to the pool of fluorescein that has leaked from them. Prominent fluorescein leakage along the superonasal vein at the upper edge of the figure is from new vessels there. An area of capillary dropout is located nasal to the disc. (Courtesy of Early Treatment Diabetic Retinopathy Study Research Group.)

NATURAL COURSE OF PROLIFERATIVE DIABETIC RETINOPATHY

Proliferation and regression of new vessels

Initially, new vessels may be barely visible. Later their caliber is commonly one-eighth to one-fourth that of a major retinal vein at the disc margin, and occasionally they are as large as such veins (Fig. 68-4). New vessels frequently form networks that often resemble part or all of a carriage wheel. The vessels radiate like spokes from the center of the patch to a circumferential vessel bounding its periphery (see Figs 68-2A and 68-7, below). New vessel networks may also be irregular in shape, without a distinct radial pattern. New vessel patches often lie over retinal veins and appear to drain into them. The superotemporal vein is involved somewhat more frequently than others.[14,15] In the 1158 DRS control-group eyes that had NVEs in at least one of the five photographic fields in which they were graded (fields 3 to 7 in Fig. 68-3), the number of times each field was involved was assessed. In each eye a count of one was divided equally among all fields containing NVEs, and the counts for each field were totaled for all eyes. Field 4, which usually includes a major portion of the superotemporal vein, had a score of 308 (27% of 1158), whereas other scores ranged from 194 (17%) for field 5 to 242 (21%) for field 7.[19]

At times new vessels grow for several disc diameters across the retina without forming prominent networks. They appear much like normal retinal vessels but are easily recognized as new vessels because of their unique capability of crossing both arterioles and veins in the underlying retina (Figs 68-4 and 68-5). New vessels of this type commonly arise on the disc and are often accompanied during their actively growing phase by mild-to-moderate thickening (presumably edema) of the disc and surrounding retina (Fig. 68-6). This appearance is similar to typical cases of diabetic papillopathy,[20] in which all or most of the dilated small vessels on and adjacent to the disc are intraretinal and characteristically do not leak on fluorescein angiography. The disc swelling and intraretinal vessels always regress spontaneously, and associated new vessels often also do so.

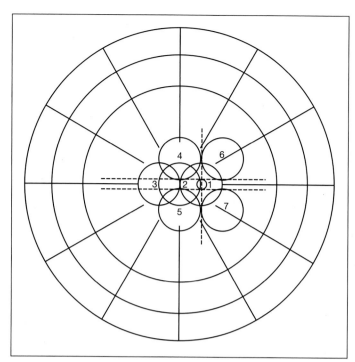

Fig. 68-3 Modified Airlie House classification. Seven standard photographic fields are shown for the right eye. Field 1 is centered on the disc, field 2 on the macula, and field 3 temporal to the macula so that its nasal edge passes through the center of the macula. Fields 4 to 7 are tangent to a vertical line passing through the center of the disc and to horizontal lines passing through its upper and lower poles, as shown. (Reproduced with permission from Diabetic Retinopathy Study Research Group. A modification of the Airlie House classification of diabetic retinopathy. DRS report no. 7. Invest Ophthalmol Vis Sci 1981; 21:210–226.[18])

The rate of growth of new vessels is extremely variable. In some patients a patch of vessels may show little change over many months, whereas in others a definite increase may be seen in 1 or 2 weeks. Early in their evolution new vessels appear bare, but later delicate white fibrous tissue usually becomes visible adjacent to them. The common clinical convention of referring to such tissue as "fibrous" is adhered to in this chapter, even though it has been shown to contain both fibrocytes and glial cells.[21,22] New vessels characteristically follow a cycle of proliferation followed by partial or complete regression.[14,23,24] Regression of a wheel-shaped net of new vessels typically begins with a decrease in the number and caliber of the vessels at the center of the patch, followed by their partial replacement with fibrous tissue. Simultaneously, the peripheral vessels tend to become more narrow, although they may still be growing in length and the patch may still be enlarging (Fig. 68-7). At times, regressing new vessels appear to become sheathed. The width of the sheath, which presumably represents opacification and thickening of the vessel wall, increases until only a network of white lines without visible blood columns remains (see Fig. 68-10, below). At times certain new vessels seem to become preferential channels, enlarging while adjacent vessels regress and disappear. Fresh, active new vessels are commonly seen emerging from the edges of partially regressed patches, and new vessels are frequently seen at different stages of development in different areas of the same eye. Early in their evolution the fibrous components of fibrovascular proliferations tend to be translucent and are easily underestimated. Subsequently, with increasing growth, contraction, or separation from the retina, they become more prominent. If contraction of the vitreous and fibrovascular proliferations does not occur, new vessels may pass through all the stages described here without causing any visual symptoms. Concurrently, a decrease in intraretinal lesions and in the caliber of major retinal vessels may occur as retinopathy enters the burned-out stage. Occasionally, new vessels appear to regress completely, leaving no trace of their previous presence.[25]

Contraction of the vitreous and fibrovascular proliferations

Before the onset of posterior vitreous detachment, neovascular networks appear to be on or slightly anterior to the retina, both by biomicroscopy and in stereophotographs. At this stage slit-lamp examination of new vessel patches that appear to be slightly elevated shows no change in the vitreous adjacent to them nor any separation between them and the retina. This suggests that mild thickening of the retina is responsible for the slightly elevated appearance of the new vessels. Typically, the edges of such a new vessel patch are tightly apposed to the retina, and its center appears slightly elevated, giving the patch as a whole a mildly convex curvature. Nearly all new-vessel patches are adherent to the posterior vitreous surface. This adhesion becomes apparent when posterior vitreous detachment occurs adjacent to the patch, pulling its edge forward. If vitreous detachment surrounds the patch, all its edges become more elevated than its center, giving its anterior surface a concave appearance.

Before the beginning of posterior vitreous detachment, new vessels are usually asymptomatic.[14,24,26] Small hemorrhages in the posterior vitreous are occasionally seen near the growing ends of the new vessels, but they usually remain subhyaloid or hang suspended in the most posterior portion of the vitreous without becoming apparent to the patient. When symptomatic vitreous hemorrhages do occur, some evidence of localized posterior vitreous detachment can usually be found. When only a small area of the posterior vitreous surface is detached, it appears flat and very close to the retina; but as detachment becomes more extensive, this surface moves forward and assumes a curved contour more or less parallel to the retina and about 0.5 to 2 DD anterior to it. This otherwise smoothly curved surface is held posteriorly by vitreoretinal adhesions at the sites of new vessels. The new vessels in turn tend to be pulled forward in these same areas. Vitreous strands and opacities can usually be seen anterior to the posterior vitreous surface, whereas posteriorly the vitreous cavity is optically empty or contains red blood cells.[14,27] The principal force pulling the posterior vitreous surface forward usually appears to be the forward vector resulting from contraction of this surface and the fibrovascular proliferations growing along it. In explaining this process to students and patients, it helps to use the analogy of a bowl lined with a piece of cloth attached to the rim of the bowl: if the cloth shrinks, it eventually becomes tightly stretched across the top of the bowl.

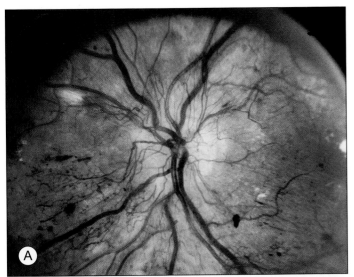

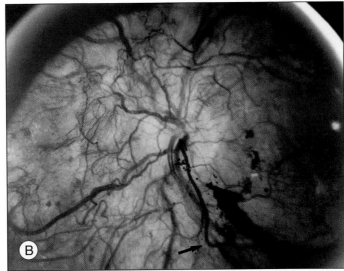

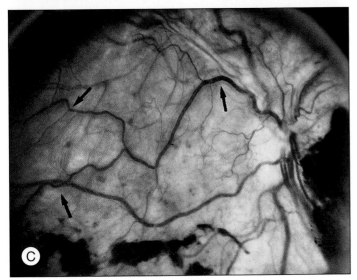

Fig. 68-4 Rapid development of large-caliber new vessels from the disc. A, In the left eye of this 21-year-old white woman, whose age at diagnosis of diabetes was 7 years, new vessels arose on the disc and extended across its margins in all quadrants. The disc margins were blurred. There were soft and hard exudates, intraretinal microvascular abnormalities, and hemorrhages in the retina and on its surface. Blood pressure was 126/96 mmHg. B, Two months later, new vessels had grown remarkably, and preretinal hemorrhage had increased. Arrow indicates large new vessel that crosses the inferotemporal artery and vein. C, Three months later, one of the new vessels (arrows) had become as large as a major retinal vein and extended nasally beyond the edge of the figure. The new vessels on and adjacent to the disc had regressed partially. Two months later, the patient died suddenly of a myocardial infarction.

The thickness of the posterior vitreous surface varies, as indicated by three different appearances. Immediately adjacent to the site of new vessels, the surface is often thick enough to be easily seen with the ophthalmoscope. Presumably this increased opacity is due to proliferation of fibrous tissue along the posterior vitreous surface. In other areas some distance from any visible new vessels, the surface is also sometimes thick enough to be detected ophthalmoscopically or in stereoscopic fundus photographs. In these areas the surface is usually somewhat shiny, with thinner and thicker areas alternating to give a "Swiss-cheese" effect but without actual holes; presumably a thin layer of fibrous tissue is also present here. In still other areas the posterior vitreous surface is so thin that it can be appreciated only by mentally integrating many separate slit-lamp sections. Only the portion directly illuminated by the slit beam is visible, and the impression of a continuous surface is gained by watching the slit beam glide along smoothly over the surface as the slit lamp is moved. Frequently in the same eye all these various appearances can be seen in different areas of the same surface, the general course of the surface continuing without change as its thickness varies (Fig. 68-8).

Posterior vitreous detachment usually begins near the posterior pole, the most common locations being the region of the superotemporal vessels, temporal to the macula, and above or below the disc.[14] Detachment often spreads fairly rapidly (within hours, days, or weeks) to the periphery of the quadrant in which it begins, unless such spread is impeded by vitreoretinal adhesions associated with patches of new vessels. Extension circumferentially into other quadrants of the fundus tends to be slower, sometimes requiring months or years to reach completion. Detachment of the vitreous from the disc is usually prevented by adhesions between the vitreous and fibrovascular proliferations arising there. Vitreous detachment is not a smoothly progressive process. It occurs in abrupt steps, usually halting whenever its advancing edge meets a patch of active or regressed new vessels. If contraction continues, the patch is pulled forward, with or without the underlying retina, and vitreous detachment spreads beyond it. At times the peripheral spread of posterior vitreous detachment is halted temporarily by invisible adhesions to the retina in areas where no new vessels are present. This is indicated by a subtle linear

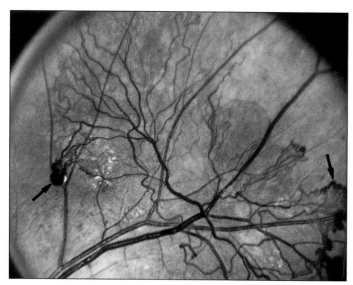

Fig. 68-5 New vessels elsewhere (NVEs) without prominent network formation. Over much of their course, these new vessels did not form networks. Large aneurysmal dilations were present at the end of a long new-vessel loop (left arrow) and at the circumference of a partial wheel-like network (right arrow). (Courtesy of Diabetic Retinopathy Study Research Group.)

within weeks or several months, retaining its red color until absorbed. Hemorrhage in the formed vitreous tends to lose its red color and become white before absorption is complete. Absorption of a large hemorrhage from the formed vitreous is usually slow, requiring many months and often not reaching completion before fresh hemorrhage occurs, except as PDR enters the burned-out stage.

The arrangement and movement of blood in the posterior fluid vitreous often make it possible to define the limits of posterior vitreous detachment ophthalmoscopically.[14,26] In areas of vitreous detachment, the presence of fresh blood in the posterior fluid vitreous obscures fundus details, distinguishing these areas from adjacent ones in which the vitreous remains attached and details of the retina are clear. In the upper quadrants of the fundus, blood tends to become deposited in thin meridional streaks on the detached posterior vitreous surface, identifying its position. Inferiorly, blood pools between the detached vitreous and attached retina, outlining the inferior extent of vitreous detachment and often forming a fluid-level or boat-shaped hemorrhage. At times, even when posterior vitreous detachment cannot definitely be identified with slit lamp and contact lens, a thin, curving line of subhyaloid hemorrhage parallel to and behind the inferior equator can be seen, presumably marking the lower edge of an area of vitreous detachment. When posterior vitreous detachment is complete, blood in the posterior fluid vitreous can be made to flow into the periphery of any quadrant by positioning the patient's head to make that quadrant dependent.

Occasionally the posterior vitreous surface can be traced across the macula on slit-lamp examination, but usually its continuity is lost in this region. In some of these cases a round or oval hole with sharp edges can be detected in the posterior vitreous surface, occupying an area 2 to 4 DD wide in the posterior pole. The posterior vitreous surface in this area appears broken, with solid vitreous protruding back through the hole and coming into contact with the retina. At times the surface of a bulging mushroom of vitreous can be seen extending posteriorly through such a hole, occasion-

elevation of the inner surface of the retina at the junction of posteriorly detached and anteriorly attached vitreous. After several weeks or months vitreous detachment usually spreads farther peripherally, and the subtle retinal fold flattens.

Traction exerted on the new vessels appears to be a factor contributing to the recurrent vitreous hemorrhages that often coincide with extension of vitreous detachment. Hemorrhages also occur independently, sometimes apparently in relation to bouts of severe coughing or vomiting and occasionally at the time of insulin reactions. More often they occur during sleep and are unrelated to any obvious factor.[28,29] Blood in the fluid vitreous posterior to the detached vitreous framework usually absorbs

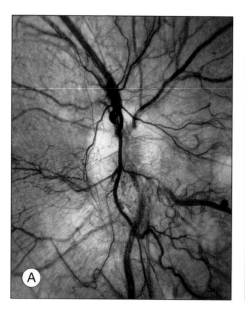
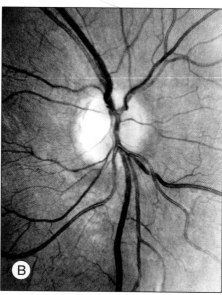

Fig. 68-6 Optic disc swelling. This 20-year-old man, whose diabetes had been diagnosed at age 14, sought ophthalmologic attention because of the sudden onset of floaters, first in the left eye and several days later in the right eye. A, The disc was swollen, had blurred margins, and was partially obscured by extensive new vessels arising on it and extending on to the retina in all quadrants. B, Five months later, disc swelling had resolved, and all new vessels had regressed spontaneously. Vision remained 20/15. (Courtesy of Diabetic Retinopathy Study Research Group.)

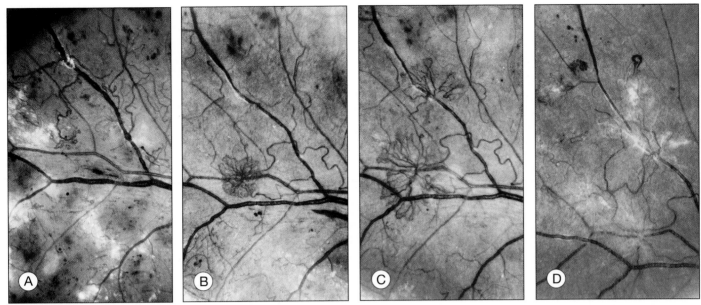

Fig. 68-7 Proliferation and regression of new vessels elsewhere (NVEs). A, Severe nonproliferative diabetic retinopathy in a patient with newly diagnosed type 2 diabetes (superotemporal quadrant of the right eye). Present were many microaneurysms, hemorrhages, and hard exudates, as well as extensive retinal edema and venous beading. Most of the tortuous small vessels appeared to be within the retina (large intraretinal microvascular abnormalities), but some may have been on its surface (NVEs). B, Eight months later, marked improvement in the intraretinal abnormalities was noted, but a wheel-like network of new vessels had appeared on the surface of the retina. Venous beading had decreased, and venous sheathing had increased. C, Three months later, the new vessel patch had enlarged, and a second patch had developed above it. During the next 2 years, the new vessels continued to grow slowly at the edges of the patches, while regressing at their centers. D, Three years after they had appeared, most of the new vessels had regressed, although there was still one dilated loop at the upper edge of the upper patch. No contraction of fibrous proliferation or vitreous had occurred, no vitreous hemorrhage was present, and vision remained good.

ally with hemorrhage suspended within its lower part (Fig. 68-9). If fresh blood is present in the posterior fluid vitreous in such cases, it can be made to flow across the macula by positioning the patient's head, indicating that the vitreous is indeed detached from the retina throughout the posterior pole.

Retinal distortion and detachment

With contraction of an extensive sheet of fibrovascular proliferations, distortion or displacement ("dragging") of the macula may occur.[30] In some cases the central, more intensely pigmented area of the retinal pigment epithelium (RPE) appears to be dragged with the neurosensory macula toward the major focus of contracted tissue, whereas in other cases only the neurosensory macula appears displaced. Since the most common site of extensive fibrovascular proliferations is on and near the disc, the macula is usually dragged nasally and often also somewhat vertically (Figs 68-10 and 68-11).

Contraction of the vitreous or fibrovascular proliferations may also lead to retinal detachment. This may be limited to avulsion of a retinal vessel, usually a vein, sometimes accompanied by vitreous hemorrhage. Alternatively, a relatively thin fold of retina may become elevated, with only a narrow zone of retinal detachment adjacent to its base, sometimes outlined by a pigmented demarcation line. In other cases retinal detachment may be more extensive, but the concave shape that is typical of traction detachment is generally maintained. At times, small, apparently full-thickness retinal holes may be seen near the

proliferations; these sometimes, but not always, lead to rhegmatogenous detachment. When such detachment does occur, it tends to have a flat or convex anterior surface and be more extensive, often reaching the ora serrata. The occurrence and severity of retinal detachment are influenced by the timing and degree of shrinkage of the vitreous and fibrovascular proliferations and by the type, extent, and location of the new vessels responsible for vitreoretinal adhesions. Extensive nets of large-caliber new vessels accompanied by heavy fibrous tissue produce broad, tight vitreoretinal adhesions. Contraction of such proliferations is often followed by extensive retinal detachment (Fig. 68-12). New vessels with little accompanying fibrous tissue tend to produce less extensive vitreoretinal adhesions and less risk of retinal detachment, particularly when posterior vitreous detachment begins soon after the onset of neovascularization (Fig. 68-13). At times, new vessels that extend for a considerable distance along the surface of the retina appear to be adherent to the retina only at their sites of origin and to the vitreous only near their distal ends. In this case the posterior vitreous surface can pull away from the retina by a distance equal to the length of the vessels before exerting traction on the retina. When new vessels are confined to the surface of the disc, vitreous detachment can reach completion without producing traction on the retina, since there are no vitreoretinal adhesions. Retinal detachment does not occur in such eyes, but recurrent vitreous hemorrhage from the new vessels is common.

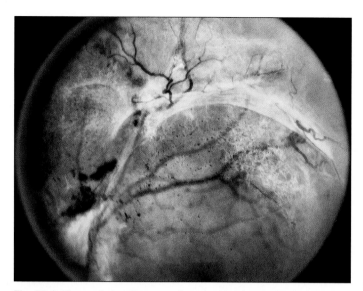

Fig. 68-8 The posterior vitreous surface. In this left eye fibrovascular proliferations were present at the disc and above the superotemporal vascular arcade. The posterior vitreous surface was adherent to these proliferations but was detached elsewhere. In the center of the figure the posterior vitreous surface was thin (visible only with slit illumination), but its position is marked by fine dots of hemorrhage deposited on it. Temporal to this area, the posterior vitreous surface has the typical "Swiss-cheese" appearance, that is, the surface can be seen as a semiopaque sheet in which there are round and oval clear areas. This same appearance is present 1 to 2 disc diameters above the disc, near the left edge of the figure. The retina was attached but is blurred, in part because the camera was focused on the elevated proliferations and also because of blood present in the posterior fluid vitreous. (Courtesy of Diabetic Retinopathy Vitrectomy Study Research Group.)

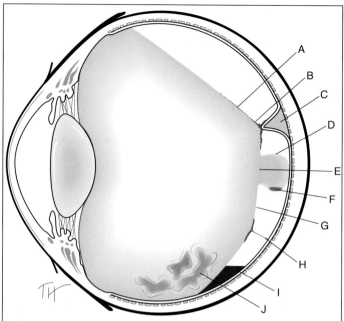

Fig. 68-9 Vitreous detachment in proliferative diabetic retinopathy. A, Blood deposited on the detached posterior surface of the formed vitreous after hemorrhage into the posterior fluid vitreous. B, Neovascular and fibrous proliferations creating a tight vitreoretinal adhesion, which pulls the retina forward and holds the formed vitreous posteriorly. C, Localized collection of subretinal fluid. D, Curved upper surface of a "mushroom" of formed vitreous extending posteriorly to reach the retina through a "hole" in the posterior vitreous surface. E, Hole in the posterior vitreous surface. F, Blood collected in the dependent portion of the mushroom of vitreous after hemorrhage into the formed vitreous. G, Posterior vitreous surface. H, A single new vessel stretching between the retina and proliferations on the detached posterior vitreous surface without traction retinal detachment. I, Blood with fluid level pooling between the retina and the posterior vitreous surface above the inferior limit of vitreous detachment after hemorrhage into the posterior fluid vitreous. J, Blood settled out in the inferior part of the formed vitreous.

Burned-out proliferative diabetic retinopathy

When vitreous contraction has reached completion (i.e., when the vitreous has detached from all areas of the retina except those where vitreoretinal adhesions associated with new vessels prevent such detachment), proliferative retinopathy tends to enter the burned-out, or "involutional," stage.[14,24,31,32] Vitreous hemorrhages decrease in frequency and severity and may stop entirely, although many months may elapse before substantial vitreous clearing occurs. Some degree of retinal detachment is usually present at this stage. If the detachment is localized and the macula remains intact, visual acuity may be good. Frequently, however, dragging or distortion of the macula or long-standing macular edema leads to substantial reduction in vision. In many cases retinal detachment involves the entire posterior pole, with resultant severe loss of vision. Although spontaneous partial reattachment occasionally occurs, if the macula has been detached for months or years, usually no significant return of vision occurs. A marked reduction in the caliber of retinal vessels is characteristic of this stage. Previously dilated or beaded veins return to normal caliber or become narrower and often appear sheathed; fewer small venous branches are visible. Changes in the arterioles are often even more striking, with decreased caliber and marked reduction of the number of visible branches. Some small arterioles now appear to be white threads without visible blood columns. Characteristically, only occasional retinal hemorrhages and microaneurysms are present. New vessels are usually reduced in caliber and number and are quiescent; at times no patent new vessels can be seen. Fibrous tissue may become thinner and more transparent, allowing the retina to be seen more clearly. Marked loss of vision at this stage often seems best explained by severe retinal ischemia.

RELATIONSHIP OF PROLIFERATIVE DIABETIC RETINOPATHY TO TYPE AND DURATION OF DIABETES

For many years it has been generally recognized that the factor most closely related to prevalence of PDR is duration of diabetes, at least in the type caused by loss of the capacity to produce insulin, characterized by sudden, symptomatic onset in nonobese patients in the first two or three decades of life and requiring the use of insulin beginning soon after diagnosis to avoid ketosis and sustain life.[33] This type of diabetes has been termed *juvenile-onset, insulin-dependent,* or *type 1 diabetes* and is contrasted with *adult-onset, noninsulin-dependent,* or *type 2 diabetes.* Adult-onset diabetes is typically discovered in older patients who are often overweight,

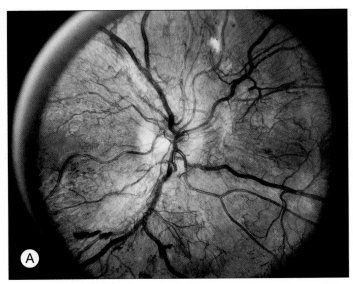
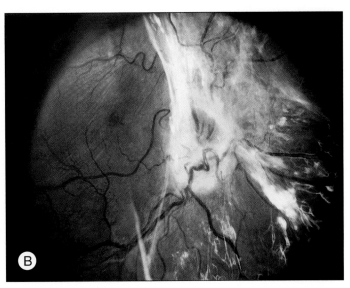

Fig. 68-10 Dragging of the macula by contraction of fibrovascular proliferations; regression of new vessels. A, In the right eye of this 21-year-old woman, whose age at diagnosis of diabetes was 10 years, extensive new vessels were present on the surface of the disc and retina, as well as many dilated intraretinal vessels (intraretinal microvascular abnormalities). A soft exudate was noted about 1 disc diameter (DD) superonasally to the disc, and several small preretinal hemorrhages were found (near bottom left). The macula was in its normal position, centered at or just temporal to the left edge of the figure. Fibrous tissue accompanying the new vessels was visible adjacent to the temporal vascular arcades and nasal to the disc. Fibrous proliferations were actually much more extensive but were transparent and difficult to detect. Visual acuity was 20/20. Contraction of the proliferations occurred within the next several months, dragging the retina nasally and superiorly, and new vessels regressed. B, Four years later, the center of the macula was above the disc and about 1 DD temporal to it. The central dark retinal pigment epithelial pigmentation appeared to coincide with the neurosensory macula. The first major bifurcation of the inferotemporal vein had been pulled upward to the disc margin from its previous position. New vessels had regressed completely, some of them now appearing as networks of white lines. Visual acuity was 20/30. (Courtesy of Diabetic Retinopathy Vitrectomy Study Research Group.)

may be asymptomatic at the time of diagnosis, and appear to have a deficiency in the regulation of insulin secretion or in its action in the liver and peripheral tissues or a combination of these defects. Typical patients are easily placed in the appropriate category, but for others classification is difficult. Many patients with type 2 diabetes take insulin, and it is incorrect to refer to all insulin-taking patients as insulin-dependent. Similarly, some patients who are without symptoms at diagnosis and for a while clearly seem to have type 2 diabetes ultimately appear to become insulin-dependent. The most accurate means of classifying patients by diabetes type is to measure plasma levels of C peptide, a polypeptide secreted from the beta cell in equimolar concentrations with insulin. C peptide is not significantly metabolized by the liver and is measurable by radioimmunoassay without interference from exogenous insulin; it thus provides a useful measure of endogenous insulin secretion.[34] In the absence of C-peptide determinations, most reports describing retinopathy characteristics either have not analyzed patients separately by diabetes type or have classified them mainly by age at diagnosis and by insulin use, sometimes taking into consideration factors such as type of onset, history of ketosis, and body weight. Comparisons of retinopathy features in type 1 and type 2 diabetes have been hampered by the difficulty in classifying diabetes type, by the scarcity of studies that have evaluated patients of both types with the same methods, and by the even greater rarity of population-based studies.

In a population-based stereophotographic study carried out by Klein et al.,[35] the prevalence of PDR in insulin-taking patients younger than 30 at diagnosis (exclusively or mainly type 1) was near zero when duration of diabetes was less than 10 years and then rose rapidly to about 50% in persons with 20 years or more of diabetes. In an older-onset (30 years or more) insulin-taking group, which included both diabetes types, prevalence of PDR rose fairly steadily, from 2% in persons with less than 5 years of diabetes to about 25% in those with 20 years or more. In the older-onset, noninsulin-taking (type 2) group, prevalence of PDR increased only slightly with duration, from less than 5% before 20 years to about 5% thereafter (Fig. 68-14). Among patients with PDR, its severity did not appear to differ between the younger-onset and the combined older-onset groups: in each case in the worse eye about 25% of patients had DRS high-risk characteristics and 15% had retinopathy severity ungradable because of extensive vitreous hemorrhage, phthisis bulbi, or enucleation secondary to complications of diabetic retinopathy. In patients with PDR, macular edema was more common in the combined older-onset group; retinal thickening or scars of previous focal photocoagulation were present in at least one eye in about 45% (versus 30% in the younger-onset group).[35]

The Diabetic Retinopathy Vitrectomy Study (DRVS) found a substantial variation in severity of PDR by diabetes type among persons with vitreous hemorrhage severe enough to reduce visual acuity to 5/200 or less for a period of at least 1 month.[36] In this study the severity of new vessels, fibrous proliferations, and vitreoretinal adhesions decreased significantly

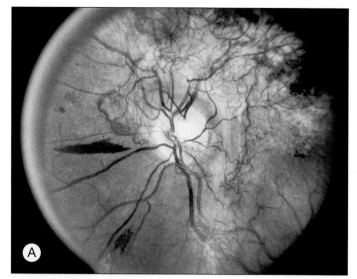

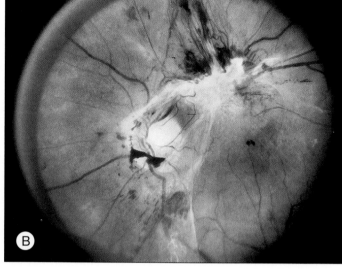

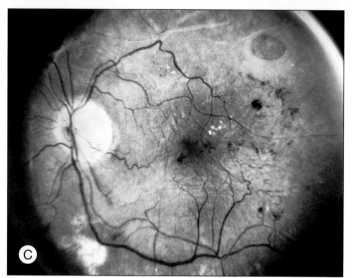

Fig. 68-11 Dragging of the macula. A, In the left eye of this 39-year-old white woman, whose age at diagnosis of diabetes was 10 years, extensive fibrovascular proliferations were present on and adjacent to the disc, centered superotemporally. The temporal edge of the patch of proliferations was tightly apposed to the retina, and the nasal edge was elevated about one-third of a disc diameter by localized posterior vitreous detachment, the lower edge of which was marked by a preretinal hemorrhage. Visual acuity was 20/60. Scatter photocoagulation was initiated. B, Three weeks after photocoagulation, the patient noted a marked decrease in visual acuity and returned for examination. There had been marked regression of the new vessels. Contraction of the proliferations had pulled the neurosensory macula (but not the corresponding, more deeply pigmented retinal pigment epithelium) up and nasally. Vitrectomy was carried out. C, Two months later, visual acuity had improved to 20/30, and the neurosensory macula had returned to near-normal position. There appeared to be a rather large, full-thickness retinal break (near upper right corner), but this did not lead to retinal detachment during the remaining 3 years of follow-up. At 4-year follow-up, vision had improved to 20/20. (Courtesy of Diabetic Retinopathy Vitrectomy Study Research Group.)

as diabetes type shifted from type 1 to type 2 (Table 68-1). The implications of this finding in regard to indications for vitrectomy are discussed at the end of this chapter.

Diabetes with onset after age 30 is more common than the younger-onset type, and in clinical practice PDR is seen with about equal frequency in the younger- and older-onset groups. Klein et al.[35] estimated that, in the population they surveyed, 43% of patients with PDR were in the younger-onset group, 42% were in the older-onset insulin-taking group, and 15% were in the noninsulin-taking group. In the DRS, in which more than 90% of the 1742 patients examined had PDR in at least one eye, 44% were classified as juvenile-onset (younger than 20 years at diagnosis and taking insulin at entry into the study); 28% as adult-onset, possibly insulin-dependent (age 20 years or older at diagnosis, not overweight, and taking insulin); and 26% as classic adult-onset (mild symptomatic or asymptomatic onset at age 20 years or older and either overweight or not taking insulin at study entry). The remaining 2% were not classifiable.[16] Aiello et al.[37] found the distribution of age at diagnosis of diabetes among 244 patients with

PDR who attended the Eye Unit at the Joslin Clinic during a 5-month period to be as follows: less than 20 years, 53%; 20 to 39 years, 25%; and 40 years or older, 22%.

PROLIFERATIVE DIABETIC RETINOPATHY AND BLOOD GLUCOSE CONTROL

On the basis of observational epidemiologic studies[35,38–43] and studies in animal models,[4,44,45] it has long been suspected that poorer glycemic control fosters development of more severe retinopathy. However, despite several clinical trials, most of which were small and of short duration,[44,47–52] this relationship remained unproved until 1993, when the Diabetes Control and Complications Trial (DCCT), a large multicenter trial in which patients with type 1 diabetes were followed up for as long as 9 years, demonstrated conclusively that the long-term risks both for the development of diabetic retinopathy and for its progression from very early to later stages can be dramatically reduced by improving blood glucose control with intensive

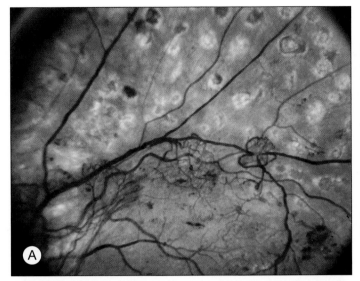

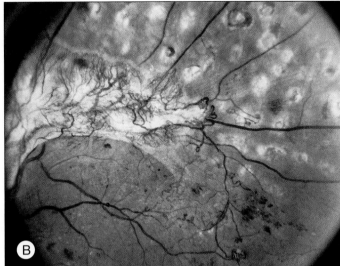

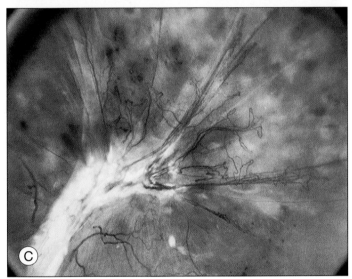

Fig. 68-12 Contraction of fibrovascular proliferations leading to extensive retinal detachment. A, In the left eye of this 35-year-old man, whose age at diagnosis of diabetes was 14 years, networks of new vessels extended over the surface of the retina along the superotemporal vein. Scars were typical of initial scatter photocoagulation, with space between scars available for additional treatment. B, Four months later, new vessels had increased, and dense fibrous tissue had appeared. C, Seven months later, fibrous proliferations had contracted. Broad adhesions prevented them from pulling away from the retina. Instead, the retina was pulled forward (detached) throughout the area shown in the figure. The photocoagulation scars were blurred by the overlying detached retina (and are out of focus). (Courtesy of Diabetic Retinopathy Vitrectomy Study Research Group.)

insulin treatment.[53-56] At this time the Stockholm Diabetes Intervention Study also reported a substantial reduction in the 9-year rate of progression to severe retinopathy with intensive insulin treatment (having previously found little difference between conventional and intensive treatment after 5 years of follow-up).[57] In addition to this long-term beneficial effect, improving blood glucose control with intensive treatment has a short-term harmful effect ("early worsening").[58-61] Early worsening is usually of little clinical importance when retinopathy is absent or mild, but it can become important when retinopathy is in the moderate to severe nonproliferative stage or the proliferative stage.[59,62-64] Both effects are discussed later.

Long-term benefit of improved glycemic control

In the DCCT a total of 1441 patients aged 13 to 39 with insulin-dependent diabetes (evidenced by deficient C-peptide secretion) of 1 to 15 years' duration were randomly assigned to either conventional or intensive insulin treatment and followed up for 4 to 9 years.[53] Conventional treatment was characterized by one

or two daily insulin injections, daily self-monitoring of urine or blood glucose, and diet and exercise education. Hemoglobin A_{1c} (HbA_{1c}) values were not used to guide treatment, unless an upper limit of 13% was exceeded. Intensive treatment consisted of insulin administered three or more times daily by injection or an external pump, with dose adjusted according to self-monitored blood glucose results performed at least four times per day, as well as anticipated dietary intake and exercise, and with the goal of lowering HbA_{1c} (measured monthly) to within the non-diabetic range (< 6.05%). Seven-field stereoscopic color fundus photographs were taken at baseline and every 6 months thereafter, and they were graded (masked to treatment) centrally using the Early Treatment of Diabetic Retinopathy Study (ETDRS) protocol.[65,66]

Of the 1441 patients, 726 patients, who were designated as the primary prevention cohort, had diabetes of 1 to 5 years' duration, no retinopathy by seven-field stereoscopic color photographs, and 24-h urinary albumin < 40 mg. The remaining 715 patients, designated the secondary intervention cohort, had diabetes of 1 to

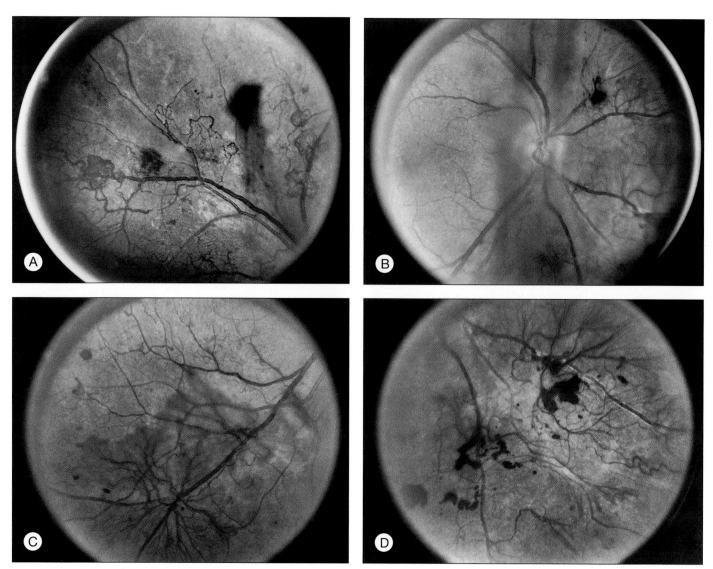

Fig. 68-13 Contraction of fibrovascular proliferations with limited vitreoretinal adhesions, leading to pulled-up retinal vessels and localized retinal detachment, and spontaneous regression of new vessels. A, In the superotemporal quadrant of the right eye of this 25-year-old man, whose age at diagnosis of diabetes was 8 years, several small, wheel-shaped networks of new vessels on the surface of the retina, venous beading, intraretinal microvascular abnormalities, and localized hemorrhage far anterior to the retina in the formed vitreous were noted. Several small, white, threadlike arterioles were present superiorly, where the retina appeared featureless, indicating loss of much of the retinal capillary bed. B, The disc and new vessels nasal to it are blurred by vitreous hemorrhage. The macula is visible in its normal position at the left edge of the figure. C, New vessels along the inferior temporal vein were in focus inferiorly, where they were on the surface of the retina, but were out of focus above the vein, where they were about a half disc diameter (DD) anterior to the retina, growing along the detached posterior vitreous surface. D, New vessels and thin fibrous proliferations inferonasal to the disc. Inferiorly, the new vessels were flat on the surface of the retina; superiorly, they were elevated about a half DD in front of the retina, on the detached posterior vitreous surface. Preretinal hemorrhages marked the inferior extent of posterior vitreous detachment. Visual acuity was 20/20.

15 years' duration, very mild (microaneurysms only) to moderate nonproliferative retinopathy, and 24-h urinary albumin < 200 mg. In each cohort baseline risk factors were balanced between the conventional and intensive treatment groups, except that in the secondary cohort retinopathy severity was slightly greater in the conventional management group, an imbalance that was adjusted for in the analyses.

Mean HbA$_{1c}$ at baseline was 8.9% in each treatment group (non-diabetic mean, 5.1; SD = 0.5). Over the entire study period, means were 9.1% and 7.2%, respectively, in the conventional and inten-

sive treatment groups, and mean blood glucose levels, assessed by quarterly seven-point capillary profiles, averaged 231 and 155 mg/dl, respectively (12.8 and 8.6 mmol/l). Compliance and follow-up were excellent; 95% of scheduled visits were completed. As in the earlier, small studies, during the first year of follow-up retinopathy progression (worsening) was observed more frequently in the intensive treatment group, but after the second year progression was more frequent in the conventional treatment group.

One of the principal outcome measures analyzed was the prevalence of progression by three or more steps on the ETDRS

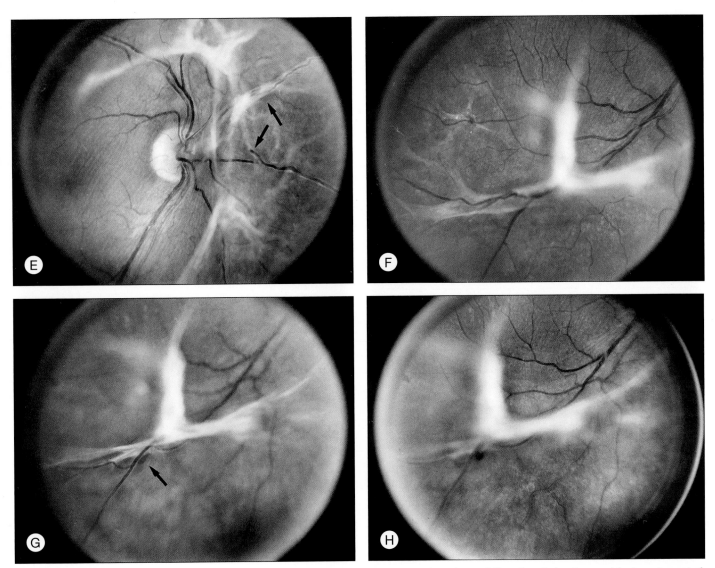

Fig. 68-13—cont'd E, One year later, following spontaneous regression of the new vessels and completion of posterior vitreous detachment, most of the proliferations were far anterior to the retina and out of focus. The inferonasal vein had been pulled upward to the horizontal meridian, and a loop of it had been pulled forward (lower arrow) without adjacent retinal detachment. The superonasal vein was also pulled forward, together with a narrow fold of retina (upper arrow). Tension lines ran through the macula, which had been displaced somewhat downward. F, The inferotemporal vein had been pulled forward, together with a narrow fold of retina, but the adjacent retina was flat. Visual acuity was 20/30. G (focused on the elevated inferotemporal vein), Three years later, a small oval retinal hole (arrow) could be seen just below the point where the inferotemporal vein was most highly elevated. Retinal detachment extended inferotemporally past the edge of the figure. H (focused on the attached posterior retina), The retina above the superotemporal vein remained flat, and visual acuity had improved to 20/20. G and H may be viewed stereoscopically by relaxing convergence (or using a base-out prism). (Courtesy of Diabetic Retinopathy Vitrectomy Study Research Group.)

retinopathy severity scale at each visit[54] (Fig. 68-15). In both cohorts progression was more common in the intensive treatment group at the 6-, 12-, and 18-month visits, but after 2 years prevalence increased more rapidly in the conventional than in the intensive treatment groups. After 4 years there was about a fivefold reduction in the risk of progression.

The DCCT demonstrated similar large risk reductions for progression from NPDR to PDR, which became evident after 3 years of follow-up and exceeded 80% (crude relative risk, 0.17) in the 5.5- to 9-year interval[54] (Table 68-2). Because most of the patients entering the trial with NPDR had microaneurysms only, it could be argued that the slowing of progression shown in

Table 68-2 represents slowing of progression from milder to more severe NPDR, not from severe NPDR to PDR. DCCT data cannot provide a convincing counterargument because patients with severe NPDR were not included in the trial. Moreover, there was a (nonsignificant) trend toward lesser treatment effect in the most severe category included in the DCCT, a small group of patients with "moderate NPDR," defined as mild IRMA or moderate to severe retinal hemorrhages and microaneurysms (Table 68-3).

Two randomized trials have reported results consistent with those of the DCCT in patients with type 2 diabetes. The Kuwamoto study, a DCCT-like study of 110 nonobese, insulin-taking Japanese patients with noninsulin-dependent diabetes who had no or mild

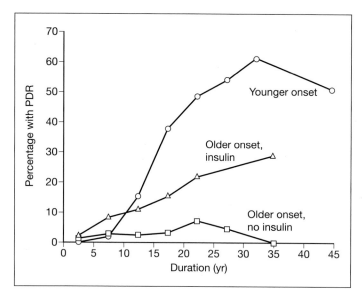

Fig. 68-14 Percentage of people with proliferative diabetic retinopathy (PDR) by duration of diabetes in each of the three groups. (Reproduced with permission from Klein R, Davis M, Moss S et al. The Wisconsin Epidemiologic Study of Diabetic Retinopathy: a comparison of retinopathy in younger and older onset diabetic persons. In: Vranic M, Hollenberg C, Steiner G, eds. Comparison of type I and II diabetes. New York: Plenum Press; 1985.[35])

Table 68-1 Percentage of Diabetic Retinopathy Vitrectomy Study (DRVS) group H eyes assigned to early vitrectomy with specified severity level of new vessels, fibrous proliferations, and vitreoretinal adhesions, by diabetes type

Fundus abnormality	Diabetes type*		
	Type 1	Mixed	Type 2
New vessels ≥ 1 disc area	81.1	58.2	42.2
Fibrous proliferations ≥ 2 disc areas	68.2	47.7	44.5
(no. of eyes)	(85)	(67)	(83)
Vitreoretinal adhesions ≥ 4 disc areas	47.8	34.5	23.6
(no. of eyes)	(115)	(84)	(106)

Reproduced with permission from Diabetic Retinopathy Vitrectomy Study (DRVS) Research Group: report no 2. Arch Ophthalmol 1985; 103:1644–1652.[36] Copyright © (1985) American Medical Association. All rights reserved.
*Type I, Age at diagnosis 20 years or younger and taking insulin at study entry; Mixed, Age at diagnosis 21 to 39 years and taking insulin at study entry; Type II, Age at diagnosis 40 years or older, or not taking insulin at study entry.

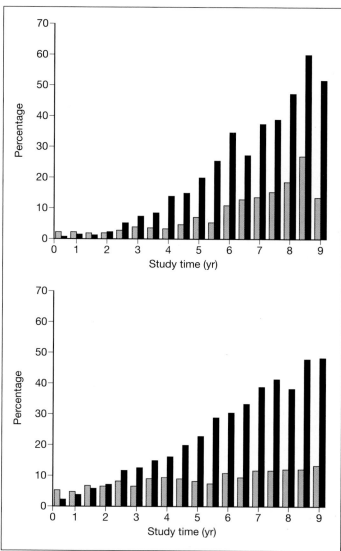

Fig. 68-15 Percentage of participants with progression of three or more steps at each semiannual visit for the conventional (solid bars) and intensive (shaded bars) treatment groups in the primary prevention (top) and secondary intervention (bottom) cohorts (P < 0.001 for intensive versus conventional treatment). (Reproduced with permission from Diabetes Control and Complications Research Group. Arch Ophthalmol 1995; 113:36–51. Copyright © (1995) American Medical Association. All rights reserved.[54])

nonproliferative retinopathy, found a reduction in the 6-year incidence of retinopathy progression from 38% in patients assigned to conventional insulin treatment to 13% in those assigned to intensive treatment (P = 0.007) and estimated the average risk reduction to be 69%. This reduction accompanied a difference in HbA$_{1c}$ that averaged 2.3 percentage points (9.4% versus 7.1%) over the 6 years (representing roughly a fourfold decrease in risk with a decrease in HbA$_{1c}$ from 10 to 7%).[67] The UK Prospective Diabetes Study (UKPDS) enrolled 3867 patients with newly diagnosed type 2 diabetes and assigned them to intensive treatment with a sulfonylurea or insulin or to conventional treatment beginning with diet only. The HbA$_{1c}$ levels of the intensively and conventionally treated cohorts (medians 7.0 and 7.9%, respectively, over 10 years of follow-up) were separated by about one-half the amount observed in the DCCT. Retinopathy progression over a 9-year period was observed in 31% of 1171 patients assigned to intensive treatment versus 38% of 459 patients assigned to conventional treatment (P = 0.012). Photocoagulation (mainly for macular edema) was also carried out less frequently in the intensively treated cohort (7.9 events per 1000 patient-years of follow-up versus 11 in the conventionally

Table 68-2 Diabetes Control and Complications Trial: rates of progression from nonproliferative diabetic retinopathy to proliferative diabetic retinopathy and crude relative risks (RRs), by follow-up time period

Time period (years)	Conventional (C) rate (cases/person-years)*	Intensive (I) rate (cases/person-years)*	Crude RR, I:C
0–1	0.86 (3/351)	0.55 (2/362)	0.65
1.5–3	1.60 (11/688)	1.41 (10/711)	0.88
3.5–5	1.86 (12/646)	0.88 (6/681)	0.47
5.5–9	3.97 (20/504)	0.69 (4/580)	0.17

Modified from Diabetes Control and Complications Trial Research Group. The effect of intensive diabetes treatment on the progression of diabetic retinopathy in insulin-dependent diabetes mellitus. Arch Ophthalmol 1995; 113:36–51.[54]
*Rates in cases per 100 person-years at risk.

treated cohort; $P = 0.0031$.[68] Neither of these trials reported rates of progression to PDR, and neither provided subgroup analyses by baseline retinopathy severity.

Hyperglycemia as a risk factor for further progression in eyes with severe NPDR or early PDR

Although no trial of intensive treatment has included patients with severe NPDR or early PDR, results of two studies support extrapolation of DCCT results to these groups. The Epidemiology of Diabetes Intervention and Complications (EDIC) study was initiated at the close of the DCCT to provide longer-term obser-

vations of these patients.[69] Patients in the conventional-therapy group were offered intensive therapy and instructed in its use and the care of all patients was transferred back to their own physicians. Patients were evaluated in EDIC at annual intervals. The most important finding was the continuation of the strong beneficial effect in the group originally randomized to intensive treatment in spite of marked narrowing of the difference in glycemic control between the two treatment groups (HbA$_{1c}$ 8.2 and 7.9%, respectively, in the conventional and intensive treatment groups, versus 9.1 and 7.2% during the DCCT). In addition, the increasing duration of diabetes in the cohort during the DCCT provided more patients with moderate NPDR or worse than had been available at the beginning of the DCCT (Table 68-3) and at the EDIC 4-year visit 42% of 110 such patients in the original conventional treatment group versus 22% of 58 patients in the conventional treatment group had progressed (by at least three steps on the ETDRS severity scale and in most cases to PDR), representing an odds reduction of 60% (95% confidence interval 18, 80; $P = 0.012$).

Additional evidence that better glycemic control in patients with severe NPDR or early PDR reduces their risk of further progression is provided by ETDRS multivariable analyses of risk factors for progression to high-risk PDR in such patients, in which HbA$_{1c}$ at baseline was a strong factor, with odds ratios ranging from 1.6 to 1.9 for patients in the highest versus the lowest categories, > 12% and > 8.3%, respectively ($P > 0.0001$).[70] Even in the lowest category the 5-year rate of high-risk PDR was high (50%), so large odds ratios were not to be expected. These analyses suggest that the benefits of better control continue to be manifest even after severe NPDR or PDR has

Table 68-3 Diabetes Control and Complications Trial: rates of progression to severe nonproliferative diabetic retinopathy (NPDR) or proliferative diabetic retinopathy (PDR) and crude relative risks (RRs), by baseline retinopathy severity and follow-up time period, and average RR over entire study time

Baseline retinopathy level	Time period (years)	Conventional (C)		Intensive (I)		Crude RR, I:C	RR†	Entire study time
		No.	Rate (cases/person-years)	No.	Rate (cases/person-years)*			% Change in risk from C (95% confidence interval)‡
MA only, 1 eye	0–3	100	(0/300)	140	(0/419)	—	—	—
	3.5–9	100	1.52 (5/328)	138	0.19 (1/521)	0.13	0.12	–88.2 (1.8 to –98.6)
MA only, both eyes	0–3	103	0.65 (2/308)	109	0.62 (2/322)	0.96	—	—
	3.5–9	100	3.05 (11/361)	105	0.53 (2/381)	0.17	0.29	–70.6 (–9.6 to –90.5)
Mild NPDR	0–3	110	1.85 (6/325)	82	1.24 (3/241)	0.67	—	—
	3.5–9	103	6.77 (23/340)	79	0.72 (2/279)	0.11	0.19	–80.7 (–49.7 to –92.6)
Moderate NPDR	0–3	38	13.68 (13/95)	32	17.61 (14/80)	1.29	—	—
	3.5–9	24	11.59 (8/69)	18	3.20 (2/63)	0.28	0.86	–14.1 (69.0 to –56.4)

Modified from Diabetes Control and Complications Trial Research Group. The effect of intensive diabetes treatment on the progression of diabetic retinopathy in insulin-dependent diabetes mellitus. Arch Ophthalmol 1995; 113:36–51.[54]
MA, Microaneurysms.
*Rates in cases per 100 person-years at risk.
†Average RR (I:C) over entire study time.
‡Percent change in risk was obtained as follows: 100 × [RR(I:C) – 1]. Negative values represent percent decrease in risk from C; positive values, percent increase.

developed, but they do not indicate what risk may be involved in improving control at this stage. What little information there is on this question is discussed later.

Early worsening of retinopathy with improved glycemic control

In the late 1970s, shortly after glycated hemoglobin assays and home blood glucose monitoring became available as aids to assess and control glycemia, several small trials of relatively short duration were initiated in persons with insulin-dependent diabetes, most of whom had mild to moderate NPDR. These trials compared intensive treatment, that is, home blood glucose monitoring combined with either continuous subcutaneous insulin infusion or multiple daily insulin injections, with conventional treatment, generally two insulin injections per day without home blood glucose monitoring.[44,46,49–51,58,60,61,71] A striking and unexpected finding in three of these trials was an initial worsening of retinopathy after 3 to 12 months of intensive treatment.[4,60,61] This worsening consisted mainly of the development of cottonwool spots in eyes free of such spots at baseline. In most cases the spots disappeared again after 6 to 12 months, and after 2 to 3 years the trend for retinopathy progression to be more frequent in intensively treated patients had reversed and now favored (but generally not to a statistically significant degree) the intensive treatment group.[47,49,50] However, occasionally PDR developed; in some cases it regressed again spontaneously, but in others photocoagulation was required. At about the same time as these early trials were done, several small uncontrolled case series in which intensive treatment was initiated in patients with severe NPDR or early PDR also reported early worsening, but in these cases it was not transient and was followed by visual loss.[62–64] These case series suggest that the risk of progression from early PDR or very severe NPDR to high-risk PDR, which is already substantial (about 25% in 4 to 6 months) without any change in glycemic control, may be doubled by intensive treatment, and the risk of macular edema may also be increased.[72] The pathogenesis of early worsening is poorly understood; one intriguing possibility is an increase in insulin-like growth factor or other growth factors.[73,74]

The occurrence of early worsening in the DCCT is summarized in Table 68-4.[59] Cottonwool spots or IRMA, or both, developed in only 1% of 348 patients entering the trial with no retinopathy. This proportion increased to 48% in the 60 patients with *mild nonproliferative retinopathy*, defined as the presence of microaneurysms plus mild retinal hemorrhages and/or hard exudates. *Clinically important early worsening* (defined as development of PDR, severe NPDR, or clinically significant macular edema) was not observed in patients with no retinopathy or with microaneurysms involving only one eye, but it occurred in 19% of the 32 patients with moderate NPDR. DCCT patients were followed up closely, and early worsening did not lead to serious visual loss, but DCCT findings support the conclusion that early worsening may be more common and more sight-threatening in patients with more severe retinopathy.

The most important risk factors for early worsening in the DCCT were the level of HbA_{1c} at baseline and the magnitude of its decrease during the first 6 months of intensive treatment. These factors were closely correlated because the higher HbA_{1c} was at baseline, the more likely it was that the decrease would be large. In multivariable models only the decrease remained significant; the risk of early worsening increased 1.6-fold for each percentage point decrease in HbA_{1c}. Many observers have speculated that a more gradual improvement in glycemic control might carry a lower risk of early worsening, but a comparison of DCCT patients whose HbA_{1c} reduction occurred over shorter versus longer periods did not support this point of view.[59]

Several case reports and small case series have also reported sight-threatening worsening following intensive treatment in patients with long-standing poor control and only mild to moderate NPDR.[75–80] Agardh et al.[75] reported 14 patients with type 1 diabetes who showed progression from no or minimal background retinopathy

Table 68-4 Early* worsening (EW) in Diabetes Control and Complications Trial patients assigned to intensive treatment

Baseline retinopathy severity	CWS/IRMA EW†		Clinically important EW‡	
	No. of patients	No. (%) with EW	No. of patients	No. (%) with EW
No retinopathy	348	4 (1.1)	348	0 (0.0)
MA only, one eye	140	14 (10.0)	140	0 (0.0)
MA only, both eyes	109	24 (22.0)	109	2 (1.8)
Mild NPDR	60	29 (48.3)	82	6 (7.3)
Moderate NPDR	NA§	NA	32	6 (18.8)

Modified from Diabetes Control and Complications Trial Research Group. Early worsening of diabetic retinopathy in the diabetes control and complications trial. Arch Ophthalmol 1998; 116:874–886.[59]
CWS, Cottonwool spot; IRMA, intraretinal microvascular abnormalities; MA, microaneurysms; NPDR, nonproliferative diabetic retinopathy.
*Within 6 to 12 months of beginning intensive treatment.
†Cottonwool spots or intraretinal microvascular abnormalities.
‡Development of macular edema or of proliferative diabetic retinopathy or severe NPDR.
§Not applicable; CWS/IRMA at baseline.

to retinopathy considered severe enough to warrant photocoagulation during a 1-year interval. In these cases mean HbA$_{1c}$ fell by 3.4%, compared to 0.4% in a control group of 17 patients matched for age and diabetes duration whose retinopathy did not worsen. Moskalets et al.[80] followed 122 patients with poorly controlled type 1 diabetes and no or nonproliferative retinopathy after they were admitted to hospital for initiation of intensive treatment. In 6 of the 122 patients (all women) visual acuity decreased in one or both eyes because of macular edema, and in 5 of the 6 patients vitreous hemorrhage subsequently caused loss of all useful vision (in 2 patients this occurred in both eyes). Mean decrease in HbA$_{1c}$ for these 6 patients was 4.5 percentage points, compared with 2 percentage points for 8 other patients who were matched for sex, age, duration of diabetes, blood pressure, microalbuminuria, retinal status, and visual acuity at baseline and in whom retinopathy progressed slightly or not at all. Gudat & Chantelau[78] reported 5 women with very poorly controlled type 1 diabetes in whom improved control was initiated because of painful polyneuropathy and who developed severe macular edema (all 5 patients) and proliferative retinopathy (3 of 5 patients) within 6 months. In these patients HbA$_{1c}$ fell about 5% to 6% within 8 to 12 weeks.

Early worsening has also been reported in patients with type 2 diabetes following decreases in HbA$_{1c}$ of 2 to 3 percentage points or more after treatment was switched to insulin because of inadequate control with oral agents.[81,82]

General considerations

In general, the substantial benefits of better glycemic control in reducing the long-term risks of sight-threatening retinopathy, as well as nephropathy and neuropathy, surely outweigh the risks of early worsening. However, patients with long-standing poor control should be evaluated ophthalmologically before intensive treatment is initiated. If PDR or very severe NPDR is already present, photocoagulation of at least one eye before beginning intensive treatment should be considered. Even if retinopathy is mild, follow-up at 2- to 4-month intervals for 6 to12 months after initiation of intensive treatment is advisable.

OTHER RISK FACTORS FOR PROLIFERATIVE DIABETIC RETINOPATHY

Most studies seeking to identify risk factors for the development of PDR begin with patients who have all degrees of NPDR, or no visible retinopathy at all, and make comparisons of baseline factors between those who do and do not develop PDR, usually over long periods. If risk factors for development of NPDR, or those for progression from less to more severe NPDR, differ from those for progression from severe NPDR to PDR, such studies would have little opportunity to identify these differences. Results of the ETDRS multivariable analyses of risk factors for progression to high-risk PDR mentioned earlier suggest that such differences, if any, are not of great importance, since the factors identified in this study (in which a majority of outcomes occurred, and occurred sooner, in patients entering with severe NPDR or non-high-risk PDR) differ little from those of previous studies.[70,83] As expected, the strongest factor was retinopathy severity; decreased visual acuity

was also a strong factor, as was HbA$_{1c}$. Additional significant factors were the presence of diabetic neuropathy, decreased hematocrit, increased serum triglyceride, and decreased plasma albumin (odds ratios for highest versus lowest categories of each factor ranged from 1.2 to 1.6).[70]

The association of elevated serum lipids with increased risk of progression to high-risk PDR, as well as their association with increased hard exudates and decreased visual acuity,[84] should provide additional motivation for lowering the frequently elevated lipid levels of diabetic patients. Severe anemia is a less frequently encountered problem in diabetic patients, but its association with increased risk of severe retinopathy may be important to these patients, as suggested by these ETDRS analyses and three other reports. In a multivariable cross-sectional analysis of 1386 patients in Finland, the relative risk of severe retinopathy (among all patients with retinopathy) was 5 for those with hemoglobin < 12 g/dl versus those with higher levels.[85] One small case series reported progression to florid PDR in 3 patients concurrently with the development of severe anemia[86] and another reported improvement in hard exudates and visual acuity in 3 patients after successful treatment of severe anemia with erythropoietin.[87]

Hypertension was not a risk factor for development of high-risk PDR in the ETDRS, and findings in previous studies have been variable.[70,83] In the UKPDS, patients with hypertension were randomized between more and less intensive regimens of blood pressure control, and retinopathy progression was significantly less common in the former, as was the incidence of photocoagulation and of a three or more line decrease in visual acuity, with risk reductions after 7.5 years ranging from 35 to 45% for these outcomes. Progression to PDR was too infrequent for analysis. These findings provide strong support for inclusion of intensive blood pressure control in the management of diabetes and diabetic retinopathy.

MANAGEMENT OF PROLIFERATIVE DIABETIC RETINOPATHY

Familiarity with the natural course of PDR suggests two principal therapeutic approaches: first, to discourage the proliferation of new vessels, and, second, to prevent or relieve the effects of contraction of the posterior vitreous surface and fibrovascular proliferations. This section deals mainly with the first aim; the second is considered in Volume 3. Among the treatments attempting to discourage proliferation of new vessels, good glycemic control has the longest history, and its remarkable efficacy has at last been proved.[53–57,67] The next promising treatment to appear was suppression of anterior pituitary function. Although no longer in use, a brief discussion of this approach is in order before taking up today's principal treatment, photocoagulation.

Pituitary ablation

Building on the fundamental discovery of Houssay & Biasotti[88] that hypophysectomy reduced the severity of diabetes in pancreatectomized dogs, Luft et al.[89] carried out hypophysectomy in the hope of ameliorating the vascular complications of diabetes. Further impetus was provided by Poulsen's report[90,91] of remission of diabetic retinopathy in a woman with postpartum anterior pituitary insufficiency (Sheehan's syndrome). Over the next 25 years, various types of pituitary suppression were used, ranging from external irradiation to transfrontal hypophysectomy, and consensus developed among advocates of these procedures that complete or nearly complete suppression of anterior pituitary function (pituitary ablation) produced rapid improvement in eyes with the intraretinal lesions characteristic of severe NPDR and actively growing new vessels not yet accompanied by extensive fibrous proliferations. Although only two randomized trials have been reported,[92,93] both small and neither in itself compelling, the weight of evidence supports the strongly held opinion of those most experienced with this procedure that it is beneficial. Particularly persuasive are comparisons between patients in whom transsphenoidal implantation of radioactive yttrium was followed by complete or nearly complete anterior pituitary suppression and similar patients in whom little or no suppression was achieved; substantially better outcome was observed in the former group.[94] Additional support is provided by a nonrandomized comparison of eyes with very extensive new vessels and IRMAs, in which outcome was better in the eyes of patients undergoing pituitary ablation than in similar eyes receiving photocoagulation or no treatment.[95] Pituitary ablation is now of only theoretical and historical interest because photocoagulation is probably at least equally effective and is free of the many substantial disadvantages of achieving and living with the hypopituitary state (i.e., operative and immediate postoperative risks, increased susceptibility to severe insulin reactions, need for continuing replacement of adrenal corticosteroids, with increased doses during infections or other stress, and sterility).

However, the favorable effect of pituitary ablation on retinopathy, which is thought to be mediated by suppression of growth hormone activity, provides rationale for medical interventions designed to achieve this effect. In one such study, daily subcutaneous injections of a genetically engineered growth hormone receptor antagonist, pegvisomant, were given for 3 months in 25 patients with non-high-risk PDR. Regression of new vessels did not occur in any patient, although the serum level of insulin-like growth factor 1 (IGF-1), a growth factor whose secretion is stimulated by growth hormone, did decrease, on an average, by 55% compared to baseline levels.[96] In a small randomized clinical trial, multiple daily subcutaneous injections of octreotide, a somatostatin analog that inhibits both growth hormone and insulin-like growth factor, were given to 11 patients with severe NPDR or non-high-risk PDR. During 15 months' follow-up, 1 out of 22 of these patients' eyes required scatter laser photocoagulation compared to 9 out of 24 eyes of 12 patients randomly assigned to an untreated control group. A placebo-controlled phase III trial of a long-acting octreotide given every 4 weeks intramuscularly is currently underway.

Inhibition of angiogenesis

A great deal of work has been done in seeking to identify growth factors, to understand their interactions, and to develop inhibitors that may be useful in slowing the progression of retinopathy to the proliferative stage. Detailed discussion of this information is beyond the scope of this chapter, but it is available in several recent reviews and in Chapter 65 of this textbook.[97–102]

Photocoagulation

The initial use of the xenon arc photocoagulator developed by Meyer-Schwickerath[103] in the treatment of PDR involved direct treatment of new vessels on the surface of the retina, particularly those that appeared to be the source of vitreous hemorrhage.[104–110] Large, slow, moderately intense burns were used, turning the retina white adjacent to the new vessels and sometimes causing them to narrow and the flow within them to slow. These effects were the result of heat generated when light was absorbed by the RPE or by hemorrhage within the retina or on its surface. Direct destruction of new vessels required burns of this strength, which usually involved the full thickness of the retina and often led to nerve fiber bundle field defects, particularly if hemorrhages were present in or on the retina. When new vessels were located some distance from the RPE, either in the vitreous or on the optic disc, they could not be treated directly with the xenon arc photocoagulator because it was not possible to concentrate enough energy in a short enough time to coagulate the rapidly flowing blood within them. The hope that this would be possible with the narrow, intense, blue-green beam of the argon laser was part of the rationale for its development.

Even before the argon laser became widely available, and before recognition of the tendency for NVDs and elevated NVEs to regrow after apparently successful direct treatment, the possibility of a much more exciting effect of extensive photocoagulation began to emerge: regression of new vessels and diminution of retinal edema and vascular congestion at some distance from the areas of retina directly treated.[111–113] Based on this observation and earlier descriptions of a remarkable asymmetry of retinopathy favoring the involved eye in diabetic patients who had unilateral disseminated chorioretinal scarring, high myopia, or optic atrophy, Beetham et al.[111] and Aiello et al.[114] began a study in which ruby laser burns were scattered across the retina from the posterior pole to the midperiphery. The long wavelength and very brief exposure time of the ruby laser limited burns mainly to the outer layers of the retina, without immediately visible effects in new vessels on its surface. The rationale initially proposed for regression of new vessels after this indirect treatment was that ischemic retina, which was postulated to be producing a vasoformative factor, was destroyed; hence the term *retinal ablation*, paralleling pituitary ablation.

It has also been proposed that photocoagulation may improve oxygenation of the ischemic inner retinal layers by destroying some of the metabolically highly active photoreceptor cells and allowing the oxygen normally diffusing from the choriocapillaris to supply these cells to continue into the inner layers of the retina, relieving hypoxia and removing the stimulus for expression of angiogenic factors.[52,115–118] This theory is appealing because it is principally the photoreceptor cells that are destroyed by mild argon laser burns, but it fails to explain why stronger burns sometimes seem more effective clinically. Additional support for the theory is provided by reports that retinal blood flow decreases and the autoregulatory response to breathing pure oxygen improves following scatter photocoagulation, as might be expected if more oxygen were reaching the inner retina from the choroid.[119,120] However, the choriocapillaris, which presumably is an important source of the oxygen postulated to be relieving inner retinal ischemia, has been found to be destroyed beneath at least some scatter burns.[121] An additional possibility is that the cells of the RPE may produce growth-stimulating and/or growth-inhibiting factors and that the response of these cells to photocoagulation injury may change the balance of these factors.[122,123] Although the mechanism of photocoagulation remains uncertain, its efficacy has been thoroughly documented in randomized clinical trials.

Clinical trials

All the early reports concerning photocoagulation suffered from small numbers of patients, brief periods of follow-up, or lack of a randomly selected control group.[124] Randomized clinical trials were needed to evaluate the possible benefits and risks of this treatment, and two collaborative studies were initiated in the early 1970s: the British multicenter trial using xenon arc photocoagulation[125] and the National Eye Institute's DRS, which compared xenon arc and argon laser photocoagulation.[126] Much of the remainder of this discussion is based on DRS reports.

Patients entering the DRS had PDR in at least one eye or severe NPDR in both eyes. Visual acuity of 20/100 or better was present in each eye. Each patient was randomly assigned to either the argon or xenon treatment group; one eye was randomly assigned to photocoagulation treatment and the other to indefinite deferral of treatment (i.e., no treatment ever), unless the protocol were to be modified because of evidence that treatment was beneficial. Patients were followed at 4-month intervals according to a protocol that provided for measurement of best-corrected visual acuity under standard lighting conditions, with separate charts for each eye. The examiners did not know the identity of the treated eye or type of treatment and attempted to reduce patient bias by urging the patient to read as far down the chart as possible with each eye, guessing at letters until more than one in a line was missed. All patients gave written informed consent and understood that the information being collected would be analyzed at frequent intervals and used, if possible, for their benefit.[127]

DRS treatment techniques are summarized in Table 68-5. Both techniques included scatter treatment with burns spaced about one-half to one burn-width apart, extending from the posterior pole to the equator and often completed in a single sitting. The argon treatment technique specified 800 to 1600 500-mm scatter burns of 0.1 s duration and direct treatment of new vessels on the disc and elsewhere, whether flat or elevated. Direct treatment was also applied to microaneurysms or other lesions thought to be causing macular edema. Follow-up treatment was applied as needed at 4-month intervals. The xenon technique was similar, but burns were fewer, of longer duration, and stronger, and direct treatment was not applied to elevated new vessels or those on the surface of the disc.

As its principal outcome variable, the DRS chose visual acuity of < 5/200 at each of two consecutively completed follow-up visits, scheduled at 4-month intervals, using for this the term *severe visual loss*. Visual acuity of < 5/200 was chosen as the level at which vision becomes too poor to be useful for walking about or for other self-care activities; the requirement of two consecutive visits was included because the rate of recovery to better visual acuity after a single visit at the < 5/200 level was 29% in the control group and 49% in the treated group; after two visits it was 12% and 29%, respectively, and after three visits, 8% and 21%.[127] Because recovery was somewhat more common in treated eyes, the endpoint chosen tends to underestimate the treatment benefit.

Table 68-6 presents 2-year cumulative rates of severe visual loss for subgroups defined by retinopathy severity in baseline stereoscopic color fundus photographs, by treatment assignment, with argon and xenon groups combined.[128] For severe visual loss to be present at the 2-year visit, visual acuity had to be < 5/200 no later than the 20-month visit. For all eyes in the untreated control group, the risk of severe visual loss within 2 years was 15.9%, and this was reduced to 6.4% by treatment. The risk was greatest in group J (36.9% in the control group). These eyes had preretinal or vitreous hemorrhage and NVD exceeding those in standard photograph 10A of the modified Airlie House classification (Fig. 68-16). The risk appeared somewhat lower for eyes with NVD of this severity without hemorrhage (group I, 26.2% in the control group). Similar risks (25.6 and 29.7%, respectively) were observed for untreated eyes in groups H and F, eyes with vitreous or preretinal hemorrhage, and less severe new vessels. Eyes in these four groups were referred to in the DRS as eyes with *high-risk characteristics* or, alternatively, eyes with three or four *new vessel–vitreous hemorrhage (NV-VH) risk factors*, these factors being: (1) new vessels present, (2) new vessels located on or within 1 DD of the disc (NVD), (3) new vessels moderate to severe (NVD equaling or exceeding those in standard photograph 10A or, for eyes without NVD, NVE equaling or exceeding one-half disc area in at least one photographic field), and (4) vitreous or preretinal hemorrhage (or both) present. In counting risk factors, the presence and severity of NVE were

Table 68-5 Diabetic retinopathy study photocoagulation techniques		
	Argon laser	Xenon arc
Scatter treatment		
No. of burns	800–1600 (500 µm) or 500–1000 (1000 µm)	400–800 (3 degrees) or 200–400 (4.5 degrees)
Exposure time	0.1 s	Not specified
Direct treatment*		
Surface NVE	+	+
Elevated NVE	+	−
NVD	+	−
Macular edema	+	+
Follow-up treatment	+	+

Reproduced with permission from Diabetic Retinopathy Study Research Group. Photocoagulation treatment of proliferative diabetic retinopathy: clinical application of Diabetic Retinopathy Study (DRS) findings. DRS report no. 8. Ophthalmology 1981; 88:583–600.[130]
*NVE, New vessels elsewhere (more than 1 disc diameter (DD) from the disc); NVD, new vessels on or within 1 DD of the disc.

Table 68-6 Cumulative 2-year rates of severe visual loss in eyes grouped by baseline retinopathy severity and treatment assignment

Retinopathy severity group	NVE	NVD	VH/PRH	No. of NV-VH risk factors	Control SVL (%)	Control No. at risk†	Treated SVL (%)	Treated No. at risk†	z-Value
A	0	0	0	0	3.6	195	3.0	182	0.4
B	0	0	+	1	4.2	11	0.0	16	1.0
C	<½ DA	0	0	1	6.8	120	2.0	96	1.8
D	<½ DA	0	+	2	6.4	18	0.0	19	1.1
E	≥½ DA	0	0	2	6.9	125	4.3	141	1.0
F	≥½ DA	0	+	3	29.7	40	7.2	41	3.0
G	+ or 0	<10A	0	2	10.5	114	3.1	126	2.4
H	+ or 0	<10A	+	3	25.6	39	4.3	35	2.9
I	+ or 0	≥10A	0	3	26.2	150	8.5	174	4.7
J	+ or 0	≥10A	+	4	36.9	76	20.1	107	3.2
All eyes				15.9	897	6.4	946	7.2	

Reproduced with permission from Diabetic Retinopathy Study Research Group. Indications for photocoagulation treatment of diabetic retinopathy. DRS report no. 14. Int Ophthalmol Clin 1987; 27:239–253.[128]
*NVD, New vessels on or within 1 disc diameter of the optic disc; NVE, new vessels elsewhere (i.e., outside the area defined as NVD); VH/PRH, vitreous/preretinal hemorrhage; NV-VH risk factors, new vessel–vitreous hemorrhage risk factors (see text); SVL, severe visual loss (visual acuity < 5/200 at two or more consecutively completed follow-up visits scheduled at 4-month intervals); DA, disc area (NVE < ½ DA indicates that NVE do not equal or exceed one-half the area of the disc in any of the standard photographic fields, NVE ≥ ½ DA indicates that NVE equal or exceed this area in at least one of these fields); 10A, standard photograph 10A of the modified Airlie House classification (Fig. 73-3).
†In the 20- to 24-month interval.

considered only in eyes without NVD because a subgroup analysis indicated that in eyes with NVD the presence of moderate or severe NVE did not further increase the risk of severe visual loss.[129] In the remaining groups (A through E and

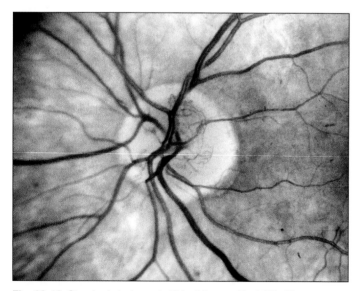

Fig. 68-16 Standard photograph 10A of the modified Airlie House classification, defining the lower limit of moderate new vessels on or within 1 disc diameter of the disc. (Reproduced with permission from Diabetic Retinopathy Study Research Group. A modification of the Airlie House classification of diabetic retinopathy. DRS report no. 7. Invest Ophthalmol Vis Sci 1981; 21:210–226.[18])

G), the risk without treatment varied from 3.6 to 10.5%. Treatment reduced the rate of severe visual loss in each group, most impressively in groups F through J. On the basis of a similar analysis conducted when somewhat fewer patients had been followed up for 2 years and estimates that in 10 to 20% of eyes treatment might cause a small permanent reduction in visual acuity, the DRS investigators concluded in 1976 that prompt photocoagulation treatment was usually desirable for eyes with high-risk characteristics. The protocol was therefore modified to allow treatment of eyes originally assigned to the untreated control group, if they had high-risk characteristics then or developed them in the future.[127]

In Table 68-7 the retinopathy severity groups presented in Table 68-6 have been combined, and observations from follow-up visits completed after the 1976 protocol change have been included.[105] Forty-three percent of the 2-year visits and all the 4-year visits included in this analysis were carried out after the 1976 protocol change. At the 2-year visit, 12% of control-group eyes had been treated, and by the 4-year visit 35% had been treated. All eyes were classified in the group to which they were originally randomly assigned, without reference to treatment of control-group eyes. In the control group the 2-year risk of severe visual loss increased from 3.2% in eyes with NPDR to 7% in eyes with PDR without high-risk characteristics, and to 26.2% in eyes with high-risk characteristics. The 4-year rates in these groups were, respectively, 12.8, 20.9, and 44.0%. Treatment reduced the risk of severe visual loss by 50% to 65% in all three groups at both 2 and 4 years, except for the NPDR group at 2 years.

Table 68-7 Cumulative 2- and 4-year rates of severe visual loss in eyes grouped by baseline retinopathy severity and treatment assignment*

Retinopathy severity	Table 67.6 groups	No. of NV-VH risk factors		Control		Treated		z-Value
				SVL (%)	No. at risk†	SVL (%)	No. at risk†	
Nonproliferative	A	0	2-year	3.2	297	2.8	303	0.3
			4-year	12.8	183	4.3	188	3.6
Proliferative without high-risk characteristics	B-E, G	1 or 2	2-year	7.0	603	3.2	615	3.1
			4-year	20.9	332	7.4	390	6.5
Proliferative with high-risk characteristics	F, H–J	3 or 4	2-year	26.2	473	10.9	570	7.1
			4-year	44.0	238	20.4	324	8.5
All eyes			2-year	14.0	1278	6.2	1489	7.4
			4-year	28.5	754	12.0	903	11.0

Reproduced with permission from Diabetic Retinopathy Study Research Group. Indications for photocoagulation treatment of diabetic retinopathy. DRS report no. 14. Int Ophthalmol Clin 1987; 27:239–253.[128]
*NV-VH risk factors, new vessel–vitreous hemorrhage risk factors (see text); SVL, severe visual loss (visual acuity < 5/200 at two or more consecutively completed follow-up visits scheduled at 4-month intervals).
†In the 20- to 24-month interval for the 2-year rates at the 44- to 48-month interval for the 4-year rates.

Fig. 68-17 depicts cumulative rates of severe visual loss by treatment assignment (argon and xenon groups combined) for up to 6 years. Two separate analyses are summarized, one excluding and the other including visits made after the 1976 protocol change. The curves for control-group eyes are very similar over the first 20 months of follow-up, and those for treated eyes are similar over at least the first 28 months. The difference between the two control-group curves is probably due, at least in part, to the beneficial effect of treatment experienced by some of these eyes after the protocol change, and the long-term analysis probably underestimates treatment effect. In each of these analyses, treatment reduced the risk of severe visual loss by 50% or more at and after the 16-month visit.[130] In Fig. 68-18, the Fig. 68-17 plots including all visits are presented separately for the argon and xenon groups. The treatment effect (i.e., the difference between treatment and control groups) appeared somewhat greater in the xenon group, but this difference was small, its statistical significance was borderline, and its clinical importance was outweighed by the greater harmful effects of DRS xenon treatment.

A temporary decrease in visual acuity is frequently noted after extensive scatter photocoagulation, with recovery to the pretreatment level in most cases within several weeks. In the DRS, visual acuity decreases of one or more lines from which recovery did *not* occur were attributed to treatment in 14% of argon-treated and 30% of xenon-treated eyes. Visual field losses were also more common in the xenon group[130,131] (Table 68-8). In a small subgroup of eyes with severe fibrous proliferations or localized traction retinal detachment, or both, visual acuity decreases of five lines or more were attributed to xenon treatment in 18% of eyes but were not significantly more frequent in argon-treated than in control eyes.[132]

In Fig. 68-19, the Fig. 68-17 plots including all visits are presented separately for the three subgroups shown in Table 68-7. In each subgroup treatment reduced the risk of severe visual loss to about one-half of that observed in control-group eyes, but this effect became apparent later, and the percentage of eyes treated that benefited (the arithmetic difference between treated and

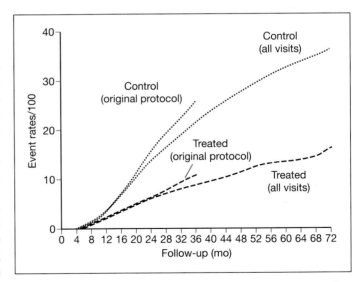

Fig. 68-17 Cumulative rates of severe visual loss, including and excluding observations made after the 1976 protocol change, for argon and xenon groups combined. (Reprinted from photocoagulation treatment of proliferative diabetic retinopathy: clinical application of Diabetic Retinopathy Study (DRS) findings. DRS report no. 8. The Diabetic Retinopathy Study Research Group. Ophthalmology 1981; 88:583–600. Copyright 1981, with permission from the American Academy of Ophthalmology.[130])

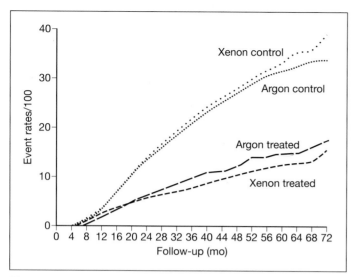

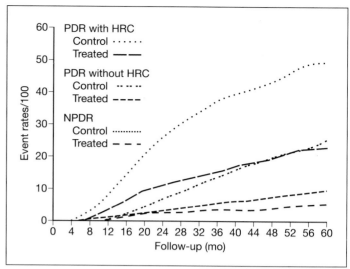

Fig. 68-18 Cumulative rates of severe visual loss by treatment group. (Reprinted from photocoagulation treatment of proliferative diabetic retinopathy: clinical application of Diabetic Retinopathy Study (DRS) findings. DRS report no. 8. The Diabetic Retinopathy Study Research Group. Ophthalmology 1981; 88:583–600. Copyright 1981, with permission from the American Academy of Ophthalmology.[130])

Fig. 68-19 Cumulative rates of severe visual loss for eyes classified by the presence of proliferative retinopathy (PDR) and high-risk characteristics (HRC) in baseline fundus photographs, argon and xenon groups combined. NPDR, Nonproliferative diabetic retinopathy. (Reprinted from photocoagulation treatment of proliferative diabetic retinopathy: clinical application of Diabetic Retinopathy Study (DRS) findings. DRS report no. 8. The Diabetic Retinopathy Study Research Group. Ophthalmology 1981; 88:583–600. Copyright 1981, with permission from the American Academy of Ophthalmology.[130])

Table 68-8 Estimated percentages of eyes with harmful effects attributable to diabetic retinopathy study treatment

	Argon (%)	Xenon (%)
Constriction of visual field (Goldmann IVe4 test object) to an average of		
≤ 45 degree, > 30 degree per meridian		
≤ 30 degree per meridian	5	25
Decrease in visual acuity	0	25
1 line	11	19
≥ 2 lines	3	11

Reproduced with permission from Diabetic Retinopathy Study Research Group. Photocoagulation treatment of proliferative diabetic retinopathy: clinical application of Diabetic Retinopathy Study (DRS) findings. DRS report no. 8. Ophthalmology 1981; 88:583–600.[130]

control groups) was smaller as retinopathy severity decreased. On the basis of this analysis and the estimates of the harmful effects of treatment summarized in Table 68-8, the DRS confirmed its previous conclusion that, for eyes with high-risk characteristics, the chance of benefit from treatment clearly outweighed its risk and recommended prompt photocoagulation for most such eyes.[130]

For eyes with severe NPDR or PDR without high-risk characteristics, the DRS concluded that either prompt treatment or careful follow-up with prompt treatment if high-risk characteristics developed was satisfactory and that DRS results were not helpful in choosing between these strategies. In univariate analyses of DRS control-group eyes that had PDR without high-risk characteristics, the severity of each of three retinopathy characteristics was associated with risk of visual loss: retinal

hemorrhages or microaneurysms, arteriolar abnormalities, and venous caliber abnormalities. These lesions – and soft exudates and IRMAs – were also risk factors for visual loss in control-group eyes with NPDR.[18] A multivariable analysis that included all DRS control-group eyes found baseline visual acuity; extent of NVD; elevation of NVD (a measure of contraction of vitreous and fibrous proliferations); and severity of hemorrhages or microaneurysms, arteriolar abnormalities, venous caliber abnormalities, and vitreous or preretinal hemorrhage all to be risk factors for visual loss. Neither in this analysis nor in a similar one confined to DRS control-group eyes that were free of NVD was the extent of NVE found to be a risk factor.[133] These findings support clinical impressions that NVE on the surface of the retina often proliferate and regress over a period of years, remaining asymptomatic unless contraction of vitreous and fibrous proliferations begins, and that the severity of intraretinal lesions may be of greater prognostic importance than the extent of NVE.

When the DRS first reported evidence of a beneficial treatment effect and modified its protocol to encourage treatment of control-group eyes with high-risk characteristics, it also modified its treatment protocol. Because the harmful effects of the DRS argon treatment were less than those observed with the xenon treatment used in the DRS, argon was given preference and, in the hope of further reducing harmful side-effects, scatter treatment was more often divided between two or more episodes several days apart. However, because the beneficial treatment effect in the xenon group, in which no focal treatment had been applied to NVD or elevated NVE, had been at least as great as that in the argon group, these technically difficult parts of the argon protocol were dropped.

Two smaller randomized trials reported beneficial treatment effects similar to those found in the DRS. The British multicenter study enrolled 107 patients with PDR of similar severity in both eyes, with visual acuity difference between eyes no greater than two lines on a Snellen chart and with visual acuity no less than 6/60 in either eye.[134] In each patient one randomly selected eye was assigned to an untreated control group, and the other was treated with mild xenon arc photocoagulation. The treatment protocol required scatter treatment for new vessels arising from the disc and direct treatment of new vessels on the surface of the retina; in eyes with NVE only, scatter treatment was optional. The numbers of scatter burns to be used were not specified, nor were indications for follow-up treatment. In 77 patients observed at the 5-year follow-up visit, 27 untreated eyes (35%) were blind (visual acuity 6/60 or less), compared with 8 treated eyes (10%). The effectiveness of photocoagulation was most impressive in eyes with NVD, and there was some suggestion that results were better when more burns were used. Hercules et al.[135] randomly assigned one eye of each of 94 patients with visual acuity no less than 6/24 and NVD of similar severity in each eye, and with difference in visual acuity between eyes no greater than two lines, to mild argon laser scatter photocoagulation. From 800 to 3000 burns (usually more than 2000) were applied, mostly with 500-mm spot size, in four to six sittings over a 1-week period with topical anesthesia used. Retreatment of untreated retina between scars was carried out when new vessels persisted or recurred. Complete or nearly complete regression of NVD occurred in 36% of treated eyes. During a follow-up period of 1 to 3 years, 36 of 94 untreated eyes became blind (visual acuity worse than 6/60 at two consecutive visits), compared with 7 of 94 treated eyes.

Two large case series reported outcome in treated eyes similar to that observed in the controlled trials previously discussed. About 2700 eyes treated for PDR with xenon arc photocoagulation by Okun et al.[136] were reviewed in a format designed to facilitate comparison with DRS results. These workers treated new vessels on the surface of the retina directly, and when such treatment was not required, they scattered mild 4.5-degree burns about one burn diameter apart, paying particular attention to cottonwool spots, surface hemorrhages, and abnormal capillaries. In the great majority of cases all four quadrants were treated in one sitting with retrobulbar anesthesia used. The number of burns was adjusted to the extent of new vessels and varied from 100 to 500. Sixty-three percent of eyes had a single treatment over the entire follow-up period, 20% had two treatments, 8% had three treatments, and 9% had four or more treatments. Follow-up ranged from 4 months to 10 years, with about 1200 eyes observed at the 4-year follow-up visit. Cumulative rates of severe visual loss were almost identical to those observed in DRS-treated eyes, both in eyes with high-risk characteristics and in those with less severe PDR. Decreases in visual acuity of one to four lines were similar to those observed with DRS xenon treatment, but the decreases of five or more lines attributable to DRS xenon treatment were not observed, a difference thought by these authors to be the result of their custom of using less intense burns, tailoring the number of burns to the severity of retinopathy, and withholding treatment from eyes with severe fibrous proliferations.[136]

Little[137] reported results in 457 eyes with NVD exceeding one-fourth disc area treated with 2000 to 4000 500-mm argon laser burns of moderate intensity placed adjacent to one another or one-half burn diameter apart and applied with topical anesthesia in four sittings over a period of 10 to 14 days.[137] New vessels regressed completely in 50% of eyes and showed some decrease in nearly all the remainder. If new vessels failed to regress within 2 months or recurred, additional treatment was applied (usually with retrobulbar anesthesia), avoiding deeply pigmented scars. Last recorded visual acuity was < 20/200 in about 18% of 241 eyes followed for 5 or more years, an outcome similar to that observed in the DRS.

Indications for photocoagulation

On the basis of the studies discussed here, as well as others, there is wide agreement that treatment should be carried out promptly in most eyes with PDR that have well-established NVD or vitreous or preretinal hemorrhage. Treatment is particularly urgent when localized fresh vitreous or preretinal hemorrhage is present because of the risk that dispersion of the hemorrhage throughout the vitreous or recurrent bleeding may soon make treatment more difficult or impossible. In the great majority of such eyes, new vessels of sufficient extent to fulfill the definition of DRS high-risk characteristics can either be seen ophthalmoscopically or be presumed to be present behind the hemorrhage. When visible or suspected new vessels seem insufficient to explain the hemorrhage, special consideration should be given to other possible causes, such as fresh retinal tears, partially avulsed retinal veins, or small patches of new vessels that have been completely avulsed from the disc or retina. Fresh horseshoe tears should generally be treated with photocoagulation or cryotherapy. Scatter photocoagulation in the area drained by an avulsed retinal vein (in the hope of reducing flow through it) or direct treatment to occlude it, or both, as has been recommended for similar problems in non-diabetic persons,[138] may be helpful. Complete avulsion of a small new vessel patch from its connections to the disc or retina should be considered as a possible explanation of a recent vitreous hemorrhage when the detached posterior vitreous surface can be seen anterior to the disc or retina and contains a subtle opacity, suggesting a small patch of empty new vessels. This occurrence is uncommon, but not rare, and has a good prognosis.[139] Usually no trace can be seen on the disc or retina of the previous new vessel patch and no treatment is necessary.

Progressive contraction of fibrous proliferations leading to displacement or detachment of the macula sometimes follows scatter photocoagulation for high-risk characteristics in eyes with extensive fibrous proliferations (see Fig. 68-11). Experience with such cases has led to some reluctance to advise photocoagulation in this situation. Few such eyes were included in the DRS, but analyses of them indicated that outcome was better with photocoagulation than without it and suggested that it is only excessively heavy treatment that should be avoided. Only in the xenon group was an adverse treatment effect found in these eyes, and even there the benefit of treatment outweighed its risks.[132] When high-risk characteristics are definitely present, scatter photocoagulation should usually be carried out, despite the presence of fibrous proliferations or localized traction retinal detachment. Areas of fibrous proliferations and retinal detachment should be avoided, and treatment strength should be mild to moderate. It may be desirable to divide treatment between several episodes. Of course, photocoagulation is not indicated when PDR is entering the stage of regression, with few or no new vessels and extensive fibrous proliferations.

Extensive neovascularization in the anterior chamber angle is a strong indication for scatter photocoagulation, if it is feasible, regardless of the presence of high-risk characteristics. Remarkable regression of these new vessels often occurs soon after scatter photocoagulation; if this treatment is carried out before extensive closure of the angle has occurred, full-blown neovascular glaucoma can be prevented. When opacities of the media preclude retinal photocoagulation, cryoapplications or vitrectomy with endophotocoagulation may be used, with or without additional direct photocoagulation of the new vessels in the anterior chamber angle.[64,140–145]

The presence of extensive retinal hemorrhages, IRMAs, venous beading, and opaque small arteriolar branches, often accompanied by prominent soft exudates, suggests rapidly progressive closure of the retinal capillary bed and severe retinal ischemia. New vessels are usually present in such eyes but may be relatively unimpressive. Severe retinal ischemia increases the urgency to initiate scatter photocoagulation, whether or not DRS high-risk characteristics are present, since eyes so affected appear to be at greater risk of anterior segment neovascularization.[146] Patients should be aware of this risk and the risk of a sudden decrease in central vision, which may occur with occlusion of the remaining arterioles supplying the macula. The clinical impression that scatter photocoagulation may precipitate such an occlusion has led to the suggestion that initial scatter treatment be divided between three or four episodes in the hope of reducing this risk.

As mentioned previously for eyes with severe NPDR or early (not high-risk) PDR, DRS results were not helpful in determining which of two treatment strategies would be attended by a more favorable visual outcome: (1) immediate photocoagulation or (2) frequent follow-up and prompt initiation of photocoagulation only if high-risk PDR developed. One of the goals of the ETDRS, a randomized clinical trial sponsored by the National Eye Institute, was to compare these alternatives (designated "early photocoagulation" and "deferral of photocoagulation," respectively) in patients with mild to severe NPDR or early PDR, with or without macular edema.[147] Other goals were to evaluate photocoagulation for diabetic macular edema and to determine the possible effects of aspirin on diabetic retinopathy. Between 1980 and 1985, 3711 patients were enrolled and assigned randomly to aspirin 650 mg/day or placebo. One eye of each patient was randomly assigned to early photocoagulation and the other to deferral. Follow-up ranged from 3 to 8 years. Eyes assigned to early photocoagulation were randomly assigned to either of two scatter treatment protocols, full or mild. The full scatter protocol called for 500 mm, 0.1-s argon blue-green or green laser burns of moderate intensity, placed one-half burn apart, extending from the posterior pole to the equator. Between 1200 and 1600 burns were applied, divided between two or more episodes. The mild scatter protocol was the same, except that 400 to 650 more widely spaced burns were applied to the same area in a single episode. Direct (local) treatment was specified for patches of surface NVE that were two disc areas or less in extent (the area of a circle about 1.4 times the diameter of the disc), using confluent, moderately intense burns that extended 500 mm beyond the edges of the patch. For larger patches or several small ones close together, full scatter alone to this area was an acceptable alternative. No direct treatment was carried out for NVD.[148]

One important outcome measure used in the ETDRS was the first occurrence of either severe visual loss, as defined in the DRS, or vitrectomy.[147] These events were combined because progression to a stage requiring vitrectomy may rightly be considered a bad outcome for ETDRS-eligible eyes and because presumably most eyes selected for vitrectomy before the occurrence of severe visual loss (68% of the 243 ETDRS eyes undergoing vitrectomy) would have developed severe visual loss within several months if vitrectomy had not been done. Five-year life-table rates of severe visual loss or vitrectomy, and relative risks for early photocoagulation compared to deferral over the entire follow-up period, are shown in Table 68-9. The first two rows include eyes with macular edema, subdivided by retinopathy severity. As anticipated, the outcome was more frequent in eyes with more severe retinopathy (in the deferral group, 10% in eyes with severe NPDR or early PDR versus 4% in eyes with mild to moderate NPDR). In both of these retinopathy subgroups, early treatment reduced the event rate to about one-half that of the deferral group, but the percentage of eyes treated that benefited was only 2% to 4%. The third row of the table includes all eyes without macular edema regardless of retinopathy severity (eyes with mild NPDR were not eligible unless macular edema was present), and, as might be expected, outcome here was intermediate between that in rows 1 and 2. Some harmful effects of scatter photocoagulation were also observed in the ETDRS: an early decrease in visual acuity (a doubling or more of the visual angle at the 4-month visit in about 10% of eyes assigned to early full scatter, compared to about 5% of eyes assigned to deferral) and some decrease in visual field. Both beneficial and harmful effects were somewhat greater with full than with mild scatter.

Fig. 68-20 presents cumulative incidence rates of high-risk PDR in ETDRS eyes assigned to deferral of photocoagulation, by severity of retinopathy at baseline. Table 68-10 shows the ETDRS retinopathy severity scale. It is of interest that high-risk PDR developed at about equal rates in eyes with moderate PDR or very severe NPDR, with rates of about 50% after 18 months. Figs 68-16, 68-21, and 68-22 present the standard photographs used in the definitions of high-risk PDR and very severe NPDR, the most important severity levels for application to clinical practice. It is convenient to express the approximate definitions of severe and very severe NPDR with the 4-2-1 rule (Table 68-10).

Table 68-9 Cumulative 5-year rates of severe visual loss or vitrectomy, and relative risks for the entire period of follow-up, by baseline retinopathy status and treatment group*

Baseline retinopathy	Treatment group				Relative risk (99% CI)
	Early photocoagulation		Deferral		
	No. at baseline	5-year rate (%)	No. at baseline	5-year rate (%)	
Mild to moderate NPDR with macular edema	1448	2	1429	4	0.55 (0.33–0.94)
Severe NPDR or early PDR with macular edema	1090	6	1103	10	0.68 (0.47–0.99)
Moderate to severe NPDR or early PDR without macular edema	1173	4	1179	5	0.78 (0.47–1.29)

Reprinted from early photocoagulation for diabetic retinopathy. Early Treatment of Diabetic Retinopathy Study report no. 9. Early Treatment of Diabetic Retinopathy Study Group. Ophthalmology 1991; 98:766–785. Copyright 1991, with permission from the American Academy of Ophthalmology.[147]
*CI, Confidence interval; NPDR, nonproliferative diabetic retinopathy; PDR, proliferative diabetic retinopathy.

The ETDRS recommended that scatter treatment not be used in eyes with mild to moderate NPDR but that it be considered for eyes approaching the high-risk stage (i.e., eyes with very severe NPDR or moderate PDR) and that it usually should not be delayed when the high-risk stage is present. The recommendation to consider photocoagulation for eyes approaching the high-risk stage was made because, although both the benefits and risks of treatment were small and roughly in balance, the risk/benefit ratio was approaching a clearly favorable range. A policy of continued observation would be expected to spare only a minority of eyes from the risks of treatment, while increasing the risk that rapid progression might occur between follow-up visits and that entry into the high-risk stage might be marked by occurrence of a large vitreous hemorrhage, making satisfactory treatment difficult. In choosing between prompt treatment and deferral, the commitment of the patient to careful follow-up and the state of the fellow eye are important factors. If visual function decreased in the fellow eye after scatter photocoagulation, deferral of treatment in the second eye may be desirable. On the other hand, in a patient whose first eye had an unfortunate outcome without photocoagulation or one with photocoagulation only after PDR was advanced, prompt treatment may be preferable, particularly if close follow-up will be difficult.

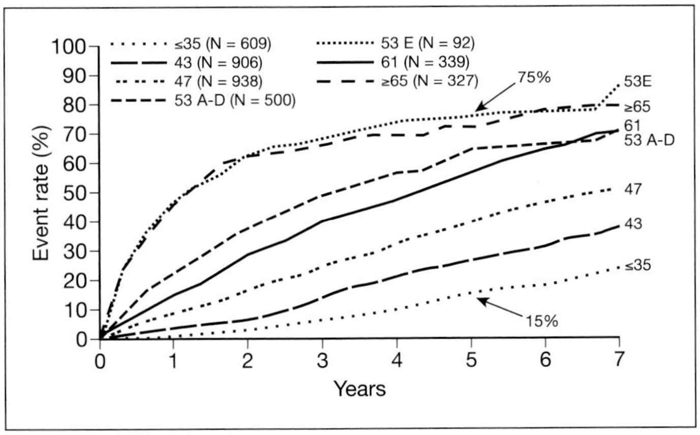

Fig. 68-20 Cumulative incidence of high-risk proliferative diabetic retinopathy in the eyes of Early Treatment Diabetic Retinopathy Study (ETDRS) patients assigned to deferral of photocoagulation. The 5-year rate for eyes with mild nonproliferative diabetic retinopathy (NPDR: level 35) was 15%. For eyes with very severe NPDR (level 53E) or moderate PDR (level 65), the 5-year rate was about 75% and the 1-year rate was almost 50%. Levels 43 and 47 represent moderate NPDR; level 53A–D, severe NPDR; and level 61, mild PDR (nVE less than half disc area or fibrous proliferation only). (Reprinted from early photocoagulation for diabetic retinopathy. Early Treatment of Diabetic Retinopathy Study report no. 9. Early Treatment of Diabetic Retinopathy Study Group. Ophthalmology 1991; 98:766–785. Copyright 1991, with permission from the American Academy of Ophthalmology.[147])

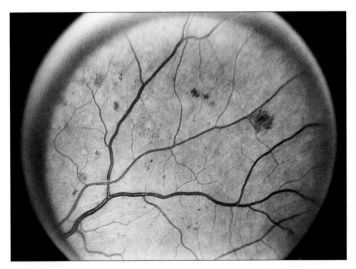

Fig. 68-21 Standard photograph 2A of the modified Airlie House classification, defining lower margin of the "severe" category for retinal hemorrhages and microaneurysms. (Reproduced with permission from Diabetic Retinopathy Study Research Group. A modification of the Airlie House classification of diabetic retinopathy. DRS report no. 7. Invest Ophthalmol Vis Sci 1981; 21:210–226.[18])

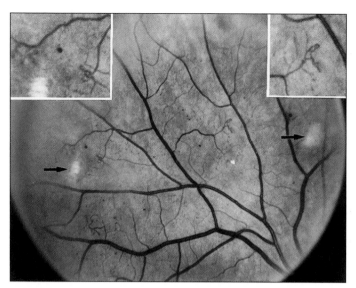

Fig. 68-22 Standard photograph 8A of the modified Airlie House classification, defining the lower margin of the "moderate" category for intraretinal microvascular abnormalities (IRMAs) (and for soft exudates, indicated by arrows). IRMAs are prominent in three areas, two of which are shown in insets. Additional IRMAs can be seen when the color transparencies used in grading are viewed stereoscopically with ×5 magnification. (Reproduced with permission from Diabetic Retinopathy Study Research Group. A modification of the Airlie House classification of diabetic retinopathy. DRS report no. 7. Invest Ophthalmol Vis Sci 1981; 21:210–226.[18])

These initial ETDRS recommendations were made without regard to patient age or type of diabetes. Subsequent analyses of ETDRS data suggest that, among patients whose retinopathy is in the severe NPDR to non-high-risk PDR range, the benefit of prompt treatment is greater in those who have type 2 diabetes (or are older than 40; these characteristics are highly correlated, and analyses using either gave almost identical results).[149] In the type 2 group, the 5-year rate of severe visual loss or vitrectomy was about 5% in eyes assigned to early photocoagulation versus 13% in eyes assigned to deferral, whereas in the type 1 group the rates were about 8% in both treatment groups (Fig. 68-23). In eyes assigned to deferral, severe visual loss or vitrectomy developed over the first 3 years at about the same rate in both diabetes types; apparently the greater treatment effect in type 2 diabetes resulted mainly from greater responsiveness to early treatment. Greater responsiveness to photocoagulation in older versus younger patients

has also been observed in other studies. In multivariable regression analyses, the Krypton Argon Regression Neovascularization Study (KARNS)[150] found that older age and management without insulin (and longer duration of diabetes and presence of fibrous proliferations) were associated with greater regression of NVD in eyes with NVD, equaling or exceeding those in Fig. 68-16 at baseline. Meyer-Schwickerath & Gerke[151] also found that regression of new vessels was achieved more often and with less extensive photocoagulation in patients with type 2 diabetes (after 3 years' complete regression in 59% versus 37% in patients with type 1 diabetes). The DRS also found greater photocoagulation treatment benefit in patients with type 2 diabetes.[149] These studies are consistent with the clinical impression that, in patients with type 2 diabetes, high-risk PDR is often first detected on the basis of a symptomatic vitreous hemorrhage in an eye in which new vessels had not been observed on previous visits, whereas in patients with type 1 diabetes, NVD are more often the first sign of high-risk PDR, an occurrence more easily managed with photocoagulation.

In summary, in older patients with type 2 diabetes who have very severe NPDR or early PDR, ETDRS results and clinical impression suggest that prompt photocoagulation is probably safer than deferral. In younger patients with type 1 diabetes, ETDRS results suggest that there is little to lose from deferring scatter photocoagulation until high-risk PDR develops. However, even in younger patients, when early NVD (less than shown in Fig. 68-16) is accompanied by the intraretinal signs of severe or very severe NPDR (see Fig. 68-2), we are inclined to recommend prompt treatment. On the other hand, when younger patients have only mild intraretinal lesions and NVE (only) that appear to be stable (i.e., that extend for some distance across the retina without prominent network formation or show partial regression), we are inclined to recommend an initial period of observation. If new vessels are demonstrated

Table 68-10 The 4-2-1 rule
Severe NPDR (any one of the following)
• H/MA ≥ Fig. 68-21 in four quadrants
• VB definitely present in ≥ two quadrants
• IRMA ≥ Fig. 68-22 in ≥ one quadrant
Very severe NPDR (two or more of the above)

H/MA, Hemorrhage/microaneurysms; *VB*, venous bleeding; *IRMA*, intraretinal microvascular abnormalities.

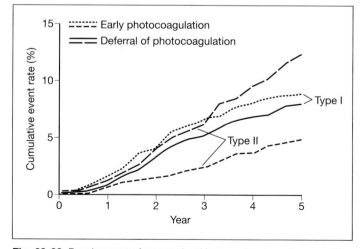

Fig. 68-23 Development of severe visual loss or vitrectomy in eyes with severe nonproliferative or early proliferative retinopathy at baseline. Early treated eyes compared with deferred eyes, for those with type I ($P = 0.43$) and type 2 ($P = 0.0001$) diabetes. Test for interaction of treatment and type ($P = 0.0002$). (Reproduced with permission from Ferris F. Early photocoagulation in patients with either type I or type 2 diabetes. Trans Am Ophthalmol Soc 1996; 94:505–537.[149])

to be growing, photocoagulation is usually recommended. However, many of these eyes remain asymptomatic for many years, with little growth and often substantial spontaneous regression of the new vessels. In such eyes vitreoretinal adhesions tend to be delicate, and when posterior vitreous detachment occurs, there is less tendency for traction retinal detachment. When the process of posterior vitreous detachment has reached completion in such an eye, new vessels are likely to be few, narrow, elevated, and partially replaced by fibrous proliferations, and there may be little to be gained from photocoagulation at this stage unless vitreous hemorrhages are occurring.

Systemic factors should also be considered in deciding whether to initiate treatment in patients with very severe NPDR or moderate PDR. Clinical impression suggests that progression of retinopathy may accelerate during pregnancy[84,152,153] or with the development of renal failure. If photocoagulation is deferred until high-risk characteristics develop, and this occurs in the later stages of pregnancy or when renal transplantation or dialysis is required, these more pressing problems may make it difficult to complete photocoagulation according to a schedule considered optimal from the ophthalmologic point of view. As already mentioned, if measures to improve long-standing poor glycemic control are planned when retinopathy is already at this stage, photocoagulation of at least one eye should be considered.

Scatter photocoagulation and macular edema

Macular edema sometimes increases, at least temporarily, after scatter photocoagulation, and this may be followed by transient or persistent reduction of visual acuity.[154–156] As mentioned above, the ETDRS documented small early harmful effects of scatter photocoagulation, particularly full scatter, in eyes with macular edema, as well as in those without. The DRS also found early harmful effects, which were greater in the xenon group. At the 6-week posttreatment visit, 21% of argon-treated and 46% of xenon-treated eyes that had macular edema and were free of high-risk characteristics at baseline had a decrease in visual acuity of two or more lines, compared with 9% of untreated eyes. Comparable percentages for eyes with neither macular edema nor high-risk characteristics were 9, 18, and 3%, respectively. After 1 year of follow-up, the greater progression of retinopathy in untreated eyes had led them to catch up with treated eyes; in the group having macular edema without high-risk characteristics at baseline, the percentages with a decrease in visual acuity of two or more lines were 32, 33, and 34%, respectively, in the argon-treated, xenon-treated, and control groups.[128] A multivariable analysis confirmed the independent effects of macular edema and treatment and provided no evidence of any interaction.[157] Both the ETDRS and the DRS support the clinical impression that eyes with macular edema requiring scatter treatment are at less risk of visual acuity loss when focal or grid treatment to reduce the macular edema precedes scatter photocoagulation. If a delay of scatter treatment seems undesirable, the ETDRS protocol can be used, combining focal/grid treatment for macular edema with scatter treatment in the nasal quadrants at the first episode of photocoagulation and adding scatter in the temporal quadrants at one or more subsequent episodes.[148] Certainly, scatter treatment should not be delayed

when the risks of vitreous hemorrhage or neovascular glaucoma seem high, regardless of the status of the macula.

TREATMENT TECHNIQUES

Direct (local) treatment of NVE

In the ETDRS, investigators had the option of applying direct photocoagulation (referred to as "local treatment") to new vessels on the retina. Confluent argon laser burns of 200- to 1000-μm spot size and a 0.1 to 0.5-s duration were specified with the resulting appearance (Fig. 68-24) very similar to that obtained with mild xenon arc photocoagulation. Local treatment was usually limited to small patches of NVE, in order to avoid large scotomas or nerve fiber bundle field defects. Because there is no good evidence that the combination of local and scatter treatment is any better than scatter treatment alone, most retina specialists avoid local treatment entirely.

Location and strength of scatter treatment

A common feature of most scatter treatment protocols is the location of burns beginning about 2 to 3 DD from the center of the macula and extending peripherally to the equator. Most of the proposed alternatives appear to aim at about the same amount of treatment, although the number, size, duration, and intensity of the exposures vary widely, from the 100 to 500, 4.5-degree, 0.2- to 0.5-s xenon burns used by Okun et al.[136] to the 2000 to 4000, 500-mm, 0.1-s argon burns advocated by Little.[137]

It is important to realize that the size of the burn produced depends not only on the spot-size setting used, but also on power and duration, so it is difficult to compare techniques, even those using the same wavelength and spot-size setting, on the basis of

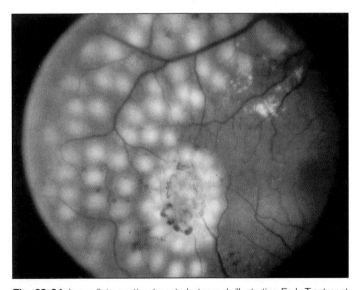

Fig. 68-24 Immediate posttreatment photograph illustrating Early Treatment Diabetic Retinopathy Study full scatter treatment and local confluent treatment of a patch of new vessels everywhere (NVE). (Reproduced with permission from Early Treatment of Diabetic Retinopathy Study Research Group. Techniques for scatter and local photocoagulation treatment of diabetic retinopathy: the Early Treatment of Diabetic Retinopathy Study report no. 3. Int Ophthalmol Clin 1987; 27:254–264.[148])

number and theoretical size of burns. It is also difficult to describe burn strength; power level is not very helpful, since the required power for a burn of given strength depends on the clarity of the media and the pigmentation of the fundus, even if spot-size setting and duration are kept constant. One useful measure of burn strength is the need for retrobulbar anesthesia. What we consider to be optimal burn strength with the argon laser is just below the level at which treatment under topical anesthesia with 500-μm, 0.1-s burns becomes painful for most patients. With topical anesthesia only, it is usually difficult or impossible to obtain burns of adequate strength when their duration is longer than 0.1 or 0.15 s or their size is >500 μm. The ETDRS protocol for full scatter treatment provides useful guidelines for initial treatment, calling for a total of 1200 to 1600 500-μm, 0.1-s argon laser burns of moderate intensity placed one-half to one burn apart and divided between two or more episodes (at least 2 weeks apart, if two episodes; at least 4 days apart, if three or more episodes). Burns usually appear to enlarge slightly within several minutes after their application, resulting in the closer spacing of the scatter burns shown in Fig. 68-24.

Blankenship[158] suggested that keeping the posterior limit of scatter treatment farther from the posterior pole may reduce harmful treatment effects. He randomly assigned 50 eyes with DRS high-risk characteristics to argon laser scatter photocoagulation with either a peripheral or a posterior treatment protocol, each carried out in a single episode with retrobulbar anesthesia. Blankenship's peripheral protocol consisted of two parts: (1) about 450 burns of moderate intensity placed with the Rodenstock pantoscopic lens and 500-μm spot-size setting in a zone bounded posteriorly by an oval passing through points 4 DD below, nasal to, and above the disc and 4 DD temporal to the center of the macula and extending peripherally to the vortex vein ampullae; and (2) 400 to 500 500-μm burns placed more peripherally with the Goldmann three-mirror lens. In his posterior protocol, treatment with the Rodenstock lens was the same but was combined with 400 to 470 500-μm burns placed more posteriorly with the Goldmann lens, up to the disc margin nasally and to within about 1.5 DD above, temporal to, and below the center of the macula. All eyes were followed up without retreatment for 6 months. Although there were trends at the 6-month follow-up visit for less visual acuity decrease and less worsening of macular edema in the peripheral treatment group, this study was too small for conclusive results. The peripheral treatment protocol may provide a useful alternative for initial treatment of eyes with macular edema in which the urgency of treatment for severe PDR is thought to preclude division of scatter treatment between two or more episodes.

Number of episodes used for scatter treatment

The new technique of optical coherence tomography was used in a recent study comparing shorter versus longer spacing between episodes of scatter photocoagulation.[159] Among the techniques currently in use, the number of episodes in which initial scatter treatment is carried out varies from one to four or more. Those techniques using a smaller number of larger burns tend toward a single episode with retrobulbar anesthesia, whereas those using

a larger number of smaller burns nearly always divide treatment into two or more episodes. Multiple episodes make it easier to avoid retrobulbar anesthesia and its occasional complications, but they may cause delays and inconvenience for patients who must travel long distances for treatment. Angle-closure glaucoma secondary to serous detachment of the peripheral choroid and ciliary body is less common when scatter treatment is carried out in two or more sessions over a period of 1 or 2 weeks,[160] and some observers believe that small losses in visual acuity may also be less common.

Doft & Blankenship[161] addressed this question in a small randomized trial. They randomly assigned one eye from each of 50 patients with DRS high-risk characteristics to scatter photocoagulation with 1200 0.1-s 500-μm argon laser burns of moderate intensity applied in either of two ways: (1) at a single episode or (2) in three episodes at 1-week intervals. Retrobulbar anesthesia was used in the single-episode group and for the first of the multiple episodes. In the latter group at the first episode, several rows of burns were placed surrounding the posterior pole, and treatment was extended temporally and nasally to the periphery, leaving the remainder of the upper quadrants (from the 10 o'clock to the 2 o'clock position) for the second episode and the remainder of the lower quadrants (from the 4 o'clock to the 8 o'clock position) for the third. Patients were examined 3, 7, 14, 21, 60, and 180 days after completion of the initial treatment episode. Peripheral choroidal detachment was noted more frequently at the 3-day visit in the single than in the multiple-episode group (17 of 25 and 10 of 25 eyes, respectively), and three eyes in the former group developed angle closure, which resolved spontaneously without any adverse effect. Transient (present at the 3-day and 7-day visit but not at the 14-day visit) exudative retinal detachment involving the macula was noted in 7 of 25 eyes treated in a single episode and in 2 of 25 eyes treated in three episodes. These eyes with exudative macular detachment had, on average, a visual acuity decrease of about five lines at the 3-day visit, but at the 6-month visit they had recovered to about the same level as eyes without such transient detachments. At the 6-month visit the numbers of eyes with a one-line, a two- to four-line, and a five- or more line decrease in visual acuity from the baseline visit were, respectively, three, six, and one in the single-episode group, compared with four, four, and one in the multiple-episode group. These differences were not significant, but the power of this small study to find differences was low. Moreover, completely surrounding the posterior pole with treatment at the initial episode in the multiple episode protocol was unlike many other multiple episode protocols, in which the more posterior burns are divided between two or more episodes.

The new technique of optical coherence tomography was used in a recent study comparing shorter versus longer spacing between episodes of scatter photocoagulation. Thirty-six patients with severe nonproliferative or early proliferative retinopathy and 20/20 vision in each eye at baseline received scatter photocoagulation in the following manner: in one eye, one quadrant was treated every week for 4 weeks and in the other eye, one quadrant was treated every other week for 8 weeks. OCT assessment of macular thickness was performed at baseline, before each session of photocoagulation, and at 16 weeks, the end of the follow-up period. Four of 36 eyes in the weekly treatment group and 3 of 36 in the biweekly group developed center-involved macular edema with decreased visual acuity (from 20/40 to 20/200), which was treated with photocoagulation. Additional photocoagulation for residual neovascularization was carried out in 35 to 40% of eyes in each group. The response of the remaining eyes is shown in Fig. 68-25. At baseline, mean retinal thickness was 191 μm in the central zone of the macular grid (1000 μm in diameter) in both groups. Thickness increased progressively after each weekly treatment to a maximum of 275 μm at week 4 and then decreased to 225 μm at 16 weeks. The increase was less after the biweekly treatments and at 16 weeks was closer to, but had not reached, the baseline value. There was little change in retinal thickness outside the central zone with either treatment technique. This study is consistent with the observations mentioned earlier of development of center-involved macular edema following scatter photocoagulation and suggests subclinical occurrence of this problem in a majority of eyes.

Wavelength

The KARNS randomly assigned 907 eyes (of 696 patients) that had NVD equaling or exceeding those in Fig. 68-16 to scatter photocoagulation (1600 to 2000 moderate-intensity 500-mm burns) with either blue-green argon or red krypton wavelengths.[150] If, after the initial treatment, NVD increased by more than 0.5 disc area, retreatment was recommended (and could also be applied for other reasons, such as increasing NVE or vitreous hemorrhage). Retreatment was carried out in 36% and 33%, respectively, of the argon and krypton groups; increased NVD was the reason for the retreatment in about 40% of retreated eyes in each group. Regression of NVD to less than

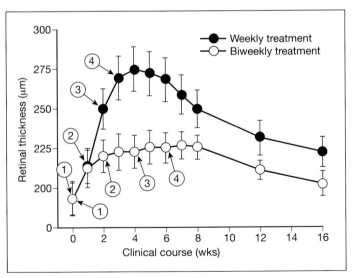

Fig. 68-25 Comparison of retinal thickness in the central zone between the weekly treated eyes and biweekly treated eyes. Each point and vertical bar indicates mean retinal thickness ± standard error of the mean. Arrows indicate each session of weekly treatment at 0-, 1-, 2-, and 3-week time points and biweekly treatment at 0-, 2-, 4-, and 6-week time points. (Reprinted from Shimura M, Yasuda K, Nakazawa T et al. Quantifying alterations of macular thickness before and after panretinal photocoagulation in patients with severe diabetic retinopathy and good vision. Ophthalmology 2003; 110:2386–2394. Copyright 2003, with permission from the American Academy of Ophthalmology.[176])

that shown in Fig. 68-16 was observed in almost identical proportions of the two groups (41.4 and 41.8%, respectively, at 3 months and 55 and 52.8%, respectively, at 1 year). No differences were found in the effectiveness of argon versus krypton treatment, but retrobulbar anesthesia was used more frequently with krypton. In two small randomized trials diode (810 nm) and double-frequency Nd:YAG (532-nm) lasers gave results similar to those of the argon green laser.[162,163]

Regression of new vessels after initial photocoagulation and indications for retreatment

There is general agreement that substantial regression of new vessels usually occurs within days or weeks after the initial application of scatter photocoagulation and that eyes in which new vessels continue to grow despite initial treatment or recur after partial or complete regression usually respond well to additional treatment. However, data documenting the rapidity and completeness of regression are sparse, and many reports do not clearly separate results after initial treatment and results after initial treatment plus retreatment as needed. Table 68-11 summarizes much of the available information. Doft & Blankenship[164] combined the single- and multiple-treatment groups previously discussed and described the course of new-vessel regression over a 6-month period without retreatment. At the 3-day posttreatment visit 10 (20%) of the 50 eyes had regressed from the high-risk stage; at 2 weeks, 25 (50%); at 3 weeks, 36 (72%); and at 6 months, 31 (62%). About one-third of the eyes that were still in the high-risk stage at 3 weeks no longer were at 6 months, whereas about one-third of those with regression at 3 weeks had progressed to the high-risk stage again at 6 months. Blankenship[158] reported similar findings in his study comparing peripheral and posterior treatment. In both groups combined there were 31 eyes with NVD greater than or equal to one-fourth disc area at baseline. In all but one of these 31 eyes, NVD was less than one-fourth disc area at the 1-month follow-up visit; at the 6-month visit, 24 of the 31 (77%) met this criterion. Vander et al.[165] reported that 59% of 59 eyes with high-risk PDR had a satisfactory response (retinopathy no longer in the high-risk category) 3 months after initial full scatter photocoagulation. In the KARNS, 3 months after the initial treatment (with or without retreatment), NVD had decreased to less than 50% of the baseline area in 54% of eyes and had decreased by a lesser amount in an additional 19%.[150] Among DRS eyes with NVD equaling or exceeding those in Fig. 68-16 at baseline (with or without NVE), all new vessels had regressed completely 1 year after the initial treatment in 20% of argon-treated eyes, and regression of NVD to less than those in Fig. 68-16 had occurred in an additional 34%; results after xenon arc photocoagulation were similar.[13] Because the DRS protocol did not emphasize or specify guidelines for retreatment, and because treatment was being compared with no treatment in that study, these results probably represent outcome to be expected after initial treatment only.

Information on the efficacy of retreatment is also sparse and difficult to compare between studies. After applying 1100 to 1500

Table 68-11 Regression of neovascularization after scatter photocoagulation

Author (year)	No. of eyes	Initial photocoagulation				Retreatment			
		Pretreatment retinopathy severity (no. of burns)	Response criterion	Time to evaluation	No. (%) with favorable response	No. retreated / no. eligible	Timing (no. of burns)	Response criterion	No. with favorable response
Doft & Blankenship (1984)[163]	50	High-risk PDR (1200 one episode)	Absence of high-risk PDR	3 days	10 (20%)	–	–	–	–
				2 weeks	25 (50%)				
				3 weeks	36 (72%)				
				6 months	31 (62%)				
Blankenship (1988)[158]	31	NVD ≥ ¼ disc area	NVD < ¼ disc area	1 month	30 (97%)	–	–	–	–
				6 months	24 (77%)				
Vander et al. (1991)[164]	59	High-risk PDR ("full scatter")	Absence of high-risk PDR	3 months	35 (59%)	–	–	–	–
Krypton Argon Regression Neovascularization Study (KARNS: 1993)[150]	907	NVD ≥ standard standard 10A (1600–2000)	NVD < 50% of baseline	3 months	490 (54%)	–	–	–	–
			NVD 50–99% of baseline		172 (19%)				
Diabetic Retinopathy Study (1978)[13]		NVD ≥ standard 10A		1 year		–	–	–	–
	188	Argon (800–1600)	No NVD or NVE		38 (20%)				
			NVD < standard 10A		64 (34%)				
	163	Xenon arc (200–800)	No NVD or NVE		36 (22%)				
			NVD < standard 10A		62 (38%)				
Rogell (1983)[165]	55	PDR (1100–1500 total in two episodes)	"Substantial regression"	1 month	21 (38%)	34/34	Monthly (300–400)	Substantial regression	30 (88%)
Reddy et al. (1995)[166]	294	≥ 2 risk factors ("full scatter")	Decrease in risk factors	6–8 weeks	177 (60%)	117/117	71 PC only 46 PC + cryo		98 (84%)
Vine (1985)[167]	Not stated	High-risk PDR (~3000)	Absence of high-risk PDR	8 weeks	Not stated	23/23	Q 6–8 week 1000–2000	< High-risk PDR	12 (52%)

PC, Photocoagulation; PDR, proliferative diabetic retinopathy; NVD, neovascularization of disc; NVE, neovascularization elsewhere.

500-μm, moderately intense argon laser burns, divided between two episodes about 1 week apart, Rogell[166] followed patients at monthly intervals, applying 300 to 400 additional burns at each visit until "substantial regression" of new vessels had occurred. In 21 of 55 eyes (38%) with PDR, the initial treatment was sufficient. Additional photocoagulation was carried out once or twice in 29 eyes and three to five times in 5 eyes; peripheral retinal cryotherapy was added in two eyes. Response to retreatment was considered satisfactory in 30 of 34 eyes (88%). In a retrospective case review of 182 patients (294 eyes), Reddy et al.[167] assessed the need for retreatment after initial full scatter photocoagulation in patients with two or more NV-VH risk factors. In 177 of 294 eyes (60%), the response to initial treatment was considered satisfactory. The remaining 117 eyes were retreated, 71 with photocoagulation alone and 46 with a combination of photocoagulation and anterior retinal cryotherapy. Retreatment was successful in 98 of 117 eyes (84%). Among an unspecified number of eyes with high-risk PDR treated initially with extensive argon laser scatter photocoagulation during a 2-year period, 23 eyes remained in the high-risk stage 8 weeks after completion of the initial treatment and were given follow-up treatment by Vine.[168] Eyes were observed at 6- to 8-week intervals, and follow-up treatment (1000 to 2000 low-intensity burns placed between scars) was applied until regression from the high-risk stage occurred or further treatment was not feasible. Retreatment was successful in 12 of 23 eyes (52%).

From these studies it appears that, on average, about two-thirds of eyes have a satisfactory response to initial scatter treatment. As mentioned earlier, this ratio tends to be more favorable in patients with type 2 diabetes. Patients with severe intraretinal lesions and actively growing new vessels, who typically have type 1 diabetes, often need multiple treatments. In most cases retreatment gives gratifying results.[139]

The ETDRS protocol contains guidelines for follow-up treatment that seem suitable for general use. Six factors are considered: (1) change in new vessels since the last visit or last photocoagulation treatment; (2) appearance of the new vessels (caliber, degree of network formation, extent of accompanying fibrous tissue); (3) frequency and extent of vitreous hemorrhage since the last visit or last photocoagulation treatment; (4) status of vitreous detachment; (5) extent of photocoagulation scars; and (6) extent of traction retinal detachment and fibrous proliferations.[148] If new vessels appear to be active, as suggested by formation of tight networks, paucity of accompanying fibrous tissue, and increase in extent in comparison to the previous visit, additional photocoagulation is considered. The case for additional treatment is stronger if the extent of new vessels is substantially greater than it was at the time of initial treatment for high-risk characteristics or if vitreous or preretinal hemorrhages are occurring repeatedly. If the caliber of new vessels has decreased and fibrous proliferations are developing, this suggests that retinopathy is entering a quiescent stage in which additional treatment may be unnecessary. A single episode of vitreous hemorrhage coincident with the occurrence of extensive posterior vitreous detachment, particularly if the only vitreoretinal adhesion remaining is at the disc, argues less for additional photocoagulation than do recurrent hemorrhages unrelated to such an occurrence. Additional photocoagulation may be less urgent after occurrence of extensive posterior vitreous detachment because additional growth of new vessels (whether along the detached posterior hyaloid surface or, much less commonly, along the surface of the retina) does not increase the extent of vitreoretinal adhesions. The extent and location of photocoagulation scars may also influence the decision regarding additional photocoagulation treatment. If the previous scatter burns appear widely spaced, or if there are areas where scatter was omitted, additional photocoagulation is considered more seriously. If repeated scatter treatment has been done and additional treatment would need to be done over old scars, clear indications are necessary before advising additional treatment, since extensive loss of visual field may occur. In such cases indefinite deferral of photocoagulation may sometimes be the best alternative, even though there are extensive new vessels on the detached posterior vitreous surface and small vitreous hemorrhages are occurring occasionally. If severe vitreous hemorrhage occurs, vitrectomy can be done, with a good chance of restoration of both central and peripheral vision.

When additional scatter treatment is carried out under the ETDRS protocol, burns are placed between treatment scars, anterior to them, or in the posterior pole, individually or severally, sparing the area within 500 μm of the center of the macula and using burns no larger than 200 μm in the zone between 500 and 1500 μm from the center. The areas chosen for treatment are generally those in which new vessels are present (or toward which they appear to be growing) or in which scars are less tightly spaced. Some experienced observers believe that priority should be given to the posterior pole, particularly the area temporal to the center of the macula, where extensive capillary loss is common and small new-vessel patches sometimes occur, and where the posterior extent of the original scatter treatment is sometimes more than the prescribed 2 DD from the center of the macula. Fig. 68-26 provides an example of follow-up treatment.

Indications for vitrectomy

When vitrectomy was initially introduced in 1970 by Machemer et al.,[11] the major indications in eyes with PDR were severe vitreous hemorrhage that had failed to clear spontaneously after a year and traction retinal detachment involving the center of the macula. As this procedure came into widespread use, it was recognized that it might be of value earlier in the course of very severe PDR.[169] A clinical trial, the DRVS, was established by the National Eye Institute to explore this possibility. In one part of the DRVS, eyes with recent severe vitreous hemorrhage (hemorrhage sufficient to obscure completely the posterior pole and to reduce visual acuity to 5/200 or less for at least 1 month) were randomly assigned to either early vitrectomy or conventional management (i.e., follow-up without vitrectomy unless retinal detachment involving the center of the macula occurred or the hemorrhage failed to clear during a 1-year waiting period).[170] After 2 years of follow-up, recovery of good vision (visual acuity of 10/20 or better) was observed more frequently in the early vitrectomy group (24.5% versus 15.2% in the conventional management group, $P = 0.01$). Loss of light perception tended to occur more frequently in the early vitrectomy group (24.9% versus 19.3% in the conventional

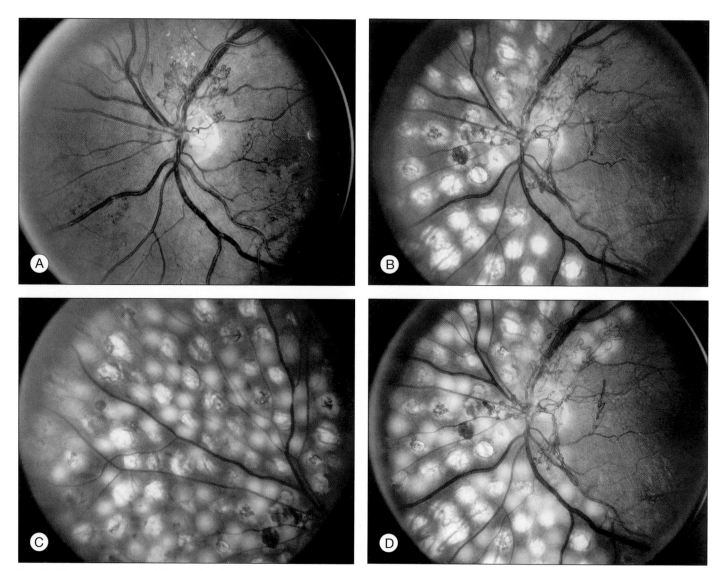

Fig. 68-26 Retreatment after initial scatter photocoagulation. A, At his initial visit in 1978, this 28-year-old man, whose age at diagnosis of diabetes was 13 years, had new vessels on disc (NVD) exceeding those in Diabetic Retinopathy Study standard photograph 10A in his left eye. Venous beading, intraretinal microvascular abnormalities, hemorrhages, and microaneurysms met the "severe" nonproliferative diabetic retinopathy criteria. Visual acuity was 20/25. Full scatter photocoagulation was applied in two episodes that were 4 weeks apart, with retrobulbar anesthesia used. NVD regressed only approximately 25% and then gradually increased. B, Two years after the initial photocoagulation, new vessels had extended along the temporal vascular arcades, nasal to the disc, and over the papillomacular bundle. Fibrous proliferations had become more prominent, and fine retinal tension lines radiated temporally from them. C and D, With topical anesthesia, 800 burns of 500-μm spot size, 0.1-s duration were applied between scars in all quadrants, with one additional row posterior to the superotemporal and inferotemporal veins and three rows between 2 and 3 disc diameters temporal to the center of the macula, where treatment had been omitted initially.

management group, $P = 0.16$). A subgroup analysis was carried out by diabetes type, as shown in Table 68-12. Patients were classified as having type 1 diabetes if the diabetes had been diagnosed at or before age 20 years and if the patients were receiving insulin at the time of entry into the study. Patients age 40 years or older at diagnosis (regardless of insulin use) were classified as having type 2 diabetes, as were patients with diabetes diagnosed at a younger age, if they were not receiving insulin at the time of entering the study. Those patients receiving insulin whose diabetes was diagnosed between age 21 and 39 (inclusive) were assigned to an intermediate group, presumably containing a mixture of type 1 and type 2 patients. The mean age at study

entry of type 1 patients was 33 years, compared to 59 years in the mixed and type 2 groups combined. Early vitrectomy appeared to be clearly advantageous only in the type 1 group, in which good vision was attained by 35.6% of patients undergoing early vitrectomy, versus 11.7% of those conventionally managed. It was suggested that this interaction might be related both to better potential of the macula for good vision in these younger patients and to the more extensive new vessels, fibrous proliferations, and vitreoretinal adhesions characterizing this group (see Table 68-1). Eyes with the most severe proliferations would be expected to be at greatest risk for distortion, dragging, or detachment of the macula while waiting for the hemorrhage to clear.

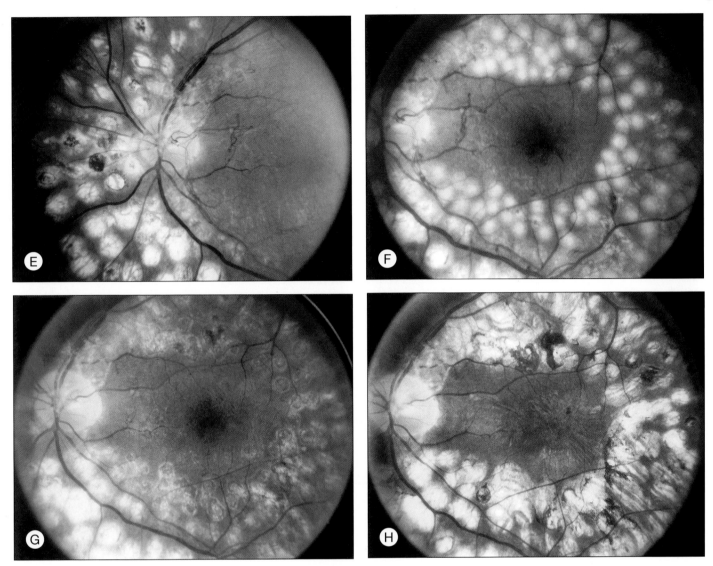

Fig. 68-26—cont'd E, One month later, new vessels had undergone partial regression, but some remained on the temporal side of the disc, along the temporal vascular arcades and over the papillomacular bundle. F, Four months later, new vessels had increased slightly and, with topical anesthesia, 150 additional 500-μm, 0.1-s burns were applied, 75 posteriorly, extending to within about 1 disc diameter of the center of the macula, and 75 temporally between scars. G, Three months later, almost complete regression of the new vessels had occurred. Retinal vessels had narrowed (compare with A and B). Visual acuity remained 20/25. Visual field was full to an IV4E Goldmann test object and averaged approximately 10 degrees in each meridian with a 13e test object. The patient was not aware of any visual loss, except for decreased night vision. H, Visual acuity and fine residual NVD remained unchanged over the next 5 years. Photocoagulation scars have increased in area and reflexes suggesting epiretinal membrane formation have developed in the macula.

In the subgroup of type 1 patients whose severe vitreous hemorrhage occurred when diabetes had been present for less than 20 years, deferral of vitrectomy appeared to be particularly disadvantageous, with good vision achieved in only 1.9% (Table 68-12); and this subgroup tended to have more severe PDR. Results after 4 years were similar.[171] These results suggest that early vitrectomy should be considered in eyes with recent severe diabetic vitreous hemorrhage when it is known from prior examination that fibrovascular proliferations are severe, particularly if it appears that macular potential is good. Older patients with severe vitreous hemorrhage sometimes have surprisingly mild PDR, and in such patients it is usually preferable to allow more time for spontaneous clearing of vitreous hemorrhage

before considering vitrectomy, particularly if vision in the fellow eye is good.

As vitrectomy techniques improved and the frequency of serious complications decreased, additional indications were suggested. These included traction on the disc, peripapillary retina, or macula that distorts these structures and leads to substantial reduction in visual acuity; opaque fibrous proliferations in front of the macula; and extensive preretinal hemorrhage.[172–175]

In a second study the DRVS compared early vitrectomy versus conventional management in eyes that had extensive active neovascular or fibrovascular proliferations and useful vision, 65% of which had had previous photocoagulation. In the conventional

Table 68-12 Percentages of eyes with visual acuities of 10/20 or better and no light perception (NLP) at the 2-year follow-up visit, by type and duration of diabetes and treatment group*

Baseline factor	No. of eyes E	No. of eyes D	≥ 10/20 E	≥ 10/20 D	Difference (E – D)	NLP E	NLP D	Difference (D – E)†
Diabetes type								
Type 1	101	103	35.6	11.7	23.9	27.7	26.2	−1.5
Mixed	70	69	18.6	17.4	1.2	24.3	15.9	−8.4
Type 2	82	72	15.9	18.1	−2.2 (P = .4007)	22.0	12.5	−9.5 (P = 0.48)
Duration of diabetes (years)								
All diabetes types								
< 20	131	129	21.4	10.1	11.3	28.2	24.8	−3.4
≥ 20	122	115	27.9	20.9	7.0 (P = .29)	21.3	13.0	−8.3 (P = 0.36)
Type 1 only								
< 20	50	53	34.0	1.9	32.1	34.0	35.8	1.8
≥ 20	51	50	37.3	22.0	15.3 (P = .007)	21.6	16.0	−5.6 (P = 0.50)

Reproduced from Diabetic Retinopathy Vitrectomy Study (DRVS) Research Group: report no 2. Arch Ophthalmol 1985; 103:1644–1652. Copyright © (1985) American Medical Association. All rights reserved.[36]
*E, Early vitrectomy group: D, deferral group.
†D minus E rather than E minus D (as for visual acuity ≥ 10/20), so that a positive value is a difference in favor of early vitrectomy, as is the case for visual acuity ≥ 10/20.

Table 68-13 Percentage of eyes with specified visual acuity at the 4-year follow-up visit for early vitrectomy and conventional management groups, and differences between groups, by severity of new vessels in baseline stereoscopic color fundus photographs*

	No. of eyes E	No. of eyes C	≥ 10/20 (%) E	≥ 10/20 (%) C	Difference (E – C)	NLP (%) E	NLP (%) C	Difference (C – E)
All eyes	145	138	44.14	28.26	15.88	22.8	18.8	−3.0
New vessels combined								
Least severe	35	34	42.9	41.2	1.7	20.0	5.9	−14.1
Moderately severe	46	36	50.0	36.1	13.9	23.9	13.9	−10.0
Severe†	39	49	43.6	20.4	23.2	17.9	22.4	4.5
Very severe†	25	19	36.0	10.5	25.5	32.0	42.1	10.1
P (for interaction)					0.0784			0.0419

Reprinted from early vitrectomy for severe proliferative diabetic retinopathy in eyes with useful vision: results of a randomized trial, Diabetic Retinopathy Vitrectomy Study report no. 3. Diabetic Retinopathy Vitrectomy Study Research Group. Ophthalmology 1988; 95:1307–1320. Copyright 1988, with permission from American Academy of Ophthalmology.[169]
*NLP, No light perception; E, early vitrectomy; C, conventional management; NVD, new vessels on or within 1 disc diameter of the disc; NVE, new vessels elsewhere.
†Eyes with either NVD 1.5 disc areas or more in extent or NVE 2.5 disc areas or more in extent in at least one of the seven standard photographic fields were classified as "severe"; eyes with both NVD and NVE of this extent were classified as "very severe."

management group, early vitrectomy was allowed if retinal detachment involving the center of the macula developed, if severe vitreous hemorrhage reducing visual acuity to 5/200 or worse occurred and persisted for 6 months or more, or if visual acuity decreased from 10/50 or better at study entry to 10/100 or worse during follow-up as a result of dense fibrous proliferations in front of the macula or traction on the optic disc, peripapillary retina, or macula. Table 68-13 summarizes the principal results after 4 years of follow-up.[170,176] In eyes with the most severe new vessels (the "severe" and "very severe" categories), early vitrectomy appeared to provide a greater chance of good vision with no increase in risk of NLP. These results are consistent with those of the earlier DRVS study and support the use of vitrectomy in cases with very severe PDR that do not respond promptly to scatter photocoagulation or in which it cannot be applied because of vitreous hemorrhage. More details concerning vitreous surgery for complications of PDR are included in Volume 3.

ACKNOWLEDGMENT

This study was supported in part by an unrestricted grant from Research to Prevent Blindness, Inc., and by a Research to Prevent Blindness Senior Scientific Investigator Award (M.D.D.).

REFERENCES

1. Cogan D, Toussaint D, Kuwabara T. Retinal vascular patterns. IV. Diabetic retinopathy. Arch Ophthalmol 1961; 66:366–378.
2. Davis M, Myers F, Engerman R et al. Clinical observations concerning the pathogenesis of diabetic retinopathy. In: Goldberg M, Fine S, eds. Symposium on the treatment of diabetic retinopathy. US Public Health Service publication no. 1890. Washington, DC: US Government Printing Office; 1969.
3. deVenecia G, Davis M, Engerman R. Clinicopathologic correlations in diabetic retinopathy. I. Histology and fluorescein angiography of microaneurysms. Arch Ophthalmol 1976; 94:1766–1773.
4. Engerman R, Bloodworth JJ. Experimental diabetic retinopathy in dogs. Arch Ophthalmol 1965; 73:205–210.
5. Kohner E, Henkind P. Correlation of fluorescein angiogram and retinal digest in diabetic retinopathy. Am J Ophthalmol 1970; 69:403–414.
6. Muraoka K, Shimizu K. Intraretinal neovascularization in diabetic retinopathy. Ophthalmology 1984; 91:1440–1446.
7. Ashton N. Pathogenesis of diabetic retinopathy. In: Little H, Jack R, Patz A et al., eds. Diabetic retinopathy. New York: Thieme-Stratton; 1983.
8. Michelson I. The mode of development of the vascular system of the retina, with some observations on its significance for certain retinal diseases. Trans Ophthalmol Soc UK 1948; 68:137–180.
9. Shimizu K, Kobayashi Y, Muraoka K. Midperipheral fundus involvement in diabetic retinopathy. Ophthalmology 1981; 88:601–612.
10. Wise G. Retinal neovascularization. Trans Am Ophthalmol Soc 1956; 54:729–826.
11. Machemer R, Buettner H, Norton E et al. Vitrectomy: a pars plana approach. Trans Am Acad Ophthalmol Otolaryngol 1971; 75:813–820.
12. Patz A. Clinical and experimental studies on retinal neovascularization. Am J Ophthalmol 1982; 94:715–743.
13. Diabetic Retinopathy Study Research Group. Photocoagulation treatment of proliferative diabetic retinopathy: the second report of the Diabetic Retinopathy Study findings. Ophthalmology 1978; 85:82–106.
14. Davis M. Vitreous contraction in proliferative diabetic retinopathy. Arch Ophthalmol 1965; 74:741–751.
15. Taylor E, Dobree J. Proliferative diabetic retinopathy: site and size of initial lesions. Br J Ophthalmol 1970; 54:11–18.
16. Diabetic Retinopathy Study Research Group. Design, methods and baseline results, DRS report no 6. Invest Ophthalmol Vis Sci 1981; 21:149–209.
17. Davis M. Methods of fundus examination. In: Kimura S, Caygill W, eds. Vascular complications of diabetes mellitus. St Louis: Mosby; 1967.
18. Diabetic Retinopathy Study Research Group. A modification of the Airlie House classification of diabetic retinopathy. DRS report no. 7. Invest Ophthalmol Vis Sci 1981; 21:210–226.
19. Prud'homme G, Rand L. The Diabetic Retinopathy Study Research Group: distribution of maximum grade of lesions in proliferative diabetic retinopathy. Invest Ophthalmol Vis Sci 1981; 20(suppl):59.
20. Schwartz J, Pavan P. Optic disc edema. Int Ophthalmol Clin 1984; 24:83–91.
21. Kampik A, Kenyon K, Michels R et al. Epiretinal and vitreous membranes: comparative study of 56 cases. Arch Ophthalmol 1981; 99:1445–1454.
22. Nork T, Wallow I, Sramek S et al. Mueller's cell involvement in proliferative diabetic retinopathy. Arch Ophthalmol 1987; 105:1424–1429.
23. Davis M. Natural history of diabetic retinopathy. In: Kimura S, Caygill W, eds. Vascular complications of diabetes mellitus. St Louis: Mosby; 1967.
24. Dobree J. Proliferative diabetic retinopathy: evolution of the retinal lesions. Br J Ophthalmol 1964; 48:637–649.
25. Bandello F, Gass J, Lattanzio R et al. Spontaneous regression of neovascularization at the disk and elsewhere in diabetic retinopathy. Am J Ophthalmol 1996; 122:494–501.
26. Larsen H. Diabetic retinopathy: an ophthalmoscopic study with a discussion of the morphologic changes and the pathogenetic factors in the disease. Acta Ophthalmol 1960; 60 (Suppl.):1–89.
27. Tolentino F, Lee P, Schepens C. Biomicroscopic study of vitreous cavity in diabetic retinopathy. Arch Ophthalmol 1966; 75:238–246.
28. Anderson BJ. Activity and diabetic vitreous hemorrhages. Ophthalmology 1980; 87:173–175.
29. Tasman W. Diabetic vitreous hemorrhage and its relationship to hypoglycemia. Mod Probl Ophthalmol 1979; 20:413–414.
30. Bresnick G, Haight B, deVenecia G. Retinal wrinkling and macular heterotopia in diabetic retinopathy. Arch Ophthalmol 1979; 97:1890–1895.
31. Beetham W. Visual prognosis of proliferating diabetic retinopathy. Br J Ophthalmol 1963; 47:611–619.
32. Ramsay W, Ramsay R, Purple R et al. Involutional diabetic retinopathy. Am J Ophthalmol 1977; 84:851–858.
33. Caird F, Pirie A, Ramsell T. Diabetes and the eye. Oxford: Blackwell Scientific; 1969.
34. Polonsky K, Rubeinstein A. C-peptide as a measure of the secretion and hepatic extraction of insulin: pitfalls and limitations. Diabetes 1984; 33:486–494.
35. Klein R, Davis M, Moss S et al. The Wisconsin Epidemiologic Study of Diabetic Retinopathy: a comparison of retinopathy in younger and older onset diabetic persons. In: Vranic M, Hollenberg C, Steiner G, eds. Comparison of type I and II diabetes. New York: Plenum Press; 1985.
36. Diabetic Retinopathy Vitrectomy Study Research Group. Early vitrectomy for severe vitreous hemorrhage in diabetic retinopathy: two-year results of a randomized clinical trial. Diabetic Retinopathy Vitrectomy Study report no 2. Arch Ophthalmol 1985; 103:1644–1652.
37. Aiello L, Rand L, Briones J et al. Diabetic retinopathy in Joslin Clinic patients with adult onset diabetes. Ophthalmology 1981; 88:619–623.
38. Bodansky H, Cudworth S, Drury P et al. Risk factors associated with severe proliferative retinopathy in insulin-dependent diabetes mellitus. Diabetes Care 1982; 5:97–100.
39. Dornan T, Mann JI, Turner R. Factors protective against retinopathy in insulin-dependent diabetics free of retinopathy for 30 years. Br Med J 1982; 285:1073–1077.
40. Klein R, Klein B, Moss S et al. Glycosylated hemoglobin predicts the incidence and progression of diabetic retinopathy. JAMA 1988; 260:2864–2871.
41. Krolewski A, Rand L, Warram J et al. Proliferative diabetic retinopathy (PDR) risk is closely related to hemoglobin A_{1c} (A_{1c}) level. Diabetes 1985; 34:71.
42. Krolewski A, Warram J, Rand L et al. Risk of proliferative diabetic retinopathy in juvenile-onset type I diabetes: a 40-year follow-up study. Diabetes Care 1986; 9:443–452.
43. Rand L, Krolewski A, Aiello L et al. Multiple factors in the prediction of risk of proliferative diabetic retinopathy. N Engl J Med 1985; 313:1433–1438.
44. Beck-Nielsen H, Richelsen B, Mogensen CE et al. Effect of insulin pump treatment for one year on renal function and retinal morphology in patients with IDDM. Diabetes Care 1985; 8:585–589.
45. Engerman R, Bloodworth JJ, Nelson S. Relationship of microvascular disease in diabetes to metabolic control. Diabetes 1977; 26:760–769.
46. Engerman R, Kern T. Progression of incipient diabetic retinopathy during good glycemic control. Diabetes 1987; 36:808–812.
47. Brinchmann-Hansen O, Dahl-Jorgensen K, Hannsen K et al. The response of diabetic retinopathy to 41 months of multiple insulin injections, insulin pumps, and conventional insulin therapy. Arch Ophthalmol 1988; 106:1242–1246.
48. Knatterud GL, Klimt CR, Levin ME et al. Effects of hypoglycemic agents on vascular complications in patients with adult-onset diabetes. VII. Mortality and selected nonfatal events with insulin treatment. JAMA 1978; 240:37–42.
49. Kroc Collaborative Study Group. The Kroc Study patients at two years: a report on further retinal changes. Diabetes 1985; 34:39.
50. Lauritzen T, Frost-Larsen K, Larsen H et al. Two-year experience with continuous subcutaneous insulin infusion in relation to retinopathy and neuropathy. Diabetes 1985; 34(Suppl.):74–79.
51. Reichard P, Berglund B, Britz A et al. Intensified conventional insulin treatment retards microvascular complications of insulin-dependent diabetes mellitus (IDDM): The Stockholm Diabetes Intervention Study (SDIS) after 5 years. J Intern Med 1991; 230:101–108.
52. Stefansson E, Hatchell D, Fisher B et al. Panretinal photocoagulation and retinal oxygenation in normal and diabetic cats. Am J Ophthalmol 1986; 101:657–664.
53. Diabetes Control and Complications Trial Research Group. The effect of intensive treatment of diabetes on the development and progression of long-term complications in insulin-dependent diabetes mellitus. N Engl J Med 1993; 329:977–936.

54. Diabetes Control and Complications Trial Research Group. The effect of intensive diabetes treatment on the progression of diabetic retinopathy in insulin-dependent diabetes mellitus. Arch Ophthalmol 1995; 113:36–51.

55. Diabetes Control and Complications Trial Research Group. Progression of retinopathy with intensive versus conventional treatment in diabetes control and complications trial. Ophthalmology 1995; 102:647–661.

56. Diabetes Control and Complications Trial Research Group. Perspectives in diabetes: the relationship of glycemic exposure (HbA$_{1c}$) to the risk of development and progression of retinopathy in the Diabetes Control and Complications Trial. Diabetes 1996; 44:968–983.

57. Reichard P, Nilsson B, Rosenqvist U. Retardation of the development of microvascular complications after long-term intensified insulin treatment: the Stockholm Diabetes Intervention Study. N Engl J Med 1993; 329:304–309.

58. Dahl-Jorgensen K, Brinchmann-Hansen O, Hanssen K et al. Rapid tightening of blood glucose control leads to transient deterioration of retinopathy in insulin-dependent diabetes mellitus: the Oslo study. Br Med J 1985; 290:811–815.

59. Diabetes Control and Complications Trial Research Group. Early worsening of diabetic retinopathy in the diabetes control and complications trial. Arch Ophthalmol 1998; 116:874–886.

60. Kroc Collaborative Study Group. Blood glucose control and the evolution of diabetic retinopathy and albuminuria: a preliminary multicenter trial. N Engl J Med 1984; 311:365–372.

61. Lauritzen T, Frost-Larsen K, Larsen H et al. Effect of 1 year of near-normal blood glucose levels on retinopathy in insulin-dependent diabetics. Lancet 1983; 1:200–204.

62. Lawson P, Champion M, Canny C et al. Continuous subcutaneous insulin infusion (CSII) does not prevent progression of proliferative and pre-proliferative retinopathy. Br J Ophthalmol 1982; 66:762–766.

63. Puklin J, Tamborlane W, Felig P et al. Influence of long-term insulin infusion pump treatment of type I diabetes on diabetic retinopathy. Ophthalmology 1982; 89:735–747.

64. Simmons R, Dueker D, Kimbrough R et al. Goniophotocoagulation for neo-vascular glaucoma. Trans Am Acad Ophthalmol Otolaryngol 1977; 83:80–89.

65. Early Treatment of Diabetic Retinopathy Study Research Group (ETDRS). Manual of operations. National Technical Information Service PB85 223006/AS. Washington, DC: National Public Information Service; 1985.

66. Early Treatment of Diabetic Retinopathy Study Research Group (ETDRS). Early treatment Diabetic Retinopathy Study design and baseline patient characteristics. ETDRS report no. 7. Ophthalmology 1991; 98(Suppl. 5):741–756.

67. Ohkubo Y, Kishikawa H, Araki E et al. Intensive insulin therapy prevents the progression of diabetic microvascular complications in Japanese patients with noninsulin-dependent diabetes mellitus: a randomized prospective 6-year study [see comments]. Diabetes Res Clin Pract 1995; 28:103–117.

68. UK Prospective Diabetes Study (UKPDS) Group. Intensive blood-glucose control with sulphonylureas or insulin compared with conventional treatment and risk of complications in patients with type2 diabetes (UKPDS 33). Lancet 1998; 352:837–853.

69. The Diabetes Control and Complications Trial/Epidemiology of Diabetes Interventions and Complications Research Group. Retinopathy and nephropathy in patients with type 1 diabetes four years after a trial of intensive therapy. N Engl J Med 2000; 342:381–389.

70. Davis M, Fisher M, Gangnon R et al. Risk factors for high-risk proliferative diabetic retinopathy and severe visual loss: Early Treatment of Diabetic Retinopathy Study report no. 18. Invest Ophthalmol Vis Sci 1998; 39:233–252.

71. Verillo A, de Teresa A, Martino C et al. Long-term improvement of metabolic control does not affect progression of background retinopathy. Transplant Proc 1986; 18:1569–1570.

72. Davis MD. Diabetic retinopathy: a clinical overview [see comments]. Diabetes Care 1992; 15:1844–1874.

73. Chantelau E, Eggert H. Acceleration of diabetic retinopathy following improved glycaemic control: a report on 13 cases. Diabetologia 1997; 40(Suppl. 1):501.

74. Chantelau E, Kohner E. Why some cases of retinopathy worsen when diabetic control improves: worsening retinopathy is not a reason to withhold intensive insulin treatment. Br Med J 1997; 315:1105–1106.

75. Agardh CD, Eckert B, Agardh E. Irreversible progression of severe retinopathy in young type I insulin-dependent diabetes mellitus patients after improved metabolic control. J Diabetes Complications 1992; 6:96–100.

76. Dandona P, Bolger J, Boag F et al. Rapid development and progression of proliferative retinopathy after strict diabetic control. Br Med J 1985; 290:895–896.

77. Daneman D, Drash A, Lobes L et al. Progressive retinopathy with improved control in diabetic dwarfism (Mauriac's syndrome). Diabetes Care 1981; 4:360–365.

78. Gudat U, Chantelau E. Rapid-progressive diabetische Retino-pathie bei Stoffwechselnormalisierung: wer ist gefahrdet? Z Klin Med 1992; 4:108–113.

79. Lawrence J, Bedford G, Thomson R. Rapid development during puberty of proliferative retinopathy after strict diabetic control. Lancet 1985; 2:322.

80. Moskalets E, Galstyan G, Starostina E et al. Association of blindness to intensification of glycemic control in insulin-dependent diabetes mellitus. J Diabetes Compl 1994; 8:45–50.

81. Henricsson M, Nilsson A, Janzon L et al. The effect of glycaemic control and the introduction of insulin therapy on retinopathy in noninsulin-dependent diabetes mellitus [see comments]. Diabetes Med 1997; 14:123–131.

82. Roysarkar TK, Gupta A, Dash RJ et al. Effect of insulin therapy on progression of retinopathy in noninsulin-dependent diabetes mellitus. Am J Ophthalmol 1993; 115:569–574.

83. Klein R, Klein B, Moss S. Epidemiology of proliferative diabetic retinopathy. Diabetes Care 1992; 15:1875–1891.

84. Chew EY, Klein ML, Ferris FL III et al. Association of elevated serum lipid levels with retinal hard exudate in diabetic retinopathy. Early Treatment Diabetic Retinopathy Study (ETDRS) report no. 22. Arch Ophthalmol 1996; 114:1079–1084.

85. Qiao Q, Keinanen-Kiukaanniemi S, Laara E. The relationship between hemoglobin levels and diabetic retinopathy. J Clin Epidemiol 1997; 50:153–158.

86. Shorb SR. Anemia and diabetic retinopathy. Am J Ophthalmol 1985; 100:434–436.

87. Berman DH, Friedman EA. Partial absorption of hard exudates in patients with diabetic end-stage renal disease and severe anemia after treatment with erythropoietin. Retina 1994; 14:1–5.

88. Houssay B, Biasotti A. La diabetes pancreatica de los perros hipofisoprivos. Rev Soc Argent Biol 1930; 6:251–296.

89. Luft R, Olivecrona H, Sjogren B. Hypophysectomy in man. Nord Med 1952; 47:351–354.

90. Poulsen J. The Houssay phenomenon in man: recovery from retinopathy in a case of diabetes with Simmonds' disease. Diabetes 1953; 2:7–12.

91. Poulsen J. Diabetes and anterior pituitary insufficiency: final course and postmortem study of a diabetic patient with Sheehan's syndrome. Diabetes 1966; 15:73–77.

92. Kohner E, Joplin G, Blach R et al. Pituitary ablation in the treatment of diabetic retinopathy. Trans Ophthalmol Soc UK 1972; 92:79–90.

93. Lundbaek K, Malmros R, Andersen H et al. Hypophysectomy for diabetic retinopathy: a controlled clinical trial. In: Goldberg M, Fine S, eds. Symposium on the treatment of diabetic retinopathy. US Public Health report no. 1890. Washington, DC: US Government Printing Office; 1969.

94. Panisset A, Kohner E, Cheng H et al. Diabetic retinopathy: new vessels arising from the optic disc. II. Response to pituitary ablation by yttrium 90 implant. Diabetes 1971; 20:824–833.

95. Kohner E, Hamilton A, Joplin G et al. Florid diabetic retinopathy and its response to treatment by photocoagulation or pituitary ablation. Diabetes 1976; 25:104–110.

96. Growth hormone antagonist for proliferative diabetic retinopathy study group. The effect of a growth hormone receptor antagonist drug on proliferative diabetic retinopathy. Ophthalmology 2001; 108:2266–2272.

97. Aiello LP. Clinical implications of vascular growth factors in proliferative retinopathies. Curr Opin Ophthalmol 1997; 8:19–31.

98. Casey R, Li WW. Perspective: factors controlling ocular angiogenesis. Am J Ophthalmol 1997; 124:521–529.

99. Clermont A, Aiello L, Mori F et al. Vascular endothelial growth factor and severity of nonproliferative diabetic retinopathy mediate retinal hemodynamics in vivo: a potential role for vascular endothelial growth factor in the progression of diabetic retinopathy. Am J Ophthalmol 1997; 124:433–446.

100. Frank RN. Diabetic retinopathy. N Engl J Med 2004; 350:48–58.

101. Miller JW, Adamis AP, Aiello LP. Vascular endothelial growth factor in ocular neovascularization and proliferative diabetic retinopathy. Diabetes Metab Rev 1997; 13:37–50.

102. Sönksen PH, Russell-Jones D, Jones RH. Growth hormone and diabetes mellitus: a review of 63 years of medical research and a glimpse into the future? Horm Res 1993; 40:68–79.

103. Meyer-Schwickerath G. Light coagulation. St Louis: Mosby; 1960.

104. Dobree J. Light coagulation in proliferative diabetic retinopathy. In: Goldberg M, Fine S, eds. Symposium on the treatment of diabetic retinopathy. US Public Health Service publication no. 1890. Washington, DC: US Government Printing Office; 1969.

105. Harris G, Rentiers P. The role of photocoagulation in the therapy of proliferative diabetic retinopathy. In: Goldberg M, Fine S, eds. Symposium on the treatment of diabetic retinopathy. US Public Health Service publication no. 1890. Washington, DC: US Government Printing Office; 1969.

106. Larsen H. Photocoagulation in proliferative diabetic retinopathy: a preliminary report. In: Goldberg M, Fine S, eds. Symposium on the treatment of diabetic retinopathy. US Public Health Service publication no. 1890. Washington, DC: US Government Printing Office; 1969.

107. McMeel J, Van Hueven W. Photocoagulation as a treatment of diabetic retinopathy. In: Goldberg M, Fine S, eds. Symposium on the treatment of diabetic retinopathy. US Public Health Service publication no. 1890. Washington, DC: US Government Printing Office; 1969.

108. Okun E, Cibis P. The role of photocoagulation in the therapy of proliferative diabetic retinopathy. Arch Ophthalmol 1966; 75:337–352.

109. Wetzig P, Jepson C. Treatment of diabetic retinopathy by light coagulation. Am J Ophthalmol 1966; 62:459–465.

110. Wetzig P, Worlton J. Treatment of diabetic retinopathy by light coagulation: a preliminary study. Br J Ophthalmol 1963; 47:539–541.

111. Beetham W, Aiello L, Balodimos M et al. Ruby laser photocoagulation of early diabetic neovascular retinopathy: preliminary report of a long-term controlled study. Arch Ophthalmol 1970; 83:261–272.

112. Meyer-Schwickerath G, Schott K. Diabetic retinopathy and photocoagulation. Am J Ophthalmol 1968; 66:597–603.

113. Okun E. The effectiveness of photocoagulation in the therapy of proliferative diabetic retinopathy (PDR) (a controlled study in 50 patients). Trans Am Acad Ophthalmol Otolaryngol 1968; 72:246–252.

114. Aiello L, Beetham W, Balodimos M et al. Ruby laser photocoagulation in treatment of diabetic proliferating retinopathy: preliminary report. In: Goldberg M, Fine S, eds. Symposium on the treatment of diabetic retinopathy. US Public Health Service publication no. 1890. Washington, DC: US Government Printing Office; 1969.

115. Gerstein D, Dantzker D. Retinal vascular changes in hereditary visual cell degeneration. Arch Ophthalmol 1969; 81:99–105.

116. Molnar J, Poitry S, Tsacopoulos M et al. Effect of laser photocoagulation on oxygenation of the retina in miniature pigs. Invest Ophthalmol Vis Sci 1985; 26:1410–1414.

117. Weiter J, Zuckerman R. The influence of the photoreceptor–RPE complex on the inner retina: an explanation for the benefit of special effects of photocoagulation. Ophthalmology 1980; 87:1133–1139.

118. Wolbarsht M, Landers MI. The rationale of photocoagulation therapy for proliferative diabetic retinopathy: a review and a model. Ophthalm Surg 1980; 11:235–245.

119. Grunwald J, Riva C, Brucker A et al. Altered retinal vascular response to 100% oxygen breathing in diabetes mellitus. Ophthalmology 1984; 91:1477–1452.

120. Patel V, Rassam S, Newsom R et al. Retinal blood flow in diabetic retinopathy. Br Med J 1992; 305:678–683.

121. Wilson D, Green W. Argon laser panretinal photocoagulation for diabetic retinopathy: scanning electron microscopy of human choroidal vascular casts. Arch Ophthalmol 1987; 105:239–242.

122. Adamis AP, Shima DT, Yeo KT et al. Synthesis and secretion of vascular permeability factor/vascular endothelial growth factor by human retinal pigment epithelial cells. Biochem Biophys Res Commun 1993; 193:631–638.

123. Glaser B, Campochiaro P, Davis JJ et al. Retinal pigment epithelial cells release an inhibitor of neovascularization. Arch Ophthalmol 1985; 103:1870–1875.

124. Ederer F, Hiller R. Clinical trials, diabetic retinopathy, and photocoagulation: a reanalysis of five studies. Surv Ophthalmol 1975; 19:267–286.

125. Cheng H. Multicentre trial of xenon-arc photocoagulation in the treatment of diabetic retinopathy: a randomized controlled study: interim report. Trans Ophthalmol Soc UK 1975; 95:351–357.

126. Aiello L, Berrocal J, Davis M et al. The Diabetic Retinopathy Study. Arch Ophthalmol 1973; 90:347–348.

127. Diabetic Retinopathy Study Research Group. Preliminary report on effects of photocoagulation therapy. Am J Ophthalmol 1976; 81:383–396.

128. Diabetic Retinopathy Study Research Group. Indications for photocoagulation treatment of diabetic retinopathy. DRS report no. 14. Int Ophthalmol Clin 1987; 27:239–253.

129. Diabetic Retinopathy Study Research Group. Four risk factors for severe visual loss in diabetic retinopathy: the third report from the Diabetic Retinopathy Study. Arch Ophthalmol 1979; 97:654–655.

130. Diabetic Retinopathy Study Research Group. Photocoagulation treatment of proliferative diabetic retinopathy: clinical application of Diabetic Retinopathy Study (DRS) findings. DRS report no. 8. Ophthalmology 1981; 88:583–600.

131. Diabetic Retinopathy Study Group. Photocoagulation treatment of proliferative diabetic retinopathy: a short report on long-range results. DRS report no. 4. In: Waldhausl W, ed. Proceedings of the Tenth Congress of the International Diabetes Foundation. Amsterdam: Excerpta Medica; 1980.

132. Diabetic Retinopathy Study Research Group. Photocoagulation of proliferative diabetic retinopathy: relationship of adverse treatment effects to retinopathy severity. DRS report no. 5. Dev Ophthalmol 1981; 2:248–261.

133. Rand L, Prud'homme G, Ederer F et al. Factors influencing the development of visual loss in advanced diabetic retinopathy. Diabetic Retinopathy Study (DRS) report no. 10. Invest Ophthalmol Vis Sci 1985; 26:983–991.

134. British Multicentre Study Group. Photocoagulation for proliferative diabetic retinopathy: a randomised controlled clinical trial using the xenon-arc. Diabetologia 1984; 26:109–115.

135. Hercules B, Gayed I, Lucas S et al. Peripheral retinal ablation in the treatment of proliferative diabetic retinopathy: a three-year interim report of a randomised controlled study using the argon laser. Br J Ophthalmol 1977; 61:555–563.

136. Okun E, Johnston G, Boniuk I et al. Xenon arc photocoagulation of proliferative diabetic retinopathy: a review of 2688 consecutive eyes in the format of the Diabetic Retinopathy Study. Ophthalmology 1984; 91:1458–1463.

137. Little H. Proliferative diabetic retinopathy: pathogenesis and treatment. In: Little H, Patz A, Forsham P, eds. Diabetic retinopathy. New York: Thieme-Stratton, 1983

138. Folk JC, Ma C, Blodi CF et al. Occlusion of bridging or avulsed retinal vessels by repeated photocoagulation. Ophthalmology 1987; 94:1610–1613.

139. Early Treatment of Diabetic Retinopathy Study Group. Case reports to accompany Early Treatment of Diabetic Retinopathy Study reports 3 and 4. Int Ophthalmol Clin 1987; 27:273–333.

140. Hilton G. Panretinal cryotherapy for diabetic rubeosis. Arch Ophthalmol 1979; 97:776.

141. Little H, Rosenthal A, Dellaporta A et al. The effect of panretinal photocoagulation on rubeosis iridis. Am J Ophthalmol 1976; 81:804–809.

142. May D, Bergstrom T, Parmet A et al. Treatment of neovascular glaucoma with transscleral panretinal cryotherapy. Ophthalmology 1980; 87:1106–1111.

143. Murphy R, Egbert P. Regression of iris neovascularization following panretinal photocoagulation. Arch Ophthalmol 1979; 97:700–702.

144. Pavan P, Folk J. Anterior neovascularization. Int Ophthalmol Clin 1984; 24:61–70.

145. Pavan P, Folk J, Weingeist T et al. Diabetic rubeosis and panretinal photocoagulation: a prospective, controlled, masked trial using iris fluorescein angiography. Arch Ophthalmol 1983; 101:882–884.

146. Bresnick GH, deVenecia G, Myers FL et al. Retinal ischemia in diabetic retinopathy. Arch Ophthalmol 1975; 93:1300–1310.

147. Early Treatment of Diabetic Retinopathy Study Group. Early photocoagulation for diabetic retinopathy. Early Treatment of Diabetic Retinopathy Study report no. 9. Ophthalmology 1991; 98:766–785.

148. Early Treatment of Diabetic Retinopathy Study Research Group. Techniques for scatter and local photocoagulation treatment of diabetic retinopathy: the Early Treatment of Diabetic Retinopathy Study report no. 3. Int Ophthalmol Clin 1987; 27:254–264.

149. Ferris F. Early photocoagulation in patients with either type I or type 2 diabetes. Trans Am Ophthalmol Soc 1996; 94:505–537.

150. KARNS. Randomized comparison of krypton versus argon scatter photocoagulation for diabetic disc neovascularization. The Krypton Argon Regression Neovascularization Study report no. 1. Ophthalmology 1993; 100:1655–1664.

151. Meyer-Schwickerath G, Gerke E. Treatment of diabetic retinopathy with photocoagulation: results of photocoagulation therapy of proliferative retinopathy in childhood-onset and maturity-onset and an approach to the dosage in photocoagulation. Acta Ophthalmol 1983; 61:756–768.

152. Chew E, Mills J, Metzger B et al. Metabolic control and progression of retinopathy. The Diabetes in Early Pregnancy Study. Diabetes Care 1995; 18:631–667.

153. Klein B, Moss S, Klein R. Effect of pregnancy on progression of diabetic retinopathy. Diabetes Care 1990; 13:34–40.

154. McDonald H, Schatz H. Macular edema following panretinal photocoagulation. Retina 1985; 5:5–10.

155. McDonald H, Schatz H. Visual loss following panretinal photocoagulation for proliferative diabetic retinopathy. Ophthalmology 1985; 92:388–393.

156. Meyers S. Macular edema after scatter laser photocoagulation for proliferative diabetic retinopathy. Am J Ophthalmol 1980; 90:210–216.

157. Ferris FI, Podgor M, Davis M et al. Macular edema in Diabetic Retinopathy Study patients. DRS report no. 12. Ophthalmology 1987; 94:754–760.

158. Blankenship G. A clinical comparison of central and peripheral argon laser panretinal photocoagulation for proliferative diabetic retinopathy. Ophthalmology 1988; 95:170–177.

159. Shimura M, Yasuda K, Nakazawa T et al. Quantifying alterations of macular thickness before and after panretinal photocoagulation in patients with severe diabetic retinopathy and good vision. Ophthalmology 2003; 110:2386–2394.

160. Liang H, Huamonte F. Reduction of immediate complications after panretinal photocoagulation. Retina 1984; 4:166–170.

161. Doft B, Blankenship G. Single versus multiple treatment sessions of argon laser panretinal photocoagulation for proliferative diabetic retinopathy. Ophthalmology 1982; 89:772–779.

162. Bandello F, Brancato R, Lattanzio R et al. Double-frequency Nd:YAG laser vs. argon-green laser in the treatment of proliferative diabetic retinopathy: randomized study with long-term follow-up. Lasers Surg Med 1996; 19:173–176.

163. Bandello F, Brancato R, Trabucchi G et al. Diode versus argon-green laser panretinal photocoagulation in proliferative diabetic retinopathy: a randomized study in 44 eyes with a long follow-up time. Graefes Arch Clin Exp Ophthalmol 1993; 231:491–494.

164. Doft B, Blankenship G. Retinopathy risk factor regression after laser panretinal photocoagulation for proliferative diabetic retinopathy. Ophthalmology 1984; 91:1453–1457.

165. Vander JF, Duker JS, Benson WE et al. Long-term stability and visual outcome after favorable initial response of proliferative diabetic retinopathy to panretinal photocoagulation. Ophthalmology 1991; 98:1575–1579.

166. Rogell G. Incremental panretinal photocoagulation: results in treating proliferative diabetic retinopathy. Retina 1983; 3:308–311.

167. Reddy VM, Zamora RL, Olk RJ. Quantitation of retinal ablation in proliferative diabetic retinopathy. Am J Ophthalmol 1995; 119:760–766.

168. Vine A. The efficacy of additional argon laser photocoagulation for persistent, severe, proliferative diabetic retinopathy. Ophthalmology 1985; 92:1532–1537.

169. Blankenship G, Machemer R. Prophylactic vitrectomy in proliferative diabetic retinopathy. Mod Probl Ophthalmol 1977; 18:236–241.

170. Diabetic Retinopathy Vitrectomy Study Research Group. Early vitrectomy for severe proliferative diabetic retinopathy in eyes with useful vision: results of a randomized trial, Diabetic Retinopathy Vitrectomy Study report no. 3. Ophthalmology 1988; 95:1307–1320.

171. Diabetic Retinopathy Vitrectomy Study Research Group. Early vitrectomy for severe vitreous hemorrhage in diabetic retinopathy: four-year results of a randomized trial. Diabetic Retinopathy Study report no. 5. Arch Ophthalmol 1990; 108:958–964.

172. deBustros S, Thompson J, Michels R et al. Vitrectomy for progressive proliferative diabetic retinopathy. Arch Ophthalmol 1987; 105:196–199.

173. O'Hanley G, Canny C. Diabetic dense premacular hemorrhage: a possible indication for prompt vitrectomy. Ophthalmology 1985; 92:507–511.

174. Ramsay R, Knobloch W, Cantrill H. Timing of vitrectomy for active proliferative diabetic retinopathy. Ophthalmology 1986; 93:283–289.

175. Shea M. Early vitrectomy in proliferative diabetic retinopathy. Arch Ophthalmol 1983; 101:1204–1205.

176. Diabetic Retinopathy Vitrectomy Study Research Group. Early vitrectomy for severe proliferative diabetic retinopathy in eyes with useful vision: clinical application of results of a randomized trial. Diabetic Retinopathy Study report no. 4. Ophthalmology 1988; 95:1321–1334.

177. Shimura M, Yasuda K, Nakazawa T et al. Quantifying alterations of macular thickness before and after panretinal photocoagulation in patients with severe diabetic retinopathy and good vision. Ophthalmology 2003; 110:2386–2394.

Chapter

69

Retinal Artery Obstruction

Sanjay Sharma
Gary C. Brown

In 1859, von Graefe[1] described an embolic central retinal artery obstruction in a patient with endocarditis and multiple systemic emboli. Knapp,[2] however, mentions that several years earlier Virchow had suggested that an embolus might be seen directly in a retinal artery with the ophthalmoscope. Duke-Elder nicely elaborates further history on this entity. Within five years after von Graefe's report, Sweiger described the histopathologic correlate of central retinal artery obstruction.[3] In 1868 Mauthner suggested that spasmodic contractions could lead to retinal arterial obstruction, and in 1874 Loring implicated focal obstructive disease within the retinal vessels as a cause. By the turn of the twentieth century, over two dozen reports of retinal arterial obstruction were present in the ophthalmic literature.[3]

Retinal arterial obstructive (occlusive) disease can be manifest in a number of different clinical fashions. The arbitrary classification given below is followed in this chapter.

1. Central retinal artery obstruction.
2. Branch retinal artery obstruction.
3. Cilioretinal artery obstruction.
4. Combined central retinal artery and vein obstruction.
5. Cotton-wool spots.

CENTRAL RETINAL ARTERY OBSTRUCTION

Incidence and demographics

Data concerning the incidence of central retinal artery obstruction (occlusion) are not readily available, but from information gathered at Wills Eye Hospital it has been estimated to occur with a frequency of about one per 10 000 outpatient visits. The abnormality is most commonly encountered in older adults, but can also be seen in children.[4] The mean age at the time of presentation is the early sixties. There appears to be no predilection for one eye over the other, and men are affected more frequently than women. In approximately 1–2% of cases there is bilateral involvement.[5] When both eyes are simultaneously affected by retinal artery obstruction, the differential diagnosis should include cardiac valvular disease, giant cell arteritis, and other vascular inflammations.[6]

Clinical features

Patients with acute central retinal artery obstruction usually relate a history of painless visual loss occurring over several seconds.

In some instances, there is a preceding history of amaurosis fugax. While amaurosis typically is suggestive of an embolic cause of occlusion, it has been recently reported in a case of giant cell arteritis.[7]

The anterior segment examination is most often initially normal in eyes with acute central retinal artery obstruction. If rubeosis iridis is present at the time the obstruction occurs, the presence of concomitant carotid artery obstruction should be considered. Under these circumstances, increased intraocular pressure resulting from the rubeosis iridis induced by the carotid artery obstruction can exceed the perfusion pressure in the central retinal artery and predispose to its occlusion.

An afferent pupillary defect usually develops within seconds after obstruction of the central retinal artery.[8] During the early phases of the obstruction the fundus appearance can be normal, but an afferent pupillary defect will still be present unless the obstruction has spontaneously resolved.

Acutely, the superficial retina in the posterior pole becomes opacified and assumes a yellow-white appearance, except in the region of the foveola, where a cherry-red spot is present (Fig. 69-1). The latter may vary is size, probably depending upon the width of the fovea (Fig. 69-2). Both cloudy swelling and cherry-red spot formation are clinical signs for which there exists a high degree of agreement among ophthalmologists.[9] Ischemic necrosis in the affected inner half of the retina corresponds to the whitening seen clinically. The size of the cherry-red spot is variable, depending upon the width of the foveola. A cherry-red spot develops because the retina in this region is extremely thin, allowing a view of the underlying retinal pigment epithelium and choroid. Furthermore, the foveolar retina is probably nourished, to an extent, by the underlying choroid, thereby preventing complete hypoxia when the central retinal artery is occluded. The retinal opacification diminishes rapidly once outside the macular area. The opacification can require hours to become apparent, although we have been able to induce it in the subhuman primate model following complete retinal arterial obstruction within 10–15 minutes. In most cases the retinal opacification resolves over a period of 4–6 weeks, usually leaving a pale optic disc, narrowed retinal vessels and visible absence of the nerve fiber layer in the affected region of the optic disc. Resultant pigmentary changes are usually absent unless there is also involvement of the choroidal circulation. In cases of severe obstruction, segmentation or "boxcarring" of the blood column can be seen in both the arteries and the veins.

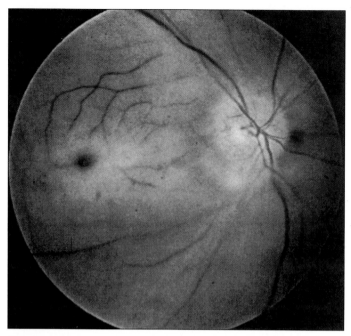

Fig. 69-1 A, Acute central retinal artery obstruction. Whitening, or opacification, of the superficial retina is present, and a cherry-red spot can be seen centrally. The opacification is most pronounced in the peripheral fovea, where the retina is the thickest. Narrowing of the retinal arteries is also present.

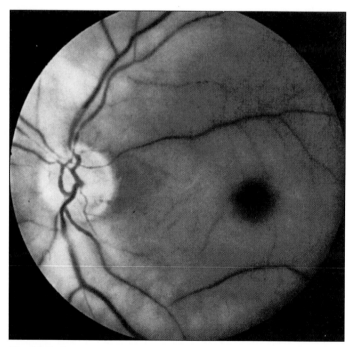

Fig. 69-2 Central retinal artery obstruction with a large cherry-red spot, probably because the fovea is broader than the usual eye.

At the time of initial examination, the visual acuity in eyes with central retinal artery obstruction ranges between counting fingers and light perception in 90% of eyes.[5] Connolly et al. were able to note a trend toward better visual acuities in patients with monocular CRAO secondary to giant cell arteritis

as compared to those with CRAO alone (OR = 2.22; 95% CI 0.37–13.2).[10] The presence of an embolus in the fundus is usually associated with poorer vision.[5] Absence of light perception is rarely encountered. In such instances, the clinician should suspect the presence of concomitant choroidal circulatory compromise or damage to the optic nerve.[5]

Approximately 25% of eyes with an acute central retinal artery obstruction have a patent cilioretinal artery that supplies part or all of the papillomacular bundle.[11] If only a part of the papillomacular bundle is spared (Figs 69-3 and 69-4), the resultant visual acuity is still usually no better than 20/100. In about 10% of eyes the cilioretinal artery spares foveolar involvement (Figs 69-5 and 69-6), in which case the visual acuity improves to 20/50 or better in 80% of eyes over a two week period. Only a small island of central vision may remain, but in some eyes a surprising amount of peripheral visual field returns.

Emboli are visible within the retinal arterial system in about 20–40% of eyes with central retinal artery obstruction.[5,12] The most common variant is the glistening, yellow cholesterol embolus (Hollenhorst plaque). This type of embolus is believed to most commonly arise from atherosclerotic deposits in the carotid arteries,[6] but certainly can also originate from the aortic arch, ophthalmic artery, or even the more proximal central retinal artery. Cholesterol emboli are often small and may not totally obstruct retinal arteries. They frequently occur asymptomatically (Fig. 69-7). In some eyes with central retinal artery obstruction, a large, nonglistening embolus is seen within the central retinal artery on the optic disc, while numerous small cholesterol emboli are present in the more peripheral retinal arteries. It is likely that the larger embolus on the disc is of the same origin, but appears

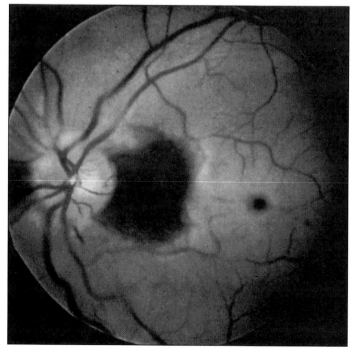

Fig. 69-3 Cilioretinal artery sparing approximately one-half of the papillomacular bundle in this left eye with a CRAO. Despite the sparing, the vision remained finger counting.

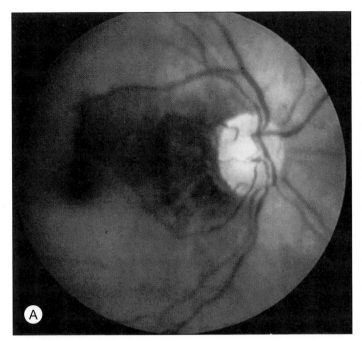
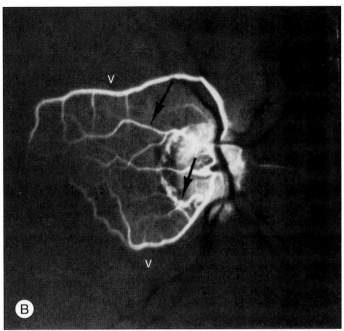

Fig. 69-4 A, Cilioretinal sparing almost to the fovea in an eye with CRAO. Vision was 20/200 in the eye. B, Fluorescein angiogram of A at 40 seconds after injection. The cilioretinal arteries are designated by the arrows; the veins that drain the region of the retina supplied by the cilioretinal arteries are labeled V.

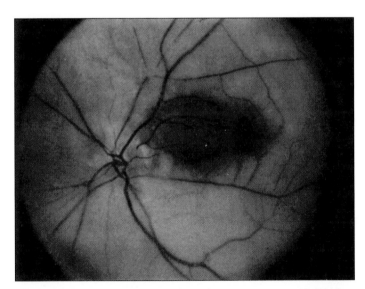

Fig. 69-5 Cilioretinal sparing reaching the foveola in an eye with CRAO. The acuity improved from hand motions to 20/30 over a period of weeks, although the patient was left with only a small central island of vision.

different ophthalmoscopically because it is surrounded by a fibrin-platelet thrombus. Calcific emboli (Fig. 69-8) are less common than cholesterol emboli, but tend to be larger and cause more severe obstructions. They usually originate from the cardiac valves.[6] Ophthalmologists, however, have a low degree of agreement on the qualitative assessment of visible retinal emboli.[13] In fact, when 42 observers were presented a series of photographs of various morphological forms of emboli, they agreed on the clinical type, only slightly more than chance alone would

predict.[13] Accordingly, we do not recommend that one should allow the qualitative features of an embolus to influence decisions regarding the systemic evaluation of acute retinal arterial occlusion.

The presence of a visible retinal arterial embolus is associated with increased mortality. Savino and associates[14] found a mortality rate of 56% over nine years in such patients, as compared to a rate of 27% during the same time in an age-matched control group without arterial emboli. Similar to what has been noted with the ocular ischemic syndrome,[15] the leading cause of death was cardiac disease. The presence of a retinal embolus does not, however, increase the likelihood of either hemodynamically significant carotid artery stenosis,[16] or of cardiac pathology which requires anticoagulation or cardiac surgery,[12] in the setting of acute retinal arterial occlusion.

The Beaver Dam Study, a large population-based study ($n = 4926$) recently determined the 10-year incidence of retinal emboli. The 10-year incidence of retinal emboli in this population was 1.5% (48 retinal embolic events occurred in 3488 at-risk participants). After controlling for age, gender, and systemic factors, a significantly higher hazard of dying with a mention of stroke on the death certificate was found in people with retinal emboli (hazard ratio, 2.40; 95% CI, 1.16–4.99).[17]

Nearly 20% of eyes with acute central retinal artery obstruction progress to develop rubeosis iridis.[18,19,20] Unlike eyes with central retinal vein obstruction, in which the new iris vessels develop at a mean time of five months after the obstruction,[21] with central retinal artery obstruction they develop at a mean of four to five weeks after the event, with a range of one to fifteen weeks.[18,19] Eyes in which the obstruction is both severe and prolonged for a period for over a week appear to be at greater

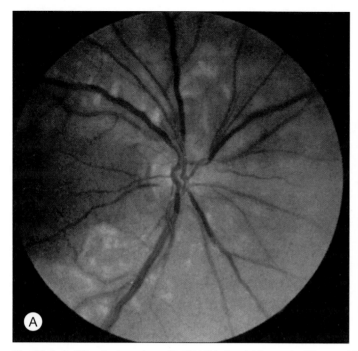

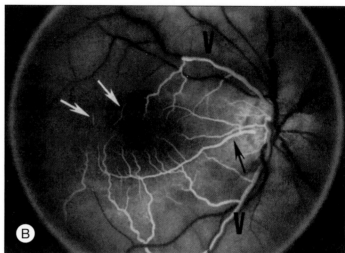

Fig. 69-6 A, Cilioretinal sparing with CRAO in the right eye of a 53-year-old woman. The visual acuity at presentation was 20/30 but improved over a 2-week period to 20/15. B, Fluorescein angiogram of A discloses the patent cilioretinal artery (black arrow) and draining retinal veins (v) that are filled with dye. Retrograde filling, via the cilioretinal artery, of arterioles normally supplied by the obstructed central retinal artery can be seen (white arrows).

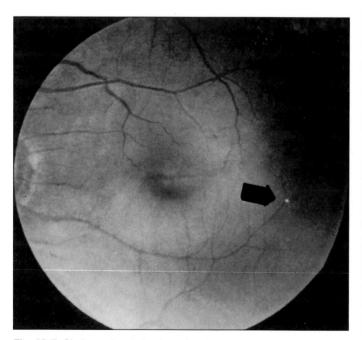

Fig. 69-7 Cholesterol embolus (arrow) in the fundus of an asymptomatic woman. As is usually the case, the embolus is present at the bifurcation, since it is trapped as the lumen of the artery narrows.

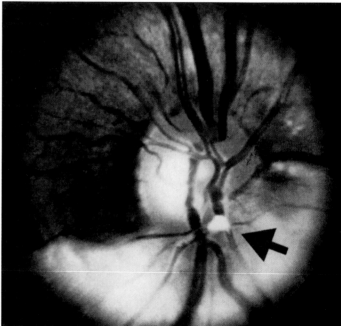

Fig. 69-8 Large calcific plaque (arrow) causing a branch retinal artery obstruction in a woman with cardiac valvular disease.

risk for the development of rubeosis iridis, when compared to those whose obstruction is reversed within the first few days following its occurrence. Laser panretinal photocoagulation is effective in causing regression of the new iris vessels in about 65% of eyes.[22]

Neovascularization of the optic disc has also been noted to occur after acute central retinal artery obstruction, and develops in about 2–3% of eyes.[23,24]

Similar to the case with neovascularization of the iris, if optic disc neovascularization is already present at the time of development of acute obstruction of the central retinal artery, the clinician should suspect a cause other than the acute blockage. In particular, underlying carotid artery obstruction should be considered.[25]

Ancillary studies

Intravenous fluorescein angiography (Fig. 69-9) may reveal a delay in retinal arterial filling or the presence of an arterial dye front (the angiographic finding with the highest *specificity*). However, the most commonly seen fluorescein angiographic sign with acute central retinal artery obstruction (the finding with the highest *sensitivity*) is a delay in retinal arteriovenous transit time (time elapsed from the appearance of dye within the arteries of the temporal vascular arcade until the corresponding veins are completely filled; normal is less than or equal to 11 seconds).[5] Late staining of the optic disc is variable, but staining of the retinal vessels is unusual. Complete lack of filling of the retinal arteries is distinctly unusual[26] and probably occurs in less than 2% of cases.[5]

The choroidal vascular bed in eyes with central retinal artery obstruction usually fills normally, although delays of five seconds or greater are seen in about 10% of cases.[5] In a normal eye the choroid generally begins to fill one to two seconds prior to filling of the retinal arteries, and is completely filled within five seconds of the first appearance of dye. A marked prolongation of choroidal filling in the presence of a cherry-red spot should arouse suspicion of an ophthalmic artery obstruction[27] or a concomitant carotid artery obstruction.[25]

The retinal circulation has a marked propensity to re-establish the circulation following an acute central retinal artery obstruction. Therefore, arterial narrowing and visual loss may persist, but the fluorescein angiogram can revert to normal at varying times after the insult.[6]

Electroretinography (Fig. 69-10) typically discloses a diminution in the amplitude of the b-wave (corresponding to the function of the Muller and/or bipolar cells) secondary to inner layer retinal ischemia (Figs 69-10 and 69-11). The a-wave, which corresponds to photoreceptor function, is generally unaffected. In some eyes the study is normal in the presence of decreased vision, possibly because of the re-establishment of retinal blood flow.

Visual field studies frequently demonstrate a remaining temporal island of vision, presumably because the choroid nourished the corresponding nasal retina. In the presence of a patent cilioretinal artery, small areas of central vision are preserved. Depending upon the degree and the extent of the obstruction, varied portions of the peripheral field may remain.[11]

Systemic associations and etiology

In many instances it is impossible to ascertain the exact pathophysiologic process responsible for a central retinal artery obstruction. Those that probably account for the majority of cases include the following: emboli,[4,5,6,28,12,16] intraluminal thrombosis,[29] hemorrhage under an atherosclerotic plaque,[29] vasculitis,[4,6,28] spasm,[4,30,31,32] circulatory collapse,[6] dissecting aneurysm[33] and hypertensive arterial necrosis.[34]

A consideration of the causes of central retinal artery obstruction is intimately related to the associated systemic abnormalities. Numerous conditions have been associated with acute retinal arterial occlusion. Systemic arterial hypertension is found in about two-thirds of patients with central retinal artery obstruction and diabetes mellitus is present in approximately one-fourth.[5]

The Retinal Emboli of Cardiac Origin Study Group, a multicenter study, reported on the cardiac findings associated with acute retinal arterial occlusion.[12,35–37] Structural cardiac pathology was seen in nearly 50% of patients with acute retinal arterial occlusion.[36] However, only 10% of these patients had pathology severe enough to warrant anticoagulation or cardiac surgery. Patients who were of high cardio-embolic risk (based on a review of systems and cardiac ausculatory examination) were 25 times more likely to receive anticoagulation or cardiac surgery for abnormalities detected by transthoracic echocardiography.[36] Only 1.5% of low cardio-embolic risk patients received anticoagulation or cardiac surgery.[123] Inatomi et al. retrospectively reviewed the usefulness of transesophageal echocardiography (TEE) for detecting cardiac lesions in patients with acute retinal artery occlusion.

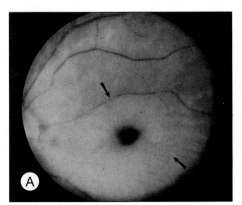
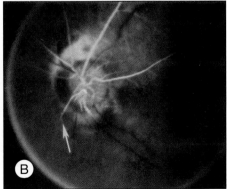
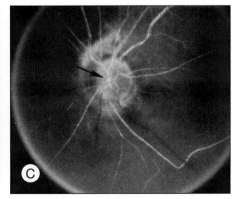

Fig. 69-9 A, Severe left central retinal artery obstruction with segmentation of the blood column in the retinal vessels (arrows). B, Fluorescein angiogram of A at 52 seconds after injection reveals poor filling. The leading edge of dye (arrow) within the inferior retinal arterial system is distinctly abnormal and indicates hypoperfusion. C, At nearly 6 minutes after injection, the retinal vessels are still poorly filled. The hypofluorescent focus (arrow) on the optic disc corresponds to staining of an embolus within the central retinal artery. (From Brown GC, Magargal LE. Ophthalmology 1982; 89:14.)

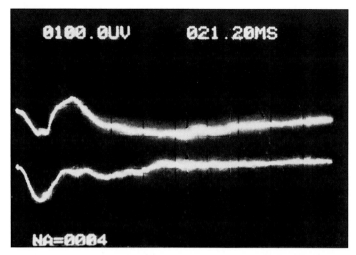

Fig. 69-10 Electroretinograms of a normal right eye (upper tracing) and a left eye (lower tracing) affected by a CRAO. The "b" wave is diminished in the lower tracing of the CRAO eye, but the "a" wave is normal.

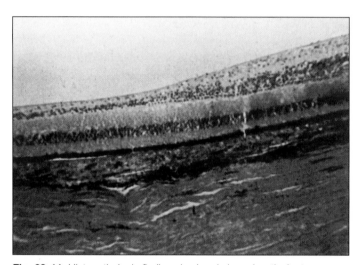

Fig. 69-11 Histopathologic findings in chronic branch retinal artery obstruction elucidate the damage to the inner retina with arterial obstructive disease. The retina on the right is unaffected, whereas on the left the inner layers have atrophied to the inner nuclear layer. (Courtesy of Dr Jerry A. Shields, Philadelphia and the Armed Forces Institute of Pathology, Washington D.C.)

While transthoracic echocardiography detected lesions in 27% of patients, TTE was able to detect lesions in 59%.[38]

Carotid atherosclerosis, in the form of an ipsilateral plaque or stenosis, is seen in 45% of cases.[39] Numerous multicenter studies have recently demonstrated the benefit of carotid endarterectomy for the management of hemodynamically significant carotid artery stenosis.[40–42] We recently reviewed 256 consecutive patients with acute retinal arterial occlusion to determine the prevalence of hemodynamically significant carotid artery stenosis.[16] Eighteen percent of acute retinal arterial occlusion of patients had carotid artery stenosis of 60% or greater.[16]

Recchia et al. have recently reviewed thrombogenicity as a risk factor for the development of retinal artery occlusion. The authors note that, while "the body normally maintains a compli-

cated but well regulated balance between thrombosis and fibrinolysis, the balance may be shifted towards thrombosis through: (a) increased levels or activity of procoagulant compounds (prothrombin, factor V, thrombin, fibrogen); (b) decreased levels or activity of endogenous anticoagulants (protein C, protein S, antithrombin III); (c) decreased levels or activity of fibrinolytic compounds (plasminogen, plasmin); (d) increased level or activity of lipoprotein a. The most common of these mutations is called the Leiden mutation."[43]

Systemic and ocular abnormalities that have been associated with retinal arterial obstruction are listed in Box 69.1. The site of the pathologic process determines whether the occlusion will be at the level of the central retinal artery (CRAO), branch retinal artery (BRAO), cilioretinal artery obstruction (cilioretinal artery occlusion) or retinal arteriole (cotton-wool spot). In some cases there is an overlap between the mechanisms and specific disease entities that cause the blockage. It should also be noted that the list is constantly enlarging as more associations are discovered.

The causes of retinal arterial obstruction in patients under the age of 30 years often differ from those found in older adults.[4,35] While carotid artery atherosclerosis can be seen in the thirties, it is very unusual for it to cause retinal arterial obstructive disease prior to this age. Disease entities that more commonly cause retinal arterial obstructive disease in the young include migraine, cardiac disorders, trauma, sickling hemoglobinopathies, and ocular abnormalities such as optic nerve drusen and prepapillary arterial loops[4] (Fig. 69-12). The Retinal Emboli of Cardiac Origin Study Group demonstrated that 45% of patients under the age of 45 have abnormalities on transthoracic echocardiography.[37] Twenty-seven percent of young patients suffering from acute retinal arterial occlusion received anticoagulation or cardiac surgery.[37] Overall, acute retinal arterial occlusion patients who are less than 45 years of age are three times more likely to have cardiac pathology which requires anticoagulation or cardiac surgery, when compared to those over the age of 45 years. Although coagulopathies are traditionally associated with venous occlusive disease,[97] abnormalities of protein C and S,[77,79] and antithrombin III[12] can be causes of acute retinal arterial occlusion in the young population.

Long-term survival seems to be decreased in people with retinal arterial obstruction. Lorentzen[98] noted a survival time of 5.5 years in people with central retinal artery obstruction, as compared to an expected survival of 15.4 years in an age matched population. The finding of a retinal arterial obstruction generally merits a complete systemic workup to look for etiologic factors, as up to 90% of affected patients have evidence of systemic disease.[4,5]

Although some believe that the presence of an embolus increases the likelihood of cardiac or carotid pathology,[99] the presence of a visible retinal embolus does not significantly alter the likelihood of either hemodynamically significant carotid artery stenosis, or cardiac pathology which requires anticoagulation or cardiac surgery.[12,16] In fact, given that physical findings, themselves can act as "diagnostic tests" by influencing the probability of disease,[100] visible emboli can be considered to be very poor "tests," as they have the ability to only minimally alter the

Box 69-1 Systemic and ocular abnormalities that have been associated with retinal arterial obstruction

Abnormalities contributing to embolus formation

Systemic arterial hypertension (via atherosclerotic plaque formation)[6,5,44]

Carotid atherosclerosis[16,34,45]

Cardiac valvular disease (including: rheumatic,[5,45] mitral valve prolapse,[12,46,47] aortic stenosis,[12,36] mitral annular calcification[36])

Left ventricular hypertrophy,[36] and segmental left wall motion abnormalities[36]

Thrombus after myocardial infarction[12,38]

Cardiac myxoma[12,36,49,50,50a]

Tumors[51]

Intravenous drug abuse[4,52]

Lipid emboli (pancreatitis)[53]

Purtscher's retinopathy (trauma)[54]

Loiasis[55,56]

Radiologic studies (carotid angiography,[57] lymphangiography,[58] hysterosalpingography,[59] head and neck corticosteroid injection,[60] retrobulbar injection[61,62])

Deep vein thrombosis (via paradoxical embolus through cardiac wall defect) (Wills Eye Hospital Retina Vascular Unit files)[62a]

Trauma (via compression, spasm, or direct vessel damage)

Retrobulbar injection[63]

Orbital fracture repair[64,65]

Anesthesia[66]

Penetrating injury[67]

Drug and/or alcohol induced stupor[27,45]

Nasal surgery[68,69]

Eyelid capillary hemangioma injection[70]

Coagulopathies

Sickle cell disease[3,71,72]

Homocystinuria[73,74]

Oral contraceptives[4,75]

Platelet abnormalities[4]

Pregnancy[4]

Lupus anticoagulants[76]

Protein S deficiency[77]

Protein C deficiency[78]

Antithrombin III deficiency[78]

Activated protein C resistance

Factor V Leiden abnormalities[79,79a]

Ocular conditions associated with retinal arterial obstruction

Prepapillary arterial loops[80,81]

Optic disc drusen[4,82]

Increased intraocular pressure (with sickling hemoglobinopathy)[4]

Toxoplasmosis[83]

Optic neuritis[84]

Collagen vascular diseases

Systemic lupus erythematosus[4,85,86]

Polyarteritis nodosa[6]

Giant cell arteritis[87,88]

Wegener's granulomatosis[89]

Liebow's lymphoid granulomatosis[90]

Other vasculitides

Orbital mucormycosis[27]

Radiation retinopathy[91]

Behçet's disease[92]

Box 69-1 Systemic and ocular abnormalities that have been associated with retinal arterial obstruction—cont'd

Miscellaneous associations

Ventriculography[65]

Fabry's disease[9]

Sydenham's chorea[93]

Migraine[4,3,31,32]

Hypotension[6]

Fibromuscular hyperplasia[94]

Nasal oxymethazolone use[95]

Lyme disease[96,96a,96b]

probability of systemic disease.[12,16] In our practices, we perform a thorough history and cardiac auscultatory examination on all patients with acute retinal arterial occlusion. If patients have any historical risk factor (past or current history of: subacute bacterial endocarditis, rheumatic heart disease, mitral valve prolapse, recent myocardial infarction, cardiac tumor, intravenous drug abuse, congenital heart disease, or any valvular heart disease) or have an audible murmur, we obtain screening transthoracic echocardiography. Carotid Doppler ultrasonography is obtained on all patients over the age of 30 years, again, regardless of embolic status.

Patients over the age of 55 years without emboli in the fundus should have an erythrocyte sedimentation rate drawn on an urgent basis to screen for giant cell arteritis. On the Retina Vascular Unit at Wills Eye Hospital, giant cell arteritis accounts for approximately 1–2% of cases of retinal arterial occlusion. If the disease is suspected, aggressive treatment with systemic corticosteroids should be instituted without delay, since we have seen the second eye become involved within hours. Unfortunately, this therapy rarely helps the vision in the affected eye.

Our recommendations regarding the main diagnostic evaluations, which are currently ordered for patients with acute retinal arterial occlusion at the Retina Vascular Unit at Wills Eye Hospital are listed in Table 69-1.

Treatment

Work in young healthy rhesus monkeys suggests that the retina sustains irreversible damage when the central retinal artery has been obstructed for 90 to 100 minutes.[101] Hayreh and Jonas have demonstrated that central retinal artery occlusion of greater than 240 minutes in middle aged or elderly atherosclerotic and arterial hypertensive rhesus monkeys produced total or almost total optic nerve atrophy and nerve fibre damage.[102]

While this may be the case in the experimental model, the central retinal artery is rarely completely obstructed in the human clinical situation. Additionally, in the animal model the obstruction was created at the point of entrance of the central retinal artery into the optic nerve; in the human the obstruction probably does not routinely occur at this location. Recovery of good vision has been noted to occur as long as three days after central retinal arterial obstruction.[103] For the above reasons, it has been

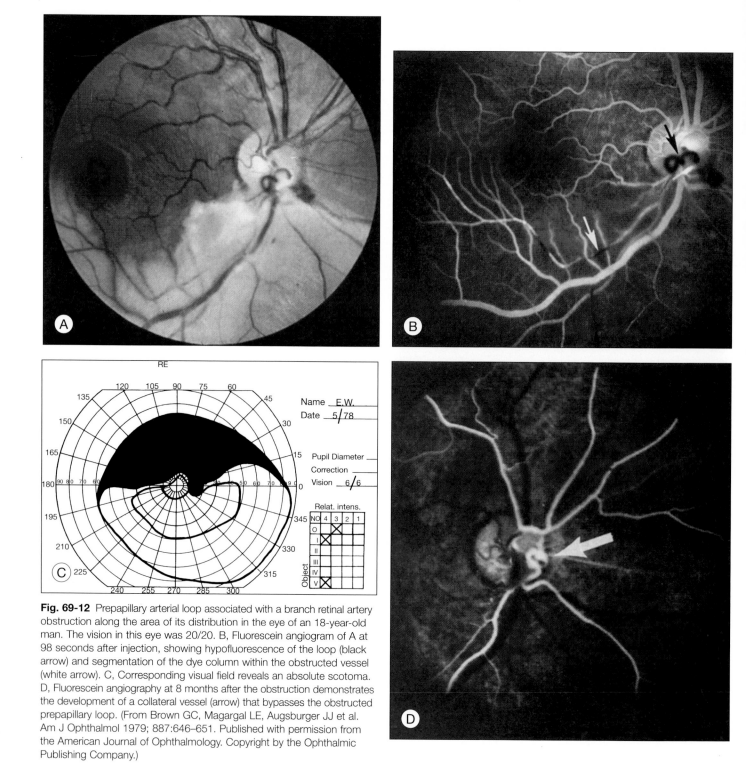

Fig. 69-12 Prepapillary arterial loop associated with a branch retinal artery obstruction along the area of its distribution in the eye of an 18-year-old man. The vision in this eye was 20/20. B, Fluorescein angiogram of A at 98 seconds after injection, showing hypofluorescence of the loop (black arrow) and segmentation of the dye column within the obstructed vessel (white arrow). C, Corresponding visual field reveals an absolute scotoma. D, Fluorescein angiography at 8 months after the obstruction demonstrates the development of a collateral vessel (arrow) that bypasses the obstructed prepapillary loop. (From Brown GC, Magargal LE, Augsburger JJ et al. Am J Ophthalmol 1979; 887:646–651. Published with permission from the American Journal of Ophthalmology. Copyright by the Ophthalmic Publishing Company.)

recommended that ocular treatment be given if a patient with an acute central retinal artery obstruction is seen within 24 hours after the onset of visual loss.

Ocular massage can be attempted with an in-and-out movement using a Goldmann contact lens or via digital massage. In rare instances, this manipulation can dislodge an obstructing embolus. Repeated manipulations to increase the pressure for 10–15 seconds, followed by a sudden release, has been recommended.[104] This technique can produce retinal arterial dilation, theoretically improving retinal perfusion as well. Russell[105] demonstrated a 16% increase in retinal arterial diameter, probably secondary to autoregulation, when the intraocular pressure was

Table 69-1 Recommended systemic evaluation of patients with acute retinal arterial occlusion

Study	Which patients	Quality of evidence
Echocardiography	High cardio-embolic risk, all young patients	Diagnostic studies[12,36,37]
Carotid ultrasonography	All adult patients, regardless of emboli	Diagnostic studies[16]
Homocysteine	Young patients with no other identifiable cause	Case series[73]
ESR to rule out GCA	Older patients with a reasonable suspicion	Case report[87]
Anticoagulation studies (routine anticoagulation studies, protein C and S, antithrombin III)	Higher suspicion in young patients, consider as a secondary screen in older patients	Case series[78]

ESR, erythrocyte sedimentation rate; GCA, giant cell arteritis.

raised to 60 mmHg. When a sudden increase in intraocular pressure was followed by a sudden decrease, Ffytche and associates[106] demonstrated an 86% increase in volume of flow.

The use of an oxygen and carbon dioxide (95% oxygen, 5% carbon dioxide) mixture has been applied systemically in some cases.[107] Although higher oxygen concentrations can lead to retinal arterial vasoconstriction,[108,109] it has been shown that inspiration of 100% oxygen can, in the presence of acute central retinal artery obstruction, produce a normal pO_2 at the surface of the retina via diffusion from the choroid.[87] There is also clinical evidence to suggest that a high dose of oxygen can improve visual function in eyes with central retinal artery obstruction.[110] Carbon dioxide, on the other hand, is a vasodilator and can produce increased retinal blood flow.[109,111] In the absence of a carbon dioxide mixture, rebreathing into a paper bag can be considered in the office.

Anterior chamber paracentesis has also been advocated for the treatment of acute central retinal artery obstruction. Augsburger and Magargal,[107] reporting on the results of an uncontrolled series, found a three gradation improvement in vision using the Snellen classification at one month after the acute event in eyes that initially underwent an anterior chamber paracentesis. This maneuver causes a sudden decrease in intraocular pressure, with the hope that the arterial perfusion pressure behind the obstruction will force an obstructing embolus downstream. Atebara and Brown[112] recently reviewed the results of 40 patients treated with anterior chamber paracentesis and carbogen inhalation, and compared them to 47 patients who received neither therapy. From this study, there was no significant difference in the visual outcomes between these two groups.[112] It is, however, possible that given the small sample of patients involved in the study, that it had insufficient power to detect a clinically relevant difference.

Treatment with antifibrinolytic agents has been reported.[113,114] Schmidt and coworkers described the benefit of thrombolytic therapy for the treatment of acute retinal arterial occlusion.[114] Although patients who received therapy were more likely to have an improvement in visual acuity, their treatment allocation was not randomized. Given that evidence supporting therapeutic claims can be graded (varying from level I – the highest, which is provided by way of randomized clinical trials to level V evidence – the lowest, which is provided though case reports),[115] we can classify the work of Schmidt et al. as level III evidence. Unfortunately, therapeutic recommendations should generally not be based on trials demonstrating effects derived from non-random allocation (level III evidence),[115] as treatment effects may in fact be due to confounding factors and not the treatment itself. Furthermore, systemic complications, such as cerebrovascular accident can occur with this treatment. In fact, Fraser and Siriwardena recently reviewed the peer-reviewed literature in order to complete a systematic review for the Cochrane Database and determined that, "there is currently not enough evidence to decide which, if any, interventions for acute non-arteritic central retinal artery occlusion would result, in any beneficial or harmful effect. Well-designed randomized controlled trials are needed to establish the most effective treatment."[116]

Fibrinolytic agents have also been delivered through the supraorbital artery in eyes with acute central retinal artery obstruction.[117] With injection into the supraorbital artery, the drug travels retrograde into the ophthalmic artery and allows doses into the central retinal artery that are over 100 times greater than those which would be achieved if a similar amount of drug was injected intravenously. Watson noted that 50% of patients with acute retinal arterial occlusion developed visual improvement with this technique.[117]

Other treatment modalities that have been described include a retrobulbar injection or systemic administration of vasodilators such as papaverine or tolazaline.[6] A possible pitfall with retrobulbar injection is the development of a retrobulbar hemorrhage, which could further compromise retinal arterial flow. Sublingual nitroglycerin, a potent vasodilating agent has been reported to re-establish flow in some cases.[118,119] Systemic anticoagulants have generally not been employed for the treatment of central retinal artery obstruction.[6]

Laser therapy has been suggested as a mechanism of obliterating emboli,[120] but its clinical usefulness remains to be seen.

Additionally, we have caused a retinal arterial embolus to move further peripherally via manipulation during a pars plana vitrectomy. Again, it is uncertain whether this technique will have clinical applicability.

BRANCH RETINAL ARTERY OBSTRUCTION

Funduscopically, a branch retinal artery obstruction appears as a localized region of superficial retinal whitening. The whitening is most prominent in the posterior pole, along the distribution of the obstructed vessel (Fig. 69-13). Areas of more intense whitening are often seen at the borders of the area of ischemia. These probably occur secondary to blockage of axoplasmic flow in the nerve fiber layer as it reaches the hypoxic retina.

Among cases of acute retinal arterial obstruction, central retinal artery obstructions accounts of approximately 57%, branch retinal artery obstruction for 38% and cilioretinal artery obstruction for 5%.[121] Over 90% of branch retinal artery obstructions involve the temporal retinal vessels.[121] It is unclear whether indeed the temporal arteries are more commonly affected, or whether nasal branch retinal artery obstructions are often asymptomatic, and thus, go undetected.

The visual prognosis in eyes with symptomatic branch retinal artery obstruction is usually quite good unless the foveola is completely surrounded by retinal whitening. About 80% of eyes eventually improve to 20/40 or better,[4] although residual field defects generally remain.

Occasionally, posterior segment neovascularization can arise after branch retinal artery obstruction (Fig. 69-14), particularly in patients with diabetes mellitus.[121,122] Shah and associates have recently reported that the rare event of iris neovascularization can also occur in patients with branch retinal arterial occlusion.[123] Artery to artery collateral vessels may also develop in the retina and are pathognomonic for branch retinal artery obstruction.

The causes of branch retinal arterial obstruction are similar to those seen with central retinal artery obstruction; thus, the systemic workup is often the same.[4,6,16,36] In cases in which the obstruction occurs at an arterial bifurcation, the cause is more likely to be embolic than when a vessel is obstructed elsewhere along its course.

Since the visual prognosis is substantially better with branch retinal artery obstruction than with central retinal artery obstruction,[124] aggressive therapy is usually not undertaken unless all of the perifoveolar capillaries are involved.

CILIORETINAL ARTERY OCCLUSION

Cilioretinal arteries usually enter the retina from the temporal aspect of the optic disc, separate from the central retinal artery, and can be seen clinically in about 20% of eyes. Fluorescein angiographically, they are visible in approximately 32% of eyes.[125] In a normal fluorescein angiographic sequence they usually fill concomitantly with the choroidal circulation, about one to two seconds before filling of the retinal arteries.

Ophthalmoscopically, a cilioretinal artery obstruction appears as an area of superficial retinal whitening along the course of the vessel. Three clinical variants have been described[126]: (1) isolated cilioretinal artery obstruction; (2) cilioretinal artery obstruction associated with central retinal vein obstruction; and (3) cilioretinal artery obstruction associated with anterior ischemic optic neuropathy.

Isolated cilioretinal artery obstruction usually has good visual prognosis[126] (Fig. 69-15). Ninety percent of affected eyes improve to 20/40 or better vision, with 60% returning to 20/20. Even when the papillomacular bundle is severely damaged, the eye has potentially excellent vision, presumably due to intact superior and inferior nerve fiber layer bundles that course above and below to supply the fovea. This variant accounts for greater than 40% of eyes with cilioretinal artery obstruction.

Cilioretinal artery obstruction in conjunction with central retinal vein obstruction (Fig. 69-16) also comprises just greater than 40% of cases of cilioretinal artery obstruction.[126] The venous obstructions are generally nonischemic, and therefore do not usually lead to rubeosis iridis and neovascular glaucoma.[126–128] It is possible, however, that a cilioretinal artery obstruction is difficult to detect in the presence of an ischemic central retinal vein obstruction, causing the incidence of rubeosis iridis to be falsely low in this subgroup with cilioretinal artery obstruction. Approximately 70% of eyes achieve 20/40 or better vision,[126] with the venous obstructive component probably accounting for the greatest degree of visual loss. From the venous point of view, Fong and associates[129] have noted that 5% of patients with central retinal vein obstruction also have a cilioretinal artery obstruction. The reasons for the association of cilioretinal artery obstruction with central retinal obstruction are unclear. Reduced hydrostatic pressure in the cilioretinal artery, as compared to the central retinal artery, may predispose the cilioretinal artery to stasis and thrombosis in the setting of increased hydrostatic pressure within the retinal venous system.[127,128] Additionally, swelling of the optic disc may compromise the cross sectional

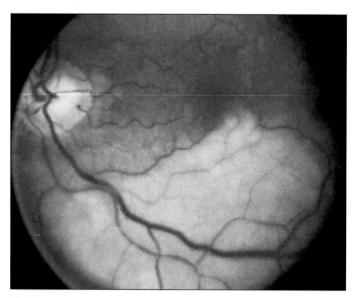

Fig. 69-13 Inferotemporal branch retinal artery obstruction.

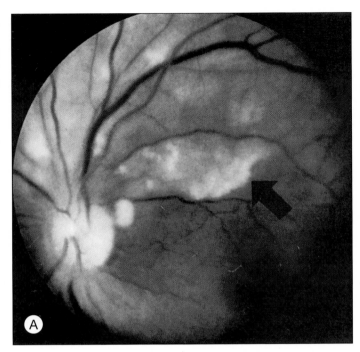
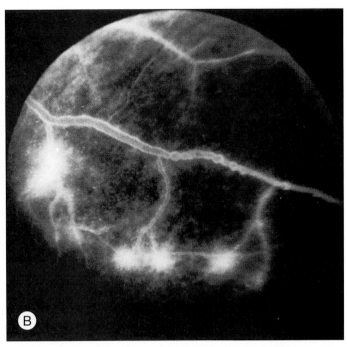

Fig. 69-14 A, Superior papillary branch retinal artery obstruction in the left eye on a 61-year-old woman. Visual acuity in the eye at this time was 20/25 but later improved to 20/20. Retinal whitening is most pronounced at the edge of the hypoxic retina (arrow) because of blocking axoplasmic flow. B, At 13 months after A, fluorescein angiography reveals multiple hyperfluorescent areas corresponding to retinal neovascularization associated with superotemporal veins.

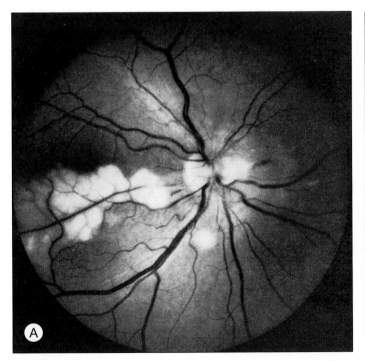
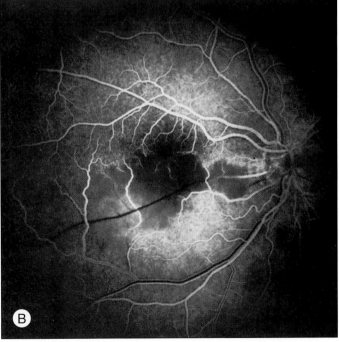

Fig. 69-15 A, Isolated cilioretinal artery obstruction. The vision was initially 20/40 but improved to 20/20 over several weeks. B, Fluorescein angiogram of A demonstrates poor filling of the obstructed cilioretinal artery and retinal capillary nonperfusion within the area of distribution of the vessel.

area of the cilioretinal artery and lead to reduced flow. According to Poiseuille's law, the flow within a blood vessel is proportional to the fourth power of the radius of the vessel. Thus, flow within a vessel with twice the radius of a second vessel will be sixteen times that within the smaller vessel.

In the group of eyes with cilioretinal artery obstruction in association with anterior ischemic optic neuropathy (Fig. 69-17) the visual prognosis is typically quite poor (20/400 to no light perception), primarily due to the optic nerve damage.[126] Hyperemic or pale swelling of the optic disc is seen in conjunction with

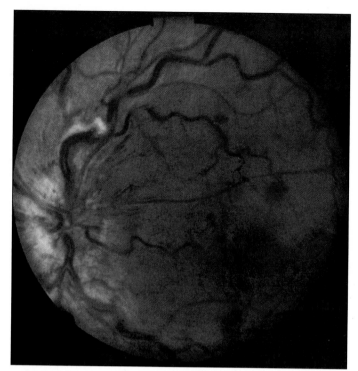

Fig. 69-16 Cilioretinal artery obstruction in association with a mild, or nonischemic, central retinal vein obstruction.

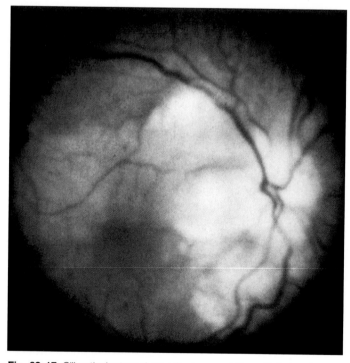

Fig. 69-17 Cilioretinal artery obstruction in association with ischemic optic neuropathy. The visual acuity was no light perception. (From Brown GC, Moffat K, Cruess AF, et al. Retina 1983; 3:184).

superficial retinal whitening along the course of the obstructed cilioretinal artery. Acute pale swelling of the optic disc is suggestive of the giant cell arteritis as the underlying cause, and is usually associated with more severe visual loss than hyperemic

swelling. It is not surprising that cilioretinal artery obstruction and anterior ischemic optic neuropathy occur together, since both appear to be manifestations of posterior ciliary insufficiency.[130,131] This variant comprises approximately 15% of all cilioretinal artery obstructions.[126]

The systemic workup for causes of cilioretinal artery obstruction is similar to that for central retinal artery obstruction. An extensive workup for embolic sources is probably not indicated, however, for cases associated with central retinal vein obstruction. Ocular treatment is generally not given for isolated cilioretinal artery obstruction or cilioretinal artery obstruction associated with central retinal vein obstruction. For cases associated with anterior ischemic optic neuropathy, the possibility of underlying giant cell arteritis as a cause should be investigated.

COMBINED RETINAL ARTERY AND VEIN OCCLUSION

Combined central retinal artery/vein obstruction demonstrates clinical features that are common to both entities.[132,133] There is usually a history of sudden visual loss. The fundus examination discloses superficial retinal opacification with a cherry-red spot in the posterior pole, similar to that seen with acute central retinal artery obstruction. The signs suggestive of venous obstruction often include dilated and tortuous retinal veins, retinal hemorrhages, a swollen optic disc, and marked thickening of the retina in the posterior pole (Fig. 69-18).

Fluorescein angiography typically shows severe retinal capillary nonperfusion, as well as the sudden termination of the mid-sized retinal vessels. Despite the marked retinal thickening seen clinically in the posterior pole, there is often a minimal amount of leakage of dye into the macular area, probably because of shutdown of the retinal vessels.[132]

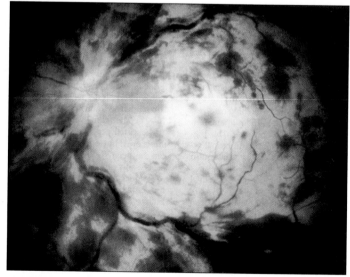

Fig. 69-18 Combined obstruction of the central retinal artery and central retinal vein. A cherry-red spot is present, as well as a swollen optic disc and intraretinal hemorrhages.

The visual prognosis is generally very poor in these eyes,[132] but occasionally spontaneous improvement can be seen.[134] The mean acuity of these cases is in the hand motions range. Approximately 80% of these eyes will progress to develop rubeosis and neovascular glaucoma. This complication can develop as rapidly as one to two weeks or at greater than one year after the obstruction, with a median time of about six weeks.[132] Aggressive pan-retinal laser photocoagulation should be considered in an attempt to prevent neovascular glaucoma, although it can still develop after such treatment is administered.[132]

The causes of combined central retinal artery/central retinal vein obstruction are probably similar to those seen with central retinal artery obstruction. Richards[133] noted associated systemic diseases that cause vasculitis, although this was not the case in a larger series.[132] Retrobulbar injection can produce this entity, and probably accounts for about one fourth of cases.[132]

Although the entity has clinical features suggestive of both central retinal artery and central retinal vein obstruction, it is uncertain whether simultaneous obstructions of both vessels are necessary to induce this abnormality. A similar funduscopic appearance has been produced experimentally in the subhuman primate model by occluding both vessels at their point of entrance into and exit from the retrobulbar nerve.[135] Nonetheless, complete blockage of the central retinal vein on the optic nerve head in the same model has also reproduced this ophthalmoscopic picture.[136] To our knowledge, the human histopathologic correlate of an acute, combined central retinal artery/vein obstruction is lacking at the time of this writing. At several months after the onset of visual loss, histopathologic features in the retina consistent with the hemorrhagic necrosis of central retinal vein obstruction and the inner retinal atrophy seen after central retinal artery obstruction have been demonstrated.[132]

Included in the differential of central retinal artery/central retinal vein obstruction is the entity of aminoglycoside toxicity.[137]

COTTON-WOOL SPOTS

A cotton-wool spot, or soft exudate, is a yellow-white lesion in the superficial retina that usually occupies an area less than one fourth that of the optic disc (Fig. 69-19). A cotton-wool spot can occur singly or in conjunction with many others (Fig. 69-20). Fluorescein angiographically, these lesions correspond to focal areas of retinal capillary nonperfusion. In some cases they are bordered by microaneurysmal abnormalities.

A cotton-wool spot is believed to develop secondary to obstruction of a retinal arteriole and resultant ischemia.[138,139] The focal hypoxia leads to blockage of axoplasmic flow within the nerve fiber layer of the retina, with the subsequent deposition of intra-axonal organelles.[140] Light microscopy of a cotton-wool spot reveals cytoid bodies (Fig. 69-21), cellular appearing bodies with a "pseudonucleus," within the nerve fiber layer. Transmission electron microscopy has shown that cytoid bodies are composed largely of mitochondria, and that they appear to have a major lipid component.[141]

Cotton-wool spots usually do not cause visual loss, but many patients relate a history of seeing "spots" in their visual field.

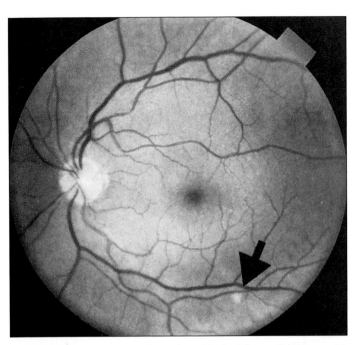

Fig. 69-19 Single cotton-wool spot (arrow) in the left eye of a 57-year-old woman discovered to have diabetes.

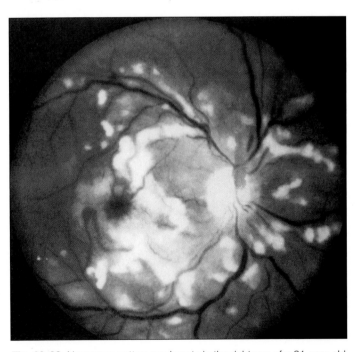

Fig. 69-20 Numerous cotton-wool spots in the right eye of a 31-year-old woman with systemic lupus erythematosus.

Most resolve within 5–7 weeks,[142] although in diabetics they can remain for longer periods of time.[143]

Diabetes mellitus is the most common cause of cotton-wool spots. When known diabetics are excluded, the most common causes of a fundus appearance in which there is a predominance of cotton-wool spots or a single cotton-wool spot are undiscovered diabetic retinopathy (20% of cases) and systemic arterial hypertension (20% of cases).[142]

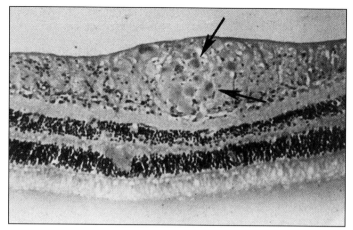

Fig. 69-21 Light microscopic section of a cotton-wool spot in the retina shown cytoid bodies (arrows) in the nerve fiber layer. (Hematoxylin–eosin ×25, courtesy of Dr Jerry A. Shields, Philadelphia.)

An increasingly common cause of cotton-wool spots is the acquired immunodeficiency syndrome (AIDS). Clinically, cotton-wool spots have been observed in as many as 50% of AIDS patients.[144] In an autopsy group this figure was 71%,[145] suggesting that the true incidence may be higher than that seen on clinical examination. The suggestion has been made that deposition of immune complexes in the blood vessels of the retina are responsible for the formation of cotton-wool spots in AIDS patients.[146,147]

The finding of even one cotton-wool spot in a nondiabetic patient with an otherwise normal fundus examination necessitates a systemic workup for possible etiologies. In approximately 95% of cases, a serious underlying systemic disorder can be found.[142] The blood pressure should be measured very soon after noting such a fundus finding, since cotton-wool spots rarely develop unless the diastolic pressure is at least 110–115 mmHg.

In theory, almost any abnormality that can cause an obstruction of the central retinal artery or a branch retinal artery (see "Central retinal artery obstruction", p. 1323) could also cause a cotton-wool spot. A list of many of the abnormalities that have been associated with cotton-wool spots is shown in Box 69-2.

Box 69-2 Abnormalities associated with cotton-wool spots in the fundus

1. Diabetic retinopathy
2. Systemic arterial hypertension
3. Collagen vascular disease
   - Systemic lupus erythematosus
   - Dermatomyositis
   - Polyarteritis nodosa
   - Scleroderma
   - Giant cell arteritis
4. Cardiac valvular disease
   - Mitral valve prolapse
   - Rheumatic heart disease
   - Endocarditis

Box 69-2 Abnormalities associated with cotton-wool spots in the fundus—cont'd

5. Acquired immunodeficiency syndrome (AIDS)
6. Central and branch retinal vein obstruction
7. Partial central retinal artery obstruction
8. Leukemia
9. Trauma
10. Radiation retinopathy
11. Metastatic carcinoma
12. Leptospirosis
13. Rocky Mountain spotted fever
14. High-altitude retinopathy
15. Severe anemia
16. Acute blood loss
17. Papilledema
18. Papillitis
19. Carotid artery atherosclerosis
20. Dysproteinemias
21. Septicemia
22. Aortic arch syndrome (pulseless disease)
23. Intravenous drug abuse
24. Acute pancreatitis
25. Onchocerciasis
26. Systemic alpha interferon administration

REFERENCES

1. Von Graefe A. Ueber Embolie der arteria centralis retinae als Urscahe plotzlicher Erblindung. Arch fur Ophthalmol 1859;5:136–157.
2. Knapp H. Embolism of a branch of the retinal artery with hemorrhage infraretus in the retina. Arch Ophthalmol 1869;1:64–84.
3. Duke-Elder S, Dobree H. System of ophthalmology, vol 10. Saint Louis: Mosby; 1967:66–97.
4. Brown GC, Magargal LE, Shields JA et al. Retinal arterial obstruction in children and young adults. Ophthalmology 1981;88:18–25.
5. Brown GC, Magargal LE. Central retinal artery obstruction and visual acuity. Ophthalmology 1982;89:14–19.
6. Gold D. Retinal arterial occlusion. Trans Am Acad Ophthalmol Otolaryngol 1977; 83:392–408.
7. Alwitry A, Holden R. One hundred transient monocular central retinal artery occlusions secondary to giant cell arteritis. Arch Ophthalmol 2003; 121:1802–1803.
8. Brown GC, Shields JA. Amaurosis fugax secondary to presumed cavernous hemangioma of the orbit. Ann Ophthalmol 1981; 12:1205–1209.
9. Sharma S, ten Hove MW, Pinkerton RMH et al. Interobserver agreement in the evaluation of acute retinal artery occlusion. Can J Ophthalmol 1997; 32:441–444.
10. Connolly BP, Krishnan A, Shah GK et al. Can J Ophthalmol 2000; 35:379–384.
11. Brown GC, Shields JA. Cilioretinal arteries and retinal arterial occlusion. Arch Ophthalmol 1979; 97:84–92.
12. Sharma S, Grown GC, Cruess AF for the RECO Study Group. The accuracy of visible retinal emboli for the detection of cardio-embolic lesions requiring anticoagulation or cardiac surgery. Br J Ophthalmol 1998; 82:655–658.
13. Sharma S, Pater JL, Lam M, Cruess AF. Can different types of retinal emboli be reliably differentiated from one another? An inter- and intraobserver agreement study. Can J Ophthalmol 1998; 33:144–148.
14. Savino PJ, Glaser JS, Cassady J. Retinal stroke. Is the patient at risk? Arch Ophthalmol 1997; 95:1185–1189.
15. Sivalingam A, Brown GC, Magargal LE et al. The ocular ischemic syndrome II. Mortality and systemic morbidity. Int Ophthalmol 1989; 13:187–191.
16. Sharma S, Brown GC, Pater JL et al. Does a visible retinal emboli increase the likelihood of hemodynamically significant carotid artery stenosis in patients with acute retinal artery occlusion? Arch Ophthalmol 1998; 116:1602–1606.
17. Klein R, Klein BEK, Moss SE et al. Retinal emboli and cardiovascular disease. The Beaver Dam Eye Study. Arch Ophthalmol 2003; 121:1446–1451.
18. Duker JS, Brown GC. Iris neovascularization associated with obstruction of the central retinal artery. Ophthalmology 1988; 95:1244–1249.

19. Duker JS, Sivalingham A, Brown GC et al. A prospective study of acute central retinal artery obstruction. The incidence of secondary ocular neovascularization. Arch Ophthalmol 1991: 109:339–342.
20. Hayreh SS, Podhajsky P. Ocular neovascularization with retinal vascular occlusion. II. Occurrence in central and branch retinal artery occlusion. Arch Ophthalmol 1982: 100:1585–1596.
21. Magargal LE, Brown GC, Augsburger JJ et al. Neovascular glaucoma following central retinal vein obstruction. Ophthalmology 1981; 88:1095–1011.
22. Duker JS, Brown GC. The efficacy of panretinal photocoagulation for neovascularization of the iris after central retinal artery obstruction. Ophthalmology 1988; 95:1244–1249.
23. Brown GC. Central retinal vein obstruction. Diagnosis and management. In: Reinecke R, ed. Ophthalmology review. Norwalk, CT: 1985:65–97.
24. Duker JS, Brown GC. Neovascularization of the optic disc associated with obstruction of the central retinal artery. Ophthalmology 1989; 96:87–91.
25. Brown GC, Magargal LE. The ocular ischemic syndrome. Clinical, fluorescein angiographic and carotid angiographic features. Int Ophthalmol 1988; 11:239–251.
26. David NJ, Norton EWD, Gass JD et al. Fluorescein angiography in central retinal artery occlusion. Arch Ophthalmol 1967; 77:619–629.
27. Brown GC, Magaral LE, Sergott R. Acute obstruction of the retinal and choroidal circulations. Ophthalmology 1986; 93:1373–1382.
28. Karjalainen K. Occlusion of the central retinal artery and retinal branch arterioles. Acta Ophthalmol (suppl) 1971; 109:1–95.
29. Perraut LE, Zimmerman LE. The occurrence of glaucoma following occlusion of the central retinal artery. A clinicopathologic report of six cases with a review of the literature. Arch Ophthalmol 1959; 61:845–865.
30. Carroll D. Retinal migraine. Headache 1970; 10:9–13.
31. Graveson GS. Retinal arterial occlusion in migraine. Br Med J 1949; 2:838–840.
32. Silberberg DH, Laties AM. Occlusive migraine. Trans Pa Acad Ophthalmol Otolaryngol 1974; 27:34–38.
33. Wolter JR, Hansen KD. Intimo-intimal intussusception of the central retinal artery. Am J Ophthalmol 1981; 92:486–491.
34. Leishman R. The eye in general vascular disease. Hypertension and arteriosclerosis. Br J Ophthalmol 1957; 41:641–701.
35. Sanborn GE. Retinal artery obstruction in young patients. Arch Ophthalmol 1997; 115:942.
36. Sharma S, Naqvi A, Sharma SM et al. for RECO. Transthoracic echocardiographic findings in patients with acute retinal arterial obstruction. Arch Ophthalmol 1996; 114:1189–92.
37. Sharma S, Sharma SM, Cruess AF et al. for the RECO Study Group. Transthoracic echocardiography in young patients with acute retinal arterial occlusion. Can J Ophthalmol 1997; 32:38–41.
38. Inatomi Y, Hino H, Hashimoto Y et al. Transesophageal echocardiography for detection of cardiac diseases in patients with retinal artery occlusion. Int Med 2001; 40:475–478.
39. Shah HG, Brown GC, Goldberg RE. Digital subtraction carotid angiography and retinal arterial obstruction. Ophthalmology 1985; 92:68–72.
40. Anonymous. Beneficial effect of carotid endarterectomy in symptomatic patients with high-grade carotid stenosis. North American Symptomatic Carotid Endarterectomy Trial Collaborators. N Engl J Med 1991; 325:445–453.
41. Anonymous. MRC European Carotid Surgery Trial: Interim results for symptomatic patients with severe (70–99%) or with mild (0–29%) carotid stenosis. European Carotid Trialists' Collaborative Group. Lancet 1991; 337:1235–1243.
42. Asymptomatic Carotid Atherosclerosis Study Group. Carotid endarterectomy for patients with symptomatic internal carotid artery stenosis. JAMA 1995; 273:1421–1428.
43. Recchia FM, Brown GC. Systemic disorders associated with retinal vascular occlusion. Curr Opin Ophthalmol 2000; 11:462–467.
44. Dahrling BE. The histopathology of early central retinal artery occlusion. Arch Ophthalmol 1965;78:506–510.
45. Appen RE, Wray SH, Cogan DG. Central retinal artery occlusion. Am J Ophthalmol 1975;79:374–381.
46. Wilson LA, Keeling PWN, Malcolm AD et al. Visual complications of mitral leaf prolapse. Br Med J 1977; 2:86–88.
47. Woldoff HS, Gerber M, Desser KB et al. Retinal vascular lesions in two patients with prolapsed mitral valve leaflets. Am J Ophthalmol 1975; 79:382–385.
48. Zimmerman LE. Embolism of central retinal artery secondary to myocardial infarction with mural thrombus. Arch Ophthalmol 1955; 73:822–826.
49. Cogan DG, Wray SH. Vascular occlusions in the eye from cardiac myxomas. Am J Ophthalmol 1975; 80:396–403.
50. Jampol LM, Wong AS, Albert DM. Atrial myxoma and central retinal artery occlusion. Am J Ophthalmol 1973; 75:242–249.
50a. Lee S, Loo JL, Ang CL. Ischemic oculopathy as a complication of surgery for an atrial myxoma. Arch Ophthalmol 2004; 122:130–131.
51. Tarkkanen A, Merenmies L, Makinen J. Embolism of the central retinal artery secondary to metastatic carcinoma. Acta Ophthalmol 1973;51:25–33.
52. Atlee WE. Talc and cornstarch emboli in eyes of drug abusers. JAMA 1972; 219:49–51.
53. Inkeles DM, Walsh JB. Retinal fat emboli as a sequelae to acute pancreatitis. Am J Ophthalmol 1975; 80:935–938.
54. Madsen PH. Traumatic retinal angiopathy (Purtscher). Ophthalmologica 1972; 165:453–458.
55. Corrigan MJ, Hill DW. Retinal artery occlusion in loaisis. Br J Ophthalmol 1968; 52:477–470.
56. Toussaint D, Danis P. Retinopathy in generalized loa-loa filariasis. A clinicopathologic study. Arch Ophthalmol 1965; 74:470–476.
57. Carlson MR, Pilger IS, Rosenbaum AL. Central retinal artery occlusion after carotid angiography. Am J Ophthalmol 1976; 81:103–104.
58. Rasmussen KE. Retinal and cerebral fat emboli following lymphangiography With oily contrast media. Acta Radiol 1970; 10:199–202.
59. Charawanamuttu AM, Hughes-Nurse J, Hamlett JD. Retinal embolism after hysterosalpingography. Br J Ophthalmol 1973; 57:166–169.
60. Wilson RS, Havener WH, McGrew RN. Bilateral retinal artery and choriocapillaris occlusion following the injection of long acting corticosteroid suspensions in combination with other drugs. I. Clinical studies. Ophthalmology 1978; 85:967–974.
61. Ellis PP. Occlusion of the central retinal artery after retrobulbar corticosteroid injection. Am J Ophthalmol 1978; 85:352–356.
62. Roth SE, Magargal LE, Kimmel AS et al. Central retinal artery occlusion in proliferative sickle-cell retinopathy after retrobulbar injection. Ann Ophthalmol 1988; 20:221–224.
62a. Nakagawa T, Hirata A, Inoue N et al. A case of bilateral central retinal artery obstruction with patent foramen ovale. Acta Ophthalmol Scand 2004; 82:111–112.
63. Kraushar MF, Seelenfeund MH, Freilich DB. Central retinal artery closure during orbital hemorrhage after retrobulbar injection. Trans Am Acad Ophthalmol Otolaryngol 1974; 78:65–70.
64. Emery JM, Huff JD, Justice J Jr. Central retinal artery occlusion after blow-out fracture repair. Am J Ophthalmol 1974; 78:538–540.
65. Nicholson DH, Guzak SV Jr. Visual loss complicating repair of orbital floor fractures. Arch Ophthalmol 1971; 86:369–375.
66. Hollenhorst RW, Svien RJ, Benoit CF. Unilateral blindness occurring during anesthesia for neurosurgical operations. Arch Ophthalmol 1954; 52:819–830.
67. Brown GC, Magargal LE. Sudden occlusion of the retinal and posterior choroidal circulations in a youth. Am J Ophthalmol 1979; 88:690–693.
68. Lee DH, Yang HN, Kim JC et al. Sudden unilateral visual loss and brain infarction after autologous fat injection into the nasolabial groove. Br J Ophthalmol 1996; 80:1026–1027.
69. Ros MA, Magargal LE, Uram M. Branch retinal artery obstruction: a review of 201 eyes. Ann Ophthalmol 1989; 21:103–107.
70. Egbert JE, Schwartz GS, Walsh AW. Diagnosis and treatment of an ophthalmic artery occlusion during intralesional injection of corticosteroids into an eyelid capillary hemangioma. Am J Ophthalmol 1996; 121:638–642.
71. Michelson PE, Pfaffenbach D. Retinal arterial occlusion following ocular trauma in youths with sickle-trait hemoglobinopathy. Am J Ophthalmol 1972; 74:494–497.
72. Sorr EM, Goldberg RE. Traumatic central retinal artery occlusion with sickle cell trait. Am J Ophthalmol 1975; 80:648–652.
73. Wenzler EM, Rademakers AJ, Boers GH et al. Hyperhomocysteinemia in retinal artery and vein occlusion. Am J Ophthalmol 1993; 115:162–167.
74. Wilson RS, Ruiz RS. Bilateral central retinal artery occlusion in homocystinuria. A case report. Arch Ophthalmol 1969; 82:267–268.
75. Friedman S, Golan A, Shoenfeld A et al. Acute ophthalmologic complications during the use of oral contraceptives. Contraception 1974; 10:685–692.
76. Kleiner R, Najarian LV, Schatten S et al. Vaso-occlusive retinopathy associated with anti-phospholipid antibodies (lupus anticoagulant retinopathy). Ophthalmology 1989; 96:896–904.
77. Keane JR. Sudden blindness after ventriculography. Bilateral retinal vascular occlusion superimposed on papilledema. Am J Ophthalmol 1974; 78:275–278.
78. Bertram B, Remky A, Arend O et al. Protein S, protein C, and antithrombin III in acute ocular occlusive disease. Ger J Ophthalmol 1995; 4:332–335.
79. Vignes S, Wilchser B, Elmaleh C et al. Retinal arterial occlusion associated with resistance to activated protein C. Br J Ophthalmol 1996; 80:1111.
79a. Kondamudi V, Reddy R, Kondamudi N et al. Sudden painless unilateral vision loss caused by branch retinal artery occlusion; implications for the primary care physician. Am J Med Sci 2004; 327:44–46.
80. Brown GC, Magargal LE, Augsburger JJ et al. Preretinal arterial loops and retinal arterial occlusion. Am J Ophthalmol 1979;87:646–651.
81. Degenhart W, Brown GC, Augsburger JJ et al. Prepapillary vascular loops. Ophthalmology 1981; 88:1126–1131.
82. Purcell JJ, Goldberg RE. Hyaline bodies of the optic papilla and bilateral acute vascular occlusions. Ann Ophthalmol 1974;6:1069–1074.

83. Braunstein RA, Gass JD. Branch artery obstruction caused by acute toxoplasmosis. Arch Ophthalmol 1980; 98:512–513.

84. Brown GC, Tasman WS. Retinal arterial obstruction in association with presumed *Toxocara canis* neuroretinitis. Ann Ophthalmol 1981; 13:1385–1387.

85. Gold DH, Morris DA, Henkind P. Ocular findings in systemic lupus erythematosus. Br J Ophthalmol 1972; 56:800–804.

86. Wong K, Ai E, Jones JV, Young D. Visual loss as the initial symptom of systemic lupus erythematosus. Am J Ophthalmol 1981; 92:238–244.

87. Fineman MS, Savino PJ, Federman JL et al. Branch retinal artery occlusion as the initial sign of giant cell arteritis. Am J Ophthalmol 1996;122:428–430.

88. Eagling EM, Sanders MD, Miller SJH. Ischaemic papillopathy. Clinical and fluorescein angiographic review of forty cases. Br J Ophthalmol 1974; 58:990–1008.

89. Artero Mora A, Serrano-Comino M, Melano A et al. Obstruction of the central artery of the retina in Wegener's granulomatosis. Med Clin 1986; 87:736–737.

90. Saurax H, Krulik M, Laroche L. Retinal arteritis in Liebow's lymphomatoid granulomatosis. J Fr Ophthalmol 1983; 6:565–569.

91. Shulovsky LJ, Fletcher GH. Retinal and optic nerve complications in a high dose irradiation technique of ethmoid sinus and nasal cavity. Radiology 1972;104:629–634.

92. Colvard DM, Robertson DM, O'Duffy D. The ocular manifestations of Behçet's disease. Arch Ophthalmol 1977; 95:1813–1817.

93. Ling W, Oftedal G, Simon T. Central retinal artery occlusion in Sydenham's chorea. Am J Dis Child 1969; 118:525–527.

94. Milch F. Personal communication. Baltimore; 1985.

95. Magargal Le, Sanborn GE, Donoso LA, et al. Branch retinal artery occlusion after excessive use of nasal spray. Ann Ophthalmol 1985; 17:500–501.

96. Lightman DA, Brod RD. Branch retinal artery occlusion associated with lyme disease. Arch Ophthalmol 1991; 109:1198–1199.

96a. Khairallah M, Ladjimi A, Chakroun M et al. Posterior segment manifestations of *Rickettsia conorii* infection. Ophthalmology 2004; 111:529–534.

96b. Gray AV, Michels KS, Lauer AK et al. *Bartonella henselae* infection associated with neuroretinitis, central retinal artery and vein occlusion, neovascular glaucoma, and severe vision loss. Am J Ophthalmol 2004; 137:187–189.

97. Comp PC, Esmon CT. Recurrent venous thromboembolism in patients with a partial deficiency of protein S. N Engl J Med 1984; 311:1525–1528.

98. Lorentzen SE. Occlusion of the central retinal artery. A follow up. Acta Ophthalmol 1969; 47:690–703.

99. Ciulla TA, Volpe NA. Retinal arterial occlusions in young adults. Am J Ophthalmol 1996; 22:134–136.

100. Sharma S. The likelihood ratio and ophthalmology: a review of how to critically appraise diagnostic studies. Can J Ophthalmol 1997; 32:475–478.

101. Hayreh SS, Kolder HE, Weingeist TA. Central retinal artery occlusion and retinal tolerance time. Ophthalmology 1980; 87:75–78.

102. Hayreh SS, Jonas JB. Optic disk and retinal nerve fiber layer damage after transient central retinal artery occlusion: an experimental study in rhesus monkeys. Am J Ophthalmol 2000; 129:786–795.

103. Duker JS, Brown GC. Recovery following acute obstruction of the retinal and choroidal circulations. A case history. Retina 1988; 8:257–260.

104. Ffytche TJ. A rationalization of treatment of central retinal artery occlusion. Trans Ophthal Soc UK 1974; 94:468–479.

105. Russell RWR. Evidence for autoregulation in human retinal circulation. Lancet 1973; 2:1048–1050.

106. Ffytche TJ, Pulpitt CJ, Hohner EM et al. Effects of changes in intraocular pressure on the retinal microcirculation. Br J Ophthalmol 1974; 58:514–522.

107. Augsburger JJ, Magargal LE. Visual prognosis following treatment of acute retinal artery obstruction. Br J Ophthalmol 1980; 64:913–917.

108. Eperon G, Johnson M, David NJ. The effect of arterial PO_2 on relative retinal blood flow in monkeys. Invest Ophthalmol 1975; 13:342–352.

109. Frayser R, Hickham JB. Retinal vascular response to breathing increased carbon dioxide and oxygen concentrations. Invest Ophthalmol 1964;3:427–431.

110. Patz A. Oxygen inhalation in retinal arterial occlusion. A preliminary report. Am J Ophthalmol 1955; 40:789–795.

111. Tsacopoulos D, David NJ. The effect of arterial PCO_2 on relative retinal blood flow in monkeys. Invest Ophthalmol 1973; 12:335–347.

112. Atebara NH, Brown GC, Cater J. Efficacy of anterior chamber paracentesis and Carbogen in treating nonarteritic central retinal arterial occlusion. Am J Ophthalmol 1995; 102:2029–2034.

113. Leydhecker W, Krieglstein GK, Brunswig D. Indications and limitations of fibrinolytic therapy for central retinal artery occlusion. Klin Monats Augen 1978; 172:43–46.

114. Schmidt D, Schumacher M, Wakhloo AK. Microcatheter urokinase infusion in central retinal artery occlusion. Am J Ophthalmol 1992; 113:429–434.

115. Sharma S. Levels of evidence and interventional ophthalmology. Can J Ophthalmol 1997; 32:359–362.

116. Fraser S, Siriwardena D. Interventions for acute non-arteritic central retinal artery occlusion. Cochrane Database Syst Rev 2002; 1:CD001989.

117. Watson PG. The treatment of acute central retinal artery occlusion. In: Can JS, ed. The ocular circulation in health and disease. St Louis: Mosby; 1969:234–245.

118. Charness ME, Liu GT. Central retinal artery occlusion in giant cell arteritis: treatment with nitroglycerin. Neurology 1991; 41:1698–1699.

119. Kuritzky S. Nitroglycerin to treat acute loss of vision. N Engl J Med 1990; 323:1428.

120. Dutton GN, Craig G. Treatment of a retinal embolus by photocoagulation. Br J Ophthalmol 1989; 73:580–581.

121. Brown GC, Reber R. An unusual presentation of branch retinal artery obstruction in association with ocular neovascularization. Can J Ophthalmol 1986; 21:103–106.

122. Kraushar MF, Brown GC. Retinal neovascularization after branch retinal arterial obstruction. Am J Ophthalmol 1987; 104:294–296.

123. Shah GK, Sharma S, Brown GC. Iris neovascularization following branch retinal artery occlusion. Can J Ophthalmol 1998; 33:389–390.

124. Rossazza C, Ployet MJ, Garant G et al. Obstruction of the central retinal artery after resection-repositioning under the nasal septum mucosa. Rev Otoneuroophthalmol 1977; 49:161–162.

125. Justice J Jr, Lehmann RP. Cilioretinal arteries. A study based on review of stereo fundus photographs and fluorescein angiographic findings. Arch Ophthalmol 1976; 94:1355–1358.

126. Brown GC, Moffat K, Cruess AF et al. Cilioretinal artery obstruction. Retina 1983; 3:182–187.

127. McLeod D, Rig CP. Cilio-retinal infarction after retinal vein occlusion. Br J Ophthalmol 1976; 60:419–427.

128. Schatz H, Fong AO, McDonald HR et al. Cilioretinal artery occlusion in young adults with central retinal vein occlusion. Ophthalmology 1991; 98:594–601.

129. Fong AC, Schatz H, McDonald HR et al. Central retinal vein occlusion in young adults (papillophlebitis). Retina 1992; 12:3–11.

130. Hayreh SS. The cilio-retinal arteries. Br J Ophthalmol 1963; 47:71–89.

131. Henkind P, Charles NC, Pearson J. Histopathology of ischemic optic neuropathy. Am J Ophthalmol 1979; 69:78–90.

132. Brown GC, Duker JS, Lehman R et al. Combined central retinal artery–central vein obstruction. Int Ophthalmol 1993;17:9–17.

133. Richards RD. Simultaneous occlusion of the central retinal artery and vein. Trans Am Ophthalmol Soc 1979; 77:191–209.

134. Jorizzo PA, Klein Ml, Shults WT et al. Visual recovery in combined central retinal artery and central retinal vein occlusion. Am J Ophthalmol 1987; 104:358–363.

135. Hayreh SS, van Heuven WAJ, Hayreh MS. Experimental retinal vascular occlusion. I. Pathogenesis of central retinal vein occlusion. Arch Ophthalmol 1978; 96:311–323.

136. Fujino T, Curtin VT, Norton EWD. Experimental central retinal vein occlusion. Arch Ophthalmol 1969;81:395–406.

137. Brown GC, Eagle RC Jr, Shakin E et al. Retinal toxicity of gentamicin. Arch Ophthalmol 1990; 108:1740–1744.

138. Ashton N. Pathological and ultrastructural aspects of the cotton-wool spot. Proc Roy Soc Med 1969; 62;1271–1276.

139. Ashton N. Henkind P. Experimental occlusion of retinal arterioles (using graded glass ballotini). Br J Ophthalmol 1965; 49:225–234.

140. McLeod D, Marshall J, Hohner EM et al. The role of axoplasmic transport in the pathogenesis of retinal cotton-wool spots. Br J Ophthalmol 1977; 61;177–191.

141. Ashton N. Pathophysiology of retinal cotton-wool spots. Br Med Bull 1970; 26:143–150.

142. Brown GC, Brown MM, Hiller T et al. Cotton-wool spots. Retina 1985; 5:206–214.

143. Kohner EM, Dollery CT, Bulpitt CJ. Cotton-wool spots in diabetic retinopathy. Diabetes 1969; 18:691–704.

144. Freeman WR, Lerner CW, Mines JA et al. A prospective study of the ophthalmologic findings in the acquired immune deficiency syndrome. Am J Ophthalmol 1984; 97:133–142.

145. Pepose JS, Holland GN, Nestor MS et al. An analysis of retinal cotton-wool spots in the acquired immunodeficiency syndrome. Am J Ophthalmol 1983; 95:118–120.

146. Freeman WR, Helm M. Retinal and ophthalmologic manifestations of AIDS. In: Ryan SJ, ed. Retina, vol. 2. Baltimore: Mosby; 1989:597–615.

147. Seligmann M, Chess L, Fahey JL et al. AIDS: an immunologic reevaluation. N Engl J Med 1984; 311:1286–1292.

Chapter

70

Central Retinal Vein Occlusion

Prithvi Mruthyunjaya
Sharon Fekrat

Central retinal vein occlusion (CVO) is a retinal vascular condition that may cause significant ocular morbidity. It commonly affects men and women equally and occurs predominantly in persons over the age of 65 years.[1-3] Younger individuals who present with a clinical picture of CVO may have an underlying inflammatory etiology.[4-6] Individuals with CVO demonstrate a significant decrease in vision-related quality of life as compared to a reference group without ocular disease.[7] CVO may impact a person's ability to perform activities of daily living, especially in cases of bilateral CVO or when concurrent ocular disease limits vision in the fellow eye.

Population-based studies report the prevalence of CVO at 0.1 to 0.4%.[2,8] In larger noncontrolled, clinical studies, the frequency of CVO is 25–42%.[1,2,8] Central retinal vein occlusion is usually a unilateral disease; however, the annual risk of developing any type of retinal vascular occlusion in the fellow eye is approximately 1% per year and is estimated that up to 7% of persons may develop a similar CVO in the fellow eye within 5 years from the onset in the first eye.[1,9,10]

CLINICAL FEATURES

A CVO usually presents as a sudden painless loss of vision, but it may also present with a history of a gradual decline of vision which may correlate with less severe occlusions. The typical clinical constellation in CVO includes retinal hemorrhages (both superficial flame-shaped and deep blot type) in all four quadrants of the fundus with a dilated, tortuous retinal venous system. The hemorrhages radiate from the optic nerve head and are variable in quantity and may result in the classic "blood and thunder" appearance (Fig. 70-1). Optic nerve head swelling, cotton-wool spots, splinter hemorrhages, and macular edema are present to varying degrees (Figs 70-2 and 70-3). Breakthrough vitreous hemorrhage may also be observed.[11] Rarely, a retinal arterial occlusion may accompany a CVO.[11,12]

With time, the extent of retinal hemorrhage may decrease or resolve completely with resultant retinal pigment epithelium alterations. The time course for resolution of the hemorrhages varies and is dependent on the amount of hemorrhage produced by the occlusion. Macular edema often persists despite resolution of the retinal hemorrhage with reported serous retinal detachments (Fig. 70-4).[13] Epiretinal membranes may also

develop. Optociliary shunt vessels can develop on the optic nerve head, a sign of newly formed collateral channels with the choroidal circulation (Fig. 70-5). Neovascularization of the optic disc (NVD) may develop as a response to secondary retinal ischemia. The vessels that comprise NVD are typically of smaller caliber than optociliary shunt vessels, branch into a vascular network resembling a net, and will leak on fluorescein angiography. In the Central Vein Occlusion Study (CVOS), a randomized multicentered clinical trial of 728 eyes with CVO evaluating natural history and treatment outcomes from laser photocoagulation, retinal neovascularization (NVE) developed in 12% of eyes receiving prophylactic panretinal photocoagulation (PRP) compared to 18% of eyes not receiving PRP.[9] Fibrovascular proliferation from NVD or NVE may result in vitreous hemorrhage or traction retinal detachment.

Visual acuity at the time of presentation is variable, but an important prognostic indicator of final visual outcome. In the CVOS, baseline visual acuity was 20/40 or better in 29%, 20/50 to 20/200 in 43%, and 20/250 or worse in 28% of persons with a median baseline acuity of 20/80.[3] Of those with initially good visual acuity (20/40 or better), the majority maintains this acuity. Individuals with intermediate visual acuity (20/50 to 20/200) had a variable outcome: 21% improved to better than 20/50, 41% stayed in the intermediate group, and 38% were worse than 20/200. Persons with poor visual acuity at onset (less than 20/200) had only a 20% chance of improvement.[9]

Anterior segment findings may include iris and angle neovascularization (INV/ANV). Iris neovascularization typically begins at the pupillary border but may extend across the iris surface. Angle neovascularization is detected during undilated gonioscopy and can be detected as fine branching vessels bridging the scleral spur. Angle neovascularization may develop without any INV in 6–12% of eyes with CVO.[3,9,14] Elevated intraocular pressure associated with INV/ANV is the hallmark of neovascular glaucoma. Longstanding ANV may lead to secondary angle closure from peripheral anterior synechiae formation. The CVOS used an index of any two clock hours of INV or any ANV as significant anterior segment neovascularization, which was found in 16% of eyes with 10 to 29 disc areas of angiographic nonperfusion and 52% of eyes with 75 disc areas or more of angiographic nonperfusion.[9] In the CVOS, worse initial visual acuity correlated with the development of INV/ANV:

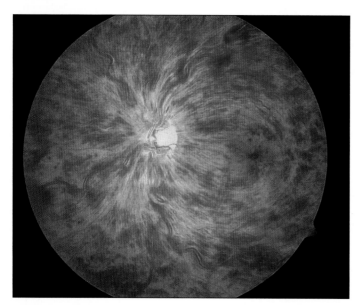

Fig. 70-1 Fundus photograph of a CVO with extensive intraretinal hemorrhage. Extensive blocking on fluorescein angiography in such an occlusion precludes accurate determination of perfusion status.

5% in eyes with 20/40 or better, 14.8% in eyes with 20/50 to 20/200, and 30.8% in eyes with worse than 20/200 acuity. In an incipient cohort of 187 patients with recent (within 1 month) onset of CVO, 56% of 36 eyes that developed INV/ANV presented with acuity of 20/200 or worse.[9]

PERFUSION STATUS

The CVOS classified the perfusion status of a CVO as perfused, nonperfused or indeterminate based on the fluorescein angiographic characteristics. Angiographic assessment of perfusion status in CVO is based on the photographic protocol from the CVOS which used a wide-angle fundus camera with sweeps of the mid periphery 30 seconds after injection of sodium fluorescein.[15]

A perfused CVO (also termed nonischemic, incomplete or partial) demonstrates less than 10 disc areas in diameter of retinal capillary nonperfusion on angiography (Fig. 70-2). These eyes typically had a lesser degree of intraretinal hemorrhage on presentation. Generally, eyes with perfused CVO had better initial and final visual acuity. A nonperfused CVO (also termed ischemic, hemorrhagic, or complete) demonstrates 10 or more disc areas in diameter of retinal capillary nonperfusion on angiography (Fig. 70-3). Acutely, these eyes demonstrate a greater degree of intraretinal hemorrhage, macular and disc edema and capillary nonperfusion than perfused CVOs. A CVO is categorized as indeterminate when there is sufficient intraretinal hemorrhage to prevent angiographic determination of the perfusion status. Other examination features that may help in determining the perfusion status in the acute phase of a CVO include baseline visual acuity, presence of an afferent pupillary defect, electroretinography, and Goldmann perimetry.[5,9,10]

The CVOS classification of initial perfusion status of the CVO was important for determining the natural history of the disease. In eyes initially categorized as perfused, 10% (56/538) developed INV/ANV, compared to 35% (61/176) of eyes initially characterized as nonperfused or indeterminate. Poor visual acuity and large areas of retinal capillary nonperfusion were significant factors associated with an increased risk of developing INV/ANV. Overall, 34% of initially perfused eyes converted to nonperfused status after 3 years. In the CVOS, 38 eyes (83%) with an indeterminate CVO at baseline were ultimately determined to be nonperfused. Initial visual acuity was

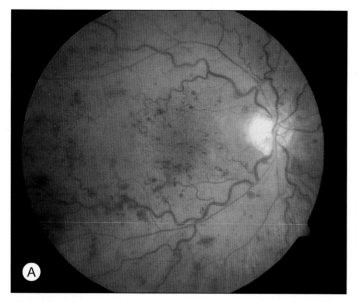

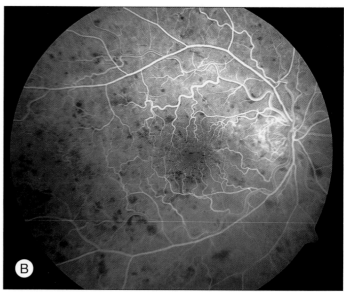

Fig. 70-2 A, Fundus photograph of an eye with central retinal vein occlusion (CVO) demonstrating typical features of venous tortuosity, macular thickening and intraretinal hemorrhage in all four quadrants of the fundus. B, Early phase angiograms of the fundus depicted in A, demonstrating an intact parafoveal capillary network in this perfused CVO.

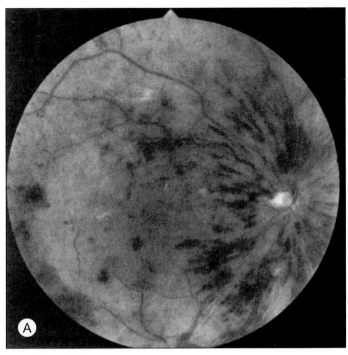
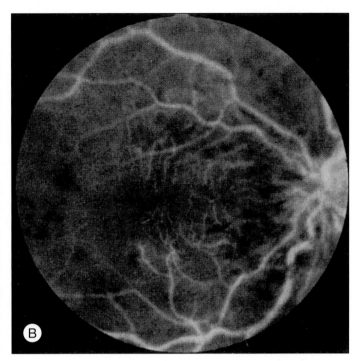

Fig. 70-3 A, Fundus photographs of an eye with recent onset of symptoms resulting from central vein occlusion. Scattered retinal hemorrhages, optic nerve swelling, and venous engorgement are present. B, Midphase fluorescein angiogram of the eye shown in "A", demonstrating capillary nonperfusion involving the inferotemporal paramacular region, including the parafoveal capillaries. This is an example of the nonperfused form of central retinal vein occlusion.

highly correlated with degree of nonperfusion ($P < 0.001$).[9] In a prospective study of 550 nonischemic, untreated CVO (determined by clinical parameters including visual acuity and fluorescein angiography), 61 (11%) converted to the ischemic type with a cumulative chance of conversion of 13% within 18 months of onset of nonischemic CVO.[1] At 3 years, there is a 45% chance of developing neovascular glaucoma after onset of ischemic CVO.[1] Electroretinography, with reduction to 60% or less of normal mean b-wave amplitude, and the presence of a relative afferent pupillary defect (greater than 0.70 log units) have been used to differentiate ischemic from nonischemic CVO in up to 97% of 140 eyes in one series.[16]

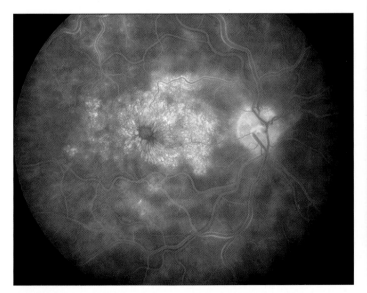

Fig. 70-4 Fluorescein angiograms of chronic CVO with resolution of intraretinal hemorrhage but persistence of cystoid macular edema demonstrated by petaloid leakage in the late phase angiograms.

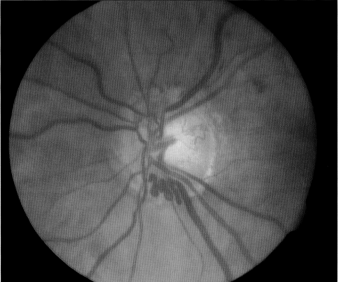

Fig. 70-5 Fundus photograph demonstrating optociliary shunt vessels at the inferior border of the optic nerve head in this patient with a chronic central retinal vein occlusion. These vessels do not leak on fluorescein angiography.

PATHOGENESIS

The clinical picture of CVO may be explained by the occlusion of the main trunk of the central retinal vein; however, the pathophysiology of CVO is not clearly understood. Histopathologic studies of eyes enucleated for CVO demonstrated a thrombus occluding the lumen of the central retinal vein at or just proximal to the lamina cribrosa.[17] This finding suggests that the anatomic variations at the level of the lamina cribrosa may be responsible for the development of a CVO. Within the retrolaminar portion of the optic nerve, the central retinal artery and vein are aligned parallel to each other in a common tissue sheath. The central retinal artery and vein are naturally compressed as they cross through the rigid sieve-like openings in the lamina cribrosa, but typically give off branching collateral vessels just before piercing the lamina. These vessels may be subject to compression from mechanical stretching of the lamina from increases in intraocular pressure, causing a posterior shift or bowing of the lamina with subsequent impingement on the central retinal vein. Furthermore, local factors may predispose to occlusion of the central retinal vein, including compression by an atherosclerotic central retinal artery or primary occlusion of the central retinal vein from inflammation.

Hemodynamic alterations may produce stagnant flow and subsequent thrombus formation in the central retinal vein, including diminished blood flow, increased blood viscosity, and an altered lumen wall (also known as Virchow's triad). Experimentally, occlusion of both the retrolaminar central retinal artery and central retinal vein, posterior to the lamina cribrosa and before collateral channels branch from the main trunk, was required to produce the clinical appearance of a hemorrhagic (ischemic) CVO. This implies that concurrent retinal artery insufficiency or occlusion may play a role in an ischemic CVO. A less hemorrhagic CVO (more likely nonischemic), it is hypothesized, may be due to occlusion of the central retinal vein proximal to the branching of the collateral channels, providing alternative routes of flow of venous blood to drain into patent areas of the central retinal vein within the optic nerve.[10]

In the largest histopathologic study of eyes with CVO, 29 eyes enucleated for acute (within 6 hours) and chronic (up to 10 years) were reviewed,[17] some of which had concurrent neovascular glaucoma. In acute occlusions, a thrombus at the level of the lamina cribrosa was adherent to a portion of the vein wall devoid of an endothelial lining. Subsequently, there was endothelial cell proliferation within the vein and secondary inflammatory cell infiltrates. Recanalization of the thrombus was demonstrated in eyes 1 to 5 years after the documented occlusion.

Anterior segment neovascularization is modulated by growth factors released from the ischemic retina. Green and colleagues demonstrated inner retinal ischemic changes in 25% of eyes enucleated for CVO. Vascular endothelial growth factor (VEGF) has been implicated in the development of neovascular complications from CVO. In a study of enucleated eyes with CVO and neovascular glaucoma, intraretinal VEGF production from areas of ischemic retina was demonstrated.[18] Aqueous VEGF levels increase prior to the development of NVI and decrease with the regression of NVI after panretinal laser photocoagulation.[19]

RISK FACTORS AND ASSOCIATIONS

> **Box 70-1** Risk factors and associations with CVO[5,13,20]
>
> - **Systemic vascular diseases:** Diabetes mellitus, hypertension, carotid insufficiency
> - **Ocular diseases:** Open angle glaucoma, ischemic optic neuropathy, pseudotumor cerebri, tilted optic nerve heads, optic nerve head drusen
> - **Hematologic alterations:** Hyperviscosity syndromes: dysproteinemias (multiple myeloma), blood dyscrasias (polycythemia very, lymphoma, leukemia, sickle cell disease or trait). Anemia, elevated plasma homocysteine, factor XII deficiency, anti-phospholipid antibody syndrome, activated protein C resistance, protein C deficiency, protein S deficiency
> - **Inflammatory/autoimmune vasculitis:** Systemic lupus erythematosus
> - **Medications:** Oral contraceptives, diuretics, hepatitis B vaccine
> - **Infectious vasculitis:** HIV, syphilis, herpes zoster, sarcoidosis
> - **Other:** After retrobulbar block, dehydration, pregnancy

Concurrent systemic vascular disease is a risk factor for CVO. The Eye Disease Case-Control Study found an increased risk of any type of CVO in those with systemic hypertension and diabetes mellitus.[20] Persons with a nonperfused CVO had a greater odds-ratio, implicating systolic and diastolic hypertension as a risk factor compared to perfused CVO. Similar associations with systemic hypertension were found in other prospective and retrospective cross-sectional studies.[21,22] Diabetes mellitus was more prevalent in individuals with a nonperfused CVO than matched controls from large population databases.[21,22] Although mortality was not increased in a clinic population with CVO compared to published United States mortality rates, an increase in calculated cardiovascular disease risk is present in persons with CVO.[21,23]

Hematologic abnormalities, particularly conditions that predispose to a hypercoagulable state, have been identified in persons with CVO. Individuals less than 60 years of age may have a greater association with hypercoagulable states and inflammatory conditions, compared to older persons with a higher incidence of systemic vascular disease risk factors.[5,6] Lahey and colleagues found one abnormal laboratory value in 27% of 55 patients younger than 56 years of age, suggesting systemic hypercoagulability.[24] Studies have demonstrated an increased incidence of coagulation cascade abnormalities, including protein C deficiency, protein S deficiency, activated protein C resistance, presence of factor V Leiden, presence of antiphospholipid antibodies, and abnormal fibrinogen levels.[25–29] In a meta-analysis of published studies, an association with elevated plasma homocysteine and low serum folate levels, but not serum vitamin B_{12} and the thermolabile methyltetrahydrofolate reductase genotype, was observed in eyes with retinal vein occlusion.[30] Hyperviscosity from blood dyscrasias, dysproteinemias, and dehydration have also been reported with CVO.[13,31]

An increased risk of CVO is present in eyes with open angle glaucoma.[20] Other ocular conditions causing deformation or mechanical pressure on the optic nerve head and lamina cribrosa, including ischemic optic neuropathy, tilted optic nerve head, optic nerve head drusen, optic disc traction syndrome and pseudotumor cerebri,[13,32] have also been associated with CVO. External compression of the globe and optic nerve from thyroid related ophthalmopathy or mass lesion and head trauma with orbital fracture may also result in CVO.[5]

CLINICAL EVALUATION

At the time of initial presentation, a careful assessment of the CVO duration and the degree of retinal ischemia will determine treatment options and the follow-up schedule. An ocular history will determine the onset of the occlusion, although individuals may not have noted the vision loss if the fellow eye has maintained good acuity. One can assume a recent onset if the historical information is unclear. A history of systemic diseases, such as hypertension, diabetes, and heart disease, and a personal or family history of thrombosis or hypercoagulable state should be determined.

The ophthalmic examination should be performed on both eyes and include visual acuity, pupillary reaction, and intraocular pressure. Undilated slit lamp examination is performed to detect INV or ANV. Atypical iris stromal vessels may be confused for INV; however, comparison with the fellow eye may help to differentiate abnormal iris vessels. Undilated gonioscopy is essential to determine the presence of ANV or evidence of angle closure from peripheral anterior synechiae, as ANV may be present without any INV.[14] Ophthalmoscopic examination will help differentiate a CVO from intraretinal hemorrhage associated with carotid occlusive disease.[33]

In general, a systemic work-up is not indicated in persons older than 60 years of age with known systemic vascular risk factors for CVO. Younger patients are more likely to have predisposing conditions resulting in thrombotic disease.[6,24] A limited systemic work up may be considered in those with a prior occlusion in the fellow eye, prior systemic thrombotic disease, family history of thrombosis, or other symptoms suggestive of a hematologic or rheumatologic condition. An initial laboratory investigation may include an erythrocyte sedimentation rate, anti-nuclear antibody, antiphospholipid antibody, and fasting plasma homocysteine levels. An elevated plasma homocysteine level may uncover a correctable etiology of CVO, which may also influence cardiovascular health.[30] Individuals with bilateral, simultaneous CVO or mixed type retinal vascular occlusions should have a detailed evaluation for a hypercoagulable condition, as these persons may be at risk for future, non-ocular thrombotic events.[9]

FOLLOW-UP

The visual acuity at initial presentation helps guide follow-up of eyes with CVO. If the initial acuity is 20/40 or better, an examination should be performed every 1–2 months for 6 months, then annually if stable. Eyes with initial acuity worse than 20/200 should be seen monthly for the initial 6 months, then bimonthly for the next 6 months, as these eyes have a greater degree of nonperfusion and a higher risk of developing INV/NVA.

Eyes with acuity between 20/50 and 20/200 should also be examined monthly for the first 6 months as they have an intermediate risk of developing INV/ANV. These examinations assess visual acuity and include undilated slit lamp examination looking for INV/ANV. Laser photocoagulation is performed if INV and/or ANV is detected to prevent neovascular glaucoma (see laser photocoagulation below). If at any time in the follow-up period the visual acuity drops below the 20/200 level, an evaluation with assessment of perfusion status and anterior segment examination is required, and monthly follow-up for an additional 6 months is recommended.[9]

THERAPEUTIC OPTIONS

Medical therapy

Identification and treatment of systemic vascular risk factors, such as systemic hypertension and diabetes mellitus, is important in individuals with CVO. Coordination with the internist is recommended. The role of systemic anticoagulation in CVO is unclear as there is no evidence that agents, such as aspirin or heparin, can prevent or alter the natural history of CVO; patients taking warfarin sodium (Coumadin) can still develop CVO despite maintaining therapeutic levels of anticoagulation.[34,35] Prophylactic use of these medications, however, may help prevent non-ocular thrombotic events, especially in individuals with known systemic vascular disease.

Oral pentoxifylline is used in systemic vascular diseases to improve perfusion to occluded vessels, enhance the development of collateral circulation, and is a potent vasodilator. Limited trials in retinal vein occlusion patients demonstrated a significant increase in retinal vein flow velocity.[36] Park et al. found, in a retrospective series of 12 patients treated with oral pentoxifylline (400 mg three times a day) for an average of 5 months, a mean reduction by 10% in macular thickening by volumetric optical coherence tomography with only one patient demonstrating worsening of macular edema. Although there was no change in visual acuity or perfusion status, pentoxiphylline may help to reduce macular edema in CVO (Carl Park MD, unpublished data, 2002). The reported increased plasma viscosity in persons with CVO has prompted interest in systemic hemodilution to increase oxygen supply to the retina. In a prospective, randomized, trial comparing the combined therapy of hemodilution and pentoxifylline administration with saline infusions alone, a significant improvement in mean visual acuity (a 1.5 line increase compared to a 1.5 line decrease in control eyes) at one year was observed and was attributed to improved blood flow from the decreased blood viscosity.[37]

Shaikh and Blumenkranz reported treating two patients with CVO associated with inflammatory features with a combination of systemic steroids (either intravenous methylprednisolone or oral prednisone) and nonsteroidal immunosuppressive medications (either cyclophosphamide or methotrexate). In both cases, transient improvement in visual acuity and reduction in macular edema were attributed to reduction of both local and systemic inflammatory disease, suggesting a role of systemic immunosuppression in select cases of CVO.[38]

Medical therapy may be used to treat sequela of CVO, especially neovascular glaucoma. Topical or systemic anti-glaucoma agents can help to reduce intraocular pressure typically by reducing aqueous humor production and enhancing outflow in sections of the anterior chamber outflow tract not occluded by anterior synechiae. Topical corticosteroids can reduce anterior segment inflammation by stabilizing tight junctions in neovascular tissue, thereby reducing vascular exudation. Cycloplegic agents prevent posterior synechiae formation between the iris and lens. Failure of medical therapy to control intraocular pressure may require surgical intervention (e.g. trabeculectomy or seton placement).

Laser photocoagulation

The CVOS was designed to answer three questions about the role of laser photocoagulation in managing CVO-associated macular edema and anterior segment neovascularization.[3] First, does early panretinal photocoagulation prevent anterior segment neovascularization in eyes with nonperfused CVO? Second, is early panretinal photocoagulation (PRP) more effective than delaying treatment until anterior segment neovascularization is first seen in preventing neovascular glaucoma in eyes with nonperfused CVO? Third, does macular grid pattern laser photocoagulation improve visual acuity in eyes with vision loss from macular edema?

Ocular neovascularization

The CVOS Group N report compared the efficacy of PRP placement at the time of study entry in eyes with non-perfused CVO that did not have evidence of INV/ANV (early treatment group, $n = 90$) with delayed, but prompt, PRP application (no early treatment group, $n = 91$) only when INV/ANV was detected. INV/ANV developed in 20% of early treatment and 34% of no early treatment eyes. There was greater resolution of INV/ANV by one month after PRP in no early treatment eyes (18/32 eyes) compared with early treatment eyes (4/18 eyes).

Panretinal photocoagulation should therefore by delivered promptly after the development of INV/ANV, not prophylactically, in eyes with nonperfused CVO. In approximately 90%, the regression of INV/ANV occurs within 1–2 months. Persistent neovascularization after PRP should be followed closely, and additional PRP may be applied in attempts to halt its progression. Persons presenting with NVD/NVE without INV/ANV should be treated with PRP, as performed in eyes with proliferative diabetic retinopathy or branch retinal vein occlusion, to prevent anterior segment neovascularization. Prophylactic placement of PRP may be considered in eyes with nonperfused CVO and risk factors for developing INV/ANV (male gender, short duration of CVO, extensive retinal non-perfusion, and extensive retinal hemorrhage) or in cases where frequent ophthalmologic follow-up is not possible.

Macular edema

The CVOS Group M report studied the effect of grid pattern argon laser photocoagulation to improve visual acuity in eyes with perfused macular edema and 20/50 acuity or worse (77 treated and 78 untreated eyes). Laser treatment involved a grid pattern in the area of leaking capillaries within 2 disc diameters of the foveal center but not within the foveal avascular zone. At 36 months, there was no significant difference in mean visual acuity between treated (20/200) and untreated (20/160) eyes. Although there was resolution of angiographic macular edema by one year in 31% of treated eyes (compared to 0% of untreated eyes), widespread damage to the perifoveal capillary network is hypothesized to contribute to the lack of visual recovery. Therefore, the CVOS did not recommend grid laser photocoagulation for CVO-associated macular edema.

Chorioretinal venous anastomosis

In eyes with perfused CVO, investigators have bypassed the occluded central retinal vein by creating a chorioretinal anastomosis (CRA) between a nasal branch retinal vein with the choroidal circulation. Successful creation of an anastomosis may allow trans-retinal retrograde flow of venous blood from the eye and prevent the development of retinal ischemia. Visual acuity may improve as a result of the reduction or resolution of macular edema and/or maintenance of retinal perfusion. CRA have been created surgically through a trans-retinal venipuncture technique[39] or, more commonly, laser energy delivered through argon or Nd-YAG systems, is directed directly at a branch retinal vein to rupture the posterior vein wall and Bruch's membrane.[40] In successful cases, the treated site along the vein demonstrates a retinal vessel diving into the choroid with dilation of the proximal portion and narrowing of the distal portion of the treated vessel. Successful CRA creation is reported in 10–54% of perfused CVO with subsequent conversion to ischemic CVO in 0–8% of eyes.[39,41–43]

Complications from this technique may include immediate intraretinal, subretinal or vitreous hemorrhage. Long-term complications include nonclearing vitreous hemorrhage, epiretinal avascular proliferation, fibrovascular proliferation, secondary neovascularization (choroidal, retinal, choroidovitreal, anterior segment), and traction retinal detachment.[39,41–44] Visual recovery may be limited in spite of successful anastomosis creation due to thrombosis of the treated vein with progressive retinal ischemia and development of macular pigment abnormalities related to resolution of chronic macular edema. Leonard and colleagues successfully created chorioretinal anastomoses by applying laser energy to rupture Bruch's membrane directly adjacent to the candidate branch vein site, avoiding laser-associated trauma to the retinal vein. Kwok reported the inability to create a successful CRA in nonperfused CVO suggesting widespread endothelial damage from the CVO limits anastomosis formation.[45] Because of an increased risk of fibrovascular complications in eyes with a nonperfused CVO, laser chorioretinal anastomosis is not a recommended treatment option in these eyes.

Surgical treatments

Pars plana vitrectomy techniques are used to address complications of CVO and, in investigational studies, to attempt to alter the natural course of the disease. Eyes with nonclearing vitreous hemorrhage from secondary retinal neovascularization may require surgical evacuation. At the time of vitrectomy, clearing of the hemorrhage can be combined with removal of epiretinal membranes and removal of fibrovascular proliferations, if present, and the placement of complete endolaser PRP.[46] Although this technique may prevent or aid in regression of anterior segment neovascularization, visual outcomes may be limited due to the extent of underlying retinal nonperfusion.[47] In eyes with extensive anterior segment neovascularization and neovascular glaucoma, pars plana vitrectomy and endolaser PRP may be combined with pars plana placement of a seton glaucoma drainage device to avoid anterior chamber hemorrhage at the time of tube placement.

Radial optic neurotomy

Opremcak and colleagues have proposed combining pars plana vitrectomy with transvitreal incision of the nasal scleral ring to release pressure on the central retinal vein at the level of the scleral outlet.[48] The procedure addresses the "compartment syndrome" that may exist in these eyes where the central retinal artery, central retinal vein and optic nerve traverse through a 1.5 mm diameter area. Vascular factors, as discussed earlier, as well as rigidity of the scleral ring may also decrease venous lumen diameter and incite a thrombotic event. Previous attempts at external decompression of the orbital portion of the optic nerve by optic nerve sheath fenestration and sectioning of the posterior scleral ring have not been validated as effective treatments for CVO.[49,50] RON is performed by pars plana vitrectomy followed by use of a 20-gauge microvitreoretinal (MVR) blade to incise the lamina cribrosa and adjacent retina. Care is taken to avoid major retinal vessels, and a radial incision orientation is used to avoid transecting nerve fibers. Intraoperative hemorrhage is typically controlled by transient elevation of intraocular pressure.

In the initial retrospective report of 11 eyes by Opremcak and colleagues, successful RON was performed with no complications. There was clinical improvement in retinal hemorrhages and venous congestion. With a mean follow up of 9 months, 73% of patients had improved Snellen acuity; however, two eyes with preoperative INV had worsening of acuity associated with the development of neovascular glaucoma.[48] Weizer and coworkers reported their experience with RON in five eyes (one with hemiretinal vein occlusion). Mean visual acuity improved from 4/200 to 20/400 with 80% demonstrating a rapid resolution of intraretinal hemorrhage and disc congestion as compared to the known natural history of CVO. Perfusion status was not significantly altered and macular edema significantly improved (by volumetric optical coherence tomography) in one eye. Two eyes developed neovascular complications (choroidovitreal and INV) but responded to PRP.[51] Garcia-Arumi and colleagues reported, in a prospective interventional trial, successful RON surgery in 14 eyes.[52] Overall, 57% gained one line of distance visual acuity, and visual recovery was significantly related to reduction in macular edema. Six (43%) developed a postoperative chorioretinal anastomosis at the RON site with a trend towards better final acuity compared to those without anastomosis formation (20/60 vs. 20/110). The CRA seen at

RON sites may allow for more active drainage of retinal edema and hemorrhage compared to laser-induced CRA. Neovascular complications were not reported. Williamson and coworkers questioned the role of vitrectomy, limited endolaser photocoagulation, and fluid to intraocular gas exchange with and without RON in ischemic CVO.[53] The rationale of vitrectomy alone was to increase retinal oxygenation while providing a postoperative oxygen rich environment with intraocular gas may enhance resolution of CVO as well as including RON to the surgical procedure. In their pilot study of eight eyes, there was equivocal benefit from RON by visual acuity and funduscopic appearance. However, segmental temporal visual field loss was demonstrated in one eye in the RON group corresponding to nasal RON site.

Tissue plasminogen activator

Thrombolytic agents have been proposed as a treatment against a suspected thrombus in the central retinal vein. Recombinant tissue plasminogen activator (r-tPA) is a synthetic fibrinolytic agent that converts plasminogen to plasmin and destabilizes intravascular thrombi. Reduction in clot size may facilitate dislodging of the entire thrombus or recanalization of the occluded retinal vein. Recombinant tissue plasminogen activator, as therapy against CVO, has been administered by several routes: systemic, intravitreal, and by endovascular cannulation of retinal vessels.

Systemic administration of low dose (50 mg) front loaded r-tPA has been attempted in two pilot studies with visual acuity improvement in 30% to 73% of patients.[54,55] Lahey reported, in a prospective clinical trial of 96 persons with CVO, a mean improvement of five lines of acuity in 42% of individuals.[56] One person in this study died from an intracranial hemorrhage following r-tPA administration which has limited enthusiasm for the systemic administration of r-tPA for CVO.

Intravitreal delivery of r-tPA has potential advantages including less risk of systemic complications, directed delivery to the vitreous cavity and subsequent access to the retinal vessels, and low risk of ocular morbidity from the procedure. Of 47 persons in three studies of intravitreal r-tPA for both ischemic and nonischemic CVO of less than 21 days duration, 28–44% had three lines of visual acuity improvement with 6 months follow-up.[56–58] Administration of r-tPA did not significantly alter final perfusion status, especially in pre-treatment ischemic eyes. Although there were no significant treatment related complications, differences in inclusion criteria and dosage of r-tPA used (between 66 and 100 μg) limits generalizations from these studies. Ghazi and colleagues reported using a standard dose of 50 μg of intravitreal r-tPA in 12 eyes with acute CVO of less than three days duration.[59] In all patients, perfusion status remained unchanged at last follow-up, however marked improvement (20/50 or better) was demonstrated in eyes with perfused CVO. This report suggests prompt use of intravitreal r-tPA, especially in perfused CVO, may provide significant visual benefit.

Endovascular delivery of r-tPA involves cannulation of retinal vessels, either through a neuroradiologic or a vitreoretinal approach, and delivery of minute quantities of r-tPA directly to the occluded vessels to release the suspected thrombus.[60,61]

Weiss and Bynoe have reported their technique of pars plana vitrectomy followed by cannulation of a branch vein and, with the aid of a stabilization arm, injecting a bolus (average 3.4 ml) of 200 µg/ml r-tPA towards the optic nerve head.[62] Of 28 eyes with CVO of greater than 1 month duration and worse than 20/400 preoperative acuity, 50% recovered more than three lines of acuity by a mean follow up of 12 months. There was a trend towards increased perfusion by fluorescein angiography attributed in part to the resolution of intraretinal hemorrhages after the procedure. Complications included vitreous hemorrhage in seven eyes and treated retinal detachment in one eye. This technique has been combined with intravitreal triamcinolone acetonide injection, hypothesized to target retinal edema, following endovascular r-tPA administration in two patients with CVO under the age of 40 with resultant improvement of 8–11 lines of acuity.[63]

Corticosteroid therapy

The role of corticosteroids has been explored in CVO with particular interest to improve visual acuity by reducing macular edema. The exact mechanism of action of corticosteroids in modulating retinal edema is unknown, but it is believed that a combination of anti-inflammatory effects with modulation of cytokine and growth factor production and stabilization of the blood–retinal barrier with reduction in vascular permeability may be involved. There is little evidence for using oral corticosteroids to treat macular edema from CVO. Oral corticosteroids, however, may be utilized to treat underlying systemic inflammatory diseases responsible for the CVO.

Intravitreal delivery of corticosteroids provides targeted delivery of the drug to the retinal vessels and macular tissue while limiting potential systemic toxicity. An intravitreal sustained release fluocinolone acetonide device (Retisert, Bausch and Lomb) is being implanted, via a pars plana incision, in clinical trials. Intravitreal injection of triamcinolone acetonide (Kenalog, TA) to treat macular edema associated with CVO has gained popularity due to the reported improvements in visual acuity, safety profile of the drug, ease of single or repeated administration and low complication rates from the delivery method (Fig. 70-6).[64-66] Park et al. retrospectively reported using a 4 milligram intravitreal injection of TA in 10 eyes with chronic perfused CVO. There was ophthalmoscopic reduction in macular edema which corresponded to significant improvement in visual acuity and macular thickness by volumetric optical coherence tomography at last follow up.[67] Although there were no complications from the procedure, including the acute sterile endophthalmitis reported in other series of intravitreal steroid injections, 40% of patients had elevated intraocular pressure requiring topical aqueous suppressants. Potential complications from these intravitreal TA injections include cataract progression, sterile endophthalmitis, elevated intraocular pressure, and retinal detachment.[67] (Please refer to Chapter 55 for further information.)

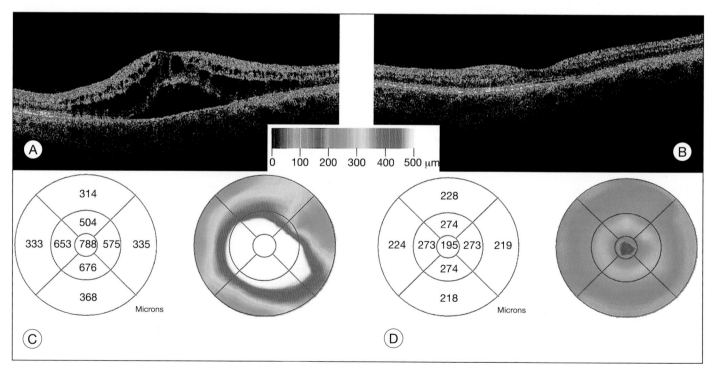

Fig. 70-6 67-year-old male with 5-month history of vision loss from a central retinal vein occlusion who received a single intravitreal injection of triamcinolone acetonide (4 mg) to treat the persistent cystoid macular edema. A, Pre-injection optical coherence tomogram (OCT) demonstrating prominent retinal thickening in the macular region with inner and outer retinal cysts and subretinal fluid accumulation. B, Retinal thickness map and corresponding color map from "A". C, 4-month post-injection OCT demonstrating dramatic resolution of retinal thickening and return of normal foveal contour. D, Retinal thickness map and corresponding color map from "C" with normal retinal thickness measurements.

CONCLUSION

CVO is a sight threatening disease with significant ocular morbidity from its known natural history including macular edema and ocular neovascularization. The prompt diagnosis and identification of complications may help limit visual loss. New treatment modalities may provide important treatment options in the future.

REFERENCES

1. Hayreh SS, Zimmerman MB, Podhajsky P. Incidence of various types of retinal vein occlusion and their recurrence and demographic characteristics. Am J Ophthalmol 1994; 117:429–441.
2. Mitchell P, Smith W, Chang A. Prevalence and associations of retinal vein occlusion in Australia. The Blue Mountains Eye Study. Arch Ophthalmol 1996; 114:1243–1247.
3. Group TCVOS. Baseline and early natural history report: the Central Vein Occlusion Study. Arch Ophthalmol 1993;111:1087–1095.
4. Fekrat S, Finkelstein D. Venous Occlusive Disease. In: Regillo CD, Brown GC, Flynn HW, eds. Vitreoretinal disease: the essentials, 1st edn. New York: Thieme, 1999.
5. Gutman FA. Evaluation of a patient with central retinal vein occlusion. Ophthalmology 1983; 90:481–483.
6. Fong AC, Schatz H. Central retinal vein occlusion in young adults. Surv Ophthalmol 1993; 38:88.
7. Deramo VA, Cox TA, Syed AB et al. Vision-related quality of life in people with central retinal vein occlusion using the 25-item National Eye Institute Visual Function Questionnaire. Archives of Ophthalmology. 2003; 121: 1297–1302.
8. Klein R, Klein BE, Moss SE, Meuer SM. The epidemiology of retinal vein occlusion: the Beaver Dam Eye Study. Trans Am Ophthalmol Soc 2000; 98:133–41; discussion 41–43.
9. Group TCVOS. Natural history and clinical management of central retinal vein occlusion. The Central Vein Occlusion Study Group. Arch Ophthalmol 1997; 115:486–491.
10. Hayreh SS. Central retinal vein occlusion. Ophthalmol Clin North Am 1998; 11:559–590.
11. Browning DJ. Patchy ischemic retinal whitening in acute central retinal vein occlusion. Ophthalmology 2002; 109:2154–2159.
12. Brown GC, Duker JS, Lehman R et al. Combined central retinal artery–central vein occlusion. Int Ophthalmol 1993; 17:9–17.
13. Ciardella AP, Clarkson JG, Guyer DR et al. Central retinal vein occlusion: a primer and review. In: Yannuzzi LA, ed. Retina–Vitreous–Macular. New York: W.B. Saunders, 1999.
14. Browning DJ, Scott AQ, Peterson CB et al. The risk of missing angle neovascularization by omitting screening gonioscopy in acute central retinal vein occlusion. Ophthalmology 1998; 105:776–784.
15. Clarkson JG. Central Vein Occlusion Study: photographic protocol and early natural history. Trans Am Ophthalmol Soc 1994; 92:203–13; discussion 13–15.
16. Hayreh SS, Klugman MR, Beri M et al. Differentiation of ischemic from non-ischemic central retinal vein occlusion during the early acute phase. Graefes Arch Clin Exp Ophthalmol 1990; 228:201–217.
17. Green W, Chan C, Hutchins G et al. Central retinal vein occlusions: a prospective histopathologic study of 29 eyes in 28 cases. Retina 1981; 1:27–55.
18. Pe'er J, Folberg R, Itin A et al. Vascular endothelial growth factor upregulation in human central retinal vein occlusion. Ophthalmology 1998; 105: 412–416.
19. Boyd SR, Zachary I, Chakravarthy U et al. Correlation of increased vascular endothelial growth factor with neovascularization and permeability in ischemic central vein occlusion. Arch Ophthalmol 2002; 120:1644–1650.
20. The Eye Disease Case-Control Study Group. Risk factors for central retinal vein occlusion. Arch Ophthalmol 1996; 114:545–554.
21. Elman MJ, Bhatt AK, Quinlan PM et al. The risk for systemic vascular diseases and mortality in patients with central retinal vein occlusion. Ophthalmology 1990; 97:1543–1548.
22. Hayreh SS, Zimmerman B, McCarthy MJ et al. Systemic diseases associated with various types of retinal vein occlusion. Am J Ophthalmol 2001; 131:61–77.
23. Martin SC, Butcher A, Martin N et al. Cardiovascular risk assessment in patients with retinal vein occlusion [comment]. Br J Ophthalmol 2002; 86: 774–776.
24. Lahey JM, Tunc M, Kearney J et al. Laboratory evaluation of hypercoagulable states in patients with central retinal vein occlusion who are less than 56 years of age. Ophthalmology 2002; 109:126–131.
25. Williamson TH, Rumley A, Lowe GD. Blood viscosity, coagulation, and activated protein C resistance in central retinal vein occlusion: a population controlled study. Br J Ophthalmol 1996; 80:203–208.
26. Abu El-Asrar AM, Abdel Gader AG, Al-Amro S et al. Hypercoagulable states in patients with retinal venous occlusion. Doc Ophthalmol 1998; 95:133–143.
27. Hayreh SS, Zimmerman MB, Podhajsky P. Hematologic abnormalities associated with various types of retinal vein occlusion. Graefes Arch Clin Exp Ophthalmol 2002; 240:180–196.
28. Gottlieb JL, Blice JP, Mestichelli B et al. Activated protein C resistance, factor V Leiden, and central retinal vein occlusion in young adults. Arch Ophthalmol 1998; 116:577–579.
29. Hvarfner C, Hillarp A, Larsson J. Influence of factor V Leiden on the development of neovascularisation secondary to central retinal vein occlusion. Br J Ophthalmol 2003; 87:305–306.
30. Cahill MT, Stinnett SS, Fekrat S. Meta-analysis of plasma homocysteine, serum folate, serum vitamin B, and thermolabile MTHFR genotype as risk factors for retinal vascular occlusive disease. Am J Ophthalmol 2003; 136: 1136–1150.
31. Francis PJ, Stanford MR, Graham EM. Dehydration is a risk factor for central retinal vein occlusion in young patients. Acta Ophthalmol Scand 2003; 81:415–416.
32. Rumelt S, Karatas M, Pikkel J et al. Optic disc traction syndrome associated with central retinal vein occlusion. Arch Ophthalmol 2003; 121: 1093–1097.
33. Kearnes TP. Differential diagnosis of central retinal vein obstruction. Ophthalmology 1983; 90:475–480.
34. Lai JC, Mruthyunjaya P, Fekrat S. Central retinal vein occlusion in patients on chronic Coumadin® anticoagulation. Invest Ophthalmol Vis Sci 2002; 42:ARVO E-Abstract 519.
35. Browning DJ, Fraser CM. Retinal vein occlusions in patients taking warfarin. Ophthalmology 2004; 111:1196–1200.
36. De Sanctis MT, Cesarone MR, Belcaro G et al. Treatment of retinal vein thrombosis with pentoxifylline: a controlled, randomized trial. Angiology 2002; 53(Suppl 1):S35–38.
37. Wolf S, Arend O, Bertram B et al. Hemodilution therapy in central retinal vein occlusion. One-year results of a prospective randomized study. Graefes Arch Clin Exp Ophthalmol 1994; 232:33–39.
38. Shaikh S, Blumenkranz MS. Transient improvement in visual acuity and macular edema in central retinal vein occlusion accompanied by inflammatory features after pulse steroid and anti-inflammatory therapy. Retina. 2001; 21:176–178.
39. Fekrat S, de Juan E, Jr. Chorioretinal venous anastomosis for central retinal vein occlusion: transvitreal venipuncture. Ophthal Surg Lasers 1999; 30: 52–55.
40. Fekrat S, Goldberg MF, Finkelstein D. Laser-induced chorioretinal venous anastomosis for nonischemic central or branch retinal vein occlusion [comment]. Arch Ophthalmol 1998; 116:43–52.
41. Browning DJ, Antoszyk AN. Laser chorioretinal venous anastomosis for nonischemic central retinal vein occlusion. Ophthalmology 1998; 105:670–677; discussion 7–9.
42. McAllister IL, Constable IJ. Laser-induced chorioretinal venous anastomosis for treatment of nonischemic central retinal vein occlusion [comment]. Arch Ophthalmol 1995; 113:456–462.
43. McAllister IL, Douglas JP, Constable IJ et al. Laser-induced chorioretinal venous anastomosis for nonischemic central retinal vein occlusion: evaluation of the complications and their risk factors. Am J Ophthalmol 1998; 126:219–229.
44. Browning D, Rotberg M. Vitreous hemorrhage complicating laser-induced chorioretinal anastomosis for central retinal vein occlusion. Am J Ophthalmol 1996; 122:588–589.
45. Kwok AK, Lee VY, Lai TY et al. Laser induced chorioretinal venous anastomosis in ischaemic central retinal vein occlusion. Br J Ophthalmol 2003; 87:1043–1044.
46. Lam HD, Blumenkranz MS. Treatment of central retinal vein occlusion by vitrectomy with lysis of vitreopapillary and epipapillary adhesions, subretinal peripapillary tissue plasminogen activator injection, and photocoagulation. Am J Ophthalmol 2002; 134:609–611.
47. Yeshaya A, Treister G. Pars plana vitrectomy for vitreous hemorrhage and retinal vein occlusion. Ann Ophthalmol 1983; 15:615–617.
48. Opremcak EM, Bruce RA, Lomeo MD et al. Radial optic neurotomy for central retinal vein occlusion: A retrospective pilot study of 11 consecutive cases. Retina 2001; 21:408–415.
49. Dev S, Buckley EG. Optic nerve sheath decompression for progressive central retinal vein occlusion. Ophthal Surg Lasers 1999; 30:181–184.
50. Vasco-Posada J. Modification of the circulation in the posterior pole of the eye. Ann Ophthalmol 1972; 4:48–59.
51. Weizer JS, Stinnett SS, Fekrat S. Radial optic neurotomy as treatment for central retinal vein occlusion. Am J Ophthalmol 2003; 136:814–819.

52. Garcia-Arumi J, Boixadera A, Martinez-Castillo V et al. Chorioretinal anastomosis after radial optic neurotomy for central retinal vein occlusion. Arch Ophthalmol 2003; 121:1385–1391.

53. Williamson TH, Poon W, Whitefield L et al. A pilot study of pars plana vitrectomy, intraocular gas, and radial neurotomy in ischaemic central retinal vein occlusion. Br J Ophthalmol 2003; 87:1126–1129.

54. Hattenbach LO, Steinkamp G, Scharrer I et al. Fibrinolytic therapy with low-dose recombinant tissue plasminogen activator in retinal vein occlusion. Ophthalmologica 1998; 212:394–398.

55. Hattenbach LO, Wellermann G, Steinkamp GW et al. Visual outcome after treatment with low-dose recombinant tissue plasminogen activator or hemodilution in ischemic central retinal vein occlusion. Ophthalmologica 1999; 213:360–366.

56. Lahey JM, Fong DS, Kearney J. Intravitreal tissue plasminogen activator for acute central retinal vein occlusion. Ophthal Surg Lasers 1999; 30:427–434.

57. Glacet-Bernard A, Kuhn D, Vine AK et al. Treatment of recent onset central retinal vein occlusion with intravitreal tissue plasminogen activator: a pilot study. Br J Ophthalmol 2000; 84:609–613.

58. Elman MJ, Raden RZ, Carrigan A. Intravitreal injection of tissue plasminogen activator for central retinal vein occlusion. Trans Am Ophthalmol Soc 2001; 99:219–221; discussion 22–23.

59. Ghazi NG, Noureddine BN, Haddad RS et al. Intravitreal tissue plasminogen activator in the management of central retinal vein occlusion. Retina 2003; 23:780–784.

60. Weiss JN. Treatment of central retinal vein occlusion by injection of tissue plasminogen activator into a retinal vein. Am J Ophthalmol 1998; 126: 142–144.

61. Paques M, Vallee JN, Herbreteau D et al. Superselective ophthalmic artery fibrinolytic therapy for the treatment of central retinal vein occlusion. Br J Ophthalmol 2000; 84:1387–1391.

62. Weiss JN, Bynoe LA. Injection of tissue plasminogen activator into a branch retinal vein in eyes with central retinal vein occlusion. Ophthalmology 2001; 108:2249–2257.

63. Bynoe LA, Weiss JN. Retinal endovascular surgery and intravitreal triamcinolone acetonide for central vein occlusion in young adults. Am J Ophthalmol 2003; 135:382–384.

64. Jonas JB, Kreissig I, Degenring RF. Intravitreal triamcinolone acetonide as treatment of macular edema in central retinal vein occlusion. Graef Arch Clin Exp Ophthalmol 2002; 240:782–783.

65. Ip MS, Kumar KS. Intravitreous triamcinolone acetonide as treatment for macular edema from central retinal vein occlusion. Arch Ophthalmol 2002; 120:1217–1219.

66. Greenberg PB, Martidis A, Rogers AH et al. Intravitreal triamcinolone acetonide for macular oedema due to central retinal vein occlusion. Br J Ophthalmol 2002; 86:247–248.

67. Park CH, Jaffe GJ, Fekrat S. Intravitreal triamcinolone acetonide in eyes with cystoid macular edema associated with central retinal vein occlusion. Am J Ophthalmol 2003; 136:419–425.

Branch Retinal Vein Occlusion

Stephen Phillips
Sharon Fekrat
Daniel Finkelstein

Branch retinal vein occlusion (BRVO) is a common cause of retinal vascular disease.[1] It affects males and females equally and occurs most frequently between the ages of 60 and 70. The interruption of venous flow in these eyes almost always occurs at a retinal arteriovenous intersection, where a retinal artery crosses a retinal vein.[2] However, a BRVO may rarely occur at a site other than at an arteriovenous crossing in eyes with ocular inflammatory disease. The most common risk factors associated with BRVO are systemic hypertension, diabetes, hyperlipidemia, glaucoma, smoking and age-related atherosclerosis.[3] Antiphospholipid antibodies, elevated plasma homocysteine levels, and low serum folate levels have also been associated with increased risk of vein occlusion.[4-6] A decreased risk is present in those with higher serum levels of high density lipoprotein (HDL) and greater alcohol consumption.[3] Other studies have suggested an increased risk of BRVO in eyes with shorter axial lengths.[7-10]

CLINICAL FEATURES

Branch retinal vein occlusion is almost always of sudden onset. The patient presents with blurred vision or a field defect and segmentally distributed intraretinal hemorrhage. Generally, intraretinal hemorrhage is less marked if the occlusion is perfused or nonischemic and is much more marked if the occlusion is nonperfused or ischemic and associated with retinal capillary nonperfusion.

The location of the venous block determines the distribution of the intraretinal hemorrhage; if the venous obstruction is at the optic nerve head, two quadrants of the fundus may be involved, whereas if the occlusion is peripheral to the disc, one quadrant or less may be involved with the intraretinal hemorrhage. If the venous blockage is peripheral to tributary veins draining the macula, there may be no macular involvement and no decrease in visual acuity. Fig. 71-1 demonstrates the typical acute appearance of a BRVO involving the superotemporal quadrant of the right eye; the macula is involved, and visual acuity has been reduced to 20/100. Rarely, a patient initially may present with very little intraretinal hemorrhage, which then becomes more extensive in succeeding weeks to months. In these instances, it is presumed that an incomplete block at the arteriovenous crossing has progressed to more complete occlusion.

One year or more after a BRVO has occurred, the intraretinal hemorrhage may have completely reabsorbed. Without the charac-

teristic segmental distribution of intraretinal hemorrhage, the ophthalmoscopic diagnosis may be more difficult, but the segmental distribution of retinal vascular abnormalities that occurred during the acute phase will persist and be apparent on fluorescein angiography. Consequently, in the chronic phase of the disease, after the intraretinal hemorrhage has been absorbed, the diagnosis may depend on noting a segmental distribution of retinal vascular abnormalities that may include capillary nonperfusion, dilation of capillaries, microaneurysms, and collateral vessel formation.

PATHOGENESIS

Because BRVO almost occurs at arteriovenous crossings,[2,11,12] underlying arterial disease may play a causative role. In 99% of 106 eyes with BRVO, the artery was located anterior to the vein at the obstructed site.[2] Histopathologically, the retinal artery and vein share a common adventitial sheath, and in some cases, a common medium.[13] The lumen of the vein may be compressed up to 33% at the crossing site.[14,15] The vitreous may also play a role in compression of susceptible arteriovenous crossing sites as evidenced by studies demonstrating that eyes with decreased axial length and higher likelihood of vitreomacular attachment at the arteriovenous crossing are at increased risk of BRVO.[16,17]

Some have postulated that turbulent blood flow at the crossing site causes focal swelling of the endothelium and deeper vein wall tissue leading to venous obstruction.[13,17,18] Other reports have demonstrated actual venous thrombus formation at the point of occlusion.[15,19]

The resulting venous obstruction leads to elevation of venous pressure that may overload the collateral drainage capacity[20] and lead to macular edema and ischemia by mechanisms that are still under investigation. Unrelieved venous pressure can also result in rupture of the vein wall with intraretinal hemorrhage.[13]

MEDICAL TREATMENT

Anticoagulant therapy has not been shown to be beneficial in either the prevention or the management of BRVO. Since the systemic administration of anticoagulants can be associated with systemic complications, and since anticoagulants could, in theory, increase the severity of intraretinal hemorrhage occurring in the acute

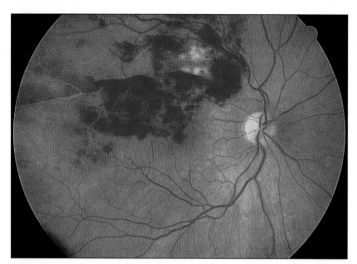

Fig. 71-1 Fundus photograph of acute, superotemporal branch vein occlusion demonstrating the segmental pattern of intraretinal hemorrhage. Hemorrhage also is present in the foveal center.

phase, such therapy is not recommended. Treatment of BRVO has focused on management of vision-limiting complications.

VISION-LIMITING COMPLICATIONS

There are three common vision-limiting complications of branch vein occlusion: macular edema, macular nonperfusion, and vitreous hemorrhage from neovascularization. It is important to appreciate the variability of these complications before considering the benefits of treatment.[21–24]

Neovascularization and vitreous hemorrhage

The Branch Vein Occlusion Study demonstrated that prophylactic scatter laser photocoagulation can lessen subsequent neovascularization and, if neovascularization already exists, that peripheral scatter laser photocoagulation can lessen subsequent vitreous hemorrhage.[1] Only eyes with the type of branch vein occlusion that shows large areas (greater than five disc diameters in diameter) of retinal capillary nonperfusion are at risk for developing neovascularization. About 40% of these eyes develop neovascularization, and of this 40%, about 60% will experience periodic vitreous hemorrhage. Retinal or disc neovascularization, or both, may develop at any time within the first 3 years after an occlusion but are most likely to appear within the first 6 to 12 months after the occlusion. If peripheral scatter laser photocoagulation is applied in eyes with large areas of nonperfusion, the incidence of neovascularization can be reduced from about 40% to 20%. However, if one were to treat prophylactically, many eyes (60%) that would never develop neovascularization would receive peripheral scatter laser photocoagulation. For this reason, it is recommended that laser photocoagulation be applied only after neovascularization is documented.

Iris neovascularization is a rare complication of BRVO; it appears, however, that diabetes (with or without retinopathy) may increase this risk. Retinal neovascularization is particularly difficult to recognize in BRVO because the collaterals that develop frequently

may mimic neovascularization. Arising presumably from pre-existing capillaries, these collaterals occur as vein-to-vein channels around the blockage site, across the temporal raphe, and in other locations to bypass the blocked retinal segment. These collaterals frequently become quite tortuous, mimicking the appearance of neovascularization if they are evaluated by ophthalmoscopy alone. When it is unclear whether an abnormal vascular pattern represents collateral formation or true neovascularization, the fluorescein angiogram (Fig. 71-2) can be helpful because leakage from neovascularization is more prominent than from collateral vessels.

The Branch Vein Occlusion Study data strongly suggest that photocoagulation after the development of neovascularization is as effective in preventing vitreous hemorrhage as is photocoagulation before the development of neovascularization.[1] When neovascularization is unequivocally confirmed by fluorescein angiography, peripheral scatter laser photocoagulation can reduce from about 60% to 30% the likelihood of vitreous hemorrhage. The scatter laser photocoagulation is applied, as demonstrated in Fig. 71-3, with argon blue-green laser photocoagulation applied to achieve "medium" white burns (200 to 500 microns in diameter) spaced one burn width apart and covering the entire area of capillary nonperfusion, as defined by fluorescein angiography, but extending no closer than two disc diameters from the center of the fovea and extending peripherally at least to the equator. Retrobulbar anesthesia is used as needed for discomfort associated with the scatter photocoagulation.

Of patients who develop neovascularization, approximately 60% experience episodes of vitreous hemorrhage if the condition is left untreated. The short- and long-term visual consequences of vitreous hemorrhage in BRVO have not been carefully studied. In some cases, the hemorrhage may be mild or may clear spontaneously without causing permanent visual impairment. However, in some patients, vitreous hemorrhage from neovascularization

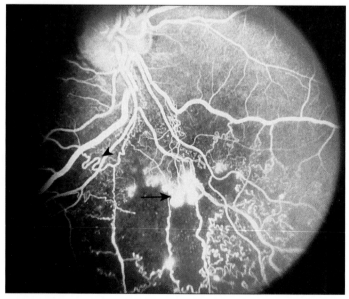

Fig. 71-2 Fluorescein angiogram demonstrating retinal neovascularization with leakage (arrow) to differentiate from collaterals that are not leaking (arrowhead).

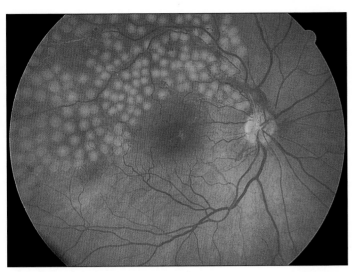

Fig. 71-3 Immediate post-treatment fundus photograph showing pattern of peripheral scatter photocoagulation.

can lead to prolonged visual disability in the affected eye. When the hemorrhage is dense, B-scan ultrasonography may help rule out an associated traction retinal detachment. Most eyes can be observed. If the vitreous hemorrhage does not spontaneously clear in a few months, a pars plana vitrectomy with sector endolaser photocoagulation should be considered.

Macular edema

In the acute phase (i.e. the first 3 to 6 months) after a branch vein occlusion, there is often extensive intraretinal hemorrhage that may involve the macula and the foveal center. Under these circumstances it is impossible to evaluate the vascular perfusion status by fluorescein angiography because the hemorrhage itself blocks the view of the retinal vessels. Additionally, hemorrhage in the foveal center may reduce visual acuity; visual acuity that is reduced by hemorrhage may recover completely if there is no other cause for the visual loss, such as macular edema or macular capillary nonperfusion. Thus, in the acute phase of the disease, when there is substantial intraretinal hemorrhage, it may be impossible to evaluate potential vision; under these circumstances, the

patient should be followed every 2 to 3 months until there is sufficient clearing of hemorrhage to allow evaluation by fluorescein angiography. Although it may be difficult to provide a prognosis in the acute phase, it is helpful to recognize that about one third to one half of patients with BRVO have a return of vision to 20/40 or better without therapy.

After the acute phase of the BRVO has passed and intraretinal hemorrhage has mostly reabsorbed, which usually takes 3 to 6 months, fluorescein angiography should be obtained to delineate the retinal vascular characteristics that may have prognostic significance: macular edema, macular nonperfusion, and large segments of capillary nonperfusion that may portend eventual neovascularization. Fluorescein angiography is the only technique that will accurately define the capillary abnormalities in BRVO; it is therefore particularly important that high-quality angiography be obtained (Fig. 71-4, A and B). When fluorescein angiography demonstrates macular edema with cystoid involvement of the fovea, but no capillary nonperfusion, it is presumed that the macular edema is the cause of vision loss. Under these circumstances, about one third of patients will spontaneously regain some vision. However, patients who have had decreased vision for over 1 year as a result of macular edema are much less likely to regain vision spontaneously. When macular edema is present ophthalmoscopically within the first 6 months after a BRVO and there is little or no leakage on fluorescein angiography, macular ischemia may be the cause of the macular edema. In such circumstances, the edema almost always spontaneously resorbs in the first year after the occlusion, often with return of vision.[25]

While contact lens biomicroscopy remains a useful tool for qualitative identification of macular edema, recent widespread availability of optical coherence tomography imaging has made it possible to acquire a quantitative measure of macular edema and change in macular edema over time and after treatment.

Grid-pattern laser photocoagulation

The Collaborative Branch Vein Occlusion Study,[26] a multicenter randomized clinical trial supported by the National Eye Institute, reported that argon laser photocoagulation may reduce visual loss from macular edema for those eyes that meet study eligibility criteria and are treated according to that protocol. Important

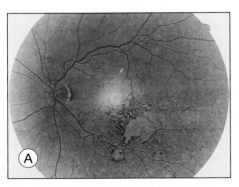
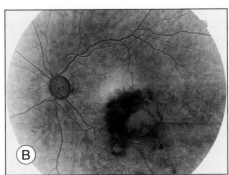
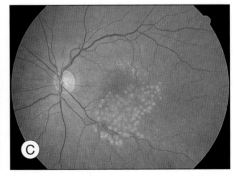

Fig. 71-4 A, Fluorescein angiogram, transit phase, demonstrating perifoveal capillary dilation with adjacent capillary nonperfusion. B, Fluorescein angiogram, late phase, demonstrating cystoid edema with foveal involvement (same case as A). C, Immediate posttreatment fundus photograph showing grid pattern of laser photocoagulation (same case as A).

eligibility criteria included fluorescein-proven perfused macular edema involving the foveal center, absorption of intraretinal hemorrhage from the foveal center, recent branch retinal vein occlusion (usually 3 to 18 months' duration), no diabetic retinopathy, and vision reduced to 20/40 or worse after best refraction.

In the Collaborative Branch Vein Occlusion Study,[26] argon laser photocoagulation was applied in a grid pattern throughout the leaking area demonstrated by fluorescein angiography (Fig. 71-4, B and C). Coagulation extended no closer to the fovea than the edge of the capillary-free zone and no farther into the periphery than the major vascular arcade. Recommended treatment parameters included a duration of 0.1 second, a 100 micron diameter spot size, and a power setting sufficient to produce a "medium" white burn. Fluorescein angiography was repeated 2 to 4 months after the treatment, and additional photocoagulation was applied to residual areas of leakage if reduced visual acuity persisted. Improvement in visual acuity was assessed in several ways.[26] When improvement was defined as reading two or more Snellen lines (beyond baseline) at two consecutive visits, treated eyes showed visual improvement more often than untreated eyes. After 3 years of follow-up, 63% of treated eyes gained two or more lines of vision, compared to 36% of untreated eyes. The average gain in visual acuity for treated eyes was one more Snellen line than in untreated eyes.

Before laser photocoagulation is performed, it is important to obtain high-quality fluorescein angiograms of the macula; the fluorescein angiogram must demonstrate that the macular edema involves the center of the fovea and that there is not a large amount of capillary nonperfusion adjacent to the capillary-free zone that could explain the visual loss. In addition, it is important to follow patients for a length of time sufficient to ascertain that macular edema is not resolving spontaneously. During this period of follow-up, it should be demonstrated that there is clearing of intraretinal hemorrhage and that there is no hemorrhage in the center of the fovea that could account for a spontaneously reversible cause of visual loss. In the application of the grid photocoagulation, laser absorption occurs at the level of the pigment epithelium; photocoagulation is not applied to directly and immediately close the leaking and dilated capillary vasculature. Although it is not understood how the laser treatment may act in lessening edema, it is interesting to note that preliminary experimental studies in the normal primate have shown a decrease in capillary diameter when this form of therapy is used and when laser absorption occurs at the level of the pigment epithelium.[27] One explanation for the effect of grid-pattern photocoagulation is that it produces a thinning of the retina so that the choroidal vasculature supplies some of the inner retinal needs, producing a consequent autoregulatory constriction of the retinal vasculature in the leaking area and thereby decreasing the edema.

In the application of grid-pattern laser photocoagulation, it is crucial to obtain good definition of landmarks so that the center of the fovea can be identified and avoided. Since landmarks frequently may be obscured in the macula after BRVO, such cases can be managed more effectively and safely by treating well peripheral to the capillary-free zone in the first sitting. When the patient returns in 2 months for follow-up evaluation, a fluorescein angiogram may identify more clearly the amount of further treatment that needs to be applied closer to the edge of the capillary-free zone, because the pigmentation of the previous treatment is then visible. Consequently, treatment in this next sitting may be brought closer to the edge of the capillary-free zone, if that is deemed necessary because of continued edema with foveal involvement and continued visual loss. The placement of grid laser treatment in this repetitively staged fashion may be safer and appears to be just as effective as a single treatment. It has never been established that macular edema must be treated quickly or that long-standing edema produces irreversible macular damage in the first 2 to 3 years.

For the grid treatment used in the Collaborative Branch Vein Occlusion Study, the argon blue-green wavelength was employed.[26] This is the only wavelength that has been proved effective; it is not known whether argon green or krypton red photocoagulation would be as effective. In other diseases when laser treatment is applied inside the capillary-free zone, it is recognized that krypton red and argon green laser photocoagulation are absorbed less than blue-green by the xanthophyll pigment of the inner retina that is present close to the foveal center. However, because the grid treatment never comes closer to the fovea than the capillary-free zone, the Branch Vein Occlusion Study did not encounter any problems with the argon blue-green laser in this region; consequently, this laser continues to be recommended.

The summary recommendations for management of acute branch vein occlusion from the Branch Vein Occlusion Study emphasize waiting at least 3 to 6 months before considering laser therapy.[2] If the vision is reduced to 20/40 or worse, wait 3 to 6 months for sufficient clearing of retinal hemorrhage to permit high-quality fluorescein angiography and then evaluate fluorescein angiography for macular edema and macular nonperfusion. If perfused macular edema accounts for the visual loss, and vision continues to be 20/40 or worse without spontaneous improvement, consider grid macular photocoagulation. If macular nonperfusion accounts for the visual loss, no laser treatment is recommended to improve vision.

Photocoagulation considerations

Familiarity with the laser treatment technique is required to individualize the treatment. Important variables, such as residual intraretinal hemorrhage, thickness of the retina from edema, location of collaterals, and presence of retinal traction influence the exact mode of therapy within the above general treatment guidelines for the management of macular edema and neovascularization. There are numerous complications of laser photocoagulation; however, it is generally recognized that with proper attention to detail, complications are infrequent. Side effects of treatment, including scotoma production, merit careful consideration and discussion with the patient before initiation of treatment. It is particularly important to recognize that laser photocoagulation should never be placed over extensive intraretinal hemorrhage in the acute phase of branch vein occlusion because the laser energy will be absorbed by the intraretinal hemorrhage rather than at the level of the pigment epithelium, probably damaging the nerve fiber layer and possibly producing preretinal fibrosis.

Vitrectomy – with and without sheathotomy

The majority of the venous lesions in BRVO occur downstream from the A-V crossing site. In a retrospective review of color photographs and fluorescein angiograms of patients with BRVO, Kumar and associates identified venous narrowing at the crossing site, and in the majority of cases, evidence of downstream hemodynamic changes on angiogram including venous phase leakage, abnormal flow, and presumed thrombi. The authors also suggested that removal of the compressive factor by sectioning the adventitial sheath (sheathotomy) may be an effective treatment for BRVO. In the first report of sheathotomy for BRVO, Osterloh and Charles[29] reported significant visual improvement in the one case presented (20/200 to 20/25+ over 8 months). In the second report, Opremcak and Bruce[30] reported equal or improved visual acuity in 12 of 15 patients (80%). Ten of those patients (67%) had improved postoperative visual acuities, with an average gain of four lines of vision. Three patients had a decline in visual acuity, with an average of two lines of vision lost. All patients had marked resolution of the intraretinal hemorrhage and edema. Visual symptoms from BRVO ranged from 1 to 12 months, with an average of 3.3 months. In two patients, intraoperative retinal vascular bleeding was controlled with intraocular diathermy. No patient in their series developed worsening edema, ischemia, retinal neovascularization, or secondary vitreous hemorrhage. Mester and colleagues reported 43 cases of BRVO treated with sheathotomy with similar results. In 16 of the cases, removal of the internal limiting membrane in the area of the arteriovenous crossing was also performed.[31] In contrast, Cahill and colleagues reported 27 cases of BRVO treated with vitrectomy and sheathotomy without a statistically significant improvement in postoperative median visual acuity.[32]

Other authors have experienced difficulty in separating the artery from the vein at the crossing site. Han and colleagues reported 20 cases of vitrectomy and attempted sheathotomy. While the visual outcome results were similar to those reported by Opremcak, in 19 of the 20 cases, the authors were unable to separate the artery from the vein.[33] No randomized, controlled study evaluating the benefit of sheathotomy has been published.[34]

There is evidence that vitreomacular attachment itself may contribute to the development of macular edema in BRVO.[35] In a study of seven patients with macular edema from BRVO, Kurimoto and coworkers found that vitrectomy with separation of the posterior hyaloid resulted in reduced macular edema in all eyes as measured by retinal thickness analysis. Six of the seven eyes had improved visual acuity at 3 months follow-up.[36] Saika and coworkers reported similar results, with reduction in macular edema and restoration of normal foveal contour in 10 of 19 eyes after vitrectomy, posterior hyaloid separation and intraocular gas tamponade.[37] Possible explanations for the clinical improvements in these studies include removal of vitreous traction, increased oxygenation of the macula, and tamponade of the macula by intraocular gas.

Intraocular corticosteroids

A recent addition to the options for treatment of macular edema has been intraocular injection of corticosteroids. The exact mechanism of macular edema development from BRVO has not been elucidated, but breakdown of the blood–retinal barrier is thought to play a role. Triamcinolone acetonide, a corticosteroid suspension, has been shown experimentally to reduce breakdown of the blood–retinal barrier when injected intravitreally.[38] Animal studies have shown intravitreal injection of triamcinolone to be nontoxic and to maintain a depot lasting 16 to 41 days. The depot is maintained longer in eyes not having undergone vitrectomy.[39–41] A human pharmacokinetics study of nonvitrectomized eyes found a single 4 mg injection of triamcinolone to have a mean elimination half-life of 18.6 days with measurable concentrations expected to last approximately 3 months.[42]

Studies of intravitreal triamcinolone treatment of macular edema in diabetes and CRVO have set a precedence for this corticosteroid's potential benefit in treating edema from BRVO. In a study by Martidis and colleagues of 16 eyes with diabetic macular edema refractory to laser treatment, the authors reported an average decrease in central macular thickness measured by OCT after intravitreal injection of triamcinolone acetonide.[43]

In a study of 10 eyes with cystoid macular edema from CRVO, Park and coworkers reported clinical improvement in macular edema in all 10 eyes, a statistically significant improvement in mean visual acuity, and improvement in mean macular volume on OCT.[44] Greenberg (one case), and Ip (two cases) had previously reported improvement in acuity and edema on OCT after intravitreal injection of triamcinolone in patients with edema from CRVO.[45,46] Injection of corticosteroids carries with it the risk of accelerated cataract development, the risk of elevated intraocular pressure, and the risk of endophthalmitis, sterile or infectious. The rate and extent of these complications are not yet clear. All studies of intravitreal triamcinolone as treatment for macular edema have relatively short follow-up.[44–46] Anecdotal reports of the return of edema after the initial response to therapy, particularly in cases involving BRVO, has tempered enthusiasm for this treatment. A multicenter, randomized, Phase 3 trial sponsored by the National Eye Institute is currently underway to assess the efficacy and safety of standard care versus intravitreal triamcinolone acetonide injection for treatment of macular edema associated with central retinal vein occlusion or branch retinal vein occlusion. Because of the limited duration of effect of intravitreal injection, human trials studying the safety and efficacy of sustained-release corticosteroids in the treatment of macular edema from BRVO are currently underway.

REFERENCES

1. Branch Vein Occlusion Study Group. Argon laser scatter photocoagulation for prevention of neovascularization and vitreous hemorrhage in branch vein occlusion, Arch Ophthalmol 1986; 104:34–41.
2. Zhao J, Sastry, SM, Sperduto, RD et al. Arteriovenous crossing patterns in branch retinal vein occlusion: The Eye Disease Case–Control Study Group. Ophthalmology 1993; 100:423–428.
3. Eye Disease Case–Control Study Group. Risk factors for branch retinal vein occlusion. Am J Ophthalmol 1993; 116:286–296.
4. Lahey JM, Tunc M, Kearney J et al. Laboratory evaluation of hypercoagulable states in patients with central retinal vein occlusion who are less than 56 years of age. Ophthalmology 2002; 109:126–131.
5. Lahey JM, Kearney JJ, Tunc M. Hypercoagulable states and central retinal vein occlusion. Curr Opin Pulm Med 2003; 9:385–392.

6. Cahill MT, Stinnett SS, Fekrat S. Meta-analysis of plasma homocysteine, serum folate, serum vitamin B$_{12}$, and thermolabile MTHFR genotype as risk factors for retinal vascular occlusive disease. Am J Ophthalmol 2003; 136:1136–1150.

7. Ariturk N, Oge Y, Erkan D et al. Relation between retinal vein occlusions and axial length. Br J Ophthalmol 1996; 80:633–636.

8. Majji AB, Janarthanan M, Naduvilath TJ. Significance of refractive status in branch retinal vein occlusion: a case–control study. Retina 1997; 17:200–204.

9. Simons BD, Brucker AJ. Branch retinal vein occlusion: axial length and other risk factors. Retina 1997; 17:191–195.

10. Timmerman EA, de Lavalette VW, van den Brom HJ. Axial length as a risk factor to branch retinal vein occlusion. Retina 1997; 17:196–199.

11. Weinberg D, Dodwell DG, Fern SA. Anatomy of arteriovenous crossings in branch retinal vein occlusion. Am J Ophthalmol 1990; 109:298–302.

12. Duker JS, Brown GC. Anterior location of the crossing artery in branch retinal vein occlusion. Arch Ophthalmol 1989; 107:998–1000.

13. Seitz R. The retinal vessels. St Louis: CV Mosby; 20–74: 1964.

14. Frangieh GT, Green WR, Barraquer-Somers E. Histopathological study of nine branch retinal vein occlusions. Arch Ophthalmol 1982; 100:1132–1140.

15. Bandello F, Tavola A, Pierro L et al. Axial length and refraction in retinal vein occlusions. Ophthalmologica 1998; 212:133–135.

16. Majii AB, Janarthnan M, Naduvilath TJ. Significance of refractive status in branch retinal vein occlusion: a case–control study. Retina 1997; 17:200–204.

17. Kumar B, Yu DY, Morgan WH et al. The distribution of angioarchitectural changes within the vicinity of the arteriovenous crossing in branch retinal vein occlusion. Ophthalmology 1998; 105:424–427.

18. Clemett RS. Retinal branch vein occlusion: changes at the site of obstruction. Br J Ophthalmol 1974; 58:548–554.

19. Bowers DK, Finkelstein D, Wolff SM et al. Branch retinal vein occlusion: a clinicopathological case report. Retina 1987; 7:252–259.

20. Christoffersen NLB, Larsen M. Pathophysiology and hemodynamics of branch retinal vein occlusion. Ophthalmology 1999; 106:2054–2062.

21. Finkelstein D, Clarkson JG and The Branch Vein Occlusion Study Group. Branch and central retinal vein occlusions. Focal points 1987: Clinical modules for ophthalmologists 5 (module 12), no 3. American Academy of Ophthalmology.

22. Gutman FA, Zegarra H. Macular edema secondary to occlusion of the retinal veins. Surv Ophthalmol 1984; 28:462–470.

23. Hayreh SS, Rojas P, Podhajsky P et al. Ocular neovascularization with retinal vascular occlusion. III. Incidence of ocular neovascularization with retinal vein occlusion. Ophthalmology 1983; 90:488–506.

24. Joffe L, Goldberg RE, Magargal LE et al. Macular branch vein occlusion, Ophthalmology 1980; 87:91–98.

25. Finkelstein D. Ischemic macular edema: recognition and favorable natural history in branch vein occlusion. Arch Ophthalmol 1992; 110:1427–1434.

26. Branch Vein Occlusion Study Group. Argon laser photocoagulation for macular edema in branch vein occlusion. Am J Ophthalmol 1984; 98:271–282.

27. Wilson DJ, Finkelstein D, Quigley HA et al. Macular grid photocoagulation: an experimental study on the primate retina. Arch Ophthalmol 1988; 106:100–105.

28. Kumar B, Yu DY, Morgan WH et al. The distribution of angioarchitectural changes within the vicinity of the arteriovenous crossing in branch retinal vein occlusion. Ophthalmology 1998; 105:424–427.

29. Osterloh MD, Charles S. Surgical decompression of branch retinal vein occlusions. Arch Ophthalmol 1988; 106:1469–1471.

30. Opremcak EM, Bruce RA. Surgical decompression of branch retinal vein occlusion via arteriovenous crossing sheathotomy: a prospective review of 15 cases. Retina 1999; 19:1–5.

31. Mester U, Dillinger P. Vitrectomy with arteriovenous decompression and internal limiting membrane dissection in branch retinal vein occlusion. Retina 2002; 22:740–746.

32. Cahill MT, Kaiser PK, Sears JE et al. The effect of arteriovenous sheathotomy on cystoid macular oedema secondary to branch retinal vein occlusion. Br J Ophthalmol 2003; 87:1329–1332.

33. Han DP, Bennett SR, Williams DF et al. Arteriovenous crossing dissection without separation of the retina vessels for treatment of branch retinal vein occlusion. Retina 2003; 23:145–151.

34. Cahill MT, Fekrat S. Arteriovenous sheathotomy for branch retinal vein occlusion. Ophthalmol Clin N Am 2002; 15:417–423.

35. Takahashi M, Hikichi T, Akiba J et al. Role of the vitreous and macular edema in branch retinal vein occlusion. Ophthalmic Surg Lasers 1997; 28:294–299.

36. Kurimoto M, Takagi H, Suzuma K et al. Vitrectomy for macular edema secondary to retinal vein occlusion: evaluation by retinal thickness analyzer. Jpn J Clin Ophthalmol 1999; 53:717–720.

37. Saika S, Tanaka T, Miyamoto T et al. Surgical posterior vitreous detachment combined with gas/air tamponade for treating macular edema associated with branch retinal vein occlusion: retinal tomography and visual outcome. Graefes Arch Clin Exp Ophthalmol 2001; 239:729–732.

38. Wilson CA, Berkowitz BA, Sato Y et al. Treatment with intravitreal steroid reduces blood–retinal barrier breakdown due to retinal photocoagulation. Arch Ophthalmol 1992; 110:1155–1159.

39. McCuen BW, Bessler M, Tano Y et al. The lack of toxicity of intravitreally administered triamcinolone acetonide. Am J Ophthalmol 1981; 91: 785–788.

40. Hida T, Chandler D, Arena J et al. Experimental and clinical observations of the intraocular toxicity of commercial corticosteroid preparations. Am J Ophthalmol 1986; 101:190–195.

41. Schindler R, Chandler D, Thresher R et al. The clearance of intravitreal triamcinolone acetonide. Am J Ophthalmol 1982; 93: 415–417.

42. Beer PM, Bakri SJ, Singh RJ et al. Intraocular concentration and pharmacokinetics of triamcinolone acetonide after a single intravitreal injection. Ophthalmology 2003; 110:681–686.

43. Martidis A, Duker JS, Greenberg P et al. Intravitreal triamcinolone for refractory diabetic macular edema. Ophthalmology 2002; 109:920–927.

44. Park CH, Jaffe GJ, Fekrat S. Intravitreal triamcinolone acetonide in eyes with cystoid macular edema associated with central retinal vein occlusion. Am J Ophthalmol 2003; 136:419–425.

45. Greenberg PB, Martidis A, Rogers AH et al. Intravitreal triamcinolone acetonide for macular oedema due to central retinal vein occlusion. Br J Ophthalmol 2002; 86:247–248.

46. Ip MS, Kumar KS. Intravitreous triamcinolone acetonide as treatment for macular edema from central retinal vein occlusion. Arch Ophthalmol 2002; 120:1217–1219.

Chapter

72

Pregnancy and Retinal Disease

Justin C. Brown
Janet S. Sunness

Pregnancy is associated with maternal hormonal, metabolic, hematologic, cardiovascular, and immunologic alterations that can affect the ocular tissues. No significant retinal changes occur in most normal pregnancies. However, pregnancy can be associated with the development of new ocular conditions such as serous retinal detachment related to pre-eclampsia, or with an exacerbation of pre-existing disease processes such as diabetic retinopathy. These ocular changes are usually transient, but can cause permanent visual disability. This chapter presents current state of knowledge about the relationship between pregnancy and maternal retinal and choroidal disorders. It also includes a brief summary of some considerations regarding diagnostic testing during pregnancy.

RETINAL AND CHOROIDAL DISORDERS ARISING IN PREGNANCY

Pre-eclampsia and eclampsia

Pre-eclampsia typically develops in the second half of pregnancy and is characterized by hypertension, edema, and proteinuria. Eclampsia is pre-eclampsia with convulsions that usually occurs late in pregnancy.

In healthy women pre-eclampsia is generally seen in first pregnancies with an incidence estimated at 5%. Risk factors for pre-eclampsia include very young or advanced maternal age, multi-fetal pregnancy, hemolytic disease of the newborn, diabetes mellitus, chronic systemic hypertension, and renal disease.

Pre-eclampsia and eclampsia place the fetus at risk due to placental vascular insufficiency. In the first half of the twentieth century, severe changes in retinal arteriolar caliber were believed to reflect placental vascular insufficiency and be an indication for pregnancy termination. Therefore, a great deal of attention was paid to retinal findings in pre-eclampsia. With improved medical and obstetrical management of hypertension and other aspects of pre-eclampsia, retinal findings are no longer used to assess this disease. In addition, retinal changes in pre-eclampsia may be significantly less frequent than they were in the past.

Early reports gave an impressive rate of visual disturbances. Scotoma, diplopia, dimness of vision, and photopsias were noted in 25% of patients with severe pre-eclampsia and up to 50% of patients with eclampsia.[1] Recent studies, discussed below, suggest that the rate of visual disturbance has decreased markedly with improved medical management of pre-eclampsia. Although photic stimuli may predispose to seizures in susceptible patients, the benefits of an ophthalmoscopic examination outweigh the small risk of seizure when an examination is indicated.[2]

Pre-eclampsia and eclampsia have been associated with a retinopathy similar to hypertensive retinopathy; serous retinal detachments; yellow, opaque retinal pigment epithelium (RPE) lesions; and cortical blindness. Arterial and venous occlusive disease can also occur and may contribute to visual loss. Early studies of retinal disorders in pre-eclampsia have been discussed in previous reviews.[3]

Retinopathy in pre-eclampsia and eclampsia

Focal or generalized retinal arteriolar narrowing is the most common ocular change seen in pre-eclampsia, but its frequency is declining. Early studies reported arteriolar attenuation in 40% to 100% of pre-eclamptic patients.[4] Recently, a retrospective study of fluorescein angiograms in pre-eclamptic patients by Schreyer identified normal retinal vessel caliber in 16 of 16 patients. In contrast, four of 14 patients with pre-existing chronic systemic hypertension had retinal vascular changes.[5] Jaffe prospectively demonstrated a statistically significant difference in arteriolar caliber between 56 study participants with severe pre-eclampsia and 25 healthy controls but no difference between 17 patients with mild pre-eclampsia and controls.[6] These studies suggest that arteriolar narrowing may be more common in pregnant patients with chronic pre-existing hypertension than those with mild pre-eclampsia. The difference in the reported prevalence of retinopathy between the early and recent literature is probably related to better medical management of pre-eclampsia and its complications.

The cause of retinal arteriolar narrowing seems to be central retinal artery vasospasm suggested by increased central retinal artery blood flow velocity.[7] When present, the retinal arteriolar attenuation associated with pre-eclampsia generally resolves after delivery, presumably due to normalization of central retinal artery blood flow. Other typical hypertensive retinopathy changes such as hemorrhages, cotton-wool spots, lipid deposits, diffuse retinal edema, and papilledema are generally not seen in pre-eclampsia[6] and should raise suspicion about additional concurrent systemic disease.

Choroidopathy in pre-eclampsia and eclampsia

Choroidal dysfunction is a common ocular complication of pre-eclampsia and eclampsia that manifests clinically as serous retinal detachments or yellow RPE lesions. The serous retinal detachments usually are bilateral and bullous but occasionally are cystic.[2,10] In the early twentieth century, serous retinal detachments were seen in 1% of severely pre-eclamptic patients and about 10% of eclamptic patients.[8–9] More recently, Saito retrospectively evaluated 31 women with severe pre-eclampsia or eclampsia and found that 40/62 (65%) eyes had serous retinal detachments and 36/62 (58%) had RPE lesions. RPE lesions were usually located in the macular or peripapillary regions, 33/36 (92%) were solitary or grouped, and 3/36 (8%) were large and geographic. After delivery, all serous retinal detachments and RPE lesions resolved. The three eyes with geographic RPE lesions all developed significant chorioretinal atrophy.[11] The apparent historical increase in the incidence of serous detachments and RPE lesions is almost certainly due to improved examination instrumentation and diagnostic testing such as fluorescein angiography.

The etiology of choroidal dysfunction is thought to be ischemia based on fluorescein angiography, limited histopathologic study, the presence of Elschnig's spots on resolution[12] and indocyanine green angiography.[13] This is further supported by the observation that posterior ciliary artery blood flow velocity is increased in pre-eclampsia suggesting vasospasm.[7] The primary choriocapillaris ischemia presumably leads to RPE ischemia manifest as yellow opacification and/or fluid pump dysfunction allowing subretinal fluid accumulation.

Although serous retinal detachment and RPE dysfunction can cause marked loss of visual acuity, these changes fully resolve postpartum and most patients return to normal vision within a few weeks. Some patients have residual RPE changes in the macula. Years later, these changes can mimic a macular dystrophy or tapetoretinal degeneration.[14] Rare patients may develop optic atrophy if chorioretinal atrophy is extensive.[15]

Saito has suggested that serous detachments are more specific to pre-eclampsia and eclampsia, whereas retinopathy is seen more often in pre-eclampsia superimposed on pre-existing hypertension.[16] Retinopathy is associated with higher levels of blood pressure than is serous detachment.[17] Although retinopathy was believed to be a reflection of possible placental insufficiency and possible adverse neonatal outcome, serous retinal detachment is not an additional risk factor.[18]

Postpartum serous detachments have been reported in pre-eclamptic patients,[19,20] and there are rare reports of exudative detachments in patients without pre-eclampsia.[21–22] While these serous retinal detachments may be mechanistically distinct, they also resolve over several weeks.

The HELLP syndrome consists of hemolysis, elevated liver enzymes, and low platelets, and it is generally associated with severe pre-eclampsia or eclampsia. Bilateral serous retinal detachments and yellow-white subretinal opacities have been seen in two patients with this disorder.[23,24]

Other ocular changes seen in pre-eclampsia and eclampsia

Cortical blindness that appears late in pregnancy or shortly after delivery is an uncommon complication of severe pre-eclampsia and eclampsia. The etiology of vision loss may be occipital ischemia in watershed areas from vasospasm[25–28] possibly related to extracellular hypercalcemia,[29] ischemia from antiphospholipid antibody related vascular occlusion,[30] vasogenic edema,[31–38] petechial[37] or larger hemorrhages,[38,39] hypertensive encephalopathy,[40,41] ischemia from hypotension during delivery,[42] or as part of a postictal state.[43] Most patients recover normal vision over several weeks. A prospective study by Cunningham showed that 15/15 women with cortical blindness underwent complete recovery over 4 hours to 8 days. CT scanning was obtained in 13/15 and MRI scanning in 5/15 revealing edema and petechial hemorrhages in the occipital cortex.[37]

The presence of large intracranial hemorrhages may portend a worse prognosis in terms of both mortality and visual recovery. Akan evaluated CT scans from 22 patients with neurologic complications from eclampsia and found that two of the three patients who died had massive intracranial hemorrhages.[38] Drislane found that among four patients with severe pre-eclampsia and multifocal cerebral hemorrhages, one died and the three others developed prolonged cognitive deficits.[39]

Cortical vision loss has been reported in five patients with HELLP syndrome. One had postictal cortical dysfunction,[43] one had venous sinus thrombosis,[44] two had signs of cortical ischemia or edema,[45,46] and one was idiopathic.[47]

Retinal arterial and venous occlusions have been reported in patients with pre-eclampsia. These may be a cause of irreversible visual loss and will be discussed later. Other ocular disorders reported associated with pre-eclampsia and eclampsia include ischemic optic neuropathy[48] and optic neuritis,[49,50] ischemic papillophlebitis,[51] peripheral retinal neovascularization,[52] choroidal neovascularization,[53] macular edema,[54] macular ischemia,[55] and a tear of the retinal pigment epithelium.[56] One patient with HELLP syndrome was reported to have developed a vitreous hemorrhage.[57]

Central serous chorioretinopathy

Central serous chorioretinopathy (CSC) is caused by localized RPE dysfunction resulting in the accumulation of subretinal fluid. People between the ages of 20 and 50 years are typically affected and there is an 8:1 male predominance.[58] Pregnancy may predispose some women to CSC. The limited amount of information available concerning CSC in pregnancy makes it difficult to determine whether CSC during pregnancy is typical CSC coincident with pregnancy or if it is a separate disorder possibly related to the hormonal hypercoagulability or hemodynamic changes of pregnancy.

Only 23 cases of CSC associated with pregnancy are reported in the medical literature.[59–67] Unlike the serous retinal detachments observed in pre-eclampsia and eclampsia, CSC is generally unilateral. The women were all previously healthy and no cases were associated with pre-eclampsia or eclampsia. No patients had antecedent eye disease other than refractive error. Primiparas and multiparas were both represented. Most of the cases developed in the third trimester and all resolved spontaneously within a few months after delivery. There were no cases of significant visual sequelae.

Pregnancy-associated CSC may recur in the context or outside of subsequent pregnancy. CSC recurred in two women, always in the same eye, in subsequent pregnancies. One patient had four successive pregnancies with CSC.[65] and one had two successive pregnancies complicated by CSC.[66] There is also one case report of a woman developing CSC 1 month postpartum in two successive pregnancies.[67] However, there is also a report of a woman with CSC in her third pregnancy who did not experience a recurrence during a subsequent pregnancy.[62] So the occurrence of CSC during one pregnancy does not necessarily mean that it will recur with future pregnancies. There is a report of one patient who experienced a recurrence of CSC outside the context of pregnancy.[62]

There is an increased incidence of subretinal white exudates (presumed to be fibrin) in pregnancy associated CSC (approximately 90%) compared to CSC in males and nonpregnant women (approximately 10%). Sunness reported that three of four patients with pregnancy related CSC had subretinal exudates.[62] Gass found that 6/6 cases of pregnancy related CSC had subretinal exudates compared to only 6/50 (12%) of nonpregnancy related cases.[63] The cause of this higher prevalence of subretinal exudates in pregnant women is unknown.

Occlusive vascular disorders

An increase in the level of clotting factors and clotting activity occurs during pregnancy.[68] Several pathologic sources of thrombosis and embolic events can also occur. One review of ischemic cerebrovascular disease suggested that pregnancy is associated with a 13-fold increase in the risk of cerebral infarctions compared to nonpregnant women.[69] This increased risk of vasoocclusive disease may also manifest as retinal or choroidal vascular occlusions.

Retinal artery occlusion

Two cases of unilateral central retinal artery occlusion (CRAO),[70,71] one case of bilateral CRAO,[72] two cases of unilateral branch retinal artery occlusion (BRAO),[73–74] and three cases of bilateral multiple BRAO[75] have been reported in association with pregnancy and in the absence of additional risk-factors. Three cases of arteriolar occlusion were associated with pre-eclampsia[72,75] and one was associated with disc edema.[74] Five of the eight (63%) cases occurred within 24 hours of delivery suggesting that this is a particularly susceptible period.

Blodi reported that multiple retinal arteriolar occlusions were seen within 24 hours after childbirth in four women. Two patients were pre-eclamptic and required cesarean section. One of the two also had evidence of cerebral infarctions. The third patient had hypertension, pancreatitis, and premature labor. The fourth was a previously healthy 16-year-old who had an oxytocin-induced labor and had a generalized seizure 2 hours after delivery. The patients reported decreased vision and all had fundus findings characterized by retinal patches characteristic of ischemia and intraretinal hemorrhages that were similar to Purtscher's retinopathy. After resolution, patients were left with focal arteriolar narrowing and optic disc pallor. The visual acuities ranged from 20/20 to 4/200 and visual field defects were compatible with the areas of occlusion. The authors suggest that complement-induced leukoemboli could have caused the retinal arteriolar occlusions.[75]

Eight additional cases of pregnancy-associated BRAO have been reported in the literature.[76–81] However, all of these cases had significant additional risk factors for vascular occlusion. Since pregnancy is a common condition, it is difficult to know whether these cases represent true pregnancy associations, multifactorial or synergistic etiologies, or just chance occurrences. One case was associated with intramuscular progestogen therapy for a threatened abortion.[76] Three cases that occurred postpartum were associated with hypercoagulability from protein C[77] or protein S[75,78] deficiency. Two cases were associated with thromboembolic occlusions attributed to mitral valve prolapse[79] and amniotic fluid embolism.[80] The final two cases developed BRAO in the first trimester in association with migraine headaches.[81]

Retinal vein occlusion

Retinal vein occlusion associated with pregnancy is exceedingly rare. Only four pregnancy-related central retinal vein occlusions (CRVO) have been reported to date[82–84] and we are not aware of any branch retinal vein occlusions. A study of central retinal vein occlusions with diurnal intraocular pressure determination in young adults included a 33-year-old pregnant woman in her third trimester who had unilateral venous dilation and tortuosity with two subretinal hemorrhages and mild foveal edema.[82] Gabsi reported the case of a 27-year-old who was 6 months pregnant when she developed a unilateral CRVO. The authors suggested impaired fibrinolysis after venous stasis as a possible mechanism.[83] A 30-year-old woman presented in the 28th week of her second pregnancy with HELLP syndrome. She developed a unilateral CRVO 10 days after emergency caesarean section.[84] The final case is that of a mild bilateral CRVO that developed early in pregnancy and resolved over several months (J. Wroblewski, personal communication). The paucity of reported cases linking pregnancy to retinal vein occlusion makes the strength of this association suspect.

Disseminated intravascular coagulopathy

Disseminated intravascular coagulation (DIC) is an acute pathological process with widespread thrombus formation in small vessels. It can occur in obstetrical complications such as abruptio placentae and intrauterine fetal death that release placental thromboplastin into maternal circulation and activate the extrinsic coagulation system. This process has a tendency to occlude the posterior choroidal vessels leading to RPE ischemia, dysfunction of the retinal pigment epithelial pump mechanism, and subsequent serous retinal detachments in the macular and peripapillary regions.[85–88] The development of serous retinal detachments in pregnancy, especially late pregnancy, may be an early ocular sign of DIC.[88] We are aware of case reports of only two patients with DIC causing serous retinal detachments.[85,88] These detachments tend to be bilateral and symptomatic. With recovery from the systemic disorder, vision generally returns to normal with only residual pigmentary change.[87,88]

Thrombotic thrombocytopenic purpura

Thrombotic thrombocytopenic purpura (TTP) is a rare, idiopathic, acute, systemic coagulopathy characterized by platelet consumption and thrombus formation in small vessels. TTP occurs at any age with a peak incidence in the third decade of life and a female to male preponderance of 3:2. Visual changes occur in approximately 8% of cases[89] due to thrombus formation in the choriocapillaris and secondary RPE ischemia. Clinical findings are usually bilateral and include serous retinal detachments, yellow spots at the level of the RPE, and localized arteriolar narrowing. We are aware of 32 reported cases of TTP in association with pregnancy. Sequelae include RPE pigmentary changes and Elschnig spots with a return to baseline vision over several weeks in most cases.[89–91]

Amniotic fluid embolism

Amniotic fluid embolism is a serious complication of pregnancy with high mortality, second only to pulmonary thromboembolism as a cause of death during pregnancy and the postpartum period. Those patients who survive the initial event usually develop DIC[92] with the potential ocular complications described above. Two patients developed multiple branch retinal arteriolar occlusions presumably related to particulate material from the amniotic fluid.[93,94] Another patient had massive blood loss from an amniotic fluid embolism leading to severe retinal and choroidal ischemia and blindness in one eye.[95]

Uveal melanoma

Pregnancy is heralded by a hormone-dependent tendency to hyperpigmentation and well-known cutaneous changes like chloasma and an increase in pigmentation of pre-existing nevi owing to increased levels of melanocyte-stimulating hormone in pregnancy.[96] Although estrogen and progesterone may stimulate melanogenesis, there is no evidence that this can cause malignant transformation of melanocytic cells.

A case-control study by Holly et al. found a decreased risk of uveal melanoma for women who had ever been pregnant with an increase in protective effect with more live births. The largest effect was observed between nulliparous and parous women.[97] However, others have reported a trend toward a larger than expected number of ocular melanomas presenting during pregnancy.[98] There are also a number of anecdotal reports of uveal melanomas presenting or growing rapidly during pregnancy.[99–103] These reports lead to speculation that uveal melanoma may be hormone-responsive but two studies have failed to show any estrogen or progesterone receptor expression in ocular melanomas.[102,104] It is possible that other hormones may be involved[102] or that tumor growth may be related to pregnancy-associated immune modulation.

Pregnancy-related uveal melanoma does not seem to differ histologically from uveal melanoma not associated with pregnancy. Shields reported that among 10 pregnancy-related choroidal melanomas evaluated after enucleation, the tumors did not differ in cell type, mitotic activity, and other features when compared to a matched group of tumors in nonpregnant women.[105]

The treatment of pregnancy-associated uveal melanoma has been described in two studies. Among 16 cases reported by Shields, 10 eyes were enucleated, four received plaque radiotherapy during or after pregnancy, and two cases were observed. Among 14 of 16 patients who elected to carry the pregnancy to term, all delivered healthy babies with no infant or placental metastases.[105] Romanowska-Dixon reported eight cases in which there were no treatment-related pregnancy complications. The authors do suggest that brachytherapy is safer towards the end of pregnancy or after delivery.[106]

Childbearing may be associated with improved survival in choroidal melanoma. Egan et al. performed a large prospective cohort study in which death rates from metastasis were 25% higher in nulliparous women and men than women who had given birth. The protective influence of parity was greatest in the first 3 years of follow-up and increased with the number of live births.[107] These results contradict a small earlier study by the same group that concluded rates of metastasis were not lower among women who reported pregnancies or oral contraceptive use.[108] A much smaller study by Shields also showed similar 5-year survival between pregnant and nonpregnant women with posterior uveal melanoma.[105]

Other changes arising in pregnancy

A choroidal osteoma has been reported that presented in the ninth month of pregnancy with visual loss due to choroidal neovascularization.[109] Cases of acute macular neuroretinopathy,[110,111] Valsalva maculopathy,[112] and cystoid macular edema[113] have been observed in the immediate postpartum period. Placental metastases from orbital rhabdomyosarcoma[114] and primary ocular melanoma have been reported.[115]

PRE-EXISTING CONDITIONS

Diabetic retinopathy

The modern medical, ophthalmologic, and obstetrical management of pregnant diabetic patients has greatly improved the outcome of pregnancy for both the fetus and the mother. Laser photocoagulation has reduced the risk of vision loss from diabetic retinopathy and improved glucose control has improved the likelihood of good fetal outcomes. Well-controlled blood glucose and adequate glycosylated hemoglobin (HbA_{1c}) before conception and throughout the pregnancy may reduce the risk of spontaneous abortion,[116,117] congenital anomalies, and fetal morbidity.[118] A recent study suggested that the severity of diabetic retinopathy may be a significant factor in predicting adverse fetal outcomes, even after correcting for blood glucose control.[119] However, another study suggested that blood glucose control may counteract adverse fetal effects associated with maternal retinopathy and nephropathy.[120]

Diabetic women who may become pregnant should establish excellent glucose control before conception, since the major period of fetal organogenesis may take place before the mother is even aware that she is pregnant. In addition, a diabetic woman's retinopathy status should be evaluated and stabilized prior to conception. This is particularly important for patients with severe nonproliferative or proliferative retinopathy because scatter laser photocoagulation may reduce progression during pregnancy.[121] Laser treatment of diabetic macular edema before pregnancy may also be important, although the effects of pregnancy on macula edema have not been adequately studied.

The Diabetes in Early Pregnancy Study (DIEP), a study of 155 insulin-dependent diabetic pregnancies,[122] as well as the data from the Diabetic Control and Complications Trial[123] and the previous data summarized by Sunness,[119] all provide evidence that better metabolic control before pregnancy diminishes the progression of diabetic retinopathy. Recent studies have found a strong correlation between the glycosylated hemoglobin level in the first month and the degree of deterioration once tight metabolic control is achieved.[122] Nerve fiber layer infarctions commonly are associated with the institution of tight metabolic control of chronic hyperglycemic patients. One study described the retinopathy status of 13 patients managed by insulin pump during pregnancy. Two patients who had rapid decrease in the HbA_{1c} level developed acute ischemic changes and ultimately proliferative retinopathy.[134] However, the long-term benefits of adequate blood glucose control outweigh concerns about the transient worsening of retinopathy that has been associated with the sudden imposition of tight metabolic control.[123–125]

The frequency of ophthalmic follow-up of a diabetic patient during pregnancy is determined by her baseline retinopathy status. Guidelines for eye care in diabetic patients recommend that a diabetic woman planning pregnancy within 12 months should be under the care of an ophthalmologist, undergo repeat evaluation in the first trimester, and after that at intervals dependent on the initial findings.[119,126]

Progression of diabetic retinopathy during pregnancy

The interpretation of changes in diabetic retinopathy as being caused by pregnancy is confounded by changes related to blood glucose levels. As medical advances continue to improve glycemic control, changes in blood glucose control that occur at the onset of pregnancy will be minimized and it may be easier to obtain a more direct understanding of the role of pregnancy in the progression of diabetic retinopathy. In the meantime, several mechanisms have been proposed as possible etiologic factors contributing to diabetic retinopathy during pregnancy.

Retinal hemodynamics may play an important role. The increase in cardiac output combined with decreased peripheral vascular resistance during pregnancy,[127] have been suggested as pathogenic factors for the development or progression of diabetic retinopathy. Three studies suggest that retinal hyperperfusion may exacerbate pre-existing microvascular damage.[128,161,162] In contrast, two studies report a reduction in retinal capillary blood flow that may exacerbate ischemia and lead to retinopathy progression.[163,164] Other studies have suggested a possible role for various growth factors found at increased concentrations during pregnancy such as IGF-1,[165] phosphorylated IGF binding protein,[166] placenta growth factor,[167,168] endothelin-1,[169] and fibroblast growth factor-2.[170] These factors may exert additive or synergistic effects.[171]

Short and long-term effects of pregnancy on diabetic retinopathy

Since there is a high rate of regression of retinopathy during the postpartum period, one must consider short-term and long-term changes separately. The DCCT research group reported that pregnant women in the conventional treatment group were 2.9 times more likely to progress three or more levels from baseline retinopathy status than nonpregnant women. The odds ratio peaked during the second trimester and persisted as long as 12 months after delivery.[178] One study of short-term effects included 16 women with no retinopathy or nonproliferative retinopathy. Progression during pregnancy was compared to progression between 6 and 15 months postpartum in the same women. The number of microaneurysms showed a rapid increase between the 28th and 35th weeks of pregnancy. Six months postpartum the number of microaneurysms decreased but in most cases remained higher than the baseline level. The number of microaneurysms remained stable over the subsequent nine-month postpartum period.[150]

Three other studies compared short-term progression of retinopathy between separate control groups of nonpregnant women and pregnant women over the same time period. The first compared the course of diabetic retinopathy in 93 pregnant women and 98 nonpregnant women. Progression was observed in 16% of the pregnant group compared to only 6% in the nonpregnant patients. Furthermore, 32% of the nonpregnant group had retinopathy at baseline compared to only 22% of the pregnant cohort. Therefore, one might have expected more progression in the nonpregnant group due to worse baseline disease, making these findings more significant.[151] A second study compared 39 nonpregnant women, 46% of whom had retinopathy at baseline, with 53 pregnant diabetic women, 57% of whom had retinopathy at baseline. In the nonpregnant group the microaneurysms remained stable, streak or blob hemorrhages appeared in three patients (8%), and no nerve fiber layer infarctions developed over 15 months. In the pregnant group, microaneurysms increased moderately, and streak and blob hemorrhages and nerve fiber layer infarctions increased markedly over the same follow-up period. One patient with nonproliferative diabetic retinopathy from the pregnant group developed proliferative retinopathy.[129] In the third study, there were 133 pregnant and 241 nonpregnant women. The groups were statistically equivalent in terms of baseline retinopathy levels. Within each quartile of glycosylated hemoglobin, pregnant women had a greater tendency to have worsening of retinopathy and the nonpregnant women had a greater tendency to have improvement in their level of diabetic retinopathy during the follow-up interval.[152]

There are four studies concerning the long-term effects of pregnancy on diabetic retinopathy. The first included 40 women followed for 12 months postpartum. Among 19 study participants with no retinopathy at baseline, 30% developed mild nonproliferative retinopathy during the second and third trimester. By one year postpartum none had clinically detectable retinopathy. Among the 21 women with retinopathy at baseline, 11 worsened during pregnancy and two developed proliferative disease. None of these 11 women had regressed to her initial retinopathy status by 1 year postpartum.[144] The second study reported changes at 12 months postpartum. Among 10 patients with no initial retinopathy who developed mild retinopathy during pregnancy, half experienced total postpartum regression, 30% had partial regression, and 20% had no change. Among five patients with initial mild retinopathy who progressed to moderate nonproliferative retinopathy, 40% experienced complete regression, 40% partial regression, and 20% no regression. However, among 12 who progressed from mild initial retinopathy to severe nonproliferative retinopathy, only 17% had total regression, 58% had partial regression, and 25% had no regression. The third study compared 28 diabetic women to 17 nulliparous matched controls over a 7-year period. Only five of 26 (19.2%) of women who had been pregnant experienced progression of retinopathy compared to eight of 16 (50%) nulliparous women suggesting that pregnancy does not affect long-term progression and may even afford a protective effect.[156] A final study of 80 women who had completed at least one successful pregnancy found no increase in the risk of proliferative retinopathy later in life compared to matched controls.[182]

Two studies suggest that the number of prior pregnancies does not appear to be a long-term factor in the severity of retinopathy present when duration of diabetes is taken into account.[153,154] In fact, a cross-sectional European study reported lower levels of retinopathy in diabetics with multiple pregnancies compared with women matched for age and duration of diabetes.[155] It is not clear if this improved status was caused by a prolonged period of tight metabolic control and better patient education, or if pregnancy confers a long-term protective effect. Another possibility involves the bias that only women with better metabolic control may have undergone the stress of multiple pregnancies.

The role of baseline retinopathy status, duration of diabetes, and metabolic control

The major determinants of the progression of diabetic retinopathy in a pregnant woman are the duration of diabetes and the degree of retinopathy at the onset of pregnancy.[121,122,129–132] Therefore, women with diabetes are strongly encouraged to complete childbearing early in their adult life.[133]

The baseline level of retinopathy at conception is the major risk factor for progression of retinopathy, according to the DIEP. When a logistic regression model was used to separate the influence of diabetes duration (shorter duration being less than 15 years, longer duration being more than 15 years) from the effect of a worse baseline level of nonproliferative diabetic retinopathy, the baseline retinopathy was highly significant but the duration of retinopathy was not. Analysis of patients with moderate or more severe retinopathy in the DIEP showed deterioration (defined as a two-step or more worsening determined on the final scale of the modified Airlie House Diabetic Retinopathy Classification) in 55% of patients with shorter duration and 50% of patients with longer duration of diabetes. However, the rates of development of proliferative retinopathy were 39% of patients with longer duration of diabetes and only 18% of patients with shorter duration of diabetes. The HbA$_{1c}$ level at the beginning of pregnancy was used in the DIEP as a measure of metabolic control. Women with an HbA$_{1c}$ level of 6 standard deviations (SD) or more from the control mean had a statistically significant higher risk of progression of retinopathy compared with patients with an HbA$_{1c}$ baseline level within 2 SD of the control mean.[122]

A longitudinal analysis of the effect of pregnancy on microvascular complications in the Diabetes Control and Complications Trial (DCCT) was recently published. Pregnant women in the intensive treatment group had a 1.63-fold greater risk of retinopathy progression during pregnancy than nonpregnant women, compared to a 2.48-fold greater risk in the conventional treatment group.[178]

A prospective study of 179 pregnancies in 139 women with type-1 diabetes reported a 10% progression rate of retinopathy in women with duration of diabetes 10–19 years compared to 0% in women with duration less than 10 years. Furthermore, women with moderate to severe retinopathy experienced progression in 30% of cases compared to only 3.7% with less severe retinopathy.[157]

Lauszus prospectively followed 112 pregnant women with insulin-dependent diabetes and found an association between the severity of retinopathy and poor glycemic control before and after pregnancy. However, no such correlation was found with intensive glycemic control during pregnancy. Those women who had progression of retinopathy during or after pregnancy had an average diabetes onset at age 14 years compared to 19 years in women whose retinopathy remained stable.

The following discussion of the progression of retinopathy during pregnancy is subdivided according to the baseline level of retinopathy present. Many of the studies did not use the more recent classification recommended by the Early Treatment Diabetic Retinopathy Study (ETDRS). Whenever possible, the results have been organized according to this classification.[135]

No initial retinopathy

Sunness summarized nine studies that included 484 diabetic pregnancies with no initial retinopathy. Twelve percent of these patients developed some background change during pregnancy, and one patient (0.2%) developed proliferative retinopathy. In 23 cases with progression for which postpartum follow-up was available, there was some regression of the nonproliferative changes in 57%.[121] The DIEP reported a 10.3% progression to mild nonproliferative diabetic retinopathy for this group of patients.[122] Four other studies of eyes with no initial retinopathy reported progression rates of 0%, 7%, 26%, and 28% respectively.[132,136,137,158]

A 12-year prospective study of patients with gestational diabetes did not demonstrate an increased risk of diabetic retinopathy.[138] However, retinal vascular tortuosity in gestational diabetics has been reported, and some degree of tortuosity persisted at 5 months postpartum.[139] There is one case report of a previously healthy nulliparous woman with gestational diabetes diagnosed at 8 weeks gestation. Glycemic control was instituted and the patient developed bilateral proliferative retinopathy by 31 weeks gestation. The patient had a markedly elevated HbA_{1c} at initial diagnosis suggesting that she may have been diabetic before becoming pregnant.[140] Puza reported a retrospective review of 100 gestational diabetics and concluded that routine examinations have little utility in these patients.[160]

Mild nonproliferative diabetic retinopathy

In two studies that included 24 pregnant women with fewer than 10 microaneurysms and dot hemorrhages in both eyes, 8% developed additional microaneurysms and 0% developed proliferative retinopathy.[121] A more recent study showed that microaneurysm counts increase during pregnancy, peak at 3 months postpartum, and then decline to baseline levels.[159] The DIEP study found that 18.8% of patients with mild nonproliferative retinopathy showed a 2-step progression on the modified Airlie House classification through the end of pregnancy. Only 6% progressed from mild nonproliferative to proliferative retinopathy.[122] A study that included seven patients with minimal retinopathy reported progression in only one during pregnancy that improved after delivery.[158]

Moderate to severe nonproliferative diabetic retinopathy

The DIEP found that 54.8% of patients with moderate retinopathy showed a two-step progression on the modified Airlie House diabetic retinopathy classification and 29% developed proliferative retinopathy by the end of pregnancy.[122] In addition, 25% of those who developed proliferative retinopathy had high-risk characteristics as defined by the Diabetic Retinopathy Study.[141]

The results of ten studies published before 1988 that included 259 pregnant women with nonproliferative diabetic retinopathy were summarized by Sunness. The analysis of this information showed that 47% of patients had an increase in the severity of nonproliferative changes during pregnancy. Differences in the scale of measurements of diabetic retinopathy among the studies caused wide variations in progression rates. Most of the studies included mild and moderate retinopathy in the wider group of nonproliferative retinopathy. Only 5% of patients in this analysis developed proliferative retinopathy during pregnancy.[121]

Four studies after 1988 reported progression rates of nonproliferative retinopathy ranging from 12% to 55%.[132,136,137,142] Two of these studies reported rates of proliferative retinopathy development at 8% and 22% during pregnancy.[137,142]

Proliferative retinopathy

Sunness summarized 12 studies including 122 women with proliferative retinopathy at baseline. Of these 122 women, 46% had some increase in neovascularization that developed during pregnancy.[121] A more recent study reported a 63% rate of progression in eyes with proliferative retinopathy at baseline.[132]

Optimal treatment of proliferative disease before pregnancy reduces the risk of progression during pregnancy. In the 1988 Sunness review, those patients who had scatter laser photocoagulation before pregnancy showed a 26% rate of progression of their proliferative disease and visual loss compared to 58% of patients without prior treatment. Those patients with complete regression of proliferative disease before pregnancy did not demonstrate progression of proliferative disease during pregnancy.[121] Somewhat different results were found in a later study by Reece. In this analysis, half of the patients with proliferative disease who underwent scatter laser photocoagulation prior to pregnancy required additional scatter treatment during pregnancy. In addition, 65% of patients who had proliferative disease during pregnancy required photocoagulation postpartum. No patient had proliferative disease that did not respond to laser photocoagulation.[143]

Proliferative retinopathy may regress near the end of pregnancy or in the postpartum period. One study found that four out of five women who developed proliferative retinopathy during pregnancy had spontaneous regression to nonproliferative status within 2 months postpartum.[144] In contrast, another study of eight women with proliferative disease reported no spontaneous regression by 3 months postpartum.[132] The possibility of spontaneous regression is a factor to consider when determining if laser photocoagulation is indicated. Most retina specialists would aggressively treat patients who have high-risk proliferative retinopathy; some retinal specialists would treat one eye or both in cases that are not high risk, given the problem of rapid progression during pregnancy. After consideration of high-risk factors such as high initial HbA_{1c} and duration of diabetes, these decisions must be made on a case-by-case basis.

Vitreous hemorrhage during labor and delivery has been reported in a few cases.[145] Currently, no evidence justifies performing a cesarean section on the basis of proliferative retinopathy alone, given the availability of vitrectomy for the treatment of nonclearing vitreous hemorrhage.[121]

Diabetic macular edema in pregnancy

Diabetic macular edema that involves or threatens the fovea is currently treated with focal laser photocoagulation outside the context of pregnancy in order to reduce the risk of moderate vision loss. Patients who develop macular edema during pregnancy frequently have different prognoses than nonpregnant patients. Spontaneous resolution after pregnancy is a common occurrence and is associated with improvement of visual acuity more frequently than in nonpregnant patients.[142]

Sinclair and Nessler reported that 16 (29%) of 56 eyes of diabetic pregnant women with initial proliferative or nonproliferative retinopathy developed diabetic macular edema during pregnancy. Of these 16 eyes, 14 (88%) had improvement in visual acuity and resolution of macular edema postpartum without laser treatment.[146]

In general, pregnant women with diabetic macular edema should not be treated during pregnancy because of the high rate of spontaneous improvement postpartum. Possible exceptions include cases in which lipid is threatening the fovea or severe progressive macular edema develops early in pregnancy. However, more detailed and systematic study of diabetic macular edema is required to allow scientifically based management recommendations.

Other risk factors for progression of diabetic retinopathy during pregnancy

Nephropathy and systemic hypertension are additional risk factors for the progression of diabetic retinopathy during pregnancy. A well-known association exists between nephropathy and retinopathy in nonpregnant patients. One study in pregnant diabetics showed that eight of nine patients in whom macular edema developed during pregnancy had proteinuria of more than 1 g per day.[147] Two studies report elevated systolic blood pressure is a risk factor for the progression of diabetic retinopathy.[132,148] Systolic blood pressure within the normal range but over 115 mmHg has been associated with an increased risk retinopathy progressed among pregnant patients.[136] The DIEP found a 1.3 odds ratio for two-step progression of retinopathy for every 10 mmHg increase in systolic blood pressure.[122]

Diabetic retinopathy and maternal and fetal well-being

Advanced diabetic retinopathy has been considered a risk factor for adverse fetal outcomes because it may reflect more widespread systemic disease. Pregnancies associated with nonproliferative diabetic retinopathy may not be at higher risk for adverse fetal outcomes.[149] However, Klein reported an adverse fetal outcome in 43% of 28 women with proliferative retinopathy compared to only 13% of 131 women with nonproliferative retinopathy.[119] Another study of 20 pregnancies of 17 women with proliferative retinopathy reported spontaneous abortion in two cases (10%), stillbirth in one case (5%), and three had major congenital anomalies.[143] Sameshima reported that among 60 pregnant patients with diabetes, the seven with proliferative retinopathy had a significantly higher incidence of fetal distress.[172] A final study of 26 women with proliferative retinopathy reported serious neonatal morbidity in 19% and mortality in 12%.[175]

One prospective study of 205 women with type-1 diabetes found that low birth weight was associated with retinopathy progression. However, retinopathy progression was not associated with earlier delivery, macrosomia, respiratory distress syndrome, neonatal hypoglycemia, or neonatal death.[174]

Improved medical and obstetrical management has improved the outcome of diabetic pregnancies. In a study of 22 pregnancies complicated by retinopathy and nephropathy in which good glycemic control was present antepartum and throughout pregnancy, there were no infant deaths and only one case of mild respiratory distress syndrome.[120] A retrospective study of 482 diabetic pregnancies reported only three perinatal deaths

which was statistically equivalent to nonpregnant deliveries over the same period.[173]

Two studies suggest an association between diabetic retinopathy and the development of pre-eclampsia. Hiilesmaa followed 683 consecutive pregnancies with type-1 diabetes and found that retinopathy was a statistically significant independent predictor of pre-eclampsia.[176] A second study looked retrospectively at 65 pregnant type-1 diabetic patients and reported that deterioration of retinopathy occurred more frequently in those with pre-eclampsia (4/8) than those without pre-eclampsia (5/65).[177] Perhaps central retinal artery vasospasm associated with pre-eclampsia exacerbates retinal ischemia.

Toxoplasmic retinochoroiditis

The likelihood of congenital toxoplasmosis occurring in the offspring of a mother with active retinochoroiditis or chorioretinal scars is often a concern. However, this usually is unfounded since congenital toxoplasmosis in the fetus results only from infection of the mother that occurs during the pregnancy itself. The presence of focal toxoplasmic retinochoroiditis or scars in a patient reflects congenital infection of that patient in essentially all cases and not new infection of the mother.[181]

Therefore the fetus of a woman with active retinochoroiditis or scars should not be at risk for contracting congenital toxoplasmosis. A study of 18 pregnant patients with active toxoplasmosis or scars, some with high stable toxoplasmosis titer, found that no infants developed congenital toxoplasmosis.[180]

Noninfectious uveitis

Uveitis disease activity may be altered during pregnancy and the postpartum period. Rabiah retrospectively evaluated 76 pregnancies of 50 women with noninfectious uveitis. The pregnancies were associated with Vogt–Koyanagi–Harada (VKH) syndrome in 33 women, Behçet's disease in 19, and idiopathic uveitis in 24. A worsening of uveitis occurred within the first 4 months of pregnancy in 49/76 (64%) pregnancies and later in pregnancy in 17 (22%). No flare-up occurred in 21 cases (28%). An early pregnancy worsening was typical of VKH and idiopathic uveitis. Postpartum worsening occurred in 38/59 cases (64%) and was characteristic of Behçet disease.[196]

Six patients with pre-existing Vogt–Koyanagi–Harada (VKH) syndrome who improved during pregnancy have been reported.[189,190,197] All patients had flare-ups of their disease postpartum. Sarcoid uveitis may also improve during pregnancy[197] or develop de novo during the postpartum period.[198] Some authors speculate that elevated endogenous free cortisol levels associated with pregnancy may suppress uveitis.[198-199] However, two cases of VKH syndrome arising de novo in the second half of otherwise normal pregnancies have also been reported, with full remission occurring postpartum.[191] In addition, one study of three patients with sarcoid uveitis showed no change in the course of the disease during pregnancy.[92]

Other retinal disorders

The stress of labor and delivery does not appear to pose a risk for rhegmatogenous retinal detachment in high myopes. This conclusion is based on three studies. The first examined 50 women with high myopia late in pregnancy and again in the first 2 weeks postpartum and reported no postpartum changes.[183] A study of 10 asymptomatic women during 19 pregnancies who gave a history of high myopia, retinal detachment, or retinal holes or lattice degeneration did not develop any new retinal pathology after delivery.[184] The final study examined 42 high myopes and four high myopes with previous retinal detachments before and after delivery and documented no progressive retinal changes.[185]

Rapid growth of choroidal hemangiomas has been reported during pregnancy.[186] Another case report described the development of exudative retinal detachments associated with choroidal hemangiomas during pregnancy.[187] The hemangioma may regress postpartum.[188] These changes have been attributed to pregnancy-related hormonal perturbations.

Two previously healthy women developed unilateral endogenous candida endophthalmitis after undergoing surgically induced abortions. One eye underwent vitrectomy and intravitreal amphotericin B injection with a final visual acuity of 20/200. The other eye had a retinal detachment after delayed diagnosis resulting in count fingers visual acuity.[192]

Retinitis pigmentosa is sometimes characterized by a sudden pregnancy-associated deterioration in visual fields after a period of relative stability. It is difficult to determine whether changes are related to pregnancy or are just coincidental. Five to ten percent of women with retinitis pigmentosa who have been pregnant reported worsening during pregnancy[193,194] and did not return to baseline after delivery.[193] There is one report in the literature of visual field deterioration during pregnancy, which resolved postpartum.[195] One case of pericentral retinal degeneration that worsened during pregnancy has been reported.[200]

DIAGNOSTIC TESTING

Fluorescein crosses the placenta and enters the fetal circulation in humans.[201] No reports of teratogenic effects in humans have been reported to the National Registry of Drug-Induced Ocular Side Effects.[121] European investigators have performed research studies involving the administration of fluorescein to 22 pregnant diabetic women and noticed no adverse effects on the fetus.[202] Another study of neonatal outcome of 105 patients who underwent fluorescein angiography (IVFA) during pregnancy showed no increased rate of adverse neonatal outcomes.[204] However, this study included only 41 cases of fluorescein angiography during the first trimester, the time when teratogenic effects are more likely to take place and are more severe. Nevertheless, one survey reported that 77% of retinal specialists never perform IVFA on a patient they know is pregnant.[203] In another survey, 89% of retina specialists who had seen a pregnant woman who required fluorescein angiography withheld testing out of fear of teratogenicity or lawsuit.[207] We recommend that fluorescein angiography in pregnant women can be considered if the results would change the management of a vision-threatening problem and appropriate informed consent is obtained.

Indocyanine green does not cross the placenta, is highly bonded to plasma proteins, and is metabolized by the liver. Reports of only six cases of the use of indocyanine green angiography (ICGA) during pregnancy have been published.[205,206] In a survey of 520 retina specialists, 105 had withheld ICGA out of fear of teratogenicity or lawsuit during pregnancy and only 24% thought it was safe to use ICGA in a pregnant patient. The authors suggest that current practice patterns concerning the use of ICGA in pregnancy may be unnecessarily restrictive.[207] Like IVFA, we recommend that ICGA in pregnant women can be considered if the results would change the management of a vision-threatening problem and appropriate informed consent is obtained.

Photodynamic therapy

We are not aware of any studies concerning the safety of photodynamic therapy during pregnancy. Caution is recommended.

SUMMARY

Information about the effects of pregnancy on the course of retinal disease is limited. In most cases the direct cause of pregnancy effects is only speculative and based on what is known about systemic changes in the mother. As our understanding of the natural course of retinal and choroidal diseases and of the effects of pregnancy on the eye improves, the ophthalmic management of both pregnant and nonpregnant patients will improve.

REFERENCES

1. Dieckmann WJ. The toxemias of pregnancy, 2nd edn. St Louis: Mosby, 1952.
2. Folk JC, Weingeist TA. Fundus changes in toxemia. Ophthalmology 1981; 88:1173–1174.
3. Sunness JS, Gass JDM, Singerman U et al. Retinal and choroidal changes in pregnancy. In: Singerman U, Jampol LM, eds. Retinal and choroidal manifestations of systemic disease. Baltimore: Williams & Wilkins, 1991.
4. Wagener HP. Arterioles of the retina in toxemia of pregnancy. JAMA 1933; 101:1380–1384.
5. Schreyer P, Tzadok J, Sherman DJ et al. Fluorescein angiography in hypertensive pregnancies. Int J Gynecol Obstet 1991; 34:127–132.
6. Jaffe G, Schatz H. Ocular manifestations of pre-eclampsia. Am J Ophthalmol 1987; 103:309–315.
7. Belfort MA. The effect of magnesium sulphate on blood flow velocity in the maternal retina in mild pre-eclampsia: a preliminary color flow Doppler study. Br J Obstet Gynaecol 1992; 99:641–645.
8. Fry WE. Extensive bilateral retinal detachment in eclampsia with complete reattachment. Arch Ophthalmol 1929; 1:609–614.
9. Hallum AV. Eye changes in hypertensive toxemia of pregnancy. JAMA 1936; 106:1649–1651.
10. Gitter HA, Heuser BP, Sarin LK et al. Toxemia of pregnancy: an angiographic interpretation of fundus changes. Arch Ophthalmol 1968; 80:449–454.
11. Saito Y, Tano Y. Retinal pigment epithelial lesions associated with choroidal ischemia in pre-eclampsia. Retina 1999; 19:262–263.
12. Oliver M, Uchenik D. Bilateral exudative retinal detachment in eclampsia without hypertensive retinopathy. Am J Ophthalmol 1980; 90:792–796.
13. Valluri S, Adelberg DA, Curtis RS et al. Diagnostic indocyanine green in pre-eclampsia. Am J Ophthalmol 1996; 122:672–677.
14. Gass JDM, Pautler SE. Toxemia of pregnancy: pigment epitheliopathy masquerading as a heredomacular dystrophy. Trans Am Ophthalmol Soc 1985; 83:114–130.
15. Fry WE. Extensive bilateral retinal detachment in eclampsia with complete reattachment. Arch Ophthalmol 1929; 1:609–614.

16. Saito Y, Omoto T, Kidoguchi K et al. The relationship between ophthalmoscopic changes and classification of toxemia in toxemia of pregnancy. Acta Soc Ophthalmol Jpn 1990; 94:870–874.

17. Sadowsky A, Serr DM, Landau J. Retinal changes and fetal prognosis in the toxemias of pregnancy. Obstet Gynecol 1956; 8:426–431.

18. Oliver M, Uchenik D. Bilateral exudative retinal detachment in eclampsia without hypertensive retinopathy. Am J Ophthalmol 1980; 90:792–796.

19. Bos AM, van Loon AJ, Ameln JG. Serous retinal detachment in pre-eclampsia. Ned Tijdschr Geneesjd 1999; 143:2430–2432.

20. Chatwani A, Oyer R, Wong S. Postpartum retinal detachment. J Reprod Med 1989; 34:842–844.

21. Bosco JAS. Spontaneous nontraumatic retinal detachments in pregnancy. Am J Obstet Gynecol 1961; 82:208–212.

22. Brismar C, Schimmelpfennig W. Bilateral exudative retinal detachment in pregnancy. Acta Ophthalmol 1989; 67:699–702.

23. Sanchez JL, Ruiz J, Nanwani K et al. Retinal detachment in pre-eclampsia and HELLP syndrome. Arch Soc Esp Oftalmol 2003; 78:335–338.

24. Burke JP, Whyte I, MacEwen CJ. Bilateral serous retinal detachments in the HELLP syndrome. Acta Ophthalmol 1989; 67:322–324.

25. Yamaguchi K, Fukuuchi Y, Nogawa S et al. Recovery of decreased local cerebral blood flow detected by the xenon/CT CBF method in a patient with eclampsia. Keio J Med 2000; 49:71–4.

26. Neihaus L, Meyer BU, Hoffmann KT. Transient cortical blindness in EHP caused by cerebral vasospasm. Nervenartz 1999; 70:931–934.

27. Kesler A, Kaneti H, Kidron D. Transient cortical blindness in pre-eclampsia with indication of generalized vascular endothelial damage. J Neuroophthalmol 1998; 18:163–165.

28. Duncan R, Hadley D, Bone I et al. Blindness in eclampsia: CT and MRI imaging. J Neurol Neurosurg Psychiat 1989; 52:899–902.

29. Kaplan PW. Reversible hypercalcemic vasoconstriction with seizure and blindness: a paradigm for eclampsia. Clin Electroencephalogr 1998; 29:120–123.

30. Branch DW, Andres R, Digre KB et al. The association of antiphospholipid antibodies with severe pre-eclampsia. Obstet Gynecol 1989; 73:541–545.

31. Do DV, Rismondo V, Nguyen QD. Reversible cortical blindness in pre-eclampsia. Am J Ophthalmol 2002; 134:916–918.

32. Hiruta M, Fukuda H, Hiruta A et al. Emergency cesarean section in a patient with acute cortical blindness and eclampsia. Masui 2002; 51: 670–672.

33. Apollon KM, Robinson JN, Schwartz RB et al. Cortical blindness in severe pre-eclampsia: CT, MRI, SPECT findings. Obstet Gynecol 2000; 95: 1017–1019.

34. Davila M, Pensado A, Rama P et al. Cortical blindness as symptom of pre-eclampsia. Rev Esp Anestesiol Reanim 1998; 45:189–200.

35. Shieh T, Kosasa TS, Tomai E et al. Transient blindness in a pre-eclamptic patient secondary to cerebral edema. Hawaii Med J 1996; 55:116–117.

36. Beeson JH, Duda EE. CT scan demonstration of cerebral edema in eclampsia preceded by blindness. Obstet Gynecol 1982; 60:529–532.

37. Cunningham FG, Fernandez CO, Hemandez C. Blindness associated with pre-eclampsia and eclampsia. Am J Obstet Gynecol 1995; 172:1291–1298.

38. Akan H, Kucac M, Bolat O et al. The diagnostic value of cranial CT in complicated eclampsia. J Belge Radiol 1993; 76:304–306.

39. Drislane FW, Wang AM. Multifocal cerebral hemorrhage in eclampsia and severe pre-eclampsia. J Neurol 1997; 244:194–198.

40. Wijman CA, Beijer IS, van Dijk GW et al. Hypertensive encephalopathy: does not only occur at high blood pressure. Ned Tijdschr Geneeskd 2002; 146:969–973.

41. Leibowitz HA, Hall PE. Cortical blindness as a complication of eclampsia. Ann Emerg Med 1984; 13:365–367.

42. Borromeo CJ, Blike GT, Wiley CW et al. Cortical blindness in a pre-eclamptic patient after a cesarean delivery complicated by hypotension. Anesth Analg 2000; 91:609–611.

43. Levavi H, Neri A, Zoldan J et al. Pre-eclampsia, "HELLP" syndrome and postictal cortical blindness. Acta Obstet Gynecol Scand 1987; 66:91–92.

44. Ertan AK, Kujat CH, Jost WH et al. HELLP syndrome – amaurosis in sinus thrombosis with complete recovery. Geburtshilfe Frauenheilkd 1994; 54:646–648.

45. Ebert AD, Hopp HS, Entezami M, et al. Acute onset of blindness during labor: report of a case of transient cortical blindness in association with HELLP syndrome. Eur J Obstet Gynecol Reprod Biol 1999; 84:111–113.

46. Crosby ET, Preston R. Obstetrical anesthesia for a parturient with pre-eclampsia. HELLP syndrome and acute cortical blindness. Can J Anaesth 1998; 45:452–459.

47. Tung CF, Peng YC, Chen Gh et al. HELLP syndrome with acute cortical blindness. Zhonghua Yi Xue Za Zhi 2001; 64:482–485.

48. Beck RW, Gamel JW, Willcourt RJ et al. Acute ischemic optic neuropathy in severe pre-eclampsia. Am J Ophthalmol 1980; 90:342–346.

49. Sommerville-Lange LB. A case of permanent blindness due to toxemia of pregnancy. Br J Ophthalmol 1950; 34:431–434.

50. Wagener H. Lesions of the optic nerve and retina in pregnancy. JAMA 1934; 103:1910–1913.

51. Price J, Marouf L, Heine MW. New angiographic findings in toxemia of pregnancy. Ophthalmology 1986; 93(suppl):125.

52. Brancato P, Menchini U, Bandello F. Proliferative retinopathy and toxemia of pregnancy. Ann Ophthalmol 1987; 19:182–183.

53. Curi AL, Jacks A, Pevisio C. Choroidal neovascular membrane presenting as a complication of pre-eclampsia in a patient with antiphospholipid syndrome. Br J Ophthalmol 2000; 84:1080.

54. Theodossiadis PG, Kollia AK, Gogas P et al. Retinal disorders in pre-eclampsia studied with optical coherence tomography. Am J Ophthalmol 2002; 133:707–709.

55. Shaikh S, Ruby AJ, Piotrowski M. Pre-eclampsia related chorioretinopathy with Purtscher's-like findings and macular ischemia. Retina 2003; 23:247–250.

56. Menchini U, Lanzetta P, Virgili G et al. Retinal pigment epithelium tear following toxemia of pregnancy. Eur J Ophthalmol 1995; 5:139–141.

57. Leff SR, Yarian DR, Masciulli L et al. Vitreous hemorrhage as a complication of HELLP syndrome. Br J Ophthalmol 1990; 74:498.

58. Todd KC, Hainsworth DP, Lee LR et al. Longitudinal analysis of central serous chorioretinopathy and sex. Can J Ophthalmol 2002; 37:405–408.

59. Normalina M, Zainal M, Alias D. Central serous choroidopathy in pregnancy. Med J Malaysia 1998; 53:439–441.

60. Khairallah M, Nouira F, Gharsallah R et al. Central serous chorioretinopathy in a pregnant woman. J Fr Ophthalmol 1996; 19:216–221.

61. Quillen DA, Gass DM, Brod RD et al. Central serous chorioretinopathy in women. Ophthalmology 1996; 103:72–79.

62. Sunness JS, Haller JA, Fine SL. Central serous chorioretinopathy and pregnancy. Arch Ophthalmol 1993; 111:360–364.

63. Gass JD. Central serous chorioretinopathy and white subretinal exudation in pregnancy. Arch Ophthalmol 1991; 109:677–681.

64. Fastenberg DM, Ober RR. Central serous choroidopathy in pregnancy. Arch Ophthalmol 1983; 101:1055–1058.

65. Chumbley LC, Frank RN. Central serous retinopathy and pregnancy. Am J Ophthalmol 1974; 77:158–160.

66. Cruysberg JR, Deutman AF. Visual disturbances during pregnancy caused by central serous choroidopathy. Br J Ophthalmol 1982; 66:240–241.

67. Bedrossian RH. Central serous retinopathy and pregnancy. Am J Ophthalmol 1974; 78:152.

68. Cunningham GF, MacDonald PC, Grant NF. Williams obstetrics, 19th edn. Norwalk, Conn: Appleton & Lange, 1993; 224–225.

69. Wiebers DO. Ischemic cerebrovascular complications of pregnancy. Arch Neurol 1985; 42:1106–1113.

70. Ayaki M, Yokoyama N, Furukawa Y. Postpartum CRAO simulating Purtscher's retinopathy. Ophthalmologica 1995; 209:37–39.

71. LaMonica CB, Foye GJ, Silberman L. A case of sudden CRAO and blindness in pregnancy. Obstet Gynecol 1987; 69:433–435.

72. Lara-Torre E, Lee MS, Wolf MA et al. Bilateral retinal occlusion progressing to longlasting blindness in severe pre-eclampsia. Obstet Gynecol 2002; 100:940–942.

73. Gull S, Prentice A. BRAO in pregnancy. Br J Obstet Gynaecol 1994; 101:77–78.

74. Humayun M, Kattah J, Cupps TR et al. Papillophlebitis and arteriolar occlusion in a pregnant woman. J Clin Neuroophthalmol 1992; 12:226–229.

75. Blodi BA, Johnson MW, Gass JD et al. Purtscher's-like retinopathy after childbirth. Ophthalmology 1990; 97:1654–1659.

76. Lanzetta P, Crovato S, Pirrachio A et al. Retinal arteriolar obstruction with progestin treatment of threatened abortion. Acta Ophthalmol Scand 2002; 80:667–669.

77. Nelson ME, Talbot JF, Preston FE. Recurrent multiple branch retinal arteriolar occlusions in a patient with protein C deficiency. Graefes Arch Clin Exp Ophthalmol 1989; 227:443–447.

78. Greven CM, Weaver RG, Owen J et al. Protein S deficiency and bilateral branch retinal artery occlusion. Ophthalmology 1991; 98:33–34.

79. Bergh PA, Hollander D, Gregori CA et al. Mitral valve prolapse and thromboembolic disease in pregnancy: a case report. Int J Gynaecol Obstet 1988; 27:133–137.

80. Kim IT, Choi JB. Occlusions of branch retinal arterioles following amniotic fluid embolism. Ophthalmologica 2002; 21:305–308.

81. Brown GC, Magargal LE, Shields JA. Retinal arterial obstruction in children and young adults. Ophthalmology 1981; 88:18–25.

82. Chew EY, Trope GE, Mitchell BJ. Diurnal intraocular pressure in young adults with central retinal vein occlusion. Ophthalmology 1987; 94: 1545–1549.

83. Gabsi S, Rekik R, Gritli N et al. Occlusion of the central retinal vein in a 6-month pregnant woman. J Fr Ophthalmol 1994; 17:350–354.

84. Gonzalvo FJ, Abecia E, Pinilla I et al. Central retinal vein occlusion and HELLP syndrome. Acta Ophthalmol Scand 2000; 78:596–598.

85. Bjerknes T, Askvik J, Albrechtsen S et al. Retinal detachment in association with pre-eclampsia and abruptio placentae. Eur J Obstet Gynecol Reprod Biol 1995; 60:91–93.

86. Cogan DG. Fibrin clots in the choriocapillaris and serous detachment of the retina. Ophthalmologica 1976; 172:298–307.

87. Martin VA. Disseminated intravascular coagulopathy. Trans Ophthalmol Soc UK 1978; 98:506–507.

88. Hoines J, Buettner H. Ocular complications of disseminated intravascular coagulation (DIC) in abruptio placentae. Retina 1989; 9:105–109.

89. Benson DO, Fitzgibbons JF, Goodnight SH. The visual system in thrombotic thrombocytopenic purpura. Ann Ophthalmol 1980; 12:413–417.

90. Larcan A, Lambert H, Laprevote-Heully MC et al. Acute choriocapillaris occlusions in pregnancy and puerperium. J Mal Vasc 1985; 10:213–219.

91. Coscas G, Gaudric A, Dhermy P et al. Choriocapillaris occlusion in Moschowitz's disease. J Fr Ophtalmol 1981; 4:101–111.

92. Sperry K. Amniotic fluid embolism. JAMA 1986; 255:2183–2203.

93. Chang M, Herbert WN. Retinal arteriolar occlusions following amniotic fluid embolism. Ophthalmology 1984; 91:1634–1637.

94. Kim IT, Choi JB. Occlusions of branch retinal arterioles following amniotic fluid embolisms. Ophthalmologica 2000; 214:305–308.

95. Fischbein FI. Ischemic retinopathy following amniotic fluid embolization. Am J Ophthalmol 1969; 67:351–357.

96. Cunningham GF, MacDonald PC, Grant NF. Williams obstetrics, 19th edn. Norwalk, Conn: Appleton & Lange, 1993; 215.

97. Holly EA, Aston DA, Ahn DK et al. Uveal melanoma, hormonal and reproductive factors in women. Cancer Res 1991; 51:1370–1372.

98. Reese AB. Tumors of the eye, 2nd edn. New York: Hoeber Medical Division, Harper & Row, 1963; 366–370.

99. Borner R, Goder G. Melanoblastoma der uvea and schwangerschaft. Klin Monatsbl Augenheilkd 1966; 149:684.

100. Frenkel M, Klein HZ. Malignant melanoma of the choroids in pregnancy. Am J Ophthalmol 1966; 62:910.

101. Pack GT, Scharnagel IM. The prognosis for malignant melanoma in the pregnant woman. Cancer 1951; 4:324.

102. Seddon JM, MacLaughlin DT, Albert DM et al. Uveal melanomas presenting during pregnancy and the investigation of oestrogen receptors in melanomas. Br J Ophthalmol 1982; 66:695.

103. Siegel R, Amslie WH. Malignant ocular melanoma during pregnancy. JAMA 1963; 185:542.

104. Foss AJ, Alexander RA, Guille MJ et al. Estrogen and progesterone receptor analysis in ocular melanomas. Ophthalmology 1995; 102:431–435.

105. Shields CL, Shields JA, Eagle RC et al. Uveal melanoma and pregnancy. A report of 16 cases. Ophthalmology 1991; 98:1667–1673.

106. Romanowska-Dixon B. Melanoma of choroids during pregnancy: case report. Klin Oczna 2002; 104:395–397.

107. Egan KM, Quinn JL, Gragoudas ES. Childbearing history associated with improved survival in choroidal melanoma. Arch Ophthalmol 1999; 117:939–942.

108. Egan KM, Walsh SM, Seddon JM et al. An evaluation of reproductive factors on the risk of metastases from uveal melanoma. Ophthalmology 1993; 100:1160–1166.

109. Gass JDM. Stereoscopic atlas of macular diseases: a funduscopic and angiographic presentation, 4th edn. St Louis: Mosby, 1997; 218–219.

110. Gass JDM. Stereoscopic atlas of macular diseases: a funduscopic and angiographic presentation, 4th edn. St Louis: Mosby, 1997; 693–695.

111. Gass JDM. Stereoscopic atlas of macular diseases: a funduscopic and angiographic presentation, 3rd edn. St Louis: Mosby, 1987; 512–513.

112. Gass JDM. Stereoscopic atlas of macular diseases: a funduscopic and angiographic presentation, 4th edn. St Louis: Mosby, 1997; 752–754.

113. Gass JDM. Stereoscopic atlas of macular diseases: a funduscopic and angiographic presentation, 3rd edn. St Louis: Mosby, 1987; 380–383.

114. Oday MP, Nielsen P, Al Bozom I. Orbital rhabdomyosarcoma metastatic to the placenta. Am J Obstet Gynecol 1994; 171:1382–1383.

115. Marsh RW, Chu NM. Placental metastasis from primary ocular melanoma: a case report. Am J Obstet Gynecol 1996; 174:1654–1655.

116. Bendon RW, Mimouni F, Khouri J et al. Histopathology of spontaneous abortion in diabetic pregnancies. Am J Perinatol 1990; 7:207–210.

117. Mills J, Simpson JL, Driscoll SG et al. Incidence of spontaneous abortion among normal women and insulin-dependent diabetic women whose pregnancies were identified within 21 days of conception. N Engl J Med 1988; 319:1617–1623.

118. Miller E, Hare JW, Cloherty JP et al. Elevated maternal hemoglobin A1c in early pregnancy and major congenital anomalies in infants of diabetic mothers. N Engl J Med 1981; 304:1331–1334.

119. Klein BK, Klein RK, Meuer SM et al. Does the severity of diabetic retinopathy predict pregnancy outcome? Diabetic Compl 1988; 2:179.

120. Jovanovic R, Jovanovic L. Obstetric management when normoglycemia is maintained in diabetic pregnant women with vascular compromise. Am J Obstet Gynecol 1984; 149:617–623.

121. Sunness JS. The pregnant woman's eye. Surv Ophthalmol 1988; 32:219–238.

122. Diabetes in Early Pregnancy Study Group. Chew EY, James LM, Metzger BE. Metabolic control and progression of retinopathy. Diabetes Care 1995; 18:631–637.

123. The Diabetes Control and Complications Trial Research Group. The effect of intensive diabetes treatment on the progression of diabetic retinopathy in insulin-dependent diabetes mellitus. Arch Ophthalmol 1995; 113:36.

124. Chang S, Fuhrmann M, the Diabetes in Early Pregnancy Study Group. Pregnancy, retinopathy, normoglycemia: a preliminary analysis. Diabetes 1985; 34(suppl):39.

125. KROC Collaborative Study Group. Blood glucose control and the evaluation of diabetic retinopathy and albuminuria. N Engl J Med 1984; 311:365.

126. Kentucky Diabetic Retinopathy Group. Guidelines for eye care in patients with diabetes mellitus. Arch Intern Med 1989; 149:769–770.

127. Cunningham GF, MacDonald PC, Grant NF. Williams obstetrics, 19th edn. Norwalk, Conn: Appleton & Lange, 1993; 763–807.

128. Chen HC, Newsom RSB, Patel V. Retinal blood flow changes during pregnancy in women with diabetes. Invest Ophthalmol Vis Sci 1994; 35:3199–3208.

129. Moloney JM, Drury MI. The effect of pregnancy on the natural course of diabetic retinopathy. Am J Ophthalmol 1982; 93:745.

130. Aiello LM, Rand LI, Briones JC et al. Nonocular clinical risk factors in the progression of diabetic retinopathy. In: Little HL, Jack RL, Patz A et al., eds. New York: Thieme-Stratton, 1983; 21–32.

131. Dibble CM, Kochenour NK, Wocley RJ et al. Effect of pregnancy on diabetic retinopathy. Obstet Gynecol 1982; 59:699.

132. Rosenn B, Miodovnik M, Kranias G et al. Progression of diabetic retinopathy in pregnancy: association with hypertension. Am J Obstet Gynecol 1992; 166:1214.

133. Beetham WP. Diabetic retinopathy in pregnancy. Trans Am Ophthalmol Soc 1950; 48:205.

134. Laatikainen L, Teramo K, Hieta-Heikurainen H et al. A controlled study of the influence of continuous subcutaneous insulin infusion treatment on diabetic retinopathy during pregnancy. Acta Med Scand 1987; 221:367–376.

135. Early Treatment Diabetic Retinopathy Study Research Group: Fundus photographic risk factors for the progression of diabetic retinopathy. Ophthalmology 1991; 98:823.

136. Berk MA, Miodovnik M, Mimouni F. Impact of pregnancy on complications of insulin-dependent diabetes mellitus. Am J Perinatol 1988; 5:359.

137. Axer-Sieger R, Hod M, Fink-Cohen S et al. Diabetic retinopathy during pregnancy. Ophthalmology 1996; 103:1815.

138. Horvat M, MacLean H, Goldberg L et al. Diabetic retinopathy in pregnancy: a 12-year prospective study. Br J Ophthalmol 1980; 64:398.

139. Boone MI, Farber ME, Jovanovic-Peterson L et al. Increased retinal vascular tortuosity in gestational diabetes mellitus. Ophthalmology 1989; 96:251.

140. Hagay Z, Schachter M, Pollack A et al. Development of proliferative retinopathy in a gestational diabetes patient following rapid metabolic control. Eur J Obstet Gynecol Reprod Biol 1994; 57:211.

141. Diabetic Retinopathy Study Research Group. Four risk factors for severe visual loss in diabetic retinopathy. Arch Ophthalmol 1979; 97:654–655.

142. Stoessel KM, Liao PM, Thompson JT et al. Diabetic retinopathy and macular edema in pregnancy. Ophthalmology 1991; 98:146.

143. Reece E, Lockwood C, Tuck S et al. Retinal and pregnancy outcomes in the presence of diabetic proliferative retinopathy. J Reprod Med 1994; 39:799.

144. Serup L. Influence of pregnancy on diabetic retinopathy. Acta Endocrinol 1986; 277:122.

145. Kitzmiller JL, Aiello LM, Kaldany LM et al. Diabetic vascular disease complicating pregnancy. Clin Obstet Gynecol 1981; 24:107.

146. Sinclair SH, Nesler C, Foxman B et al. Macular edema and pregnancy in insulin-dependent diabetes. Am J Ophthalmol 1984; 97:154.

147. Chang S, Fuhrmann M et al. Pregnancy, retinopathy, normoglycemia: a preliminary analysis. Diabetes 1985; 34:39A.

148. Teuscher A, Schnell H, Wilson PWF. Incidence of diabetic retinopathy and relationship to baseline plasma glucose and blood pressure. Diabetes Care 1988; 11:246–251.

149. Rodman HM, Singerman LJ, Aiello LM et al. Diabetic retinopathy and its relationship to pregnancy. In: Merkatz IR, Adams PJ, eds. The diabetic pregnancy: a perinatal perspective. New York: Grune and Stratton, 1979; 73–91.

150. Soubrane G, Canivet J, Coscas G. Influence of pregnancy on the evolution of background retinopathy: preliminary results of a prospective fluorescein angiography study. In: Ryan JJ, Dawson AK, Little HL, eds. Retinal diseases. New York: Grune and Stratton, 1985; 15–20.

151. Ayed S, Jeddi A, Dagfous F et al. Aspects evolutifs de la retinopathie diabetique pendant la grosse. J Fr Ophtalmol 1992; 15:474.

152. Klein BK, Mosse SE, Klein R. Effect of pregnancy on progression of diabetic retinopathy. Diabetes Care 1990; 13:34.

153. Klein BK, Klein R. Gravity and diabetic retinopathy. Am J Epidemiol 1984; 119:564.

154. Lipman MJ, Kranias G, Bene CH et al. The effect of multiple pregnancies on diabetic retinopathy. Ophthalmology 1993; 100:141.

155. Chaturvedi N, Stephenson JM, Fuller JH. The relationship between pregnancy and long-term maternal complications in the EURODIAB IDDM complications study. Diabetic Med 1995; 18:950–954.

156. Kaaja R, Sjoberg L, Hellsted T et al. Long-term effects of pregnancy on diabetic complications. Diabet Med 1996; 13:165–169.

157. Temple RC, Aldridge VA, Sampson MJ et al. Impact of pregnancy on the progression of diabetic retinopathy in type 1 diabetes. Diabet Med 2001; 18:573–577.

158. Lapolla A, Cardone C, Negrin P et al. Pregnancy does not induce or worsen retinal and peripheral nerve dysfunction in insulin-dependent diabetic women. J Diabetes Complic 1998; 12:74–80.

159. Hellstedt T, Kaaja R, Teramo L et al. The effect of pregnancy on mild diabetic retinopathy. Graefes Arch Clin Exp Ophthalmol 1997; 235:437–441.

160. Puza SW, Malee MP. Utilization of routine ophthalmologic examinations in pregnant diabetic patients. J Matern Fetal Med 1996; 5:7–10.

161. Loukovaara S, Kaaja R, Immonen I. Macular capillary blood flow velocity by blue-field entoptoscopy in diabetic and healthy women during pregnancy and the postpartum period. Graefes Arch Clin Exp Ophthalmol 2002; 240:977–982.

162. Loukovaara S, Harju M, Kaaja R et al. Retinal capillary blood flow in diabetic and nondiabetic women during pregnancy and postpartum period. Invest Ophthalmol Vis Sci 2003; 44:1486–1491.

163. Hellstedt T, Kaaja R, Teramo K et al. Macular blood flow during pregnancy in patients with early diabetic retinopathy measured by blue-field entoptic stimulation. Graefes Arch Clin Exp Ophthalmol 1996; 234:659–663.

164. Schocket LS, Grunwald JE, Tsang AF et al. The effect of pregnancy on retinal hemodynamics in diabetic versus nondiabetic mothers. Am J Ophthalmol 1999; 128:477–484.

165. Lauszus FF, Klebe JG, Bek T et al. Increased serum IGF-1 during pregnancy is associated with progression of diabetic retinopathy. Diabetes 2002; 52:852–856.

166. Gibson JM, Westwood M, Lauszus FF et al. Phosphorylated insulin-like growth factor binding protein 1 is increased in pregnant diabetic subjects. Diabetes 1999; 48:321–326.

167. Khaliq A, Foreman D, Ahmed A et al. Increased expression of placenta growth factor in proliferative diabetic retinopathy. Lab Invest 1998; 78:109–116.

168. Spirin KS, Saghizadeh M, Lewin SL et al. Basement membrane and growth factor gene expression in normal and diabetic human retinas. Curr Eye Res 1999; 18:490–499.

169. Best RM, Hayes R, Hadden DR et al. Plasma levels of endothelin-1 in diabetic retinopathy in pregnancy. Eye 1999; 13:179–182.

170. Hill DJ, Flyvbjerg A, Arany E et al. Increased levels of serum fibroblast growth factor-2 in diabetic pregnant women with retinopathy. J Clin Endocrinol Metab 1997; 82:1452–1457.

171. Castellon R, Hamdi HK, Sacerio I et al. Effects of angiogenic growth factor combinations on retinal endothelial cells. Exp Eye Res 2002; 74:523–535.

172. Sameshima H, Kai M, Kajiya S et al. Retinopathy and perinatal outcome in diabetic pregnancy. Nippon Sanka Fujinka Gakkai Zasshi 1995; 47:1048–1054.

173. Zhu L, Nakabayashi M, Takeda Y. Statistical analysis of perinatal outcomes in pregnancy complicated with diabetes mellitus. J Obstet Gynaecol Res 1997; 23:555–563.

174. McElvy SS, Demarini S, Miodovnik M et al. Fetal weight and progression of diabetic retinopathy. Obstet Gynecol 2001; 97:587–592.

175. Lauszus FF, Gron PL, Klebe JG. Pregnancies complicated by diabetic proliferative retinopathy. Acta Obstet Gynecol Scand 1998; 77:814–818.

176. Hiilesmaa V, Suhonen L, Teramo K. Glycaemic control is associated with pre-eclampsia but not with pregnancy-induced hypertension in women with type 1 diabetes mellitus. Diabetologia 2000; 43:1534–1539.

177. Lovestam-Adrian M, Agardh CD, Aberg A et al. Pre-eclampsia is a potent risk factor for deterioration of retinopathy during pregnancy in type 1 diabetic patients. Diabet Med 1997; 14:1059–1065.

178. Diabetes Control and Complications Trial Research Group. Effect of pregnancy on microvascular complications in the diabetes control and complications trial. Diabetes Care 2000; 24:1084–1091.

179. Lauszus F, Klebe JG, Bek T. Diabetic retinopathy in pregnancy during tight metabolic control. Acta Obstet Gynecol Scand 2000; 79:367–370.

180. Oniki S. Prognosis of pregnancy in patients with toxoplasmic retinochoroiditis. Jpn J Ophthalmol 1983; 27:166–174.

181. Perkins ES. Ocular toxoplasmosis. Br J Ophthalmol 1973; 57:1–17.

182. Hemachandra A, Ellis D, Lloyd CE et al. The influence of pregnancy on IDDM complications. Diabetes Care 1995; 18:950–954.

183. Neri A, Grausbord R, Kremer I et al. The management of labor in high myopic patients. Eur J Obstet Gynecol Reprod Biol 1985; 19:277–279.

184. Landau D, Seelenfreund MH, Tadmor O et al. The effect of normal childbirth on eyes with abnormalities predisposing to rhegmatogenous retinal detachment. Graefes Arch Clin Exp Ophthalmol 1995; 233:598–600.

185. Prost M. Severe myopia and delivery. Klin Oczna 1996; 98:129–130.

186. Reese AB. Tumors of the eye, 2nd edn. New York: Hoeber Medical Division, Harper & Row, 1963; 366–370.

187. Cohen VM, Rundle PA, Rennie IG. Choroidal hemangiomas with exudative retinal detachments during pregnancy. Arch Ophthalmol 2002; 120:862–864.

188. Pitta C, Bergen R, Littwin S. Spontaneous regression of a choroidal hemangioma following pregnancy. Ann Ophthalmol 1979; 11:772–774.

189. Snyder DA, Tessler HH. Vogt–Koyanagi–Harada syndrome. Am J Ophthalmol 1980; 90:69–75.

190. Steahly LP. Vogt–Koyanagi–Harada syndrome and pregnancy. Am J Ophthalmol 1990; 22:59–62.

191. Friedman Z, Granat M, Neumann E. The syndrome of Vogt–Koyanagi–Harada and pregnancy. Metab Pediatr Ophthalmol 1980; 4:147–149.

192. Chen SJ, Chung YM, Liu JH. Endogenous Candida endophthalmitis after induced abortion. Am J Ophthalmol 1998; 125:873–875.

193. Sunness JS. The pregnant woman's eye. Surv Ophthalmol 1988; 32:219–238.

194. Yoser SL, Heckenlively JR, Friedman L et al. Evaluation of clinical findings and common symptoms in retinitis pigmentosa. Invest Ophthalmol Vis Sci 1987; 28(suppl):112.

195. Wagener H. Lesions of the optic nerve and retina in pregnancy. JAMA 1934; 103:1910–1913.

196. Rabiah PK, Vitale AT. Noninfectious uveitis and pregnancy. Am J Ophthalmol 2003; 136:91–98.

197. Taguchi C, Ikeda E, Hikita N et al. A report of two cases suggesting positive influence of pregnancy on uveitis activity. Nippon Ganka Gakkai Zasshi 1999; 103:66–71.

198. Hyman BN. Postpartum uveitis. Ann Ophthalmol 1976; 8:677–680.

199. Scott JS. Immunological diseases and pregnancy. Br Med J 1966; 1:1559–1567.

200. Hayaska S, Ugomori S, Kanamori M et al. Pericentral retinal degeneration deteriorates during pregnancies. Ophthalmologica 1990; 200:72–76.

201. Samples JR, Meyer SM. Use of ophthalmic medications in pregnant and nursing women. Am J Ophthalmol 1988; 106:616–623.

202. Soubrane G, Canivet J, Coscas G. Influence of pregnancy on the evolution of background retinopathy: preliminary results of a prospective fluorescein angiography study. In: Ryan SJ, Dawson AK, Little HL, eds. Retinal diseases. New York: Grune & Stratton, 1985.

203. Halperin LS, Olk RJ, Soubrane G et al. Safety of fluorescein angiography during pregnancy. Am J Ophthalmol 1990; 109:563–566.

204. Greenberg F, Lewis RA. Safety of fluorescein angiography during pregnancy (Letter). Am J Ophthalmol 1990; 110:323–324.

205. Valluri S, Adelberg DA, Curtis RS et al. Diagnostic indocyanine green angiography in pre-eclampsia. Am J Ophthalmol 1996; 122:672–677.

206. Iida T, Hagimura N, Otani T et al. Choroidal vascular lesions in serous retinal detachment viewed with indocyanine green angiography. Nippon Ganka Gakkai Zasshi 1996; 100:817–824.

207. Fineman MS, Maguire JI, Fineman SW et al. Safety of indocyanine green angiography during pregnancy: a survey of the retina, vitreous, macula societies. Arch Ophthalmol 2001; 119:353–355.

Chapter

73

Preeclampsia–Eclampsia Syndrome
Richard R. Ober

TERMINOLOGY

The American College of Obstetricians and Gynecologists now prefers a modified version of a clinical classification of hypertensive disorders in pregnancy that was first proposed in 1972 and recently endorsed by the US National High Blood Pressure Education Program (Box 73-1).[1,2] The term *gestational hypertension* has recently replaced the term *pregnancy-induced hypertension* to describe cases in which elevated blood pressure without proteinuria develops in a woman after 20 weeks of gestation and blood pressure levels return to normal postpartum.[2,3] In pregnant women, hypertension is defined as a systolic pressure of 140 mmHg or higher or a diastolic pressure of 90 mmHg or higher that occurs after 20 weeks of gestation in a woman with previously normal blood pressure.[2,3] Although earlier reports suggested that an increase in blood pressure of 30 mmHg systolic or 15 mmHg diastolic from second-trimester values was also of diagnostic value, this concept is no longer considered valid.[2,3]

As many as one-fourth of women with gestational hypertension will develop proteinuria, i.e., preeclampsia.[3] Preeclampsia is a pregnancy-specific syndrome defined by hypertension and proteinuria that may also be associated with myriad other signs and symptoms, such as edema, visual disturbances, headache, and epigastric pain (Box 73-2).[2–4] This multisystem disorder may include coagulation and/or liver function abnormalities. If seizures that cannot be attributed to other causes occur in a woman with preeclampsia, the disorder is termed *eclampsia*.[2–4] Although the phrase "toxemia of pregnancy" was used for over a century to describe preeclampsia–eclampsia, its use is now discouraged because the term was also used for a variety of other poorly understood conditions and because it erroneously implies that a toxin circulating in the blood is the cause of the disorder.

Preeclampsia is classified as mild or severe depending on the extent of blood pressure elevation and proteinuria and the presence of other signs and symptoms of end-organ involvement or fetal growth restriction (Box 73-3).[3] Importantly, the differentiation between mild and severe preeclampsia cannot be rigidly pursued because apparently mild disease may rapidly progress to severe disease.[4,5]

Women with severe preeclampsia and hepatic involvement may develop HELLP syndrome.[6,7] Manifestations include hemolysis (H), elevated liver enzymes (EL), and low platelet counts (LP). In one study, HELLP syndrome occurred in approximately 20%

of women with severe preeclampsia–eclampsia.[6] As with severe preeclampsia, HELLP syndrome is associated with an increased risk of adverse outcomes, and even fetal or maternal death.

SYSTEMIC MANIFESTATIONS

The incidence of preeclampsia is commonly cited to be about 5%, although remarkable variations are reported.[4,5] The incidence of eclampsia between 1990 and 2000 in Dallas, Texas, at Parkland Hospital was approximately 1 in 2300 deliveries.[5] Factors that are associated with an increased risk of preeclampsia include nulliparity, multiple gestation, extremes of age, family history of preeclampsia–eclampsia, African-American heritage, obesity, diabetes mellitus, chronic hypertension, chronic renal disease,

---

Box 73-1 Classification of hypertensive disorders in pregnancy

- Chronic hypertension
- Preeclampsia–eclampsia
- Preeclampsia superimposed on chronic hypertension
- Gestational hypertension
  - o Transient
  - o Chronic

Data from Report of the National High Blood Pressure Education Program Working Group on High Blood Pressure in Pregnancy. Am J Obstet Gynecol 2000; 183:S1–S22.[2]

Box 73-2 Criteria for diagnosis of preeclampsia

- Blood pressure of 140 mmHg systolic or higher or 90 mmHg diastolic or higher that occurs after 20 weeks of gestation in a woman with previously normal blood pressure
- Proteinuria, defined as urinary excretion of 0.3 g protein or higher in a 24-h urine specimen
- Preeclampsia is a pregnancy-specific syndrome that usually occurs after 20 weeks of gestation

Data from American College of Obstetricians and Gynecologists. Diagnosis and management of preeclampsia and eclampsia. ACOG practice bulletin no. 33. Obstet Gynecol 2002; 99:159–167.[3]

antiphospholipid syndrome, hydatidiform mole, and fetal hydrops.[3–5] The etiology of preeclampsia remains unknown; theories include alterations in the immune response, genetic predisposition, increased free radical formation, endothelial cell dysfunction, incomplete invasion by the trophoblast, increased pressor responses, or inflammatory factors.[2–5]

Ordinarily, the onset of preeclampsia is after the 20th week of gestation, and hypertension is the most significant primary sign. Fluid retention may occur, initially causing edema in the lower legs; progression to massive edema, anasarca, or pulmonary edema may occur in severe preeclampsia. Although it is a major traditional criterion, edema is such a common finding in pregnant women that many authorities now feel that its presence should not validate the diagnosis of preeclampsia any more that its absence should preclude the diagnosis.[3–5] However, proteinuria is an important sign of preeclampsia, and the diagnosis is questionable in its absence.[5] Headache is unusual in milder cases but is increasingly frequent in more severe disease. Other symptoms indicating severe preeclampsia are epigastric or right-upper-quadrant pain, vomiting, and visual disturbances (Box 73-3).

Preeclampsia may progress rapidly without warning to the convulsive phase (eclampsia), which is a life-threatening complication of pregnancy.[5] Single or multiple seizures, each lasting approximately 1 min, may be followed by a coma of varying duration. Convulsions are usually preceded by an unrelenting severe headache or visual disturbances; thus these symptoms are considered ominous.

Multiple organs can be involved in the preeclampsia–eclampsia syndrome.[3–5] Cardiovascular effects include systemic vasospasm, abnormal pressor responses to angiotensin II, increased cardiac output, and hemoconcentration. Hematologic consequences include hemolysis, thrombocytopenia, and coagulation abnormalities. Renal function abnormalities include decreased glomerular filtration rate, oliguria, proteinuria, and sodium retention. Other possible abnormal manifestations include hepatic dysfunction, abnormal placental perfusion, and abnormal eicosanoid metabolism.

Box 73-3 Diagnosis of severe preeclampsia

Preeclampsia is considered severe if one or more of the following criteria is present:
- Blood pressure of 160 mmHg systolic or higher or 110 mmHg diastolic or higher on two occasions at least 6 h apart while the patient is on bed rest
- Proteinuria of 5 g or higher in a 24-h urine specimen or 3+ or greater on two random urine samples collected at least 4 h apart
- Oliguria of less than 500 ml in 24 h
- Cerebral or visual disturbances
- Pulmonary edema or cyanosis
- Epigastric or right-upper-quadrant pain
- Impaired liver function
- Thrombocytopenia
- Fetal growth restriction

Data from American College of Obstetricians and Gynecologists. Diagnosis and management of preeclampsia and eclampsia. ACOG practice bulletin no. 33. Obstet Gynecol 2002; 99:159–167.[3]

Neurologic and cerebral manifestations vary from diffuse symptoms such as headache, drowsiness, and confusion to more severe signs and symptoms including hyperreflexia, visual disturbance, blindness, hemiparesis, quadriparesis, grand mal seizures, and coma.[3–5,8] Cerebral involvement is the most frequent cause of death in preeclampsia–eclampsia.[3–5]

OCULAR MANIFESTATIONS

Visual disturbances may occur in 40% of patients with the preeclampsia–eclampsia syndrome, and, on rare occasions, may be the initial symptom.[8] Blurred vision is the most common symptom; other less common symptoms include amaurosis, photopsia, scotomata, diplopia, chromatopsia, and homonymous hemianopsia. The visual system may be affected in 30% to 100% of patients with preeclampsia–eclampsia.[9] Although abnormalities of the retina and retinal vasculature are most frequent, the conjunctiva, choroid, optic nerve, and visual cortex can also be affected in preeclampsia–eclampsia.

Conjunctiva

Mild arteriolar spasm involving the bulbar conjunctival vessels has been observed in normal pregnancy, but in preeclampsia–eclampsia the vasospasm may be severe and can result in local ischemia.[10] Capillary tortuosity, conjunctival hemorrhage, and intravascular thrombi have also been observed.[10]

Retina

Retinal vascular changes occur in 40% to 100% of cases and are the most common abnormality seen in the preeclampsia–eclampsia syndrome.[11–19] The most common retinal abnormality is spasm and narrowing of retinal vessels. Wagener[11] reported spastic lesions of the retinal arterioles in about 70% of cases of preeclampsia–eclampsia. The earliest finding is focal constriction of retinal arterioles (Fig. 73-1), which may progress to generalized narrowing (Fig. 73-2) as the preeclampsia becomes more severe.[9] The retinal vascular abnormalities involve predominantly the posterior pole and may be associated with peripapillary or focal areas of retinal edema. The retinal capillaries may be dilated, and areas of capillary nonperfusion may be present (Fig. 73-3).[12] The retinal vascular changes generally, but not always, correlate with the severity of the systemic hypertension. The vasospastic manifestations are reversible, and the retinal vessels rapidly return to normal after delivery.

Earlier reports[11,13–15] noted the frequent occurrence of retinal hemorrhages and cottonwool spots. However, background changes are probably much more infrequent than would appear from these reports, and if present, suggest the presence of underlying vascular disease, such as diabetes and hypertension, which occur frequently in preeclamptic patients.[9] If permanent organic changes of the retinal vessels develop, they will be manifested by sclerosis of the vessel walls with associated arteriovenous crossing changes and an increased arteriole-to-vein ratio.

Visual loss as a result of retinal vascular involvement is unusual; however, temporary or permanent blindness may result.[20,21] Temporary decrease in vision to the light perception level,

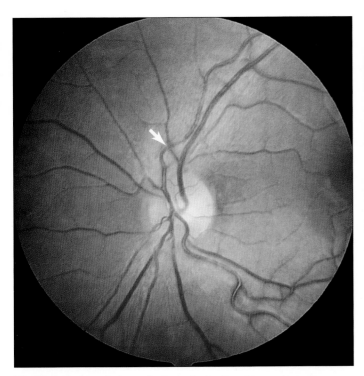

Fig. 73-1 Fundus photograph of a patient with mild preeclampsia demonstrating focal arteriolar constriction (arrow). (Courtesy of G Jaffe and H Schatz.)

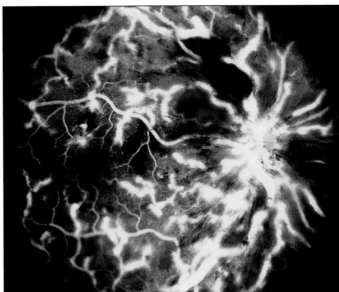

Fig. 73-3 Fluorescein angiogram in preeclamptic patient, showing widespread capillary nonperfusion, perivascular staining, and staining of optic nerve head. (Courtesy of J Price, L Marouf, W Heine, and R Young.)

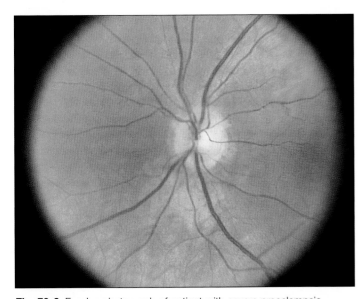

Fig. 73-2 Fundus photograph of patient with severe preeclampsia, showing generalized retinal arteriolar narrowing with increased arteriole-to-vein ratio. (Courtesy of G Jaffe and H Schatz.)

secondary to severe retinal arteriolar spasm and retinal edema, was reported in one patient.[20] Severe central retinal artery angiospasm and secondary optic atrophy were reported as the cause of permanent blindness in another patient.[21]

Other retinal vascular abnormalities in preeclamptic patients involving either retinal capillaries or arterioles have been reported.[22–24] Unilateral visual loss from white-centered retinal hemorrhages was the first clinical feature noted in a normotensive pregnant patient who developed severe preeclampsia within 48 h of the examination.[22] Severe vasospasm with anoxic damage to retinal capillaries was speculated as the cause. Another report described bilateral peripheral retinal neovascularization after resolution of preeclampsia.[23] The pathogenesis was attributed to microthrombus formation, possibly secondary to low-grade disseminated intravascular coagulation. Severe visual loss with findings simulating Purtscher's retinopathy was reported within hours of childbirth in three young women with labor complicated by preeclampsia.[24] Ophthalmoscopy and fluorescein angiography revealed multiple superficial peripapillary and macular patches of ischemic retinal whitening, suggesting a microembolic phenomenon. Complement-activated leukoemboli formed during parturition may be the pathogenesis of this disorder (Fig. 73-4). A more recent report described a preeclamptic patient with bilateral permanent blindness secondary to arteriole occlusions consistent with a Purtscher's-like retinopathy.[25] Another recent report described a bilateral chorioretinopathy with Purtscher's-like findings and macular ischemia in a preeclamptic woman developing one day after delivery.[26]

Branch et al.[27] reported the occurrence of unilateral transient vision loss (amaurosis fugax) in two preeclamptic women with antiphospholipid antibodies. Presumably, the visual disturbances in these patients were secondary to a retinal thrombotic event from a hypercoagulable state, since visual symptoms in collagen-vascular diseases associated with the presence of a lupus anticoagulant have been well documented.[28] However, fundus examination was not performed to document the presence of retinal occlusive disease. Color flow Doppler ultrasonography showed absent or minimal central retinal artery blood flow in a preeclamptic patient with visual disturbances characterized by photopsia.[29] However, no funduscopic documentation was obtained.

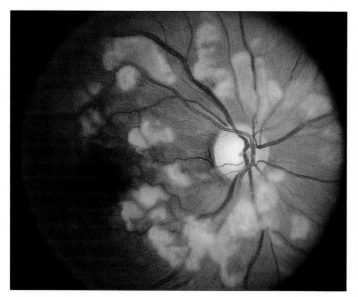

Fig. 73-4 Fundus photograph of preeclamptic patient showing multiple superficial peripapillary and macular patches of ischemic retinal whitening simulating Purtscher's retinopathy.

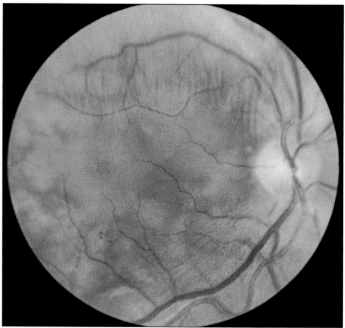

Fig. 73-5 Fundus photograph of a patient with severe preeclampsia demonstrating retinal edema and striae and yellow-white opaque lesions at the level of retinal pigment epithelium. (Courtesy of DM Fastenberg.)

Visual symptoms have been associated with retinal vascular abnormalities in HELLP syndrome.[30–32] Blurred central vision and a central field defect were reported in association with mild constriction of the lower temporal artery in a patient with preeclampsia and HELLP syndrome.[30] A spontaneous vitreous hemorrhage has been reported in a woman in her last trimester of pregnancy who was later diagnosed as having severe preeclampsia and HELLP syndrome.[31] The hemorrhage was thought to be related to a clotting abnormality originating from a small branch arteriole. Unilateral central retinal vein occlusion was noted 10 days after delivery in a woman with severe preeclampsia with HELLP syndrome.[32]

Choroid

First described by von Graefe[33] in 1855, serous retinal detachment is an unusual, but well-documented, cause of visual loss in the preeclamptic–eclamptic syndrome. This complication occurs in less than 1% of preeclamptic patients, with a slightly higher incidence in eclamptic patients.[34–36] The detachments usually occur in patients with severe preeclampsia or eclampsia, and although they rarely may be associated with retinal vascular changes,[37] they are usually observed in the absence of significant retinal vascular abnormalities.[38–41]

Retinal striae may be the first sign of a detachment, followed by generalized retinal edema in the posterior pole. Focal detachments may occur in the posterior pole, which may progress to involve the entire retina. The detachments are usually associated with yellow-white focal lesions at the level of the retinal pigment epithelium[38,42,43] (Fig. 73-5). These mosaic, deep opaque lesions are probably a manifestation of choroidal ischemia, since they reflect the lobular pattern of the choriocapillaris.[42,43] A recent report using optical coherence tomography in a preeclamptic woman showed macular edema persisting for 2 months after

delivery and depicted the characteristic alterations of retinal pigment epithlium and choriocapillaris associated with Elschnig spots.[44]

Bilateral serous retinal detachments have also been reported in a pregnant woman with HELLP syndrome and preeclampsia.[45,46] In both reports, investigators postulated that the pathogenesis of retinal pigment epithelium ischemia in this disorder is lobular choroidal ischemia. Experimental and clinical evidence confirms that serous retinal detachments in patients with preeclampsia–eclampsia result from choroidal vascular damage.[38,40,47,48] Soon after delivery, spontaneous retinal reattachment occurs, and return of vision is complete in most cases, despite the development of permanent pigment epithelial alteration (Elschnig spots).[38,40,41,49] These nonprogressive pigmentary disturbances, if discovered later in life, may be mistaken for a heredomacular dystrophy or a diffuse tapetoretinal dystrophy.[50]

A unilateral choroidal neovascular membrane was recently reported in a 35-year-old preeclamptic woman with the antiphospholipid syndrome.[51] The authors postulated that preeclampsia and antiphospholipid antibodies were both risk factors for choroidal ischemia that led to damage to the choriocapillaris–Bruch's membrane–retinal pigment epithelium complex and secondary choroidal neovascular membrane formation.

Optic nerve

Optic nerve involvement may accompany the retinal vascular changes, and optic atrophy can be the end result and also a cause of visual disability.[45] Papilledema may be observed and is a manifestation of malignant arterial hypertension. Visual loss was described in two preeclamptic patients and occurred as a result of widespread capillary occlusion in which the optic nerve was also involved[12] (Fig. 73-3). Background changes consisting of hemorrhages and cottonwool spots were also present in these patients.

Selective optic nerve involvement is rare in preeclampsia; however, temporary bilateral blindness was reported in one patient who presented with chalky-white nerve heads.[52] The visual loss was thought to be secondary to acute ischemic optic neuropathy as a result of impairment of the blood supply to the prelaminar portion of the optic nerve head. Earlier reports[21,53] of optic neuritis observed in patients with preeclampsia were probably descriptions of hypertensive optic neuropathy, since inflammation is not a manifestation of ocular involvement.

NEUROLOGIC MANIFESTATIONS

Neurologic manifestations of preeclampsia–eclampsia vary from diffuse symptoms such as headaches and confusion to focal signs such as diplopia, visual loss, and paralysis.[8] Transient diplopia secondary to a sixth-nerve palsy has been reported as an unusual manifestation of preeclampsia in one patient.[54] Extensive investigation, including brain scan and cranial angiography, revealed no evidence of other pathology; therefore, intense vasospasm of the vessels supplying the abducens nerve was postulated as the cause for the diplopia.

Severe bilateral visual loss in preeclampsia–eclampsia, occurring in association with normal fundi and pupillary responses and absent optokinetic nystagmus, suggests the diagnosis of cortical blindness.[55–60] Complete visual recovery usually occurs within days, even if light perception is lost. A case of transient cortical blindness following several brief seizures was reported in one patient with preeclampsia and HELLP syndrome.[55] The diagnosis of cortical blindness has been supported by abnormal electroencephalography in preeclamptic patients,[56,57] which, despite visual recovery, may remain abnormal, suggesting persistent cortical dysfunction.[56] The transient nature of the visual loss suggests that cortical blindness originates from cerebral anoxia caused by either vascular spasm or cerebral edema.[56–59]

Cerebral angiographic studies of eclamptic women have been consistent with evidence of cerebral vasospasm.[61,62] Other evidence supports the concept that cortical blindness is induced by vascular changes.[63,64] Using Doppler velocimetry, Williams & McLean[63] showed that cerebral blood flow velocity is increased in patients with preeclampsia, suggesting an increased resistance to flow. Torres et al.[64] also used Doppler velocimetry to demonstrate findings consistent with vasospasm of the posterior cerebral artery in a preeclamptic patient with cortical blindness. However, other investigators[65] using neuroimaging studies in a preeclamptic patient with reversible cortical blindness showed that the blindness resulted from cerebral edema and not cerebral vasospasm.

Recent advances in neuroradiologic imaging, including the use of computed tomography (CT) scans and magnetic resonance imaging (MRI), have greatly enhanced our understanding of the correlation between neurologic complaints and neuroanatomic pathologic changes characteristic of preeclampsia–eclampsia.[56,58–61,66–68] CT scans may demonstrate the presence of cerebral edema in patients with acute visual loss and can confirm postpartum resolution of the edema.[56,58,59,51] CT scans in preeclamptic–eclamptic women with cortical blindness typically show low-density areas predominantly in the occipital lobes.[59,61,66] These areas are nonenhancing and have been attributed to localized areas of decreased perfusion associated with arterial spasm, infarction, or cerebral edema. MRI will probably soon become the imaging method of choice to evaluate the brain in patients with preeclampsia–eclampsia.[59,64,67–69] MRI shows increased signal intensities in the occipital lobes of preeclamptic–eclamptic patients with cortical blindness and is considerably more sensitive than CT scans in the detection of white-matter lesions. Hysteria, intracranial venous thrombosis, and other causes of cortical blindness must also be considered in pregnant patients with visual loss and normal fundi.[70]

FLUORESCEIN AND INDOCYANINE GREEN ANGIOGRAPHY

Fluorescein angiographic studies, although limited, have been helpful in interpreting the abnormal retinal and choroidal vascular changes that occur in preeclampsia. Price et al.[12] described two preeclamptic patients, without retinal detachment, in whom angiography demonstrated retinal vascular decompensation manifested by dilated capillaries, widespread capillary occlusion, and perivascular and optic nerve head staining (Fig. 73-3). Another study[37] demonstrated abnormal retinal capillary filling in a preeclamptic patient with retinal detachment. In contrast, most fluorescein angiographic studies[38–41,71] have emphasized the absence of retinal vascular abnormalities and demonstrated choroidal vascular abnormalities in preeclamptic patients with retinal detachment. Reports[38,40] have demonstrated delayed perfusion of the choriocapillaris in the early phase of the angiogram (Fig. 73-6) and in the middle- and late-phase areas of nonperfusion with foci of gradual fluorescein leakage and coalescence of dye in the subpigment epithelial and subretinal space (Fig. 73-7).

These observations provided clinical evidence that retinal detachment in preeclampsia was secondary to choroidal arteriole and choriocapillaris occlusion. After resolution of the exudative retinal detachment, irregular alterations of the pigment epithelium are usually noted in the macula and posterior pole (Fig. 73-8). These focal areas of depigmentation or hyperpigmentation are the result of healed ischemic infarcts of the choriocapillaris (Elschnig spots) and account for the transmission or blockage of fluorescein dye.[49]

Valluri et al.[72] reviewed postpartum fluorescein and indocyanine green angiographic findings for four patients with preeclampsia. They showed nonperfusion in the early phases of the angiogram (Fig. 73-9) and staining of the choroidal vasculature with subretinal leakage in the late phases of the angiogram (Fig. 73-10). Their results provided direct evidence of choroidal ischemia and suggested that choroidal vascular damage in preeclampsia may not be limited to the choriocapillaris but may also affect the small- to medium-sized vessels in the choroid.

Abnormal multifocal electroretinographic (MERG) changes were reported in a preeclamptic patient with choroidal ischemia 3 months post partum when repeat fluorescein and indocyanine green angiography were unremarkable.[73] The authors concluded

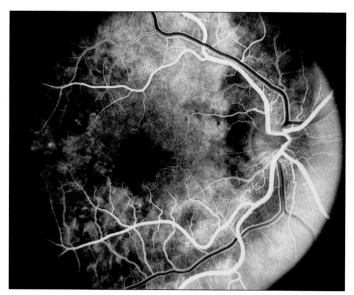

Fig. 73-6 Fluorescein angiogram in arteriovenous phase in a preeclamptic patient 14 days after delivery, showing delayed filling of choriocapillaris. (Reproduced from Mabie WC, Ober RR. Fluorescein angiography in toxaemia of pregnancy. Br J Ophthalmol 1980; 64:666–671.[41])

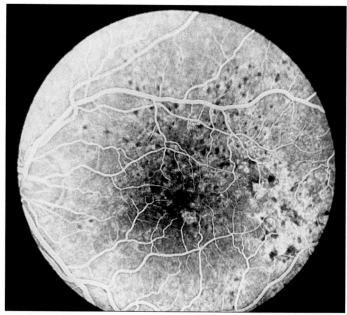

Fig. 73-8 Mid-phase fluorescein angiogram 2 months after delivery in preeclamptic patient showing retinal pigment epithelial disturbance and focal nonfluorescent areas with surrounding hyperfluorescence (Elschnig spots). (Reproduced from Fastenberg DM, Fetkenhour CL, Choromokos E et al. Choroidal vascular changes in toxemia of pregnancy. Am J Ophthalmol 1980; 89:362–368.[38])

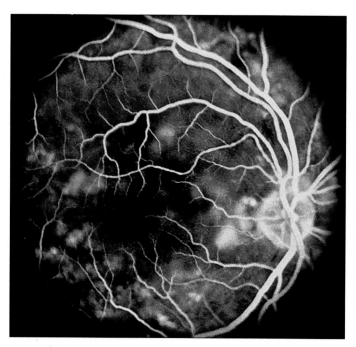

Fig. 73-7 Mid-phase fluorescein angiogram of eclamptic patient 2 days after delivery, showing foci of active fluorescein leakage with pooling of dye in the subpigment epithelial and subretinal spaces. (Reproduced from Fastenberg DM, Fetkenhour CL, Choromokos E et al. Choroidal vascular changes in toxemia of pregnancy. Am J Ophthalmol 1980; 89:362–368.[38])

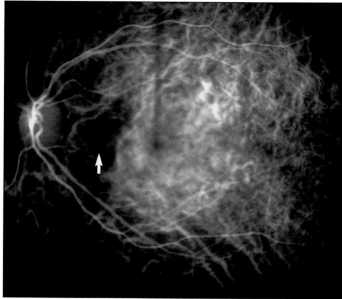

Fig. 73-9 Early-phase indocyanine green angiogram of a patient with severe preeclampsia showing peripapillary choroidal hypoperfusion (arrow). (Reproduced from Valluri S, Adelberg DA, Curtis RS et al. Diagnostic indocyanine green angiography in preeclampsia. Am J Ophthalmol 1996; 122:672–677.72)

that MERG had the advantage of being noninvasive and more sensitive than angiography in the evaluation of macular choroidal ischemia in preeclampsia.

Ocular fluorophotometry was performed in patients with either preeclampsia or eclampsia, and fluorescein concentrations in the aqueous and posterior vitreous increased significantly compared to those in normal subjects.[74] The blood–aqueous barrier and blood–retinal barrier were only disrupted in patients with fluorescein angiograms demonstrating focal or diffuse retinal arteriolar constriction.

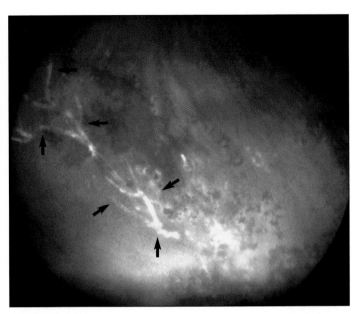

Fig. 73-10 Late-phase indocyanine green angiogram of a patient with severe preeclampsia demonstrating staining of medium-sized choroidal vessels (arrows). (Reproduced from Valluri S, Adelberg DA, Curtis RS et al. Diagnostic indocyanine green angiography in preeclampsia. Am J Ophthalmol 1996; 122:672–677.72)

PATHOPHYSIOLOGY

Systemic

Vasospasm is basic to the pathophysiology of preeclampsia–eclampsia.[3,5] Most effects on the mother in preeclampsia–eclampsia can be categorized as cardiovascular, hematologic, and regional perfusion abnormalities.[3] Vascular constriction causes resistance to blood flow and accounts for the development of arterial hypertension.[5] It is likely that vasospasm itself exerts a damaging effect on blood vessels. An increased sensitivity to angiotensin II, and other pressor agents, results in endothelial cell damage. The vascular changes, together with local hypoxia of the surrounding tissues, lead to hemorrhage, necrosis, and other end-organ disease. Fibrin deposition may be prominent, as seen in fatal cases. The pathophysiology of arterial hypertension is still poorly understood and is probably a multifactorial disease secondary to the interaction of many abnormalities, including genetic effects.[48] Abnormalities may occur in cell membranes, calcium, sodium, and potassium metabolism, the central nervous system, prostaglandins, vascular endothelial-derived vasoactive agents, and the renin–angiotensin–aldosterone system.[48]

Ocular

Experimental and clinical data have improved our understanding of the effects of systemic hypertension on the posterior segment of the eye.[48,75–79] The differing regulatory mechanisms of the retina and choroidal vasculature help to explain the pathogenesis of the fundus abnormalities in preeclampsia and the apparently unrelated manifestations of hypertensive choroidopathy and retinopathy.[48] The retinal circulation has no sympathetic innervation and is largely under the influence of autoregulatory mecha-

nisms. The exact mechanism and site of autoregulation are still unclear, except that autoregulation probably operates by altering the vascular resistance. An abrupt rise in blood pressure excites normal retinal vessels to increase their vascular tone (vasoconstriction) by autoregulatory mechanisms. If elevated blood pressure is controlled, the retinal vessels return to a normal state without permanent vascular damage. However, if elevated blood pressure is prolonged, autoregulation fails and dilation of terminal arterioles with disruption of the blood–retinal barrier occurs. The capillary bed is exposed to higher pressures, and subsequently, occlusion of terminal arterioles occurs, causing capillary nonperfusion and ischemia with associated hemorrhages, cottonwool spots, and retinal edema. Finally, permanent sclerotic changes in the vessels may develop.

Studies have suggested that vascular endothelial-derived vasoactive agents modulate local vascular tone and thereby may play a role in autoregulation.[48] Interestingly, Hayreh's experimental studies[48] in hypertensive rhesus monkeys revealed no "spasm" of retinal arterioles by fluorescein angiography in acute phases of hypertension, contradicting classical teaching. He referred to the ophthalmoscopic findings of arteriolar narrowing as an artifact produced by retinal edema partially masking the arterioles from the sides.

The choroidal vascular tone is primarily controlled by the sympathetic nervous system.[48,67,68] The choroidal arterioles undergo constriction in response to systemic hypertension; however, increased blood pressure can overcome the compensatory tone of the sympathetic response, and vascular damage can result. The cause of choroidal occlusion noted in patients with hypertensive choroidopathy is poorly understood; in addition to ocular sympathetic derangement, other mechanisms have been proposed. Leaking vasoconstrictor agents, including angiotensin II, epinephrine (adrenaline), and vasopressin, may act on the walls of choroidal vessels, resulting in choroidal vasoconstriction and ischemia.[48]

Collier[47] reproduced choroidal ischemia by retrograde injection of latex microspheres into feline vortex veins. He postulated that occlusion of the choriocapillaris led to increased hydrostatic pressure, with subsequent vasodilation of the choriocapillaris and fluid seepage into the subretinal space. Fibrin–platelet occlusion of the choroidal arteries and choriocapillaris may occur as part of disseminated intravascular coagulopathy, which is seen in a variety of disease states, including preeclampsia.[80] The predilection for fibrin–platelet intravascular coagulopathy to occur in the macular area may be related to the rapid deceleration of blood flow as it empties from the short posterior ciliary arteries into the large sinusoidal network of the choriocapillaris.[80] Finally, emboli may originate in the products of conception on an immunologic basis.[38] Klein[49] showed that multifocal areas of choroidal vascular occlusion produced ischemic changes in the overlying retinal pigment epithelium and outer retinal layers, leading to acute exudative retinal detachment and subsequent late pigmentary alterations (Elschnig spots).

The pathogenesis of hypertensive optic neuropathy is controversial.[48,75,78,79] The optic nerve head has a complicated blood supply; it is supplied anteriorly by branches of the central retinal artery, with the primary source being the posterior ciliary artery circulation, and peripapillary choroid, a major source. In addition, the optic nerve head is under the influence of intraocular pressure anteriorly and intracranial pressure in the subarachnoid space posteriorly. Evidence suggests that the optic disc swelling seen in malignant hypertension is a distinct entity and not simply a manifestation of elevated intracranial pressure, hypertensive retinopathy, or hypertensive encephalopathy.[75] Hypertensive optic neuropathy is postulated to represent a form of anterior ischemic optic neuropathy. Ischemia of axons results in axoplasmic flow stasis and axonal swelling of the optic disc.[79] The cause of optic nerve head ischemia in malignant hypertension is probably a combination of vasoconstriction and vaso-occlusive changes of the peripapillary choroid and diffusion of angiotensin II and other endogenous vasoconstrictors into the optic nerve head from the peripapillary choroid.[48]

HISTOPATHOLOGY

Systemic

Almost every organ in the body can be affected in severe preeclampsia–eclampsia. Most of the pathologic changes noted can be attributed to hypoxia resulting from severe abnormal vasospasm, leading to ischemia, hemorrhage, thrombosis, and necrosis of tissues.[5] The histopathologic lesions may resolve, but if ischemia is severe enough, extensive infarction of organs can occur. Organs frequently affected by the ischemic process include placenta, kidney, liver, brain, heart, and lung.

Ocular

The ocular histopathologic changes in preeclampsia–eclampsia are similar to those seen in other severe hypertensive disorders. Experimental studies[76–79] demonstrated the vascular changes in severe systemic hypertension that were characterized by acute ischemia. In hypertensive retinopathy, retinal capillaries showed narrowed lumina, degeneration of pericytes, and vascular leakage resulting from disruption of the blood–retinal barrier.[79] Fibrinoid necrosis of retinal arterioles occurred in the most severe cases. In the sclerotic stage of hypertensive retinopathy, the retinal vessels showed thickening and hyperplasia of muscle cells. As degeneration progressed, the retinal vessels developed hyalinized walls with loss of muscle cells. In hypertensive choroidopathy, severe vascular narrowing or fibrin–platelet occlusion of choroidal arterioles and choriocapillaris caused fibrinoid necrosis of the vessel walls.[76,77,79] The acute ischemia of the overlying retinal pigment epithelium resulted in retinal detachment and subretinal exudate. As recovery occurred, small characteristic scars (Elschnig spots) with central pigment spots developed in the posterior pole and represented healed ischemic infarcts of the retinal pigment epithelium and choriocapillaris.[49] Experimental clinicopathologic studies[78] to elucidate the pathogenesis of hypertensive optic neuropathy demonstrated severe vasoconstriction that resulted in optic nerve changes ranging from optic disc edema to optic atrophy. Optic disc edema appeared to result from axonal hydropic swelling secondary to ischemic infarcts, and this was followed by eventual loss of axons and by gliosis.

MANAGEMENT PRINCIPLES

Maternal and fetal

No single screening test for preeclampsia has been found to be reliable and cost-effective.[3] Whereas several reports suggest that, although administration of low-dose aspirin (60 to 80 mg) may be an appropriate option in women at high risk for developing preeclampsia, aspirin use is not currently recommended for preeclampsia prophylaxis.[3–5] A preliminary report suggested that antioxidant-loading with vitamins E and C prevents preeclampsia.[3–5] These results need to be confirmed in larger randomized trials. Daily calcium supplementation has not been shown to prevent preeclampsia and therefore is not recommended.[3–5]

Delivery is the only definitive treatment for preeclampsia.[3–5] The mother with preeclampsia benefits by immediate delivery, since the signs and symptoms of preeclampsia are reversible after delivery. However, the fetus benefits if allowed to remain in utero as long as possible, since this reduces complications associated with prematurity. Therefore a decision regarding the timing of delivery is critical in the preeclamptic patient. For a preterm patient with mild preeclampsia, conservative management is generally indicated.[3–5] Medical management is directed towards correcting the specific abnormal manifestations, such as reduction of hypertension and correction of electrolyte imbalances. If preeclampsia fails to improve in response to medical management, delivery by either induction of labor or cesarean section is usually advisable. Delivery should be considered in women who have signs and symptoms of severe preeclampsia at 32 to 34 weeks of gestation. When delivery is indicated, parenteral magnesium sulfate is generally administered to prevent seizures. Women with eclampsia require prompt intervention. Treatment of eclampsia consists of: (1) control of convulsions; (2) correction of hypoxia and acidosis; (3) blood pressure control; and (4) delivery after control of convulsions.[3–5]

Ocular

The fundus abnormalities in preeclampsia generally improve in response to appropriate medical management or upon spontaneous or elective delivery. Many earlier reports[11,13–17,19,81,82] stressed the value of the fundus examination in the diagnosis, prognosis, and management of the preeclamptic patient. Strong emphasis was placed on the importance of the degree of retinal arteriolar narrowing (vasospasm) and its prognostic implication for the survival of the newborn. Termination of the pregnancy was advocated in cases of severe retinal vascular involvement to reduce fetal mortality and to prevent permanent damage to the mother's vascular system. However, these studies were retrospective and uncontrolled, and many of the patients had underlying vascular disease, such as diabetes and hypertension.

Jaffe & Schatz[9] performed a prospective, controlled, masked study in 56 pregnant women, and divided them into normal, mild preeclamptic, and severe preeclamptic groups. They concluded that the arteriole-to-vein ratio and the number of focal constrictions did not differ significantly between the normal pregnant group and the mild preeclamptic group. Although they could differentiate the severe preeclamptic patient from the normal patient and the mild preeclamptic patient, since the diagnosis is clinically obvious in severe preeclampsia, they concluded that the role of the ophthalmologist in the diagnosis and management of preeclampsia is limited. They suggested that, rather than using retinal arteriolar caliber as a screening test, a more useful test might be a simple estimate of visual acuity, which could be performed by the obstetrician using a Snellen card. Amsler grid testing could provide a similar simple screening test. Patients with visual loss or distortion could then be referred, if necessary, for ophthalmic evaluation.

Fluorescein and indocyanine green angiography have been useful in limited studies[38–41,72] in elucidating the pathogenesis of retinal detachment in preeclamptic patients and could possibly provide information for recognizing early preeclampsia, such as subclinical choriocapillaris damage. However, it is unlikely that sufficient information could be obtained to provide useful guidelines for the termination of pregnancy, and although there is no evidence to suggest that fluorescein is toxic to the fetus, some investigators[38,40,72] have expressed concern over this possibility.

PROGNOSIS

Maternal and perinatal

The preeclampsia–eclampsia syndrome is a major cause of maternal death and obstetric morbidity. Fortunately, maternal mortality due to eclampsia has decreased in the past three decades from 5% to 10% to less than 3% of cases.[5] Maternal mortality is mainly due to cerebrovascular lesions. Other causes of death include pulmonary edema and cardiac, liver, or renal failure. Deaths from preeclampsia alone are rare. The perinatal mortality rate has ranged from 13% to 30%, although comparisons of perinatal mortality rates are difficult to make because of different definitions of stillbirths and neonatal deaths in different countries.[83]

Visual

Despite the common occurrence of visual symptoms, blindness in preeclampsia–eclampsia is uncommon and usually temporary and reversible, with generally complete recovery of vision.[60] Dieckmann[84] cited an incidence of amaurosis from 1% to 3% in eclampsia. Cunningham et al.,[59] claiming blindness to be more common, recently reported an incidence of 15% in women with severe preeclampsia or eclampsia. Blindness subsequently resolved in all patients, 14 out of 15 patients having had cortical blindness. Although cortical blindness, associated with cerebral edema and normal fundi, is generally reversible, persistent visual field deficits have been reported.[56–59,61,66]

Temporary blindness with subsequent complete visual recovery has been explained on the basis of reversible severe retinal arteriolar vasospasm.[20,52] Isolated cases of permanent total blindness as a result of retinal arteriolar occlusion have been reported in the literature but are extremely rare.[21,26,70] A case of permanent blindness was recently reported in a preeclamptic patient with both retinal (Purtscher's-like retinopathy) and brain (MRI findings consistent with bilateral lateral geniculate infarcts) abnormalities.[85] The authors emphasized the importance of a multidisciplinary approach to the evaluation of blindness in the preeclamptic women. Optic atrophy secondary to retinal vascular involvement or selective ischemia of the optic nerve is unusual but may cause visual impairment.[21,52,70] Visual loss secondary to retinal detachment is usually temporary, with visual recovery occurring within days after delivery.[38–41] However, despite spontaneous retinal reattachment, focal pigmentary macular disturbances with some visual impairment may persist.[35]

REFERENCES

1. Hughes EC, ed. Obstetric-gynecologic terminology. Philadelphia: FA Davis; 1972:422.
2. Report of the National High Blood Pressure Education Program Working Group on High Blood Pressure in Pregnancy. Am J Obstet Gynecol 2000; 182:S1–S22.
3. American College of Obstetricians and Gynecologists. Diagnosis and management of preeclampsia and eclampsia. ACOG practice bulletin no. 33. Obstet Gynecol 2002; 99:159–167.
4. Barron WM. Hypertension. In: Barron WM, Lindheimer MD, eds. Medical disorders during pregnancy, 4th edn. St Louis: Mosby; 2000:1–38.
5. Cunningham FG, Gant NF, Leveno KJ et al. Hypertensive disorders in pregnancy. In: Williams obstetrics, 21st edn. New York: McGraw-Hill; 2001:567–618.
6. Sibai BM, Ramadan MK, Usta I et al. Maternal morbidity and mortality in 442 pregnancies with hemolysis, elevated liver enzymes, and low platelets (HELLP syndrome). Am J Obstet Gynecol 1993; 169:1000–1006.
7. Weinstein L. Syndrome of hemolysis, elevated liver enzymes and low platelet count: a severe consequence of hypertension in pregnancy. Am J Obstet Gynecol 1982; 142:159–163.
8. Royburt M, Seidman DS, Serr DM et al. Neurologic involvement in hypertensive disease of pregnancy. Obstet Gynecol Surv 1991; 46:656–664.
9. Jaffe G, Schatz H. Ocular manifestations of preeclampsia. Am J Ophthalmol 1987; 103:309–315.
10. Landesman R, Douglas RG, Holze E. The bulbar conjunctival vascular bed in the toxemias of pregnancy. Am J Obstet Gynecol 1954; 68:170–183.
11. Wagener HP. Arterioles of the retina in toxemia of pregnancy. JAMA 1933; 101:1380–1384.
12. Price J, Marouf L, Heine MW et al. New angiographic findings in toxemia of pregnancy: evidence for retinal and choroidal vascular decompensation. Poster presentation at American Academy of Ophthalmology annual meeting, New Orleans, November 9–13, 1986.
13. Hallum AV. Eye changes in hypertensive toxemia of pregnancy: a study of three hundred cases. JAMA 1936; 106:1649–1651.
14. Hallum AV. Changes in retinal arterioles associated with the hypertensions of pregnancy. Arch Ophthalmol 1947; 37:472–490.
15. Wagener HP. Lesions of the optic nerve and retina in pregnancy. JAMA 1934; 103:1910–1913.
16. Landesman R, Douglas RG, Snyder SS. Retinal changes in the toxemias of pregnancy. I. History, vomiting of pregnancy, mild and severe pre-eclampsia, and eclampsia. Am J Obstet Gynecol 1951; 62:1020–1033.
17. Landesman R, Douglas RG, Snyder SS. Retinal changes in the toxemias of pregnancy. II. Mild and severe hypertension, renal disease, and diabetes mellitus. Am J Obstet Gynecol 1952; 63:16–27.
18. Sadowsky A, Serr DM, Landau J. Retinal changes and fetal prognosis in the toxemias of pregnancy. Obstet Gynecol 1956; 8:426–431.
19. Schultz JF, O'Brien CS. Retinal changes in hypertensive toxemia of pregnancy: a report of 47 cases. Am J Ophthalmol 1938; 21:767–774.
20. Gandhi J, Ghosh S, Pillari VT. Blindness and retinal changes with preeclamptic toxemia. NY State J Med 1978; 78:1930–1932.
21. Somerville-Large LB. A case of permanent blindness due to toxaemia of pregnancy. Br J Ophthalmol 1950; 34:431–434.
22. Capoor S, Goble RR, Wheatley T et al. White-centered retinal hemorrhages as an early sign of preeclampsia. Am J Ophthalmol 1995; 119:804–806.
23. Brancato R, Menchini U, Bandello F. Proliferative retinopathy and toxemia of pregnancy. Ann Ophthalmol 1987; 19:182–183.
24. Blodi BA, Johnson MW, Gass JDM et al. Purtscher's-like retinopathy after childbirth. Ophthalmology 1990; 97:1654–1659.
25. Lara-Torre E, Lee MS, Wolf MA et al. Bilateral retinal occlusion progressing to long-lasting blindness in severe preeclampsia. Obstet Gynecol 2002; 100:940–942.
26. Shaikh S, Ruby AJ, Piotrowski M. Preeclampsia-related chorioretinopathy with Purtscher's-like findings and macular ischemia. Retina 2003; 23:247–250.
27. Branch DW, Andres R, Digre KB et al. The association of antiphospholipid antibodies with severe preeclampsia. Obstet Gynecol 1989; 73:541–545.
28. Levine SR, Crofts JW, Lesser GR et al. Visual symptoms associated with the presence of a lupus anticoagulant. Ophthalmology 1988; 95:686–692.

29. Belfort MA, Saade GR. Retinal vasospasm associated with visual disturbance in preeclampsia: color flow Doppler findings. Am J Obstet Gynecol 1993; 169:523–525.

30. Wentzel M, Lehnen H. A case of mild ocular manifestations in pregnancy-induced hypertension with HELLP syndrome. Acta Ophthalmol (Copenh) 1994; 72:391–392.

31. Leff SR, Yarian DL, Masciulli L et al. Vitreous hemorrhage as a complication of HELLP syndrome. Br J Ophthalmol 1990; 74:498.

32. Gonzalo FJ, Abecia E, Pinilla I et al. Central retinal vein occlusion and HELLP syndrome. Acta Ophthalmol Scand 2000; 78:596–598.

33. von Graefe A. Ueber eine Krebsablagerung im Innern des Auges, deren ursprunglicher Sitz zwischen Sclera und Choroidea war. Graefes Arch Klin Ophthalmol 1855; 2:214–224.

34. Bosco JAS. Spontaneous nontraumatic retinal detachment in pregnancy. Am J Obstet Gynecol 1961; 82:208–212.

35. Dornan KJ, Mallek DR, Wittmann BK. The sequelae of serous retinal detachment in preeclampsia. Obstet Gynecol 1982; 60:657–663.

36. Fry WE. Extensive bilateral retinal detachment in eclampsia, with complete reattachment: report of two cases. Arch Ophthalmol 1929; 1:609–614.

37. Kenny GS, Cerasoli JR. Color fluorescein angiography in toxemia of pregnancy. Arch Ophthalmol 1972; 87:383–388.

38. Fastenberg DM, Fetkenhour CL, Choromokos E et al. Choroidal vascular changes in toxemia of pregnancy. Am J Ophthalmol 1980; 89:362–368.

39. Gitter KA, Houser BP, Sarin KL et al. Toxemia of pregnancy: an angiographic interpretation of fundus changes. Arch Ophthalmol 1968; 80:449–454.

40. Mabie WC, Ober RR. Fluorescein angiography in toxaemia of pregnancy. Br J Ophthalmol 1980; 64:666–671.

41. Oliver M, Uchenik D. Bilateral exudative retinal detachment in eclampsia without hypertensive retinopathy. Am J Ophthalmol 1980; 90:792–796.

42. Saito Y, Omoto T, Fukuda M. Lobular pattern of choriocapillaris in pre-eclampsia with aldosteronism. Br J Ophthalmol 1990; 74:702–703.

43. Saito Y, Tano Y. Retinal pigment epithelial lesions associated with choroidal ischemia in preeclampsia. Retina 1998; 18:103–108.

44. Theodossiadis MD, Kollia AK, Gogas DP et al. Retinal disorders in preeclampsia studied with optical coherence tomography. Am J Ophthalmol 2002; 133:707–709.

45. Burke JP, Whyte I, MacEwen CJ. Bilateral serous retinal detachments in the HELLP syndrome. Acta Ophthalmol (Copenh) 1989; 67:322–324.

46. Tranos PG, Wickremashinghe SS, Hundal KS et al. Bilateral serous retinal detachment as a compilation of HELLP syndrome. Eye 2002; 16:491–492.

47. Collier RH. Experimental embolic ischemia of the choroids. Arch Ophthalmol 1967; 77:683–692.

48. Hayreh SS. Systemic arterial blood pressure and the eye. Eye 1996; 10:5–28.

49. Klein BA. Ischemic infarcts of the choroid (Elschnig spots): a cause of retinal separation in hypertensive disease with renal insufficiency – a clinical and histopathologic study. Am J Ophthalmol 1968; 66:1069–1091.

50. Gass JDM, Pautler SE. Toxemia of pregnancy pigment epitheliopathy masquerading as a heredomacular dystrophy. Trans Am Ophthalmol Soc 1985; 83:114–130.

51. Curi AL, Jacks A, Pavesio C. Choroidal neovascular membrane presenting as a complication of preeclampsia in a patient with the antiphospholipid syndrome. Br J Ophthalmol 2000; 84:1080.

52. Beck RW, Gamel JW, Willcourt RJ et al. Acute ischemic optic neuropathy in severe preeclampsia. Am J Ophthalmol 1980; 90:342–346.

53. Mathew M, Rajani CK, Gulati N. Amaurosis in toxaemia of pregnancy. Ind J Ophthalmol 1975; 23:25–26.

54. Barry-Kinsella C, Milner M, McCarthy N et al. Sixth nerve palsy: an unusual manifestation of preeclampsia. Obstet Gynecol 1994; 83:849–851.

55. Levavi H, Neri A, Zoldan J et al. Pre-eclampsia, "HELLP" syndrome, and postictal cortical blindness. Acta Obstet Gynecol Scand 1987; 66:91–92.

56. Grimes DA, Ekbladh LE, McCartney WH. Cortical blindness in preeclampsia. Int J Gynaecol Obstet 1980; 17:601–603.

57. Nishimura RN, Koller R. Isolated cortical blindness in pregnancy. West J Med 1982; 137:335–337.

58. Beeson JH, Duda EE. Computed axial tomography scan demonstration of cerebral edema in eclampsia preceded by blindness. Obstet Gynecol 1982; 60:529–532.

59. Cunningham FG, Fernandez CO, Hernandez C. Blindness associated with preeclampsia and eclampsia. Am J Obstet Gynecol 1995; 172:1291–1298.

60. Do DV, Rismondo V, Nguyen QD. Reversible cortical blindness in preeclampsia. Am J Ophthalmol 2002; 134:916–918.

61. Lewis LK, Hinshaw DB, Will AD et al. CT and angiographic correlation of severe neurological disease in toxemia of pregnancy. Neuroradiology 1988; 30:59–64.

62. Will AD, Lewis KL, Hinshaw DB Jr et al. Cerebral vasoconstriction in toxemia. Neurology 1987; 37:1555–1557.

63. Williams KP, McLean C. Peripartum changes in maternal cerebral blood flow velocity in normotensive and preeclamptic patients. Obstet Gynecol 1993; 82:334–337.

64. Torres P, Antolin E, Gratacos E et al. Cortical blindness in preeclampsia: diagnostic evaluation by transcranial Doppler and magnetic resonance imaging techniques. Acta Obstet Gynecol Scand 1995; 74:642–644.

65. Apollon KM, Robinson JN, Schwartz RB et al. Cortical blindness in severe preeclampsia: computed tomography, magnetic resonance imaging and single-photon-emission computed tomographic findings. Obstet Gynecol 2000; 95:1017–1019.

66. Lau SPC, Chan FL, Yu YL et al. Cortical blindness in toxaemia of pregnancy: findings on computed tomography. Br J Radiol 1987; 60:347–349.

67. Digre KB, Varner MW, Osborn AG et al. Cranial magnetic resonance imaging in severe preeclampsia vs eclampsia. Arch Neurol 1993; 50:399–406.

68. Sanders TG, Clayman DA, Sanchez-Ramos L et al. Brain in eclampsia: MR imaging with clinical correlation. Radiology 1991; 180:475–478.

69. Herzog TI, Angel OH, Karram MM et al. Use of magnetic resonance imaging in the diagnosis of cortical blindness in pregnancy. Obstet Gynecol 1990; 76:980–982.

70. Carpenter F, Kava HL, Plotkin D. The development of total blindness as a complication of pregnancy. Am J Obstet Gynecol 1953; 66:641–647.

71. Schreyer P, Tzadok J, Sherman DJ et al. Fluorescein angiography in hypertensive pregnancies. Int J Gynecol Obstet 1990; 34:127–132.

72. Valluri S, Adelberg DA, Curtis RS et al. Diagnostic indocyanine green angiography in preeclampsia. Am J Ophthalmol 1996; 122:672–677.

73. Kwok AK, Li JZ, Chan WM et al. Multifocal electroretinographic and angiographic changes in pre-eclampsia. Br J Ophthalmol 2001; 85:111–112.

74. Chaine G, Attali P, Gaudric A et al. Ocular fluorophotometric and angiographic findings in toxemia of pregnancy. Arch Ophthalmol 1986; 104:1632–1635.

75. Hayreh SS, Servais GE, Virdi PS. Fundus lesions in malignant hypertension. V. Hypertensive optic neuropathy. Ophthalmology 1986; 93:74–87.

76. Hayreh SS, Servais GE, Virdi PS. Fundus lesions in malignant hypertension. VI. Hypertensive choroidopathy. Ophthalmology 1986; 93:1383–1400.

77. Kishi S, Tso MOM, Hayreh SS. Fundus lesions in malignant hypertension. I. A pathologic study of experimental hypertensive choroidopathy. Arch Ophthalmol 1985; 103:1189–1197.

78. Kishi S, Tso MOM, Hayreh SS. Fundus lesions in malignant hypertension. II. A pathologic study of experimental hypertensive optic neuropathy. Arch Ophthalmol 1985; 103:1198–1206.

79. Tso MOM, Jampol LM. Pathophysiology of hypertensive retinopathy. Ophthalmology 1982; 89:1132–1145.

80. Cogan DG. Ocular involvement in disseminated intravascular coagulopathy. Arch Ophthalmol 1975; 93:1–8.

81. Cheney RC. The toxemias of pregnancy from an ophthalmologic standpoint. JAMA 1924; 83:1383–1390.

82. Mussey RD, Mundell BJ. Retinal examinations: a guide in the management of the toxic hypertensive syndrome of pregnancy. Am J Obstet Gynecol 1939; 37:30–36.

83. Cunningham FG, MacDonald PC, Gant NF et al. Hypertensive disorders in pregnancy. In: Williams obstetrics, 20th edn. Stamford, CT: Appleton & Lange; 1997:693–744.

84. Dieckmann WJ. The toxemias of pregnancy, 2nd edn. St Louis: Mosby; 1952:240–249.

85. Museman CP, Shelton S. Permanent blindness as a complication of pregnancy-induced hypertension. Obstet Gynecol 2002; 100:943–945.

Chapter

74

Hypertension

Robert P. Murphy
Linda A. Lam
Emily Y. Chew

Hypertension has been ranked as the fourth largest mortality risk factor in the world, accounting for 6% of all deaths. Mild hypertension accounts for the largest proportion of cardiovascular deaths in the USA because of its high prevalence.[1] As many as an estimated 58 million adults in the USA have elevated blood pressure (systolic blood pressure ≥ 140 mmHg or diastolic blood pressure ≥ 90 mmHg) or are taking antihypertensive medication.[2]

Although improvement in the diagnosis and treatment of systemic hypertension in the past several decades has reduced the morbidity and mortality rates due to this disease, the management of hypertension and its complications challenges all physicians.

Systemic hypertension may accelerate the progression of diabetic retinopathy and may be associated with an increased risk of retinal arterial and venous occlusion.[3-5] Hypertensive disease, in which there is persistent pathologic elevation of arterial pressure and increased total peripheral resistance, is associated with vascular lesions in the brain, heart, kidneys, and eyes. Although the causes of hypertension are as varied as they are numerous, in more than 90% of patients the cause is not known.

Elevation of systemic blood pressure causes both focal and generalized retinal arteriolar constriction, presumably mediated by autoregulation. These findings are relatively common in longstanding hypertension. A prolonged duration of particularly high blood pressure can be associated with a breakdown of the inner blood–retinal barrier, with extravasation of plasma and red blood cells. Retinal hemorrhages, cottonwool spots, intraretinal lipid, and, in severe cases, the development of a macular star configuration of intraretinal lipid can be seen.[6] In severe hypertension, closure of retinal capillaries can be observed. When the choroidal vessels are severely affected by elevated blood pressure, as in acute hypertension, fibrinoid necrosis of choroidal arterioles can cause occlusion of areas of choriocapillaris, with a subsequent breakdown of the outer blood–retinal barrier. In severe cases the optic nerve can be involved.

In most cases the hypertensive changes are not extensive enough to induce breakdown of either the inner or outer blood–retinal barriers. Instead, the chronic effects of hypertension on the retinal vessels become intimately associated with arteriolosclerotic changes in the retina characterized by vascular thickening. The complex relationship between pure hypertensive vascular changes and the changes of arteriolosclerosis, coupled with the great variation of expression of these changes, makes it difficult to describe a classification of retinal vascular changes due to hypertension alone.

Recently, for research purposes, a method of objectively evaluating the retinal vessel calibers from digitized fundus photographs provided information regarding the association of microvascular characteristics with macrovascular disease, such as cardiovascular disease and strokes.[7] In the Beaver Dam Eye Study, a population-based study, the calibers of retinal vessels were measured using this technique. The results showed that narrowed retinal arterioles were associated with long-term risk of hypertension, suggesting that structural alterations of the microvasculature may be linked to the development of hypertension.[8] However, in the Blue Mountain Eye Study, another population-based study, past and current hypertension was felt to be a direct cause of significant arteriolar narrowing of the retinal vessels when these methods of vessel diameters were applied.[9] Nevertheless, these results point to the association of hypertension to retinal vascular changes. Unfortunately, these techniques are not easily applied in clinical practice.

In a prospective study, the presence of hypertensive retinopathy diagnosed clinically was correlated with a doubling of the risk of coronary heart disease events.[10] The possible role of systemic risk factors, such as hyperlipidemia, in the development of retinal arteriolar changes has been implicated in previous clinical studies.[11] A study performed on a small number of patients has concluded that lipidemia by itself is not a risk factor for the development of retinal changes.[12] Racial differences exist in the prevalence of diabetic retinopathy, as the prevalence of hypertensive retinopathy in African Americans has been found to be twice that in whites.[13]

ARTERIOSCLEROSIS AND HYPERTENSION

Traditionally, the arteriolar changes of hypertension have been considered to result primarily from vasospasm, whereas the arteriolosclerotic changes result from thickening of the arteriolar wall. Because hypertension has such an important effect on the development of arteriolosclerotic changes, it is impossible to consider them entirely separately. This relationship must be considered when any of the existing classifications of hypertensive or arteriolosclerotic changes are used.

Arteriolar narrowing

Diffuse arteriolar narrowing is a hallmark of hypertensive retinopathy. Although it can be seen as an acute vasospastic response to acute hypertension, it is more commonly seen in chronic hypertension. This reduction in the caliber of arterioles is largely responsible for the reduction of the arteriole-to-venule ratio associated with hypertension. The normal ratio is 2:3.

Focal arteriolar narrowing is attributed to localized areas of spasm of the arteriolar wall and can be reversible. Persistent focal arteriolar narrowing may be due to edema in the wall of the arteriole or to localized areas of fibrosis.

Arteriolosclerosis and atherosclerosis

Hypertensive arteriolosclerosis refers to the progressive increase in the elastic and muscular components of the wall of the arteriole induced by hypertension. With long-standing hypertension, elastic tissue forms multiple concentric layers in the intima of the arteriole. The muscular layer can be replaced by collagen fibers, and the intima can be replaced by hyaline thickening. These changes result in the "onion-skin" appearance described by Ashton & Harry.[14] With advancing age, similar changes can develop in the absence of systemic hypertension; such changes are termed *senile* or *involutional arteriolosclerosis*. These changes are accelerated by hypertension.

The changes in the walls of the arterioles induce a change in the character of the light reflex from the vessels. Grading of these arteriolosclerotic changes by observing the changes in the light reflex is a major component of the Scheie classification.[15]

Atherosclerosis refers to the changes that develop in the intima of larger vessels, the medium and large arteries. Lipid deposition in the intima is often associated with calcification and fibrosis, which can compromise the lumen and predispose the artery to thrombosis. Atheromatous changes have been described in the peripapillary retinal arteries and in the ciliary and choroidal arteries.[16] Occlusion of atherosclerotic choroidal arteries is one of the causes of outer retinal ischemic atrophy.

Sclerotic changes

Increasing thickening of the arteriolar wall caused by the arteriolosclerotic process causes progressive changes in the appearance of the light reflex from the arteriole. Normally, the arteriolar wall is invisible; only the column of red blood cells in the lumen is visible, and this appears as the red line we recognize as the vessel. Reflection of the incident light from the convex surface of the normal arteriolar wall causes a thin line of reflected light to appear in the middle of the blood column – the normal light reflex. As the wall becomes thickened, the light reflex loses its brightness and becomes somewhat broader, duller, and more diffuse in appearance. This is the earliest sign of arteriolosclerosis.

With increasing thickening of the arteriolar wall and decreasing lumen, there is further diffusion of the light from the arteriole, and the light reflex takes on the reddish-brown hue of the "copper wire" reflex. With good control of hypertension, however, this finding is relatively uncommon.

As the process continues, there is further thickening of the arteriolar wall with associated reduction in the lumen. The arteriole

assumes the appearance of a "silver wire," when the column of blood can no longer be visualized. Although these vessels do not appear to be carrying blood, fluorescein angiographic examination reveals that they are often perfused. This scenario is an uncommon finding in controlled systemic hypertension.

Arteriolosclerotic thickening of the vessel wall also affects the appearance of the arteriolovenous crossing. The arteriole and venule usually share a common adventitial sheath where they cross, with the venule lying anteriorly. Both vascular sclerosis and perivascular glial cell proliferation contribute to the compression of the venule and constriction of its lumen, causing the appearance of arteriolovenous "nicking"[16] (Fig. 74-1). This venous compression (Gunn's sign) varies in severity from a very mild tapering of the venous blood column to more severe tapering, to interruption of the visible blood column.

The sclerotic changes can also cause deflection of the venule as it crosses the arteriole (Salus' sign). Normally the venule crosses the arteriole at an acute angle. With increasing sclerotic changes, the venule assumes a more obtuse angle with respect to the arteriole at the common crossing, and in some cases it crosses the arteriole at a right angle.

Retinal microaneurysms occur in a wide variety of retinal vascular diseases, including hypertension, and represent a nonspecific finding (Fig. 74-2). Ashton[17] noted the association of microaneurysms, cottonwool spots, and nonperfusion of retinal capillaries in hypertension (Fig. 74-3). Retinal macroaneurysms may also be associated with hypertension (Fig.74-4). In a review of 120 patients with retinal arterial macroaneurysms, 75% of patients in the series were women and 67% had hypertension.[16]

Accelerated hypertension

Acute hypertension of any cause can enter an accelerated or malignant stage, characterized by fibrinoid necrosis of the

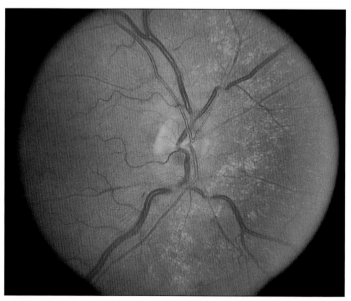

Fig. 74-1 Right fundus of a patient with hypertensive retinopathy with generalized diffuse arteriolar narrowing. Arteriovenous crossings in the superior and inferior nasal areas show mild nicking of the vein.

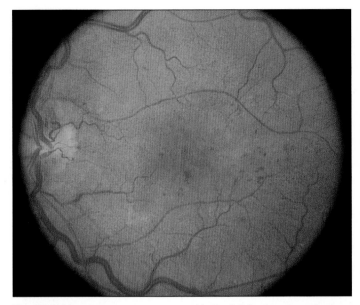

Fig. 74-2 Microaneurysms are apparent in the left fundus of a patient with chronic hypertension.

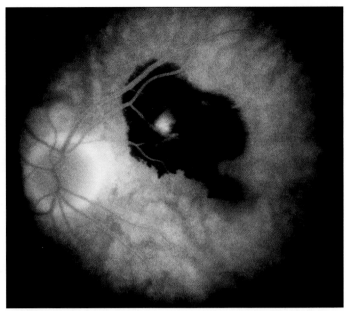

Fig. 74-4 Acquired macroaneurysm occurs in patients with hypertension.

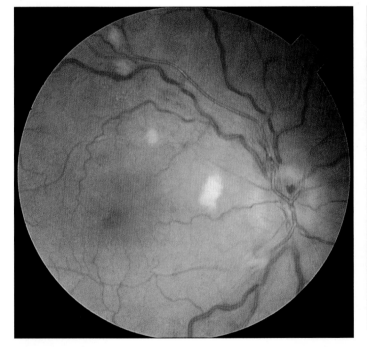

Fig. 74-3 Cottonwool spots associated with hypertensive retinopathy are seen in the right fundus.

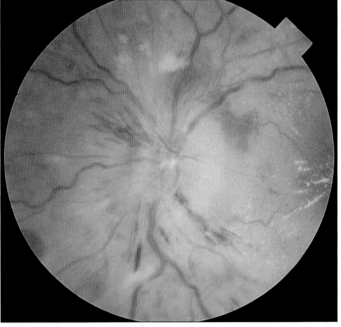

Fig. 74-5 Marked optic disc swelling with retinal hemorrhages associated with malignant hypertension.

arterioles with papilledema[14] (Fig. 74-5). Fibrinoid necrosis is not common in retinal arterioles and is usually observed in the arteries and arterioles of the choroid. However, with decompensation of the inner blood–retinal barrier, retinal edema with microcystic formation can occur.[16] A case report showed that accelerated hypertensive retinopathy could simulate Leber stellate neuroretinitis with a macular star exudate, in the absence of the other retinal findings[18] (Figs 74-5 to 74-7). Retinal hemorrhages can occur, as can cottonwool spots and retinal capillary occlusion.[19]

HYPERTENSIVE CHOROIDOPATHY

Numerous investigators have described the changes that accelerated hypertension can induce in the retinal pigment epithelium and choroid. Fibrinoid necrosis of the choroidal vessels can cause patchy nonperfusion of areas of choriocapillaris. These are most easily seen with fluorescein angiographic examination. This type of outer ischemic retinal atrophy with ischemic necrosis of the retinal pigment epithelium can also be caused by prolonged increases in intraocular pressure from external sources (e.g., a Honan balloon) or from increased intraocular pressure.

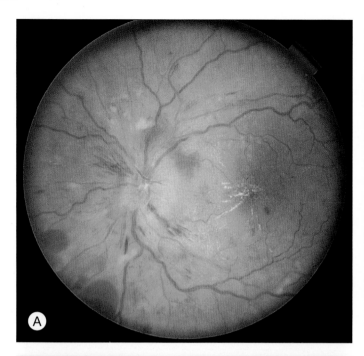

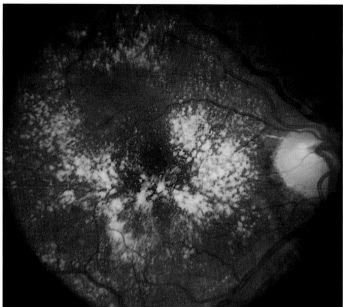

Fig. 74-7 Marked lipid deposition in the right macula of a black woman following acute changes of malignant hypertension.

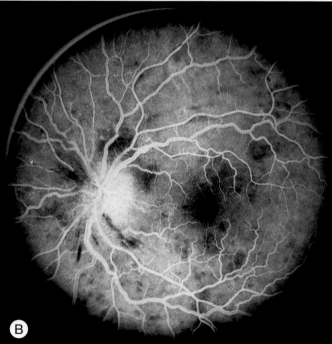

Fig. 74-6 A, This 65-year-old man with malignant hypertension has optic disc swelling and stellate lipid deposition in the left macular area. B, The fluorescein angiogram shows dilated capillaries over the disc, which leaks fluorescein. There are areas of capillary nonperfusion.

Patches of retinal pigment epithelium overlying occluded choriocapillaris appear yellow and profusely leak fluorescein (acute Elschnig's spots). As these heal, the retinal pigment epithelium becomes hyperpigmented directly over the occluded choriocapillaris, with a margin of hypopigmentation. These healed Elschnig's spots no longer leak fluorescein, but there is transmission fluorescence through the hypopigmented halo.

Localized bullous detachments of the neurosensory retina or retinal pigment epithelium are occasionally observed (Fig. 74-8). Some of these are attributed to a breakdown of the inner blood–retinal barrier with retinal endothelial cell decompensation. However, most are considered to result from retinal pigment epithelial decompensation due to fibrinoid necrosis of choroidal arteries with occlusion of the choriocapillaris. The outer retina and subretinal space in these cases contain a protein-rich exudate.

Siegrist's streaks are linear configurations of hyperpigmentation that develop over choroidal arteries in chronic hypertension.[16] In this unusual finding, the retinal pigment epithelium directly overlying the sclerotic choroidal arteries becomes hyperplastic, and the choriocapillaris becomes attenuated in this zone.

HYPERTENSIVE OPTIC NERVE CHANGES

Accelerated hypertension can also cause optic disc edema, with swelling of the optic nerve head and dilation of the capillaries of the optic nerve.[6] The cause of these changes remains controversial. In some cases, hypertensive encephalopathy with elevated intracranial pressure may play a role, as can ischemic and mechanical factors.

CLASSIFICATION OF HYPERTENSIVE AND ARTERIOSCLEROTIC CHANGES

Numerous attempts have been made to organize the morphologic retinal changes of hypertension and arteriolosclerosis into a clinically useful classification. The work of Keith et al.[20] in 1939 was an important step in identifying and classifying the changes of hypertension. The Keith–Wagener–Barker classification is based on the level of severity of retinal findings of a

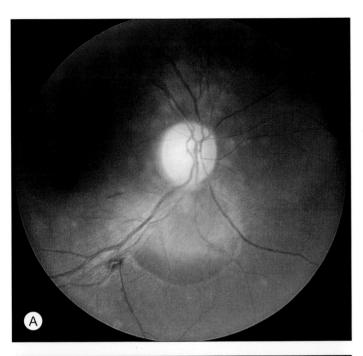

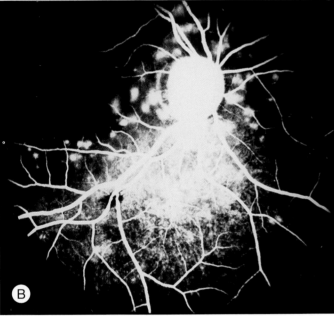

Fig. 74-8 A, Hypertensive choroidopathy is demonstrated by the pigment epithelial detachment inferior to the right optic disc. B, Fluorescein angiography showed the marked fluorescence from the deep layers of the retinal pigment epithelium in the peripapillary area.

group of patients with known hypertension. Their classification defines four groups:

1. Group I: there is minimal constriction of the retinal arterioles with some tortuosity in patients with mild hypertension.
2. Group II: retinal abnormalities include those of group I, with more definite focal narrowing and arteriolovenous nicking in patients with minimal or no other systemic involvement.

3. Group III: abnormalities include those of groups I and II and also hemorrhages and exudates and vasospastic changes, including focal arteriolar constriction and cottonwool spots. Many of these patients have identifiable cardiac, cerebral, or renal dysfunction.
4. Group IV: the abnormalities listed above are present and are usually more severe, and there is optic disc edema. Elschnig's spots are present in some. The cardiac, cerebral, and renal diseases are more severe.

Perhaps the classification that is used more commonly is that described by Scheie[15] in 1953. Scheie attempted to quantify the changes of hypertension and arteriolosclerosis separately in a five-stage classification, ranging from normal to the most severe changes visible in the retina:

1. Stage 0: although the patient has diagnosed hypertension, there are no visible retinal vascular abnormalities.
2. Stage I: diffuse arteriolar narrowing is seen, especially in the smaller vessels. Arteriolar caliber is uniform, with no focal constriction.
3. Stage II: arteriolar narrowing is more pronounced, and there can be focal areas of arteriolar constriction.
4. Stage III: both focal and diffuse arteriolar narrowing is more obvious and severe, and retinal hemorrhages may be present.
5. Stage IV: all of the previously listed abnormalities may be present, along with retinal edema, hard exudates, and optic disc edema.

In the Scheie classification, the arteriolosclerotic changes are attributed to thickening of the arteriolar wall, with concomitant changes in the arteriolar light reflexes and the color and appearance of the arterioles. The thickening also causes changes in the appearance of the arteriolovenous crossings due to increasing compression of the point where they share a common adventitial sheath. The stages of these differences are as follows:

1. Stage 0: normal.
2. Stage 1: there is broadening of the light reflex from the arteriole, with minimal or no arteriolovenous compression.
3. Stage 2: light reflex changes and crossing changes are more prominent.
4. Stage 3: the arterioles have a "copper wire" appearance, and there is more arteriolovenous compression.
5. Stage 4: the arterioles have a "silver wire" appearance, and the arteriolovenous crossing changes are most severe.

REFERENCES

1. Julius S. Current trends in the treatment of hypertension: a mixed picture. Am J Hypertens 1997; 10:300–305.
2. Hypertension prevalence and the status of awareness, treatment, and control in the United States: final report of the subcommittee on definition and prevalence by the 1984 Joint National Committee. Hypertension 1985; 7:457–468.
3. Bonnet S, Marechal G. Influence of arterial hypertension on diabetic retinopathy (in French). J Mal Vasc 1992; 17:308–310.

4. Sperduto RD, Hiller R, Chew E et al. Risk factors for hemiretinal vein occlusion: comparison with risk factors for central and branch retinal vein occlusion, The Eye Disease Case-Control Study. Ophthalmology 105:765, 1998.

5. Mitchell P, Wang JJ, Smith W. Risk factors and significance of finding asymptomatic retinal emboli. Clin Exp Ophthalmol 2000; 28:13–17.

6. Lee AG, Beaver HA. Acute bilateral optic disk edema with a macular star figure in a 12-year-old girl. Surv Ophthalmol 2002; 47: 42–49.

7. Knudtson MD, Lee KE, Hubbard LD et al. Revised formulas for summarizing retinal vessel diameters. Curr Eye Res 2003; 27:143–149.

8. Wong TY, Shankar A, Klein R et al. Prospective cohort study of retinal vessel diameters and risk of hypertension. Br Med J 2004; 329:79.

9. Leung H, Wang JJ, Rochtchina E et al. Impact of current and past blood pressure on retinal arteriolar diameter in an older population. J Hypertens 2004; 22:1543–1549.

10. Duncan BB, Wong TY, Tyroler HA et al. Hypertensive retinopathy and incident coronary heart disease in high risk men. Br J Ophthalmol 2002; 86:1002–1006.

11. Dodson PM, Galton DJ, Winder AF. Retinal vascular abnormalities in the hyperlipidaemias. Trans Ophthalmol Soc UK 1981; 101:17–21.

12. Orlin C, Lee K, Jampol L et al. Retinal arteriolar changes in patients with hyperlipidemias. Retina 1988; 8:6–9.

13. Wong TY, Klein R, Duncan BB et al. Racial differences in the prevalence of hypertensive retinopathy. Hypertension 2003; 41: 1086–1091.

14. Ashton N, Harry J. The pathology of cotton-wool spots and cytoid bodies in hypertensive retinopathy and other diseases. Trans Ophthalmol R Soc UK 1963; 83:91–114.

15. Scheie HG. Evaluation of ophthalmoscopic changes of hypertension and arteriolar sclerosis. Arch Ophthalmol 1953; 49:117.

16. Green WR. Systemic diseases with retinal involvement. In: Spencer WH, ed. Ophthalmic pathology: an atlas and textbook. Philadelphia: WB Saunders; 1985.

17. Ashton N. Pathological and ultrastructural aspect of the cotton-wool spot. Proc R Soc Med 1969; 62:1271–1276.

18. Noble KG. Hypertensive retinopathy simulating Leber stellate neuroretinitis. Arch Ophthalmol 1997; 115:1594–1595.

19. de Venecia G, Jampol LM. The eye in accelerated hypertension. II. Localized serous detachments of the retina in patients. Arch Ophthalmol 1984; 102:68–73.

20. Keith NM, Wagener HP, Barker NW. Some different types of essential hypertension: their cause and prognosis. Am J Med Sci 1939; 197:332.

Chapter

75

Rheumatic Diseases

Jennifer E. Thorne
Douglas A. Jabs

The rheumatic diseases are a heterogeneous collection of immuno-logically mediated, multisystem diseases that are loosely grouped into three general categories: (1) the arthritides; (2) the connective tissue diseases; and (3) the vasculitides (Box 75-1). The diagnosis of each of the rheumatic disorders is based on a clinical diagnosis. The American College of Rheumatology (ACR) developed criteria for most of the rheumatic diseases in order to create homogeneity in clinical research and reporting in the literature. Although these criteria are for research purposes, they provide a useful description of the clinical features of the disease.

Ocular involvement is common and varies with the rheumatic disease in question.[1] The major ophthalmic manifestations of the rheumatic diseases include scleritis, Sjögren's syndrome, uveitis, retinal vascular disease, and neuro-ophthalmic lesions.[1] The pattern of ocular involvement varies among the different rheumatic disorders. Scleritis is most often seen with rheumatoid arthritis (RA) and the vasculitides, acute anterior uveitis (AAU) with the seronegative spondyloarthropathies, and retinal vascular and neuro-ophthalmic lesions with disorders having either a vaso-occlusive (e.g., systemic lupus erythematosus or SLE) or vasculitic component.

RHEUMATOID ARTHRITIS

General considerations

RA is the most common rheumatic disorder. Affecting approximately 1% to 2% of adults, it is classically an additive, symmetric, deforming, peripheral polyarthritis.[2-6] Although all joints may be involved, it primarily affects the small joints of the hands and feet. As with all inflammatory arthritides, RA is associated with the gel phenomenon, a stiffness at rest that improves with use; patients often complain of morning stiffness. Eighty-five to 90% of patients with RA are positive for RF, which is an autoantibody directed against immunoglobulin G (IgG).[6,7]

Extra-articular disease is common in RA and may affect a wide variety of nonarticular tissues.[8] Rheumatoid nodules occur in approximately 25% of patients with RA, are located subcutaneously on extensor surfaces, and have a characteristic histologic picture consisting of central necrosis with a surrounding palisade of inflammatory cells. The lungs may be affected with rheumatoid pleural effusions, pleural nodules, pulmonary nodules, and occasionally interstitial fibrosis. Caplan's syndrome consists of RA and pneumoconiosis resulting in a particularly severe interstitial fibrosis. Cardiac disease includes pericarditis and rheumatoid nodules involving the conducting system or heart valves, or both.[6,8,9]

Rheumatoid vasculitis affects fewer than 1% of patients with RA and is typically seen in patients with severe arthritis and high titers of RF. It generally presents as either a peripheral polyneuropathy or as refractory skin ulcers. Patients may develop digital gangrene or, occasionally, visceral ischemia.[6,8,10,11] Felty's syndrome is a triad of RA, splenomegaly, and leukopenia, and may be seen in up to 3% of patients with RA. In addition, patients with Felty's syndrome often have hyperpigmentation, chronic leg ulcers, and recurrent infections.

Treatment

The goals of treatment for RA include the reduction of pain, control of joint damage, and prevention of loss of function. Before 1990, the treatment of RA was approached in a stepwise fashion, first with nonsteroidal anti-inflammatory drugs (NSAIDs) and followed by disease-modifying antirheumatic drugs (DMARDs) in refractory or more severe cases.[12] Studies have suggested, however, that joint destruction occurs soon after the onset of synovitis.[12] It is estimated that 50% of joint destruction seen over an 8-year period occurs in the first 2 years.[13] Therefore, DMARDs are now instituted within the first 3 months of diagnosis of RA in addition to NSAID therapy.[12] Therapy with NSAIDs includes salicylates, older nonselective cyclo-oxygenase (COX) inhibitors, and the newer COX-2 inhibitors. These NSAIDs are used to control pain and swelling and to improve the joint function but typically do not alter disease course long-term. Remittive agents or DMARDs include hydroxychloroquine, sulfasalazine, methotrexate, and several biologic agents. Hydroxychloroquine and sulfasalazine are effective for milder disease.[14,15] Hydroxychloroquine is often used first because of its relative lack of toxicity. Chloroquine is slightly more efficacious than hydroxychloroquine in the treatment of RA but is also more toxic; therefore, it is used infrequently.[16] Methotrexate, an antimetabolite, is typically the first choice of remittive agents for more severe or advanced disease and has been found to be efficacious in the treatment of RA in multiple randomized clinical trials.[17-19] Methotrexate was found to improve clinical

---

Box 75-1 The rheumatic diseases

Arthritides
Rheumatoid arthritis
Seronegative (HLA-B27-associated) spondyloarthropathies
  Ankylosing spondylitis
  Reiter's syndrome and reactive arthritis
  Inflammatory bowel disease
  Psoriatic arthritis
Juvenile rheumatoid arthritis (juvenile idiopathic arthritis)

Connective tissue diseases
Systemic lupus erythematosus
Scleroderma
Overlap syndromes – mixed connective tissue disease
Polymyositis and dermatomyositis
Sjögren's syndrome
Relapsing polychondritis

Systemic vasculitides
Giant-cell arteritis
Takayasu's arteritis
Polyarteritis nodosa
Churg–Strauss syndrome
Wegener's granulomatosis
Behçet's disease
Hypersensitivity vasculitis
Henoch–Schönlein purpura
Vasculitis with connective tissue disease
Lymphomatoid granulomatosis
Essential mixed cryoglobulinemia associated with hepatitis C
Hypocomplementemic urticarial vasculitic syndrome (HUVS)

---

signs and symptoms of RA, improve functional status, and slow radiographic disease progression. Biologics are engineered agents designed to block cytokines or cytokine receptors. Biologic agents, including etanercept, infliximab, adalimumab, and anakinra, have been found to be effective remittive agents in randomized clinical trials.[12,20–22]

Immunosuppressive drugs, such as azathioprine,[23] ciclosporin,[24] or cyclophosphamide,[25] are also efficacious in the treatment of RA but are used less frequently because of their toxicity. Occasionally they may be used in the treatment of rheumatoid vasculitis. Although effective, intramuscular and oral gold and D-penicillamine are rarely used due to more efficacious and better-tolerated newer drugs. Minocycline has been shown to be modestly effective in a randomized trial and is used for mild disease, although infrequently.[26] Traditionally, low-dose prednisone (5 mg every other day to 10 mg/day) was used in selected patients to decrease stiffness and increase mobility.

Ocular manifestations

Anterior segment manifestations are the most common ocular problems in patients with RA. These include Sjögren's syndrome, scleritis, and marginal corneal ulcers. Sjögren's syndrome affects approximately 11% to 13% of patients with RA.[27] Scleral disease may be classified as episcleritis or scleritis. Episcleritis presents with discomfort rather than pain, more superficial ocular inflammation, less frequent ocular complications, and typically has a less frequent association with systemic disease.[28] Scleritis is often characterized by pain, presents with deeper inflammation and edema in the sclera, often has ocular complications, and is associated with systemic disease in approximately 50% of cases.[28,29] Episcleritis may be self-limited and spontaneously remitting, whereas scleritis typically requires therapy. Scleritis may be classified as diffuse anterior, nodular, posterior, or necrotizing. Scleromalacia perforans is a separate category, in which there is an insidious but destructive scleral process, and is seen in patients with long-standing RA. Any of the above types of scleritis may be seen in association with RA, although diffuse anterior scleritis is most common.[28]

Scleritis is a common ocular manifestation of RA, affecting an estimated 1% to 6% of patients with RA and 14% of patients with rheumatoid vasculitis.[30,31] Although estimates of the frequency of scleritis in patients with RA have been as high as 6%, large series have shown that approximately 1% of patients with RA have scleritis.[31] Patients with RA and scleritis tend to have a longer and more severe disease and a higher prevalence of extra-articular disease.[27,32] Retrospective studies have also suggested a higher frequency of rheumatoid vasculitis and Felty's syndrome among patients with scleral disease.[10] One study of patients with necrotizing scleritis or necrotizing keratitis and RA suggested an increased mortality among these patients.[30]

Rheumatoid corneal melts, also known as marginal corneal ulcers, may be either bland (not inflammatory) or necrotizing (peripheral ulcerative keratitis or PUK) in nature. Noninflammatory marginal keratitis can often be treated with local measures. Necrotizing keratitis requires aggressive medical therapy with systemic corticosteroids and immunosuppressive drugs. Patients with PUK and RA have a high mortality rate, possibly due to an underlying rheumatoid vasculitis.[30–33] Brown's syndrome has been described in a few patients with RA and is due to a stenosing tenosynovitis of the superior oblique tendon.[34]

Posterior segment lesions

Posterior segment lesions due to RA are uncommon and have included a retinal microangiopathy with cottonwool spots, which is probably related to rheumatoid vasculitis.[31] Posterior scleritis has also been described in patients with RA. The most commonly encountered reason for ophthalmic evaluation of the posterior segment in a patient with RA is to monitor for antimalarial drug therapy. The antimalarial drugs chloroquine and hydroxychloroquine have an anti-inflammatory effect and, because of their relative lack of toxicity, are commonly used as first-line remittive agents in the treatment of RA. Hydroxychloroquine is now used almost exclusively because of its lesser toxicity.[35] Both drugs accumulate in pigmented tissues, such as the retinal pigment epithelium, and may cause a "bull's-eye" pigmentary retinopathy[35–37] (Fig. 75-1). The retinopathy of the antimalarial drugs is said to be reversible when discovered early, but irreversible, despite discontinuation of the drug, when allowed to progress. For this reason, patients taking antimalarial drugs are often referred for screening ophthalmic examinations in order to detect the earliest signs of antimalarial toxicity. Our practice is that all patients receiving hydroxychloroquine therapy have a

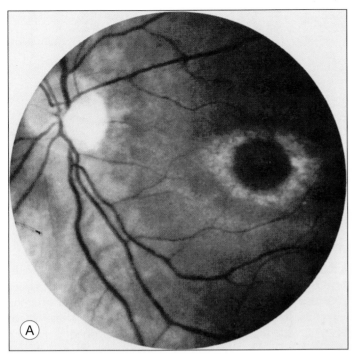 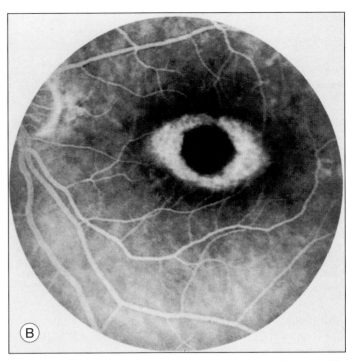

Fig. 75-1 Fundus photograph (A) and fluorescein angiogram (B) of a patient with chloroquine retinopathy. (Reproduced from Cruess AF, Schachat AP, Nicholl J et al. Chloroquine retinopathy. Is fluorescein angiography necessary? Ophthalmology 1985; 92:1127–1129.)

baseline ophthalmic examination including visual acuity, Amsler grid testing, color vision testing, dilated fundus examination, fundus photography, and visual field testing with the Humphrey automated perimetry 10-2 test. The timing of follow-up examinations to screen for signs of toxicity is controversial. Studies have suggested that the frequency of retinopathy is less than 5% when dosages of less than 6.5 mg/kg per day of hydroxychloroquine are used (generally less than 400 mg/day).[37] Patients can be treated with large total doses without evidence of toxicity when these daily doses are used.[38] However, the risk for patients taking less than 6.5 mg/kg per day of hydroxychloroquine remains greater than zero over long-term follow-up.[39] Cost-effectiveness analyses have suggested that annual ophthalmic examinations may be the most cost-effective approach.[40] However, a study in which rheumatologists and ophthalmologists were surveyed revealed that the majority recommended monitoring every 6 months.[41] Therefore, our practice has been to follow patients who are taking hydroxychloroquine at a dose of 400 mg daily every 6 months. These patients are followed with eye examinations, including visual acuity, color vision, Amsler grid testing, and dilated fundus examination. Automated perimetry is performed on any patient with visual symptoms such as decreased vision or glare, Amsler grid changes, or color vision changes.

SERONEGATIVE SPONDYLOARTHROPATHIES

The seronegative spondyloarthropathies (outlined in Box 75-1) include ankylosing spondylitis (AS), Reiter's syndrome, arthritis with inflammatory bowel disease (IBD), and psoriatic arthritis.

They are linked by statistical association with the tissue type human leukocyte antigen (HLA)-B27 and by overlapping features, but are distinguished by somewhat different clinical patterns.[42] Each of these diseases has as its most common ophthalmic manifestation nongranulomatous AAU (Table 75-1). Indeed, AAU shares with the seronegative spondyloarthropathies a statistical association with HLA-B27, as approximately 50% of patients with nongranulomatous AAU will be HLA-B27-positive.[42,43]

Ankylosing spondylitis
General considerations
AS is characterized by involvement of the axial skeleton and bony fusion (ankylosis). The cause is unknown, but the strong association with HLA-B27 suggests a genetic predisposition. Over 90% of white patients with AS are HLA-B27-positive, whereas only 6% to 8% of the general population are HLA-B27-positive. AS affects 0.1% to 0.2% of the general population and 2% of patients who are HLA-B27-positive.[44] Although young adult men are mostly affected, women may have a mild form or atypical disease.[42,45,46]

The classic features of AS are chronic low-back pain, fusion of the axial skeleton (spinal ankylosis), and sacroiliitis. The demonstration of sacroiliitis on radiographic examination of the sacroiliac joints is the sine qua non for the diagnosis of spondylitis. The end-stage of this process is a completely fused and immobilized spine, also known as a "bamboo" or "poker" spine. In addition to the spinal arthritis, which is the hallmark of the disease, patients may develop arthritis of the shoulders and hips, limited chest expansion, and restrictive lung disease.

	Table 75-1 Seronegative spondyloarthropathies	
Disorder	Frequency of HLA-B27 (%)	Frequency of uveitis (%)
Ankylosing spondylitis	90–100	25
Reiter's syndrome	70–90	20–40
Inflammatory bowel disease	6	2–12
(with sacroiliitis)	(50–70)	(50)
Psoriatic arthritis	18–22	7
(with sacroiliitis)	(50–60)	–

HLA, human leukocyte antigen.

Other extra-articular features include apical pulmonary fibrosis, aortic insufficiency due to aortitis, and heart block.[42,46]

Treatment

The treatment of AS relies on the judicious use of NSAIDs and a program of physical therapy and exercise. Indometacin appears to be more effective in the treatment of spondylitis than many of the others. Anti-inflammatory medications do not reverse and generally do not prevent the ultimate spinal ankylosis. However, they relieve symptoms and allow the patient to participate in an exercise program. The program of physical therapy and exercise allows the patient to maximize the mobility of the spine and to allow spinal fusion to occur in a posture most advantageous to the patient.[42,46] Methotrexate and infliximab have been reported to be effective in the management of more severe disease.[42,47,48]

Ocular manifestations

The primary ocular manifestation of AS is recurrent, nongranulomatous AAU.[43,46,49] Generally one eye at a time is affected, although both eyes may suffer attacks.[43,49] Occasionally the anterior chamber inflammation may be so severe as to produce hypopyon, fibrin deposition, and posterior synechiae.[46] AAU occurs in 25% to 40% of patients with AS.[44,46,49] Conversely, studies of patients with AAU have demonstrated AS as the underlying disease in 18% to 34% of patients.[50,51]

Posterior segment lesions

Posterior segment lesions are rare in patients with AS. Occasionally, a "spillover" inflammation extending into the vitreous has been described.[52] Perkins reported that spondylitis was a cause of acute panuveitis in 6% of cases and was a cause of panuveitis in 11% of men.[53] This more severe ocular involvement is considerably less common than the typical anterior uveitis.

Reiter's syndrome and reactive arthritis
General considerations

Reiter's syndrome is characterized by the classic triad of arthritis, urethritis, and conjunctivitis. In 1981, the original set of criteria were expanded to: (1) the presence of a peripheral arthritis with a duration of 1 month; and (2) an associated urethritis, cervicitis, or diarrhea.[54] The increased scope of the disease encompasses "reactive arthritis" in which a sterile arthritis ensues after the infection has resolved.[54] Typically it is rare for a patient to present with the classic triad originally described as Reiter's syndrome. Historically, Reiter's syndrome has existed in two forms: epidemic and endemic. Epidemic Reiter's syndrome occurs after infectious gastroenteritis with a limited number of organisms, including *Shigella*, *Salmonella*, and *Yersinia*. The subsequent arthritis occurs well after the infectious gastroenteritis has resolved and is a sterile arthritis. It appears to represent an immunologic response to the infectious organism, which triggers the arthritis and extra-articular inflammation, but the mechanism by which this occurs has not yet been fully explained.[42,54,55] Although a "triggering" agent can be identified for epidemic Reiter's syndrome, none has been identified for endemic Reiter's syndrome. Because patients with Reiter's syndrome often developed urethritis and presented to venereal disease clinics, it was initially believed that endemic Reiter's syndrome was due to *Chlamydia*, but studies have not demonstrated a higher prevalence of chlamydial infection in patients with Reiter's syndrome than in controls, and the role of *Chlamydia* remains debated.[42,54] Like AS, Reiter's syndrome has a genetic predisposition, in that 63% to 95% of patients will be HLA-B27-positive.

The arthritis of Reiter's syndrome is an asymmetric, episodic, oligoarthritis affecting primarily the lower extremities, particularly large joints such as the knees or ankles. Other articular features include periostitis, such as heel pain, interphalangeal arthritis of the toes and fingers producing "sausage digits," and sacroiliitis. Mucocutaneous lesions include urethritis in men and cervicitis in women, circinate balanitis, painless oral ulcers, nail lesions, and keratoderma blennorrhagicum. Patients may also have systemic symptoms including fever and weight loss. The disease tends to follow an episodic and relapsing course, but 15% to 30% of patients develop chronic arthritis over 10 to 20 years of follow-up.[42,54,56]

Ocular manifestations

Conjunctivitis is one of the hallmarks of the disease and is one of the original triad described by Reiter. It tends to be a feature of early disease, in particular of the initial attack, and can be missed if patients are only seen during subsequent attacks. The more serious ocular manifestation is uveitis. As in AS, this is a nongranulomatous, recurrent AAU. AAU is said to occur in 5% to 20% of patients with the initial attack and in as many as 50% of Reiter's patients with long-term follow-up.[44,49,57] An unusual keratitis with punctate epithelial lesions progressing to a central loss of the corneal epithelium and subepithelial infiltrates has rarely been described.[57–59]

Posterior segment lesions

Posterior segment lesions are unusual in patients with Reiter's syndrome, although spillover vitritis and cystoid macular edema secondary to anterior uveitis have been described. Perkins[53] found that 23% of patients with acute panuveitis had Reiter's syndrome, all of whom were men. Rarely, multifocal choroiditis has been reported in Reiter's syndrome.[60–62] Occasional optic disc edema secondary to the anterior uveitis has been reported. Lee et al.,[57] in a series of 113 patients with Reiter's syndrome, reported no cases of posterior segment disease, a result which emphasizes the relative infrequency of these complications compared with the anterior segment ones.

Inflammatory bowel disease
General considerations

IBD consists of two distinct diseases: ulcerative colitis and Crohn's disease. Ulcerative colitis is an inflammatory disorder of the gastrointestinal mucosa with diffuse involvement of the colon. Crohn's disease is a focal granulomatous disease involving all areas of the bowel and affecting both the large and small bowel. Crohn's disease is also known as regional enteritis, granulomatous ileocolitis, and granulomatous colitis. Extraintestinal manifestations of IBD include dermatitis, mucous membrane disease, ocular inflammation, and arthritis. Skin disorders occur in 6% to 15% of patients with IBD and include erythema nodosum and pyoderma gangrenosum.[63,64]

Arthritis occurs in up to 22% of patients and occurs as two distinct variants. Enteropathic ("colitic") arthritis is a large-joint, lower-extremity, nondeforming oligoarthritis. The activity of enteropathic arthritis parallels the activity of the bowel disease. The prevalence is said to be 15% in Crohn's disease and up to 10% in ulcerative colitis.[65] The second form of arthritis associated with IBD is AS. The activity of the spondylitis is unrelated to the activity of the bowel disease. It is said to occur in 20% of patients with Crohn's disease and in 10% to 15% in ulcerative colitis.[65] Multiple series have shown that 50% to 70% of patients with spondylitis and IBD are HLA-B27-positive.[65] Of the HLA-B27-positive patients with IBD, 50% will develop AAU.[42,63,65]

Treatment

Treatment of IBD is dependent on the extent and severity of the disease. Typically treating the underlying bowel disease improves the peripheral joint disease. Localized proctitis may be treated with corticosteroid enemas, but more extensive bowel disease may require systemic therapy. Sulfasalazine is used first

in an effort to minimize steroid complications and is often used to decrease the dose of corticosteroids needed. Severe IBD can also be treated with corticosteroid-sparing agents, such as azathioprine or methotrexate.[65] Infliximab may induce remissions in Crohn's disease and is effective in the treatment of Crohn's-related fistulas.[66] However, infliximab appears to be ineffective in treatment of ulcerative colitis.[65] Because of the risk of colonic malignancy with long-standing ulcerative colitis, a colectomy is sometimes performed. After colectomy the extraintestinal manifestations may resolve.[65]

Ocular manifestations

Ocular inflammation occurs in approximately 4% to 6% of patients with IBD.[49,64,67–69] The ocular manifestations of this disease include anterior uveitis, scleritis and, occasionally, keratitis. The most common ocular manifestation is anterior uveitis and most often presents as a nongranulomatous, recurrent AAU. This type of uveitis is seen in association with spondylitis and HLA-B27. Chronic and bilateral uveitis also occurs occasionally and may be seen more frequently in women with IBD.[49,70,71] All types of scleritis have been associated with IBD, including necrotizing scleritis and posterior scleritis.[67,69,72,73] The scleral inflammation may parallel the activity of the underlying bowel disease.[69,73] Rarely, keratitis[73] and Brown's syndrome[74] may be seen in association with IBD.

Posterior segment lesions

Occasionally, posterior segment inflammation has been associated with the uveitis of IBD, and it generally consists of vitritis and retinitis. There have been occasional case reports of retinal vascular disease, including retinal artery occlusion and retinal vasculitis, papillitis and neuroretinitis, and ischemic optic neuropathy (ION) in patients with IBD.[10,75–78] It has been suggested that these retinal vascular lesions are due to a thrombic diathesis seen in some patients with IBD.[77] Posterior scleritis has been reported in patients with IBD.[73,76] Knox et al.[73] have reported posterior scleritis with exudative detachments or optic disc edema (Fig. 75-2) in patients with Crohn's disease.

Psoriatic arthritis
General considerations

Psoriatic arthritis is a syndrome in which psoriasis is associated with an inflammatory arthritis and, usually, a negative RF test. Psoriasis is a cutaneous disorder affecting 1% to 3% of the general population characterized by erythematous, well-demarcated macules with silvery scales. It occurs on extensor surfaces, particularly the elbows and scalp, but also the chest and back. Up to 20% of patients with psoriasis will develop arthritis.[79,80] In patients with psoriatic arthritis, the skin disease may be quite mild or occult. The skin disease generally precedes the onset of arthritis by several years, but in 15% of patients the arthritis precedes the onset of skin disease.[79] Nail changes are common and include pitting, transverse ridges, crumbling, and onycholysis.

Psoriatic arthritis has been divided into five groups on the basis of the clinical presentation. "Classic" psoriatic arthritis is

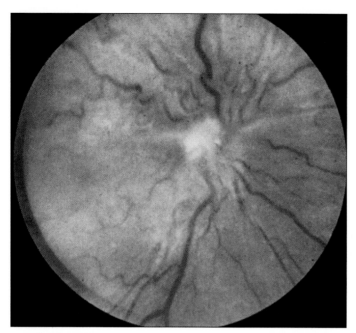

Fig. 75-2 Papillopathy in a patient with Crohn's disease. (Reproduced from Knox DL, Schachat AP, Mustonen E. Primary, secondary, and coincidental ocular complications of Crohn's disease. Ophthalmology 1984; 91:163–173.)

manifested by involvement of the distal interphalangeal joints. Arthritis mutilans is a severely deforming, usually widespread arthritis with ankylosis and characteristic erosive radiologic changes. A symmetric, additive, deforming polyarthritis similar to RA is another form. The most common presentation is a monoarthritis or asymmetric oligoarthritis, usually affecting distal interphalangeal, proximal interphalangeal, or metatarsal interphalangeal joints. Psoriatic spondylitis is the fifth type. Multiple studies have demonstrated an association of HLA-B27 with psoriatic spondylitis, and approximately 60% of patients with psoriatic spondylitis are HLA-B27-positive.[79]

Ocular manifestations

Conjunctivitis occurred in approximately 20% to 33% of patients with psoriatic arthritis, anterior uveitis in 7%, and scleral disease in 2%.[49,79,80] The uveitis is often recurrent, nongranulomatous AAU and associated with HLA-B27 and spondylitis, but chronic uveitis may occur.[49] Brown's syndrome has also been reported in patients with psoriatic arthropathy.[81]

JUVENILE RHEUMATOID ARTHRITIS

General considerations

Juvenile RA (JRA), also called juvenile chronic arthritis (JCA) or juvenile idiopathic arthritis (JIA), is defined as arthritis of greater than 3 months' duration with an onset at less than 16 years of age. The traditional classification of JRA developed by the ACR depends on the pattern of presentation of the arthritis and consists of three categories: (1) polyarthritis; (2) oligoarthritis; and (3) systemic disease. *Polyarthritis* is defined as presentation with more than five joints involved, whereas *oligoarthritis* has

four or less. *Systemic disease* is the disorder originally described by Still and has prominent systemic features with a variable arthritis.[82] *Juvenile chronic arthritis* was the term used by the European League against Rheumatism classification system, a system that was used primarily in Europe and has been replaced by the classification system proposed by the International League of Associations for Rheumatology (ILAR).[83] Because only one subset of children have RF-positive polyarthritis, which is similar to the adult form of RA, the term *juvenile rheumatoid arthritis* was thought not to encompass the full spectrum of disease and therefore, the ILAR classification system uses the term *juvenile idiopathic arthritis* instead of JRA.[84] The ACR has not adopted the ILAR classification system or the term JIA as yet, though this classification is similar to the one used by the ACR. The ACR and ILAR classification systems are listed in Table 75-2.[83,84]

The systemic variant of JRA and JIA is known as Still's disease. The male-to-female ratio is approximately 1:1 and it usually affects young children less than 5 years of age. The arthritis has a variable relation to the onset of disease but generally presents as polyarthritis. The systemic features predominate and include fever, a salmon-colored evanescent, maculopapular rash, lymphadenopathy, hepatosplenomegaly, serositis, an elevated erythrocyte sedimentation rate (ESR), and leukocytosis. Ocular disease is not generally associated with this variant.[82]

Two types of polyarticular disease have been described in both classification systems. Children over 10 years of age may develop a seropositive (RF-positive), RA-like polyarthritis. Among this subgroup, girls are more commonly affected than boys. The arthritis is an additive, symmetric, deforming polyarthritis identical to adult RA. The arthritis tends to be persistent and results in severe morbidity. As in adult RA, these patients often are HLA-DR4-positive. Ocular disease is uncommon in this subgroup.[82,84] In the second type of polyarticular disease, the children are older and tend to present with an additive, symmetric, deforming polyarthritis. However, patients are RF-negative but are HLA-

Table 75-2 Comparison of ACR and ILAR classification systems

Classification system	ACR (JRA)	ILAR (JIA)
Types of arthritis	Systemic	Systemic
	Oligoarticular	Oligoarticular
	ANA+	ANA+
	ANA–, HLA-B27+	Enthesitis-related
	RF+ polyarthritis	RF+ polyarthritis
	RF– polyarthritis	RF– polyarthritis
		Psoriatic
		Undefined

ACR, American College of Rheumatology; ILAR, International League of Associations for Rheumatology; JRA, juvenile rheumatoid arthritis; JIA, junvenile idiopathic arthritis; ANA, antinuclear antibody; HLA, human leukocyte antigen; RF, rheumatoid factor; +, positive; –, negative

B27-positive. Sacroiliitis and spondylitis are common, and a characteristic fusion of the posterior spines of the C2 and C3 vertebrae in the cervical spine can be seen. Micrognathia occurs in approximately 25%. A recurrent AAU occurred in 25% and was indistinguishable from other B27-associated anterior uveitides.[82,84]

Two types of oligoarticular disease have also been defined in the ACR classification system. Juvenile AS occurs in older boys, with 12 years as the mean age of onset, and has a male-to-female ratio of 5:1. The arthritis is an oligoarthritis affecting the large joints and lower extremities. Sacroiliitis is common, and these children progress to classic AS with time. Ninety percent of these children are HLA-B27-positive, and 25% develop a recurrent, nongranulomatous AAU. The disease appears to share the clinical and immunogenetic features of the seronegative spondylo-arthropathies in adults, including the same types of arthritis and uveitis. This type of arthritis is classified as enthesitis-related arthritis using the ILAR classification system.[42,82,84] A second type of oligoarticular disease, antinuclear antibody (ANA)-positive oligoarticular disease, is similarly defined in both classification systems. It is generally seen in young girls under age 5, although boys may also be affected. The arthritis is an oligoarticular, large-joint, lower-extremity arthritis that tends to remit spontaneously and not leave significant articular deformities. Over 80% of these patients have a positive ANA.[82,84,85] This subgroup of patients is associated with the HLA antigens HLA-DR5, DR6, DR8, DQ1, and DQ2, and chronic anterior uveitis is the most severe ocular manifestation.[85–87]

Treatment

The goal of treatment for JRA is to control clinical symptoms and to limit joint deformity using the safest therapy available.[82] First-line therapy typically begins with either aspirin or NSAIDs. Because of the potential association between aspirin use and Reye syndrome, any aspirin or NSAID should be discontinued in a sick child who potentially has influenza or varicella. Systemic corticosteroids are avoided except in severe systemic disease because of the potential for growth retardation with long-term use. If the patient fails to respond to NSAIDs alone, methotrexate is typically used. Methotrexate has been shown to be effective in the treatment of JRA in a randomized clinical trial, and there is extensive experience with the drug over long-term follow-up.[88–90] Methotrexate also effectively treats JRA-associated uveitis.[91–93] Other immunosuppressive drug therapies, including ciclosporin and azathioprine, have been used to treat JRA that is refractory to treatment with methotrexate.[82] Etanercept has also been shown to be effective in the treatment of polyarticular JRA in a multicenter randomized clinical trial.[94]

Ocular manifestations

Approximately 12% to 17% of children with JRA have uveitis.[95–97] A population-based study performed in Finland reported the mean annual incidence and prevalence rates for JRA-associated uveitis as 0.2 and 2.4 cases per 100 000 population respectively.[98] The ocular manifestation of JRA is generally an anterior uveitis. Recurrent AAU is seen with B27-associated subgroups. Chronic anterior uveitis is seen with ANA-positive oligoarticular disease where frequencies have been reported to range from 20% to 56%.[85,99–102] Although traditionally it has been said that cases of chronic uveitis occur primarily in girls, one retrospective study of 90 children with JRA found no gender difference in the risk of developing uveitis.[95] The chronic anterior uveitis tends to be asymptomatic or minimally symptomatic; therefore, it is recommended that patients with ANA-positive oligoarticular JRA be evaluated every 3 months for screening in an effort to detect the uveitis early.[96,103] Two-thirds of patients have bilateral disease, and in patients with unilateral disease, the majority will develop uveitis in the fellow eye within 1 year of presentation.[82] The chronic uveitis typically requires chronic therapy.

Sight-threatening ocular complications may develop in patients with chronic uveitis with band keratopathy and cataracts occurring in up to one-third of patients.[82,95] Secondary glaucoma occurs in 10% to 20% of patients with JRA-associated uveitis and is a poor prognostic finding.[97,99,101,102,104] Posterior synechiae are common. Other complications include macular edema in 8% to 10% of cases and phthisis in 4% to 10% of patients. Although blindness developed in 40% of patients reported in early series, more recent series have reported a better prognosis.[97,99,101,105–107] The improved prognosis appears to be due to earlier detection, better treatment, and better surgical management of the complications. Although pars plana lensectomy with vitrectomy and aphakic correction had traditionally been considered the best method of cataract surgery in these patients,[100,108] more recent case series suggest that intraocular lenses can be placed in these patients with good visual outcome.[109,110] Posterior segment lesions other than macular edema due to chronic anterior uveitis are not common.[97]

FAMILIAL JUVENILE SYSTEMIC GRANULOMATOSIS

General considerations

Familial juvenile systemic granulomatosis (Mendelian inheritance in man (MIM) 186580), also known as Jabs syndrome, Blau syndrome, and autosomal dominant granulomatous disease of childhood, is an uncommon autosomal dominant genetic disease with polyarthritis and uveitis.[111–115] The joint disease is a granulomatous, deforming, nonerosive polysynovitis. Other features of the syndrome may include rash, cranial nerve palsies, and vasculopathy.[111–115] The syndrome is caused by mutations in the CARD15 gene, which is involved in apoptosis.[116]

Children with this syndrome are often misdiagnosed as having either JRA or sarcoidosis. Familial juvenile systemic granulomatosis is distinguished from JRA by the presence of polyarthritis on presentation, the absence of ANA antibodies, and the pattern of inheritance. Familial juvenile systemic granulomatosis differs from sarcoidosis by the pattern of arthritis, the absence of pulmonary involvement and adenopathy, and the inheritance pattern.[115]

Ocular manifestations

The uveitis associated with familial juvenile systemic granulomatosis may be a chronic anterior uveitis or a chronic panuveitis with multifocal choroiditis. Patients may require aggressive medical therapy to control the uveitis, including immunosuppressive drugs. Ocular complications such as cataract and macular edema are common.[115]

SYSTEMIC LUPUS ERYTHEMATOSUS

General considerations

SLE is generally regarded as the prototypic autoimmune disease. The cause of SLE is unknown, but a genetic predisposition has been suggested. Pathogenetically, SLE is characterized by B-cell hyperreactivity, polyclonal B-cell activation, hypergammaglobulinemia, autoantibody formation, and abnormal T cells. Autoantibodies include ANA, antibodies to DNA, both single-stranded DNA (anti-ssDNA) and double-stranded, or native, DNA (anti-dsDNA or anti-nDNA), and antibodies to cytoplasmic components (anti-Sm, anti-Ro, and anti-La). Studies have demonstrated multiple defects in T-cell signaling pathways in patients with SLE that are thought to lead to autoreactivity and hyperactivated T lymphocytes. Classically SLE has been regarded as an immune complex disease, in which circulating immune complexes are deposited in tissue and incite an inflammatory response, which may lead to end-organ damage. Immunoregulatory abnormalities in SLE lead to an inadequate clearing of immune complexes and further hyperactivation of both B and T cells causing further inflammation and tissue damage.[117–120]

Almost any organ system may be affected by SLE. Cutaneous disease occurs in approximately 85% of patients and is most often manifested by the characteristic butterfly rash across the nose and cheeks, known as a malar flush. Other cutaneous lesions include discoid lupus erythematosus, vasculitic skin lesions such as cutaneous ulcers or splinter hemorrhages, purpuric skin lesions, and alopecia. Less common skin lesions include a maculopapular eruption, lupus profundus, bullous skin lesions, and urticarial skin lesions. Mucosal lesions occur in 30% to 40% of patients and characteristically are painless oral ulcers. Photosensitivity is a common feature of the skin lesions in SLE, and patients may be extremely sun-sensitive.[121–123]

Between 80% and 85% of patients with SLE will have articular disease at some point, either polyarthralgias or a nondeforming, migratory polyarthritis. Cutaneous nodules, myalgias, and myositis are less common. Systemic features occur in over 80% of patients with SLE and include fatigue, fever, and weight loss. Renal disease is present in approximately 50% of patients. Clinically this presents as either proteinuria with a nephrotic picture or glomerulonephritis. Lupus nephritis is a major cause of the morbidity and mortality of SLE.[121–123]

Raynaud's phenomenon occurs in 20% of patients. Cardiac disease includes pericarditis, occasionally myocarditis, and Libman–Sacks endocarditis. Pleuropulmonary lesions include pleuritic chest pain and, less commonly, pneumonitis. Hepatosplenomegaly and adenopathy can be seen in over 50% of patients with SLE.[121–123] Involvement of the central nervous system (CNS) by lupus occurs in over 35% of patients with SLE. Peripheral neuropathy and cranial nerve palsies are less common. The most common manifestations of CNS lupus are seizures, an organic brain syndrome, and psychosis. Transverse myelitis is an uncommon manifestation occurring in only 4% of patients with SLE but is often seen in association with optic neuritis.[121–124]

The hematologic system may frequently be affected by SLE. Patients often have a chronic anemia but also may develop an autoimmune hemolytic anemia. Leukopenia, in particular lymphopenia, is a characteristic feature. Thrombocytopenia occurs in approximately one-third of patients.[122] A circulating anticoagulant (the "lupus anticoagulant") may be demonstrated in 28% to 34% of patients with SLE.[121,123,125,126] The lupus anticoagulant is a member of a family of antiphospholipid antibodies, which also includes the anticardiolipin antibodies. These antibodies are found in combination with clinical features, including arterial or venous thrombosis and pregnancy morbidity in patients with antiphospholipid antibody syndrome (APS), which may be a primary disease unassociated with other autoimmune diseases or may be secondary to SLE. Approximately 15% of patients with SLE have APS.[126–129] The APS is associated with occlusive disease, which can lead to tissue ischemia and end-organ damage, and with thrombotic disorders, such as deep-vein thrombophlebitis and strokes.[126,128–134] The mechanism(s) by which antiphospholipid antibodies cause thrombosis is not clear, but two possible mechanisms are induction of platelet aggregation by the antibody or inhibition of prostacyclin production by the vascular endothelium.[122,129,130,131,135]

Because of the diffuse manifestations of SLE, criteria for the diagnosis have been established and are outlined in Box 75-2. To establish a diagnosis of SLE, four or more criteria must be met.[136] It should be emphasized that these criteria were designed for use by clinical investigators.

Treatment

Because SLE is a multisystem disease with highly variable features in different patients, treatment is directed at the specific organs

---

Box 75-2 The 1982 revised criteria for the classification of systemic lupus erythematosus*

1. Malar rash
2. Discoid lupus
3. Photosensitivity
4. Oral ulcers
5. Arthritis
6. Serositis (pleuritis, pericarditis)
7. Renal disorder (proteinuria, nephritis)
8. Neurologic disorder (seizures, psychosis)
9. Hematologic disorder (hemolytic anemia, or leukopenia, lymphopenia, or thrombocytopenia)
10. Immunologic disorder (positive lupus erythematosus cell preparation or anti-DNA test or anti-Sm or false-positive test for syphilis)
11. Antinuclear antibody

*A person shall be said to have systemic lupus erythematosus if he or she has four or more of the 11 criteria.

involved. NSAIDs or low-dose prednisone are used for the treatment of arthritis and serositis.[137] Hydroxychloroquine is often used for the treatment of the skin disease or as a corticosteroid-sparing agent for mild systemic disease, although it may require 3 to 6 months of therapy before a response is noted.[137,138] High-dose corticosteroids, either alone or in combination with immunosuppressive drugs, are necessary for severe end-organ or life-threatening disease, such as severe hematologic abnormalities, lupus nephritis, or CNS lupus.[137,139,140]

Cytotoxic drugs have proven to be effective in the treatment of patients with severe lupus nephritis. Monthly intravenous cyclophosphamide at a dose of 0.5 to 1.0 g/m^2 and daily oral cyclophosphamide 1 to 2 mg/kg per day have been used alone or in combination with oral corticosteroids to control life-threatening active lupus nephritis.[137,141,142] However, because pulse intravenous cyclophosphamide causes fewer side-effects than oral cyclophosphamide, pulse intravenous cyclophosphamide is the preferred treatment for lupus nephritis. For severe, refractory disease, bone marrow immunoablation with or without autologous stem cell transplantation has been successful in inducing remission in a small number of patients over 1 to 2 years of follow-up.[143] Anticoagulation therapy is often used in patients with SLE and APS.[144,145]

Ocular manifestations

The major ocular manifestations of SLE are: (1) involvement of the skin of the eyelids with cutaneous disease; (2) secondary Sjögren's syndrome; (3) scleritis; (4) retinal vascular lesions; and (5) neuro-ophthalmic lesions. Eyelid disease is most often discoid lupus erythematosus involving the margin of the lids.[146] Secondary Sjögren's syndrome occurs in approximately 20% of patients with SLE and is indistinguishable from the sicca complex seen in other patients with connective tissue diseases.[125]

Posterior segment manifestations

Retinal vascular manifestations are the most common form of ophthalmic involvement in patients with SLE. Most frequently these consist of cottonwool spots with or without intraretinal hemorrhages (Fig. 75-3). The prevalence of retinopathy varies widely depending on the patient population studied, from 3% of ambulatory outpatients to 28% of hospitalized patients with SLE having retinal vascular findings.[147–149] These retinal vascular changes occur independently of hypertension and are thought to be related to the underlying microangiopathy of SLE. The histopathologic picture of CNS lupus is that of a microangiopathic disease with small-vessel vaso-occlusion, and the process is presumed to be similar in the retina. Studies of autopsy material have demonstrated immunoreactants, primarily immunoglobulin and complement, in the vessel walls, and these may be responsible for the microangiopathy.[150] Fluorescein angiographic studies[151] have suggested that a mild background retinopathy with microaneurysms and telangiectatic vessels may be relatively common.

Although it is clear that the finding of retinal vascular changes in patients with SLE correlates with active disease,[152] the

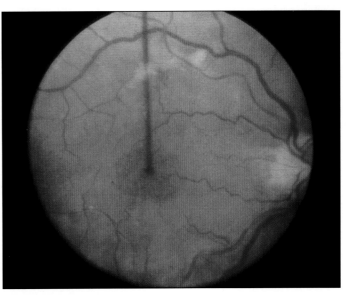

Fig. 75-3 Cottonwool spots in a patient with active systemic lupus erythematosus.

relationship of cottonwool spots alone to CNS lupus remains enigmatic. To date, this relationship has been debated and has not been established. Most experts believe that the finding of cottonwool spots alone does not indicate the presence of CNS lupus.

Although this milder microangiopathy retinopathy is more common, an occasional severe retinal vaso-occlusive disease has been described.[153–159] This more severe retinal vaso-occlusive disease appears to be associated with CNS lupus, and, in particular, diffuse CNS dysfunction, such as an organic brain syndrome.[160] The more severe retinal vascular disease includes central retinal artery occlusion, central retinal vein occlusion, branch artery occlusion, and a diffuse retinal vaso-occlusive disease (Fig. 75-4). Although this process has been called "retinal vasculitis" by some, the pathogenesis may well not be a true vasculitis. Cases of severe retinal vaso-occlusive disease in SLE in association with the lupus anticoagulant have been reported (Fig. 75-5), and the retinal disease is thought to be related to this autoantibody.[161]

With severe retinal vascular disease, the prognosis for vision is poor, and retinal neovascularization commonly develops. Panretinal photocoagulation may be of value in the treatment of the neovascularization of severe lupus retinopathy.[159,160] Even less common than retinopathy is lupus choroidopathy.[153,159,161,162] Early histologic studies demonstrated the frequent occurrence of mononuclear inflammatory cells in the choroid of patients with untreated SLE.[153] The clinical changes seen in patients with lupus choroidopathy involve serous elevations of the retina, most often of the neurosensory retina; serous elevations of the retinal pigment epithelium and combined elevations may also be seen (Figs 75-6 and 75-7). These clinical findings are associated with a systemic vascular disease, either hypertension from lupus nephritis or systemic vasculitis.[162] Treatment of the underlying disease with systemic corticosteroids, immunosup-

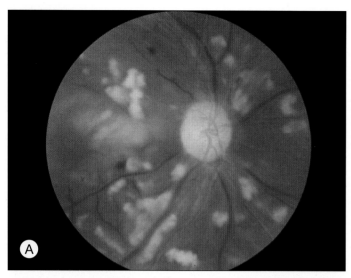
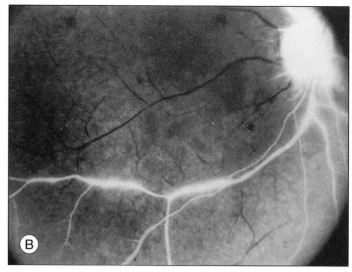

Fig. 75-4 Fundus photograph (A) and fluorescein angiogram (B) demonstrating diffuse vaso-occlusive disease in a patient with systemic lupus erythematosus. Fluorescein angiogram shows extensive nonperfusion of the retina. (Reproduced from Jabs DA, Fine SL, Hochberg MC et al. Severe retinal vaso-occlusive disease in systemic lupus erythematosus. Arch Ophthalmol 1986; 104:558–563.)

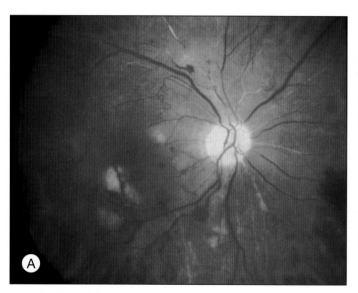
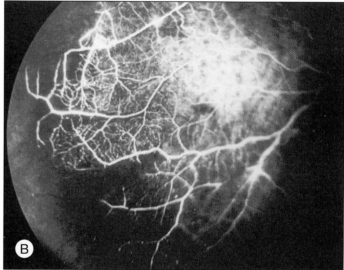

Fig. 75-5 Fundus photograph (A) and fluorescein angiogram (B) demonstrating diffuse vaso-occlusive disease in a patient with systemic lupus erythematosus. Note peripheral nonperfusion of the retina. The patient had anticardiolipin antibodies. (Reproduced from Jabs DA, Fine SL, Hochberg MC et al. Severe retinal vaso-occlusive disease in systemic lupus erythematosus. Arch Ophthalmol 1986; 104:558–563.)

pressive agents if needed, and control of the hypertension can lead to resolution of the serous retinal detachments.[162]

Neuro-ophthalmic involvement in SLE includes cranial nerve palsies from lupus microangiopathy, lupus optic neuropathy, and central, retrochiasmal disorders of vision.[163–169] The cerebral disorders of vision include hallucinations and visual field loss. The optic nerve lesions seen in SLE are most often reported as retrobulbar optic neuritis.[169] However, other optic nerve lesions can be seen, including anterior optic neuritis with optic disc edema, ION, and a slowly progressive visual loss from lupus optic neuropathy.[163–169,170] Histopathologic studies have suggested a microangiopathic process as the pathogenesis of the lupus optic neuropathy. Focal demyelination can be seen, but more severe lesions with axonal damage and even optic nerve infarcts have also been demonstrated.[164–166] One case demonstrated both demyelination and loss of axons with foci of total destruction of the optic nerve.[166] Transverse myelitis is seen in over 50% of patients with lupus optic neuropathy, compared with its overall prevalence of 4% in patients with SLE.[169] The prevalence of clinical optic neuropathy in SLE has been estimated at 1% to 2% of patients with SLE[121,124,125]; however, lupus optic neuropathy may be more frequent, as visual evoked response testing has suggested that optic nerve abnormalities are common in patients with CNS lupus.[171]

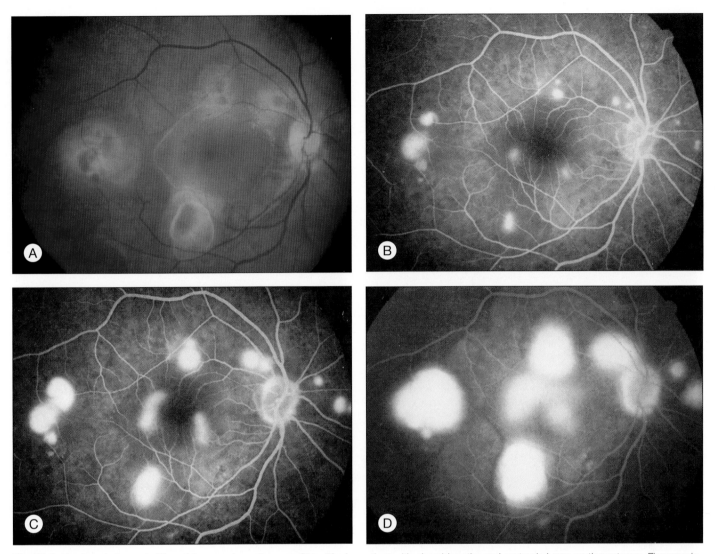

Fig. 75-6 Fundus photograph (A) and fluorescein angiograms (B to D) of a patient with choroidopathy and systemic lupus erythematosus. Fluorescein angiogram demonstrates multiple "smokestack" areas of fluorescein leakage. (Reproduced from Jabs DA, Hanneken AM, Schachat AP et al. Choroidopathy in systemic lupus erythematosus. Arch Ophthalmol 1988; 106:230–234.)

SCLERODERMA

General considerations

Scleroderma is a systemic connective tissue disease of unknown etiology characterized by fibrous and degenerative changes in the skin and viscera. In addition to the thickening and fibrous replacement of the dermis of the skin, there are vascular insufficiency and vasospasm. Scleroderma typically affects middle-aged women, with an onset of disease in the fourth to fifth decade of life. The hallmarks of scleroderma are the skin changes, which consist of thickening, tightening, induration, and subsequent loss of mobility and contracture. The disease most characteristically begins peripherally and involves the fingers and hands with a subsequent centripetal spread up the arms to involve the face and body. Telangiectasia and calcinosis are common. Over 95% of scleroderma patients will have Raynaud's phenomenon, and some will develop digital ulcers.[172–174]

Organ involvement is common and includes esophageal dysmotility with gastroesophageal reflux in over 90% of patients. The small bowel and large bowel may be involved with decreased motility, malabsorption, and diverticulosis. Cardiopulmonary disease is manifested primarily by pulmonary fibrosis, which results in restrictive lung disease with a decreased diffusing capacity. The consequences of the interstitial fibrosis include pulmonary hypertension and right heart failure. As the management of scleroderma-related renal disease has improved, cardiopulmonary complications in scleroderma have become the leading cause of mortality. Musculoskeletal features include polyarthralgias, tendon friction rubs, and, occasionally, myositis.[172]

Renal disease has been the major cause of mortality and is often associated with the onset of malignant hypertension and a rapid progression to renal failure. This process is sometimes known as "scleroderma renal crisis" or "scleroderma kidney."

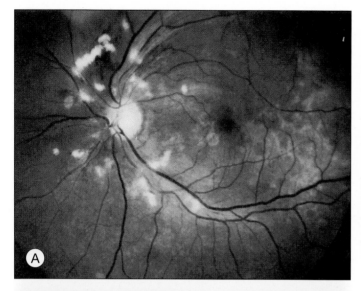

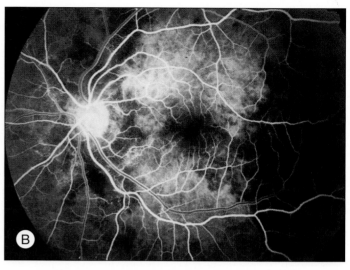

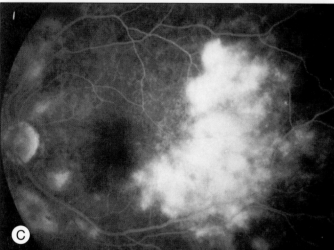

Fig. 75-7 Fundus photograph (A) and fluorescein angiograms (B and C) of a patient with systemic lupus erythematosus. The patient had an exudative retinal detachment, which resolved with treatment. Fluorescein angiograms demonstrate delayed choroidal perfusion with late leakage. (Reproduced from Jabs DA, Hanneken AM, Schachat AP et al. Choroidopathy in systemic lupus erythematosus. Arch Ophthalmol 1988; 106:230–234.)

This complication was considered fatal up until the late 1970s; however, aggressive antihypertensive therapy may sometimes reverse the scleroderma renal crisis.[175–178]

There is a spectrum of disease to scleroderma. The CREST syndrome is named for its features of calcinosis, Raynaud's phenomenon, esophageal dysmotility, sclerodactyly, and telangiectasia. This syndrome appears to have a more benign and more slowly progressive course than systemic scleroderma.[179] Systemic scleroderma is a more rapidly progressive skin disease with more severe visceral involvement.[172] Overlap syndromes occur between scleroderma and other diseases. The best-known overlap syndrome is mixed connective tissue disease (MCTD), which has features of SLE, systemic scleroderma, and myositis. It was originally characterized by antibodies to ribonuclear protein, and it had been suggested that some of the clinical features responded to corticosteroids.[180] Long-term follow-up studies have suggested that MCTD generally evolves into systemic scleroderma, and some experts no longer consider MCTD a separate entity.[181]

Treatment

No specific treatment has been shown to alter the progression of scleroderma effectively, and traditionally treatment has been directed towards management of the complications and symptomatic relief. Corticosteroids are ineffective in the treatment of scleroderma itself, but occasionally may be used to treat the complications of lung disease and myositis.[172,182] Immunosuppressive agents have not shown any consistent value in the treatment of scleroderma.[172]

Scleroderma renal crisis can often be controlled by aggressive treatment of the hypertension and dialysis for renal failure.[175,176,178] Raynaud's phenomenon is most often treated with calcium channel antagonists, such as nifedipine. These agents are effective in symptomatic relief and reducing the number of attacks of Raynaud's phenomenon.[183,184]

Ocular manifestations

Studies of ocular involvement have suggested that the anterior segment is most commonly affected. The skin disease may cause the eyelids to develop tightness, blepharophimosis, and lagophthalmos. Lid involvement occurs in 30% to 65% of patients. Despite the frequent involvement of the eyelids, corneal exposure is not common. Conjunctival vascular abnormalities, including telangiectasia and vascular sludging, can occur in up to 70% of patients, and keratoconjunctivitis sicca with a Sjögren's-like picture has been described.[185,186] Minor salivary gland biopsy studies have suggested that two different pathogenetic mechanisms may be present. Some patients have inflammation of the glands, similar to Sjögren's syndrome, and this mechanism seems to associate more often with the CREST syndrome. The other mechanism appears to be glandular fibrosis, which is seen more often in patients with diffuse systemic scleroderma.[187,188] Periorbital edema,[189] cranial nerve palsies,[190,191] scleral pits,[192] and restrictive ophthalmopathy[193,194] have also been reported.

Posterior segment lesions

The most commonly described retinal lesion in patients with scleroderma is the retinopathy of malignant hypertension, including cottonwool spots, intraretinal hemorrhages, and optic disc edema. Both clinical and histologic studies have documented that the picture is identical to that of idiopathic malignant hypertension. These patients have malignant hypertension due to scleroderma renal crisis. Pathologic studies have shown early hyalinization of the ciliary arteries, microinfarcts in the nerve fiber layer with multiple cytoid bodies, neuroretinal edema, subretinal exudates, optic disc edema, and fibrinoid changes with fibrin plugs in the choroidal arterioles and choriocapillaris.[185,195–200]

In contrast to the infrequent findings of retinopathy in patients with scleroderma, small case series of fluorescein angiographic studies have suggested more frequent abnormalities of the choroidal vasculature in patients with systemic scleroderma, including patchy and irregular perfusion of the choroid and variable hyperfluorescence of the retinal pigment epithelium in one-third to one-half of the patients. Clinically these lesions were silent, and ophthalmoscopy results were normal.[198,200,201] There have been occasional case reports of other rare ocular complications in patients with systemic scleroderma, including branch and central retinal vein occlusions and retinal hemorrhages.[185,186,200,202]

POLYMYOSITIS AND DERMATOMYOSITIS

General considerations

Polymyositis and dermatomyositis are inflammatory diseases of skeletal muscle characterized by pain and weakness in the involved muscle groups. In the typical case, weakness begins insidiously and involves the proximal muscle groups, particularly those of the shoulders and hips. Dermatomyositis is distinguished from polymyositis by the presence of cutaneous lesions. The skin lesions of dermatomyositis are an erythematous to violaceous rash, variably affecting the eyelids (heliotrope rash), cheeks, nose, chest, and extensor surfaces. The knuckles of the fingers may develop plaques known as Gottron's papules.[203–205]

The diagnosis of myositis is based on the characteristic clinical features and abnormal laboratory tests. Laboratory abnormalities include an elevated ESR, elevated skeletal muscle enzymes released into the serum as a consequence of skeletal muscle damage, abnormal electromyography, and a muscle biopsy revealing muscle damage and inflammation. The potentially abnormal muscle enzymes include creatinine phosphokinase, aldolase, aspartate transferase, alanine transferase, and lactic dehydrogenase.[203–206]

Bohan & Peter[204] have classified polymyositis and dermatomyositis into five groups: (1) primary idiopathic polymyositis; (2) primary idiopathic dermatomyositis; (3) dermatomyositis (or polymyositis) associated with neoplasia; (4) childhood dermatomyositis (or polymyositis) associated with vasculitis; and (5) polymyositis or dermatomyositis associated with collagen-vascular disease (overlap group). Dermatomyositis with neoplasia is most often seen in patients over age 50 and rarely in young patients.[203,206] Vasculitis is common in patients with childhood dermatomyositis. Inflammatory myositis with a defined connective tissue disease is most often associated with SLE, primary Sjögren's syndrome, or scleroderma.

Ocular manifestations

Other than the heliotrope rash of dermatomyositis, ocular involvement by inflammatory myositis is relatively uncommon. Occasionally, ophthalmoplegia due to involvement of the extraocular muscles by the myositis may occur.[194,207]

Posterior segment lesions

Cottonwool spots have occasionally been reported in association with dermatomyositis.[208–213] The majority of these reports are in children with dermatomyositis, and this association may be due to the vasculitis commonly seen in these children.[208–213] However, a microangiopathy has also been reported in an occasional dermatomyositis patient without demonstrable systemic vasculitis.[213] The retinal vasculopathy may be due to the presence of inflammatory mediators in the microvasculature.

SJÖGREN'S SYNDROME

General considerations

Sjögren's syndrome was originally described as a triad of dry eyes, dry mouth, and RA. Subsequently, it became apparent that Sjögren's syndrome could exist with several other connective tissue diseases, including SLE and scleroderma (secondary Sjögren's syndrome) or without a definitive connective tissue disease (primary Sjögren's syndrome).[214–216]

The cause of the dry eyes and dry mouth in patients with Sjögren's syndrome is a mononuclear inflammatory infiltrate into the lacrimal and salivary glands resulting in glandular destruction and dysfunction. Several studies have demonstrated that the minor salivary gland biopsy is a useful tool for documenting the presence of this inflammatory infiltrate.[214–216] Immunohistologic studies have suggested that the majority of cells in this infiltrate are CD4+ T cells, with lesser numbers of CD8+ T cells and B cells.[215,217,218]

Although several classification systems for the diagnosis of Sjögren's syndrome have been proposed, no uniform system has become widely accepted. Two diagnostic criteria, the San Diego criteria and the original criteria proposed by the European Economic Community (EEC) Study group, have been used in the USA and Europe respectively.[219,220] The San Diego criteria differ from the EEC criteria in that the presence of an inflammatory infiltrate seen on minor salivary gland biopsy or the presence of autoantibodies is required for the diagnosis of Sjögren's syndrome.[219,220] The San Diego criteria, however, have been used more typically for research purposes. For clinical diagnosis, most investigators use a simple system in which two of the following three elements are present: (1) keratoconjunctivitis sicca; (2) evidence of salivary gland dysfunction such as a positive minor salivary gland biopsy or abnormal salivary flow study; and (3) presence of a defined connective tissue disease, such as RA, SLE, or scleroderma.[219] Secondary Sjögren's syndrome is diagnosed when a defined connective tissue disease is present, and primary Sjögren's syndrome when no definable connective tissue disease is present. There appears to be a subgroup of patients with primary Sjögren's syndrome who have an aggressive systemic illness associated with serologic abnormalities, cutaneous vasculitis, CNS disease, and hematologic abnormalities.[221] Patients with Sjögren's syndrome frequently have multiple autoantibodies, including ANA, RF, and antibodies to the two Sjögren's syndrome antigens, Ro (SSA) and La (SSB). Antibody studies using enzyme-linked immunosorbent assay techniques have shown antibodies to Ro in 96% of patients and to La in 87% of patients with Sjögren's syndrome, but other detection methods, such as immunodiffusion, give lower percentages.[222]

Ocular manifestations

The finding of keratoconjunctivitis sicca is the ocular hallmark of Sjögren's syndrome. This disorder is most often documented by an abnormal Schirmer's test demonstrating decreased tear production and by demonstrating damage to the ocular surface using rose Bengal staining. Occasionally, patients with RA and secondary Sjögren's syndrome may develop a corneal melting disorder.

Posterior segment lesions

Posterior segment lesions are usually not intrinsic to Sjögren's syndrome itself. However, among that group of patients with primary Sjögren's syndrome and other systemic autoimmune features, ION, presumably as a consequence of a CNS vasculitis, has been described.[221] Rosenbaum & Bennett[223] reported a series of patients with primary Sjögren's syndrome and anterior and intermediate uveitis.

RELAPSING POLYCHONDRITIS

General considerations

Relapsing polychondritis is a disorder characterized by recurrent, widespread, potentially destructive inflammation of cartilage, the cardiovascular system, and the organs of special sense.[224] The most common clinical features are outlined in Table 75-3 and include auricular inflammation, arthropathy, and nasal cartilage inflammation. Laryngotracheobronchial disease occurs in approximately one-half of the patients with relapsing polychondritis and may lead to death from laryngeal collapse. Involvement of the internal ear, cardiovascular system, and skin is less common.[1,224–228]

The arthropathy is a migratory, asymmetric, nondeforming polyarticular disease often affecting the parasternal articular surfaces. Cardiovascular lesions include aortic insufficiency, due to progressive dilation of the aortic ring. Skin lesions, which are most often due to cutaneous vasculitis, include palpable purpura and livedo reticularis. Auricular chondritis and nasal chondritis are the features that most often suggest the diagnosis. On biopsy of cartilaginous structures, such as the ear, there is loss of basophilic staining of the cartilage matrix, as well as perichondral inflammation. Eventually there is cartilage destruction and replacement by fibrous tissue. Approximately 20% of patients will have an associated connective tissue disease, including systemic vasculitis, SLE, or RA.[1,224–228]

Ocular manifestations

Ocular manifestations are common in relapsing polychondritis and occur in 50% to 54% of patients.[221,229–232] The most common ocular manifestations are conjunctivitis, scleritis, and uveitis. In patients with an associated vasculitis, optic nerve involvement and cranial nerve palsies may be seen. Scleral involvement is the most common ocular manifestation of relapsing polychondritis and occurs in approximately 35% to 41% of patients.[221,229] Most often diffuse anterior scleritis is the type present, but recurrent episcleritis, necrotizing scleritis, or posterior scleritis can also be

Table 75-3 Features of relapsing polychondritis	
Feature	Frequency (%)
Auricular inflammation	85
Arthropathy	76
Nasal cartilage inflammation	66
Ocular inflammation	59
Laryngotracheobronchial disease	51
Vestibuloauditory disease	42
Cardiovascular disease	24
Systemic vasculitis	11
Cutaneous disease	16

seen. The occasional reports of chorioretinitis in patients with relapsing polychondritis appear to represent posterior scleritis. Uveitis occurs in approximately 17% to 25% of patients with relapsing polychondritis and most often represents an anterior uveitis, which may occur alone or in conjunction with scleritis (sclerouveitis). Keratitis, including marginal corneal ulceration, has been seen in 10% to 15% of patients with relapsing polychondritis.[221,229–232]

Posterior segment manifestations

The most commonly reported posterior segment manifestation in relapsing polychondritis is posterior scleritis, which may be complicated by exudative retinal detachment.[232–234] Another posterior segment manifestation of relapsing polychondritis is ION, which has been reported as part of their disease in patients with a systemic vasculitis. Isaak and co-workers[225] have reported retinopathy in 10% of their patients with relapsing polychondritis. Most often this retinopathy consisted of a few cottonwool spots and intraretinal hemorrhages, but branch retinal vein and central retinal vein occlusions have also been described.

SYSTEMIC VASCULITIDES

The systemic vasculitides are listed in Box 75-3. Each of the different vasculitides is characterized by its clinical pattern of vessel involvement and the histopathologic features of the vasculitis.[235–238] The classification system for the systemic vasculitides was modified in 1994 by the Chapel Hill Consensus Conference, and categorizes the vasculitides by the size of the vessels involved: large-, medium-, or small-sized blood vessels.[239] Ocular manifestations are common in vasculitis and generally fall into two categories: (1) scleritis; and (2) vasculitis-related damage to the retina, optic nerve, or other cranial nerves. The frequency of ocular involvement and the pattern of ocular involvement are dependent on the size and pattern of blood vessels involved by a given type of vasculitis.

Box 75-3 Systemic vasculitides

Large-vessel disease
Giant-cell arteritis
Takayasu's arteritis

Medium-vessel disease
Polyarteritis nodosa

Small-vessel disease
Churg–Strauss syndrome
Wegener's granulomatosis
Behçet's disease
Hypersensitivity vasculitis
Henoch–Schönlein purpura
Vasculitis with connective tissue disease
Lymphomatoid granulomatosis
Essential mixed cryoglobulinemia associated with hepatitis C
Hypocomplementemic urticarial vasculitic syndrome (HUVS)

Large-vessel vasculitides

Giant-cell arteritis

General considerations   Giant cell arteritis (GCA) or temporal arteritis has been described in all races, although whites are affected most often. It is particularly common in northern climates such as Scandinavia, the UK, and the northern USA. Autopsy studies have estimated the prevalence of GCA at 1.1% of the population.[240]

The clinical features of GCA are listed in Table 75-4.[163] They include headache, polymyalgia rheumatica, jaw claudication, constitutional symptoms such as fever and malaise, and ophthalmic symptoms. The signs include tenderness over the temporal artery, a pulseless temporal artery, scalp tenderness, fever, and loss of vision.[241–244]

The most commonly abnormal laboratory test is the ESR. Over 90% of patients will have an elevated ESR. Keltner[245] has stated that only 2% will have a normal ESR; however, frequencies of normal ESR in patients with polymyalgia rheumatica and suspected GCA have been reported to range from 6% to 22%.[242–244] Care must be taken in interpreting the ESR, because the method used must be known. Markedly elevated ESRs are obtained with a Westergren method. In patients with GCA, the

Table 75-4 Features of giant-cell arteritis

Symptoms	Frequency (%) (range)
Headache	60 (36–100)
Polymyalgia rheumatica	47 (20–86)
Jaw claudication	36 (4–67)
Anorexia	36 (15–69)
Malaise	29 (12–97)
Extremity claudication	8 (3–43)
Depression	25 (4–46)
Facial neuralgia	21 (2–41)
Blurred vision	16 (6–23)
Vertigo	12 (3–20)
Amaurosis fugax	12 (2–19)
Diplopia	12 (2–43)
Temporal artery tenderness	55 (28–91)
Nodular artery	35 (8–48)
Pulseless artery	51 (23–72)
Scalp tenderness	57 (28–97)
Fever	48 (71–98)
Weight loss	45 (16–76)
Blindness	36 (7–66)

Modified from Goodman BW Jr. Temporal arteritis. Am J Med 1979; 67:839–852.

Westergren method yields a median ESR of 96 mm/h, with a range of 50 to 132 mm/h. Studies stating that the normal ESR in elderly patients can be as high as 40 mm/h have used the Westergren method. The Wintrobe method uses a closed-ended tube. The mean ESR in patients with GCA using the Wintrobe method is 51 mm/h, with a range of 38 to 59 mm/h.[241,244,246,247] C-reactive protein has been suggested as a good marker since it is a more sensitive marker of the acute-phase response, and a normal C-reactive protein has been reported in only 1% of patients with suspected or confirmed GCA.[241,248]

The definitive test for the diagnosis of GCA is the temporal artery biopsy. The characteristic features in a temporal artery biopsy are occlusion of the vessel lumen with either thrombus or subintimal edema and cellular proliferation. There is fragmentation of the internal elastic lamina and a patchy degeneration of smooth-muscle cells. Granulomatous inflammation of the vessel wall affects the media, adventitia, and subintima and is composed of lymphocytes, plasma cells, histiocytes, epithelioid cells, and giant cells.[241] Temporal artery biopsies can occasionally be negative on one side and positive on the second side. Two studies have suggested that the prevalence of false-negative unilateral biopsies is in the 4% to 5% range, but one study reported the frequency of false-negative biopsies as high as 15%. These false-negative results are due to the presence of "skip areas" in the temporal artery biopsy.[243,249–254]

Treatment The treatment of GCA is with systemic corticosteroids. The dose of prednisone for patients with GCA is in the range of 1 mg/kg per day (60 to 80 mg/day). Generally the symptoms respond promptly within several days. Treatment with corticosteroids is prophylactic for loss of vision. Every-other-day steroids are ineffective in the initial treatment of GCA.[241,255,256]

Some studies have suggested that GCA is a self-limited disease that will "burn itself out" at the end of 1 to 2 years. These studies have recommended treatment for 1 to 2 years. Treatment is generally instituted at the initial high dose and slowly tapered, utilizing the ESR and clinical symptoms to monitor disease. Occasionally, longer-lasting disease will be seen, as well as patients who will require longer-term treatment.[257,258] Corticosteroid-sparing agents, such as methotrexate, azathioprine, ciclosporin, and cyclophosphamide, as well as hydroxychloroquine and dapsone, have been tried in the treatment of GCA, with mixed results. Methotrexate has been the most extensively and rigorously studied, but data from randomized placebo-controlled clinical trials do not support its use.[259,260]

Ocular manifestations The most frequent ocular manifestation is ION. This can present either as anterior ION or retrobulbar ION. Visual loss from GCA has occurred in over 36% of patients reported. Early series generally reported 50% to 70% of patients with visual loss, but the most recent series have reduced this to 13%.[255,256,258] This reduction in visual loss presumably represents earlier recognition of the disease and the institution of corticosteroid treatment.[243,245,258,261] The characteristic clinical features of ION are a painless, sudden, and profound

loss of vision, loss of color vision, and the characteristic altitudinal field defect. This may sometimes be a Bjerrum-type scotoma rather than complete altitudinal loss. When optic disc edema is present, anterior ION is diagnosed. When optic disc edema is not present, retrobulbar ION is the diagnosis. ION is due to involvement by the arteritic process of the posterior ciliary arteries supplying the optic nerve. Central retinal artery occlusion and branch retinal artery occlusions have also been seen, although less frequently.[243,245,258,261] Amaurosis fugax has been reported in a variable number of patients, ranging from 2% to 19%, depending on the series. Amaurosis is believed to be a "pre-ION" symptom and an indication for immediate corticosteroid treatment. In one series almost 40% of patients with amaurosis fugax and GCA developed ION and another 15% developed central retinal artery occlusions.[255]

Ischemic retinopathy with cottonwool spots or hemorrhages, or both, is present in a small number of patients.[262–264] Several series have reported occasional diplopia or ophthalmoplegia.[265–269] The ophthalmoplegic pattern fluctuates with time and is thought to represent ischemia to the extraocular muscles. These patients are also said to be at high risk for the development of ION and to require prompt corticosteroid treatment.[267–269] Other ocular complications reported include the ocular ischemic syndrome,[270] hypotony,[271] choroidal ischemia,[272] and cortical blindness. These other forms of ophthalmic involvement occur in 5% to 7% of patients with GCA.[245]

Although the use of corticosteroids in a patient who has developed ION is said to be prophylactic for the second eye and not to bring about improvement in the involved eye, there have been case reports of reversal of ION with the immediate institution of high-dose "pulse" intravenous corticosteroids.[256,273] This treatment involves the use of 1 g methylprednisolone daily as an intravenous infusion for 1 to 3 days. A response was seen when patients were treated within the first 24 h of presentation. A similar beneficial response was reported with pulse corticosteroids for central retinal artery occlusion due to GCA.[274]

Takayasu's arteritis

General considerations Takayasu's arteritis affects large arteries, particularly branches of the aorta. It occurs primarily in children and young women. The disease is rare in the western world but is common in Asia. Other names for Takayasu's arteritis include *aortic arch arteritis, aortitis syndrome,* and *pulseless disease.* The disease may be localized to any segment of the aorta or its primary branches or involve the entire aorta. The inflammatory process primarily affects the large elastic arteries and is characterized by a panarteritis with a granulomatous inflammation. The involved vessels may ultimately become narrowed or obliterated, resulting in ischemia to the supplied tissues. Areas of weakened vascular wall may develop dissections or aneurysms.[238,275–279]

Clinically the course of the disease is divided into pre-pulseless and pulseless phases. Systemic features such as fatigue, weight loss, and low-grade fever are common in the pre-pulseless phase. Abnormalities in circulation, such as claudication of the extremities, syncope, Raynaud's phenomenon, and angina, may occur during the pre-pulseless phase. Evidence of vascular insufficiency due to large-artery narrowing or reduction leads to the characteristic pulseless phase. The disease is most often diagnosed using arteriography, which shows vascular segments with smooth-walled, tapered, and focal or generalized narrowing, as well as other areas with dilation.[275–279]

Treatment Takayasu's arteritis may be rapidly progressive and fatal. Treatment is generally with systemic corticosteroids at a dose of prednisone of 1 mg/kg per day, which may successfully suppress the disease and reverse absent pulses.[276,278] Cyclophosphamide, methotrexate, ciclosporin, and mycophenolate mofetil have been used with some benefit in corticosteroid-resistant cases or in cases in which the corticosteroid could not be tapered to appropriately low maintenance doses. Surgical arterial reconstruction may be necessary.[280]

Ocular manifestations The most characteristic ocular findings are hypertensive retinopathy and Takayasu's retinopathy. In a series of 78 patients with Takayasu's arteritis, 30.8% of patients had hypertensive retinopathy and 13.5% had Takayasu's retinopathy.[281] Takayasu's retinopathy may be categorized into four stages: (1) stage 1 is dilation of small vessels; (2) stage 2 is capillary microaneurysm formation; (3) stage 3 is retinal arteriovenous anastomoses; and (4) stage 4 is arteriovenous anastomoses with other ocular complications.[281,282] The arteriovenous anastomoses are generally seen around the disc and in the midperiphery, and they are thought to be due to ocular ischemia from narrowing of the common carotid and vertebral arteries. The retinal changes can be best demonstrated by fluorescein angiography. More severe ischemia may result in peripheral retinal nonperfusion, neovascularization, and vitreous hemorrhage.[282]

Medium-vessel vasculitides
Polyarteritis nodosa
General considerations Polyarteritis nodosa (PAN) is characterized by necrotizing vasculitis of the medium- and small-sized muscular arteries. The lesions are segmented and in various stages of development. Histologic findings are characterized by infarction and the formation of microaneurysms.[235,236]

The mean age of onset of PAN is 40 to 50 years. Constitutional symptoms are seen in approximately 70% of patients with PAN. Renal involvement is common, affecting 40% of patients, and either related to vasculitis or glomerulonephritis. Hypertension may develop as a result of renal disease and affects one-third of patients. Gastrointestinal disease with infarction of the viscera also occurs infrequently. Neurologic disease is common, often presenting with mononeuritis multiplex in 42% to 70% of patients with PAN. Involvement of the CNS is rare.[283–285] Approximately 10% of patients are hepatitis B antigen-positive, and hepatitis B has been associated as an etiologic agent in the development of PAN. Circulating immune complexes composed of hepatitis B antigen and antibodies to hepatitis B antigen in vessel walls have been demonstrated in the early stage of the disease. Hepatitis B-induced PAN probably represents one of the few documented examples of an immune complex-mediated vasculitis.[286–288]

Treatment Survival in patients with untreated PAN was poor, with only 55% of patients still alive 5 years after the initial diagnosis. The most common causes of death were renal failure, gastrointestinal infarction or hemorrhage, and cerebral vasculitis. High-dose oral corticosteroid therapy has prolonged survival and often quiets the disease.[289] However, because of the poor long-term outcome with corticosteroid therapy alone, patients are often treated with corticosteroids and immunosuppressive drugs such as cyclophosphamide. This therapy appears to improve disease control and long-term outcome.[235,284,290] The initial dose of cyclophosphamide is generally 2 mg/kg per day. The corticosteroids are continued until the disease is controlled and then tapered over a period of 2 to 3 months. The cyclophosphamide is continued for a period of 1 year and then tapered and discontinued. Long-term remissions may be induced by this type of treatment.[284,290] As an alternative, intravenous cyclophosphamide has been used at 10 to 15 mg/kg monthly and may be less toxic.[291] Azathioprine, methotrexate, and mycophenolate mofetil may be effective for milder disease.[285]

Ocular manifestations Ocular manifestations occur in approximately 10% to 20% of patients with PAN. Older series reporting ocular disease and PAN did not distinguish between PAN and other forms of vasculitis. In particular, Wegener's granulomatosis was often confused with PAN. The most common ocular manifestations of PAN are related to the vascular disease, and include hypertensive retinopathy in patients with renal disease, cottonwool spots from the vasculitis, retinal artery occlusive disease, central lesions resulting in visual loss (e.g., homonymous hemianopsia, visual hallucinations), cranial nerve palsies, scleritis, and marginal corneal ulceration. Posterior scleritis and serous retinal detachments due to choroidal ischemia have been reported.[285,292–304]

Small-vessel vasculitides
Churg–Strauss syndrome (allergic granulomatosis)
General considerations Churg–Strauss syndrome, also called allergic granulomatosis or Churg–Strauss angiitis, is a syndrome of a necrotizing vasculitis affecting small arteries and veins, an allergic diathesis (particularly asthma), and extravascular granulomas. Lung disease is the sine qua non for the diagnosis of Churg–Strauss syndrome. Pulmonary infiltrates and pleural effusions have been reported. Eosinophilia is present, and the cell count may be greater than 15 000 cells/μl. On pathologic examination, granulomas are often seen with eosinophilic tissue infiltration. A mononeuropathy or polyneuropathy attributed to the vasculitis frequently occurs.[305–310]

Treatment Treatment for Churg–Strauss syndrome typically is with high-dose oral corticosteroids either alone or in combination with oral cyclophosphamide. The 5-year survival rate is 79%. The presence of renal, gastrointestinal, or cardiac disease predicts poorer outcome and typically mandates more aggressive treatment.[310]

Ocular manifestations In addition to the vasculitis-related ocular complications seen in classic PAN, conjunctival granulomas have been reported in patients with Churg–Strauss syndrome. Case reports have described uveitis, marginal corneal ulcers, scleritis, and neuro-ophthalmic lesions, including cranial nerve palsies, papilledema, and optic neuropathy in association with the disease.[310–314]

Wegener's granulomatosis

General considerations Wegener's granulomatosis was originally described as the triad of necrotizing granulomatous lesions of the upper and lower respiratory tracts, focal necrotizing vasculitis, and glomerulitis.[235,310,315–319] Subsequently, limited Wegener's granulomatosis was described, which consisted of upper- and lower-airway granulomatous disease without involvement of the kidneys.[320,321] Later studies employing renal biopsy have demonstrated that often there are subclinical renal lesions in patients with limited Wegener's granulomatosis. The clinical features of Wegener's granulomatosis are outlined in Table 75-5.[315-319,322]

Sinus disease 'is the most characteristic feature clinically, although biopsy specimens of sinus tissue may show only necrotic material without characteristic histologic features. Superinfection of the sinuses due to the presence of necrotic material commonly occurs. Pulmonary disease is also frequent and lung biopsy specimens are often diagnostic. Renal disease may be present on biopsy, even when it is not clinically evident. Early detection of renal disease is essential since up to 85% of patients with Wegener's granulomatosis will develop renal disease during the course of the disease, and, if left untreated, the mean survival time in a patient with Wegener's-associated renal disease is 5 months.[315–318,322,323]

Treatment Before the use of immunosuppressive drugs for treatment, Wegener's granulomatosis was considered a fatal disease with a mean untreated survival of 5 months. The 1-year mortality was 82%.[322] With corticosteroid treatment, the mean

survival was increased to 12.5 months, but long-term survival was only seen in patients with limited Wegener's granulomatosis.[322–324] Combination therapy with prednisone 1 mg/kg per day and oral cyclophosphamide 2 mg/kg per day improved the survival rate to greater than 80% at 5 years.[310,318,323,324] Typically the corticosteroids are used until the disease is controlled and then subsequently tapered and discontinued. Treatment is continued for 1 year after a complete remission has been achieved, and patients are then tapered off their cyclophosphamide. The best results with this treatment regimen have been reported by the US National Institutes of Health, where 93% of patients successfully achieve a remission.[317,318,323] In one study in which 158 patients with Wegener's granulomatosis were treated with combination prednisone and cyclophosphamide, 91% of patients had an improvement in their disease and 75% had complete remission.[323] Although some patients relapse when the cyclophosphamide is discontinued, a second remission can be achieved with reinduction therapy. Complications of this treatment include leukopenia, hemorrhagic cystitis, gonadal dysfunction, alopecia, and a 2.4-fold increase in the risk of neoplasia.[323] In a randomized controlled trial of patients taking oral cyclophosphamide, 30% developed *Pneumocystis carinii* pneumonia.[325] For this reason, *P. carinii* prophylaxis is recommended in patients taking daily oral cyclophosphamide. Although pulse intravenous cyclophosphamide therapy has fewer side-effects than oral cyclophosphamide, intravenous cyclophosphamide is less effective in inducing a sustained remission than daily oral cyclophosphamide.[324] Other therapies for Wegener's granulomatosis have included methotrexate, mycophenolate mofetil, and biologics such as etanercept and infliximab, which are used either for milder disease or for remission maintenance.

Ocular manifestations Ocular disease occurs in 29% to 58% of patients with Wegener's granulomatosis.[318,323,326–328] The three main categories of ocular involvement are: (1) orbital disease; (2) scleritis with or without peripheral keratitis; and (3) vasculitis-mediated vascular complications. Orbital involvement is common, ranging from 15% to 50% of patients, and in some series is the most common form of ophthalmic involvement.[318,327] Orbital disease may be an extension of the granulomatous inflammation from the sinus into the orbit. This inflammation can lead to a compartment syndrome within the orbit, proptosis, orbital apex syndrome, compressive optic neuropathy, and subsequent irreversible vision loss. Orbital pseudotumor, separate from the sinus inflammation, may also be seen.[329] In addition to orbital pseudotumor, orbital cellulitis may occur as sinus inflammation extends into the orbit, and dacryocystitis may occur from involved and superinfected nasal mucosa.[326,327]

Scleritis is common in Wegener's granulomatosis, occurring in 16% to 38% of patients, and is either the first or second most frequent ocular feature, depending on the series.[313,318,330] The scleritis can be of any type, particularly diffuse anterior or necrotizing scleritis. Marginal corneal ulcers are often seen in association with the scleritis (necrotizing sclerokeratitis), and occasionally without scleritis.[326–328,330] Posterior scleritis has also been reported.[331]

Table 75-5 Features of Wegener's granulomatosis	
Organ system	Frequency (%)
Paranasal sinuses	89–91
Lung	48–94
Kidney	25–85
Joints	34–67
Nasopharynx	65
Ear	60
Eye	29–58
Skin	45–46
Nervous system	22–29

Posterior segment lesions Retinal vascular and optic nerve manifestations occur in 10% to 18% of patients with ocular involvement from Wegener's granulomatosis.[326–328,332] The lesions may be merely cottonwool spots with or without intraretinal hemorrhages, or a more severe vaso-occlusive disease of the retina. Several cases of branch or central retinal artery occlusion have been reported, as has branch retinal vein occlusion. Optic nerve disease is even more common than is retinal vascular disease and includes ION and "optic disc vasculitis." In patients with retinal vasculitis, neovascularization, vitreous hemorrhage, and rubeotic glaucoma may develop.[326–328,331,332] Vision loss in Wegener's granulomatosis has been reported in approximately 8% of patients.[323] Occasionally, the ocular disease in Wegener's granulomatosis will be active despite apparent control of the systemic disease.[330] Although the ocular disease typically responds to treating the underlying disease, some patients, particularly those with severe orbital involvement, may require more aggressive therapy than that required to control other involved organs.[31]

Behçet's disease

General considerations Behçet's disease was initially described by Behçet in 1937 as a triad of oral ulcers, genital ulcers, and hypopyon uveitis. The disease is most common in the Middle and Far East, particularly Japan. In these populations the disease is associated with the HLA type HLA-B51.[333] The clinical features of Behçet's disease are outlined in Table 75-6.[334–337]

Oral ulcers are the most common clinical feature. They are painful, ranging from 2 to 10 mm, and often come in crops. The genital ulcers have similar features but are less often diagnosed. Ocular disease is common and occurs in 68% to 85% of patients. The skin disease can be erythema nodosum, superficial thrombophlebitis, pyoderma, or the phenomenon of *pathergy*, which is defined as the presence of a pustule after breaking the skin by a needle, as in drawing blood. The arthritis is an asymmetric, nondeforming, large-joint polyarthritis that is frequently corticosteroid-responsive. Vascular disease is common and can present as a migratory superficial thrombophlebitis, major vessel thrombosis, arterial aneurysms, or even peripheral gangrene. The CNS disease has been classically divided into three types: (1) brainstem syndrome; (2) meningoencephalitis; and (3) confusional states; most often patients present with combinations of the three. The greatest mortality in Behçet's disease comes from CNS involvement.[334–345]

The diagnosis of Behçet's disease is established clinically on the basis of the presence of various clinical features. A variety of criteria have been proposed for Behçet's disease, but the 1990 criteria, published by an International Study Group for Behçet's Disease, are most commonly used to establish the diagnosis.[346] Using these criteria, the definition of Behçet's disease requires recurrent oral ulceration plus two of the following: recurrent genital ulceration, eye lesions, skin lesions, or a positive pathergy test. These criteria have been found to be 91% sensitive and 96% specific for the diagnosis of Behçet's disease.[346]

Treatment The natural history of ocular Behçet's disease is poor. The majority of patients will lose all or part of their vision within 5 years. Seventy-four percent of the eyes in the series described by Mamo[347] had vision worse than 20/200. Of the 25 eyes that deteriorated to no light perception, vision declined to this level over a period of 3.6 years. The clinical impression was that corticosteroid therapy delayed the progression of the disease but did not alter the ultimate outcome.

Immunosuppressive drugs have been used in the treatment of Behçet's disease since the early 1970s. Initially, chlorambucil was used, typically at a dose of 0.1 to 0.2 mg/kg per day.[348–356] Other studies have used cyclophosphamide at a dose of 1 to 2 mg/kg per day.[356] As with alkylating agent therapy for other diseases, the dose is generally adjusted to keep the white blood cell count over 2500 cells/μl. Systemic corticosteroids, at an initial dose of 1 mg/kg per day of oral prednisone, are used in combination with an immunosuppressive agent to control the acute disease.[356] Once the disease has been controlled, the corticosteroids are tapered and discontinued, and the immunosuppressive drug is continued for 12 to 18 months, then tapered and discontinued. Uncontrolled case series of chlorambucil therapy for Behçet's disease have shown long-term, drug-free remissions after 2 years of treatment.[349,350,356] Less published data are available using cyclophosphamide in the treatment of ocular Behçet's disease; however, some clinicians have found it equally effective as chlorambucil and easier to use.[356]

Ciclosporin has been reported to be effective in the treatment of ocular Behçet's disease.[357–359] A randomized clinical trial of 96 patients found that 50% of patients treated with ciclosporin at a dose of 10 mg/kg per day had a 75% to 100% reduction in the frequency and severity of attacks of their ocular disease.[358] However, nearly 25% of patients treated with ciclosporin had no benefit in terms of the frequency and severity of ocular attacks. Ciclosporin does have the problem of nephrotoxicity, which occurs to some degree in nearly all patients if high doses (10 mg/kg per day) are used.[360] Lower doses of ciclosporin (4 to 5 mg/kg per day) are now used in conjunction with systemic corticosteroids. Azathioprine has also been used in the treatment of Behçet's disease and, in a randomized controlled

Table 75-6 Features of Behçet's disease

Feature	Frequency (%)
Oral ulcers	98–99
Genital ulcers	80–87
Ocular disease	68–79
Skin disease	69–90
Arthritis	44–59
Thrombophlebitis	24–30
Central nervous system disease	14–18

clinical trial, was found to prevent contralateral eye involvement in patients with unilateral disease and to prevent any eye involvement in those patients with Behçet's disease without ocular disease.[361] However, as with ciclosporin, not all patients responded well, as 22% required additional therapy.[361]

Ocular manifestations The most common ocular manifestations are uveitis and retinal vasculitis.[338,339,362] Conjunctivitis, keratitis, and scleritis have occasionally been described but are less common. Neuro-ophthalmic lesions due to the vascular involvement of Behçet's disease have been described. These include cranial nerve palsies, papilledema, and ION.[363,364] The most frequent ocular manifestation is anterior uveitis. This presents either with or without a hypopyon.[362] Early series commonly described hypopyon uveitis, but later series have decreased the frequency of hypopyon uveitis from as high as 88% to as low as 9%. This decrease likely represents earlier diagnosis and more aggressive therapy.[338,339,362]

Posterior segment lesions The characteristic posterior segment lesion is retinal vasculitis (Fig. 75-8), which may involve both veins and arteries with arterial occlusion and retinal necrosis. Occasionally, secondary neovascularization and retinal detachment develop.[338,339,362,365] The disease is most often bilateral; Dinning & Perkins[351] found that 81% of cases were bilateral in 1 year and 93% within 2 years. They also found a frequency of neovascularization of 17%.

The pathologic finding is a perivascular infiltrate with lymphocytes and plasma cells associated with retinal necrosis. Early lesions show a sparse round cell infiltrate of the retina, choroid, and chamber angle, whereas later lesions show extensive loss of retinoarchitecture with neovascularization. The endstage of the disease is a blind, painful eye with secondary glaucoma, rubeosis, and retinal detachment.

Other small-vessel vasculitides

Several other small-vessel vasculitides exist and are listed in Box 75-3. Of these, three vasculitic syndromes have associated ocular complications: (1) vasculitis related to connective tissue disease such as RA or SLE; (2) essential mixed cryoglobulinemia typically associated with hepatitis C infection; and (3) hypocomplementemic urticarial vasculitis syndrome (HUVS).

Vasculitis associated with connective tissue disease
Small-vessel vasculitis may be a clinical manifestation of connective tissue diseases such as RA and SLE. In RA, vasculitis is typically seen in patients with long-standing disease who have severe joint disease, rheumatoid nodules, and high titers of RF.[6,10,11,31] Small-sized arteries in the extremities are affected and may result in skin lesions and peripheral neuropathy.[6,31] Pathologic examination reveals a fibrinoid necrosis with a mixed inflammatory cell infiltrate within the vessels.[6,10,11,31] In SLE, small-vessel vasculitis may cause skin lesions, including skin ulcers and livedo reticularis, a reticular reddish-purple skin rash most commonly seen on the legs.[31,366] Pathologic changes are nonspecific and may include fibrinoid necrosis of small vessels and capillaries, with deposition of immunoglobulin and complement.[31] Ocular manifestations of RA and SLE have been described above.

Essential mixed cryoglobulinemia
Essential mixed cryoglobulinemia or type II cryoglobulinemia is a small-vessel vasculitis, which may result in palpable purpura, arthralgias or arthritis, lymphadenopathy, hepatosplenomegaly, peripheral neuropathy, and hypocomplementemia.[367] Renal disease may also be seen in up to 60% of patients with essential mixed cryoglobulinemia.[367] Most cases of essential mixed cryoglobulinemia are associated with hepatitis C virus infection. In essential mixed cryoglobulinemia, an estimated 85% to 95% of patients have circulating antibodies to hepatitis C virus.[368-370] The serum cryoglobulins consist of immune complexes containing polyclonal IgG antibodies to hepatitis C viral RNA.[368,369] In one prospective study, 54% of patients with hepatitis C virus and chronic liver disease had serum cryoglobulins.[370] Diagnosis is made by the presence of a cutaneous small-vessel vasculitis

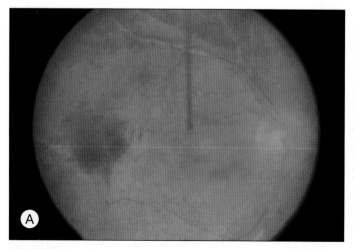
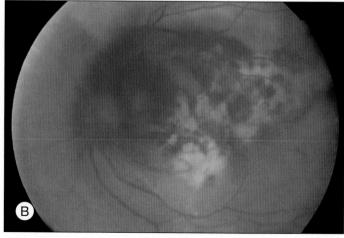

Fig. 75-8 A and B, Fundus photographs from a patient with Behçet's disease demonstrating retinal vasculitis. A demonstrates early macular lesion, and B, progressive disease 1 month later.

confirmed by biopsy and the presence of serum cryoglobulins in a patient with typical clinical features. Hypocomplementemia, elevated liver function tests, and evidence of hepatitis C virus infection also aid in the diagnosis of essential mixed cryoglobulinemia. Ocular disease is unusual, but cases of nongranulomatous anterior uveitis associated with essential mixed cryoglobulinemia have been reported.[371]

Hypocomplementemic urticarial vasculitis syndrome

An uncommon systemic, small-vessel vasculitis, HUVS is characterized by recurrent urticarial lesions associated with a cutaneous vasculitis, constitutional symptoms, arthralgias or arthritis, angioedema, and glomerulonephritis.[372,373] The joint and kidney disease may be indistinguishable from that found in SLE and, in fact, the presence of low titers of ANA autoantibodies is often found in patients with HUVS.[373] Serum levels of the third and fourth component of complement (C3 and C4 respectively) may range from low-normal to undetectable in patients with HUVS.[373] Diagnosis of HUVS is suggested in a patient with recurrent urticarial accompanied by a leukocytoclastic vasculitis, constitutional symptoms, arthralgias, and hypocomplementemia. A continuous granular deposition of immunoreactants along the basement membrane zone seen on skin biopsy using direct immunofluorescence technique helps to confirm the diagnosis.[374] Ocular findings in HUVS have been reported and include conjunctivitis, episcleritis, nongranulomatous anterior uveitis, and diffuse anterior scleritis.[372–377] Posterior ophthalmic manifestations have not been reported. Treatment with oral corticosteroids may improve constitutional symptoms as well as treat the vasculitis and ocular inflammation. In cases of severe vasculitis or ocular disease, corticosteroid-sparing immunosuppressive therapy may be required.[374]

REFERENCES

1. Henkind P, Gold DH. Ocular manifestations of rheumatic disorders: natural and iatrogenic. Rheumatology 1973; 4:13–59.
2. Hochberg MC. Adult and juvenile rheumatoid arthritis: current epidemiologic concepts. Epidemiol Rev 1981; 3:27–44.
3. Gabriel SE, Crowson CS, O'Fallon W. The epidemiology of rheumatoid arthritis in Rochester, MN, 1955–1985. Arthritis Rheum 1999; 42:415–422.
4. Drosos AA, Alamanos I, Voulgari PV et al. Epidemiology of adult rheumatoid arthritis in northwest Greece 1987–1995. J Rheumatol 1997; 24:2129–2135.
5. Doran MF, Pond GR, Crowson CS et al. Trends in incidence and mortality in rheumatoid arthritis in Rochester, Minnesota, over a forty-year period. Arthritis Rheum 2002; 46:625–640.
6. Harris ED. Clinical features of rheumatoid arthritis. In: Ruddy S, Harris ED, Sledge CB et al., eds. Kelly's textbook of rheumatology, 6th edn. Philadelphia: Saunders; 2001:967–1000.
7. Smith JB, Haynes MK. Rheumatoid arthritis: a molecular understanding. Ann Intern Med 2002; 136:908–921.
8. Hurd ER. Extra-articular manifestations of rheumatoid arthritis. Semin Arthritis Rheum 1979; 8:151–176.
9. MacDonald WJ Jr, Crawford MH, Klippel JH et al. Echocardiographic assessment of cardiac structure and function in patients with rheumatoid arthritis. Am J Med 1977; 63:890–896.
10. Scott DGI, Bacon PA, Tribe CR. Systemic rheumatoid vasculitis: a clinical and laboratory study of 50 cases. Medicine 1981; 60:288–297.
11. Schneider HA, Yonker RA, Katz P et al. Rheumatoid vasculitis: experience with 13 patients and review of literature. Semin Arthritis Rheum 1985; 14:280.
12. American College of Rheumatology Subcommittee on Rheumatoid Arthritis Guidelines. Guidelines for the management of rheumatoid arthritis: 2002 update. Arthritis Rheum 2002; 46:328–346.
13. Plant MJ, Jones PW, Saklatvala J. Patterns of radiological profession in early rheumatoid arthritis: results of an 8 year prospective study. J Rheumatol 1998; 25:417–422.
14. Clark P, Casas E, Tugwell P et al. Hydroxychloroquine compared with placebo in rheumatoid arthritis: a randomized controlled trial. Ann Intern Med 1993; 119:1067–1071.
15. Hannonen P, Möttönen T, Hakola M et al. Sulfasalazine in early rheumatoid arthritis: a 48-week double-blind, prospective, placebo-controlled study. Arthritis Rheum 1993; 36:1501–1509.
16. Landewe RBM, Goei Thè HS, van Rijthoven AW. A randomized, double-blind, 24-week controlled study of low-dose ciclosporin versus chloroquine for early rheumatoid arthritis. Arthritis Rheum 1994; 37:637–643.
17. Williams HJ, Wilkens RF, Samuelson CO et al. Comparison of low-dose oral pulse methotrexate and placebo in the treatment of rheumatoid arthritis: a controlled clinical trial. Arthritis Rheum 1985; 28:721–730.
18. Weinblatt ME, Coblyn JS, Fox DA et al. Efficacy of low-dose methotrexate in rheumatoid arthritis. N Engl J Med 1985; 312:818–822.
19. Kremer JM. Safety, efficacy, and mortality in a long-term cohort of patients with rheumatoid arthritis taking methotrexate: followup after a mean of 13.3 years. Arthritis Rheum 1997; 40:984–985.
20. Moreland LW, Schiff MH, Baumgartner SW et al. Etanercept therapy in rheumatoid arthritis: a randomized controlled trial. Ann Intern Med 1999; 130:478–486.
21. Lipsky PE, van der Heijde DM, St Clair EW et al. Infliximab and methotrexate in the treatment of rheumatoid arthritis. N Engl J Med 2000; 343:1594–1602.
22. Cohen S, Hurd E, Cush J et al. Treatment of rheumatoid arthritis with anakinra, a recombinant human interleukin-1 receptor antagonist, in combination with methotrexate. Results of a twenty-four-week, multicenter, randomized, double-blind, placebo-controlled trial. Arthritis Rheum 2002; 46:614–624.
23. Woodland J, Chaput de Saintongue DM, Evans SJ et al. Azathioprine in rheumatoid arthritis: double-blind study of full versus half doses versus placebo. Ann Rheum Dis 1981; 40:355–359.
24. Van Rijthoven AW, Dijkmans BA, Goei Thè HS et al. Cyclosporin treatment for rheumatoid arthritis: a placebo-controlled, double blind, multicentre study. Ann Rheum 1986; 45:726–731.
25. Townes AS, Sowa JM, Shulman LE. Controlled trial of cyclophosphamide in rheumatoid arthritis. Arthritis Rheum 1976; 19:563–572.
26. O'Dell JR, Paulsen G, Haire CE et al. Treatment of early seropositive rheumatoid arthritis with minocycline: four-year follow up of a double blind, placebo-controlled trial. Arthritis Rheum 1999; 42:1691–1695.
27. Williamson J. Incidence of eye disease in cases of connective tissue disease. Trans Ophthalmol Soc UK 1974; 94:742–752.
28. Jabs DA, Mudun A, Dunn JP et al. Episcleritis and scleritis: clinical features and treatment results. Am J Ophthalmol 2000; 130:469–476.
29. Sainz de la Maza M, Jabbur NS, Foster CS. Severity of scleritis and episcleritis. Ophthalmology 1994; 101:389–396.
30. Foster CS, Forstot SL, Wilson LA. Mortality rate in rheumatoid arthritis patients developing necrotizing scleritis or peripheral ulcerative keratitis. Ophthalmology 1984; 91:1253–1263.
31. Thorne JE, Jabs DA. Ocular manifestations of vasculitis. Rheum Dis Clin North Am 2001; 27:761–779.
32. Watson PG, Hazelman BL. The sclera and systemic disorders. Philadelphia: WB Saunders; 1976.
33. Sainz de la Maza M, Foster CS, Jabbur NS. Scleritis associated with rheumatoid arthritis and with other systemic immune-mediated diseases. Ophthalmology 1994; 101:1281–1286.
34. Killian PJ, McClain B, Lawless OJ. Brown's syndrome. An unusual manifestation of rheumatoid arthritis. Arthritis Rheum 1977; 20:1080–1081.
35. Finbloom DS, Silver K, Newsome DA et al. Comparison of hydroxychloroquine and chloroquine use and the development of retinal toxicity. J Rheumatol 1985; 12:692–694.
36. Scherbel AL, Mackenzie AH, Nousek JE et al. Ocular lesions in rheumatoid arthritis and related disorders with particular reference to retinopathy: a study of 741 patients treated with and without chloroquine drugs. N Engl J Med 1965; 273:360–366.
37. Tobin DR, Krohel GB, Rynes RI. Hydroxychloroquine: seven-year experience. Arch Ophthalmol 1982; 100:81–83.
38. Johnson MW, Vine AK. Hydroxychloroquine therapy in massive total doses without retinal toxicity. Am J Ophthalmol 1987; 104:139–144.
39. Thorne JE, Maguire AM. Resolution of hydroxychloroquine maculopathy. Br J Ophthalmol 1999; 83:1201–1203.
40. Prashker MJ, Meenan RF. The total costs of drug therapy for rheumatoid arthritis. A model based on costs of drug, monitoring, and toxicity. Arthritis Rheum 1995; 138:318–325.
41. Mazzuca SA, Yung R, Brandt KD et al. Current practices for monitoring ocular toxicity related to hydroxychloroquine (Plaquenil) therapy. J Rheumatol 1994; 21:59–63.

42. Arnett FC. Seronegative spondyloarthropathies. Bull Rheum Dis 1988; 37:1–12.

43. Rosenbaum JT. Acute anterior uveitis and spondyloarthropathies. Rheum Dis Clin North Am 1992; 18:143–151.

44. Khan MA. Update on spondyloarthropathies. Ann Intern Med 2002; 136:896–907.

45. Jimenez-Balderas FJ, Mintz G. Ankylosing spondylitis: clinical course in women and men. J Rheumatol 1993; 20:2069–2072.

46. van der Linden S, van der Heijde D. Ankylosing spondylitis. In: Ruddy S, Harris ED, Sledge CB et al., eds. Kelly's textbook of rheumatology, 6th edn. Philadelphia: Saunders; 2001:1039–1053.

47. Creemers MCW, Franssen MJAM, van de Putte LBA et al. Methotrexate in severe ankylosing spondylitis: an open study. J Rheumatol 1995; 22:1104–1110.

48. Braun J, Brandt J, Listing J et al. Treatment of active ankylosing spondylitis with infliximab: a randomized controlled multicenter trial. Lancet 2002; 359:1187–1195.

49. Tay-Kearney ML, Schwam BL, Lowder C et al. Clinical features and associated systemic diseases of HLA-B27 uveitis. Am J Ophthalmol 1996; 121:47–56.

50. Hogan MJ, Kimura SJ, Thygeson P. Uveitis in association with rheumatism. Arch Ophthalmol 1957; 57:400–413.

51. Kimura SJ, Hogan MJ, O'Connor GR et al. Uveitis and joint diseases: a review of 191 cases. Trans Am Ophthalmol Soc 1966; 64:291–310.

52. Belmont JB, Michelson JB. Vitrectomy in uveitis associated with ankylosing spondylitis. Am J Ophthalmol 1982; 94:300–304.

53. Perkins ES. Uveitis and toxoplasmosis. London: Churchill; 1966.

54. Yu DTY, Fan PT. Reiter's syndrome and undifferentiated spondyloarthropathy. In: Ruddy S, Harris ED, Sledge CB et al., eds. Kelly's textbook of rheumatology, 6th edn. Philadelphia: Saunders; 2001:1055–1069.

55. Saari KM, Vilppula A, Lassus A et al. Ocular inflammation in Reiter's disease after salmonella enteritis. Am J Ophthalmol 1980; 90:63–68.

56. Leirisalo-Repo M. Prognosis, course of disease, and treatment of the spondyloarthropathies. Rheum Dis Clin North Am 1998; 24:737–752.

57. Lee DA, Barker SM, Su WPD et al. The clinical diagnosis of Reiter's syndrome: Ophthalmic and non-ophthalmic aspects. Ophthalmology 1986; 93:350–356.

58. Ostler HB, Dawson CR, Schachter J et al. Reiter's syndrome. Am J Ophthalmol 1971; 71:986–991.

59. Rowson NJ, Dart JK. Keratitis in Reiter's syndrome. Br J Ophthalmol 1992; 76:126.

60. Mattsson R. Recurrent retinitis in Reiter's disease. Acta Ophthalmol 1955; 33:403–408.

61. Needham AD, Harding SP, Carey P. Bilateral multifocal choroiditis in Reiter syndrome. Arch Ophthalmol 1997; 115:684–685.

62. Conway RM, Graham SL, Lassere M. Incomplete Reiter's syndrome with focal involvement of the posterior segment. Aust NZ J Ophthalmol 1995; 23:63–66.

63. Greenstein J, Janowitz HD, Sachar DB. The extraintestinal complications of Crohn's disease and ulcerative colitis: A study of 700 patients. Medicine (Baltimore) 1976; 55:401–412.

64. Bernstein CN, Blanchard JF, Rawsthorne P et al. The prevalence of extaintestinal diseases in inflammatory bowel disease: a population-based study. Am J Gastroenterol 2001; 96:1116–1122.

65. Wollheim FA. Enteropathic arthritis. In: Ruddy S, Harris ED, Sledge CB et al., eds. Kelly's textbook of rheumatology, 6th edn. Philadelphia: Saunders; 2001:1081–1085.

66. Baert FJ, D'Haens GR, Peters M et al. Tumor necrosis factor-antibody (infliximab) therapy profoundly down-regulates the inflammation in Crohn's ileocolitis. Gastroenterology 1999; 116:22–29.

67. Billson FA, Dombal FTD, Watkinson G et al. Ocular complications of ulcerative colitis. Gut 1967; 8:102–106.

68. Edwards FC, Truelove SC. The course and prognosis of ulcerative colitis. III. Complications. Gut 1964; 5:1–15.

69. Hopkins DJ, Horan E, Burton IL et al. Ocular disorders in a series of 332 patients with Crohn's disease. Br J Ophthalmol 1974; 58:732–737.

70. Lyons JL, Rosenbaum JT. Uveitis associated with inflammatory bowel disease compared with uveitis associated with spondyloarthropathy. Arch Ophthalmol 1997; 115:61–64.

71. Banares A, Hernandez-Garcia C, Fernandez-Gutierrez B et al. Eye involvement in the spondyloarthropathies. Rheum Dis Clin North Am 1998; 24:771–784.

72. Crohn BB. Ocular lesions complicating ulcerative colitis. Am J Med Sci 1925; 169:260–267.

73. Knox DL, Schachat AP, Mustonen E. Primary, secondary, and coincidental ocular complications of Crohn's disease. Ophthalmology 1984; 91:163–173.

74. Bradshaw DJ, Bray VJ, Enzenauer RW et al. Acquired Brown syndrome associated with enteropathic arthropathy: a case report. J Pediatr Ophthalmol Strabismus 1994; 31:118–119.

75. Duker JS, Brown GC, Brooks L. Retinal vasculitis in Crohn's disease. Am J Ophthalmol 1987; 102:664–668.

76. Ellis PP, Gentry JH. Ocular complications of ulcerative colitis. Am J Ophthalmol 1964; 58:779–785.

77. Schneiderman JH, Sharpe JA, Sutton DMC. Cerebral and retinal vascular complications of inflammatory bowel disease. Ann Neurol 1979; 5:331–334.

78. Heuer DK, Gager WE, Reeser FH. Ischemic optic neuropathy associated with Crohn's disease. J Clin Neuro Ophthalmol 1982; 2:175–177.

79. Gladman DD, Rahman P. Psoriatic arthritis. In: Ruddy S, Harris ED, Sledge CB et al., eds. Kelly's textbook of rheumatology, 6th edn. Philadelphia: Saunders; 2001:1071–1079.

80. Gladman DD, Shuckett R, Russell ML et al. Psoriatic arthritis: clinical and laboratory analysis of 220 patients. Q J Med 1987; 62:127–138.

81. Thorne JE, Volpe NJ, Lui GT. Magnetic resonance imaging of acquired Brown syndrome in a patient with psoriasis. Am J Ophthalmol 1999; 127:233–235.

82. Cassidy JT. Juvenile rheumatoid arthritis. In: Ruddy S, Harris ED, Sledge CB et al., eds. Kelly's textbook of rheumatology, 6th edn. Philadelphia: Saunders; 2001:1297–1313.

83. Petty RE, Southwood TR, Baum J et al. Revision of the proposed classification criteria for juvenile idiopathic arthritis: Durban 1997. J Rheumatol 1998; 25:1991–1994.

84. Petty RE, Smith JR, Rosenbaum JT. Arthritis and uveitis in children: a pediatric rheumatology perspective. Am J Ophthalmol 2003; 135:879–884.

85. Schaller JG, Johnson GD, Holborow EJ et al. The association of antinuclear antibodies with the chronic iridocyclitis of juvenile rheumatoid arthritis (Still's disease). Arthritis Rheum 1974; 17:409–416.

86. Melin-Aldana H, Giannini EH, Taylor J et al. Human leukocyte antigen-DR1*1104 in the chronic iridocyclitis of pauciarticular juvenile rheumatoid arthritis. J Pediatr 1992; 121:56–59.

87. Malagon C, Van Kerckhove C, Giannini EH et al. The iridocyclitis of early onset pauciarticular juvenile rheumatoid arthritis: outcome in immunogenetically characterized patients. J Rheumatol 1992; 19:160–167.

88. Giannini EH, Brewer EJ, Kuzmina N et al. Methotrexate in resistant juvenile rheumatoid arthritis: results of the USA–USSR double-blind placebo-controlled trial. N Engl J Med 1992; 326:1043–1049.

89. Lovell DJ. Ten years of experience with methotrexate. Past, present and future. Rev Rheum Engl Ed 1997; 64:186S–189S.

90. Rose CD, Singsen BH, Eichenfield AH et al. Safety and efficacy of methotrexate therapy for juvenile rheumatoid arthritis. J Pediatr 1990; 117:653–659.

91. Shetty AK, Zganjar BE, Ellis GS Jr et al. Low-dose methotrexate in the treatment of severe juvenile rheumatoid arthritis and sarcoid iritis. J Pediatr Ophthalmol Strabismus 1999; 36:125–128.

92. Weiss AH, Wallace CA, Sherry DD. Methotrexate for resistant chronic uveitis in children with juvenile rheumatoid arthritis. J Pediatr 1998; 133:266–268.

93. Samson CM, Waheed N, Foster CS. Methotrexate therapy for chronic noninfectious uveitis: analysis of a case series of 160 patients. Ophthalmology 2001; 108:1134–1139.

94. Lovell DJ, Giannini EH, Reiff A. Etanercept in children with polyarticular juvenile rheumatoid arthritis. N Engl J Med 2000; 342:763–769.

95. Berk AT, Kocak N, Unsal E. Uveitis in juvenile arthritis. Ocul Immunol Inflamm 2001; 9:243–251.

96. Boone MI, Moore TL, Cruz OA. Screening for uveitis in juvenile rheumatoid arthritis. J Pediatr Ophthalmol Strabismus 1998; 35:41–43.

97. Chylack LT. The ocular manifestations of juvenile rheumatoid arthritis. Arthritis Rheum 1977; 20:217–223.

98. Paivonsalo-Hietanen T, Tuominen J, Vaahtoranta-Lehtonen H et al. Incidence and prevalence of different uveitis entities in Finland. Acta Ophthalmol Scand 1997; 75:76–81.

99. Key SN, Kimura SJ. Iridocyclitis associated with juvenile rheumatoid arthritis. Am J Ophthalmol 1975; 80:425–429.

100. Kanski JJ. Anterior uveitis in juvenile rheumatoid arthritis. Arch Ophthalmol 1977; 95:1794–1797.

101. Rosenberg AM, Oen KG. The relationship between ocular and articular disease activity in children with juvenile rheumatoid arthritis and associated uveitis. Arthritis Rheum 1986; 29:797–800.

102. Gori S, Broglia AM, Ravelli A et al. Frequency and complications of chronic iridocyclitis in ANA-positive pauciarticular juvenile chronic arthritis. Int Ophthalmol 1994; 18:225–228.

103. Section on Rheumatology and Section on Ophthalmology. Guidelines for ophthalmologic examinations in children with juvenile rheumatoid arthritis. Pediatrics 1993; 92:295–296.

104. Merayo-Lloves J, Power WJ, Rodriguez A et al. Secondary glaucoma in patients with uveitis. Ophthalmologica 1999; 213:300–304.

105. Kanski JJ. Juvenile arthritis and uveitis. Surv Ophthalmol 1990; 34:253–267.

106. Sherry DD, Mellins ED, Wedgwood RJ. Decreasing severity of chronic uveitis in children with pauciarticular arthritis. Am J Dis Child 1991; 145:1026–1028.

107. Cabral DA, Petty RE, Malleson PN et al. Visual prognosis in children with chronic anterior uveitis and arthritis. J Rheumatol 1994; 21:2370–2375.

108. Paikos P, Fotopoulou M, Papathanassiou M et al. Cataract surgery in children with uveitis. J Pediatr Ophthalmol Strabismus 2001; 38:16–20.

109. Probst LE, Holland EJ. Intraocular lens implantation in patients with juvenile rheumatoid arthritis. Am J Ophthalmol 1996; 122:161–170.

110. Benezra D, Cohen E. Cataract surgery in children with chronic uveitis. Ophthalmology 2000; 107:1255–1260.

111. Jabs DA, Houk JL, Bias WB et al. Familial granulomatous synovitis, uveitis, and cranial neuropathies. Am J Ophthalmol 1985; 78:801–806.

112. Blau EB. Familial granulomatous arthritis, iritis, and rash. J Pediatr 1985; 107:689–693.

113. McKusick VA. Mendelian inheritance in man. Catalogs of human genes and genetic disorders, 12th edn. Baltimore: Johns Hopkins University Press; 1998:1730.

114. Miller JJ II. Early-onset "sarcoidosis" and "familial granulomatous arthritis (arteritis)": the same disease. J Pediatr 1986; 109:387–388.

115. Latkany PA, Jabs DA, Smith JR et al. Multifocal choroiditis in patients with familial juvenile systemic granulomatosis. Am J Ophthalmol 2002; 134:897–904.

116. Miceli-Richard C, Lesage S, Rybojad M et al. CARD15 mutations in Blau syndrome. Nature Genetics 2001; 29:19–20.

117. Hahn BH. Pathogenesis of systemic lupus erythematosus. In: Ruddy S, Harris ED, Sledge CB et al., eds. Kelly's textbook of rheumatology, 6th edn. Philadelphia: Saunders; 2001:1089–1103.

118. Seligman VA, Suarez C, Lum R et al. The Fc receptor IIIA-158F allele is a major risk factor for the development of lupus nephritis among Caucasians but not non-Caucasians. Arthritis Rheum 2001; 44:618–625.

119. Kammer GM. High prevalence of T cell type I protein A deficiency in systemic lupus erythematosus. Arthritis Rheum 1999; 42:1458–1465.

120. Deng C, Kaplan MJ, Yang J et al. Decreased ras-mitogen-activated protein kinase signaling may cause DNA hypomethylation in T lymphocytes from lupus patients. Arthritis Rheum 2001; 44:397–407.

121. Estes D, Christian CL. The natural history of systemic lupus erythematosus by prospective analysis. Medicine 1971; 50:85–95.

122. Edworthy SM. Clinical manifestations of systemic lupus erythematosus. In: Ruddy S, Harris ED, Sledge CB et al., eds. Kelly's textbook of rheumatology, 6th edn. Philadelphia: Saunders; 2001:1105–1123.

123. Dubois EL, Tuffanelli DL. Clinical manifestations of systemic lupus erythematosus. JAMA 1964; 190:104–116.

124. Feinglass EJ, Arnett FC, Dorsch CA et al. Neuropsychiatric manifestations of systemic lupus erythematosus: diagnosis, clinical spectrum, and relationship to other features of the disease. Medicine 1976; 55:323–339.

125. Hochberg MC, Boyd RE, Aheran JM et al. Systemic lupus erythematosus: a review of clinico-laboratory features and immunogenetic markers in 150 patients with emphasis on demographic subsets. Medicine (Baltimore) 1985; 64:285–295.

126. Harris EN, Boey ML, Mackworth-Young CG et al. Anti-cardiolipin antibodies: detection by radioimmunoassay and association with thrombosis in systemic lupus erythematosus. Lancet 1983; 2:1211–1217.

127. Perez-Vazquez ME, Villa AR, Drenkard C et al. Influence of disease duration, continued follow-up and further antiphospholipid testing on the frequency and classification category of antiphospholipid syndrome in a cohort of patients with SLE. J Rheumatol 1993; 20:437–442.

128. Simioni P, Prandoni P, Zanon E et al. Deep venous thrombosis and lupus anticoagulant. A case-control study. Thromb Haemost 1996; 76:187–189.

129. Durrani OM, Gordon C, Murray PI. Primary anti-phospholipid antibody syndrome (APS): current concepts. Surv Ophthalmol 2002; 47:215–238.

130. Glueck HI, Kant KS, Weiss MA et al. Thrombosis in systemic lupus erythematosus: relation to the presence of circulating anticoagulants. Arch Intern Med 1985; 145:1389–1395.

131. Petri M, Rheinschmidt M, Whiting-O'Keefe Q et al. The frequency of lupus anticoagulant in systemic lupus erythematosus: a study of sixty consecutive patients by activated partial thromboplastin time. Russell viper venom time and anti-cardiolipin antibody level. Ann Intern Med 1987; 106:524–531.

132. Love PE, Santoro SA. Antiphospholipid antibodies: anti-cardiolipin and the lupus anticoagulant in systemic lupus erythematosus (SLE) and in non-SLE disorders. Ann Intern Med 1990; 112:682–698.

133. Dunn JP, Noorily SW, Petri M et al. Antiphospholipid antibodies and retinal vascular disease. Lupus 1996; 5:313–322.

134. Kleiner RC, Nigerian LV, Schattten S et al. Vaso-occlusive retinopathy associated with anti phospholipid antibodies (lupus anticoagulant retinopathy). Ophthalmology 1989; 96:896–904.

135. Boey ML, Colaco CB, Gharavi AE et al. Thrombosis in systemic lupus erythematosus: striking association with the presence of circulating lupus anticoagulant. Br Med J 1983; 287:1021–1023.

136. Tan EM, Cohen AS, Fries JF et al. The 1982 revised criteria for the classification of systemic lupus erythematosus. Arthritis Rheum 1982; 25:1271–1277.

137. Hahn BH. Management of systemic lupus erythematosus. In: Ruddy S, Harris ED, Sledge CB et al., eds. Kelly's textbook of rheumatology, 6th edn. Philadelphia: Saunders; 2001:1125–1143.

138. Canadian Hydroxychloroquine Study Group. A randomized study of the effect of withdrawing hydroxychloroquine sulfate in systemic lupus erythematosus. N Engl J Med 1991; 324:150–157.

139. Isenberg DA, Morrow WJW, Snaith ML. Methylprednisolone pulse therapy in the treatment of systemic lupus erythematosus. Ann Rheum Dis 1982; 41:347–350.

140. Felson DT, Anderson J. Evidence for the superiority of immunosuppressive drugs and prednisone alone in lupus nephritis. N Engl J Med 1984; 311:1528–1533.

141. Gourley MF, Austin HA III, Scott D et al. Methylprednisolone and cyclophosphamide, alone or in combination, in patients with lupus nephritis. Ann Intern Med 1996; 125:549–555.

142. Bansal VK, Beto JA. Treatment of lupus nephritis. A meta-analysis of clinical trials. Am J Kidney Dis 1997; 29:193–202.

143. Brodsky RA, Petri M, Smith BD et al. Immunoablative high-dose cyclophosphamide without stem-cell rescue for refractory, severe autoimmune disease. Ann Intern Med 1998; 129:1031–1035.

144. Khamashta MA, Cuadrado MJ, Mujic F et al. The management of thrombosis in the antiphospholipid–antibody syndrome. N Engl J Med 1995; 332:993–997.

145. Rosove MH, Brewer PMC. Antiphospholipid thrombosis: clinical course after the first thrombotic event in 70 patients. Ann Intern Med 1992; 117:303–308.

146. Huey C, Jakobiec FA, Iwamoto T et al. Discoid lupus erythematosus of the eyelids. Ophthalmology 1983; 90:1389–1398.

147. Gold DH, Morris DA, Henkind P. Ocular findings in systemic lupus erythematosus. Br J Ophthalmol 1972; 56:800–804.

148. Lanham JG, Barrie T, Kohner EM et al. SLE retinopathy: evaluation of fluorescein angiography. Ann Rheum Dis 1982; 41:473–478.

149. Shearn MA, Pirofsky B. Disseminated lupus erythematosus: analysis of thirty-four cases. Arch Intern Med 1952; 90:790–807.

150. Karpik AG, Schwartz MM, Dickey LE et al. Ocular immune reactants in patients dying with systemic lupus erythematosus. Clin Immunol Immunopathol 1985; 35:295–312.

151. Santos R, Barojas E, Alarcon-Segovia D et al. Retinal microangiopathy in systemic lupus erythematosus. Am J Ophthalmol 1975; 80:249–252.

152. Klinkhoff AV, Beattie CW, Chalmers A. Retinopathy in systemic lupus erythematosus: relationship to disease activity. Arthritis Rheum 1986; 29:1152–1156.

153. Maumenee AE. Retinal lesions in lupus erythematosus. Am J Ophthamol 1940; 23:971–981.

154. Aronson A, Ordinis NG, Diddle KR et al. Immune-complex deposition in the eye in systemic lupus erythematosus. Arch Intern Med 1979;139: 1312–1313.

155. Klinkhoff AV, Beattie CW, Chalmers A. Retinopathy in systemic lupus erythematosus: relationship to disease activity. Arthritis Rheum 1986; 29:1152–1156.

156. Appen RE, Wray SH, Cogan DG. Central retinal artery occlusion. Am J Ophthalmol 1975; 79:374–381.

157. Gold D, Feiner L, Heinkind P. Retinal arterial occlusive disease in systemic lupus erythematosus. Arch Ophthalmol 1977; 95:1580–1585.

158. Silverman M, Lubeck MJ, Brimey WG. Central retinal vein occlusion complicating systemic lupus erythematosus. Arthritis Rehem 1978; 21:839–843.

159. Kayazawa F, Honda A. Severe retinal vascular lesions in systemic lupus erythematosus. Ann Ophthalmol 1981; 13:1291–1294.

160. Jabs DA, Fine SL, Hochberg MC et al. Severe retinal vaso-occlusive disease in systemic lupus erythematosus. Arch Ophthalmol 1986; 104:558–563.

161. Hall S, Buettner H, Luthra HS. Occlusive retinal vascular disease in systemic lupus erythematosus. J Rheumatol 1984; 11:846–850.

162. Jabs DA, Hanneken AM, Schachat AP et al. Choroidopathy in systemic lupus erythematosus. Arch Ophthalmol 1988; 106:230–234.

163. Graham EM, Spalton DJ, Barnard RO et al. Cerebral and retinal vascular changes in systemic lupus erythematosus. Ophthalmology 1985; 92:444–448.

164. Hackett ER, Martinez RD, Larson PF et al. Optic neuritis in systemic lupus erythematosus. Arch Neurol 1974; 31:9–11.

165. Shepherd DI, Downie AW, Best PV. Systemic lupus erythematosus and multiple sclerosis. Arch Neurol 1974; 30:423–426.

166. April RS, Vansonnenberg E. A case of neuromyelitis optic (Devic's syndrome) in systemic lupus erythematosus: clinicopathologic report and review of the literature. Neurology 1976; 26:1066–1070.

167. Allen IV, Miller JHD, Kirk J et al. Systemic lupus erythematosus clinically resembling multiple sclerosis and with unusual pathological and ultrastructural features. J Jeurol Neurol Neuosurg Psychiatry 1979; 42:392–401.

168. Lessell S. The neuro-ophthalmology of systemic lupus erythematosus. Doc Ophthalmol 1979; 47:13–42.

169. Jabs DA, Miller NR, Newman SA et al. Optic neuropathy in systemic lupus erythematosus. Arch Ophthalmol 1986; 104:564–568.

170. Hayreh SS. Posterior ischemic optic neuropathy. Ophthalmologica 1981; 182:29–41.

171. Billingsley LM, Yannakakis GD, Stevens MB. Evoked potentials (EPs): a sensitive test for CNS-SLE. Arthritis Rheum 1985; 28:522–525.

172. Seibold JR. Scleroderma. In: Ruddy S, Harris ED, Sledge CB et al., eds. Kelly's textbook of rheumatology, 6th edn. Philadelphia: Saunders; 2001: 1211–1239.

173. Ruffanelli DL, Winkelmann RK. Systemic scleroderma: a clinical study of 727 cases. Arch Dermatol 1961; 84:359–368.

174. Rodnan GP. The natural history of progressive systemic sclerosis (diffuse scleroderma). Bull Rheum Dis 1963; 13:301–309.

175. Lopez-Overjero JA, Saal D, D'Angelo WA et al. Reversal of vascular and renal crises of scleroderma by oral angiotensin-converting-enzyme blockade. N Engl J Med 1979; 300:1417–1419.

176. Mitnick PD, Feig PU. Control of hypertension and reversal of renal failure in scleroderma. N Engl J Med 1978; 299:871–875.

177. Sorensen LB, Paunicka K, Harris M. Reversal of scleroderma renal crisis for more than two years in a patient treated with captopril. Arthritis Rheum 1983; 26:797–800.

178. Thurm RH, Alexander JC. Captopril in the treatment of scleroderma renal crisis. Arch Intern Med 1984; 144:733–735.

179. McCarty GA, Rice JR, Bembe ML et al. Anticentromere antibody: clinical correlations and association with favorable prognosis in patients with scleroderma variants. Arthritis Rheum 1983; 26:1–7.

180. Sharp GC, Irvin WS, Tan EM et al. Mixed connective tissue disease – an apparently distinct rheumatic disease syndrome associated with a specific antibody to an extractable nuclear antigen (ENA). Am J Med 1972; 52:148–159.

181. Nimelstein SH, Brody S, McShane D et al. Mixed connective tissue disease: a subsequent evaluation of the original 25 patients. Medicine 1980; 59:239–248.

182. Silver RM, Miller KS, Kinsella MB et al. Evaluation and management of scleroderma lung disease using bronchoalveolar lavage. Am J Med 1990; 88:470–473.

183. Rodeheffer RJ, Rommer JA, Wigley F et al. Controlled double-blind trial of nifedipine in the treatment of Raynaud's phenomenon. N Engl J Med 1983; 308:880–888.

184. White CJ, Phillips WA, Abrahams LA et al. Objective benefit of nifedipine in the treatment of Raynaud's phenomenon. Am J Med 1986; 80:623–629.

185. Horan EC. Ophthalmic manifestations of progressive systemic sclerosis. Br J Ophthalmol 1969; 53:388–392.

186. West RH, Barnett AJ. Ocular involvement in scleroderma. Br J Ophthalmol 1979; 63:845–847.

187. Cipoletti JF, Buckingham RB, Barnes EL et al. Sjögren's syndrome in progressive systemic sclerosis. Ann Intern Med 1977; 87:535–541.

188. Osial TA, Whiteside TL, Buckingham RB et al. Clinical and serologic study of Sjögren's syndrome in patients with progressive systemic sclerosis. Arthritis Rheum 1983; 26:500–505.

189. Dorwart BB. Periorbital edema in progressive systemic sclerosis. Ann Intern Med 1974; 80:273–274.

190. Teasdall RD, Frayha RA, Shulman LE. Cranial nerve involvement in systemic sclerosis (scleroderma): a report of ten cases. Medicine (Baltimore) 1980; 59:149–153.

191. Rush JA. Isolated superior oblique paralysis in progressive systemic sclerosis. Ann Ophthalmol 1981; 13:217–218.

192. Mabon M, Whitcher JP, Anderson R. Bilateral scleral pit associated with systemic sclerosis. Am J Ophthalmol 1999; 128:521–522.

193. Campbell WW, Bajandas FJ. Restrictive ophthalmopathy associated with linear scleroderma. J Neuroophthalmol 1995; 15:95–97.

194. Arnett FC, Michels RG. Inflammatory ocular myopathy in systemic sclerosis (scleroderma). Arch Intern Med 1973; 132:740–743.

195. Pollack IP, Becker B. Cytoid bodies of the retina in a patient with scleroderma. Am J Ophthalmol 1962; 54:655–660.

196. Ashton N, Coomes EN, Garner A et al. Retinopathy due to progressive systemic sclerosis. J Pathol Bacteriol 1968; 96:259–261.

197. MacLean H, Guthrie W. Retinopathy in scleroderma. Trans Ophthalmol Soc UK 1969; 139:209–220.

198. Farkas TG, Sylvester V, Archer D. The choroidopathy of progressive systemic sclerosis (scleroderma). Am J Ophthalmol 1972; 74:875–886.

199. Grennan DM, Forrester J. Involvement of the eye in SLE and scleroderma. Ann Rheum Dis 1977; 36:152–156.

200. Heese RJ, Slagle DF. Scleroderma choroidopathy: report of an unusual case. Ann Ophthalmol 1982; 14:524–525.

201. Serup L, Serup J, Hagdrup H. Fundus fluorescein angiography in generalized scleroderma. Ophthalm Res 1987; 19:303–306.

202. Saari KM, Rudenburg HA, Laitinen O. Bilateral central retinal vein occlusion in a patient with scleroderma. Ophthalmologica 1981; 182:7.

203. Wortmann RL. Inflammatory diseases of muscle and other myopathies. In: Ruddy S, Harris ED, Sledge CB et al., eds. Kelly's textbook of rheumatology, 6th edn. Philadelphia: Saunders; 2001:1273–1296.

204. Bohan A, Peter JB. Polymyositis and dermatomyositis (first of two parts). N Engl J Med 1975; 292:344–350.

205. Bohan A, Peter JB. Polymyositis and dermatomyositis (second of two parts). N Engl J Med 1975; 292:403–407.

206. Bohan A, Peter JB, Bowman RL et al. A computer-assisted analysis of 153 patients with polymyositis and dermatomyositis. Medicine 1977; 56:255–261.

207. Susac JO, Garcia-Mullin R, Glaser JS. Ophthalmoplegia in dermatomyositis. Neurology 1973; 23:305–309.

208. Bruce GM. Retinitis in deramatomyositis. Trans Am Ophthalmol Soc 1938; 36:282–303.

209. Lisman JV. Dermatomyositis with retinopathy: report of a case. Arch Ophthalmol 1947; 37:155–156.

210. Devries S. Retinopathy in dermatomyositis. Arch Ophthalmol 1951; 46:432–435.

211. Munro S. Fundus appearances in a case of acute dermatomyositis. Br J Ophthalmol 1958; 43:548.

212. Liebman S, Cook C. Retinopathy with dermatomyositis. Arch Ophthalmol 1965; 74:704–705.

213. Zamora J, Pariser K, Hedges T et al. Retinal vasculitis in polymyositis-dermatomyositis. Arthritis Rheum 1987; 30:S106.

214. Bloch KJ, Buchanan WW, Wohl MJ et al. Sjögren's syndrome: a clinical, pathological, and serological study of sixty-two cases. Medicine 1965; 44:187–231.

215. Whaley K, Webb J, McAvoy BA et al. Sjögren's syndrome. II. Clinical associations and immunological phenomen. Q J Med 1973; 42:513–548.

216. Whaley K, Williamson J, Chisholm DM et al. Sjögren's syndrome. I. Sicca components. Q J Med 1973; 42:279–304.

217. Adamson TC III, Fox RI, Frisman DM et al. Immunohistologic analysis of lymphoid infiltrates in primate Sjögren's syndrome using monoclonal antibodies. J Immunol 1983; 130:203–208.

218. Fox RI, Carstens SA, Fong S et al. Use of monoclonal antibodies to analyze peripheral blood and salivary gland lymphocyte subsets in Sjögren's syndrome. Arthritis Rheum 1982; 25:419–426.

219. Fox RI, Michelson P, Törnwall J. Approaches to the treatment of Sjögren's syndrome. In: Ruddy S, Harris ED, Sledge CB et al., eds. Kelly's textbook of rheumatology, 6th edn. Philadelphia: Saunders; 2001:1027–1038..

220. Fox RI, Törnwall J, Michelson P. Current issues in the diagnosis and treatment of Sjögren's syndrome. Curr Opin Rheumatol 1999; 11:364–371.

221. Alexander EL, Provost TT, Stevens MB et al. Neurologic complications in primary Sjögren's syndrome. Medicine (Baltimore) 1982; 61:247–257.

222. Harley JB, Alexander EL, Bias WB et al. Anti-Ro (SSA) and anti-La (SSB) in patients with Sjögren's syndrome. Arthritis Rheum 1986; 29:196–200.

223. Rosenbaum JT, Bennett RM. Chronic anterior and posterior uveitis and primary Sjögren's syndrome. Am J Ophthalmol 1987; 104:346–352.

224. Hochberg MC. Relapsing polychondritis. In: Ruddy S, Harris ED, Sledge CB et al., eds. Kelly's textbook of rheumatology, 6th edn. Philadelphia: Saunders; 2001:1463–1467.

225. Isaak BL, Liesegang TJ, Michel CJ. Ocular and systemic findings in relapsing polychondritis. Ophthalmology 1986; 93:681–689.

226. McAdam LP, O'Hanlan MA, Bluestone R et al. Relapsing polychondritis: prospective study of 23 patients and a review of the literature. Medicine 1976; 55:193–215.

227. Pearson CM, Kline HM, Newcomer VD. Relapsing polychondritis. N Engl J Med 1960; 263:51–58.

228. Trentham DE, Le CH. Relapsing polychondritis. Ann Intern Med 1998; 129:114–120.

229. Michel CJ, McKenna CH, Luthra HS et al. Relapsing polychondritis: survival and predictive role of early disease manifestations. Ann Intern Med 1986; 104:74–78.

230. Hoang-Xuan T, Foster CS, Rice BA. Scleritis in relapsing polychondritis: response to therapy. Ophthalmology 1990; 97:892–897.

231. Zeuner M, Straub RH, Rauh G et al. Relapsing polychondritis: clinical and immunogenetic analysis of 62 patients. J Rheumatol 1997; 24:96–101.

232. Anderson B. Ocular lesions in relapsing polychondritis and other rheumatoid syndromes. Trans Am Acad Ophthalmol Otol 1967; 71:227–242.

233. McKay DAR, Watson PG, Lyne AJ. Relapsing polychondritis and eye disease. Br J Ophthalmol 1974; 58:600–605.

234. Magargal LE, Donoso LA, Goldberg RE et al. Ocular manifestations of relapsing polychondritis. Retina 1981; 1:96–99.

235. Fauci AS, Haynes BF, Katz P. The spectrum of vasculitis: clinical, pathologic, immunologic, and theraputic considerations. Ann Intern Med 1978; 89:660–676.

236. DeRemee RA, Weiland LH, McDonald TJ. Respiratory vasculitis. Mayo Clin Proc 1980; 55:492–498.

237. Sergent JS. Classification of vasculitis. In: Ruddy S, Harris ED, Sledge CB et al., eds. Kelly's textbook of rheumatology, 6th edn. Philadelphia: Saunders; 2001:1153–1154.

238. Lie JT. Illustrated histopathologic classification criteria for selected vasculitis syndromes. Arthritis Rheum 1990; 33:1074–1087.

239. Jennette JC, Falk RP, Andrassy K et al. Nomenclature of systemic vasculitides. Proposal of an international consensus conference. Arthritis Rheum 1994; 37:187–192.

240. Ostberg, G. Temporal arteritis in a large necropsy series. Ann Rheum Dis 1971; 30:224–235.

241. Hunder GG. Giant cell arteritis and polymyalgia rheumatica. In: Ruddy S, Harris ED, Sledge CB et al., eds. Kelly's textbook of rheumatology, 6th edn. Philadelphia: Saunders; 2001:1155–1164.

242. Fauchald P, Rygvold O, Oystese B. Temporal arteritis and polymyalgia rheumatica. Ann Intern Med 1972; 77:845–852.

243. Huston KA, Hunder GG, Lie JT et al. Temporal arteritis: a 25-year epidemiologic, clinical, and pathologic study. Ann Intern Med 1978; 88:162–167.

244. Goodman BW Jr. Temporal arteritis. Am J Med 1979; 67:839–852.

245. Keltner JL. Giant cell arteritis: signs and symptoms. Ophthalmology 1982; 89:1101–1110.

246. Klein SM. Erythrocyte sedimentation rate in the elderly. Arch Ophthalmol 1972; 88:617–620.

247. Hayes GS, Stinson IN. Erythrocyte sedimentation rate and age. Arch Ophthalmol 1976; 94: 939–950.

248. Cantini F, Salvarani C, Olivieri I et al. Erythrocyte sedimentation rate and C-reactive protein in the evaluation of disease activity and severity in polymyalgia rheumatica: a prospective follow-up study. Semin Arthritis Rheum 2000; 30:17–24.

249. Albert DM, Ruchman MC, Keltner JL. Skip areas in temporal arteritis. Arch Ophthalmol 1976; 94:2072–2077.

250. Klein RG, Campbell RJ, Carney JA. Skip lesions in temporal arteritis. Mayo Clin Proc 1976; 51:504–510.

251. McDonnell PJ, Moore GW, Miller NR et al. Temporal arteritis: a clinicopathologic study, Ophthalmology 1986; 93:518–530.

252. Kansu T, Corbett JJ, Savino P et al. Giant cell arteritis with normal sedimentation rate. Arch Neurol 1977; 34:624–625.

253. Biller J, Asconape J, Weinblatt ME et al. Temporal arteritis associated with normal sedimentation rate. JAMA 1982; 274:486–487.

254. Gonzalez-Gay MA, Garcia-Porrua C, Llorca J et al. Biopsy-negative giant cell arteritis: clinical spectrum and predictive factors for positive temporal artery biopsy. Semin Arthritis Rheum 2001; 30:249–256.

255. Hunder GG, Sheps SG, Allen GL et al. Daily and alternate-day corticosteroid regimens in treatment of giant cell arteritis. Ann Intern Med 1975; 82:613–618.

256. Rosenfeld SI, Kosmorsky GS, Klingele TG et al. Treatment of temporal arteritis with ocular involvement. Am J Med 1986; 80:143–145.

257. Cullen JF. Temporal arteritis: occurrence of ocular complications 7 years after diagnosis. Br J Ophthalmol 1972; 56:584–588.

258. Cullen JF, Coleiro JA. Ophthalmic complications of giant cell arteritis. Surv Ophthalmol 1976; 20:247–260.

259. Hoffman G, Cid M, Hellmann D et al. A multicenter placebo controlled study of methotrexate in giant cell arteritis. Arthritis Rheum 2002; 46:1309–1318.

260. Jover JA, Hernandez-Garcia C, Morado IC et al. Combined treatment of giant-cell arteritis with methotrexate and prednisone. Ann Intern Med 2001; 134:106–114.

261. Wang FM, Henkind P. Visual system involvement in giant cell (temporal) arteritis. Surv Ophthalmol 1979; 23:264–271.

262. McLeod D, Kohner EM, Marshall J. Fundus signs in temporal arteritis. Br J Ophthalmol 1978; 62:591–594.

263. Tang RA, Kaldis LC. Retinopathy in temporal arteritis. Ann Ophthalmol 1982; 14:652–654.

264. Wagener HP, Hollenhorst RW. The ocular lesions of temporal arteritis. Am J Ophthalmol 1958; 45:617–630.

265. Barricks ME, Traviesa DB, Glaser JS et al. Ophthalmoplegia in cranial arteritis. Brain 1977; 100:209–221.

266. Dimant J, Grob D, Brunner NG. Ophthalmoplegia, ptosis, and miosis in temporal arteritis. Neurology 1980; 30:1054–1058.

267. Lockskin MD. Diplopia as early sign of temporal arteritis: report of two cases. Arthritis Rheum 1970; 13:419–421.

268. Verdick M, Nielsen NV. Acute transient ophthalmomalacia in giant-cell arteritis: report of a case. Acta Ophthalmol 1975; 53:875–878.

269. Miller NR. Visual manifestations of temporal arteritis. Rheum Dis Clin North Am 2001; 27:781–797.

270. Zion VM, Goodside V. Anterior segment ischemia with ischemic optic neuropathy. Surv Ophthalmol 1974; 19:19–30.

271. Radda TM, Bardach H, Riss B. Acute ocular hypotony: a rare complication of temporal arteritis. Ophthalmologica 1981; 182:148–152.

272. Spolaore R, Gaudric A, Coscas G et al. Acute sectorial choroidal ischemia. Am J Ophthalmol 1984; 98:707–716.

273. Model DG. Reversal of blindness in temporal arteritis with methylprednisolone. Lancet 1978; 1:340.

274. Matzkin DC, Slamovits TL, Sachs R et al. Visual recovery in two patients after intravenous methylprednisolone treatment of central retinal artery occlusion secondary to giant-cell arteritis. Ophthalmology 1992; 99:68–71.

275. Arend WP, Michel BA, Bloch DA et al. The American College of Rheumatology 1990 criteria for the classification of Takayasu arteritis. Arthritis Rheum 1990; 33:1129–1134.

276. Fraga A, Mintz G, Valle L et al. Takayasu's arteritis: frequency of systemic manifestations (study of 22 patients) and favorable response to maintenance steroid therapy with adrenocorticosteroids (12 patients). Arthritis Rheum 1972; 15:617–624.

277. Lupi-Herrera E, Sanchez-Torres G, Marcushamer J. Takayasu's arteritis: clinical study of 107 cases. Am Heart J 1977; 93:94–103.

278. Shelhamer JH, Volkman DJ, Parrillo JE et al. Takayasu's arteritis and its therapy. Ann Intern Med 1985; 103:121–126.

279. Ishikawa K. Natural history and classification of occlusive thromboaortopathy (Takayasu's disease). Circulation 1978; 57:27–35.

280. Fraga A, Medina F. Takayasu's arteritis. Curr Rheum Rep 2002; 4:30–38.

281. Chun YS, Park SJ, Park IK et al. The clinical and ocular manifestations of Takayasu arteritis. Retina 2001; 21:132–140.

282. Tanaka T, Shimizu K. Retinal arteriovenous shunts in Takayasu's disease. Ophthalmology 1987; 94:1380–1388.

283. Lightfoot RW Jr, Michel BA, Bloch DA et al. The American College of Rheumatology 1990 criteria for the classification of polyarteritis nodosa. Arthritis Rheum 1990; 33:1088–1093.

284. Cohen RD, Conn DI, Ilstrup DM. Clinical features, prognosis, and response to treatment in polyarteritis. Mayo Clin Proc 1980; 55:146–155.

285. Sergent JS. Polyarteritis and related disorders. In: Ruddy S, Harris ED, Sledge CB et al., eds. Kelly's textbook of rheumatology, 6th edn. Philadelphia: Saunders; 2001:1185–1195.

286. Duffy J, Lidsky MD, Sharp JT et al. Polyarthritis, polyarteritis, and hepatitis B. Medicine 1976; 55:19–37.

287. Gocke DJ, Hsu K, Morgan C et al. Association between polyarteritis and Australia antigen. Lancet 1970; 2:1149–1153.

288. Sergent JS, Lockshin MD, Christian CI et al. Vasculitis with hepatitis B antigenemia: long-term observations in nine patients. Medicine 1976; 55:1–18.

289. Medical Research Council. Treatment of polyarteritis nodosa with cortisone: results after three years. Br Med J 1960; 1:1399–1400.

290. Fauci AS, Doppmann JL, Wolff SM. Cyclophosphamide-induced remissions in advanced polyarteritis nodosa. Am J Med 1978; 64:890–894.

291. Gayraud M, Guillevin L, Cohen P et al. Treatment of good prognosis polyarteritis nodosa and Churg–Strauss syndrome: comparison of steroids and oral or pulse cyclophosphamide in 25 patients. Br J Rheumatol 1997; 36:1290–1296.

292. Gaynon IE, Asbury MK. Ocular findings in a case of periarteritis nodosa. Am J Ophthalmol 1943; 26:1072–1076.

293. Goldsmith J. Periarteritis nodosa with involvement of the choroidal and retinal arteries. Am J Ophthalmol 1946; 29:435–446.

294. Goar EL, Smith LS. Polyarteritis nodosa of the eye. Am J Ophthalmol 1952; 35:1619–1625.

295. Sheehan B, Harriman DGF, Bradshaw JPP. Polyarteritis nodosa with ophthalmic and neurological complications. Arch Ophthalmol 1958; 60:537–547.

296. Blodi FC, Sullivan PB. Involvement of the eyes in periarteritis nodosa. Trans Am Acad Sci 1959; 63:161–165.

297. Moore R, Sevel D. Corneo-scleral ulceration in periarteritis nodosa. Br J Ophthalmol 1966; 50:651–655.

298. Kimbrell OC, Wheliss JA. Polyarteritis nodosa complicated by bilateral optic neuropathy. JAMA 1967; 201:139–140.

299. Rosen ES. The retinopathy in polyarteritis nodosa. Br J Ophthalmol 1968; 52:903–906.

300. Kielar RA. Exudative retinal detachment and scleritis in polyarteritis. Am J Ophthalmol 1976; 82:694–698.

301. Stefani FH, Brandt F, Pielsticker K. Periarteritis nodosa and thrombotic thrombocytopenic pupura with serous retinal detachment in siblings. Br J Ophthalmol 1978; 62:402–407.

302. Purcell JJ, Birkenkamp R, Tsai CC. Conjunctival lesions in periarteritis nodosa. Arch Ophthalmol 1984; 102:736–738.

303. Kinyoun JL, Kalina RE, Klein ML. Choroidal involvement in systemic necrotizing vasculitis. Arch Ophthalmol 1987; 105:939–942.

304. Akova YA, Jabbur NS, Foster CS. Ocular presentation of polyarteritis nodosa. Clinical course and management with steroid and cytotoxic therapy. Ophthalmology 1993; 100:1775–1781.

305. Churg J, Strauss L. Allergic granulomatosis, allergic angiitis, and periarteritis nodosa. Am J Pathol 1951; 27:277–281.

306. Chumbley LC, Harrison EG, DeRemee RA. Allergic granulomatosis and angiitis (Churg–Strauss syndrome): report and analysis of 30 cases. Mayo Clin Proc 1977; 52:477–480.

307. Cooper BJ, Bacal E, Patterson R. Allergic angiitis and granulomatosis. Arch Intern Med 1978; 138:367–374.

308. Finan MC, Winkelmann RK. The cutaneous extravascular necrotizing granuloma (Churg–Strauss granuloma) and systemic disease: a review of 27 cases. Medicine (Baltimore) 1983; 62:142–146.

309. Masi AT, Hunder GG, Lie JT et al. The American College of Rheumatology 1990 criteria for the classification of Churg–Strauss syndrome (allergic granulomatosis and angiitis). Arthritis Rheum 1990; 33:1094–1100.

310. Calabrese LH, Duna G. Vasculitis associated with antineutrophil cytoplasmic antibody. In: Ruddy S, Harris ED, Sledge CB et al., eds. Kelly's textbook of rheumatology, 6th edn. Philadelphia: Saunders; 2001:1165–1184.

311. Cury D, Breakey AS, Payne BF. Allergic granulomatosis angiitis associated with uveoscleritis and papilledema. Arch Ophthalmol 1956; 55:261–266.

312. Miesler DM, Stock EL, Wertz RD et al. Conjunctival inflammation and amyloidosis in allergic granulomatosis and angiitis (Churg–Strauss syndrome). Am J Ophthalmol 1981; 91:216–219.

313. Robin JB, Schanzlin DJ, Meisler DM et al. Ocular involvement in the respiratory vasculitides. Surv Ophthalmol 1985; 30:127–140.

314. Weinstein JM, Chui H, Lane S et al. Churg–Strauss syndrome (allergic granulomatous angiitis): neuroophthalmologic manifestations. Arch Ophthalmol 1983; 101:1217–1220.

315. Brandwein S, Esdaile J, Danoff D et al. Wegener's granulomatosis: clinical features and outcome in 13 patients. Arch Intern Med 1983; 143:476–479.

316. Wolff SM, Fauci AS, Horn RG et al. Wegener's granulomatosis. Ann Intern Med 1974; 81:513–525.

317. Fauci AS, Wolff SM. Wegener's granulomatosis: studies in eighteen patients and a review of the literature. Medicine (Baltimore) 1973; 52:535–542.

318. Fauci AS, Haynes BF, Katz P et al. Wegener's granulomatosis: prospective clinical and therapeutic experience with 85 patients for 21 years. Ann Intern Med 1983; 98:76–85.

319. Leavitt RY, Fauci AS, Bloch DA et al. The American College of Rheumatology 1990 criteria for the classification of Wegener's granulomatosis. Arthritis Rheum 1990; 33:1101–1107.

320. Cassan SM, Coles DT, Harrison EG. The concept of limited forms of Wegener's granulomatosis. Am J Med 1970; 49:366–379.

321. Coutu RE, Klein M, Lessell S et al. Limited form of Wegener granulomatosis: eye involvement as a major sign. JAMA 1975; 233:868–871.

322. Harman LE, Margo CE. Wegener's granulomatosis. Surv Ophthalmol 1998; 42:458–480.

323. Hoffman GS, Kerr GS, Leavitt RY et al. Wegener's granulomatosis: an analysis of 158 patients. Ann Intern Med 1992; 116:488–498.

324. Hollander D, Manning RT. The use of alkylating agents in the treatment of Wegener's granulomatosis. Ann Intern Med 1967; 67:393–398.

325. Lacki JK, Schochat T, Sobieska M et al. Immunological studies in patients with rheumatoid arthritis treated with methotrexate or cyclophosphamide. Z Rheumatol 1994; 53:76–82.

326. Bullen CL, Liesegang TJ, McDonald TJ et al. Ocular complications of Wegener's granulomatosis. Ophthalmology 1983; 90:279–290.

327. Haynes BF, Fishman ML, Fauci AS et al. The ocular manifestations of Wegener's granulomatosis: fifteen years experience and review of the literature. Am J Med 1977; 63:131–141.

328. Straatsma BR. Ocular manifestations of Wegener's granulomatosis. Am J Ophthalmol 1957; 44:789–799.

329. Blodi FC, Gass JDM. Inflammatory pseudotumor of the orbit. Br J Ophthalmol 1968; 52:579–583.

330. Sainz de la Maza M, Foster CS, Jabbur NS. Scleritis associated with systemic vasculitic diseases. Ophthalmology 1995; 102:687–692.

331. Jaben SL, Norton EWD. Exudative retinal detachment in Wegener's granulomatosis: case report. Ann Ophthalmol 1982; 14:717–720.

332. Greenberger MH. Central retinal artery closure in Wegener's granulomatosis. Am J Ophthalmol 1967; 63:515–516.

333. Ohno S, Ohguchi M, Hirose S et al. Close association of HLA-Bw51 with Behçet's disease. Arch Ophthalmol 1982; 100:1455–1458.

334. Chajek T, Fainaru M. Behçet's disease: report of 41 cases and a review of the literature. Medicine 1975; 54:179–196.

335. Chamberlain MA. Behçet's syndrome in 32 patients in Yorkshire. Ann Rheum Dis 1977; 36:491–499.

336. Ghate JV, Jorizzo JL. Behçet's disease. In: Ruddy S, Harris ED, Sledge CB et al., eds. Kelly's textbook of rheumatology, 6th edn. Philadelphia: Saunders; 2001:1205–1209.

337. Sakane T, Takeno M, Suzuki N et al. Behçet's disease. N Engl J Med 1999; 341:1284–1301.

338. Mamo JG, Baghdassarian A. Behçet's disease: a report of 28 cases. Arch Ophthalmol 1964; 71:4–14.

339. Michelson JB, Chisari FV. Behçet's disease. Surv Ophthalmol 1982; 26:190–203.

340. Mason RM, Barnes CG. Behçet's syndrome with arthritis. Ann Rheum Dis 1969; 28:95–103.

341. Zizic TM, Stevens MB. The arthropathy of Behçet's disease. Johns Hopkins Med J 1975; 136:243–248.

342. Schotland DL, Wolf SM, White HH et al. Neurologic aspects of Behçet's disease. Am J Med 1963; 34:544–548.

343. Kalbain VV, Challis MT. Behçet's disease. Report of twelve cases with three manifesting as papilledema. Am J Med 1970; 49:823–828.

344. O'Duffy JD, Golstein NP. Neurologic involvement in seven patients with Behçet's disease. Am J Med 1976; 61:17–18.

345. Shimizu T, Mishima S, Miyoshi K et al. Behçet's disease. Jpn J Opthalmol 1974; 18:93–102.

346. International Study Group for Behçet's Disease. Criteria for diagnosis of Behçet's disease. Lancet 1990; 335:1078–1080.

347. Mamo JG. The rate of visual loss in Behçet's disease. Arch Ophthalmol 1970; 84:451–452.

348. O'Duffy JD, Robertson DM, Goldstein NP. Chlorambucil in the treatment of uveitis and meningoencephalitis of Behçet's disease. Am J Med 1984; 76:75–84.

349. Abdalla MI, Baghat NED. Long-lasting remission of Behçet's disease after chlorambucil therapy. Br J Ophthalmol 1973; 57:706–711.

350. Tessler HH, Jennings T. High-dose short-term chlorambucil for intractable sympathetic ophthalmia and Behçet's disease. Br J Ophthalmol 1990; 74:353–357.

351. Dinning WJ, Perkins ES. Immunosuppressive agents in uveitis: a preliminary report of experience with chlorambucil. Br J Ophthalmol 1975; 59:397–403.

352. Mamo JG, Azzam SA. Treatment of Behçet's disease with chlorambucil. Arch Ophthalmol 1970; 84:446–450.

353. Mamo JG. Treatment of Behçet's disease with chlorambucil. Arch Ophthalmol 1976; 94:580–583.

354. Tricoulis D. Treatment of Behçet's disease with chlorambucil. Br J Ophthalmol 1976; 60:55–57.

355. Tabbara KF. Chlorambucil in Behçet's disease: a reappraisal. Ophthalmology 1983; 90:906–908.

356. Jabs DA, Rosenbaum JT, Foster CS et al. Guidelines for the use of immunosuppressive drugs in patients with ocular inflammatory disorders: recommendations of an expert panel. Am J Ophthalmol 2000; 130:492–513.

357. Nussenblatt RB, Palestine AG, Chan CC et al. Effectiveness of cyclosporin therapy for Behçet's disease. Arthritis Rheum 1985; 28:671–679.

358. Masuda K, Nakajima A, Urayama A et al. Double-masked trial of ciclosporin versus colchicine and long-term open study of ciclosporin in Behçet's disease. Lancet 1989; 1:1093–1096.

359. Whitcup SM, Salvo EC, Nussenblatt RB. Combined ciclosporin and corticosteroid therapy for sight-threatening uveitis in Behçet's disease. Am J Ophthalmol 1994; 118:39–45.

360. Palestine AG, Austin HA, Balow JE et al. Renal histopathologic alterations in patients treated with cyclosporin for uveitis. N Engl J Med 1986; 314:1293–1298.

361. Yazici J, Pazarli H, Barnes CG et al. A controlled trial of azathioprine in Behçet's syndrome. N Engl J Med 1990; 322:281–285.

362. Colvard DM, Robertson DM, O'Duffy JD. The ocular manifestations of Behçet's disease. Arch Ophthalmol 1977; 95:1813–1817.

363. Kalbian VV, Challis MT. Behçet's disease: report of twelve cases with three manifesting as papilledema. Am J Med 1970; 49:823–829.

364. Scouras J, Koutroumanos J. Ischaemic optic neuropathy in Behçet's syndrome. Ophthalmologica 1976; 173:11–18.

365. Michelson JB, Michelson PE, Chisari FV. Subretinal neovascular membrane and disciform scar in Behçet's disease. Am J Ophthalmol 1980; 90:182–183.

366. Nguyen QD, Foster CS. Systemic lupus erythematosus and the eye. Int Ophthalmol Clin 1998; 38:33–60.

367. Gonzalez EB, Conn DL. Hypersensitivity vasculitis (small-vessel cutaneous vasculitis). In: Ruddy S, Harris ED, Sledge CB et al., eds. Kelly's textbook of rheumatology, 6th edn. Philadelphia: Saunders; 2001:1197–1203.

368. Misiani R, Bellavita P, Fenili D et al. Hepatitis C virus infection in patients with essential mixed cryoglobulinemia. Ann Intern Med 1992; 117:573–579.

369. Agnello V, Chung RT, Kaplan LM. A role for hepatitis C virus infection in type II cryoglobulinemia. N Engl J Med 1992; 327:1490–1495.

370. Lunel F, Musset L, Cacoub P et al. Cryoglobulinemia in chronic liver disease: role of HCV and liver damage. Gastroenterology 1994; 106:1291–1296.

371. Corwin JM, Baum J. Iridocyclitis in two patients with hypocomplementemic cutaneous vasculitis. Am J Ophthalmol 1982; 94:111–113.

372. Wisnieski JJ, Baer AN, Christensen J et al. Hypocomplementemic urticarial vasculitis syndrome. Clinical and serologic findings in 18 patients. Medicine (Baltimore) 1995; 74:24–41.

373. Wisnieski JJ. Urticarial vasculitis. Curr Opin Rheumatol 2000; 12:24–31.

374. Thorne JE, Hernandez MI, Rencic A et al. Severe scleritis and urticarial lesions. Am J Ophthalmol 2002; 134:932–934.

375. Corwin JM, Baum J. Iridocyclitis in two patients with hypocomplementemic cutaneous vasculitis. Am J Ophthalmol 1982; 94:111–113.

376. Sanchez NP, Winkelmann RK, Schroeter AL et al. The clinical and histopathologic spectrums of urticarial vasculitis: study of 40 cases. J Am Acad Dermatol 1982; 7:599–605.

377. Davis MD, Daoud MS, Kirby B et al. Clinicopathologic correlation of hypocomplementemic and normocomplementemic urticarial vasculitis. J Am Acad Dermatol 1998; 38:899–905.

Chapter

76

Parafoveal Telangiectasis

Emily Y. Chew

Retinal telangiectasis, a term proposed by Reese,[1] refers to a developmental retinal vascular disorder characterized by an ectasia of capillaries of the retina, in which irregular capillary dilation and incompetence occur in the retinal periphery or the macula. Funduscopic and fluorescein angiographic findings in patients with macular dysfunction secondary to retinal telangiectasis have been well described.[2] If only the capillaries of the foveal avascular zone are involved, it is known as *parafoveal telangiectasia*, a rather nonspecific term that describes the presence of dilated capillaries in the juxtafoveal area. The cause of this condition is unknown and it was originally called *idiopathic juxtafoveolar retinal telangiectasis* by Gass & Oyakawa.[3] Parafoveal telangiectasis can be considered as having two basic forms: (1) a developmental or congenital vascular anomaly, which may be part of the larger spectrum of Coats disease; and (2) a presumably acquired form found in middle-aged and older persons. A modification of this classification by Gass & Blodi[4,5] has further subdivided this group of patients into three categories (Table 76-1).

CONGENITAL PARAFOVEAL TELANGIECTASIS

Group 1A: Unilateral congenital parafoveal telangiectasis

Patients with unilateral congenital parafoveal telangiectasis are typically men whose mean age at onset of the disease is 40 years. The telangiectasis is usually confined unilaterally to the temporal half of the macula, occurring in an area of one to two disc diameters, with equal areas superior and inferior to the horizontal raphe involved (Fig. 76-1). Macular edema and exudation are the main causes of visual loss in these patients. Visual acuity at presentation usually ranges from 20/25 to 20/40, although 20/200 may occur.

A limited number of cases with group 1A disease have experienced improvement in visual acuity after treatment of the area of telangiectasis with laser photocoagulation.[3,6] However, spontaneous resolution has also occurred.[3] Therapy for such a rare disease is difficult to assess in a controlled, randomized clinical trial. Photocoagulation may indeed be helpful in improving or stabilizing central visual acuity.

Table 76-1 Parafoveal telangiectasis classification according to Gass and Oyakawa[3]				
	Group 1A Unilateral congenital parafoveal telangiectasis	Group 1B Unilateral idiopathic parafoveal telangiectasis	Group 2 Bilateral acquired parafoveal telangiectasis	Group 3 Bilateral idiopathic perifoveal telangiectasis and capillary obliteration
Mean age (years)	40	40	50–60	50
Sex	Males	Males	Males and females	–
Perifoveal area involved	Temporal 1 to 2 disc diameters	One clock-hour area only	Temporal or the entire perifoveal network	Progressive obliteration of the entire perifoveal network
Other retinal features			Eventual retinal pigment epithelial hyperplasia, right-angle venule, yellow lesion at the center of the fovea avascular zone, subretinal neovascularization	Optic disc pallor

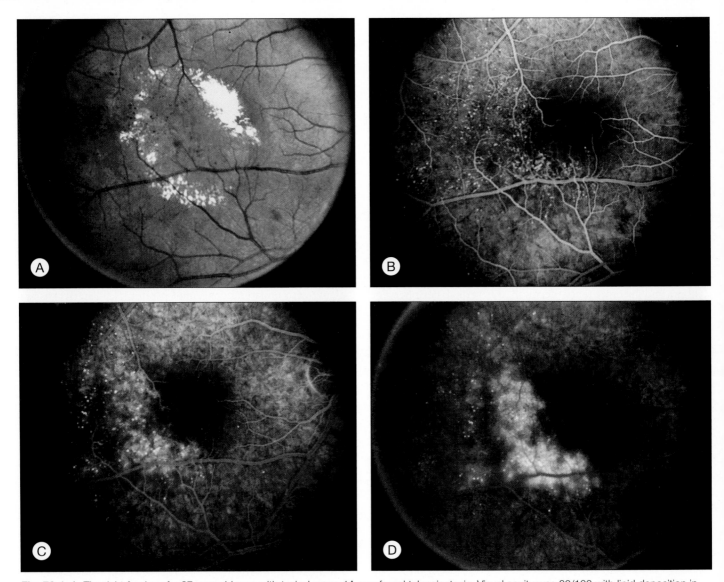

Fig. 76-1 A, The right fundus of a 37-year-old man with typical group 1A parafoveal telangiectasis. Visual acuity was 20/100 with lipid deposition in the foveal avascular zone. He was found to have an abnormal glucose tolerance test. His left eye was normal. B, Telangiectasis of the retinal capillaries temporal to the fovea involving approximately two disc diameters. C, Leakage from the microaneurysms and the telangiectasis. D, Late leakage of fluorescein.

ACQUIRED PARAFOVEAL TELANGIECTASIS

Group 1B: Unilateral idiopathic parafoveal telangiectasis

Unilateral idiopathic parafoveal telangiectasis, according to Gass,[2] is found in middle-aged men who have a very small area of capillary telangiectasis confined to one clock-hour at the edge of the foveal avascular zone. This may or may not be accompanied by hard exudates. Rarely does this area of telangiectasis have much leakage on fluorescein angiography. Visual acuity is rarely less than 20/25. Because of the excellent visual acuity and the close proximity of the telangiectasis to the center of the fovea, it is probably not advisable to photocoagulate such lesions. Although this is considered an acquired condition, it may very well be part of the spectrum of congenital telangiectasis occurring in a small localized area of the retina.

Group 2: Bilateral acquired parafoveal telangiectasis

Patients in group 2A are a combination of groups 2 and 3 from the former classification proposed by Gass & Oyakwa.[3] This is the most common group of all patients with parafoveal telangiectasis. These patients are typically diagnosed in their fifth or sixth decade of life. Both sexes may be affected. A familial incidence has also been reported.[4,7]

In this condition, there is microaneurysmal and saccular dilation and capillary nonperfusion of the parafoveal capillaries. Usually the parafoveal telangiectasis is symmetric, bilateral, and involves an area of less than one disc diameter. This often involves the area temporal to the fovea (Fig. 76-2), or it may involve the entire perifoveal capillary network. Minimal macular edema without lipid exudation is associated with this early form of parafoveal telangiectasis. Biomicroscopy reveals minimal-to-mild dilation of retinal capillaries with slight graying of the retinal area involved. Refractile deposits of unknown substance, located in the superficial layers of the retina, have been described in areas overlying or adjacent to the telangiectasis.[8] Visual decline may occur secondary to serous exudation, accompanied by hard exudates and macular edema. Right-angle retinal venules are commonly seen in this group of patients with parafoveal telangiectasis, and they appear, on stereoscopic viewing, to be draining the outer retinal capillary plexus. A characteristic feature of this group is the eventual development of hyperplasia of the retinal pigment epithelium (RPE) along these right-angle venules.

The typical fluorescein angiographic features show dilated, ectatic perifoveal capillaries (Fig. 76-2, C to F). These incompetent vessels display hyperfluorescence, whereas the areas of RPE hyperplasia routinely block fluorescence. On initial presentation, the level of visual loss is usually minimal, 20/30 or better. Mild visual disturbance can be seen when there is light-gray loss of transparency with or without thickening of the parafoveal retina. Optical coherence tomography (OCT) has provided further insight into the retinal thickness at the different stages of the natural course of the disease. It appears that, in the presence of retinal staining with fluorescein angiography, there may be no associated retinal thickening. In addition, photocoagulation given to these leaking vessels appears to have minimal beneficial effects. Two reports of intravitreal injections of steroids for cases with retinal edema showed a gain of two lines on the visual acuity chart with short-term follow-up.[9,10] Central visual loss may be gradual over many years with progressive atrophy of the central foveal areas.

Acute central visual loss occurs in some patients with the development of neovascularization, which may begin as intraretinal neovascularization. Later follow-up of such cases shows the presence of retinochoroidal anastomosis with the development of choroidal neovascularization, which often involves the center of the foveal avascular zone.[11] (Figs 76-3A and 76-4). Photodynamic therapy administered twice was reported to result in short-term success of 7 months with an improvement of 20/70 to 20/50.[12] Others have reported favorable results in a case series in which a number of cases of classic choroidal neovascularization, including parafoveal telangiectasis, were treated with photodynamic therapy.[13]

Treatment with intravitreal delivery of drugs targeting the decrease in vascular endothelial growth factor in these lesions may be beneficial but has not been reported. Such therapy may be conducted in the near future. Photocoagulation for the parafoveal telangiectasis itself is also not recommended because the amount of exudation is minimal and the area of retinal capillary involvement is often within one disc diameter of the center of the foveola. A small case series showed no beneficial effects of laser.[14] The limited natural history available on these patients suggests that long-term prognosis for preservation of central visual acuity in those patients who do not develop neovascularization is good.

In an update of the classification, Gass & Blodi[4] added the category 2B of juvenile occult familial idiopathic juxtafoveolar retinal telangiectasis in two brothers, 9 and 12 years of age. They had subretinal neovascularization and subtle retinal juxtafoveolar telangiectasis with no evidence of superficial retinal refractile deposits, hyperpigmented plaques, or right-angle venules.

Group 3: Bilateral idiopathic perifoveal telangiectasis and capillary obliteration

According to Gass & Blodi,[5] two patients in their fifth decade of life lost central vision to the level of legal blindness bilaterally

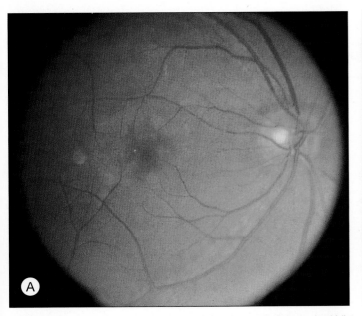
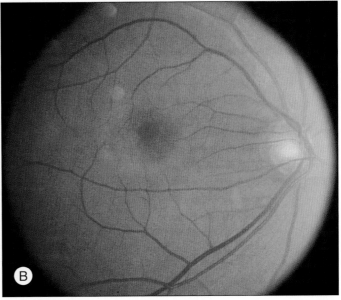

Fig. 76-2 A and B, This 51-year-old woman with type 2 diabetes had bilateral group 2 perifoveal telangiectasis involving the temporal perifoveal capillaries. She had 20/30 vision bilaterally. At the level of the posterior vitreous in the temporal macular area, both eyes were glistening; note refractile deposits with minimal pigmentary changes at the level of the retinal pigment epithelium temporal to the foveal avascular zone.

Continued

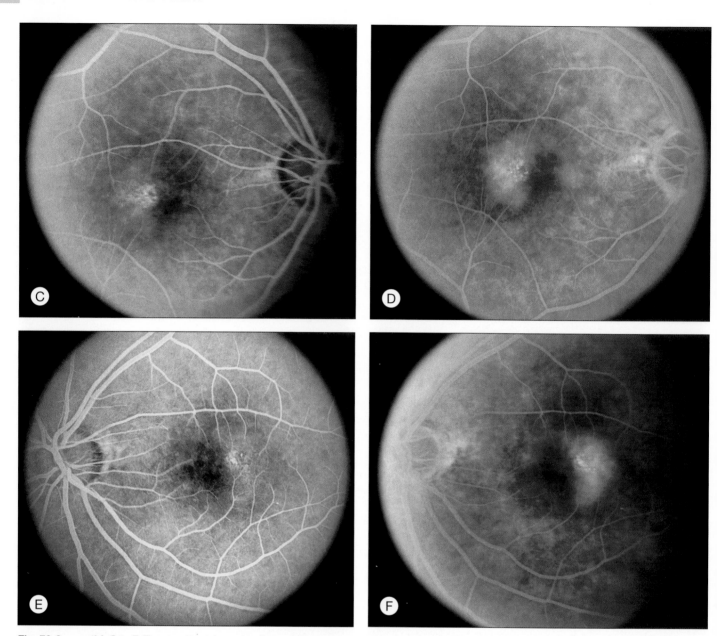

Fig. 76-2—cont'd C to F, Fluorescein angiography showed the typical temporal involvement of the perifoveal capillaries and the late leakage of fluorescein bilaterally.

secondary to telangiectasis and progressive obliteration of the vessels with enlargement of the foveal avascular zone. There was no evidence of fluorescein leakage from these telangiectatic vessels. Additional clinical features included optic disc pallor and hyperactive deep tendon reflexes with an otherwise normal neurologic examination and investigation. This macular change is similar to that found in patients with sickle-cell retinopathy.

DIFFERENTIAL DIAGNOSIS

Parafoveal telangiectasis is a clinical entity that is distinctly different from secondary telangiectasis, which can result from various other diseases. A common condition is the branch retinal vein obstruction, which leads to a segmental picture of capillary

changes, including telangiectasis and microaneurysmal and saccular dilation, as well as capillary obliteration. This can be distinguished from parafoveal telangiectasis in that the area involved in branch retinal vein occlusion affects the entire capillary bed distal to the arteriolar–venular crossing. The capillary dilation may extend slightly into the region drained by neighboring venules. This dilation is caused by the development of collateral pathways of venous outflow.

Radiation retinopathy also results in secondary telangiectasis with similar macular capillary abnormalities. However, radiation retinopathy tends to have multiple abnormal retinal areas with evidence of other features such as cottonwool spots and retinal neovascularization. The history of irradiation to the eye or head area will also help to distinguish this disease from parafoveal

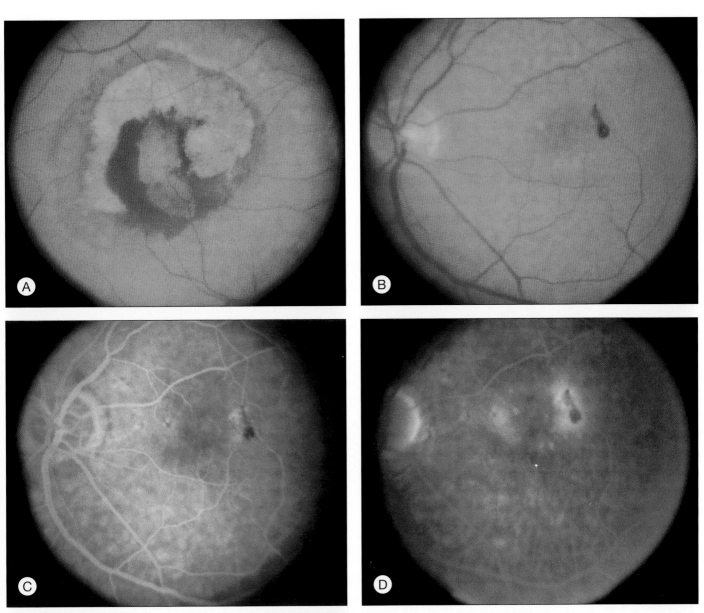

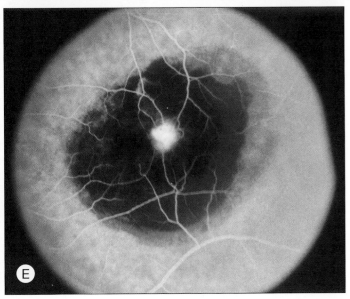

Fig. 76-3 A, This 57-year-old woman with a 17-year history of type 2 diabetes had central vision loss (5/200) in the right eye with a large submacular hemorrhage, which consisted of fresh red and old white blood, and a serous detachment of the neurosensory retina overlying the macula. B, The left eye had 20/50 visual acuity with hyperpigmentation of the retinal pigment epithelium temporal to the foveal avascular zone with minimal macular edema. C and D, The fluorescein angiogram of the left eye showed perifoveal telangiectasia, which increased in fluorescence during the study, and blocked fluorescence was noted in the area of the pigmentation. E, The right eye showed blocked fluorescein from the submacular hemorrhage, whereas the subfoveal area showed hyperfluorescence, which was evidence of choroidal neovascularization, associated with perifoveal telangiectasis.

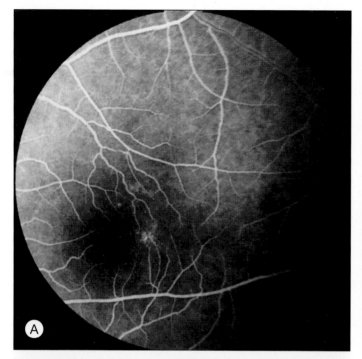

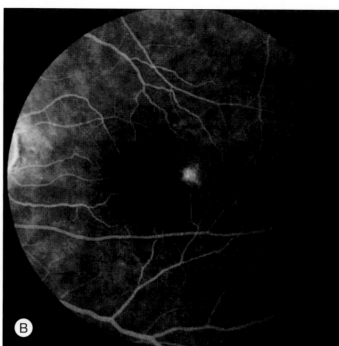

Fig. 76-4 A, A 56-year-old woman with group 2 parafoveal telangiectasis. B, Late leakage with good visual acuity of 20/20. C, Eight months later, visual acuity dropped acutely to 20/100 with subfoveal choroidal neovascularization. The patient was also diagnosed with diabetes mellitus with an abnormal glucose tolerance test.

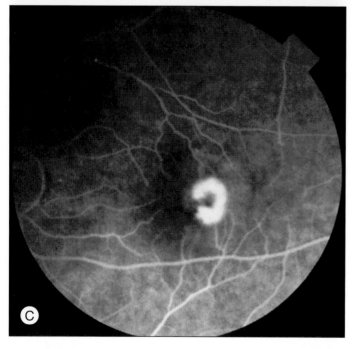

telangiectasis. However, in a case-control study of patients with and without typical parafoveal telangiectasis and in the absence of radiation retinopathy, radiation to the head was found to be a risk factor associated with the presence of parafoveal telangiectasia.[15]

An inflammatory process that produces vitreous cellular infiltration may also result in dilated perifoveal capillaries and macular edema. Primary parafoveal telangiectasis occurs in the absence of any signs of inflammation. Because of the common occurrence of the retinal pigment hyperplasia, especially in group

2A of parafoveal telangiectasis, the diagnosis of focal choroiditis with the chorioretinal scar may be erroneously made.

Age-related macular degeneration is another entity for which parafoveal telangiectasis may be mistaken. Good-quality stereo fluorescein angiography is essential in differentiating the two entities. Parafoveal telangiectasis has fluorescein at the level of the retinal vasculature, whereas leakage associated with choroidal neovascularization involves the deeper retina, the RPE. High-speed indocyanine green angiography may also be useful in distinguishing between intraretinal and choroidal (subretinal) neovascularization. In age-related macular degeneration, the choroidal neovascularization is accompanied by drusen and RPE abnormalities with no evidence of retinal capillary disease. The yellow lesion sometimes seen in parafoveal telangiectasis may be very similar in appearance to foveomacular dystrophy. However, fluorescein angiography will delineate the lack of telangiectasis and perifoveal capillary fluorescein leakage in patients with foveomacular dystrophy.

ASSOCIATION WITH DIABETES MELLITUS

Green et al.[16,17] described the clinical and histopathologic features of parafoveal telangiectasis (group 2) in two separate reports. In the first report,[17] the investigators reported on the findings of a 58-year-old woman. On light and electron microscopic study, however, the investigators were unable to demonstrate telangiectatic capillaries. The capillary lumina were, in fact, narrowed. Localized endothelial defects were found in the temporal parafoveal area and, to a lesser extent, in the mid-periphery. There was also degeneration of pericytes with accumulation of lipid within the capillary walls and the presence of multilaminated basement membrane. These retinal capillary changes were similar to those observed in the diabetic and prediabetic state. However, this patient had no history of diabetes mellitus. Although her fasting blood glucose levels on two occasions were normal, a diagnostic glucose tolerance test was not performed. This case does indeed suggest a possible relationship of diabetes mellitus with parafoveal telangiectasis.

One group of investigators has raised the hypothesis that parafoveal telangiectasis may be caused by abnormal glucose metabolism.[18] Twenty-eight patients with this entity underwent glucose tolerance testing. Although the number of cases was small, there was a suggestion of an association, with 35% of the patients showing abnormal glucose tolerance tests. This view is also supported by the description of patients with long-standing diabetes and parafoveal telangiectasis.[19] Further studies are required to evaluate the true relationship of parafoveal telangiectasis with diabetes mellitus. Another systemic disease that has been reported to be associated with cases of parafoveal telangiectasis is celiac sprue.[20]

A histopathological study by Eliassi-Rad & Green[16] showed dilation and proliferation of retinal capillaries into the outer retinal and subretinal space. There was migration of the retinal pigment epithelium within the retina along the telangiectatic vessels. Preretinal neovascularization was also found. Interestingly, there was a sharp demarcation between the edematous and nonedematous retina. The edema was seen throughout all the layers of the retina, including the nerve fiber layer as well as the ganglion cell layer. With the staining of the retina with fluorescein in eyes with minimal edema, Gass has postulated that it

is possible that the primary abnormality may be found in the parafoveal retinal neural or Mueller cells.[11]

SUMMARY

The pathogenesis of parafoveal telangiectasis is unknown. There are speculations that the unilateral group 1A may be a developmental retinal vascular anomaly. In group 2A patients, the telangiectasis is most commonly located temporal to the foveal avascular zone, which is considered to be a watershed zone between the superotemporal and inferotemporal arcade. This may predispose this area to chronic low-grade congestion, which may be important in the pathogenesis of parafoveal telangiectasis.[4] The hypothesis that there may be a primary defect in the neural or Mueller cells is also intriguing.[11] The role of abnormal glucose metabolism remains to be studied further.

REFERENCES

1. Reese AB. Telangiectasis of the retina and Coats' disease. Am J Ophthalmol 1956; 42:1–8.
2. Gass JDM. A fluorescein angiographic study of macular dysfunction secondary to retinal vascular disease. V. Retinal telangiectasis. Arch Ophthalmol 1968; 80:592–605.
3. Gass JD, Oyakawa RT. Idiopathic juxtafoveolar retinal telangiectasis. Arch Ophthalmol 1982; 100:769–780.
4. Gass JDM, Blodi BA. Idiopathic juxtafoveolar retinal telangiectasis: update of classification and follow-up study. Ophthalmology 1993; 100:1536–1546.
5. Gass JDM, Blodi BA. Idiopathic juxtafoveolar retinal telangiectasis: update of classification and follow-up study. Ophthalmology 1993; 100:1536–1546.
6. Chopdar A. Retinal telangiectasis in adults: fluorescein angiographic findings and treatment by argon laser. Br J Ophthalmol 1978; 62:243–250.
7. Hutton WL, Snyder WB, Fuller D et al. Focal parafoveal retinal telangiectasis. Arch Ophthalmol 1978; 96:1362–1367.
8. Moisseiev J, Lewis H, Bartov E et al. Superficial retinal refractile deposits in juxtafoveal telangiectasis. Am J Ophthalmol 1990; 109:604–605.
9. Alldredge CD, Garretson BR. Intravitreal triamcinolone for the treatment of idiopathic juxtafoveal telangiectasis. Retina 2003; 23:113–116.
10. Martinez J. Intravitreal triamcinolone acetonide for bilateral acquired parafoveal telangiectasis. Arch Ophthalmol 2003; 121:1658–1659.
11. Gass JDM. Histological study of presumed parafoveal telangiectasia. Retina 2000; 20:226–227.
12. Potter MJ, Szabo SM, Chan EY et al. Photodynamic therapy of a subretinal neovascular membrane in type 2A idiopathic juxtafoveolar retinal telangiectasis. Am J Ophthalmol 2002; 133:149–151.
13. Muller-Velten R, Michels S, Schmidt-Erfurth U et al. Photodynamic therapy: extended indication. Ophthalmologe 2003; 100:384–390.
14. Park DW, Schatz H, McDonald HR et al. Grid laser photocoagulation for macular edema in bilateral juxtafoveal telangiectasis. Ophthalmology 1997; 104:1838–1846.
15. Maberley DA, Yannuzzi LA, Gitter K et al. Radiation exposure: a new risk factor for idiopathic perifoveal telangiectasis. Ophthalmology 1999; 106:2248–2253.
16. Eliassi-Rad B, Green WR. Histologic study of presumed parafoveal telangiectasis. Retina 1999; 19:332–335.
17. Green WR, Quigley HA, de la Cruz Z et al. Parafoveal retinal telangiectasis: light and electron microscopy studies. Trans Ophthalmol Soc UK 1980; 100:162–170.
18. Millay RH, Klein ML, Handelman IL et al. Abnormal glucose metabolism and parafoveal telangiectasia. Am J Ophthalmol 1986; 102:363–370.
19. Chew EY, Murphy RP, Newsome DA et al. Parafoveal telangiectasis and diabetic retinopathy. Arch Ophthalmol 1986; 104:71–75.
20. Lee HC, Liu M, Ho AC. Idiopathic juxtafoveal telangiectasis in association with celiac sprue. Arch Ophthalmol 2004; 122:411–413.

Coats' Disease

Diana V. Do
Julia A. Haller

HISTORY

Coats' disease, an idiopathic condition characterized by telangiectatic and aneurysmal retinal vessels with intraretinal and subretinal exudates,[1] was first described by George Coats[2] in 1908. In his initial classification, Coats separated this new entity into three distinct groups. Eyes with massive subretinal exudate and no demonstrable vascular abnormalities were included in group I. Group II consisted of eyes with massive subretinal exudate and multiple retinal vascular abnormalities with intraretinal hemorrhage. Coats separated eyes with massive subretinal exudate and frank retinal arteriovenous malformations into group III.[2] Eugen von Hippel later demonstrated that this third category represented the distinctly separate entity of angiomatosis retinae, leading Coats to drop this group from his classification. In 1912, and again in 1915, Theodor Leber described a disease with similar vascular findings that lacked the massive subretinal exudates described by Coats. This syndrome was later named *Leber's multiple miliary aneurysm disease*. In a 1915 paper, Leber concluded that what he had described was merely an earlier stage of the disease process identified by Coats.[3–8] This conclusion was later reinforced by Reese,[9] who described an eye with Leber's miliary aneurysms that progressed into a classic case of Coats' disease during long-term follow-up. Although some authors have disagreed, most authorities today classify Leber's disease as an early or nonprogressive form of Coats' disease.[3–5,10–17]

ETIOLOGY

Early descriptions of Coats' disease focused primarily on the morphology of the disease and attempted to explain the disease process solely on the basis of funduscopic and histologic changes.[3,14,18–22] Because he often found hemorrhages associated with subretinal exudates in his cases, Coats suggested that the exudates were secondary to organization and partial resorption of the hemorrhages. Coats also postulated that the primary process might be infectious in light of the mononuclear infiltrate found on histologic examination (Coats' first papers were based on histologic examination of enucleated eyes received from various colleagues).[2] This conclusion was supported by a number of other authors, including Straub, Müller, and Francois, who all suspected toxoplasmosis as the underlying cause.[7] Subsequent investigations and the failure of antiinflammatory adreno-

corticotropic hormone (ACTH) and steroid therapies have refuted early theories of a primary infectious or inflammatory etiology.[3,7,18–20,22]

Several authors have suggested a primary vascular etiology for the disease. Reese[23] demonstrated marked thickening of endothelial basement membrane of the characteristic telangiectatic vessels due to the deposition of periodic acid–Schiff (PAS)-positive material. Because of some histologic similarities to diabetic retinopathy and some isolated case reports of disease exacerbation at the time of pregnancy, Imre[7,24] and others have speculated on an endocrinologic basis for Coats' disease, although this has never been documented.

Recently, genetic mutations have been implicated in the development of Coats' disease. Cremers et al. found that 55% of cases with retinitis pigmentosa and Coats'-like exudative vasculopathy contained a mutation in the CRB1 gene.[25] This report suggests that the CRB1 gene may be involved in Coats' disease as well as other retinal diseases and dystrophies.

In addition, several reports have implicated a deficiency of norrin, a retinal protein, in the pathogenesis of Coats' disease.[26,27] In one case report, a female with unilateral Coats' disease gave birth to a son affected by Norrie disease.[26] Both carried a missense mutation within the NDP gene on chromosome Xp11.2. Further analysis on archival tissue from nine enucleated eyes from males with unilateral Coats' disease revealed a mutation in the NDP gene in one subject. Shastry and colleagues have isolated the norrin protein, cloned it into an expression vector, and are studying its structure and function.[27] Interestingly, a prior study also has implicated the norrin protein in retinal developmental vasculogenesis. Berger et al.[28] developed a mutant mouse line with the Norrie disease model and demonstrated that abnormalities of the retinal vessels, including telangiectasis, bulb-like dilatations, and underdevelopment of the capillary bed, are present. These reports suggest a genetic basis for Coats' disease and that a mutation in the NDP gene may be responsible.

CLINICAL PICTURE

Coats' disease is painless, affects males three times as often as females, has no reported racial or ethnic predilection, and is clinically unilateral in 80% or more of cases.[3,5] Age at diagnosis has been as young as 4 months in one case,[12] and there has been speculation, so far unsubstantiated, that the disease may be present at birth in at least some instances.[3,4,7] Approximately two-thirds of the juvenile cases have been reported to present before 10 years of age, most often with complaints of poor vision, strabismus, or the development of leukocoria. Adult cases, although generally not accompanied by strabismus, are essentially identical in both clinical presentation and disease course. Although the adult form of the disease has been described as frequently associated with hypercholesterolemia, such an association does not appear to occur in the juvenile form.[3,5,22,29]

Isolated case reports have described a number of other disorders occurring concurrently with Coats' disease, including retinitis pigmentosa,[30,31] Senior–Loken syndrome,[32] the ichthyosis hystrix variant of epidermal nevus syndrome,[33] Turner's syndrome,[3] diffuse central nervous system venous abnormality,[34] and Hallermann–Streiff syndrome.[35] Small,[36] in 1968, reported the combination of mental retardation, muscular dystrophy, and an exudative vasculopathy in four siblings. Egerer et al.[37] noted histologic evidence of rosettes characteristic of retinal dysplasia in a series of nine enucleated eyes carrying the diagnosis of Coats' disease. Fogle et al.[38] noted an exudative vasculopathy with a clinical picture similar to that of Coats' disease arising from abnormal choroidal vessels in both eyes of a patient with retinitis pigmentosa. Despite these reports, no definite connection has been made between other systemic or ocular conditions and Coats' disease. Although there is no conclusive evidence to suggest genetic transmission, a missense mutation within the NDP gene on chromosome Xp11.2 was found both in a female with unilateral Coats' disease and her son who had Norrie disease.[26]

The typical ophthalmoscopic picture in Coats' disease is that of a localized, lipid-rich, yellow subretinal exudate (Fig. 77-1) associated with vascular anomalies including sheathing, telangiectasia, tortuosity, aneurysmal dilations, zones of capillary dropout, and occasionally neovascularization. Much variability may exist in this clinical picture, however. Exudate, hemorrhage, or a combination of the two may be minimal during less active stages of the disease and may be so massive as to obscure the overlying retinal vasculature during the progressive stages of the disease. The vascular abnormalities may be too subtle for identification by even the most careful ophthalmoscopic examination or may be the dominant part of the clinical picture. The clinical course is variable but generally progressive. Acute exacerbations of the disease may be separated in time by more quiescent stages. Spontaneous remissions have been reported but are the exception.[39] Subretinal choroidal neovascularization may occur in areas of lipid deposition. As subretinal exudation increases, serous retinal detachment develops and progresses until the affected retina becomes visible behind the lens. Hemorrhagic retinal macrocysts may ensue.[40] Secondary complications such as iridocyclitis, cataract, and secondary neovascular glaucoma can lead to phthisis bulbi in severe cases.[2,41–44]

FLUORESCEIN ANGIOGRAPHY

Fluorescein angiography is largely responsible for our current understanding of Coats' disease as a pathologic process secondary to the idiopathic loss of the blood–retinal barrier. Investigators in the pre-angiogram era attempted to explain the disease and its etiology in terms of the visible lesions and their similarity to other diseases such as diabetic retinopathy or Eales' disease. It is now understood that exudates, hemorrhages, and neovascularization in these diseases are expressions of a common loss of vascular integrity and not of a common etiology. The typical fluorescein angiographic picture of Coats' disease is one of numerous localized anomalies of the retinal vasculature (Figs 77-2 to 77-4). Telangiectasia, aneurysms, beading of vessel walls, and various vascular communicating channels are seen in the larger vessels involved. These vessels show early and persistent leakage, which verifies their role as the source of exudation and hemorrhage. This leakage, which represents breakdown of the blood–retinal barrier, also can

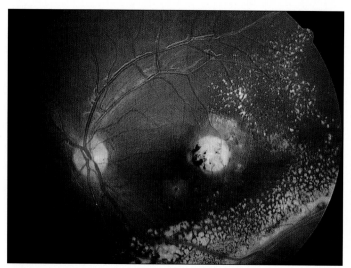

Fig. 77-1 Macular lipid deposition with subretinal fibrosis and pigmentation and an inferotemporal exudative retinal detachment in a boy with Coats' disease.

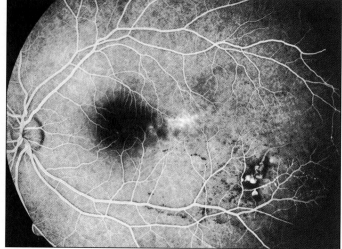

Fig. 77-2 Early-phase fluorescein angiogram demonstrates filling of telangiectatic and aneurysmal vascular channels along the inferotemporal arcade. Vessel wall beading is seen.

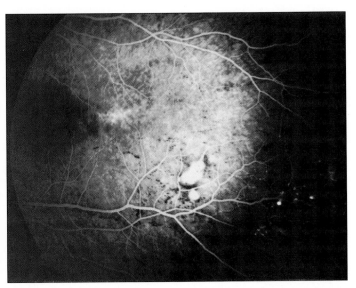

Fig. 77-3 In the later phase of the angiogram, centered more temporally, leakage of dye from abnormal vessels is seen. The sectoral vascular anomalies extend into the periphery.

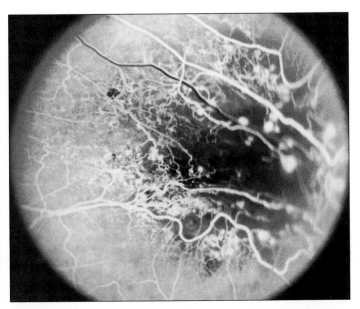

Fig. 77-4 Early-phase fluorescein angiogram frame from a peripheral sweep shows numerous characteristic vascular changes in a patient with Coats' disease. There is diffuse loss of the capillary bed, widespread venular and arteriolar anomalies with numerous communicating channels, telangiectasia, and aneurysmal formations.

be detected by vitreous fluorophotometry.[45] Microvascular involvement is reflected in fluorescein angiograms by areas of diffuse loss of the capillary bed or areas of complete capillary nonperfusion. Zones of microvascular involvement are typically surrounded by areas of arteriolar and venular anomalies. Although some early authors described cases of massive exudation or hemorrhage without areas of obvious vascular involvement, fluorescein angiography and histologic specimens invariably show unsuspected anomalous vessels. The ability to identify all anomalous vessels,

especially those with the greatest degree of leakage, has made adequate treatment of Coats' disease a possibility.[3,5,6,10,46–49]

HISTOPATHOLOGY

Pathologic samples of eyes with Coats' disease were once abundant owing to enucleations for suspected intraocular tumors.[44] Recognition and description of the disease, as well as improved diagnostic techniques, have now reduced the number of available pathologic specimens.

Examination of pathologic specimens by light and electron microscopy has revealed loss of both vascular endothelium and pericytes with subsequent mural disorganization, resulting in loss of the blood–retinal barrier.[1,3,10,13,16,20,41,45,46,49–53]

As in diabetic retinopathy, retinal vessels are primarily involved, subretinal lipid and hemorrhage may accumulate, and aneurysms of the retinal vessels may be found. In contrast to diabetic retinopathy, subretinal lipid exudation is typically massive, intraretinal exudation and hemorrhage are not common, vessel abnormalities include telangiectasia, and all levels of the retinal vascular circuit are involved.[2,3,10,13,41,48,54] Proteinaceous subretinal exudates are characteristic, with prominent cholesterol clefts and foamy histiocytes. Senft et al.[55] reported a case in which intraocular bone formation occurred in a late stage of Coats' disease, confusing clinicians because of calcification consistent with retinoblastoma seen on echography and CT scanning.

DIFFERENTIAL DIAGNOSIS

The differential diagnosis of the juvenile form of Coats' disease includes other conditions that produce leukocoria or strabismus,[41] including retinoblastoma,[43–45] retinal detachment, persistent hyperplastic primary vitreous, congenital cataract, Norrie's disease, and familial exudative vitreoretinopathy,[57] among other diagnoses. Coats' disease at any age may be confused with Eales' disease, vasculitis, collagen-vascular disease,[58] tumor accompanied by exudation,[59] conditions associated with retinal hemorrhage,[60] diabetic vasculopathies with lipid deposition, branch retinal vein occlusion or epiretinal membrane with secondary vascular leakage,[61] idiopathic juxtafoveal telangiectasis,[62] or any vasculopathy producing exudation.[4,57,59,63–68]

DIAGNOSIS AND ANCILLARY TESTING

Ancillary testing may be useful when the diagnosis of Coats' disease is suspected, but other clinical entities must be ruled out, most notably retinoblastoma.[69] Particularly when retinal detachment with subretinal exudate and dilated retinal vessels coexist, even an experienced clinician may have difficulty differentiating these entities ophthalmoscopically. Echography can allow differentiation between Coats' disease and retinoblastoma on the basis of features such as the character of the retinal detachment and the presence or absence of subretinal calcifications. Echography is less useful when the retinoblastoma is poorly calcified and also has shortcomings in detecting optic nerve or extraocular extension of retinoblastoma when heavy calcification exists.[70]

Computed tomography (CT) is valuable because of its ability to characterize intraocular morphology, quantify subretinal densities, identify vascularities within the subretinal space through the use of contrast enhancement, and detect other abnormalities that may be associated in the orbital or intracranial space. Spiral CT has the advantage of reducing anesthesia risk in small children and also decreases acquisition time and staff and equipment monitoring requirements.[71]

Magnetic resonance imaging (MRI) as an auxiliary test is useful because it permits multiplanar imaging and superior contrast resolution and yields biochemical insight into the structure and composition of tissues.[24,72,73] It is less useful in detecting calcium than either ultrasound or CT scanning.[70] An MRI study of 28 patients with leukocoria or intraocular mass, or both,[74] found that retinoblastomas could be reliably distinguished from Coats' disease, toxocariasis, and persistent hyperplastic primary vitreous. Calcification could not be reliably detected on MRI scanning.

High-resolution Doppler ultrasound has been suggested[75] as a diagnostic adjunct, providing unique information with real-time imaging and duplex pulse Doppler evaluation. This technique may delineate structural abnormalities not shown by CT or MRI.

Aqueous lactic dehydrogenase (LDH) and isoenzyme levels have not proved valuable in distinguishing between Coats' disease and retinoblastoma. Examination of subretinal fluid, although rarely used, is accurate in confirming the diagnosis of Coats' disease on the basis of cholesterol crystal and pigment-laden macrophages in the absence of tumor cells.[70]

TREATMENT

Early, unsuccessful attempts were made to treat Coats' disease with ACTH, steroids, specific antibiotics, and even intravenous serum. In 1943, Guyton and McGovern[76] reported some success with transscleral diathermy of the abnormal vessels. In the 1950s Paufique and Etienne, as well as Reese, reported partial success with X-ray radiation.[3,6,7]

After Meyer-Schwickerath applied photocoagulation techniques to the treatment of Coats' disease with an 80% cure rate, this became the treatment of choice. Xenon arc rapidly became the preferred method of photocoagulation, with authors such as Zweng advocating this over the early ruby pulse lasers. The development of fluorescein angiography and advances in photocoagulation techniques led to improved treatment results.[3,6,17,43,47,49,77–79]

The goal of treatment in Coats' disease is preservation or improvement in visual acuity, or preservation of retinal attachment and ocular integrity if vision is irreparably lost. Treatment is indicated if exudate is extensive and progressive, threatens central acuity, or produces significant retinal detachment. Intervention is directed at closing areas of vascular leakage to allow resorption of exudate. Visual results are variable, depending on the degree of initial exudate. If the macula is extensively involved by lipid, vision remains poor even with successful resolution of exudates.

In less severe cases of exudation due to Coats' disease, laser photocoagulation is the treatment of choice. Fluorescein angiographic guidance assists focal treatment of vascular leakage. Most wavelengths of laser light are adequate for treatment, although those near the yellow portion of the spectrum have better absorption by blood in the target vascular channels and may be particularly useful if the vessels are in detached retina. Leaking lesions are treated directly with moderate to large (100 to 500 microns, depending on size and location of the target lesions) applications of moderate-intensity light. Scatter photocoagulation to areas of extensive nonperfusion is of unproven value but may decrease the risk of later neovascularization (Figs 77-5 to 77-7) If lesions are too peripheral to be reached with the slit-lamp delivery system, the indirect ophthalmoscope-mounted laser, transscleral laser, or cryotherapy may be used.[80] These methods may be particularly useful in children, who usually require general anesthesia for treatment. If the retina is exudatively detached, cryotherapy can be applied directly to the anomalous vessels, using a freeze–refreeze technique. In some cases it may be necessary to drain subretinal fluid to obtain sufficient retinal vascular freezing. Diathermy or laser also may be used as an alternative to cryotherapy. Transpupillary laser can also be used, particularly after drainage of subretinal fluid. When drainage of extensive subretinal fluid is necessary, a pediatric infusion cannula placed in the anterior chamber works well for maintaining the globe (Fig. 77-8).

Egerer and co-workers[5] reported treatment results in 1974 using xenon arc photocoagulation and cryotherapy in nondetached eyes and diathermy in detached eyes. In four of the 22 eyes in their series, surgical reattachment with scleral bed dissection, diathermy, and scleral buckling was used, and exudates resorbed in all four eyes after treatment. The 18 eyes in their series that were not detached were treated with xenon arc photocoagulation to posterior anomalous vessels and cryotherapy to more peripherally located areas. Of these eyes, 15 had resolution of exudates.

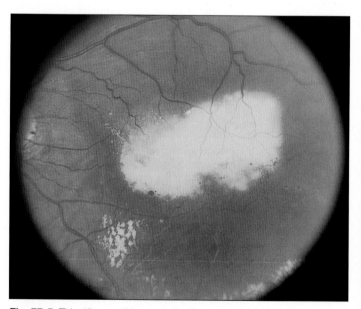

Fig. 77-5 This 40-year-old woman had noted some drop in vision in her left eye a few months previously. Examination disclosed thick lipid accumulation in the macula, with numerous vascular anomalies in the inferior and temporal fundus. (From Haller JA. Coats' disease and retinal telangiectasia. In: Yanoff M, Duker JS, eds. Ophthalmology. London: Mosby; 1999.)

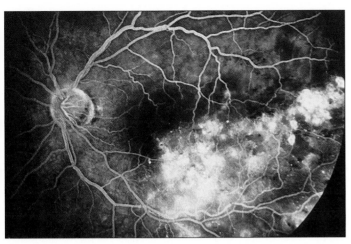

Fig. 77-6 A fluorescein angiogram highlights areas of vascular abnormalities and leakage in the posterior pole.

The authors noted a correlation between unsuccessful treatment and involvement of three or more quadrants by vascular change. As the disease reappeared in three eyes at intervals of up to 5 years after initial treatment, the authors recommended twice-yearly follow-up of patients treated for Coats' disease[1] (Fig. 77-9).

Siliodor et al.[81] have used intraocular infusion, drainage of subretinal fluid, and cryotherapy with success in eyes with advanced bullous retinal detachments. In their series of 13 children, all with blind eyes, the six eyes followed without surgery developed painful neovascular glaucoma necessitating enucleation. None of these seven eyes treated surgically developed neovascular glaucoma, and all eyes remained cosmetically acceptable.

Ridley and co-workers[47] reported stabilization or improvement in 21 of 28 eyes treated with a cryotherapy, photocoagulation, and, in severe cases, subretinal fluid drainage and vasoablation, with or without a scleral buckle.

Pauleikhoff et al.[82] reported a series of 292 eyes, 197 of which were treated either by photocoagulation, cryotherapy, diathermy, or retinal detachment surgery (6.3%). Complete scarring of vascular lesions and resorption of exudates occurred in 52.1% of the overall cases and in 67.3% of the cases with no retinal detachment. The success rate decreased to 33% in eyes with exudative retinal detachment. Final visual acuity was less than 20/400 in 45.3%, between 20/200 and 20/30 in 39.4%, and better than 20/30 in 15.3%.

Machemer and Williams[74] reported improvement in the clinical course of selected cases of Coats' disease with vitreous surgery consisting of removal of vitreal and preretinal membranes to eliminate traction detachment and destruction of leaking vessels. Other authors have advocated use of vitrectomy with internal drainage of subretinal fluid to flatten the retina, before vasoablative procedures, and intraocular tamponade with gas or silicone oil.[29]

Shields and colleagues[83] conducted a large retrospective review of 150 patients with Coats' disease to determine risk factors for poor visual outcome and enucleation. Among the 150 patients, 117 individuals (124 eyes) were followed exclusively by the authors for a minimum of 6 months and had a median follow-up period of 23 months (range 6 months to 24 years). Initial management in these 124 eyes included observation in 22 eyes (18%), photocoagulation in 16 (13%), cryotherapy in 52 (42%), retinal detachment repair with drainage of subretinal fluid and cryotherapy or photocoagulation in 20 (17%), and enucleation in 14 (11%). A second treatment was necessary in 60 eyes, and a third treatment was undertaken in 27 eyes. One-hundred and three eyes were able to be followed ophthalmoscopically and the median interval time from initial treatment to complete resolution of telangiectasia was 10 months (range 2 to 123 months). Exudation resolved after treatment of telangiectasias in 46 cases (45%) over a median of 12 months. Among the 88 eyes with retinal detachment that underwent surgical intervention, 50 eyes (57%) had complete

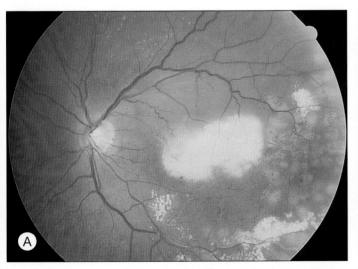
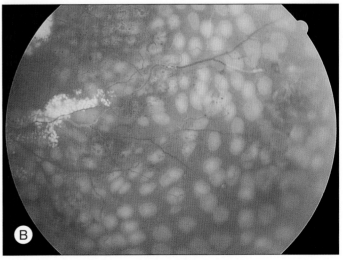

Fig. 77-7 Laser photocoagulation was used to treat focal areas of leakage in the posterior pole (A) and peripheral retina (B) with a modified scatter pattern to zones of capillary nonperfusion. Burns were 100 to 500 microns and of moderate intensity applied through a fundus contact lens. (B from Haller JA. Coats' disease and retinal telangiectasia. In: Yanoff M, Duker JS, eds. Ophthalmology. London: Mosby; 1999.)

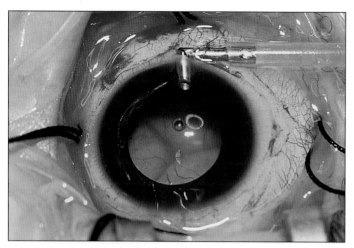

Fig. 77-8 In this eye of an 18-month-old boy with total exudative retinal detachment, anatomic stability was achieved by infusion into the anterior chamber, posterior drainage of subretinal fluid, and cryotherapy to 11 clock hours of peripheral vascular anomalies. (From Haller JA. Coats' disease and retinal telangiectasia. In: Yanoff M, Duker JS, eds. Ophthalmology. London: Mosby; 1999.)

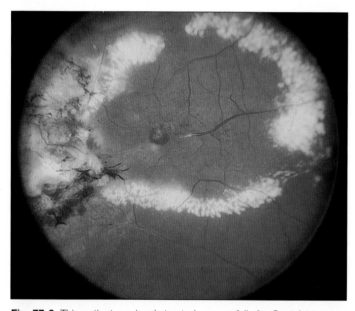

Fig. 77-9 This patient previously treated successfully for Coats'-type exudative retinopathy (see old scarring and fibrosis to the left of the photograph) has now developed a new adjacent area of vascular malformation and aneurysmal dilation, with a circinate lipid exudate.

resolution of the detachment. Visual outcome at the last follow-up visit revealed a visual acuity of 20/50 or better in 16%, between 20/60 and 20/100 in 8%, from 20/200 to finger counting in 29%, and hand motions to no light perception in 47%. In their series, risk factors predictive of poor visual outcome (20/200 or worse) were postequatorial ($P = 0.01$), diffuse ($P = 0.01$), or superior ($P = 0.04$) location of the telangiectasis and exudation, failed resolution of subretinal fluid after treatment ($P = 0.02$), and presence of retinal macrocysts ($P = 0.02$). Significant risk factors for enucleation included elevated intraocular pressure

(greater than 22 mmHg; $P < 0.001$) and iris neovascularization ($P < 0.001$).

Complications of photocoagulation in Coats' disease include inflammation, choroidal detachment, progressive exudation, creation of chorioretinal and vitreochoroidal anastomoses, epiretinal membrane formation, sympathetic ophthalmia, and hemorrhage. Even with resolution of exudates, extensive subretinal fibrosis and pigmentation often limits visual recovery. Intraocular surgical intervention carries the added risks of endophthalmitis, retinal tear formation, rhegmatogenous retinal detachment, and proliferative vitreoretinopathy.[2,3,5,6,48,85–88]

REFERENCES

1. Egbert PR, Chan C, Winter FC. Flat preparations of the retinal vessels in Coats' disease. J Pediatr Ophthalmol 1976; 13:336–339.
2. Coats G. Forms of retinal dysplasia with massive exudation. R Lond Ophthalmol Hosp Rep 1908; 17:440.
3. Asdourian G. Vascular anomalies of the retina. In: Peyman GA, Sanders DR, Goldberg MF, eds. Principles and practices of ophthalmology, vol. 2. Philadelphia: WB Saunders, 1980.
4. Campbell FP. Coats' disease and congenital vascular retinopathy. Trans Am Ophthalmol Soc 1976; 24:365–424.
5. Egerer I, Tasman W, Tomer TL. Coats' disease. Arch Ophthalmol 1974; 92:109–112.
6. Harris GS. Coats' disease: diagnosis and treatment. Can J Ophthalmol 1970; 5:311–320.
7. Imre G. Coats' disease. Am J Ophthalmol 1962; 54:175.
8. Spadavecchia V. Retinite di Coats. Ann Ottal 1939; 67:321.
9. Reese AB. Telangiectasis of the retina and Coats' disease. Am J Ophthalmol 1956;42:1–8.
10. Blodi FC. Vascular anomalies of the fundus. In: Duane T, ed. Clinical ophthalmology, vol. 3. Hagerstown, MD: Harper & Row, 1980.
11. Bonnet M. Le syndrome de Coats. J Fr Ophtalmol 1980; 3:57–66.
12. Dow DS. Coats' disease: occurrence in a four-month-old. South Med J 1973; 66:836–838.
13. Hogan MJ, Zimmerman LE. Ophthalmic pathology, an atlas and textbook, 2nd edn. Philadelphia: WB Saunders, 1962.
14. Hopper KD, Boal DK, Eggli KD. CT and MR imaging of the pediatric orbit. Radiographics 1992; 12:485–503.
15. Speiser P. Die Hamangiome des Augenhintergrundes. Klinisches Bild und Behandlung, Klin Montasbl Augenheilkd 1981; 178:313–322.
16. Theodossiadis GP, Bairaktaris-Kouris E, Kouris T. Evolution of Leber's miliary aneurysms: a clinicopathological study. J Pediatr Ophthalmol Strabismus 1979; 16:364–370.
17. Turut P, Constantinides G, Woillez M. Formes mixtes-hemangiome caverneux de la retine-anopathie de Leber–Coats (a propos de 2 observations). Bull Soc Ophtalmol Fr 1978; 78:663–666.
18. Bito LZ, Baroody RA. The penetration of exogenous prostaglandin and arachidonic acid into, and their distribution within, the mammalian eye. Curr Eye Res 1981–1982; 1:659–669.
19. Sugar HS. Coats' disease: telangiectatic or multiple vascular origin. Am J Ophthalmol 1958; 45:508–517.
20. Tripathi R, Ashton N. Electron microscopical study of Coats' disease. Br J Ophthalmol 1971; 55:289–301.
21. Wise GN. Coats' disease. Arch Ophthalmol 1957; 58:735–746.
22. Woods AC, Duke J. Coats' disease. I. Review of the literature, diagnostic criteria, clinical findings, and plasma lipid studies. Br J Ophthalmol 1963; 47:385–412.
23. Reese AB. Massive retinal fibrosis in children. Am J Ophthalmol 1936; 19:576.
24. Imre G. Coats' disease and hyperlipemic retinitis. Am J Ophthalmol 1967; 64:726–733.
25. Cremers FP, Maugeri A, den Hollander AI et al. The expanding roles of ABCA4 and CRB1 in inherited blindness. Novartis Found Symp 2004; 255:68–79.
26. Black GC, Perveen R, Bonshek R et al. Coats' disease of the retina (unilateral retinal telangiectasis) caused by somatic mutation in the NDP gene: a role for norrin in retinal angiogenesis. Hum Mol Genet 1999; 8:2031–2035.
27. Shastry BS, Trese MT. Overproduction and partial purification of the Norrie disease gene product, norrin, from a recombinant baculovirus. Biochem Biophys Res Commun 2003; 312:229–234.

28. Berger W, van de Pol D, Bachner D et al. An animal model for Norrie disease (ND): gene targeting of the mouse ND gene. Hum Mol Genet 1996; 5:51–59.

29. Yeung JWS, Harris GS. Coats' disease: a study of cholesterol transport in the eye. Can J Ophthalmol 1976; 11:61–68.

30. Khan JA, Ide CH, Strickland MP. Coats'-type retinitis pigmentosa. Surv Ophthalmol 1988; 32:317–332.

31. Pruett RC. Retinitis pigmentosa: clinical observations and correlations. Trans Am Ophthalmol Soc 1983; 81:693–735.

32. Schuman JS, Lieverman KV, Friedman AH et al. Senior–Loken syndrome (familial retinal dystrophy) and Coats' disease. Am J Ophthalmol 1985; 100:822–827.

33. Burch JV, Leveille AS, Morse PH. Ichthyosis hystrix (epidermal nevus syndrome) and Coats' disease. Am J Ophthalmol 1980; 89:25–30.

34. Robitaille JM, Monsein L, Traboulsi EI. Coats' disease and central nervous system venous malformation. Ophthalmic Genet 1996; 17:215–218.

35. Newell SW, Hall BD, Anderson CW et al. Hallermann–Streiff syndrome with Coats' disease. J Pediatr Ophthalmol Strabismus 1994; 31:123–125.

36. Small RG. Coats' disease and muscular dystrophy. Trans Am Acad Ophthalmol Otolaryngol 1968; 72:225–231.

37. Egerer I, Rodrigues MM, Tasman WS. Retinal dysplasia in Coats' disease. Can J Ophthalmol 1975; 10:79–85.

38. Fogle JA, Welch RB, Green WR. Retinitis pigmentosa and exudative vasculopathy. Arch Ophthalmol 1978; 96:696–702.

39. Deutsch TA, Rabb MF, Jampol LM. Spontaneous regression of retinal lesions in Coats' disease. Can J Ophthalmol 1982; 17:169–172.

40. Gobel SD, Augsburger JJ. Hemorrhagic retinal macrocysts in advanced Coats' disease. Retina 1991; 11:437–440.

41. Chang M, McLean IW, Merritt JC. Coats' disease: a study of 62 histologically confirmed cases. J Pediatr Ophthalmol Strabismus 1984; 21:163–168.

42. Friedenwald H, Friedenwald JS. Terminal stage in a case of retinitis with massive exudation. Trans Am Ophthalmol Soc 1929; 27:188.

43. Morales AG. Coats' disease: natural history and results of treatment. Am J Ophthalmol 1965; 60:855.

44. Naumann GO, Portwich E. Atiologie and letzer Anlass zu 1000 Enukleationen. Klin Monatsbl Augenheilkd 1976; 168:622.

45. Cunha-Vaz JG. The blood–retinal barriers. Doc Ophthalmol 1976; 41:287–327.

46. Kuwabara T, Cogan DG. Studies of retinal vascular patterns. I. Normal architecture. Arch Ophthalmol 1960; 64:904–911.

47. Ridley ME, Shields JA, Brown GC et al. Coats' disease: evaluation of management. Ophthalmology 1982; 89:1381–1387.

48. Schatz H, Burton TC, Yanuzzi LA et al. Abnormal retinal and disc vessels and retinal leak. In: Schatz H, ed. Interpretation of fundus fluorescein angiography. St Louis: Mosby, 1978.

49. Tarkkanen A, Laatikainen L. Coats' disease: clinical, angiographic, histopathological findings and clinical management. Br J Ophthalmol 1983; 67:766–776.

50. Duke JR, Woods AC. Coats' disease. II. Studies on the identity of the lipids concerned, and the probable role of mucopolysaccharides in its pathogenesis. Br J Ophthalmol 1963; 47:413–434

51. Farkas TG, Potts AM, Boone C. Some pathologic and biochemical aspects of Coats' disease. Am J Ophthalmol 1973; 75:289–301.

52. Takei Y. Origin of ghost cells in Coats' disease. Invest Ophthalmol 1976; 15:677–681.

53. Yannuzzi LA, Gitter KA, Schatz H. The macula: a comprehensive text and atlas. Baltimore: Williams & Wilkins, 1979.

54. Elwyn H. The place of Coats' disease among the diseases of the retina. Arch Ophthalmol 1940; 23:507.

55. Senft SH, Hidayat AA, Cavender JC. Atypical presentation of Coats' disease. Retina 1994; 14:36–38.

56. Jaffe MS, Shields JA, Canny CL et al. Retinoblastoma simulating Coats' disease: a clinicopathologic report. Ann Ophthalmol 1977; 9:863–868.

57. Plager DA, Orgel IK, Ellis FD et al. X-linked recessive familial exudative vitreoretinopathy. Am J Ophthalmol 1992; 114:145–148.

58. Green WR. Bilateral Coats' disease. Arch Ophthalmol 1967; 77:378–383.

59. Guthoff R, Berger RW, Draeger J. Measurements of ocular coat dimensions by means of combined A- and B-scan ultrasonography. Ophthalmol Res 1984; 16:289–291.

60. Kakur B, Taylor D. Fundus hemorrhage in infancy. Surv Ophthalmol 1992; 37:1–17.

61. Scimeca G, Magargal LE, Augsburger JJ. Chronic exudative ischemic superior temporal-branch retinal-vein obstruction simulating Coats' disease. Ann Ophthalmol 1986; 18:118–120.

62. Gass JDM, Oyakawa RT. Idiopathic juxtafoveal retinal telangiectasis. Arch Ophthalmol 1982; 100:769–780.

63. Benson WE, Shields JA, Tasman W et al. Posterior scleritis: a cause of diagnostic confusion. Arch Ophthalmol 1979; 97:1482–1486.

64. Boynton JR, Purnell EW. Bilateral microphthalmos without microcornea associated with unusual papillomacular retinal folds and high hyperopia. Am J Ophthalmol 1975; 79:820–826.

65. Gass JD, Blodi BA. Idiopathic juxtafoveolar retinal telangiectasis: update of classification and follow-up study. Ophthalmology 1993; 100:1536–1546.

66. Jalkh AE, Avila MP, Trempe CL et al. Diffuse choroidal thickening detected by ultrasonography in various ocular disorders. Retina 1983; 3:277–283.

67. Sherman JL, McLean IW, Brallier DR. Coats' disease: CT-pathologic correlation in two cases. Radiology 1983; 146:77–78.

68. Swayne LC, Garfinkle WB, Bennett RH. CT of posterior ocular staphyloma in axial myopia. Arch Otolaryngol 1975; 101:251.

69. Smirniotopoulos JG, Bargallo N, Maffee MG. Differential diagnosis of leukokoria: radiologic-pathologic correlation. Radiographics 1994; 14:1059–1079.

70. Haik BG. Advanced Coats' disease. Trans Am Ophthalmol Soc 1991; 89:371–476.

71. O'Brien JM, Char DH, Tucker N et al. Efficacy of unanesthetized spiral computed tomography scanning initial evaluation of childhood leukocoria. Ophthalmology 1995; 102:1345–1350.

72. Beets-Tan RG, Hendriks MJ, Ramos LM et al. Retinoblastoma: CT and MRI. Neuroradiology 1994; 36:59–62.

73. Lai WW, Edward DP, Weiss RA et al. Magnetic resonance imaging findings in a case of advanced Coats' disease. Ophthalmic Surg Lasers 1996; 27:234–238.

74. Machemer R, Williams JM Sr. Pathogenesis and therapy of traction detachments in various retinal vascular diseases. Am J Ophthalmol 1988; 105:173–181.

75. Glasier CM, Brodsky MC, Leithiser RE Jr. et al. High-resolution ultrasound with Doppler: a diagnostic adjunct in orbital and ocular lesions in children. Pediatr Radiol 1992; 22:174–178.

76. Guyton JS, McGovern FH. Diathermy coagulation in the treatment of angiomatosis retinae and of juvenile Coats' disease: report of two cases. Am J Ophthalmol 1943; 26:675.

77. Haye C, Haut J, Aubry JP et al. Traitement d'un cas de maladie de Coats par photocoagulation. Bull Soc Ophtalmol Fr 1968; 68:711–714.

78. Taillanter-Francoz A, Bonnet M, Baserer T. Formes mineures du syndrome de Leber–Coats (observations cliniques). Bull Soc Ophtalmol 1981; 81:523–525.

79. Turut P, Francois P. Hemangiome caverneux de la retine. J Fr Ophtalmol 1979; 2:393–404.

80. Sneed SR, Blodi CF, Pulido JS. Treatment of Coats' disease with the binocular indirect argon laser photocoagulator (Letter). Arch Ophthalmol 1989; 107:789–790.

81. Siliodor SW, Augsburger JJ, Shields JA et al. Natural history and management of advanced Coats' disease. Ophthalmic Surg 1988; 19:89–93.

82. Pauleikhoff D, Kruger K, Heinriech T et al. Epidemiologic features and therapeutic results in Coats' disease. Invest Ophthalmol Vis Sci 1988; 29:335.

83. Shields JA, Shield CL, Honavar SG et al. Classification and management of coats disease: the 2000 Proctor Lecture. Am J Ophthalmol 2001; 131:572–583.

84. Bechrakis NE, Müller-Stolzenberg NW, Helbig H et al. Sympathetic ophthalmia following laser cyclocoagulation. Arch Ophthalmol 1994; 112: 80–84.

85. de Guillebon HF, End D, Elzeneiny I. Electrical impedance of ocular coats during diathermy applications. Arch Ophthalmol 1970; 83:489.

86. Mondon H, Hammard H, Girard P et al. A propos d'un cas de gliose retinienne au cours d'une maladie de Coats. Bull Soc Ophtalmol Fr 1970; 70:881–883.

87. Theodossiadis GP. Some clinical, fluorescein-angiographic, and therapeutic aspects of Coats' disease. J Pediatr Ophthalmol Strabismus 1979; 16:257–262.

88. Tolentino FI, Refojo MF, Schepens CL. A hydrophilic acrylate implant for scleral buckling. Retina 1981; 1:281–286.

Chapter

78

Disseminated Intravascular Coagulopathy and Related Vasculopathies

James P. Bolling

Disseminated intravascular coagulopathy (DIC) is an excessive formation of fibrin clots within small vessels throughout the body. DIC may vary considerably in severity. It is often a terminal event in life, possibly the most frequent cause of death, and a complication of many diseases. DIC can also present in a chronic or subacute form compatible with life. Since characteristic changes may occur in the eye, it behoves ophthalmologists to know something about the disease and its clinical implications.

GENERAL CONSIDERATIONS

The hypercoagulable state leading to DIC may be due to sepsis, antigen–antibody complexes, "foreign" proteins associated with massive tissue necrosis, malignancies, crush injuries, obstetric complications (including toxemia of pregnancy and retained gestational products), body burns, or widespread hemolysis.

The suggested pathogenesis is damage to vascular endothelial cells leading to activation of the coagulation cascade.[1–5] What begins as a hypercoagulable state at the local level becomes a hypocoagulable state for the rest of the circulation. The result is a drop in the platelet count (thrombocytopenia) to less than 100 000/mm^3 and low levels of fibrinogen, whereas the fibrin split products are elevated. The most reliable laboratory tests are the platelet count, D-dimer (fibrin degradation product or FDP), prothrombin time, partial thromboplastin time, and fibrinogen. Widespread hemorrhage is common.

DIC may occur at any age. The literature cites many cases in the neonatal period.[6] At whatever age it occurs, the course of DIC is usually acute, characterized by fever, ecchymoses in the skin and mucous membranes, massive hemorrhage from various areas (epistaxis, hemoptysis, or melena), and ischemic necrosis at the sites of vascular obstruction. Renal and cardiac lesions are the usual causes of death, but the brain and lungs are also frequently involved. An exception to this abrupt dénouement is the case with carcinomatosis, in which the course is apt to be chronic and fibrinolytic products in the blood are minimal. DIC is the lethal mechanism in Ebola virus infections.[7]

Treatment of DIC mandates removal of the cause, such as selection of appropriate antibiotics, but to be effective also must address the coagulopathy. Platelet transfusions are necessary along with management of shock, steroids, heparin, and antithrombin III infusion.[2] Recently it has been suggested that infusion of activated protein C may be helpful.[8]

Related to DIC, and sometimes considered an idiopathic form of the disease, is thrombotic thrombocytopenic purpura (TTP). The basic lesion in TTP is a subendothelial thrombus occurring in the wake of an acute infection. A procoagulant substance is believed to be released from the endothelial cells; some patients have been shown to have a unique circulating protein that induces platelet aggregation. Classic symptoms of TTP are fever, hemolytic anemia, renal failure, and fluctuating central nervous system signs. The disease may run a fulminant course, indistinguishable from DIC, or may run a chronic course, waxing and waning over months or years. In the latter case, it may simulate lupus erythematosus or vasculitis clinically, but differs in not having the characteristic gamma-globulins in the blood. The treatment of choice is plasmapheresis.

Also related to DIC (and to TTP) is idiopathic thrombocytopenic purpura (ITP). This is believed to be an autoimmune platelet disease and is apt to occur in persons with a past history of easy bruisability. In children it may develop explosively with hemorrhage or petechiae following a viral exanthem or upper respiratory tract infection. Nevertheless, it usually resolves within a few months and does not have the serious implications of DIC or TTP. In adults it is relatively rare and then often occurs in association with lupus erythematosus, rheumatoid arthritis, or other steroid-sensitive autoimmune diseases. The treatment of choice is corticosteroids.

One subset of patients with toxemia of pregnancy are patients with the HELLP syndrome. This entity includes hemolysis (H), elevated liver enzymes (EL), and a low platelet count (LP).[9–11]

MANIFESTATIONS IN THE OCULAR FUNDI

The characteristic fundus manifestations of any of the foregoing processes are bilateral serous detachment of the retina or hemorrhage in the submacular choroid, or both. The pathologic basis is occlusive disease in the choriocapillaris and adjacent vessels by fibrin–platelet clots.[12–15] Hemorrhages in the retina and hemorrhagic extension into the vitreous[16] (perhaps especially common in the neonate) have been reported, but surprisingly, the retinas are usually normal unless there is significant coexisting hypertension or anemia.

Although the literature on chorioretinal changes with DIC is scanty, pathologic changes in the eyes of patients dying with this complication are frequent. Most cases are thus diagnosed in retrospect. Ocular manifestations of DIC may also be overlooked in the setting of life-threatening illness.

The literature on ocular complications with TTP and ITP is considerably more extensive,[17,18] but since the ocular signs and symptoms are similar in the three entities, they will be considered together as a unit. The minimal sign is a patchy delay in filling of the choroidal vessels on fluorangiography. Vision becomes reduced, often varying with posture, as serous detachment develops in the overlying retina. Further extension of the process may result in an extensive detachment of the retina, as occurs with choroidal infarcts regardless of etiology, or there may be a relatively flat elevation of the retina against a dark background associated with choroidal hemorrhage. The latter appearance has rarely been described in conditions other than DIC and TTP. It presents not only a dark reflex from the central fundus by ophthalmoscopy, but also has superimposed white streaks that probably represent thromboses of the larger vessels in the choroid[19] (Fig. 78-1A and B). On fluorangiography the dark central area, which is due to the choroidal hemorrhage, may be misinterpreted as an absent

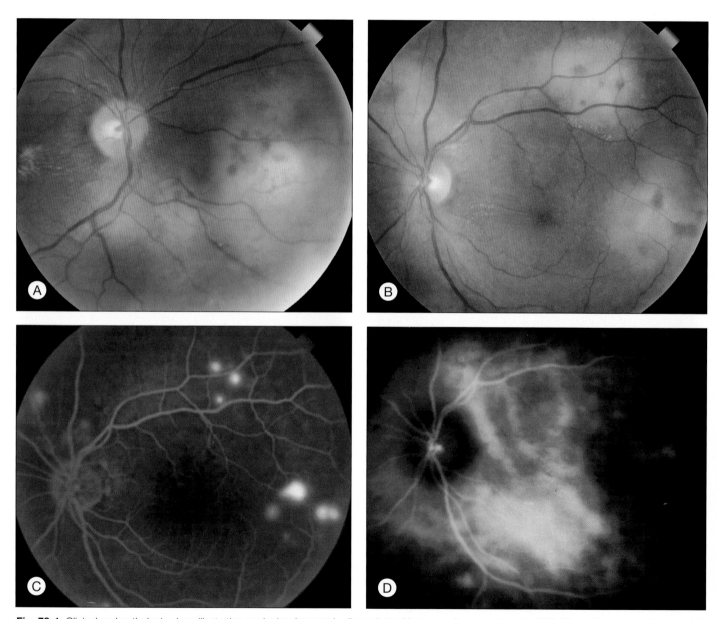

Fig. 78-1 Clinical and pathologic signs illustrating ocular involvement in disseminated intravascular coagulopathy (DIC). The patient was a 42-year-old woman with systemic lupus erythematosus who developed DIC in the wake of bacterial pneumonia. A, Fundus photo of the right eye shows large fibrin deposits under the retina. An exudative retinal detachment can be seen inferiorly in this eye. B, Color fundus photograph of the left eye of the same patient shows a large fibrin deposit at the temporal limit of the macula. C, Fluorescein angiogram, mid-phase of the left eye in the same patient, shows multiple areas of hyperfluorescence confirming leakage through the retinal pigment epithelium into the subretinal space. D, Indocyanine green angiogram of the left eye in the same patient shows the area of hypofluorescence consistent with the fibrin deposit and leakage on fluorescein angiography.

filling of the vessels. The fundus changes are bilaterally symmetric and found almost exclusively in the submacular areas.

Major pathologic changes in the adult eye are fibrin clots in the submacular choriocapillaris and in adjacent vessels (Fig. 78-1C and D). In mild cases, these clots may be the sole abnormality and produce no clinically evident signs. More severe abnormalities are cystoid macular edema, serous detachment of the central retina, vacuolation and disruption of the pigment epithelium, choroidal hemorrhage, and cytodegenerative clumping of the choroidal melanocytes. Infiltration is minimal or absent. Rarely do the intravascular thromboses extend to the peripheral choroid or to the anterior segment of the eye.

The ocular manifestations of toxemia of pregnancy are discussed in Chapter 79. It should be mentioned that toxemia of pregnancy involves a low-grade DIC. Serous retinal detachments in the macular area have been reported in pregnancy in the absence of hypertensive retinopathy.[4] Similar findings are reported in the HELLP syndrome. There are numerous reports on the association of central serous retinopathy in pregnancy.[20-23] A unique feature of central serous retinopathy in pregnancy is an increased level of fibrin deposited under the retina. The same finding can occur in systemic lupus erythematosus.[24] It is interesting to speculate on the relationship between central serous retinopathy in pregnancy and lupus, and how it is similar to the retinal findings in toxemia of pregnancy.

Manifestations of DIC and TTP in the neonate have been reported frequently in the pediatric literature and occasionally in the ophthalmic literature.[9] The occurrence may be a complication of placenta previa, hyaline membrane disease, sepsis, hepatocellular failure, or trauma. Unlike the adult counterpart, some neonatal eyes are reported to show hyphema with thrombi in the iris and ciliary body in addition to the choriocapillary involvement.

The reason for the preferential localization of thromboses in the submacular region is unclear. Suggested possibilities are as follows: sudden deceleration of the blood flow as the ciliary arteries merge with the large choriocapillary bed, natural leakiness of the choriocapillary vessels, anatomic holes in Bruch's membrane,[21] and the abundance of ciliary vessels that penetrate the sclera in the submacular region.[9,25-27] Of relevance is the experimental evidence that labeled microspheres injected into the circulation show a similar tendency to localize in the posterior pole of the eye. Whatever the reason, there is general agreement that the subretinal exudate derives from the obstructed choriocapillaris, with consequent disruption of the overlying pigment epithelium.

The frequency of ocular complications is unknown. Occasionally they constitute the initial symptoms. Undoubtedly many cases go unrecognized, since the seriousness of the cardiac, pulmonary, cerebral, and renal changes overshadows the ocular manifestations. The pathognomonic clots in the choriocapillaris are a frequent incidental finding in postmortem examinations, but there is nothing in the eye lesions to alter the treatment or prognosis of the systemic disease. The ocular changes are simply a local manifestation of a widespread process involving small vessels throughout the body.

REFERENCES

1. Hoines J, Buettner H. Ocular complications of disseminated intravascular coagulation (DIC) in abruptio placentae. Retina 1989; 9:105–109.
2. Howes EL, McKay DG. Circulating immune complexes: effects on ocular vascular permeability in the rabbit. Arch Ophthalmol 1975; 93:365–370.
3. Levi M, Keller TT, van Gorp E et al. Infection and inflammation and the coagulation system. Cardiovasc Res 60:26–39.
4. Mabie WC, Ober RR. Fluorescein angiography in toxaemia of pregnancy. Br J Ophthalmol 1980; 64:666–671.
5. Meyer PA. The observation of immune complex formation and deposition in the eyes of living rabbits. Clin Exp Immunol 1987; 69:166–178.
6. Ortiz JM, Yanoff M, Cameron JD et al. Disseminated intravascular coagulation in infancy and in the neonate: ocular findings. Arch Ophthalmol 1982; 100:1413–1415.
7. Geisbert TW, Young HA, Jahrling PB et al. Mechanisms underlying coagulation abnormalities in Ebola hemorrhagic fever: overexpression of tissue factor in primate monocytes/macrophages is a key event. J Infect Dis 2003; 188:1618–1629.
8. Toh CH, Dennis M. Disseminated intravascular coagulation: old disease, new hope. Br Med J 2003; 327:974–977.
9. Moresco RN, Vargas LC, Voegeli CF et al. D-dimer and its relationship to fibrinogen/fibrin degradation products (FDPs) in disorders associated with activation of coagulation or fibrinolytic systems. J Clin Lab Anal 2003; 17:77–79.
10. Weinstein L. Syndrome of hemolysis, elevated liver enzymes, and low platelet count: a severe consequence of hypertension in pregnancy. Am J Obstet Gynecol 1982; 142:159–167.
11. Weinstein L. Preeclampsia/eclampsia with hemolysis, elevated liver enzymes, and thrombocytopenia. Obstet Gynecol 1985; 66:657–660.
12. Cogan DG. Ocular involvement in disseminated intravascular coagulopathy. Arch Ophthalmol 1975; 93:1–8.
13. Cogan DG. Fibrin clots in the choriocapillaris and serous detachment of the retina. Ophthalmologica 1976; 172:298–307.
14. Gass DM. Central serous chorioretinopathy and white subretinal exudation during pregnancy. Arch Ophthalmol 1991; 109:677–681.
15. Gaudric A, Coscas G, Bird AC. Choroidal ischemia. Am J Ophthalmol 1982; 94:489–498.
16. Wiznia RA, Price J. Vitreous hemorrhages and disseminated intravascular coagulation in the newborn. Am J Ophthalmol 1976; 82:222–226.
17. Benson DO, Fitzgibbons JF, Goodnight SH. The visual system in thrombocytopenic purpura. Ann Ophthalmol 1980; 12:413–417.
18. Lambert SR, High KA, Cotlier E et al. Serous retinal detachments in thrombotic thrombocytopenic purpura. Arch Ophthalmol 1985; 103:1172–1174.
19. Brancato R, Menchini U, Bandello F. Proliferative retinopathy and toxemia of pregnancy. Ann Ophthalmol 1987; 19:182–183.
20. Fastenberg DM, Fetkenhour CL, Choromokos E et al. Choroidal vascular changes in toxemia of pregnancy. Am J Ophthalmol 1980; 89:362–368.
21. Fastenberg DM, Ober RR. Central serous choroidopathy in pregnancy. Arch Ophthalmol 1983; 101:1055–1058.
22. Gass DM, Pautler SE. Toxemia of pregnancy pigment epitheliopathy masquerading as a heredomacular dystrophy. Trans Am Ophthalmol Soc 1985; 83:114–130.
23. Sunness JS, Haller JA, Fine SL. Central serous chorioretinopathy and pregnancy. Arch Ophthalmol 1993; 111:360–364.
24. Cunningham ET, Alfred PR, Irvine AR. Central serous chorioretinopathy in patients with systemic lupus erythematosus. Ophthalmology 1996; 103:2081–2090.
25. Klien BA. Ischemic infarcts of the choroid (Elschnig spots): a cause of retinal separation in hypertensive disease with renal insufficiency – a clinical and histopathologic study. Am J Ophthalmol 1968; 66:1069–1074.
26. Oliver M, Uchenik D. Bilateral exudative retinal detachment in eclampsia without hypertensive retinopathy. Am J Ophthalmol 1980; 90:792–796.
27. Young NJA, Bird AC, Sehmi K. Pigment epithelial diseases with abnormal choroidal perfusion. Am J Ophthalmol 1980; 90:607–618.

Chapter

79

Hemoglobinopathies

Geoffrey G. Emerson
Joseph B. Harlan, Jr.
Sharon Fekrat
Gerard A. Lutty
Morton F. Goldberg

Sickle-cell hemoglobinopathies all share the common feature of an abnormal globin protein chain, which can lead to sickling of erythrocytes and obstruction of the microcirculation. Sickle vaso-occlusive events are insidious and affect virtually every vascular bed in the eye, often with visually devastating consequences.

Hemoglobin is the oxygen-carrying protein present in all human erythrocytes. It is a tetrameric molecule made up of iron-containing porphyrin (heme) groups surrounded by globin chains, which serve to shelter the central heme groups from noxious interactions. Inherited disturbances of hemoglobin stem from mutations in the genes that code for the individual globin subunits of the molecule. These mutations may result in specific structural aberrations in the globin subunits themselves, or they may result in reduced synthesis of structurally normal globin polypeptides. In the former case, the disturbance is termed a *hemoglobinopathy*. In the latter case, the disturbance is termed a *thalassemia*. In the case of sickle-cell and related hemoglobinopathies, the culprit is a point mutation affecting the amino-acid sequence of the beta-globin subunit. The substitution of valine for glutamic acid in the 6-position of the beta-chain produces hemoglobin S; the substitution of lysine at the same position yields hemoglobin C. Since an individual inherits one chromosome from each parent, the hemoglobin C and S mutations can each occur in a purely homozygous form or in a heterozygous form in combination with hemoglobin A, or they may occur with each other in a "compound" heterozygous form. The resulting hemoglobinopathies include hemoglobin CC (homozygous C disease), hemoglobin SS (sickle-cell disease or anemia), hemoglobin SC (sickle-cell hemoglobin C disease), hemoglobin AS (sickle-cell trait), and hemoglobin AC (hemoglobin C trait). Beta-thalassemia, which involves markedly diminished production of the beta-globin subunit, may also occur in conjunction with hemoglobin S, resulting in the compound heterozygous state termed "sickle-cell beta-thalassemia," or "HbSThal disease."

POPULATION STATISTICS

It is estimated that, of the population of African descendants in North America, approximately 8.5% possess sickle-cell trait (HbAS), 2.5% have hemoglobin C trait (HbAC), 0.14% have sickle-cell disease (HbSS), 0.016% have homozygous C disease (HbCC), 0.2% have sickle-cell hemoglobin C disease (HbSC), and 0.03% have sickle-cell thalassemia (HbSThal).[1–4]

SYSTEMIC FEATURES

In general, systemic effects are most severe in those patients with HbSS disease. Hemoglobin S usually accounts for more than 90% of the total hemoglobin in these individuals, creating a more fertile environment for the propagation of sickling and erythrostasis in the face of triggering factors such as hypoxia, acidosis, inflammation, and increased viscosity. The vicious cycle of sickling, increased viscosity, reduced flow, vaso-occlusion, deoxygenation of hemoglobin, and further sickling occurs in the microvascular circulation and may lead to large-scale erythrocytic sludging, end-organ damage, and hemolytic anemia. Occlusion of precapillary arterioles leads to painful crises involving the joints, chest, abdomen, and long bones. Pulmonary infarcts, cerebrovascular accidents, hematuria secondary to microrenal infarcts, and infarction of the renal cortex, spleen, intestines, liver, and bone marrow may all occur.[5] Bony infarcts may be evident on skull, long bone, and vertebral X-rays showing regions of sclerosis and bony trabeculation. Repeated ischemic insults to the femoral head may cause severe disability from aseptic necrosis.[6]

Systemic manifestations occur less frequently in HbSThal and HbSC patients and are extremely rare in HbAS patients. Mild anemia and a tendency for a relatively smooth systemic course with only a few crises per year are usually the rule for HbSC and HbSThal heterozygotes. The paradox, however, is that, despite the less dramatic systemic consequences of their disease, it is the HbSC and HbSThal subjects who are more likely to have retinal manifestations. Systemic and/or ocular manifestations[7,8] are very rarely present in HbAS heterozygotes, in whom only 50% of the total hemoglobin is abnormal hemoglobin S, except under conditions of extreme hypoxia.[9] One important exception occurs in the case of hyphema in HbAS heterozygotes, in which the ocular morbidity may approach that found in the compound heterozygotes or in the homozygous states.[10] Research has not yet been able to explain the reason for the profound discrepancy in the severity of the retinal and systemic manifestations in the various hemoglobinopathies.

PATHOPHYSIOLOGY

The central event in the pathogenesis of sickle-cell disease is the polymerization of deoxygenated hemoglobin S, which results in the transformation of the normal erythrocyte into the elongated sickled cell first described by Herrick in 1910.[11] Polymerization of hemoglobin S occurs as red cells pass through a deoxygenated, hyperosmolar, or acidotic capillary bed. The extent and rate of this polymerization depend on the red cell's initial degree of oxygenation, as well as the intracellular concentration of hemoglobin S.[12] Low flow and high oxygen extraction predispose a given vascular bed to sickling and secondary occlusion. In most instances, however, the transit time of red cells through the microcirculation is much shorter than the time required for polymerization to produce sickling of the erythrocyte. If these times were equal, virtually all red cells would contain polymer, resulting in sickling and generalized vaso-occlusion and death. In reality, polymerization only occurs in about 20% of the cells transiting capillary beds in HbSS disease.[13] In addition, an astonishing heterogeneity exists among the circulating red cells in sickle patients.[14] Density gradient separation of blood from human sickle-cell patients reveals several different subpopulations of red cells. The densest cells include both irreversibly sickled cells and very dense nonsickled cells, termed *dense discocytes*, whereas less dense subgroups include normal-density discocytes and low-density reticulocytes.[14–16] Reticulocytes are immature red-cell precursors forced into the circulation in states of chronic hemolytic anemia. These cells are deformable and contain a relatively low concentration of intracellular hemoglobin, which polymerizes and depolymerizes rapidly.

The generation of dense cells in HbSS disease involves a defect in red-cell membrane potassium chloride co-transport, which leads to cellular dehydration, cellular volume contraction, and a corresponding rise in the concentration of intracellular hemoglobin S. Under hypoxic conditions, these changes favor hemoglobin polymerization, which ultimately leads to further cell membrane damage, dysregulation of cell volume, cellular dehydration, and higher cell density. The final stage is the irreversibly sickled cell, which has a distorted and elongated shape under both hypoxic and fully oxygenated conditions.[14] Abnormally enhanced membrane potassium chloride co-transport has also been demonstrated in HbSC and HbCC erythrocytes,[17–20] leading to accelerated cellular dehydration, increased intracellular hemoglobin concentration, and increased cell density.

Although dense cells have traditionally been implicated in vaso-occlusive events in the sickle hemoglobinopathies, there is emerging evidence that the pathophysiology of vaso-occlusion involves more than simple mechanical obstruction by rigid, dense, irreversibly sickled erythrocytes. Leukocytes[21] and low-density circulating reticulocytes[14,22–25] both express adhesion molecules that promote abnormal adherence to the vascular endothelium. Some young reticulocytes express integrin $\alpha_4\beta_1$ (VLA-4), enabling the cells to bind to vascular cell adhesion molecule-1 (VCAM-1) found on the surface of activated endothelial cells. Sickle reticulocytes also express the nonintegrin glycoprotein IV (CD 36), which may mediate binding to vascular endothelial cells.[22] Red cell–endothelial adhesion is further promoted by the direct activation of endothelial cells, leading to the expression of adhesion molecules such as intercellular adhesion molecule-1 (ICAM-1), VCAM-1, E-selectin, and P-selectin.[26] Sickle reticulocyte adherence to the vascular endothelium creates microvascular stasis, which in turn leads to prolonged red-cell transit time, increased oxygen extraction, further polymerization of hemoglobin S, and complete vessel occlusion. Dense, irreversibly sickled cells do not adhere well to the vascular endothelium, because they lack the adhesion molecules present on low-density reticulocytes, and because their rigidity prohibits large areas of surface contact with endothelial cells.[26]

Other research has examined the role of inflammatory cytokines, such as tumor necrosis factor-alpha (TNF-α) and interleukin-1 (IL-1), which may contribute to vaso-occlusion by accelerating the production of adhesion molecules on the vascular endothelium and by activating polymorphonuclear leukocytes.[27] These cytokines may be released under conditions of stress, such as systemic infection or tissue hypoxia. Other investigators have theorized that some form of imbalance in the fibrinolytic system may also contribute to microvascular occlusions through enhanced deposition of fibrin and increased thrombin activity.[28–30] Perhaps activation of the vascular endothelium is the critical event in the initiation of the clotting cascade.

Hematocrit also plays a role in vaso-occlusion by affecting the blood viscosity.[31] This may provide a partial explanation for the discrepancy in the severity of ocular and systemic manifestations in the various sickling hemoglobinopathies. HbSC and HbSThal subjects tend to have substantially higher hematocrits than HbSS subjects, contributing to higher viscosity with potentially more pronounced vaso-occlusion in the retinal microvasculature during any given sickling event. Even though HbSS patients have a larger number of circulating sickled red cells, their overall lower hematocrit may provide relative protection from vaso-occlusion in the small-caliber vessels of the retina.[5] An alternative theory proposes that the retinal vascular occlusions in HbSS disease may actually be so complete that total infarction and retinal necrosis occur, with no viable tissue remaining that is capable of initiating an angiogenic response. In contrast, the occlusions in HbSC disease may be less severe, resulting in chronic ischemia, but less complete infarction, and therefore with continuous secretion of angiogenic substances by the damaged tissues.[1]

Lutty and co-workers propose a third theory. Using a rat model, they demonstrated that high-density HbSS erythrocytes (dehydrated dense discocytes and irreversibly sickled cells) are easily trapped in retinal capillaries and precapillary arterioles under hypoxic conditions, whereas HbSC cells (normal- and high-density cells) show very little retention in the retinal microvasculature, regardless of oxygen concentration.[32] Retention of HbSC cells did occur, however, after stimulation of the vascular endothelium with cytokines. Perhaps vaso-occlusion in HbSC disease actually depends more on extraerythrocytic factors, such as abnormalities in the fibrinolytic system, leukocyte interactions, activation of vascular endothelium, and the induction of adhesion molecules, than on the mechanical trapping of dense, rigid, sickled cells. This subtle difference in pathophysiology may provide an explanation for the discrepancy in the severity of systemic and ocular findings seen in subjects with HbSC and HbSS disease.

CLINICAL FEATURES

Clinical manifestations of sickle hemoglobinopathies may be grouped according to the presence or absence of vasoproliferative changes.

Nonproliferative manifestations

Nonproliferative ocular manifestations of the sickle hemoglobinopathies have been well described and include altered conjunctival vasculature, iris atrophy, retinal "salmon-patch" hemorrhages, retinal "iridescent spots," retinal "black sunbursts," and various abnormalities of the retinal vasculature, macula, choroid, optic disc, and vitreoretinal interface.

Conjunctival vasculature

Clinical evidence of vaso-occlusion may be seen in the conjunctival vasculature in the form of dark red, comma-shaped, or corkscrew-shaped vascular fragments that appear to be isolated from other neighboring vessels.[33] The anomalous vascular segments (Fig. 79-1) are most obvious in the inferior bulbar conjunctiva. Interestingly, SS subjects show more prominent conjunctival changes than SC subjects. Patients possessing sickle-cell trait (AS) almost never have conjunctival findings. The radiant heat of the slit-lamp beam may induce vasodilatation, reversing the anomalous vascular changes.[34,35] The characteristic comma-shape pattern may also disappear after oxygen inhalation or after blood transfusion.[33] In contrast, pharmacologic agents inducing vasoconstriction, such as phenylephrine, may serve to enhance the conjunctival sign.[36] Histopathologic examination of the aberrant conjunctival vessels reveals endothelial proliferation, aggregation of red cells in distal portions of capillaries, and dilatation and thinning of the proximal segments of the vessels.[37] Nagpal and co-workers[38] reported a positive correlation between the severity of conjunctival sickling and the number of irreversibly sickled cells in HbAS, HbSC, and HbSS subjects.

Iris atrophy

Segmental iris atrophy has been demonstrated in subjects with HbSC disease[39,40] and is thought to be caused by sectorial ischemic necrosis (Fig. 79-2). Galinos and co-workers[40] have also described neovascularization of the iris stroma, using intravenous fluorescein angiography. In one case, the neovascular pattern resembled the classic sea fan of proliferative sickle-cell retinopathy.[40]

Salmon-patch hemorrhage

The salmon-patch hemorrhage (Fig. 79-3) is a round to oval sequestrum of blood located either in the preretinal space or within the superficial retina. The lesion may be up to one disc diameter or more in size, with well-defined boundaries and either a flattened or a dome-shaped configuration. Such hemorrhages, which usually occur in the midperiphery adjacent to an intermediate arteriole, are thought to result from blowout of vascular walls weakened by prior episodes of occlusion and ischemia. Although the hemorrhage is initially red, it may turn a red-orange or salmon color over time because of progressive hemolysis. The local collection of blood may remain beneath the internal limiting lamina, enter the neurosensory retina itself, dissect internally into the vitreous, or dissect externally into the subretinal space.[41,42]

Iridescent spots

After resorption of the salmon-patch hemorrhage, the retina may appear entirely normal, without any evidence of residual

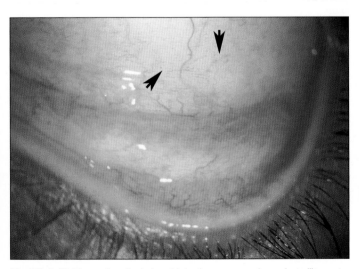

Fig. 79-1 Sickle conjunctival sign. Note the comma-shaped capillary segments, some of which appear to be isolated from the remaining circulation (arrows).

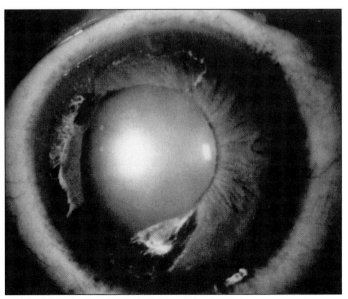

Fig. 79-2 Slit-lamp photograph demonstrating extensive iris atrophy resulting from sickling in the iris vessels.

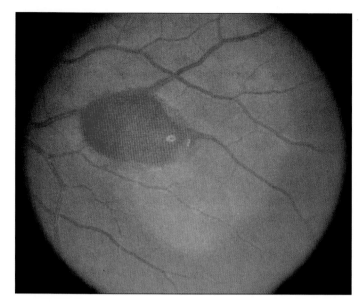

Fig. 79-3 Retinal and preretinal orange-red hemorrhage obscuring the retinal vasculature.[42]

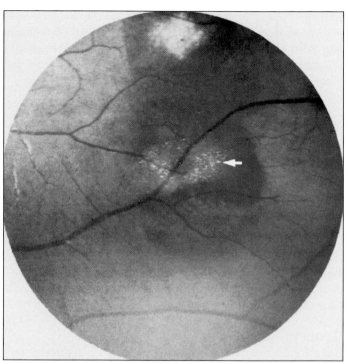

Fig. 79-4 Iridescent spot. Note the schisis cavity containing refractile granules (arrow).

preretinal, intraretinal, or subretinal blood. In the location of the hemorrhage, however, there may also be a faint indentation or depression representing thinning of the inner retina. This appears on ophthalmoscopy as a dimple outlined by the internal limiting membrane's light reflex. In addition, a small schisis cavity may develop after resorption of the intraretinal portion of the hemorrhage. The cavity may contain multiple glistening, refractile, yellowish granules or iridescent spots (Fig. 79-4), which represent collections of hemosiderin-laden macrophages. Histopathologic study discloses the presence of both intracellular and extracellular iron in the small retinoschisis cavity. The cavity is lined anteriorly by the internal limiting lamina and posteriorly by the neurosensory retina.[41] The finding of iridescent spots was observed in 33% of HbSC subjects, 18% of HbSThal subjects, and 13% of HbSS subjects.[43–45] These percentages vary among different patient series.[4,46,47]

Black sunburst

The black sunburst lesion[4] appears as a flat, round to oval black patch, about one-half to two disc diameters in size (Fig. 79-5). Glistening, refractile granules, similar to those observed in iridescent spots, may be present. The black sunburst represents intraretinal migration of hyperplastic retinal pigment epithelium (RPE) in response to blood that had dissected between the RPE and neurosensory retina.[41] Perivascular RPE pigment accumulation gives the lesion's borders a stellate or spiculated appearance. Histopathologic study discloses focal hypertrophy of the RPE along with areas of RPE hyperplasia and migration. Also present are diffuse iron deposits, hemosiderin-laden macrophages, and pigment deposition. Thinning and degeneration of the neurosensory retina overlying the sunburst lesion are also observed. Black sunbursts are found in 41% of HbSC patients,[43] 35% of HbSS patients,[44] and 20% of HbSThal patients.[45]

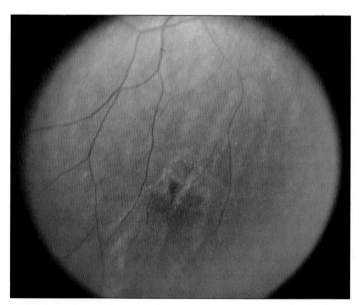

Fig. 79-5 Fundus photograph of a black sunburst surrounded by iridescent spots.

Black sunbursts are thought to have an alternative pathogenesis. The lesion may evolve directly from the salmon-patch hemorrhage, if the blood dissects deeply into the retina or into the subretinal space, stimulating migration and hyperplasia of RPE cells.[41,48,49] Direct evolution of salmon-patch lesions into a black sunburst has been documented in a 17-year-old man with SC disease over a 6-year period.[48] Some investigators have shown choroidal neovascularization (CNV) within black sunbursts, suggesting that the RPE hyperplasia may occur in response to the underlying CNV.[50,51] Others have even suggested that the black sunburst represents an RPE response to a localized occlusion in the choroidal vasculature.[52,53]

Retinal vasculature

The major vessels of the posterior pole usually appear normal, although nonspecific increased tortuosity may be observed in up to 47% of SS and 32% of SC patients.[4] Posterior pole vascular tortuosity is very rare in AS and SThal subjects. Although the cause of the tortuosity is not known, some hypothesize that it is due to peripheral arteriovenous shunting. Other posterior pole changes range from subtle perifoveal capillary dropout to arteriolar silver wiring (Fig. 79-6) to central retinal artery occlusion.[5,54] Central, branch, and macular retinal artery occlusions have been reported.[44,49,55–66] Although peripheral retinal arterial occlusions are very common, central and branch retinal vein occlusions are extremely rare in sickle-cell hemoglobinopathies.[5]

A common area of the retina for occlusive events is in the periphery, where vessels may end abruptly, sometimes in hairpin-shaped loops. Occlusions of the peripheral retinal microvasculature have been documented in HbSS subjects as early as 20 months of age.[67] Although retinal capillaries appear to be the initial site of occlusion early in life, larger-caliber vessels eventually become nonperfused with age. With repeated vaso-occlusive events in the peripheral retina over a prolonged time, centripetal recession of the most peripheral vascular arcades, away from the ora serrata and toward the equator, occurs. The end result is a totally ischemic retina in the pre-equatorial region.[5]

Macula

Fluorescein angiographic studies of HbSS subjects have demonstrated enlargement of the foveal avascular zone with perifoveal capillary dropout resulting from arteriolar occlusion.[54] This nonperfusion causes degeneration and thinning of the inner retina, producing a concave dimple or depression in the macula known as the macular depression sign (Fig. 79-7). The depression is highlighted on ophthalmoscopy by the surrounding light reflex coming from the internal limiting lamina at the border between healthy and atrophic retina. The depression stands out darkly from the normal internal light reflexes and usually contains a single central bright spot or streak. The macular depression may or may not be accompanied by diminution of visual acuity.[68] Roy and associates[69] suggested that the tremendous range of red-blood-cell density present in sickle-cell patients correlates with slowing of the blood flow in macular capillaries and increased erythrocyte transit time. Diminished macular blood flow velocity increases the chances of stasis, sickling, and vaso-occlusion.

Vascular irregularities may occur at the macula, the temporal raphe, or both. They include microaneurysmal dots, dilated precapillary arterioles and capillary segments, nerve fiber layer infarcts, loss of capillaries in the foveal avascular zone with dynamic vascular remodeling, and hairpin-shaped venous loops with adjacent capillary dropout.[36,54,70] Approximately 32% of HbSS patients, 36% of HbSC patients, and 20% of HbSThal patients have one or more of these findings.[54,70,71] Interestingly, the chronic remodeling of the parafoveal vasculature, with subsequent enlargement of the foveal avascular zone, does not correlate well with reduction in visual acuity.[72] The temporal horizontal raphe, an imaginary line that extends from the fovea to the temporal periphery, contains terminal arteriolar branches similar to those found in the peripheral retina. Both the temporal raphe and the peripheral retina represent watershed areas, and, as such, both are subject to the same process of terminal arteriolar occlusions. For reasons that are unknown, however, no strong correlation has been demonstrated between the amount of nonperfusion along the temporal raphe and the amount of nonperfusion in the peripheral retina.[70]

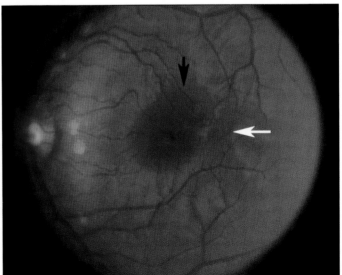

Fig. 79-7 Macular depression sign. Note the areas of macular thinning superotemporal to the fovea (black arrow) and along the temporal raphe (white arrow).

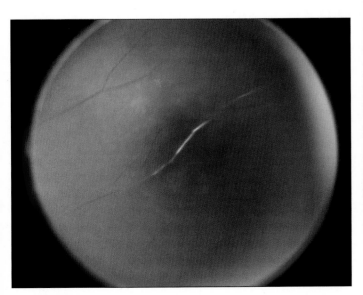

Fig. 79-6 Arteriolar silver wiring.

Choroidal occlusions

Described numerous times in patients with sickling hemoglobinopathies,[67,73–75] choroidal nonperfusion is thought to result from occlusive events in the posterior ciliary arterial circulation. As in the retinal circulation, interaction of adhesion molecules (VLA-4) on dense reticulocytes to the endothelium appears to play a role.[25] Some investigators have suggested that vaso-occlusive events in the choroidal vasculature may be involved in the formation of the black sunburst lesion,[52,53] CNV,[50,51] or both. Histopathologic features associated with choroidal vaso-occlusion include impacted erythrocytes, increased fibrin, and platelet fibrin thrombi.[30,67] Although the inner retina is spared in choroidal occlusion, RPE hypertrophy, pigment migration, and atrophy of the outer retina may occur. Ischemic necrosis and atrophy of the uveal tract have also been shown to occur after scleral buckling surgery in patients with HbSC disease.[76]

Abnormalities of the vitreoretinal interface

Peripheral retinal whitening, comparable to white-without-pressure, has been described in patients with sickle hemoglobinopathies[43–45,77,78] and has been shown to occur in up to 93% of HbSS subjects,[44] 83% of HbSC subjects,[43] and 82% of HbSThal subjects.[45] This finding, which seems to correlate inversely with the severity of changes in the peripheral vasculature,[77] may represent abnormal or stronger than usual vitreoretinal adherence. It is unclear whether this finding is truly unique to sickle hemoglobinopathy or is simply a vitreoretinal interface change similar to white-without-pressure seen in the general population.[36]

Well-demarcated, round to oval, mottled brown lesions in the retina have been documented in patients with SS and SC disease.[36,44,79] The lesions, termed "dark-without-pressure," may be found in the posterior pole and midperiphery and tend to be one to three disc diameters in size, with an uneven, mottled brown surface. Flat, geographical, and homogeneous in appearance, they may appear to be outlined by a rim of slightly paler retina. Fluorescein angiography is unremarkable, and the underlying choroid has a normal appearance on ophthalmoscopy. The lesions are also relatively transient phenomena, appearing and disappearing without any residual traces of their existence. For these reasons, it has been speculated that the dark-without-pressure zones are associated with hemorrhage, but this is unlikely, and the true etiology is unclear.[44,79]

Vascular changes at the optic nerve head

Vascular changes at the optic disc are transient and consist of dilated, dark capillary vessels that demonstrate occlusion on fluorescein angiography.[36,44,72] These vessels, which appear as small red dots with either a linear or a Y-shaped configuration on highly magnified ophthalmoscopy (Fig. 79-8), are essentially precapillary arterioles plugged with sickled erythrocytes. The involved vessels intermittently open and close, and the ischemic insult is apparently not severe enough to have an impact on visual function.

Neovascularization of the optic disc has been reported in four HbSC subjects[80–83] and one HbSS subject.[44]

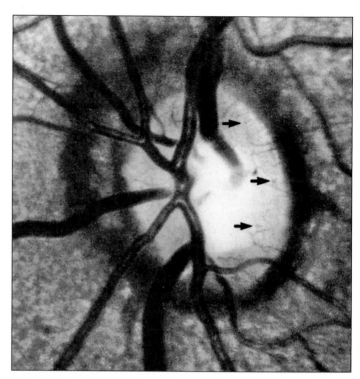

Fig. 79-8 A magnified view of the optic disc, demonstrating the sickle-cell disc sign. Note the tiny dark spots, which represent segments of blood within small vessels on the disc surface (arrows).

Angioid streaks

Angioid streaks, evident on ophthalmoscopy as dark red to brown subretinal bands of irregular contour that often radiate from the optic disc, represent discontinuities or breaks in thickened and calcified Bruch's membrane. Angioid streaks have been reported to occur in roughly 1% to 2% of patients with sickle hemoglobinopathy,[44,84,85] and may be more common in HbSS subjects. Condon & Serjeant[44] noted angioid streaks in 22% of Jamaican SS subjects over age 40 and in only 2% of Jamaican HbSS subjects under 40 years of age. In the majority of cases the clinical course is benign, and CNV in the streaks is apparently rare.

Proliferative sickle retinopathy

Peripheral retinal arteriolar occlusion is the initiating event in the pathogenesis of proliferative sickle retinopathy. Arteriolar closure preferentially occurs at or near Y-shaped bifurcations,[70] producing local ischemia and stimulating the production of vascular growth factors. The end result is the emergence of sea fan-shaped neovascular fronds that predispose to vitreous hemorrhage, subsequent tractional vitreous membrane formation, and ultimately tractional and/or rhegmatogenous retinal detachment.[5,86]

Goldberg has developed the following widely recognized classification scheme detailing the stages of proliferative sickle retinopathy.

Goldberg stage I

The hallmark of stage I retinopathy (Fig. 79-9) is peripheral arteriolar occlusion.[36] Presumably, sickled erythrocytes function

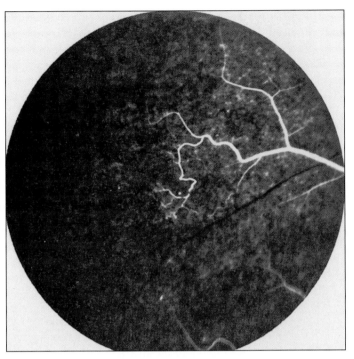

Fig. 79-9 Stage I sickle retinopathy. Midphase angiogram of occluded peripheral retinal vessels and peripheral capillary dropout.

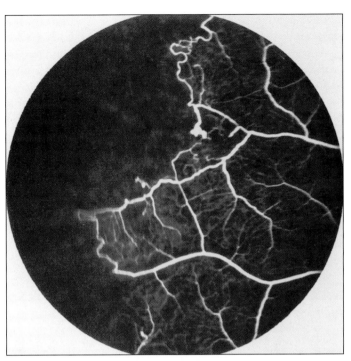

Fig. 79-10 Stage II sickle retinopathy. Arteriolar-venular anastomoses are apparent at the border of the perfused and nonperfused retina.

as microemboli in capillaries and precapillary arterioles, impeding flow and turning the arteriolar segment a dark-red cyanotic color. Peripheral retinal nonperfusion results. Vaso-occlusion occurs preferentially in the peripheral retina, presumably because of longer arteriovenous transit times, decreased blood flow, and possibly an increased number of occludable bifurcation sites. Eventually, "silver wires" may develop in permanently occluded arterioles (Fig. 79-6).

Goldberg stage II

In stage II, vascular remodeling occurs at the boundary between perfused and nonperfused peripheral retina. Connections form between occluded arterioles and adjacent terminal venules by way of pre-existing capillaries, resulting in arteriovenous anastomoses at the border separating the vascularized postequatorial retina and the ischemic pre-equatorial peripheral retina (Fig. 79-10). The anastomoses do not show leakage on fluorescein angiography, confirming that they indeed represent enlargement of pre-existing vessels with intact blood–retinal barrier properties, rather than true neovascularization. Angiography also demonstrates sluggish blood flow through the arteriovenous connections, theoretically enhancing deoxygenation, sickling, and additional vaso-occlusion. This environment of chronic ischemia sets the stage for true neovascular proliferation.[36,83,87]

Goldberg stage III

Peripheral retinal neovascularization often assumes a frond-like configuration, resembling the marine invertebrate *Gorgonia flabellum*, known in common parlance as the sea fan (Fig. 79-11). The majority of neovascular sea fan formations are found at the

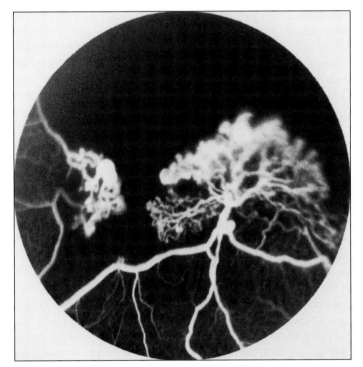

Fig. 79-11 Fundus angiogram demonstrating stage III sickle retinopathy. Note the large peripheral areas of capillary dropout and the sea fans extending toward the nonperfused retina.

interface between perfused and nonperfused peripheral retina (Fig. 79-12), growing toward the ischemic pre-equatorial retina.[5,83] Arising from the venous side of the arteriovenous anastomoses, sea fans develop an average of 18 months after the formation of

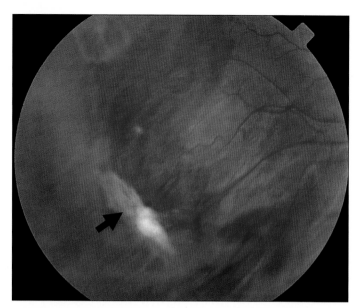

Fig. 79-12 Stage III sickle retinopathy. Note the blood vessels within an area of preretinal fibrovascular proliferation (sea fan, arrow) adjacent to ischemic retina.

the arteriovenous connections and have a predilection for the superotemporal quadrant of the fundus.[5] The chronic ischemic environment of the peripheral retina may induce the production of local vasogenic factors that promote and sustain neovascular tissue. Elevated levels of vascular endothelial growth factor (VEGF) and basic fibroblast growth factor (bFGF) have been demonstrated in direct association with sea fan neovascularization.[30,88–90]

Further analyses of preretinal neovascularization in sickle-cell subjects, using a dual-perspective microscopic technique, suggest a possible mechanical basis for sea fan evolution.[67] Specifically, occlusive events create hydrostatic back-pressure that leads to focal extrusion of the upstream segment of the occluded vessel into the preretinal space. Over time, the elevated intraluminal pressure causes continued expansion of the extruded vessel, stretching the endothelial cells and pericytes within venules. This, in turn, could stimulate endothelial cell proliferation,[91] along with the formation of neovascular tissue.[48] Traction from adherent vitreous strands could contribute to elevation and growth of sea fans.

Sea fans may begin as nothing more than a delicate, flat preretinal neovascular carpet, which may be easily overlooked against the reddish coloration of the underlying fundus. The fine, neovascular capillaries may eventually grow into a fan shape, spreading across the retinal surface in a plane between the posterior hyaloid and the internal limiting lamina. Sea fan formation is most common at sites of arteriovenous anastomoses and crossings.[92] One possible explanation is that the thickened, less compliant vessel walls present at the arteriovenous crossing site may give rise to whirl-like eddy currents, which in turn create intraluminal forces driving the vessel or a segment of the vessel toward the retinal surface and eventually into the vitreous.

Classically, each sea fan has at least one major nutrient arteriole and one major draining venule, although Lutty & McLeod have demonstrated multiple feeding arterioles and multiple draining venules for most sea fans.[92] Side-to-side anastomoses may develop, along with additional nutrient and draining vessels. The net effect is a larger, arborizing neovascular proliferation more likely to form peripheral traction bands in the vitreous. With time, a proliferative mantle of whitish tissue may envelop the sea fan, often in association with adherent vitreous bands, resulting in a tractional membrane composed of a collagenous, acellular matrix that may drag the neovascular frond off the internal limiting lamina. Tractional elevation is presumed to be due to retraction of atrophic collagenous tubes[92] or could be due to ordinary vitreous collapse with tugging on adherent preretinal neovascular tissue.

Statistically, sea fans are most commonly found in the superotemporal quadrant, followed, in order, by the inferotemporal, superonasal, and inferonasal quadrants. They are usually limited to the equatorial retina, rarely extending to the posterior pole or to the ora serrata. Sea fans represent true neovascular tissue and thus show profuse leakage of intravascular fluorescein dye, indicating loss of the blood–retinal barrier. The clinician can take advantage of this property by using intravenous fluorescein angiography or angioscopy to detect subtle patches of neovascularization not evident during standard ophthalmoscopy, as well as to reveal advanced sea fans hidden beneath whitish "pseudoglial" proliferation or blood clots.[5] The lack of an adequate blood–retinal barrier gives rise to chronic transudation into the vitreous from the neovascular tissue, which in turn accelerates vitreous degeneration, collapse, and traction, creating the basis for hemorrhage and retinal detachment.[5,36]

Goldberg stage IV

Stage IV is defined by the presence of vitreous hemorrhage. As sea fans grow into the vitreous cavity, traction on their delicate vascular channels results in bleeding at irregular intervals for years. Traction-induced hemorrhage may occur in the setting of minor ocular trauma, vitreous syneresis, normal vitreous movement, or contraction of vitreous bands induced by previous hemorrhage. Vitreous hemorrhage may be entirely asymptomatic, if it remains localized to the region adjacent to the sea fan. Visually devastating consequences may occur, however, when the hemorrhage dissects centrally into the vitreous gel. True fibroglial membranes and vitreous strands may arise in the setting of chronic hemorrhage and neovascular plasma transudation, providing a scaffold for future tractional and/or rhegmatogenous retinal detachment.[5]

Stage IV retinopathy occurs more commonly in HbSC subjects (21% to 23%) and is found less commonly in HbSS subjects (2% to 3%).[4,44,84] The incidence of vitreous hemorrhage may be even lower in other sickle hemoglobinopathies.[4,84] Studies of untreated sickle retinopathy by Condon and co-workers revealed three significant risk factors for subsequent vitreous hemorrhage: (1) hemoglobin SC disease; (2) the presence of any vitreous hemorrhage in the eye on the initial examination; and (3) greater than 60 degrees of active neovascularization in the retinal periphery.[93]

Goldberg stage V

Vitreous bands and condensed contractile membranes are common sequelae of chronic vitreous hemorrhage and plasma transudation from incompetent neovascular tissue. They serve as key mechanical players in the progression to stage V retinopathy, defined as the presence of tractional and/or rhegmatogenous retinal detachment. Retinal breaks, which may be either round or horseshoe-shaped, usually occur in the immediate vicinity of the tractional vascular proliferations. The extensive nature of the perivascular tissue matrix, combined with adjacent hemorrhage, can make the retinal break extremely difficult to detect. Retinal breaks may occur even in the absence of direct vitreoretinal traction and are usually due to localized retinal atrophy and thinning from chronic ischemia and vaso-occlusion.[5,41]

As one would expect, retinal detachment is found most frequently in SC subjects,[4] since these are the patients most plagued by proliferative disease. Retinal detachment is rarely present in HbAS[94] or HbSS[44,95] subjects.

Autoinfarction

Sea fan fronds may regress over time with an eventual rate as high as 60% because of the process of autoinfarction.[42,80,96–98] Although not completely understood, the pathophysiology of autoinfarction is probably multifactorial. In a milieu of chronic hypoxia and ischemia, multiple recurrent episodes of thromboses and sickling within sea fans may eventually lead to permanent infarction of the lesion. Major nutrient vessels may also become kinked or even avulsed by vitreous traction, resulting in complete interruption of feeder flow. Histopathologic studies by McLeod and co-workers have demonstrated that the process of auto-infarction may begin with preretinal capillaries rather than in the larger feeding arterioles, and may occur side by side with new vessel formation in the same sea fan formation.[92] Finally, reduced production and release of vasogenic factors[97–99] or increased production of pigment epithelium-derived factor (PEDF)[100] may also contribute to the spontaneous regression of neovascular tissue. It should be remembered that neovascular formations are, by nature, more prone to severe vaso-occlusion and thrombosis than normal retinal vessels, given their intrinsically low flow rates. Although sea fans may autoinfarct in one region of the eye, they may continue to flourish in other regions of the same eye. For this reason, most neovascular lesions are considered potentially dangerous and ordinarily should be treated and obliterated.

DIFFERENTIAL DIAGNOSIS OF PERIPHERAL RETINAL NEOVASCULARIZATION

Peripheral retinal neovascularization is not unique to the sickle hemoglobinopathies and may occur in a host of systemic and purely ocular disease processes[99,101] (Box 79-1). The diagnostic evaluation of peripheral retinal neovascularization should include a detailed patient and family history in conjunction with rigorous clinical examination. If a sickle hemoglobinopathy is suspected, a rapid sickle screening test should be performed. If the test result is positive, formal hemoglobin electrophoresis is then used to make the definitive diagnosis.

Box 79-1 Differential diagnosis of peripheral retinal neovascularization

Central and branch retinal vein occlusion
Chronic myelogenous leukemia
Chronic retinal detachment
Diabetic retinopathy
Dominantly inherited peripheral retinal neovascularization
Eales disease
Familial exudative vitreoretinopathy
Hyperviscosity syndromes
Idiopathic occlusive arteriolitis
Incontinentia pigmenti
Pars planitis syndrome
Posterior uveitis
Radiation retinopathy
Retinopathy of prematurity
Rheumatic fever
Sarcoidosis
Sickle-cell retinopathy
Talc embolization

TREATMENT

Indications

Given the high rate of spontaneous regression and/or lack of progression of sea fan neovascularization in some eyes, indications for treatment of retinal neovascularization are not always clear. Nevertheless, therapeutic intervention is usually undertaken in cases of bilateral proliferative disease, spontaneous hemorrhage, large elevated sea fans, or rapid growth of neovascular tissue, or cases in which one eye has already been lost to proliferative retinopathy. On the other end of the spectrum, a single eye containing one small sea fan frond may be conservatively followed until expansion of the lesion or hemorrhage occurs.

The usual goal of management is the early treatment of stage III lesions, before progression to substantial hemorrhage and/or retinal detachment occurs. If early treatment is successful, the need for pars plana vitrectomy and/or scleral buckling will be obviated, with avoidance of the concomitant surgical complications that often occur in sickle-cell patients.[86,97,102,103] Techniques such as diathermy, cryotherapy, and laser photocoagulation have all been employed to achieve involution of neovascular lesions. Of these techniques, laser photocoagulation has the fewest side-effects. Specific methods of laser application include direct coagulation of feeder vessels, local scatter photocoagulation with and without focal treatment of the sea fan, and 360-degree peripheral scatter delivery.

Laser photocoagulation
Feeder vessel photocoagulation

Direct, heavy laser treatment of nutrient arterioles and subsequently draining venules (Fig. 79-13) has been shown to cause closure of sea fans in 88% of eyes studied in a controlled clinical trial.[104] With effective closure of sea fans comes a reduced likelihood of vitreous hemorrhage and concomitant

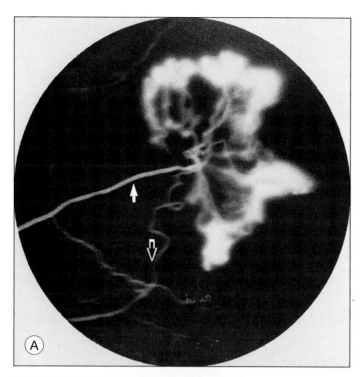

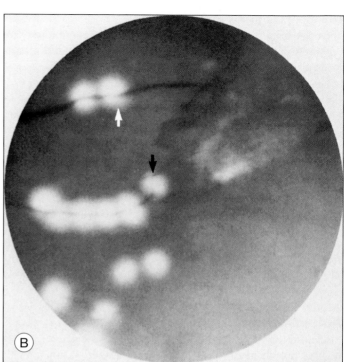

Fig. 79-13 A, Fundus angiogram demonstrating leakage from a perfused sea fan before feeder vessel treatment. The open arrow shows the feeding arteriole, and the white arrow shows the draining vein. B, Fundus photograph demonstrating fresh feeder vessel treatment to the same sea fan as in A. Note the segmentation of the blood column at the treatment sites (arrows). C, Fundus angiogram demonstrating closure of the sea fan depicted in B, 3 months after feeder vessel treatment.

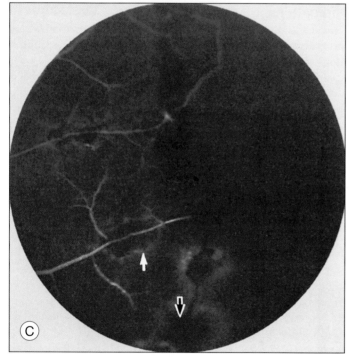

secondary visual loss. Although both xenon arc and argon lasers have been effective in achieving sea fan closure, the argon laser is currently the most widely used for this purpose.

Although different laser treatment protocols have never been formally compared, one recommended protocol uses argon laser slit-lamp delivery, beginning with a spot size of about 500 μm, 0.2 s duration, and a power sufficient to achieve closure of the nutrient arteriole (usually starting at 500 mW).[105] If photocoagulation at the initial settings fails to bring about complete interruption of flow, the power level may be increased in 50- to 100-mW steps until complete segmentation of the blood column is achieved. If the feeder arteriole still does not segment, retreatment is immediately initiated within the original white laser burn, using a smaller (50-μm) spot size at higher power settings. Alternatively, one can bring the patient back 2 weeks later and initiate retreatment at lower power settings, taking advantage of the retinal thinning and pigmentary changes that have occurred within the original laser burn.[97] Once segmentation of the feeder arteriole has been accomplished, the same steps are used to treat the draining venule. Given the requirement for relatively high power settings, it is not surprising that significant complications have been observed, including chorioretinal neovascularization (Fig. 79-14), choroidovitreal neovascularization, and retinal detachment[93,104–112] (Box 79-2). One study documented complications in 32% of treated patients in the 6 months after treatment.[104] The effectiveness of the treatment may be evaluated immediately after treatment, using fluorescein angiography or fluorescein angioscopy for more peripheral lesions. If one or more neovascular fronds remain perfused, repeated treatment of the feeder vessels may be attempted, or the clinician may elect to pursue supplemental methods such as scatter photocoagulation[113] or cryotherapy.[114,115] Most therapists have abandoned feeder vessel treatment in favor of scatter photocoagulation, except in recalcitrant cases with repetitive bleeding.

Scatter photocoagulation

Scatter photocoagulation (Fig. 79-15), which has also been shown to be effective in reducing the chances of vitreous hemorrhage and secondary visual loss in patients with proliferative disease,[96] is preferred by many clinicians over feeder vessel photocoagulation because of the lower rate of complications. One important advantage of feeder vessel photocoagulation over local scatter, however, is that direct feeder vessel treatment seems to be more successful in promoting closure if the sea fan is elevated.[113]

In local scatter treatment, the spots are placed approximately one burn width apart and are applied up to one disc diameter anterior to and posterior to the sea fan, with treatment extending 1 clock-hour to either side of the sea fan. Beginning with a spot size of 500 μm and a duration of 0.2 s, power should be appropriately titrated to achieve a modest-intensity, gray-white burn.[105] Local scatter photocoagulation is thought to cause involution of sea fans by reducing the retinal production of angiogenic factors initially triggered in the milieu of ischemia created by prior vaso-occlusion. The laser scar itself enhances chorioretinal adhesion, theoretically preventing or minimizing the extent of subsequent retinal detachment. If the sea fan is not elevated, direct treatment may be performed in conjunction with local scatter applications. Failure to induce regression of the neovascular tissue, especially in the context of developing vitreous hemorrhage, may prompt the clinician to pursue aggressive feeder vessel photocoagulation.

In the case of an eye with a lone sea fan or in any eye that contains 60 degrees or less of circumferential neovascularization, the risk of vitreous hemorrhage and secondary visual loss is relatively low,[93] and therefore the indications for treatment are less clear. Many clinicians believe, however, that since the risks of scatter treatment are also low, it should probably be performed whenever neovascularization is detected.[96] A possible exception may be the subset of SS subjects over 40 years of age, 86% of whom tend to remain stable or demonstrate regression of neovascular tissue.[116]

Regular follow-up is necessary to monitor the regression or progression of neovascular disease. Thus, the reliable patient is the preferred candidate for local scatter photocoagulation. Despite previous scatter treatment, new fronds of neovascularization may still develop in up to 34% of eyes.[96] With regular follow-up, however, new sea fans may be detected early and receive proper treatment in a timely fashion.

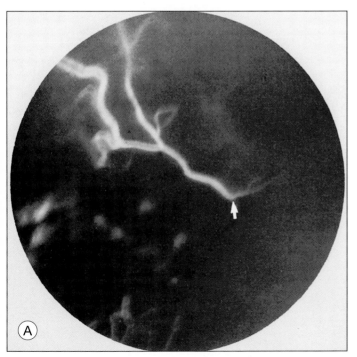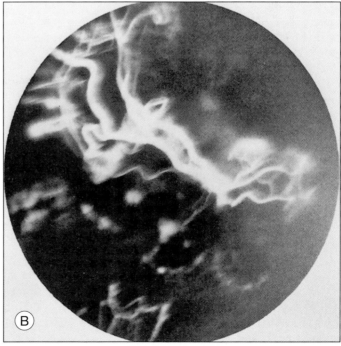

Fig. 79-14 Fundus angiograms of chorioretinal neovascularization. A, Early-phase angiogram demonstrating choroidal origin of new blood vessels within the previous feeder vessel photocoagulation scars (arrow). B, Late-phase angiogram demonstrating further perfusion and leakage.

Box 79-2 Complications of sea fan feeder vessel photocoagulation

Choroidal ischemia
Choroidal hemorrhage
Choroidal neovascularization
Choroidovitreal neovascularization
Epiretinal membrane
Macular hole
Retinal breaks
Rhegmatogenous retinal detachment
Subretinal fibrosis
Tractional retinal detachment
Vitreous hemorrhage

For an unreliable patient who is not likely to comply with follow-up, a 360-degree peripheral scatter technique may be considered, but there is no clear evidence that the outcome from this technique is any better than either the natural course of untreated disease or sector scatter photocoagulation to individual sea fans.[97,113] Some investigators also suspect that extensive 360-degree peripheral laser may foster the development of macular pucker and vitreous traction, which may contribute to significant visual loss.[105]

Cryotherapy

If lenticular or vitreous opacities preclude an adequate view of the retina on contact lens biomicroscopy, and if laser photocoagulation is thus impossible, transconjunctival cryotherapy may be necessary to treat neovascularization. If the view is still poor with indirect ophthalmoscopy, fluorescein angioscopy may be employed for visualization of neovascular fronds.[97] The single freeze–thaw technique has been successful in approximately 70% of treated sea fans.[115] During cryotherapy application, care should be taken to surround the neovascular tissue completely and to avoid overlap of neighboring applications. Retreatment in the same area (e.g., triple freeze–thaw technique) may create retinal breaks and detachment and should be avoided.[117]

Laser vitreolysis

The neodymium:yttrium-aluminum-garnet (Nd:YAG) laser has been used in patients with proliferative sickle retinopathy to transect localized avascular vitreous traction bands that are elevating the retina and/or sea fans or that are causing hemorrhage from neovascular tissue. Used initially in the treatment of vitreous bands in diabetic retinopathy,[118–120] YAG vitreolysis appears to offer a less invasive alternative to surgical vitrectomy for relieving moderate vitreous traction in sickle retinopathy. Potential complications include choroidal hemorrhage, breaks in Bruch's membrane, damage to the RPE, preretinal hemorrhage, and diffuse vitreous hemorrhage from transected fibrovascular tissues. The likelihood of these complications is minimized when the traction bands are narrow, avascular, or minimally perfused, and located at least 3 mm from the retinal surface. Treatment closer than 3 mm from the retinal surface increases the risk of direct damage to the RPE, Bruch's membrane, and choroid. In the case of extensive vitreoretinal traction that is in proximity to the retinal surface or that is threatening the fovea, conventional vitrectomy surgery is usually preferred.[121]

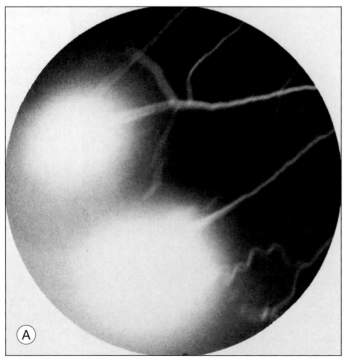
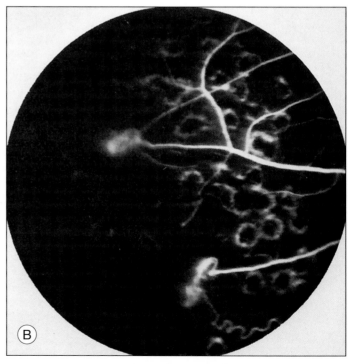

Fig. 79-15 Late-phase fundus angiograms. A, A perfused sea fan before scatter photocoagulation. B, The sea fan in A 4 months after scatter photocoagulation. Note the marked regression following treatment.

Pars plana vitrectomy

Vitrectomy surgery carries a significantly higher risk of intraoperative and postoperative complications in patients with sickle hemoglobinopathies as compared to patients with normal hemoglobin.[102,122] As a result, indications for proceeding with vitrectomy are stringent.[103,123] Patients with new visually significant vitreous hemorrhages are usually followed for at least 6 months to allow clearing of the media. If the view permits, cryotherapy or laser treatment is initiated. If no view of the fundus is possible, the patient is followed with approximately monthly ultrasound examinations in order to detect retinal detachments, for which early surgery is indicated. If visual acuity improves to a level permitting the patient to function to his or her satisfaction, vitrectomy is deferred. Pars plana vitrectomy, in combination with endolaser photocoagulation, may be considered, however, in cases of long-standing vitreous hemorrhage (duration usually greater than 6 months) in which the view is inadequate for laser or cryotherapy.

The primary goal of vitrectomy surgery in sickle patients with severe hemorrhage is to clear the media well enough to visualize and treat the offending neovascular lesions. The surgery can be very challenging, often requiring manipulation in the far retinal periphery, a region that may be so thinned and atrophic from chronic ischemia that the slightest amount of iatrogenic traction may create retinal breaks and possible retinal detachment. Another hazard of far peripheral surgical manipulation is inadvertent lens trauma. Traction on sea fans during surgery may also initiate fresh bleeding, which may be difficult to control. This can be minimized or prevented with preoperative photocoagulation or cryotherapy, assuming a reasonable view is possible. If, at the conclusion of vitrectomy, there is no residual traction, retinal break, or detachment, scleral buckling is unnecessary. Unfortunately, one or more of these features are often present, often necessitating buckle placement immediately after the vitrectomy.[5,102,124]

After combined vitrectomy/lensectomy or vitrectomy in an aphakic patient, sickled erythrocytes may migrate forward from the vitreous cavity into the anterior chamber, clogging the trabecular meshwork and creating secondary glaucoma. The aqueous humor, with its relatively low oxygen tension, low pH, and high ascorbate (a reducing agent) concentration serves to enhance sickling, which, in turn, leads to sequestration of blood cells in the aqueous humor and further acidification and deoxygenation of the anterior chamber, fueling a vicious cycle of sickling and erythrostasis.[125] Only a moderate increase in intraocular pressure may cause a reduction in perfusion of the optic nerve head and retina, putting the eye at risk for optic atrophy and artery occlusion.[126] The intraocular pressure should be maintained at an average of less than 25 mmHg.[9,127,128] Repeated use of mannitol and acetazolamide is contraindicated because they increase hemoconcentration and blood viscosity, predisposing the patient to further occlusive events. Acetazolamide also interferes with the recapturing of bicarbonate in the kidney, lowering the pH of the blood, and increasing the chances of further sickling. Methazolamide, which produces less of a systemic acidosis and may even raise the pH somewhat, is the most appropriate of the systemic intraocular pressure-lowering agents to use in this setting. Most topical intraocular pressure-lowering agents may be used to treat glaucoma resulting from outflow obstruction by sickled erythrocytes, with the exception of compounds that contain frank vasoconstricting agents such as epinephrine (adrenaline). Anterior chamber paracentesis is indicated in cases in which the topical and systemic therapies fail to achieve the desired target pressure (usually 24 mmHg or lower).[102]

Expansile gases are another source of unpredictable postoperative intraocular pressure elevation and should be avoided if possible.[97]

Scleral buckling

As with pars plana vitrectomy, scleral buckling surgery in sickle-cell patients carries with it an increased risk of intraoperative and postoperative complications compared with nonsicklers.[97] Complications are similar to those seen in pars plana vitrectomy, including persistent intraocular hemorrhage, hyphema with secondary glaucoma, infarctions of the macula and optic nerve from elevated intraocular pressure, and the potential for intraoperative sickling crises.[97,129] Buckle placement may also cause anterior segment ischemia, as demonstrated by Ryan & Goldberg.[76] For these reasons, scleral buckling surgery is usually avoided unless absolutely necessary. Rhegmatogenous detachments usually require immediate buckling, but tractional detachments are only buckled when definite progression has been documented. In cases of extensive traction and vitreous hemorrhage, a combined buckle/vitrectomy may be performed.

To lower the risk of intraoperative vaso-occlusion and ischemia, an exchange blood transfusion may be considered before surgery to achieve a target hemoglobin A level of 50% to 60% (measured by electrophoresis) and a target hematocrit of 35% to 40%.[130] The transfusion takes place over a 3- to 5-day interval and involves direct replacement of the patient's whole blood with washed and packed donor erythrocytes. An alternative method, called *erythropheresis*, makes use of an automated blood cell separator to replace sickle red cells with donor erythrocytes.[129] Exchange transfusion is not without its own serious risks, however, including various immune-mediated transfusion reactions as well as transmission of infectious diseases such as human immunodeficiency virus (HIV) and hepatitis. When an exchange transfusion is being considered, the risks and benefits should be thoroughly discussed with the patient. An alternative to exchange transfusion is the use of a hyperbaric chamber[131] to increase blood oxygenation, but such equipment is neither convenient nor widely available. The advent of modern vitrectomy techniques, particularly the ability to soften the eye and promote vasoperfusion, has minimized the need for exchange transfusion in most cases, although anterior segment ischemia is still a risk.[122]

Local anesthesia should be used whenever possible, because it is less likely than general endotracheal anesthesia to cause systemic hypotension and lowered vascular perfusion within the eye. When local anesthetic preparations are chosen, care should be taken to avoid mixtures containing epinephrine or similar sympathomimetic agents to minimize regional vasoconstriction and ischemia. Similarly, topical phenylephrine should be used sparingly, with increased reliance on topical anticholinergic agents, such as atropine and homatropine, for pupillary dilation, to lessen the likelihood of anterior segment ischemia.[129] Maintaining a low intraocular pressure postoperatively helps to maximize intraocular perfusion, but overzealous use of systemic agents actually may enhance sickling by causing hemoconcentration and acidosis. Methazolamide is preferable to recurrent use of mannitol or acetazolamide in the setting of elevated intraocular pressure (see discussion above).

Additional prophylactic measures include the use of supplemental oxygen; the avoidance of surgical techniques that threaten the anterior and long posterior ciliary arteries, such as removal of or excessive traction on the rectus muscles and transscleral coagulation in the horizontal meridians; the use of transscleral cryotherapy instead of diathermy, which can cause scleral shrinkage with secondary intraocular pressure elevation and decreased perfusion of ocular tissues; drainage of subretinal fluid during buckling to minimize intraocular pressure elevation and maximize tissue perfusion; preoperative laser closure of sea fans to reduce the risks of intraoperative hemorrhage; and preoperative consultation with an experienced hematologist.[129]

Desferrioxamine

Desferrioxamine (diethylenetriamine penta-acetic acid) is an iron chelator given to many sickle-cell patients to combat iatrogenic iron overload from chronic transfusion therapy.[132] Since its introduction in 1963,[133] various case reports have documented ocular side-effects of the drug, including lens opacities,[134] degenerative changes in the RPE,[135] and a toxic optic neuropathy featuring disc swelling, abnormal color vision, and central scotomas.[133,136] Abnormalities in the electroretinogram, electro-oculogram, and visual evoked response have all been reported.[133] Unfortunately, no controlled clinical trials investigating the ocular toxicity of desferrioxamine exist.

Although the mechanism of desferrioxamine toxicity is not known, the toxic effects are thought to be dose-dependent and partially reversible with cessation of therapy.[137] Our current recommendation is that sickle-cell patients receiving the drug should, in addition to the usual rigorous surveillance of proliferative retinopathy with serial dilated examinations, undergo formal kinetic and/or static perimetry, with the possible addition of color vision testing, every 6 months to 1 year.

FUTURE INVESTIGATIONS

Current investigations into the pathophysiology of vaso-occlusion in the sickle-cell retina have provided insights on a molecular level. An evolving body of research continues to reinforce the notion that vaso-occlusion is not simply a mechanical plugging of capillaries by rigid cells, but may also involve enhanced adhesion of reticulocytes to endothelial cells,[21–26,138] altered cytokine production, which drives the expression of adhesion molecules and the activation of polymorphonuclear leukocytes,[27,139] imbalances in the fibrinolytic system, which

may predispose the microvasculature to fibrin deposition,[28–30] and membrane channel regulation of red-cell volume and intracellular hemoglobin concentration.[14,140] With the further delineation of these subtler molecular mechanisms, specific pharmacologic therapies may be developed to provide an effective solution to vascular occlusion.

Photodynamic therapy with Visudyne may prove useful in treating neovascularization without damaging adjacent tissues,[141] although there are no comprehensive data yet to support this application.

Finally, efforts continue to be directed toward the search for agents that will block the production of or inhibit the action of angiogenic factors (e.g., bFGF, VEGF) that are crucial to the growth of neovascular tissue.[88,100,142,143]

Systemic therapy

Pneumococcal sepsis is a leading cause of death in young patients with sickle-cell disease because a spleen that is damaged by sickle-cell disease cannot clear pneumococcus from the blood. Children over the age of 2 with sickle-cell disease should be vaccinated against *Streptococcus pneumoniae* at age 2 with boosters every 5 years thereafter.[3]

Another therapeutic avenue involves drugs capable of stimulating the production of fetal hemoglobin, which has a higher oxygen affinity than hemoglobin A. Hydroxyurea is currently the only drug being widely used for this purpose,[12,144–147] but there has been growing interest in butyric acid,[148,149] butyrate analogues,[150] and other short-chain fatty-acid derivatives[151] as pharmacologic stimuli for fetal hemoglobin production. Hydroxyurea may also reduce adhesion of sickled erythrocytes to the endothelium,[152,153] and has been shown to reduce pain crises, acute chest syndrome, blood transfusions, and hospitalizations in sickle-cell patients in a double-blind, placebo-controlled trial.[154] Therapy with hydroxyurea should be closely monitored, as it can cause neutropenia and thrombocytopenia.

Recent attention has also centered on drugs that inhibit potassium and water loss from SS red cells, thus preventing formation of "dense" cells with a high intracellular hemoglobin concentration. One promising candidate is the antifungal agent clotrimazole, which has been shown to reduce the number of dense and irreversibly sickled cells in several HbSS subjects.[17] Other investigators have proposed bone marrow transplantation as a potential cure for sickle-cell disease.[155–157] Finally, antibodies that inhibit binding of sickle erythrocytes to the endothelium are currently being tested.[158,159]

REFERENCES

1. Gagliano DA, Jampol L, Rabb M. Sickle cell disease. In: Tasman WS, Jaeger E, eds. Duane's clinical ophthalmology. Philadelphia: Lippincott-Raven, 1996; vol 3:1–40.
2. Jandl J. Blood. In: Pathophysiology. Cambridge: Blackwell Scientific Publications, 1991.
3. Steinberg M. Management of sickle cell disease. N Engl J Med 1999; 340:1021–1030.
4. Welch RB, Goldberg MF. Sickle-cell hemoglobin and its relation to fundus abnormality. Arch Ophthalmol 1966; 75:353–362.
5. Goldberg MF. Retinal neovascularization in sickle cell retinopathy. Trans Am Acad Ophthalmol Otolaryngol 1977; 83:OP409–OP431.

6. Bloch R. Hematologic disorders. In: Duane T, Jaeger E, eds. Clinical ophthalmology. Philadelphia: Harper & Row, 1994;5.

7. Nia J, Lam WC, Kleinman DM et al. Retinopathy in sickle cell trait: does it exist? Can J Ophthalmol 2003; 38:46–51.

8. Mehta JS, Whittaker KW, Tsaloumas MD. Latent proliferative sickle cell retinopathy in sickle cell trait. Acta Ophthalmol Scand 2001; 79:81–82.

9. Serjeant G. Sickle cell disease. Oxford: Oxford University Press, 1985.

10. Goldberg MF. Sickled erythrocytes, hyphema, and secondary glaucoma: I. The diagnosis and treatment of sickled erythrocytes in human hyphemas. Ophthalmol Surg 1979; 10:17–31.

11. Herrick J. Peculiar elongated and sickle-shaped red blood corpuscles in a case of severe anemia. Arch Intern Med 1910; 6:517–621.

12. Bunn HF. Pathogenesis and treatment of sickle cell disease. N Engl J Med 1997; 337:762–769.

13. Mozzarelli A, Hofrichter J, Eaton WA. Delay time of hemoglobin S polymerization prevents most cells from sickling in vivo. Science 1987; 237:500–506.

14. Kaul DK, Fabry ME, Nagel RL. The pathophysiology of vascular obstruction in the sickle syndromes. Blood Rev 1996; 10:29–44.

15. Fabry ME, Nagel RL. Heterogeneity of red cells in the sickler: a characteristic with practical clinical and pathophysiological implications. Blood Cells 1982; 8:9–15.

16. Kaul DK, Fabry ME, Windisch P et al. Erythrocytes in sickle cell anemia are heterogeneous in their rheological and hemodynamic characteristics. J Clin Invest 1983; 72:22–31.

17. Brugnara C, Gee B, Armsby CC et al. Therapy with oral clotrimazole induces inhibition of the Gardos channel and reduction of erythrocyte dehydration in patients with sickle cell disease. J Clin Invest 1996; 97:1227–1234.

18. Brugnara C, Kopin AS, Bunn HF et al. Regulation of cation content and cell volume in hemoglobin erythrocytes from patients with homozygous hemoglobin C disease. J Clin Invest 1985; 75:1608–1617.

19. Canessa M, Spalvins A, Nagel RL. Volume-dependent and NEM-stimulated K+,Cl– transport is elevated in oxygenated SS, SC and CC human red cells. FEBS Lett 1986; 200:197–202.

20. Fabry ME, Romero JR, Buchanan ID et al. Rapid increase in red blood cell density driven by K:Cl cotransport in a subset of sickle cell anemia reticulocytes and discocytes. Blood 1991; 78:217–225.

21. Mathews M, McLeod DS, Merges C et al. Neutrophils and leucocyte adhesion molecules in sickle cell retinopathy. Br J Ophthalmol 2002; 86:684–690.

22. Joneckis CC, Ackley RL, Orringer EP et al. Integrin alpha 4 beta 1 and glycoprotein IV (CD36) are expressed on circulating reticulocytes in sickle cell anemia. Blood 1993; 82:3548–3555.

23. Setty BN, Stuart MJ. Vascular cell adhesion molecule-1 is involved in mediating hypoxia-induced sickle red blood cell adherence to endothelium: potential role in sickle cell disease. Blood 1996; 88:2311–2320.

24. Swerlick RA, Eckman JR, Kumar A et al. Alpha 4 beta 1-integrin expression on sickle reticulocytes: vascular cell adhesion molecule-1-dependent binding to endothelium. Blood 1993; 82:1891–1899.

25. Lutty GA, Otsuji T, Taomoto M et al. Mechanisms for sickle red blood cell retention in choroid. Curr Eye Res 2002; 25:163–171.

26. Solovey A, Lin Y, Browne P et al. Circulating activated endothelial cells in sickle cell anemia. N Engl J Med 1997; 337:1584–1590.

27. Francis RB Jr, Haywood LJ. Elevated immunoreactive tumor necrosis factor and interleukin-1 in sickle cell disease. J Natl Med Assoc 1992; 84:611–615.

28. Francis RB Jr. Elevated fibrin D-dimer fragment in sickle cell anemia: evidence for activation of coagulation during the steady state as well as in painful crisis. Haemostasis 1989; 19:105–111.

29. Kunz M, Cao J, Merges C et al. Adhesion molecules, neutrophils and imbalance in the fibrinolytic system in sickle cell retinopathy. Invest Ophthalmol Vis Sci 1997; 38 (suppl):1117.

30. Lutty GA, Merges C, Crone S et al. Immunohistochemical insights into sickle cell retinopathy. Curr Eye Res 1994; 13:125–138.

31. Horne MK 3rd. Sickle cell anemia as a rheologic disease. Am J Med 1981; 70:288–298.

32. Lutty GA, Phelan A, McLeod DS et al. A rat model for sickle cell-mediated vaso-occlusion in retina. Microvasc Res 1996; 52:270–280.

33. Paton D. The conjunctival sign of sickle-cell disease. Arch Ophthalmol 1961; 66:90–94.

34. Fink AI, Funahashi T, Robinson M et al. Conjunctival blood flow in sickle-cell disease. Preliminary report. Arch Ophthalmol 1961; 66:824–829.

35. Paton D. The conjunctival sign of sickle-cell disease. Further observations. Arch Ophthalmol 1962; 68:627–632.

36. Nagpal KC, Goldberg MF, Rabb MF. Ocular manifestations of sickle hemoglobinopathies. Surv Ophthalmol 1977; 21:391–411.

37. Funahashi T, Fink A, Robinson M et al. Pathology of conjunctival vessels in sickle-cell disease. A preliminary report. Am J Ophthalmol 1964; 57:713–718.

38. Nagpal KC, Asdourian GK, Goldbaum MH et al. The conjunctival sickling sign, hemoglobin S, and irreversibly sickled erythrocytes. Arch Ophthalmol 1977; 95:808–811.

39. Chambers J, Puglisi J, Kernitsky R et al. Iris atrophy in hemoglobin SC disease. Am J Ophthalmol 1974; 77:247–249.

40. Galinos S, Rabb MF, Goldberg MF et al. Hemoglobin SC disease and iris atrophy. Am J Ophthalmol 1973; 75:421–425.

41. Romayanada N, Goldberg MF, Green WR. Histopathology of sickle cell retinopathy. Trans Am Acad Ophthalmol Otolaryngol 1973; 77:OP642–OP676.

42. Gagliano DA, Goldberg MF. The evolution of salmon-patch hemorrhages in sickle cell retinopathy. Arch Ophthalmol 1989; 107:1814–1815.

43. Condon PI, Serjeant GR. Ocular findings in hemoglobin SC disease in Jamaica. Am J Ophthalmol 1972; 74:921–931.

44. Condon PI, Serjeant GR. Ocular findings in homozygous sickle cell anemia in Jamaica. Am J Ophthalmol 1972; 73:533–543.

45. Condon PI, Serjeant GR. Ocular findings in sickle cell thalassemia in Jamaica. Am J Ophthalmol 1972; 74:1105–1109.

46. Goldberg MF. Natural history of untreated proliferative sickle retinopathy. Arch Ophthalmol 1971; 85:428–437.

47. Levine RA, Kaplan AM. The ophthalmoscopic findings in C + S disease. Am J Ophthalmol 1965; 59:37–42.

48. van Meurs JC. Evolution of a retinal hemorrhage in a patient with sickle cell-hemoglobin C disease. Arch Ophthalmol 1995; 113:1074–1075.

49. Asdourian G, Nagpal KC, Goldbaum M et al. Evolution of the retinal black sunburst in sickling haemoglobinopathies. Br J Ophthalmol 1975; 59:710–716.

50. Liang JC, Jampol LM. Spontaneous peripheral chorioretinal neovascularisation in association with sickle cell anaemia. Br J Ophthalmol 1983; 67:107–110.

51. Lutty GA, McLeod DS, Pachnis A et al. Retinal and choroidal neovascularization in a transgenic mouse model of sickle cell disease. Am J Pathol 1994; 145:490–497.

52. Cogan DG. Ophthalmic manifestations of systemic vascular disease. Major Probl Intern Med 1974; 3:1–187.

53. Wise G, Dollery C, Henkind P. The retinal circulation. New York: Harper & Row, 1971.

54. Asdourian GK, Nagpal KC, Busse B et al. Macular and perimacular vascular remodelling sickling haemoglobinopathies. Br J Ophthalmol 1976; 60:431–453.

55. Acacio I, Goldberg MF. Peripapillary and macular vessel occlusions in sickle cell anemia. Am J Ophthalmol 1973; 75:861–866.

56. Conrad WC, Penner R. Sickle-cell trait and central retinal-artery occlusion. Am J Ophthalmol 1967; 63:465–468.

57. Goodman G, Von Sallmann L, Holland MG. Ocular manifestations of sickle-cell disease. Arch Opthalmol 1957; 58:655–682.

58. Kabakow B, Van Weimoky SS, Lyons HA. Bilateral central retinal artery occlusion; occurrence in a patient with cortisone-treated systemic lupus erythematosus, sickle cell trait, and active pulmonary tuberculosis. Arch Opthalmol 1955; 54:670–676.

59. Klein ML, Jampol LM, Condon PI et al. Central retinal artery occlusion without retrobulbar hemorrhage after retrobulbar anesthesia. Am J Ophthalmol 1982; 93:573–577.

60. Knapp JW. Isolated macular infarction in sickle cell (SS) disease. Am J Ophthalmol 1972; 73:857–859.

61. Lieb W, Geeraets W, Guerry D. Ocular and systemic manifestions of sickle cell disease. Acta Opthalmol 1951; 58:25–45.

62. Ryan SJ Jr. Occlusion of the macular capillaries in sickle cell hemoglobin C disease. Am J Ophthalmol 1974; 77:459–461.

63. Weissman H, Nadel AJ, Dunn M. Simultaneous bilateral retinal arterial occlusions treated by exchange transfusions. Arch Ophthalmol 1979; 97:2151–2153.

64. Appen RE, Wray SH, Cogan DG. Central retinal artery occlusion. Am J Ophthalmol 1975; 79:374–381.

65. Chopdar A. Multiple major retinal vascular occlusions in sickle cell haemoglobin C disease. Br J Ophthalmol 1975; 59:493–496.

66. Condon PI, Whitelocke RA, Bird AC et al. Recurrent visual loss in homozygous sickle cell disease. Br J Ophthalmol 1985; 69:700–706.

67. McLeod DS, Goldberg MF, Lutty GA. Dual-perspective analysis of vascular formations in sickle cell retinopathy. Arch Ophthalmol 1993; 111:1234–1245.

68. Goldbaum MH. Retinal depression sign indicating a small retinal infarct. Am J Ophthalmol 1978; 86:45–55.

69. Roy MS, Gascon P, Giuliani D. Macular blood flow velocity in sickle cell disease: relation to red cell density. Br J Ophthalmol 1995; 79:742–745.

70. Stevens TS, Busse B, Lee CB et al. Sickling hemoglobinopathies; macular and perimacular vascular abnormalities. Arch Ophthalmol 1974; 92:455–463.

71. Marsh RJ, Ford SM, Rabb MF et al. Macular vasculature, visual acuity, and irreversibly sickled cells in homozygous sickle cell disease. Br J Ophthalmol 1982; 66:155–160.

72. Goldberg MF. Retinal vaso-occlusion in sickling hemoglobinopathies. Birth Defects Orig Artic Ser 1976; 12:475–515.

73. Condon PI, Serjeant GR, Ikeda H. Unusual chorioretinal degeneration in sickle cell disease. Possible sequelae of posterior ciliary vessel occlusion. Br J Ophthalmol 1973; 57:81–88.

74. Dizon RV, Jampol LM, Goldberg MF et al. Choroidal occlusive disease in sickle cell hemoglobinopathies. Surv Ophthalmol 1979; 23:297–306.

75. Stein MR, Gay AJ. Acute chorioretinal infarction in sickle cell trait. Report of a case. Arch Ophthalmol 1970; 84:485–490.

76. Ryan SJ, Goldberg MF. Anterior segment ischemia following scleral buckling in sickle cell hemoglobinopathy. Am J Ophthalmol 1971; 72:35–50.

77. Condon PI, Serjeant GR. The progression of sickle cell eye disease in Jamaica. Doc Ophthalmol 1975; 39:203–210.

78. Nagpal KC, Huamonte F, Constantaras A et al. Migratory white-without-pressure retinal lesions. Arch Ophthalmol 1976; 94:576–579.

79. Nagpal KC, Goldberg MF, Asdourian G et al. Dark-without-pressure fundus lesions. Br J Ophthalmol 1975; 59:476–479.

80. Condon PI, Serjeant GR. Behaviour of untreated proliferative sickle retinopathy. Br J Ophthalmol 1980; 64:404–411.

81. Kimmel AS, Magargal LE, Tasman WS. Proliferative sickle retinopathy and neovascularization of the disc: regression following treatment with peripheral retinal scatter laser photocoagulation. Ophthalm Surg 1986; 17:20–22.

82. Ober RR, Michels RG. Optic disk neovascularization in hemoglobin SC disease. Am J Ophthalmol 1978; 85:711–714.

83. Raichand M, Goldberg MF, Nagpal KC et al. Evolution of neovascularization in sickle cell retinopathy. A prospective fluorescein angiographic study. Arch Ophthalmol 1977; 95:1543–1552.

84. Clarkson JG. The ocular manifestations of sickle-cell disease: a prevalence and natural history study. Trans Am Ophthalmol Soc 1992; 90:481–504.

85. Nagpal K. Angioid streaks and sickle hemoglobinopathies. Br J Ophthalmol 1977; 37:325–328.

86. Jampol LM, Green JL Jr, Goldberg MF et al. An update on vitrectomy surgery and retinal detachment repair in sickle cell disease. Arch Ophthalmol 1982; 100:591–593.

87. Goldberg MF. Classification and pathogenesis of proliferative sickle retinopathy. Am J Ophthalmol 1971; 71:649–665.

88. Cao J, Mathews MK, McLeod DS et al. Angiogenic factors in human proliferative sickle cell retinopathy. Br J Ophthalmol 1999; 83:838–846.

89. Cao J, Kunz M, Merges C et al. Immunolocalization of angiogenic factors in proliferative sickle cell retinopathy. Invest Ophthalmol Vis Sci 1997; 38 (suppl.):1117.

90. Lutty GA, McLeod DS, Merges C et al. Localization of vascular endothelial growth factor in human retina and choroid. Arch Ophthalmol 1996; 114:971–977.

91. Curtis AS, Seehar GM. The control of cell division by tension or diffusion. Nature 1978; 274:52–53.

92. McLeod DS, Merges C, Fukushima A et al. Histopathologic features of neovascularization in sickle cell retinopathy. Am J Ophthalmol 1997; 124:455–472.

93. Condon P, Jampol LM, Farber MD et al. A randomized clinical trial of feeder vessel photocoagulation of proliferative sickle cell retinopathy. II. Update and analysis of risk factors. Ophthalmology 1984; 91:1496–1498.

94. Isbey H, Clifford G, Tanaka K. Vitreous hemorrhage associated with sickle-cell trait and sickle-cell hemoglobin C disease. Am J Ophthalmol 1958; 45:870–879.

95. Kearney WF. Sickle cell ophthalmopathy. NY State J Med 1965; 65:2677–2681.

96. Farber MD, Jampol LM, Fox P et al. A randomized clinical trial of scatter photocoagulation of proliferative sickle cell retinopathy. Arch Ophthalmol 1991; 109:363–367.

97. Goldberg MF, Jampol LM. Treatment of neovascularization, vitreous hemorrhage, and retinal detachment in sickle cell retinopathy. Trans New Orleans Acad Ophthalmol 1983; 31:53–81.

98. Nagpal KC, Patrianakos D, Asdourian GK et al. Spontaneous regression (autoinfarction) of proliferative sickle retinopathy. Am J Ophthalmol 1975; 80:885–892.

99. Jampol LM, Goldbaum MH. Peripheral proliferative retinopathies. Surv Ophthalmol 1980; 25:1–14.

100. Kim SY, Mocanu C, McLeod DS et al. Expression of pigment epithelium-derived factor (PEDF) and vascular endothelial growth factor (VEGF) in sickle cell retina and choroid. Exp Eye Res 2003; 77:433–445.

101. Gitter KA, Rothschild H, Waltman DD et al. Dominantly inherited peripheral retinal neovascularization. Arch Ophthalmol 1978; 96:1601–1605.

102. Cohen SB, Fletcher ME, Goldberg MF et al. Diagnosis and management of ocular complications of sickle hemoglobinopathies: Part IV. Ophthalm Surg 1986; 17:312–315.

103. Goldbaum MH, Peyman GA, Nagpal KC et al. Vitrectomy in sickling retinopathy: report of five cases. Ophthalm Surg 1976; 7:92–102.

104. Jacobson MS, Gagliano DA, Cohen SB et al. A randomized clinical trial of feeder vessel photocoagulation of sickle cell retinopathy. A long-term follow-up. Ophthalmology 1991; 98:581–585.

105. Jampol LM, Farber M, Rabb MF et al. An update on techniques of photocoagulation treatment of proliferative sickle cell retinopathy. Eye 1991; 5:260–263.

106. Carney MD, Paylor RR, Cunha-Vaz JG et al. Iatrogenic choroidal neovascularization in sickle cell retinopathy. Ophthalmology 1986; 93:1163–1168.

107. Condon PI, Serjeant GR. Choroid neovascularization. An important complication of photocoagulation for proliferative sickle cell retinopathy. Trans Ophthalmol Soc UK 1981; 101:429.

108. Condon PI, Jampol LM, Ford SM et al. Choroidal neovascularisation induced by photocoagulation in sickle cell disease. Br J Ophthalmol 1981; 65:192–197.

109. Dizon-Moore RV, Jampol LM, Goldberg MF. Chorioretinal and choriovitreal neovascularization. Their presence after photocoagulation of proliferative sickle cell retinopathy. Arch Ophthalmol 1981; 99:842–849.

110. Fox PD, Acheson RW, Serjeant GR. Outcome of iatrogenic choroidal neovascularisation in sickle cell disease. Br J Ophthalmol 1990; 74:417–420.

111. Galinos SO, Asdourian GK, Woolf MB et al. Choroido-vitreal neovascularization after argon laser photocoagulation. Arch Ophthalmol 1975; 93:524–530.

112. Goldbaum MH, Galinos SO, Apple D et al. Acute choroidal ischemia as a complication of photocoagulation. Arch Ophthalmol 1976; 94:1025–1035.

113. Rednam KR, Jampol LM, Goldberg MF. Scatter retinal photocoagulation for proliferative sickle cell retinopathy. Am J Ophthalmol 1982; 93:594–599.

114. Hanscom TA. Indirect treatment of peripheral retinal neovascularization. Am J Ophthalmol 1982; 93:88–91.

115. Lee CB, Woolf MB, Galinos SO et al. Cryotherapy of proliferative sickle retinopathy. Part I. Single freeze–thaw cycle. Ann Ophthalmol 1975; 7:1299–1308.

116. Fox PD, Vessey SJ, Forshaw ML et al. Influence of genotype on the natural history of untreated proliferative sickle retinopathy – an angiographic study. Br J Ophthalmol 1991; 75:229–231.

117. Goldbaum MH, Fletcher RC, Jampol LM et al. Cryotherapy of proliferative sickle retinopathy, II: triple freeze–thaw cycle. Br J Ophthalmol 1979; 63:97–101.

118. Aron-Rosa D, Greenspan DA. Neodymium:YAG laser vitreolysis. Int Ophthalmol Clin 1985; 25:125–134.

119. Brown GC, Benson WE. Treatment of diabetic traction retinal detachment with the pulsed neodymium-YAG laser. Am J Ophthalmol 1985; 99:258–262.

120. Fankhauser F, Kwasniewska S, van der Zypen E. Vitreolysis with the Q-switched laser. Arch Ophthalmol 1985; 103:1166–1171.

121. Hrisomalos NF, Jampol LM, Moriarty BJ et al. Neodymium-YAG laser vitreolysis in sickle cell disease. Arch Ophthalmol 1987; 105:1087–1091.

122. Leen JS, Ratnakaram R, Del Priore LV et al. Anterior segment ischemia after vitrectomy in sickle cell disease. Retina 2002; 22:216–219.

123. Ryan SJ. Role of the vitreous in the haemoglobinopathies. Trans Ophthalmol Soc UK 1975; 95:403–406.

124. Goldberg MF. Treatment of proliferative sickle retinopathy. Trans Am Acad Ophthalmol Otolaryngol 1971; 75:532–556.

125. Goldberg MF, Dizon R, Moses VK. Sickled erythrocytes, hyphema, and secondary glaucoma: VI. The relationship between intracameral blood cells and aqueous humor pH, PO_2, and PCO_2. Ophthalm Surg 1979; 10:78–88.

126. Al-Abdulla NA, Haddock TA, Kerrison JB et al. Sickle cell disease presenting with extensive peri-macular arteriolar occlusions in a nine-year-old boy. Am J Ophthalmol 2001; 131:275–276.

127. Goldberg MF. The diagnosis and treatment of secondary glaucoma after hyphema in sickle cell patients. Am J Ophthalmol 1979; 87:43–49.

128. Goldberg MF. The diagnosis and treatment of sickled erythrocytes in human hyphemas. Trans Am Ophthalmol Soc 1978; 76:481–501.

129. Cohen SB, Fletcher ME, Goldberg MF et al. Diagnosis and management of ocular complications of sickle hemoglobinopathies: part V. Ophthalm Surg 1986; 17:369–374.

130. Brazier DJ, Gregor ZJ, Blach RK et al. Retinal detachment in patients with proliferative sickle cell retinopathy. Trans Ophthalmol Soc UK 1986; 105:100–105.

131. Freilich DB, Seelenfreund MH. Long-term follow-up of scleral buckling procedures with sickle cell disease and retinal detachment treated with the use of hyperbaric oxygen. Mod Probl Ophthalmol 1977; 18:368–372.

132. Rahi AH, Hungerford JL, Ahmed AI. Ocular toxicity of desferrioxamine: light microscopic histochemical and ultrastructural findings. Br J Ophthalmol 1986; 70:373–381.

133. Orton RB, de Veber LL, Sulh HM. Ocular and auditory toxicity of long-term, high-dose subcutaneous deferoxamine therapy. Can J Ophthalmol 1985; 20:153–156.

134. Bloomfield SE, Markenson AL, Miller DR et al. Lens opacities in thalassemia. J Pediatr Ophthalmol Strabismus 1978; 15:154–156.

135. Haimovici R, D'Amico DJ, Gragoudas ES et al. The expanded clinical spectrum of deferoxamine retinopathy. Ophthalmology 2002; 109:164–171.

136. Lakhanpal V, Schocket SS, Jiji R. Deferoxamine (Desferal)-induced toxic retinal pigmentary degeneration and presumed optic neuropathy. Ophthalmology 1984; 91:443–451.

137. Dennerlein JA, Lang GE, Stahnke K et al. [Ocular findings in Desferal therapy.] Ophthalmologe 1995; 92:38–42.

138. Lubin BH. Sickle cell disease and the endothelium. N Engl J Med 1997; 337:1623–1625.

139. Malave I, Perdomo Y, Escalona E et al. Levels of tumor necrosis factor alpha/cachectin (TNF alpha) in sera from patients with sickle cell disease. Acta Haematol 1993; 90:172–176.

140. Moore CM, Ehlayel M, Leiva LE et al. New concepts in the immunology of sickle cell disease. Ann Allergy Asthma Immunol 1996; 76:385–400; quiz 403.

141. Spaide RF. Personal communication.

142. Auerbach W, Auerbach R. Angiogenesis inhibition: a review. Pharmacol Ther 1994; 63:265–311.

143. Fan TP, Jaggar R, Bicknell R. Controlling the vasculature: angiogenesis, anti-angiogenesis and vascular targeting of gene therapy. Trends Pharmacol Sci 1995; 16:57–66.

144. Charache S. Eye disease in sickling disorders. Hematol Oncol Clin North Am 1996; 10:1357–1362.

145. Charache S. Mechanism of action of hydroxyurea in the management of sickle cell anemia in adults. Semin Hematol 1997; 34 (suppl. 3):15–21.

146. Ohene-Frempong K, Smith-Whitley K. Use of hydroxyurea in children with sickle cell disease: what comes next? Semin Hematol 1997; 34 (suppl. 3):30–41.

147. Rogers ZR. Hydroxyurea therapy for diverse pediatric populations with sickle cell disease. Semin Hematol 1997; 34 (suppl. 3):42–47.

148. Constantoulakis P, Knitter G, Stamatoyannopoulos G. On the induction of fetal hemoglobin by butyrates: in vivo and in vitro studies with sodium butyrate and comparison of combination treatments with 5-AzaC and AraC. Blood 1989; 74:1963–1971.

149. Faller DV, Perrine SP. Butyrate in the treatment of sickle cell disease and beta-thalassemia. Curr Opin Hematol 1995; 2:109–117.

150. Stamatoyannopoulos G, Blau CA, Nakamoto B et al. Fetal hemoglobin induction by acetate, a product of butyrate catabolism. Blood 1994; 84:3198–3204.

151. Liakopoulou E, Blau CA, Li Q et al. Stimulation of fetal hemoglobin production by short chain fatty acids. Blood 1995; 86:3227–3235.

152. Adragna NC, Fonseca P, Lauf PK. Hydroxyurea affects cell morphology, cation transport, and red blood cell adhesion in cultured vascular endothelial cells. Blood 1994; 83:553–560.

153. Bridges KR, Barabino GD, Brugnara C et al. A multiparameter analysis of sickle erythrocytes in patients undergoing hydroxyurea therapy. Blood 1996; 88:4701–4710.

154. Charache S, Terrin ML, Moore RD et al. Effect of hydroxyurea on the frequency of painful crises in sickle cell anemia. Investigators of the Multicenter Study of Hydroxyurea in Sickle Cell Anemia. N Engl J Med 1995; 332:1317–1322.

155. Platt OS, Guinan EC. Bone marrow transplantation in sickle cell anemia – the dilemma of choice. N Engl J Med 1996; 335:426–428.

156. Vermylen C, Cornu G. Bone marrow transplantation for sickle cell anemia. Curr Opin Hematol 1996; 32:163–166.

157. Walters MC, Patience M, Leisenring W et al. Bone marrow transplantation for sickle cell disease. N Engl J Med 1996;335(6):369–376.

158. Kaul DK, Tsai HM, Liu XD et al. Monoclonal antibodies to alphaVbeta3 (7E3 and LM609) inhibit sickle red blood cell–endothelium interactions induced by platelet-activating factor. Blood 2000; 95:368–374.

159. Hebbel RP. Blockade of adhesion of sickle cells to endothelium by monoclonal antibodies. N Engl J Med 2000; 342:1910–1912.

Chapter

80

Retinopathy of Prematurity

Earl A. Palmer
Dale L. Phelps
Rand Spencer
Gerard A. Lutty

Retinopathy of prematurity (ROP) is a disease affecting the retinas of premature infants. Its key pathologic change, retinal neovascularization, has several features in common with the other proliferative retinopathies such as diabetic and sickle cell retinopathy. Each of these proliferative retinal vascular disorders appears to be associated with local ischemia and the subsequent development of neovascularization.

ROP is unique in that the vascular disease is found only in infants with immature, incompletely vascularized retinas; hence its connection with premature birth. The range of possible outcomes for patients with ROP extends from minimal sequelae with no effect on vision, in mild cases, to bilateral, irreversible and total blindness in more advanced cases. Contemporary neonatology practices in the premature infant nursery have improved the survival rate of the smallest premature infants, who are also those at highest risk of developing ROP. This disorder is a major challenge to all physicians who take care of premature infants.

HISTORICAL PERSPECTIVE

Early history

Retinopathy of prematurity, first identified by Terry in 1942,[1,2] within a decade became the primary cause of childhood blindness in the United States and a major cause of blindness throughout the technologically developed world.[3] Terry's original reports designated the condition *retrolental fibroplasia* (RLF), on the basis of his impression that it involved a proliferation of the embryonic hyaloid system, but Owens and Owens[4] found that the hyaloid system was normal at birth and that RLF developed postnatally. As the pathogenesis and clinical spectrum of manifestations became better understood, the term *retinopathy of prematurity* was generally adopted.

The discovery of the relationship between supplementary oxygen and ROP in the 1950s[5–9] led to the practice of rigid curtailment of oxygen supplementation in the nursery, and a dramatic decrease in the incidence of ROP followed. It is unfortunate that during this period, when concern for damage to the eye prompted this curtailment of oxygen in the premature nursery, no clinical monitoring systems were available to measure blood oxygenation. The relatively arbitrary restriction of oxygen supplementation had an adverse effect on premature infant morbidity and mortality rates.[10] An increase in deaths caused by respiratory distress syndrome (RDS) was reported,[11] and an increase in the incidence of cerebral palsy and neurologic disorders was also found.[12]

Retinopathy of prematurity and contemporary nursery practices

By the late 1960s and early 1970s, arterial blood gas analysis had come into general use, and the oxygen requirements of premature infants with RDS were better documented.[13,14] Even with relatively high concentrations of inspired oxygen, arterial oxygen tension values were deficient in some infants with severe RDS. In this latter group, routine restriction of oxygen in the inspired air to no more than 40% would be expected to raise morbidity and mortality rates.[15] Arterial blood gas monitoring enabled pediatricians to titrate the incubator oxygen concentration to more nearly meet the individual premature infant's oxygen needs.

More recently, transcutaneous oxygen monitoring and continuous pulse oximetry monitoring have provided additional noninvasive and continuous tools. Many problems still exist with these techniques[16] and their influence on ROP has been disappointingly weak.[17,18] Perhaps most importantly, there have been no trials to determine what the best levels of transcutaneous oxygen should be, or of what pulse oximetry saturations should be targeted in preterm or term infants.[19]

Following the advent and progress of neonatology as a subspecialty, more of the highest-risk premature infants, those with extremely low gestations, are now surviving. It is these infants, with the greatest immaturity of the retinal vasculature, who have the highest risk of ROP. In 1981, Phelps[20] estimated the incidence of ROP that was associated with an increase in survival rates of infants with birth weights less than 1000 g. Eight percent of these low-birth-weight infants survived in 1950, but with ventilators, surfactant, intravenous nutrition, and other gains in knowledge, survival has risen to 37% to 72% in this group.[21–23] Clearly, infants are surviving today who would not have survived to develop ROP in earlier years; these very low birth-weight survivors account for the substantial number of new cases of ROP occurring in recent years.[24–26] As a result, there has been renewed and mounting interest in the pathogenesis and therapy of ROP.[27–29]

THE ROLE OF OXYGEN

Clinical findings

Results of controlled nursery studies[5,8] that suggested supplementary oxygen to be the principal cause of ROP in the epidemic of the early 1950s were confirmed, and the role of prolonged oxygen was documented, in a collaborative randomized controlled trial.[9] Such observations were further supported by experimental findings.

Since the discovery that supplementary oxygen was a major cause of ROP in the 1950s, attempts to delineate the critical blood oxygen levels producing associated ROP have been fruitless so far. In a prospective study of 589 infants monitored by intermittent blood gas measurements, and where clinical goals were to avoid elevated arterial oxygen, the occurrence of ROP was not related to arterial oxygen levels.[30] Only the duration of oxygen exposure was a risk factor. Somewhat unexpectedly, continuous transcutaneous monitoring of blood oxygen levels has been of no more value in preventing visual disability in the smallest of these infants than intermittent monitoring.[17] It has been suggested by Lucey and Dangman[31] that therapeutic oxygen, although important, has been overemphasized as a cause of ROP under contemporary neonatal care practices.* They emphasized that other factors related to very low birth weight are probably quite important, especially in view of current nursery monitoring of oxygen. Kalina et al.,[32] and Johns et al.,[33] have even reported ROP in infants with cyanotic congenital heart disease. Birth weight is inversely related to risk of ROP[34] and is at least as good an indicator as is gestational age. With current nursery practices, ROP is truly a disorder of the "smallest and sickest" infants.

Experimental findings

In the early 1950s the laboratory kitten model was used extensively because it demonstrated selective response to oxygen by the immature retinal vessels.[6,7,35] Lesions closely resembling the early stages of human ROP were produced. In the full-term newborn kitten, the immature retinal vascularization is comparable to that of a human fetus at 6 months' gestation, thus providing the unique opportunity to study the response to oxygen of the immature retina, albeit in a full-term, healthy animal.[3] When hyperoxia studies were extended to other animal models, such as the young mouse and puppy,[6] the general concept of oxygen toxicity to immature retinal vessels was further established.

Investigators[36-37] have pointed out the histologic differences in the retinas of these animal models from the human but were unable to explain why progression to retinal detachment did not occur. It is noteworthy that McLeod, D'Anna, and Lutty reported

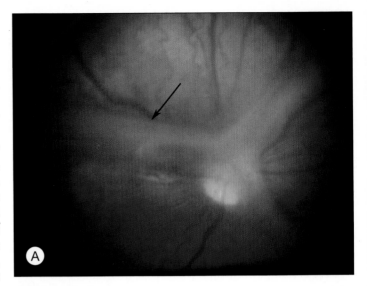

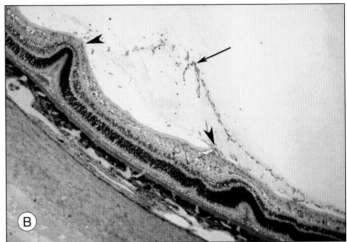

Fig. 80-1 A, Ophthalmoscopic examination of a 45-day-old dog exposed to 100% oxygen for the first 4 days of life disclosed a 2 mm wide area of retinal neovascularization (arrow) extending from the disc to the temporal midperiphery. Two similar structures are present at the 2- and 5-o'clock positions. B, Area of temporal retinal neovascularization (arrow) indicated by arrow in "A" shows mild folds in the retina (arrowheads) (periodic acid–Schiff and hematoxylin; ×50).

the production of intravitreal neovascularization with traction retinal folds in young dogs exposed to hyperoxia.[38] These findings add to the potential application of the canine model to investigate these stages of ROP (Figs 80-1 and 80-2).

The hyperoxic animal models demonstrated that only the incompletely vascularized retina was susceptible to oxygen's adverse effect, and that the more immature the vascularization, the greater the pathologic response to oxygen.[35] These findings supported the clinical observation that the infant with a less mature retina has greater susceptibility to ROP, and the infant with a fully vascularized retina has no risk of ROP. Accordingly, the temporal retina, the last part of the retina to become vascularized, remains susceptible to ROP the longest (Fig. 80-3).

---

*We agree with the conclusions in that report but do not agree with all the reasons cited by the authors. They point out that by combining data from the early clinical studies in oxygen, approximately one third of the "high-oxygen" group infants did not develop ROP. The failure to detect ROP in many of the high-oxygen group could be readily explained by the inability to view the peripheral fundus with the direct ophthalmoscope, the instrument used in studies in the early 1950s. As a result, patients with stages 1 and 2 ROP, particularly in zone III or peripheral zone II, could have been recorded as normal. Furthermore, because the majority of cases of stages 1 and 2 disease undergo spontaneous regression, ROP would not have been detected on follow-up examination.

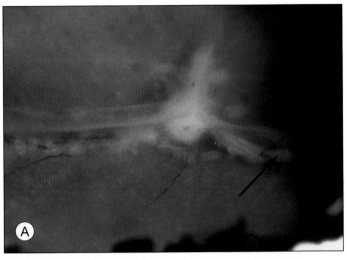
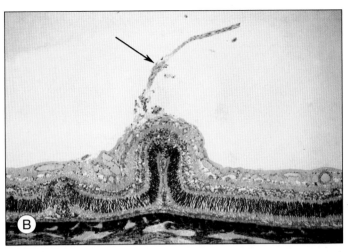

Fig. 80-2 A, Gross appearance of the areas of neovascularization extending temporally and two smaller areas in the same 45-day-old dog shown in Fig. 80-1. A denser 2 × 0.5 mm area is present inferior nasally (arrow). B, Area from "A" (marked by arrow) discloses retinal neovascularization (arrow) attached to the apex of a retinal fold (OAS and hematoxylin; ×125).

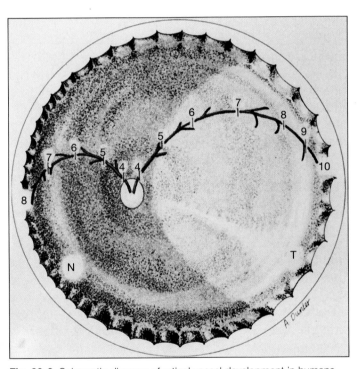

Fig. 80-3 Schematic diagram of retinal vessel development in humans. At 4 months' gestation, vessels grow from the disc to reach the ora serrata nasally at 8 months and the ora temporally shortly after term. The vascularization of the newborn kitten corresponds to the 6½-month-gestation human fetus.

MECHANISM OF OXYGEN'S EFFECTS ON THE IMMATURE RETINA

Primary stage of retinal vasoconstriction and vascular occlusion

The primary effect of elevated blood oxygen in any retina is retinal vasoconstriction, which if sustained, is followed by some degree of vascular closure.

In young kittens the initial vasoconstriction occurs within the first few minutes after oxygen exposure. The caliber of the vessels is reduced by approximately 50% initially, but then rebounds to its original dimensions. Continued oxygen exposure results in gradual vasospasm during the next 4 to 6 hours, until the vessels are approximately 80% constricted.[39] At this stage, constriction is still reversible. However, if it is sustained as a result of significantly elevated arterial oxygen partial pressure levels for an additional period (a total stay in oxygen of 10 to 15 hours), some of the more immature peripheral vessels are permanently occluded[7,40] (Fig. 80-4).

This occlusion progresses as the duration of hyperoxia increases, and local vascular obliteration is complete after 2 to 3 days of exposure. In the dog, after 4 days of exposure to hyperoxia, most capillaries are lost and only major blood vessels have survived.[41] Flower[42] suggested that the vasoconstriction might protect the neural retina from excessive oxygen pressures.

Electron microscopic observations demonstrate selective hyperoxic injury to the endothelial cells of the most immature vessels, without obvious changes in the neuronal elements of the retina.[43]

Secondary stage of retinal neovascularization

After removal of the laboratory animal to ambient air following sustained hyperoxia, a marked endothelial proliferation arises from the residual vascular complexes immediately adjacent to retinal capillaries ablated during hyperoxia (Fig. 80-5). This can be readily demonstrated on fluorescein angiography (Fig. 80-6). Nodules of proliferating endothelial cells canalize to form new vessels that not only grow within the retina, but also erupt through the internal limiting membrane to grow on its surface, similar to the neovascularization in other proliferative retinopathies (Figs 80-7 to 80-10). In the dog and cat, the initial preretinal neovascular formations are like angioblastic masses with few lumens (formations called popcorn by some), which mature

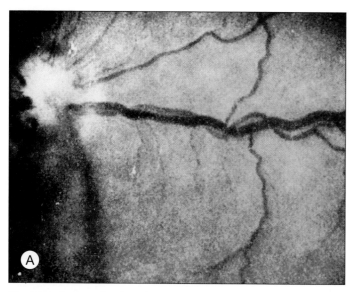
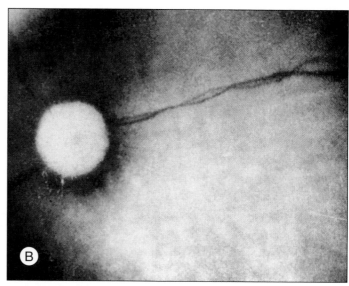

Fig. 80-4 A, Normal caliber of the retinal vessels of a 15-day-old kitten in ambient air. B, Constriction of retinal vessels in littermate of kitten in "A" after 12 hours of oxygen exposure with an arterial oxygen pressure averaging approximately 250 mm. From Patz A, Payne, JW. Retinopathy of prematurity. In: Duane TD, ed. Clinical ophthalmology. Hagerstown, Md: Lippincott, 1983

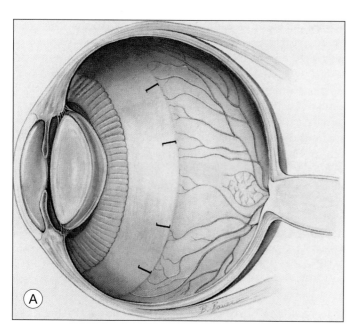
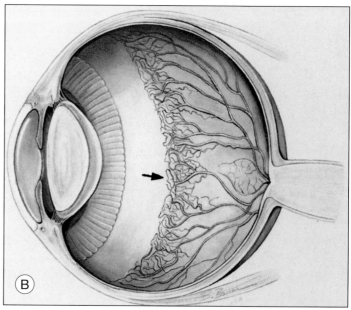

Fig. 80-5 A, Schematic diagram of vascular closure of the most anterior and immature retinal vascular bed (indicated by brackets) of a young kitten exposed to hyperoxia for a relatively short period. The posterior, more mature vessels are unaffected. B, Three weeks after removal of the subject in "A" to ambient air. Neovascularization has developed immediately posterior to the area of capillary closure (arrow). Part B from Patz A et al. Am J Ophthalmol 1954; 38:291.

into neovascular formations that include vessels invested with pericytes.[44,45] Small hemorrhages occur frequently in the area of neovascularization. Although the neovascularization may be extensive, this is generally the maximum response to oxygen in the kitten model and is followed by progressive vascular remodeling and involution of abnormalities. The preretinal neovascularization in the dog persists and can develop into tented membranes which create tractional retinal folds in the retina (Figs 80-1 and 80-2).[38] The mouse and rat preretinal neovascular formations,

however, will regress after 5 days.[39,46–48] Even though regression is rapid and spontaneous in mice, the mouse model has been very useful in evaluating topical[49] and systemic drugs,[50–52] experimental gene therapy strategies[53–55] and endogenous inhibitors like pigment epithelial growth factor.[56]

Oxygen exerts an important effect on the remodeling of the original primitive capillary network that develops in the retina.[57] Capillaries regress from areas of higher oxygen concentration and grow toward areas of lower oxygen. Penn et al.[58] have used

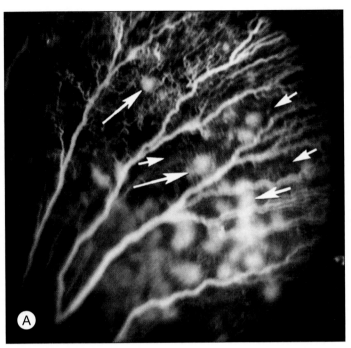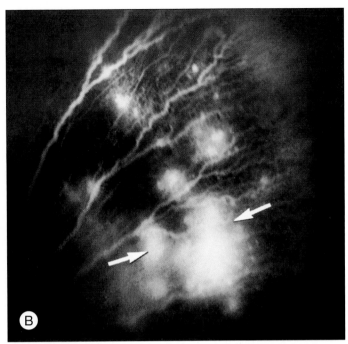

Fig. 80-6 A, Fluorescein angiogram of a young kitten with oxygen-induced retinal neovascularization (arrows); midtransit phase of angiogram. B, Late phase of angiogram of young kitten in "A". Note dye leakage from neovascularization (arrows).

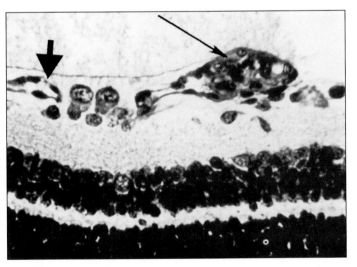

Fig. 80-7 Cross section of the eye of a 21-day-old mouse exposed to hyperoxia. Normal capillary is seen just posterior to the area of vascular closure (short arrow); an endothelial nodule proliferating from the most anterior part of the vascularized retina is erupting through the internal limiting membrane (long arrow). From Patz A, Eastham A, Higginbotham DH, Kleh T. Oxygen studies in retrolental fibroplasia. II. The production of the microscopic changes of retrolental fibroplasia in experimental animals. Am J Ophthalmol 1953; 36:1511–1522.

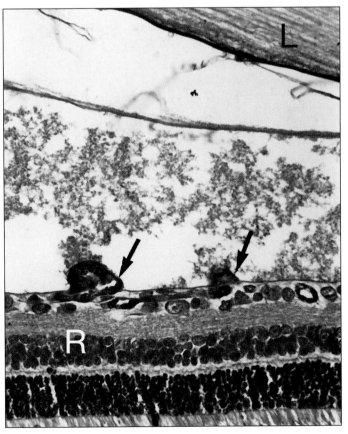

Fig. 80-8 Cross section of the eye of a young mouse exposed to hyperoxia showing neovascularization on the surface of the retina just posterior to the zone of capillary closure (arrows). R, Anterior retina; L, lens. From Patz A. Am J Ophthalmol 1982; 94:715.

experimentally alternating periods of high and low oxygen in the rat pup model to produce a more proliferative form of retinopathy. Pierce and colleagues[28] have used hyperoxia and hypoxia in a mouse pup model to demonstrate the correlation of vascular endothelial growth factor (VEGF) protein production with periods of low oxygen, as well as its disappearance after

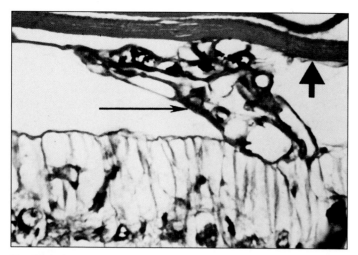

Fig. 80-9 Cross-section of the retina of a young kitten exposed to hyperoxia. Intravitreal neovascularization is seen just posterior to the zone of capillary closure (long arrow). Short arrow, lens capsule. From Patz A et al. Am J Ophthalmol 1954; 38:291.

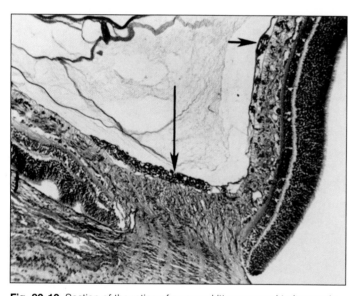

Fig. 80-10 Section of the retina of a young kitten exposed to hyperoxia. Neovascularization is seen over the surface of the disc (long arrow). Short arrow indicates small nodules of surface neovascularization. From Patz A et al. Am J Ophthalmol 1954; 38:291.

oxygenation. Although it is apparent that VEGF most closely fits the identity of Michaelson's proposed Factor X,[59,60] targeting VEGF or its receptors as a therapy for proliferative retinopathy has not yet resulted in complete inhibition of preretinal neovascularization in animal models.[61–63] This suggests that other growth factors, such as adenosine[64,65] and IGF-1,[66,67] may be involved as well.

PATHOGENESIS

Normal retinal vasculogenesis

It is appropriate to review briefly the normal vascular development of the retina as background for understanding the patho-

genesis of ROP. Michaelson[59] originally suggested that retinal capillaries arise by budding from preexistent arteries and veins that originate from the hyaloid vessels at the optic nerve head. Cogan[68,69] proposed a similar mechanism, except for the hypothesis of budding of solid endothelial cords from the hyaloid vessels. Ashton[48] suggested that the mesenchyme, the blood vessel precursor, grows from the optic disc through the nerve fiber layer to the periphery of the retina. Mesenchymal precursors have recently been observed far in advance of formed blood vessels in human fetal retinas.[69A] On the posterior edge of the advancing mesenchyme, a "chicken-wire" meshwork of capillaries develops. This fine meshwork of vessels undergoes absorption and remodeling to produce mature arteries and veins in the retina that are surrounded by the capillary meshwork.[48,57] Variations in the development of the capillaries may be species-specific. However, across all species studied to date, VEGF now appears to be a key growth factor in guiding vessel growth and, as previously stated, most closely fits the identity of Michaelson's proposed Factor X.[59,60] In the kitten, Chan-Ling and Stone have demonstrated the role of astrocytes leading to the growth of the capillary network.[70–72] In addition, Provis et al.[73] have demonstrated the expression of VEGF message in the predicted location in the developing normal human retina, just anterior to the developing vessels (Fig. 80-11).

Fig. 80-12 shows the normal rate of progression of the retinal vessels into the far retinal periphery in human premature infants without ROP according to their "postconceptional age (gestational age at birth plus chronologic age)." More than 80% of prematurely born infants have been observed to develop this relatively mature retinal vasculature by the time they reach their due date. In contrast, only about half of them will have matured to this degree 4 weeks earlier in their development.[34]

Pathogenesis of ROP

The description of the mechanism of oxygen's effects given previously points out the initial changes in the developing vessels, and that historically this was believed to be an injury caused by "excess" oxygen. Alon et al. demonstrated that hyperoxia caused downregulation of VEGF and death of endothelial cells, suggesting that VEGF is an endothelial survival factor.[74] In the time that follows closure of these growing vessels, the differentiating retina becomes increasingly ischemic and hypoxic and VEGF is upregulated[75–77] driving the neovascularization.[71]

Theoretically the provision of increased oxygen should downregulate the release of such growth factor(s) and permit the neovascularization to remodel and regress in an orderly fashion. Szewczyk[77] proposed just this; he treated infants with significant ROP by returning them to oxygen and gradually weaning it thereafter. With no controls, it is difficult to know from his report if this success was due to the well-known propensity for spontaneous involution of ROP. This hypothesis was tested in the kitten model of oxygen-induced retinopathy. Systemic mild hypoxia (lowered oxygen) was found to worsen the retinopathy,[78] whereas mild hyperoxia improved it.[79] Similar results have been demonstrated in a mouse model,[28] where VEGF is clearly one of the major growth factors involved. With NIH sponsorship, a

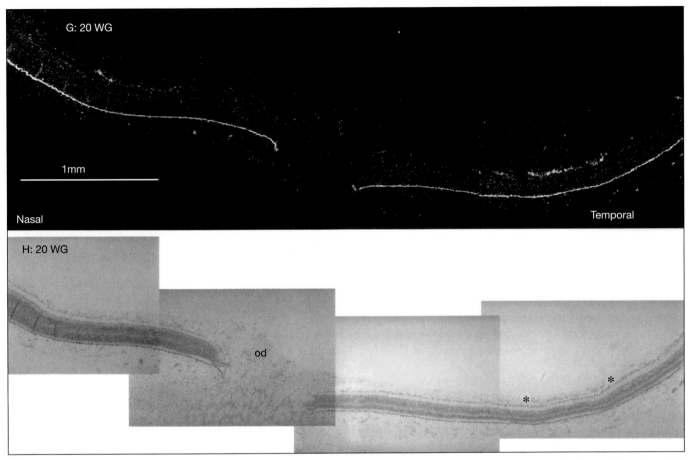

Fig. 80-11 VEGF mRNA expression in the human fetal retina. Bright (H) and dark-field (G) views of the retina in cross-section from a 20-week gestation human fetus. In dark-field illumination the RPE is prominent. Note the greater differentiation of the retinal layers in the section to the right (temporal) of the optic disc. The vascular layer lies superficially, VEGF mRNA expression being limited to the most distal portion of that vasculature (G), indicated in the light-field image (H) by asterisks. From Provis JM, Leech J, Diaz CM et al. Exp Eye Res 1997; 65:555–568.

multicenter clinical trial chaired by Dale L. Phelps studied this concept in the nursery. Results showed that once the ROP was established, raising the oxygen saturation mildly did not harm the ROP, but neither was it of clear benefit.[80] In general, the study showed no statistical difference in the progression to severe ROP between the two oxygen treatment regimens that were tested.[80]

The clinical and histopathologic observations of Flynn and co-workers[81–86] led them to postulate the following sequence of events in the development of ROP in human infants:

1. Injury to the endothelium occurs where it has just differentiated from mesenchyme to form the primitive capillary meshwork. This is reminiscent of the animal studies in which a short duration of hyperoxia resulted in capillary damage limited to the most recently differentiated vascular complexes (see Fig. 80-5A). It is currently believed that environmental factors other than oxygen also are involved. Recent work from Brooks and associates suggests that nitric oxide and subsequent formation of peroxynitrite can contribute to the vaso-obliterative stage of ROP.[87] The work of Alon et al. suggests that reduced VEGF

results in death of endothelial cells[74] because of its role as a survival factor. It is probable that all of these contribute to the vaso-attenuation that occurs in hyperoxia.

2. After injury to the vascular endothelium by some noxious agent(s), the mesenchyme and the mature arteries and veins survive and merge via the few remaining vascular channels to form a mesenchymal arteriovenous shunt. The shunt replaces the destroyed or damaged capillary bed.

3. The mesenchymal arteriovenous shunt is located at the demarcation between the avascular anterior retina and the vascularized posterior retina. It consists of a nest of primitive mesenchymal and maturing endothelial cells that are fed by mature arteries and veins. No capillaries are found in the region of the shunt. Flynn[83] suggested that this structure represents the pathognomonic lesion of acute ROP.

Flynn described a dormant period after the injury, which may last from several days to months, during which the retinal findings are relatively stable. The tissues comprising the shunt may thicken, and the gray-white initial color of the structure turns from pink to salmon to red. He stated: ". . . during this period when

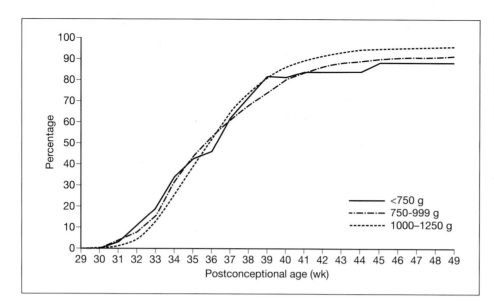

Fig. 80-12 Cumulative proportion of infants with no retinopathy of prematurity whose vessels end in zone III, by postconceptional age. From Palmer EA, Flynn JT, Hardy RJ et al. for the Cryotherapy for Retinopathy of Prematurity Cooperative Group. Incidence and early course of retinopathy of prematurity. Ophthalmology 1991; 98:1628–1640.

vasculogenic activity resumes in the retina, the fate of the eye is decided."[83] Flynn pointed out that when the cells inside the shunt divide and differentiate into normal capillary endothelium, they form primitive endothelial tubes that send forth a "brush" border of capillaries that grows anteriorly into the avascular retina. This represents involution of ROP, which he observed to occur in more than 90% of cases at this early stage.

In progressive disease, however, the primitive cells inside the shunt proliferate and erupt through the internal limiting membrane, growing on the surface of the retina and into the vitreous body. Flynn stated: "it is this lack of differentiation and destructive proliferation of cells and their invasion into spaces and tissues where they do not belong that is the chief event in the process of membrane proliferation leading to traction detachment."[83]

Foos[88–90] suggested a pathogenesis of ROP based on examination of histopathologic material. He used the terms *vanguard* and *rearguard* to describe the cellular components of the developing retina. The vanguard, or anterior component, contains spindle-shaped cells thought to be glia, which play a role in nourishing the immature retina during its development.[69,91–93] The rearguard

contains primitive endothelial cells. As the retina matures, the endothelial cells aggregate into cords that, according to Foos,[90] subsequently lumenize and become the primordial capillaries of the retina. It is from the rearguard and primitive endothelial cells that the neovascularization of ROP will develop (Figs 80-13 and 79-14). Foos noted that as the developing vasculature reaches its most anterior extent and matures, the spindle cells of the vanguard disappear. The work of Chan-Ling et al.,[69A] Kretzer et al.,[94] McLeod et al.,[95] and Provis et al.[73] showed that spindle cells are endothelial precursors and, in fetal human and neonatal dog retina,[95] the precursors organize and differentiate to form the initial retinal vasculature.[69A]

INTERNATIONAL CLASSIFICATION

The international classification of ROP clinically divides the retina into three anteroposterior zones and describes the extent of disease by the 30-degree meridians (hours of the clock) involved (Fig. 80-15). Retinal changes are divided into stages of severity, based on descriptive and photographic standards.[96]

Zones of involved retina

Each of the three zones of the retina is centered on the optic disc, instead of the macula, as is the usual practice for standard retinal drawings (Fig. 80-15). Zone I is the posterior pole, or inner zone. It is a circle, centered on the disc, whose radius is twice the distance from the disc to the macula. It subtends an arc of about 60 degrees (Fig. 80-16). Zone II extends from the peripheral border of zone I to a concentric circle tangential to the nasal ora serrata. Temporally, this imaginary boundary corresponds approximately to the anatomic equator. Once the nasal vessels have reached the ora serrata, zone III is the remaining temporal crescent of retina anterior to zone II. Zone III, which is the farthest from the disc, is the last zone to become vascularized. It is clinically very important to continue classifying ROP as zone II as long as there remains any active ROP or any nonvascularized retina

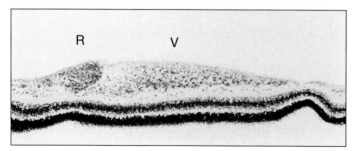

Fig. 80-13 Retinopathy of prematurity, stage 2, in a 27-week stillborn infant, showing meridional section through the retinal ridge, with a thick layer of spindle cells that tapers anteriorly (to the right), representing the proliferative vanguard zone (V). Nodule of proliferating endothelial cells is seen in the rearguard zone (R). From Foos RY. Retinopathy of prematurity – pathologic correlation of clinical stages. Retina 1987; 7:260–276.

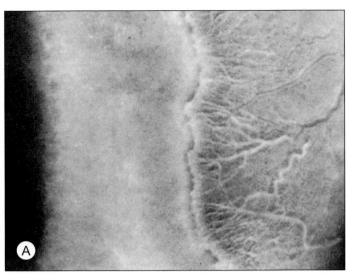
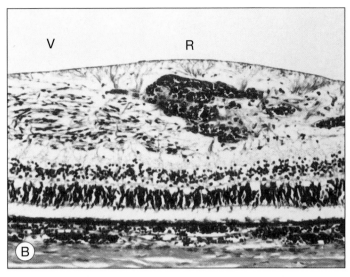

Fig. 80-14 A, Retinopathy of prematurity, stage 2 specimen from a 29-week-old infant. Photomicrograph shows moderately elevated ridge, with tortuosity of retinal vessels posterior to ridge. B, Photomicrograph of ridge in eye from "A" with posterior aspect of a thickened vanguard zone (V) and conspicuous vasodilation of rearguard zone (R), which has been characterized clinically as an arteriovenous shunt. From Foos RY. Retinopathy of prematurity – pathologic correlation of clinical stages. Retina 1987; 7:260–276.

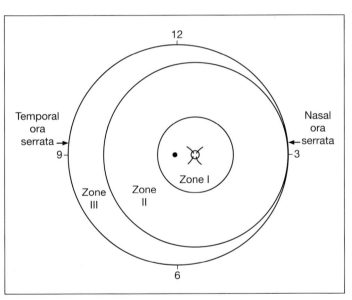

Fig. 80-15 Schematic diagram of a right eye, showing zones of the retina and clock hours used to describe the location and extent of retinopathy of prematurity.

on the nasal side near the horizontal meridian. As a precaution, the clinician should *always err on the side of more posterior zoning* because the more posterior the zone of involvement, the worse the prognosis.[97]

Extent of retinopathy of prematurity

The extent of the ROP changes is described according to the twelve 30-degree sectors involved, labeled as hours of the clock (Fig. 80-15): the nasal side of the right eye is at 3:00, and the nasal side of the left eye is at 9:00.

Staging

The abnormal vascular changes are divided into three stages (Fig. 80-17), and may progress to retinal detachment (Stages 4 and 5) (Fig. 80-18).

Stage 1: Demarcation line

Stage 1 is characterized by the presence of a demarcation line, the first pathognomonic ophthalmoscopic sign of ROP (Fig. 70-17A).

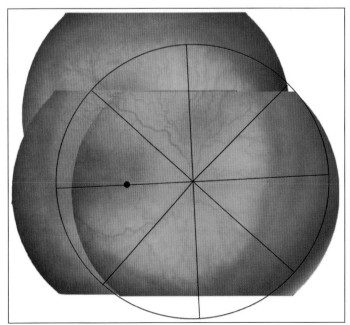

Fig. 80-16 Zone 1 grid overlaid on a montage of RetCam photos: black dot represents foveal center. Diameter of circle is twice the distance from the disc to the fovea. This illustration demonstrates how ROP may involve both Zones I and II in the same eye.

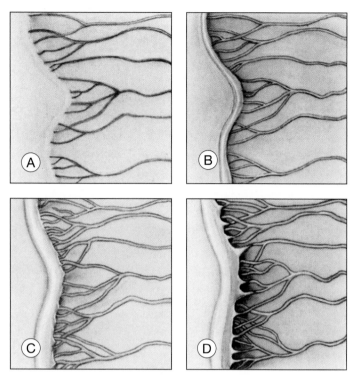

Fig. 80-17 Diagrams modified from color photographs of the international classification of retinopathy of prematurity. Vascularized, more mature retina is seen to the right and avascular retina to the left in the diagrams. A, The demarcation line of stage 1. B, The characteristic ridge of stage 2 is noted. C, Extraretinal fibrovascular proliferative tissue of "mild" stage 3. D, "Moderate" proliferation of extraretinal fibrovascular tissue from the ridge in more advanced stage 3. Modified from Reference 96.

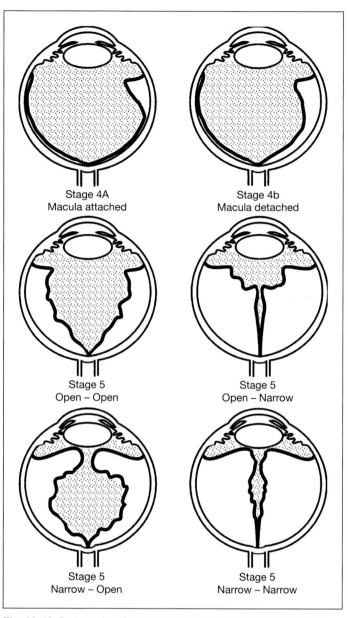

Fig. 80-18 Retinopathy of prematurity detachment configurations. Top two = 4a and b detachments. Bottom four = stage 5. Courtesy Rand Spencer, MD.

This line represents a structure separating the anterior, avascular retina from the posterior, vascularized retina. It is essentially flat and white and lies within the plane of the retina. Abnormal branching or arcading of vessels leads up to the line in many cases. (Stage 1 is relatively evanescent, generally either progressing to stage 2 or involuting to normal vascularization within a week or so.)

Stage 2: Ridge

In stage 2, the demarcation line of stage 1 has grown. It now has height and width, occupies a volume, and extends centripetally within the globe (Fig. 80-17B). The ridge may be white or pink and, rarely, vessels may even leave the surface of the retina to enter it. Small tufts of new vessels ("popcorn" lesions) may be seen located posterior to the ridge structure but not attached to the ridge. The absence of fibrovascular growth from the surface of the ridge separates this stage from stage 3.

Stage 3: Ridge with extraretinal fibrovascular proliferation

Stage 3 is characterized by the addition of extraretinal, fibrovascular tissue proliferating from the formerly stage 2 ridge (Fig. 80-17C and D). This proliferating tissue is localized continuous with the posterior and interior aspect of the ridge, causing a ragged appearance of the ridge as proliferation increases

into the vitreous. As in stage 2, vessels may leave the surface of the retina to enter the ridge and could be mistaken for retinoschisis or even detachment. The presence of elevated retinal vessels coursing from the retinal surface to the height of the ridge does not alone constitute a retinal detachment[96]; however, this could signify the presence of vitreous traction.

Stage 4: Subtotal retinal detachment

Stage 4 is characterized by the presence of a partial but definite retinal detachment (Fig 80-18, top pair) added to the findings of stage 3 ROP. Most commonly the retinal elevation is tractional in nature, although occasionally there may be some exudative effusion of fluid, or traction, or both, from active adjacent stage 3 neovascularization. The further classification of retinal detachment follows the next sections on the international classification.

"Plus" disease

Plus disease signifies a more florid form of ROP. Increasing dilation and tortuosity of the retinal vessels, iris vascular engorgement, pupillary rigidity, and vitreous haze indicate progressive vascular incompetence. When the vascular changes are so marked that the posterior veins are enlarged and the arterioles tortuous, this represents plus disease, and a plus sign is added to the ROP stage number. This finding is a key sign of worse prognosis.[98] The only standard photograph, which has been used in four multicenter clinical trials, is shown in Fig. 80-19A.

Zone 1 ROP

The appearance of ROP that is located in zone I can be dangerously deceptive, in that the proliferation signifying stage 3 can be spread out "flat" on the retina posterior to the ridge, rather than elevated.[34] In severe plus disease cases inside zone I, centripetal proliferation from the ridge may occur virtually simultaneously with detachment of the retina.

Classification of retinal detachment

In 1987, ophthalmologists and pathologists established a second international committee for the classification of the late stages of ROP.[99] This supersedes an earlier classification of Reese et al.,[100] and expands the basic international classification published in 1984. The classification of retinal detachment is based on an understanding of the development of the more severe stages of ROP gained from surgical experience[101,102] and from the study of pathologic material.[90] The features of the retinal detachment (stage 4 and 5) of the 1984 classification are elaborated. The term *cicatricial* from Reese's[100] classification is eliminated because traction detachment of the retina may have exudative features. The classification employs the same parameters of location and extent of disease described earlier. The focus is on the morphology, location, and extent of the retinal detachment (see Fig. 80-18).

Stage 4A: Extrafoveal retinal detachment

Typically this is a concave, traction type of detachment that occurs in the periphery without involvement of the central macula (Fig. 80-20). Generally, these detachments are located at the sites of extraretinal fibrovascular proliferation (EFP) where there is vitreous traction. These areas of elevation may start in any zone where there was stage 3 disease that incompletely involuted following ablative treatment with laser photocoagulation or cryotherapy, and they may become circumferential. On occasion they may extend for 360 degrees in the periphery without elevation of the macula, or they may be segmental, occupying only a portion of the circumference of the periphery. The prognosis anatomically and visually is relatively good in the absence of posterior extension. Frequently these areas of peripheral detachment will reattach spontaneously and not affect macular function.

Stage 4B: Partial retinal detachment including the fovea

This can follow extension of stage 4A, or may appear as a fold from the disc through zone I to zones II and III (Fig. 80-21). Once a stage 4 detachment involves the fovea, the prognosis for recovery of good visual acuity is poor.

Stage 5: Total retinal detachment

This is virtually always funnel shaped. The classification of stage 5 detachments divides the funnel into an anterior and a posterior part (refer to Fig. 80-18). When open both anteriorly and posteriorly, the detachment has a concave configuration and extends to the optic disc. An alternative configuration is one in which the funnel is narrow in both its anterior and posterior aspects, and the detached retina is located just behind the lens. A third, less common type is one in which the funnel is open anteriorly but narrowed posteriorly. Least common is a funnel that is

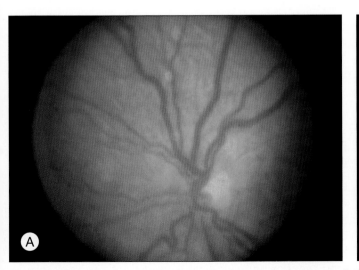
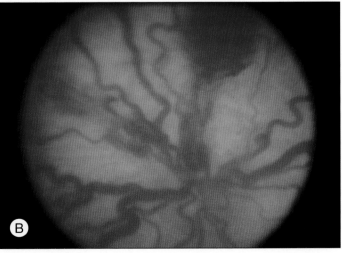

Fig. 80-19 Plus disease examples. A, Fundus photograph of minimum dilation and tortuosity of retinal vessels considered as plus disease in NIH studies of ROP. B, Fundus appearance of an extremely severe degree of posterior pole plus disease in an eye that soon developed total retinal detachment. Part A from Cryotherapy for Retinopathy of Prematurity Cooperative Group: Multicenter trial of cryotherapy for retinopathy of prematurity: preliminary results. Arch Ophthalmol 1988; 106:471–479; Part B courtesy Ophthalmic Photography, Oregon Health & Science University, Portland.

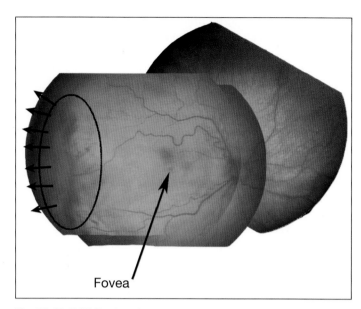

Fig. 80-20 ROP Fundus photo montage of right eye showing elevation of retina posterior to incompletely regressed stage 3 ROP with vitreous traction (arrows). Oval approximates area of retinal detachment.

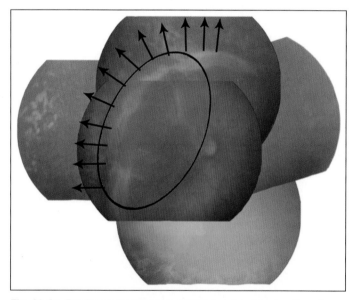

Fig. 80-21 Fundus photo montage of right eye showing elevation of retina posterior to fibrotic ridge of incompletely regressed stage 3 ROP. Arrows away from ridge indicate vectors of vitreous traction elevating ridge and adjacent retina, including the macula. Oval approximates area of retinal detachment.

narrow anteriorly and open posteriorly. The configuration of the funnel-shaped detachment can sometimes be appreciated by ultrasonography.

Other factors

The classification of retinal detachment in ROP focuses attention on certain physical findings in stages 4 and 5.

1. The appearance of the retrolenticular space. This space may be occupied by heavily vascularized translucent tissue, which represents disease activity. As the disease subsides, the tissue occupying this space becomes white, with a scarcity of blood vessels. This is the appearance that gave rise to the term "retrolental fibroplasia" formerly used to describe ROP.

2. Peripheral trough. The presence of a peripheral red reflex in combination with apparent narrow funnel stage 5 retinal detachment indicates the presence of attached or shallowly detached avascular, stretched, and nonfunctioning peripheral retina. Occasionally, we have seen a peripheral red reflex coming from choroid beneath detached retina that has become adherent to the posterior lens capsule.

3. Anterior segment. The anterior segment may be involved in the more severe stages of ROP. The changes in the anterior segment are described as follows:

    (a) Shallow anterior chamber and corneal edema. A relatively shallow anterior chamber may be a normal early finding in a premature infant's eye; however, when a progressively shallow anterior chamber develops along with a retinal detachment in ROP, it has serious implications. Some cases progress to acute angle-closure glaucoma or to a flat chamber and corneal decompensation. Even in eyes with only partial retinal detachment, we have seen angle-closure glaucoma occur over the years after the acute phases of ROP have involuted. (See later section on glaucoma.)

    (b) Iris abnormalities. Posterior synechiae, iris atrophy, and ectropion uveae are common formations in eyes with stage 4 or 5 ROP. Particularly in eyes with stage 5 disease, the iris may become rigid and the pupil difficult to dilate because of adhesions to the anterior lens capsule and persistence of the pupillary membrane with retention of its vascular network. Rarely, the pupil can seclude, leading to iris bombé and angle closure. (See later section on glaucoma.) Posterior synechiae are less common and usually less extensive in eyes with stage 4 disease.

4. Other tissues. Subretinal blood and exudate may be identifiable by ultrasonographic examination but can be difficult to distinguish from one another. Subretinal fibrotic membranes may be present but usually are recognized only during surgery.

PATHOGENESIS CORRELATED WITH CLINICAL CLASSIFICATION

Garner[103] reviewed the pathology of ROP, considering the observations of Flynn and Foos, to provide a useful correlation of the histopathologic changes with the clinical description of the stages of ROP. According to Garner, the demarcation line of stage 1 ROP morphologically comprises two relatively distinct zones. The more anterior vanguard zone is formed by a mass of spindle-shaped cells, which are the progenitors of the differentiated vascular endothelium. As such it corresponds to the primitive mesenchyme (spindle cells) seen in normal fetal development but with a considerable increase in the number of cells. It is this hyperplasia, involving both thickening and widening, that makes the demarcation line visible.[103]

The demarcation line, according to Garner, is "devoid of functioning capillaries."[103] As already mentioned, the rearguard zone of endothelial cells will be the source of the subsequent neovascularization (vasoproliferation).

According to Garner, the retinal ridge that characterizes stage 2 results from the proliferation of endothelial cells "with some evidence of organization into recognizable vascular channels."[103] Flynn et al.[85] demonstrated that in this stage these channels leak fluorescein on angiographic examination.

According to Foos,[90] the stage 3 "extraretinal vascularization" may appear histologically as placoid, polypoid, or pedunculated. The placoid pattern is the most common and also the most important because it correlates with subsequent development of retinal detachment. Foos demonstrated that these extraretinal vessels are apparently derived from proliferating endothelial cells and not from the vasoformative mesenchymal "spindle" cells based on his factor VIII preparations. He also observed significant synchisis and condensation of the vitreous body in stage 3. Foos suggested that a condensation of the vitreous body over the ridge is related to depolymerization of hyaluronic acid and collapse of the collagenous framework into optically visible structures.[90]

INVOLUTION OF RETINOPATHY OF PREMATURITY

Involution of ROP typically begins at 38.6 weeks postconceptional/postmenstrual age, and may be characterized by a downgrading of staging and/or growth of retinal vessels into a more peripheral zone.[104]

Regressed ROP

Although active ROP usually involutes without progressing to retinal detachment, cicatricial sequelae can remain even in those cases.[97,105] The relatively stable state of the eye that exists after retinopathy has run its course is referred to as regressed ROP. In Box 80-1 the residual changes have been classified into those affecting the retinal periphery and those affecting the posterior fundus. Each location has been further subdivided to describe separately the vascular alterations and the residual retinal changes. The retinal pigmentary changes can be mistaken for side effects of treatment.[105a]

The most serious complications of regressed ROP are the late development of retinal detachment and angle-closure glaucoma. At almost any age after the neonatal period, but especially several years after birth, retinal detachment remains a definite risk in eyes with sequelae from ROP. Eyes with high myopia, peripheral retinal pigmentary changes or lattice-like degeneration, vitreoretinal interface changes, vitreous condensation, and stretching and folding of the retina are at special risk of developing retinal breaks and detachment. Eyes with partial retinal detachment present at about 3 months after threshold retinopathy remain at risk for progression of the detachment.[106] The greater the detachment at 3 months, the worse outcomes tended to be.

Box 80-1 Regressed retinopathy of prematurity

Peripheral changes

Vascular
Failure to vascularize peripheral retina
Abnormal, nondichotomous branching of retinal vessels
Vascular arcades with circumferential interconnection
Telangiectatic vessels

Retinal
Pigmentary changes
Vitreoretinal interface changes
Thin retina
Peripheral folds
Vitreous membranes with or without attachment to retina
Lattice-like degeneration
Retinal breaks
Traction or rhegmatogenous retinal detachment

Posterior changes

Vascular
Vascular tortuosity
Straightening of blood vessels in temporal arcade
Abnormal narrowing or widening in the angle of insertion of major temporal arcade

Retinal
Pigmentary changes
Distortion and ectopia of macula
Stretching and folding of retina in macular region leading to periphery
Vitreoretinal interface changes
Vitreous membrane
Dragging of retina over disc

Overall visual outcomes for 61 eyes studied were poor; only six eyes had better than 20/200 visual acuity.[106] As a precautionary measure, these patients and their parents should be alert to the symptoms of retinal detachment as soon as the child is old enough to appreciate and report them.

As discussed previously, the ophthalmologist should be aware of the risk of angle-closure glaucoma developing later in life in patients with regressed ROP. These patients, too, should be advised of this risk and alerted to the possible symptoms.

Patients with regressed ROP are at risk for developing strabismus and amblyopia early in life.[107–112] In the CRYO-ROP study, 200 (6.6%) of 3030 infants who had weighed less than 1251 g at birth were strabismic at the 3-month examination. (An additional 206 infants who had been examined at 3 months had developed strabismus by the 12-month examination, so the total prevalence of strabismus in the first year of life was 14.7%.) When the group of infants with no ROP was compared with those with ROP, ROP was found to be a significant predictor of strabismus at 3 months. Subgroup analysis determined that the risk for strabismus increased as the zone of ROP became more posterior and the stage more severe. Irrespective of ROP history, strabismus at 3 months strongly predicted the presence of strabismus at 12 months. Regular examinations and attention to refractive, visual, and extraocular muscle status are indicated for all infants who have had ROP until about age 18 months, and thereafter as clinically indicated.[113]

History of prematurity

Whenever there is a history of prematurity, especially with very low birth weight, careful examination is recommended to rule out any evidence of regressed ROP. This should be done regardless of the presenting age of the patient. Particular attention should be given to the temporal periphery of the retina in view of its predilection for ROP changes and its relatively greater potential effects on macular vision. When the patient has significant myopia – especially dating back to early childhood – and a history of prematurity, the diagnosis of regressed ROP should be considered; the following section is relevant to this.

Other ocular findings of regressed retinopathy of prematurity

Myopia

In very low birth weight infants who are born weighing less than 1251 g, 20% develop myopia in the first 2 years of life. The lower the birth weight, the higher the chance of myopia. In addition, among infants with ROP, the incidence of myopia increases in direct relationship to the severity of ROP; for example, in patients who develop zone II, stage 3 ROP (without plus disease), 44% to 45% are myopic at 12 and 24 months postterm. In contrast, infants of this same birth weight group who never develop ROP have a 13% incidence of myopia.[114]

The exact mechanism of the myopia remains somewhat obscure. Fletcher and Brandon[115] suggested that it might be due to an elongation of the globe, alteration of the lens or the corneal curvature, or a combination of these factors. Between 6% to 7% of patients with ROP have high myopia of 5 D or more, compared with about 1% of otherwise comparable premature infants with no ROP.[114] Tasman[116,117] noted that patients with the highest degree of myopia had a significantly greater complication rate of retinal detachments in later years. We have adopted the practice of questioning every new patient with moderate to high degrees of myopia regarding a past history of prematurity and have detected several previously unsuspected cases of regressed ROP.

Other refractive and binocular defects

Kushner[107,118] reported an increase in astigmatism and anisometropia in regressed ROP. In the multicenter trial of cryotherapy for ROP (CRYO-ROP), 2518 infants born weighing less than 1251 g were refracted 12 months postterm, and 3.3% had anisometropia. Of the 1548 who had ROP of some degree, 4.8% had anisometropia.[114] Approximately 20% of ROP cases are asymmetric at the time they reach threshold for treatment, and this asymmetry may well contribute to anisometropia. Amblyopia, nystagmus, and strabismus are also common after ROP has regressed.[107,109,113,118,119]

Lens and corneal changes

At the 12-month examination of the CRYO-ROP study, there was an overall incidence of cataract of 0.3% in the natural history population. The incidence of cataract among eyes with a history of zone I ROP or zone II stage 3+ ROP was approximately 2.5%.[120] Kushner[118] pointed out that the early development of cataract may seriously compromise vision in the presence of retinal abnormalities. Furthermore, the development of a cataract, if left unoperated because of the associated impaired vision resulting from retinal changes, could produce phacolytic glaucoma if allowed to mature. Results can be quite satisfactory from cataract surgery in adults with a history of ROP.[120A] Patients with ROP also have an increased risk of developing keratoconus, irregularities of corneal curvature, band keratopathy, and acute hydrops.[121,122]

GLAUCOMA IN RETINOPATHY OF PREMATURITY

Glaucoma is a serious complication of ROP in both the acute and regressed phases of the disease. The glaucoma in many of these patients is amenable to treatment, and in some instances, preventable.

Glaucoma in patients with advanced retinopathy

Patients with advanced retinopathy who develop a shallow anterior chamber occasionally develop acute or subacute glaucoma later. In the CRYO-ROP study,[123] it was found that 20.3% of 195 patients who developed ROP of the threshold severity for entry into the randomized trial developed shallow anterior chambers in the control eye that did not receive cryotherapy, compared with 12% in the eye that received cryotherapy, when examined at about 12 months postterm. By this time, 1.5% of those control eyes had been noted to have glaucoma.[124]

In some cases these patients may respond to topical steroids and cycloplegic agents.[125] This complication, which does not always look typical of iris bombé, may occur at any time: in the nursery, shortly after discharge, and throughout childhood. Because of this complication, parents should be cautioned to consult an ophthalmologist if the child appears to be having sudden discomfort and apparent irritation of the eye. Where feasible, the parents also may be instructed to recognize the appearance of corneal haze and episcleral injection.

Diagnosis and management of glaucoma in advanced ROP is a major challenge, and ophthalmologists and the patient's family should realize that this complication could occur. There is the possibility that subacute glaucoma can go unrecognized and result in total loss of useful vision. We should strive to alert the family to this possibility without imposing a burden of anxiety on them. They should be encouraged to seek ophthalmic consultation without hesitation, because the change in appearance of the eye may be fairly subtle even when the pressure is markedly elevated. Major loss of vision could occur as a result of the glaucoma in patients who still have some useful vision with partial retinal detachment. A trial of topical steroids and cycloplegic agents is recommended in suitable cases of glaucoma in the setting of ocular damage from ROP,[125] and further glaucoma management may be required.

Angle-closure glaucoma in regressed retinopathy of prematurity

Johnson and Swan[126] reported that eyes with regressed ROP are at increased risk of developing acute angle-closure glaucoma.

This complication was also reported by Pollard[127] and by Smith, and Shivitz.[128] The risk extends into adulthood. We have observed several of these cases and have followed children and young adults with regressed ROP who, between regular ophthalmic examinations, developed angle-closure glaucoma. In the previous edition of this chapter, Arnall Patz MD, described two separate cases of adult patients, 20 and 30 years old respectively, who had had uneventful, full dilation of the pupils accomplished repeatedly over a period of several years. For each of these patients, laser iridotomy was used successfully in the eye with elevated pressure, and prophylactic iridotomy was done uneventfully in each patient's fellow eye (Figs 80-22 and 80-23). Rarely, lensectomy is required to resolve the angle closure.[129]

Kushner[125,130] pointed out that certain patients with mild degrees of regressed ROP have a predilection for developing ciliary block glaucoma. Because this form of glaucoma may be treatable by surgery in selected cases, the ophthalmologist should be aware of this potential complication and of its management. Many patients are unaware of the risk and are not receiving regular ophthalmologic care.[118] Patients and their families should be advised of this risk and also alerted to the symptoms of acute angle-closure glaucoma.

DIFFERENTIAL DIAGNOSIS

Since the turn of the century, diagnosing ROP is rarely a problem in an infant or child with a history of premature birth and/or

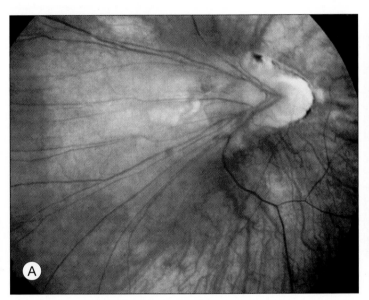
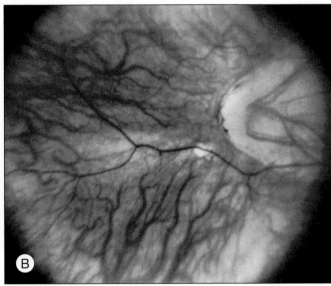

Fig. 80-22 A, Fundus photograph of the right eye of a 33-year-old patient with regressed retinopathy of prematurity. Note dragging of disc and heterotopia of the macula. B, Left eye of patient in "A" with similar findings. At age 33 years the patient developed acute narrow-angle glaucoma in the left eye, which was successfully treated by laser iridotomy. Prophylactic iridotomy was performed on the right eye.

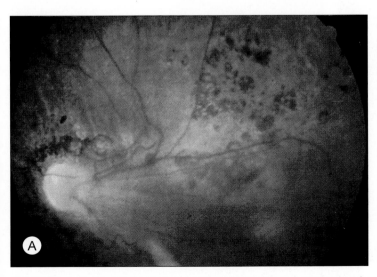
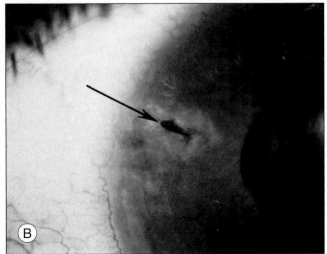

Fig. 80-23 A, Fundus photograph of a patient with regressed retinopathy of prematurity. Note dragging of vessels across the disc and heterotopia of the macula. The patient developed acute narrow-angle glaucoma at the age of 20 years. B, Laser iridotomy (arrow) controlled the acute angle-closure attack, and a prophylactic iridotomy also was performed successfully in the fellow eye.

low birth weight, because of the ophthalmological consultations that likely would have been performed during the newborn period. Differential diagnosis remains an issue in eyes of patients with ROP-like fundus findings, but who did not undergo newborn eye consultation.

Stages 1 to 3

Because it may resemble stages 1, 2, or 3 of ROP, the principal condition to be considered in the differential diagnosis is familial exudative vitreoretinopathy (FEVR). Indeed, in older children it is impossible to make the correct diagnosis without a careful family history and/or examination of family members.[131–136]

Familial exudative vitreoretinopathy (FEVR) is most commonly an autosomal dominant disease although recessive and X-linked pedigrees have been described.[137,138] In its acute form, it is characterized by peripheral areas of avascularity in the temporal retina. The neovascularization associated with the disease is very similar to that seen in acute ROP (Figs 80-14, 80-24 and 80-25). The changes in FEVR may progress, as in ROP, to dragging of the retina temporally, subretinal exudation, cicatrization, and retinal detachment. The severe changes usually are asymmetric and generally detected anywhere from birth to 10 years of age. Asymptomatic affected older family members often exhibit only avascularity of the peripheral temporal retina. In contrast

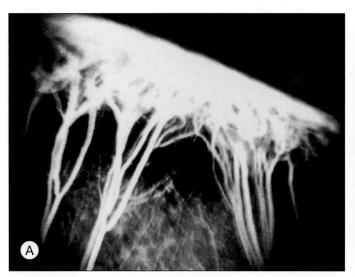
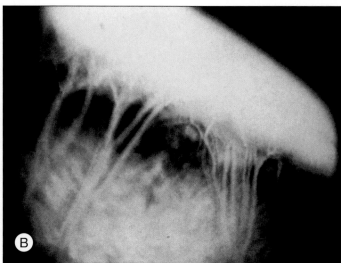

Fig. 80-24 Familial exudative vitreoretinopathy. A, Fluorescein angiogram (early transit) of a patient with familial exudative vitreoretinopathy. Note leakage from neovascularization at the border of the vascularized and avascular retina. B, Photograph of late transit of dye showing extensive leakage from neovascularization. Courtesy Robert E. Kalina.

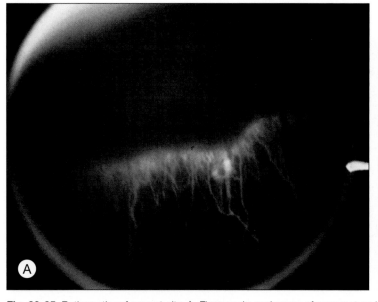
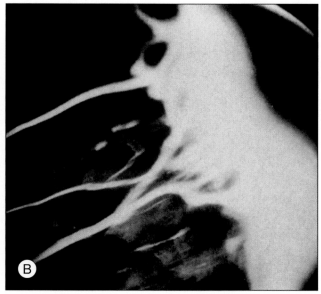

Fig. 80-25 Retinopathy of prematurity. A, Fluorescein angiogram of a premature infant with mild stage 3 retinopathy of prematurity. Leakage from neovascularization is noted. B, Extensive dye leakage from neovascularization in the late phase of an angiogram of a patient with more severe stage retinopathy of prematurity. Note similarity to patient in Fig. 80-21.

to its usual course in ROP, neovascular growth may occur several years after birth in FEVR.

A history of prematurity with a negative family history militates against the diagnosis of FEVR, as does a normal peripheral retinal examination of both parents.

We have noted that atypical cases of Coats' disease, Eales' disease, and retinoschisis occasionally resemble ROP. The absence of the history of prematurity usually eliminates these cases from consideration as ROP.

Stages 4 and 5

Other conditions associated with retinal detachment and/or leukocoria, most importantly retinoblastoma, must be differentiated from the advanced stages of ROP. Those conditions also include persistent fetal vasculature, congenital cataracts, incontinentia pigmenti, FEVR and Norrie's disease. Premature birth does not, of course, exclude these other disorders.

Retinoblastoma
History
In general, patients with retinoblastoma have a history of full-term birth. The exception, retinoblastoma occurring in a premature infant, is extremely rare. Fortunately, premature infants routinely receive examinations during the newborn period, so later diagnostic confusion between ROP and retinoblastoma is unlikely.

Family history
Another important clue in the differential diagnosis is a positive family history. About one-third to one-fourth of retinoblastoma cases are genetically inherited as autosomal dominant mutations. The family history for ROP is negative unless there have been other family members with a history of prematurity.

Clinical features
Retinoblastoma usually is more advanced in one eye, in contrast to ROP, which is usually bilateral and fairly symmetric. However, the examiner should recognize that retinal detachment in ROP may also be asymmetric, and that retinoblastoma may be advanced in both eyes at diagnosis. The small retinoblastoma that presents as a localized white nodule is not a problem in differential diagnosis. Large retinoblastomas with tumor in the vitreous are more likely to present a confusing picture and may require further study.

Ultrasonography
Ultrasonographic examinations can be helpful in differentiating the tumefaction of a large retinoblastoma from the retinal detachment of advanced ROP. Retinoblastomas are frequently posterior mass lesions and often demonstrate highly reflective echoes due to calcification. In ROP, common examination findings are multiple echoes and complex ultrasound patterns that usually are located just behind the lens or in the retinal periphery.

Computed tomographic (CT) scans
CT scans in retinoblastoma will show a tumor mass, as opposed to retina and membranes. Calcium is frequently present in retinoblastoma.

Persistent fetal vasculature

Persistent fetal vasculature (PFV), formerly known as persistent hyperplastic primary vitreous (PHPV), is a congenital anomaly, usually unilateral and occurring in the full-term infant.[139,140] Microcornea and microphthalmia are usually present, and the ciliary processes appear to be dragged by traction toward the center of the pupil. The lens may be cataractous and the membrane behind the lens in PFV is grayish white and may be vascularized. Frequently, no retinal vessels are visible. Ultrasonography most often shows attached retina and a stalk extending from the optic nerve through the central vitreous cavity.

Congenital cataracts

The diagnosis of congenital cataracts is easily made by slit-lamp examination. When the cataracts are not dense, some areas of normal retina can be visualized posteriorly and peripherally. Even in advanced stage 5 ROP with a narrow–narrow detachment configuration, there is rarely lens clouding during infancy.

Incontinentia pigmenti

Incontinentia pigmenti (IP) is an X-linked dominant disorder manifesting pigmentary skin abnormalities with ocular, central nervous system and dental abnormalities. The disease is confined almost exclusively to females and there is usually no history of preterm birth. Skin abnormalities are present within the first two weeks of life. Ocular involvement occurs in about one third of cases and is typically bilateral but frequently asymmetric. Ocular findings include avascularity of the peripheral retina which, as in ROP, may lead to fibrovascular proliferation, hemorrhage and traction retinal detachment. RPE abnormalities are also reported in IP that are not typical of changes seen with ROP.

Familial exudative vitreoretinopathy (FEVR)

Advanced stages of FEVR with retinal detachment and vitreous hemorrhage may simulate stage 4 or 5 ROP. Differentiating factors include the lack of history of low birth weight, and often a family history positive for FEVR. Also, fundus changes in FEVR tend to be more asymmetric than those that usually occur with ROP.

Norrie's disease

Norrie's disease is a congenital retinal dysplasia that can exactly mimic the clinical appearance of advanced ROP. It is an X-linked recessive syndrome and therefore occurs in males, being only very rarely manifested in heterozygotic females. There is no causative connection with prematurity, which can be the crucial factor in making a distinction. An examination at 4 to 6 weeks of age would be a great aid in making the differential diagnosis. Patients with Norrie's disease demonstrate leukocoria considerably earlier than those with ROP. Norrie's disease is generally associated with deafness and mental retardation.

RISK FACTORS

In general, prematurity, low birth weight, a complex hospital course, and prolonged supplemental oxygen are today's established risk factors for the development of ROP.[10,70,103,141,142] Supplemental oxygen given for a period of weeks, without specific indication, was abundantly documented to be a major cause of ROP during the epidemic of the 1950s but is no longer the predominant factor in cases of ROP seen since the mid-1970s. Life-support systems now found in neonatal intensive care units include blood gas monitoring and have resulted in the survival of extremely low birth-weight infants – those with the most immature retinas who are thus at the highest risk of ROP. Cases of ROP still occur in this group of infants despite the most meticulous monitoring of arterial blood oxygen levels. Supplemental oxygen, although clearly a major risk factor in the past, is now believed largely to be a marker for immaturity of organ systems, neonatal illness, and stress.

The role of blood carbon dioxide levels in the development of ROP is controversial. Bauer and Widmayer,[143] following Flower's observation[144] that carbon dioxide enhanced the oxygen-induced retinal changes in beagles, conducted a retrospective analysis of infants with low birth weights. They reported that higher arterial carbon dioxide values were the most important variable in separating those infants of equal gestation who developed ROP from those without disease. Biglan et al.[145] and Brown et al.[141,146] failed to confirm this association and, indeed, found that infants with "scarring retinopathy of prematurity" had lower carbon dioxide blood levels. It is likely that this parameter, like many others, is associated with an unstable clinical course – as is ROP – but not necessarily linked with it causally.

Numerous other neonatal health factors have been reported to be associated with ROP, including cyanosis, apnea, mechanical ventilation, intraventricular hemorrhages, seizures, transfusions, septicemia, in utero hypoxia, anemia, patent ductus arteriosus, and vitamin E deficiency.[13,14,31,43,57,90,103,108,111,118,120,136,142,145–149,150,151–159] These associations require further investigation to identify causal relationships. In a study of 4099 infants born weighing less than 1251 g significant additional factors were identified, including white race, multiple birth, and being transported elsewhere for intensive care. Once ROP develops, greater risk is associated with ROP located in Zone I, the presence of plus disease, the severity of stage, and the extent of circumferential involvement.[98] The risk factors studied during the CRYO-ROP study were consolidated into a mathematical model that can predict the risk of an unfavorable outcome for a particular eye that reaches prethreshold severity.[160]

EXAMINATION PROCEDURES IN THE NURSERY

General aspects and timing of the examination

During the 1970s there was increasing attention to the clinical findings in ROP that were revealed through examination with the binocular indirect ophthalmoscope. Nursery examination techniques were developed that have continued through the end of the century. It was increasingly appreciated that many infants develop early peripheral vascular changes of ROP that

regress and leave no apparent damage.[82,86,147,161,162–165] Furthermore, it was noted that the timing of the examination in the nursery would determine the results of incidence studies on ROP,[166] because mild-to-moderate forms of the disorder could be transient. The nursery surveillance carried out in the CRYO-ROP study produced definitive information concerning the early course of ROP. The "natural history" portion of this study recorded data from 4099 infants born weighing less than 1251 g. One finding changed the way we think about the timing of events in ROP: these events occur on a schedule according to the infant's corrected age (postmenstrual age since mother's last menstrual period, or "postconceptional age"), rather than the time since birth, the so-called chronologic age[34] (Fig. 80-26).

For infants in the birth weight category studied, it was found that those who develop stage 1 ROP (and no worse) do so at a median of 34.3 postmenstrual weeks. The median time for onset of stage 2 ROP that progresses no further is 35.4 weeks, and 95% of these cases have the onset at 32 weeks or later. For patients with eyes that reached the treatment randomization "threshold" severity of stage 3+ ROP (at least 5 contiguous or 8 interrupted clock hours in zones I or II), the threshold was reached at a median of 36.9 weeks (90% of cases were in the range of 33.6 to 42.0 weeks) (Table 80-1). From these data it appears that if premature infants can be examined by 32 weeks postmenstrual age, and those found to have ROP are followed, there is a low probability that severe ROP will go undetected. By 2 weeks post-term, or 42 weeks postmenstrual age, 95% of patients who will develop threshold ROP will have done so.[34] Presumably, virtually all the rest will have at least developed ROP and will have been placed under serial observation. Thus the 10-week interval from 32 to 42 weeks postconception can now be identified as the crucial window during which acute ROP usually runs its course. As the disease regresses, further problems may arise from cicatricial sequelae.

It is established that birth weight and gestational age are inversely related to the risk of ROP.[34] For screening or case finding, the upper "limit" of birth weight indicating the need for fundus examination must be tempered by several facts. Although rare cases of ROP-like conditions have been reported in full-term infants, no author has proposed screening fundus examinations for all newborn infants. Since the risk of ROP increases inversely with birth weight, at what point on the risk-by-birth-weight curve do we find that risk is sufficient to justify routine screening fundus examinations? Upper limit birth weight guidelines vary around the world, because of variations in newborn care and behavior of ROP in higher birth weight infants. The neonatologist may identify special risk factors (see Risk factors, above) that motivate examination of selected infants with birth weights greater than the guideline weight.

Screening guidelines

Because ROP can progress to blindness during the first 3 months of life[166] and treatment is available to arrest it in many cases, a protocol has been recommended for examining the eyes of premature infants during that time span. In 2001, the American Academies of Ophthalmology and Pediatrics and the Association

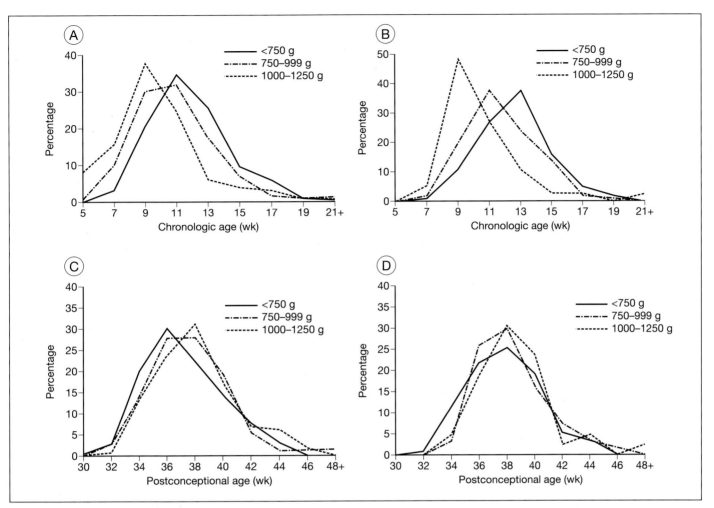

Fig. 80-26 A, Distribution of onset of prethreshold retinopathy of prematurity (ROP) by chronologic age and by birth weight. B, Comparable data for threshold ROP. C, Prethreshold data by postconceptional age, for comparison with "A" (by chronologic age). D, Threshold data by postconceptional age, for comparison with "B" (by chronologic age). From Palmer EA, Flynn JT, Hardy RJ et al. for the Cryotherapy for Retinopathy of Prematurity Cooperative Group. Incidence and early course of retinopathy of prematurity. Ophthalmology 1991; 98:1628–1640.

for Pediatric Ophthalmology and Strabismus issued a joint statement. It calls for at least two screening fundus examinations for all infants born weighing 1500 g or less or with gestational age of 28 weeks or less, as well as for other premature infants up to 2000 g believed to be at high risk by the attending pediatrician. The responsibility inherent in these examinations mandates that the ophthalmologists have prior experience in examining preterm

Table 80-1 Onset of retinopathy of prematurity events in postconceptional age (weeks)

Stage	5th percentile	Median	95th percentile
1	*	34.3	39.1
2	32	35.4	40.7
Threshold	33.6	36.9	42

*Not available; 17% of infants had stage 1 ROP on the first examination. (From Reference 34.)

infants. Each infant's first examination should be done 4 to 6 weeks from birth, or by 31 to 33 weeks postconceptional (postmenstrual) age, whichever is later. Examinations prior to age 4 weeks are not considered necessary.

The subsequent examination schedule is determined by findings on the initial examination, as shown at the end of this chapter.

In November 2002, Reynolds et al. reported an analysis of combined data from the CRYO-ROP study (n = 4099) and the LIGHT-ROP study (n = 361) to develop screening criteria based on the evidence from those two clinical trials. The authors concluded that the initial eye examination should be performed by 31 weeks postmenstrual age or 4 weeks from birth, whichever is later, in order to detect prethreshold retinopathy in a timely fashion. Prethreshold ROP is defined as ROP of less severity than the threshold severity in the CRYO-ROP trial, but with any ROP in Zone I, or Zone II ROP of Stage 2+ or Stage 3 with or without plus disease. It appeared that most risk had passed not only whenever full vascularization had been achieved, but also whenever vessels reached the nasal ora serrata without any ROP development prior to that. (It may be very difficult to get a good view of the physical relationship between the nasal ora serrata and the retinal vessels. Consequently, for eyes that can only be deemed *probably* to have reached to zone III, we see them again in 2 weeks to gain confidence in our previous determination.) If the infant reaches 45 weeks gestational age without developing prethreshold ROP or worse, the risk of visual loss from ROP is minimal.[168] The authors caution that recommendations for infants born prior to 24 weeks are by extrapolation. They also point out that the database excluded infants born weighing more than 1250 g, and some of those larger infants are at risk for ROP. Guidelines for those larger infants would need to be derived from different studies. It should also be noted that these are data from the USA, and the natural history of ROP may be different in other parts of the world. Follow-up screening schedule advice, in light of more recent research, is given at the end of this chapter.

The only substitute for experience and expertise is caution. After performing 50 to 100 ROP examinations, the ophthalmologist begins to develop a sense of when it is safe to extend intervals between examinations.

Side effects of the examination

Very low birth weight infants, while they are still in a precarious general condition, are best left undisturbed except for life-sustaining activities. The stress of an indirect ophthalmoscopic examination is necessary, however, whenever the risk of treatable disease capable of progressing to blindness exists or when information is needed to assist in the general medical evaluation (e.g. seeking chorioretinitis or evidence of chromosomal defect).[169] Screening programs must be designed around the consideration that the procedure may be stressful for the infant.

Techniques of eye examination

Eye examinations should be performed at the request of, or with the approval of, an attending neonatologist. Pupils may be effectively dilated in most infants with Cyclomydril eye drops (cyclopentolate 0.2% and phenylephrine 1%) instilled twice 1 to 5 minutes apart, with the excess drops immediately blotted from the lids to minimize systemic side effects such as hypertension and intestinal ileus.[169] The examination is performed about 25 to 30 minutes later using a binocular indirect ophthalmoscope and a 28 D lens. More heavily pigmented infants sometimes fail to respond adequately to the mydriatic drops, in which case 0.5% cyclopentolate or 1% tropicamide, or both, and 2.5% phenylephrine may be substituted and instilled twice. Most examiners generally use a lid speculum, and there are now a variety of designs suitable for premature infants. Among these are the Cook, Sauer, and Schaefer specula. The infant's hands almost always must be physically restrained, and a nurse is ordinarily available to assist with this. As a precaution against viral or chlamydial transfer, the lid speculum must be sterile for each infant and the examination lens should be wiped with an alcohol sponge between cases whenever it has touched the infant's face. Many ophthalmologists wear gloves during the examination, and this universal precaution is recommended.

Fortunately, the least mature infants do not have an active Bell's reflex. However, an active doll's-eye reflex provides a means to move the eyes to the sides by rotating the infant's head toward the side, to allow the retinal periphery to be examined. In general, ROP severe enough to cause serious concern will be visible far enough posteriorly in the fundus to bring it into view without scleral indentation. However, to determine the final maturity of retinal vascularization requires either serial examinations well past full term or, preferably, examination of the nasal retina to the ends of the growing vessels to determine whether vascularization has advanced into zone III.[34,99] For this far-nasal peripheral retinal examination, scleral indentation or eye positioning is generally needed. An aluminum-wired Calgiswab nasopharyngeal culture swab (Inolex Corp., Glenwood, Ill.) can be used as an inexpensive, sterile, and relatively gentle tool for this (Fig. 80-27). The tip can be bent to any desired angle, even to resemble a fine muscle hook. Because the fiber tip is water soluble, prolonged examinations can soften it so that the swab needs to be replaced. Scleral depressors designed for infant examinations (e.g. the Flynn depressor) are also commercially available. For scleral depression, instillation of topical anesthetic, such as proparacaine, is indicated if the infant seems unusually disturbed during the examination. It is recommended that a member of the nursery staff be present during the entire examination to monitor the infant's airway, vital signs, and behavior and to deal with any apnea or other adverse reactions that may occur.

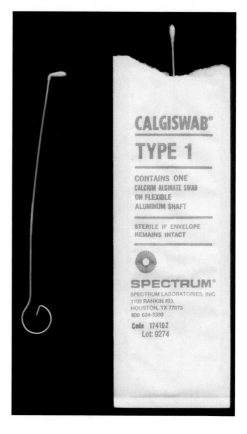

Fig. 80-27 Malleable and delicate nasopharyngeal culture swab used to rotate the globe by inserting the tip into the conjunctival sac. Left, The swab has been bent to resemble a muscle hook.

Informing the patient's family

Often ROP becomes severe just as the infant is achieving medical stability, making it an especially hard blow to the parents who have already experienced much anxiety. The ophthalmologist or neonatologist should keep families informed of the results of eye examinations. The ophthalmologist should contact the parents at the time it is first realized that the ROP is becoming severe, for example, when it develops in zone I or when zone II ROP reaches stage 3. If the parents are kept apprised of the eye condition as it develops, it may soften the emotional impact if the ROP ultimately causes vision damage, and it helps pave the way for discussion of possible surgical intervention.

PROPHYLAXIS AND THERAPY

The role of vitamin E

Vitamin E, a recognized antioxidant, is a logical agent for consideration in the prevention of ROP. Owens and Owens[4,170] investigated the role of vitamin E supplements in the late 1940s, before the implication of oxygen in this disorder and without consideration of the antioxidant effects of vitamin E. Some two decades later the antioxidant property of vitamin E and its possible prophylactic role in ROP were examined by Johnson et al.[171,172] Subsequent controlled clinical trials tested the role of large doses of vitamin E in the prevention of ROP.[173–180] It is difficult to evaluate the published data because of the different routes of administration and time of initiating of vitamin E supplements. The management of stage 3+ disease also differed in some of the studies.

Kretzer et al.[37,94,148] examined ocular specimens obtained at autopsy from vitamin E-treated infants and controls from the nursery study of Hittner et al.[173] They postulated the following series of events in the pathogenesis of ROP:

1. Activation of spindle cells results initially in the increase in gap junctions between adjacent spindle cells, secondarily in the increase in cytoplasmic volume of rough endoplasmic reticulum, and ultimately in the synthesis and secretion of angiogenic factors.
2. Maturation of spindle cells is associated with a decrease in gap junctions, a diminished cytoplasmic volume of rough endoplasmic reticulum, and a cessation of synthesis and secretion of angiogenic factors.
3. Myofibroblasts invade the vitreous concomitantly with spindle cell maturation and provide the tractional force that can produce retinal separation.[94]

A report from the Institute of Medicine published in 1986[181] provides the following conclusion and recommendation of the special committee assigned to review the vitamin E results: "Vitamin E as prophylaxis for retinopathy of prematurity was subject to a detailed analysis. This committee found no conclusive evidence either of benefit or harm from vitamin E administration. Risks from vitamin E appear to be minimal for premature infants provided that doses are kept moderate to achieve a blood level no higher than 3 mg/dl."[181] We believe there is ample evidence that vitamin E deficiency should be avoided in premature infants.

The role of light

Historically there has been a long-standing interest in a possible relationship between light and ROP. In his original descriptions of retrolental fibroplasia, Terry[182,183] considered premature exposure of the eye to light as an important etiologic possibility.

Before the importance of the role of inspired oxygen levels was recognized in ROP, two studies addressed the question of the effect of light. In the late 1940s, Hepner et al.[184] patched the eyes of five premature infants from birth until they weighed 2000 g. They found that four of the five infants developed ROP and they concluded that light was not a factor in its development. In 1952, Locke and Reese[185] reported on a series of 22 premature infants (birth weight less than 2000 g) in which they had patched one eye of each baby. Both found that there was no difference in the incidence of ROP between the patched eyes and the unpatched eyes.[184,185]

During the 1980s and 1990s there were conflicting reports about the effect of light on ROP.[186–188] In 1985, Glass conducted a cohort study of reduced lighting, which was not a randomized, controlled trial, but suggested that reducing ambient light could reduce ROP, particularly in infants of less than 1000 g birth weight.[187] With a similar approach, Ackerman also reduced light exposure but saw no effect on ROP; however, she did not shield the infants from the day of birth.[186]

Although pioneering and innovative, these clinical studies of light and ROP fell short of the design and statistical criteria necessary to test this relationship.[188] Because of this, a feasibility trial of the use of light-reducing goggles (the LIGHT-ROP Study), chaired by James D. Reynolds, was sponsored by the National Eye Institute in 1995 at three nurseries in the United States. Half of 409 infants with birth weights of less than 1250 g were randomly selected to either wear goggles containing 97% near neutral density filters until 31 weeks postconceptional age or undergo no extraordinary light reduction. There were 173 control patients and 188 treated patients. The study concluded that there is no clinically important effect of light on the occurrence or severity of ROP.[189]

Neither the American Academy of Ophthalmology nor the American Academy of Pediatrics have made any recommendations about restricting ambient light from the eyes of premature infants.

Cryotherapy

From 1968, reports suggested that ablative treatment of the peripheral retina of premature infants with ROP may ameliorate the course of the disease. Those early reports suggested that photocoagulation[190–193] or cryotherapy[194,195] may accomplish this goal. Further reports through 1982 have been tabulated elsewhere.[196] Based on personal experience, Kingham,[197] in 1978, expressed skepticism that cryotherapy was of value. Indeed, in 1980 Kalina[198] concluded that "no treatment is of proven value for the proliferative stages of RLF [ROP]." Yet in the same year, Ben-Sira et al.[199] expressed the opinion, based on their clinical experience, that cryotherapy is "safe and effective." Reports continued to appear through the early 1980s with conflicting results and conclusions.[197–199,200–204] A former advocate of cryotherapy published a revised opinion that "the benefits . . . do not seem to warrant the risks involved in these tiny patients,"[150] while simultaneously others were advocating it.[152,202]

Small controlled trials continued to show mixed but encouraging results.[151,204] The need for a full scale, formal clinical trial was apparent.

The multicenter trial of cryotherapy

The CRYO-ROP study was organized in 1985 under the chairmanship of Earl A. Palmer. Supported by the National Eye Institute, the study began enrolling premature infants weighing 1250 g or less at birth in 1986. Although enrollment was scheduled to continue until mid-1988, it was stopped in January 1988 because preliminary results showed a compelling favorable effect of cryotherapy in improving the anatomic outcome for the macula of treated eyes.[123] The study has been continued for longer-term follow-up, and a final examination was carried out when the children were about 15 years old.[123a]

Treatment

Infants eligible for the cryotherapy trial had stage 3 ROP, involving five or more clock hours of retina posterior to zone III in the presence of a standardized plus disease.[96,123] Outlines of the protocol have been published,[34,124,205–207] as well as the manual of procedures.[208] In brief, contiguous, non-overlapping spots of transscleral cryotherapy were directed at the entire anterior cuff of avascular retina (Fig. 80-28). No infant received cryotherapy to both eyes during the study, and the eye to receive cryotherapy was randomly determined. Laser photocoagulation was not studied, since no practical laser delivery instrument had been developed at the time of this study.

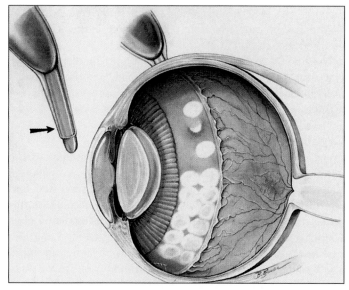

Fig. 80-28 Schematic diagram of cryotherapy for stage 3+ retinopathy of prematurity. The freeze applications extend posteriorly to the ridge but do not spread through the ridge. Treatment inferiorly is complete and is in progress superiorly. Schematic of protective sleeve around the tip of the cryoprobe is indicated by arrow.

Results

The results of the CRYO-ROP study were evaluated through a masked comparison by fundus photographs of the incidence of objectively visible macular fold, retinal detachment, or retrolental mass in the eyes that received cryotherapy, with those eyes not receiving it.[205] Age-appropriate visual acuity outcomes were performed as the children grew and developed.[105,124,209] Cryotherapy was found to reduce the listed unfavorable fundus outcomes over the serial examination visits. At the 10-year outcome assessment, 247 of the original randomized cohort were examined and total retinal detachments had continued to occur in control eyes that had received cryotherapy, increasing from 38.6% at 5½ years to 41.4% at 10 years, while treated eyes remained stable at 22%. Unfavorable fundus outcomes were present in 27% of treated eyes vs. 48% of control eyes, and visual acuity was 20/200 or worse in 44% of treated eyes vs. 62% of control eyes.[209] By the close of the 20th century, level 3 and level 2 neonatal intensive care units had become organized to provide screening ophthalmic examinations for all high-risk infants and to provide peripheral retinal ablative therapy for cases of severe ROP.

Current concepts in management of retinopathy of prematurity
Treatment techniques

Cryotherapy – special considerations   Cryotherapy was performed during the CRYO-ROP study with the use of general anesthesia in 27.5% of the patients; for the rest, cryotherapy was performed in a room within or adjacent to the neonatal intensive care unit (NICU) using local or even topical anesthesia.[123] The average number of individual freezes used in the CRYO-ROP study was 50. As with other forms of eye surgery, a number of factors are considered in determining the method of analgesia or anesthesia, including the physical arrangement of the nursery, proximity to operating or procedure rooms, experience of the anesthesiologist, current medical stability of the infant, "track record" of the infant in tolerating previous stressful procedures, experience of the cryosurgeon, and posterior extent of retinopathy.

Laser – special considerations   In an effort to reduce the time and stress accompanying cryotherapy, refinements of ablative therapeutic technique were studied–in particular, laser therapy, using the binocular indirect ophthalmoscope delivery system (LIO).[210–212] During the early 1990s laser ablation gained acceptance as an alternative to cryotherapy.[149,211] In general, ophthalmologists have found that the LIO delivery system is technically easier than cryotherapy and creates fewer postoperative sequelae related to the treatment (inflammation and swelling) than cryotherapy. Furthermore, it seemed apparent that the outcomes of treatment of threshold disease in zone I and posterior zone II were superior to cryotherapy, and at least equivalent to cryotherapy results for zone II disease.[211,213–220]

When LIO delivery systems became available around 1990, the only laser offered was an Argon photocoagulator (488–532 nm). Subsequently, the Diode laser (810 nm) photocoagulator was introduced. It has become more popular than the Argon because of its portability and a lower incidence of postoperative cataract formation. Although circumstances may require taking patients to the operating suite for ROP laser therapy, it can also be done in the NICU, with the patient under local anesthesia and with or without the aid of conscious sedation.

A technique of laser treatment in the NICU is to place the infant swaddled in a blanket in an open warmer. Mydriatic drops are instilled about an hour before beginning surgery. Treatment is performed with the aid of the infant's nurse, and a neonatologist is always available in the nursery should resuscitation be necessary. A heart rate monitor, apnea monitor and pulse oximeter are used throughout the procedure to alert the surgeon and nurse about any systemic problems. Topical anesthesia is instilled in the eye(s) to be treated and then a lid speculum is placed. Lidocaine 2% is injected subconjunctivally in each quadrant (0.25–0.3 cc) for local anesthesia. Approximately 10 minutes is allowed for the anesthetic to take effect. Treatment is then begun with the LIO delivery system, generally with a 28D-condensing lens for viewing. Appropriate laser safety precautions must be taken for the protection of all personnel within line-of-sight of the laser beam.

Photocoagulation burns are distributed 0.5–1 burn width apart. The objective of the treatment is to scatter burns throughout the entire peripheral, non-vascularized retina. This can usually be accomplished in one treatment session. Treatment is generally started at the anterior edge of the vascularized retina and applied out to the ora serrata utilizing a Calgiswab or like instrument for eye positioning and scleral depression when necessary to treat the peripheral retina. Initial settings for the Diode laser are a power of 0.15 watts and a pulse duration of 0.3–0.4 seconds. This power setting is usually subthreshold for photocoagulation. Power is then titrated up in increments of 50 milliwatts until a yellowish-grey reaction is observed in the retina. The power and/or pulse duration often need to be varied from one area to another in the avascular retina.

The total number of laser applications necessary to treat a given eye will depend primarily on the size of the avascular zone in the eye; eyes with vascularization only into Zone I will require a larger number of laser spots than those with disease in Zone II. In the authors' experience, if the ROP is in mid-to-peripheral Zone II, then 600–1000 laser spots may be sufficient to cover the entire nonvascularized retina for 360 degrees. However, if the eye to be treated has vessel growth only in Zone I, then it is not unusual to apply 1500–2000 laser spots for adequate coverage. Although the desire is to perform all the necessary treatment for each eye in one session, circumstances such as reduced visibility or patient distress may necessitate more than one treatment session. Occasionally, inadvertently skipped areas near the ROP ridge require supplementary treatment in 10–14 days, in the absence of signs of involution.

Recommendations for patient selection

Laser or cryotherapy should be considered for both eyes whenever both eyes meet treatment criteria (see next section). In occasional cases the added stress of treating the second eye at the same session may not be justifiable.

A conservative approach in patients with symmetrically involved eyes, who are medically capable of withstanding treatment, is as follows:

For cases in which disease is not progressing very rapidly or barely meets treatment criteria, it is reasonable to observe both eyes for a week or so after treating one eye only. If the process in the treated eye begins regressing while that of the untreated eye continues to worsen, and the medical condition of the patient is satisfactory, then treat the second eye. If the ROP in the untreated eye begins to subside spontaneously, treatment may not be necessary. If the procedure is performed under general anesthesia, it may be considered appropriate to treat both eyes, even in the presence of marginal indications, to eliminate the possible increased risk inherent in a second anesthetic induction. This decision should be individualized in light of all clinical information and in consultation with the parents.

The early treatment for retinopathy of prematurity trial (ETROP)

In 1999, under the chairmanship of William V. Good, the National Eye Institute funded a clinical trial to study optimal ROP treatment indications. In this trial, called the ETROP study, eyes were randomized to early peripheral retinal ablation or conventional management (observation until threshold criteria developed) once they achieved a high-risk level of prethreshold ROP. The ETROP study showed a significant benefit of earlier treatment intervention as measured by visual acuity outcome at a corrected age of 9 months and in the structural outcome of the retina at corrected ages of 6 and 9 months.[221] In the selected high-risk eyes that were studied, unfavorable acuity results were reduced by earlier treatment intervention to 14.5%, from 19.5% in the conventionally treated control group ($P = 0.01$). Unfavorable structural outcomes were reduced from 15.6% in the control group to 9.1% in the early treatment eyes ($P =$ less than 0.001).

The ETROP study results, published in December 2003, produced a new clinical algorithm as a guide for treatment intervention in eyes with severe ROP.[221] Prompt treatment is indicated for eyes with Type 1 ROP and continued serial observations without treatment is recommended for eyes with Type 2 ROP, as explained in Table 80-2.

Table 80-2 The ETROP indications for treatment

Type 1 ROP ("new threshold") Administer peripheral ablation treatment	Type 2 ROP Wait and watch for progression
Zone II: plus disease with stage 2 or 3 Zone I: plus disease with stage 1, 2 or 3 disease stage 3 without plus disease	Zone II: stage 3 without plus disease Zone I: stage 1 or 2 without plus

The ETROP Group cautions that plus disease should involve at least 2 quadrants of the fundus (usually 6 or more clock hour segments) with dilation and tortuosity of the posterior retinal blood vessels meeting the published standard (Fig. 80-19A).

Zone III

Currently, treatment is rarely, if ever, needed for such far-peripheral ROP. Keep in mind that the strict definition of zone III holds that the nasalmost part of the retina must be fully vascularized to the ora serrata, without ROP.

Retinal detachment

There is a need for randomized trials of treatment approaches for retinal detachment from ROP. Current clinical thinking about the treatment of retinal detachment from ROP is discussed in Chapter 144.

The ETROP Study: better outcomes, changing clinical strategy

In the ETROP trial, only 66% of the high-risk eyes selected at random to be treated conventionally went on to receive laser therapy (cryotherapy was rarely used). Secondary analysis of the large database produced a simplified revision of the indications for treatment, which was a great practical improvement over the computer generated algorithm used to select the research subjects for the study.[160] (see Table 80-2).

Some of the advantages of an earlier treatment policy may be lost if newborn eye examinations do not occur as in the ETROP study. Careful reading of the methods used in the trial[222] reveals a real impact on an intensive care unit's policy for serial ROP examinations. Therefore, consider the following schedule for infants who do not meet criteria for treatment:

Twice a week if there is type 2 ROP (see Table 80-2)
Zone II no plus, stage 3 (or with plus, stage 1)
Zone I no plus, stage 1 or 2
Every week if the ROP is near type 2
Zone II no plus, stage 2
Zone I immature, no ROP
Every 2 weeks if less concerning
Zone II no plus, immature or stage 1

Favorable signs, with respect to progression or involution of ROP, include attainment of postmenstrual age of 45 weeks without developing at least type 2 (as defined above) ROP, and either the completion of full retinal vascularization or progression of retinal vascularization into zone III without previous zone II ROP.[168]

Until ROP can be prevented, it behooves us, the physicians caring for premature infants, to detect cases that need treatment through coordinated and timely methods, in order to benefit each of our recovering preterm patients. Neonatologists, ophthalmologists, discharge coordinators and ROP coordinators must collaborate in adhering to local policies that are developed for the benefit of these infants.

REFERENCES

1. Terry TL. Extreme prematurity and fibroblastic overgrowth of persistent vascular sheath behind each crystalline lens. I. Preliminary report. Am J Ophthalmol 1942; 25:203–204.
2. Terry TL. Fibroblastic overgrowth of persistent tunica vasculosa lentis in premature infants. II. Report of cases – clinical aspects. Arch Ophthalmol 1943; 29:36–53.
3. Patz A. The role of oxygen in retrolental fibroplasias. Trans Am Ophthalmol Soc 1968; 66: 940–985.
4. Owens WC, Owens EU. Retrolental fibroplasia in premature infants. Am J Ophthalmol 1949; 32:1–29.
5. Patz A, Hoeck LE, De La Cruz, E. Studies on the effect of high oxygen administration in retrolental fibroplasia. I. Nursery observations. Am J Ophthalmol 1952; 35:1248–1253.
6. Patz A, Eastham A, Higginbotham DH, Kleh T. Oxygen studies in retrolental fibroplasia. II. The production of the microscopic changes of retrolental fibroplasia in experimental animals, Am J Ophthalmol 1953; 36:1511–1522.
7. Ashton N, Ward B, Serpell G. Role of oxygen in the genesis of retrolental fibroplasia: a preliminary report. Br J Ophthalmol 1953; 37:513–520.
8. Lanman JT, Guy LP, Dancis J. Retrolental fibroplasia and oxygen therapy. JAMA 1954; 55:223–226.
9. Kinsey VE. Retrolental fibroplasia: cooperative study of retrolental fibroplasia and the use of oxygen. Arch Ophthalmol 1956; 56:481–543.
10. Bolton DPG, Cross KW. Further observations on cost of preventing retrolental fibroplasias. Lancet 1974; 1:445–448.
11. Avery ME, Oppenheimer EH. Recent increase in mortality from hyaline membrane disease, J Pediatr 1960; 57:553–559.
12. McDonald AD. Cerebral palsy in children of very low birth weight. Arch Dis Child 1963; 38:579–588.
13. Strang LB, MacLeish MH. Ventilatory failure and right-to-left shunt in newborn infants with respiratory distress. Pediatrics 1961;28:17–27.
14. Warley MA, Gairdner D. Respiratory distress syndrome of the newborn – principles in treatment. Arch Dis Child 1962;37:455–465.
15. Patz A. Retrolental fibroplasias. Surv Ophthalmol 1969;14:1–29.
16. Horbar JD. Monitoring and controlling neonatal oxygen therapy. In: Silverman WA, Flynn JT, eds. Retinopathy of prematurity. Boston: Blackwell, 1985; 153–180.
17. Flynn JT, Bancalari E, Bawol R et al. Retinopathy of prematurity: a randomized, prospective trial of transcutaneous oxygen monitoring. Ophthalmology 1987; 94:630–638.
18. Flynn JT, Bancalari E, Snyder ES. A cohort study of transcutaneous oxygen tension and the incidence and severity of retinopathy of prematurity. N Engl J Med 1992; 326:1050–1054.
19. Tin W. Oxygen therapy: 50 years of uncertainty. Pediatrics 2002; 110:615–616.
20. Phelps DL. Retinopathy of prematurity: an estimate of vision loss in the United States, 1979. Pediatrics 1981; 67:924–926.
21. Finnstrom O, Olausson PO, Sedin G et al. The Swedish national prospective study on extremely low birth weight (ELBW) infants – incidence, mortality, morbidity and survival in relation to level of care. Acta Paediat 1998; 86:503–511.
22. National NeoKnowledge Network. Multi-institutional comparative analysis for births in 1996. Based on 1810 liveborn infants <1000 g birth weight. Wayne, Penn: MDS, 1997.
23. Strebel R, Bucher HU. Improved chance of survival for very small premature infants in Switzerland. Schweiz Med Wochenschr 1994; 124:1653–1659 [in German].
24. Gibson DL, Sheps SB, Hong Uh S et al. Retinopathy of prematurity-induced blindness: birth weight-specific survival and the new epidemic. Pediatrics 1990; 86:405–412.
25. Kennedy J, Todd DA, Watts J et al. Retinopathy of prematurity in infants less than 29 weeks' gestation: 3½ years pre- and postsurfactant. J Pediatr Ophthalmol Strabismus 1997; 34:289–292.
26. Palmer E. The continuing threat of retinopathy of prematurity. Am J Ophthalmol 1996; 122:420–423.
27. Aiello LP. Vascular endothelial growth factor and the eye – biochemical mechanisms of action and implications for novel therapies. Ophthalmic Res 1997; 29:354–362.
28. Pierce EA, Foley ED, Smith LEH. Regulation of vascular endothelial growth factor by oxygen in a model of retinopathy of prematurity. Arch Ophthalmol 1996; 114:1219–1228. (note: see correction of errata in Arch Ophthalmol 115:427, 1997).
29. Stone J, Maslim J. Mechanisms of retinal angiogenesis. Prog Ret Eye Res 1996; 16:157–181.
30. Kinsey VE, Arnold HJ, Kalina RE. PaO_2 levels and retrolental fibroplasia: a report of the cooperative study. Pediatrics 1977; 60:655–668.

31. Lucey JF, Dangman B. A reexamination of the role of oxygen in retrolental fibroplasias. Pediatrics 1984; 73:82–96.

32. Kalina RE, Hodson WA, Morgan BC. Retrolental fibroplasia in a cyanotic infant. Pediatrics 1972; 50:765–768.

33. Johns KJ, Johns JA, Feman SS et al. Retinopathy of prematurity in infants with cyanotic congenital heart disease. Am J Dis Child 1991; 145:200–203.

34. Palmer EA, Flynn JT, Hardy RJ et al. for the Cryotherapy for Retinopathy of Prematurity Cooperative Group. Incidence and early course of retinopathy of prematurity. Ophthalmology 1991; 98:1628–1640.

35. Ashton N, Ward B, Serpell G. Effect of oxygen on developing retinal vessels with particular reference to the problem of retrolental fibroplasias. Br J Ophthalmol 1954; 38:397–432.

36. Gole GA. Animal models of retinopathy of prematurity. In: Silverman WA, Flynn JT, eds. Retinopathy of prematurity. Boston: Blackwell;1985; 53–96.

37. Kretzer FL, Hittner HM. Initiating events in the development of retinopathy of prematurity. In: Silverman WA, Flynn JT, eds. Retinopathy of prematurity. Boston: Blackwell, 1985; 121–152.

38. McLeod DS, D'Anna SA, Lutty GA. Clinical and histopathologic features of canine oxygen-induced proliferative retinopathy. Invest Ophthalmol Vis Sci 1998; 39:1918–1932.

39. Ashton N, Cook C. Direct observation of the effect of oxygen on developing vessels: a preliminary report. Br J Ophthalmol 1954; 38:433–440.

40. Patz A. Current concepts of the effect of oxygen on the developing retina. Curr Eye Res 1984; 3:159–163.

41. McLeod DS, Brownstein R, Lutty GA. Vaso-obliteration in the canine model of oxygen-induced retinopathy. Invest Ophthalmol Vis Sci 1996; 37:300–311.

42. Flower RW. Perinatal retinal vascular physiology. In: Silverman WA, Flynn JT, eds. Retinopathy of prematurity. Boston: Blackwell Scientific Publishers, 1985; 97–120.

43. Ashton N, Pedler C. Studies on developing retinal vessels. IX. Reaction of endothelial cells to oxygen. Br J Ophthalmol 1962; 16:257–276.

44. Chan-Ling T, Stone J. Degeneration of astrocytes in feline retinopathy of prematurity causes failure of the blood–retinal barrier. Invest Ophthalmol Vis Sci 1992; 33:2148–2152.

45. McLeod DS, Crone SN, Lutty GA. Vasoproliferation in the neonatal dog model of oxygen-induced retinopathy. Invest Ophthalmol Vis Sci 1996; 37:1322–1333.

46. Penn JS, Henry MM, Tolman BL. Exposure to alternating hypoxia and hyperoxia causes severe proliferative retinopathy in the newborn rat. Pediatric Res 1994; 36:724–731.

47. Smith LEH, Wesolowski E, McLellan A et al. Oxygen-induced retinopathy in the mouse. Invest Ophthalmol Vis Sci 1994; 35:101–111.

48. Ashton N. Oxygen and the growth and development of retinal vessels: in vivo and in vitro studies. Am J Ophthalmol 1966; 62:412–435.

49. Riecke B, Chavakis E, Bretzel R et al. Topical application of integrin antagonists inhibits proliferative retinopathy. Horm Metab Res 2001; 33:307–311.

50. Sharma J, Barr S, Geng Y et al. Ibuprofen improves oxygen-induced retinopathy in a mouse model. Curr Eye Res 2003; 27:309–314.

51. Wilkinson-Berka J, Alousis N, Kelly D et al. COX-2 inhibition and retinal angiogenesis in a mouse model of retinopathy of prematurity. Invest Ophthalmol Vis Sci 2003; 44:974–979.

52. Higgins RD, Hendricks-Munoz KD, Caines VV et al. Hyperoxia stimulates endothelin-1 secretion from endothelial cells; modulation by captopril and nifedipine. Curr Eye Res 1998; 17:487–493.

53. Raisler BJ, Berns KI, Grant MB et al. Adeno-associated virus type-2 expression of pigmented epithelium-derived factor or Kringles 1–3 of angiostatin reduce retinal neovascularization. Proc Natl Acad Sci USA 2001; 99:8909–8914.

54. Afzal A, Shaw L, Caballero S. Reduction in preretinal neovascularization by ribozymes that cleave the A2b adenosine receptor mRNA. Circ Res 2003; 93:500–6.

55. Aurricchio A, Maguire A et al. Inhibition of retinal neovascularization by intraocular viral-mediated delivery of anti-angiogenic agents. Mol Ther 2002;6:490–494.

56. Stellmach V, Crawford SE, Zhou W et al. Prevention of ischemia-induced retinopathy by the natural ocular antiangiogenic agent pigment epithelium-derived factor. Proc Nat Acad Sci 2001; 98:2593–2597.

57. Phelps DL. Oxygen and developmental retinal capillary remodeling in the kitten. Invest Ophthalmol Vis Sci 1990; 31:2194–2200.

58. Penn JS, Tolman BAL, Henry MM. Oxygen-induced retinopathy in the rat: relationship of retinal nonperfusion to subsequent neovascularization. Invest Ophthalmol Vis Sci 1994; 35:3429–3435.

59. Michaelson IC. The mode of development of the vascular system of the retina with some observations on its significance for certain retinal diseases. Trans Ophthalmol Soc UK 1948; 68:137–180.

60. Miller JW. Vascular endothelial growth factor and ocular neovascularization. Am J Pathol 1997; 151:13–23.

61. Aiello LP, Pierce EA, Foley ED et al. Suppression of retinal neovascularization in vivo by inhibition of vascular endothelial growth factor (VEGF) using soluble VEGF-receptor chimeric proteins. Proc Natl Acad Sci USA 1995; 92:10457–10461.

62. McLeod DS, Taomoto M, Cao J et al. Localization of VEGF receptor-2 (KDR/FLK-1) and effects of blocking it in oxygen-induced retinopathy. Invest Ophthalmol Vis Sci 2002;43:474–482.

63. Sone H, Kawakami Y, Segawa T et al. Effects of intraocular or systemic administration of neutralizing antibody against vascular endothelial growth factor on the murine experimental model of retinopathy. Life Sci 1999;65:2573–2580.

64. Lutty GA, McLeod DS. Retinal vascular development and oxygen-induced retinopathy: a role for adenosine. Prog Ret Eye Res 2003;22:95–111.

65. Mino RP, Spoerri PE, Caballero S et al. Adenosine receptor antagonists and retinal neovascularization in vivo. Invest Ophthalmol Vis Sci 2001; 42:3320–3324.

66. Hellstrom A, Engstrom E, Hard AL et al. Postnatal serum insulin-like growth factor I deficiency is associated with retinopathy of prematurity and other complications of premature birth. Pediatrics. 2003; 112:1016–1920.

67. Hellstrom A, Peruzzi C, Ju M et al. Low IGF-I suppresses VEGF-survival signaling in retinal endothelial cells: direct correlation with clinical retinopathy of prematurity. Proc Natl Acad Sci USA 2001; 98:5804–5808.

68. Cogan DG. Development and senescence of the human retinal vasculature. Trans Ophthalmol Soc UK 1963; 83:465–489.

69. Cogan DG, Kuwabara T. Accessory cells in vessels of the perinatal human retina. Arch Ophthalmol 1986; 104:747–752.

69A. Chan-Ling T, McLeod DS, Hughes S et al. Astrocyte–endothelial cell relationships during human retinal vascular development. Invest Ophthalmol Vis Sci 2004; 45:2020–2032.

70. Chan-Ling T, Tout S, Hollander H et al. Vascular changes and their mechanisms in the feline model of retinopathy of prematurity. Invest Ophthalmol Vis Sci 1992; 33:2128–2147.

71. Stone J, Itin A, Chan-Ling T et al. The roles of endothelial growth factor (VEGF) and neuroglia in retinal vascularization during normal development and in retinopathy of prematurity. J Neurochem 1995; 65:121.

72. Stone J, Chan-Ling T, Pe'er J et al. Roles of vascular endothelial growth factor and astrocyte degeneration in the genesis of retinopathy of prematurity. Invest Ophthalmol Vis Sci 1996; 37:290–299.

73. Provis JM, Leech J, Diaz CM et al. Development of the human retinal vasculature–cellular relations and VEGF expression. Exp Eye Res 1997; 65:555–568.

74. Alon T, Hemo I, Itin, A et al. Vascular endothelial growth factor acts as a survival factor for newly formed retinal vessels and has implications for retinopathy of prematurity. Nature Medicine 1995; 1:1024–1028.

75. Donahue ML, Phelps DL, Watkins RH et al. Retinal vascular endothelial growth factor (VEGF) mRNA expression is altered in relation to neovascularization in oxygen-induced retinopathy. Curr Eye Res 1996; 15:175–184.

76. Dorey CK, Aouididi S, Reynaud X et al. Correlation of vascular permeability factor/vascular endothelial growth factor with extraretinal neovascularization in rat. Arch Ophthalmol 1996; 114:1210–1217.

77. Szewczyk TS. Retrolental fibroplasia and related ocular diseases: classification, etiology, and prophylaxis. Am J Ophthalmol 1953; 36:1333–1361.

78. Phelps DL, Rosenbaum A. Effects of marginal hypoxemia on recovery from oxygen-induced retinopathy in the kitten model. Pediatrics 1984; 73:1–10.

79. Phelps DL. Reduced severity of oxygen-induced retinopathy in kittens recovered in 28% oxygen. Pediatr Res 1988; 24:106–109.

80. STOP-ROP Multicenter Study Group. Supplemental therapeutic oxygen for prethreshold retinopathy of prematurity (STOP-ROP), a randomized, controlled trial. I. Primary outcomes. Pediatrics 2000; 105:295–310.

81. Cantolino SJ, O'Grady GE, Herrera JA et al. Ophthalmoscopic monitoring of oxygen therapy in premature infants: fluorescein angiography in acute retrolental fibroplasias. Am J Ophthalmol 1971; 72:322–331.

82. Flynn JT. Acute proliferative retrolental fibroplasia: evolution of the lesion. Graefes Arch Clin Exp Ophthalmol 1975; 195:101–111.

83. Flynn JT. Retinopathy of prematurity. Pediatr Clin North Am 1987; 34:1487–1515.

84. Flynn JT, Bancalari E, Bachynski BN et al. Retinopathy of prematurity: diagnosis, severity, and natural history. Ophthalmology 1987; 94:620–629.

85. Flynn JT, Cassady J, Essner D et al. Fluorescein angiography in retrolental fibroplasia: experience from 1969–1977. Ophthalmology 1979; 86:1700–1723.

86. Flynn JT, O'Grady GE, Herrera, J. Retrolental fibroplasia: I. Clinical observations. Arch Ophthalmol 1977; 95:217–223.

87. Brooks SE, Gu X, Samuel S et al. Reduced severity of oxygen-induced retinopathy in eNOS-deficient mice. Invest Ophthalmol Vis Sci 2001; 42:222–228.

88. Foos RY. Acute retrolental fibroplasias. Graefes Arch Clin Exp Ophthalmol 1975; 95:87–100.

89. Foos RY. Chronic retinopathy of prematurity. Ophthalmology 1985; 92:563–574.

90. Foos RY. Retinopathy of prematurity – pathologic correlation of clinical stages. Retina 1987; 7:260–276.

91. Friedenwald JS, Owens WC, Owens EU. Retrolental fibroplasia in premature infants. III. The pathology of the disease. Trans Am Ophthalmol Soc 1952; 49:207–234.

92. Reese AB, Blodi F. Retrolental fibroplasia. Am J Ophthalmol 1951; 34:1–24.

93. Reese AB, Blodi FC, Locke JC. The pathology of early retrolental fibroplasia with an analysis of the histologic findings in the eye of newborn and stillborn infants. Am J Ophthalmol 1952; 35:1407–1426.

94. Kretzer FL, McPherson AR, Hittner, HM. An interpretation of retinopathy of prematurity in terms of spindle cells: relationship to vitamin E prophylaxis and cryotherapy. Graefes Arch Clin Exp Ophthalmol 1986; 224:205–214.

95. McLeod DS, Lutty GA, Wajer SD et al. Visualization of a developing vasculature. Microvasc Res 1987; 33:257–269.

96. Committee for the Classification of Retinopathy of Prematurity. An international classification of retinopathy of prematurity. Arch Ophthalmol 1984; 102:1130–1134.

97. Cryotherapy for Retinopathy of Prematurity Cooperative Group: The natural ocular outcome of premature birth and retinopathy: status at one year. Arch Ophthalmol 1994; 112:903–912.

98. Schaffer DB, Palmer EA, Plotsky DF et al. Prognostic factors in the natural course of retinopathy of prematurity. Ophthalmology 1993; 100:230–236.

99. International Committee for Classification of the Late Stages of Retinopathy of Prematurity: An international classification of retinopathy of prematurity: II. The classification of retinal detachment. Arch Ophthalmol 1987; 105:906–912.

100. Reese AB, King MJ, Owens WC. A classification of retrolental fibroplasia. Am J Ophthalmol 1953; 36:1333–1335.

101. McPherson AR, Hittner HM, Lemos R. Retinal detachment in young premature infants with acute retrolental fibroplasia: thirty-two new cases. Ophthalmology 1982;89:1160–1169.

102. Machemer R. Description and pathogenesis of late stages of retinopathy of prematurity. Ophthalmology 1985; 92:1000–1004.

103. Garner A. The pathology of retinopathy of prematurity. In: Silverman WA, Flynn JT, eds. Retinopathy of prematurity. Boston: Blackwell, 1985; 19–52.

104. Repka MX, Palmer, EA. Involution of retinopathy of prematurity. Arch Ophthalmol 2000; 118:645–649.

105. Cryotherapy for Retinopathy of Prematurity Cooperative Group: Multicenter trial of cryotherapy for retinopathy of prematurity: Snellen acuity and structural outcome at 5½ years. Arch Ophthalmol 1996; 114:417–424.

105a. Fishburne BC, Winthrop KL, Robertson JE. Atrophic fundus lesions associated with untreated retinopathy of prematurity. Amer J Ophthalmol 1997; 124:247–249.

106. Gilbert WS, Quinn GE, Dobson V et al. Partial retinal detachment at 3 months after threshhold retinopathy of prematurity. Arch Ophthalmol 1996; 114:1085–1091.

107. Kushner BJ. Strabismus and amblyopia associated with regressed retinopathy of prematurity. Arch Ophthalmol 1982; 100:256–261.

108. Laws D, Shaw DE, Robinson J et al. Retinopathy of prematurity: a prospective review at six months. Eye 1996; 6:477–483.

109. Schaffer DB, Quinn GE, Johnson L. Sequelae of arrested mild retinopathy of prematurity. Arch Ophthalmol 1984; 102:373–376.

110. Cats BP, Tan, KEWP. Prematures with and without regressed retinopathy of prematurity: comparison of long-term (6–10 years) ophthalmological morbidity. J Pediatr Ophthalmol Strabismus 1989; 26:271–275.

111. Robinson R, O'Keefe M. Follow-up study on premature infants with and without retinopathy of prematurity. Br J Ophthalmol 1993; 77:91–94.

112. Snir M, Nissenkorn I, Sherf I et al. Visual acuity, strabismus, and amblyopia in premature babies with and without retinopathy of prematurity. Ann Ophthalmol 1988; 20:256–258.

113. Bremer L, Fellows RR, Palmer EA et al. Strabismus in premature infants in the first year of life. Arch Ophthalmol 1998; 116:329–333.

114. Quinn GE, Dobson V, Repka MX et al. Development of myopia in infants with birth weights less than 1251 grams. Ophthalmology 1992; 99:329–40.

115. Fletcher MC, Brandon S. Myopia of prematurity. Am J Ophthalmol 1955; 40:474–481.

116. Tasman W. Vitreoretinal changes in cicatricial retrolental fibroplasia. Trans Am Ophthalmol Soc 1970; 68:548–594.

117. Tasman W. Late complications of retrolental fibroplasia. Ophthalmology 1979; 86:1724–1740.

118. Kushner BJ. The sequelae of regressed retinopathy of prematurity. In: Silverman WA, Flynn JT, eds. Retinopathy of prematurity. Boston: Blackwell, 1985; 239–248.

119. Foster RS, Metz HS, Jampolsky A. Strabismus and pseudostrabismus with retrolental fibroplasias. Am J Ophthalmol 1975; 79:985–989.

120. Summers GC, Phelps DL, Tung B et al. Ocular cosmesis in retinopathy of prematurity. Arch Ophthalmol 1992; 110:1092–1097.

120a. Krolicki TJ, Tasman W. Cataract extraction in adults with retinopathy of prematurity. Arch Ophthalmol 1995; 113:173–177.

121. Hittner HM, Rhodes LM, McPherson AR. Anterior segment abnormalities in cicatricial retinopathy of prematurity. Ophthalmology 1979; 86:803–816.

122. Lorfel RS, Sugar HS. Keratoconus associated with retrolental fibroplasia. Ann Ophthalmol 1976; 8:449–450.

123. Cryotherapy for Retinopathy of Prematurity Cooperative Group: Multicenter trial of cryotherapy for retinopathy of prematurity: preliminary results. Arch Ophthalmol 1988; 106:471–479.

123a. Cryotherapy for Retinopathy of Prematurity Cooperative Group: Fifteen-year Outcomes Following Threshold Retinopathy of Prematurity. Final Results From the Multicenter Trial of Cryotherapy for Retinopathy of Prematurity. Arch Ophthalmol 2005; 123:311–318.

124. Cryotherapy for Retinopathy of Prematurity Cooperative Group: Multicenter trial of cryotherapy for retinopathy of prematurity: one-year outcome-structure and function. Arch Ophthalmol 1990; 108:950–955.

125. Kushner BJ. Ciliary block glaucoma in retinopathy of prematurity. Arch Ophthalmol 1982; 100:1078–1079.

126. Johnson DR, Swan KC. Retrolental fibroplasia – a continuing problem. Trans Pac Coast Oto Ophthalmol Soc 1966; 47:129–133.

127. Pollard ZF. Secondary angle-closure glaucoma in cicatricial retrolental fibroplasia. Am J Ophthalmol 1980; 89:651–653.

128. Smith J, Shivitz I. Angle-closure glaucoma in adults with cicatricial retinopathy of prematurity. Arch Ophthalmol 1984; 102:371–372.

129. Pollard ZF. Lensectomy for secondary angle-closure glaucoma in advanced cicatricial retrolental fibroplasia. Ophthalmology 1984; 91:395–398.

130. Kushner BJ, Sondheimer S. Medical treatment of glaucoma associated with cicatricial retinopathy of prematurity. Am J Ophthalmol 1982; 94:313–317.

131. Canny CLB, Oliver GL. Fluorescein angiographic findings in familial exudative vitreoretinopathy. Arch Ophthalmol 1976; 94:1114–1120.

132. Criswick VG, Schepens CL. Familial exudative vitreoretinopathy. Am J Ophthalmol 1969; 68:578–594.

133. Gow J, Oliver GL. Familial exudative vitreoretinopathy: an expanded view. Arch Ophthalmol 1971; 86:150–155.

134. Ober RR, Bird AC, Hamilton AM et al. Autosomal dominant exudative vitreoretinopathy. Br J Ophthalmol 1980; 64:112–120.

135. Slusher MM, Hutton WE. Familial exudative vitreoretinopathy. Am J Ophthalmol 1979; 87:152–156.

136. Miyakubo H, Hashimoto K, Miyakubo S. Retinal vascular pattern in familial exudative vitreoretinopathy. Ophthalmology 1984; 91:1524–1530.

137. DeCrecchio G, Simonelli F, Nunziata G et al. Autosomal recessive familial exudative vitreoretinopathy: evidence for genetic heterogeneity. Clin Genet 1998; 54:315–320.

138. Fullwood P, Jones J, Bundey S et al. X-linked exudative vitreoretinopathy: clinical features and genetic linkage analysis. Br J Ophthalmol 1993; 77:168–170.

139. Payne JW, Patz A. Current status of retrolental fibroplasia: the retinopathy of prematurity. Ann Clin Res 1979; 11:205–221.

140. Pruett RC, Schepens CL. Posterior hyperplastic primary vitreous. Am J Ophthalmol 1970; 69:535–543.

141. Brown DR, Biglan AW, Stretavsky MAM. Screening criteria for the detection of retinopathy of prematurity in patients in a neonatal intensive care unit. J Pediatr Ophthalmol Strabismus 1987; 24:212–214.

142. Clark C, Gibbs JAH, Maniello R et al. Blood transfusions: a possible risk factor in retrolental fibroplasias. Acta Paediatr Scand 1981; 70:535–539.

143. Bauer CR, Widmayer SM. A relationship between $PaCO_2$ and retrolental fibroplasia (RLF). Pediatr Res 1981; 15:649.

144. Flower RW. A new perspective on the pathogenesis of retrolental fibroplasia: the influence of elevated arterial CO_2. Retinopathy of Prematurity Conference, Dec 4–6, 1981.

145. Biglan AW, Brown DR, Reynolds JD et al. Risk factors associated with retrolental fibroplasias. Ophthalmology 1981; 91:1504–1511.

146. Brown DR, Milley JR, Ripepi U et al. Retinopathy of prematurity – risk factors in a five-year cohort of critically ill premature neonates. Am J Dis Child 1987; 141:154–160.

147. Kalina RE, Karr DJ. Retrolental fibroplasia: experience over two decades in one institution. Ophthalmology 1982; 89:91–95.

148. Kretzer FL, Hittner HM, Johnson AT et al. Vitamin E and retrolental fibroplasia: ultrastructural support of clinical efficacy. Ann NY Acad Sci 1982; 393:145–166.

149. Laser ROP Study Group. Laser therapy for retinopathy of prematurity (Letter). Arch Ophthalmol 1994; 112:154–156.

150. Mousel DK. Cryotherapy for retinopathy of prematurity: a personal retrospective, Ophthalmology 1985; 92:375–378.

151. Tasman W, Brown GC, Schaffer DB et al. Cryotherapy for active retinopathy of prematurity. Ophthalmology 1986; 93:580–585.

152. Topilow HW, Ackerman AL, Wang FM. The treatment of advanced retinopathy of prematurity by cryotherapy and scleral buckling surgery. Ophthalmology 1985; 92:379–387.

153. Quinn GE, Dobson V, Barr CC et al. Visual acuity of eyes after vitrectomy for ROP: follow-up at 5+ years. Ophthalmology 1996; 103:595–600.

154. Aranda JV, Clark TE, Maniello R et al. Blood transfusions (BT): possible potentiating risk factor in retrolental fibroplasia (RLF). Pediatr Res 1975; 9:362.

155. Bossi E, Koerner F, Zulauf M. Retinopathy of prematurity (ROP): risk factors – a statistical analysis with matched pairs. Retinopathy of Prematurity Conference, Dec 4–6, 1981.

156. Mittelman D, Cronin C. Relationship of blood transfusion and retrolental fibroplasia. Retinopathy of Prematurity Conference, Dec 4–6, 1981.

157. Procianoy RS, Garcia-Prats JA, Hittner HM et al. An association between retinopathy of prematurity and interventricular hemorrhage in very low birth weight infants. Acta Paediatr Scand 1981; 70:473–477.

158. Sacks M, Schaffer DB, Anday EK et al. Retrolental fibroplasia and blood transfusion in very low birth-weight infants. Pediatrics 1981; 68:770–744.

159. Hammer ME, Mullen PW, Ferguson JG et al. Logistic analysis of risk factors in acute retinopathy of prematurity. Am J Ophthalmol 1986; 102:1–6.

160. Hardy RJ, Palmer EA, Dobson V et al. Risk analysis of prethreshold retinopathy of prematurity. Arch Ophthalmol 2003; 121:1697–1701.

161. Kalina RE. Normal and pathologic anatomy of the immature eye. Trans Pac Coast Oto Ophthalmol Soc 1970; 51:185–193.

162. Kingham JD. Acute retrolental fibroplasia. Arch Ophthalmol 1977; 95:39–47.

163. McCormick AQ. Retinopathy of prematurity. Curr Probl Pediatr 1977; 7:1–28.

164. O'Grady GE, Flynn JT, Herrera JA. The clinical course of retrolental fibroplasia in premature infants. South Med J 1972; 65:655–658.

165. O'Grady GE, Flynn JT, Clarkson J et al. Retrolental fibroplasia: clinical fluorescein angiographic and pathological correlation. Mod Probl Ophthalmol 1974; 12:144–151.

166. Palmer EA. Optimal timing of examination for acute retrolental fibroplasia. Ophthalmology 1981; 88:662–668.

167. Fierson WM, Palmer EA, Petersen RA et al. Screening examination of premature infants for retinopathy of prematurity. Pediatrics 2001; 108:809–811.

168. Reynolds JD, Dobson V, Quinn GE et al. Evidence-based screening criteria for retinopathy of prematurity: natural history data from the CRYO-ROP and LIGHT-ROP studies. Arch Ophthalmol 2002; 120:1470–1476.

169. Palmer EA. Risks of dilating a child's pupils. Trans Pac Coast Oto Ophthalmol Soc 1982; 63:141–145.

170. Owens WC, Owens EU. Retrolental fibroplasia in premature infants. II. Studies on the prophylaxis of the disease: the use of alpha tocopherol acetate. Am J Ophthalmol 1949; 32:1631–1637.

171. Johnson L, Schaffer D, Boggs TR. The premature infant, vitamin E deficiency, and retrolental fibroplasia. Am J Clin Nutr 1974; 27:1158–1171.

172. Johnson LH, Schaffer DB, Goldstein DE et al. Influence of vitamin E treatment (Rx) and adult blood transfusions on mean severity of retrolental fibroplasia (MS-RLF) in premature infants. Pediatr Res 1977; 11:535.

173. Hittner HM, Godio LB, Rudolph AJ et al. Retrolental fibroplasia: efficacy of vitamin E in a double-blind clinical study of preterm infants. N Engl J Med 1981; 305:1365–1371.

174. Phelps DL. Vitamin E and retinopathy of prematurity. In: Silverman WA, Flynn JT, eds. Retinopathy of prematurity. Boston: Blackwell, 1985; 181–206.

175. Phelps DL, Rosenbaum AL, Isenberg SJ et al. Tocopherol efficacy and safety for preventing retinopathy of prematurity: a randomized, controlled, double-masked trial. Pediatrics 1987; 79:489–500.

176. Finer NN, Schindler RF, Peters KL et al. Vitamin E and retrolental fibroplasia: improved visual outcome with early vitamin E. Ophthalmology 1983; 90:428–435.

177. Puklin JE, Simon RM, Ehrenkranz RA. Influence on retrolental fibroplasia of intramuscular vitamin E administration during respiratory distress syndrome. Ophthalmology 1982; 89:96–103.

178. Milner RA, Watts JL, Paes B et al. Retrolental fibroplasia in 1500 gram neonates: part of a randomized clinical trial of the effectiveness of vitamin E. Retinopathy of Prematurity Conference, Dec 4–6, 1981.

179. Johnson L, Bowen F, Herman N et al. The relationship of prolonged elevation of serum vitamin E levels to neonatal bacterial sepsis (SEP) and necrotizing enterocolitis (NEC). Pediatr Res 1983; 17:319.

180. Schaffer DB, Johnson L, Quinn GE et al. Vitamin E and retinopathy of prematurity: follow-up at one year. Ophthalmology 1985; 92:1005–1011.

181. Institute of Medicine. Report of a study: vitamin E and retinopathy of prematurity. Washington, DC: National Academy; 1986.

182. Terry TL. Fibroplastic overgrowth of the persistent tunica vasculosa lentis in premature infants. IV. Etiologic factors. Arch Ophthalmol 1943; 29:54–65.

183. Terry TL. Retrolental fibroplasia in premature infants. V. Further studies on fibroplastic overgrowth of persistent tunica vasculosa lentis. Arch Ophthalmol 1945; 33:203–208.

184. Hepner WR, Krause AC, Davis ME. Retrolental fibroplasia and light. Pediatrics 1949; 3:824–828.

185. Locke JC, Reese AB. Retrolental fibroplasia: the negative role of light, mydriatics, and the ophthalmoscopic examinations in its etiology. Arch Ophthalmol 1952; 48:44–47.

186. Ackerman B, Sherworit E, Williams J. Reduced incidental light exposure: effect on the development of retinopathy of prematurity in low birth weight infants. Pediatrics 1989; 83:958–962.

187. Glass P, Avery GB, Subramianian KNS et al. Effect of bright light in the hospital nursery on the incidence of retinopathy of prematurity. N Engl J Med 1985; 313:410–414.

188. Phelps DL, Watts JL. Early light reduction to prevent ROP. The Cochrane Library, Neonatal Module 1997.

189. Reynolds JD, Hardy RJ, Kennedy KA et al. Lack of efficacy of light reduction in preventing retinopathy of prematurity. N Engl J Med 1998; 338:1572–1576.

190. Nagata M, Kobayashi Y, Fukuda H. Photocoagulation for the treatment of the retinopathy of prematurity (first report). J Clin Ophthalmol 1968; 22:419.

191. Nagata M, Tsuruoka Y. Treatment of acute retrolental fibroplasia with xenon arc photocoagulation. Jpn J Ophthalmol 1972; 16:131–142.

192. Oshima K, Ikui H, Kano M et al. Clinical study and photocoagulation of retinopathy of prematurity. Folia Ophthalmol Jpn 1971; 22:700–707.

193. Tanabe Y, Ikema M. Retinopathy of prematurity and photocoagulation therapy. Acta Soc Ophthalmol Jpn 1972; 76:260–266.

194. Payne JW, Patz A. Treatment of acute proliferative retrolental fibroplasia. Trans Am Acad Ophthalmol Otolaryngol 1972; 76:1234–1246.

195. Yamashita Y. Studies on retinopathy of prematurity. III. Cryocautery for retinopathy of prematurity. Rinsho Ganka 1972; 26:385–393.

196. Palmer EA, Biglan AW, Hardy RJ. Retinal ablative therapy for active proliferative retinopathy of prematurity: history, current status, and prospects. In: Silverman WA, Flynn JT, eds. Retinopathy of prematurity. Boston: Blackwell, 1985; 207–228.

197. Kingham JD. Acute retrolental fibroplasia. II. Treatment by cryosurgery. Arch Ophthalmol 1978; 96:2049–2053.

198. Kalina RE. Treatment of retrolental fibroplasia. Surv Ophthalmol 1980; 24:229–236.

199. Ben-Sira I, Nissenkorn I, Grunwald E et al. Treatment of acute retrolental fibroplasias by cryopexy. Br J Ophthalmol 1980; 64:758–762.

200. Bert MD, Friedman MW, Ballard R. Combined cryosurgery and scleral buckling in acute proliferative retrolental fibroplasias. J Pediatr Ophthalmol Strabismus 1981; 18:9–12.

201. Fritch CD. Early management of retinal problems associated with prematurity: cryotherapy treatment. Ann Ophthalmol 1983; 15:565–566.

202. Hindle NW. Cryotherapy for retinopathy of prematurity to prevent retrolental fibroplasias. Can J Ophthalmol 1982; 17:207–212.

203. Keith CG. Visual outcome and effect of treatment in stage III developing retrolental fibroplasia. Br J Ophthalmol 1982; 66:446–449.

204. Palmer EA, Goodman S. A pilot randomized trial of cryotherapy for retinopathy of prematurity (ROP). Invest Ophthalmol Vis Sci 1987; 28(suppl):105.

205. Cryotherapy for Retinopathy of Prematurity Cooperative Group: Multicenter trial of cryotherapy for retinopathy of prematurity: three-month outcome. Arch Ophthalmol 1990; 108:195–204.

206. Palmer EA. The multicenter trial of cryotherapy for retinopathy of prematurity. J Pediatr Ophthalmol Strabismus 1986; 23:56–57.

207. Palmer EA, Phelps DL. Multicenter trial of cryotherapy for retinopathy of prematurity. Pediatrics 1986; 77:428–429.

208. Cryotherapy for Retinopathy of Prematurity Cooperative Group: Manual of Procedures. Archived at the National Technical Information Service, Springfield, Va: US Department of Commerce, NTIS Accession No. PB88-16350; 1988.

209. Cryotherapy for Retinopathy of Prematurity Cooperative Group. Multicenter trial of cryotherapy for retinopathy of prematurity: ophthalmological outcomes at 10 years. Arch Ophthalmol 2001; 119:1110–1118.

210. Landers MB, Semple HC, Ruben JB et al. Argon laser photocoagulation for advanced retinopathy of prematurity. Am J Ophthalmol 1990; 110:429–431.

211. Landers MB III, Toth CA, Semple CS et al. Treatment of retinopathy of prematurity with argon laser photocoagulation. Arch Ophthalmol 1992; 110:44–47.

212. McNamara JA, Tasman WS, Brown GC et al. Laser photocoagulation for retinopathy of prematurity. Ophthalmology 1991; 98:576–580.

213. O'Keefe M, Burke J, Algawi K et al. Diode laser photocoagulation to the vascular retina for progressively advancing retinopathy of prematurity. Br J Ophthalmol 1995; 79:1012–1014.

214. Hammer ME, Pusateri TJ, Hess JB et al. Threshold retinopathy of prematurity. Transition from cryopexy to laser treatment. Retina 1995; 15:486–489.

215. Capone A Jr, Diaz-Rohena R, Sternberg P Jr. et al. Diode-laser photocoagulation for zone 1 threshold retinopathy of prematurity. Am J Ophthalmol 1993; 116:444–450.

216. Hunter DG, Repka MX. Diode laser photocoagulation for threshold retinopathy of prematurity. A randomized study. Ophthalmology 1993; 100:238–244.

217. McNamara JA, Tasman W, Vander JF et al. Diode laser photocoagulation for retinopathy of prematurity. Preliminary results. Arch Ophthalmol 1992; 110:1714–1716.

218. Fleming TN, Runge PE, Charles ST. Diode laser photocoagulation for prethreshold, posterior retinopathy of prematurity. Am J Ophthalmol 1992; 114:589–592.

219. DeJoyce MH, Ferrone PJ, Trese MT. Diode laser ablation for threshold retinopathy of prematurity. Arch Ophthalmol 2000; 118:365–367.

220. White JE, Repka MX. Randomized comparison of diode laser photocoagulation versus cryotherapy for threshold retinopathy of prematurity. 3-year outcome. J Pediatr Ophthalmol Strabismus 1997; 34:83–87.

221. Early Treatment for Retinopathy of Prematurity Cooperative Group: Revised indications for treatment of retinopathy of prematurity: results of the early treatment for retinopathy of prematurity randomized trial. Arch Ophthalmol 2003; 121:1684–1696.

222. Early Treatment for Retinopathy of Prematurity Cooperative Group. Multicenter trial of early treatment for retinopathy of prematurity: study design. Controlled Clinical Trials 2004; 25:311–325.

Chapter

81

Acquired Retinal Macroaneurysms

Emily Y. Chew
Robert P. Murphy

Acquired retinal macroaneurysms are fusiform or round dilations of the retinal arterioles that occur in the posterior fundus within the first three orders of arteriolar bifurcation. Often they are located at the site of an arteriolar bifurcation or an arteriovenous crossing (Fig. 81-1). The supratemporal artery is the most commonly reported site of involvement because patients with such involvement are more likely to have visual impairment. Women make up the majority of reported cases. Most cases are unilateral, while 10% may be bilateral.

This clinical entity usually is unrelated to any other retinal disease, although macroaneurysms have been described in angiomatosis retinae, Eales' disease, Leber's miliary aneurysms, Coats' disease,[1] branch retinal artery occlusion (Fig. 81-2), branch retinal vein occlusion,[2] and hypertensive retinopathy with idiopathic polypoidal choroidal vasculopathy (posterior uveal bleeding syndrome).[3] Most commonly, retinal macroaneurysm affects patients in the sixth and seventh decades of life. Often associated are vascular problems such as hypertension and general arteriosclerotic cardiovascular disease, as noted by Robertson,[4] who first coined the term *retinal macroaneurysm*. Uncontrolled hypertension can present with a retinal artery macroaneurysm and its accompanying vitreous hemorrhage.[5] A large collaborative series by Schatz et al. described the findings in 130 eyes of 120 patients with retinal macroaneurysms. These authors found two thirds of these patients to be hypertensive.[6] Serum lipid and lipoprotein abnormalities have also been reported in patients with this condition.[7]

Although a patient with a retinal arteriolar macroaneurysm may be asymptomatic if the macula is not involved (Fig. 81-3), the most common clinical symptom is decline in central visual acuity as a result of retinal edema, exudation, or hemorrhage.[8,9] Bleeding from macroaneurysms can occur in the subretinal space, into the retina, beneath the internal limiting membrane, or into the vitreous. So-called hourglass hemorrhages are typical. If a pulsatile macroaneurysm is present, some investigators speculate that a greater risk of vitreous hemorrhage exists.[10]

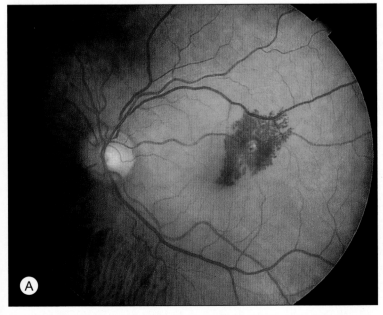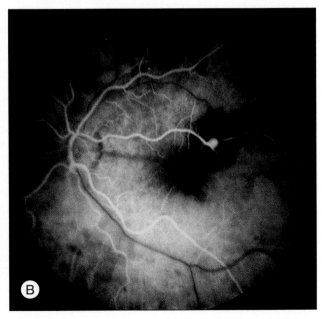

Fig. 81-1 A, A 62-year-old woman with hypertension had a subretinal hemorrhage associated with a macroaneurysm in her left supratemporal artery. B, The fluorescein angiogram demonstrated hypofluorescence from blockage from the retinal hemorrhage and hyperfluorescence of the retinal macroaneurysm itself, apparent as a round dilation located at the arteriolar bifurcation.

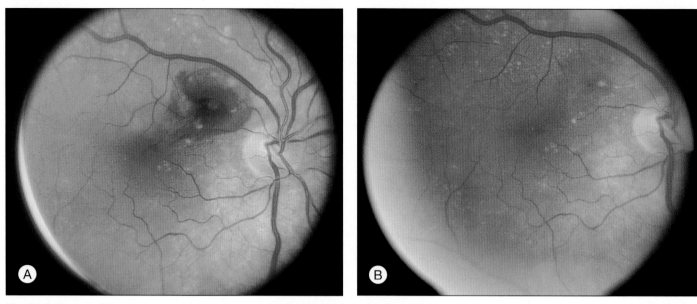

Fig. 81-2 The retinal macroaneurysm in the right eye was associated with a branch retinal artery occlusion.

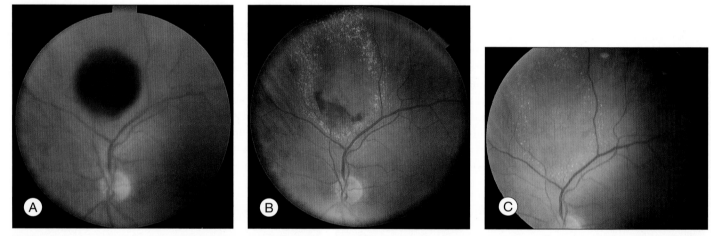

Fig. 81-3 A, The retinal hemorrhage superior to the optic disc, associated with a retinal macro–aneurysm, caused no ocular symptoms. B, Six months later, the retinal macroaneurysm is partially obstructed by the resolving retinal hemorrhage, with a surrounding ring of lipid. C, Eight months later, the macroaneurysm spontaneously involuted, with a complete resolution of the hemorrhage and a decrease in the lipid.

Hemorrhage in the space beneath the retinal pigment epithelium may produce a dark lesion simulating an ocular tumor such as malignant melanoma[11] or a lesion associated with age-related macular degeneration.

The hemorrhage may also partially or completely obscure the aneurysm (Fig. 81-4). In such cases, the use of indocyanine green angiography has been helping establishing the diagnosis and influencing the management of these patients who present with submacular or premacular hemorrhage.[12]

Occasionally, multiple macroaneurysms occur. Other retinal microvascular changes associated with macroaneurysms include widening of the periarterial capillary-free zone around the area of the aneurysm, capillary dilation and nonperfusion, microaneurysms, and artery-to-artery collaterals.

Fluorescein angiography initially may fail to demonstrate the macroaneurysm because of blockage by the surrounding hemor-

rhage. Dense hemorrhage in the retina can cause marked hypofluorescence. In such cases of dense hemorrhage, indocyanine green angiography may be useful because its absorption and emission peak in the near-infrared range allowing the light to penetrate the hemorrhage to a greater extent than fluorescein angiography. A small case series using indocyanine green angiography has demonstrated these lesions to be pulsatile and contiguous with the arterial wall, pathognomonic of an insolated retinal artery macroaneurysm.[13] The macroaneurysm typically fills in the early arterial phase of the angiogram. The appearance of the late phase of the fluorescein angiogram varies, ranging from little staining of the vessel wall to marked leakage. Leakage of surrounding dilated capillaries also may be seen. The lipid often present in the macular area fails to block fluorescein unless the amount of lipid is massive. Macular hole formation following rupture of a retinal arterial macroaneurysm has been reported.[14]

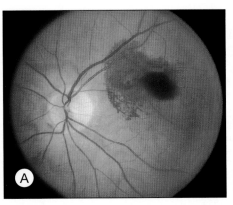
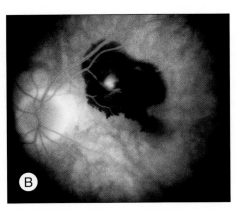
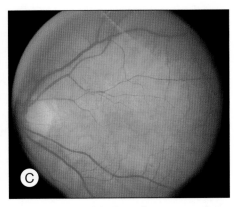

Fig. 81-4 A, A preretinal hemorrhage partially obscures the retinal macroaneurysm. B, The fluorescein angiogram showed the hyperfluorescence that corresponded to the hemorrhage and the hyperfluorescence of the retinal macroaneurysm. C, At 20 months later, there is spontaneous resolution of the hemorrhage and the retinal macroaneurysm.

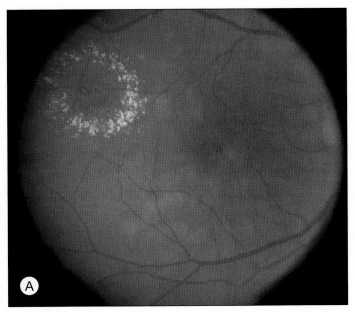
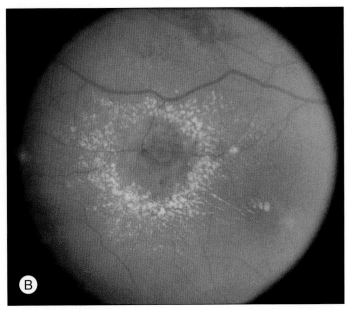

Fig. 81-5 A, The retinal macroaneurysm caused a progressive increase in the retinal hard exudate, resulting in a visual acuity decrease to 20/25 in the right eye over a period of 22 months. B, The edema and lipid were threatening the macula. The patient was offered treatment.

Histopathologic studies of macroaneurysms have shown gross distention of the involved retinal arteriole. Surrounding this are fibroglial proliferation, dilated capillaries, extravasated blood, lipoidal exudates, and hemosiderin deposits.

Several series have reported on the natural history and treatment response of macroaneurysms.[7,15–18] The yellow dye laser has been considered for treatment because of its theoretical advantages.[19–21] Some investigators believe the visual prognosis is excellent in most patients who have macroaneurysms and do not have treatment because the lesions can thrombose and undergo spontaneous involution with clearing of the macular exudate.[16] However, the exudative process may progress in some patients and cause structural damage to the macula with loss of vision (Fig. 81-5). Moderate visual loss also may occur if bleeding causes secondary morphologic changes in the macula.

No clear indication for treatment with laser photocoagulation has been established, and the beneficial effects of such treatments have not been proved. Vitrectomy was performed for clearing the macular hemorrhage associated with the rupture of a macroaneurysm.[22]

Many investigators consider direct laser photocoagulation of the macroaneurysm if the lipid exudate coming from it threatens the fovea. Treatment when hemorrhage is present is fraught with difficulties. There is also the danger of occluding the retinal arteriole during treatment. This potential complication must always be considered when the distal portion of the arteriole being considered for treatment supplies the macula.

The differential diagnoses of retinal macroaneurysms include other retinal vascular abnormalities, including diabetic retinopathy, retinal telangiectasis, retinal capillary angioma, cavernous hemangioma, malignant melanoma,[23] and the hemorrhagic pigment epithelial detachment of age-related macular degeneration.[24]

Systemic investigations for hypertension and cardiovascular disease should be conducted in patients who have a retinal arteriolar macroaneurysm. Usually it is not difficult to distinguish acquired retinal macroaneurysms from the microaneurysms associated with diabetes mellitus, venous occlusive disease of the retina, or the various other retinal vascular diseases.

REFERENCES

1. Nadel AJ, Gupta KK. Macroaneurysms of the retinal arteries. Arch Ophthalmol 1976; 94:1092–1096.
2. Cousins SW, Flynn HE Jr, Clarkson JG. Macroaneurysms associated with retinal branch vein occlusion. Am J Ophthalmol 1990; 109:567–570.
3. Ross RD, Gitter KA, Cohen G et al. Idiopathic polypoidal choroidal vasculopathy associated with retinal macroaneurysm and hypertensive retinopathy. Retina 1996; 16:105–111.
4. Robertson DM. Macroaneurysms of the retinal arteries. Trans Am Acad Ophthalmol Otolaryngol 1973; 77:55–67.
5. Sekuri C, Kayikcioglu M, Kaykcioglu O. Retinal artery macroaneurysm as initial presentation of hypertension. Int J Cardiol 2004; 93:87–88.
6. Green WR. Retinal ischemia: vascular and circulatory conditions and diseases. In: Spencer WH, ed. Ophthalmic pathology. Philadelphia: WB Saunders, 1985.
7. Cleary PE, Kohner EM, Hamilton AM et al. Retinal macroaneurysms. Br J Ophthalmol 1975; 59:355–361.
8. Lavin MJ, Marsh RJ, Peart S et al. Retinal arterial macroaneurysms: a retrospective study of 40 patients. Br J Ophthalmol 1987; 71:817–825.
9. Rabb MF, Gagliano DA, Teske MP. Retinal arterial macroaneurysms. Surv Ophthalmol 1988; 33:73–96.
10. Shults WT, Swan KC. Pulsatile aneurysms of the retinal arterial tree. Am J Ophthalmol 1974; 77:304–309.
11. Perry HD, Zimmerman LE, Benson WE. Hemorrhage from isolated aneurysm of a retinal artery: report of two cases simulating malignant melanoma. Arch Ophthalmol 1977; 95:281.
12. Townsend-Pico WA, Meyers SM, Lewis H. Am J Ophthalmol 2000; 129:33–37.
13. Schneider U, Wagner AL, Kreissig I. Indocyanine green videoangiography of hemorrhagic retinal arterial macroaneurysms. Ophthalmologica 1997; 211:115–118.
14. Mitamura Y, Terashima H, Takeuchi S. Macular hole formation following rupture of retinal arterial macroaneurysm. Retina 2002; 22:113–115.
15. Abdel-Khalek MN, Richardson J. Retinal macroaneurysm: natural history and guidelines for treatment. Br J Ophthalmol 1986; 70:2–11.
16. Asdourian GK, Goldberg MJ, Jampol L et al. Retinal macroaneurysms. Arch Ophthalmol 1977; 95:624–628.
17. Lewis RA, Norton EWD, Gass JDM. Acquired arterial macroaneurysms of the retina. Br J Ophthalmol 1976; 60:21–30.
18. Palestine AG, Robertson DM, Goldstein BG. Macroaneurysms of the retinal arteries. Am J Ophthalmol 1982; 93:164–171.
19. Joondeph BC, Joondeph HC, Blair NP. Retinal macroaneurysms treated with the yellow dye laser. Retina 1989; 9:187–192.
20. Mainster MA, Whitacre MM. Dye yellow photocoagulation of retinal arterial macroaneurysms. Am J Ophthalmol 1988; 105:97–98.
21. Russell SR, Folk JC. Branch retinal artery occlusion after dye yellow photocoagulation of an arterial macroaneurysm. Am J Ophthalmol 1987; 104:186–187.
22. Zhao P, Hayashi H, Oshima K et al. Ophthalmology 2000; 107:613–617.
23. Fritsche PL, Flipsen E, Polak BC. Subretinal hemorrhage from retinal arterial macroaneurysm simulating malignancy. Arch Ophthalmol 2000; 118:1704–1705.
24. Hochman MA, Seery CM, Zarbin MA. Pathophysiology and management of subretinal hemorrhage. Surv Ophthalmol 1997; 42:195–213.

Eales Disease

Mohammed K. Barazi
Robert P. Murphy

In 1880 Henry Eales noted abnormal retinal veins in healthy young men with recurrent vitreal hemorrhages.[1] He did not observe any signs of inflammation preceding or accompanying the hemorrhages and did not describe neovascularization. Furthermore, he believed that epistaxis was associated with the retinal hemorrhages and that constipation and elevated venous pressure were underlying causes of this condition. In the century that followed, he was honored with the eponym for the disease characterized by idiopathic recurrent vitreal hemorrhage.

Duke-Elder[2] thought that Eales disease was not a distinct clinical entity, but instead represented the clinical manifestation of many diseases. Indeed, the etiologies of many of the so-called idiopathic hemorrhages were elucidated with refined diagnostic techniques and laboratory tests. However, after eliminating cases in which other diagnoses were determined, a group of patients with idiopathic retinal perivasculitis and peripheral nonperfusion remained. Investigators now generally agree that Eales disease is a distinct entity comprising certain characteristic funduscopic and fluorescein angiographic findings.[3] However, it remains a diagnosis by exclusion, and retinal diseases with other causes of inflammation or neovascularization must be excluded. These other diseases include primary branch vein occlusion (BVO), diabetic retinopathy, sickle retinopathy, sarcoidosis, systemic lupus erythematosus, and other collagen-vascular diseases.

Eales disease is an idiopathic obliterative vasculopathy that primarily affects the peripheral retina of adults. Retinal changes include extensive peripheral nonperfusion, perivascular sheathing, and neovascularization. Visual loss is characteristically caused by bilateral recurrent vitreous hemorrhages. While uncommon in North America, Eales disease is widespread in India and portions of the Middle East.

CLINICAL FINDINGS

Eales disease predominantly affects healthy young adults. The peak age of onset of symptoms is 20 to 30 years. Most investigators note a male predominance.[4,5] Murphy and colleagues,[3] however, in their study of 55 patients in the USA, found that men and women were equally affected. Most patients' symptoms include those of vitreal hemorrhage, such as floaters, cobwebs, blurring, or decreased visual acuity. Others have blurring secondary to retinal vasculitis or uveitis, but without hemorrhage. Many patients complain of symptoms in only one eye, but detailed ophthalmologic examination of the other eye reveals the early changes of Eales disease, such as peripheral nonperfusion and vascular sheathing. Between 80% and 90% of patients eventually develop bilateral involvement.

Inflammation

Ocular inflammation is the initial manifestation of Eales disease. Signs and symptoms of inflammation occur at varying times in the course of the disease but are less common in late stages. Vascular sheathing is found in up to 80% of patients, with involvement ranging from thin white lines limiting the blood column on both sides to heavy exudative sheathing (Fig. 82-1). The thin white lines tend to be continuous, and the heavy exudative sheathing is usually segmental. Superficial flame-shaped hemorrhages are often located in the areas of sheathed vessels.

On fluorescein angiography, areas of vascular sheathing frequently leak dye. However, the sheathing does not always correspond to the staining. In addition, the intensity of the dye leakage seen with fluorescein angiography is not always proportional to the activity of the inflammatory process.

Many investigators report that Eales disease is a primary disease of the retinal veins. Elliot & Harris[6] have suggested that the disease be called "periphlebitis retinae." However, Murphy el al.[3] documented approximately the same prevalence of arteriolar as venular sheathing. Because the retinal arterioles are involved, these authors maintain that it is more accurate to describe the disease as a retinal vasculitis or vasculopathy, since the vessel wall itself appears to be involved, and both arteriolar and venular vessels are affected.[3]

Anterior uveitis is uncommon in Eales disease, although spillover manifesting as nongranulomatous inflammation may occur in cases with severe retinal periphlebitis. The vitritis in Eales is rarely dense. A mild vitreous haze overlying the areas of vasculitis is more common. Active or healed choroiditis has not been noted in Eales disease and should raise suspicion of a different disease process. Macular edema occurs in the eyes with sheathing, and cystoid changes can often be seen with fluorescein angiography. Macular edema is common when epiretinal membranes are present. Although the exact cause of the macular edema is unknown, it may be associated with low-grade inflammation.

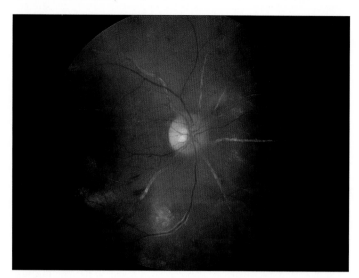

Fig. 82-1 Arteriolar and venous sheathing. Note the spectrum of both continuous and segmental sheathing of both arteries and veins.

Nonperfusion

All patients with Eales disease have varying degrees of peripheral retinal nonperfusion. The nonperfusion is generally confluent, with the temporal quadrant most commonly affected. Intraretinal hemorrhages often first appear in the affected area, followed by an increase in vascular tortuosity with frequent collateral formation around occluded vessels. Occasionally the microvascular abnormalities are so severe that areas of the fundus resemble the vascular pattern seen in Coats disease. Fine, solid white lines representing the remains of obliterated large vessels are commonly seen in the area of nonperfusion. These fine lines retain the configuration of the normal retinal vasculature.

The junction between the anteroperipheral nonperfusion and the posterior perfused retina is usually sharply demarcated (Fig. 82-2). Elliot[4] and Spitznas et al.[7] have carefully documented the vascular abnormalities at the junction between the perfused and the nonperfused zones. These include microaneurysms, arteriovenous shunts, venous beading, and, occasionally, hard exudates and cottonwool spots. Stumps of obliterated vessels stain with fluorescein during angiography.

Despite extensive peripheral nonperfusion, the macula is usually spared, preserving central vision. However, in some patients the nonperfusion extends to the macula (Fig. 82-3). Visual acuity in these eyes is usually less than 20/400.

Patients with Eales disease can also develop BVO, which can be either solitary or multiple. These patients can be differentiated from patients with primary BVO because the pathologic changes in BVO are usually confined to the affected quadrant of the retina.

In contrast, Eales disease affects more extensive areas of the peripheral retina and does not respect either the anatomic distribution of venules in the retina or the horizontal midline. These two conditions can occur together, and Eales disease may predispose to the development of BVO (Fig. 82-4).

Neovascularization

Neovascularization is observed in up to 80% of patients with Eales disease. The new vessels can form either on the disc (NVD) or elsewhere within the retina (NVE). The NVE is usually located at the junction between perfused and nonperfused retina. Rubeosis iridis can also develop in these patients. Vitreous hemorrhage from the neovascularization is common and is one of the major causes of visual loss. While this hemorrhage may often clear within 4 to 8 weeks, it often remains unresolved. The retinal neovascularization is frequently associated with a prominent fibrous component. Occasionally patients have extensive retinal and vitreal proliferation of relatively avascular interlocking strands and sheets of fibrous scar tissue (Fig. 82-5). These eyes have associated anteroposterior vitreoretinal traction and are at risk of developing retinal detachment.

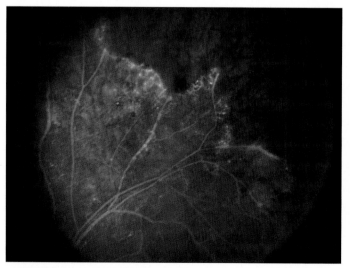

Fig. 82-2 Peripheral nonperfusion. Microaneurysms, venous beading, and arteriovenous shunting can be noted at the margin of perfused and nonperfused retina.

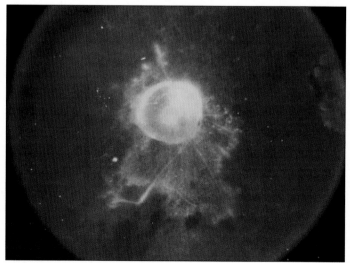

Fig. 82-3 An example of severe nonperfusion which began peripherally and extended posteriorly to involve the macula and peripapillary retina.

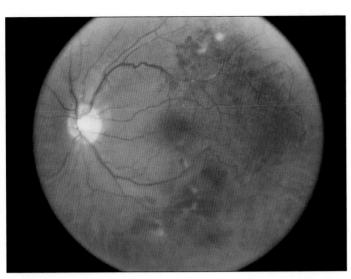

Fig. 82-4 Secondary branch vein occlusion as a sequel to vascular inflammation in an Eales patient.

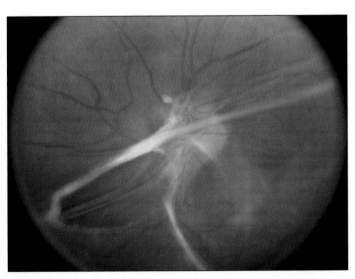

Fig. 82-5 Hypovascular fibroproliferation emanating from the disc.

Other vitreoretinal abnormalities

Murphy et al.[3] documented posterior vitreous detachment (PVD) in 27% of their patients with Eales disease. All these patients with PVD except one, experienced vitreous hemorrhage. Four of these patients had macular holes. The age range of the patients with PVD was from 13 to 63 years, with a mean age of 35 years. The PVD in the younger patients could have been due to a low-grade, chronic inflammation of the vitreous. The macular holes may represent a complication of posterior vitreous separation from the retina secondary to premature vitreous degeneration.

Anteroposterior contraction of fibrovascular tissue adherent to both retina and posterior vitreous can cause both traction and rhegmatogenous retinal detachments, though the former are much more common.

TREATMENT AND PROGNOSIS

Various treatments have been proposed for Eales disease. Henry Eales treated his patients with a mixture of laxative, digitalis, and belladonna. Other medications have included vitamin C, thyroid extract, osteogenic hormones, and androgenic hormones. Systemic steroid therapy in massive doses has also been used. None of these treatments has demonstrated a clear-cut benefit.

Meyer-Schwickerath[8] used light coagulation treatment in 1954 and reported good results. Since that time, laser photocoagulation has evolved to become the treatment of choice for patients with neovascularization.[7,9] Murphy et al.[3] found favorable results in eyes that were treated with fairly light, full-scatter photocoagulation to the nonperfused retina and the junction of perfusion and nonperfusion. Both NVD and NVE often regress with relatively light photocoagulation intensity[7] (Fig. 82-6). Prophylactic peripheral laser to nonperfused retina in asymptomatic eyes has also been advocated.[10] Because retinal nonperfusion can be progressive in this disease, new areas of neovascularization can develop and should be treated with supplemental photocoagulation.

The major cause of visual loss in Eales disease is recurrent vitreal hemorrhage. Usually the hemorrhage settles to the lower portion of the vitreous and is reabsorbed within several weeks or months, with the return of normal central vision. Although the visual acuities of patients with Eales disease range from normal to no light perception, most eyes retain good acuity. Murphy et al.[3] reported that 67% of their patients had a final visual acuity of the better eye that ranged from 20/15 to 20/40, 24% ranged from 20/50 to 20/200, and 9% were worse than 20/250. Long-term data have also been presented by Atmaca et al.,[11] who in 185 eyes noted improved vision in 20% and stabilized vision in 43% of 185 eyes with at least 5 years' follow-up.

Severe visual loss usually results from complications of neovascularization, such as persistent vitreous hemorrhage, retinal detachment, and anterior segment neovascularization with secondary glaucoma. Photocoagulation, properly applied, may prevent the development of these complications. Vitrectomy techniques can often be employed for removing persistent vitreal hemorrhage and scar tissue. Recently, the use of systemic steroids and antituberculous medications, combined with aggressive laser and early vitrectomy, has been advocated.[12] No treatment is known to prevent or reverse the nonperfusion itself or to prevent visual loss from capillary nonperfusion of the macula.

SYSTEMIC ABNORMALITIES

Many investigators have emphasized the relationship between Eales disease and tuberculosis. One study reported a prevalence of either tuberculosis or history of exposure to tuberculosis in 48% of patients with Eales disease. Another used nested polymerase chain reaction to search for tubercular antigen, finding a statistically significant difference between Eales and control eyes.[13] This association suggests that immune mechanisms, including perhaps immune responses to tuberculin protein, may play a role in the pathogenesis of Eales disease. However, with various authors implicating human leukocyte antigen, free

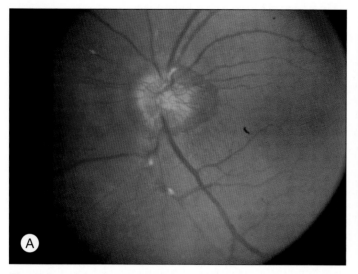
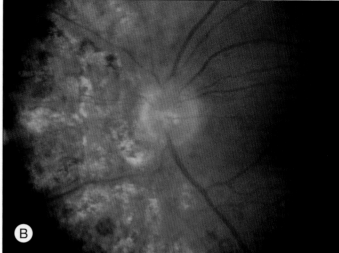

Fïg. 82.6 A, Neovascularization of the disc. Note the segmental exudative arteriolar sheathing. B, Approximately 2½ years later the patient has had total regression of the neovascularization after treatment with full-scatter photocoagulation. Note that the former area of the arteriolar sheathing has resorbed.

radical damage, vascular endothelium growth factor expression, and retinal autoimmunity as well as possible mycobacterial links, Eales disease appears to be of multifactorial etiology.[14,15]

Eales disease is increasingly associated with neurologic sequelae, with vascular infarction implicated as the causative factor in these patients. Cerebrovascular accidents, seizures, and migraine headaches, among other manifestations, have all been reported.[16]

Some patients with Eales disease appear to have a concomitant vestibuloauditory dysfunction. The prevalence of bilateral hearing loss in persons aged 17 years or older in the general population is only about 17%. Renie et al.[17] reported an overall rate of 48% bilateral hearing loss in their survey of patients with Eales disease. The cause of hearing decrease in these patients is not known with certainty; however, it may have a vascular basis. The cochlea receives its entire blood supply through a small cochlear capillary. The hair cells of the organ of Corti are known to be very sensitive to hypoxia; therefore any form of vascular occlusion could result in cochlear dysfunction.

Eales disease has long been recognized, but much remains unknown. The concomitant vestibuloauditory and neurologic abnormalities indicate that the pathologic expression of this disease is not confined to the eye. The association of Eales disease with both ocular inflammation and hypersensitivity to tuberculin protein suggests that this disease may be associated with immunologic phenomena whose mechanism remains unknown.

REFERENCES

1. Eales H. Cases of retinal hemorrhage associated with epistaxis and constipation. Birmingham Med Rev 1880; 9:262.

2. Duke-Elder WS. Diseases of the retina, vol. 10. System of ophthalmology. St Louis: Mosby; 1967.

3. Murphy RP, Renie WA, Proctor LR et al. A survey of patients with Eales disease. In: Fine SL, Owens SL, eds. Management of retinal vascular and macular disorders. Baltimore: Williams & Wilkins; 1983.

4. Elliot AJ. Thirty-year observation of patients with Eales disease. Am J Ophthalmol 1985; 80:404–408.

5. Spitznas M, Meyer-Schwickerath GT, Stephan B. The clinical picture of Eales disease. Graefes Arch Clin Exp Ophthalmol 1975; 194:73–85.

6. Elliot AJ, Harris GS. The present status of the diagnosis and treatment of periphlebitis retinae (Eales disease). Can J Ophthalmol 1969; 4:117–122.

7. Spitznas M, Meyer-Schwickerath G, Stephan B. Treatment of Eales disease with photocoagulation. Graefes Arch Clin Exp Ophthalmol 1975; 194:193–198.

8. Meyer-Schwickerath G. Eales disease: treatment with light-coagulation. Mod Probl Ophthalmol 1966; 4:10–18.

9. Fine SL, Patz A, Orth DH. Retinal vascular disorders: diagnosis and management, vol. 2. Sights and sounds in ophthalmology. St Louis: Mosby; 1976.

10. Ishaq M, Niazi MK. Usefulness of laser photocoagulation in managing asymptomatic eyes of Eales disease. Journal of Ayub Medical College, Abbottabad: JAMC 2002; 14:22–25.

11. Atmaca LS, Batioglu B, Atmaca Sonmez P. A long-term follow-up of Eales disease. Ocul Immunol Inflamm 2002; 10:213–221.

12. El-Asrar AM, Al-Kharashi SA. Full panretinal photocoagulation and early vitrectomy improve prognosis of retinal vasculitis associated with tuberculoprotein hypersensitivity (Eales disease). Br J Ophthalmol 2002; 86:1248–1251.

13. Madhavan HN, Therese KL, Doraiswamy K. Further investigations on the association of *Mycobacterium tuberculosis* with Eales disease. Ind J Ophthalmol 2002; 50:35–39.

14. Biswas J, Sharma T, Gopal L et al. Eales disease – an update. Surv Ophthalmol 2002; 47:197–214.

15. Perentes Y, Chan CC, Bovey E et al. Massive vascular endothelium growth factor (VEGF) expression in Eales disease. Klin Monatsbl Augenheilkd 2002; 219:311–314.

16. Biswas J, Raghavendran R, Pinakin G et al. Presumed Eales disease with neurologic involvement: report of three cases. Retina 2001; 21:141–145.

17. Renie WA, Murphy RP, Anderson KC et al. The evaluation of patients with Eales disease. Retina 1983; 3:243–248.

Chapter

83

Radiation Retinopathy

Albert M. Maguire
Andrew P. Schachat

Radiation retinopathy is characterized by delayed onset of slowly progressive occlusive vasculopathy that may lead to capillary non-perfusion, large-vessel occlusion, retinal vascular incompetence, neovascularization, and other sequelae. These changes may cause loss of visual function. Radiation retinopathy is not a "complication" of radiation; it is a manifestation of a tissue-limiting toxicity of treatment. Just as blindness can be anticipated following enucleation, if the eyes are included in the field of radiation treatment, damage to the visual system may be anticipated at some time after radiation therapy.

The first report of posterior-segment complications following radiation therapy appeared in 1933, when Stallard[1] reported exudates, hemorrhages, pigment epithelial changes, optic disc edema, and optic atrophy in patients who had been treated with radon seeds for retinal capillary hemangioma and retinoblastoma. Moore,[2] in 1935, expanded on Stallard's observations in his presidential address to the UK Ophthalmological Society.

PATHOLOGY AND PATHOGENESIS

Irvine & Wood[3] reported an animal model for radiation retinopathy. Monkeys were treated with up to 30 Gy to the eye and were then examined periodically. The first changes were seen 12 to 24 months after treatment. These involved focal loss of capillary endothelial cells and pericytes. As areas of capillary loss became confluent, cottonwool spots were seen clinically. These subsequently faded as large areas of retinal capillary nonperfusion developed. Histopathologic studies showed that the first changes involved deep, small retinal vessels. Larger vessels were involved later in the course of the condition. Occlusion of the choriocapillaris developed but was much less pronounced than the retinal capillary nonperfusion. Intraretinal neovascularization was seen, but in this model there was no preretinal or disc neovascularization. After 2½ to 3½ years, the monkeys developed iris neovascularization and neovascular glaucoma.

Archer et al.[4] studied the effects of ocular radiation in rats. Six months after single ocular exposures of 15 to 20 Gy, endothelial cell loss and capillary closure were observed. Thymidine labeling studies demonstrated a fivefold to 10-fold increase in the number of microvascular cells undergoing DNA synthesis, suggesting that accelerated cell division was taking place to compensate for endothelial cell loss. Neovascularization was not seen in rats treated with radiation alone. However, when streptozocin-induced diabetic rats underwent ocular irradiation, new intraretinal and preretinal vessels sometimes developed.

Archer and colleagues[4,5] have proposed a model for the pathophysiology of radiation retinopathy that emphasizes the role of the vascular endothelial cell. Presumably, endothelial cell damage initially occurs in the arterial circulation as a result of free radical generation in this high-oxygen environment. After an initial wave of cell death, the remaining viable endothelial cells replicate and migrate to maintain vascular architecture. Later cycles of endothelial cell death occur during mitosis as a result of radiation-induced damage to chromosomal DNA. After a variable latency period, the depleted pool of replicating cells is unable to compensate for cell loss. The vascular endothelium becomes discontinuous, resulting in intraluminal coagulation and capillary closure characteristic of radiation retinopathy.

Archer and colleagues[4] performed a clinicopathologic study on seven human eyes enucleated after teletherapy irradiation with high-energy photons, gamma-rays, or X-rays. Retinal capillary changes were frequently seen, including fusiform dilations, microaneurysms, and acellularity. In contradistinction to diabetic retinopathy, in which pericyte loss predominates, a predilection for endothelial cell loss was identified in cases with radiation injury. Ultrastructural examination demonstrated that new intraretinal vessels had fenestrated endothelium. Histopathologic studies of eyes receiving proton beam therapy for intraocular melanoma have demonstrated retinopathy in areas directly adjacent to the irradiated tumor. The lack of radiation damage in areas outside the proton beam has been emphasized.[6] The postmitotic neural retina, like neurons in the central nervous system, is highly resistant to radiation damage.[7] Pathologic changes in the neural retina are secondary to radiation-induced vasculopathy. As demonstrated in animal models, damage to mitotically active endothelial cells eventually leads to occlusive vascular disease and its sequelae. Studies in humans have shown loss of ganglion cells secondary to neovascular glaucoma, cystic changes in the outer plexiform and inner nuclear layers, and thickening of the vessel walls from deposition of fibrillary or hyaline material. There may be myointimal proliferation in larger vessels.[8] In general, there appears to be preferential damage to inner retinal layers. Photoreceptors appear to be relatively resistant to radiation damage.[9,10] It has been shown in animal studies that rods can be damaged by single doses of 20 Gy, but that cones require doses of 100 Gy or more before significant changes are seen.[11] Clinically, patients with ocular irradiation do not suffer from night blindness or other symptoms of photoreceptor degeneration.[12]

Although most authors agree that radiation damage to the retina is mediated primarily through damage to retinal vessels, involvement of the choroidal vasculature may be seen as well.[13] Midena and colleagues[14] used fluorescein and indocyanine green angiography to study the effects of external beam radiation on the choroidal circulation. In eyes with radiation retinopathy, areas of choriocapillaris perfusion defects were evident in areas remote from retinal ischemia. Large choroidal vessels were largely unaffected. Loss of vision was not attributable to choroidal hypoperfusion.

Subretinal and choroidal neovascularization (CNV) has been reported as a rare complication of ocular irradiation.[14,15] Choriovitreal neovascular complexes have been observed at sites of severe chorioretinal atrophy after radon seed brachytherapy.[16]

CLINICAL FEATURES

Flick,[17] in 1948, described acute ocular lesions in survivors of the atomic blasts at Hiroshima and Nagasaki. Retinal abnormalities, including exudates (cottonwool spots), intraretinal and preretinal hemorrhages, and Roth's spots, were documented. The frequency with which these lesions occurred correlated with white blood cell counts. Presumably, the retinal lesions were largely the result of pancytopenia caused by radiation exposure, not direct radiation-induced retinal injury.

Delayed radiation damage to retinal blood vessels causes vascular incompetence and occlusion. The earliest changes typically seen in radiation retinopathy include capillary dilation, telangiectasias, microaneurysm formation, and capillary closure. Cottonwool spots occur transiently, with later evolution of large areas of capillary nonperfusion. Exudative phenomena resulting from retinal vascular incompetence may occur. Retinal edema with preferential involvement of the macula is often seen.[18] However, a localized retinopathy corresponding to the radiation field may develop.[19]

The occlusive microangiopathy in radiation retinopathy may be slowly and inexorably progressive.[20] Although spontaneous improvement may occur, this is an infrequent event. In a study of 218 patients after proton beam irradiation of paramacular choroidal melanomas, 87% of the patients were found to have macular edema by postirradiation year 3, with spontaneous resolution in only 5% of cases.[21] In a long-term follow-up study of eyes with radiation retinopathy, Kinyoun et al. found that eyes with proliferative retinopathy had a poor visual prognosis despite successful treatment with panretinal photocoagulation. Eyes with nonproliferative disease had a relatively benign course, with most eyes maintaining reading vision (see Prognosis).[22]

Widespread capillary closure and retinal ischemia may lead to retinal and disc neovascularization, vitreous hemorrhage, and retinal detachment.[11,23,24] Anterior-segment neovascularization may also occur, leading to neovascular glaucoma. Other late changes include retinal pigment epithelial atrophy and, in some cases, generalized dispersion of the retinal pigment epithelium, leading to a "salt-and-pepper" fundus appearance.[8] In addition to the ubiquitous microangiopathic changes, central retinal artery obstruction[24,25] and central retinal vein obstruction[26] have been reported following radiation therapy, although a causative relation is not certain. An association between radiation exposure and idiopathic parafoveal telangiectasis has likewise been reported.[27] In one case-control series, a history of therapeutic head and neck irradiation or of environmental radiation exposure increased the risk of patients developing parafoveal telangiectasis.

Spaide and colleagues[28] reported an unusual choroidal vascular anomaly in patients receiving external beam radiation to treat subfoveal CNV secondary to age-related macular degeneration. In this retrospective analysis, 193 patients were evaluated: these patients underwent treatment with either 10 to 12 Gy or 20 Gy external beam photons. Nineteen patients (9.8%) developed round to oval vascular blebs along the periphery of the CNV that showed marked leakage of fluorecein dye on angiography. These lesions, termed radiation-induced choroidal neovasculopathy, were best imaged using indocyanine green angiography. Patients who developed this finding tended to have a poor visual prognosis.

In the 1982 report by Brown and colleagues[8] involving 36 eyes with radiation retinopathy, 20 patients had received radioactive cobalt plaques (brachytherapy) for the treatment of intraocular tumors. Eighty-five percent of these patients developed hard exudates, 75% showed microaneurysm formation, 65% had intraretinal hemorrhages, 35% had retinal vascular telangiectasia, 30% had cottonwool spots, and 20% showed vascular sheathing. The 16 patients who received external beam irradiation (teletherapy) showed hard exudates in 38% of cases, microaneurysms in 81%, and intraretinal hemorrhage in 88%. Retinal vascular telangiectasia and cottonwool spots were seen in 38% of these patients, and vascular sheathing was apparent in 25% of cases. Brown and co-workers[8] postulate that the increased frequency of hard exudate formation in patients treated with brachytherapy rather than teletherapy may have been connected with vascular leakage related to the intraocular neoplasm, and not simply the radiation therapy alone (Fig. 83-1). One of the 20 plaque-treated patients developed posterior-segment neovascularization, as compared with seven of 16 patients treated with external beam radiation. Four of the 16 patients subsequently developed neovascular glaucoma. Presumably, neovascularization is more frequent in patients who are treated with external beam radiation, as the entire retinal area receives the dose as opposed to a localized area following radioactive plaque therapy.[8]

Guyer and colleagues[21] reported the largest series of patients following irradiation of choroidal melanomas. Of 218 patients receiving proton beam therapy for paramacular tumors, 89% developed some manifestation of radiation retinopathy within a follow-up period of 5 months to 15 years (median, 40 months). The earliest and most common finding was macular edema, present in 87% of patients within 3 years of radiation treatment. Other features of radiation-induced microangiopathy were seen with high frequency, including microaneurysms and telangiectasia, intraretinal hemorrhages, capillary nonperfusion, and cottonwool spots. Retinal neovascularization was relatively rare after proton beam treatment, occurring in only 6% of patients.

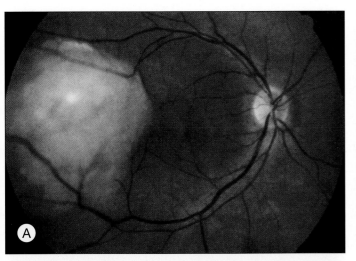

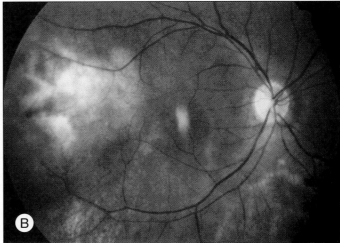

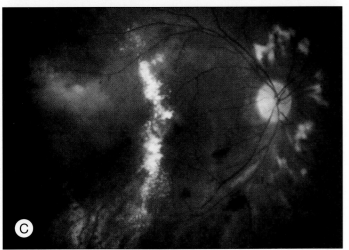

Fig. 83-1 A, Pretreatment appearance of a 6 mm elevated choroidal melanoma. B, Twelve months after iodine-125 plaque irradiation, the tumor has almost flattened out completely. Notice a small hemorrhage and cottonwool spot inferior to the disc. These are the earliest clinical signs of radiation retinopathy. C, Thirty-six months after treatment, there is marked lipid exudation. The peripapillary cottonwool spots are much more prominent.

Microangiographic changes may become apparent 6 months or more after treatment, but in some cases are not detected for several years. Amoaku & Archer[19] found the interval between external beam radiation treatment and the detection of radiation retinopathy to be between 1.0 and 8.5 years (mean, 4.7 years). They emphasized the need for long-term follow-up in patients receiving ocular irradiation, since retinopathy has a variable and delayed onset. In the report of Brown et al.,[8] the time of onset of radiation retinopathy after radioactive plaque therapy ranged from 4 to 32 months (mean, 14.6 months), and after external beam radiation the onset ranged from 7 to 36 months (mean, 18.7 months). The possibility of persistent toxicity after radiation exposure is suggested by the long latency between incidental environmental or therapeutic exposure and development of idiopathic parafoveal telangiectasia. In this circumstance, the average time to onset from exposure to diagnosis of retinal changes was determined to be 42 years![27]

INCIDENCE AND DOSIMETRY

The frequency with which radiation-related retinal changes are seen varies from report to report. Methodology varies considerably between various studies, making meaningful comparisons problematic. Data for radiation doses to the retina are unreliable in many instances and are often not calculated for teletherapy methods. In most studies, the occurrence of retinopathy is determined retrospectively by using ambiguous criteria, such as onset of symptoms, various fundus changes, or angiographic abnormalities. In addition, the length of follow-up varies considerably. As discussed earlier, the length of follow-up is critical in assessing the prevalence of radiation retinopathy.[19]

It is generally accepted that the incidence of radiation retinopathy depends on both the total radiation dose and fraction size. Using precise dosimetry data, Parsons and co-workers[29] determined the risk of radiation retinopathy according to these parameters. Using both retrospective and prospective data, these authors analyzed 68 eyes of 64 patients receiving teletherapy for extracranial tumors. They found that doses in the 45 to 55 Gy range delivered to half or more of the retina produced a 53% rate of retinopathy, with the risk increased by diabetes, chemotherapy, and high dose per fraction. Patient age was not correlated with the risk of developing retinopathy. Median time to onset of symptoms was 2.5 years (range 1 to 6.5 years), with vision worse than 20/200 in 27 eyes of 26 patients as a result of ischemia.

Rubeosis iridis and/or glaucoma were first detected a median of 28 months (17 months to 5.5 years) after irradiation. No eye developed retinopathy below 45 Gy, and the authors concluded that doses to the retina less than 45 Gy given in 1.8 to 2 Gy fractions rarely cause significant retinopathy in the absence of coexisting factors. Using data from the literature, the authors constructed a sigmoid dose–response curve for the development of radiation retinopathy.

Several independent studies[5] have corroborated the findings of Parsons and co-workers. Most studies report that, under normal conditions, a minimum exposure of 30 to 35 Gy of cephalic radiation is needed before retinopathy can be expected. In two reports, after 60 Gy, 50% of patients had retinal changes, and after 70 to 80 Gy, 85% to 95% of eyes had retinal changes within several months.[7,12] On the other hand, in a report of patients who received radiation for sinus cancer, all patients who received more than 45 to 50 Gy showed retinal changes, although they did not usually have visual loss. Mild decreased vision was seen following 65 Gy, however, and severe visual loss was seen in patients treated with 68 Gy or more.

In reviewing data from patients treated with brachytherapy using cobalt plaques, Brown et al.[8] observed that foveal damage was seen after a mean of 150 Gy, with a range of 45 to 220 Gy; patients who had no foveal damage had received a mean dose to the fovea of 50 Gy (range, 35 to 90 Gy). One patient who had diabetes showed foveal damage after 45 Gy, but otherwise no patient who received less than 100 Gy to the fovea showed changes. After external beam radiation, the mean dose to the fovea that produced damage was 49 Gy, with a range of 35 to 72 Gy. Brown et al.[8] concluded that much higher doses of local therapy must be delivered to an area to produce damage than appears to be needed after external beam radiation.

Similar results have been reported for the development of retinopathy after brachytherapy with other radioactive isotopes. In a study of 64 patients receiving iodine-125 brachytherapy for uveal melanoma, Packer and colleagues[30] observed a 23.4% incidence of radiation retinopathy and a 18.8% incidence of rubeosis iridis after a mean follow-up of 64.9 months. Radiation doses for the iodine-125 plaque were calculated at between 80 and 100 Gy. Finger et al.[31] observed a low rate of retinopathy, 8.7%, following palladium-103 brachytherapy after a limited follow-up of 13.5 months. In this study, patients were treated for uveal melanoma with either high-dose radiation (80 to 100 Gy) or low-dose radiation (40 to 50 Gy) combined with microwave hyperthermia. It is expected that the frequency of retinopathy will increase as longer-duration follow-up becomes available.

The incidence of radiation retinopathy after helium ion or proton beam irradiation has also been reported (Fig. 83-2). Eighty-nine percent of patients receiving 70 Gy of proton beam radiation in five fractions over 7 to 10 days developed radiation maculopathy.[21]

Several studies support the findings of Parsons and colleagues that radiation-induced side-effects increase with increased fraction size. In one series, 22% of patients treated with 250 cGy fractions developed optic nerve damage, as opposed to 12.5% of

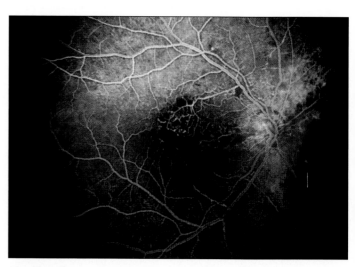

Fig. 83-2 Three years after proton beam radiation for a nasal choroidal melanoma (not shown), fluorescein angiography highlights areas of capillary nonperfusion. There are marked intraretinal microvascular abnormalities.

patients who were treated with 200 cGy fractions.[32] Larger daily dose fractions used in bone marrow transplantation may significantly lower the threshold for radiation retinopathy.[33,34]

It is difficult to establish definitively the threshold radiation dose required to produce retinopathy. Changes have been seen after as little as 11 to 15 Gy of external beam radiation to the retina.[35,36] Reports continue to appear in the literature documenting retinopathy after incrementally smaller doses of radiation. The development of retinopathy may be multifactorial in some cases, thereby confounding the determination of the radiation threshold dose. Indeed, a case of occlusive retinal microvasculopathy identical to radiation retinopathy has been observed in a bone marrow transplant recipient in the absence of prior radiation therapy.[33] Lopez and co-workers[34] found that five of eight bone marrow transplant recipients undergoing total-body irradiation with high-dose chemotherapy developed an occlusive microangiographic characteristic of radiation retinopathy. Two of the five patients with retinopathy received a total radiation dose of 12 Gy, suggesting that high-dose chemotherapy lowered the threshold for radiation-induced damage. Although the occurrence of this ischemic retinopathy has been designated "bone marrow transplant retinopathy" by many authors, the retinal findings are indistinguishable from those of radiation retinopathy. Significantly, histopathologic examination in two cases of bone marrow transplant retinopathy has revealed changes similar to those seen in radiation retinopathy, with endothelial cell loss and relative preservation of vascular pericytes.[37] Numerous studies examining the effect of low-dose external beam or plaque radiotherapy on subfoveal CNV in age-related macular degeneration have failed to show radiation retinopathy (versus choroidopathy[28]) as a complication.[38–40] In studies examining the effect of external beam therapy,[39,40] total dose delivered to the macula ranged from 8 to 16 Gy in divided fractions. In a study[38] where ophthalmic plaque was used, apex dose delivered to the macula ranged from 1250 to 2362 cGy in a single application. Follow-up in these studies was typically limited to less than 2 years, thereby limiting the sensitivity of detection of radiation-related complications.

DIFFERENTIAL DIAGNOSIS AND DIAGNOSTIC EVALUATION

Radiation retinopathy may be indistinguishable from changes seen in patients with diabetic retinopathy. Patients who have had multiple-branch retinal artery obstructions or multiple episodes of venous occlusive disease, or who have retinal telangiectasia from other causes, may have a similar picture as well. The diagnosis can usually be confirmed by questioning the patient and determining if there has been radiation therapy in the past. A review of the treatment records will permit the ophthalmologist to determine whether the eyes were included in the field of radiation. In some cases the etiology of an occlusive retinopathy may be multifactorial and the role of radiation indeterminate.

The diagnosis of radiation retinopathy should be considered following cephalic radiation for any reason. Radiation retinopathy has been reported after orbital treatment for thyroid disease[41,42] and for orbital pseudotumor, as well as after intracranial radiation therapy for both primary and metastatic central nervous system tumors.[43] It is well known to occur after paranasal sinus radiation therapy[7] and can occur after radiation therapy for skin tumors of the face and lids.

The diagnosis can usually be made clinically, and the fluorescein angiographic findings can lend support to the clinical diagnosis (Fig. 83-3). Areas of capillary nonperfusion are so consistent that it is difficult to make the diagnosis without this finding.[8] Retinal capillaries appear to be affected before the larger vessels. Hayreh[24] has reviewed the angiographic findings and has documented the occurrence of obliteration of retinal vessels, microaneurysm formation, telangiectasia and retinal neovascularization,

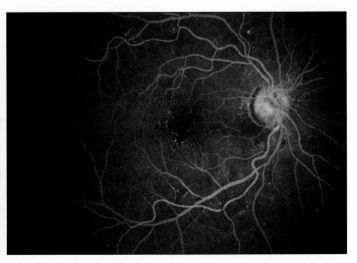

Fig. 83-3 Typical mid-phase angiographic appearance of radiation retinopathy. Note microaneurysms, areas of capillary nonperfusion, and intraretinal microvascular abnormalities. This patient had been treated for an orbital tumor.

cottonwool spots, hard exudates, retinal hemorrhage, cystoid macular edema, vascular sheathing and perivasculitis, optic disc edema, and disc neovascularization.

TREATMENT

Visual loss related to macular nonperfusion probably cannot be reversed. However, several groups[44,45] have applied treatment guidelines of the Early Treatment Diabetic Retinopathy Study (ETDRS) to eyes with macular edema and posterior-segment neovascularization, with favorable results. In one study, 12 eyes with clinically significant macular edema secondary to radiation were treated with focal and grid photocoagulation;[45] eight of 12 (67%) eyes showed improvement in macular edema after laser therapy, with six (50%) eyes having complete resolution of clinically significant edema after a mean follow-up of 39 months. Vision improved from a median preoperative level of 20/100 to 20/75 at the time of final examination. Macular ischemia, cataract, and radiation optic neuropathy were noted in all eyes and contributed to vision loss in some cases. It is of interest that clinically significant edema developed 87 months after radiation treatment.

Hykin and co-workers[46] examined the efficacy of ETDRS-type treatment for eyes with clinically significant radiation macular edema (CSRME) secondary to scleral plaque radiotherapy for choroidal melanoma. In this retrospective study, 19 cases treated once with focal laser were compared to a matched group of 23 eyes with CSRME receiving no treatment. Treated eyes showed significant benefit with respect to vision improvement at 6 months, with 8/19 (42%) gaining ≥ 1 Snellen line versus no cases in the untreated group. A trend was noted in the treated group towards resolution of macular edema at 6 months and towards less vision loss at 12 months following focal laser. However, early improvement in vision and edema in the treated group was not sustained. Both groups showed equivalent degrees of vision loss at 2-year follow-up, with both 68% of cases and of controls experiencing doubling of the visual angle. No significant difference between treated and untreated eyes in visual acuity was seen at 2 years. The authors concluded that a single treatment with focal laser will not result in sustained benefit and that additional treatments may be indicated for persistent or recurrent CSRME.

In an earlier report, Kinyoun et al.[44] described treatment of six eyes with high-risk neovascularization by panretinal photocoagulation. Three eyes had regression of new vessels, with no recurrent vitreous hemorrhages within 19 to 66 months' follow-up. Pars plana vitrectomy was performed in three eyes with nonclearing hemorrhages, with improvement in vision. Kinyoun et al. later reported a success rate of 91% in 11 eyes treated with panretinal photocoagulation for proliferative radiation retinopathy.[22] However, long-term visual outcome in this group was poor, with few eyes retaining vision better than 20/200.

Kwok et al.[47] analyzed the occurrence of neovascular glaucoma in a group of 50 eyes undergoing cataract surgery after external beam radiation. Panretinal photocoagulation significantly reduced the incidence of neovascular glaucoma after cataract surgery, with 5 of 15 without laser and 0 of 35 eyes with laser developing neovascular glaucoma. Several other authors[18,20,34,48,49] have reported favorable results using similar photocoagulation techniques to treat radiation-induced clinically significant macular edema or high-risk neovascularization.

Hyperbaric oxygen has been proposed as a treatment for radiation retinopathy, but its benefit remains unproved, and it may even exacerbate the disease.[50] One study analyzed the use of corticosteroids and hyperbaric oxygen in the treatment of radiation optic neuropathy and showed no beneficial effect.[51]

PROGNOSIS

Radiation retinopathy may lead to visual loss from foveal nonperfusion, macular edema, vitreous hemorrhage, retinal detachment, or neovascular glaucoma. Retinopathy appears to be slowly progressive, although spontaneous regression has been seen. In patients treated with proton beam irradiation for paramacular choroidal melanomas, 67% maintained vision of 20/200 or better at 3 years after irradiation.[21] Fifty-nine percent of patients receiving cobalt irradiation for choroidal melanomas maintained vision of 20/200 or better.[52] Kinyoun et al. reported the long-term follow-up of patients with nonproliferative and proliferative forms of radiation retinopathy. Eyes with proliferative retinopathy had a poor visual prognosis despite successful treatment with panretinal photocoagulation. In 14 eyes with proliferative retinopathy, median visual acuity dropped from 20/90 to 20/400 after 75 months of follow-up, with only two eyes maintaining better than 20/200 vision. Eyes with nonproliferative retinopathy showed a modest decline in vision, from 20/25 to 20/50 over 51 months of follow-up, with 7 of 27 eyes developing 20/200 or worse.[22]

Three situations appear to exacerbate radiation retinopathy:[5,29] (1) patients who have a pre-existing microangiopathy appear to be more prone to developing severe changes; (2) diabetic patients are more likely to show changes following lower doses of radiation than are nondiabetic patients[8,53,54] (Fig. 83-4); and (3) patients who receive certain chemotherapeutic agents may show more marked or severe changes, even if the chemotherapy is not administered concomitantly.[55] Chan & Shukovsky[56] reported that patients who received simultaneous 5-fluorouracil showed more frequent loss of vision. Similarly, the lower threshold for radiation-induced retinopathy in bone marrow transplant recipients appears to be related to high-dose chemotherapy.[34] Concomitant use of hyperbaric oxygen may also exacerbate the condition, with severe disease seen following only 36 Gy.[50]

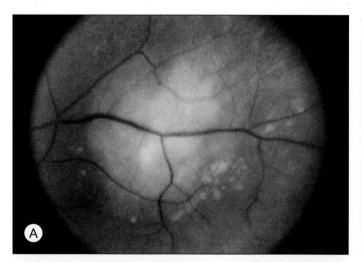

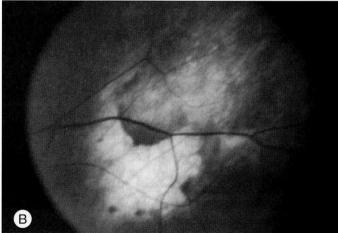

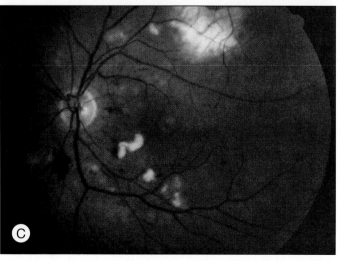

Fig. 83-4 A, Choroidal metastasis from adenocarcinoma of the lung is present along the superotemporal arcade. The patient has diabetes but does not have any diabetic retinopathy. B, Four weeks after 35 Gy of external beam radiation, the tumor has regressed completely. C, Twelve months later, there are multiple hemorrhages and cottonwool spots. The inferior aspect of the regressed tumor is visible at the top of the photograph.

REFERENCES

1. Stallard HB. Radiant energy as (a) a pathogenic and (b) a therapeutic agent in ophthalmic disorders. Br J Ophthalmol Suppl 1933; 6:1–126.
2. Moore RF. Presidential address. Trans Ophthalmol Soc UK 1935; 55:3–26.
3. Irvine AR, Wood IS. Radiation retinopathy as an experimental model for ischemic proliferative retinopathy and rubeosis iridis. Am J Ophthalmol 1987; 103:790–797.
4. Archer DB, Amoaku WMK, Gardner TA. Radiation retinopathy: clinical, histopathological, ultrastructural, and experimental correlations. Eye 1991; 5:239–251.
5. Archer DB. Doyne lecture: responses of retinal and choroidal vessels to ionizing radiation. Eye 1993; 7:1–13.
6. Ferry AP, Blair CJ, Gragoudas ES et al. Pathologic examination of ciliary body melanoma treated with proton beam irradiation. Arch Ophthalmol 1985; 103:1849–1853.
7. Nakissa N, Rubin P, Strohl R et al. Ocular and orbital complications following radiation therapy of paranasal sinus malignancies and review of literature. Cancer 1983; 51:980–986.
8. Brown GC, Shields JA, Sanborn G et al. Radiation retinopathy. Ophthalmology 1982; 89:1494–1501.
9. Egbert PR, Fajardo LF, Donaldson SS et al. Posterior ocular abnormalities after irradiation for retinoblastoma: a histopathological study. Br J Ophthalmol 1980; 64:660–665.
10. Ross HS, Rosenberg S, Friedman AH. Delayed radiation necrosis of the optic nerve. Am J Ophthalmol 1973; 76:683–686.
11. Cibis PA, Noell WK, Eichel B. Ocular effects produced by high-intensity X-radiation. Arch Ophthalmol 1955; 53:651–663.
12. Merriam GR Jr, Szechter A, Focht EF. The effects of ionizing radiations on the eye. Front Radiat Ther Oncol 1972; 6:346–385.
13. Elmassri A. Radiation chorioretinopathy. Br J Ophthalmol 1986; 70:326–329.
14. Midena E, Segato T, Valenti M et al. The effect of external eye irradiation on choroidal circulation. Ophthalmology 1996; 103:1651–1660.
15. Boozalis GT, Schachat AP, Green WR. Subretinal neovascularization from the retina in radiation retinopathy. Retina 1987; 7:156–161.
16. Archer DB, Amoaku WMK, Kelly G. Choroidoretinal neovascularisation following radon seed treatment of retinoblastoma in two patients. Br J Ophthalmol 1993; 77:95–99.
17. Flick JJ. Ocular lesions following the atomic bombing of Hiroshima and Nagasaki. Am J Ophthalmol 1948; 31:137–154.
18. Chaudhuri PR, Austin DJ, Rosenthal AR. Treatment of radiation retinopathy. Br J Ophthalmol 1981; 65:623–625.
19. Amoaku WMK, Archer DB. Cephalic radiation and retinal vasculopathy. Eye 1990; 4:195–203.
20. Amoaku WMK, Archer DB. Fluorescein angiographic features, natural course, and treatment of radiation retinopathy. Eye 1990; 4:657–667.
21. Guyer DR, Mukai S, Egan KM et al. Radiation maculopathy following proton beam irradiation for choroidal melanoma. Ophthalmology 1992; 99:1278–1285.
22. Kinyoun JL, Lawrence BS, Barlow WE. Proliferative radiation retinopathy. Arch Ophthalmol 1996; 114:1097–1100.
23. Chee PHY. Radiation retinopathy. Am J Ophthalmol 1968; 66:860–865.
24. Hayreh SS. Post-radiation retinopathy: a fluorescence fundus angiographic study. Br J Ophthalmol 1970; 54:705–714.
25. Shukovsky LJ, Fletcher GH. Retinal and optic nerve complications in a high dose irradiation technique of ethmoid sinus and nasal cavity. Radiology 1972; 104:629–634.
26. Cogan DG. Lesions of the eye from radiant energy. JAMA 1950; 142:145–151.
27. Maberley DAL, Yanuzzi LA, Gitter K et al. Radiation exposure: a new risk factor for idiopathic perifoveal telangiectasis. Ophthalmology 1999; 106:2248–2253.
28. Spaide RF, Leys A, Herrmann-Delemazure B et al. Radiation-associated choroidal neovasculopathy. Ophthalmology 1999; 106:2254–2260.
29. Parsons JT, Bova FJ, Fitzgerald CR et al. Radiation retinopathy after external beam irradiation: analysis of time–dose factors. Int J Radiat Oncol Biol Phys 1994; 30:765–773.
30. Packer S, Stoller S, Lesser ML et al. Long-term results of iodine 125 irradiation of uveal melanoma. Ophthalmology 1992; 99:767–774.
31. Finger PT, Buffa A, Mishra S et al. Palladium 103 plaque radiotherapy for uveal melanoma: clinical experience. Ophthalmology 1994; 101:256–263.
32. Harris JR, Levene MB. Visual complications following irradiation for pituitary adenomas and craniopharyngiomas. Radiology 1976; 120:167–171.
33. Cunningham ET, Irvine AR, Rugo HS. Bone marrow transplantation retinopathy in the absence of radiation therapy. Am J Ophthalmol 1996; 122:268–270.
34. Lopez PF, Sternberg P, Dabbs CK et al. Bone marrow transplant retinopathy. Am J Ophthalmol 1991; 112:635–646.
35. Elsas T, Thorud E, Jetne V et al. Retinopathy after low dose irradiation for an intracranial tumor of the frontal lobe. Acta Ophthalmol (Copenh) 1988; 66:65–68.
36. Perrers-Taylor M, Brinkley D, Reynolds T. Choroido-retinal damage as a complication of radiotherapy. Acta Radiol Ther Phys Biol 1965; 3:431–440.
37. Webster AR, Anderson JR, Richards EM et al. Ischaemic retinopathy occurring in patients receiving bone marrow allografts and campath-IG: a clinico-pathological study. Br J Ophthalmol 1995; 79:687–691.
38. Finger PT, Berson A, Ng T et al. Ophthalmic plaque radiotherapy for age-related macular degeneration associated with subretinal neovascularization. Am J Ophthalmol 1999; 127:170–177.
39. The Radiation Therapy for Age-related Macular Degeneration (RAD) Study Group. A prospective, randomized, double-masked trial on radiation therapy for neovascular age-related macular degeneration. Ophthalmology 1999; 106:2239–2247.
40. Valmaggia C, Ries G, Ballinari P. Radiotherapy for subfoveal choroidal neovascularization in age-related macular degeneration: a randomized clinical trial. Am J Ophthalmol 2002; 133:521–529.
41. Kinyoun JL, Kalina RE, Brower SA. Radiation retinopathy after orbital irradiation for Graves' ophthalmopathy. Arch Ophthalmol 1984; 102:1473–1476.
42. Kinyoun JL, Orcutt JC. Radiation retinopathy. JAMA 1987; 258:610–611.
43. Bagan SM, Hollenhorst RW. Radiation retinopathy after irradiation of intracranial lesions. Am J Ophthalmol 1979; 88:694–697.
44. Kinyoun JL, Chittum ME, Wells CG. Photocoagulation treatment of radiation retinopathy. Am J Ophthalmol 1988; 105:470–478.
45. Kinyoun JL, Zamber RW, Lawrence BS et al. Photocoagulation treatment for clinically significant radiation macular oedema. Br J Ophthalmol 1995; 79:144–149.
46. Hykin PG, Shields CL, Shields JA et al. The efficacy of focal laser therapy in radiation-induced macular edema. Ophthalmology 1998; 105:1425–1429.
47. Kwok SK, Leung SF, Ho PCP et al. Neovascular glaucoma developing after uncomplicated cataract surgery for heavily irradiated eyes. Ophthalmology 1997; 104:1112–1115.
48. Gass JDM. A fluorescein angiographic study of macular dysfunction secondary to retinal vascular disease. IV. X-irradiation, carotid artery occlusion, collagen vascular disease, and vitritis. Arch Ophthalmol 1968; 80:606–617.
49. Thompson GM, Migdal CS, Whittle RJM. Radiation retinopathy following treatment of posterior nasal space carcinoma. Br J Ophthalmol 1983; 67:609–614.
50. Stanford MR. Retinopathy after irradiation and hyperbaric oxygen. J R Soc Med 1984; 77:1041–1043.
51. Roden D, Bosley TM, Fowble B et al. Delayed radiation injury to the retrobulbar optic nerves and chiasm: clinical syndrome and treatment with hyperbaric oxygen and corticosteroids. Ophthalmology 1990; 97:346–351.
52. Haye C, Desjardins L, Bouder P et al. Maculopathies par radiations chez les patients traités pour melanomeschoroidiens. Ophtalmologie 1990; 4:229–231.
53. Viebahn M, Barricks ME. Potentiating effect of diabetes in radiation retinopathy. Int J Radiat Oncol Biol Phys 1993; 25:379–380.
54. Wara WM, Irvine AR, Neger RE et al. Radiation retinopathy. Int J Radiat Oncol Biol Phys 1979; 5:81–83.
55. Chacko DC. Considerations in the diagnosis of radiation injury. JAMA 1981; 245:1255–1258.
56. Chan RC, Shukovsky LJ. Effects of irradiation on the eye. Radiology 1976; 120:673–675.

Chapter

84

Ocular Ischemic Syndrome

Sanjay Sharma
Gary C. Brown

In 1963, Kearns and Hollenhorst[1] reported on the ocular symptoms and signs occurring secondary to severe carotid artery obstructive disease. They called the entity "venous stasis retinopathy" and noted that it occurred in approximately 5% of patients with severe carotid artery insufficiency or thrombosis. Some confusion has since arisen with this term because it has also been used to designate mild central retinal vein obstruction.[2] A number of additional alternative nomenclatures have been proposed, including ischemic ocular inflammation,[3] ischemic coagulopathy,[4] and the ocular ischemic syndrome.[5,6] Histopathologic examination of eyes with the entity generally does not reveal inflammation,[7,8] and therefore the descriptive term that we prefer is the ocular ischemic syndrome.

DEMOGRAPHICS AND INCIDENCE

The mean age of patients with the ocular ischemic syndrome is about 65 years, with a range generally from the fifties to the eighties. No racial predilection has been identified, and males are affected more than females by a ratio of about 2:1. Either eye can be affected, and in approximately 20% of patients ocular involvement is bilateral. The incidence of the disease has not been extensively studied, but from the work of Sturrock and Mueller[9] an annual estimate of 7.5 cases/million persons can be made. This number may be falsely low, since it is possible that a number of cases are misdiagnosed.

ETIOLOGY

In general, a 90% or greater stenosis of the ipsilateral carotid arterial system is present in eyes with the ocular ischemic syndrome.[5] It has been shown that a 90% carotid stenosis reduces the ipsilateral central retinal artery perfusion pressure by about 50%.[10,11] The obstruction can occur within the common carotid or internal carotid artery. In about 50% of cases the affected vessel is 100% occluded.[5]

Occasionally, obstruction of the ipsilateral ophthalmic artery can also be responsible.[5,12,13] Rarely, an isolated obstruction of the central retinal artery alone can mimic the dilated retinal veins and retinal hemorrhages seen in eyes with the ocular ischemic syndrome.[14]

Atherosclerosis within the carotid artery is the cause for the great majority of cases of the ocular ischemic syndrome.[5] Dissecting aneurysm of the carotid artery has been reported as a cause,[15] as has giant cell arteritis.[16] Hypothetically, entities such as fibromuscular dysplasia,[17] Behçet's disease,[18] trauma,[19] and inflammatory entities that cause carotid artery obstruction could lead to the ocular ischemic syndrome.

CLINICAL PRESENTATION

Visual loss

Greater than 90% of patients with the ocular ischemic syndrome relate a history of visual loss in the affected eye(s).[5] In two-thirds of these it occurs over a period of weeks; it is abrupt in approximately 12%. In this latter group with sudden visual loss there is often a cherry-red spot present on funduscopic examination (Fig. 84-1).

Prolonged recovery following exposure to a bright light has been described in patients with severe carotid artery obstruction.[20] Concurrent attenuation of the visual evoked response has also been observed in these cases after light exposure. The phenomenon has been attributed to ischemia of the macular retina. In cases of bilateral, severe carotid artery obstruction, the visual loss after exposure to bright light occurs in both eyes, mimicking occipital lobe ischemia due to vertebrobasilar disease.[21]

Dissection of the internal carotid artery has been reported to cause scintillating scotomata that resemble a migraine aura.[22] While these could theoretically be associated with the classic ocular ischemic syndrome, they have not been observed by the authors.

A history of amaurosis fugax is elicited in about 10% of ocular ischemic syndrome patients.[5] Amaurosis fugax, or fleeting loss of vision for seconds to minutes, is thought to be most commonly caused by emboli to the central retinal arterial system, although vasospasm may also play a role.[23] Although the majority of people with amaurosis fugax alone do not have the ocular ischemic syndrome, it can be an indicator of concomitant, ipsilateral carotid artery obstructive disease. About one-third of patients with amaurosis fugax have an ipsilateral carotid artery obstruction of 75% or greater.[24] Rarely, it has been associated with a stenosis of the ophthalmic artery.[24]

Pain

Pain is present in the affected eye or orbital region in about 40% of cases,[5] and has been referred to as "ocular angina." Most often, it is

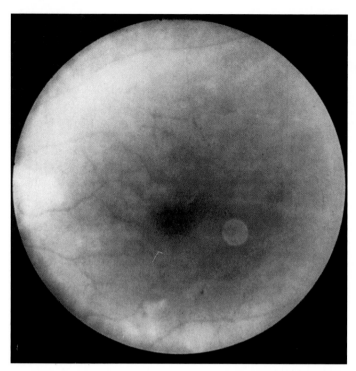

Fig. 84-1 Cherry-red spot in the left eye of a 66-year-old man with rubeosis iridis, a 100% ipsilateral common carotid artery obstruction and a history of rapid visual loss.

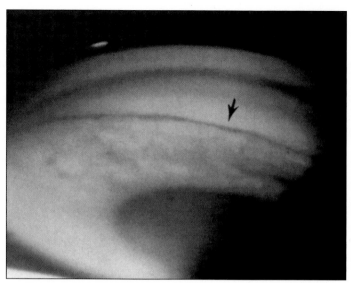

Fig. 84-2 Rubeosis iridis in an eye with the ocular ischemic syndrome. Fibrovascular tissue is present within the anterior chamber angle (arrow).

described as a dull ache. It can occur secondary to neovascular glaucoma, but in those cases in which the intraocular pressure is normal the cause may be ischemia to the globe and/or ipsilateral dura.

Visual acuity

The presenting visual acuities of patients with the ocular ischemic syndrome are bimodally distributed with 43% of affected eyes having vision ranging from 20/20 to 20/50, and 37% having counting fingers or worse vision.[25] Absence of light perception is generally not seen early, but can develop in the later stages of the disease, usually secondary to neovascular glaucoma. Among all eyes with the ocular ischemic syndrome at the end of one year of follow-up, including those with and without treatment, approximately 24% remain in the 20/20–20/50 group and 58% have counting fingers or worse vision.

Anterior segment changes

Rubeosis iridis is encountered in approximately two thirds of eyes with the ocular ischemic syndrome at the time of presentation[5] (Fig. 84-2). Nevertheless, only slightly over half of these eyes have or develop an increase in intraocular pressure, even if the anterior chamber angle is closed by fibrovascular tissue. Impaired ciliary body perfusion, with a subsequent decrease in aqueous production, probably accounts for this phenomenon.

Flare in the anterior chamber is usually present in most eyes with rubeosis iridis. An anterior chamber cellular response is seen in almost one fifth of eyes with the ocular ischemic syndrome,[5] but it rarely exceeds grade 2, as per the Schlaegel classification.[26] Keratic precipitates can be present, but are unusual.

In unilateral cases, there is generally little difference between the degree of lens opacification in each eye. As the disease advances, however, cataractous lens changes can develop. In advanced cases, the lens may become mature.

Although not an anterior segment sign, prominent collateral vessels are occasionally seen on the forehead. These vessels connect the external carotid system on one side of the head to that of the other. These vascular collaterals should not be mistaken for the enlarged tender vessels seen with giant cell arteritis and considered for temporal artery biopsy.

Posterior segment findings

The retinal arteries are usually narrowed and the retinal veins are most often dilated, but not tortuous (Fig. 84-3). The venous dilation may be accompanied by beading, but usually not to the extent seen in eyes with marked preproliferative or proliferative diabetic retinopathy. Dilation of the veins is probably a nonspecific response to the ischemia from the inflow obstruction. Nevertheless, in some eyes both the retinal arteries and veins are narrowed. In contrast, eyes with central retinal vein obstruction usually also have dilated retinal veins, but they are often tortuous. The fact that the ocular ischemic syndrome occurs secondary to impaired inflow, while central retinal vein obstruction is usually associated with compromised outflow resulting from thrombus formation at or near the lamina cribrosa, may account for this difference.[27]

Retinal hemorrhages are seen in about 80% of affected eyes. They are most commonly present in the mid-periphery,[27a] but can also extend into the posterior pole (Figs 84-4 and 84-5). While dot and blot hemorrhages are the most common variant, superficial retinal hemorrhages in the nerve fiber layer are occasionally seen. The hemorrhages probably arise secondary to leakage from the smaller retinal vessels, which have sustained endothelial damage as a result of the ischemia. Similar to the case with diabetic retinopathy, they may also result from the rupture of

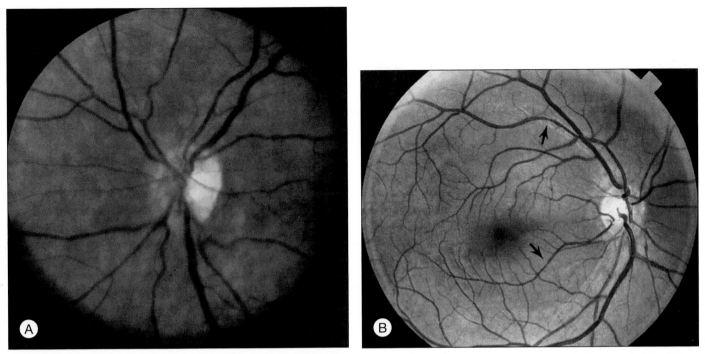

Fig. 84-3 A, Narrowed retinal arteries and dilated, but not tortuous, retinal veins in an eye with ocular ischemic syndrome. B, Focal narrowing of the retinal arteries (arrows) in the right eye of a 55 year old man with ocular ischemic syndrome and bilateral internal carotid artery obstructions. (B from Brown GC, Magargal LE. Int Ophthalmol 1988; 11:239–51.)

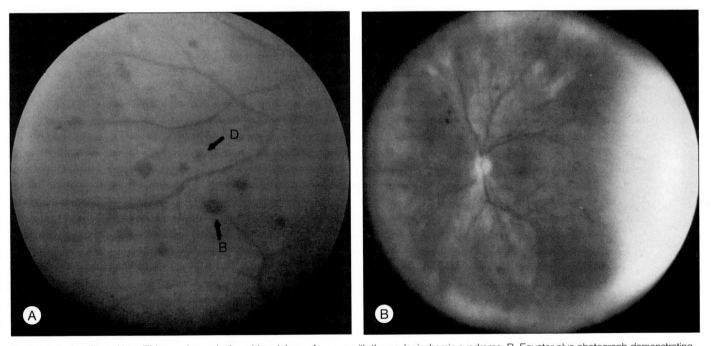

Fig 84-4 A, Dot (D) and blot (B) hemorrhages in the mid-periphery of an eye with the ocular ischemic syndrome. B, Equator plus photograph demonstrating retinal hemorrhages in the midperiphery in an ocular ischemic syndrome. (From Brown GC, Magargal LE. Int Ophthalmol 1988; 11:239–51.)

microaneurysms. In general, the hemorrhages seen with the ocular ischemic syndrome are less numerous than those accompanying central retinal vein obstruction. They are almost never confluent.

Microaneurysms are frequently observed outside the posterior pole, but can be seen in the macular region also. Hyperfluorescence with fluorescein angiography (Fig. 84-6) differentiates these abnormalities from hypofluorescent retinal hemorrhages. Retinal telangiectasia has also been described.[28]

Posterior segment neovascularization can occur at the optic disc or on the retina. Neovascularization of the disc (Fig. 84-7) is

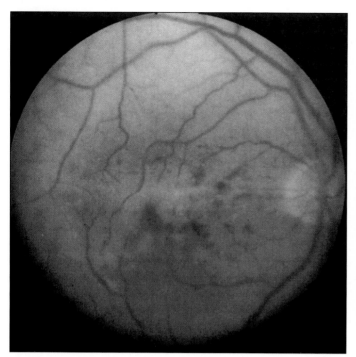

Fig. 84-5 Right fundus of a 35-year-old man with a cherry-red spot, rubeosis iridis, and retinal hemorrhages in the macula. A 95% right internal carotid artery obstruction was present.

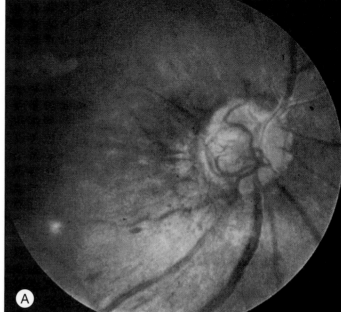

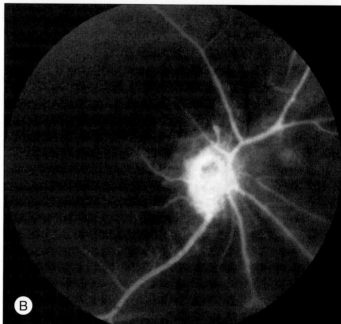

Fig. 84-7 A, Neovascularization of the disc in an eye with the ocular ischemic syndrome. B, Fluorescein angiogram of 'A' reveals marked hyperfluorescence resulting from leakage of dye from new vessels. (Reprinted from Brown GC, Magargal LE, Simeone FA et al. Arterial obstruction and ocular neovascularization. Ophthalmology 1982; 89:139–46. Copyright 1982, with permission from the American Academy of Ophthalmology.)

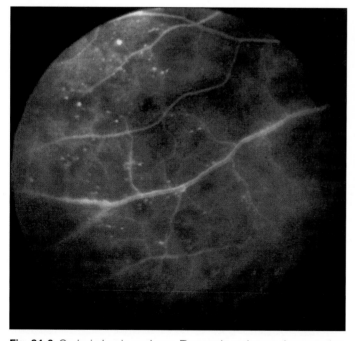

Fig. 84-6 Ocular ischemic syndrome. Fluorescein angiogram demonstrating numerous hyperfluorescent microaneurysms in the midperipheral retina. (From Brown GC, Magargal LE. Int Ophthalmol 1988; 11:239–51.)

encountered in about 35% of eyes, while neovascularization of the retina is seen in about 8%.[5] Vitreous hemorrhage arising from traction upon the neovascularization by the vitreous gel has been reported to occur in 4% of eyes with the ocular ischemic syndrome in a retrospective study.[5] Rarely, the neovascularization can

progress to severe preretinal fibrovascular proliferation (Fig. 84-8). Neovascularization of the retina (Fig. 84-9) is encountered in 8% of eyes with ocular ischemia. It is usually present concomitant with neovascularization of the disc.

A cherry-red spot is seen in approximately 12% of eyes with the ocular ischemic syndrome (Fig. 84-1).[5] It can occur secondary to inner layer retinal ischemia from embolic obstruction of the central retinal artery, but probably more often develops when the intraocular pressure exceeds the perfusion pressure within the central retinal artery, particularly in eyes with neovascular glaucoma.

Additional posterior segment signs[5] include cotton-wool spots (Fig. 84-10) in 6% of eyes, spontaneous retinal arterial pulsations in 4% (Fig. 84-11), and cholesterol emboli within the retinal arteries in 2%. In contrast to spontaneous retinal venous pulsations, which are a normal variant and located at the base of the large veins on the optic disc, the arterial pulsations are usually more pronounced, and may extend a disc diameter or more out from the optic disc into the surrounding retina. Anterior ischemic optic neuropathy (Fig. 84-12) has also been reported in ocular ischemic syndrome eyes.[5,29,30] Acquired arteriovenous communications of the retina are rarely seen.[31]

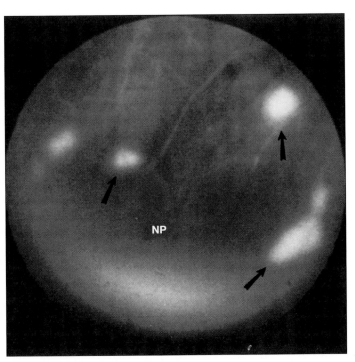

Fig. 84-8 Fibrovascular proliferation overlying the optic disc and causing retinal traction in an eye with the ocular ischemic syndrome. (From Brown GC, Magargal LE. Int Ophthalmol 1988; 11:239–51.)

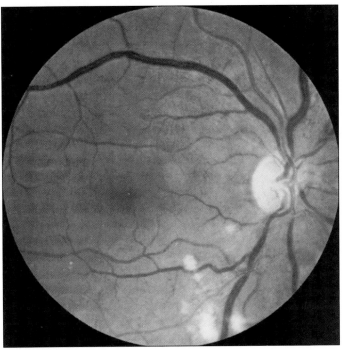

Fig. 84-10 Cotton-wool spots in the fundus of a man with the ocular ischemic syndrome. Irregularly dilated retinal veins are also evident.

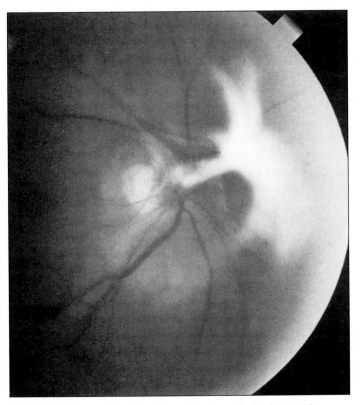

Fig. 84-9 Neovascularization of the retina (arrows) with fluorescein angiography in a nondiabetic person affected by the ocular ischemic syndrome. Retinal capillary nonperfusion (NP) can also be seen. (Reprinted from Brown GC, Magargal LE, Simeone FA et al. Arterial obstruction and ocular neovascularization. Ophthalmology 1982; 89:139–46. Copyright 1982, with permission from the American Academy of Ophthalmology.)

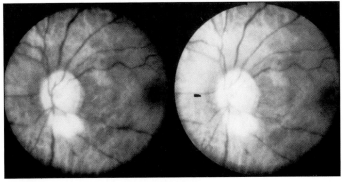

Fig. 84-11 Photographs taken several seconds apart in a fundus affected by the ocular ischemic syndrome. Closure of the retinal arteries can be seen below. (From Brown GC, Magargal LE. Int Ophthalmol 1988; 11:239–51.)

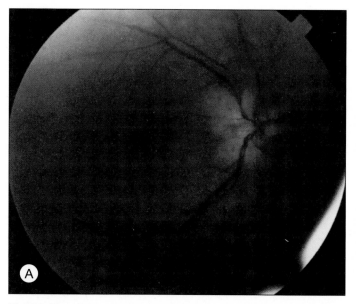
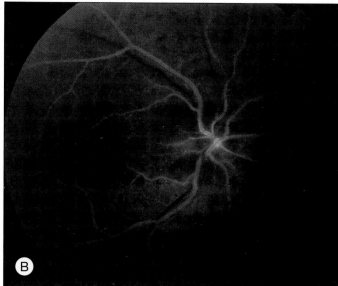

Fig. 84-12 A, Pale optic disc resulting from ischemic optic neuropathy in a 67-year-old man with a 100% right internal carotid artery obstruction. Midperipheral retinal hemorrhages and rubeosis iridis were also present. B, Fluorescein angiogram of 'A' at 81 seconds after injection. The nerve head is hypofluorescent. (From Brown GC. J Clin Neuro Ophthalmol 1986; 6:39–42.)

A list of the anterior and posterior segment signs found with the ocular ischemic syndrome is shown in Table 84-1.[1–5,9]

ANCILLARY STUDIES

Fluorescein angiography

The intravenous fluorescein angiographic signs[5] associated with the ocular ischemic syndrome are listed in Table 84-2.

Delayed arm-to-choroid and arm-to-retina circulation times are frequently observed in the ocular ischemic syndrome. However, these measurements may be difficult to assess, since they depend upon whether the dye was injected in the antecubital fossa or hand, and also on the rate of injection. The observation of a well-demarcated, leading edge of fluorescein dye within a retinal artery after an intravenous injection is a distinctly unusual finding. It can be seen in eyes with the ocular ischemic syndrome, secondary to hypoperfusion (Fig. 84-13).

Normally, the choroidal filling is completed within five seconds after the first appearance of dye. Sixty percent of eyes with the ocular ischemic syndrome demonstrate patchy and/or delayed choroidal filling (Fig. 84-14). In some instances, the filling is delayed for a minute or longer. Although not the most sensitive sign, an abnormality in choroidal filling is the most specific fluorescein angiographic sign in ocular ischemic eyes.

Prolongation of the retinal arteriovenous transit time is seen in 95% of eyes with the ocular ischemic syndrome (highly sensitive), but can also be seen in eyes with central retinal artery obstruction and central retinal vein obstruction (low specificity). Normally, the major retinal veins in the temporal vascular arcade are completely filled within 10–11 seconds after the first appearance of dye within the corresponding retinal arteries. In extreme cases of the ocular ischemic syndrome, the retinal veins fail to fill throughout the study.

Table 84-1 Anterior and posterior segment signs seen in eyes with the ocular ischemic syndrome

Anterior segment	
Rubeosis iridis	67%
Neovascular glaucoma	35%
Uveitis (cells and flare)	18%
Posterior segment	
Narrowed retinal arteries	Most
Dilated retinal veins	Most
Retinal hemorrhages	80%
Neovascularization	37%
Optic disc	35%
Retina	8%
Cherry red spot	12%
Cotton-wool spot(s)	6%
Spontaneous retinal arterial pulsations	4%
Vitreous hemorrhage	4%
Cholesterol emboli	2%
Ischemic optic neuropathy	2%

(Adapted from Brown GC, Magargal LE. The ocular ischemic syndrome. Clinical, fluorescein angiographic and carotid angiographic features. Int Ophthalmol 1988; 11:239–251.)

Table 84-2 Fluorescein angiographic signs seen in eyes with the ocular ischemic syndrome

Delayed and/or patchy choroidal filling	60%
Prolonged retinal arteriovenous transit time	95%
Retinal vascular staining	85%
Macular edema	17%
Other signs	
Retinal capillary nonperfusion	
Optic nerve head hyperfluorescence	
Microaneurysmal hyperfluorescence	

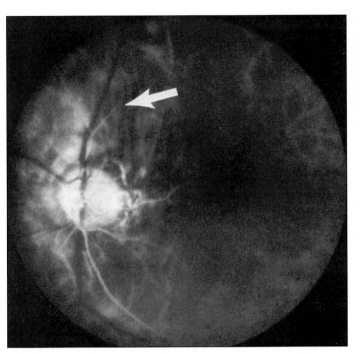

Fig. 84-13 Fluorescein angiogram of an eye with the ocular ischemic syndrome at 38 seconds after injection. A leading edge of the dye (arrow) is present within a retinal artery. (Reprinted from Brown GC, Magargal LE, Simeone FA et al. Arterial obstruction and ocular neovascularization. Ophthalmology 1982; 89:139–46. Copyright 1982, with permission from the American Academy of Ophthalmology.)

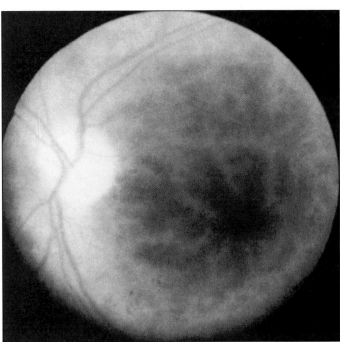

Fig. 84-15 Staining of the macular vessels in the ocular ischemic syndrome. (From Brown GC, Magargal LE. Int Ophthalmol 1988; 11:239–51.)

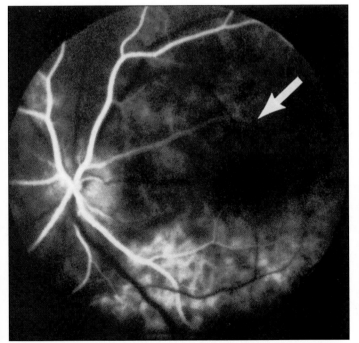

Fig. 84-14 Fluorescein angiogram of an ocular ischemic syndrome eye at 44 seconds after injection shows patchy choroidal filling. A leading edge of dye (arrow) can again be seen within a retinal artery. (From Brown GC, Magargal LE. Int Ophthalmol 1988; 11:239–51.)

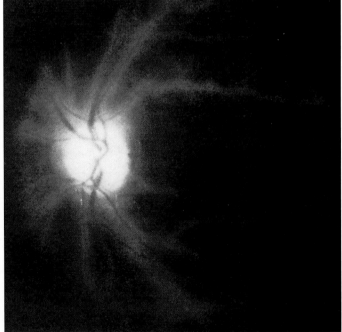

Fig. 84-16 Prominent staining of the retinal arteries in the later phases of fluorescein angiography in an eye with the ocular ischemic syndrome.

Staining of the retinal vessels in the later phases of the study is seen in about 85% of eyes (Figs 84-15 and 84-16). Both larger and smaller vessels can be involved, the arteries generally more so than the veins. Chronic hypoxic damage to endothelial cells may account for the staining. In contrast, staining of the retinal vessels is uncommon with central retinal artery obstruction alone.

With central retinal vein obstruction, the veins can demonstrate late staining, but the retinal arteries are generally not affected.

Macular edema with fluorescein angiography is seen in about one sixth of eyes with the ocular ischemic syndrome[32] (Fig. 84-17). Hypoxia, and subsequent endothelial damage, within the smaller retinal vessels, as well as leakage from microaneurysms, may account for this phenomenon (Fig. 84-18). Dye accumulation may be mild or severe, and is usually associated with hyperfluorescence of the optic disc. The disc, however, is typically not swollen. Despite the prominent leakage with fluorescein angiography, the ophthalmoscopic cystic changes of macular edema are generally not as pronounced as those seen after ocular surgery or those associated with diabetic retinopathy.

Retinal capillary nonperfusion can be seen in some eyes (Fig. 84-19). The histopathologically observed absence of endothelial cells and pericytes within the retinal capillaries most likely corresponds to the areas of nonperfusion seen with fluorescein angiography.[7,8,33]

Bilateral, simultaneous, intravenous fluorescein angiography is a technique that has been reported to be helpful diagnostically in patients with a unilateral ocular ischemic syndrome.[34] However, the technique requires specialized equipment and is not generally available.

Electroretinography

The electroretinogram often discloses a diminution of the amplitude, or absence, of both the a- and b-waves in eyes with the ocular ischemic syndrome[5,6] (Fig. 84-20). The b-wave corresponds to activity of the Mueller and/or bipolar cells, and therefore to inner layer retinal function, while the a-wave correlates with activity of the photoreceptors in the outer retina.[35,36] Therefore, with central retinal artery obstruction, in which there is essentially inner layer retinal ischemia, the b-wave amplitude is characteristically decreased. With the ocular ischemic syndrome there is both retinal vascular and choroidal compromise, leading to ischemia of the inner and outer retina, respectively. Thus, both the b-wave and a-waves are affected.

Reduction in the amplitude of the oscillatory potential of the b-wave has been noted in eyes with retinal ischemia secondary to carotid artery stenosis.[37] This can be seen in patients with proven carotid artery disease, even in the presence of a normal fluorescein angiogram.

Carotid artery imaging

Carotid angiography typically discloses a 90% or greater obstruction of the ipsilateral internal or common carotid artery in persons with the ocular ischemic syndrome (Fig. 84-21). Given that noninvasive tests, such as duplex ultrasonography and oculoplethysmography, have an accuracy of approximately between 88 and 95% in detecting carotid stenosis of 75% or greater,[38–40] and that angiography has a potential for serious complications, angiography is obtained only in select surgical cases.

Others

Visual evoked potentials have been used to study eyes with severe carotid artery stenosis. The recovery time of the amplitude of the major positive peak after photostress has been shown to improve in patients with severe stenosis after endarterectomy.[41]

Ophthalmodynamometry can be of benefit in detecting decreased ocular perfusion in cases of unilateral ocular ischemic syndrome.[10,42]

In the absence of an ophthalmodynamometer, Kearns[42] has advocated light digital pressure on the upper lid of the affected eye during ophthalmoscopy. Retinal arterial pulsations can usually be readily induced in eyes with the ocular ischemic syndrome. This is generally not the case in eyes with central retinal vein obstruction, an entity that can be confused with the ocular ischemic syndrome.

SYSTEMIC ASSOCIATIONS

Diseases associated in one way or another with atherosclerosis are frequently seen in conjunction with the ocular ischemic syndrome. Systemic arterial hypertension has been reported in 73%

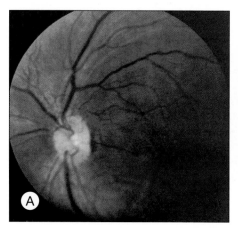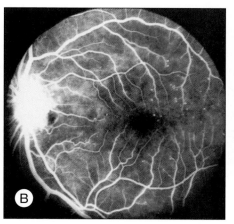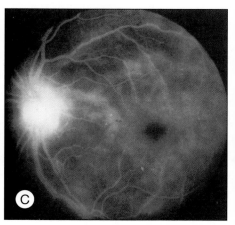

Fig. 84-17 A, Left fundus of a 60-year-old woman with a 100% left internal carotid artery obstruction. The retinal veins are dilated, but not tortuous. B, Fluorescein angiogram of 'A' at over a minute after injection. A number of microaneurysms are present and the optic disc is hyperfluorescent. C, At 6½ minutes after injection, prominent leakage of dye is evident. (From Brown GC. Am J Ophthalmol 1986; 102:442. Published with permission from the American Journal of Ophthalmology. Copyright by the Ophthalmic Publishing Group.)

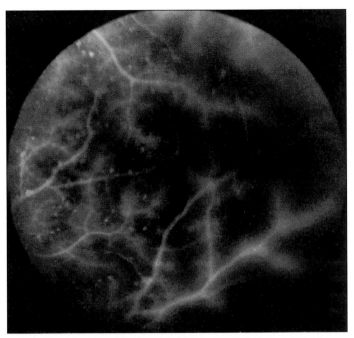

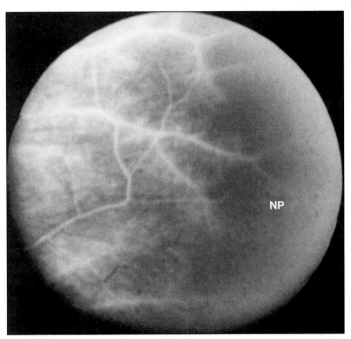

Fig. 84-18 Peripheral fluorescein angiogram of the same eye shown in Fig. 84-17. Many hyperfluorescent microaneurysms are seen, as is staining of the retinal vessels. (From Brown GC. Am J Ophthalmol. 1986; 102:442. Published with permission from the American Journal of Ophthalmology. Copyright by the Ophthalmic Publishing Group.)

Fig. 84-19 Fluorescein angiography reveals retinal capillary nonperfusion (NP) in an ocular ischemic syndrome eye. (From Brown GC, Magargal LE. Int Ophthalmol. 1988; 11:239–51.)

of ocular ischemic syndrome patients and concomitant diabetes mellitus has been observed in 56%.[43] In an age matched historical control population from the Framingham Study,[44] the corresponding prevalences for systemic arterial hypertension and diabetes mellitus were 26% and 6%.

At the time of presentation, almost one fifth of patients relate a history of having peripheral vascular disease for which previous bypass surgery was required.[43] The stroke rate for patients for people with the ocular ischemic syndrome is approximately 4% per year.[45]

A rare but serious cause of OIS is giant cell arteritis.[46] This condition has been reported to cause bilateral loss of vision in which may occur despite treatment with steroids.[47]

Mortality data[43] have shown that the five-year death rate for patients with the ocular ischemic syndrome is 40%. The leading cause of death is cardiovascular disease, which accounts for about two thirds of cases. Stroke is the second leading cause of death. Thus, most patients with the ocular ischemic syndrome should probably be referred for cardiac evaluation, as well as a carotid workup. It is also important to note that Mizener et al. noted that in 69% of their patients, OIS was the first clinical manifestation of carotid occlusive disease, a fact that only further

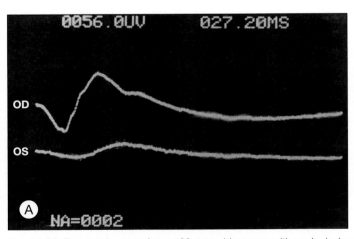

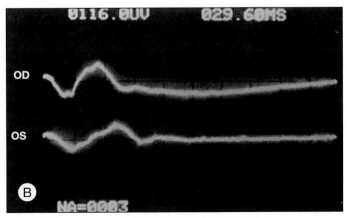

Fig. 84-20 Electroretinogram from a 62-year-old woman with ocular ischemic syndrome and a severe left carotid artery stenosis. The tracing of the right eye (OD) is seen above, and that of the left eye (OS) is seen below. A, The a and the b-waves are markedly diminished in the left eye before endarterectomy. B, After left endarterectomy the amplitudes of the a and b waves have increased in the left eye. The vision correspondingly improved from counting fingers to 20/70.

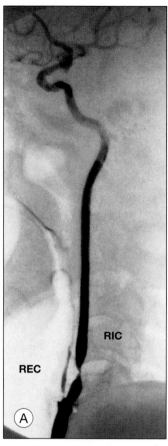
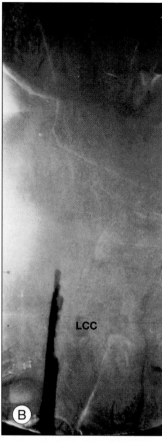

Fig. 84-21 Carotid angiography in a patient with bilateral ocular ischemic syndrome. A, A marked stenosis is visible within the right internal carotid artery (RIC), as well as in the right external carotid artery (REC). B, A 100% obstruction of the left common carotid artery (LCC) is present. (From Brown GC, Magargal LE. Int Ophthalmol 1988; 11:239–51.)

underscores the importance of timely systemic evaluation in these patients.[48]

DIFFERENTIAL DIAGNOSIS

The entities that are most commonly confused with the ocular ischemic syndrome include mild central retinal vein obstruction and diabetic retinopathy. Features that differentiate these abnormalities are listed in Table 84.3. In contrast to the ocular ischemic syndrome, the veins in eyes with mild, or nonischemic, central retinal vein obstruction are often dilated and tortuous. Additionally, with light digital pressure on the lid it is difficult to induce retinal arterial pulsations in eyes with central retinal vein obstruction. While both entities usually have a prolonged retinal arteriovenous transit time, choroidal filling defects and prominent retinal arterial staining are usually absent on fluorescein angiography in eyes with central retinal vein obstruction.

Diabetic retinopathy can exist concomitantly with the ocular ischemic syndrome. The presence of hard exudate in the posterior pole usually suggests diabetic retinopathy, rather than the ocular ischemic syndrome.

As is the case with central retinal vein obstruction, choroidal filling defects and retinal arterial staining are generally absent on fluorescein angiography in eyes with diabetic retinopathy.

In some cases of diabetic retinopathy, the ocular ischemic syndrome can exacerbate the proliferative changes. It has not been proven that carotid stenosis is protective against the development of proliferative diabetic retinopathy.[45]

TREATMENT

With regard to vision, the natural course of the ocular ischemic syndrome is uncertain. Nonetheless, most eyes with the fully developed entity probably have a poor long-term outcome. When rubeosis iridis is present, well over 90% of eyes become legally blind within a year of discovery.[25]

When a carotid artery is 100% obstructed, endarterectomy is usually ineffective since a thrombus often propagates distally to the next major vessel. In these cases, extracranial to intracranial bypass surgery, usually from the superficial temporal artery to the middle cerebral artery, has been attempted to alleviate the obstruction. Although case reports suggest that this procedure can be of benefit initially in salvaging vision in eyes with the ocular ischemic syndrome,[49,50–54] as well as causing regression of neovascular glaucoma,[55] the visual prognosis at one year after the surgery is almost universally poor.[25] Additionally, the procedure has not been shown in a large randomized study to be of benefit in preventing the risk of ischemic stroke.[56]

That being said, some authors have offered objective support of improvement in perfusion following endarterectomy. Costa et al. were able to demonstrate increased mean peak systolic flow velocities and end diastolic velocities in the orbital vessels following surgery, with a significant reduction of the mean resistance indices in the central retinal and posterior ciliary arteries.[57]

Kawaguchi et al. recently evaluated the effects of superficial temporal to middle cerebral artery (STA-MCA) bypass in a series of patients with the OIS. These authors compared a number of clinical parameters including carotid Doppler flow imaging in 32 patients who received STA-MCA as compared to nine patients with OIS who did not have STA-MCA. Prior to surgery all 32 patients had reversal of flow in their ophthalmic arteries. The mean peak systolic flow improved to 0.15 m/s at 3 months as compared to –0.26 at baseline. In addition, whereas all patients had reversal of flow in the ophthalmic artery preoperatively, 56% developed antegrade flow at the 3-month period. In the final analysis, 47% developed visual improvement following surgery and the remainder visual stability.[58]

Although there are no randomized studies that compare the natural history of the disease to the course after carotid endarterectomy, this surgery may also stabilize or improve vision in the eyes of patients who undergo successful endarterectomy prior to the development of rubeosis iridis.[25,59] Not withstanding, the visual results associated with this treatment are fair at best. In the series of Sivalingam et al.[25] at the end of one year, 7% of eyes with the ocular ischemic syndrome that underwent endarterectomy had visual improvement, 33% were unchanged, and 60% had worse vision. Among the sixty total ocular ischemic syndrome

Table 84-3 Features that differentiate the ocular ischemic syndrome (OIS), central retinal vein obstruction (CRVO) and diabetic retinopathy

	OIS	CRVO	Diabetic retinopathy
Laterality	80% Unilateral	Usually unilateral	Bilateral
Age	50s to 80s	50–80s	Variable
Fundus signs			
Venous status	Dilated (not tortuous), beaded	Dilated and tortuous	Dilated and beaded
Hemorrhages	Peripheral, dot and blot	Nerve fibre layer, posterior pole	Posterior pole, dot and blot
Microaneurysms	In midperiphery	Variable	Present in posterior pole
Exudate	Absent	Rare	Common
Optic disc	Normal	Swollen	Affected in papillopathy
Retinal arterial perfusion pressure	Decreased	Normal	Normal
Fluorescein angiography			
Choroidal filling	Delayed, patchy	Normal	Normal
Arteriovenous transit time	Prolonged	Prolonged	May be prolonged
Retinal vessel staining	Arterial	Venous	Usually absent

eyes in the group, an endarterectomy was performed for only three without rubeosis. At the end of one year follow-up the vision was better in one, stable in one, and worse in the third. Endarterectomy appears to rarely cause regression of iris neovascularization in eyes with the ocular ischemic syndrome.[60]

It should be noted that eyes with the ocular ischemic syndrome will occasionally develop a severe increase in intraocular pressure after ipsilateral carotid endarterectomy.[61,62] This is most likely to occur in eyes with rubeosis iridis and anterior chamber angle compromise from fibrovascular tissue formation. Although aqueous outflow is impaired in such eyes, ciliary body perfusion and aqueous humor formation are also decreased secondary to the carotid stenosis. When the carotid obstruction is suddenly reversed, ciliary body perfusion and aqueous humor formation increase, but the outflow obstruction in the anterior chamber angle is still present. Thus, the intraocular pressure rises drastically. Ciliary body destructive procedures or glaucoma filtering surgery may be required in these cases.

Several large randomized studies have recently been published concerning the indications for carotid endarterectomy in general.[63–65,66] Carotid endarterectomy has been proven to be efficacious in both symptomatic patients with high-graded (70–99%) carotid stenosis, and in asymptomatic patients with greater than (or equal to) 60% stenosis. Specifically, the investigators of the North American Symptomatic Carotid Endarterectomy Trial noted a 17% absolute risk reduction in the cumulative 2-year risk of ipsilateral stroke, and a 10% absolute risk reduction in fatal ipsilateral stroke when those randomized to endarterectomy were compared to those who were treated medically.[64] The European Carotid Surgery Trialists' Collaborative Group[63] also were able to demonstrate a similar treatment effect of carotid endarterectomy for patients with 70–99% stenosis (6-fold reduction in 3-year risk of ipsilateral stroke), but also found that in the 0–29% stenosis group the early risks of surgery (2.3% died or had a disabling stroke within 30 days of surgery) outweighed the three year benefit when compared to medical therapy. The investigators

of the Asymptomatic Carotid Atherosclerosis Study[65] were able to demonstrate an aggregate risk reduction of 53% in the incidence of death or stroke, when those randomized to surgery were compared to those who received medical treatment. Asymptomatic patients with carotid artery stenosis of 60% or greater reduction in diameter were eligible to benefit. Accordingly, any patient with the ocular ischemic syndrome and severe carotid artery stenosis should be considered for carotid endarterectomy.

Full scatter panretinal laser photocoagulation has been advocated for ocular ischemic eyes with rubeosis iridis and/or posterior segment neovascularization.[59,67] This generally consists of 1500–2000 500-micron burns with the argon green laser. Unlike the situation when rubeosis iridis occurs secondary to diabetic retinopathy, in which there is regression in a majority of cases with full scatter panretinal photocoagulation, approximately 36% of ocular ischemic syndrome eyes will demonstrate regression of the iris neovascularization after full scatter treatment.[44] If the anterior chamber angle is completely closed by fibrovascular tissue and there is no posterior segment neovascularization, panretinal photocoagulation is probably not indicated unless a glaucoma filtering procedure is being considered, as higher success rates of filtration surgery have been reported when PRP has been performed.[68] While there is little in the reported literature regarding the management of macular edema secondary to this condition, Klais and Spaide recently reported excellent clinical resolution of fluid and dramatic improvement in vision in a patient treated with vitreal triamcinolone acetonide.[69]

REFERENCES

1. Kearns TP, Hollenhorst RW. Venous stasis retinopathy of occlusive disease of the carotid artery. Proc Mayo Clin. 1963; 38:304–312.
2. Hayreh SS. So-called "central retinal vein occlusion." Venous-stasis retinopathy. Ophthalmologica 1976; 172:14–37.
3. Knox DL. Ischemic ocular inflammation. Am J Ophthalmol 1965; 60:995–1002.
4. Young LHY, Appen RE. Ischemic oculopathy, a manifestation of carotid artery disease. Arch Neurol 1981; 38:358–361.

5. Brown GC, Magargal LE. The ocular ischemic syndrome. Clinical, fluorescein angiographic and carotid angiographic features. Int Ophthalmol 1988; 11:239–251.

6. Brown GC, Magargal LE, Simeone FA et al. Arterial obstruction and ocular neovascularization. Ophthalmology 1982; 89:139–146.

7. Kahn M, Green WR, Knox DL et al. Ocular features of carotid occlusive disease. Retina 1986; 6:239–252.

8. Michelson PE, Knox DL, Green WR. Ischemic ocular inflammation. A clinicopathologic case report. Arch Ophthalmol 1971; 86:274–280.

9. Sturrock GD, Mueller HR. Chronic ocular ischaemia. Br J Ophthalmol 1984; 68:716–723.

10. Kearns TP. Ophthalmology and the carotid artery. Am J Ophthalmol 1979; 88:714–722.

11. Kobayashi S, Hollenhorst RW, Sundt TM Jr. Retinal arterial pressure before and after surgery for carotid artery stenosis. Stroke 1971; 2:569–575.

12. Bullock J, Falter RT, Downing JE et al. Ischemic ophthalmia secondary to an ophthalmic artery occlusion. Am J Ophthalmol 1972; 74:486–493.

13. Madsen PH. Venous-stasis insufficiency of the ophthalmic artery. Acta Ophthalmol 1965; 40:940–947.

14. Magargal LE, Sanborn GE, Zimmerman A. Venous stasis retinopathy associated with embolic obstruction of the central retinal artery. J Clin Neuro-ophthalmol 1982; 2:113–118.

15. Duker JS, Belmont JB. Ocular ischemic syndrome secondary to carotid artery dissection. Am J Ophthalmol 1988; 106:750–752.

16. Hamed LM, Guy JR, Moster ML, Bosley T. Giant cell arteritis in the ocular ischemic syndrome. Am J Ophthalmol 1992; 113:702–705.

17. Effeney DJ, Krupski WC, Stoney RJ et al. Fibromuscular dysplasia of the carotid artery. Austral & New Zeal J Surg 1983; 53:527–531.

18. Dhobb M, Ammar F, Bensaid Y et al. Arterial manifestations in Behçet's disease: four new cases. Ann Vasc Surg 1986; 1:249–252.

19. Sadun AA, Sebag J, Bienfang DC. Complete bilateral internal carotid artery occlusion in a young man. J Clin Neuro-ophthalmol 1983; 3:63–66.

20. Donnan GA, Sharbrough FW. Carotid occlusive disease. Effect of bright light on visual evoked response. Arch Neurol 1982; 39:687–689.

21. Wiebers DO, Swanson JW, Cascino TL et al. Bilateral loss of vision in bright light. Stroke 1989; 20:554–558.

22. Ramadan NM, Tietjen GE, Levine SR et al. Scintillating scotomata associated with internal carotid artery dissection: report of three cases. Neurology 1991; 41:1084–1087.

23. Winterkorn JM, Teman AJ. Recurrent attacks of amaurosis fugax treated with calcium channel blocker. Ann Neurol 1991; 30:423–425.

24. Aasen J, Kerty E, Russell D et al. Amaurosis fugax: clinical, Doppler and angiographic findings. Acta Neurol Scand 1988; 77:450–455.

25. Sivalingam A, Brown GC, Magargal LE. The ocular ischemic syndrome. III. Visual prognosis and the effect of treatment. Int Ophthalmol 1991; 15:15–20.

26. Schlaegel T. Symptoms and signs of uveitis. In: Duane TD, ed. Clinical Ophthalmology, vol. 4. Hagerstown, Harper and Row; 1983:1–7.

27. Green WR, Chan CC, Hutchins GM, Terry JM. Central retinal vein occlusion. A prospective histopathologic study of 29 eyes in 28 cases. Retina 1981; 1:27–55.

27a. Foncea Beti N, Mateo I, Diaz La Calle V et al. The ocular ischemic syndrome. Clin Neurol Neurosurg 2003; 106:60–62.

28. Campo RV, Reeser FH. Retinal telangiectasia secondary to bilateral carotid artery occlusion. Arch Ophthalmol 1983; 101:1211–1213.

29. Brown GC. Anterior ischemic optic neuropathy occurring in association with carotid artery obstruction. J Clin Neuro-Ophthalmol 1986; 6:39–42.

30. Waybright EA, Selhorst JB, Combs J. Anterior ischemic optic neuropathy with internal carotid artery occlusion. Am J Ophthalmol 1982; 93:42–47.

31. Bolling JP, Buettner H. Acquired retinal arteriovenous communications in occlusive disease of the carotid artery. Ophthalmology 1990; 97:1148–1152.

32. Brown GC. Macular edema in association with severe carotid artery obstruction. Am J Ophthalmol 1986; 102:442–448.

33. Dugan JD, Green WR. Ophthalmic manifestations of carotid occlusive disease. Eye 1991; 5:226–238.

34. Choromokos EA, Raymond LA, Sacks JG. Recognition of carotid stenosis with bilateral simultaneous retinal fluorescein angiography. Ophthalmology 1982; 89:1146–1148.

35. Carr RE, Siegel JM. Electrophysiologic aspects of several retinal diseases. Am J Ophthalmol 1964; 58:95–107.

36. Henkes HE. Electroretinography in circulatory disturbances of the retina. II. The electroretinogram in cases of occlusion of the central retinal artery or one of its branches. Arch Ophthalmol 1954; 51:42–53.

37. Coleman K, Fitzgerald D, Eustace P et al. Electroretinography, retinal ischaemia and carotid artery disease. Eur J Vasc Surg 1990; 4:569–573.

38. Bosley TM. The role of carotid noninvasive tests in stroke prevention. Semin Neurol 1986; 6:194–203.

39. Castaldo JE, Nicholas GG, Gee W et al. Duplex ultrasound and ocular pneumoplethysmography concordance in detecting severe carotid stenosis. Arch Neurol 1989; 46:518–522.

40. Neale ML, Chambers JL, Kelly AT et al. Reappraisal of duplex criteria to assess significant carotid artery stenosis with special reference to reports of the North American Symptomatic Carotid Endarterectomy Trial and the European Carotid Surgery Trial. J Vasc Surg 1994; 20:642–9.

41. Banchini E, Franchi A, Magni R et al. Carotid occlusive disease. An electrophysiological investigation. J Cardiovasc Surg 1987; 28:524–527.

42. Kearns TP. Differential diagnosis of central retinal vein obstruction. Ophthalmology 1983; 90:475–480.

43. Sivalingham A, Brown GC, Magargal LE et al. The ocular ischemic syndrome II. Mortality and systemic morbidity. Int Ophthalmol 1989; 13:187–191.

44. Kannel WB, Gordon T (eds). The Framingham Study. Public Health Service Publication No. NIH 77-1247, Section 6, Tables 6–9, Section 29, Tables A-22 and A-23, Section 32, pp. 84–85.

45. Duker J, Brown GC, Bosley TM et al. Asymmetric proliferative diabetic retinopathy and carotid artery disease. Ophthalmology 1990; 97:869–874.

46. Casson RJ, Fleming FK, Shaikh A et al. Bilateral ocular ischemic syndrome secondary to giant cell arteritis. Arch Ophthalmol 2001; 119:306–307.

47. Hwang JM, Girkin CA, Perry JD et al. Bilateral ocular ischemic syndrome secondary to giant cell arteritis progressing despite corticosteroid treatment. Am J Ophthalmol 1999; 127:102–104.

48. Mizener JB, Podhajsky P, Hayreh SS. Ocular ischemic syndrome. Ophthalmology 1997; 104:859–864.

49. Edwards MS, Chater NL, Stanley JA. Reversal of chronic ischaemia by extracranial–intracranial arterial by-pass. Neurosurgery 1980; 7:480–483.

50. Higgins RA. Neovascular glaucoma associated with ocular hypoperfusion secondary to carotid artery disease. Austral J Ophthalmol 1984; 12:155–162.

51. Katz B, Weinstein PR. Improvement of photostress recovery testing after extracranial–intracranial bypass surgery. Br J Ophthalmol 1986; 70:277–280.

52. Kearns TP, Younge BR, Peipgras PG. Resolution of venous stasis retinopathy after carotid artery bypass surgery. Proc Mayo Clin 1980; 55:342–346.

53. Kiser WD, Gonder J, Magargal LE et al. Recovery of vision following treatment of the ocular ischemic syndrome. Ann Ophthalmol 1983; 15:305–310.

54. Shibuya M, Suzuki Y, Takayasu M et al. Effects of STA–MCA anastomosis for ischaemic oculopathy due to occlusion of the internal carotid artery. Acta Neurochir 1990; 103:71–75.

55. Kearns TP, Siebert RG. The ocular aspects of carotid artery surgery. Tr Am Ophthalmol Soc 1978; 76:247–265.

56. The EC/IC Bypass Study Group. Failure of extracranial–intracranial arterial bypass to reduce the risk of ischemic stroke. Results of an international randomized trial. N Eng J Med 1985; 313:1191–1200.

57. Costa VP, Kuzniec S, Molnar LJ et al. The effects of carotid endarterectomy on the retrobulbar circulation of patients with severe occlusive carotid artery disease. An investigation by color Doppler imaging. Ophthalmology 1999; 106:306–310.

58. Kawaguchi S, Sakaki T, Kamada K et al. Effects of superficial temporal to middle cerebral artery bypass for ischaemic retinopathy due to internal carotid artery occlusion/stenosis. Acta Neurochir (Wien) 1994; 129:166–70.

59. Johnston ME, Gonder JR, Canny CL. Successful treatment of the ocular ischemic syndrome with panretinal photocoagulation and cerebrovascular surgery. Can J Ophthalmol 1988; 23:114–119.

60. Hauch TL, Busuttil RW, Yoshizumi MO. A report of iris neovascularization. An indication for carotid endarterectomy. Surgery 1984; 95:358–362.

61. Coppeto JR, Wand M, Bear L et al. Neovascular glaucoma and carotid artery obstructive disease. Am J Ophthalmol 1985; 99:567–570.

62. Melamed S, Irvine J, Lee DA. Increased intraocular pressure following endarterectomy. Ann Ophthalmol 1987; 19:304–306.

63. European Carotid Surgery Trialists' Collaborative Group. MRC European carotid surgery trial: interim results for symptomatic patients with severe (70–99%) or with mild carotid stenosis. Lancet 1991; 337:1235–1243.

63. North American Symptomatic Carotid Endarterectomy Trial Collaborators. Beneficial effect of carotid endarterectomy in symptomatic patients with high-grade carotid stenosis. N Eng J Med 1991; 325:445–453.

64. Asymptomatic Carotid Atherosclerosis Study Group. Carotid endarterectomy for patients with asymptomatic internal carotid artery stenosis. JAMA 1995; 273:1421–1428.

65. Mayberg MR, Wilson SE, Yatsu F et al. for the Veterans Affairs Cooperative Studies Program 309 Trialist Group. Carotid endarterectomy and prevention of cerebral ischemia in symptomatic carotid stenosis. JAMA 1991; 266:3289–3294.

66. Carter JE. Panretinal photocoagulation for progressive ocular neovascularization secondary to occlusion of the common carotid artery. Ann Ophthalmol 1984; 16:572–576.

67. Eggleston TF, Bohling CA, Eggleston HC et al. Photocoagulation for ocular ischemia associated with carotid artery occlusion. Ann Ophthalmol 1980; 12:84–87.

68. Allen RC, Bellows AR, Hutchinson BT et al. Filtration surgery in the treatment of neovascular glaucoma. Ophthalmology 1982; 89:1181–1187.

69. Klais CM, Spaide RF. Intravitreal triamcinolone acetonide injection in ocular ischemic syndrome. Retina 2004; 24:459–61.

Chapter

85

The Epidemiology of Diabetic Retinopathy

Ronald Klein
Barbara E. K. Klein

INTRODUCTION

Despite the efficacy of photocoagulation, retinopathy remains an important cause of visual loss in people with diabetes. Epidemiological studies over the past 25 years have described the natural history of retinopathy in the population and its associated risk factors.[1] Clinical trials have demonstrated the efficacy of intensive glycemic and blood pressure control and a spate of new medical interventions are being developed and tested in ongoing randomized controlled clinical trials.[2–5] Findings from these studies have been applied to developing guidelines for care for persons with diabetes.[6] However, considerable loss of vision associated with diabetic retinopathy remains. The purpose of this chapter is to provide an overview of the epidemiology of diabetic retinopathy and application of findings from these studies to the clinical management of persons with diabetes mellitus.

PREVALENCE OF DIABETIC RETINOPATHY

A growing number of population-based studies have provided estimates of the prevalence of diabetic retinopathy. One such study, the Wisconsin Epidemiologic Study of Diabetic Retinopathy (WESDR),[7–9] using stereoscopic fundus photographs of seven standard photographic fields and objective grading by standard protocols, provided estimates of prevalence and severity of retinopathy in both persons with younger-onset taking insulin (diagnosis before 30 years, type 1 diabetes) and older-onset persons (diagnosis at 30 years of age or older) whether or not persons were taking insulin (type 2 diabetes, Table 85-1). In the WESDR, 71% of younger-onset persons had retinopathy, 23% had proliferative retinopathy, and 6% had clinically significant macular edema.[8,10] In older-onset persons in the WESDR, 39% of those persons who did not take insulin and 70% of those who did take insulin had retinopathy; 3% of the former and 14% of the latter had proliferative retinopathy, and 4% of the former and 11% of the latter had clinically significant macular edema.[9,10]

These prevalence estimates are from data collected approximately 25 years ago in an 11-county area of southern Wisconsin (99.4% white). More recent prevalence data have been reported in other population-based studies with frequencies varying from that found in the WESDR (Table 85-1, see Table 14.14 in reference 1).[1,11–51] Even though standardized protocols for detecting and classifying diabetic retinopathy were used in the WESDR, comparisons with other studies must be made cautiously because of possible differences in the definitions of diabetes, its component complications, in the methods used to detect and classify retinopathy, and the age, sociodemographic, and genetic differences among groups under study which may influence prevalence (see below). In addition, without adjusting for duration of diabetes, age, level of glycemia and blood pressure, and other factors associated with the prevalence of retinopathy, comparisons among populations are of limited usefulness.

With these caveats in mind, a recent effort to provide more up-to-date estimates of prevalence involved pooled data from eight studies including the WESDR.[52] These pooled analyses included 615 individuals who were black and 1415 who were Hispanic. The prevalence estimates were limited to persons 40 years of age and older. The estimates of retinopathy were higher in the WESDR group compared to the seven other studies, all of which were performed at least 10 years after the WESDR. Based on pooled analyses from these studies, it was estimated that, among persons with diabetes, the crude prevalence of diabetic retinopathy was 40% and the crude prevalence of severe retinopathy (preproliferative and proliferative retinopathy or macular edema) was 8%. Projection of these rates to the diabetic population 40 years of age or older in the USA resulted in an estimate of 4 million persons with retinopathy, of whom 900 000 have signs of vision-threatening retinopathy.

INCIDENCE AND PROGRESSION OF DIABETIC RETINOPATHY

There are fewer reports of incidence of retinopathy in population-based studies.[12,25,53–64] The incidence of retinopathy in a 4-year interval in the entire WESDR population was 40.3%.[53,54] The 4-year incidence and rates of progression of diabetic retinopathy in the WESDR are presented in Table 85-2. The younger-onset group using insulin had the highest 4-year incidence, rate of progression, and progression to proliferative retinopathy, while the older-onset group not using insulin had the lowest rates. The older-onset group taking insulin had the highest 4-year incidence of macular edema (Table 85-3).[55] While the incidence of proliferative retinopathy was higher in the younger-onset group, the estimates of the number of incident cases in the 4-year period were higher in the group with older-onset age than in the group with younger-onset age (120 versus 83 persons) due to the higher frequency of people with older-onset diabetes.

Table 85-1 Prevalence and severity of retinopathy and macular edema at the baseline examination in the Wisconsin Epidemiologic Study of Diabetic Retinopathy

Retinopathy status	Younger-onset, taking insulin (n = 996)	Older-onset, taking insulin (n = 673)	Older onset, not taking insulin (n = 692)
None	29.3	29.9	61.3
Early nonproliferative	30.4	30.6	27.3
Moderate to severe nonproliferative	17.6	25.7	8.5
Proliferative without DRS high-risk characteristics	13.2	9.1	1.4
Proliferative with DRS high-risk characteristics or worse	9.5	4.8	1.4
Clinically significant macular edema	5.9	11.6	3.7

Modified from Klein R. Diabetes mellitus: oculopathy. In: Degroot LJ, Jameson JL, eds. Endocrinology, 4th edn. Philadelphia, PA: WB Saunders; 1995:857–867.[220]
DRS, Diabetic Retinopathy Study.

Table 85-2 Four-year incidences of any retinopathy, improvement or progression of retinopathy, and progression to proliferative diabetic retinopathy (PDR) in younger-onset diabetic patients, by sex, Wisconsin Epidemiologic Study of Diabetic Retinopathy 1980–1986

Retinopathy	Younger-onset		Older-onset taking insulin		Older-onset not taking insulin	
	No. at risk	%	No. at risk	%	No. at risk	%
Any retinopathy	271	59.0	154	47.4	320	34.4
Improvement	376	6.9	215	15.3	101	19.8
No change	713	55.1	418	58.1	486	71.0
Progression	713	41.2	418	34.0	486	24.9
Progression to PDR	713	10.5	418	7.4	486	2.3

Modified from Klein R, Klein BE, Moss SE et al. The Wisconsin Epidemiologic Study of Diabetic Retinopathy. IX. Four-year incidence and progression of diabetic retinopathy when age at diagnosis is less than 30 years. Arch Ophthalmol 1989; 107:237–243;[53] and Klein R, Klein BE, Moss SE et al. The Wisconsin Epidemiologic Study of Diabetic Retinopathy. X. Four-year incidence and progression of diabetic retinopathy when age at diagnosis is 30 years or more. Arch Ophthalmol 1989; 107:244–249.54
Note: Number at risk for incidence of any retinopathy refers to group that had no retinopathy (level 10/10) at baseline exam and were at risk of developing retinopathy at follow-up exam. Number at risk for improvement in retinopathy refers to those with retinopathy levels of 21/21 to 51/51 at baseline exam who could have a decrease in their retinopathy severity by at least two steps or more at follow-up exam. Number at risk for no change, progression, or progression to PDR refers to those with retinopathy levels of 10/10 to 51/51 who either did not change by two or more steps or progressed by two or more steps.

Table 85-3 Four-year incidences of macular edema and clinically significant macular edema (CSME), by diabetes group, Wisconsin Epidemiologic Study of Diabetic Retinopathy 1980–1986

Group	No. of patients	No. with macular edema	Incidence (%)	No. with CSME	Incidence (%)
Younger-onset	610	50	8.2	26	4.3
Older-onset	652	34	5.2	19	2.9
Taking insulin	273	23	8.4	14	5.1
Not taking insulin	379	11	2.9	5	1.3
Oral hypoglycemic agents	243	9	3.7	4	1.6
Diet only	102	1	1.0	1	1.0
None	34	1	2.9	0	0

Reprinted from Klein R, Moss SE, Klein BE et al. The Wisconsin Epidemiologic Study of Diabetic Retinopathy XI. The incidence of macular edema. Ophthalmology 1989; 96:1501–1510.[55] Copyright © 1989 with permission from American Academy of Ophthalmology.

In the WESDR, the estimated annual incidence and rates of progression of retinopathy were compared for the first 4 years of the study with the next 6 years of the study.[56] There were few differences in the estimated annual incidence or rates of progression between these two periods. However, the estimated annual incidence of proliferative diabetic retinopathy was higher in the last 6 years compared to the first 4 years of the study. While adjusting for the severity of retinopathy or duration of diabetes at baseline and the 4-year follow-up, the estimated annual incidence of proliferative retinopathy remained higher over the last 6 years of the study only in the older-onset groups. These data suggest that incidence and progression of retinopathy remained unchanged or worsened despite improvements in glycemic control in people taking insulin over the first 4 years of the study. There are few other population-based incidence data collected over a long period of time using objective measures to detect retinopathy to compare with these findings.

Based on the WESDR data, it is estimated that each year, of the 10 million Americans with known diabetes mellitus, 96 000 will develop proliferative retinopathy, and 48 000 will develop proliferative retinopathy with Diabetic Retinopathy Study (DRS) high-risk characteristics for severe loss of vision. Each year, 121 000 people with diabetes are estimated to develop macular edema.

THE RELATIONSHIP OF RACE/ETHNICITY TO DIABETIC RETINOPATHY

In 1990, based on clinical observations, Raab et al. wrote: "The rate of blindness from diabetic eye disease is higher in blacks than in whites. Severe macular edema ... appears to be more common in blacks ... Virtually no data exist on the prevalence and natural history of diabetic retinopathy in the black population compared directly with the white population."[65] Contrary to his observations, data from a study of a clinic-based cohort showed that African Americans with type 1 diabetes, despite higher frequencies of hyperglycemia and hypertension, had a lower rate of progression of retinopathy than a group of whites.[66]

At present, there are few published data available on the prevalence of retinopathy and macular edema in black and Hispanic populations of diabetic persons living in the USA. Data from the New Jersey 725 study cohort, using similar methods to detect and classify retinopathy severity as in the WESDR cohort, showed a similar frequency and severity of retinopathy in African Americans with type 1 diabetes as found in whites with type 1 diabetes in the WESDR.[50,51]

In three population-based studies, the National Health and Nutrition Examination Survey III (NHANES III),[41] the Atherosclerosis Risk in Communities (ARIC) study,[67] and the Cardiovascular Health Study (CHS),[68] retinopathy was more prevalent in African Americans with type 2 diabetes than in whites. In the NHANES III, compared to whites, African Americans had a higher frequency of people: in poor control (glycosylated hemoglobin greater than 8.3%, 37% versus 30%); with high systolic blood pressure (>142 mmHg, 42% versus 32%); with a longer duration of diabetes (>14 years, 29% versus 23%); and on insulin therapy (43% versus 24%). There was no difference (odds ratio (OR) 0.94, 95%, confidence interval (CI) 0.54–1.66) in the prevalence of retinopathy between African Americans and whites while controlling for these factors.[41] In addition, there were no statistically significant interactions of race with diabetes severity variables or systolic blood pressure, suggesting that the effect of risk factors was similar in both racial groups. Similarly, after correction for glycemia and other risk factors, Cruickshank & Alleyne[69] reported no difference in the frequency of nonproliferative retinopathy in black Jamaicans with type 2 diabetes compared to whites with type 2 diabetes. Higher prevalence of retinopathy in African Americans with type 2 diabetes appears due, in part, to poorer glycemic and blood pressure control. These data suggest that programs designed to better control blood sugar and blood pressure in diabetic African Americans might be beneficial.

Findings regarding ethnic differences between Mexican Americans and non-Hispanic whites have not been consistent. Haffner et al.[26] found that, after controlling for all measured risk factors, the frequency of retinopathy in Mexican Americans in San Antonio was 2.4 times as high as the frequency of retinopathy in non-Hispanic whites studied in the WESDR. Similarly, in the NHANES III, retinopathy was more prevalent in Mexican Americans compared to non-Hispanic whites 40 years of age or older.[41] Retinopathy was more prevalent in Mexican Americans (OR 2.15, 95%, CI 1.15, 4.04) compared to non-Hispanic whites even while controlling for duration of diabetes, glycosylated hemoglobin level, blood pressure, and type of antihyperglycemic medication used. However, Hamman et al.[28] did not find a difference in the frequency of retinopathy between Hispanics and non-Hispanic whites examined in the San Luis Valley Study. The crude prevalence of proliferative diabetic retinopathy in Hispanic groups in Colorado (7%) was slightly but not significantly higher than the frequency of proliferative retinopathy in non-Hispanic whites with known type 2 diabetes in Colorado (5%). West et al.[35] also reported a similar prevalence of retinopathy in Mexican Americans with type 2 diabetes living in Arizona (of whom 48% had any retinopathy, 6% had proliferative retinopathy, and 5% had clinically significant macular edema) as in Caucasian populations, suggesting no excess risk of diabetic retinopathy attributable to Hispanic origin. However, a recent comparison of the Proyecto VER data with data from other groups of whites, excluding the WESDR, showed a higher prevalence of diabetic retinopathy in Arizona Mexican Americans than in non-Hispanic whites with type 2 diabetes.[52] A higher prevalence of proliferative retinopathy and macular edema was found in a population-based study of Mexican Americans living in Los Angeles than in Caucasians living in Beaver Dam.[36] These variations in prevalence among ethnic groups may be a result of differences in how long it takes to diagnose diabetes after its onset, how it was defined, and levels of glycemia and blood pressure. Differences among Hispanic whites may be due to the degree of gene sharing with Native Americans, a group with a high prevalence of retinopathy (see below).

Some Native American groups have been found to have among the highest prevalence of type 2 diabetes in the world. They have also been reported to have higher rates of severe retinopathy for a given duration of type 2 diabetes compared to whites.[13,14] The reason for this difference is not clear. Native Americans such as the Pima and Oklahoma Indians may have been exposed to longer periods of more severe hyperglycemia at a younger age than whites with type 2 diabetes. However, among different Native American groups, the prevalence and severity of retinopathy appear to vary.[16,46,70–72] This may reflect different levels of the same risk factors, different relative importance of those risk factors, or genetic differences.

There are few data on the prevalence of retinopathy in Asian Americans and other racial ethnic groups.[31,42,48] Prevalence of retinopathy in second-generation Japanese American males (Nisei), 12%, was significantly lower than that reported in the diabetes clinic at Tokyo University Hospital (49% among patients with an onset of diabetes from 20 to 59 years of age and 47% among those with an onset after 59 years of age) and in whites reported in the WESDR (36%).[9,31] There is a need for more data on the prevalence and incidence of retinopathy in Chinese and other Asian American groups.

GENETIC FACTORS

Data from early studies were not consistent regarding the role of genetic factors and the prevalence and incidence of retinopathy.[73–76] Data from a number of newer studies that have examined familial clustering have suggested that genetic factors may be involved more strongly in the susceptibility to diabetic retinopathy.[77,78] One such study, the Diabetes Control and Complications Trial (DCCT), investigated clustering of diabetic retinopathy in families of 372 participants with type 1 diabetes.[77] Data from this study showed an increased risk of severe retinopathy among relatives of retinopathy-positive versus retinopathy-negative DCCT participants at baseline (OR 3.1, 95% CI 1.2–7.8). They also reported correlations for the severity of retinopathy of 0.187 (all family members), 0.327 (parent–offspring), 0.249 (father–child), 0.391 (mother–child), and 0.060 (sib–sib) that were all significant except for sib–sib pairs. They concluded that the severity of retinopathy is influenced by familial factors. In a recent study in India, the odds ratio for retinopathy in the siblings of probands with type 2 diabetes with retinopathy while adjusting for age, glycosylated hemoglobin, duration of diabetes, proteinuria, and other factors was 3.37 (95% CI 1.56–7.29, $P = 0.002$).[78] These findings are consistent with twin study data showing that retinopathy occurs more often among concordant identical twin pairs where both have diabetes than in dizygotic twins where both have diabetes.[79–81] In addition, the time of appearance of retinopathy, as well as its severity, are more correlated among diabetic identical twins than dizygotic twins, suggesting that the tendency to develop diabetic retinopathy and possibly its progression are influenced by genetic factors.

Clinical studies have reported a positive association between retinopathy severity and the presence of human leukocyte antigen (HLA)-B8, HLA-B15, or HLA-DR4 in people with type 1 diabetes. In a case–control study of Joslin Clinic patients with type 1 diabetes, Rand et al.[75] reported that patients with DR 3/0 and 4/0 or where the DR was X/X were more likely to have proliferative diabetic retinopathy than patients with 3/X, 4/X, or 3/4. However, antigens of the BF locus, located on chromosome 6, have not been found by others to be related to proliferative retinopathy.[76]

In a subset of the WESDR younger-onset group, while adjusting for factors associated with proliferative retinopathy, the presence of DR4 and the absence of DR3 were associated with a 5.4-times increase in the odds of having proliferative retinopathy compared to the absence of both DR4 and DR3.[82] No other genetic factors were statistically significantly associated with the presence of proliferative retinopathy. However, based on analyses of the 10-year follow-up data from this study, DR4 appeared to have a statistically significant protective effect for the incidence of proliferative diabetic retinopathy.[83] Further analyses of the 14-year data showed no relation of HLA-DR3 and DR4 status with incidence and progression of diabetic retinopathy, progression to proliferative retinopathy, and incidence of macular edema.[84] The pattern of associations was similar irrespective of duration or age at diagnosis of diabetes. Mortality and nephropathy rates did not differ by HLA-DR3/DR4 status, suggesting that selective mortality did not explain the lack of associations seen. The discrepancy between cross-sectional findings and the 14-year incidence was postulated to be due to increasing homogeneity of retinopathy and diminishing power to detect small differences.

Fine mapping has revealed an insertion deletion polymorphism in the promoter region of the plasminogen activator inhibitor 1 gene, which maps at 7q21.3-q22, to be associated with diabetic retinopathy ($P = 0.016$) in Pima Indians with type 2 diabetes.[85] In other genetic analyses in Pima Indians, linkage to retinopathy on chromosome 3 and 9 and linkage to both retinopathy and nephropathy on chromosomes 3 and 9 were found. Angiotensin II (type 1) receptor gene (AGTR1) is known to be located on chromosome 3q21-25. The investigators suggested that these loci could presumably influence susceptibility to the complications by influencing the microvasculature directly, by influencing the severity of hyperglycemia, or by other unknown mechanisms.[86] There was no evidence of linkage to retinopathy at the site of the angiotensin-converting enzyme (ACE) gene on chromosome 17q23, and the angiotensin gene on chromosome 1q42-43, sites previously found to be inconsistently associated with retinopathy in other studies.[87,88]

Study of specific genetic factors associated with the hypothesized pathogenetic factors for retinopathy, such as aldose reductase activity, collagen formation, inflammatory processes, protein kinase activity, glycosylation, and platelet adhesiveness and aggregation, may yield a better understanding of the possible causal relationships between genetic factors and diabetic retinopathy. There are already a number of new studies that have reported associations between retinopathy and mitochondrial DNA mutations,[89] and polymorphisms of the aldose reductase gene,[90,91] tumor necrosis factor-beta NcoI gene,[92] epsilon4 allele of apolipoprotein E gene,[93] paraoxonase (an enzyme that prevents oxidation of low-density lipoprotein-cholesterol) gene,[94] endothelial nitric oxide synthase gene,[95] intercellular adhesion molecule-1 (ICAM-1),[96] alpha2beta1 integrin gene (involved with platelet function),[97] and cytokine vascular endothelial growth factor (VEGF) gene.[98]

SEX

In the WESDR, higher frequencies of proliferative retinopathy were present in younger-onset males compared to females.[8] However, there were no significant differences in the 4-, 10-, or 14-year incidence or progression of diabetic retinopathy between the sexes.[53,56,61] There were no significant differences in the prevalence, 10-year incidence of retinopathy, or rates of progression to proliferative retinopathy between the sexes in people with older-onset diabetes in the WESDR.[9,54,56]

AGE AND PUBERTY

The prevalence and severity of diabetic retinopathy increased with increasing age in younger-onset persons in the WESDR.[8] Prior to

13 years of age, diabetic retinopathy was infrequent, irrespective of the duration of the disease. The 4-year incidence of retinopathy increased with increasing age, with the sharpest increase occurring in persons who were 10 to 12 years old at baseline.[53] Four-year rates of progression of retinopathy in younger-onset persons rose steadily with increasing age until 15 to 19 years of age, after which there was a gradual decline. No child younger than 13 years of age at baseline was found to have proliferative retinopathy at the 4-year follow-up. These findings have formed the rationale for guidelines for not screening for retinopathy in children with type 1 diabetes.[6]

In the WESDR, menarchal status, a crude marker of puberty, at the time of the baseline examination was related to the prevalence and severity of retinopathy.[99] While controlling for other risk factors, those who were postmenarchal were three times as likely to have retinopathy as those who were premenarchal. In a follow-up study of 60 children with type 1 diabetes, Frost-Larsen & Starup[100] found the incidence of retinopathy to be higher after puberty than before, independent of duration or metabolic control of diabetes or type of treatment. These findings have been observed in other studies.[101,102] Increases in growth hormone, insulin-like growth factor I, sex hormones, and blood pressure and poorer glycemic control (due to increased insulin resistance, poorer compliance, and/or inadequate insulin dosage) have been hypothesized to explain the higher risk of developing retinopathy after puberty.

In the WESDR older-onset persons taking insulin, the 4-year incidence of retinopathy and progression of retinopathy had a tendency to decrease with age.[54] The 4-year frequency of improvement tended to increase with age. For those not taking insulin, the 4-year rate of progression to proliferative retinopathy decreased with age. Few people 75 years of age or older with type 2 diabetes developed proliferative retinopathy over the 10 years of follow-up. These findings are consistent with data from other population-based studies.[12,25] In one such study of people with type 2 diabetes in Rochester, Minnesota, Ballard et al.[18] reported a lower incidence of retinopathy with increasing age in diabetic people older than 60 years of age. These findings might reflect a less severe disease in the older-old or selective survival, that is, older persons who develop severe retinopathy are at higher risk of dying and not being seen at follow-up in these studies.

DURATION OF DIABETES

Perhaps the most consistent relationship found in persons with diabetes is the increase in the frequency and severity of diabetic retinopathy and macular edema with increasing duration of diabetes (Fig. 85-1).[8] The prevalence of retinopathy 3 to 4 years after diagnosis of diabetes in the WESDR younger-onset group with type 1 diabetes was 14% in males and 24% in females. However, in persons with diabetes for 19 to 20 years, 50% of males and 33% of females had proliferative retinopathy. Shortly after diagnosis of diabetes, retinopathy was more frequent in the older-onset groups compared with the younger-onset group (Figs 85-1 and 85-2).[9] In the first 3 years after diagnosis of diabetes, 23% of the older-onset group not taking insulin had retinopathy, and 2% had proliferative retinopathy.

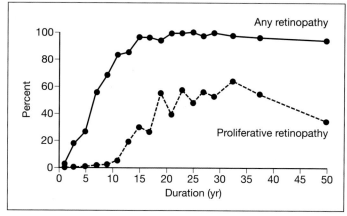

Fig. 85-1 Prevalence of any retinopathy and of proliferative diabetic retinopathy in insulin-taking patients diagnosed with diabetes at age < 30 years, by duration of diabetes. Data are from Wisconsin Epidemiologic Study of Diabetic Retinopathy 1980–1982. (Reproduced with permission from Klein R, Klein BE, Moss SE. Risk factors for retinopathy. In: Feman SS, ed. Ocular problems in diabetes mellitus. Boston: Blackwell Scientific Publications; 1992:39. With permission from Blackwell Publishing Ltd.[218])

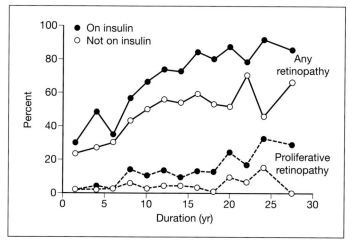

Fig. 85-2 Prevalence of any retinopathy and of proliferative diabetic retinopathy in patients diagnosed with diabetes at age 30 years, by duration of diabetes. Data are from Wisconsin Epidemiologic Study of Diabetic Retinopathy 1980–1982. (Reproduced with permission from Klein R, Klein BE, Moss SE. Risk factors for retinopathy. In: Feman SS, ed. Ocular problems in diabetes mellitus. Boston: Blackwell Scientific Publications; 1992:39. With permission from Blackwell Publishing Ltd.[218])

Harris et al.,[103] using data regarding retinopathy prevalence at different durations of diabetes from older-onset participants in the WESDR and from a study in Australia, extrapolated to the time when retinopathy prevalence was estimated to be zero. They estimated that the onset of detectable retinopathy occurred approximately 4 to 7 years before diagnosis of type 2 diabetes in these populations.

In the WESDR, the 4- and 10-year incidence of diabetic retinopathy increased with increasing duration of diabetes at baseline.[53,54,56] The risk of developing retinopathy in the younger-onset group was high (74%) after 10 years of diabetes. The 4-year incidence of proliferative retinopathy varied from 0% during the first 3 years after diagnosis of diabetes to 28% in those with 13 to 14 years of diabetes. Thereafter, the incidence remained stable.[53] A similar trend was found in a cohort of patients with type 1 diabetes followed at the Joslin Clinic.[104] In the older-onset WESDR group, 2% of those with less than 5 years' duration and 5% of those with 15 or more years of diabetes who were not taking insulin at baseline developed signs of proliferative retinopathy at the 4-year follow-up.[54]

AGE AT DIAGNOSIS

Age at diagnosis was not related to incidence or progression of diabetic retinopathy in any of the diabetes groups followed in the WESDR.[53,54] In contrast, while controlling for other risk factors, in a cohort with type 2 diabetes in Rochester, Minnesota, the development of retinopathy was significantly associated with younger age at diagnosis.[18]

GLYCEMIA

In 1978, Kelly West in his textbook on the epidemiology of diabetes and its complications wrote: "The extent to which hyperglycemia determines the risk of retinopathy is not at all clear. This is the most important issue at hand and deserves high priority in epidemiologic research."[105] In part, this question was raised by inconclusive results regarding the effects of glycemic control on the incidence of diabetic retinopathy from the University Group Diabetes Program (UGDP).[106] This long-term prospective clinical trial, initiated in 1960, was designed to evaluate the effects of four methods of treatment (oral hypoglycemic agents, insulin in fixed or variable doses, and diet only) on mortality and vascular complications in type 2 diabetes. No significant differences were found in the incidence or progression of retinopathy in the groups studied at 5 years or at 12 years (for the insulin and diet groups), despite differences in levels of glycemic control as measured by fasting blood glucose values.

While data from the UGDP did not show a benefit of differences in therapy for glycemic control in persons with type 2 diabetes, evidence from animal studies by Engerman et al.[107] and from epidemiological studies in populations of diabetic persons showed that glycemic control was associated with lower risk of incidence and progression of retinopathy. In a prospective trial of "good" and "'poor'" control in alloxan-induced diabetes in dogs, Engerman et al. demonstrated fewer and less severe retinal microangiopathic changes (microaneurysms, capillary dropout, etc.) in "well"-controlled than in "poorly" controlled animals.

Over the past 25 years there has been a remarkable shift to an emphasis on the need for strict glycemic control in an effort to prevent diabetic retinopathy and other microvascular complications associated with diabetes. At baseline in the WESDR, the mean glycosylated hemoglobin in persons with type 1 diabetes was 10.6% and the mean random blood sugar was 260 mg/dl. Only 3.6% of the younger-onset population took insulin more than twice a day.

Epidemiologic studies have consistently demonstrated an association between good glycemic control and the incidence and progression of diabetic retinopathy.[13,14,16–18,21,22,25–31,108,109] Data from the WESDR showed that lower glycosylated hemoglobin

at any stage of retinopathy prior to the proliferative phase and at any duration of diabetes was associated with lower incidence and progression of retinopathy (Figs 85-3–85-5).[60,108,109] However, the WESDR and other epidemiologic studies could not address the question of underlying severity of the diabetes, independently leading to both poorer control and more severe retinopathy. This could only be addressed by randomized therapeutic trials of metabolic control.

In the 1980s, with the advent of continuous subcutaneous insulin infusion (CSII) systems, the wider acceptance of multidose (three or four doses per day) treatment regimens, and the development of newer means of determining control using home blood glucose monitoring and glycosylated hemoglobin, randomized therapeutic trials comparing differences in metabolic control in persons with type 1 diabetes became feasible. Data from early small randomized therapeutic trials in people with type 1 diabetes showed few differences in the progression of retinopathy between those in the experimental group under strict glycemic control and those in the control group under conventional treatment.[110–114] In the Steno Study, progression of retinopathy was found in 67% of patients on CSII compared to 33% in conventional-treated (CT) patients after 1 year.[112] This was unexpected because of clinical observations of the benefits of intensive insulin treatment. However, after 2 years, progression of retinopathy was similar between the CSII and CT groups.[113] In most cases, the early worsening of retinopathy was associated with the appearance of cotton-

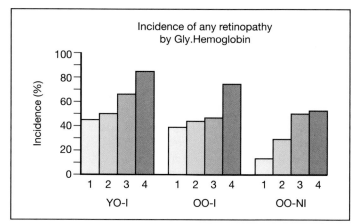

Fig. 85-3 Relation of 4-year incidence of diabetic retinopathy by quartiles of glycosylated hemoglobin at baseline in younger-onset persons taking insulin and older-onset persons taking and not taking insulin at baseline in the Wisconsin Epidemiologic Study of Diabetic Retinopathy. The ranges for baseline glycosylated hemoglobin in the younger-onset group (YO-I) are first quartile: 6.0–10.8%; second quartile: 10.9–12.2%; third quartile: 12.3–14.1%; and fourth quartile: 14.2–23.3%. The ranges for baseline glycosylated hemoglobin in the older-onset group taking insulin (OO-I) are first quartile: 6.9–10.1%; second quartile: 10.2–11.8%; third quartile: 11.9–13.4%; and fourth quartile: 13.5–19.2%. The ranges for baseline glycosylated hemoglobin in the older-onset group not taking insulin (OO-NI) are first quartile: 6.2–8.5%; second quartile: 8.6–9.8%; third quartile: 9.9–11.6%; and fourth quartile: 11.7–23.6%. (Reproduced with permission from Klein R. Retinopathy and other ocular complications in diabetes. In: Porte D Jr, Sherwin RS, Baron A, eds. Ellenberg and Rifkin's diabetes mellitus, 6th edn. New York: McGraw-Hill; 2003:676–677. With permission of The McGraw-Hill Companies.[219])

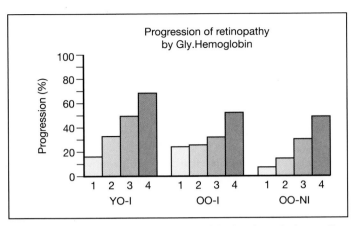

Fig. 85-4 Relation of 4-year progression of diabetic retinopathy by quartiles of glycosylated hemoglobin at baseline in younger-onset persons taking insulin (YO-I) and older-onset persons taking (OO-I) and not taking (OO-NI) insulin at baseline in the Wisconsin Epidemiologic Study of Diabetic Retinopathy. (Reproduced with permission from Klein R. Retinopathy and other ocular complications in diabetes. In: Porte D Jr, Sherwin RS, Baron A, eds. Ellenberg and Rifkin's diabetes mellitus, 6th edn. New York: McGraw-Hill; 2003:676–677. With permission of The McGraw-Hill Companies.[219])

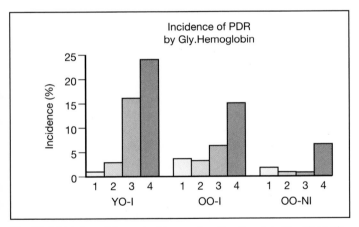

Fig. 85-5 Relation of 4-year incidence of proliferative diabetic retinopathy by quartiles of glycosylated hemoglobin at baseline in younger-onset persons taking insulin (YO-I) and older-onset persons taking (OO-I) and not taking (OO-NI) insulin at baseline in the Wisconsin Epidemiologic Study of Diabetic Retinopathy. (Reproduced with permission from Klein R. Retinopathy and other ocular complications in diabetes. In: Porte D Jr, Sherwin RS, Baron A, eds. Ellenberg and Rifkin's diabetes mellitus, 6th edn. New York: McGraw-Hill; 2003:676–677. With permission of The McGraw-Hill Companies.[219])

wool spots or retinal hemorrhages. Similarly, in the Kroc Study, a multicentered therapeutic trial involving 69 insulin-dependent patients who were randomly assigned to either CSII or CT, progression of retinopathy was reported for both groups over an 8-month period, despite significant improvement in metabolic control in the CSII group.[110,111] Those in the CSII group tended to show slightly faster progression of retinopathy (between-group differences were of borderline significance). Progression in the CSII group was associated with the appearance of cottonwool spots. Similar findings have been reported from a small trial in

Oslo.[114,115] The appearance of cottonwool spots in the well-controlled experimental group in all three studies has been hypothesized to have resulted directly from the abruptly decreased supply of glucose and changes in retinal blood perfusion or indirectly from elevations in other factors (e.g., somatomedin C) that have been reported to cause enhanced intravascular platelet aggregation and intravascular coagulation. The results of these trials suggested that achievement of glycemic control in individuals with type 1 diabetes, previous poor control, and nonproliferative retinopathy should be done slowly to minimize the risk of progression to the more severe preproliferative or proliferative phase of the disease. Similar worsening was reported in the pilot phase of a randomized controlled clinical trial of intensive treatment in Veterans Administration patients with type 2 diabetes but the difference between treatment groups was not statistically significant.[116]

Meta-analyses of these and 14 other small clinical trials showed that after 2 or more years of intensive glycemic control, the risk of retinopathy progression was significantly lower (OR 0.49, 95% CI 0.28, 0.85) in those in the intensively treated group compared to those on conventional treatment.[117] These studies included only patients with retinopathy, and thus the question of preventing the initial development of retinopathy by metabolic control was not answered.

The DCCT was "designed to compare intensive with conventional diabetes therapy with regard to their effects on the development and progression of the early vascular and neurologic complications of IDDM."[2] Two of the main questions asked in the study were: "Will intensive therapy prevent the development of diabetic retinopathy in patients with no retinopathy (primary prevention)?" and "Will intensive therapy affect the progression of early retinopathy (secondary intervention)?" In addition, the DCCT examined the magnitude of the effect of intensive insulin treatment on progression of retinopathy, the degree to which this effect changes over time, and the relation of the effect to the level of severity of the retinopathy at baseline.[118–120]

Subjects included persons with type 1 diabetes who were C-peptide-deficient, 13 to 39 years of age, who were in general good health except for the presence of type 1 diabetes and did not have hypertension, hypercholesterolemia, or other severe medical conditions. There were two groups. In the primary prevention group, subjects had to have had type 1 diabetes for 1 to 5 years, have no retinopathy as detected by stereoscopic fundus photography of seven fields of both eyes, a best corrected visual acuity of 20/25 or better in each eye, and a urinary excretion rate of < 40 mg of albumin in 24 h. In the secondary prevention group, subjects had to have had type 1 diabetes for 1 to 15 years, minimal to moderate nonproliferative retinopathy in at least one eye, best corrected visual acuity of 20/32 or better in each eye, and a urinary excretion rate of < 200 mg of albumin per 24 h.

Randomization was used to assign conventional or intensive insulin therapy.[2] Conventional therapy consisted of one or two daily injections of insulin per day, daily self-monitoring of urine or blood glucose, and education about exercise and diet. No attempts were made to adjust the insulin dosage on a daily basis. Intensive therapy consisted of administration of insulin three or more times daily by injections or an external pump. In addition, there was adjustment of the insulin dosage under the direction of an expert team taking into account self-monitoring of blood glucose performed four times per day, dietary intake, and anticipated exercise.[118]

From 1983 through 1989, 1441 patients were randomized. The primary outcome measure was a sustained (at two consecutive 6-month visits) three-step progression of diabetic retinopathy. This was based on an ordinal severity scale based on retinopathy scores in both eyes determined by grading of stereoscopic color fundus photographs of the seven standard fields. Nonocular outcomes measured in the study were development of urinary albumin excretion (mg/24 h) > 40 (microalbuminuria) or albumin > 300 (gross proteinuria), and the incidence of clinical neuropathy. Adverse events included mortality, incidence of severe hypoglycemia, gain in weight, myocardial infarction, and stroke.

The average follow-up in the study was 6.5 years (range 3 to 9 years) after randomization. The average difference in glycosylated hemoglobin between the intensive and conventional treatment groups for both the primary and secondary prevention was nearly 2%. Fewer than 5% of the cohort in the intensively treated group were able to maintain their glycosylated hemoglobin level at 6.0% or less over the course of the study.

An important finding of the trial was the statistically significant reduction in risk of sustained progression of retinopathy by three or more steps by 76% (Table 85-4 and Fig. 85-6). In the secondary-intervention cohort, the intensive-therapy group had a reduction of average risk of progression by 54% during the entire study period compared to the patients assigned to the conventional-therapy group. In addition, when both cohorts were combined, the intensive-therapy group also had a reduction in risk for development of severe nonproliferative retinopathy or proliferative retinopathy by 47% and of treatment with photocoagulation by 51% (Table 85-4). There was a decrease in the incidence of clinically significant macular edema in the group assigned to intensive therapy compared to those assigned to conventional therapy. However, this difference did not reach statistical significance.

Early worsening of retinopathy in the first year of treatment of the intensive therapy group in the secondary-intervention cohort was observed as had been reported previously.[111,113,115] On average, it took about 3 years to demonstrate the beneficial effect of intensive treatment. After 3 years, the beneficial effect of intensive insulin treatment increased over time.

The DCCT investigators also examined whether there was an association of glycosylated hemoglobin values < 8% versus those > 8% for progression of retinopathy. When they combined the two groups (conventional and intensive treatment groups), they found no evidence to support the concept of a glycemic threshold regarding progression of retinopathy, as had been described by others.[121]

Intensive insulin treatment reduced but did not prevent the incidence and progression of retinopathy in persons without signs of retinopathy at the baseline examination. The 9-year cumulative incidence of one microaneurysm or more severe retinopathy in eyes with no retinopathy present at baseline was 70% in persons with < 2.5 years' type 1 diabetes and 62% in persons with > 2.5 years' duration at baseline. Approximately 40% of these individuals developed a three-step progression of their retinopathy.[119]

The DCCT examined whether intensive therapy was more beneficial when started earlier in the course of type 1 diabetes. They found that the 9-year cumulative incidence of sustained three-step progression in persons without retinopathy with type 1 diabetes for fewer than 2.5 years in the intensive therapy group was 7% compared to 20% in those with more than 2.5 years. The 9-year cumulative incidence of sustained three-step progression in the intensive therapy group was lower in eyes with minimal to early nonproliferative retinopathy at baseline compared to eyes with more severe nonproliferative retinopathy at baseline (11.5 to 18.2% versus

Table 85-4 Development and progression of long-term complications of diabetes in the study cohorts and reduction in risk with intensive as compared with conventional therapy*

| Complications | Primary prevention | | | Secondary intervention | | | Both cohorts† |
	Conventional therapy Rate/100 patient-years	Intensive therapy	Risk reduction % (95% CI)	Conventional therapy Rate/100 patient-years	Intensive therapy	Risk reduction % (95% CI)	Risk reduction % (95% CI)
≥ 3-step sustained retinopathy	4.7	1.2	76 (62–85)‡	7.8	3.7	54 (39–66)‡	63 (52–71)‡
Macular edema§	–	–	–	3.0	2.0	23 (13–48)	26 (8–50)
Severe nonproliferative or proliferative retinopathy§	–	–	–	2.4	1.1	47 (14–67)¶	47 (15–67)¶
Laser treatment**	–	–	–	2.3	0.9	56 (26–74)‡	51 (21–70)¶

*Rates shown are absolute rates of the development and progression of complications per 100 patient-years. Risk reductions represent the comparison of intensive with conventional treatment, expressed as a percentage and calculated from the proportional-hazards model with adjustment for baseline values as noted, except in the case of neuropathy. CI denotes confidence interval.
† Stratified according to the primary-prevention and secondary-prevention cohorts.
‡P ≤ 0.002 by the two-tailed rank-sum test.
§Too few events occurred in the primary-prevention cohort to allow meaningful analysis of this variable.
¶P < 0.04 by the two-tailed rank-sum test.
**Denotes the first episode of laser therapy for macular edema or proliferative retinopathy.

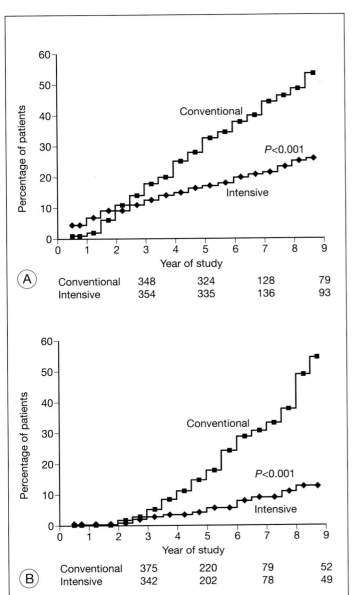

Fig. 85-6 Cumulative incidence of a sustained change in retinopathy in patients with type 1 diabetes mellitus receiving intensive or conventional therapy in A, the primary-prevention and B, the secondary-intervention arms of the Diabetes Control and Complications Trial. The effect of intensive treatment of diabetes on the development and progression of long-term complications in insulin-dependent diabetes. The Diabetes Control and Complications Trial Research Group. N Engl J Med 1993; 329:977–986.[2] Copyright © 1992 Massachusetts Medical Society. All rights reserved.)

43.8%). These data suggested a benefit of beginning intensive treatment earlier in the course of diabetes, prior to the onset of diabetic retinopathy.[119]

The most important adverse event was a two- to threefold increase in severe hypoglycemia in the intensive insulin treatment group compared to the conventional group. There was a 33% increase in the mean adjusted risk of becoming overweight (body weight more than 120% above the ideal) in persons in the intensive compared to the conventional insulin treatment group, also considered an adverse outcome.

From the trial, it was estimated that intensive therapy would result in a "gain of 920 000 years of sight, 691 000 years free from end-stage renal disease, 678 000 years free from lower extremity amputation, and 611 000 years of life at an additional cost of $4.0 billion over the lifetime" of the 120 000 persons with insulin-dependent diabetes mellitus in the USA who meet DCCT eligibility criteria.[122] The incremental cost per year of life gained was $28 661, and when adjusted for quality of life, intensive therapy costs $19 987 per quality-of-life-year gained. These findings were similar to cost-effectiveness ratios for other medical interventions in the USA.

Four years of additional follow-up of the DCCT cohort after the study was stopped revealed that, despite convergence of glycosylated hemoglobin levels in the intensive and conventional groups, the protective effect of glycemic control was maintained in the intensive group.[123]

THE UK PROSPECTIVE DIABETES STUDY (UKPDS)

The UK Prospective Diabetes Study (UKPDS) was a randomized controlled clinical trial involving 3867 newly diagnosed patients with type 2 diabetes.[3,124,125] After 3 months of diet treatment, patients with a mean of two fasting plasma glucose concentrations of 6.1 to 15.0 mmol/l were randomly assigned to intensive glycemic control with a sulfonylurea or insulin or conventional glycemic control. The latter group was further divided into those who were overweight or not. Metformin was included as one of the treatment arms for 1704 overweight patients, and analyses included comparison of the effect of metformin against conventional therapy in overweight patients. After 12 years of follow-up, there was a reduction in rate of progression of diabetic retinopathy of 21% and reduction in need for laser photocoagulation of 29% in the intensive versus the conventional treatment group. In addition, there were no differences in reduction in the incidence of the retinopathy endpoints among the three agents used in the intensive treatment group (chlorpropamide, glibenclamide, and insulin) but the chlorpropamide treatment group failed to show a reduced rate of retinopathy requiring photocoagulation. Furthermore, there was no difference in vision outcomes between conventional and intensive treatments. It was concluded that metformin was preferred as the first-line pharmacological therapy in newly diagnosed type 2 diabetic patients who were overweight based on their finding of a significant (39%) reduction in myocardial infarction compared to the conventional treatment group. However, when metformin was added to sulfonylureas (in both obese and nonobese patients), it was associated with increased diabetes-related (96%) and all-cause mortality (60%) compared to conventional therapy. The intensive treatment group suffered significantly more major hypoglycemic episodes and weight gain than patients in the conventional group. Economic analyses of the clinical trial data suggested that intensive glucose control increased treatment costs but substantially reduced complication costs and increased the time free of such complications.[125]

The development of new treatment modalities for glycemic control has resulted in two new clinical trials which permit evaluation of near normalization of glycemic level on the incidence of cardiovascular disease and retinopathy. The first, the Glycemic Control and Complications in Diabetes Mellitus Type 2, is an ongoing 7-year randomized controlled parallel-treatment trial, and its secondary objective is the evaluation of glycemic control on the incidence and progression of diabetic retinopathy in American war veterans 41 years of age or older whose glycemia is inadequately controlled on maximal therapy.[126] The approach used in this trial is an intensification of combination therapy and frequent blood glucose monitoring to achieve HbA_{1c} levels within normal limits (≤ 6.0%). Another new large randomized controlled clinical trial that began in February 2003, the Action to Control Cardiovascular Risk in Diabetes (ACCORD), is studying the effect of near normalization of blood glucose (defined as keeping HbA_{1c} levels close to 6.0%) on the incidence and progression of retinopathy in persons with type 2 diabetes. Both studies should provide additional information regarding the risks and benefits of intensive treatment resulting in near normalization of glycemic level in persons with type 2 diabetes, a level of control not achieved in the UKPDS.

Based on the results of the DCCT and the UKPDS, it appears that intensive therapy should be the primary public health care strategy aimed at reducing the risk of visual loss from diabetic retinopathy in persons with both type 1 and 2 diabetes. The data from these clinical trials provided further support for the American Diabetes Association guidelines of a target goal of glycosylated hemoglobin of 7.0% for persons with diabetes.[127] However, data from the NHANES III[128] and the WESDR[129] suggest that few persons with diabetes reach this targeted level of glycemic control.

C-PEPTIDE STATUS

The relationship of endogenous insulin secretion to diabetic retinopathy independent of glycemic control is uncertain.[130–133] In the WESDR, the highest prevalence and most severe retinopathy were found in individuals with undetectable or low plasma C-peptide (< 0.3 nmol/l), whereas the lowest frequencies and least severe retinopathy were found in older-onset individuals not using insulin who were overweight.[134] Older- and younger-onset individuals who were using insulin and who had no detectable C-peptide had similar frequencies of proliferative retinopathy. While controlling for other risk factors associated with the incidence and progression of diabetic retinopathy, there was no relationship of C-peptide level to incident or progressed retinopathy in persons with type 1 diabetes in the WESDR.[135] However, in the DCCT, higher C-peptide levels at entry were associated with reduced incidence of retinopathy and lower incidence of hypoglycemic episodes.[136] In the WESDR, while controlling for characteristics associated with retinopathy in older-onset people who were not taking insulin (type 2 diabetes), there was no protection associated with higher levels of C-peptide.[134,135] These findings suggest that the level of glycemia, and not the level of endogenous insulin secretion as indicated by C-peptide level, is more important in determining the presence and severity of retinopathy in individuals with type 2 diabetes.

EXOGENOUS INSULIN

It has been suggested that exogenous insulin may be a possible cause of atherosclerosis and retinopathy in people with type 2 diabetes.[137] In the WESDR, there was no association between the amount or type of exogenous insulin used and the presence, severity, incidence, or progression of retinopathy in the older-onset group using insulin whose C-peptide was 0.3 nmol/l. or greater.[134,135] These data suggest that exogenous insulin itself is unlikely to be causally related to retinopathy in diabetic people with normal C-peptide levels.

BLOOD PRESSURE

Anecdotal observations from clinical studies have long suggested a relationship between hypertension and the severity of diabetic retinopathy.[138] Increased blood pressure, through an effect on blood flow, has been hypothesized to damage the retinal capillary endothelial cells resulting in the development and progression of retinopathy.[139] While epidemiologic data from cross-sectional studies suggest a positive relation of prevalence of retinopathy and hypertension, data from cohort studies regarding the relationship between high blood pressure or hypertension and the development and progression of retinopathy have not yielded consistent findings.[8-11,13,14,16–18,21,22,25,26,28-30,61,70,71,140,141] Some of the earlier studies were limited by small sample size, selection of patients, failure to control for possible confounders, selective dropout of patients, and insensitive measures of detecting retinopathy.

In the WESDR, blood pressure was a significant predictor of the 14-year incidence of diabetic retinopathy in people with younger-onset type 1 diabetes.[61] While controlling for other risk factors such as retinopathy severity, glycosylated hemoglobin, and duration of diabetes at baseline, the relationships between blood pressure and the incidence or progression of retinopathy remained in the younger-onset group. However, in the WESDR, neither the systolic nor the diastolic blood pressure was found to be related to the 10-year incidence and progression of retinopathy in either of the older-onset groups.[140] The UKPDS did find that the incidence of retinopathy was associated with systolic blood pressure. For each 10 mmHg decrease in mean systolic blood pressure, a 13% reduction was found for microvascular complications. No threshold was found for any endpoint.[142] In the WESDR, a 10-mmHg rise in diastolic blood pressure was found to be associated with a 330% increased 4-year risk of developing macular edema in those with type 1 diabetes and a 210% increased risk in those with type 2 diabetes.[143]

The EURODIAB Controlled Trial of Lisinopril in Insulin-Dependent Diabetes Mellitus (EUCLID) study sought to examine the role of an ACE inhibitor in reducing the incidence and progression of retinopathy in a group of largely normotensive type 1 diabetic patients, of whom 85% did not have microalbuminuria at baseline.[144] This study showed a statistically significant 50% reduction in the progression of retinopathy in those taking lisinopril over a 2-year period after adjustment for glycemic control. Progression to proliferative retinopathy was also reduced, although the relation was not statistically significant. There was no significant interaction with blood glucose control. It was postulated that

ACE inhibitors might have an effect independent of blood pressure lowering.[145]

The UKPDS sought to determine whether lowering blood pressure was beneficial in reducing macrovascular and microvascular complications associated with type 2 diabetes.[4] One thousand forty-eight patients with hypertension (mean blood pressure 160/94 mmHg) were randomized to a regimen of tight control with either captopril (an ACE-inhibitor) or atenolol (a beta-blocker) and another 390 patients to less tight control of their blood pressure. The aim in the group randomized to tight control of blood pressure (by the standards at the beginning of the clinical trial) was to achieve blood pressure values < 150/<85 mmHg. If these goals were not met with maximal doses of a beta-blocker or ACE inhibitor, additional medications were prescribed, including a loop diuretic, a calcium channel blocker, and a vasodilator. The aim in the group randomized to less tight control was to achieve blood pressure values <180/< 105 mmHg. Tight blood pressure control resulted in a 35% reduction in retinal photocoagulation compared to conventional control, presumably due to a lower incidence of macular edema. After 7.5 years of follow-up, there was a 34% reduction in the rate of progression of retinopathy by two or more steps using the modified Early Treatment Diabetic Retinopathy Study (ETDRS) severity scale and a 47% reduction in the deterioration of visual acuity by three lines or more using the ETDRS charts (for example, a reduction in vision from 20/30 to 20/60 or worse on a Snellen chart). Atenolol and captopril were equally effective in reducing the risk of developing these microvascular complications, suggesting that blood pressure reduction was more important than the type of medication used to reduce it. The effects of blood pressure control were independent of those of glycemic control. These findings support the recommendations for blood pressure control in patients with type 2 diabetes as a means of preventing visual loss from diabetic retinopathy.

The Appropriate Blood Pressure Control in Diabetes (ABCD) trial consisted of two randomized masked clinical trials comparing the effects of intensive and moderate blood pressure control in persons with type 2 diabetes. The first trial included a diastolic blood pressure goal of 75 mmHg in the intensive group and a diastolic blood pressure of 80 to 89 mmHg in the moderate group in 470 hypertensive subjects (baseline diastolic blood pressure of > 90 mmHg) with type 2 diabetes.[5,146] After a 7- to 11-week run-in period with placebo, persons were randomized to either nisoldipine (a calcium channel blocker) 10 mg/day (titrated up to 60 mg/day as needed) versus placebo or enalapril (an ACE inhibitor) 5 mg/day (titrated up to 40 mg/day as needed) versus placebo for nisoldipine as the initial antihypertensive medication.[5] If a single-study medication alone did not achieve the target blood pressure, then metoprolol followed by hydrochlorothiazide were added until the target blood pressure was achieved. The mean blood pressure achieved was 132/78 mmHg in the intensive group and 138/86 mmHg in the moderate-control group. Over a 5-year follow-up period, there was no difference between the intensive and moderate groups with regard to progression of diabetic retinopathy. There was no difference in nisoldipine versus enalapril in progression of retinopathy. The authors concluded that the lack of efficacy in their study compared to the UKPDS might have

resulted from the shorter time period of the ABCD trial (5 years versus 9 years on average for the UKPDS), lower average blood pressure control in the ABCD trial (144/82 mmHg versus 154/87 mmHg in the UKPDS), and poorer glycemic control in the ABCD trial than the UKPDS.[4,5] These data also suggest the possibility of a threshold effect below which there is minimal reduction in the risk of progression of retinopathy by further reduction of blood pressure.

However, results from a second clinical trial from the same ABCD group suggested otherwise.[146] In the second ABCD trial, the question was whether lowering blood pressure in normotensive (blood pressure < 140/90 mmHg) patients with type 2 diabetes offered any beneficial results on vascular complications. The effect of intensive versus moderate diastolic blood pressure control on diabetic vascular complications in 480 normotensive type 2 diabetic patients was examined in a prospective, randomized controlled trial. Subjects randomized to the intensive therapy were treated with either nisoldipine 10 mg/day titrated to 20, 40, and then 60 mg/day (plus placebo for enalapril) or enalapril 5 mg/day titrated to 10, 20, and then 40 mg/day (plus placebo for nisoldipine) as the initial medication to achieve a diastolic blood pressure 10 mmHg below the baseline diastolic blood pressure. The subjects randomized to the moderate-therapy group were initially randomized to a placebo with a diastolic blood pressure goal of 80 to 89 mmHg. If those in the moderate-therapy group became hypertensive (systolic blood pressure ≥ 160 mmHg or diastolic blood pressure ≥ 90 mmHg on two consecutive visits), they were given either nisoldipine or enalapril. Over the 5-year period, the intensive blood pressure control group showed less progression of diabetic retinopathy (34% versus 46%, $P = 0.019$) than the moderate-therapy group with no difference whether enalapril or nisoldipine was used as the initial antihypertensive agent. There was no difference in the incidence of retinopathy between the moderate and the intensive groups (39% versus 42%, respectively). Proliferative retinopathy developed in 0% of the intensive group and 3.9% of the moderate group. In addition, there was a significantly lower rate of development or progression of microalbuminuria, and there was a 70% reduction in the incidence of stroke in the intensive compared to the moderate-therapy group. The authors concluded that "over a five-year follow-up period, intensive (approximately 128/75 mmHg) control of blood pressure in normotensive type 2 diabetic patients decreased the progression of diabetic retinopathy." They concluded that the specific initial agent used (calcium channel blocker versus ACE-inhibitor) appears to be less important than the achievement of the lower blood pressure values in normotensive type 2 diabetic patients.

The ACCORD is also examining whether, in the context of good glycemic control, a "therapeutic strategy that targets a systolic blood pressure of < 120 mmHg will reduce the rate of cardiovascular disease events compared to a strategy that targets a systolic blood pressure of < 140 mmHg" in persons with type 2 diabetes. In that trial, the effect of blood pressure control on the incidence and progression of retinopathy will be examined. The aim of another clinical trial that is underway, the Diabetic Retinopathy Candesartan Trials (DIRECT), consisting of three randomized double-masked, parallel, placebo-controlled studies, is to determine the impact of treatment with candesartan, an angiotensin II type 1 receptor blockade on the incidence and progression of diabetic retinopathy.[147] Persons with type 1 diabetes ($n = 1700$) without retinopathy have been randomized into a primary prevention study and 1200 with nonproliferative retinopathy into a secondary prevention study. In a third arm in persons with type 2 diabetes, 1600 persons with nonproliferative retinopathy have been randomized and will be followed for 3 years.

PROTEINURIA AND DIABETIC NEPHROPATHY

Data from most studies suggest a strong association between the prevalence of diabetic nephropathy, as manifest by microalbuminuria or gross proteinuria, and the incidence and progression of retinopathy.[8,9,16,21,26,27,30,56,148,149] There are anecdotal reports of patients with renal failure having more severe macular edema that improves after dialysis or renal transplantation. Lipid, rheological, and platelet abnormalities associated with nephropathy may be involved in the pathogenesis of retinopathy. In the WESDR, in the younger-onset group taking insulin, the relative risk of proliferative retinopathy developing over 4 years in those with gross proteinuria at baseline was 2.32 (95% CI 1.40, 3.83) compared with those without gross proteinuria.[149] However, while controlling for other relevant risk factors, the relationship was of borderline significance. For the older-onset group taking insulin, the relative risk was 2.02 (95% CI 0.91, 4.44), and for those not taking insulin, it was 1.13 (95% CI 0.15, 8.50).

A greater proportion of those with type 1 diabetes participating in a cohort study in Pittsburgh who had microalbuminuria or overt nephropathy at entry in the study progressed to proliferative disease over a 2-year follow-up.[150] However, in the same study, nephropathy at baseline was not associated with overall progression of retinopathy. Data from these studies suggest that, in those with type 1 diabetes, gross proteinuria is a risk indicator for proliferative retinopathy. These nephrotic patients might benefit from having regular ophthalmologic evaluation.

In the study of Oklahoma Indians with type 2 diabetes, gross proteinuria was associated with retinopathy at baseline but was not found to be a risk factor for the development of retinopathy.[70,71] In Pima Indians with type 2 diabetes, after controlling for other risk factors, the presence of proteinuria or renal insufficiency predicted the development of proliferative retinopathy.[72] The incidence-rate ratio was 4.8. However, in people with type 2 diabetes in Rochester, Minnesota, persistent proteinuria was not an independent predictor of subsequent incidence of retinopathy.[18]

There are no clinical trial data to show that interventions that prevent or slow diabetic nephropathy will reduce the incidence and progression of retinopathy.

SERUM LIPIDS AND LIPID-LOWERING

Macular edema is an important cause of loss of vision in people with diabetes.[151] Hard exudate, a lipoprotein deposit, is often associated with macular edema. Data from early clinical studies showed an association of elevated plasma triglycerides and lipids with hard exudate.[152] Clinical trials of clofibrate showed that treatment with this drug with reduction of lipid levels reduced the incidence of hard exudate but failed to restore vision to eyes with established macular edema at the onset of the trial.[152] Clofibrate was associated with liver toxicity and is no longer used.

In the WESDR, higher total serum cholesterol was associated with higher prevalence of retinal hard exudates in both the younger- and the older-onset groups taking insulin but not in those with type 2 diabetes using oral hypoglycemic agents.[153] In the ETDRS, higher levels of serum lipids (triglycerides, low-density lipoproteins, and very-low-density lipoproteins) at baseline were associated with increased risk of developing hard exudates in the macula and decreased visual acuity.[154] In a study of Mexican patients with type 2 diabetes, Santos et al.[93] showed the frequency of severe retinal hard exudates was higher in those with e4 allele polymorphism of the apolipoprotein E gene.

Very small pilot studies have been undertaken to examine the efficacy of statin therapy in preventing or reducing the severity of macular edema and have suggested a possible short-term benefit.[155–157] To our knowledge, there are no completed large clinical trials showing the efficacy of lipid-lowering agents in reducing the progression of retinopathy, the incidence of macular edema, or the loss of vision. In persons with type 2 diabetes, the ACCORD will permit examination of whether a "therapeutic strategy that raises the serum HDL [high-density lipoprotein]-cholesterol and lowers triglyceride levels in the context of desirable levels of serum LDL [low-density lipoprotein] cholesterol and good glycemic control reduces the incidence of macular edema and progression of retinopathy compared to a strategy that only achieves desirable levels of LDL-cholesterol and glycemic control."

CIGARETTE SMOKING

Smoking would be expected to be associated with retinopathy because it is known to cause tissue hypoxia by increasing blood carbon monoxide levels, causing vasoconstriction of the small blood vessels.[158] Additionally, smoking may lead to increased platelet aggregation and adhesiveness.[159] However, most epidemiologic data show no relationship between cigarette smoking and the incidence or progression of diabetic retinopathy.[16,18, 27,30,71,160–162] In the WESDR, cigarette smoking was not associated with the 4- or 10-year incidence or progression of diabetic retinopathy or of macular edema.[161,162] Despite this, diabetic patients should be advised not to smoke because of an increased risk of cardiovascular and respiratory disease to which persons with diabetes are already prone, as well as cancer. In the WESDR, after controlling for other risk factors, younger-onset people who smoked were 2.4 times and older-onset people were 1.6 times as likely to die as those who did not smoke.[163]

ALCOHOL

Because alcohol is associated with decreased platelet aggregation and adhesiveness, one might anticipate a possible protective effect in reducing the incidence and progression of retinopathy.[164] Data from one study suggested such a beneficial effect, while that from another study suggested an increased risk of proliferative retinopathy.[165,166] No relation between alcohol consumption and diabetic retinopathy was found in a population-based study in Australia.[37] In the UKPDS, a relation of increased alcohol consumption to increased severity of retinopathy was found only in newly diagnosed men with type 2 diabetes.[43] In the WESDR, alcohol consumption was associated with a lower frequency of proliferative retinopathy in the younger-onset group.[167] However, there was no relationship between alcohol consumption at the 4-year examination and the incidence and progression of retinopathy in either the younger- or older-onset groups at the 10-year follow-up.[168] Of interest in the WESDR was an association of reduction in cardiovascular disease mortality in persons with type 1 diabetes who drank on average one drink of alcohol per day.[169]

BODY MASS INDEX

The relationship between diabetic retinopathy and body mass index is inconsistent among various studies investigating this.[8,16,18,72,170–173] In the WESDR, body mass was inversely related to the presence or severity of diabetic retinopathy only in the older-onset people not using insulin.[173] While controlling for other risk factors, older-onset persons in the WESDR who were underweight at baseline (body mass index < 20 kg/m^2 for both men and women) were three times as likely to develop retinopathy as those who were of normal weight (body mass index of 20 to 27.7 kg/m^2 for men and 20 to 27.2 kg/m^2 for women). It has been speculated that underweight older-onset subjects are more likely to be in a "severe" phase of their type 2 diabetes or have a late-onset type 1 diabetes. Persons obese at baseline (body mass index > 31.0 kg/m^2 for men and 32.1 kg/m^2 for women) were 35% more likely to have progression of retinopathy and 41% more likely to develop proliferative retinopathy than those who were of normal weight at baseline. However, these associations were not statistically significant.

PHYSICAL ACTIVITY

Few epidemiologic data are available describing the relationship between diabetic retinopathy and physical activity.[174–177] One study found no relationship between participating in team sports in high school or college and a history of laser treatment or blindness in people with type 1 diabetes.[176] The same group reported that physical activity in youth did not relate to complications of diabetes.[174,175] In the WESDR, women diagnosed to have diabetes before 14 years of age who participated in team sports were less likely to have proliferative diabetic retinopathy than those who did not.[177] There was no association between physical activity or leisure-time energy expenditure and the presence and severity of diabetic retinopathy in men.

SOCIOECONOMIC STATUS

Inconsistent relationships between socioeconomic status and retinopathy severity have been reported.[16,35,178,179] Hanna et al.[178] reported a significant correlation between proliferative retinopathy and occupational status (working class) or a lower income in a case–control study of 49 people with type 1 diabetes.

Haffner et al.[179] did not find a relationship between socioeconomic status, measured using a combination of the Duncan Index, educational attainment, or income and severe retinopathy in 343 Mexican Americans and 79 non-Hispanic whites with type 2 diabetes in San Antonio. West et al.[16] also did not observe a relationship between retinopathy severity and education level in a population of Oklahoma Indians with type 2 diabetes. In the Proyecto Vision and Eye Research (VER) cohort of Mexican-Americans, low income, once adjusted for other factors, was related to proliferative retinopathy (OR 3.93, 95% CI 1.31, 11.80).[35]

In the WESDR, with the exception of an association of lower incidence of proliferative retinopathy in those with more education in younger-onset women 25 years of age or older, socioeconomic status (education level and Duncan Socioeconomic Index score) was not associated with risk of developing proliferative retinopathy.[180] It may be that the absence of a relationship of socioeconomic status and retinopathy severity in the WESDR and San Antonio Study is related to the lack of an association of glycemia to socioeconomic status in these populations.

HORMONE AND REPRODUCTIVE EXPOSURES IN WOMEN

In the WESDR, menarchal status at the baseline examination was related to the prevalence and severity of retinopathy.[99] Sex hormones have been hypothesized to explain the higher risk of developing retinopathy after puberty. However, it seems unlikely that increased estrogen associated with the onset of puberty is responsible for the increase in retinopathy. Use of oral contraceptives, which contain estrogens as well as progestins, does not appear to increase the risk of retinopathy.[181]

Pregnancy, a condition associated with high levels of estrogens, is associated with more rapid progression of retinopathy. When pregnant women were compared with nonpregnant diabetic women of similar age and duration of diabetes, the pregnant women were more likely to develop retinopathy if they had not had it or to have greater likelihood of progression of their retinopathy when the groups were followed for a time interval about equal to the length of the pregnancy.[182] This remained true after controlling for level of glycemia and blood pressure. Similar findings have been reported by others.[183,184] A complementary finding was reported by Lovestam-Adria et al.,[185] who found that progression of retinopathy was more likely to occur in pre-eclamptic diabetic women than in those without pre-eclampsia. Similarly, Rosenn et al.[186] found that glycemia and blood pressure were important determinants of progression of retinopathy during pregnancy. While these are important factors in those not pregnant, the fact of pregnancy in all likelihood accelerates the process. Other investigators have found that progression of retinopathy was related to prior duration of diabetes.[187,188] Because duration of diabetes is a risk factor for progression of retinopathy irrespective of pregnancy status, this is also not a novel finding. However, it may be useful information in tailoring a follow-up plan for eye care during pregnancy.

There are limited data to suggest that serum insulin-like growth factor 1 levels are associated with progression of retinopathy during pregnancy.[189] A small study was performed to determine whether the vasoconstrictor endothelin-1 (ET-1) which is elevated in hypertension and diabetes was associated with severity of retinopathy in pregnancy. While diabetic women had higher levels of ET-1 in pregnancy than nondiabetic women in the same trimester, there was no relationship to severity of diabetic retinopathy.[190] The study was hampered by its small number of patients and so must be regarded as inconclusive.

However, despite the apparent deleterious effect of pregnancy on retinopathy, the number of past pregnancies was unrelated to the severity of diabetic retinopathy in younger-onset women in the WESDR.[191] Similarly, in a study in Oulu, Finland, there appeared to be little influence on retinopathy of second and subsequent pregnancies.[192] These data may be interpreted to suggest that pregnancy imparts a transient increased risk for incidence or progression of retinopathy. However, since there may be decreased fertility that results from more severe or more complicated diabetes, it may be that those who sustain repeated pregnancies are more robust, and this is reflected in relative protection against more severe or more progressive retinopathy.

Another source of exposure to estrogens is hormone replacement therapy. Although this treatment has come under intense scrutiny, there is no evidence to suggest that exposure to these medicines increases the risk of diabetic retinopathy.[191]

CO-MORBIDITY AND MORTALITY

In the WESDR, the risk of developing a heart attack, stroke, diabetic nephropathy, and amputation was higher in those with proliferative diabetic retinopathy compared to those with no or minimal nonproliferative retinopathy at baseline (Table 85-5).[193] In persons with type 1 diabetes, while controlling for age and sex, retinopathy severity was associated with all-cause and ischemic heart disease mortality and in persons with type 2 diabetes with all-cause, ischemic heart disease mortality, and stroke.[194] After controlling for systemic factors, the relations remained only for all-cause and stroke mortality in persons with type 2 diabetes. These data suggest that the presence of more severe retinopathy in diabetic patients is an indicator for increased risk of ischemic heart disease death and may identify individuals who should be under care for cardiovascular disease. This had been reported by others.[195–197] The higher risk of cardiovascular disease in persons with more severe retinopathy may be due, in part, to the association of severe retinopathy with cardiovascular disease risk factors such as increased fibrinogen, increased platelet aggregation, hyperglycemia, and hypertension.

The ETDRS demonstrated that aspirin, when needed for the prevention of myocardial infarction or stroke, did not increase the risk of vitreous hemorrhage or loss of vision in people with proliferative retinopathy.[198] Aspirin was not found to prevent the progression of retinopathy in the ETDRS and the WESDR.[198,199] Treatment with aspirin has been found to be associated with a significant reduction in heart attack.[200] Results from this and other studies have led to a recommendation of use of enteric-coated aspirin in low doses (81 to 325 mg/day) in people with diabetes who have a history of angina, myocardial infarction, stroke or transient ischemic attacks, and peripheral vascular disease.

NEW MEDICAL INTERVENTIONS

Aside from glycemic and blood pressure control, no other medical intervention has been demonstrated to reduce the incidence and progression of diabetic retinopathy. All randomized controlled clinical trials of aldose reductase inhibitors have not shown efficacy of this intervention in preventing the incidence and progression of retinopathy in people with diabetes.[201] A number of new clinical trials are currently underway to evaluate the efficacy of various new agents, including protein kinase C (PKC) inhibitors, vascular endothelial growth factor inhibitors, and metalloproteinase inhibitors in preventing the incidence or progression of diabetic retinopathy.

Table 85-5 The relative risk for the prevalence and 4-year incidence of myocardial infarction, stroke, and amputation of lower extremities associated with the presence of proliferative retinopathy, corrected for age in the Wisconsin Epidemiologic Study of Diabetic Retinopathy

	Myocardial infarction		Stroke		Amputation of lower extremity	
	RR	95% CI	RR	95% CI	RR	95% CI
Younger-onset group						
Prevalence	3.5	1.5–7.9	2.6	0.7–9.7	7.1	2.6–19.7
Incidence	4.5	1.3–15.4	1.6	0.4–5.7	6.0	2.1–16.9
Older-onset group taking insulin						
Prevalence	0.8	0.4–1.4	1.2	0.6–2.4	4.2	2.3–7.9
Incidence	1.2	0.5–3.4	2.9	1.2–6.8	3.4	0.9–13.2
Older-onset group not taking insulin						
Prevalence	0.3	0–2.4	2.9	0.9–9.4	5.2	0.6–45.0
Incidence	1.5	0.2–12.5	6.0	1.1–32.6	7.0	0.8–64.4

In addition, a large multicenter randomized controlled clinical trial has recently begun to examine the efficacy of intravitreal injection of steroids in the treatment of severe diabetic macular edema. However, pilot data from such trials have shown a significant number of complications, including cataract and a rise in intraocular pressure, and in some cases requiring trabeculectomy.[202]

Clinical trials are currently in progress to examine the efficacy of PKC inhibitors. One isoform of the PKC family, PKCβ has been linked to increased angiogenesis, permeability, and inflammatory responses, all thought to be involved in the pathogenesis of diabetic retinopathy.[203] Data from a phase II/III randomized controlled clinical trial in persons with moderate to severe nonproliferative retinopathy showed no efficacy in preventing the incidence of proliferative retinopathy or macular edema.[204]

PUBLIC HEALTH APPLICATIONS OF EPIDEMIOLOGICAL DATA

Based on the observation that many diabetic patients with severe retinopathy were not receiving dilated eye examinations, guidelines for these examinations were developed and implemented using epidemiological data.[6,205,206] The guidelines recommended that, after the initial screening examination, "subsequent examinations for both type 1 and type 2 diabetic patients should be repeated annually by an ophthalmologist or optometrist who is knowledgeable and experienced in diagnosing the presence of diabetic retinopathy, and is aware of its management."[6] However, a number of reports have demonstrated poor compliance with these guidelines.[207–209] In one study, only 16% of diabetic patients who received primary care in upstate New York received an annual ophthalmic examination using funduscopy by an optometrist or ophthalmologist in two consecutive years.[210] Reasons for poor compliance with the recommended American Diabetes Association guidelines have been provided by others.[207,211,212] Physician factors may explain the reasons why patients may not be receiving optimal care. In one study, 52% of primary care physicians reported that they performed in-office ophthalmoscopy, 90% of which were through undilated pupils, an approach shown to have limited sensitivity to detecting vision-threatening retinopathy in other studies.[211] Moss et al.[212] studied persons with type 1 and type 2 diabetes for 10 or more years who were participating in WESDR. In those not having a dilated eye examination in the previous year, 31 and 35% of those with type 1 diabetes and type 2 diabetes, respectively, reported not having been told by their primary care doctors that they needed one.

Patient factors also explain some of the reasons why guidelines for dilated eye examinations are not being followed. In the WESDR, among those not having a dilated eye examination in the previous year, 79 and 71% of those with type 1 diabetes and type 2 diabetes, respectively, reported not having had one because they had no problems with their eyes, and 32 and 11% said they were too busy. These data suggest the importance of educating patients with diabetes about the asymptomatic nature of diabetic retinopathy, and the benefits of a dilated-eye examination. This has become an important priority of the National Eye Institute (National Eye Health Education Program) and other specialty organizations.[213] Of course, patients may elect not to follow the advice given or deny its importance. Another reason is that of cost. Moss et al.[212] found that the ability to afford eye care was also a reason patients gave for not having such care. In that study, 30% of persons with type 1 diabetes and 12% of those with type 2 diabetes said they could not afford an examination.

Re-examination of WESDR data by Batchhelder & Barricks[214] led them to conclude, based on the "remarkably low incidence of treatable conditions over 4 years for patients with retinopathy levels 21 or less and over 10 years for patients with no retinopathy at their baseline examination" that "these data do not suggest any difference in effectiveness for screening intervals of 1, 2, 3 or even 4 years for this group of low-risk patients." Others, also using models, have suggested in those with type 2 diabetes without retinopathy examinations every 2 years rather than yearly would be adequate to detect vision-threatening retinopathy.[215] The National Committee for Quality Assurance[216] released the Health Plan Employer Data and Information Set (HEDIS) 1999 draft which suggested every-other-year examinations for retinopathy if there was no evidence of retinopathy in the previous year's eye exam, persons were not taking insulin, and if the glycosylated HbA_{1c} was less than 8% (unpublished). However, the WESDR data showed that, in individuals with type 2 diabetes with no retinopathy present at baseline, 4 per 1000 developed proliferative retinopathy and 10 per 1000 persons developed clinically significant macular edema over a 4-year period.

There is a need to examine the issue of the sensitivity of the screens in detecting the presence of retinopathy. The epidemiologic data are based on detection of retinopathy by skilled graders using standardized protocols under study conditions to grade stereoscopic color fundus photographs of the DRS seven standard fields. Studies have demonstrated a variable sensitivity, in practice as low as 33%, in the detection of retinopathy by ophthalmoscopy in people with diabetes.[217] Newer screening approaches, including digital cameras with central reading centers, are being considered for the screening of diabetic patients not under the care of an ophthalmologist. There is a need to conduct epidemiological studies and controlled clinical trials to evaluate the interval and type of ophthalmic screening in persons with diabetes and no retinopathy in various health care settings to provide better evidence of efficacy of specific approaches before developing new eye care guidelines for people with diabetes as proposed by HEDIS. All of the accumulated data should be reconsidered when guidelines are revised.

CONCLUSIONS

Prevention of diabetes remains an important goal in reducing the complications and costs of this disease. Until approaches for primary prevention of diabetes itself become available, clinical trial data have shown that secondary prevention through medical interventions designed to control blood pressure and glycemia will reduce the incidence and progression of retinopathy and loss of vision. However, the success of these interventions has been limited, in part due to inability to achieve normalization of blood sugar with current drug delivery systems. While new interventions (e.g., reduction of lipids) may be of further benefit, tertiary prevention of visual loss (screening examination through a dilated pupil by skilled eye care providers on a regular basis for early detection and subsequent treatment, when indicated, of vision-threatening retinopathy with photocoagulation) remains an important approach to care for diabetic patients.

REFERENCES

1. Klein R, Klein BE. Vision disorders in diabetes. In: National Diabetes Data Group. Diabetes in America, 2nd edn. NIH publication no. 95–1468. Bethesda, MD: National Institutes of Health, National Institute of Diabetes and Digestive and Kidney Diseases; 1995:293–338.
2. The Diabetes Control and Complications Trial (DCCT) Research Group. The effect of intensive treatment of diabetes on the development and progression of long-term complications in insulin-dependent diabetes. N Engl J Med 1993; 329:977–986.
3. UK Prospective Diabetes Study Group (UKPDS). Intensive blood-glucose control with sulphonylureas or insulin compared with conventional treatment and risk of complications in patients with type 2 diabetes. (UKPDS 33). Lancet 1998; 352:837–853.
4. UK Prospective Diabetes Study Group (UKPDS). Tight blood pressure control and risk of macrovascular and microvascular complications in type 2 diabetes (UKPDS 38). Br Med J 1998; 317:703–713.
5. Schrier RW, Estacio RO, Esler A et al. Effects of aggressive blood pressure control in normotensive type 2 diabetic patients on albuminuria, retinopathy, and strokes. Kidney Int 2002; 61:1086–1097.
6. Fong DS, Aiello L, Gardner TW et al. Diabetic retinopathy. Diabetes Care 2003; 26(suppl. 1):S99–S102.
7. Klein R, Klein BEK, Moss SE et al. Prevalence of diabetes mellitus in southern Wisconsin. Am J Epidemiol 1984; 119:54–61.
8. Klein R, Klein BEK, Moss SE et al. The Wisconsin Epidemiologic Study of Diabetic Retinopathy. II. Prevalence and risk of diabetic retinopathy when age at diagnosis is less than 30 years. Arch Ophthalmol 1984; 102:520–526.
9. Klein R, Klein BEK, Moss SE et al. The Wisconsin Epidemiologic Study of Diabetic Retinopathy. III. Prevalence and risk of diabetic retinopathy when age at diagnosis is 30 or more years. Arch Ophthalmol 1984; 102:527–532.
10. Klein R, Klein BEK, Moss SE et al. The Wisconsin Epidemiologic Study of Diabetic Retinopathy. IV. Diabetic macular edema. Ophthalmology 1984; 91:1464–1474.
11. Houston A. Retinopathy in the Poole area: an epidemiological inquiry. In: Eschwege E, ed. Advances in diabetes epidemiology. Amsterdam: Elsevier; 1982:199–206.
12. Dwyer MS, Melton LJ 3rd, Ballard DJ et al. Incidence of diabetic retinopathy and blindness: a population-based study in Rochester, Minnesota. Diabetes Care 1985; 8:316–322.
13. Dorf A, Ballintine EJ, Bennett PH et al: Retinopathy in Pima Indians. Relationships to glucose level, duration of diabetes, age at diagnosis of diabetes, and age at examination in a population with a high prevalence of diabetes mellitus. Diabetes 1976; 25:554–560.
14. Bennett PH, Rushforth NB, Miller M et al. Epidemiologic studies of diabetes in the Pima Indians. Recent Prog Horm Res 1976; 32:333–376.
15. Kahn HA, Leibowitz HM, Ganley JP et al. The Framingham Eye Study. I. Outline and major prevalence findings. Am J Epidemiol 1977; 106:17–32.
16. West KM, Erdreich LJ, Stober JA. A detailed study of risk factors for retinopathy and nephropathy in diabetes. Diabetes 1980; 19:501–508.
17. King H, Balkau B, Zimmet P et al. Diabetic retinopathy in Nauruans. Am J Epidemiol 1983; 117:659–667.
18. Ballard DJ, Melton LJ 3rd, Dwyer MS et al. Risk factors for diabetic retinopathy: a population-based study in Rochester, Minnesota. Diabetes Care 1986; 9:334–342.
19. Danielsen R, Jonasson F, Helgason T. Prevalence of retinopathy and proteinuria in type 1 diabetics in Iceland. Acta Med Scand 1982; 212: 277–280.
20. Constable IJ, Knuiman MW, Welborn TA et al. Assessing the risk of diabetic retinopathy. Am J Ophthalmol 1984; 97:53–61.
21. Knuiman MW, Welborn TA, McCann VJ. Prevalence of diabetic complications in relation to risk factors. Diabetes 1986; 35:1332–1339.
22. Sjolie AK. Ocular complications in insulin treated diabetes mellitus. An epidemiological study. Acta Ophthalmol 1985; 172(suppl.):1–72.
23. Nielsen NV. Diabetic retinopathy. II. The course of retinopathy in diabetics treated with oral hypoglycaemic agents and diet regime alone. A one year epidemiologic cohort study of diabetes mellitus. The Island of Falster, Denmark. Acta Ophthalmol (Copenh) 1984; 62:266–273.
24. Nielsen NV. Diabetic retinopathy. I. The course of retinopathy in insulin-treated diabetics. A one year epidemiological cohort study of diabetes mellitus. The Island of Falster, Denmark. Acta Ophthalmol (Copenh) 1984; 62:256–265.
25. Teuscher A, Schnell H, Wilson PW. Incidence of diabetic retinopathy and relationship to baseline plasma glucose and blood pressure. Diabetes Care 1988; 11:246–251.
26. Haffner SM, Fong D, Stern MP et al. Diabetic retinopathy in Mexican Americans and non-Hispanic whites. Diabetes 1988; 37:878–884.
27. Jerneld B. Prevalence of diabetic retinopathy. A population study from the Swedish island of Gotland. Acta Ophthalmol 1988; 188:3–32.
28. Hamman RF, Mayer EJ, Moo-Young GA et al. Prevalence and risk factors of diabetic retinopathy in non-Hispanic whites and Hispanics with NIDDM. San Luis Valley Diabetes Study. Diabetes 1989; 38:1231–1237.
29. McLeod BK, Thompson JR, Rosenthal AR. The prevalence of retinopathy in the insulin-requiring diabetic patients of an English county town. Eye 1988; 2:424–430.
30. Kostraba JN, Klein R, Dorman JS. The Epidemiology of Diabetes Complications Study. IV. Correlates of diabetic background and proliferative retinopathy. Am J Epidemiol 1991; 133:381–391.
31. Fujimoto W, Fukuda M. Natural history of diabetic retinopathy and its treatment in Japan. In: Baba S, Goto Y, Fukui I, eds. Diabetes mellitus in Asia. Amsterdam: Excerpta Med; 1976:225–231.
32. Kullberg CE, Abrahamsson M, Arnqvist HJ et al. The VISS Study Group. Prevalence of retinopathy differs with age at onset of diabetes in a population of patients with type 1 diabetes. Diabetes Med 2002; 19:924–931.
33. Lopez IM, Diez A, Velilla S et al. Prevalence of diabetic retinopathy and eye care in a rural area of Spain. Ophthalm Epidemiol 2002; 9:205–214.
34. Broadbent DM, Scott JA, Vora JP et al. Prevalence of diabetic eye disease in an inner city population: the Liverpool Diabetic Eye Study. Eye 1999; 13:160–165.
35. West SK, Klein R, Rodriguez J et al. Diabetes and diabetic retinopathy in a Mexican-American population: Proyecto VER. Diabetes Care 2001; 24:1204–1209.
36. Varma R, Torres M, Pena F et al. Prevalence of diabetic retinopathy in adult Latinos: the Los Angeles Latino Eye Study. Ophthalmology 2004; 111:1298–1306.
37. McKay R, McCarty CA, Taylor HR. Diabetic retinopathy in Victoria, Australia: the Visual Impairment Project. Br J Ophthalmol 2000; 84:865–870.
38. Toeller M, Buyken AE, Heitkamp G et al. Prevalence of chronic complications, metabolic control and nutritional intake in type 1 diabetes: comparison between different European regions. EURODIAB Complications Study group. Horm Metab Res 1999; 31:680–685.
39. Leske MC, Wu SY, Hyman L et al. Diabetic retinopathy in a black population: the Barbados Eye Study. Ophthalmology 1999; 106:1893–1899.
40. Rajala U, Laakso M, Qiao Q et al. Prevalence of retinopathy in people with diabetes, impaired glucose tolerance, and normal glucose tolerance. Diabetes Care 1998; 21:1664–1669.
41. Harris MI, Klein R, Cowie CC et al. Is the risk of diabetic retinopathy greater in non-Hispanic blacks and Mexican Americans than in non-Hispanic whites with type 2 diabetes? A US population study. Diabetes Care 1998; 21:1230–1235.
42. Dowse GK, Humphrey AR, Collins VR et al. Prevalence and risk factors for diabetic retinopathy in the multiethnic population of Mauritius. Am J Epidemiol 1998; 147:448–457.
43. Kohner EM, Aldington SJ, Stratton IM et al. United Kingdom Prospective Diabetes Study, 30: diabetic retinopathy at diagnosis of non-insulin-dependent diabetes mellitus and associated risk factors. Arch Ophthalmol 1998; 116:297–303.
44. Mitchell P, Smith W, Wang JJ et al. Prevalence of diabetic retinopathy in an older community. The Blue Mountains Eye Study. Ophthalmology 1998; 105:406–411.
45. Gonzalez Villalpando ME, Gonzalez Villalpando C, Arredondo Perez B et al. Moderate-to-severe diabetic retinopathy is more prevalent in Mexico City than in San Antonio, Texas. Diabetes Care 1997; 20:773–777.
46. Berinstein DM, Stahn RM, Welty TK et al. The prevalence of diabetic retinopathy and associated risk factors among Sioux Indians. Diabetes Care 1997; 20:757–759.
47. Kernell A, Dedorsson I, Johansson B et al. Prevalence of diabetic retinopathy in children and adolescents with IDDM. A population-based multicentre study. Diabetologia 1997; 40:307–310.
48. Collins VR, Dowse GK, Plehwe WE et al. High prevalence of diabetic retinopathy and nephropathy in Polynesians of Western Samoa. Diabetes Care 1995; 18:1140–1149.
49. Klein R, Klein BE, Moss SE et al. The Beaver Dam Eye Study. Retinopathy in adults with newly discovered and previously diagnosed diabetes mellitus. Ophthalmology 1992; 99:58–62.
50. Roy MS. Diabetic retinopathy in African Americans with type 1 diabetes: The New Jersey 725: I. Methodology, population, frequency of retinopathy, and visual impairment. Arch Ophthalmol 2000; 118:97–104.

51. Roy MS, Klein R. Macular edema and retinal hard exudates in African Americans with type 1 diabetes: The New Jersey 725. Arch Ophthalmol 2001; 119:251–259.
52. Eye Diseases Prevalence Research Group. The prevalence of diabetic retinopathy in the United States. Arch Ophthalmol 2004; 122:522–563.
53. Klein R, Klein BE, Moss SE et al. The Wisconsin Epidemiologic Study of Diabetic Retinopathy. IX. Four-year incidence and progression of diabetic retinopathy when age at diagnosis is less than 30 years. Arch Ophthalmol 1989; 107:237–243.
54. Klein R, Klein BE, Moss SE et al. The Wisconsin Epidemiologic Study of Diabetic Retinopathy. X. Four-year incidence and progression of diabetic retinopathy when age at diagnosis is 30 years or more. Arch Ophthalmol 1989; 107:244–249.
55. Klein R, Klein BE, Moss SE et al. The Wisconsin Epidemiologic Study of Diabetic Retinopathy XI. The incidence of macular edema. Ophthalmology 1989; 96:1501–1510.
56. Klein R, Klein BE, Moss SE et al. The Wisconsin Epidemiologic Study of Diabetic Retinopathy. XIV. Ten-year incidence and progression of diabetic retinopathy. Arch Ophthalmol 1994; 112:1217–1228.
57. Henricsson M, Nystrom L, Blohme G et al. The incidence of retinopathy 10 years after diagnosis in young adult people with diabetes: results from the nationwide population-based Diabetes Incidence Study in Sweden (DISS). Diabetes Care 2003; 26:349–354.
58. Lloyd CE, Becker D, Ellis D et al. Incidence of complications in insulin-dependent diabetes mellitus: a survival analysis. Am J Epidemiol 1996; 143:431–441.
59. Klein R, Palta M, Allen C et al. Incidence of retinopathy and associated risk factors from time of diagnosis of insulin-dependent diabetes. Arch Ophthalmol 1997; 115:351–356.
60. Tudor SM, Hamman RF, Baron A et al. Incidence and progression of diabetic retinopathy in Hispanics and non-Hispanic whites with type 2 diabetes. San Luis Valley Diabetes Study, Colorado. Diabetes Care 1998; 21:53–61.
61. Klein R, Klein BE, Moss SE et al. The Wisconsin Epidemiologic Study of Diabetic Retinopathy: XVII. The 14-year incidence and progression of diabetic retinopathy and associated risk factors in type 1 diabetes. Ophthalmology 1998; 105:1801–1815.
62. Porta M, Sjoelie AK, Chaturvedi N et al. EURODIAB Prospective Complications Study Group. Risk factors for progression to proliferative diabetic retinopathy in the EURODIAB Prospective Complications Study. Diabetologia 2001; 44:2203–2209.
63. Ling R, Ramsewak V, Taylor D et al. Longitudinal study of a cohort of people with diabetes screened by the Exeter Diabetic Retinopathy Screening Programme. Eye 2002; 16:140–145.
64. Younis N, Broadbent DM, Vora JP et al. Liverpool Diabetic Eye Study. Incidence of sight-threatening retinopathy in patients with type 2 diabetes in the Liverpool Diabetic Eye Study: a cohort study. Lancet 2003; 361:195–200.
65. Rabb MF, Gagliano DA, Sweeny NE: Diabetic retinopathy in blacks. Diabetes Care 1990; 13:1202–1206.
66. Arfken CL, Reno PL, Santiago JV et al. Development of proliferative retinopathy in African Americans and whites with type 1 diabetes. Diabetes Care 1998; 21:792–795.
67. Klein R, Sharrett AR, Klein BE et al. The association of atherosclerosis, vascular risk factors, and retinopathy in adults with diabetes: the Atherosclerosis Risk in Communities Study. Ophthalmology 2002; 109:1225–1234.
68. Klein R, Marino EK, Kuller LH et al. The relation of atherosclerotic cardiovascular disease to retinopathy in people with diabetes in the Cardiovascular Health Study. Br J Ophthalmol 2002; 86:84–90.
69. Cruickshank JK, Alleyne SA. Black West Indian and matched white diabetics in Britain compared with diabetics in Jamaica: body mass, blood pressure, and vascular disease. Diabetes Care 1987; 10:170–179.
70. Lee ET, Lee VS, Lu M et al. Development of proliferative retinopathy in NIDDM, a follow-up study of American Indians in Oklahoma. Diabetes 1992; 41:359–367.
71. Lee ET, Lee VS, Kingsley RM et al. Diabetic retinopathy in Oklahoma Indians with NIDDM. Incidence and risk factors. Diabetes Care 1992; 15:1620–1627.
72. Nelson RG, Newman JM, Knowler WC et al. Incidence of end-stage renal disease in type 2 (non-insulin-dependent) diabetes mellitus in Pima Indians. Diabetologia 1988; 31:730–736.
73. Barbosa J, Ramsay RC, Knobloch WH et al. Histocompatibility antigen frequencies in diabetic retinopathy. Am J Ophthalmol 1980; 90:148–153.
74. Dornan TL, Ting A, McPherson CK et al. Genetic susceptibility to the development of retinopathy in insulin-dependent diabetics. Diabetes 1982; l31:226–231.
75. Rand LI, Krolewski AS, Aiello LM et al. Multiple factors in the prediction of risk of proliferative diabetic retinopathy. N Engl J Med 1985; 113:1433–1438.
76. Jervell J, Solheim B. HLA-antigens in long standing insulin dependent diabetics with terminal nephropathy and retinopathy with and without loss of vision [letter]. Diabetologia 1979; 17:391.

77. The Diabetes Control and Complications Trial Research Group. Clustering of long-term complications in families with diabetes in the diabetes control and complications trial. Diabetes 1997; 46:1829–1839.
78. Rema M, Saravanan G, Deepa R et al. Familial clustering of diabetic retinopathy in South Indian type 2 diabetic patients. Diabetes Med 2002; 19:910–916.
79. Tattersall RB, Pyke DA. Diabetes in identical twins. Lancet 1972; 2:1120–1125.
80. Pyke DA, Tattersall RB. Diabetic retinopathy in identical twins. Diabetes 1973; 22:613–618.
81. Leslie RD, Pyke DA. Diabetic retinopathy in identical twins. Diabetes 1982; 31:19–21.
82. Cruickshanks KJ, Vadheim CM, Moss SE et al. Genetic marker associations with proliferative retinopathy in persons diagnosed with diabetes before 30 years of age. Diabetes 1992; 41:879–885.
83. Cruickshanks KJ, Klein R, Klein BE et al. HLA-DR4 and the incidence of proliferative retinopathy. Diabetes 1993; 42:33A.
84. Wong TY, Cruickshanks KJ, Klein R et al. HLA-DR3and DR4 and their relation to the incidence and progression of diabetic retinopathy. Ophthalmology 2002; 109:275–281.
85. Nagi DK, McCormack LJ, Mohamed-Ali V et al. Diabetic retinopathy, promoter (4G/5G) polymorphism of PAI-1 gene, and PAI-1 activity in Pima Indians with type 2 diabetes. Diabetes Care 1997; 20:1304–1309.
86. Imperatore G, Hanson RL, Pettitt DJ et al. Sib-pair linkage analysis for susceptibility genes for microvascular complications among Pima Indians with type 2 diabetes. Diabetes 1998; 47:821–830.
87. Marre M, Bernadet P, Gallois Y et al. Relationships between angiotensin I converting enzyme gene polymorphism, plasma levels, and diabetic retinal and renal complications. Diabetes 1994; 43:384–388.
88. Tarnow L, Cambien F, Rossing P et al. Lack of relationship between an insertion/deletion polymorphism in the angiotensin I-converting enzyme gene and diabetic nephropathy and proliferative retinopathy in IDDM patients. Diabetes 1995; 44:489–494.
89. Fukuda M, Nakano S, Imaizumi N et al. Mitochondrial DNA mutations are associated with both decreased insulin secretion and advanced microvascular complications in Japanese diabetic subjects. J Diabetes Compl 1999; 13:277–283.
90. Demaine A, Cross D, Millward A. Polymorphisms of the aldose reductase gene and susceptibility to retinopathy in type 1 diabetes mellitus. Invest Ophthalmol Vis Sci 2000; 41:4064–4068.
91. Yamamoto T, Sato T, Hosoi M et al. Aldose reductase gene polymorphism is associated with progression of diabetic nephropathy in Japanese patients with type 1 diabetes mellitus. Diabetes Obes Metab 2003; 5:51–57.
92. Kankova K, Muzik J, Karaskova J et al. Duration of non-insulin-dependent diabetes mellitus and the TNF-beta NcoI genotype as predictive factors in proliferative diabetic retinopathy. Ophthalmologica 2001; 215:294–298.
93. Santos A, Salguero ML, Gurrola C et al. The epsilon4 allele of apolipoprotein E gene is a potential risk factor for the severity of macular edema in type 2 diabetic Mexican patients. Ophthalm Genet 2002; 23:13–19.
94. Kao Y, Donaghue KC, Chan A et al. Paraoxonase gene cluster is a genetic marker for early microvascular complications in type 1 diabetes. Diabetes Med 2002; 19:212–215.
95. Taverna MJ, Sola A, Guyot-Argenton C et al. eNOS4 polymorphism of the endothelial nitric oxide synthase predicts risk for severe diabetic retinopathy. Diabetes Med 2002; 19:240–245.
96. Kamiuchi K, Hasegawa G, Obayashi H et al. Intercellular adhesion molecule-1 (ICAM-1) polymorphism is associated with diabetic retinopathy in type 2 diabetes mellitus. Diabetes Med 2002; 19:371–376.
97. Matsubara Y, Murata M, Maruyama T et al. Association between diabetic retinopathy and genetic variations in alpha2beta1 integrin, a platelet receptor for collagen. Blood 2000; 95:1560–1564.
98. Yang B, Cross DF, Ollerenshaw M et al. Polymorphisms of the vascular endothelial growth factor and susceptibility to diabetic microvascular complications in patients with type 1 diabetes mellitus. J Diabetes Compl 2003; 17:1–6.
99. Klein BE, Moss SE, Klein R. Is menarche associated with diabetic retinopathy? Diabetes Care 1990; 13:1034–1038.
100. Frost-Larsen K, Starup K. Fluorescein angiography in diabetic children. A follow-up. Acta Ophthalmol (Copenh) 1980; 58:355–360.
101. Murphy RP, Nanda M, Plotnick L et al. The relationship of puberty to diabetic retinopathy. Arch Ophthalmol 1990; 108:215–218.
102. Kostraba JN, Dorman JS, Orchard TJ et al. Contribution of diabetes duration before puberty to development of microvascular complications in IDDM subjects. Diabetes Care 1989; 12:686–693.
103. Harris MI, Klein R, Welborn TA et al. Onset of NIDDM occurs at least 4–7 years before clinical diagnosis. Diabetes Care 1992; 15:815–819.
104. Aiello LM, Rand LI, Briones JC et al. Diabetic retinopathy in Joslin Clinic patients with adult-onset diabetes. Ophthalmology 1981;88:619–623.
105. West KM. Epidemiology of diabetes and its vascular lesions. New York: Elsevier; 1978:415.

106. University Group Diabetes Program. Effects of hypoglycemic agents on vascular complications in patients with adult-onset diabetes. VIII. Evaluation of insulin therapy: final report. Diabetes 1982; 31(suppl. 5):1–81.

107. Engerman R, Bloodworth JM Jr, Nelson S. Relationship of microvascular disease in diabetes to metabolic control. Diabetes 1977; 26:760–769.

108. Klein R, Klein BE, Moss SE et al. Glycosylated hemoglobin predicts the incidence and progression of diabetic retinopathy. JAMA 1988; 260:2864–2871.

109. Klein R, Klein BE, Moss SE et al. The relationship of hyperglycemia to the long-term incidence and progression of diabetic retinopathy. Arch Intern Med 1994; 154:2169–2178.

110. The Kroc Collaborative Study Group. Blood glucose control and the evolution of diabetic retinopathy and albuminuria. A preliminary multicenter trial. N Engl J Med 1984; 311:365–372.

111. The Kroc Collaborative Study Group. Diabetic retinopathy after two years of intensified insulin treatment. Follow-up of the Kroc Collaborative Study. JAMA 1988; 260:37–41.

112. Lauritzen T, Frost-Larsen K, Larsen HW et al. Effect of 1 year of near-normal blood glucose levels on retinopathy in insulin-dependent diabetics. Lancet 1983; 1:200–204.

113. Lauritzen T, Frost-Larsen K, Larsen HW et al. Two-year experience with continuous subcutaneous insulin infusion in relation to retinopathy and neuropathy. Diabetes 1985; 34(suppl. 3):74–79.

114. Dahl-Jorgensen K, Brinchmann-Hansen O, Hanssen KF et al. Effect of near normoglycaemia for two years on progression of early diabetic retinopathy, nephropathy, and neuropathy: the Oslo study. Br Med J 1986; 293:1195–1199.

115. Dahl-Jorgensen K, Brinchmann-Hansen O, Hanssen KF et al. Rapid tightening of blood glucose control leads to transient deterioration of retinopathy in insulin dependent diabetes mellitus: the Oslo study. Br Med J 1985; 290:811–815.

116. Emanuele N, Klein R, Abraira C et al. Evaluations of retinopathy in the VA Cooperative Study on glycemic control and complications in type II diabetes (VA CSDM). A feasibility study. Diabetes Care 1996; 19:1375–1381.

117. Wang PH, Lau J, Chalmers TC. Meta-analysis of effects of intensive blood-glucose control on late complications of type I diabetes. Lancet 1993; 341:1306–1309.

118. The Diabetes Control and Complications Trial Research Group. The effect of intensive diabetes treatment on the progression of diabetic retinopathy in insulin-dependent diabetes mellitus: The Diabetes Control and Complications Trial. Arch Ophthalmol 1995; 113:36–51.

119. The Diabetes Control and Complications Trial Research Group. Progression of retinopathy with intensive versus conventional treatment in the Diabetes Control and Complications Trial. Ophthalmology 1995; 102:647–661.

120. The Diabetes Control and Complications Trial Research Group. The absence of a glycemic threshold for the development of long-term complications: the perspective of the Diabetes Control and Complications Trial. Diabetes 1996; 45:1289–1298.

121. Warram JH, Manson JE, Krolewski AS. Glycosylated hemoglobin and the risk of retinopathy in insulin-dependent diabetes mellitus. N Engl J Med 1995; 332:1305–1306.

122. The Diabetes Control and Complications Trial Research Group. Lifetime benefits and costs of intensive therapy as practiced in the Diabetes Control and Complications Trial. JAMA 1996; 276:1409–1415.

123. The Diabetes Control and Complications Trial/Epidemiology of Diabetes Interventions and Complications Research Group. Retinopathy and nephropathy in patients with type 1 diabetes four years after a trial of intensive therapy. N Engl J Med 2000; 342:381–389.

124. UK Prospective Diabetes Study Group. Effect of intensive blood-glucose control with metformin on complications in overweight patients with type 2 diabetes (UKPDS 34). Lancet 1998; 352:854–865.

125. Gray A, Raikou M, McGuire A et al. Cost effectiveness of an intensive blood glucose control policy in patients with type 2 diabetes: economic analysis alongside randomised controlled trial (UKPDS 41). United Kingdom Prospective Diabetes Study Group. Br Med J 2000; 320:1373–1378.

126. Duckworth WC, McCarren M, Abraira C; VA Diabetes Trial. Glucose control and cardiovascular complications: the VA Diabetes Trial. Diabetes Care 2001; 24:942–945.

127. American Diabetes Association. Position statement: standards of medical care for patients with diabetes mellitus. Diabetes Care 1994; 17:616–623.

128. Harris MI. Health care and health status and outcomes for patients with type 2 diabetes. Diabetes Care 2000; 23:754–758.

129. Klein R, Klein BE, Moss SE et al. The medical management of hyperglycemia over a 10-year period in people with diabetes. Diabetes Care 1996; 19:744–750.

130. Smith RB, Pyke DA, Watkins PJ et al. C-peptide response to glucagon in diabetics with and without complications. NZ Med J 1979; 89:304–306.

131. Sjoberg S, Gunnarsson R, Gjotterberg M et al. Residual insulin production, glycaemic control and prevalence of microvascular lesions and polyneuropathy in long-term type I (insulin dependent) diabetes mellitus. Diabetologia 1987; 30:208–213.

132. Sjoberg S, Gjotterberg M, Lefvert AK et al. Significance of residual insulin production in long-term type I diabetes mellitus. Transplant Proc 1986; 18:1498–1499.

133. Madsbad S, Lauritzen E, Faber OK et al. The effect of residual beta-cell function on the development of diabetic retinopathy. Diabetes Med 1986; 3:42–45.

134. Klein R, Moss SE, Klein BE et al. Wisconsin Epidemiologic Study of Diabetic Retinopathy. XII. Relationship of C-peptide and diabetic retinopathy. Diabetes 1990; 39:1445–1450.

135. Klein R, Klein BE, Moss SE. The Wisconsin Epidemiologic Study of Diabetic Retinopathy. XVI. The relationship of C-peptide to the incidence and progression of diabetic retinopathy. Diabetes 1995; 44:796–801.

136. Steffes MW, Sibley S, Jackson M et al. Beta-cell function and the development of diabetes-related complications in the Diabetes Control and Complications Trial. Diabetes Care 2003; 26:832–836.

137. Serghieri G, Bartolomei G, Pettenello C et al. Raised retinopathy prevalence rate in insulin-treated patients: A feature of obese type II diabetes. Transplant Proc 1986; 18:1576–1577.

138. Davis MD. Diabetic retinopathy, diabetes control, and blood pressure. Transplant Proc 1986; 18:1565–1568.

139. Kohner EM. Diabetic retinopathy. Br Med Bull 1989; 45:148–173.

140. Klein R, Klein BE, Moss SE et al. Is blood pressure a predictor of the incidence or progression of diabetic retinopathy? Arch Intern Med 1989; 149:2427–2432.

141. Klein BE, Klein R, Moss SE et al. A cohort study of the relationship of diabetic retinopathy to blood pressure. Arch Ophthalmol 1995; 113:601–606.

142. Adler A, Stratton IM, Neil HA et al. Association of systolic blood pressure with macrovascular and microvascular complications of type 2 diabetes (UKPDS 36): prospective observational study. Br Med J 2000; 321:412–419.

143. Klein R, Klein BE, Moss SE et al. The Wisconsin Epidemiologic Study of Diabetic Retinopathy. XV. The long-term incidence of macular edema. Ophthalmology 1995; 102:7–16.

144. Chaturvedi N, Sjolie AK, Stephenson JM et al. Effect of lisinopril on progression of retinopathy in normotensive people with type 1 diabetes: the EUCLID Study Group. EURODIAB controlled trial of lisinopril in insulin-dependent diabetes mellitus. Lancet 1998; 351:28–31.

145. Chaturvedi N. Modulation of the renin–angiotensin system and retinopathy. Heart 2000; 84(suppl. 1):i29–i31.

146. Estacio RO, Jeffers BW, Gifford N et al. Effect of blood pressure control on diabetic microvascular complications in patients with hypertension and type 2 diabetes. Diabetes 2000; 23(suppl. 2):B54–B64.

147. Chaturvedi N, Sjoelie AK, Svensson A et al. The Diabetic Retinopathy Candesartan Trials (DIRECT) programme, rationale and study design. J Renin Angiotensin Aldosterone Syst 2002; 3:255–261.

148. Cruickshanks KJ, Ritter LL, Klein R et al. The association of microalbuminuria with diabetic retinopathy. The Wisconsin Epidemiologic Study of Diabetic Retinopathy. Ophthalmology 1993; 100:862–867.

149. Klein R, Moss SE, Klein BE. Is gross proteinuria a risk factor for the incidence of proliferative diabetic retinopathy? Ophthalmology 1993; 100:1140–1146.

150. Lloyd CE, Klein R, Maser RE et al. The progression of retinopathy over 2 years: the Pittsburgh Epidemiology of Diabetes Complications (EDC) Study. J Diabetes Complications 1995; 9:140–148.

151. Moss SE, Klein R, Klein BE. The incidence of vision loss in a diabetic population. Ophthalmology 1988; 95:1340–1348.

152. Duncan LJP, Cullen JF, Ireland JT et al. A three-year trial of Atromid therapy in exudative diabetic retinopathy. Diabetes 1968; 17:458–467.

153. Klein BE, Moss SE, Klein R et al. The Wisconsin Epidemiologic Study of Diabetic Retinopathy. XIII. Relationship of serum cholesterol to retinopathy and hard exudate. Ophthalmology 1991; 98:1261–1265.

154. Chew EY, Klein ML, Ferris FL 3rd et al. Association of elevated serum lipid levels with retinal hard exudate in diabetic retinopathy. Early Treatment Diabetic Retinopathy Study (ETDRS) Report 22. Arch Ophthalmol 1996; 114:1079–1084.

155. Gordon B, Chang S, Kavanagh M et al. The effects of lipid lowering on diabetic retinopathy. Am J Ophthalmol 1991; 112:385–391.

156. Freyberger H, Schifferdecker E, Schatz H. [Regression of hard exudates in diabetic background retinopathy in therapy with etofibrate antilipaemic agent.] Med Klin (Munich) 1994; 89:594–597, 633.

157. Dale J, Farmer J, Jones AF et al. Diabetic ischaemic and exudative maculopathy: are their risk factors different? Diabetes Med 2000; 17:47.

158. Goldsmith JR, Landaw SA. Carbon monoxide and human health. Science 1968; 162:1352–1359.

159. Hawkins RI. Smoking, platelets and thrombosis. Nature 1972; 236:450–452.

160. Klein R, Klein BE, Davis MD. Is cigarette smoking associated with diabetic retinopathy? Am J Epidemiol 1983; 118:228–238.

161. Moss SE, Klein R, Klein BE. Association of cigarette smoking with diabetic retinopathy. Diabetes 1991; 14:119–126.

162. Moss SE, Klein R, Klein BE. Cigarette smoking and ten-year progression of diabetic retinopathy. Ophthalmology 1996; 103:1438–1442.

163. Klein R, Moss SE, Klein BE et al. Relation of ocular and systemic factors to survival in diabetes. Arch Intern Med 1989; 149:266–272.

164. Jakubowski JA, Vaillancourt R, Deykin D. Interaction of ethanol, prostacyclin, and aspirin in determining human platelet reactivity in vitro. Arteriosclerosis 1988; 8:436–441.

165. Kingsley LA, Dorman JS, Doft BH et al. An epidemiologic approach to the study of retinopathy: the Pittsburgh diabetic morbidity and retinopathy studies. Diabetes Res Clin Pract 1988; 4:99–109.

166. Young RJ, McCulloch DK, Prescott RJ et al. Alcohol: Another risk factor for diabetic retinopathy? Br Med J 1984; 288:1035–1037.

167. Moss SE, Klein R, Klein BE. Alcohol consumption and the prevalence of diabetic retinopathy. Ophthalmology 1992; 99:926–932.

168. Moss SE, Klein R, Klein BE. The association of alcohol consumption with the incidence and progression of diabetic retinopathy. Ophthalmology 1994; 101:1962–1968.

169. Valmadrid CT, Klein R, Moss SE et al. Alcohol intake and the risk of coronary heart disease mortality in persons with older-onset diabetes mellitus. JAMA 1999; 282:239–246.

170. Diabetes Drafting Group. Prevalence of small vessel and large vessel disease in diabetic patients from 14 centres. The World Health Organization multinational study of vascular disease in diabetes. Diabetologia 1985; 28(suppl.):615–640.

171. LaPorte RE, Dorman JS, Tajima N et al. Pittsburgh insulin-dependent diabetes mellitus morbidity and mortality study: physical activity and diabetic complications. Pediatrics 1986; 78:1027–1033.

172. van Leiden HA, Dekker JM, Moll AC et al. Risk factors for incident retinopathy in a diabetic and nondiabetic population: the Hoorn study. Arch Ophthalmol 2003; 121:245–251.

173. Klein R, Klein BE, Moss SE. Is obesity related to microvascular and macrovascular complications in diabetes? The Wisconsin Epidemiologic Study of Diabetic Retinopathy. Arch Intern Med 1997; 157:650–656.

174. Orchard TJ, Dorman JS, Maser RE et al. Factors associated with avoidance of severe complications after 25 yr of IDDM. Pittsburgh Epidemiology of Diabetes Complications Study I. Diabetes Care 1990; 13:741–747.

175. Kriska AM, LaPorte RE, Patrick SL et al. The association of physical activity and diabetic complications in individuals with insulin-dependent diabetes mellitus: the Epidemiology of Diabetes Complications Study – VII. J Clin Epidemiol 1991; 44:1207–1214.

176. LaPorte RE, Dorman JS, Tajima N et al. Pittsburgh insulin-dependent diabetes mellitus morbidity and mortality study: physical activity and diabetic complications. Pediatrics 1986; 78:1027–1033.

177. Cruickshanks KJ, Moss SE, Klein R et al. Physical activity and proliferative retinopathy in people diagnosed with diabetes before age 30 years. Diabetes Care 1992; 15:1267–1272.

178. Hanna AK, Roy M, Zinman B et al. An evaluation of factors associated with proliferative diabetic retinopathy. Clin Invest Med 1985; 8:109–116.

179. Haffner SM, Hazuda HP, Stern MP et al. Effects of socioeconomic status on hyperglycemia and retinopathy levels in Mexican Americans with NIDDM. Diabetes Care 1989; 12:128–134.

180. Klein R, Klein BE, Jensen SC et al. The relation of socioeconomic factors to the incidence of proliferative diabetic retinopathy and loss of vision. Ophthalmology 1994; 101:68–76.

181. Klein BE, Moss SE, Klein R. Oral contraceptives in women with diabetes. Diabetes Care 1990; 13:895–898.

182. Klein BE, Moss SE, Klein R. Effect of pregnancy on progression of diabetic retinopathy. Diabetes Care 1990; 13:34–40.

183. Chew EY, Mills JL, Metzger BE et al. Metabolic control and progression of retinopathy. The diabetes in early pregnancy study. National Institute of Child Health and Human Development diabetes in early pregnancy study. Diabetes Care 1995; 18:631–637.

184. Hemachandra A, Ellis D, Lloyd CE et al. The influence of pregnancy on IDDM complications. Diabetes Care 1995; 18:950–954.

185. Lovestam-Adrian M, Agardh CD, Aberg A et al. Pre-eclampsia is a potent risk factor for deterioration of retinopathy during pregnancy in type 1 diabetic patients. Diabetes Med 1997; 14:1059–1065.

186. Rosenn B, Miodovnik M, Kranias G et al. Progression of diabetic retinopathy in pregnancy: association with hypertension in pregnancy. Am J Obstet Gynecol 1992; 166:1214–1218.

187. Temple RC, Aldridge VA, Sampson MJ et al. Impact of pregnancy on the progression of diabetic retinopathy in type 1 diabetes. Diabetes Med 2001; 18:573–577.

188. Lauszus F, Klebe JG, Bek T. Diabetic retinopathy in pregnancy during tight metabolic control. Acta Obstet Gynecol Scand 2000; 79:367–370.

189. Lauszus FF, Klebe JG, Bek T et al. Increased serum IGF-1 during pregnancy is associated with progression of diabetic retinopathy. Diabetes 2003; 52:852–856.

190. Best RM, Hayes R, Hadden DR et al. Plasma levels of endothelin-1 in diabetic retinopathy in pregnancy. Eye 1999; 13(Pt 2):179–182.

191. Klein BE, Klein R, Moss SE. Exogenous estrogen exposures and changes in diabetic retinopathy. The Wisconsin Epidemiologic Study of Diabetic Retinopathy. Diabetes Care 1999; 22:1984–1987.

192. Vaarasmaki M, Anttila M, Pirttiaho H et al. Are recurrent pregnancies a risk in type 1 diabetes? Acta Obstet Gynecol Scand 2002; 81:1110–1115.

193. Klein R, Klein BE, Moss SE. Epidemiology of proliferative diabetic retinopathy. Diabetes Care 1992; 15:1875–1891.

194. Klein R, Klein BE, Moss SE et al. Association of ocular disease and mortality in a diabetic population. Arch Ophthalmol 1999; 117:1487–1495.

195. Davis MD, Hiller R, Magli YL et al. Prognosis for life in patients with diabetes: relation to severity of retinopathy. Trans Am Ophthalmol Soc 1979; 77:144–170.

196. Hanis CL, Chu HH, Lawson K et al. Mortality of Mexican Americans with NIDDM. Retinopathy and other predictors in Starr county, Texas. Diabetes Care 1993; 16:82–89.

197. Neil A, Hawkins M, Potok M et al. A prospective population-based study of microalbuminuria as a predictor of mortality in NIDDM. Diabetes Care 1993; 16:996–1003.

198. Early Treatment Diabetic Retinopathy Study Research Group. Effects of aspirin treatment on diabetic retinopathy. ETDRS report no. 8. Early Treatment Diabetic Retinopathy Study Research Group. Ophthalmology 1991; 98(suppl.):757–765.

199. Klein BE, Klein R, Moss SE. Is aspirin usage associated with diabetic retinopathy? Diabetes Care 1987; 10:600–603.

200. Hennekens CH, Jonas MA, Buring JE. The benefits of aspirin in acute myocardial infarction. Still a well-kept secret in the United States. Arch Intern Med 1994; 154:37–39.

201. Sorbinil Retinopathy Trial Research Group. A randomized trial of sorbinil, an aldose reductase inhibitor in diabetic retinopathy. Arch Ophthalmol 1990; 108:1234–1244.

202. Pearson P, Baker CW, Eliott D et al. Fluocinolone acetonide intravitreal implant in patients with diabetic macular edema: 12 month results. Invest Ophthalmol 2003; 44:4288.

203. Aiello LP. The potential role of PKC beta in diabetic retinopathy and macular edema. Surv Ophthalmol 2002; 47(suppl. 2):S263–S269.

204. Milton RC, Aiello LP, Davis MD et al. PKC-DRS Study Group. Initial results of the Protein Kinase C ß Inhibitor Diabetic Retinopathy Study (PKC-DRS). Diabetes 2003; 52(suppl. 1):A114.

205. Witkin SR, Klein R. Ophthalmologic care for persons with diabetes. JAMA 1984; 251:2534–2537.

206. American College of Physicians, American Diabetes Association, and American Academy of Ophthalmology. Screening guidelines for diabetic retinopathy. Ann Intern Med 1992; 116:660–671.

207. Sprafka JM, Fritsche TL, Baker R et al. Prevalence of undiagnosed eye disease in high-risk diabetic individuals. Arch Intern Med 1990; 150:857–861.

208. Brechner RJ, Cowie CC, Howie LJ et al. Ophthalmologic examination among adults with diagnosed diabetes mellitus. JAMA 1993; 270:1714–1718.

209. Weiner JP, Parente ST, Garnick DW et al. Variation in office-based quality. A claim-based profile of care provided to Medicare patients with diabetes. JAMA 1995; 273:1503–1508.

210. Kraft SK, Marrero DG, Lazaridis EN et al. Primary care physicians' practice patterns and diabetic retinopathy. Current levels of care. Arch Fam Med 1997; 6:29–37.

211. Bresnick GH, Mukamel DB, Dickinson JC et al. A screening approach to the surveillance of patients with diabetes for the presence of vision-threatening retinopathy. Ophthalmology 2000; 107:19–24.

212. Moss SE, Klein R, Klein BE. Factors associated with having eye examinations in persons with diabetes. Arch Fam Med 1995; 4:529–534.

213. The National Eye Institute, The National Eye Health Education Program (NEHEP). Planning the partnership: from vision research to health education. Bethesda, MD: National Institutes of Health; 1990.

214. Batchelder T, Barricks M. The Wisconsin Epidemiologic Study of Diabetic Retinopathy. Arch Ophthalmol 1995; 113:702–703.

215. Vijan S, Hofer TP, Hayward RA. Cost–utility analysis of screening intervals for diabetic retinopathy in patients with type 2 diabetes mellitus. JAMA 2000; 283:889–896.

216. National Committee for Quality Assurance. Health Plan Employers Data and Information Set (HEDIS) 2.5. Washington DC: National Committee for Quality Assurance; 1996.

217. Valez R, Haffner S, Stern MP et al. Ophthalmologist versus retinal photographs in screening for diabetic retinopathys. Clin Res 1987; 35:363A.

218. Klein R, Klein BE, Moss SE. Risk factors for retinopathy. In: Feman SS, ed. Ocular problems in diabetes mellitus. Boston: Blackwell Scientific Publications; 1992:39.

219. Klein R. Retinopathy and other ocular complications in diabetes. In: Porte D Jr, Sherwin RS, Baron A, eds. Ellenberg and Rifkin's diabetes mellitus, 6th edn. New York: McGraw-Hill; 2003:676–677.

220. Klein R. Diabetes mellitus: oculopathy. In: Degroot LJ, Jameson JL, eds. Endocrinology, 4th edn. Philadelphia, PA: WB Saunders; 1995:857–867.

Clinical Applications of Diagnostic Indocyanine Green Angiography

Nicole E. Gross
Lawrence A. Yannuzzi

The past decade has witnessed the emergence and evolution of indocyanine green (ICG) angiography as a useful diagnostic adjunct and investigative tool for chorioretinal diseases.[1–3] In spite of enhanced imaging of the choroidal circulation, practical clinical applications for this imaging system have not fulfilled earlier expectations. The principal limiting factor is the inability to image clearly the small capillaries in the choriocapillaris with high levels of spatial and temporal resolution. With the use of serial sequential subtraction techniques, the capillaries of the choriocapillaris can be imaged with ICG angiography; but this sophisticated technique has only been suitable within investigative models, not for practical clinical application.[4,5] Essentially, the clinical use for ICG angiography is of value in only a few, selective degenerative and inflammatory abnormalities, and rarely, for the evaluation of a mass lesion of the fundus. Yet, when clinical examination with slit-lamp biomicroscopy is not adequate for a definitive diagnosis and neither ultrasound nor fluorescein angiography provides sufficient additional information, ICG may be of practical value to the clinician in the diagnosis and management of selective patients with fundus abnormalities, including neovascular maculopathies, certain tumors, inflammatory conditions, and vascular disorders.

NEOVASCULAR MACULOPATHIES

Neovascular maculopathies associated with focal disease, such as pathological myopia, hereditary disorders, idiopathic and inflammatory choroidopathies, and even trauma, are generally composed of well-demarcated or so-called classic choroidal neovascularization (CNV). These small capillaries are not as well discriminated with a large ICG molecule and its dye–protein bioconjugate. Accordingly, fluorescein angiography is preferred in evaluating those instances. However, in age-related macular degeneration (AMD), there is generally a predominance of ill-defined or so-called "occult" CNV;[2,6,7] the appearance of these vessels is enhanced by the ICG molecule, which can be used to identify two specific occult CNV variants, retinal angiomatous proliferation (RAP), and polypoidal CNV,[8,9] as well as nonspecific plaques of occult CNV.

ICG is very helpful in establishing a full delineation of the extent of the neovascularization and the particular vascular components consisting of the neovascularization itself. Although there is

evidence that ICG angiography can differentiate a cluster of soft drusen from occult CNV (Fig. 86-1), there is still no management consideration or form of therapy to justify the use of this diagnostic adjunct in the routine evaluation of such patients. Nonetheless, patients with soft drusen and occult CNV not evident on fluorescein angiography, but demonstrable with ICG, have been known to be at greater risk of future neovascularized events.[10–13] So, there is an indication to perform ICG angiography in patients with soft drusen and suspected choroidal neovascularization, since the evaluation of the fellow eyes via ICG angiography is important for determining the risk of a neovascularized event and the associated visual prognosis in such high-risk patients (Fig. 86-2).

In RAP, there is not much in the way of subretinal hemorrhage, but there is often preretinal hemorrhage in front of the proliferating intraretinal neovascularization.[8] An additional feature of RAP is that most patients present with a pigment epithelial detachment (PED).[8,14] The hemorrhage and the PED obscure the precise nature of the neovascularization on fluorescein angiography while ICG angiography preferentially identifies the new vessels while emitting fluorescence within serous spaces, such as detached pigment epithelium or neurosensory retina (Fig. 86-3). RAP has its own set of clinical features, natural course, and visual prognosis.[8,14] As well, there may be future therapeutic implications that are specific to each of these forms of neovascularization, compared to the more typical choroidal proliferation.

While other neovascular maculopathies are most predominantly associated with classic CNV, ICG angiography is sometimes useful to ascertain whether indeed there are new vessels or simply hemorrhages beneath the retina. In pathologic myopia, this is a particularly useful application (Fig. 86-4). One other possible application is the identification of polypoidal CNV in some of these other degenerative maculopathies. Polypoidal CNV has now been described in patients with angioid streaks and pathological myopia.[15]

ICG angiography is also useful in the study of peripheral subretinal or intraretinal hemorrhages. Such lesions may occur spontaneously, in other conditions, or even following surgery (Fig. 86-5). Invariably, the most common cause of peripheral neovascularization is polypoidal CNV, which is best imaged with ICG angiography.

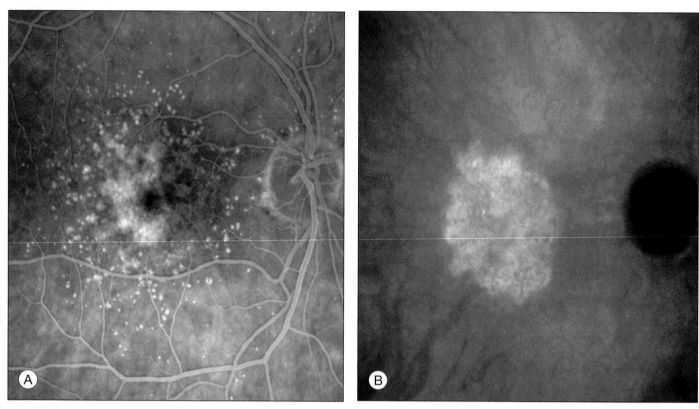

Fig. 86-1 A, The fluorescein angiogram reveals areas of hyperfluorescence that seem to be staining, confluent drusen. B, The indocyanine green study was essential in the identification of a hyperfluorescent plaque of choroidal neovascularization.

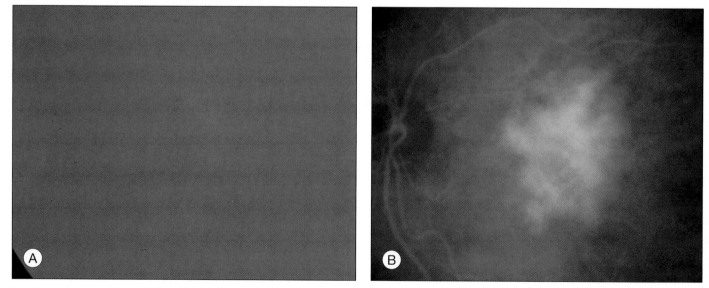

Fig. 86-2 A, This fluorescein angiogram was taken through the cataract of a patient followed for choroidal neovascularization in the other eye, and reveals some indistinct hyperfluorescence that was interpreted as staining, confluent drusen. B, An indocyanine green study was obtained, despite the dense cataract, which interfered with the fluorescein angiogram. A distinct plaque of choroidal neovascularization was identified in the patient's previously uninvolved fellow eye with indocyanine green angiography.

The most common and perhaps most definitive use of ICG angiography for patients with occult CNV is for polypoidal CNV. In these cases, the near infrared light that excites the ICG dye penetrates the pigment epithelium and the associated serosanguineous complications with a higher level of efficiency to determine the presence of these abnormal vessels.[16–26] This is particularly true when the polypoidal vascular abnormality is not of a particularly large dimension and the overlying pigment epithelium is relatively intact, obscuring the clinical identification of the vascular components (Fig. 86-6).

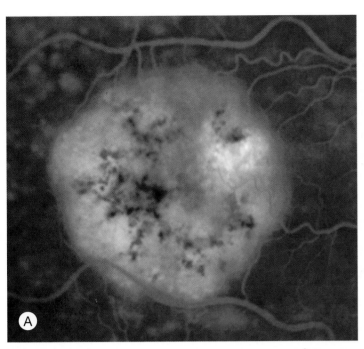
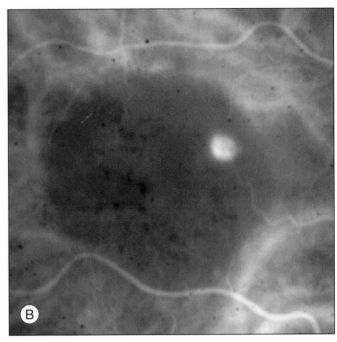

Fig. 86-3 A, Fluorescein angiogram shows a hyperfluorescent pigment epithelial detachment (PED) with some overlying hypofluorescent pigment figures. B, Only an indocyanine green angiogram demonstrates the retinal angiomatous proliferation lesion that is hyperfluorescent at the nasal margin of the hypofluorescent PED in this patient.

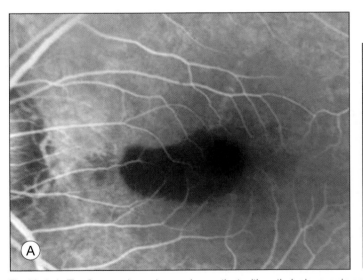
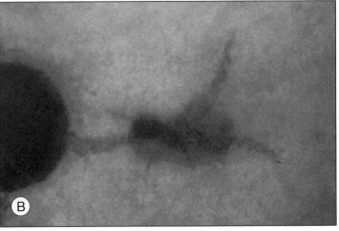

Fig.86-4 A, The fluorescein angiogram in a patient with pathologic myopia and a subretinal hemorrhage cannot determine the nature of the hemorrhage since imaging beneath the blood is not possible. B, Indocyanine green (ICG) angiogram of the patient reveals that the subretinal blood, which is hypofluorescent on the study, is not a choroidal neovascular membrane. The hypofluorescent lacquer cracks, better identified with ICG imaging, are seen beneath the blood.

Patients with this form of neovascularization also commonly have serous PED associated with the lesions.[16–26] ICG angiography can distinguish the serous from the vascular component of the PED in the determination of the precise composition of the neovascularization. The same is true for blood, which is common and more severe in this form of neovascular AMD (Fig. 86-7).

CHRONIC CENTRAL SEROUS CHORIORETINOPATHY

ICG angiography has become an established way to identify the chronic state of central serous chorioretinopathy (CSC).[27,28] Commonly, the diagnosis of CSC is made in eyes with neurosensory detachments and focal pinpoint leaks at the level of the retinal pigment epithelium on fluorescein angiography.[29]

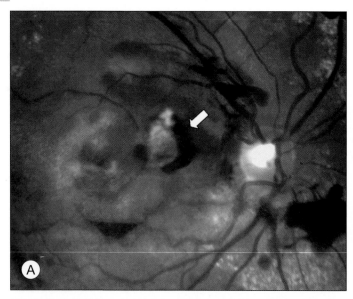

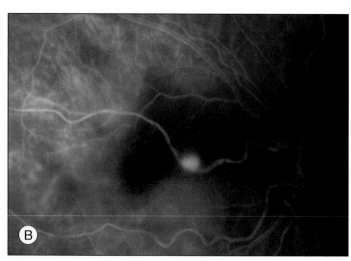

Fig. 86-5 A, Red-free photograph captures multiple hemorrhages, subretinal fluid, and an area presumed to be choroidal neovascularization (CNV) in a patient with drusen. B, The indocyanine green angiogram demonstrates two hyperfluorescent retinal arterial macroaneurysms not detected on fluorescein angiography due to the overlying hemorrhage; these macroaneurysms were misidentified as CNV.

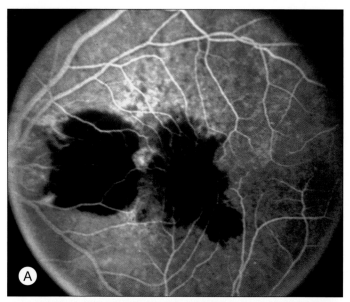

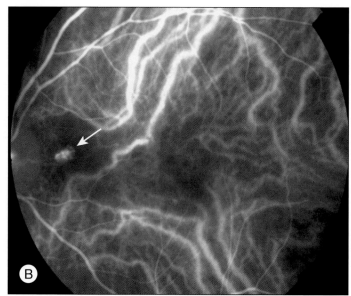

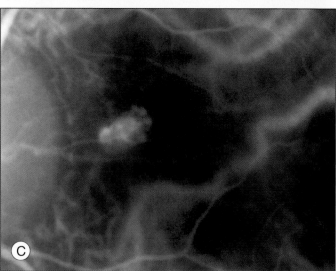

Fig. 86.6 A, Fluorescein angiogram of a patient reveals two large areas of hypofluorescence, with a hyperfluorescent area, believed to be a choroidal neovascular membrane, between the two hypofluorescences. B, The indocyanine green (ICG) angiogram demonstrates an area of peripapillary hypofluorescence (arrow) within a larger hypofluorescent area that was not seen on the fluorescein angiogram. C, Close-up of the ICG reveals that a small cluster of active, hyperfluorescent peripapillary polypoidal choroidal neovascularization is responsible for the hemorrhages and decreased vision in this patient.

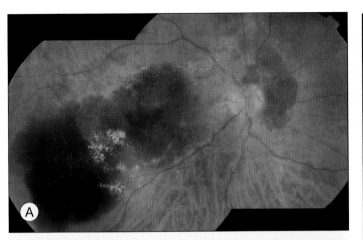

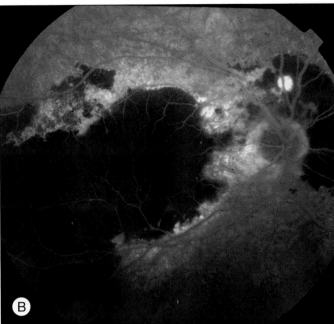

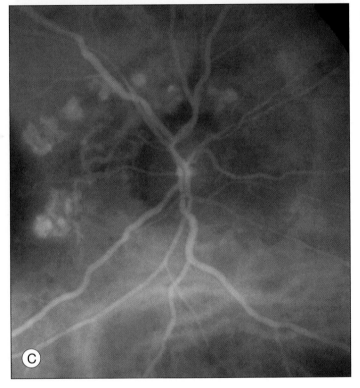

Fig. 86-7 A, Color composite photograph of a patient with decreased vision and large subretinal hemorrhages in the macula and peripapillary area. B, Fluorescein angiogram demonstrates an area of hyperfluorescence around the disc that is not well delineated. C, Indocyanine green angiogram exhibits a large polypoidal network surrounding the disc in this patient with polypoidal choroidal vaculopathy.

These characteristic findings, however, are not always present in the chronic stage of the disease. Instead, there is diffuse decompensation to the retinal pigment epithelium with slow or gradual leakage – a so-called ooze.[27,28,30] In virtually all of these eyes, there is inner choroidal staining with ICG angiography, a marker for the disease. With ICG angiography guidance, these inner choroidal leaking areas can be identified and treated with ICG-guided photodynamic therapy to resolve chronic detachments[31] (Fig. 86-8). In addition, the use of ICG guidance for the treatment of focal leaks in patients with CSC is currently under clinical investigation. In some patients with CSC, the chronic detachments are actually due to polypoidal CNV masquerading as CSC[25] (Fig. 86-9). Only with ICG angiography can this proper diagnosis be made and

appropriate treatment instituted, either thermal laser to the leaking polypoidal vascular element or ICG-guided photodynamic therapy.

CHOROIDAL TUMORS

ICG angiography is seldom of practical value in the evaluation of a choroidal tumor. However, the evaluation of eyes suspected of choroidal hemangiomas is an exception.[32–37] The characteristic findings of ICG angiography confirm the nature of the disorder, and above all, now serve as a guide for photodynamic therapy, which is the standard approach to management of these lesions when associated with chronic detachment and visual loss[38–40] (Fig. 86-10).

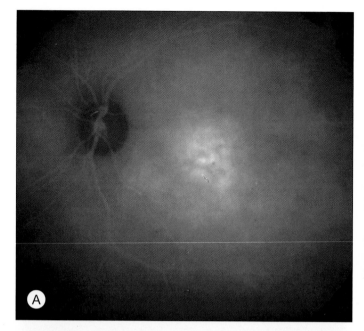

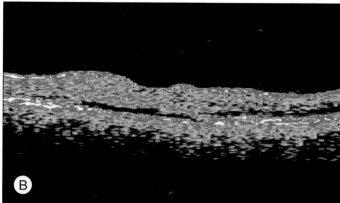

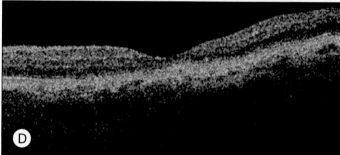

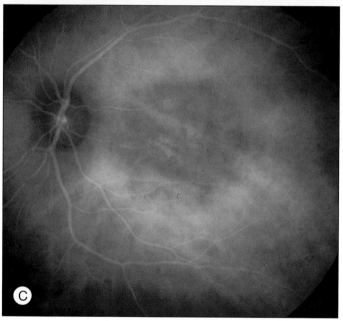

Fig. 86-8 A, Indocyanine green (ICG) angiogram of a patient with chronic central serous chorioretinopathy reveals an area of central hyperfluorescence that corresponds to choroidal hyperpermeability and a chronic neurosensory retinal detachment. This study was used to identify and guide the treatment of the patient with photodynamic therapy (PDT). B, The pretreatment optical coherence tomography (OCT) image captures the chronic neurosensory detachment below the thickened retina. C, Three weeks post-PDT, the ICG angiogram reveals the circular hypofluorescence of the treatment area with resolution of the choroidal hyperpermeability and chronic neurosensory retinal detachment. D, An OCT image confirms resolution of the chronic neurosensory retinal detachment, with restoration of the foveal contour.

Choroidal nevi, in the posterior pole or even in the peripheral fundus, may become associated with overlying hemorrhages. Invariably, there is blockage by the blood, making fluorescein angiography of little value in studying these eyes. However, ICG angiography is useful in identifying the underlying neovascularization and possibly in guiding thermal laser treatment if indicated. The neovascularization in such eyes has been reported to be polypoidal CNV in nature.[41]

Some ophthalmologists believe that choroidal melanomas have a dual circulation that can only be appreciated with ICG angiography.[33,34] Of more importance, perhaps, is the identification of a vascular network with ICG angiography within an amelonotic choroidal mass to distinguish a melanoma from an inflammatory or granulomatous lesion.[33,34]

CHOROIDAL INFLAMMATIONS

Usually, ICG angiography and fluorescein angiography alike are not necessary in making the diagnosis of chorioretinal inflammatory or infectious diseases. However, there are some exceptions when the specific diagnosis is uncertain. For example, in birdshot chorioretinopathy, ICG angiography has a characteristic pattern with a choroidal vasotropic distribution of late hypofluorescence in these eyes[42] (Fig. 86-11). There is no specific pattern in the

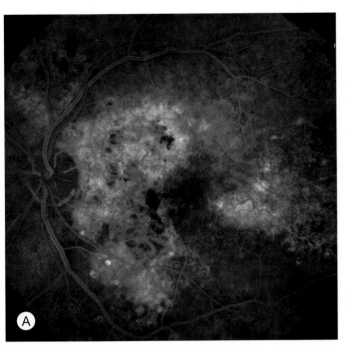

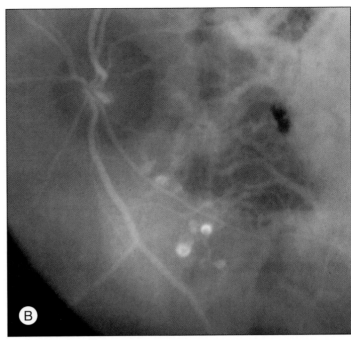

Fig. 86-9 A, A fluorescein angiogram (FA) in a patient with chronic central serous chorioretinopathy (CSC) depicting areas of hyperfluorescent stippling or "oozing" with some overlying hypofluorescent areas. B, The indocyanine green (ICG) angiogram demonstrates that this patient has a hyperfluorescent chain of polypoidal choroidal neovascularization. ICG was necessary to diagnose this patient as having polypoidal choroidal neovascularization masquerading as CSC.

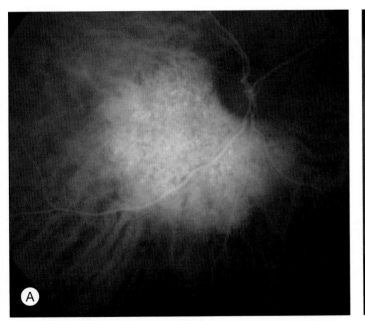

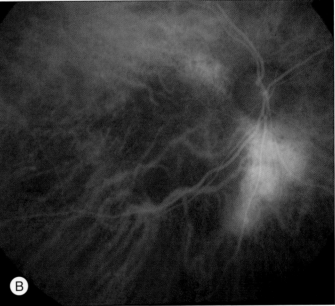

Fig. 86-10 A, Indocyanine green (ICG) angiogram of a 36-year-old female with a recent decline in vision to 20/400 due to progression of her choroidal hemangioma, which is hyperfluorescent and abuts the temporal side of the optic nerve. Treatment of the lesion with photodynamic therapy (PDT) was performed, avoiding the optic nerve. B, The ICG study 2 weeks following PDT reveals a hypofluorescent area corresponding to the treatment spot in the macula with a good response and visual improvement to 20/80. The residual hyperfluorescent area corresponds to the untreated area of the hemangioma.

peripapillary area, although an irregular area of late hypofluorescence may occur on ICG studies.

In multifocal choroiditis, numerous hypofluorescent lesions may be seen in the late phases of the studies that exceed any correlating clinical or fluorescein angiographic changes.[43] In addition, there is a zone of peripapillary hypofluorescence, which often corresponds to field loss in these eyes.[44] Following the use of anti-inflammatory therapy, the circumpapillary hypofluorescence diminishes, although not completely, leaving a ring of permanent atrophy which is best delineated with ICG angiography.

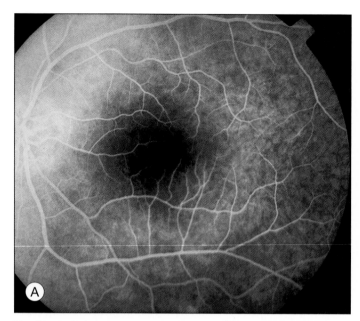

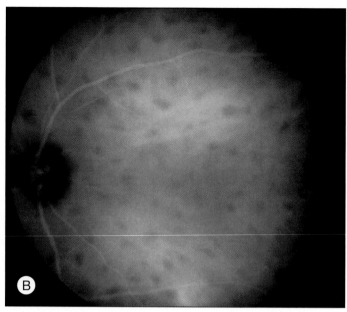

Fig. 86-11 A, A fluorescein angiogram of a patient with birdshot choroidopathy is virtually unremarkable. B, The indocyanine green study, however, demonstrates multiple hypofluorescent lesions aligned along the choroidal vessels.

In multiple evanescent white-dot syndrome (MEWDS),[45,46] ICG angiography can be useful in cases where the diagnosis is not certain. A number of ICG patterns have been described,[47–50] two of which appear to be pathognomonic. A peripapillary area surrounding the disc with a lace-like border circumferentially corresponds to an enlargement of the blind spot in this disease.[51–53] On resolution of the acute manifestations, the hypofluorescence and associated blind spot diminish dramatically, but some eyes maintain some degree of peripapillary atrophy. The other specific or pathognomonic ICG manifestation in a subset of these patients is a so-called dots-on-spots configuration[50] (Fig. 86-12). This dual-layer change, evident in the late stages of the ICG angiogram as hypofluorescent lesions overlying other larger lesions, is not known to occur in any other disorder of the fundus. In addition, there are segmental areas of choroidal staining on the ICG angiogram indicative of a significant choroidal inflammatory component to MEWDS.[49,50] The choroidal involvement documented with ICG in patients with MEWDS is not evident clinically, or with fluorescein angiography.

In patients suspected of having acute zonal occult outer retinopathy (AZOOR), the ICG angiogram can be helpful by delineating very well-demarcated zonal abnormalities[42] (Fig. 86-13). Sometimes, these abnormalities do not appear on either clinical examination or fluorescein angiography. ICG angiogram abnormalities occur prior to those on the fluorescein study, in part due to progressive atrophy of both the pigment epithelium and choriocapillaris. Multiple hyperfluorescent ICG spots in the fundus are also characteristic of the disorder, differentiating it from other mimicking entities, including dominant retinal dystrophies.

A number of other choroidal inflammatory diseases have been studied with ICG angiography. For example, in serpiginous choroidopathy, Giovannini et al. have described occult satellite lesions in clinically uninvolved fellow eyes.[54] The exudative detachments seen in Vogt–Koyanagi–Harada syndrome have been described as having characteristic ICG changes consisting of hypofluorescence;[55] and granulomatous diseases like sarcoidosis, tuberculosis, and even toxoplasmosis are associated with hyperfluorescent nodular lesions on the ICG angiogram.[42] Nonetheless, ICG angiography itself is seldom needed to make these clinical diagnoses in patients.

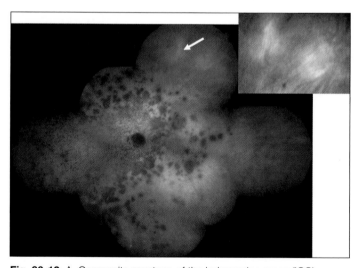

Fig. 86-12 A, Composite montage of the indocyanine green (ICG) angiogram in a patient with multiple evanescent white-dot syndrome. Note the numerous large hypofluorescent spots with overlying smaller hypofluorescent dots. These lesions evident on the ICG study far outnumbered the clinically apparent ones. The arrow demonstrates the enlarged area in Figure 85-12B. B, An interesting finding on the ICG corresponds to these areas of relative hyperfluorescence of the choroidal vessels, which indicate a localized inflammatory reaction.

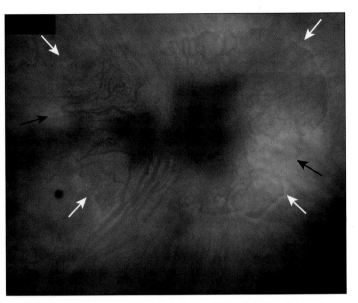

Fig. 86-13 A composite indocyanine green (ICG) angiogram in a patient with acute zonal occult outer retinopathy reveals a peripapillary area of hypofluorescence (outlined by white arrows) that represents the involved zones. Interestingly, at some of the margins of the hypofluorescent area, areas of relative hyperfluorescence to the surrounding retina exist (black arrows). These hyperfluorescent areas may represent active sites of progressive inflammation that are only evident with ICG angiography.

CHOROIDAL VASCULAR ISCHEMIA

Choroidal ischemia may be present in patients with diabetes, Takayasu's disease, sickle-cell disease, radiation retinopathy, and other disorders that can be imaged with ICG angiography. However, there are as yet no known applications for the treatment of such changes documented with ICG angiography.

CONCLUSIONS

In summary, ICG angiography has provided new and interesting information with respect to a number of choroidal abnormalities. Its greatest impact and application have been in the area of occult CNV and inflammatory disorders. ICG angiography has led to a better understanding of these conditions and, in some cases, has become a diagnostic-imaging adjunct for clinical management and treatment. As a result of the increased use of ICG angiography, new identifying features of the natural course of many disorders, as well as novel therapeutic approaches, have surfaced. In particular, patients with occult CNV secondary to AMD have benefited from ICG imaging since clinical trials have included ICG angiography and thus provided us with more definitive information about this devastating condition, especially with regard to treatment. With greater clinical experience and study, ICG angiography promises to provide new information for more specific diagnoses, a better understanding of the pathophysiologic mechanisms, and new approaches to the treatment of choroidal diseases.

ACKNOWLEDGMENT

This work was supported by the Macula Foundation, New York, NY, USA.

REFERENCES

1. Macular Photocoagulation Study Group. Argon laser photocoagulation of neovascular maculopathy. Arch Ophthalmol 1991; 109:1109–1114.
2. Freund KB, Yannuzzi LA, Sorenson JA. Age-related macular degeneration and choroidal neovascularization. Am J Ophthalmol 1993; 115:786–791.
3. Destro M, Puliafito CA. Indocyanine green videoangiography of choroidal neovascularization. Ophthalmology 1989; 96:846–853.
4. Flower RW, Klein GJ. Pulsatile flow in the choroidal circulation: a preliminary investigation. Eye 1990; 4:310–318.
5. Flower R. Extraction of choriocapillaris hemodynamic data from ICG fluorescence angiograms. Invest Ophthalmol Vis Sci 1993; 34:2720–2729.
6. Lim SI, Sternberg P, Capone A et al. Selective use of indocyanine green angiography for occult choroidal neovascularization. Am J Ophthalmol 1995; 120:75–82.
7. Destro M, Puliafito CA. Indocyanine green videoangiography of choroidal neovascularization. Ophthalmology 1988; 96:846–853.
8. Yannuzzi LA, Negrao S, Iida T et al. Retinal angiomatous proliferation in age-related macular degeneration. Retina 2001; 21:416–434.
9. Moorthy RS, Lyon AT, Rabb MF et al. Idiopathic polypoidal choroidal vasculopathy of the macula. Ophthalmology 1998; 105:1380–1385.
10. Chang B, Yannuzzi LA, Ladas ID et al. Choroidal neovascularization in second eyes of patients with unilateral exudative age-related macular degeneration. Ophthalmology 1995; 102:1380–1386.
11. Pieramici DJ, Bressler SB. Age-related macular degeneration and risk factors for the development of choroidal neovascularization in the fellow eye. Curr Opin Ophthalmol 1998; 9:38–46.
12. Pauleikhoff D, Radermacher M, Spital G et al. Visual prognosis of the second eyes in patients with unilateral late exudative age-related macular degeneration. Graefes Arch Clin Exp Ophthalmol 2002; 240:539–542.
13. Guyer DR, Yannuzzi LA, Ladas I et al. Indocyanine green guided laser photocoagulation of focal spots at the edge of plaques of choroidal neovascularization: a pilot study. Arch Ophthalmol 1996; 114:693–697.
14. Lafaut BA, Aisenbrey S, van den Broecke C et al. Polypoidal choroidal vasculopathy pattern in age-related macular degeneration. Retina 2000; 20:650–654.
15. Lafaut BA, Leyes AM, Snyers B et al. Polypoidal choroidal vasculopathy in Caucasians. Graefes Arch Clin Exp Ophthalmol 2000; 238:752–759.
16. Lip PL, Hope-Ross MW, Gibson JM. Idiopathic polypoidal choroidal vasculopathy: a disease with diverse clinical spectrum and systemic associations. Eye 2000; 5:695–700.
17. Lois N. Idiopathic polypoidal choroidal vasculopathy in a patient with atrophic age-related macular degeneration. Br J Ophthalmol 2001; 85:1011–1012.
18. Mohand-Said M, Nodarian M, Salvanet-Bouccara A. Idiopathic polypoidal choroidal vasculopathy: 2 case reports. J Franc Ophthalmol 2002; 25:517–521.
19. Ross RD, Gitter KA, Cohen G et al. Idiopathic polypoidal choroidal vasculopathy associated with retinal arterial macroaneurysm and hypertensive retinopathy. Retina 1996; 16:105–111.
20. Spaide RF, Yannuzzi LA, Slakter JS et al. Indocyanine green videoangiography of idiopathic polypoidal choroidal vasculopathy. Retina 1995; 15:100–110.
21. Yannuzzi LA, Ciardella AP, Spaide RF et al. The expanding clinical spectrum of idiopathic polypoidal choroidal vasculopathy. Arch Ophthalmol 1999; 115:478–485.
22. Yannuzzi LA, Freund KB, Goldbaum M et al. Polypoidal choroidal vasculopathy masquerading as central serous chorioretinopathy. Ophthalmology 2000; 107:767–777.
23. Yannuzzi LA, Sorenson JS, Spaide RF et al. Idiopathic polypoidal choroidal vasculopathy. Retina 1990; 10:1–8.
24. Gross NE, Aizman A, Brucker A et al. The nature and risk of neovascularization in the fellow eye of patients with unilateral retinal angiomatous proliferation. In Press.
25. Yannuzzi LA. Myopic staphyloma. Presented at the Macula Society Meeting, Las Vegas, NV February 23, 2004.
26. Staurenghi G, Orzalesi N, La Capria A et al. Laser treatment of feeder vessels in subfoveal choroidal neovascular membranes: a revisitation using dynamic indocyanine green angiography. Ophthalmology 1998; 105:2297–2305.
27. Sorenson JA, Yannuzzi LA, Slakter JS et al. A pilot study of indocyanine-green videoangiography-guided laser treatment of recurrent occult choroidal neovascularization in age-related macular degeneration. Arch Ophthalmol 1994; 112:473–479.

28. Flower RW. Optimizing treatment of choroidal neovascularization feeder vessels associated with age-related macular degeneration. Am J Ophthalmol 2002; 134:228–39.

29. Hayashi K, Hasegawa Y, Tokoro T. Indocyanine green angiography of central serous chorioretinopathy. Int Ophthalmol 1986; 9:371–374.

30. Guyer DR, Yannuzzi LA, Slakter JA et al. Digital indocyanine green videoangiography of central serous chorioretinopathy. Arch Ophthalmol 1994; 112:1057–1062.

31. Schatz H. Central serous chorioretinopathy and serous detachment of the retinal pigment epithelium. Int Ophthalmol Clin 1975; 15:159–168.

32. Yannuzzi LA, Shakin JL, Fisher YL et al. Peripheral retinal detachments and retinal pigment epithelial atrophic tracts secondary to central serous pigment epitheliopathy. Ophthalmology 1984; 91:1554–1572.

33. Yannuzzi LA, Slakter JS, Gross NE et al. Indocyanine green angiography-guided photodynamic therapy for treatment of chronic central serous chorioretinopathy: a pilot study. Retina 2003; 23:288–298.

34. Guyer DR, Gragoudas ES, Yannuzzi LA et al. Digital indocyanine green angiography of intraocular tumors. Semin Ophthalmol 1993; 8:224–229.

35. Shields C, Shields J. Indocyanine green angiography of choroidal tumors. In: Flower DW, Yannuzzi LA, Slakter JS, eds. Indocyanine green angiography. St. Louis: CV Mosby; 1997.

36. Shields CL, Shields JA, De Potter P. Patterns of indocyanine green videoangiography of choroidal tumors. Br J Ophthalmol 1995; 79:237–245.

37. Bonnet M, Habozit F, Magnard G. Valeur de l'angiographie en infra-rouge au vert d'indocyanine dans le diagnostic clinique des angiomes de la choroide. Bull Soc Ophthalmol Fr 1976; 76:713–716.

38. Quentel G, Coscas G. Angiographie en fluorescence infrarouge au vert d'indocyanine. Bull Soc Ophtalmol Fr 1984; 84:559–563.

39. Piccolino FC, Borgia L, Zinicola E. Indocyanine green angiography of circumscribed choroidal hemangiomas. Retina 1996; 16:19–28.

40. Schmidt-Erfurth UM, Kusserow C, Barbazetto IA et al. Benefits and complications of photodynamic therapy of papillary capillary hemangiomas. Ophthalmology 2002; 109:1256–1266.

41. Schmidt-Erfurth UM, Michels S, Kusserow C et al. Photodynamic therapy for symptomatic choroidal hemangioma: visual and anatomic results. Ophthalmology 2002; 109:2284–2294.

42. Porrini G, Giovannini A, Amato G et al. Photodynamic therapy of circumscribed choroidal hemangioma. Ophthalmology 2003; 110:674–680.

43. Spaide RF, Yannuzzi LA. Unpublished data 2004.

44. Slakter JS. Indocyanine green angiography of inflammatory disorders. Presented at the Macula Society Meeting, Palm Desert, CA, February 25, 1994.

45. Slakter JS, Giovannini A, Yannuzzi LA et al. Unpublished data 1996.

46. Khorram KD, Jampol LM, Rosenberg MA. Blind spot enlargement as a manifestation of multifocal choroiditis. Arch Ophthalmol 1991; 109:1403–1407.

47. Jampol LM, Sieving PA, Pugh D et al. Multiple evanescent white dot syndrome: I. Clinical findings. Arch Ophthalmol 1984; 102:671–674.

48. Sieving PA, Fishman GA, Jampol LM et al. Multiple evanescent white dot syndrome: II. Electrophysiology of the photoreceptors during retinal pigment epithelial disease. Arch Ophthalmol 1984; 102:675–679.

49. Ie D, Glaser BM, Murphy RP et al. Indocyanine green angiography in multiple evanescent white-dot syndrome. Am J Ophthalmol 1994; 117:7–12.

50. Obana A, Kusumi M, Miki T. Indocyanine green angiographic aspects of multiple evanescent white dot syndrome. Retina 1996; 16:97–104.

51. Ikeda N, Ikeda T, Nagata M et al. Location of lesions in multiple evanescent white dot syndrome and the cause of the hypofluorescent spots observed by indocyanine green angiography. Graefes Arch Clin Exp Ophthalmol 2001; 239:242–247.

52. Gross NE, Yannuzzi LA, Freund KB et al. Multiple evanescent white dot syndrome. In press.

53. Dodwell DG, Jampol LM, Rosenberg M et al. Optic nerve involvement associated with the multiple evanescent white dot syndrome. Ophthalmology 1990; 97:862–868.

54. Reddy CV, Brown J, Folk JC et al. Enlarged blind spots in chorioretinal inflammatory disorders. Ophthalmology 1996; 103:606–617.

55. Barile GR, Reppucci VS, Schiff WM et al. Circumpapillary chorioretinopathy in multiple evanescent white dot syndrome. Retina 1997; 17:75–77.

Chapter

87

Optical Coherence Tomography and Retinal Thickness Assessment for Diagnosis and Management

Andrew A. Moshfeghi
Elias C. Mavrofrides
Carmen A. Puliafito

INTRODUCTION

Ophthalmologists use slit-lamp biomicroscopy stereoscopically to evaluate the posterior pole and to detect vitreoretinal interface changes. A fundus contact lens is typically required to achieve adequate stereopsis for optimal appreciation of vitreoretinal interface changes and subtle retinal abnormalities. This technique is time-consuming, difficult for the examiner and the patient, can induce temporary corneal surface irregularities, and often results in missed pathology. In addition, clinical findings obtained in this manner are subject to interobserver variation and are not readily quantifiable. Optical coherence tomography (OCT) is an objective and versatile new tool for the adjunctive evaluation of posterior-segment disorders which rapidly provides the examiner with a quantifiable two-dimension cross-section (tomograph) of the retina.[1]

OCT has been likened to B-scan ultrasonography, but OCT relies upon differential reflections of light instead of dynamic echoes of sound to render a two-dimensional image of the retina.[2] Utilization of light instead of sound provides OCT with very high spatial resolution (approximately 8 μm) compared to conventional posterior-segment ultrasonography (approximately 150 μm).[2]

OCT is based on the principle of low-coherence interferometry wherein an infrared (approximately 830 nm wavelength) incident beam created by a superluminescent diode source is axially projected from the OCT unit on to the patient's retina in a scanning fashion.[1,2] The beam is focused on the retina by a 78-D lens, whose axial position is adjustable for fine focusing. A second beam (internal reference beam) is projected internal to the unit at a known reference distance. When the two light beams (internal reference beam and the back-scattered and back-reflected light from the retina) attempt to recombine, the reference beam must be altered in order to combine with the diagnostic beam.[1,2] The amount the reference beam is altered compared to its baseline to match the probe signal (optical path length difference) results in a signal generation.[1,2] The OCT unit employs a Michaelson interferometer in order to carry out this process. The magnitude of the back-scattered and reflected light from the target tissue is demonstrated as a false-color image in two dimensions.[1,2]

Variations in the optical characteristics of tissue account for differential reflective intensities and the associated heterogeneous false-color image appearance. Software manipulation of the raw OCT image data can result in a false-color map representing three-dimensional topographic retinal features and quantitative retinal thickness measurements.[1,2] Images are stored on digital media to enable comparison of serial evaluations and for archiving purposes.

Although retinal imaging is most common, OCT has numerous applications in ophthalmology, including anterior-segment evaluation and quantification of the peripapillary nerve fiber layer (NFL) in glaucoma patients.[3-5] In addition, several nonophthalmic applications are emerging that appear promising.[6-11] This chapter will focus on the use of OCT in the evaluation and management of patients with macular disease.

OBTAINING AN OCT IMAGE

Mydriasis aids artifact-free OCT image acquisition. A miotic pupil does not preclude OCT evaluation of the macula, but may result in a vignette artifact of the macular image in which the proximal and distal ends of the scan are clipped by pupillary block of the incident light.[2]

The patient is seated in a comfortable chair of adjustable height without wheels. The patient's head is then positioned on the machine with the chin on the chin rest and the forehead against the forehead strap in exactly the same manner as with slit-lamp biomicroscopy. Several controls are available on the OCT unit (StratusOCT, Carl Zeiss Meditec, Germany) to ensure proper patient positioning. The patient is asked to blink several times prior to image acquisition to ensure a smooth optical surface. Once properly aligned, the patient is asked to look straight ahead at a fixation target. The operator sees an infrared image of the patient's fundus on the OCT display allowing anatomic localization of the OCT scan. This also allows the fixation target to be moved appropriately to obtain scans of peripheral macular lesions or to assist macular evaluation of patients with eccentric fixation.

Image acquisition is controlled via joystick and button depression by the OCT operator. Various imaging acquisition sequences are available, but the radial lines function is the most commonly used modality for evaluation of macular disease. Six radial lines are scanned, the centers of which are concentric on the fovea. We prefer to obtain the radial lines sequence using the high-resolution 512 transverse pixel scan which takes approximately 1.3 s per radial line scan. We follow this sequence with the fast-scan option which samples the same radial lines using a 128 transverse pixel scan in approximately 0.3 s per radial line scan. The relatively fast speed of the 128 transverse pixel scan is less likely to include motion artifact (fixation loss) and is therefore ideal for creating three-dimensional renderings of the perifovea.[2] Some clinicians use this low-resolution scan as a screening tool to detect macular abnormalities. If an obvious abnormality is detected with the fast, low-resolution scan, a subsequent high-resolution scan can then be quickly and easily obtained through the area of interest. Scan length varies from 3 mm to 6 mm and this parameter is set by the OCT operator.

The second eye can then be evaluated without the need to reposition the patient. A high-magnification infrared image of the scanned region of retina is displayed on the OCT monitor and OCT printout for correlation with fundus features and scan orientation. We find it useful also to obtain formal digital fundus photographs for highly detailed correlation of fundus features with OCT findings.

It is possible to image the retina using OCT in a silicone oil-filled eye.[12] This can be extremely useful in evaluating retinal anatomy following surgery in which silicone oil has been used instead of gas tamponade. Intraocular gas covering the area of interest (e.g., parafoveal region) precludes accurate OCT scanning.[13] Dense nuclerosclerotic or posterior subcapsular cataracts do not necessarily prevent adequate OCT scans. Remarkably, the incident and reflected light from the OCT unit can penetrate quite significant media opacities from cataract, capsular opacification, vitreous hemorrhage, asteroid hyalosis,

or vitreitis.[14] In cases with more significant media opacities, image quality is correlatively degraded but a gross appreciation of macular details is typically achievable.

OCT IMAGE INTERPRETATION

A comprehensive review of OCT images of retinal disorders is beyond the scope of this chapter. The reader is referred to an excellent OCT text and atlas for a more complete collection of images and descriptions.[15] Typical examples of selected common retinal disorders are presented here. Many principles used in interpreting OCT images of the retinal diseases described below can help guide the clinician with the interpretation of disease states not specifically mentioned here. Attention is given to the OCT appearance of these disorders, as all these entities are comprehensively discussed in separate chapters throughout this text. In order to understand the OCT appearance of complex vitreoretinal pathologic states, an appreciation of the normal macular appearance with OCT is crucial.

NORMAL MACULA

The OCT image closely approximates the histological appearance of the macula and for this reason it has been referred to as an in vivo optical biopsy. Correlation with histologic retinal features in patients with ultra-high-resolution OCT has been performed and found to be quite accurate.[16,17] The currently available OCT

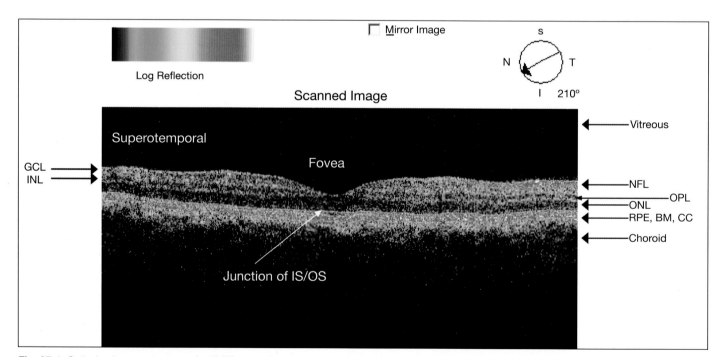

Fig. 87-1 Optical coherence tomography (OCT) scan of normal macula. Radial-line OCT scan of a normal macula. The scan was obtained by sweeping from the superotemporal (left) to the inferonasal macula (right). The foveal depression is noted centrally. The black, speckled region above the retina corresponds to the vitreous cavity. The false color scale in the upper left-hand corner corresponds to the log of reflectivity (red, high reflectivity; yellow and green, medium reflectivity; blue, low reflectivity). Histologic correlates of selected retinal layers are labeled in the figure with arrows and abbreviations. NFL, nerve fiber layer; GCL, ganglion cell layer; INL, inner nuclear layer; OPL, outer plexiform layer; ONL, outer nuclear layer; RPE, retinal pigment epithelium; BM, Bruch's membrane; CC, choriocapillaris.

product is not able to discriminate the more subtle microstructural differences, but is generally able to discriminate accurately the cellular and noncellular elements of the retina.[17] The interpretative strength of OCT derives from its ability to discriminate levels of high and low signal intensity from various tissue elements.[17]

Differences in signal intensity are represented by a false-color coding system which is represented by the colors of the visible color spectrum: highly reflective structures are represented by red, medium reflections appear yellow or green, and structures with low reflectivity are blue. A black signal designates the absence of a reflective signal. Reflected light results in signals with a magnitude ranging from 10^{-5} to 10^{-9}, or 50 to 90 dB.

The output from the OCT indicates the directionality of each scan with an arrow: inferior to superior, temporal to nasal, for all six individual radial line scans. For the OCT-3, horizontal and tangential scans always proceed in the direction towards the optic nerve, while the vertical scan always passes from inferior to superior. When evaluating an individual radial line scan, the clinician reads the left side of the scan as the beginning of the scan and the right side of the scan as the end. This ensures proper fundus correlation with the OCT images. For example, a scan which the machine labels as sweeping from temporal to nasal corresponds to a scan image whose left edge is temporal and whose right edge is nasal.

The top of the scan image corresponds to the vitreous cavity. In a normal patient (Fig. 87-1), this will be optically silent (black), without any significant reflections being noted except for perhaps identification of the posterior hyaloid face (in a patient with complete posterior vitreous detachment) or normal insertion of the posterior hyaloid near the macula in young patients. The posterior vitreous face appears as a thin horizontal or oblique line above or inserting in the retina.

The anterior surface of the retina demonstrates high reflectivity (red) and its horizontal expanse demonstrates the normal contour of the macula with the central foveal depression (Fig. 87-1). Derangement of this contour is seen in innumerable disorders, many of which are described below. The internal structure of the retina consists of heterogeneous

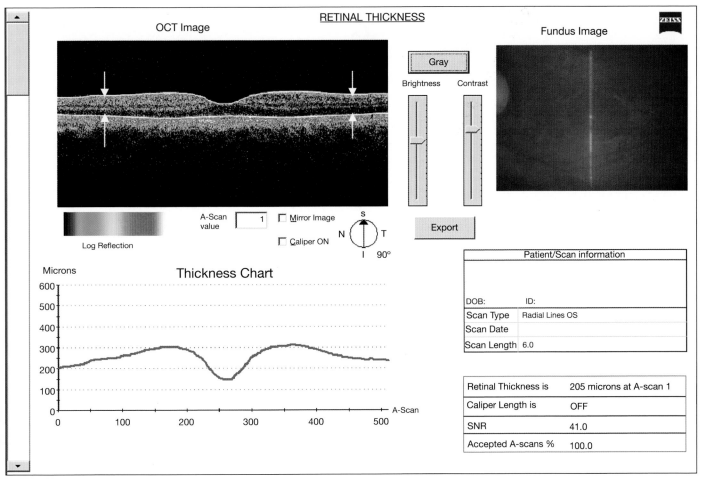

Fig. 87-2 Optical coherence tomography (OCT) retinal thickness scan of normal macula. Retinal OCT thickness analysis generated from a vertical scan through a normal macula. The anterior and posterior borders of the retina have been identified and labeled with white lines (highlighted by arrows). The distance between the lines is arithmetically determined and results in the generation of scale which plots retinal thickness for each point along the scan. In the upper right-hand corner, a gray-scale image of the patient's macula (noting the angle of the laser scan with a bright line) is seen.

reflections, corresponding to varying ultrastructural anatomy. The horizontally aligned NFL demonstrates a high tissue signal (red) that facilitates its identification (Fig. 87-1).[17] High-flow intraretinal structures such as retinal blood vessels seen in this layer can result in a focal hyperreflective spot with optical shadowing of the retinal microstructures posterior to the vessel.[17]

The retinal pigment epithelium (RPE), Bruch's membrane, and choriocapillaris complex collectively comprises the highly reflective external band. This thick band in the outer retina/anterior choroid appears as a red, linear stripe in OCT images (Fig. 87-1).[17] Just anterior to this band is another highly reflective line representing the junction between the photoreceptors' inner and outer segments. The outer retinal structures are better discriminated via ultra-high-resolution OCT, which is not yet commercially available.[16]

The axially aligned cellular layers of the retina (inner nuclear, outer nuclear, and ganglion cell layers) demonstrate less back-scattering and back-reflection of incident OCT light.[17] This manifests as relatively low tissue signals (blue, green, yellow) compared to the horizontally aligned structures (internal limiting membrane, Henle's layer, and NFL).

RETINAL THICKNESS ASSESSMENT

The OCT unit determines the anterior and posterior surface of the retina in order to calculate retinal thickness.[17] A transverse line is drawn along the anterior surface of the retina which is identified as the junction between low or absent vitreous cavity signal and very high inner retinal signals (internal limiting membrane and NFL). Similarly, the posterior extent of the highly reflective external band is identified and a second transverse line is drawn posteriorly (Fig. 87-2). A software algorithm known as segmentation uses the processes of smoothing, edge detection, and error correction to facilitate this process. Once the anterior and posterior lines are drawn, simple arithmetic

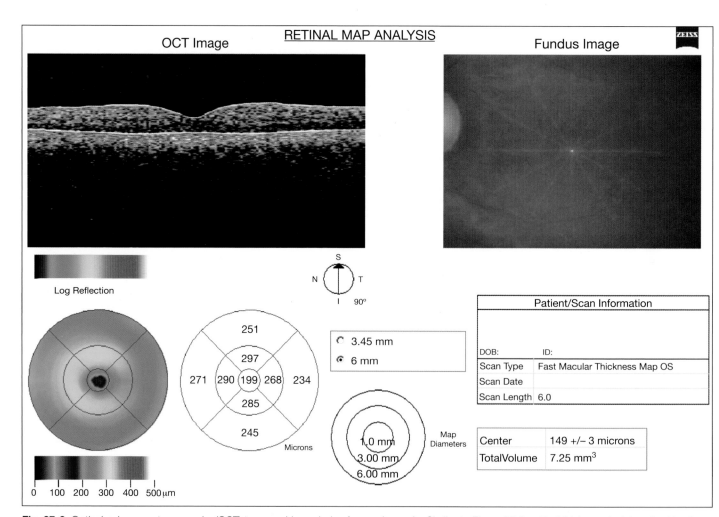

Fig. 87-3 Optical coherence tomography (OCT) topographic analysis of normal macula. Similar to Figure 87-2, retinal thickness is determined by the OCT system not just for one radial scan, but for all six scans (gray-scale image, upper right-hand corner). Averaging calculations (with compensatory extrapolation of retinal thickness for the nonscanned areas) result in the formation of a topographical thickness map of the macula. Color coding indicates relative thickness (white/red, thick; yellow/green, medium thickness; blue/black, thin) with actual numerical values given for each region of the macula in the map adjacent to the color-coded map.

results in a retinal thickness measurement that is equal to the distance between the anterior and posterior lines. Retinal thickness can be determined at any transverse location along the scan and the thickness at each point is represented on a retinal thickness graph (Fig. 87-2).[17]

Occasionally, the software protocol draws the lines incorrectly, resulting in incorrect thickness measurements. Therefore, care must be taken that high-quality, artifact-free scans are obtained before running the retinal thickness algorithm. Similarly, the clinician should not rely solely upon the retinal thickness measurements without reviewing the accuracy of the retinal outlines.[17] New retinal thickness protocols are being developed that incorporate improved retinal thickness assessment, improved error correction, and user alteration of the retinal outlines.

MACULAR TOPOGRAPHY

Information accrued from multiple retinal thickness measurements along the six sampling scans can be used to create a topographic color-coded map of the macula (Fig. 87-3). The macula is divided into nine regions. The average thickness of each region is calculated. To account for the empty space between sampling scans (places where samples were not obtained), the software allows interpolation of adjacent thickness values to fill in the gaps. The numerical averages for each of the nine macular regions is presented alongside a color-coded map (Fig. 87-3).[17] Retinal thickness is accurately calculable for thicknesses between 0 and 500 μm.[17]

OCT IMAGES OF SELECTED RETINAL DISORDERS

VITREORETINAL INTERFACE DISORDERS

Vitreomacular traction

Vitreomacular traction (VMT) syndrome is characterized by distortion of the macular contour due to anteroposterior and tangential tractional forces applied by the vitreous to the parafoveal region. There is an abnormally firm adherence by the posterior hyaloid to the retina, and decreased visual acuity can result from secondary intraretinal edema and distorted macular architecture.[18-21] The vitreous adherence can be difficult or impossible to identify directly on clinical exam, and many cases are only discovered after cataract extraction fails to result in visual improvement.

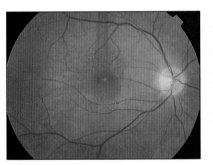

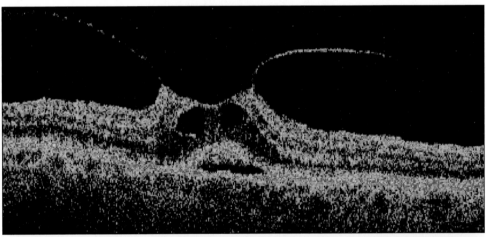

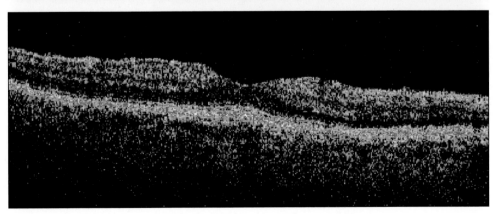

Fig. 87-4 Vitreomacular traction syndrome. This color fundus photograph (top, left) is from a 75-year-old man with a 3-week history of central visual distortion in the right eye. Visual acuity is 20/25. The photograph demonstrates loss of the foveal reflex and subretinal fluid parafoveally. No leakage was seen on the fluorescein angiogram, but the corresponding optical coherence tomography (OCT) image (top, right) demonstrates prominent insertion of the posterior hyaloid on to the parafoveal region, resulting in marked intraretinal cystic edema and a small collection of subfoveal fluid.

After 3 months of observation management, the patient's symptoms suddenly resolved and visual acuity returned to 20/20. The follow-up OCT (bottom) demonstrates restoration of the normal foveal contour with a complete posterior vitreous detachment and no subretinal or intraretinal fluid.

OCT has been extremely instrumental in confirming many cases of VMT that are clinically undetectable.[22–25] OCT demonstrates the abnormal vitreomacular tractional bands from the prominent posterior hyaloid, intraretinal edema, and distorted macular contour with or without subretinal fluid accumulation (Fig. 87-4). It has been said that the OCT-3 does not visualize the posterior hyaloid face with as high sensitivity as OCT-2 or the original product. OCT-3 is optimized to evaluate retinal tissue microstructure; however increased sensitivity for visualization of the posterior hyaloid is possible by varying the signal-to-noise ratio (operator adjustment) for patients with suspected vitreoretinal interface disorders such as VMT. Although this technique is sometimes used to create convincing images, it is not necessary; one can infer the presence of vitreous traction simply by noting the unusual peaked macular architecture that such traction creates, often in an eccentric pattern (Fig. 87-5).[25]

OCT is also important in following patients with VMT. In some cases spontaneous resolution can occur, justifying a period of observation before surgical intervention.[23–25] OCT can be used to monitor subtle changes in vitreoretinal adherence and retinal architecture, assisting the decision-making process.

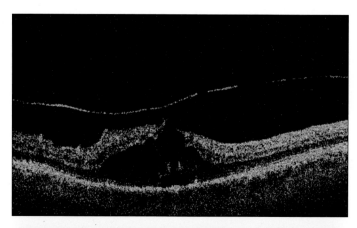

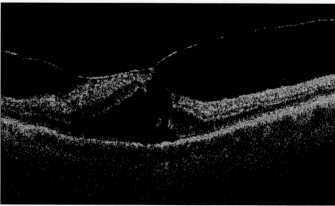

Fig. 87-5 Vitreomacular traction syndrome. This 67-year-old man had vitreomacular traction. The top OCT image demonstrates the effect of abnormal vitreomacular traction, even though actual vitreoretinal adhesion is not visualized in this particular scan. Diffuse cystic retinal thickening is noted and the retina has a "tethered" appearance eccentric to the fovea. The bottom OCT scan is from the same patient from a slightly different angle and demonstrates the abnormal vitreoretinal adhesion.

Epiretinal membrane

Glial proliferation on the surface of the retina can result in distortion of the macular vascular architecture and the development of macular edema.[26] Occasionally, epiretinal membranes can evolve into macular pseudoholes and epiretinal membranes are often seen in conjunction with idiopathic full-thickness macular holes.[26,27] Patients are either asymptomatic in occult cases or complain of visual distortion and decreased vision. Fluorescein angiography variably demonstrates macular leakage.[26]

Epiretinal membranes are often clearly delineated on OCT as a taut hyperreflective line along the retinal surface (Fig. 87-6).[25,28–30] Visualization of the membrane is enhanced when there is some separation between the membrane and inner retina. In some cases, the membrane is more tightly adherent to the retina and cannot be directly confirmed on the OCT image. In these cases, the secondary effects of the membrane, such as irregularity of the macular contour and macular thickening, are used to establish the presence of the membrane. Mild membranes often result in minimal visual distortion and loss of the normal foveal contour.[26,27] More advanced membranes show variable irregularity of the inner retinal layers and diffuse retinal thickening.[25,28]

OCT is useful in qualitatively and quantitatively establishing a baseline macular appearance and retinal thickness. This is important in monitoring changes in observational cases and for documenting response to treatment in patients undergoing vitrectomy with membrane peeling.[25] It is especially helpful for patients in that it allows the physician qualitatively to demonstrate the easily interpretable OCT appearance of their eye and the implications of the distorting epiretinal membrane.

Macular holes and pseudoholes

A full-thickness defect in the neural retina as seen with OCT can differentiate a true macular hole from a pseudohole seen clinically.[25] Pseudoholes are seen in the presence of a dense sheet of epiretinal membrane with a central defect that overlies the foveal center, giving the ophthalmoscopic appearance of a true macular hole.[25,28,29] OCT demonstrates the overlying epiretinal membrane and the absence of a true retinal defect (Fig. 87-7).[25,28,29]

An impending macular hole (Gass, stage 1) is a retinal defect in which there is detachment of the fovea with variable thinning, but no full-thickness retinal defect.[31] In a true full-thickness macular hole (Gass, stages 2 to 4), there is a complete absence of neural retinal tissue overlying the foveal center.[31] Generally, the retinal defect is accompanied by significant intraretinal fluid cysts on all sides of the hole, which is erroneously referred to clinically as a "cuff of subretinal fluid" (Fig. 87-8). Indeed, except in rare presentations of macular holes with extensive subretinal fluid accumulation,[32] there is usually minimal subretinal fluid seen by OCT with initial presentation of idiopathic macular holes. The edges of the hole can have a "curled-up" appearance, either the result of significant intraretinal fluid accumulation or due to persistent vitreofoveal traction (Gass, stages 2 and 3). OCT has been vital in identifying the role of perifoveal

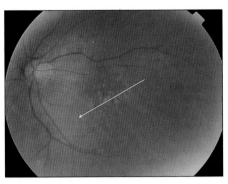
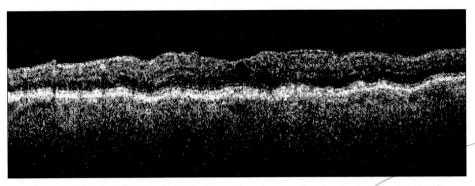

Fig. 87-6 Epiretinal membrane of an 88-year-old man who complained of difficulty driving in the previous few months. A color fundus photograph (left) demonstrates media opacity from moderate nuclear sclerotic cataracts, an epiretinal membrane distorting the macular architecture, and soft macular drusen. Visual acuity is 20/30, OS. An oblique optical coherence tomography scan through the macula (right) demonstrates a thin, well-delineated epiretinal membrane coursing over the retinal surface associated with mild cystic retinal thickening. Irregular excrescences from the highly reflective external band correspond to soft macular drusen.

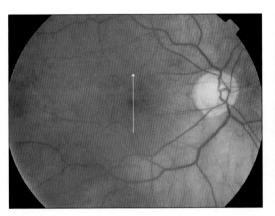
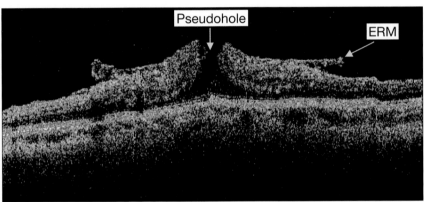

Fig. 87-7 Epiretinal membrane and macular pseudohole. Color fundus photograph (left) of a 65-year-old woman with a history of decreased visual acuity in the right eye for 2 years. Visual acuity is 20/40. Distortion of the retinal vessel architecture in the inferior macula along with the appearance of macular pseudohole is noted. Corresponding vertical optical coherence tomography scan (right) through the macula demonstrates diffuse cystic retinal thickening with foveal excavation (pseudohole) underlying a discontinuity in the prominent epiretinal membrane (ERM) that surrounds the fovea. The outer retinal elements remain intact beneath the pseudohole, explaining the relatively good visual acuity despite marked macular distortion.

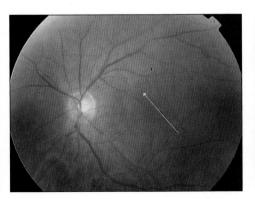
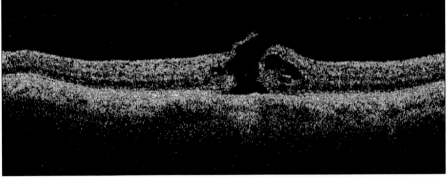

Fig. 87-8 Full-thickness macular hole. This 63-year-old man had decreased visual acuity in the left eye. The color fundus photograph (left) shows a full-thickness macular hole with an appearance of a cuff of surrounding subretinal fluid. Visual acuity is 20/80. Oblique optical coherence tomography scan (right) through the macula demonstrates a full-thickness retinal defect with an intact retinal pigment epithelium layer. In contrast to what is seen clinically, there does not appear to be a cuff of subretinal fluid. Rather, intraretinal cystic thickening is seen at the edges of the hole, which are "curled" anteriorly. There is partial separation of the posterior vitreous over the macula in this stage 2 macular hole.

posterior vitreous detachment with persistent foveal traction in the development of macular holes.[25,33,34] In full-thickness macular holes with complete separation of the posterior hyaloid (Gass, stage 4), one may be able to observe the detached hyaloid face in the radial scans.[25,33–35] Occasionally OCT will demonstrate a retinal operculum apparently floating above the foveal center.[25,34]

A better visual prognosis for macular hole repair is associated with better visual acuity at presentation, smaller diameter of macular hole, and shorter duration of visual symptoms.[33,36] OCT can accurately quantify macular hole diameter via radial scans, and future OCT parameters may provide additional predictive information.[25,37]

Following pars plana vitrectomy, membrane peeling, and long-acting tamponade (gas or silicone oil), OCT can be used to confirm complete macular hole closure and restoration of the normal foveal contour.[12,13] In cases with suboptimal postoperative visual outcomes, OCT can be used to evaluate retinal anatomy and the associated retinal contribution to this vision loss.[25,33] As noted earlier, macular OCT can be performed after the gas bubble's inferior meniscus has receded above the fovea (to a 40% to 45% fill) or immediately following vitrectomy in silicone-oil-filled eyes.[12,13]

AGE-RELATED MACULAR DEGENERATION (AMD)

Dry AMD: drusen, vitelliform lesions, and geographic atrophy

Drusen appear as irregular excrescences of the highly reflective external band indicating changes in the RPE and Bruch's membrane (Fig. 87-9).[38] In cases exhibiting large and confluent drusen or a single large druse (vitelliform lesion), OCT demonstrates a significant convex excrescence of the highly reflective external band.[38] Geographic atrophy of the RPE allows deeper penetration and increased reflectivity of the light signal from the choroid, resulting in increased intensity of the signal from this layer. This leads to irregular, posterior thickening of the highly reflective external band rather than loss of this band (as might be initially suspected with atrophy of the RPE layer).[38] OCT also effectively demonstrates thinning of the retina corresponding to areas of focal or diffuse retinal atrophy overlying these RPE changes.[38]

Neovascular AMD

In cases suspicious for exudative changes, OCT can be extremely useful in detecting suspected intraretinal, subretinal, or sub-RPE fluid when angiographic interpretation is equivocal, inconvenient,

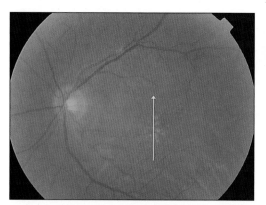
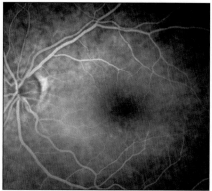
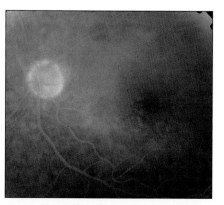

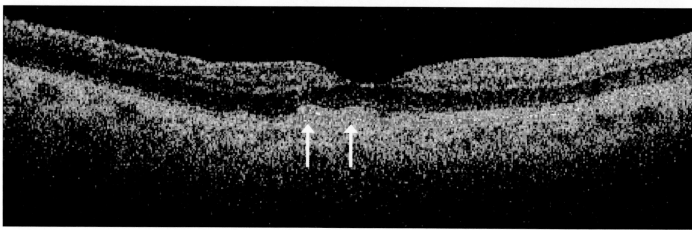

Fig. 87-9 Dry age-related macular degeneration/drusen. This 72-year-old woman had dry macular degeneration in the left eye. The color fundus photograph (top, left) demonstrates media opacity from moderate nuclear sclerotic cataracts and soft moderate to large-sized drusen in the macula. Visual acuity is 20/40. Fluorescein angiography mid-phase (top, middle) and late-phase (top, right) demonstrates staining of the drusen and absence of leakage. A vertical optical coherence tomography scan (bottom) through the foveal center demonstrates irregular excrescences from the highly reflective external band beneath the foveal center. No subretinal fluid or significant cystic retinal thickening is appreciated.

or not readily accessible. In cases with active neovascular AMD, OCT can be used as an adjunct to fluorescein angiography in helping to establish a baseline retinal thickness, volume, and extent of choroidal neovascularization (CNV) and fluid involvement. OCT is particularly helpful in identifying the location and level of CNV (intraretinal, subretinal, sub-RPE) and other lesion components (blood, fluid, pigment, and fibrosis).[38,39] Specific lesion composition as described by fluorescein angiographic appearance can often be correctly surmised by OCT evaluation, but not consistently so. Characteristic features of several common presentations of neovascular AMD are demonstrated in Figures 87.10 to 87.14.

Classic choroidal neovascularization

A well-defined pattern of early hyperfluorescence with late leakage on fluorescein angiography characterizes classic CNV secondary to exudative AMD. On OCT, the neovascular lesion appears as a highly reflective, fusiform area beneath the retina along the external reflective band (Fig. 87-10). Secondary exudation from the lesion can be seen as intraretinal or subretinal fluid accumulation. Intraretinal edema can range from mild retinal thickening to diffuse cystic edema. OCT is highly sensitive in identifying even small amounts of subretinal fluid, which is seen as a nonreflective space between the outer retinal signal and the highly reflective external band.[38,39] Extensive irregularity of the adjacent external band is common, consistent with the associated RPE/choroid changes found in these patients.

Occult choroidal neovascularization

Occult CNV is seen on fluorescein angiography as mottled hyperfluorescence in the mid-phase with associated late leakage (fibrovascular pigment epithelial detachments (PEDs)) or as late leakage of undetermined origin. On OCT, these occult lesions may show evidence of PED, irregularity of the external band, and variable subretinal or intraretinal fluid accumulation (Fig. 87-11).[38]

Pigment epithelial detachment

PEDs have a characteristic and striking OCT appearance and often accompany occult CNV. There is a clear elevation of the

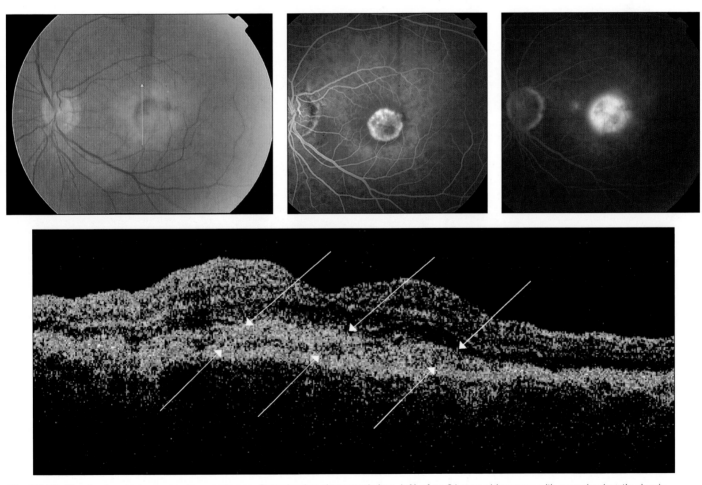

Fig. 87-10 Classic choroidal neovascular membrane. Color fundus photograph (top, left) of an 81-year-old woman with a predominantly classic subfoveal choroidal neovascular membrane. On fluorescein angiography, a well-demarcated hyperfluorescent area is delineated early (top, middle) and evolves into an intensely leaking lesion late (top, right) in the study. On optical coherence tomography evaluation through the lesion (bottom), diffuse retinal thickening with small intraretinal cysts and an outer retinal or subretinal neovascular complex with increased tissue reflectivity (between arrows) is noted. No subretinal fluid is noted in this particular lesion.

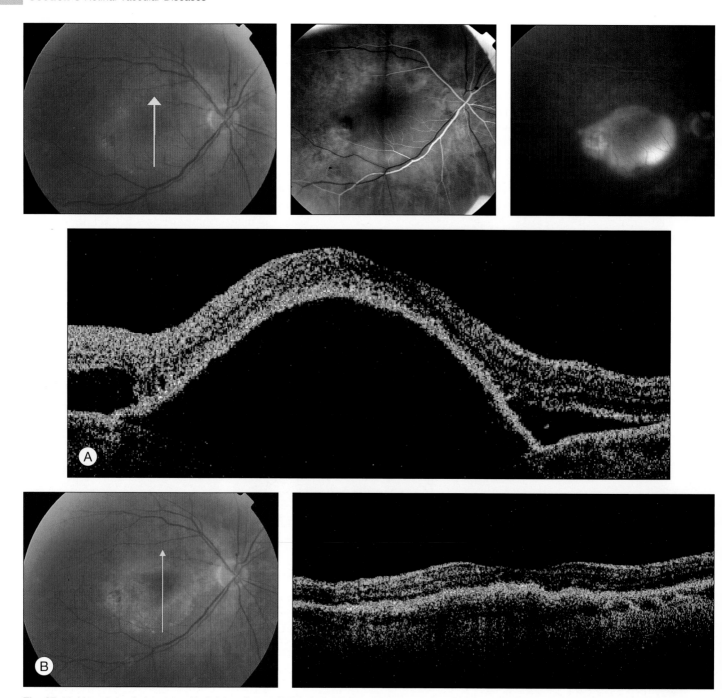

Fig. 87-11 Vascularized pigment epithelial detachment (PED). A, A 68-year-old woman presented with decreased vision to 6/200 in the right eye for 2 weeks. A PED and associated subretinal fluid is evident on the color fundus photograph (top, left). Fluorescein angiography (top, middle and right) demonstates an occult pattern of fluorescein leakage and pooling of dye within the PED. The vertical optical coherence tomography (OCT) scan (bottom) depicts quite clearly the large PED and surrounding subretinal fluid accumulation. The lack of intraretinal fluid in the retina overlying the foveal center is noticeably absent. The patient was treated with a combination of verteporfin photodynamic therapy (PDT) and intravitreal triamcinolone acetonide. B, Same patient as in Figure 87-11A. Two months later, the visual acuity improved to 20/70 along with a collapse of the PED (color fundus photograph, left) and resolution of subretinal fluid on OCT (right).

highly reflective external band which can be considered an anatomical proxy for the RPE near its posterior extent. This usually conforms to a concave smooth elevation with an optically quiet zone within the dome-shaped elevation (Fig. 87-11).[38] The highly reflective external band should be continuous on both sides of the PED; a discontinuity may raise suspicion for

an RPE tear or could be the result of blocking of the incident OCT beam by overlying exudate, blood, fibrosis, or other highly reflective pathologic retinal components.[40]

Hemorrhagic RPE detachments have a similar conformation, but there is marked attenuation of the optical reflections as they pass through the blood.[38,40] Very dense hemorrhage will block transmission of the incident light altogether and result in optical shadowing posterior to the hemorrhage.[40] The anterior face of a dense hemorrhage demonstrates extremely high optical reflectivity with posterior shadowing.

PEDs can be due to idiopathic central serous chorioretinopathy (ICSC), occult CNV, and certain ocular inflammations.[40] Those identified with OCT first should therefore be further evaluated with fluorescein angiography or indocyanine green angiography to determine if occult CNV or other etiologies are involved.

Tear of the retinal pigment epithelium

Long-standing substantial sub-RPE fluid collection due to active CNV can lead to a spontaneous tear in the RPE. RPE tears have also been described following verteporfin photodynamic therapy (PDT) or laser therapy of lesions overlying a serous PED.[41-43] It is felt that the RPE layer is put on stretch as a result of increasing or considerable subretinal fluid accumulation and this stress

leads to a tear in the RPE. A sheet of RPE cells then contracts and scrolls up upon itself in a radial fashion, leaving an area of retina without underlying RPE.[41-43] Subretinal hemorrhage frequently accompanies an RPE tear, which appears ophthalmoscopically as an area of well-demarcated hyperpigmentation immediately adjacent to an area of relative hypopigmentation. Fluorescein angiography demonstrates this as an absolute window defect, with well-circumscribed hyperfluorescence that does not increase in intensity or leak as the angiogram progresses (Fig. 87-12). The lack of fluorescein leakage distinguishes an RPE tear from a totally (100%) classic CNV membrane.[38] An OCT scan directly through the tear will show an irregular highly reflective outer band that appears thicker than the normal band due to scrolling of the RPE (Fig. 87-12).[38, 41-43] This is immediately adjacent to an area where there is increased reflectivity from the choroid (posterior thickening of the external band) from the absence of the RPE.[38, 41-43] A sharply demarcated vertical discontinuity can also be seen in some instances.

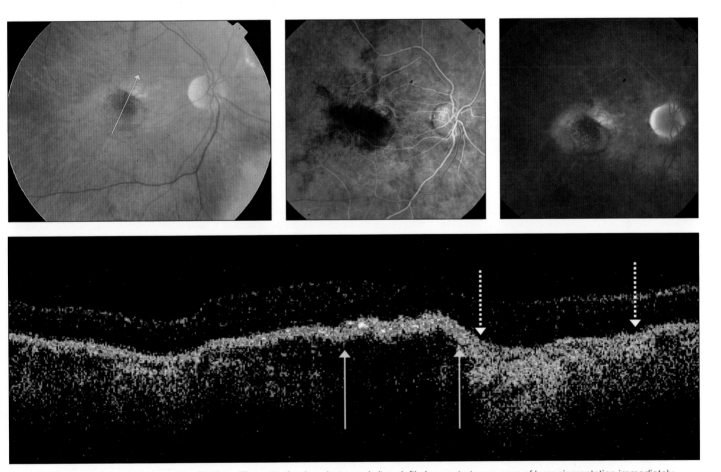

Fig. 87-12 Tear of the retinal pigment epithelium. The color fundus photograph (top, left) demonstrates an area of hypopigmentation immediately adjacent to an area of hyperpigmentation, indicative of a retinal pigment epithelium (RPE) tear in a 75-year-old woman with neovascular age-related macular degeneration. The junction between these two areas of varying pigmentation is well-delineated. Fluorescein angiography arteriovenous (top, middle) and late recirculation phases (top, right) demonstrate an absolute window defect without leakage beyond its borders with an area of adjacent relative hypofluorescence corresponding to the scrolled RPE. An optical coherence tomography scan (bottom) through these two areas demonstrates an area where the highly reflective external band is extremely attenuated (corresponding to absent RPE; noted as the area between dashed white arrows) immediately adjacent to an area where the highly reflective external band is thicker than usual (corresponding to scrolled, retracted RPE; noted as the area in between yellow arrows). Shallow sub-RPE fluid is noted. No subretinal fluid is appreciated in this particular scan, although subretinal fluid or subretinal hemorrhage is frequently seen in this setting.

Retinal angiomatous proliferation

The term *retinal angiomatous proliferation* (RAP) was coined by Yannuzzi and co-workers to describe a variant form of CNV in AMD patients.[44] RAP is typified by intraretinal neovascularization in the form of a retinal–retinal anastomosis and intraretinal hemorrhage with or without a serous PED.[44] As the RAP lesion evolves, a chorioretinal anastomosis forms. Labeling a CNV lesion as an RAP has prognostic implications insofar as they tend to fare poorer than other lesions with treatment.[44] The OCT appearance of early RAP is characterized by cystic retinal thickening, possible mild sub-RPE fluid (serous PED), and an intraretinal hyperreflective complex consistent with intraretinal CNV (Fig. 87-13).[44, 45] Subretinal fluid is not as prominent in early RAP lesions, but may also be seen. Later, these lesions progress to large PEDs with overlying cystic edema and shallow surrounding subretinal fluid accumulation.[44] OCT can be used to confirm treatment (macular photocoagulation, transpupillary thermotherapy, or combination PDT

and intravitreal triamcinolone acetonide) response, often showing reduction of the PED with resolution of the overlying fluid.[38,46,47]

Choroidal neovascularization: response to treatment

Current treatment modalities for CNV (verteporfin PDT and macular photocoagulation) employ pre- and posttreatment evaluation with intravenous fluorescein angiography (IVFA) and/or indocyanine green angiography and OCT. OCT has increasingly become a test obtained for adjunctive evaluation of CNV at baseline and as a measure of treatment response.[48–51] Current therapies for CNV rely upon visualization and angiographic characterization of CNV for direct ablation.[48–51] Future treatment strategies with vascular endothelial growth factor (VEGF) inhibition will not rely on direct physical targeting of the CNV lesion. Therefore, it is anticipated that OCT will play a major role in the evaluation of CNV lesions before and after treatment,

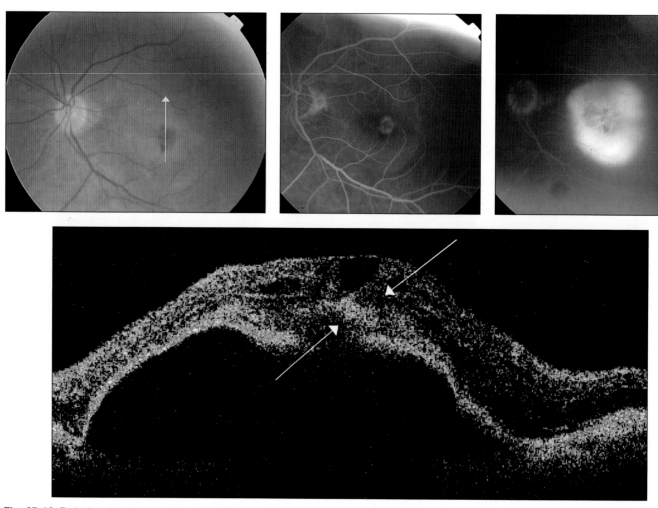

Fig. 87-13 Retinal angiomatous proliferation. A 69-year-old woman with poor vision OS for 1 year presented with visual acuity of 20/400 OS. Subretinal fluid and intraretinal hemorrhage are appreciated on the color fundus photograph (top, left). Fluorescein angiography demonstrates a minimally classic choroidal neovascular (also minimally neovascular) complex (top, middle and right). A vertical optical coherence tomography scan (bottom) through the foveal center demonstrates significant intraretinal cystic edema, large pigment epithelial detachment, and a central intraretinal neovascular complex (between white arrows). Subretinal fluid is notable peripherally.

perhaps even replacing IVFA at posttreatment (anti-VEGF therapy) follow-up visits. OCT can determine if cystic retinal thickening or subretinal fluid accumulation is present after treatment and response to therapy can thereby be determined (Fig. 87-11).[48-51]

Disciform scarring

Disciform scarring and subretinal fibrosis mark the end stage of untreated CNV and often accompany lesions treated with verteporfin PDT. This scarring appears as a smooth, elevated white or light-gray tissue in the subretinal space. Scarring often appears as an area of hyperfluorescence with intense late staining on fluorescein angiography, which can often be confused with persistent leakage.[38] The decision as to whether to re-treat with verteporfin PDT hinges on this discrimination between leakage and staining.

OCT is extremely helpful with this decision.[38] Subretinal fibrosis appears as a highly reflective outer-retinal or subretinal complex (Fig. 87-14). Whether or not it is associated with subretinal fluid or intraretinal cystic swelling is a function of the neovascular activity of the entire AMD lesion. In our experience eyes harboring intensely staining fibrosis without active leakage do not demonstrate significant intraretinal cystic thickening or subretinal fluid accumulation as an active lesion would. On the other hand, an active neovascular complex will show subretinal and intraretinal fluid accumulation in association with irregularities of the external band. With experience, OCT greatly facilitates the differentiation of an active neovascular complex from subretinal fibrosis.

It is important to note that on occasion old CNV lesions with fibrosis may demonstrate small or medium-sized cysts within the overlying retina (Fig. 87-14). We feel this represents an end-stage "burned-out" lesion whose cysts are due to chronic inflammation, not due to leakage from an active CNV complex.

IDIOPATHIC CENTRAL SEROUS CHORIORETINOPATHY

OCT is particularly helpful in diagnosing and managing patients with suspected ICSC.[52] OCT is useful in delineating the

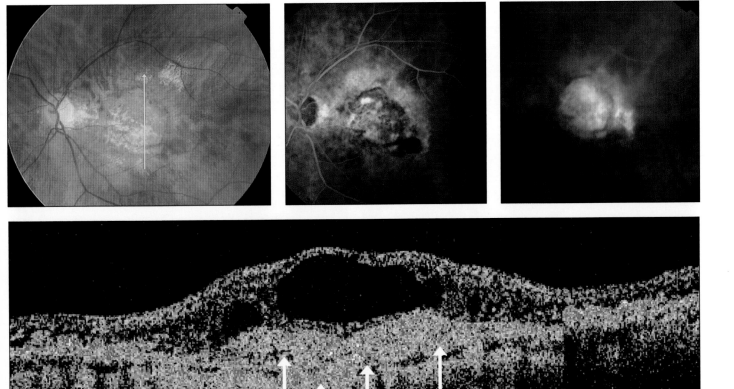

Fig. 87-14 Disciform scar. This 83-year-old woman had a history of end-stage neovascular age-related macular degeneration after multiple photodynamic therapy treatments. Subretinal fibrosis is noted in a subfoveal location on the color fundus photograph (top, left). Fluorescein angiography (top, middle, and right) demonstrates staining with minimal leakage. A vertical optical coherence tomography scan (bottom) through the fovea depicts the subretinal fibrosis as a well-delineated area of increased optical reflectivity (shown as red) below the retina and above the highly reflective external band (the outer extent of the subretinal fibrosis is noted by white arrows). Subretinal fluid is notably absent. We therefore feel the overlying cystic retinal changes are more representative of chronic end-stage disease (perhaps due to inflammation) than of active neovascular activity.

presence and extent of subretinal fluid accumulation as well as identifying any associated PED.[52] OCT is more sensitive than clinical exam and fluorescein angiography in identifying small amount of subretinal fluid (Fig. 87-15).[53] Although fluorescein angiography typically confirms the diagnosis (Fig. 87-15), certain cases can be confused with occult CNV. Assessing OCT characteristics, such as the regularity of the external band or extent of intraretinal edema, can often be used to distinguish these conditions.

OCT also has an important role in the management of patients with ICSC. Quantitative monitoring of subretinal fluid may direct decision-making. Even when symptoms are unchanged, further observation may be indicated when there has been some decrease in the subretinal fluid on OCT after a period of

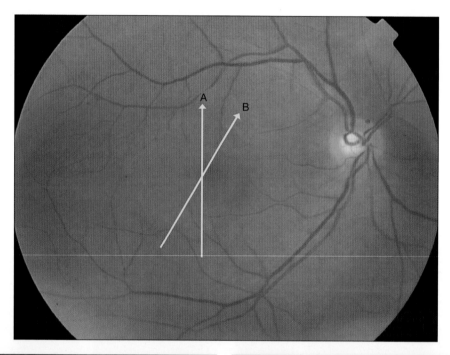

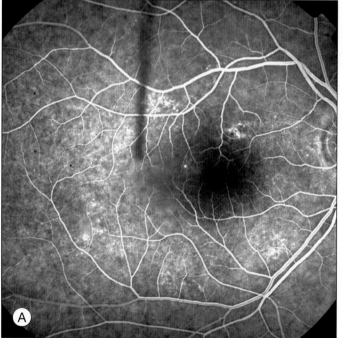

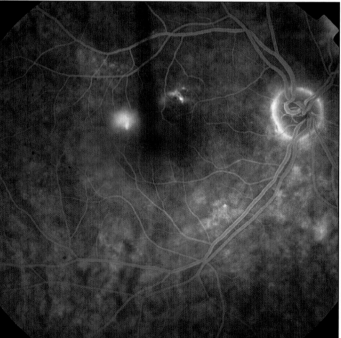

Fig. 87-15 Idiopathic central serous chorioretinopathy. A, Color fundus photograph (top) demonstrates a well-demarcated zone of subretinal fluid involving the fovea in a 53-year-old female patient with idiopathic central serous chorioretinopathy. Lettered arrows indicate the respective orientation of the optical coherence tomography (OCT) scans in Figure 87-15B. Fluorescein angiography demonstrates a focal area of intense hyperfluorescence (bottom, middle) with late pooling of dye (bottom, right).

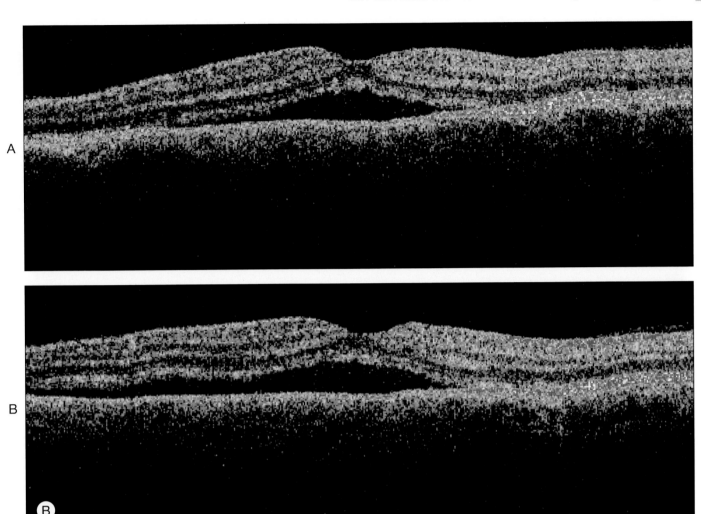

Fig. 87-15—cont'd B, Same patient as in Figure 87-15A. Vertical OCT scan through the fovea (A, top) shows a collection of shallow subretinal fluid, with a minimal overlying retinal thickening. An oblique OCT scan through the fovea (B, bottom) demonstrates the greater extent of subretinal fluid accumulation compared to the vertical scan. A focal pigment epithelial detachment is not identified in these particular OCT scans. No evidence of a choroidal neovascular membrane was identified in any of the scans.

observation. Treatment may be more likely indicated if subretinal fluid levels persist or increase over time.[54–59] Localization of the area of leakage on OCT (which usually appears as a localized PED) can be useful in cases in which thermal laser therapy or PDT is considered to hasten fluid resolution.[54–59]

DIABETIC RETINOPATHY

Nonproliferative diabetic retinopathy (NPDR) and diabetic macular edema (DME)

In the evaluation of patients with diabetic retinopathy, OCT provides valuable information about retinal thickness and extent of retinal edema.[60–62] Determination of macular edema can be difficult with biomicroscopy alone, especially when mild.[63–71] OCT can be used to distinguish patients with normal retinal contour and thickness despite extensive angiopathy from those with early retinal edema. Patients with DME will exhibit cystic retinal thickening in a diffuse or segmental manner (Fig. 87-16).[62]

Intraretinal focal hyperreflections that correspond clinically to retinal exudates are a frequent finding, especially in patients with DME (Fig. 87-16).[60] In cases where there is a vertical disparity in retinal thickness, a concomitant or occult branch retinal vein occlusion (BRVO) must be considered.[72]

The Early Treatment of Diabetic Retinopathy Study provided guidelines for laser management of patients with DME.[73,74] Although OCT was not available for use in this study, quantitative retinal thickness maps can be used to direct laser therapy and may be better than using biomicroscopy alone.[60] One must be careful not to decide to apply macular laser photocoagulation to treat DME based solely on the OCT image. Clinical exam and fluorescein angiography are essential in determining the size of the foveal avascular zone (FAZ).[60] Excessive laser near the border of the FAZ can result in worsened macular ischemia.[75] Although ischemic retina may appear thinned on OCT, this is not a reliable proxy for fluorescein angiography in patients with macular ischemia.[60]

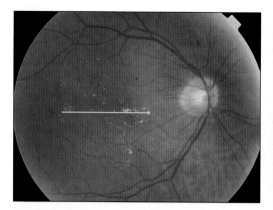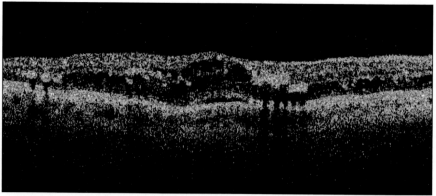

Fig. 87-16 Diabetic macular edema. Color fundus photograph (left) of a 63-year-old man with diabetic macular edema and nonproliferative diabetic retinopathy. Retinal edema is appreciated along with numerous exudates adjacent to the foveal center. Horizontal optical coherence tomography scan (right) through the fovea shows diffuse intraretinal cystic thickening with loss of the normal foveal depression. Intraretinal hyperreflective foci with posterior optical shadowing correspond to areas of retinal exudates seen clinically. A focal area of shallow subretinal fluid is noted centrally.

Increasingly, patients with refractory DME are being managed by the use of intravitreal triamcinolone acetonide.[60,76] Treatment of patients with no prior laser therapy with intravitreal triamcinolone acetonide is also considered in the setting of an enlarged FAZ.[60,76] OCT is quite helpful in monitoring the response to treatment with either or both of these treatment modalities.[60,76] The OCT response to intravitreal triamcinolone acetonide can be remarkable: some patients show significant edema reduction just days after the procedure.[60,76]

Macular traction has become increasingly recognized in patients with DME unresponsive to both laser and intravitreal triamcinolone acetonide.[77–79] These patients often show the clinical appearance of a taut posterior hyaloid with diffuse fluorescein leakage.[77–79] Recognition of this condition can be difficult by clinical exam alone. This is readily recognized in OCT scans by diffuse cystic retinal thickening, a flat-appearing foveal contour, and a thickened hyperreflective linear vitreoretinal interface.[60,80] Focal vitreoretinal adhesions that cannot be identified on clinical exam are also often evident on OCT.[60] These findings can direct the decision as to whether to proceed with vitrectomy and membrane peeling.[60,80–82]

Proliferative diabetic retinopathy and tractional retinal detachment

Once extraretinal neovascular proliferation involves the macula, stable vision may progressively deteriorate. The decision for surgery typically hinges on the progressive nature of the traction and the degree to which the macula is affected by the traction. Tractional elevation of the retina with intraretinal fluid accumulation causing retinal thickening and subretinal fluid accumulation are clearly seen by OCT evaluation (Fig. 87-17).[60] In this manner, OCT can be used to confirm tractional distortion and elevation of the macula as the cause of vision loss, thus indicating the need for surgery.[60] In other cases, OCT may show that the traction has minimal direct effect on the foveal region, and other causes for vision loss (macular ischemia) must be considered before proceeding with surgery.

MISCELLANEOUS RETINAL VASCULAR DISEASES

Retinal vein occlusion

Diffuse intraretinal cystic thickening of the retina is evident on OCT scanning of patients with central retinal vein occlusion (CRVO) complicated by macular edema.[72,83–86] The cystic spaces and retinal thickening seen on OCT are evenly distributed throughout the macula, with no predilection for the superior or inferior hemiretina (Fig. 87-18).[72,83–86] There is also often a significant component of subretinal fluid accumulation. OCT allows confirmation of macular edema as a component of vision loss in CRVO, and provides quantitative information of edema extent.[72,83–86] Prior to the advent of OCT, the Central Vein Occlusion Study showed that there was no visual benefit of laser photocoagulation in the management of CRVO-associated macular edema.[87] This has stimulated extensive research into new treatments for this condition.[88–94] OCT monitoring of treatment response has been a key part of evaluating the effectiveness of these modalities.[72,83–86]

Similar to CRVO, OCT can be used in the evaluation of patients with BRVO. In cases of macular edema due to BRVO, the vertical OCT scan through the foveal center (inferior to superior sweep) is quite helpful in identifying the horizontal demarcation of the edematous component (Fig. 87-19).[72,83,85,95] With this scan, one will often see diffuse cystic retinal thickening abutting the foveal center in one hemiretina (inferior or superior) in immediate contiguity with normal-appearing nonedematous retina in the other hemiretina.[72,95] This finding in an elderly, hypertensive patient with subacute visual loss is nearly pathognomonic for BRVO with macular edema. Confirmation of macular edema and associated foveal distortion as the cause for vision loss is an important application of OCT in these patients. The Branch Vein Occlusion Study provided guidelines for grid laser

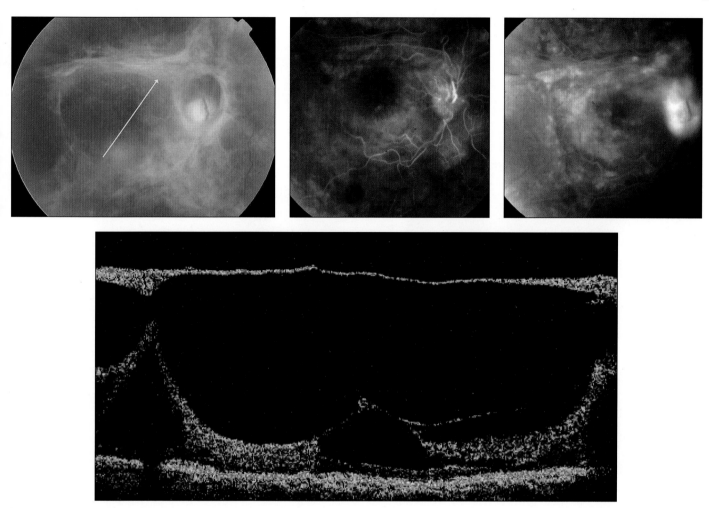

Fig. 87-17 Traction retinal detachment/proliferative diabetic retinopathy. Color fundus photograph (top, left) of a 28-year-old man with advanced proliferative diabetic retinopathy with tractional retinal detachment involving the macula. Fluorescein angiography mid and late phases (top, middle and right) demonstrate diffuse staining and leakage. An oblique optical coherence tomography scan (bottom) through the fovea demonstrates abnormal tractional bands inserting on the retinal surface, resulting in marked distortion of the retinal architecture. Diffuse cystic changes are noted.

to manage vision loss due to BRVO-associated macular edema.[96] In addition to surgical intervention, intravitreal triamcinolone acetonide has been shown to be successful at temporarily reducing persistent macular edema in patients with BRVO.[97–103] As a result, OCT can be used to establish quantitatively baseline macular thickness, to determine the need for observation versus intervention, and to monitor the subsequent response.[72]

Idiopathic juxtafoveal retinal telangiectasis (IJRT)

IJRT is a common retinal vascular disorder that typically affects young to middle-aged males.[104] The formation of telangiectatic vessels – with a predilection for the temporal macula – results in macular edema and compromised central visual acuity.[104] High-magnification evaluation of the temporal macula can demonstrate small grouped telangiectasias and in many cases retinal venules with a "right-angle" configuration.[104] Fluorescein angiogra-

phy demonstrates characteristic leakage in the macula, with a propensity for the temporal half of the macula.[104] A characteristic OCT pattern has been identified in which a relatively normal foveal contour is accompanied by the presence of horizontally oblong small intraretinal (inner retina) cysts (Fig. 87-20).[72] As expected, a horizontal OCT scan through the center of the fovea demonstrates the greatest concentration of these oblong cysts in the temporal half of the macula.[72] Subretinal fluid is typically not appreciated with OCT.[72]

Pseudophakic cystoid macular edema

Numerous conditions can result in limited visual improvement and worse than expected visual acuity following cataract surgery. In some cases, this results from pre-existing, undetected retinal pathology (see section on visually significant cataract, below). In other cases, refractive issues and transient ocular surface changes in the absence of retinal pathology cause this situation. Postoperative cystoid macular edema (CME) is

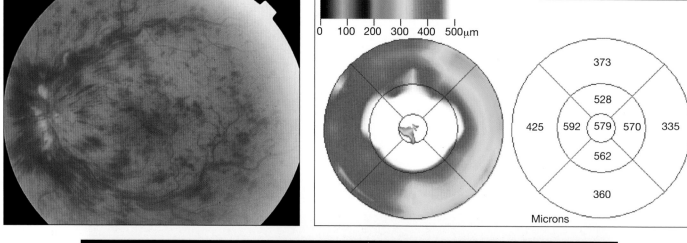

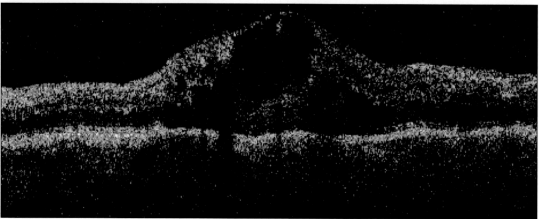

Fig. 87-18 Central retinal vein occlusion. An 81-year-old man presented with sudden and severe visual loss in the left eye. The color fundus photograph (top, left) demonstrates diffuse intraretinal hemorrhages radiating from the optic disc and in all four quadrants along with notable macular thickening. The optical coherence tomography (OCT) thickness map (top, right) demonstrates the diffuse nature of macular edema. OCT scan (bottom) through the fovea demonstrates diffuse intraretinal cystic thickening and subfoveal fluid collection.

another frequent cause of such vision loss. Since it is often difficult to distinguish CME on biomicroscopy, it may be difficult to confirm the true etiology for vision loss on exam alone.

Although fluorescein angiography was used in the past, OCT is especially useful in this situation because it provides rapid, noninvasive evaluation of retinal contour and thickness. Diffuse medium to large cystic spaces are seen in the outer nuclear layer of the central macula with maximal retinal thickness concentric on the fovea (Fig. 87-21).[105] Once the diagnosis is confirmed, response to topical therapy can be monitored. If the edema resolves on OCT without a corresponding improvement in vision, investigations for other etiologies of vision loss are indicated. In cases with persistent edema and vision loss, consideration of intravitreal triamcinolone has become increasingly popular.[106–108]

It should be noted that certain rare conditions exist that demonstrate significant intraretinal cystic spaces on OCT but do not demonstrate leakage by fluorescein angiography (nicotinic acid maculopathy, Goldmann–Favre vitreoretinal degeneration, enhanced S-cone syndrome, X-linked juvenile retinoschisis, docetaxel toxicity, and many cases of VMT).[109–112] These simulating conditions might erroneously be treated as refractory pseudophakic CME without the benefit of fluorescein angiography, further examination, or additional history. These conditions should be considered in cases with refractory CME, and appropriate evaluation should be obtained.[109–112]

RETINAL DETACHMENT

Rhegmatogenous retinal detachment

Rhegmatogenous retinal detachment involving the macula can be documented with fundus photography and OCT. OCT demonstrates an elevation of the neural retina due to extensive subretinal fluid presence.[113] Because involvement of the macula portends a poorer prognosis than macula-sparing detachments, OCT is one method that can be considered to document the advanced status of the detachment at baseline.[113,114]

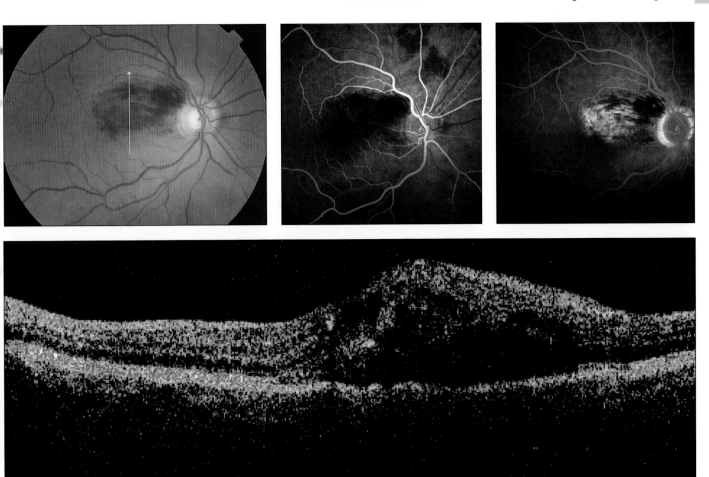

Fig. 87-19 Branch retinal vein occlusion. A 75-year-old hypertensive female patient presented with decreased vision in the right eye. The color fundus photograph (top, left) demonstrates diffuse intraretinal hemorrhages in a pattern that respects the horizontal midline. Macular edema is noted as well. Fluorescein angiography (top, middle and right) depicts blocked fluorescence due to intraretinal hemorrhages and late leakage in the macula and papillomacular bundle. Vertical optical coherence tomography scan through the fovea demonstrates a relatively normal retinal thickness in the early part of the scan (corresponding to the uninvolved inferior macula), but as the scan approaches the foveal center, diffuse intraretinal cystic thickening is noted together with some subretinal fluid accumulation. This vertical disparity between normal retinal and cystic thickened retina is nearly pathognomonic for branch retinal vein occlusion.

Exudative retinal detachment

Exudative detachments of the macula are seen in numerous inflammatory conditions that affect the posterior segment. Similar to macula-involving rhegmatogenous retinal detachments, OCT can be used to document the presence, extent, and degree of subretinal fluid.[115] Retinal infiltrates and sub-RPE lesions often accompany localized and diffuse exudative detachments, and these can be assessed more accurately for level of involvement with OCT than with clinical examination or other diagnostic modalities.[115] OCT can also be used in patients with chronic uveitis to detect CME.[116,117]

VISUALLY SIGNIFICANT CATARACT: PREOPERATIVE EVALUATION

Modern small-incision phacoemulsification techniques have resulted in rapid surgeries with few complications. Retina

specialists have always encountered the classic patient who underwent uneventful cataract extraction with intraocular lens placement without improvement in visual function postoperatively. It is difficult to convince even the most reasonable patient in this situation that their cataract surgery was not the cause of the lack of visual improvement, no matter how much explanation is offered. In our experience, the lack of visual improvement is usually due to a noncataractous entity such as coexisting but unsuspected or undetected AMD (geographic atrophy, disciform scar, or active CNV lesion), visually significant epiretinal membrane, or VMT. Cataract surgeons will often request fluorescein angiography or retinal consultation for patients they feel are at risk for a macular problem preoperatively due to fellow-eye involvement, but in many instances advanced media opacity precludes optimal evaluation in this manner.

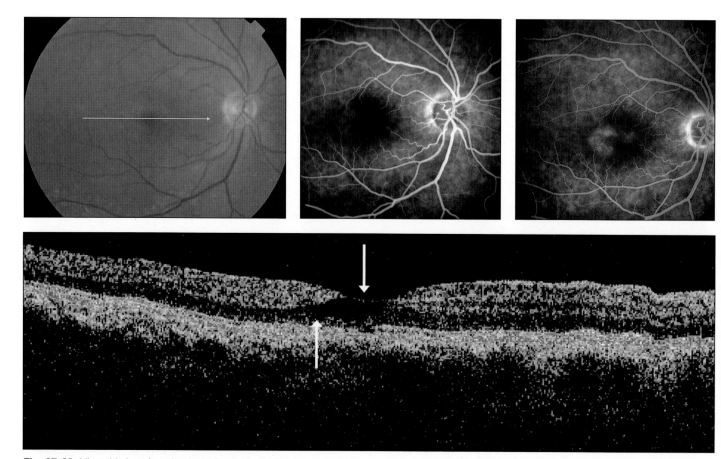

Fig. 87-20 Idiopathic juxtafoveal retinal telangiectasis. This 68-year-old woman had decreased vision in her right eye. The color fundus photograph (top, left) demonstrates loss of the foveal reflex and parafoveal retinal pigment epithelium (RPE) mottling. Fluorescein angiography (top, middle and right) shows leakage from juxtafoveolar capillaries with a temporal predilection. A horizontal optical coherence tomography (OCT) scan (bottom) shows a thin, spindle-shaped cyst in the inner retina temporal to the fovea. This OCT appearance is nearly pathognomonic for idiopathic juxtafoveal retinal telangiectasis. Notably absent on the OCT scan is diffuse cystic thickening or subretinal fluid accumulation as one might see with choroidal neovascularization.

Perhaps the best use of OCT for the anterior-segment surgeon is the preoperative evaluation of all patients with visually significant cataracts. The high-wavelength incident beam of the OCT can penetrate significant media opacity efficiently, even in instances where fluorescein angiography cannot. It saves the surgeon postoperatively from having to explain the lack of visual improvement and to demonstrate definitively that the ultimate cause of visual impairment was due to the preexisting condition (AMD, ERM, or VMT, to name a few) and not entirely due to the cataract. In this regard alone, preoperative OCT evaluation is cost-effective for the anterior-segment surgeon. Because of its noninvasive nature and rapid image acquisition, it is an ideal way of ensuring that optimal patient selection is being achieved preoperatively and cost-effectively. In patients who are found to harbor pre-existing macular pathology, appropriate preoperative counseling (explanation of the potential for lack of visual improvement), further testing, or appropriate referral to a retinal specialist can be made.

SUMMARY

OCT is a powerful and elegant new tool that has revolutionized the diagnostic approach to macular disease. In addition to providing new information to the clinician, it also helps many patients understand better their ocular disorder and the goal of medical and surgical therapy. In this chapter, we have described the technology behind OCT, its practical application, and the interpretation of OCT images of common retinal diseases. The fundoscopic and angiographic appearance of many retinal disorders is often readily identified simply by pattern recognition. The new paradigm of OCT introduces a new era of ophthalmic pattern recognition for the rapid identification of macular disease via OCT. OCT can be used to guide diagnostic and treatment algorithms in an effective and efficient manner. We eagerly anticipate the commercial availability of ultra-high-resolution OCT which will enable greater discrimination of retinal structures (approximate resolution of 2 μm to 3 μm) and improve quantitative assessment of the macula.[16] Software algorithms are continually evolving that increase analytical power and ease of operation.

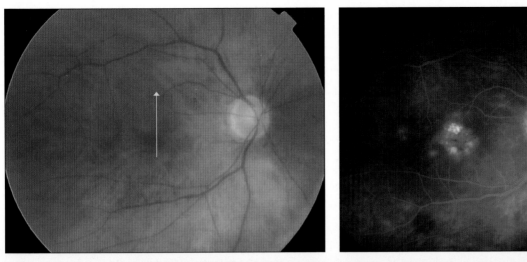
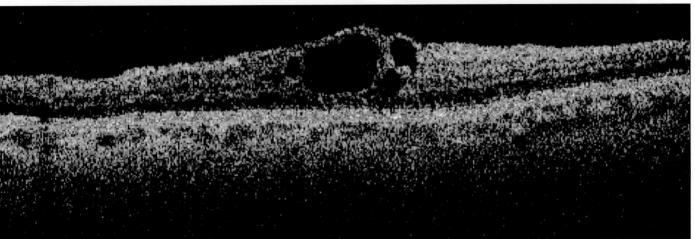

Fig. 87-21 Pseudophakic cystoid macular edema. The color fundus photograph (top, left) is from a 76-year-old pseudophakic woman with refractory cystoid macular edema 3 years after phacoemulsification and intraocular lens implantation. Visual acuity is 20/60. Late-phase fluorescein angiogram (top, right) demonstrates leakage in a petalloid pattern. Vertical optical coherence tomography scan through the macula (bottom) demonstrates intraretinal cystic spaces of varying sizes corresponding with the areas of leakage on angiography.

Inferior   Superior

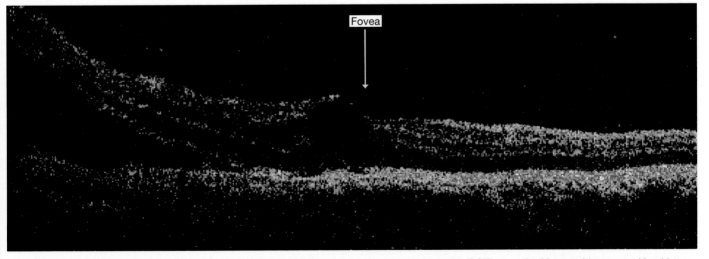

Fig. 87-22 Macula-off rhegmatogenous retinal detachment. Vertical optical coherence tomography (OCT) scan of a 32-year-old woman with a history of high myopia who presented with a macula-off inferior rhegmatogenous retinal detachment. A vertical OCT scan through the fovea demonstrates the subretinal fluid abutting the foveal center and minimal overlying cystic changes.

REFERENCES

1. Huang D, Swanson EA, Lin CP et al. Optical coherence tomography. Science 1991; 254:1178–1181.

2. Fujimoto JG, Hee MR, Duang D et al. Principles of optical coherence tomography. In: Schuman JS, Puliafito CA, Fujimoto JG, eds. Optical coherence tomography of ocular diseases. Thorofare, NJ: SLACK; 2004:3–20.

3. Pieroth L, Schuman JS, Hertzmark E et al. Evaluation of focal defects of the nerve fiber layer using optical coherence tomography. Ophthalmology 1999; 106:570–579.

4. Schuman JS, Pedut-Kloizman T, Hertzmark E et al. Reproducibility of nerve fiber layer thickness measurements using optical coherence tomography. Ophthalmology 1996; 103:1889–1898.

5. Paunescu LA, Schuman JS, Price LL et al. Reproducibility of nerve fiber thickness, macular thickness, and optic nerve head measurements using StratusOCT. Invest Ophthalmol Vis Sci 2004; 45:1716–1724.

6. Pitris C, Saunders KT, Fujimoto JG et al. High-resolution imaging of the middle ear with optical coherence tomography: a feasibility study. Arch Otolaryngol Head Neck Surg 2001; 127:637–642.

7. Boppart SA, Herrmann JM, Pitris C et al. Real-time optical coherence tomography for minimally invasive imaging of prostate ablation. Comput Aided Surg 2001; 6:94–103.

8. Aguirre AD, Hsiung P, Ko TH et al. High-resolution optical coherence microscopy for high-speed, in vivo cellular imaging. Opt Lett. 2003; 28:2064–2066.

9. Fujimoto JG. Optical coherence tomography for ultrahigh resolution in vivo imaging. Nat Biotechnol 2003; 21:1361–1367.

10. Pantanowitz L, Hsiung PL, Ko TH et al. High-resolution imaging of the thyroid gland using optical coherence tomography. Head Neck 2004; 26:425–434.

11. Rogowska J, Patel NA, Fujimoto JG et al. Optical coherence tomographic elastography technique for measuring deformation and strain of atherosclerotic tissues. Heart 2004; 90:556–562.

12. Jumper JM, Gallemore RP, McCuen BW 2nd et al. Features of macular hole closure in the early postoperative period using optical coherence tomography. Retina 2000; 20:232–237.

13. Sato H, Kawasaki R, Yamashita H. Observation of idiopathic full-thickness macular hole closure in early postoperative period as evaluated by optical coherence tomography. Am J Ophthalmol 2003; 136:185–187.

14. Browning DJ, Fraser CM. Optical coherence tomography to detect macular edema in the presence of asteroid hyalosis. Am J Ophthalmol 2004; 137:959–961.

15. Schuman JS, Puliafito CA, Fujimoto JG (eds). Optical coherence tomography of ocular diseases. Thorofare, NJ: Slack; 2004.

16. Drexler W, Sattmann H, Hermann B et al. Enhanced visualization of macular pathology with the use of ultrahigh-resolution optical coherence tomography. Arch Ophthalmol 2003; 121:695–706.

17. Hee MR, Fujimoto JG, Ko T et al. Interpretation of the optical coherence tomography image. In: Schuman JS, Puliafito CA, Fujimoto JG, eds. Optical coherence tomography of ocular diseases. Thorofare, NJ: SLACK, Inc.; 2004:21–56.

18. Smiddy WE, Michels RG, Glaser BM et al. Vitrectomy for macular traction caused by incomplete vitreous separation. Arch Ophthalmol 1988; 106:624–628.

19. Margherio RR, Trese MT, Margherio AR et al. Surgical management of vitreomacular traction syndromes. Ophthalmology 1989; 96:1437–1445.

20. McDonald HR, Johnson RN, Schatz H. Surgical results in the vitreomacular traction syndrome. Ophthalmology 1994; 101:1397–1402.

21. Hikichi T, Yoshida A, Trempe CL. Course of vitreomacular traction syndrome. Am J Ophthalmol 1995; 119:55–61.

22. Gallemore RP, Jumper JM, McCuen BW 2nd et al. Diagnosis of vitreoretinal adhesions in macular disease with optical coherence tomography. Retina 2000; 20:115–120.

23. Sulkes DJ, Ip MS, Baumal CR et al. Spontaneous resolution of vitreomacular traction documented by optical coherence tomography. Arch Ophthalmol 2000; 118:286–287.

24. Voo I, Mavrofrides EC, Puliafito CA. Clinical applications of optical coherence tomography for the diagnosis and management of macular diseases. Ophthalmol Clin North Am 2004; 17:21–31.

25. Mavrofrides EC, Rogers AH, Truong S et al. Vitreoretinal interface disorders. In: Schuman JS, Puliafito CA, Fujimoto JG, eds. Optical coherence tomography of ocular diseases. Thorofare, NJ: SLACK, Inc.; 2004:57–102.

26. Smiddy WE, Michels RG, Green WR. Morphology, pathology, and surgery of idiopathic vitreoretinal macular disorders. A review. Retina 1990; 10:288–296.

27. Gass JD. Lamellar macular hole: a complication of cystoid macular edema after cataract extraction. Arch Ophthalmol 1976; 94:793–800.

28. Wilkins JR, Puliafito CA, Hee MR et al. Characterization of epiretinal membranes using optical coherence tomography. Ophthalmology 1996; 103:2142–2151.

29. Suzuki T, Terasaki H, Niwa T et al. Optical coherence tomography and focal macular electroretinogram in eyes with epiretinal membrane and macular pseudohole. Am J Ophthalmol 2003; 136:62–67.

30. Mori K, Gehlbach PL, Sano A et al. Comparison of epiretinal membranes of differing pathogenesis using optical coherence tomography. Retina 2004; 24:57–62.

31. Gass JD. Reappraisal of biomicroscopic classification of stages of development of a macular hole. Am J Ophthalmol 1995; 119:752–759.

32. Tabandeh H, Smiddy WE, Mello M et al. Surgery for idiopathic macular holes associated with extensive subretinal fluid. Retina 2001; 21:15–9.

33. Hee MR, Puliafito CA, Wong C et al. Optical coherence tomography of macular holes. Ophthalmology 1995; 102:748–756.

34. Gaudric A, Haouchine B, Massin P et al. Macular hole formation: new data provided by optical coherence tomography. Arch Ophthalmol 1999; 117:744–751.

35. Altaweel M, Ip M. Macular hole: improved understanding of pathogenesis, staging, and management based on optical coherence tomography. Semin Ophthalmol 2003; 18:58–66.

36. Ullrich S, Haritoglou C, Gass C et al. Macular hole size as a prognostic factor in macular hole surgery. Br J Ophthalmol 2002; 86:390–393.

37. Ip MS, Baker BJ, Duker JS et al. Anatomical outcomes of surgery for idiopathic macular hole as determined by optical coherence tomography. Arch Ophthalmol 2002; 120:29–35.

38. Mavrofrides EC, Villate N, Rosenfeld PJ et al. (eds). Optical coherence tomography of ocular diseases. In: Schuman JS, Puliafito CA, Fujimoto JG (eds). Optical coherence tomography of ocular diseases. Thorofare, NJ: SLACK, Inc.; 2004:243–343.

39. Ting TD, Oh M, Cox TA et al. Decreased visual acuity associated with cystoid macular edema in neovascular age-related macular degeneration. Arch Ophthalmol 2002; 120:731–737.

40. Hee MR, Baumal CR, Puliafito CA et al. Optical coherence tomography of age-related macular degeneration and choroidal neovascularization. Ophthalmology 1996; 103:1260–1270.

41. Pece A, Introini U, Bottoni F et al. Acute retinal pigment epithelial tear after photodynamic therapy. Retina 2001; 21:661–665.

42. Gelisken F, Inhoffen W, Partsch M et al. Retinal pigment epithelial tear after photodynamic therapy for choroidal neovascularization. Am J Ophthalmol 2001; 131:518–520.

43. Srivastava SK, Sternberg P Jr. Retinal pigment epithelial tear weeks following photodynamic therapy with verteporfin for choroidal neovascularization secondary to pathologic myopia. Retina 2002; 22:669–671.

44. Yannuzzi LA, Negrao S, Iida T et al. Retinal angiomatous proliferation in age-related macular degeneration. Retina 2001; 21:416–434.

45. Zacks DN, Johnson MW. Retinal angiomatous proliferation: optical coherence tomographic confirmation of an intraretinal lesion. Arch Ophthalmol 2004; 122:932–933.

46. Borrillo JL, Sivalingam A, Martidis A et al. Surgical ablation of retinal angiomatous proliferation. Arch Ophthalmol 2003; 121:558–561.

47. Kuroiwa S, Arai J, Gaun S et al. Rapidly progressive scar formation after transpupillary thermotherapy in retinal angiomatous proliferation. Retina 2003; 23:417–420.

48. Rogers AH, Martidis A, Greenberg PB et al. Optical coherence tomography findings following photodynamic therapy of choroidal neovascularization. Am J Ophthalmol 2002; 134:566–576.

49. Giovannini A, Amato GP, Mariotti C et al. OCT imaging of choroidal neovascularisation and its role in the determination of patients' eligibility for surgery. Br J Ophthalmol 1999; 83:438–442.

50. Giovannini A, Amato G, Mariotti C et al. Optical coherence tomography in the assessment of retinal pigment epithelial tear. Retina 2000; 20:37–40.

51. Costa RA, Farah ME, Cardillo JA et al. Immediate indocyanine green angiography and optical coherence tomography evaluation after photodynamic therapy for subfoveal choroidal neovascularization. Retina 2003; 23:159–165.

52. Mavrofrides EC, Puliafito CA, Fujimoto JG. Central serous chorioretinopathy. In: Schuman JS, Puliafito CA, Fujimoto JG, eds. Optical coherence tomography of ocular diseases. Thorofare, NJ: SLACK, Inc.; 2004:215–242.

53. Wang M, Sander B, Lund-Andersen H et al. Detection of shallow detachments in central serous chorioretinopathy. Acta Ophthalmol Scand 1999; 77:402–405.

54. Gass JD. Photocoagulation treatment of idiopathic central serous choroidopathy. Trans Am Acad Ophthalmol Otolaryngol 1977; 83:456–467.

55. Robertson DM. Argon laser photocoagulation treatment in central serous chorioretinopathy. Ophthalmology 1986; 93:972–974.

56. Novak MA, Singerman LJ, Rice TA. Krypton and argon laser photocoagulation for central serous chorioretinopathy. Retina 1987; 7:162–169.

57. Brancato R, Scialdone A, Pece A et al. Eight-year follow-up of central serous chorioretinopathy with and without laser treatment. Graefes Arch Clin Exp Ophthalmol 1987; 225:166–168.

58. Burumcek E, Mudun A, Karacorlu S et al. Laser photocoagulation for persistent central serous retinopathy: results of long-term follow-up. Ophthalmology 1997; 104:616–622.

59. Cardillo Piccolino F, Eandi CM, Ventre L et al. Photodynamic therapy for chronic central serous chorioretinopathy. Retina 2003; 23:752–763.

60. Cruz-Villegas V, Flynn HW Jr. Diabetic retinopathy. In: Schuman JS, Puliafito CA, Fujimoto JG, eds. Optical coherence tomography of ocular diseases. Thorofare, NJ: SLACK, Inc., 2004:157–214.

61. Schaudig UH, Glaefke C, Scholz F et al. Optical coherence tomography for retinal thickness measurement in diabetic patients without clinically significant macular edema. Ophthalm Surg Lasers 2000; 31:182–186.

62. Hee MR, Puliafito CA, Duker JS et al. Topography of diabetic macular edema with optical coherence tomography. Ophthalmology 1998; 105:360–370.

63. Strom C, Sander B, Larsen N et al. Diabetic macular edema assessed with optical coherence tomography and stereo fundus photography. Invest Ophthalmol Vis Sci 2002; 43:241–245.

64. Sanchez-Tocino H, Alvarez-Vidal A, Maldonado MJ et al. Retinal thickness study with optical coherence tomography in patients with diabetes. Invest Ophthalmol Vis Sci 2002; 43:1588–1594.

65. Goebel W, Kretzchmar-Gross T. Retinal thickness in diabetic retinopathy: a study using optical coherence tomography (OCT). Retina 2002; 22:759–767.

66. Massin P, Duguid G, Erginay A et al. Optical coherence tomography for evaluating diabetic macular edema before and after vitrectomy. Am J Ophthalmol 2003; 135:169–177.

67. Yamaguchi Y, Otani T, Kishi S. Resolution of diabetic cystoid macular edema associated with spontaneous vitreofoveal separation. Am J Ophthalmol 2003; 135:116–118.

68. Browning DJ, McOwen MD, Bowen RM Jr et al. Comparison of the clinical diagnosis of diabetic macular edema with diagnosis by optical coherence tomography. Ophthalmology 2004; 111:712–715.

69. Brown JC, Solomon SD, Bressler SB et al. Detection of diabetic foveal edema: contact lens biomicroscopy compared with optical coherence tomography. Arch Ophthalmol 2004; 122:330–335.

70. Frank RN, Schulz L, Abe K et al. Temporal variation in diabetic macular edema measured by optical coherence tomography. Ophthalmology 2004; 111:211–216.

71. Kang SW, Park CY, Ham DI. The correlation between fluorescein angiographic and optical coherence tomographic features in clinically significant diabetic macular edema. Am J Ophthalmol 2004; 137:313–322.

72. Cruz-Villegas V, Puliafito CA, Fujimoto JG. Retinal vascular diseases. In: Schuman JS, Puliafito CA, Fujimoto JG, eds. Optical coherence tomography of ocular diseases. Thorofare, NJ: SLACK, Inc.; 2004:103–156.

73. Early Treatment Diabetic Retinopathy Study Research Group. Treatment techniques and clinical guidelines for photocoagulation of diabetic macular edema. Early Treatment Diabetic Retinopathy Study report no. 2. Ophthalmology 1987; 94:761–774.

74. Early Treatment Diabetic Retinopathy Study Research Group. Photocoagulation for diabetic macular edema. Early Treatment Diabetic Retinopathy Study report no. 1. Arch Ophthalmol 1985; 103:1796–1806.

75. Rivellese M, George A, Sulkes D et al. Optical coherence tomography after laser photocoagulation for clinically significant macular edema. Ophthalm Surg Lasers 2000; 31:192–197.

76. Martidis A, Duker JS, Greenberg PB et al. Intravitreal triamcinolone for refractory diabetic macular edema. Ophthalmology 2002; 109:920–927.

77. Lewis H, Abrams GW, Blumenkranz MS et al. Vitrectomy for diabetic macular traction and edema associated with posterior hyaloidal traction. Ophthalmology 1992; 99:753–759.

78. Harbour JW, Smiddy WE, Flynn HW Jr et al. Vitrectomy for diabetic macular edema associated with a thickened and taut posterior hyaloid membrane. Am J Ophthalmol 1996; 121:405–413.

79. Pendergast SD, Hassan TS, Williams GA et al. Vitrectomy for diffuse diabetic macular edema associated with a taut premacular posterior hyaloid. Am J Ophthalmol 2000; 130:178–186.

80. Kaiser PK, Riemann CD, Sears JE et al. Macular traction detachment and diabetic macular edema associated with posterior hyaloidal traction. Am J Ophthalmol 2001; 131:44–49.

81. Yamamoto T, Hitani K, Tsukahara I et al. Early postoperative retinal thickness changes and complications after vitrectomy for diabetic macular edema. Am J Ophthalmol 2003; 135:14–19.

82. Giovannini A, Amato G, Mariotti C et al. Optical coherence tomography findings in diabetic macular edema before and after vitrectomy. Ophthalm Surg Lasers 2000; 31:187–191.

83. Hee MR, Puliafito CA, Wong C et al. Quantitative assessment of macular edema with optical coherence tomography. Arch Ophthalmol 1995; 113:1019–1029.

84. Sekiryu T, Yamauchi T, Enaida H et al. Retina tomography after vitrectomy for macular edema of central retinal vein occlusion. Ophthalm Surg Lasers 2000; 31:198–202.

85. Lerche RC, Schaudig U, Scholz F et al. Structural changes of the retina in retinal vein occlusion-imaging and quantification with optical coherence tomography. Ophthalm Surg Lasers 2001; 32:272–280.

86. Ip M, Kahana A, Altaweel M. Treatment of central retinal vein occlusion with triamcinolone acetonide: an optical coherence tomography study. Semin Ophthalmol 2003; 18:67–73.

87. Evaluation of grid pattern photocoagulation for macular edema in central vein occlusion. The Central Vein Occlusion Study Group M report. Ophthalmology 1995; 102:1425–1433.

88. McAllister IL, Douglas JP, Constable IJ et al. Laser-induced chorioretinal venous anastomosis for nonischemic central retinal vein occlusion: evaluation of the complications and their risk factors. Am J Ophthalmol 1998; 126:219–229.

89. Browning DJ, Antoszyk AN. Laser chorioretinal venous anastomosis for nonischemic central retinal vein occlusion. Ophthalmology 1998; 105:670–677; discussion 677–679.

90. Peyman GA, Kishore K, Conway MD. Surgical chorioretinal venous anastomosis for ischemic central retinal vein occlusion. Ophthalm Surg Lasers 1999; 30:605–614.

91. Opremcak EM, Bruce RA, Lomeo MD et al. Radial optic neurotomy for central retinal vein occlusion: a retrospective pilot study of 11 consecutive cases. Retina 2001; 21:408–415.

92. Quiroz-Mercado H, Sanchez-Buenfil E, Guerrero-Naranjo JL et al. Successful erbium: YAG laser-induced chorioretinal venous anastomosis for the management of ischemic central retinal vein occlusion. A report of two cases. Graefes Arch Clin Exp Ophthalmol 2001; 239:872–875.

93. Weiss JN, Bynoe LA. Injection of tissue plasminogen activator into a branch retinal vein in eyes with central retinal vein occlusion. Ophthalmology 2001; 108:2249–2257.

94. Park CH, Jaffe GJ, Fekrat S. Intravitreal triamcinolone acetonide in eyes with cystoid macular edema associated with central retinal vein occlusion. Am J Ophthalmol 2003; 136:419–425.

95. Spaide RF, Lee JK, Klancnik JK Jr et al. Optical coherence tomography of branch retinal vein occlusion. Retina 2003; 23:343–347.

96. The Branch Vein Occlusion Study Group. Argon laser photocoagulation for macular edema in branch vein occlusion. Am J Ophthalmol 1984; 98:271–282.

97. Opremcak EM, Bruce RA. Surgical decompression of branch retinal vein occlusion via arteriovenous crossing sheathotomy: a prospective review of 15 cases. Retina 1999; 19:1–5.

98. Shah GK, Sharma S, Fineman MS et al. Arteriovenous adventitial sheathotomy for the treatment of macular edema associated with branch retinal vein occlusion. Am J Ophthalmol 2000; 129:104–106.

99. Fujii GY, de Juan E Jr, Humayun MS. Improvements after sheathotomy for branch retinal vein occlusion documented by optical coherence tomography and scanning laser ophthalmoscope. Ophthalm Surg Lasers Imaging 2003; 34:49–52.

100. Cahill MT, Kaiser PK, Sears JE et al. The effect of arteriovenous sheathotomy on cystoid macular oedema secondary to branch retinal vein occlusion. Br J Ophthalmol 2003; 87:1329–1332.

101. Mason J 3rd, Feist R, White M Jr et al. Sheathotomy to decompress branch retinal vein occlusion: a matched control study. Ophthalmology 2004; 111:540–545.

102. Yamaji H, Shiraga F, Tsuchida Y et al. Evaluation of arteriovenous crossing sheathotomy for branch retinal vein occlusion by fluorescein videoangiography and image analysis. Am J Ophthalmol 2004; 137:834–841.

103. Chen SD, Lochhead J, Patel CK et al. Intravitreal triamcinolone acetonide for ischaemic macular oedema caused by branch retinal vein occlusion. Br J Ophthalmol 2004; 88:154–155.

104. Gass JDM, Blodi BA. Idiopathic justafoveolar retinal telangiectasis: update of classification and follow-up study. Ophthalmology 1986; 100;1536–1546.

105. Mavrofrides EC, Cruz-Villegas V, Puliafito CA. Miscellaneous retinal diseases. In: Schuman JS, Puliafito CA, Fujimoto JG, eds. Optical coherence tomography of ocular diseases. Thorofare, NJ: SLACK, Inc.; 2004:457–482.

106. Conway MD, Canakis C, Livir-Rallatos C et al. Intravitreal triamcinolone acetonide for refractory chronic pseudophakic cystoid macular edema. J Cataract Refract Surg 2003; 29:27–33.

107. Benhamou N, Massin P, Haouchine B et al. Intravitreal triamcinolone for refractory pseudophakic macular edema. Am J Ophthalmol 2003; 135:246–249.

108. Jonas JB, Kreissig I, Degenring RF. Intravitreal triamcinolone acetonide for pseudophakic cystoid macular edema. Am J Ophthalmol 2003; 136:384–386.

109. Marmor MF, Jacobson SG, Foerster MH et al. Diagnostic clinical findings of a new syndrome with night blindness, maculopathy, and enhanced S cone sensitivity. Am J Ophthalmol 1990; 110:124–134.

110. Gass JD. Nicotinic acid maculopathy. Am J Ophthalmol 1973; 76:500–510.

111. Spirn MJ, Warren FA, Guyer DR et al. Optical coherence tomography findings in nicotinic acid maculopathy. Am J Ophthalmol 2003; 135:913–914.

112. Teitelbaum BA, Tresley DJ. Cystic maculopathy with normal capillary permeability secondary to docetaxel. Optom Vis Sci 2003; 80:277–279.

113. Ip M, Garza-Karren C, Duker JS et al. Differentiation of degenerative retinoschisis from retinal detachment using optical coherence tomography. Ophthalmology 1999; 106:600–605.

114. Hassan TS, Sarrafizadeh R, Ruby AJ et al. The effect of duration of macular detachment on results after the scleral buckle repair of primary, macula-off retinal detachments. Ophthalmology 2002; 109:146–152.

115. Villate N, Mavrofrides EC, Davis J. Chorioretinal inflammatory diseases. In: Schuman JS, Puliafito CA, Fujimoto JG, eds. Optical coherence tomography of ocular diseases. Thorofare, NJ: SLACK, Inc.; 2004:371–412.

116. Markomichelakis NN, Halkiadakis I, Pantelia E et al. Patterns of macular edema in patients with uveitis: qualitative and quantitative assessment using optical coherence tomography. Ophthalmology 2004; 111:946–953.

117. Antcliff RJ, Stanford MR, Chauhan DS et al. Comparison between optical coherence tomography and fundus fluorescein angiography for the detection of cystoid macular edema in patients with uveitis. Ophthalmology 2000; 107:593–599.

Chapter

88

Retina-Related Clinical Trials: a Resource Bibliography

Barbara S. Hawkins
Diana V. Do

A major initiative of the National Eye Institute undertaken almost simultaneously with its creation as one of the National Institutes of Health, US Department of Health and Human Services, was the Diabetic Retinopathy Study (DRS), a multi-center randomized clinical trial designed and conducted to evaluate the safety and effectiveness of panretinal photocoagulation with respect to reducing the risk of vision loss and blindness in patients with diabetic retinopathy. The successful completion of that clinical trial not only provided ophthalmologists with a way to reduce the blinding effects of proliferative diabetic retinopathy but also demonstrated that members of the ophthalmologic community could collaborate to evaluate promising treatments for other important ophthalmologic conditions. During the 30-year period since publication of the preliminary findings from the DRS, the National Eye Institute has sponsored many additional clinical trials, most of which concern treatments of retinal conditions or retina-related conditions. During the past decade, the number of ophthalmologic clinical trials completed or initiated in the USA and elsewhere has increased dramatically, with many of the more recent trials undertaken with full or partial support from industrial sponsors. The purpose of this chapter is to provide the retinal specialist with a bibliography of publications in peer-reviewed journals from many of the major retina-related clinical trials. Although other clinical trials in ophthalmology were conducted before the DRS, the focus is on clinical trials, and primarily multicenter clinical trials, that have had outcomes and other findings published since 1975. A brief summary of the key information has been added to the bibliographic reference to articles judged to be of most interest to retinal specialists. The organization of the citations is by specific trials or sets of trials, with clinical trials that focus on the same condition grouped together. The order of the conditions is chronologic by publication of findings from the first major clinical trial in each condition. Whenever a randomized trial was conducted as part of a larger study or preceded by a pilot study, publications from the pilot study or selected publications from the larger study have been included in the bibliography for the clinical trial or set of clinical trials.

DIABETIC RETINOPATHY

Findings from several clinical trials of treatment or prevention of diabetic retinopathy are discussed in Chapters 67 and 68.

Diabetic Retinopathy Study (DRS)

The historical importance of and other information about the DRS are described above. From 1972 through 1975, 1758 patients enrolled at DRS-participating centers.

Diabetic Retinopathy Study Research Group. Preliminary report on effects of photocoagulation therapy. Am J Ophthalmol 1976; 81:383–396.

> With 1732 patients enrolled and one eye of each patient assigned to photocoagulation, visual acuity of 5/200 or worse at two consecutive examinations 4 months apart had been observed in 9% of untreated eyes versus 4% of treated eyes. This finding led to the decision to halt enrollment of new patients, to disseminate the findings to physicians, and to offer panretinal photocoagulation to all untreated eyes deemed to be at high risk of progression and vision loss.

Diabetic Retinopathy Study Research Group. Photocoagulation treatment of proliferative diabetic retinopathy: the second report of Diabetic Retinopathy Study findings. Ophthalmology 1978; 85:82–106.

> A detailed analysis of findings for all patients enrolled confirmed that scatter photocoagulation compared to no treatment reduced severe visual acuity loss and reduced the rate of progression to more severe stages of proliferative diabetic retinopathy. Throughout 3 years of follow-up, treated eyes had approximately half the risk of having visual acuity reduced to 5/200 or worse at two or more consecutive examinations.

Diabetic Retinopathy Study Research Group. Four risk factors for severe visual loss in diabetic retinopathy: the third report from the Diabetic Retinopathy Study. Arch Ophthalmol 1979; 97:654–655.

> Four factors were identified as increasing the risk of severe visual acuity loss: (1) presence of vitreous or preretinal hemorrhage; (2) presence of new vessels; (3) location of new vessels on or near the optic disc; and (4) severity of new vessels. Risk of severe visual acuity loss increased fourfold for eyes with three or more of these factors in comparison to eyes with none of them.

Diabetic Retinopathy Study Research Group. Photocoagulation treatment of proliferative diabetic retinopathy: a short report of long range results. Diabetic Retinopathy Study (DRS) report number four. International Congress series no. 500, Diabetes 1979. In: Waldhausl WK, ed. Proceedings of the 10th Congress of the International Diabetes Federation. Amsterdam: Excerpta Medica; 1979:789–794.

Continued follow-up of DRS patients demonstrated the persistent effects of photocoagulation treatment, with a 50% reduction in severe loss of visual acuity maintained for up to 5 years.

Diabetic Retinopathy Study Research Group. Photocoagulation treatment of proliferative diabetic retinopathy: relationship of adverse treatment effects to retinopathy severity. Diabetic Retinopathy Study report no. 5. Dev Ophthalmol 1981; 2:248–261.

Both xenon arc and argon laser photocoagulation reduced the risk of severe visual loss, outweighing any harmful effects of treatment, even in eyes with severe fibrous proliferation and/or traction retinal detachment. However, xenon arc photocoagulation increased the risk of serious macular damage in eyes with severe fibrous proliferation or localized traction retinal detachment.

Diabetic Retinopathy Study Research Group. Diabetic Retinopathy Study report number 6: design, methods, and baseline results. Invest Ophthalmol Vis Sci 1981; 21:149–208.

Diabetic Retinopathy Study Research Group. Diabetic Retinopathy Study report number 7: a modification of the Airlie House classification of diabetic retinopathy. Invest Ophthalmol Vis Sci 1981; 21:210–226.

Diabetic Retinopathy Study Research Group. Photocoagulation treatment of proliferative diabetic retinopathy. Clinical application of Diabetic Retinopathy Study (DRS) findings. DRS report number 8. Ophthalmology 1981; 88:583–600.

Knatterud GL. Mortality experience in the Diabetic Retinopathy Study. Isr J Med Sci 1983; 19:424–428.

The annual mortality rate among DRS patients was approximately 5% and was higher among those with more advanced retinopathy.

Ederer F, Podgor MJ, the Diabetic Retinopathy Study Research Group. Assessing possible late treatment effects in stopping a clinical trial early: a case study. Diabetic Retinopathy Study report no. 9. Control Clin Trials 1984; 5:373–381.

Rand LI, Prud'homme GJ, Ederer F et al. Factors influencing the development of visual loss in advanced diabetic retinopathy: Diabetic Retinopathy Study (DRS) report no. 10. Invest Ophthalmol Vis Sci 1985; 26:983–991.

Neovascularization of the disc had the strongest association with severe visual acuity loss among untreated eyes.

Kaufman SC, Ferris FL, Swartz M et al. Intraocular pressure following panretinal photocoagulation for diabetic retinopathy: Diabetic Retinopathy report no. 11. Arch Ophthalmol 1987; 105:807–809.

Panretinal photocoagulation reduced the risk of elevated intraocular pressure, possibly preventing the development of neovascular glaucoma.

Ferris FL, Podgor MJ, Davis MD et al. Macular edema in Diabetic Retinopathy Study patients. Diabetic Retinopathy Study report number 12. Ophthalmology 1987; 94:754–760.

Although panretinal photocoagulation was associated with some loss of visual acuity soon after treatment, especially in eyes with pre-existing macular edema, the long-term benefits of panretinal photocoagulation outweighed the risk of visual loss.

Kaufman SC, Ferris FL, Seigel DG et al. Factors associated with visual outcome after photocoagulation for diabetic retinopathy: Diabetic Retinopathy Study report no. 13. Invest Ophthalmol Vis Sci 1989; 30:23–28.

Despite panretinal photocoagulation, the risk for severe visual loss rose with increasing neovascularization on the disc, hemorrhages/microaneurysms, retinal elevation, proteinuria, and hyperglycemia, and fell with increasing photocoagulation treatment density.

Diabetic Retinopathy Study Research Group. Indications for photocoagulation treatment of diabetic retinopathy: Diabetic Retinopathy Study report no. 14. Int Ophthalmol Clin 1987; 27:239–253.

The most important indicators for panretinal photocoagulation are the presence of high-risk characteristics of proliferative retinopathy defined earlier in DRS report number 3.

UK Multicentre Controlled Study

This randomized trial of xenon arc photocoagulation for diabetic maculopathy was conducted concurrently with the DRS; initial findings were published shortly after the first publication from the DRS. This multicenter trial was sponsored by the British Diabetic Association and the Wellcome Trust.

Multicentre Controlled Study Coordinating Committee. Photocoagulation treatment of diabetic maculopathy. Interim report of a multicentre controlled study. Lancet 1975; 2:1110–1113.

Photocoagulation with the xenon arc led to less deterioration in visual acuity than no treatment. Initiation of treatment was recommended before visual acuity was "seriously impaired."

Multicentre Controlled Study Coordinating Committee. Proliferative diabetic retinopathy: treatment with xenon-arc photocoagulation. Interim report of multicentre controlled randomised controlled trial. Br Med J 1977; 1:739–741.

Photocoagulation with the xenon arc led to less monocular blindness than no treatment. New vessels on the disc regressed more in treated eyes than in untreated eyes.

Diabetic Retinopathy Vitrectomy Study (DRVS)

The primary goal of the DRVS, a multicenter randomized clinical trial, was to compare early vitrectomy with conventional management of severe vitreous hemorrhage secondary to diabetic retinopathy. As with most other multicenter clinical trials, data regarding the natural history of patients in the control arm were of interest. Patient accrual began in October 1976 and ended in June 1983. The DRVS was sponsored by the National Eye Institute, National Institutes of Health, US Department of Health and Human Services.

Diabetic Retinopathy Vitrectomy Study Research Group. Two-year course of visual acuity in severe proliferative diabetic retinopathy with conventional management. Diabetic Retinopathy Vitrectomy Study (DRVS) report no. 1. Ophthalmology 1985; 92:492–502.

> After 2 years of follow-up, visual acuity of eyes assigned to conventional treatment was worse than 5/200 in 45% of eyes with more than four disc areas of new vessels and visual acuity of 10/30 to 10/50 at baseline.

Diabetic Retinopathy Vitrectomy Study Research Group. Early vitrectomy for severe vitreous hemorrhage in diabetic retinopathy. Two-year results of a randomized trial. Diabetic Retinopathy Vitrectomy Study report 2. Arch Ophthalmol 1985; 103:1644–1652.

> Visual acuity was 10/20 or better in 25% of the early vitrectomy group compared with 15% of the deferral group after 2 years of follow-up.

Diabetic Retinopathy Vitrectomy Study Research Group. Early vitrectomy for severe proliferative diabetic retinopathy in eyes with useful vision. Results of a randomized trial – Diabetic Retinopathy Vitrectomy Study report 3. Ophthalmology 1988; 95:1307–1320.

> After 4 years of follow-up, 44% of the early vitrectomy group versus 28% of the conventional management group had visual acuity of 10/20 or better.

Diabetic Retinopathy Vitrectomy Study Research Group. Early vitrectomy for severe proliferative diabetic retinopathy in eyes with useful vision. Clinical application of results of a randomized trial – Diabetic Retinopathy Vitrectomy Study report 4. Ophthalmology 1988; 95:1321–1334.

> Six cases illustrate when early vitrectomy should be considered in eyes with advanced, active, proliferative diabetic retinopathy.

Diabetic Retinopathy Vitrectomy Study Research Group. Early vitrectomy for severe vitreous hemorrhage in diabetic retinopathy. Four-year results of a randomized trial: Diabetic Retinopathy Vitrectomy Study report 5. Arch Ophthalmol 1990; 108:958–964, 1452.

> After 4 years of follow-up, more eyes in the early vitrectomy arm than in the deferral arm continued to have visual acuity of 10/20 or better.

Early Treatment Diabetic Retinopathy Study (ETDRS)

The ETDRS was designed to evaluate the effectiveness of laser photocoagulation and aspirin, together and singly, in delaying or preventing progression of early diabetic retinopathy to more severe stages and blindness and to determine the optimum time to initiate photocoagulation in diabetic retinopathy. This multicenter clinical trial was sponsored by the National Eye Institute, National Institutes of Health, US Department of Health and Human Services. Enrollment of patients began in December 1979 and ended in July 1985 with 3711 patients enrolled. Clinical follow-up of ETDRS patients ended in 1989.

Initiation of the ETDRS was a motivating factor in the development of a new visual acuity chart for use in prospective clinical research studies; it has been used in many subsequent clinical trials. Articles that report on the design and evaluation of the chart are included at the end of the ETDRS bibliography.

Early Treatment Diabetic Retinopathy Study Research Group. Photocoagulation for diabetic macular edema. Early Treatment Diabetic Retinopathy Study report number 1. Arch Ophthalmol 1985; 103:1796–1806.

> Eyes with clinically significant macular edema benefited from focal photocoagulation and were about half as likely to lose three or more lines of vision compared with eyes assigned to deferral of photocoagulation.

Early Treatment Diabetic Retinopathy Study Research Group. Treatment techniques and clinical guidelines for photocoagulation of diabetic macular edema. Early Treatment Diabetic Retinopathy Study report number 2. Ophthalmology 1987; 94:761–774.

Early Treatment Diabetic Retinopathy Study Research Group. Techniques for scatter and local photocoagulation treatment of diabetic retinopathy: Early Treatment Diabetic Retinopathy Study report no. 3. Int Ophthalmol Clin 1987; 27:254–264.

Early Treatment Diabetic Retinopathy Study Research Group. Photocoagulation for diabetic macular edema: Early Treatment Diabetic Retinopathy Study report no. 4. Int Ophthalmol Clin 1987; 27:265–272.

> This report summarizes ETDRS reports number 1 and number 2.

Early Treatment Diabetic Retinopathy Study Research Group. Case reports to accompany Early Treatment Diabetic Retinopathy Study reports 3 and 4. Int Ophthalmol Clin 1987; 27:273–334.

Kinyoun J, Barton F, Fisher M et al. Detection of diabetic macular edema: ophthalmoscopy versus photography – Early Treatment Diabetic Retinopathy Study report number 5. Ophthalmology 1989; 96:746–751.

There was close agreement between retinal specialists (using contact lens biomicroscopy) and photographic graders (using stereoscopic color fundus photographs) in detecting diabetic macular edema.

Prior MJ, Prout T, Miller D et al. C-peptide and the classification of diabetes mellitus patients in the Early Treatment Diabetic Retinopathy Study: report number 6. Ann Epidemiol 1993; 3:9–17.

Early Treatment Diabetic Retinopathy Study Research Group. Early Treatment Diabetic Retinopathy Study design and baseline patient characteristics. ETDRS report number 7. Ophthalmology 1991; 98:741–756.

Early Treatment Diabetic Retinopathy Study Research Group. Effects of aspirin treatment on diabetic retinopathy: ETDRS report number 8. Ophthalmology 1991; 98:757–765.

Aspirin (650 mg/day) had no clinically beneficial or harmful effects in patients with retinopathy.

Early Treatment Diabetic Retinopathy Study Research Group. Early photocoagulation for diabetic retinopathy: ETDRS report number 9. Ophthalmology 1991; 98:766–785.

Initiation of scatter photocoagulation was recommended for eyes with high-risk proliferative retinopathy. Whenever possible, scatter photocoagulation should be applied after completion of focal laser in eyes with macular edema.

Early Treatment Diabetic Retinopathy Study Research Group. Grading diabetic retinopathy from stereoscopic color fundus photographs – an extension of the modified Airlie House classification. ETDRS report number 10. Ophthalmology 1991; 98:786–806.

Early Treatment Diabetic Retinopathy Study Research Group. Classification of diabetic retinopathy from fluorescein angiograms. ETDRS report number 11. Ophthalmology 1991; 98:807–822.

Early Treatment Diabetic Retinopathy Study Research Group. Fundus photographic risk factors for progression of diabetic retinopathy: ETDRS report number 12. Ophthalmology 1991; 98:823–833.

Severity of intraretinal microvascular abnormalities, hemorrhages and/or microaneurysms, and venous beading were the most important factors in predicting progression to proliferative diabetic retinopathy.

Early Treatment Diabetic Retinopathy Study Research Group. Fluorescein angiographic risk factors for progression of diabetic retinopathy: ETDRS report number 13. Ophthalmology 1991; 98:834–840.

Fluorescein leakage, capillary loss and dilation, and various arteriolar abnormalities were associated with progression to proliferative retinopathy.

Early Treatment Diabetic Retinopathy Study Investigators. Aspirin effects on mortality and morbidity in patients with diabetes mellitus: Early Treatment Diabetic Retinopathy Study report 14. JAMA 1992; 268:1292–1300.

Fong DS, Barton FB, Bresnick GH et al. Impaired color vision associated with diabetic retinopathy: Early Treatment Diabetic Retinopathy Study report no. 15. Am J Ophthalmol 1999; 128:612–617.

Chew EY, Williams GA, Burton TC et al. Aspirin effects on the development of cataracts in patients with diabetes mellitus: Early Treatment Diabetic Retinopathy Study report 16. Arch Ophthalmol 1992; 110:339–342.

Flynn HW, Chew EY, Simons BD et al. Pars plana vitrectomy in the Early Treatment Diabetic Retinopathy Study. ETDRS report number 17. Ophthalmology 1992; 99:1351–1357.

Baseline characteristics and visual outcomes in patients who underwent vitrectomy were presented. The 5-year cumulative rate of vitrectomy was 5%; visual acuity was 20/100 or better in 48% of eyes.

Ferris FL. Early photocoagulation in patients with either type I or type II diabetes. Tr Am Ophth Soc 1996; 94:505–536.

Patients with type 2 diabetes were more likely to benefit from early scatter photocoagulation than patients with type 1 diabetes based on analysis of data from both the DRS and ETDRS.

Davis MD, Fisher MR, Gangnon RE et al. Risk factors for high-risk proliferative diabetic retinopathy and severe visual loss: Early Treatment Diabetic Retinopathy Study report no. 18. Invest Ophthalmol Vis Sci 1998; 39:233–252.

The most important risk factor for severe visual acuity loss was earlier development of high-risk proliferative diabetic retinopathy.

Early Treatment Diabetic Retinopathy Study Research Group. Focal photocoagulation treatment of diabetic macular edema. Relationship of treatment effect to fluorescein angiographic and other retinal characteristics at baseline: ETDRS report no. 19. Arch Ophthalmol 1995; 113:1144–1155.

Chew EY, Klein ML, Murphy RP et al. Effects of aspirin on vitreous/preretinal hemorrhage in patients with diabetes mellitus: Early Treatment Diabetic Retinopathy Study report no. 20. Arch Ophthalmol 1995; 113:52–55.

Use of aspirin did not increase the occurrence of vitreous or preretinal hemorrhage.

Braun CI, Benson WE, Remaley NA et al. Accommodative amplitudes in the Early Treatment Diabetic Retinopathy Study. ETDRS report number 21. Retina 1995; 15:275–281.

Chew EY, Klein ML, Ferris FL et al. Association of elevated serum lipid levels with retinal hard exudate in diabetic retinopathy: Early Treatment Diabetic Retinopathy Study (ETDRS) report 22. Arch Ophthalmol 1996; 114:1079–1084.
    Patients with elevated total serum cholesterol or serum low-density lipoprotein were twice as likely to have retinal hard exudates as patients with normal levels.

Fong DS, Segal PP, Myers F et al. Subretinal fibrosis in diabetic macular edema. ETDRS report 23. Arch Ophthalmol 1997; 115:873–877.
    Subretinal fibrosis is an infrequent complication of diabetic macular edema but developed in eyes with very severe hard exudates.

Fong DS, Ferris FL, Davis MD et al. Causes of severe visual loss in the Early Treatment Diabetic Retinopathy Study: ETDRS report no. 24. Am J Ophthalmol 1999; 127:137–141.
    Persistent severe visual loss was an infrequent occurrence and was most commonly caused by vitreous hemorrhage or preretinal hemorrhage, macular edema, or macular pigmentary changes.

Chew EY, Benson WE, Remaley NA et al. Results after lens extraction in patients with diabetic retinopathy: Early Treatment Diabetic Retinopathy Study report number 25. Arch Ophthalmol 1999; 117:1600–1606.
    Visual improvement was seen in 55% of patients at 1 year after cataract extraction. The main reasons for poor visual results after surgery were complications of macular edema and/or proliferative retinopathy.

Barton FB, Fong DS, Knatterud GL et al. Classification of Farnsworth-Munsell 100-hue test results in the Early Treatment Diabetic Retinopathy Study. Am J Ophthalmol 2004; 138:119–124.

Ferris FL, Kassoff A, Bresnick GH et al. New visual acuity charts for clinical research. Am J Ophthalmol 1982; 94:91–96.

Ferris FL, Sperduto RD. Standardized illumination for visual acuity testing in clinical research. Am J Ophthalmol 1982; 94:97–98.

Ferris FL, Freidlin V, Kassoff A et al. Relative letter and position difficulty on visual acuity charts from the Early Treatment Diabetic Retinopathy Study. Am J Ophthalmol 1993; 116:735–740.

Sorbinil Retinopathy Trial (SRT)

The SRT was sponsored by the National Eye Institute, National Institutes of Health, US Department of Health and Human Services and by Pfizer. Patient accrual began in August 1983 and ended in October 1986 with 497 patients enrolled.

Sorbinil Retinopathy Trial Research Group. A randomized trial of sorbinil, an aldose reductase inhibitor, in diabetic retinopathy. Arch Ophthalmol 1990; 108:1234–1244.
    Sorbinil, as administered in the SRT, did not have a clinically important effect on the course of diabetic retinopathy in adults with insulin-dependent diabetes.

Sorbinil Retinopathy Trial Research Group. The Sorbinil Retinopathy Trial: neuropathy results. Neurology 1993; 43:1141–1149.

Cohen RA, Hennekens CH, Christen WG et al. Determinants of retinopathy progression in type 1 diabetes mellitus. Am J Med 1999; 107:45–51.

Christen WG, Manson JE, Bubes V et al. Risk factors for progression of distal symmetric polyneuropathy in type 1 diabetes mellitus. Am J Epidemiol 1999; 150:1142–1151.

Krypton Argon Regression of Neovascularization Study (KARNS)

The KARNS was a multicenter clinical trial with the primary goal of comparing krypton red laser with argon blue-green laser for panretinal photocoagulation with respect to regression of disc neovascularization in diabetic retinopathy. KARNS was sponsored by the National Eye Institute, National Institutes of Health, US Department of Health and Human Services. Patient accrual began in December 1984 and was completed in June 1990 after 798 patients (1053 eyes) had been enrolled.

Singerman LJ, Ferris FL, Mowery RP et al. Krypton laser for proliferative diabetic retinopathy: the Krypton Argon Regression of Neovascularization Study. J Diab Complications 1988; 2:189–196.

Krypton Argon Regression of Neovascularization Study Research Group. Randomized comparison of krypton versus argon scatter photocoagulation for diabetic disc neovascularization. Ophthalmology 1993; 100:1655–1664.
    Scatter photocoagulation with either krypton red or argon blue-green laser was equally effective in the treatment of proliferative diabetic retinopathy.

Diabetes Control and Complications Trial (DCCT)

The DCCT was a multicenter randomized clinical trial designed to compare intensive with conventional diabetes therapy with respect to development and progression of early vascular and neurologic complications of insulin-dependent diabetes mellitus. Patient accrual continued from 1983 through 1989 at the 29 participating clinical centers. The DCCT was sponsored by the National Institute of Diabetes and Digestive and Kidney Diseases, the National Heart, Lung, and Blood Institute, the National Eye

Institute, and the National Center for Research Resources (National Institutes of Health, US Department of Health and Human Services) and various corporate sponsors. A follow-up study of members of the DCCT cohort, the Epidemiology of Diabetes Interventions and Complications (EDIC), was undertaken to assess the long-term effects of intensive and conventional diabetes therapy during the DCCT.

Diabetes Control and Complications Trial Research Group. The Diabetes Control and Complications Trial (DCCT): design and methodologic considerations for the feasibility phase. Diabetes 1986; 35:530–545.

Diabetes Control and Complications Trial Research Group. The Diabetes Control and Complications Trial (DCCT): results of feasibility study. Diabetes Care 1987; 10:1–10.

Diabetes Control and Complications Trial Research Group. Feasibility of centralized measurements of glycated hemoglobin in the Diabetes Control and Complications Trial, a multicenter study. Clin Chem 1987; 33:2267–2271.

Diabetes Control and Complications Trial Research Group. Implementation of a multicomponent process to obtain informed consent in the Diabetes Control and Complications Trial. Control Clin Trials 1989; 10:83–96.

Diabetes Control and Complications Trial Research Group. The effect of intensive treatment of diabetes on the development and progression of long-term complications in insulin-dependent diabetes mellitus. N Engl J Med 1993; 329:977–986.
    Relative to rates in the conventional treatment arm, intensive therapy reduced onset and progression of diabetic retinopathy by 76% and 54%, respectively, occurrence of nephropathy by 54%, and onset of neuropathy by 60%.

Diabetes Control and Complications Trial Research Group. Expanded role of the dietician in the Diabetes Control and Complications Trial: implications for clinical practice. J Am Diet Assoc 1993; 93:758–764, 767.

Diabetes Control and Complications Trial Research Group. Nutrition interventions for intensive therapy in the Diabetes Control and Complications Trial. J Am Diet Assoc 1993; 93:768–772.

Diabetes Control and Complications Trial Research Group. Effect of intensive diabetes treatment on the development and progression of long-term complications in adolescents with insulin-dependent diabetes mellitus: Diabetes Control and Complications Trial. J Pediatr 1994; 125:177–188.
    In the DCCT cohort of young patients (13 to 17 years old), intensive control reduced the risk of development and progression of retinopathy compared to conventional treatment by 53% and 70%.

Diabetes Control and Complications Trial Research Group. A screening algorithm to identify clinically significant changes in neuropsychological functions in the Diabetes Control and Complications Trial. J Clin Exp Neuropsychol 1994; 16:303–316.

Diabetes Control and Complications Trial Research Group. The effect of intensive diabetes treatment on the progression of diabetic retinopathy in insulin-dependent diabetes mellitus. The Diabetes Control and Complications Trial. Arch Ophthalmol 1995; 113:36–51.
    Intensive therapy significantly reduced the risk of a three-step progression of retinopathy to 12% compared to 54% in the conventional therapy group.

Diabetes Control and Complications Trial Research Group. Progression of retinopathy with intensive versus conventional treatment in the Diabetes Control and Complications Trial. Ophthalmology 1995; 102:647–661.
    Intensive therapy reduced the risk of development of any retinopathy to 70% from 90% in the conventional treatment arm and also reduced the risk of progression. Intensive therapy was most effective when initiated early after diagnosis of insulin-dependent diabetes mellitus.

Diabetes Control and Complications Trial Research Group. Implementation of treatment protocols in the Diabetes Control and Complications Trial. Diabetes Care 1995; 18:361–376.

Diabetes Control and Complications Trial (DCCT) Research Group. Effect of intensive diabetes management on macrovascular events and risk factors in the Diabetes Control and Complications Trial. Am J Cardiol 1995; 75:894–903.

Diabetes Control and Complications Trial Research Group. The relationship of glycemic exposure (HbA$_{1c}$) to the risk of development and progression of retinopathy in the Diabetes Control and Complications Trial. Diabetes 1995; 44:968–983.

Diabetes Control and Complications Trial (DCCT) Research Group. Effect of intensive diabetes treatment on nerve conduction in the Diabetes Control and Complications Trial. Ann Neurol 1995; 38:869–880.

Diabetes Control and Complications Trial Research Group. Influence of intensive diabetes treatment on quality-of-life outcomes in the Diabetes Control and Complications Trial. Diabetes Care 1996; 19:195–203.
    No difference between patients on conventional treatment and those on intensive treatment was found with respect to quality of life, psychiatric symptom indices, or psychosocial events.

Diabetes Control and Complications Trial Research Group. The absence of a glycemic threshold for the development of long-term complications: the perspective of the Diabetes Control and Complications Trial. Diabetes 1996; 45:1289–1298.

Diabetes Control and Complications Trial Research Group. Lifetime benefits and costs of intensive therapy as practiced in the Diabetes Control and Complications Trial. JAMA 1996; 276:1400–1415.

Diabetes Control and Complications Trial Research Group. Pregnancy outcomes in the Diabetes Control and Complications Trial. Am J Obstet Gynecol 1996; 174:1343–1353.

Diabetes Control and Complications Trial Research Group. Effect of intensive therapy on residual β-cell function in patients with type I diabetes in the Diabetes Control and Complications Trial. Ann Intern Med 1998; 128:517–523.

Diabetes Control and Complications Trial Research Group. Early worsening of diabetic retinopathy in the Diabetes Control and Complications Trial. Arch Ophthalmol 1998; 116:874–886.

> Worsening of diabetic retinopathy during the first year after entry was observed among nearly twice as many patients in the intensive treatment arm as in the conventional treatment arm. The long-term benefits of intensive treatment outweighed the early risks.

Epidemiology of Diabetes Interventions and Complications (EDIC) Research Group. Design, implementation, and preliminary results of a long-term follow-up of the Diabetes Control and Complications Trial cohort. Diabetes Care 1999; 22:99–111.

Epidemiology of Diabetes Interventions and Complications (EDIC) Research Group. Effect of intensive diabetes treatment on carotid artery wall thickness in the Epidemiology of Diabetes Interventions and Complications. Diabetes 1999; 48:383–390.

Diabetes Control and Complications Trial/Epidemiology of Diabetes Interventions and Complications Research Group. Retinopathy and nephropathy in patients with type I diabetes four years after a trial of intensive therapy. N Engl J Med 2000; 342:381–389.

> The intensive therapy group continued to demonstrate a persistent reduction in the risk of progressive retinopathy and nephropathy compared to conventional therapy group 4 years after the conclusion of the DCCT.

Diabetes Control and Complications Trial Research Group. Effect of pregnancy on microvascular complications in the Diabetes Control and Complications Trial. Diabetes Care 2000; 23:1084–1091.

Diabetes Control and Complications Trial (DCCT)/Epidemiology of Diabetes Interventions and Complications (EDIC) Research Group. Beneficial effects of intensive therapy of diabetes during adolescence: outcomes after the conclusion of the Diabetes Control and Complications Trial (DCCT). J Pediatr 2001; 139:804–812.

Diabetes Control and Complications Trials Research Group. Influence of intensive diabetes treatment on body weight and composition of adults with type 1 diabetes in the Diabetes Control and Complications Trial. Diabetes Care 2001; 24:1711–1721.

Writing Team for the Diabetes Control and Complications Trial/Epidemiology of Diabetes Interventions and Complications Research Group. Effect of intensive therapy on the microvascular complications of type 1 diabetes mellitus. JAMA 2002; 287:2563–2569.

Diabetes Control and Complications Trials/Epidemiology of Diabetes Interventions and Complications Research Group. Intensive diabetes therapy and carotid intima-media thickness in type 1 diabetes mellitus. N Engl J Med 2003; 348:2294–2303.

Lyons TJ, Jenkins AJ, Zheng D et al. Diabetic retinopathy and serum lipoprotein subclasses in the DCCT/EDIC cohort. Invest Ophthalmol Vis Sci 2004; 45:910–918.

> The severity of retinopathy was positively associated with triglycerides and negatively associated with high-density lipoprotein cholesterol. In men, retinopathy was also positively associated with low-density lipoprotein cholesterol.

UK Prospective Diabetes Study (UKPDS)

United Kingdom Prospective Diabetes Study Group. UK Prospective Study of Therapies of Maturity-Onset Diabetes. I: Effect of diet, sulphonylurea, insulin or biguanide therapy on fasting plasma glucose and body weight over 1 year. Diabetelogia 1983; 24:404–411.

United Kingdom Prospective Study Group. United Kingdom Prospective Diabetes Study. III. Prevalence of hypertension and hypotensive therapy in patients with newly diagnosed diabetes. Hypertension 1985; 7(suppl 2):8–13.

United Kingdom Prospective Study Group. United Kingdom Prospective Diabetes Study. IV. Characteristics of newly-presenting type 2 diabetic patients: male preponderance and obesity at different ages. Diabetic Med 1988; 5:154–159.

United Kingdom Prospective Diabetes Study Group. United Kingdom Prospective Diabetes Study. VI. Complications in newly diagnosed type 2 diabetic patients and their association with different clinical and biochemical risk factors. Diabetes Res 1990; 13:1–11.

United Kingdom Prospective Diabetes Study Group. UK Prospective Diabetes Study 7: Response of fasting glucose to diet therapy in newly presenting type II diabetic patients. Metabolism 1990; 39:905–912.

United Kingdom Prospective Diabetes Study Group. UK Prospective Diabetes Study (UKPDS): VIII. Study design, progress and performance. Diabetologia 1991; 34:877–890.

United Kingdom Prospective Diabetes Study Group. UK Prospective Diabetes Study IX: Relationships of urinary albumin and N-acetylglucosaminidase to glycemia and hypertension at diagnosis of type 2 (non-insulin-dependent) diabetes mellitus and after 3 months diet therapy. Diabetologia 1992; 36:835–842.

United Kingdom Prospective Diabetes Study Group. UK Prospective Diabetes Study (UKPDS) X: Urinary albumin excretion over 3 years in diet-treated type 2 (non-insulin-dependent) diabetic patients and association with hypertension, hyperglycaemia and hypertriglyceridaemia. Diabetologia 1993; 36:1021–1029.

United Kingdom Prospective Diabetes Study Group. UK Prospective Diabetes Study (UKPDS). XI: Biochemical risk factors in type II diabetic patients at diagnosis compared with age matched normal subjects. Diabetic Med 1994; 11:534–544.

United Kingdom Prospective Diabetes Study Group. UK Prospective Diabetes Study (UKPDS) XII. Differences between Asian, Afro-Caribbean, and White Caucasian type 2 diabetic patients at diagnosis of diabetes. Diabetic Med 1994; 11:670–677.

United Kingdom Prospective Diabetes Study Group. United Kingdom Prospective Diabetes Study (UKPDS) 13: relative efficacy of randomly allocated diet, sulphonylurea, insulin, or metformin in patients with newly diagnosed non-insulin dependent diabetes followed for three years. Br J Med 1995; 310:83–88.

United Kingdom Prospective Diabetes Study Group. UK Prospective Diabetes Study 16: overview of 6 years' therapy of type 2 diabetes: a progressive disease. Diabetes 1995; 44:1249–1258.

United Kingdom Prospective Diabetes Study Group. UK Prospective Diabetes Study 17: a nine-year update of a randomized, controlled trial on the effect of improved metabolic control on complications in non-insulin-dependent diabetes mellitus. Ann Intern Med 1996; 124:136–145.

United Kingdom Prospective Diabetes Study Group. UK Prospective Diabetes Study 23: risk factors for coronary artery disease in non-insulin dependent diabetes. Br Med J 1998; 316:823–828.

United Kingdom Prospective Diabetes Study Group. UK Prospective Diabetes Study 24: relative efficacy of sulfonylurea, insulin and metformin therapy in newly diagnosed non-insulin-dependent diabetes with primary diet failure followed for six years. Ann Intern Med 1998; 128:165–175.

United Kingdom Prospective Diabetes Study Group. UK Prospective Diabetes Study 26: sulphonylurea failure in non-insulin-dependent diabetic patients over 6 years. Diabet Med 1998; 15:297–303.

United Kingdom Prospective Diabetes Study Group. UK Prospective Diabetes Study 28: a randomized trial of efficacy of early addition of metformin in sylphonylurea-treated non-insulin-dependent diabetes. Diabetes Care 1998; 21:87–92.

Kohner EM, Aldington SJ, Stratton IM et al. United Kingdom Prospective Diabetes Study, 30: Diabetic retinopathy at diagnosis of non-insulin-dependent diabetes mellitus and associated risk factors. Arch Ophthalmol 1998; 116:297–303.
    Retinopathy was present in 39% of men and 35% of women with newly diagnosed noninsulin-dependent diabetes.

United Kingdom Prospective Diabetes Study Group. Intensive blood-glucose control with sulphonylureas or insulin compared with conventional treatment and risk of complications in patients with type 2 diabetes (UKPDS 33). Lancet 1998; 352:837–853.
    Over a 10 year period, a 25% risk reduction in microvascular endpoints was observed in the intensive treatment group (median hemoglobin (Hb) A_{1c} 7.0%) compared with the conventional treatment group (median HbA_{1c} 7.9%).

United Kingdom Prospective Diabetes Study Group. Effect of intensive blood glucose control with metformin on complications in overweight patients with type 2 diabetes (UKPDS 34). Lancet 1998; 352:854–865.

United Kingdom Prospective Diabetes Study (UKPDS) Group. Tight blood pressure control and risk of macrovascular and microvascular complications in type 2 diabetes: UKPDS 38. Br Med J 1998; 317:705–713.
    Tight blood pressure control (mean, 144/82 mmHg) compared to lesser control (mean, 154/87 mmHg) reduced progression rates of diabetic retinopathy and deterioration of visual acuity.

United Kingdom Prospective Diabetes Study Group. Efficacy of atenolol and captopril in reducing risk of macrovascular and microvascular complications in type 2 diabetes: UKPDS 39. Br Med J 1998; 317:713–720.
    Similar proportions of patients assigned to atenolol and to captopril had diabetic retinopathy that worsened by two grades after 9 years: 37% and 31%, respectively.

United Kingdom Prospective Diabetes Study Group. Cost effectiveness of improved blood glucose control in hypertensive patients with type 2 diabetes: UKPDS 40. Br Med J 1998; 317:720–726.

Stratton IM, Kohner EM, Aldington SJ et al. UKPDS 50: Risk factors for incidence and progression of retinopathy in type II diabetes over 6 years from diagnosis. Diabetologia 2001; 44:156–163.

Of 1216 patients without retinopathy at diagnosis of type 2 diabetes, 22% had developed retinopathy (microaneurysms or worse in both eyes) by 6 years after diagnosis. HbA_{1c} was strongly associated with incidence and, especially, progression of retinopathy. Incidence of retinopathy was also strongly associated with incidence of retinopathy. However, smoking was associated with a reduced incidence of retinopathy.

Gray A, Clarke P, Farmer A et al. Implementing intensive control of blood glucose concentration and blood pressure in type 2 diabetes in England: cost analysis (UKPDS 63). Br Med J 2002; 325:860–865.

VEIN OCCLUSIONS

Branch Vein Occlusion Study (BVOS)

The BVOS was a multicenter randomized clinical trial designed to assess in eyes with retinal branch vein occlusion whether scatter photocoagulation with the argon laser could prevent development of neovascularization and peripheral scatter photocoagulation could prevent vitreous hemorrhage, and whether macular photocoagulation could improve visual acuity in eyes with macular edema and visual acuity of 20/40 or worse. The first patient enrolled in July 1977; the last enrollment was in February 1985. The BVOS was sponsored by the National Eye Institute, National Institutes of Health, US Department of Health and Human Services. BVOS findings are discussed in Chapter 71.

Finkelstein D, Clarkson J, Diddie K et al. Branch vein occlusion: retinal neovascularization outside the involved segment. Ophthalmology 1982; 89:1357–1361.

Peripheral retinal neovascularization developed within normal retina in 4 of 366 BVOS cases.

Branch Vein Occlusion Study Group. Argon laser photocoagulation for macular edema in branch vein occlusion. Am J Ophthalmol 1984; 98:271–282.

Argon laser photocoagulation improved visual acuity in eyes with macular edema secondary to retinal branch vein occlusion, macular edema, and visual acuity of 20/40 or worse, with a gain of at least two lines of visual acuity in more laser-treated eyes compared to untreated eyes.

Branch Vein Occlusion Study Group. Argon laser scatter photocoagulation for prevention of neovascularization and vitreous hemorrhage in branch vein occlusion: a randomized clinical trial. Arch Ophthalmol 1986; 104:34–41.

Peripheral scatter argon laser photocoagulation decreased the risk of vitreous hemorrhage compared to untreated eyes. In addition, scatter treatment before development of neovascularization was shown not to be beneficial; treatment after development of neovascularization was recommended.

Central Vein Occlusion Study (CVOS)

The CVOS included two randomized trials and two observational studies in its design. The goals of the CVOS were: (1) to determine whether photocoagulation therapy could prevent iris neovascularization in eyes with central vein occlusion and evidence of ischemic retina; (2) to assess whether grid photocoagulation could reduce loss of central visual acuity due to macular edema secondary to central vein occlusion; (3) to describe the course and prognosis for eyes with central vein occlusion. Patient accrual began in August 1988 and ended in July 1992. Patients were divided into four groups at entry: (1) perfused; (2) nonperfused; (3) indeterminate perfusion; or (4) macular edema. The CVOS was sponsored by the National Eye Institute, National Institutes of Health, US Department of Health and Human Services. Findings from the CVOS are discussed in Chapter 70.

Central Vein Occlusion Study Group. Central Vein Occlusion Study of photocoagulation therapy. Baseline findings. Online J Curr Clin Trials 1993; 95:1087–1095.

Central Vein Occlusion Study Group. Baseline and early natural history report. The Central Vein Occlusion Study. Arch Ophthalmol 1993; 111:1087–1095.

Of 46 eyes in the indeterminate perfusion group, 83% had at least 10 disc areas of nonperfusion (28 eyes) or iris or angle neovascularization developed before retinal status could be assessed (10 eyes). Among 522 of 547 eyes in the perfused group with a 4-month examination, 30 eyes had iris or angle neovascularization and 51 more had evidence of at least 10 disc areas of nonperfusion.

Central Vein Occlusion Study Group. Evaluation of grid pattern photocoagulation for macular edema in central vein occlusion. The Central Vein Occlusion Study Group M report. Ophthalmology 1995; 102:1425–1433.

Macular grid photocoagulation reduced macular edema but did not provide a better visual acuity outcome than no treatment.

Central Vein Occlusion Study Group. A randomized clinical trial of early panretinal photocoagulation for ischemic central vein occlusion. The Central Vein Occlusion Study Group N report. Ophthalmology 1995; 102:1434–1444.

Prophylactic panretinal photocoagulation decreased development of angle neovascularization or 2 or more clock-hours of iris neovascularization but did not prevent neovascularization. These findings suggest that photocoagulation should be administered at the time neovascularization is detected.

Central Vein Occlusion Study Group. Natural history and clinical management of central retinal vein occlusion. Arch Ophthalmol 1997; 115:486–491.

Findings are presented for 714 of 725 patients to document the natural history and outcomes with laser photocoagulation. Baseline visual acuity was a strong predictor of 3-year visual acuity for patients with good (20/40 or better) or poor (20/200 or worse) visual acuity initially and a strong predictor for development of iris or angle neovascularization. One-third of initially perfused eyes converted to nonperfusion.

AGE-RELATED MACULAR DEGENERATION AND OTHER CONDITIONS ASSOCIATED WITH CHOROIDAL NEOVASCULARIZATION

Findings from many of the trials listed below are discussed in Chapters 61 and 99.

Macular Photocoagulation Study (MPS)

The MPS was initiated in 1979 under the sponsorship of the National Eye Institute, National Institutes of Health, US Department of Health and Human Services, to evaluate laser photocoagulation for choroidal neovascularization secondary to age-related macular degeneration and ocular histoplasmosis. In addition, small trials of laser photocoagulation for idiopathic choroidal neovascularization were conducted. The MPS consisted of three multicenter randomized trials of argon laser photocoagulation of extrafoveal choroidal neovascularization (begun in 1979), three trials of krypton laser photocoagulation for juxtafoveal neovascular lesions (begun in 1981), and two trials of laser photocoagulation (with a second randomization of eyes assigned to laser photocoagulation between argon green and krypton red laser) of subfoveal choroidal neovascularization secondary to age-related macular degeneration only (begun in 1985).

Macular Photocoagulation Study Group. Argon laser photocoagulation for senile macular degeneration: results of a randomized clinical trial. Arch Ophthalmol 1982; 100:912–918.

After fewer than half the eyes in each treatment arm had been followed for 1 year, a substantial difference between laser-treated and untreated eyes was observed with respect to severe loss of visual acuity from the baseline levels (loss of six or more lines on a logMar chart): 25% versus 60%. This trial was the first to demonstrate the effectiveness of any treatment for choroidal neovascularization with respect to delaying or preventing loss of visual acuity.

Macular Photocoagulation Study Group. Argon laser photocoagulation for ocular histoplasmosis: results of a randomized clinical trial. Arch Ophthalmol 1983; 101:1347–1357.

Laser photocoagulation of extrafoveal choroidal neovascularization was even more effective in eyes with ocular histoplasmosis than in eyes with age-related macular degeneration. By 2 years after enrollment, only 13% of laser-treated eyes versus 46% of untreated eyes had visual acuity six or more lines worse than at baseline.

Macular Photocoagulation Study Group. Argon laser photocoagulation for idiopathic neovascularization: results of a randomized clinical trial. Arch Ophthalmol 1983; 101:1358–1361.

Among a much smaller number of eyes with idiopathic extrafoveal choroidal neovascularization, the findings with respect to severe loss of visual acuity were intermediate between those of the other two MPS trials for extrafoveal lesions.

Macular Photocoagulation Study Group. Changing the protocol: a case report from the Macular Photocoagulation Study. Control Clin Trials 1984; 5:203–216.

Macular Photocoagulation Study Group. Recurrent choroidal neovascularization after argon laser photocoagulation for neovascular maculopathy. Arch Ophthalmol 1986; 104:503–512.

After more than 80% of the 284 eyes that initially had extrafoveal choroidal neovascularization had been followed for 3 years or more, 59% of eyes with age-related macular degeneration, 30% of eyes with ocular histoplasmosis, and 33% of eyes with idiopathic choroidal neovascularization had recurrent choroidal neovascularization documented at one or more follow-up examinations.

Macular Photocoagulation Study Group. Argon laser photocoagulation for neovascular maculopathy: three-year results from randomized clinical trials. Arch Ophthalmol 1986; 104:694–701.

Initial reports of the effectiveness of laser photocoagulation were confirmed with follow-up for 3 years or longer of patients in all three trials for eyes with extrafoveal choroidal neovascularization.

Macular Photocoagulation Study Group. Krypton laser photocoagulation for neovascular lesions of ocular histoplasmosis: results of a randomized clinical trial. Arch Ophthalmol 1987; 105:1499–1507.

The effect of laser photocoagulation of juxtafoveal choroidal neovascular lesions of ocular histoplasmosis was equally dramatic as when used to treat extrafoveal lesions: 6% versus 26% with severe visual acuity loss from baseline by the 3-year examination.

Macular Photocoagulation Study Group. Persistent and recurrent neovascularization after krypton laser photocoagulation for neovascular lesions of ocular histoplasmosis. Arch Ophthalmol 1989; 107:344–352.

Blackhurst DW, Maguire MG, the Macular Photocoagulation Study Group. Reproducibility of refraction and visual acuity measurement under a standard protocol. Retina 1989; 9:163–169.

Chamberlin JA, Bressler NM, Bressler SB et al. The use of fundus photographs and fluorescein angiograms in the identification and treatment of choroidal neovascularization in the Macular Photocoagulation Study. Ophthalmology 1989; 96:1526–1534.

Macular Photocoagulation Study Group. Krypton laser photocoagulation for neovascular lesions of age-related macular degeneration: results of a clinical trial. Arch Ophthalmol 1990; 108:816–824.

Three years after enrollment, 49% of laser-treated eyes versus 58% of untreated eyes that enrolled with juxtafoveal neovascular lesions had lost six or more lines of visual acuity from baseline. Laser treatment was recommended only for patients without definite hypertension.

Macular Photocoagulation Study Group. Persistent and recurrent neovascularization after krypton laser photocoagulation for neovascular lesions of age-related macular degeneration. Arch Ophthalmol 1990; 108:825–831.

Macular Photocoagulation Study Group. Krypton laser photocoagulation for idiopathic neovascular lesions: results of a randomized clinical trial. Arch Ophthalmol 1990; 108:832–837.

Bressler SB, Maguire MG, Bressler NM et al. Relationship of drusen and abnormalities of the retinal pigment epithelium to the prognosis of neovascular macular degeneration. Arch Ophthalmol 1990; 108:1442–1447.

Large drusen and focal hyperpigmentation were risk factors for development of choroidal neovascularization in the fellow eye. Also, the risk of recurrent neovascularization was nearly three times higher among study eyes after laser treatment of extrafoveal choroidal neovascularization for patients who had large drusen in the fellow eye at baseline compared to those who did not.

Folk JC, Blackhurst DW, Alexander J et al. Pretreatment fundus characteristics as predictors of recurrent choroidal neovascularization. Arch Ophthalmol 1991; 109:1193–1194.

Bressler NM, Bressler SB, Alexander J et al. Loculated fluid: a previously undescribed fluorescein angiographic finding in choroidal neovascularization associated with macular degeneration. Arch Ophthalmol 1991; 109:211–215.

Macular Photocoagulation Study Group. Argon laser photocoagulation for neovascular maculopathy: five-year results from randomized clinical trials. Arch Ophthalmol 1991; 109:1109–1114.

The benefits of laser photocoagulation of extrafoveal choroidal neovascularization due either to age-related macular degeneration or to ocular histoplasmosis and of idiopathic extrafoveal choroidal neovascularization persisted through 5 years of follow-up.

Macular Photocoagulation Study Group. Laser photocoagulation of subfoveal neovascular lesions in age-related macular degeneration: results of a randomized clinical trial. Arch Ophthalmol 1991; 109:1220–1231.

Initially, eyes with subfoveal choroidal neovascularization that were treated with laser had larger losses of visual acuity from baseline than untreated eyes. However, by 2 years after entry, 21% of laser-treated eyes versus 38% of untreated eyes had visual acuity that was six or more lines worse than at baseline.

Macular Photocoagulation Study Group. Laser photocoagulation of subfoveal recurrent neovascular lesions in age-related macular degeneration: results of a randomized clinical trial. Arch Ophthalmol 1991; 109:1232–1241.

Laser photocoagulation was particularly effective for subfoveal recurrent choroidal neovascularization, with only 10% of laser-treated eyes versus 32% of untreated eyes having visual acuity six or more lines worse at the 2-year examination than at baseline.

Macular Photocoagulation Study Group. Subfoveal neovascular lesions in age-related macular degeneration: guidelines for evaluation and treatment in the Macular Photocoagulation Study. Arch Ophthalmol 1991; 109:1242–1257.

Fine SL, Wood WJ, Singerman LJ et al. Laser treatment for subfoveal neovascular membranes in ocular histoplasmosis syndrome: results of a pilot randomized clinical trial. Arch Ophthalmol 1993; 111:19–20.

Macular Photocoagulation Study Group. Five-year follow-up of fellow eyes of patients with age-related macular degeneration and unilateral extrafoveal choroidal neovascularization. Arch Ophthalmol 1993; 111:1189–1199.

Choroidal neovascularization developed in fellow eyes initially free of such lesions at a rate of approximately 5% per year during 5 years of follow-up.

Macular Photocoagulation Study Group. Laser photocoagulation of subfoveal neovascular lesions of age-related macular degeneration. Updated findings from two clinical trials. Arch Ophthalmol 1993; 111:1200–1209.

Macular Photocoagulation Study Group. Visual outcome after laser photocoagulation for subfoveal choroidal neovascularization secondary to age-related macular degeneration: the influence of initial lesion size and initial visual acuity. Arch Ophthalmol 1994; 112:480–488.

Initial visual acuity and size of the subfoveal neovascular lesions were used to classify eyes based on pattern of visual acuity loss in laser-treated and untreated eyes. Eyes with lesions larger than 2 disc areas in eyes with visual acuity of 20/160 or better had little or no benefit from treatment.

Macular Photocoagulation Study Group. Persistent and recurrent neovascularization after laser photocoagulation for subfoveal choroidal neovascularization of age-related macular degeneration. Arch Ophthalmol 1994; 112:489–499.

Macular Photocoagulation Study Group. Laser photocoagulation for juxtafoveal choroidal neovascularization. Five-year results from randomized clinical trials. Arch Ophthalmol 1994; 112:500–509.

Macular Photocoagulation Study (MPS) Group. Evaluation of argon green vs krypton red laser for photocoagulation of subfoveal choroidal neovascularization in the Macular Photocoagulation Study. Arch Ophthalmol 1994; 112:1176–1184.

No difference was found between argon green and krypton red laser for treatment of subfoveal choroidal neovascularization with respect to any of the vision or other outcomes examined.

Macular Photocoagulation Study Group. Laser photocoagulation for neovascular lesions nasal to the fovea. Results from clinical trials for lesions secondary to ocular histoplasmosis or idiopathic causes. Arch Ophthalmol 1995; 113:56–61.

Comparison of visual acuity outcomes between laser-treated and untreated eyes in this subgroup of patients confirmed that laser photocoagulation, even in the papillomacular bundle, was beneficial.

Macular Photocoagulation Study Group. The influence of treatment extent on the visual acuity of eyes treated with krypton laser for juxtafoveal choroidal neovascularization. Arch Ophthalmol 1995; 113:190–194.

Only 5% of eyes in which the foveal margin of lesions that came to within 200 μm of the center of the foveal avascular zone and were treated in accord with the MPS protocol experienced severe loss of visual acuity in comparison to 25% of eyes in which the foveal margin was treated incompletely.

Macular Photocoagulation Study Group. Occult choroidal neovascularization. Influence on visual outcome in patients with age-related macular degeneration. Arch Ophthalmol 1995; 114:400–412.

Treatment of classic choroidal neovascularization alone in subfoveal lesions composed of both classic and occult neovascularization was not beneficial with respect to visual acuity outcomes and recurrent neovascularization.

Macular Photocoagulation Study Group. Five-year follow-up of fellow eyes of individuals with ocular histoplasmosis and unilateral extrafoveal or juxtafoveal choroidal neovascularization. Arch Ophthalmol 1996; 114:677–688.

Among fellow eyes free of choroidal neovascularization at the time patients enrolled in one of the MPS trials for eyes with ocular histoplasmosis and extrafoveal or juxtafoveal neovascularization, choroidal neovascularization developed in 9% within 5 years, a rate of approximately 2% per year. New choroidal neovascular lesions developed in areas of the macula in which "atypical" histo spots were present earlier in follow-up.

Macular Photocoagulation Study Group. Risk factors for choroidal neovascularization in the second eye of patients with juxtafoveal or subfoveal choroidal neovascularization secondary to age-related macular degeneration. Arch Ophthalmol 1997; 115:741–747.

Four independent risk factors were identified: (1) five or more drusen; (2) focal hyperpigmentation; (3) any large drusen; and (4) definite systemic hypertension. Five-year incidence of choroidal neovascularization in second eyes ranged from 7% in eyes with none of these risk factors to 87% of eyes with all four risk factors.

Other trials of laser treatment of choroidal neovascularization

Coscas G, Soubrane G, Ramahefasolo C et al. Perifoveal laser treatment for subfoveal choroidal new vessels in age-related macular degeneration. Results of a randomized clinical trial. Arch Ophthalmol 1991; 109:1258–1265.

Canadian Ophthalmology Study Group. Argon green vs krypton red laser photocoagulation of extrafoveal choroidal neovascular lesions. One-year results in age-related macular degeneration. Arch Ophthalmol 1993; 111:181–185.

Canadian Ophthalmology Study Group. Argon green vs krypton red laser photocoagulation for extrafoveal choroidal neovascularization. One-year results in ocular histoplasmosis. Arch Ophthalmol 1994; 112:1166–1173.

Trials of photodynamic therapy with verteporfin (Visudyne)

Multicenter randomized clinical trials of verteporfin were initiated in 1996 to evaluate safety and efficacy for treating subfoveal choroidal neovascularization secondary to age-related macular degeneration. The Verteporfin in Photodynamic Therapy (VIP) trial also investigated the use of verteporfin for subfoveal choroidal neovascularization secondary to pathologic myopia. These trials were sponsored by QLT (Vancouver, British Columbia) and Novartis Pharma (Basel, Switzerland).

Treatment of Age-Related Macular Degeneration with Photodynamic Therapy (TAP) Study Group. Photodynamic therapy of subfoveal choroidal neovascularization in age-related macular degeneration with verteporfin: one-year results of 2 randomized clinical trials – TAP report 1. Arch Ophthalmol 1999; 117:1329–1345.

After 1 year of follow-up, 67% of eyes with predominantly classic subfoveal lesions assigned to verteporfin compared with 39% of eyes assigned to placebo had lost fewer than 15 letters of visual acuity from baseline.

Treatment of Age-Related Macular Degeneration with Photodynamic Therapy (TAP) Study Group. Photodynamic therapy of subfoveal choroidal neovascularization in age-related macular degeneration with verteporfin: two-year results of 2 randomized clinical trials – TAP report 2. Arch Ophthalmol 2001; 119:198–207.

After 2 years of follow-up, 59% of eyes with predominantly

classic subfoveal lesions assigned to verteporfin compared with 31% of eyes assigned to placebo had lost fewer than 15 letters of visual acuity from baseline.

Treatment of Age-Related Macular Degeneration with Photodynamic Therapy (TAP) Study Group. Verteporfin therapy of subfoveal choroidal neovascularization in patients with age-related macular degeneration: additional information regarding baseline lesion composition's impact on vision outcomes – TAP report no. 3. Arch Ophthalmol 2002; 120:1443–1454.

Verteporfin therapy significantly reduced the risk of moderate and severe vision loss, with greater benefit in the absence of occult choroidal neovascularization.

Rubin GS, Bressler NM, Treatment of Age-Related Macular Degeneration with Photodynamic Therapy (TAP) Study Group. Effects of verteporfin therapy on contrast sensitivity: results from the Treatment of Age-Related Macular Degeneration with Photodynamic Therapy (TAP) investigation – TAP report no. 4. Retina 2002; 22:536–544.

After 2 years of follow-up, verteporfin-treated eyes were less likely to lose six or more and 15 or more letters on the Pelli–Robson chart compared with placebo-treated eyes (21% versus 45%, and 7% versus 12%).

Treatment of Age-Related Macular Degeneration with Photodynamic Therapy (TAP) Study Group. Verteporfin therapy for subfoveal choroidal neovascularization in age-related macular degeneration: three-year results of an open-label extension of 2 randomized clinical trials – TAP report no. 5. Arch Ophthalmol 2002; 120:1307–1314.

Vision outcomes for verteporfin-treated eyes with predominantly classic subfoveal lesions remained stable from year 2 to year 3.

Bressler SB, Pieramici DJ, Koester JM et al. Natural history of minimally classic subfoveal choroidal neovascular lesions in the Treatment of Age-Related Macular Degeneration with Photodynamic Therapy (TAP) investigation. Outcomes potentially relevant to management – TAP report no. 6. Arch Ophthalmol 2004; 122:325–329.

Among eyes with minimally classic lesions at baseline that were assigned to placebo, 40% had lesions that converted to predominantly classic lesions, more than half by the 3-month examination, and almost all by the 9-month examination.

Verteporfin in Photodynamic Therapy (VIP) Study Group. Photodynamic therapy of subfoveal choroidal neovascularization in pathologic myopia with verteporfin. 1-year results of a randomized clinical trial – VIP report no. 1. Ophthalmology 2001; 108:841–852.

After 1 year of follow-up, 72% of verteporfin-treated eyes compared with 44% of placebo-treated eyes lost fewer than eight letters, with 32% versus 15% improving at least five letters.

Verteporfin in Photodynamic Therapy Study Group. Verteporfin therapy of subfoveal choroidal neovascularization in age-related macular degeneration: two-year results of a randomized clinical trial including lesions with occult with no classic choroidal neovascularization – Verteporfin in Photodynamic Therapy report no. 2. Am J Ophthalmol 2001; 131:541–560.

After 2 years of follow-up of patients with lesions composed of occult with no classic choroidal neovascularization who had recent disease progression, 55% of verteporfin-treated eyes compared with 68% of placebo-treated eyes lost at least 15 letters.

Verteporfin in Photodynamic Therapy (VIP) Study Group. Verteporfin therapy of subfoveal choroidal neovascularization in pathologic myopia: 2-year results of a randomized clinical trial – VIP report no. 3. Ophthalmology 2003; 110:667–673.

After 2 years of follow-up, 36% of verteporfin-treated eyes compared with 51% of placebo-treated eyes lost at least eight letters on a logMAR visual acuity chart, with 40% versus 13% gaining at least five letters.

Treatment of Age-Related Macular Degeneration with Photodynamic Therapy (TAP) and Verteporfin in Photodynamic Therapy (VIP) Study Groups. Effect of baseline lesion size, visual acuity, and lesion composition on visual acuity changes from baseline with and without verteporfin therapy in choroidal neovascularization secondary to age-related macular degeneration – TAP and VIP report no. 1. Am J Ophthalmol 2003; 136:407–418.

Lesion size was a more important predictive factor for magnitude of treatment benefit than either lesion composition or visual acuity. Smaller verteporfin-treated lesions (no larger than four disc areas) had similar visual acuity outcomes to predominantly classic lesions.

Treatment of Age-Related Macular Degeneration with Photodynamic Therapy (TAP) and Verteporfin in Photodynamic Therapy (VIP) Study Groups. Photodynamic therapy of subfoveal choroidal neovascularization with verteporfin. Fluorescein angiographic guidelines for evaluation and treatment – TAP and VIP report no. 2. Arch Ophthalmol 2003; 121:1253–1268.

Treatment of Age-Related Macular Degeneration with Photodynamic Therapy (TAP) and Verteporfin in Photodynamic Therapy (VIP) Study Groups. Acute severe visual acuity decrease after photodynamic therapy with verteporfin: case reports from randomized clinical trials – TAP and VIP report no. 3. Am J Ophthalmol 2004; 137:683–696.

Acute severe visual acuity decrease after verteporfin therapy was uncommon in the TAP investigation and in the VIP trial.

Treatment of Age-Related Macular Degeneration with Photodynamic Therapy (TAP) and Verteporfin in Photodynamic Therapy (VIP) Study Groups. Verteporfin therapy of subfoveal choroidal neovascularization in age-related macular degeneration: meta-analysis of 2-year safety results in three randomized clinical trials: TAP and VIP report no. 4. Retina 2004; 24:1–12.

Although similar in safety profile to placebo, verteporfin therapy was associated with a higher incidence of visual disturbances (22% versus 16% in TAP), injection site reactions (13% versus 6%), photosensitivity reactions (2% versus 0.3%), and infusion-related back pain (2% versus 0%).

Japanese Age-Related Macular Degeneration Trial (JAT) Study Group. Japanese Age-Related Macular Degeneration Trial (JAT): 1-year results of photodynamic therapy with verteporfin in Japanese patients with subfoveal choroidal neovascularization secondary to age-related macular degeneration. Am J Ophthalmol 2003; 136:1049–1061.

After 1 year of follow-up, 50% and 77% of verteporfin-treated patients demonstrated no leakage from classic or occult choroidal neovascularization, respectively.

Houle J-M, Strong HA. Duration of skin photosensitivity and incidence of photosensitivity reactions after administration of verteporfin. Retina 2002; 22:691–697.

Photosensitivity reactions occurred in 2% of patients, all within the first 2 days of treatment.

Submacular Surgery Trials (SST)

The SST was designed to evaluate the safety and effectiveness of surgical removal of subfoveal neovascularization. This set of multicenter randomized trials was sponsored by the National Eye Institute (National Institutes of Health, US Department of Health and Human Services). The first patient enrolled in April 1997 (SST Group H trial); accrual ended in September 2001. The SST was preceded by a set of four randomized pilot trials, the SST Pilot Study.

Grossniklaus HE, Green WR, for the Submacular Surgery Trials Research Group. Histopathologic and ultrastructural findings of surgically excised choroidal neovascularization. Arch Ophthalmol 1998; 116:745–749.

Submacular Surgery Trials Pilot Study Investigators. Submacular Surgery Trials randomized pilot trial of laser photocoagulation versus surgery for recurrent choroidal neovascularization secondary to age-related macular degeneration. I. Ophthalmic outcomes. Submacular Surgery Trials Pilot Study report number 1. Am J Ophthalmol 2000; 130:387–407.

Of 31 patients in the laser treatment arm and 28 patients in the surgery arm with visual acuity measured 2 years after enrollment (89% of 70 patients enrolled in the SST Group R pilot trial), 65% of laser-treated eyes versus 50% of surgery eyes had visual acuity that was better than or no more than one line worse than at baseline.

Submacular Surgery Trials Pilot Study Investigators. Submacular Surgery Trials randomized pilot trial of laser photocoagulation versus surgery for recurrent choroidal neo-

vascularization secondary to age-related macular degeneration. II. Quality of life outcomes. Submacular Surgery Trials Pilot Study report number 2. Am J Ophthalmol 2000; 130:408–418.

SF-36 summary scores were similar for both treatment arms throughout 2 years of follow-up in the SST Group R pilot trial and were consistent with those of the general US population of similar age.

Sadda SR, Pieramici DJ, Marsh MJ et al. Changes in lesion size after submacular surgery for subfoveal choroidal neovascularization in the Submacular Surgery Trials pilot study. Retina 2004; 24:888–899.

Orr PR, Marsh MJ, Hawkins BS et al. Evaluation of the Traveling Vision Examiner Program of the Submacular Surgery Trials pilot study. Ophthalm Epidemiol 2005; 12:47–57.

Childs AL, the Submacular Surgery Trials Patient-Centered Outcomes Subcommittee for the Submacular Surgery Trials Pilot Study Investigators. Responsiveness of the SF-36 Health Survey to changes in visual acuity among patients with subfoveal choroidal neovascularization. Am J Ophthalmol 2004; 137:373–375.

Submacular Surgery Trials Research Group. Responsiveness of the National Eye Institute Visual Function Questionnaire to changes in visual acuity: findings in patients with subfoveal choroidal neovascularization. SST report no. 1. Arch Ophthalmol 2003; 121:531–539, 1513.

Submacular Surgery Trials Research Group. Clinical trial performance of community-based compared with university-based practices: lessons from the Submacular Surgery Trials. SST report no. 2. Arch Ophthalmol 2004; 122:857–863.

Submacular Surgery Trials Research Group. Effect of order of administration of health-related quality of life instruments on responses. SST report no. 3. Quad Life Res 2005; 14:493–500.

Submacular Surgery Trials Research Group. Health- and vision-related quality of life among patients with choroidal neovascularization secondary to age-related macular degeneration at time of enrollment in randomized trials of submacular surgery. SST report no. 4. Am J Ophthalmol 2004; 138:91–108.

Submacular Surgery Trials Research Group. Health- and vision-related quality of life among patients with ocular histoplasmosis or idiopathic choroidal neovascularization at time of enrollment in a randomized trial of submacular surgery. Submacular Surgery Trials report no. 5. Arch Ophthalmol 2005; 123:78–88.

Submacular Surgery Trials Research Group. Patients' perceptions of the value of current vision: assessment of preference values among patients with subfoveal choroidal neovascularization – the Submacular Surgery Trials (SST)

Vision Preference Value Scale: SST report no. 6. Arch Ophthalmol 2004; 122:1856–1867.

Submacular Surgery Trials Research Group. Histopathological and ultrastructural features of surgically-excised subfoveal choroidal neovascular lesions: SST report no. 7. Arch Ophthalmol 2005.

Submacular Surgery Trials Research Group. Guidelines for interpreting retinal photographs and coding findings in the Submacular Surgery Trials (SST): SST report no. 8. Retina 2005; 25:253–268.

Submacular Surgery Trials Research Group. Surgical removal versus observation for subfoveal choroidal neovascularization, either associated with the ocular histoplasmosis syndrome or idiopathic. I. Ophthalmic findings from a randomized clinical trial: Submacular Surgery Trials Group H Trial. SST report no. 9. Arch Ophthalmol 2004; 122:1597–1611.

> After 2 years of follow-up, 55% of eyes in the surgery arm versus 46% of eyes in the observation arm had visual acuity that was better than or within one line (seven letters) of baseline visual acuity. Within the subgroup of eyes with visual acuity worse than 20/100 at baseline, these percentages were 76% and 50%, respectively, indicating that surgery should be considered for such eyes.

Submacular Surgery Trials Research Group. Surgical removal versus observation for subfoveal choroidal neovascularization, either associated with the ocular histoplasmosis syndrome or idiopathic. II. Quality-of-life findings from a randomized clinical trial: SST Group H Trial. SST report no. 10. Arch Ophthalmol 2004; 122:1616–1628.

Submacular Surgery Trials Research Group. Surgery for subfoveal choroidal neovascularization in age-related macular degeneration: ophthalmic findings. SST report no. 11. Ophthalmology 2004; 111:1967–1980.

> Findings from the SST Group N trial showed no clinically or statistically meaningful difference in ophthalmic outcomes between eyes assigned to surgery and eyes assigned to observation.

Submacular Surgery Trials Research Group. Surgery for subfoveal choroidal neovascularization in age-related macular degeneration: quality-of-life findings. SST report number 12. Ophthalmology 2004; 111:1981–1992.

Submacular Surgery Trials Research Group. Surgery for hemorrhagic choroidal neovascular lesions of age-related macular degeneration: ophthalmic findings. SST report no. 13. Ophthalmology 2004; 111:1993–2006.

> Surgery reduced the risk of severe visual acuity loss in the SST Group B trial but the percentage of eyes that achieved stable or improved visual acuity did not differ between the surgery and observation arms. In the absence of any other effective treatment, surgery could be considered in similar eyes with relatively good visual acuity to reduce the risk of severe visual acuity loss.

Submacular Surgery Trials Research Group. Surgery for hemorrhagic choroidal neovascular lesions of age-related macular degeneration: quality-of-life findings. SST report no. 14. Ophthalmology 2004; 111:2007–2014.

Trials of other treatments of choroidal neovascularization

Chakravarthy U, Houston RF, Archer D. Treatment of age-related subfoveal neovascular membranes by teletherapy: a pilot study. Br J Ophthalmol 1993; 77:265–273.

Radiation Therapy for Age-Related Macular Degeneration (RAD) Study Group. A prospective, randomized, double-masked trial on radiation therapy for neovascular age-related macular degeneration (RAD Study). Ophthalmology 1999; 106:2239–2247.

Pharmacological Therapy for Macular Degeneration Study Group. Interferon alfa-2 is ineffective for patients with choroidal neovascularization secondary to age-related macular degeneration. Results of a randomized placebo-controlled clinical trial. Arch Ophthalmol 1997; 115:865–872.

Age-Related Eye Disease Study (AREDS)

The goal of AREDS, a multicenter prospective study of 4757 persons aged 55 to 80 years, is to assess the clinical course of age-related macular degeneration and age-related cataract. AREDS includes a placebo-controlled randomized prevention trial of high-dose vitamin and mineral supplements for patients at risk of age-related macular degeneration and of high-dose vitamin supplement for patients at risk of age-related cataract. Patient accrual began in September 1990 and ended in January 1998. AREDS is sponsored by the National Eye Institute, National Institutes of Health, US Department of Health and Human Services.

Age-Related Eye Disease Study Research Group. The Age-Related Eye Disease Study (AREDS): design implications. AREDS report no. 1. Control Clin Trials 1999; 20:573–600.

Age-Related Eye Disease Study Research Group. The Age-Related Eye Disease Study (AREDS): a clinical trial of zinc and antioxidants. AREDS report no. 2. J Nutr 2000; 130(suppl.):1516–1519.

Age-Related Eye Disease Study Research Group. Risk factors associated with age-related macular degeneration. A case-control study in the Age-Related Eye Disease Study: Age-Related Eye Disease Study report number 3. Ophthalmology 2000; 107:2224–2232.

> Smoking and hypertension were associated with the presence of large drusen and neovascular age-related macular degeneration among AREDS participants.

Age-Related Eye Disease Study Research Group. The Age-Related Eye Disease Study (AREDS) system for classifying cataracts from photographs: AREDS report no. 4. Am J Ophthalmol 2001; 131:167–175.

Age-Related Eye Disease Study Research Group. Risk factors associated with age-related nuclear and cortical cataract. A case-control study in the Age-Related Eye Disease Study, AREDS report no. 5. Ophthalmology 2001; 108:1400–1408.

Age-Related Eye Disease Study Research Group. The Age-Related Eye Diseases Study system for classifying age-related macular degeneration from stereoscopic color fundus photographs: the Age-Related Eye Disease Study report number 6. Am J Ophthalmol 2001; 132:668–681.

Age-Related Eye Disease Study Research Group. The effect of five-year zinc supplementation on serum zinc, serum cholesterol, and hematocrit in persons assigned to treatment group in the Age-Related Eye Disease Study: AREDS report no. 7. J Nutr 2002; 132:697–702.

Age-Related Eye Disease Study Research Group. A randomized, placebo-controlled clinical trial of high-dose supplementation with vitamins C and E, beta carotene, and zinc for age-related macular degeneration and vision loss. AREDS report no. 8. Arch Ophthalmol 2001; 119:1417–1436.

> With an average follow-up of the 3609 participants of 6.3 years, treatment with zinc alone or zinc in combination with antioxidants reduced the risk of advanced age-related macular degeneration among eyes at highest risk. Antioxidants plus zinc reduced the rate of moderate visual acuity loss.

Age-Related Eye Disease Study Research Group. A randomized, placebo-controlled, clinical trial of high-dose supplementation with vitamins C and E and beta carotene for age-related cataract and vision loss. AREDS report no. 9. Arch Ophthalmol 2001; 119:1439–1452.

Clemons TE, Chew EY, Bressler SB et al. National Eye Institute Visual Function Questionnaire in the Age-Related Eye Disease Study (AREDS). AREDS report no. 10. Arch Ophthalmol 2003; 121:211–217.

> As expected, AREDS participants with advanced age-related macular degeneration had the worst scores on a standard vision-targeted instrument for assessing health-related quality of life.

Age-Related Eye Disease Study Research Group. Potential public health impact of Age-Related Eye Disease Study results. AREDS report no. 11. Arch Ophthalmol 2003; 121:1621–1624.

> Based on findings from AREDS, an estimated 8 million people aged 55 and older have intermediate or monocular advanced age-related macular degeneration. Without treatment to reduce their risk, advanced age-related macular degeneration is projected to develop in 1.3 million of them. With the supplements used in AREDS, an estimated 300 000 persons would avoid progression to advanced stages.

Age-Related Eye Disease Study Research Group. Associations of mortality with ocular disorders and an intervention of high-dose antioxidants and zinc in the Age-Related Eye Disease Study. AREDS report no. 13. Arch Ophthalmol 2004; 122:716–726.

> All-cause mortality was reduced among participants assigned to zinc alone or zinc in combination with antioxidants in comparison to participants who were not assigned to a zinc-containing supplement.

Complications of AMD Prevention Trial (CAPT)

CAPT is a multicenter randomized trial designed to evaluate low-intensity laser treatment as a method of preventing vision loss among patients at risk of choroidal neovascularization and other manifestations of advanced age-related macular degeneration due to having large drusen in both eyes. Accrual of patients to CAPT began in May 1999 and was completed in March 2001 with 1052 patients enrolled. CAPT is sponsored by the National Eye Institute, National Institutes of Health, US Department of Health and Human Services.

CAPT was preceded by a pilot study, the Choroidal Neovascularization Prevention Trial (CNVPT). The CNVPT included two randomized pilot trials, one for patients whose second eyes were at risk of choroidal neovascularization (Fellow Eye Study) and one for patients who did not have choroidal neovascularization in either eye (Bilateral Drusen Study).

Choroidal Neovascularization Prevention Trial Research Group. Laser treatment in eyes with large drusen: short-term effects seen in a pilot randomized clinical trial. Ophthalmology 1998; 105:11–23.

> Although choroidal neovascularization developed with low frequency among both treated and untreated eyes in the Bilateral Drusen Study, it developed in more treated eyes in the Fellow Eye Study: 10 of 59 treated eyes versus two of 59 untreated eyes. Nevertheless, untreated eyes in the Fellow Eye Study lost more visual acuity by 18 months of follow-up.

Choroidal Neovascularization Prevention Trial Research Group. Choroidal neovascularization in the Choroidal Neovascularization Prevention Trial. Ophthalmology 1998; 105:1364–1372.

> Choroidal neovascular lesions that developed in eyes with high-risk drusen after macular laser photocoagulation were typically occult, often subfoveal, and associated with the region in which laser spots were applied.

Kaiser RS, Berger JW, Maguire MG et al. Laser burn intensity and the risk for choroidal neovascularization in the CNVPT fellow eye study. Arch Ophthalmol 2001; 119:826–832.

> Although higher-intensity prophylactic laser applications were associated with greater drusen reduction, they were

also associated with greater risk of choroidal neovascularization development.

Choroidal Neovascularization Prevention Trial Research Group. Laser treatment in fellow eyes with large drusen: updated findings from a pilot randomized clinical trial. Ophthalmology 2003; 110:971–978.

By 4 years of follow-up, the cumulative incidence of choroidal neovascularization in treated and untreated eyes was similar. The highest risk in treated eyes was during the first 1 to 2 years after prophylactic laser.

Complications of Age-Related Macular Degeneration Prevention Trial Study Group. Complications of Age-Related Macular Degeneration Prevention Trial (CAPT): rationale, design and methodology. Clin Trials 2004; 1:91–107.

Complications of Age-Related Macular Degeneration Prevention Trial Research Group. Baseline characteristics, the 25-item National Eye Institute Visual Functioning Questionnaire, and their associations in the Complications of Age-Related Macular Degeneration Prevention Trial (CAPT). Ophthalmology 2004; 111:1307–1316.

RETINOPATHY OF PREMATURITY

Initiation of the Multicenter Trial of Cryotherapy for Retinopathy of Prematurity (CRYO-ROP) was stimulated by an increase in the incidence of retinopathy of prematurity following a decline after early clinical trials demonstrated that exposure to 100% oxygen in incubators had been responsible for the epidemic of retinopathy of prematurity in the USA in the 1950s. Increased incidence in the 1970s and 1980s was attributable to advances in neonatal medicine that had increased survival among very-low-birth-weight premature infants. CRYO-ROP was designed to determine the safety and efficacy of transscleral cryotherapy of the peripheral retina in selected low-birth-weight infants with retinopathy of prematurity and to study the natural history of retinal vessel development and outcome in such children. Accrual to the trial began in January 1986 and ended in January 1988. CRYO-ROP was sponsored by the National Eye Institute, National Institutes of Health, US Department of Health and Human Services. Following completion of CRYO-ROP, three additional trials were undertaken to evaluate proposed approaches to reduce the complications of retinopathy of prematurity, all with sponsorship by the National Eye Institute, either alone or in collaboration with other institutes of the National Institutes of Health. Findings from these trials are discussed in Chapter 80.

Multicenter Trial of Cryotherapy for Retinopathy of Prematurity (CRYO-ROP)

Cryotherapy for Retinopathy of Prematurity Cooperative Group. Multicenter trial of Cryotherapy for Retinopathy of Prematurity: preliminary results. Arch Ophthalmol 1988; 106:471–479.

Among eyes of infants assigned to cryotherapy, 22% versus 43% of eyes assigned to observation had a posterior retinal detachment, retinal fold involving the macula, or retrolental tissue.

Cryotherapy for Retinopathy of Prematurity Cooperative Group. Multicenter trial of Cryotherapy for Retinopathy of Prematurity: preliminary results. Pediatrics 1988; 81:697–706.

This article is a coordinated duplicate publication of the above findings.

Phelps DL, Phelps CE. Cryotherapy in infants with retinopathy of prematurity. A decision model for treating one or both eyes. JAMA 1989; 261:1751–1756.

Findings from the CRYO-ROP trial were used to calculate utilities and suggested that the worse eye of infants with moderately severe retinopathy of prematurity and both eyes of infants with very severe disease should be treated with cryotherapy.

Palmer EA. Results of US randomized clinical trial of cryotherapy for ROP (CRYO-ROP). Doc Ophthal 1990; 74:245–251.

Cryotherapy for Retinopathy of Prematurity Cooperative Group. Multicenter trial of Cryotherapy for Retinopathy of Prematurity: three-month outcome. Arch Ophthalmol 1990; 108:195–204.

Three-month outcomes from the randomized trial for all 260 infants enrolled update the 1988 preliminary report on effectiveness of transscleral cryotherapy. Eyes treated with cryotherapy had reduced risk of posterior retinal detachment, retinal fold involving the macula, or retrolental tissue compared to untreated eyes: 31% versus 51% respectively.

Watzke RC, Robertson JE, Palmer EA et al. Photographic grading in the Retinopathy of Prematurity Cryotherapy trial. Arch Ophthalmol 1990; 108:950–955.

Features graded from photographs of the posterior fundus and assessed for severity were temporal retinal vessel traction, retinal fold, macular ectopia, retinal detachment, retrolental mass, blood vessel attenuation, retinal pigment epithelium scarring, and cataract. (The 1993 report by Evans et al. describes the technique used to photograph the posterior fundus of the eyes of these infants.)

Dobson V, Quinn GE, Biglan AW et al. Acuity card assessment of visual function in the Cryotherapy for Retinopathy of Prematurity trial. Invest Ophthalmol Vis Sci 1990; 31:1702–1708.

Monocular acuity levels were obtained at the 12-month follow-up examination for 95% of infants assessed using the acuity card procedure.

Cryotherapy for Retinopathy of Prematurity Cooperative Group. Multicenter trial of Cryotherapy for Retinopathy of

Prematurity: one-year outcome – structure and function. Arch Ophthalmol 1990; 108:1408–1416.

After 1 year of follow-up, eyes assigned to transscleral cryotherapy had reduced risk of posterior retinal detachment, retinal fold involving the macula, or retrolental tissue compared to untreated eyes: 26% versus 47%, respectively. Assessment of grating visual acuity using the Teller Acuity Card correlated with retinal findings: 35% of eyes treated with cryotherapy versus 56% of eyes not treated had an unfavorable functional outcome at 1 year.

Palmer EA, Hardy RJ, Davis BR et al. Operational aspects of terminating randomization in the Multicenter Trial of Cryotherapy for Retinopathy of Prematurity. Control Clin Trials 1991; 12:277–292.

Hardy RJ, Davis BR, Palmer EA et al. Statistical considerations in terminating randomization in the Multicenter Trial of Cryotherapy for Retinopathy of Prematurity. Control Clin Trials 1991; 12:293–303.

Palmer EA, Flynn JT, Hardy RJ et al. Incidence and early course of retinopathy of prematurity. Ophthalmology 1991; 98:1628–1640.

Incidence and early natural course of retinopathy of prematurity were monitored in the 4099 premature infants enrolled in the natural-history cohort followed in parallel with the randomized trial. The highest incidence (90%) was observed among infants who weighed less than 750 g at birth and the lowest incidence (47%) among those who weighed 1000 to 1250 g. The timing of retinal vascular events correlated more closely with postconceptional age than with postnatal age.

Phelps DL, Brown DR, Tung B et al. 28-day survival rates of 6676 neonates with birth weights of 1250 grams or less. Pediatrics 1991; 87:7–17.

Quinn GE, Dobson V, Barr CC et al. Visual acuity in infants after vitrectomy for severe retinopathy of prematurity. Ophthalmology 1991; 98:5–13.

Of 98 infants (129 eyes) enrolled in the CRYO-ROP randomized trial who had total retinal detachment before the 1-year examination, 71 eyes underwent vitrectomy and 58 were observed. Only six eyes had retinal reattachment by 1 year; only two of the six eyes had pattern vision. None of the eyes observed without further treatment had any evidence of visual function.

Gilbert WS, Dobson V, Quinn GE et al. The correlation of visual function with posterior retinal structure in severe retinopathy of prematurity. Arch Ophthalmol 1992; 110:625–631.

Grating acuity correlated well with the appearance of the posterior retinal structure in 84% of 304 eyes at the 1-year examination.

Summers G, Phelps DL, Tung B et al. Ocular cosmesis in retinopathy of prematurity. Arch Ophthalmol 1992; 110:1092–1097.

The overall incidence of adverse ocular cosmetic outcomes in the natural-history cohort was 15%, including strabismus (13%), nystagmus (3%), total retrolental membrane (1%), epiphora (0.6%), corneal opacity (0.6%), and cataract (0.3%).

Evans MS, Wallace PR, Palmer EA. Fundus photography in infants. J Ophthalm Photo 1993; 15:38–39.

Cryotherapy for Retinopathy of Prematurity Cooperative Group. Multicenter trial of Cryotherapy for Retinopathy of Prematurity: 3-year outcome – structure and function. Arch Ophthalmol 1993; 111:339–344.

Among the 256 surviving children who participated in the CRYO-ROP trial and were examined after 3.5 years, the benefits of transscleral cryotherapy persisted, as shown by better letter acuity, grating acuity, and posterior pole status among treated eyes than among untreated eyes.

Reynolds J, Dobson V, Quinn GE et al. Prediction of visual function in eyes with mild to moderate posterior pole residua of retinopathy of prematurity. Arch Ophthalmol 1993; 111:1050–1056.

Physicians were not able to predict visual acuity reliably in eyes with macular hypertropia or macular fold due to retinopathy of prematurity based on retinal appearance.

Schaffer DB, Palmer EA, Plotsky DF et al. Prognostic factors in the natural course of retinopathy of prematurity. Ophthalmology 1993; 100:230–237.

Lower birth weight, younger gestational age at birth, white race, multiple birth, and delivery other than at a study center nursery increased the risk of threshold retinopathy of prematurity by 3 months after birth in the natural history cohort.

Schaffer DB, Palmer EA, Plotsky DF et al. Prognostic factors in the natural course of retinopathy of prematurity. Ophthalmology 1993; 100:230–237.

Cryotherapy for Retinopathy of Prematurity Cooperative Group. The natural ocular outcome of premature birth and retinopathy. Status at 1 year. Arch Ophthalmol 1994; 112:903–912.

Eyes with zone I, stage 3 disease had the worst posterior fundus outcomes at 1 year in the natural-history cohort. Eyes with zone II retinopathy of prematurity without plus disease or with zone III retinopathy of prematurity had a low risk (< 1%) of an unfavorable outcome.

Dobson V, Quinn GE, Summers CG et al. Effect of acute-phase retinopathy of prematurity on grating acuity development in the very low birth weight infant. Invest Ophthalmol Vis Sci 1994; 35:4236–4244.

Untreated threshold disease resulted in moderate to severe reductions in grating acuity; less than prethreshold retinopathy of prematurity had no effect on development of grating acuity.

Quinn GE, Dobson V, Biglan A et al. Correlation of retinopathy of prematurity in fellow eyes in the Cryotherapy for Retinopathy of Prematurity study. Arch Ophthalmol 1995; 113:469–473.

During the acute-phase interval between 32 and 42 weeks' postconceptional age, a high degree of correspondence of severity and location of retinopathy of prematurity was observed between fellow eyes and study eyes. Correlation declined over time with asymmetry by 1 year of age in eyes with prethreshold retinopathy of prematurity.

Dobson V, Quinn GE, Saunders RA et al. Grating visual acuity in eyes with retinal residua of retinopathy of prematurity. Arch Ophthalmol 1995; 113:1172–1177.

Eyes with retinal folds, partial detachments, or macular hypertropia had grating visual acuity deficit at ages 1 through 4.5 years of age. Eyes with regressed retinopathy of prematurity and without retinal residua had no deficit in grating visual acuity compared to eyes that did not have retinopathy of prematurity.

Dobson V, Quinn GE, Tung B et al. Comparison of recognition and grating acuities in very-low-birth-weight children with and without retinal residua of retinopathy of prematurity. Invest Ophthalmol Vis Sci 1995; 36:692–702.

Eyes with acuity better than 20/150 to 20/300 tended to have better recognition (letter) acuity than resolution (grating) acuity, in contrast to eyes with worse acuity, which tended to have better resolution acuity than recognition acuity, at the 3.5- and 4.5-year examinations.

Cryotherapy for Retinopathy of Prematurity Cooperative Group. Multicenter trial of Cryotherapy for Retinopathy of Prematurity: Snellen visual acuity and structural outcome at 5½ years after randomization. Arch Ophthalmol 1996; 114:417–424.

At the 5.5-year follow-up examination, eyes in the cryotherapy-treated group had better outcomes than untreated eyes with respect to both visual acuity and fundus status. However, fewer treated eyes than control eyes had visual acuity of 20/40 or better.

Kivlin JD, Biglan AW, Gordon RA et al. Early retinal vessel development and iris vessel dilation as factors in retinopathy of prematurity. Arch Ophthalmol 1996; 114:150–154.

The risk of developing threshold retinopathy of prematurity was inversely related to the extent of retinal vessel development observed during early screening examinations. Dilated iris vessels were also associated with development of threshold retinopathy of prematurity.

Quinn GE, Dobson V, Barr CC et al. Visual acuity of eyes after vitrectomy for retinopathy of prematurity: follow-up at 5½ years. Ophthalmology 1996; 103:595–600.

At 5.5 years of age, 21% of eyes that earlier had vitrectomy for total retinal detachment had partial retinal reattachment. Poor visual outcomes (light perception or no light perception) were present equally in vitrectomized and nonvitrectomized eyes.

Gilbert WS, Quinn GE, Dobson V et al. Partial retinal detachment at 3 months after threshold retinopathy of prematurity. Long-term structural and functional outcome. Arch Ophthalmol 1996; 114:1085–1091.

Eyes with partial retinal detachments that involved the fovea had worse outcomes at 4.5 years than eyes with partial retinal detachments that spared the fovea. Most eyes had visual acuity of 20/200 or worse.

Quinn GE, Dobson V, Hardy RJ et al. Visual fields measured with double-arc perimetry in eyes with threshold retinopathy of prematurity from the Cryotherapy for Retinopathy of Prematurity trial. Ophthalmology 1996; 103:1432–1437.

Monocular visual fields of eyes with severe threshold disease were smaller than fields of eyes that did not develop ROP. Also, eyes treated with cryotherapy had smaller fields than control eyes.

Dobson V, Quinn GE, Abramov I et al. Color vision measured with pseudoisochromatic plates at five-and-a-half years in eyes of children from the CRYO-ROP study. Invest Ophthalmol Vis Sci 1996; 37:2467–2474.

No difference in color vision deficits was detected between treated eyes and natural-history eyes. However, increased prevalence of blue-yellow color deficit was present in preterm children compared to the general adult population.

Bartholomew PA, Chao J, Evans JL et al. Acceptance/use of the teller acuity card procedure in the clinic. Am Orthop J 1996; 46:99–105.

Saunders RA, Donahue ML, Christmann LM et al. Racial variation in retinopathy of prematurity. Arch Ophthalmol 1997; 115:604–608.

Race was a risk factor for development of threshold disease. Severe retinopathy of prematurity occurred with greater frequency in low-birth-weight white infants than in low-birth-weight black infants.

Bremer DL, Palmer EA, Fellows RR et al. Strabismus in premature infants in the first year of life. Arch Ophthalmol 1998; 116:329–333.

Quinn GE, Dobson V, Kivlin J et al. Prevalence of myopia between 3 months and 5½ years in preterm infants with and without retinopathy of prematurity. Ophthalmology 1998; 105:1292–1300.

Repka MX, Summers CG, Palmer EA et al. The incidence of ophthalmologic interventions in children with birth weights less than 1251 grams. Results through 5½ years. Ophthalmology 1998; 105:1621–1627.

> Both children who participated in the CRYO-ROP trial and those in the natural-history cohort underwent a large number of ophthalmologic treatments during the first 5.5 years of life.

Dobson V, Quinn GE, Siatkowski RM et al. Agreement between grating acuity at age 1 year and Snellen acuity at age 5.5 years in the preterm child. Invest Ophthalmol Vis Sci 1999; 40:496–503.

Harvey EM, Dobson V, Tung B et al. Interobserver agreement for grating acuity and letter acuity assessment in 1- to 5.5-year-olds with severe retinopathy of prematurity. Invest Ophthalmol Vis Sci 1997; 40:1565–1576.

Repka MX, Palmer EA, Tung B et al. Involution of retinopathy of prematurity. Arch Ophthalmol 2000; 118:645–649.

> Acute-phase retinopathy of prematurity began to involute at a mean of 38.6 weeks postmenstrual age. Zone III disease was almost always associated with a favorable outcome.

Quinn GE, Dobson V, Siatkowski RM et al. Does cryotherapy affect refractive error? Results from treated versus control eyes in the Cryotherapy for Retinopathy of Prematurity trial. Ophthalmology 2001; 108:343–347.

> Prevalence of high myopia (8 D or more) was greater among eyes treated with cryotherapy than in control eyes of participants in the CRYO-ROP trial after 10 years.

Cryotherapy for Retinopathy of Prematurity Cooperative Group. Multicenter trial of Cryotherapy for Retinopathy of Prematurity: ophthalmological outcomes at 10 years. Arch Ophthalmol 2001; 119:1110–1118.

> After 10 years, treated eyes continued to have better outcomes than control eyes with respect to visual acuity and fundus status. The proportion of eyes with visual acuity of 20/40 or better was similar in the two groups of eyes.

Cryotherapy for Retinopathy of Prematurity Cooperative Group. Effect of retinal ablative therapy for threshold retinopathy of prematurity: results of Goldmann perimetry at the age of 10 years. Arch Ophthalmol 2001; 119:1120–1125.

Cryotherapy for Retinopathy of Prematurity Cooperative Group. Contrast sensitivity at age 10 years in children who had threshold retinopathy of prematurity. Arch Ophthalmol 2001; 119:1129–1133.

Editorial Committee for the Cryotherapy for Retinopathy of Prematurity Cooperative Group. Multicenter Trial of Cryotherapy for Retinopathy of Prematurity. Natural history ROP: ocular outcome at 5½ years in premature infants with birth weights less than 1251 g. Arch Ophthalmol 2002; 120:595–599.

Hardy RJ, Palmer EA, Dobson V et al. Risk analysis of prethreshold retinopathy of prematurity. Arch Ophthalmol 2003; 121:1697–1701.

Multicenter Study of Light Reduction in Retinopathy of Prematurity (LIGHT-ROP)

Reynolds JD, Hardy RJ, Kennedy KA et al. Lack of efficacy of light reduction in preventing retinopathy of prematurity. N Engl J Med 1998; 338:1572–1576.

> Reduced nursery lighting did not decrease the incidence of retinopathy of prematurity compared to normal nursery lighting among premature infants with birth weights of 1250 g or less in this randomized trial.

LIGHT-ROP Cooperative Group. The design of the multicenter study of Light Reduction in Retinopathy of Prematurity (LIGHT-ROP). J Pediatr Ophthalmol Strabismus 1999; 36:257–263.

Kennedy KA, Fielder AR, Hardy RJ et al. Reduced lighting does not improve medical outcomes in very-low-birth-weight infants. J Pediatr 2001; 139:527–531.

Supplemental Therapeutic Oxygen for Prethreshold Retinopathy of Prematurity (STOP-ROP)

STOP-ROP Multicenter Study Group. Supplemental Therapeutic Oxygen for Prethreshold Retinopathy of Prematurity (STOP-ROP), a randomized, controlled trial. I: Primary outcomes. Pediatrics 2000; 105:295–310.

> Premature infants with prethreshold disease and median pulse oximetry less than 94% saturation were randomly assigned to conventional oxygen with pulse oximetry targeted at 89% to 94% saturation or supplemental oxygen with pulse oximetry targeted at 96% to 99% saturation. No substantive difference in rates of progression was found.

Oden NL, Phelps DL, the STOP-ROP Multicenter study group. Statistical issues related to early closure of STOP-ROP, a group-sequential trial. Control Clin Trials 2003; 24:28–38.

Early Treatment of Retinopathy of Prematurity (ETROP or EARLY-ROP)

Early Treatment for Retinopathy of Prematurity Cooperative Group. Revised indications for the treatment of retinopathy of prematurity. Results of the Early Treatment for Retinopathy of Prematurity randomized trial. Arch Ophthalmol 2003; 121:1684–1696.

> Early treatment with peripheral retinal ablation reduced unfavorable outcomes with respect to both visual acuity and structure in comparison to standard management of prethreshold retinopathy of prematurity in premature infants in this randomized trial.

OTHER RETINAL AND RETINA-RELATED CONDITIONS

Collaborative Ocular Melanoma Study (COMS)

The COMS was designed and conducted to evaluate radiotherapy for treatment of choroidal melanoma, either in comparison to enucleation (COMS randomized trial of iodine-125 brachytherapy) or in combination with enucleation (COMS randomized trial of pre-enucleation radiation). Both US and Canadian centers participated in the COMS. In addition, a nonrandomized observational study of small choroidal melanoma was conducted at a subset of COMS centers. A parallel prospective study of quality of life among patients in the brachytherapy trial (COMS-QOLS) was initiated in 1995. Accrual of patients began in November 1986 and ended in July 1988 after 2320 patients had enrolled in the randomized trials. The COMS was sponsored by the National Eye Institute and the National Cancer Institute, National Institutes of Health, US Department of Health and Human Services. The COMS and fndings published to date are discussed in more detail in Chapter 44.

Earle J, Kline RW, Robertson DM. Selection of iodine 125 for the Collaborative Ocular Melanoma Study. Arch Ophthalmol 1987; 105:763–764.

Markowitz JA, Hawkins BS, Diener-West M et al. A review of mortality from choroidal melanoma, I. Quality of published reports, 1966 through 1988. Arch Ophthalmol 1992; 110:239–244.

Diener-West M, Hawkins BS, Markowitz JA et al. A review of mortality from choroidal melanoma, II. A meta-analysis of 5-year mortality rates following enucleation, 1966 through 1988. Arch Ophthalmol 1992; 110:245–250.

> A systematic review of published rates of death following enucleation yielded estimates of 5-year mortality rates of 15% for "small" choroidal melanoma, 30% for "medium" choroidal melanoma, and 50% for "large" choroidal melanoma.

Collaborative Ocular Melanoma Study Group. Accuracy of diagnosis of choroidal melanoma in the Collaborative Ocular Melanoma Study. COMS report no. 1. Arch Ophthalmol 1990; 108:1268–1273.

Collaborative Ocular Melanoma Study Group. Complications of enucleation surgery. COMS report no. 2. In: Franklin RM, ed. Proceedings of the symposium on retina and vitreous. Amsterdam: Kugler Publications; 1993:181–190.

> Preliminary findings presented in this report have been superseded by COMS report number 11.

Collaborative Ocular Melanoma Study Group. Design and methods of a clinical trial for a rare condition: the Collaborative Ocular Melanoma Study. COMS report no. 3. Control Clin Trials 1993; 14:362–391.

Collaborative Ocular Melanoma Study Group. Mortality in patients with small choroidal melanoma. COMS report no. 4. Arch Ophthalmol 1997; 115:886–893.

> In the nonrandomized study of small choroidal melanoma, 5- and 8-year all-cause mortality rates were 6% and 15%, respectively.

Collaborative Ocular Melanoma Study Group. Factors predictive of growth and treatment of small choroidal melanoma. COMS report no. 5. Arch Ophthalmol 1997; 115:1537–1544.

> Factors predictive of time to growth of small untreated choroidal melanoma were initial tumor size, orange pigment, absence of drusen, and absence of retinal pigment epithelial changes adjacent to the tumor.

Collaborative Ocular Melanoma Study Group. Histopathologic characteristics of uveal melanomas in eyes enucleated from the Collaborative Ocular Melanoma Study. COMS report no. 6. Am J Ophthalmol 1998; 125:745–766.

Collaborative Ocular Melanoma Study Group. Sociodemographic and clinical predictors of participation in two randomized trials: findings from the Collaborative Ocular Melanoma Study. COMS report no. 7. Control Clin Trials 2001; 22:526–537.

Grossniklaus HE, Albert DM, Green R et al. Clear cell differentiation in choroidal melanoma. COMS report no. 8. Arch Ophthalmol 1997; 115:894–898.

Collaborative Ocular Melanoma Study Group. The Collaborative Ocular Melanoma Study (COMS) randomized trial of pre-enucleation radiation of large choroidal melanoma. I: Characteristics of patients enrolled and not enrolled. COMS report no. 9. Am J Ophthalmol 1998; 125:767–778.

> Within 7 years of enrollment of the first patient in the COMS, 6078 patients with choroidal melanoma had been evaluated at COMS centers, of whom 1860 had tumors that met the size criteria for the trial of pre-enucleation radiation, 1302 met all eligibility criteria, and 1003 enrolled and were assigned randomly to pre-enucleation radiation or enucleation alone.

Collaborative Ocular Melanoma Study Group. The Collaborative Ocular Melanoma Study (COMS) randomized trial of pre-enucleation radiation of large choroidal melanoma. II: Initial mortality findings. COMS report no. 10. Am J Ophthalmol 1998; 125:779–796.

> Five-year survival rates were 62% for patients assigned to pre-enucleation radiation and 57% for patients who had enucleation only. Five-year rates of death with histopathologically confirmed melanoma were 26% and 28%, respectively.

Collaborative Ocular Melanoma Study Group. The Collaborative Ocular Melanoma Study (COMS) randomized trial of pre-enucleation radiation of large choroidal melanoma.

III: Local complications and observations following enucleation. COMS report no. 11. Am J Ophthalmol 1998; 126:362–372.

The only differences between patients treated with pre-enucleation radiation and enucleation alone during the first 5 years after treatment were lower incidence rates of local tumor recurrence and severe ptosis in the pre-enucleation radiation group.

Collaborative Ocular Melanoma Study Group. Echography (ultrasound) procedures for the Collaborative Ocular Melanoma Study (COMS), report no. 12. J Ophthalm Nurs Technol 1999; 18:143–149, 219–232.

Collaborative Ocular Melanoma Study (COMS) Group. Consistency of observations from echograms made centrally in the Collaborative Ocular Melanoma Study. COMS report no. 13. Ophthalm Epidemiol 2002; 9:11–27.

Collaborative Ocular Melanoma Study Group. Cause-specific mortality coding: methods in the Collaborative Ocular Melanoma Study. COMS report no. 14. Control Clin Trials 2001; 22:248–262.

Collaborative Ocular Melanoma Study Group. Assessment of metastatic disease status at death in 435 patients with large choroidal melanoma in the Collaborative Ocular Melanoma Study (COMS). COMS report no. 15. Arch Ophthalmol 2001; 119:670–676.

Collaborative Ocular Melanoma Study Group. Collaborative Ocular Melanoma Study (COMS) randomized trial of I-125 brachytherapy for medium choroidal melanoma. I. Visual acuity after 3 years. COMS report no. 16. Ophthalmology 2001; 108:348–366.

By 3 years after treatment with iodine-125 brachytherapy, 43% of tumor eyes had visual acuity of 20/200 or worse. Similarly, 49% had lost six or more lines of visual acuity from baseline.

Collaborative Ocular Melanoma Study Group. The COMS randomized trial of iodine 125 brachytherapy for choroidal melanoma, II: Characteristics of patients enrolled and not enrolled. COMS report no. 17. Arch Ophthalmol 2001; 119:951–965.

By the end of patient accrual in July 2001, 8712 patients with choroidal melanoma had been evaluated at COMS centers; 5046 had tumors that met the size criteria for the randomized trial of iodine-125, of whom 2164 met all eligibility criteria and 1317 enrolled. The most common reason for ineligibility for this trial was unsuitable tumor location for brachytherapy as administered in the COMS.

Collaborative Ocular Melanoma Study Group. The COMS randomized trial of iodine 125 brachytherapy for choroidal melanoma, III: Initial mortality findings. COMS report no. 18. Arch Ophthalmol 2001; 119:969–982.

Among the 1317 patients enrolled in this COMS trial, 5-year all-cause mortality rates were 19% among those assigned to enucleation and 18% among those assigned to brachytherapy. Five-year rates of death with confirmed melanoma metastasis were 11% in the enucleation arm and 9% in the brachytherapy arm.

Collaborative Ocular Melanoma Study Group. The COMS randomized trial of iodine 125 brachytherapy for choroidal melanoma. IV. Local treatment failure and enucleation in the first 5 years after brachytherapy. COMS report no. 19. Ophthalmology 2002; 109:2197–2206. [Correction in Ophthalmology 2004; 111:1564.]

The 5-year rate of enucleation, primarily because of tumor growth, was 12%.

Collaborative Ocular Melanoma Study Group. Trends in size and treatment of recently diagnosed choroidal melanoma, 1987–1997. Findings from patients examined at Collaborative Ocular Melanoma Study (COMS) centers. COMS report no. 20. Arch Ophthalmol 2003; 121:1156–1162.

Collaborative Ocular Melanoma Study Group. Comparison of clinical, echographic, and histopathological measurements from eyes with medium-sized choroidal melanoma in the Collaborative Ocular Melanoma Study. COMS report no. 21. Arch Ophthalmol 2003; 121:1163–1171.

Comparisons of baseline measurements of tumor size from multiple sources showed good agreement in enucleated eyes, suggesting that very few patients treated with brachytherapy would have received inadequate radiotherapy.

Collaborative Ocular Melanoma Study Group. Ten-year follow-up of fellow eyes of patients enrolled in Collaborative Ocular Melanoma Study randomized trials. COMS report no. 22. Ophthalmology 2004; 111:966–976.

Almost all survivors retained good visual acuity in their fellow eyes for up to 10 years. There was no evidence that fellow eyes of patients whose tumor eye was treated with radiotherapy (brachytherapy or pre-enucleation radiation) were at greater risk of vision loss or other ophthalmic problems than those treated with enucleation alone.

Diener-West M, Reynolds SM, Agugliaro DJ et al. Screening for metastasis from choroidal melanoma: the Collaborative Ocular Melanoma Study Group report 23. J Clin Oncol 2004; 22:2438–2444.

Collaborative Ocular Melanoma Study Group. The Collaborative Ocular Melanoma Study (COMS) randomized trial of pre-enucleation radiation of large choroidal melanoma. IV. Ten-year mortality findings and prognostic factors. COMS report no. 24. Am J Ophthalmol 2004; 138:936–951.

By 10 years after enrollment, 32% of 436 patients were alive and cancer-free. Only baseline age and longest tumor basal diameter were predictive of time to death, whether with melanoma metastasis or from any cause.

Collaborative Ocular Melanoma Study Group. Second primary cancers after enrollment in the COMS trials for treatment of choroidal melanoma. COMS report no. 25. Arch Ophthalmol 2005; 123:601–604.

Wells CG, Bradford RH, Fish GE et al. Choroidal melanomas in American Indians. Arch Ophthalmol 1996; 114:1017–1018.

Melia BM, Moy CS, McCaffrey L. Quality of life in patients with choroidal melanoma: a pilot study. Ophthalm Epidemiol 1999; 6:19–28.

Collaborative Ocular Melanoma Study Quality of Life Study Group. Quality of life assessment in the Collaborative Ocular Melanoma Study: design and methods. COMS-QOLS report no. 1. Ophthalm Epidemiol 1999; 6:5–17.

Collaborative Ocular Melanoma Study – Quality of Life Study Group. Development and validation of disease-specific measures for choroidal melanoma. COMS-QOLS report no. 2. Arch Ophthalmol 2003; 121:1010–1020.

Collaborative Ocular Melanoma Study – Quality of Life Study Group. Quality of life after I-125 brachytherapy versus enucleation for choroidal melanoma: 5-year results from the Collaborative Ocular Melanoma Study. COMS-QOLS report no. 3. Arch Ophthalmol 2005 (in press).

Studies of the Ocular Complications of AIDS (SOCA)

In order to address issues regarding treatment of eye involvement, primarily cytomegalovirus retinitis, in patients with the acquired immune deficiency syndrome (AIDS), the National Eye Institute has sponsored a clinical trials network. Most of the SOCA clinical trials have been conducted in collaboration with the AIDS Clinical Trials Group. Several of the trials also have had industry sponsorship. Accrual of patients to the first SOCA trial began in March 1990. Clinical applications of SOCA findings are discussed in Chapters 91 and 92.

Studies of Ocular Complications of AIDS (SOCA) Research Group, in collaboration with the AIDS Clinical Trials Group (ACTG). Studies of Ocular Complications of AIDS foscarnet–ganciclovir cytomegalovirus retinitis trial: 1. Rationale, design, and methods. Control Clin Trials 1992; 13:22–39.

Studies of Ocular Complications of AIDS Research Group, in collaboration with the AIDS Clinical Trials Group. Mortality in patients with the acquired immunodeficiency syndrome treated with either foscarnet or ganciclovir for cytomegalovirus retinitis. N Engl J Med 1992; 326:213–220.
    After 19 months of treatment, the rate of mortality in the ganciclovir group was 77% higher than in the foscarnet group, leading to suspension of the treatment protocol.

Studies of Ocular Complications of AIDS Research Group, in collaboration with the AIDS Clinical Trials Group. Foscarnet–ganciclovir cytomegalovirus retinitis trial: 4. Visual outcomes. Ophthalmology 1994; 101:1250–1261.
    At 6 months after randomization, visual outcomes were similar, with 88% of the forscarnet-assigned patients and 93% of the ganciclovir-assigned patients having a best-corrected visual acuity of 20/40 or better.

Studies of Ocular Complications of AIDS Research Group, in collaboration with the AIDS Clinical Trials Group. Morbidity and toxic effects associated with ganciclovir or foscarnet therapy in a randomized cytomegalovirus retinitis trial. Arch Intern Med 1995; 155:65–74.
    Foscarnet was associated with more infusion-related symptoms, genitourinary symptoms, and a trend toward more nephrotoxic effects when compared to ganciclovir.

Studies of Ocular Complications of AIDS Research Group, in collaboration with the AIDS Clinical Trials Group. Antiviral effects of foscarnet and ganciclovir therapy on human immunodeficiency virus p24 antigen in patients with AIDS and cytomegalovirus retinitis. J Infect Dis 1995; 172:613–621.

Studies of Ocular Complications of AIDS Research Group, in collaboration with the AIDS Clinical Trials Group. Combination foscarnet and ganciclovir therapy vs monotherapy for the treatment of relapsed cytomegalovirus retinitis in patients with AIDS: the Cytomegalovirus Retreatment trial. Arch Ophthalmol 1996; 114:23–33.
    Combination therapy with foscarnet and ganciclovir resulted in a statistically significant decrease in the rate of visual field loss and in the rate of increase in retinal area involvement.

Studies of Ocular Complications of AIDS Research Group, in collaboration with the AIDS Clinical Trials Group. Clinical vs photographic assessment of treatment of cytomegalovirus retinitis: Foscarnet–Ganciclovir Cytomegalovirus Retinitis Trial report 8. Arch Ophthalmol 1996; 114:848–855.
    Progression of retinitis was difficult to recognize clinically, and movement of retinitis borders by 750 μm or more during the first 4 weeks of treatment did not necessarily represent a treatment failure.

Wu AW, Coleson LC, Holbrook J et al. Measuring visual function and quality of life in patients with cytomegalovirus retinitis: development of a questionnaire. Arch Ophthalmol 1996; 114:841–847.

Studies of Ocular Complications of AIDS Research Group, in collaboration with the AIDS Clinical Trials Group. Assessment of cytomegalovirus retinitis: clinical evaluation vs centralized grading of fundus photographs. Arch Ophthalmol 1996; 114:791–805.

Studies of Ocular Complications of AIDS Research Group, in collaboration with the AIDS Clinical Trials Group. MSL-109 adjuvant therapy for cytomegalovirus retinitis in patients with acquired immunodeficiency syndrome: the Monoclonal Antibody Cytomegalovirus Retinitis trial Arch Ophthalmol 1997; 115:1528–1536. [Correction in Arch Ophthalmol 1998; 116:296].

Studies of Ocular Complications of AIDS Research Group, in collaboration with the AIDS Clinical Trials Group. Parenteral cidofovir for cytomegalovirus retinitis in patients with AIDS: the HPMPC Peripheral Cytomegalovirus Retinitis trial. A randomized, controlled trial. Ann Intern Med 1997; 126:264–274.

> Both low and high doses of cidofovir slowed progression of cytomegalovirus retinitis. Median time to progression of retinitis was 64 days in the low-dose cidofovir group compared to 21 days in the deferral group.

Studies of Ocular Complications of AIDS (SOCA) Research Group, in collaboration with the AIDS Clinical Trials Group (ACTG). Rhegmatogenous retinal detachment in patients with cytomegalovirus retinitis: the Foscarnet–Ganciclovir Cytomegalovirus Retinitis trial. Am J Ophthalmol 1997; 124:61–70.

> The risk of rhegmatogenous retinal detachment was 19% at 6 months and 38% at 1 year and was unrelated to type of intravenous therapy used.

Studies of Ocular Complications of AIDS Research Group, in collaboration with the AIDS Clinical Trials Group. Foscarnet–Ganciclovir Cytomegalovirus Retinitis trial: 5. Clinical features of cytomegalovirus retinitis at diagnosis. Am J Ophthalmol 1997; 124:141–157.

> Visual symptoms and signs of ocular inflammation were strong indicators of the presence of cytomegalovirus retinitis.

Studies of Ocular Complications of AIDS Research Group, in collaboration with the AIDS Clinical Trials Group. Cytomegalovirus (CMV) culture results, drug resistance, and clinical outcome in AIDS patients with CMV treated with either foscarnet or ganciclovir. J Infect Dis 1997; 176:50–58.

Holbrook JT, Davis MD, Hubbard LD et al. Risk factors for advancement of cytomegalovirus retinitis in patients with acquired immunodeficiency syndrome. Arch Ophthalmol 2000; 118:1196–1204.

> In eyes with retinitis, baseline risk factors for advancement while receiving treatment were smaller area involved, active margins, and posterior location.

Holbrook JT, Meinert CL, Van Natta ML et al. Photographic measures of cytomegalovirus retinitis as surrogates for visual outcomes in treated patients. Arch Ophthalmol 2001; 119:554–563.

Silicone Study

The Silicone Study was conducted to compare postoperative tamponade effectiveness of intraocular silicone oil with that of long-acting gas for managing retinal detachment complicated by proliferative vitreoretinopathy. Patient accrual began in September 1985 and ended in June 1991. A total of 555 eyes were enrolled. The Silicone Study was sponsored by the National Eye Institute, National Institutes of Health, US Department of Health and Human Services. Clinical application of findings from the Silicone Study is discussed in Chapters 127 through 130.

Azen SP, Irvine AR, Davis MD et al. The validity and reliability of photographic documentation of proliferative vitreoretinopathy. Ophthalmology 1989; 96:352–357.

Lean JS, Stern WH, Irvine AR et al. Classification of proliferative vitreoretinopathy used in the Silicone Study. Ophthalmology 1989; 96:765–771.

Azen SP, Boone DC, Barlow W et al. Methods, statistical features, and baseline results of a standardized, multicentered ophthalmological surgical trial: the Silicone Study. Control Clin Trials 1991; 12:438–455.

Silicone Study Group. Vitrectomy with silicone oil or sulfur hexafluoride gas in eyes with severe proliferative vitreoretinopathy: results of a randomized clinical trial. Silicone Study Report 1. Arch Ophthalmol 1992; 110:770–779.

> After 24 months of follow-up, more eyes assigned to silicone oil than assigned to sulfur hexafluoride gas had visual acuity of 5/200 or better. Macular attachment was achieved more often in eyes treated with silicone oil.

Silicone Study Group. Vitrectomy with silicone oil or perfluoropropane gas in eyes with severe proliferative vitreoretinopathy: results of a randomized clinical trial. Silicone Study Report 2. Arch Ophthalmol 1992; 110:780–792.

> Visual acuity outcome did not differ between the silicone oil and perfluoropropane gas arms among eyes that had undergone prior vitrectomy and intraocular gas tamponade. However, among eyes without prior vitrectomy, perfluoropropane gas was associated with more posterior retinal attachments than silicone oil.

McCuen BW, Azen SP, Stern W et al. Vitrectomy with silicone oil or with perfluoropropane gas in eyes with severe proliferative vitreoretinopathy. Silicone Study Report No. 3. Retina 1993; 13:279–284.

> No difference was found between silicone oil and perfluoropropane gas in eyes with severe proliferative vitreoretinopathy with respect to visual acuity, macular reattachment, or retinal reattachment.

Barr CC, Lai MY, Lean JS et al. Postoperative intraocular pressure abnormalities in the Silicone Study. Silicone Study report 4. Ophthalmology 1993; 100:1629–1635.

> Chronic elevated intraocular pressure was more common in eyes treated with silicone oil than those treated with perfluoropropane gas (8% versus 2%). Furthermore, nearly twice as many eyes treated with perfluoropropane gas had chronic hypotony.

Blumenkranz MS, Azen SP, Aaberg T et al. Relaxing retinotomy with silicone oil or long-acting gas in eyes with severe proliferative vitreoretinopathy. Silicone Study Report 5. Am J Ophthalmol 1993; 116:557–564.

Eyes undergoing vitreoretinal surgery for the first time had successful visual acuity outcomes and anatomic reattachment without the need for relaxing retinotomy.

Hutton WL, Azen SP, Blumenkranz MS et al. The effects of silicone oil removal. Silicone Study Report 6. Arch Ophthalmol 1994; 112:778–785.

Eyes from which silicone oil was removed more often achieved visual acuity of 5/200 or better than eyes without silicone oil removal (63% versus 35%). However, recurrent retinal detachment developed more often in eyes after silicone oil was removed.

Abrams GW, Azen SP, Barr CC et al. The incidence of corneal abnormalities in the Silicone Study. Silicone Study report 7. Arch Ophthalmol 1995; 113:764–769.

The 2-year incidence of corneal abnormalities did not differ between eyes assigned to silicone oil versus long-acting gas.

Cox MS, Azen SP, Barr CC et al. Macular pucker after successful surgery for proliferative vitreoretinopathy. Silicone Study report 8. Ophthalmology 1995; 102:1884–1891.

No difference was found between eyes assigned to silicone oil versus long-acting gas with respect to macular pucker after 6 months.

Lean J, Azen SP, Lopez PF et al. The prognostic utility of the Silicone Study classification system. Silicone Study report 9. Arch Ophthalmol 1996; 114:286–292.

Diddie KR, Azen SP, Freeman HM et al. Anterior proliferative vitreoretinopathy in the Silicone Study. Silicone Study report number 10. Ophthalmology 1996; 103:1092–1099.

Compared to eyes that had posterior proliferative vitreoretinopathy, eyes with anterior proliferative retinopathy had worse baseline vitreoretinopathy, worse visual acuity, and more hypotony and macular pucker.

Abrams GW, Azen SP, McCuen BW et al. Vitrectomy with silicone oil or long-acting gas in eyes with severe proliferative vitreoretinopathy: results of additional and long-term follow-up. Silicone Study report 11. Arch Ophthalmol 1997; 115:335–344.

No difference in outcomes was found between silicone oil-treated eyes and perfluoropropane-treated eyes during long-term follow-up.

Macular hole

Freeman WR, Azen SP, Kim JW et al. Vitrectomy for the treatment of full-thickness stage 3 or 4 macular holes: results of a multicenter randomized clinical trial. Arch Ophthalmol 1997; 115:11–21.

Although more adverse events occurred in eyes treated surgically, those eyes had higher rates of hole closure and improvement in visual acuity than observed eyes.

Retinitis pigmentosa

Berson EL, Rosner B, Sandberg MA et al. A randomized trial of vitamin A and vitamin E supplementation for retinitis pigmentosa. Arch Ophthalmol 1993; 111:761–772.

Patients treated with vitamin A had somewhat lower rates of decline in retinal function and patients treated with vitamin E had somewhat higher rates of decline compared to placebo-treated eyes.

Sandberg MA, Weigel-DeFranco C, Rosner B et al. The relationship between visual field size and electroretinogram amplitude in retinitis pigmentosa. Invest Ophthalmol Vis Sci 1996; 37:1693–1698.

Visual field size was correlated with electroretinogram amplitude.

Berson EL, Rosner B, Sandberg MA et al. Further evaluation of docosahexaenoic acid in patients with retinitis pigmentosa receiving vitamin A treatment: subgroup analyses. Arch Ophthalmol 2004; 122:1306–1314.

Chapter

89

Ocular Toxoplasmosis

Douglas A. Jabs
Quan Dong Nguyen

Infection with *Toxoplasma gondii* is a frequent cause of retinal disease.[1–5] *T. gondii* is an obligate intracellular parasite, and infection is widespread in nature, affecting both humans and animals. Human toxoplasmosis may occur in either a congenital or an acquired form. Serologic evidence of previous *Toxoplasma* infection is present in 20% to 70% of the population of the USA.[6,7] In the infant or immunocompromised patient, toxoplasmosis may represent a life-threatening illness. Ocular toxoplasmosis is a potentially blinding necrotizing retinitis that may have a prolonged and relapsing course.[8–13]

ORGANISM AND LIFE CYCLE

T. gondii is a coccidian classified as belonging to the phylum Apicomplexa, class Sporozoea, order Eucoccidia, and suborder Eimeria. The infection is a zoonosis, and members of the cat family are the definitive hosts.[14–17] Old strains appear to be antigenically similar to new ones, and there appears to be only one species. The three forms of the parasite are tachyzoites (trophozoites), bradyzoites (tissue cysts), and sporozoites (oocysts).[6,14,18–20] Tachyzoites are crescent-shaped and are approximately 2 to 3 μm × 6 to 7 μm. The tachyzoite is the invasive form of the parasite and is responsible for the manifestations of acute infection. It can invade every form of mammalian cell except nonnucleated erythrocytes. The mechanism of cell entry is unknown but may be by either penetration or by mechanical or chemical action on the cell membrane. Once the tachyzoite becomes intracellular, it resides within a vacuole and multiplies by endodyogeny (two daughter cells are formed within each parent). The tachyzoite is susceptible to heat, freezing, desiccation, and gastric secretions.[6,18]

There appear to be three strains of *T. gondii* – types I, II, and III – and there may be recombinants as well. Type I is highly virulent in mice; types II and III are relatively avirulent. Data from small case series suggest that type II strains predominate in patients with acquired immunodeficiency syndrome (AIDS) and congenital infections, whereas ocular toxoplasmosis in immunocompetent hosts tends to involve type I strain or type I recombinants.[21,22]

Bradyzoites are the encysted form of the parasite found in tissue cysts. The cysts vary in size from 10 to 200 μm and may contain 50 to 3000 bradyzoites. Bradyzoites are formed within host cell vacuoles, and the surrounding membrane is elaborated by the organism. Because the cyst is intracellular and incorporates host elements into its wall, it is protected from the immune response of the host and may remain in tissues for years without provoking an inflammatory response.[23–26] Tissue cysts can develop in any organ and are responsible for persistence of latent infection. Rupture of tissue cysts causes reactivation of latent infection. In the immunocompromised host, this may lead to dissemination of *Toxoplasma* organisms. In the eye, cyst rupture may lead to active retinitis.

The oocyst is produced only in the cat, measures 10 to 12 μm in diameter, and has a thick and resistant wall. After a cat ingests either tissue cysts or oocysts, organisms are released and invade the epithelial cells of the cat intestine. The organisms then undergo an enteroepithelial asexual cycle of division (schizogony), followed by a sexual phase that results in the release of millions of oocysts 3 to 21 days after ingestion. The oocysts become infectious after they undergo sporogony with division into two sporocysts, each of which develops into four sporozoites. Oocysts may remain viable in moist soil for up to 2 years but are susceptible to dry heat and temperatures above 66°C. Cats are infected primarily by the ingestion of raw meat, wild birds, and mice.

Humans may become infected by ingesting inadequately cooked meat, chicken, and eggs,[11,27–33] presumably owing to contamination of these animals with oocysts from cats or from contaminated foodstuffs or pasture. Sand and soil contamination represents another source of infection for humans, particularly children. Infection in humans and other animals occurs after ingestion of either the tissue cyst or the oocyst. Digestive enzymes disrupt the cyst wall, and *Toxoplasma* organisms are released. They invade the intestinal epithelium, disseminate throughout the body, and multiply intracellularly.[6] This process leads to cell death and disruption of the cell membrane, which then releases the tachyzoites. The tachyzoites then invade adjacent cells and continue the process. The host's immune response to the infection causes the tachyzoites to transform into the slowly dividing bradyzoites, which form tissue cysts. These cysts may remain dormant in tissues throughout the life of the host but also may reactivate and cause clinical disease.

EPIDEMIOLOGY

Toxoplasma infection is a worldwide zoonosis. The organism infects many species of warm-blooded animals, both wild and domestic.[14–16] In humans, the prevalence of antibodies to *Toxoplasma* increases with increasing age. In the USA, it is estimated that approximately 20% to 70% of adults are seropositive for antibodies to *Toxoplasma*.[6] The prevalence of ocular toxoplasmosis varies throughout the world. In the USA, it has been estimated to be 0.6%.[34] The highest reported prevalence is in Rio Grande do Sol, the southernmost state of Brazil, where the prevalence of active and inactive (healed, pigmented retinal, or retinochoroidal lesions) ocular toxoplasmosis was 21.3% in individuals 13 years or older.[35] Studies from Brazil have shown that, over 7 years, 9.5% of seroconverters (those with acquired systemic toxoplasmosis) and 8.3% of baseline seropositive patients developed eye disease.[36,37] Toxoplasmosis in humans may be acquired by any of the following modes of transmission: (1) ingestion of undercooked, infected meat containing *Toxoplasma* cysts;[18,20,25] (2) ingestion of the oocyst from contaminated hands or food;[25] (3) inoculation of tachyzoites through a break in the skin;[20] (4) drinking of raw milk;[38] (5) blood transfusion or organ transplantation;[18,39] and (6) transplacental transmission.[9,40,41] The major routes of transmission are the ingestion of contaminated foodstuffs, accidental contamination of hands from disposing of cat feces, and transplacental transmission of infection from mother to fetus during gestation. Teutsch and associates[17] reported an outbreak of toxoplasmosis in a riding stable where the probable mode of transmission was inhalation of *Toxoplasma* oocysts from infected cats inhabiting the stable.

A municipal water system that used unfiltered, chloraminated surface water was the likely source of a large, community-wide outbreak of toxoplasmosis in Greater Victoria, British Columbia, Canada, in 1994.[42] One hundred individuals aged 6 to 83 years met the definition for an acute, outbreak-related case; 94 patients resided in Greater Victoria and six had visited it. Nineteen of the patients had retinitis. The epidemic curve appeared bimodal, with peaks that were preceded by increased rainfall and turbidity in the implicated reservoir.

PATHOGENESIS

Acute systemic toxoplasmosis in normal hosts is most often a subclinical infection but may present as a mild flu-like illness. The disease is controlled by the host's immune response to the acute infection. If the parasite reaches the eye, a focus of infection is established, which progresses from a retinitis to involve the choroid secondarily. The host's immune response appears to induce the conversion of the tachyzoite to the bradyzoite and encystment.[19] Tachyzoite antigens, detected by immunohistochemistry, and large numbers of T cells have been observed in the retinal lesions and in the choroid. Infiltrating T lymphocytes may play a role in early recognition of the *Toxoplasma* organism.[43] Healing of the lesion occurs with control of the acute infection and scar formation. The cyst may remain inactive in the scar or adjacent to it for a period of years. During this period there may be slow replication of the bradyzoite. Ultimately, the cyst wall may rupture, releasing organisms into the surrounding retina and resulting in a recurrence of the retinitis.[4,44]

The reasons for cyst rupture are unclear, but immunosuppression may contribute to this phenomenon. It was originally thought that the retinitis represented a hypersensitivity response to *Toxoplasma* antigens.[23] However, the occurrence of very aggressive disease in immunocompromised hosts[7,16,17,24,25,38] and the analysis of animal models of ocular toxoplasmosis† have suggested that the retinitis is due directly to *Toxoplasma* proliferation. Secondary changes such as the vitreitis and anterior uveitis may represent a hypersensitivity response.[45,46]

PATHOLOGY

The characteristic ocular lesion is an area of retinitis adjacent to an inactive retinochoroidal scar. Within the active lesion, there is necrosis of the retina and choroid with destruction of the retinal architecture, but a well-defined margin exists between the areas of necrotic and nonnecrotic retina. The inflammatory response is mononuclear in nature and consists of lymphocytes, macrophages, and epithelioid cells with plasma cells accumulating at the edge of the lesion (Fig. 89-1). Viable and intact cysts may be present either adjacent to scars or within the area of retinal necrosis (Figs 89-1 and 89-2), and rarely tachyzoites may be identified in the extracellular space.[47] Dispersed melanotic granules derived from the retinal pigment epithelium may be seen in areas of necrotic retina. Examination of retina away from the area of direct involvement demonstrates nonspecific chronic inflammatory changes, including perivascular lymphocytic infiltration, edema, gliosis, and neuronal degeneration.[33,48,49]

Histopathologic examination of the anterior segment (Fig. 89-1) reveals a nonspecific granulomatous or nongranulomatous inflammatory process. Large mutton-fat keratic precipitates consisting of an accumulation of mononuclear cells adherent to the corneal endothelium are frequently seen, and similar changes may be seen in the iris, trabecular region, and lens.

CLINICAL FINDINGS

Toxoplasmosis in humans may be conveniently considered under four general headings: (1) acquired; (2) congenital; (3) toxoplasmosis in the immunocompromised host; and (4) ocular.

Acquired toxoplasmosis

Acquired infection with *Toxoplasma* is generally a subclinical and asymptomatic infection. In 10% to 20% of acute infections, the host is symptomatic and has an acute flu-like illness. Clinically, these patients may have fever, lymphadenopathy, malaise, myalgias, and a maculopapular skin rash sparing the palms and soles; less often there may be hepatosplenomegaly, lymphocytosis, and atypical lymphocytes on blood smear.[25] In the immunocompetent host, the disease is self-limited and benign. However, in an immunocompromised host (e.g., AIDS patient) a life-threatening encephalitis, pneumonitis, or myocarditis may develop.

Although conventional dogma has been that most ocular toxoplasmosis is secondary to reactivation of congenital disease, more recent data have suggested that acquired ocular disease may account for more disease. In an analysis of available data,

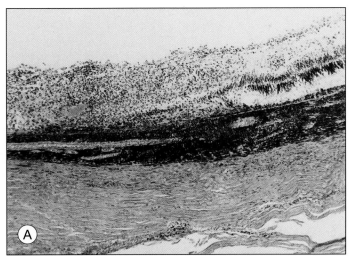

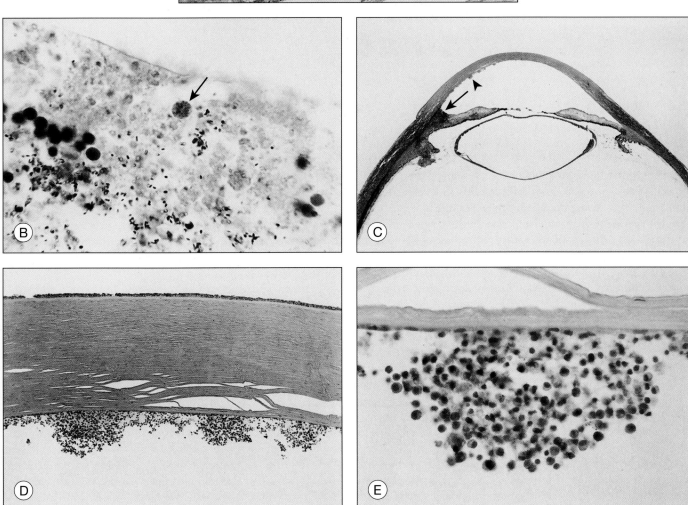

Fig. 89-1 Pathologic findings of ocular toxoplasmosis. A, An intense inflammatory reaction is present in the retina, overlying vitreous, and subjacent choroid. The retina is partially necrotic with a well-defined border between necrotic and unaffected retina (periodic acid–Schiff (PAS); ×90). (Armed Forces Institute of Pathology (AFIP) negative no. 57-1205.) B, Area of necrotic retina with *Toxoplasma* cyst (arrow) (PAS; ×600). (AFIP negative no. 57-1204.) C, Inflammatory reaction of the anterior segment with iridocyclitis, inflammatory cells occluding the inferior angle (arrow), inflammatory pupillary membrane, and mutton-fat keratic precipitates (arrowhead) (hematoxylin & eosin (HE); ×65). (AFIP negative no. 57-1208.) D, Keratic precipitates (HE; ×90). (AFIP negative no. 57-1207.) E, Higher-power view shows the keratic precipitates to be composed of histiocytes and some mononuclear cells (HE; ×460). (AFIP negative no. 57-1206; AFIP accession no. 754058.) (Reproduced from Green WR. Retina. In: Spencer WH, ed. Ophthalmic pathology: an atlas and textbook, vol. 2. Philadelphia: WB Saunders; 1985.)

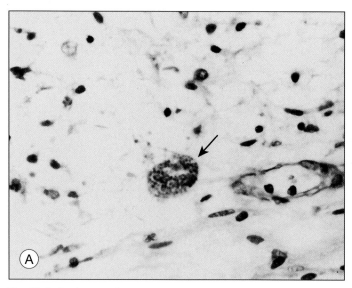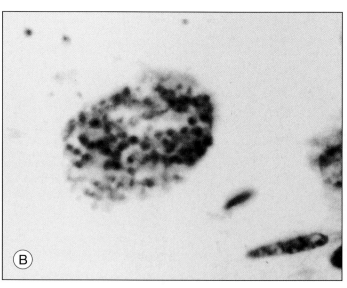

Fig. 89-2 Ocular toxoplasmosis in a neonate who died of congenital toxoplasmosis. A, At the margin of a necrotic area of retina is a spherical cyst (arrow) containing *Toxoplasma* organisms (periodic acid–Schiff; ×750). B, Higher-power view of the cyst (periodic acid–Schiff; ×2000). (Reproduced from Green WR. Retina. In: Spencer WH, ed. Ophthalmic pathology: an atlas and textbook, vol. 2. Philadelphia: WB Saunders; 1985.)

Gilbert & Stanford[51] estimated that 66% to 86% of ocular toxoplasmosis in the UK was due to postnatally acquired infection.[52] Akstein and co-workers[53] followed 37 patients for 4 years after an outbreak of acquired toxoplasmosis, the source of which was aerosolization of oocysts from infected cats in a riding stable. They found that ocular disease developed in one of 37 patients (3%) with evidence of acquired infection. Burnett et al.[54] reported an outbreak of 100 patients with acquired toxoplasmosis in Greater Victoria, Canada; 20 of the patients had retinal lesions consistent with ocular toxoplasmosis, and all had serologically proven acquired toxoplasmosis. Epidemiologic data suggested that municipal drinking water was the source of the outbreak. Silveira et al.[55] have reported acquired toxoplasmosis as the cause of retinochoroiditis in multiple families in southern Brazil. They speculated that repetitive ingestion of *Toxoplasma* organisms from raw foodstuffs during preparation resulted in the acquisition of ocular toxoplasmosis.

Congenital toxoplasmosis

Congenital toxoplasmosis results from transplacental transmission of *T. gondii* infection. The prevalence of congenital toxoplasmosis has been estimated at 1 in 10 000 live births in the USA and 1 in 1000 live births in France.[7] Only maternal infection acquired just before or during gestation endangers the fetus. Chronic maternal infection is not associated with congenital disease. The incidence and severity of congenital infection vary with the timing of infection. The lowest incidence occurs in the first trimester (15% to 20%), but the disease is usually severe and may result in spontaneous abortion or stillbirth. If *Toxoplasma* infection is acquired by the mother during the third trimester, transmission occurs in approximately 40% of cases, but it most often results in subclinical infection with few cases of clinical congenital toxoplasmosis.[54–56]

Over 80% of congenitally infected infants develop evidence of ocular disease by adolescence; 20% to 40% of the cases are bilateral. When there is bilateral involvement, 29% of the eyes have visual acuity worse than 20/40.[57] Clinical manifestations of congenital toxoplasmosis consist of retinochoroiditis, hydrocephalus, microcephaly, cerebral calcifications, seizures, psychomotor retardation, organomegaly, jaundice, rash, and fever. Congenital toxoplasmosis must be differentiated from other congenital infections, including rubella, cytomegalovirus (CMV), herpes simplex, and syphilis.

There is a spectrum of clinical disease in patients with congenital *Toxoplasma* infection. Couvreur & Desmonts[9] followed 300 cases of congenital toxoplasmosis. The findings were as follows: ocular lesions in 76%, neurologic disorders in 51%, intracranial calcification in 32%, and hydrocephalus or microcephaly in 26%. Retinochoroiditis is the most frequent abnormality in patients with congenital infection, being present in approximately 75% to 80% of cases. It is bilateral in 85% of affected persons.[9,58] Mets and associates[59] conducted a prospective, longitudinal study of 94 patients with congenital toxoplasmosis. Chorioretinal scars, found in all patients, were the most common eye finding and were often found in the periphery. Many children with congenital toxoplasmosis had substantial retinal damage at birth and associated loss of vision. Active lesions became quiescent with treatment. There is a predilection for the posterior pole of the eye to be affected by congenital toxoplasmosis, and this may be related to the end-artery anatomy of the fetal macular circulation.[60]

The diagnosis of the classic congenital toxoplasmosis syndrome is based on the clinical triad of: (1) convulsions; (2) cerebral calcification; and (3) chorioretinitis.[3] Anti-*Toxoplasma* antibodies of the immunoglobulin M (IgM) class are found in 75% of infants with congenital toxoplasmosis. IgM antibodies are produced by the fetus in response to infection with *Toxoplasma* and are specific for fetal infection, since maternal IgM cannot cross the placental barrier. Fetal IgM antibodies are not detected in 25% of cases at birth owing to delayed antibody synthesis by the fetus.[40]

In children with mild infection, the disease may become apparent only later in life when retinochoroidal scarring is detected on ophthalmoscopic examination (Fig. 89-3). This may occur during an evaluation for strabismus, as a consequence of a routine school vision check, or during a routine ocular examination.[3]

Toxoplasmosis in immunocompromised hosts

Toxoplasmosis is a major cause of morbidity and mortality in immunocompromised hosts.[8,12,13,20,61] Life-threatening encephalitis, pneumonitis, or myocarditis may develop in these patients. In patients with AIDS, cerebral toxoplasmosis is particularly common. Immunodeficient or immunosuppressed patients, such as those with Hodgkin's disease,[62] hematologic malignancies,[33,61] collagen-vascular disorders,[13] or organ transplants,[12,63] as well as those with AIDS,[27–29,31,64] may also develop retinochoroiditis from toxoplasmosis, which may be an atypical and severe necrotizing form of retinochoroiditis. Histopathologically, these lesions show focal zones of inner retinal necrosis with a minimal inflammatory cell infiltrate and multiple, viable, free *Toxoplasma* organisms[11,33] (Fig. 89-4).

CMV and *T. gondii* both cause a necrotizing retinopathy in immunocompromised hosts. The diagnosis of each of these infections is usually made on clinical findings. However, the two infections may occasionally be confused with one another because of similar clinical features. Elkins and colleagues[67] reported five cases of necrotizing retinopathy in immunosuppressed patients, which were diagnosed initially as CMV retinopathy but subsequently were found to be toxoplasmic retinochoroiditis. The correct diagnosis was based on endoretinal biopsy and/or the rapid response to antitoxoplasmic drug therapy. In addition, immunocompromised patients with more than one simultaneous retinal infection have been reported.[65,66]

Although ocular toxoplasmosis can occur in patients with AIDS, it is uncommon and affects only an estimated 1% to 2% of those patients in the USA. Higher rates have been reported in France and Brazil.[67] Jabs[68] reported a significant association between ocular toxoplasmosis and cerebral toxoplasmosis in patients with AIDS; 56% of patients with ocular disease also had cerebral involvement. Twelve percent of patients with cerebral toxoplasmosis were found to have ocular disease as well.

Serologic diagnosis of toxoplasmosis in immunocompromised patients is often difficult owing to a depressed antibody response, in which IgM antibody may not be detectable and the rise in IgG antibody titer is not present.[7]

Ocular toxoplasmosis

Ocular toxoplasmosis most often presents as a focal necrotizing retinitis; it is generally associated with a vitreitis and often a granulomatous anterior uveitis. Less commonly, ocular infection may present as a papillitis. Secondary complications of ocular toxoplasmosis include cataract, glaucoma, posterior synechiae, cystoid macular edema, retinal perivasculitis, and chorioretinal vascular anastomoses. Rarely, toxoplasmic retinochoroiditis can be associated with an overlying scleritis.[68] The age of the first attack of ocular toxoplasmosis is typically in the second decade, and 75% of cases occur between 10 and 35 years of age. With long-term follow-up, the 5-year recurrence rate is 79%,[69] and some patients may have multiple recurrences.[70]

Retinochoroiditis

Ocular toxoplasmosis most often presents as a focus of retinitis involving the inner layers of the retina and presenting as a whitish, fluffy lesion with surrounding retinal edema (Fig. 89-5). An overlying vitreitis is present and may be generalized. The retina is the primary site of infection, but the choroid[71] and sclera may be secondarily involved by the associated inflammatory response. Active lesions are classically adjacent to an old inactive scar. In elderly patients, toxoplasmosis can present as multifocal or diffuse necrotizing retinitis, which may be associated with occlusive retinal arteritis.[72] Older patients may be more susceptible to severe ocular *Toxoplasma* infections because of an age-related decline in cell-mediated immunity and chronic underlying disease.[72]

Symptoms are present in over 90% of patients with active *Toxoplasma* retinitis. The majority of patients present with a history of floaters; however, patients can also present with reduced central vision due to retinochoroiditis involving the fovea or to media opacities from the vitreitis. Patients may complain of metamorphopsia caused by serous detachment of the macula secondary to a deep retinal lesion or may develop reduced vision secondary to cystoid macular edema or cataract formation as a result of chronic disease.

Three morphologic variants of retinal *Toxoplasma* lesions have been described: (1) large destructive lesions; (2) punctate inner retinal lesions; and (3) punctate outer (or deep) retinal lesions.[73] Large destructive retinal lesions are defined as an area of active retinitis greater than one disc diameter in size. The lesion is dense, yellowish-white, elevated, surrounded by a ring of retinal edema, and associated with a severe vitreous inflammation. Over half

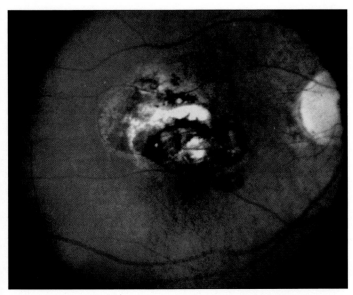

Fig. 89-3 Inactive chorioretinal scar caused by toxoplasmosis.

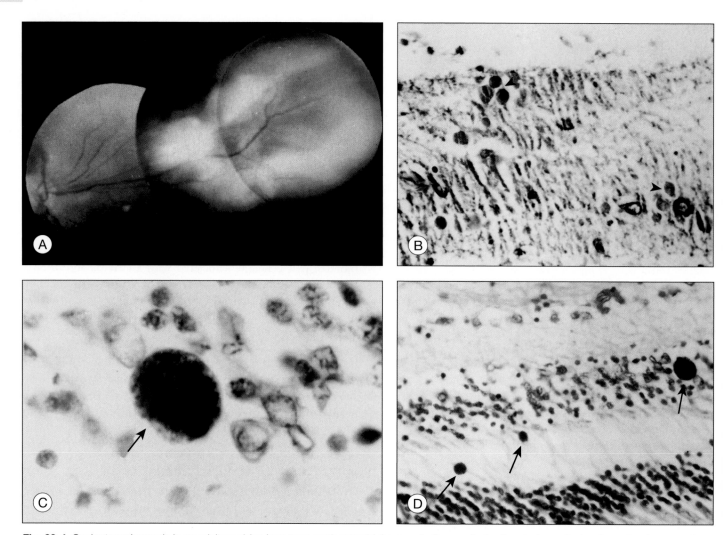

Fig. 89-4 Ocular toxoplasmosis in an adult receiving long-term corticosteroid therapy. A, Composite fundus photograph showing extensive area of *Toxoplasma* retinitis. B, Necrotic retina showing numerous *Toxoplasma* cysts (arrowhead) (periodic acid–Schiff (PAS); ×525). C, *Toxoplasma* cysts (arrow) in an area of necrotic retina (PAS; ×750). D, *Toxoplasma* cysts (arrows) in adjacent noninvolved retina (PAS; ×550). (A from Nicholson DH, Wolchok EB. Ocular toxoplasmosis in an adult receiving long-term corticosteroid therapy. Arch Ophthalmol 1976; 94:248–254. B to D from Green WR. Retina. In: Spencer WH, ed. Ophthalmic pathology: an atlas and textbook, vol. 2. Philadelphia: WB Saunders; 1985.)

of the cases have an associated anterior uveitis. The large destructive lesion is the most common and the most serious variant of active retinitis. Of patients with this type of lesion, 40% had reduced vision with the initial episode, and complications are most frequent with large destructive lesions. Regardless of their location, large destructive lesions typically require treatment. If the acute lesion is located near a major retinal vessel, a branch retinal artery or branch retinal vein occlusion can result.[74]

Punctate inner retinal lesions are single or multifocal gray areas of active retinitis associated with mild retinal edema. There is a mild overlying vitreous reaction. If located in the retinal periphery, this type of lesion may be benign, spontaneously remitting, and not need treatment. However, if this type of lesion is in the macular region, it can result in visual loss and requires treatment.

Punctate outer retinal lesions are characterized by multifocal, gray-white, punctate lesions at the level of the deep retina or retinal pigment epithelium and are associated with little or no overlying vitreous reaction. These lesions tend to resolve slowly and recur in a satellite fashion in adjacent areas. Acute punctate outer retinal toxoplasmosis must be differentiated from similar deep gray-white changes that may occur in acute posterior multifocal placoid pigment epitheliopathy, serpiginous choroiditis, and diffuse unilateral subacute neuroretinitis.[75] Kyrieleis arterialitas refers to the accumulation of periarterial exudates, which can occur either in the vicinity of the acute retinitis or elsewhere in the retina.[2]

Toxoplasmic papillitis

A minority of patients with ocular toxoplasmosis develop foci of inflammation within or directly adjacent to the optic nerve head. These patients have severe unilateral papillitis, and initially the diagnosis of toxoplasmosis is often not suspected. However, the presence of inactive *Toxoplasma* scars in the retina often suggests the appropriate diagnosis.

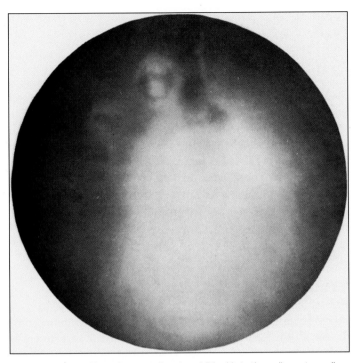

Fig. 89-5 Active *Toxoplasma* retinochoroiditis. Note the adjacent small, inactive *Toxoplasma* scars. This lesion is an example of the large destructive variant.

Choroidal neovascularization has been described as a late complication of ocular toxoplasmosis. Fine et al.[82] described three cases of choroidal neovascularization adjacent to inactive toxoplasmosis scars. They stress the importance of considering this diagnosis as a cause of sudden vision loss in patients with inactive *Toxoplasma* scars. Other retinal vascular lesions described as complicating toxoplasmosis include branch artery obstruction of a vessel passing through an area of active retinitis, periphlebitis, periarteritis during the acute stages of retinochoroiditis,[56,74,81] and retinochoroidal vascular anastomoses.[82] Toxoplasmic scleritis has been reported in patients with associated toxoplasmic retinochoroiditis.[68]

Visual prognosis
Friedmann & Knox[75] reported that 26 (41%) of their 63 patients with toxoplasmic retinochoroiditis ultimately suffered permanent unilateral visual loss to 20/100 or less. A lesion in the macular region was the cause of this severe visual loss in 88% of these cases, and large destructive lesions in the retinal periphery accounted for visual loss in the other cases. Visual loss was independent of the number of preceding episodes of active retinitis but was associated with the duration of the active episode. Mild to moderate visual loss (20/40 to 20/70) was seen in an additional 16% of cases.

Folk & Lobes[78] reported six patients with toxoplasmic papillitis. The patients were healthy young adults who had floaters, blurred vision, and occasionally pain with eye movement. There was an associated mild anterior segment reaction, but a severe vitreous inflammation was present. The optic nerve head lesion was a white inflammatory mass, sometimes in a sectorial distribution, associated with disc edema, or adjacent retinal edema, or both. There were dense visual field defects corresponding to the site of the lesion on the optic disc. Resolution of the lesion resulted in sectorial optic disc pallor and the associated visual field defect.

Some patients with toxoplasmic papillitis have a focus of inflammation adjacent to the optic nerve head in association with old *Toxoplasma* scars,[77] and the diagnosis is more obvious. However, the diagnosis is more difficult if papillitis is the only lesion. The differential diagnosis of *Toxoplasma* papillitis includes optic neuritis, anterior ischemic optic neuropathy, sarcoidosis, optic disc vasculitis,[78] tumors of the optic nerve head, and other causes of retinitis that may have an associated optic nerve involvement, such as *Candida*, CMV, herpes simplex virus, and varicella-zoster virus.

Complications of *Toxoplasma* retinochoroiditis
The complications of ocular toxoplasmosis include chronic iridocyclitis, cataract formation, secondary glaucoma, band keratopathy, cystoid macular edema, retinal detachment, and optic atrophy secondary to optic nerve involvement. Friedmann & Knox[75] reported secondary complications in one-third of their patients (21 of 63), most often in association with large destructive lesions. The most common complication was secondary glaucoma, which occurred in 12% (8 of 63) of patients.

DIAGNOSIS

The diagnosis of *Toxoplasma* retinitis is made on the basis of the appearance of the characteristic lesion (i.e., an area of active retinitis adjacent to an inactive chorioretinal scar). The results of laboratory tests for *Toxoplasma* infection are supportive of the diagnosis. In adults, other causes of retinochoroiditis such as sarcoidosis, tuberculosis, syphilis, and viral and fungal infections should be considered in the differential diagnosis. In congenital toxoplasmosis, the differential diagnosis includes other causes of macular coloboma, such as congenital herpes simplex virus, CMV, and foci of retinoblastoma.[3]

Serologic tests for demonstration of antibodies to *Toxoplasma*
Several serologic tests can demonstrate the presence of antibodies to *Toxoplasma*, including the Sabin–Feldman dye test, indirect fluorescent antibody test, indirect hemagglutination test, complement fixation test, and the enzyme-linked immunosorbent assay (ELISA) test. Indirect fluorescent antibody and ELISA tests are now used most often. However, because the prevalence of antibodies to *Toxoplasma* is high in certain communities and because high-titer antibodies can persist for years in otherwise healthy persons, the interpretation of these tests is often fraught with difficulty.[83] In humans the prevalence of seropositivity for antibodies to *Toxoplasma* increases with age. In countries such as France, the prevalence of anti-*Toxoplasma* antibodies is greater than 90% by the fourth decade of life, and in the USA it is estimated that 20% to 70% of healthy adults have been previously infected with toxoplasmosis.

In ocular toxoplasmosis, low titers of IgG antibody to toxoplasmosis are usual. If the clinical lesion is characteristic of toxoplasmosis and the serologic titer is positive, the diagnosis of *Toxoplasma* chorioretinitis can usually be made with confidence. If the retinal lesion is atypical and the serology is positive, the diagnosis of *Toxoplasma* chorioretinitis is only presumptive, owing to the high prevalence of antibodies in the general population.[7]

Aqueous humor antibody

In 1966, Desmonts[86] described a method for determining the ratio of anti-*Toxoplasma* antibody in aqueous humor to that in serum. A coefficient was calculated comparing the concentration of anti-*Toxoplasma* antibody divided by the concentration of gamma-globulin in the aqueous to that in the serum. In uninfected patients the coefficient is approximately 1, but it ranges from 0.5 to 2.0 in the normal fellow eye of patients with unilateral ocular toxoplasmosis. A coefficient of 8 or above is consistent with the intraocular production of specific anti-*Toxoplasma* antibodies and suggestive of active ocular toxoplasmosis. ELISA techniques are now used to make these measurements.[85] Since a paracentesis is required, it is not a routine diagnostic test in the USA, although it is used more often in Europe.

Polymerase chain reaction

Polymerase chain reaction (PCR) has been investigated as a useful technique to identify *Toxoplasma* on specimens obtained from ocular fluids and from paraffin-embedded retinal tissue.[86,87] Briefly, *Toxoplasma* DNA in the specimens is detected by PCR assay, in which the target is part of a ribosomal DNA (rDNA) repetitive gene. The basepair segment is amplified with the synthetic oligonucleotide primers.[86] DNA is obtained from the specimens through proper preparation. The DNA is then amplified in a reaction containing, among others, all four deoxyribonucleotide triphosphates, each of the two oligonucleotide primers, and Taq polymerase.[86] The amplification is usually done in an automated DNA thermal cycler. Identification of *Toxoplasma* by PCR is particularly helpful in cases in which the diagnosis is suspected but no organism could be seen by histology and serologic tests for anti-*Toxoplasma* antibody is negative.

IgG appears to be the major class involved in the humoral response against the *T. gondii* parasite, followed by IgA. In an analysis of 88 patients with a diagnosis of ocular toxoplasmosis, Ronday and associates noted 65% had intraocular IgG production (against *T. gondii*), 52% had intraocular IgA production, 37.5% had both IgG and IgA production, 27% had IgG production only, and 15% had IgA production only. Among the 13 patients tested, only one patient had intraocular IgM production.[90]

The combination of local antibody production and PCR analysis of intraocular fluids can aid significantly in the diagnosis of ocular toxoplasmosis.[89–91] Ongkosuwito and associates[92] showed, in a study of 22 patients with primary ocular toxoplasmosis (not from scars) and 42 patients with recurrent toxoplasmosis, that intraocular production of anti-*T. gondii* IgG was more frequently noted in patients with recurrent than in those with primary ocular toxoplasmosis (81% versus 41%), whereas intraocular *T. gondii* DNA (as detected by PCR) was more frequently found in patients with primary ocular toxoplasmosis than those with recurrent diseases (37% versus 4%).[87]

Toxoplasmic neuroretinitis

Toxoplasma gondii infection can also cause neuroretinitis, a distinct clinical entity consisting of visual loss, optic nerve head edema, and macular exudate in a stellate pattern, and variable vitreous inflammation. Fish et al.[81] described five patients with unilateral neuroretinitis and serologic evidence of *T. gondii* infection. All the patients had optic nerve edema, macular star formation, and vitreous inflammation but no other foci of active retinochoroiditis. Two patients had inactive peripheral chorioretinal scars compatible with previous ocular toxoplasmosis infection. Therapy with anti-*Toxoplasma* antibiotics and systemic corticosteroids quieted the disease and improved the visual acuity.

Treatment
Principles
Since acquired systemic toxoplasmosis in an immunocompetent host is a benign and self-limited illness, no treatment is generally given. Conversely, because of the potential for severe and sometimes life-threatening disease in an immunocompromised host, or in cases of congenital toxoplasmosis, treatment is generally given. However, in ocular toxoplasmosis the decision to treat is made on the basis of the nature and location of the lesion. Small peripheral lesions will heal spontaneously, usually without adverse sequelae, and may be observed. Conversely, lesions in the posterior pole and large destructive lesions can cause significant visual loss and are generally treated. The American Uveitis Society has conducted a survey of its members to identify the indications (relative or absolute) for initiating treatment of ocular toxoplasmosis. Results of the survey among members who replied showed that the most common indications were: zone I disease (i.e., adjacent to the optic nerve or fovea): 100%, vitreous reaction of 3+ or 4+: 95%, persistence of disease for greater than 1 month: 88%, decreased visual acuity: 77%, and lesion greater than one disc diameter in size: 70%.[93]

Several drugs have shown efficacy against the tachyzoite in animal models and clinical situations, but none has proved beneficial against the bradyzoite. The drugs clinically used in the treatment of ocular toxoplasmosis include pyrimethamine, sulfadiazine, trimethoprim-sulfamethoxazole, clindamycin, and azithromycin. Both pyrimethamine and sulfadiazine interfere with folic acid metabolism in the parasite but act at different points in the metabolic pathway. Thus the two drugs are synergistic when given together and are usually used as such.

The classic treatment regimen for ocular toxoplasmosis consists of pyrimethamine, sulfadiazine, and corticosteroids and is often known as triple drug therapy.[94] Oral corticosteroids are added to the antibiotics to minimize the damage to other ocular structures caused by the inflammatory response. Similarly, topical corticosteroids and cycloplegics are used to treat any associated anterior uveitis. Because *Toxoplasma* retinitis represents an active proliferation of organisms, oral corticosteroid treatment should not be given without antibiotic coverage. Severe fulminant ocular toxoplasmosis has been reported in patients treated with oral corticosteroids alone.[11,63,95] In a large series of patients from the Netherlands oral corticosteroid therapy alone was associated with poorer visual outcomes.[96] Clindamycin is also used in the treatment of ocular toxoplasmosis. Some authors have used it as a single agent,[97] others in combination with sulfadiazine,[98] and some have even advocated the use of quadruple drug therapy, consisting of pyrimethamine, sulfadiazine, corticosteroids, and clindamycin.[94] Although all these antibiotics have demonstrated activity in animal models, and efficacy has been reported in unmasked uncontrolled studies, there are limited randomized, controlled studies of treatment. Indeed, no consensus has been reached on the best initial treatment, as some authors prefer triple drug therapy, others prefer quadruple drug therapy, and different dosages of corticosteroids are recommended by different authors.[94] Our preference has been to use the classic triple drug therapy (Box 88-1) initially. In a survey of American Uveitis Society members, triple drug therapy was the most often cited preferred therapeutic regimen for a typical case of ocular toxoplasmosis (Table 89-1), but the diversity of opinion was wide, and the plurality of triple drug therapy was small.[93] In a study from the Netherlands, 108 patients with ocular toxoplasmosis were assigned to one of three regimens by clinic (pyrimethamine and sulfadiazine, clindamycin, or trimethoprim-sulfamethoxazole) and the results were compared to patients with peripheral lesions that were not treated. Only pyrimethamine

---

Box 89-1 Treatment of ocular toxoplasmosis

1. Pyrimethamine, two 50 mg loading doses 12 h apart, then 25 mg by mouth twice daily
2. Sulfadiazine, 2 g loading dose, then 1 g by mouth four times daily
3. Prednisone, 20 to 40 mg by mouth once daily
4. Folinic acid, 3 to 5 mg by mouth twice weekly
5. Emphasize fluid intake to minimize the possibility of sulfadiazine renal crystallization

---

Duration of treatment varies with the patient's response but may require 4 to 6 weeks.

Table 89-1 Preferred therapeutic regimens for typical cases of ocular toxoplasmosis

Regimen	Respondents (%)
Pyrimethamine, sulfadiazine, prednisone (triple drug therapy)	32
Pyrimethamine, sulfadiazine, clindamycin, prednisone (quadruple therapy)	27
Sulfadiazine, clindamycin, prednisone	16
Clindamycin, prednisone	6

Modified from Engstrom RE Jr, Holland GN, Nussenblatt RB et al. Current practices in the management of ocular toxoplasmosis. Am J Ophthalmol 1991; 111:601–610.[96]

and sulfadiazine showed a beneficial effect, as it was associated with smaller lesions.[99] However, none of these short-term regimens was associated with a decrease in the recurrence rate.

Azithromycin has also been reported to be efficacious for ocular toxoplasmosis. In a randomized clinical trial of 46 patients with active ocular toxoplasmosis, patients were randomized to azithromycin 250 mg and pyrimethamine 50 mg/day or pyrimethamine 50 mg/day and sulfadiazine 1 g four times daily. Oral prednisone was begun on day 3 in both groups. Both arms of the study showed a similar degree of improvement in visual acuity response rates, but the regimen of azithromycin and pyrimethamine had nearly 50% fewer adverse events when compared to sulfadiazine and pyrimethamine.[100]

The duration of treatment depends on the patient's response to therapy, but often it should be between 4 and 6 weeks. Corticosteroids, if given, should be tapered as soon as the eye has quieted, and the antibiotics discontinued only after the prednisone has been stopped.

In patients with AIDS, relapse of the toxoplasmosis with discontinuation of therapy is generally seen. Therefore chronic suppressive therapy to prevent relapse has been recommended.[27,94] Of respondents in the American Uveitis Society survey, 63% used such chronic suppressive therapy in patients with AIDS. The best regimen for this secondary prophylaxis remains to be determined.

In the past, short-term treatment of acute attacks has been the mainstay of therapy for immunologically normal patients. However, in a randomized controlled trial of 124 patients with ocular toxoplasmosis from Brazil, where frequent occurrences are common, prophylactic treatment with double-strength trimethoprim-sulfamethoxazole (Bactrim DS) given every 3 days led to a decrease in recurrences of disease (7% in the prophylactic group compared to 24% in the observation group).[101] As such, prophylactic trimethoprim-sulfamethoxazole may be of value in patients with frequent recurrences.

Recently, Bosch-Driessen and associates have identified a potential increase in risk of reactivation of ocular toxoplasmosis following cataract extraction, which implies that prophylactic treatment with antiparasitic drugs during and after cataract surgery may be valuable for patients who are at risk of visual loss.[103]

Drugs used in the treatment of toxoplasmosis
Pyrimethamine

Pyrimethamine (Daraprim) is a diaminopyrimidine that acts as a folic acid antagonist. Its action on *Toxoplasma* is synergistic with sulfonamides. Pyrimethamine is readily absorbed from the gastrointestinal tract, is lipid-soluble, and is distributed throughout the cells of the body. The concentration of pyrimethamine in the cerebrospinal fluid is approximately 25% of that in plasma.[103] Pyrimethamine is generally used in conjunction with sulfonamides. Pyrimethamine is started with either a single oral loading dose of 75 mg or two loading doses of 50 mg 12 h apart, followed by treatment at a dosage of 25 mg once or twice daily.

Pyrimethamine's most serious adverse effect is a dose-related and reversible bone marrow suppression, resulting in anemia, leukopenia, or thrombocytopenia.[104] Another common side-effect is gastrointestinal intolerance, manifested as anorexia and nausea. In one study[105] gastrointestinal upset occurred in half of the patients treated and marrow suppression in 12%. Because of this effect on the bone marrow, hematologic monitoring must be performed while the patient is taking pyrimethamine. Bone marrow toxicity can often be avoided by administering folinic acid (leucovorin calcium) 3 to 5 mg orally two or three times weekly. This inhibits the toxic side-effects of pyrimethamine without reducing its efficacy against toxoplasmosis. Because it is teratogenic, pyrimethamine is contraindicated in pregnant women.

Sulfadiazine

Sulfadiazine is an effective toxoplasmacidal agent that works synergistically with pyrimethamine, and combination therapy is generally used. Sulfadiazine is started with a single oral 2 to 4 g loading dose followed by treatment at a dosage of 1 g four times daily. The most common side-effect of sulfadiazine is a skin rash, but the more serious side-effect is renal crystallization, which can be avoided by a high fluid intake. Sodium bicarbonate, at a dosage of 1 teaspoon three times daily, is sometimes given to alkalinize the urine and help prevent crystallization. Sulfadiazine should be withdrawn if a skin rash, crystalluria, albuminuria, or hematuria occurs.

Clindamycin

Clindamycin has been reported to be an effective drug in the treatment of toxoplasmosis in animals,[60,106] and open-label, uncontrolled series have reported successful use in the treatment of human ocular toxoplasmosis.[97,98,107] Tabbara and associates[108] have reported a reduction in *Toxoplasma* cysts in the healed lesions of rabbits treated with clindamycin, suggesting that clindamycin may have some effect in treating the encysted form. Clindamycin appears to be concentrated in the retinal pigment epithelium and therefore may be given at the dosage of 300 mg orally four times daily.

The most serious side-effect of clindamycin is pseudomembranous colitis, which is reported to occur in 1 in 50 000 to 1 in 100 000 cases.[108] This complication has resulted in fatal outcomes, and it is therefore recommended that the drug be discontinued if diarrhea develops. Pseudomembranous colitis is due to a toxin produced by *Clostridium difficile*, and treatment with clindamycin may result in overgrowth of this organism. Treatment with oral vancomycin suppresses *C. difficile* and results in resolution of the colitis.[109]

Azithromycin

Azithromycin (Zithromax) is an azalide, a subclass of macrolide antibiotics, that is administered orally. Azithromycin is derived from erythromycin; however, it differs chemically from erythromycin. Azithromycin has emerged as a potentially effective agent in the management of ocular toxoplasmosis. In a prospective, randomized clinical trial of 46 patients with active ocular toxoplasmosis in the Netherlands, a combination of azithromycin (250 mg daily) and pyrimethamine (50 mg daily) was compared to a combination of sulfadiazine (1 g four times daily) and pyrimethamine (50 mg daily). Oral prednisone (40 mg daily) was begun on day 3 in patients in both groups. Both regimens showed similar degree in improving vitreous inflammation and visual acuity. However, the combination of azithromycin and pyrimethamine had a statistically significant lower rate of adverse events (nearly 50%) than the regimen of sulfadiazine and pyrimethamine.[100] Azithromycin may thus be an appropriate and effective alternative to sulfadiazine in the treatment of ocular toxoplasmosis, and should be used in place of sulfadiazine in patients who possess an allergy to sulfa-containing drugs.

Other antibiotics

Minocycline is a semisynthetic tetracycline that has shown promise in the treatment of murine toxoplasmosis and ocular toxoplasmosis in rabbits.[110] However, no study has reported the results of its use in human ocular toxoplasmosis. The suggested dose is 100 mg orally once or twice daily.[94] Tetracycline 250 mg four times daily has also been suggested instead of minocycline.[94]

Spiramycin is not currently available in the USA but has been used in Europe and in animal studies. Reports of its efficacy in the treatment of *Toxoplasma* retinochoroiditis have been conflicting.[62] Nolan & Rosen[110] found spiramycin to have some effect in the treatment of toxoplasmosis but less than that of pyrimethamine, and recurrences after treatment are common.[18]

Opremcak and colleagues,[111] in an uncontrolled case series of 16 patients, reported that trimethoprim-sulfamethoxazole appears to be a safe and effective alternative to sulfadiazine, pyrimethamine, and folinic acid in treating selected cases of ocular toxoplasmosis. The dosage used was 160 mg trimethoprim and 800 mg sulfamethoxazole (one Bactrim DS) orally twice daily for 4 to 6 weeks. All 16 patients in the study had resolution of active retinochoroiditis and improved vision. However, given the spontaneous resolution of most cases of ocular toxoplasmosis in immunologically normal hosts,[113] the relative efficacy of this approach is uncertain.

Atovaquone (Mepron) is a hydroxynaphthoquinone effective against *Plasmodium falciparum* and is used for treatment of mild to moderate *Pneumocystis carinii* pneumonia in patients with AIDS. Atovaquone has also been reported to be effective in the treatment of ocular and central nervous system toxoplasmosis in patients with AIDS who are intolerant to pyrimethamine, sulfa, and clindamycin.[114] Concurrent administration of food increases absorption of atovaquone twofold.[115] Gormley et al.[115] reported in an animal model that atovaquone reduces the number of cerebral *Toxoplasma* cysts after acute infection and in chronic disease. Since tissue cysts are believed to be responsible for reactivation of *Toxoplasma* retinochoroiditis, atovaquone may have the potential to reduce the risk of recurrent retinochoroidal disease. Similar beneficial effects in humans remain to be determined.

Systemic corticosteroids

Systemic corticosteroid therapy has been used as an adjunct in the treatment of ocular toxoplasmosis to suppress the inflammatory response and minimize the damage to the surrounding retina and other structures. A wide range of dosages has been suggested, from a maximum of 20 mg oral prednisone daily to doses of 1.0 to 1.5 mg/kg daily (60 to 100 mg prednisone daily in an adult).[4,94,116] It has been our practice to use moderate doses of prednisone, generally in the range of 20 to 40 mg/day.

We believe that systemic steroids should not be used as the sole agent in the treatment of ocular toxoplasmosis and should only be used with appropriate antibiotic coverage.[11,46,95,96,116,117] Since the retinitis appears to be due to the active proliferation of *Toxoplasma* organisms, treatment with steroids alone may inhibit the inflammatory response and may result in a more destructive retinitis. Nicholson & Wolchok[11] and Sabates and associates[65] have described cases of fulminant ocular toxoplasmosis with panuveitis and a severe, diffuse necrotizing retinitis in patients treated with steroids alone. As noted above, oral corticosteroid therapy alone has been reported to result in poorer visual outcomes.[96] The occurrence of an aggressive necrotizing retinitis in immunocompromised patients with ocular toxoplasmosis[27,29] underscores the need for antibiotic treatment when corticosteroids are used. In patients with ocular toxoplasmosis and AIDS, we generally have treated only with antibiotics and have not used systemic corticosteroids. In this situation, antibiotics alone have resulted in satisfactory control of the retinitis.

Surgical treatment

Photocoagulation and cryotherapy have been tried in the treatment of ocular toxoplasmosis. These methods may destroy the *Toxoplasma* cysts, as well as the tachyzoites. However, when used in the treatment of active lesions, photocoagulation may be associated with retinal hemorrhage, vitreous hemorrhage, or even retinal detachment.[118] Furthermore, *Toxoplasma* cysts may reside in ophthalmoscopically normal retina, making either of these treatments unlikely to be curative. Photocoagulation may be considered in the treatment of choroidal neovascularization, which can be a late complication of ocular toxoplasmosis.[80]

Prevention

Preventive measures to minimize human contact with infectious forms of the parasite are important in controlling acquired and congenital forms of toxoplasmosis. Adequate cooking of meat kills the tissue cyst and prevents this form of transmission. Care should be exercised in the handling of raw meat, cats, and possibly contaminated soil. Hands should be washed, or, if appropriate, gloves should be worn. Patients at risk should avoid contact with cat feces altogether. Pregnant women seronegative for *Toxoplasma* antibodies should be advised to avoid any contact with cats during their pregnancy. Sandboxes should be kept covered when not in use, and cat-litter pans should be cleaned every day to avoid sporulation.[23]

REFERENCES

1. Duke-Elder S, Perkins ES. System of ophthalmology, vol. 9. Diseases of the uveal tract. St. Louis: Mosby; 1966.
2. Gass JDM. Stereoscopic atlas of macular diseases: diagnosis and treatment, 2nd edn. St. Louis: Mosby; 1987.
3. Schlaegel TF Jr. Toxoplasmosis. In: Duane TD, Jaeger EA, eds. Clinical ophthalmology, vol. 4. Hagerstown, MD: Harper & Row; 1978.
4. Tabbara KF. Toxoplasmosis. In: Duane TD, Jaeger EA, eds. Clinical ophthalmology, vol. 4. Hagerstown, MD: Harper & Row; 1978.
5. Wilder HC. *Toxoplasma* chorioretinitis in adults. Arch Ophthalmol 1952; 48:127–136.
6. Anderson S. *Toxoplasma gondii*. In: Mandell GL, Douglas RG Jr, Bennett JE, eds. Principles and practice of infectious diseases. New York: John Wiley; 1979.
7. McCabe RE, Remington JS. *Toxoplasma gondii*. In: Mandell GL, Douglas RG Jr, Bennett JE, eds. Principles and practice of infectious diseases, 2nd edn. New York: John Wiley; 1985.
8. Cohen SN. Toxoplasmosis in patients receiving immunosuppressive therapy. JAMA 1970; 211:657–660.
9. Couvreur J, Desmonts G. Congenital and maternal toxoplasmosis: a review of 300 congenital cases. Dev Med Child Neurol 1962; 4:519–530.
10. Hoerni B, Vallat M, Durand M et al. Ocular toxoplasmosis and Hodgkin's disease: report of two cases. Arch Ophthalmol 1978; 96:62–63.
11. Nicholson DH, Wolchok EB. Ocular toxoplasmosis in an adult receiving long-term corticosteroid therapy. Arch Ophthalmol 1976; 94:248–254.
12. Reynolds ES, Walls KW, Pfeiffer RJ. Generalized toxoplasmosis following renal transplantation: report of a case. Arch Intern Med 1966; 118:401–405.
13. Ruskin J, Remington JS. Toxoplasmosis in the compromised host. Ann Intern Med 1976; 84:193–199.
14. Krick JA, Remington JS. Toxoplasmosis in the adult – an overview. N Engl J Med 1978; 298:550–553.
15. Miller NL, Frenkel JK, Dubey JP. Oral infections with *Toxoplasma* cysts and oocysts in felines, other mammals, and in birds. J Parasitol 1972; 58:928–937.
16. Swartzberg JE, Remington JS. Transmission of *Toxoplasma*. Am J Dis Child 1975; 129:777–779.
17. Teutsch SM, Juranek DD, Sulzer A et al. Epidemic toxoplasmosis associated with infected cats. N Engl J Med 1979; 300:695–699.
18. McCabe RE, Remington JS. Toxoplasmosis. In: Warren KS, Mahmoud AAF, eds. Tropical and geographical medicine. New York: McGraw-Hill; 1984.
19. Shimada K, O'Connor GR, Yoneda C. Cyst formation by *Toxoplasma gondii* (RH strain) in vitro. Arch Ophthalmol 1974; 92:496–505.
20. Shoukrey N, Tabbara KF. Eye-related parasitic diseases. In: Tabbara KF, Hyndiuk RA, eds. Infections of the eye. Boston: Little, Brown; 1986.
21. Bootroyd JC, Grigg ME. Population biology of *Toxoplasma gondii* and its relevance to human infection: do different strains cause different disease? Curr Opin Microbiol 2002; 5:438–442.
22. Grigg ME, Ganatra J, Boo JC et al. J Infect Dis 2001; 184:6533–6539.
23. Frenkel JK. Pathogenesis of toxoplasmosis with a consideration of cyst rupture in Besnoitia infection. Surv Ophthalmol 1961; 6:799–832.
24. Frenkel JK. Breaking the transmission chain of *Toxoplasma*: a program for the prevention of toxoplasmosis. Bull NY Acad Med 1974; 50:228–245.
25. Frenkel JK. Toxoplasmosis. Pediatr Clin North Am 1985; 32:917–932.
26. Frenkel JK, Jacobs L. Ocular toxoplasmosis: pathogenesis, diagnosis, and treatment. Arch Ophthalmol 1958; 59:260–279.
27. Holland GN, Engstrom RE, Glasgow BJ et al. Ocular toxoplasmosis in patients with the acquired immunodeficiency syndrome. Am J Ophthalmol 1988; 106:563–667.
28. Jabs DA, Green WR, Fox R et al. Ocular manifestations of acquired immune deficiency syndrome. Ophthalmology 1989; 96:1092–1099.
29. Parke DW II, Font RL. Diffuse toxoplasmic retinochoroiditis in a patient with AIDS. Arch Ophthalmol 1986; 104:571–575.
30. Pepose JS, Holland GN, Nestor MS et al. Acquired immune deficiency syndrome: pathogenic mechanisms of ocular disease. Ophthalmology 1985; 92:472–484.
31. Schuman JS, Orellana J, Friedman AH et al. Acquired immune deficiency syndrome (AIDS). Surv Ophthalmol 1987; 31:384–410.
32. Weiss MJ, Velazquez N, Hofeldt AJ. Serologic tests in diagnosis of presumed toxoplasmic retinochoroiditis. Am J Ophthalmol 1990; 109:407–411.
33. Yeo JH, Jakobiec FA, Iwamoto T et al. Opportunistic toxoplasmic retinochoroiditis following chemotherapy for systemic lymphoma: a light and electron microscopic study. Ophthalmology 1983; 90:852–898.
34. Maetz HM, Kleinstein RN, Federico D et al. Estimated prevalence of ocular toxoplasmosis and toxocariasis in Alabama. J Infect Dis 1987; 156:414.
35. Glasner PD, Silveira C, Kruszon-Moran D et al. An unusually high prevalence of ocular toxoplasmosis in southern Brazil. Am J Ophthalmol 1992; 114:136–144.
36. Glasner PD, Silveira C, Kruszon-Moran D et al. An unusually high prevalence of ocular toxoplasmosis in southern Brazil. Am J Ophthalmol 1992; 114:136–144.
37. Glasner PD, Silveira C, Kruszon-Moran D et al. An unusually high prevalence of ocular toxoplasmosis in southern Brazil. Am J Ophthalmol 1993; 114:136–144.
38. Silveira C, Belfort R Jr, Muccioli C et al. A follow-up study of *Toxoplasma gondii* infection in southern Brazil. Am J Ophthalmol 2001; 131:351–354.

39. Sacks JJ, Roberto RR, Brooks NF. Toxoplasmosis infection associated with raw goat's milk. JAMA 1982; 248:1728–1732.
40. Ryning FW, McLeod R, Maddox JC et al. Probable transmission of *Toxoplasma gondii* by organ transplantation. Ann Intern Med 1979; 90:47–49.
41. Desmonts G, Forestier F, Thulliez P et al. Prenatal diagnosis of congenital toxoplasmosis. Lancet 1985; 1:500–503.
42. Perkins ES. Ocular toxoplasmosis. Br J Ophthalmol 1973; 57:1–17.
43. Bowie WR, King AS, Werker DH et al. Outbreak of toxoplasmosis associated with municipal drinking water. The BC Toxoplasma Investigation Team. Lancet 1997; 350:1255–1256.
44. Brézin AP, Kasner L, Thulliez P et al. Ocular toxoplasmosis in the fetus: immunohistochemistry analysis and DNA amplification. Retina 1994; 14:19–26.
45. Tabbara KF. Ocular toxoplasmosis. In: Tabbara KF, Hyndiuk RA, eds. Infections of the eye. Boston: Little, Brown; 1986.
46. Abrahams IW, Gregerson DS. Longitudinal study of serum antibody responses to retinal antigens in acute ocular toxoplasmosis. Am J Ophthalmol 1982; 93:224–231.
47. O'Connor GR. The role of parasite invasion and of hypersensitivity in the pathogenesis of toxoplasmic retinochoroiditis. Ocular Inflamm Ther 1983; 1:37–46.
48. Brézin AP, Egwuagu CE, Burnier M Jr et al. Identification of *Toxoplasma gondii* in paraffin-embedded sections by the polymerase chain reaction. Am J Ophthalmol 1990; 110:599–604.
49. Rao NA, Font RL. Toxoplasmic retinochoroiditis: electron-microscopic and immunofluorescence studies of formalin-fixed tissue. Arch Ophthalmol 1977; 95:273–277.
50. Zimmerman LE. Ocular pathology of toxoplasmosis. Surv Ophthalmol 1961; 6:832–876.
51. Gilbert RE, Stanford MR. Is ocular toxoplasmosis caused by prenatal or postnatal infection? Br J Ophthalmol 2000; 84:224–226.
52. Gilbert RE, Stanford MR. Is ocular toxoplasmosis caused by prenatal or postnatal infection? Br J Ophthalmol 2000; 84:224–226.
53. Akstein RB, Wilson LA, Teutsch SM. Acquired toxoplasmosis. Ophthalmology 1982; 89:1299–1301.
54. Burnett AJ, Shortt SG, Isaac-Renton J et al. Multiple cases of acquired toxoplasmosis retinitis presenting in an outbreak. Ophthalmology 1998; 105:1032–1037.
55. Silveira C, Belfort R Jr, Burnier M Jr et al. Acquired toxoplasmic infection as the cause of toxoplasmic retinochoroiditis in families. Am J Ophthalmol 1988; 106:362–364.
56. Koppe JG, Kloosterman GJ, deRoerer-Bonnet H. Toxoplasmosis and pregnancy with a long-term follow-up of the children. Eur J Obstet Gynecol Reprod Biol 1974; 43:101–110.
57. Nussenblatt RB, Belfort R Jr. Ocular toxoplasmosis. JAMA 1994; 271:304–309.
58. Wilson CB, Remington JS, Stagno S et al. Development of adverse sequelae in children born with subclinical congenital *Toxoplasma* infection. Pediatrics 1980; 66:767–774.
59. Mets MB, Holfels E, Boyer KM et al. Eye manifestations of congenital toxoplasmosis. Am J Ophthalmol 1996; 122:309–324.
60. Remington JS, Desmonts G. Toxoplasmosis. In: Remington JS, Klein JO, eds. Infectious diseases of the fetus and newborn infant, 2nd edn. Philadelphia: WB Saunders; 1983.
61. Mets MB, Holfels E, Boyer KM et al. Eye manifestations of congenital toxoplasmosis. Am J Ophthalmol 1996; 122:309–324.
62. Tabbara KF, Nozik RA, O'Connor GR. Clindamycin effects on experimental ocular toxoplasmosis in the rabbit. Arch Ophthalmol 1974; 92:244–247.
63. Vietzke WM, Gelderman AH, Grimley PM et al. Toxoplasmosis complicating malignancy: experience at the National Cancer Institute. Cancer 1968; 21:816–827.
64. Harper JS III, London WT, Sever JL. Five drug regimens for treatment of acute toxoplasmosis in squirrel monkeys. Am J Trop Med Hyg 1985; 34:50–57.
65. Sabates R, Pruett RC, Brockhurst RJ. Fulminant ocular toxoplasmosis. Am J Ophthalmol 1981; 92:497–503.
66. Weiss A, Margo CE, Ledford DK et al. Toxoplasmic retinochoroiditis as an initial manifestation of the acquired immune deficiency syndrome. Am J Ophthalmol 1986; 101:248–249.
67. Elkins BS, Holland GN, Opremcak M et al. Ocular toxoplasmosis misdiagnosed as cytomegalovirus retinopathy in immunocompromised patients. Ophthalmology 1994; 101:499–507.
68. Jabs DA. Ocular manifestations of HIV infections. Trans Am Ophthalmol Soc 1995; 93:623–683.
69. Cochereau-Massin I, LeHoang P, Lautier-Frau M et al. Ocular toxoplasmosis in human immunodeficiency virus-infected patients. Am J Ophthalmol 1992; 114:130–135.
70. Schuman JS, Weinberg RS, Ferry AP et al. Toxoplasmic scleritis. Ophthalmology 1988; 95:1399–1403.

71. Bosch-Driessen LE, Berendschot TT, Ongkosuwito JV et al. Ocular toxoplasmosis: clinical features and prognosis of 154 patients. Ophthalmology 2002; 109:869–878.
72. Friedman CT, Knox DL. Variations in recurrent actoxoplasmic retinochoroiditis. Arch Ophthalmol 1969; 81:481–493.
73. Hausmann N, Richard G. Acquired ocular toxoplasmosis: a fluorescein angiography study. Ophthalmology 1991; 98:1647–1651.
74. Johnson MW, Greven CM, Jaffe GJ et al. Atypical, severe toxoplasmic retinochoroiditis in elderly patients. Ophthalmology 1997; 104:48–57.
75. Friedmann CT, Knox DL. Variations in recurrent active toxoplasmic retinochoroiditis. Arch Ophthalmol 1969; 81:481–493.
76. Braunstein RA, Gass JDM. Branch artery obstruction caused by acute toxoplasmosis. Arch Ophthalmol 1980; 98:512–513.
77. Doft BH, Gass JDH. Punctate outer retinal toxoplasmosis. Arch Ophthalmol 1985; 103:1332–1336.
78. Folk JC, Lobes LA. Presumed toxoplasmic papillitis. Ophthalmology 1984; 91:64–67.
79. Willerson D, Aaberg T, Reeser F et al. Unusual ocular presentation of acute toxoplasmosis. Br J Ophthalmol 1977; 61:693–701.
80. Hayreh SS. Optic disc vasculitis. Br J Ophthalmol 1972; 56:652–670.
81. Fish RH, Hoskins JC, Kline LB. Toxoplasmosis neuroretinitis. Ophthalmology 1993; 100:1177–1182.
82. Fine SL, Owens SL, Haller JA et al. Choroidal neovascularization as a late complication of ocular toxoplasmosis. Am J Ophthalmol 1981; 91:318–322.
83. Shepp DH, Hackman RC, Conley FK et al. *Toxoplasma gondii* reactivation identified by detection of parasitemia in tissue culture. Ann Intern Med 1985; 103:218–221.
84. Kennedy JE, Wise GN. Retinochoroidal vascular anastomosis in uveitis. Am J Ophthalmol 1971; 71:1221–1225.
85. Eichenwald HF. The laboratory diagnosis of toxoplasmosis. Ann NY Acad Sci 1956; 64:207–211.
86. Desmonts G. Definitive serological diagnosis of ocular toxoplasmosis. Arch Ophthalmol 1966; 76:839–851.
87. Rollins DF, Tabbara KF, O'Connor GR et al. Detection of toxoplasmal antigen and antibody in ocular fluids in experimental ocular toxoplasmosis. Arch Ophthalmol 1983; 101:455–457.
88. Aouizerate F, Cazenave J, Poirier L et al. Detection of *Toxoplasma gondii* in aqueous humour by the polymerase chain reaction. Br J Ophthalmol 1993; 77:107–109.
89. Chan C, Palestine AG, Li Q et al. Diagnosis of ocular toxoplasmosis by the use of immunocytology and the polymerase chain reaction. Am J Ophthalmol 1994; 117:803–805.
90. Ronday MJ, Ongkosuwito JV, Rothova A et al. Intraocular anti-*Toxoplasma gondii* IgA antibody production in patients with ocular toxoplasmosis. Am J. Ophthalmol 1999; 127:294–300.
91. Baarsma GS, Luyendijk L, Kijlstra A et al. Analysis of local antibody production in the vitreous humor of patients with severe uveitis. Am J. Ophthalmol 1991; 112:147–150.
92. Ongkosuwito JV, Bosch-Driessen EH, Kijlstra A et al. Serologic evaluation of patients with primary and recurrent ocular toxoplasmosis for evidence of recent infection. Am J. Ophthalmol 1999; 128:407–412.
93. de Boer JH, Verhagen C, Bruinenberg M et al. Serologic and polymerase chain reaction analysis of intraocular fluids in the diagnosis of infectious uveitis. Am J Ophthalmol 1996; 121:650–658.
94. Ongkosuwito JV, Bosch-Driessen EH, Kijlstra A et al. Serologic evaluation of patients with primary and recurrent ocular toxoplasmosis for evidence of recent infection. Am J Ophthalmol 1999; 128:407–412.
95. Rothova A, Meenken C, Buitenhuis HJ et al. Therapy for ocular toxoplasmosis. Am J Ophthalmol 1993; 115:517–523.
96. Engstrom RE Jr, Holland GN, Nussenblatt RB et al. Current practices in the management of ocular toxoplasmosis. Am J Ophthalmol 1991; 111:601–610.
97. O'Connor GR, Frenkel JK. Dangers of steroid treatment in toxoplasmosis: periocular injections and systemic therapy. Arch Ophthalmol 1976; 94:213.
98. Bosch-Driessen LE, Berendschot TT, Ongkosuwito JV et al. Ocular toxoplasmosis: clinical features and prognosis of 154 patients. Ophthalmology 2002; 109:869–878.
99. Lakhanpal V, Schocket SS, Nirankari VS. Clindamycin in the treatment of toxoplasmic retinochoroiditis. Am J Ophthalmol 1983; 95:605–613.
100. Tate GW Jr, Martin RG. Clindamycin in the treatment of human ocular toxoplasmosis. Can J Ophthalmol 1977; 12:188–195.
101. Rothova A, Meenken C, Buitenhuis HJ et al. Therapy for ocular toxoplasmosis. Am J Ophthalmol 1993; 115:517–523.
102. Silveira C, Belfort R Jr, Muccioli C et al. The effect of long-term intermittent trimethoprin–sulfamethoxazole treatment on recurrences of toxoplasmic retinochoroiditis. Am J Ophthalmol 2002; 134:41–46.

103. Bosch-Driessen LH, Berbraak FD, Suttorp-Schulten MS et al. A prospective, randomized trial of pyrimethamine and azithromycin vs pryimethmine and sulfadiazine for the treatment of ocular toxoplasmosis. Am J Ophthalmol 2002; 134:34–40.

104. Beverley JKA. A rational approach to the treatment of toxoplasmic uveitis. Trans Ophthalmol Soc UK 1958; 78:109–116.

105. Giles CL. The treatment of *Toxoplasma* uveitis with pyrimethamine and folinic acid. Am J Ophthalmol 1964; 58:611–617.

106. Ghosh N, Levy PN, Leopold IH. Therapy of toxoplasmic uveitis. Am J Ophthalmol 1965; 59:55–60.

107. Silveira C, Belfort R Jr, Muccioli C et al. The effect of long-term intermittent trimethoprin/sulfamethoxazole treatment on recurrences of toxoplasmic retinochoroiditis. Am J Ophthalmol 2002; 134:41–46.

108. Tabbara KF, O'Connor GR. Treatment of ocular toxoplasmosis with clindamycin and sulfadiazine. Ophthalmology 1980; 87:129–134.

109. Viteri AL, Howard PH, Dyck WP. The spectrum of lincomycin–clindamycin colitis, Gastroenterology 1974; 66:1137–1144.

110. Nolan J, Rosen ES. Treatment of active toxoplasmic retino-choroiditis. Br J Ophthalmol 1968; 52:396–399.

111. Opremcak EM, Scales DK, Sharpe MR. Trimethoprim–sulfamethoxazole therapy for ocular toxoplasmosis. Ophthalmology 1992; 99:920–925.

112. Rothova A, Meenken C, Buitenhuis HJ et al. Therapy for ocular toxoplasmosis. 1993; 115:517–523.

113. Lopez JS, de Smet MD, Masur H et al. Orally administered 566C80 for treatment of ocular toxoplasmosis in a patient with the acquired immunodeficiency syndrome. Am J Ophthalmol 1992; 113:331–332.

114. Bartlett JG. Medical management of HIV infection. Baltimore: Port City Press; 1997.

115. Gormley PD, Pavesio CE, Minnasian D et al. Effects of drug therapy on *Toxoplasma* cysts in an animal model of acute and chronic disease, Invest Ophthalmol 1998; 39:1171–1175.

116. Knox DL. Active presumed *Toxoplasma* retinochoroiditis: its treatment. S Afr Arch Ophthalmol 1974; 2:137–139.

117. Ghartey KN, Brockhurst RJ. Photocoagulation of active toxoplasmic retinochoroiditis. Am J Ophthalmol 1980; 89:858–864.

Chapter

90

Ocular Toxocariasis
C. P. Wilkinson

INTRODUCTION

Zoonotic ocular infections are unusual in adults, but invasion of the eye by the roundworm *Toxocara canis* is an important cause of reduced visual acuity in young patients. Most individuals with serologic evidence of toxocariasis are asymptomatic,[1] and in some populations, as many as 30% of asymptomatic children demonstrate serologic evidence of prior *Toxocara* infestation.[2] Although the precise incidence of ocular toxocariasis remains unknown, it is a diagnosis that appears to be made rather commonly in children. Loss of vision as a result of intraocular *Toxocara* usually occurs because of damage to the vitreous and retina, and a variety of typical clinical pictures have been described.[3-5] The systemic form of toxocariasis was described before the ocular, and an understanding of the former disorder and of the life cycle of *T. canis* is important to know. In 1952, Beaver and associates[6] first described the systemic effects of *Toxocara* infestation in the human and termed the disorder *visceral larval migrans*. Findings associated with the syndrome range from a mild-to-moderate eosinophilia in an asymptomatic patient to a fulminating and fatal disease associated with pneumonia, congestive heart failure, or convulsions.[7,8] In addition, some patients without a clinical history of the disorder and without eosinophilia may exhibit serum enzyme-linked immunosorbent assay (ELISA) titers as high as 1:32.[9] It has been hypothesized that the ingestion of large amounts of larvae may result in a more marked eosinophilia than that associated with infestation of fewer organisms, and one report correlated the degree of eosinophilia with ELISA titers.[9] Fever, irritability, pallor, anorexia, and malaise usually characterize symptomatic visceral larval migrans. Transitory infiltrates of the lungs are common, and hepatomegaly is the most frequently observed physical finding. The disorder is usually self-limited.[8] Systemic visceral larval migrans is typically a disease of young children from 6 months to 4 years of age, with an average age of 2 years. Interestingly, the systemic disorder is only rarely associated with the development of ocular toxocariasis, so the organism is responsible for two relatively distinct human diseases.[5,7,10,11]

T. canis is a common ascarid of dogs and the most frequent cause of both visceral larval migrans and ocular toxocariasis.[7,8,11] These roundworms have a life cycle that cannot be completed in the human (Fig. 90-1). Fertilized ova containing infectious larvae are deposited in the soil, from which they are ingested by both the canine and the human. In both dog and human, the larvae migrate into the wall of the small intestine, where they gain access to the lymphatic and portal circulation. Systemic dissemination of organisms to the liver, lungs, brain, kidney, heart, muscles, and eye then occurs. In the human, this completes the life cycle, and the parasites are usually enclosed by an inflammatory granulomatous response that is primarily eosinophilic (Fig. 90-2), although the larvae may remain viable for years under such conditions.[4,7,8] Similarly, in the mature canine, the organisms do not usually evolve further.[12] However, in pregnancy, the host response in the infected bitch is altered, and previously encysted larvae may resume migratory behavior[12] (Fig. 90-1). Many organisms cross the placenta and enter the developing canine fetus. In the newborn and young canine host, larvae reaching the lungs migrate via the larynx and pharynx into the intestine, where they quickly mature into adult worms (Fig. 90-1) that produce infectious ova that are passed in fecal material. Prenatal infection is the primary route of transmission to puppies.[4,11] Puppies can also become infected by ingesting infectious ova that are present in the feces and milk of nursing bitches, in the fecal material of other infected young canines, or in infected nonhosts, such as mice. Because of the inability of the parasite to mature into an adult form in humans, a search for *T. canis* ova in human feces is inevitably unrewarding. The laboratory diagnosis of *T. canis* infestation is discussed later.

Intraocular involvement by *T. canis* also tends to occur in young patients, but those who are older than individuals developing visceral larval migrans.[3-5,9] Most patients with the ocular form of the disorder do not provide a history compatible with prior visceral larval migrans, and an eosinophilia is frequently not discovered. Nevertheless, case-controlled studies of patients with ocular toxocariasis have demonstrated the historical importance of pica and exposure to puppies,[13-15] and some patients with the eye disorder provide an obvious history of concurrent or prior systemic infestations.[16] The dose and virulence of the organisms, the immune response of the host, and other factors may be important in explaining the differences between typical clinical presentations of systemic and ocular involvement by *T. canis*. In experimental studies in primates, ocular toxocariasis did not occur after gastrointestinal implantation of infectious larvae, despite an elevation of serum ELISA titers.[10] However,

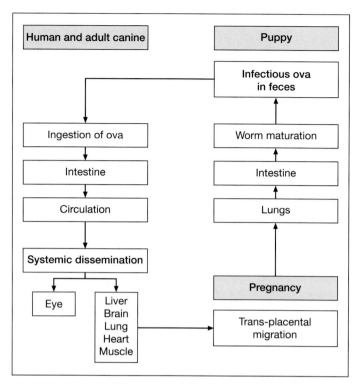

Fig. 90-1 Life cycle of *Toxocara canis* (see text).

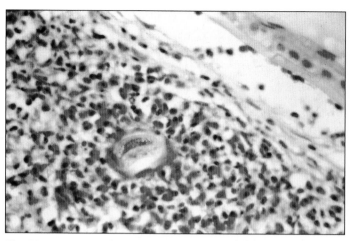

Fig. 90-2 Intraocular *Toxocara* remnants surrounded by an exuberant inflammatory reaction consisting primarily of eosinophils.

ocular involvement following similar implantation in Mongolian gerbils was observed in over half of the experimental cohort,[17] and species differences in susceptibility are obviously significant.[18]

This chapter discusses the effects of *T. canis* larval invasion of the eye and includes: (1) a historical review of the problem; (2) a description of the variety of clinical presentations associated with this syndrome; (3) the differential diagnosis; (4) current laboratory diagnostic methods; (5) therapeutic maneuvers in managing ocular toxocariasis; and (6) a brief discussion of the goals and means of preventive management.

HISTORICAL REVIEW

The evolution of thinking regarding the importance of *T. canis* as a cause of blindness has been discussed extensively elsewhere.[4,5] Wilder[16] was the first to implicate nematode larvae as an important cause of childhood blindness. She examined 46 eyes that had been enucleated for suspected retinoblastoma and that contained an intraocular inflammatory response dominated by eosinophils (Fig. 90-2). She was able to demonstrate nematode larvae or their capsules in 24 cases in this series, although the organisms were initially reported as hookworm larvae. Several of the specimens were subsequently identified as second-stage *Toxocara* larvae by Nichols,[19] who was aware of the report by Beaver and co-authors,[6] which had initially described the systemic form of toxocariasis. The cases presented by Wilder[16] were not thoroughly described clinically, but apparently most of them involved eyes with marked intravitreal inflammation, retinal detachment, and leukocoria.

In 1959 Irvine & Irvine[20] described histologic findings in an eye that had signs and symptoms different from those of the cases of Wilder.[16] This eye of a 4-year-old boy had clear media. Vision was 20/70, and the patient was referred because of blurring and strabismus. Subsequent ophthalmologic examination revealed an inferior retinal detachment, but indirect ophthalmoscopy was apparently not performed, and a distinct mass was not recognized clinically. However, the eye was removed because of the fear of retinoblastoma following a positive P-32 test and the discovery of "suspicious cells" in aqueous fluid. The gross pathologic examination revealed a white inflammatory mass in the peripheral retina and vitreous. Subsequent histologic examination revealed remnants of a *T. canis* larva in the inferior periphery.

In 1960 Ashton[21] described four cases of histologically proven *Toxocara* endophthalmitis that presented in a distinct fashion that represented a third classic form of this disorder. In each of these eyes, a large white retinochoroidal granuloma, suspected of being a retinoblastoma at that time, was observed in the posterior pole. Minimal signs of intravitreal inflammation were present, and extensive vitreous bands were present in only one of four cases. The following year, Duguid[22] described a larger series of cases of ocular toxocariasis and emphasized the difference between the solid posterior pole "retinal granuloma" and more diffuse chronic endophthalmitis. In 1965 Hogan et al.[23] documented *Toxocara* in the eye of a patient who had been followed for more than 1 year before death and who had fundus findings typical of the pars planitis syndrome.

Increased awareness of the different presentations of ocular toxocariasis resulted in a reduction in the number of eyes with histologically proven disease.[24] In 1971 Wilkinson & Welch[3] presented a series of 41 eyes with proven or presumed ocular toxocariasis. Eyes with chronic endophthalmitis and leukocoria were much more likely to have been enucleated, whereas eyes with the posterior or peripheral isolated and visible granulomas were usually diagnosed clinically, and enucleation was not performed to confirm the diagnosis. In this series, a peripheral granulomatous mass with relatively clear media but organized vitreous bands was the most common form of presentation, being seen in 18 of 41 (44%) cases.[3] However, an isolated posterior pole inflammatory mass was the most common form of presentation in a series of 100 cases subsequently reported by Hagler and co-authors.[25] Bilateral involvement with single inflammatory masses in a different portion of each eye is quite rare.[26]

A variety of other relatively unusual forms of *Toxocara* endophthalmitis have subsequently been described,[4,5,27] and these are briefly discussed later.

CLINICAL PRESENTATIONS

Toxocara endophthalmitis can usually be classified in one of four ways: (1) chronic endophthalmitis; (2) posterior pole "granuloma;" (3) peripheral granulomatous inflammatory mass; or (4) atypical presentation.

Chronic endophthalmitis

Chronic endophthalmitis (vitreous abscess) was the first form of *T. canis* endophthalmitis to be described histologically.[16] Most of the cases originally described by Wilder[16] were in this classification, and the eyes were enucleated because of the possibility of retinoblastoma. The presence of a dense vitreous inflammatory response, a profound reduction in the clarity of the media, and a major retinal detachment were documented in most cases.

Patients with this form of *Toxocara* endophthalmitis tend to be slightly younger than those with a more localized granulomatous response occurring in relatively clear media.[3] The history is usually negative for trauma, intraocular surgery, or other conditions associated with bacterial or fungal endophthalmitis. However, a history of pica may be obtained.[3,14,15] External signs of ocular inflammation are usually absent.

Acutely, this form of endophthalmitis may occasionally be associated with a granulomatous response in the anterior chamber, and a hypopyon may be observed in severe cases. Dense cellular infiltrates in the vitreous gel may make visualization of the retina exceedingly difficult. Ill-defined yellowish-white masses may be observed through this dense vitreous haze, and secondary retinal detachments may be visualized or diagnosed ultrasonographically.[28] The acute phase of inflammation may be followed by a cicatricial stage in which fibrocellular membranes develop deep within the vitreous gel or as cyclitic membranes. Alternatively, in some eyes the inflammatory reaction may subside, and the vitreous may clear dramatically. In such cases a dense white mass, representing the primary focus of intraocular inflammation and the presumed site of the parasite, may be detected. This may be visualized in the posterior pole or in the periphery, and in some cases the picture may evolve into one of the categories described below. The prognosis in this form of endophthalmitis depends primarily on the degree of intravitreal organization that occurs during the acute inflammatory episode.

Posterior pole "granuloma"

The presentation of the posterior pole granuloma form of endophthalmitis depends on the stage at which it is observed,

although these patients may be more likely to present with a secondary strabismus than those with chronic endophthalmitis.[3] This form of the infestation may initially present with relatively hazy vitreous and signs of acute inflammation, in which the posterior pole granuloma is observed as an ill-defined, hazy mass surrounding vitreous inflammation. However, the vitreous gel may become quite clear as the inflammation subsides, and the media may also be clear in the eye in which the diagnosis is delayed or in which relatively little vitreous inflammation occurs initially. Subretinal or intraretinal inflammatory masses in this form of the disorder typically become very well defined and are relatively small, ranging in size from 0.75 to 6.0 mm in diameter (Fig. 90-3). The spherical granulomatous masses are usually white or gray, and traction bands running from the mass to the surrounding retina are frequently observed if the inflammatory reaction has extended into the vitreous cavity (Fig. 90-4). Retinochoroidal vascular anastomoses may be associated with these lesions if they are present in the macular

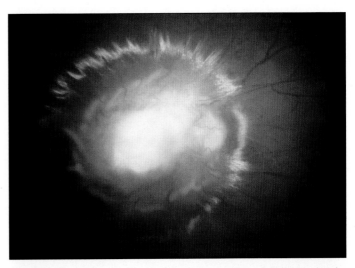

Fig. 90-3 Posterior pole *Toxocara* "granuloma." There is little intravitreal organization.

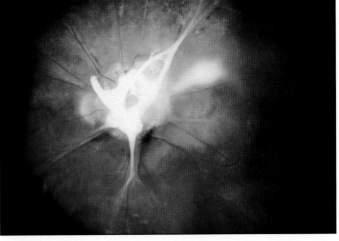

Fig. 90-4 Posterior pole "granuloma" with secondary fibrocellular membranes extending into the vitreous gel and surrounding retina.

zone,[27] and macular lesions may be observed in association with peripheral inflammatory masses.[25]

The prognosis for stability in eyes with this form of *Toxocara* endophthalmitis is relatively good. However, central vision has usually been lost by the time the diagnosis is made. Choroidal neovascularization may occur as a late complication of *Toxocara* lesions in the posterior pole.[27,29]

Peripheral inflammatory mass

The peripheral inflammatory mass form of *Toxocara* endophthalmitis may also be preceded by a more active and acute form of apparent diffuse endophthalmitis. However, as clearing in the media occurs, a dense, white inflammatory mass is visualized in the periphery of the retina. This mass may be quite localized, spherical, and similar to those observed in the posterior pole. Alternatively, the inflammation may be much more diffuse and appear as a "snow bank," as is visualized in typical severe pars planitis.[23] Fibrocellular bands may be observed running from a peripheral inflammatory mass to the more posterior retina or the optic nerve (Fig. 90-5). Localized traction on the retina may result in the production of a fold in the peripheral retina associated with the inflammatory mass[3] (Fig. 90-6). The prognosis in eyes with peripheral granulomatous inflammation is usually relatively good. By the time this diagnosis is made, active inflammation is usually not progressive.[3] However, intraretinal traction bands associated with this disorder can lead to production of both traction and rhegmatogenous retinal detachments, which are discussed later.

Atypical presentations

In addition to the above three classic forms of *Toxocara* endophthalmitis, atypical forms of posterior intraocular inflammation

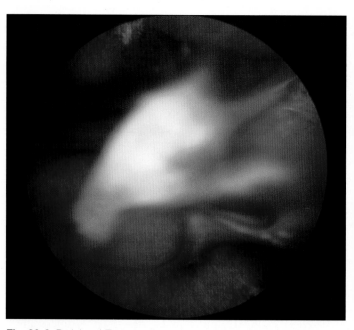

Fig. 90-6 Peripheral *Toxocara* "granuloma." A fold of retina is pulled toward the inflammatory mass.

have been observed. These include: (1) inflammation and swelling of the optic nerve head;[30] (2) motile subretinal nematode;[31] and (3) diffuse chorioretinitis.[5] Anterior segment involvement by *Toxocara* has resulted in conjunctivitis, keratitis, focal iris nodules, and lens changes.[4,5] In nearly all of these reported cases of atypical presentations, the diagnosis of *Toxocara* endophthalmitis was presumed and was not confirmed histologically.

DIFFERENTIAL DIAGNOSIS

The diagnosis of ocular toxocariasis is not difficult when discrete inflammatory masses associated with typical vitreous and epiretinal organization are observed. However, in eyes with severe vitreous opacification, it may be impossible to make the appropriate diagnosis on the basis of morphologic features alone. Important considerations in the differential diagnosis of intraocular toxocariasis include: (1) retinoblastoma; (2) other forms of endophthalmitis and uveitis; (3) retinopathy of prematurity (ROP); (4) familial exudative vitreoretinopathy; (5) Coats disease; (6) persistent hyperplastic primary vitreous; and (7) idiopathic optic neuritis.

Retinoblastoma

Retinoblastoma is the most important entity frequently confused with ocular toxocariasis.[5] Classic descriptions of ocular toxocariasis by Wilder[16] and Ashton[21] were the results of the possibility that the reported eyes might have been harboring retinoblastomas. Shields[5] reported that more than one-fourth of eyes referred for evaluation of possible retinoblastoma were subsequently discovered to have ocular toxocariasis. It should be noted, however, that this report dates from 1984. It is likely that the incorrect diagnosis rate is lower today.

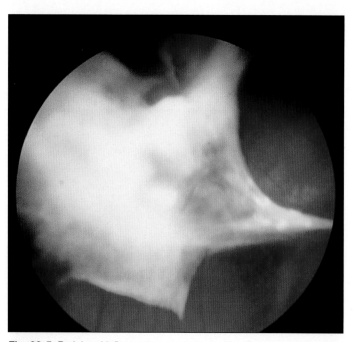

Fig. 90-5 Peripheral inflammatory mass caused by *Toxocara canis*, with typical fibrocellular stalks extending into the vitreous cavity and toward the retinal surface.

Patients with retinoblastoma are usually diagnosed before 2 years of age and are therefore younger than typical children with ocular toxocariasis. Eyes with exophytic forms of retinoblastoma typically have a clear vitreous without signs of inflammation or membrane formation. A more hazy vitreous may be observed in eyes with an endophytic type of tumor, but signs of vitreoretinal traction are typically absent, as are inflammatory cyclitic membranes and secondary cataracts.[5]

In cases in which the differential diagnosis is relatively difficult, ultrasonography and computed tomography may be very valuable in demonstrating intraocular tumors and calcium. If the differential diagnosis is particularly difficult, evaluation of intraocular fluids may be in order, and this is briefly described later.

Other forms of endophthalmitis and uveitis

A variety of forms of endophthalmitis resulting from endogenous infection or trauma may present in a fashion that closely mimics ocular toxocariasis. Typical bacterial infections produce a much more acute form of intraocular inflammation. More indolent infectious processes may be quite impossible to distinguish from nematode endophthalmitis. In such cases, laboratory diagnostic methods may be of value in differentiating a variety of forms of endophthalmitis. Pars planitis or chronic cyclitis is a condition that typically occurs in an older age group than that in which ocular toxocariasis occurs. The disorder is bilateral in approximately 80% of cases. It may be impossible to distinguish this form of inflammation from that caused by *Toxocara*. Hogan and co-authors[23] described a case of pars planitis in which subsequent histologic examination demonstrated that the inflammation observed in the inferior periphery of the eye was due to *T. canis*.

Retinopathy of prematurity

The morphologic features of ROP may closely mimic those of peripheral cicatricial ocular toxocariasis. In both conditions a peripheral white retinal mass may be associated with a fold of retina extending from the posterior pole toward the focus of inflammation. However, ROP is usually diagnosed soon after birth. A history of extreme prematurity is rare in patients with ocular toxocariasis, and the latter condition is almost always unilateral.

Familial exudative vitreoretinopathy

This disorder may be associated with vitreoretinal traction and folds of retina extending from the posterior pole to a peripheral type of mass. However, the peripheral mass is usually associated with anomalous vessels and signs of exudation, and these are usually less obvious in association with peripheral inflammatory masses resulting from *Toxocara*. In addition, familial exudative vitreoretinopathy is typically bilateral and associated with a positive family history.

Coats disease

Coats disease may present in the same age group as does toxocariasis, and it is typically unilateral. In relatively early cases, classic intraretinal telangiectatic vessels are observed in association with yellow intraretinal and subretinal exudates. In later stages, associated with a secondary retinal detachment, the diagnosis may be somewhat more difficult, but the vitreous in cases of Coats disease typically reveals no signs of marked inflammation, and intravitreal and epiretinal fibrocellular organization are characteristically absent. Vasoproliferative masses associated with ocular toxocariasis have been reported.[32]

Persistent hyperplastic primary vitreous

Persistent hyperplastic primary vitreous (PHPV) is usually diagnosed within the first few weeks of life. The involved eye is typically microphthalmic, and the condition is almost always unilateral. Although the retrolental fibrovascular mass observed in this condition may superficially resemble an inflammatory mass of ocular toxocariasis, distinguishing between the two disorders is usually not difficult.

Papillitis of unknown etiology

Inflammation and tumefaction of the optic nerve head as a result of intraocular toxocariasis are quite unusual.[27,30] Other forms of granulomatous inflammation involving the optic nerve may appear morphologically similar to cases associated with toxocariasis.[5] Laboratory studies may be required to assist in the diagnosis of this unusual problem.

LABORATORY DIAGNOSIS

As noted above, patients with ocular toxocariasis frequently do not demonstrate an increased eosinophil count. Although a variety of skin tests and immunologic evaluation of serum were employed in the past to assist in the diagnosis of ocular toxocariasis, they were of limited value.[4,5] Currently, ELISA testing of serum and intraocular fluids and cytologic evaluation of intraocular materials are employed.

Enzyme-linked immunosorbent assay

The current test of choice to document systemic or ocular infection with *T. canis* is the ELISA test.[5] In this test, second-stage larval secretory antigen is extracted in vitro and used for detection of antibodies in the human serum and intraocular fluids. Although the Centers for Disease Control and Prevention consider serum ELISA titers less than 1:32 to be insignificant in the diagnosis of systemic toxocariasis,[33] others have stated that a serum titer of 1:8 is sufficient to support a diagnosis of ocular toxocariasis if the patient has signs and symptoms compatible with that disorder.[25] In a report of Ellis and co-workers,[33] 23.1% of 333 children without signs of ocular toxocariasis exhibited a serum titer ≥ 1:32, and 31.8% had a titer ≥ 1:16. Thus a positive serum titer cannot be used to confirm absolutely a diagnosis of ocular toxocariasis, although the absence of any serologic evidence of *Toxocara* infestation may assist in reducing the odds of this organism being the cause of ocular disease. ELISA testing of intraocular fluids has been demonstrated to be of great value in diagnosing ocular toxocariasis.[5,34] Typically, higher ELISA titers have been discovered in both the aqueous humor and vitreous aspirates than in the serum of patients. Positive intraocular ELISA titers have been discovered in patients with absent serum levels of antibody.[35]

Cytology

Cytologic study of aqueous humor or vitrectomy specimens may also be helpful in confirming the diagnosis of ocular toxocariasis. The presence of eosinophils in these intraocular fluids is consistent with intraocular *Toxocara*, whereas most other forms of intraocular inflammation are associated with other types of inflammatory cells. Remnants of *Toxocara* organisms have occasionally been recovered from vitrectomy specimens obtained at surgery.[36]

THERAPY

The treatment of ocular toxocariasis depends primarily on the stage of inflammation at which the patient is initially observed and the secondary structural changes in the vitreous and retina that are associated with this infestation. (Prevention of the deposition of infectious ova in the soil by treating infected puppies remains a major goal, as mentioned later.) Specific or nonspecific medical therapy has been recommended in the treatment of ocular toxocariasis, and surgical intervention may also be indicated in selected cases.

Medical therapy

Although antihelminthic drugs such as tiabendazole and diethylcarbamazine have been recommended in selected cases of visceral larval migrans,[37] the advisability of killing an intraocular organism is questionable; the death of the larva may be theoretically associated with an enhanced inflammatory reaction similar to that observed in association with onchocerciasis.[5,37] However, other studies have demonstrated a superiority of albendazole over tiabendazole in the treatment of ocular toxocariasis.[38] And another report documented favorable responses to a combination of albendazole and oral steroids in active disease.[39] Nonspecific therapy may also be of value.

In eyes with significant intraocular inflammation, cycloplegic agents should be employed when signs of anterior segment involvement are present. In such cases, topical corticosteroids should also be used to reduce symptoms and complications of anterior chamber inflammation. In active severe inflammation of the vitreous and retina, periocular injections of corticosteroids may be helpful, and in eyes in which vision is threatened by severe inflammation, oral corticosteroids may be justified.[37,39] *T. canis* is not a self-replicating organism, and steroid therapy helps reduce the inflammatory organization without permitting the overgrowth of the infectious agent.[37] Route of administration, dose, and length of therapy should be individualized.

Ocular surgery

The most common indication for surgical intervention in cases of ocular toxocariasis is retinal detachment.[25,40,41] Intravitreal fibrocellular membrane formation and contraction are associated with the development of retinal breaks (Fig. 90-7) and

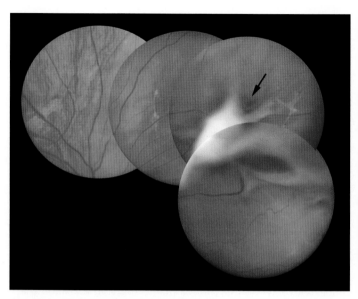

Fig. 90-7 Same case as Fig. 90-6. Vitreoretinal traction upon the inflammatory mass has caused a retinal break (arrow) and retinal detachment.

also with the production of traction types of retinal detachments. Although scleral buckling techniques may be appropriate in the management of selected cases of retinal detachment caused by *T. canis*, closed vitrectomy techniques have frequently been required to manage these cases.[25,40,41] In such eyes, vitrectomy techniques are used to eliminate transvitreal or epiretinal membranes producing traction on the retina, to cure traction detachments, or to permit settling of the retina after routine closure of responsible retinal breaks (Fig. 90-8). Vitrectomy techniques can also be employed to remove selected subretinal granulomas.[42]

Hagler and associates[25] reported 17 consecutive cases in which retinal detachment was due to ocular toxocariasis. The retina was successfully reattached in 12 (71%) cases, and vision remained stable or improved in 15 (88%) of the 17 eyes. Small et al.[41] reported 12 similar cases. The retina was completely reattached after vitreous surgery in 10 (83%), and visual acuity improved in 7 (70%) of the anatomic successes. More recent reports have documented generally successful anatomic outcomes.[40,42]

Laser therapy has been employed to eradicate motile subretinal nematodes,[5] although the precise type of organism and the value of therapy remain unknown.

PREVENTION

The dog population in the USA has been estimated to be over 52 million, and these pets are most likely to be found in homes with young children.[7] A minimum of 750 cases of ocular toxocariasis is estimated to occur in the USA each year, and systemic visceral larval migrans is significantly more common.[11] A meaningful reduction in the incidence of toxocariasis will require treatment of infected puppies at an appropriate age.[43] In untreated puppies, the prevalence of *Toxocara* infection

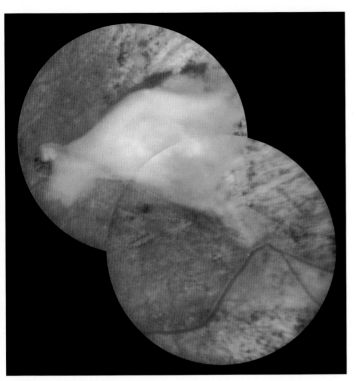

Fig. 90-8 Same case as Figs 90-6 and 90-7. Vitreous surgical techniques, without scleral buckling, have successfully reattached the retina.

approximates 100%.[7,11] Female adult worms become gravid by the time a puppy is 5 to 6 weeks old, and thousands of eggs can be released in puppy feces each day.[11] In one study, 80% of puppies less than 6 weeks of age had worms in their intestines, but only 20% had stools that were positive for *Toxocara* eggs.[11] Thus stool evaluations of puppies are unreliable, and *all* puppies should be treated with appropriate antihelminthic agents before they are 4 weeks old. Surveys have indicated that a minority of veterinarians may be aware of the importance of treating puppies at such an early age.[11]

A number of surveys have demonstrated that infectious *Toxocara* eggs can be recovered in public parks and children's playgrounds for years after they have been deposited in puppy fecal material.[7] Although there appears to be no practical method of eliminating all ova from these areas, contamination of child play sandpits can be prevented by covering the area with a clear vinyl sheet at night and on rainy days.[44]

Summary

Ocular toxocariasis is a major cause of visual loss in the young. Reduced visual acuity usually occurs because of damage to the vitreous and retina caused by an inflammatory response to the organism. A variety of relatively distinct clinical presentations have been described. The diagnosis can usually be made on the basis of intraocular findings, and ELISA testing of the serum or intraocular fluids may be of value in certain atypical cases. Medical and surgical therapy is of value in selected situations.

REFERENCES

1. Altcheh J, Nallar M, Conca M et al. Toxocariasis: clinical and laboratory features in 54 patients. An Pediatr (Barc.) 2003; 58:425–431.
2. Ellis GS Jr, Pakalnis VA, Worley G et al. *Toxocara canis* infestation: clinical and epidemiological associations with seropositivity in kindergarten children. Ophthalmology 1986; 93:1032–1037.
3. Wilkinson CP, Welch RB. Intraocular *Toxocara*. Am J Ophthalmol 1971; 71:921–930.
4. Molk R. Ocular toxocariasis: a review of the literature. Ann Ophthalmol 1983; 15:216–231.
5. Shields JA. Ocular toxocariasis: a review. Surv Ophthalmol 1984; 28:361–381.
6. Beaver PC, Snyder CH, Carrera GM et al. Chronic eosinophilia due to visceral larva migrans. Pediatrics 1952; 9:7–19.
7. Glickman LT, Magnaval J. Zoonotic roundworm infections. Infect Dis Clin North Am 1993; 7:717–732.
8. Zinkham WH. Systemic visceral larval migrans. In Ryan SJ, Smith RE, eds. Selected topics on the eye in systemic disease. New York: Grune & Stratton; 1979:167–175.
9. Bass JL, Mehta KA, Glickman LT et al. Clinically inapparent *Toxocara* infection in children. N Engl J Med 1983; 308:723–724.
10. Luxenberg MN. An experimental approach to the study of intraocular *Toxocara*. Trans Am Ophthalmol Soc 1979; 77:542–602.
11. Schantz PM. Of worms, dogs, and human hosts: continuing challenges for veterinarians in prevention of human diseases. J Am Vet Med Assoc 1994; 204:1023–1028.
12. Ottesen EA. Visceral larval migrans and other unusual helminth infections. In: Mandell GL, Douglas RG, Bennett JE, eds. Principles and practice of infectious diseases, 2nd edn. New York: John Wiley; 1979.
13. Marmor M, Glickman L, Shofer F et al. *Toxocara canis* infection of children: epidemiological and neuropsychological findings. Am J Public Health 1987; 77:554–559.
14. Schantz PM, Meyer D, Glickman LT. Clinical, serologic, and epidemiologic characteristics of ocular toxocariasis. Am J Trop Med Hyg 1979; 28:24–28.
15. Schantz PM, Weis PE, Pollard ZF et al. Risk factors for toxocaral ocular larva migrans: a case–control study. Am J Public Health 1980;70:1269–1272.
16. Wilder HC. Nematode endophthalmitis. Trans Am Acad Ophthalmol Otolaryngol 1950; 55:99–109.
17. Takayanagi TH, Akao N, Suzuki R et al. New animal model for human ocular toxocariasis: ophthalmoscopic findings. Br J Opthalmol 1999; 83:967–972.
18. Taylor MR. The epidemiology of ocular toxocariasis. J Helminthol 2001; 75:109–118.
19. Nichols RL. The etiology of visceral larva migrans. I. Diagnostic morphology of infective second-stage *Toxocara* larvae. J Parasitol 1956; 42:349–362.
20. Irvine WC, Irvine AR Jr. Nematode endophthalmitis: *Toxocara canis* – report of one case. Am J Ophthalmol 1959;47:185–191.
21. Ashton N. Larval granulomatosis of the retina due to *Toxocara*. Br J Ophthalmol 1960; 44:129–148.
22. Duguid IM. Features of ocular infestation by *Toxocara*. Br J Ophthalmol 1961; 45:789–796.
23. Hogan MJ, Kimura SJ, Spencer WH. Visceral larval migrans and peripheral retinitis. JAMA 1965; 194:1345–1347.
24. Perkins ES. Pattern of uveitis in children. Br J Ophthalmol 1966; 50:169–185.
25. Hagler WS, Pollard ZF, Jarrett WH et al. Results of surgery for ocular *Toxocara canis*. Ophthalmology 1981; 88:1081–1086.
26. Benitez-del Castillo JM, Herreros G, Guillen JL et al. Bilateral ocular toxocariasis demonstrated by aqueous humor enzyme-linked immunosorbent assay. Am J Ophthalmol 1995; 119:514–516.
27. Gass JDM: Stereoscopic atlas of macular diseases, 4th edn. St Louis: Mosby;1997.
28. Wan WL, Cano MR, Pince KJ et al. Echographic characteristics of ocular toxocariasis. Ophthalmology 1991; 98:28–32.
29. Monshizadeh R, Ashrafzadeh MT, Rumelt S. Choroidal neovascular membrane: a late complication of inactive toxocara chorioretinitis. Retina 2000; 20:219–220.
30. Bird AC, Smith JL, Curtin VT. Nematode optic neuritis. Am J Ophthalmol 1970; 69:72–77.
31. Rubin ML, Kaufman HE, Tierney JP et al. An intraretinal nematode (a case report). Trans Am Acad Ophthalmol Otolaryngol 1968; 72:855–866.
32. Shields CL, Shields JA, Barrett J et al. Vasoproliferative tumors of the ocular fundus: classification and clinical manifestations in 103 patients. Arch Ophthalmol 1995; 113:615–623.
33. Ellis GS Jr, Pakalnis VA, Worley G et al. *Toxocara canis* infestation: clinical and epidemiological associations with seropositivity in kindergarten children. Ophthalmology 1986; 93:1032–1037.
34. Biglan AW, Glickman LT, Lobes LA Jr. Serum and vitreous *Toxocara* antibody in nematode endophthalmitis. Am J Ophthalmol 1979; 88:898–901.
35. Sharkey JA, McKay PS. Ocular toxocariasis in a patient with repeatedly negative ELISA titers to *Toxocara canis*. Br J Ophthalmol 1993; 77:253–254.

36. Maguire AM, Green WR, Michels RG et al. Recovery of intraocular *Toxocara canis* by pars plana vitrectomy. Ophthalmology 1990; 97:675–680.

37. O'Connor GR. Chemotherapy of toxoplasmosis and toxocariasis. In: Srinivasan BD, ed. Ocular therapeutics. New York: Masson;1980.

38. Sturchler D, Schubarth P, Gualzata M et al. Thiabendazole vs. albendazole in treatment of toxocariasis: a clinical trial. Ann Trop Med Parasitol 1989; 83:473–478.

39. Barisan-Asenbauer T, Maca SM, Hauff W et al. Treatment of ocular toxocariasis with albendazole. J Oc Pharm Therapeut 2001; 17:287–294.

40. Amin HI, McDonald HR, Han DP et al. Vitrectomy update for macular traction in ocular toxocariasis. Retina 2000; 20:80–85.

41. Small KW, McCuen BW, de Juan E et al. Surgical management of retinal traction caused by ocular toxocariasis. Am J Ophthalmol 1989; 108:10–14.

42. Werner JC, Ross RD, Green WR et al. Pars plana vitrectomy and subretinal surgery for ocular toxocariasis. Arch Ophthalmol 1999; 117:532–534.

43. Editorial. *Toxocara canis* and human health. Br Med J 1994; 3009:5–6.

44. Uga S, Kataoka N. Measures to control *Toxocara* egg contamination in sandpits of public parks. Am J Trop Med Hyg 1995; 52:21–24.

Chapter

91

Cytomegalovirus Infections of the Retina

Jean D. Vaudaux
Gary N. Holland

Human cytomegalovirus (CMV) is an enveloped herpesvirus with a double-stranded DNA core. Infection by CMV is common, with serologic evidence of prior infection exceeding 50% in many areas of the world. In the general population of industrialized countries, seropositivity increases with advancing age and lower socioeconomic status.[1] Vertical transmission in utero can occur with either primary maternal CMV infection acquired during pregnancy or with reactivation of latent maternal CMV infection during pregnancy. Postnatal transmission can occur following contact with persons shedding virus in urine, saliva, breast milk, semen, or cervical secretions. Sexual transmission is a major source of infection in adults, particularly among men who have sex with men; seropositivity can approach 100% in homosexual and bisexual men infected with human immunodeficiency virus (HIV).[2] The virus can also be transmitted by transfusion of blood products or after solid organ (especially liver) or bone marrow transplantation at any age.

Primary CMV infection of immunocompetent adults and children is usually asymptomatic, with a mononucleosis-like syndrome developing in only 5% to 10% of infected individuals.[3] A latent infection is established thereafter, primarily involving bone marrow progenitor cells, although peripheral blood monocytes can be involved as well. In profoundly immunosuppressed individuals, latent CMV infection can reactivate and disseminate, often producing clinically apparent disease that involves many tissues, including the retina.[4–7]

CONGENITAL CYTOMEGALOVIRUS INFECTION

CMV is the most common virus to cause congenital infections. The reported prevalence of congenital CMV infection ranges from approximately 0.2% to 2.5% of all live births, depending on the populations that have been studied and on the criteria used to establish the diagnosis of congenital CMV infection.[8,9] The risk of congenital CMV infection appears highest in lower socioeconomic groups and in other populations having a high prevalence of maternal immunity,[10,11] attributable to the fact that the fetus can be infected after reactivation of latent maternal virus.

Whenever primary maternal CMV infection occurs during pregnancy, the risk of transmission to the fetus ranges from 30% to 40%.[12,13] Primary infection during the first half of pregnancy is associated with more severe disease.[14] Approximately 5% to 15% of infected infants present with symptoms or clinical signs of disease at birth,[13,15] most commonly petechiae, jaundice, hepatosplenomegaly, and thrombocytopenia.[16] Long-term central nervous system sequelae will affect more than 90% of survivors.[12,17]

Recurrent maternal CMV infection, defined as intermittent viral excretion from reactivation of latent maternal CMV infection in the presence of immunity, leads to congenital infection in up to 1% of cases.[17] Disease is less severe in such cases, probably as a consequence of pre-existing maternal immunity, which is partially protective.[18]

Retinitis is the most common ophthalmic manifestation of congenital CMV infection, with a reported prevalence of 11% to 25% in the setting of symptomatic congenital CMV infection.[15,19,20] Until the mid-1990s, it was widely accepted that retinitis was an early manifestation of congenital infection, presenting at birth or shortly thereafter, but Boppana and associates[21] have described development of retinitis later in life among children who initially had no clinical lesions on ophthalmoscopy; they also reported cases of apparent reactivation from a previously asymptomatic and inactive retinal scar.[21] They did not discriminate between the two groups of patients despite the fact that reactivation from existing scars and development of new lesions may be very different in pathogenesis. Neither of these two groups of children had evidence of systemic disease reactivation and subsequent dissemination of CMV.[21] Reactivation from virus that persists in the retina is a possible explanation for those cases with previously inactive scars, but the source of virus in patients exhibiting new retinitis lesions is less obvious; limited reactivation of nonocular infection, with viremia but without clinical disease, might be an explanation, but it is also possible that small foci of retinitis actually may have been present, but not recognized, on earlier examinations. Nevertheless, these observations suggest that even asymptomatic children with evidence of congenital infection at birth should be screened regularly for ocular involvement until later in childhood.

Perinatal infections, defined as those occurring within 1 month after birth,[22] are more common than congenital infections; they result either from contact with CMV shed by the cervical mucosa during vaginal delivery or from infected breast milk.

Perinatal infections are usually asymptomatic and do not result in any long-term clinical sequelae.

POSTNATAL CMV RETINITIS IN IMMUNOSUPPRESSED HOSTS

Postnatally acquired CMV retinitis occurs only in severely immunosuppressed individuals. It is seen most commonly in people with acquired immunodeficiency syndrome (AIDS), but transplant recipients or other individuals who receive potent immunosuppressive drug regimens are also at risk.

CMV retinitis in people with AIDS
Epidemiology

As of July 2004, it was estimated that approximately 38 million people in the world were living with HIV disease or AIDS, of whom approximately 2 million were under 15 years of age.[23] Although AIDS has now become the condition most commonly associated with CMV retinitis in children, the frequency of AIDS-related eye disease, including CMV retinitis, appears to be substantially lower in the pediatric than in the adult AIDS population,[24] which might, in part, reflect the lower CMV seroprevalence in children. CMV retinitis has been reported in approximately 5% of immunosuppressed children.[25] In Rwanda, a prevalence figure of 2% was reported for CMV retinitis in an HIV-infected pediatric population.[26]

Retinitis is the most common manifestation of CMV disease in adult individuals with AIDS,[27,28] accounting for approximately 70% to 85% of CMV-associated end-organ disease.[28–30] Before the era of highly active antiretroviral therapy (HAART), 16.5% to 34% of HIV-infected individuals eventually had reactivation of latent infection and development of clinically apparent CMV end-organ disease.[27,30–38]

At least 90% of HIV-infected individuals live in developing countries, with two-thirds of the world's HIV-infected population in sub-Saharan Africa.[23] The prevalence of CMV retinitis in HIV-infected individuals in these countries is generally lower than in North America and Western Europe. In Brazil, where there is a substantial prevalence of HIV infection, AIDS-related CMV retinitis has been reported in 25% of individuals with newly diagnosed HIV-infection in São Paulo,[39] similar to the prevalence in the United States in the early years of the AIDS epidemic. In Africa, the reported prevalence of CMV retinitis in patients with AIDS ranges from none to 8.5%.[40–44] A prospective study conducted in India revealed that 17% of patients with AIDS had CMV retinitis,[45] but few data exist regarding other parts of Asia. The lower reported prevalence of CMV retinitis in developing countries, particularly those on the African continent, may simply reflect the fact that many HIV-infected individuals die before their immune function deteriorates to the level at which CMV retinitis typically occurs.

In the first decade of the AIDS epidemic, reported median survival after diagnosis of CMV retinitis increased from 6 weeks to 12.6 months,[29,31,33,46–50] attributable to better treatment or prophylaxis of opportunistic infections, and the introduction of the first antiretroviral drugs. Nevertheless, it remained a poor prognostic sign in terms of survival until the introduction of HAART.

The effect of HAART

Epidemiologic data regarding AIDS and CMV retinitis changed dramatically following the introduction of potent antiretroviral drugs in the late 1990s.[51] Several classes of antiretroviral drugs are currently available, including nucleoside reverse-transcriptase inhibitors (nRTIs), non-nucleoside reverse transcriptase inhibitors (nnRTIs), and protease inhibitors (PIs); the latter target viral proteases involved in the assembly of new viral particles rather than the viral genome. Any combination of three or more antiretroviral drugs, or a combination containing one PI and one nnRTI, are considered HAART.

The use of HAART has been associated with reduced HIV replication and an increase in CD4+ T-lymphocyte counts,[52] as well as a marked increase in survival.[53] A reduced incidence of opportunistic infections,[54] and a drop in newly diagnosed cases of CMV retinitis by 55% to more than 90% over a period of 2 to 3 years,[51,54–56] were also reported.

Recovery of CMV-specific CD4+ T-lymphocyte responses,[57,58] and lymphoproliferative responses to CMV can be observed in people taking HAART,[58,59] suggesting that CMV-specific memory T-lymphocytes can be reconstituted during HAART. Nevertheless, if a severely immunosuppressed HIV-infected individual has no surviving CMV-specific CD4+ T-lymphocytes clones to be expanded, protective immunity against CMV may not be regained with HAART. Thus, the absolute number of CD4+ T-lymphocytes does not necessarily indicate protection against CMV retinitis.[60]

Most improvements in immune function seem to occur during the first year following initiation of HAART, and long-term immune reconstitution may not be complete.[61] Moreover, community-based studies reveal that only a low proportion of patients actually end up with undetectable HIV blood levels after 14 months of HAART,[62] and that virological failure (manifested as recurrence of elevated HIV blood levels) may occur in up to 44% of patients treated with PIs within the first 6 months following initiation of therapy.[63]

Risk factors

People with AIDS have a higher prevalence of CMV retinitis than other populations of immunosuppressed individuals. Multiple theories have been proposed to explain this observation, including specific or unique immune defects associated with HIV infection, CMV transactivation by HIV,[64,65] or HIV-induced microvascular and blood flow alterations in the retina that facilitate local infection (see Pathogenic mechanisms of ocular disease, p. 1607). Among people with AIDS, men who have sex with men are at higher risk of developing CMV retinitis,[66,67] probably because CMV seropositivity in this population approaches 100%.[2]

CD4+ T-lymphocyte count is a fairly reliable predictor of risk for developing CMV retinitis in HIV-infected individuals who have not been treated with HAART; there is an increased risk in patients with counts of 50 cells/mm³ or less[28,36,37]; the incidence of CMV retinitis in the latter group may be as high as 20% per year.[36] Additionally, it has been shown that the CD8[+] T-lymphocyte count is also predictive of CMV retinitis in patients with AIDS[38,68]; the risk appears higher when the CD8[+] T-lymphocyte count falls below 520 cells/mm[3].[38] The CD8[+] T-lymphocyte count is of no additional and independent predictive value if CD4[+] T-lymphocytes count is already known, however.[38]

CD4[+] T-lymphocyte count seems to be a less reliable predictor regarding the risk of developing CMV retinitis in patients who have initiated HAART.[69,70] In particular, individuals can still develop CMV retinitis in the early weeks of HAART, before immune reconstitution has occurred, despite rising CD4[+] T-lymphocyte counts.[71]

Zurlo and associates[72] showed that HIV-infected people with detectable CMV viremia were statistically more likely to develop CMV disease than those without, but concluded that the positive predictive value of CMV viremia was relatively low (35%), thus making it a mediocre prognostic tool. Salmon and associates[73] have reported a higher predictive value for development of CMV disease among patients with positive CMV blood cultures at the onset of AIDS; 50% developed CMV retinitis within a mean period of 7.7 months. Also, quantitation of CMV DNA in peripheral blood leukocytes has shown that a higher number of CMV DNA copies might be associated with an increased risk of developing CMV retinitis in patients with CD4[+] T-lymphocyte counts <100 cells/mm[3].[74,75] Viremia caused by glycoprotein B group 2 strains of CMV may also be associated with a higher risk.[76]

HIV-associated retinal microvasculopathy with cotton-wool spots ("HIV retinopathy," "AIDS retinopathy") has been demonstrated to be an independent risk factor for CMV retinitis (see Pathogenic mechanisms of ocular disease).[66,67]

CMV disease remains a potential problem despite the availability of HAART; HIV-infected individuals who fail to respond to HAART or in whom HIV resistance occurs can develop CMV retinitis. In some cases, survival may be prolonged by HAART, but adequate protection against CMV will not be achieved with immune reconstitution, because CMV-specific clones are not restored. Currently, it appears that the majority of HIV-infected individuals in urban areas of the United States who are diagnosed with CMV retinitis have been exposed to HAART.[70]

CMV retinitis in other immunosuppressed hosts

CMV retinitis is also associated with causes of immunosuppression other than HIV disease, including inherited immunodeficiency states, malignancies, and use of systemic immunosuppressive chemotherapy after solid organ or bone marrow transplantation. In the adult population, most cases of CMV retinitis before the AIDS epidemic were seen in the setting of iatrogenic immunosuppression following solid organ transplantation.[4,5] Currently, although solid organ and bone marrow transplant recipients account for a minority of cases, transplantation is an increasingly important risk factor, given increases in the number of procedures, improved recipient survival, and the use of more potent immunosuppressive drugs to treat recipients.[77–79]

Although a prevalence of 15% was reported for active or healed CMV retinitis among heart transplant recipients in one series,[80] the prevalence of CMV retinitis among solid organ transplant recipients is generally believed to be much lower than in HIV-infected individuals. Other reports cite a prevalence figure of 0.3% to 3.5% for solid organ transplant recipients.[81–83]

Bone marrow transplant[84,85] and hematopoietic stem cell transplant recipients[86] are also at risk for CMV disease, although CMV pneumonitis is more prevalent than CMV retinitis in these populations.[87] The main risk factors are chronic graft-versus-host disease and CMV seropositivity prior to transplantation.[86]

PATHOGENIC MECHANISMS OF OCULAR DISEASE

CMV reaches the eye through the bloodstream. Infection of retinal vascular endothelial cells, which may play a key role in the initiation of retinal infection,[88,89] has been demonstrated in people with AIDS and CMV retinitis, and inclusion bodies have been seen in endothelial cells of small retinal vessels of other immunosuppressed individuals.[5] Some autopsy studies of HIV-infected individuals have failed to demonstrate CMV infection of retinal vascular endothelial cells.[31,32] This observation may simply reflect destruction of vascular endothelial cells in areas of the retina with full-thickness necrosis.[89] Alternatively, infection of neuroretinal tissue might occur in some eyes after diapedesis of infected leukocytes through damaged vessel walls, without infection of endothelial cells. Vascular breaches and leakage around microaneurysms are frequent findings in people with AIDS; these changes might facilitate the passage of CMV through the blood–retinal barrier.[90,91]

CMV causes full-thickness necrosis of the retina, with CMV antigens detected in cells in all layers of the retina, including RPE cells.[32] Histopathologic examination of CMV retinitis typically reveals an abrupt transition between the areas of necrotic and normal-appearing retina (Fig. 91-1). Cytomegalic cells with eosinophilic intracytoplasmic or intranuclear inclusions are invariably present, and are considered pathognomonic for CMV infection.[32] Infected RPE cells appear to represent independent areas of infection, as they are generally separate from sites of prior or active viral retinitis. Similarly, CMV antigens can be found in rare cells of the choroid,[32,92] probably also representing independent sites of infection, as they can be demonstrated in areas of intact overlying RPE and retina.[32]

Infection within the retina spreads by cell-to-cell transmission, but CMV infection has not been observed to advance across the ora serrata to involve the pars plana. New lesions occur infrequently, suggesting that the initial establishment of infection is more difficult than the spread of infection within the retina.

In most cases, the cellular inflammatory response to CMV retinitis consists of a relatively sparse leukocytic infiltrate composed predominately of lymphocytes.[93,94] Isolated foci of prominent neutrophilic infiltrates can be observed in 22–50% of cases at autopsy, however.[31,32,48]

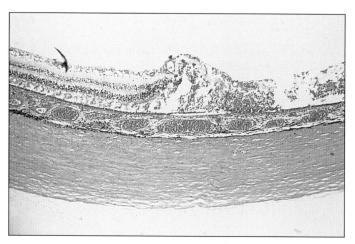

Fig. 91-1 A light micrograph showing the transition between normal retina and full-thickness necrosis associated with cytomegalovirus retinitis (hematoxylin–eosin). From Holland GN, Gottlieb MS, Yee RD et al. Am J Ophthalmol 1982; 93:393–402.

The relationship between CMV retinitis and HIV retinopathy has been the subject of debate. CMV retinitis often occurs in areas of prior or concurrent HIV retinopathy,[31,95,96] attributable to a microvasculopathy characterized by loss of pericytes, thickened and multilaminated basal lamina, swollen endothelial cells, and slitlike narrowing of lumina.[90,91] In one study, CMV DNA was identified in cotton-wool spots by polymerase chain reaction (PCR) amplification of retinal punch biopsies taken at autopsy,[97] further linking CMV infection to areas of retinal vascular injury. CMV is not a universal finding in patients with cotton-wool spots, however; another study found no evidence of CMV in individuals with HIV retinopathy alone.[32]

Isolated cases of retinal co-infection by CMV and HIV,[98] by CMV, HIV, and human herpes virus-6,[99] and by CMV, HIV, and herpes simplex virus[100] have been described. Although the

clinical relevance of such co-infection remains unknown, HIV has been shown to enhance CMV production in vitro,[64,65] suggesting that viral co-infection may contribute to greater severity of CMV retinitis in some patients.

CLINICAL FEATURES OF CYTOMEGALOVIRUS RETINITIS

CMV retinitis lesions can be unilateral or bilateral, and may be present in any part of the retina.[69,101,102] Initial examination typically reveals one or two foci of disease (Fig. 91-2); multifocal disease having three, four, or five independent lesions is uncommon. CMV retinitis lesions may develop in all areas topographically,[69] although the majority of early lesions are adjacent to blood vessels (Fig. 91-3), probably reflecting the hematogenous spread of the virus and the potential for CMV to infect retinal vascular endothelial cells.[88,89] Isolated involvement of the fovea, which is observed in 5% to 10% of eyes,[69,101] or CMV papillitis,[101,103,104] which affects less than 10% of eyes, may also occur.

Lesions are generally described as being in one or more of three zones.[105] Zone 1 encompasses that area within one disc diameter (1500 μm) of the optic disc margin or two disc diameters (3000 μm) of the fovea; lesions in zone 1 can result in immediate reduction in visual acuity with enlargement. Zone 2 extends to the vortex veins, and zone 3 represents the portion of the retina from the anterior border of zone 2 to the ora serrata. Lesions in zone 3, which underlie the vitreous base, increase the risk of subsequent retinal detachment.

CMV infection causes retinal whitening or opacification, attributable to retinal necrosis and variable amounts of edema. The hallmark feature of untreated CMV retinitis lesions is an irregular, dry-appearing, granular border, often with characteristic, small, isolated "satellites" at the advancing edge, representing early foci of retinal infection (Fig. 91-2B). Two distinct

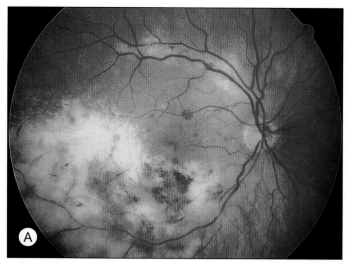

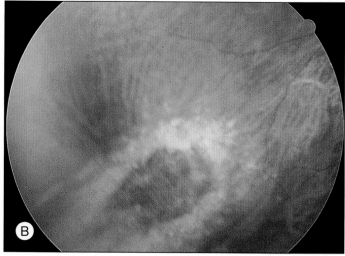

Fig. 91-2 A, The fulminant/edematous variant of cytomegalovirus (CMV) retinitis is characterized by dense retinal opacification, hemorrhage, and inflammatory retinal vascular sheathing. B, The indolent/granular variant of CMV retinitis, characterized by a granular border with small satellite lesions typical of CMV infection.

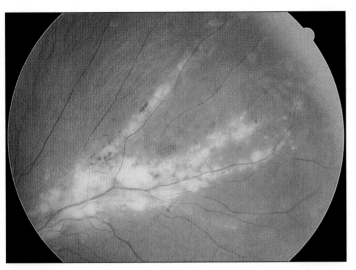

Fig. 91-3 Early cytomegalovirus retinitis observed along retinal vessels.

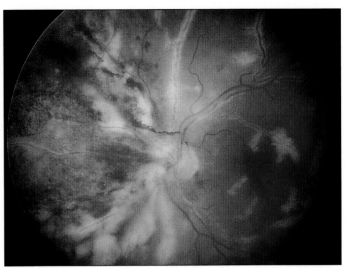

Fig. 91-4 Dense inflammatory sheathing of retinal vessels associated with cytomegalovirus retinitis. Sheathing of vessels can occur remote from foci of infection, as seen in the macula of this eye. This finding is reminiscent of "frosted branch angiitis."

types or variants of untreated CMV retinitis have been described.[102] The term "fulminant/edematous" has been used to describe those lesions with the classic features of disease, including marked edema with dense, confluent areas of retinal whitening, usually accompanied by moderate to severe retinal hemorrhage and vascular sheathing (Fig. 91-2A).[101] They tend to be irregular in shape, and associated with blood vessels. In contrast, "indolent/granular" lesions are those characterized by little edema, only faint, grainy opacification, little or no hemorrhage, and no vascular sheathing (Fig. 91-2B). This type of lesion tends to be round or oval, and may be more common in the retinal periphery.[33] These variants represent two ends of a continuous clinical spectrum, and it is often difficult to classify individual lesions as being one type or the other.[69] Types may have relevance to progression (see Course of disease),[106] but inability to classify all lesions limits the clinical utility of these designations. Opacity seems to be the major factor in assigning the terms indolent/granular or fulminant/edematous; investigators have begun to quantitate the degree of lesion opacity alone as a possible marker of disease severity.[69,70]

In some patients, retinal vascular sheathing may be a prominent finding in eyes with CMV retinitis (Fig. 91-4),[107,108] giving an appearance similar to "acute frosted branch angiitis," a form of idiopathic retinal periphlebitis, originally described in immunocompetent individuals.

Mild vitreous humor[48] and anterior chamber inflammatory reactions[69,101] are almost invariably present in patients with active CMV retinitis, but moderate to severe intraocular inflammation is uncommon.[101,109] Patients with AIDS-related CMV retinitis who begin HAART can have increased inflammation, however, as immune reconstitution occurs (see Immune recovery uveitis in course of disease).

HAART has not altered the basic clinical characteristics of CMV retinitis, although the spectrum of lesion severity may be greater at diagnosis among treated patients.[70] Because opacity is believed to reflect virus activity,[102,105] it is possible that lesions that are first diagnosed soon after initiation of HAART will be less opaque, attributable to improving immune function and suppression of CMV. HAART has occasionally been found to result in clinical inactivation of previously undiagnosed CMV retinitis lesions after immune reconstitution has occurred.[110]

Symptoms of CMV retinitis, including blurred vision, scotomata, or floaters, are present in up to 78% of patients.[101] Lesions restricted to the periphery can result in floaters or visual field defects, but may be asymptomatic. Involvement of the posterior pole, by contrast, is more frequently accompanied by both blind spots and blurred vision. Optic nerve infection will cause profound and sudden loss of vision, and will be accompanied by an afferent pupillary defect.[101,104]

COURSE OF DISEASE

The AIDS epidemic has provided an opportunity to study the natural history of untreated CMV disease. CMV retinitis generally occurs late in the course of AIDS[37]; it is the initial manifestation of AIDS in only approximately 2% of cases.[47,111,112] Prolonged survival resulting from prophylaxis against *Pneumocystis carinii* pneumonia significantly increased the risk of eventually developing CMV disease in the era before HAART became available.[113] Disease often begins in only one eye, with later involvement of the fellow eye.[114]

Enlargement of untreated CMV retinitis lesions is relentless,[31] spreading in a brushfire-like manner, with the entire retina being destroyed over a period of 6 months or less.[48] Lesion borders advance at approximately one disc diameter every 6 to 8 weeks,[106] resulting in centrifugal expansion from an initial focus of retinitis.

Egbert and associates[5] reported that infection has a tendency not to involve the macula. Subsequent experience in people with AIDS has shown that once established, lesions tend to spread more rapidly toward the ora serrata than toward the fovea; thus, within the vascular arcades, they can display a fovea-sparing pattern of enlargement (Fig. 91-5).[115] Factors contributing to the preferential anterior spread and relative tendency to spare the fovea with enlargement of lesions are unknown, although regional variations in retinal vascularity have been suggested as playing a role.[115] New lesions do not necessarily spare the anatomic macula or fovea, however.[69]

As a lesion enlarges, its older, central portion evolves into inactive gray or transparent gliotic scar tissue, as necrotic tissue is cleared. Areas of scarring can also have marked retinal and RPE atrophy with fine pigmentary mottling (Fig. 91-6). The advancing border of the lesion remains active, leaving behind it an area that undergoes the same evolution as described above. Small isolated foci of infection (satellites) at the leading edge of an active border eventually coalesce and are incorporated into the solid area of opacification.[5]

For research purposes, "progression" has been defined as enlargement of existing lesions or development of new lesions in remote areas of the retina. As a study end-point, border advancement must reach a threshold of 750 μm before progression is scored.

Various factors are related to the progression of CMV retinitis. It has been hypothesized that extensive vascular sheathing in non-HIV immunosuppressed individuals may predict rapid progression of CMV retinitis.[5] In people with AIDS, untreated lesions of the indolent/granular variant tend to advance more slowly.[106]

Spontaneous resolution of the advancing lesion border is never seen with persistence of severe immunosuppression; it has been

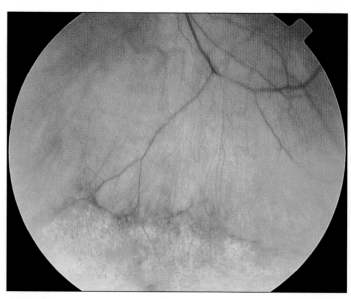

Fig. 91-6 An inactive focus of peripheral cytomegalovirus retinitis during successful maintenance therapy. The lesion is characterized by a thin gliotic scar with mottling of the underlying retinal pigment epithelium.

described, however, in heart and renal transplant recipients after reducing the dosage of, or discontinuing, immunosuppressive drug therapy.[4] Similarly, spontaneous and sustained resolution of AIDS-related CMV retinitis without specific anti-CMV therapy has been reported to accompany immune reconstitution following use of HAART (see Treatment, p. 1613).[110,116,117]

Complications

Retinal detachment

Rhegmatogenous retinal detachment is a particularly severe complication of CMV retinitis; it is present in approximately 3% of eyes at diagnosis[101] and occurs in 15% to 40% of eyes at some point during the course of disease.[46,47,118–121] In the pre-HAART era, the risk of retinal detachment in an eye with CMV retinitis has been estimated to be approximately 19% at 6 months and 38% at 1 year.[120] This risk increases with duration of CMV infection,[122–124] larger lesions,[120,125] and anterior lesions that extend to the ora serrata and the vitreous base.[118,124] Additional risk factors may include advanced patient age,[120] low CD4+ T-lymphocyte count,[120] active lesions,[125,126] and prior retinal detachment in the fellow eye.[123,125,126] The surgical management of CMV-associated retinal detachment is discussed in Chapter 145.

Exudative detachment of the macula has been observed in up to 29% of eyes with active CMV retinitis in zone 1 (Fig. 91-7); it is most common with peripapillary lesions.[32,101,127]

Immune recovery uveitis

Severe intraocular inflammatory reactions can develop in eyes with CMV retinitis following initiation of HAART,[128,129] if immune reconstitution occurs. This phenomenon, known as "immune recovery uveitis" (IRU), is attributed to immune reactions directed against CMV antigens; IRU invariably involves

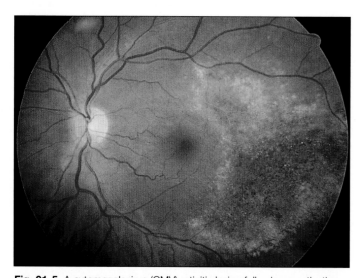

Fig. 91-5 A cytomegalovirus (CMV) retinitis lesion following reactivation during maintenance therapy. The opaque border indicates virus activity. The configuration of the lesion border suggests that border advancement is more rapid in anterior and circumferential directions than in a posterior direction, resulting in spread of disease around the fovea. This occurrence has led to the designation of CMV retinitis as a "fovea-sparing disease". From Holland GN, Tufail A, Jordan C. Cytomegalovirus diseases. In: Pepose JS, Holland GN, Wilhelmus KR, eds. Ocular Infection & Immunity. St Louis: Mosby, 1996.

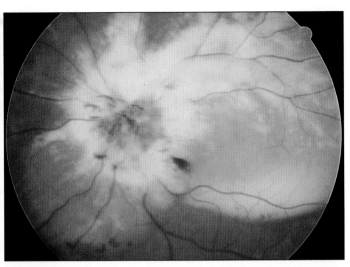

Fig. 91-7 A large exudative detachment of the macula associated with untreated peripapillary cytomegalovirus retinitis. (Reproduced from Holland GN, Sakamoto MJ, Hardy D et al. and the UCLA CMV Retinopathy Study Group: Arch Ophthalmol 1986; 104:1794–1800. Copyright © (1986) American Medical Association. All rights reserved.)

only eyes with pre-existing active or inactive CMV infection.[130,131] Prior to the HAART era, similar, severe uveitis had been described following withdrawal of immunosuppressive agents in a kidney transplant recipient with CMV retinitis,[5] attributable to a recovering immune system.

The pathogenesis of IRU is not fully understood. Nussenblatt and Lane[60] postulated that HAART causes expansion of remaining CMV-specific T-lymphocyte clones up to a threshold where there is a sufficient number to mount an inflammatory response directed against CMV antigens; thereafter, improved cellular immunity is effective again at inactivating and eliminating CMV within the eye, leading to decreased production of antigens, and a progressive decrease in the inflammatory signs. Analysis of vitreous humor from one patient with IRU identified CMV-specific CD8+ T-lymphocytes.[132] It is unclear why IRU is not observed in all individuals with CMV retinitis who experience immune reconstitution following the initiation of HAART; modulating factors might include different strains of CMV with different antigenic profiles, or the presence of extraocular sites of CMV disease that may trigger or enhance an inflammatory reaction.

Because HIV-infected individuals may exhibit low levels of inflammation without being on HAART, IRU must be defined on the basis of differences in intraocular inflammation from pre-HAART levels in individual patients, or by specific thresholds of inflammation, making it difficult to formulate precise clinical definitions of IRU. In general, though, the basic features of IRU are moderate to severe vitreous humor[128,129] and anterior chamber[116,133] inflammatory reactions, with or without papillitis, that occur during the first few weeks of HAART (Fig. 91-8).[128] Complications of IRU include cystoid macular edema (CME),[128,134,135] epiretinal membrane formation,[128,134] optic disc neovascularization,[134,136,137] retinal neovascularization,[138] vitreomacular traction syndrome,[139] proliferative vitreo-

retinopathy,[133,140] posterior and anterior subcapsular cataracts,[133,140] posterior synechiae,[133] and angle closure glaucoma.[141]

The presence of IRU also increases the risk of complications from procedures such as retinovitreous surgery and cataract extraction. Clinical evidence suggests that vitreous humor inflammation is transient in many people with IRU,[129–131] but that its complications may be chronic. Local corticosteroid injection may result in some transient improvement of IRU-associated CME, but recrudescence is common.

Patients with IRU complain of floaters and decreased, blurred, or foggy vision.[128,142] Initial vision loss from IRU is often transient, possibly because it is caused by vitreous humor haze. The complications of IRU can be associated with permanent vision loss.[128,134,143]

Reported prevalence figures for IRU vary greatly.[128,129,134,142] A prospective study identified IRU in 63% of "HAART responders" over a median follow-up period of 21.5 months.[142] The incidence of IRU ranges from 0.109/person-year to 0.83/person-year among HAART responders,[134,142] depending on the study design and the definitions used. Other factors, such as size of lesions, and possibly the type of specific anti-CMV therapy used prior to the development of IRU, might also be responsible for variations between centers. Although Arevalo and associates[144] did not find any significant difference in the surface area of involved retina between eyes with and those without IRU, Karavellas and associates[140] found that eyes with CMV retinitis involving more than 30% of retinal surface area were at significantly higher risk of developing IRU, presumably because there are more viral antigens present in larger lesions. Data suggest that more aggressive anti-CMV therapy before and early after initiation of HAART might decrease the incidence of IRU,[131,133,134] probably reflecting the fact that therapy reduces the amount of virus within the eye. The use of cidofovir after initiation of HAART is associated with a greater risk of IRU, however, probably related to its known tendency to induce inflammation (see Treatment, p. 1613).[145] Although treatment using other anti-CMV drugs during early immune reconstitution may be protective, the continuous use of anti-CMV agents *after* immune reconstitution has been achieved is not protective against IRU.[145]

Other complications

CME and epiretinal membrane formation are uncommon in the absence of IRU.[146,147] Other uncommon, vision-threatening complications of CMV retinitis have been described, including branch retinal vessel occlusion[119,148] and retinal neovascularization.[148,149] Fluorescein angiography should be considered in any patient with CMV retinitis and unexplained loss of vision.

DIAGNOSIS

Diagnosis of CMV retinitis is primarily clinical, relying on the typical features discussed above. The majority of people with AIDS are CMV seropositive[7]; thus, serologic studies or attempts to isolate CMV from extraocular sites cannot confirm a diagnosis of CMV retinitis in HIV-infected individuals.

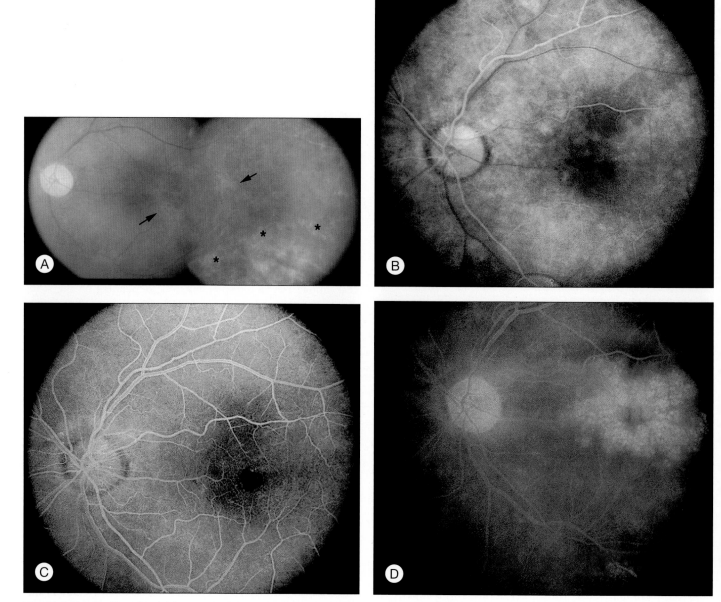

Fig. 91-8 Fundus (A) and serial fluorescein angiographic (B to D) photographs of the left eye in an individual with AIDS, who was on highly active antiretroviral therapy, including a protease inhibitor, show inactive cytomegalovirus (CMV) retinitis just beyond zone 1 (asterisks) with moderate vitreous inflammation, epiretinal membrane formation (arrows), and marked cystoid macular edema (D). The patient's CD4+ T lymphocyte count had climbed from below 40 cells/mm³ at the time of first diagnosis of CMV retinitis to above 200 cells/mm³ when macular edema was first noted.

PCR-based analysis of vitreous humor offers high diagnostic sensitivity and specificity.[150] It is usually reserved for patients with atypical lesions; for disease that is not responsive to treatment; or for those patients for whom a vitreous biopsy would carry little added risk, such as those already scheduled to undergo vitrectomy for retinal detachment repair.

DIFFERENTIAL DIAGNOSIS

Despite the distinct clinical features of CMV retinitis, other disorders are sometimes confused with this infection.[102] It is occasionally difficult to distinguish early foci of CMV retinitis from cotton-wool spots. The latter are not associated with satellite lesions or inflammation, however, and usually have sharp, well-delineated margins.[151] Repeat examination after one week may help to confirm the diagnosis of very small, early CMV retinitis lesions, which will invariably enlarge.

Some features of the clinical appearance of CMV retinitis may be mimicked by other infections of the retina, such as severe toxoplasmic retinochoroiditis in immunosuppressed individuals.[152,153] The absence of an irregular, granular lesion border; the presence of prominent vitreous humor and anterior chamber inflammatory reactions; and a paucity of intralesional hemorrhage are features that may help clinicians to diagnose toxoplasmic retinochoroiditis in immunosuppressed individuals.[152]

Other necrotizing herpetic retinopathies, including herpes simplex virus (HSV)[154] and varicella-zoster virus (VZV)[155] retinopathies, also occur in immunosuppressed individuals, but are less common than CMV retinitis. HSV and VZV infections of the retina generally present as the acute retinal necrosis (ARN) syndrome[154,156] or the progressive outer retinal necrosis (PORN) syndrome,[155] with their own distinct clinical presentations.

TREATMENT

The AIDS epidemic prompted the development of new antiviral agents with specific activity against CMV. Anti-CMV drugs that have been approved by the United States Food and Drug Administration (FDA) include ganciclovir and its valyl-ester prodrug valganciclovir; foscarnet; cidofovir; and fomivirsen. Each is virostatic only; thus, CMV retinitis lesions may eventually reactivate despite treatment in persistently immunosuppressed individuals. As a result, initial high-dose therapy to inactivate retinal lesions ("induction"; Fig. 91-9) is followed by lower dose "maintenance therapy" in an attempt to prevent progression. A number of early uncontrolled, open-labeled studies, and a group of later prospective, randomized clinical trials, have established the value of empirically derived treatment protocols based on this approach for each of the approved anti-CMV agents.[46,47,50,101,105,111,157–173] The majority of these studies were published before the HAART era.

Anti-CMV drugs
Ganciclovir
The nucleoside analog ganciclovir (Cytovene®, Roche Pharmaceuticals, Nutley, NJ) inhibits viral DNA elongation by hindering the action of the viral DNA polymerase, thus inhibiting CMV replication. To be effective, ganciclovir needs to be activated by phosphorylation that is mediated by virus-encoded enzymes. Ganciclovir can be given intravenously, orally, or via an intravitreous implant (Vitrasert®, Bausch & Lomb Surgical, Inc., San Dimas, CA; see Local therapies, below). Intravenous ganciclovir is usually administered at a dose of 5 mg/kg every 12 hours for induction and 5 mg/kg once daily for maintenance therapy. Ganciclovir is primarily eliminated by renal excretion, thus requiring dose adjustment in cases of renal insufficiency.

Oral ganciclovir[162–164,170] has poor oral bioavailability (approximately 7%), although it can be enhanced by concomitant absorption of food. Oral ganciclovir has been reported to have comparable efficacy to intravenous ganciclovir as maintenance therapy for CMV retinitis.[163,170] Caution must be exercised, however, in interpreting reported data; Holland and Tufail[174] have pointed out that the analytic techniques used in these studies can identify substantial differences in times to disease progression (as occur in studies that compare immediate treatment to deferral of treatment) but are less able to identify smaller, albeit important, differences in progression attributable to dose effects during studies of relatively short duration. In fact, it is generally accepted that oral ganciclovir is less effective for control of lesion activity than intravenously administered drug, as would be expected on the basis of its lower plasma concentrations.

Valganciclovir (Valcyte®, Roche Pharmaceuticals, Nutley, NJ) has significantly better bioavailability (61%) than oral ganciclovir; after oral administration, it is hydrolyzed to ganciclovir in the gastrointestinal mucosa, thus achieving higher plasma levels of the active drug that are comparable to those obtained with intravenous ganciclovir. Because oral valganciclovir has an efficacy and safety profile comparable to intravenous ganciclovir, it can be used for both induction (900 mg twice daily for 21 days) and maintenance therapy (900 mg once daily).[175,176]

Ganciclovir can result in severe neutropenia through bone marrow toxicity. The combination of ganciclovir and zidovudine

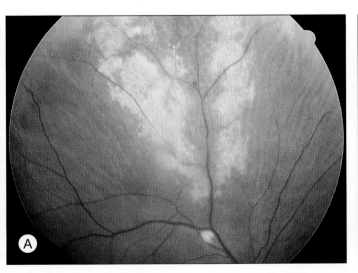 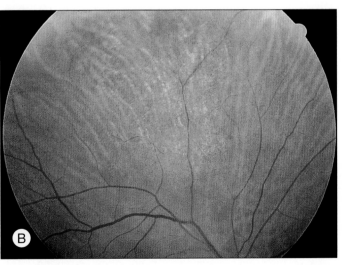

Fig. 91-9 A, An untreated focus of cytomegalovirus retinitis. B, The same eye after 2 weeks of induction using ganciclovir. The lesions have become less opacified, and the lesion borders have not advanced. The area of infected retinal tissue has been replaced by a thin gliotic scar, with fine mottling of the retinal pigment epithelium. From Holland GN. An update on AIDS-related cytomegalovirus retinitis. (Reprinted with permission from Holland GN. An update on AIDS-related cytomegalovirus retinitis. In Focal Points 1991: Clinical Modules for Opthalmologists, volume IX, module 5. San Francisco: American Academy of Opthalmology. 1991.)

can increase this risk.[177] Bone marrow toxicity can be minimized by the concurrent use of recombinant leukocyte growth factors, such as granulocyte colony-stimulating factor (filgrastim; Neupogen®, Amgen Inc., Thousand Oaks, CA).[50] Other possible side-effects of ganciclovir include nausea, diarrhea, fever, thrombocytopenia, and anemia.[175,176] Patients are also at risk for septic complications from indwelling catheters used to administer intravenous ganciclovir; secondary infections can include endogenous bacterial endophthalmitis.[178] The use of oral valganciclovir avoids these catheter-related risks, as well as avoiding the altered quality of life and cost of paraphernalia associated with intravenous drug administration.

Foscarnet

Although foscarnet (Foscavir®, AstraZeneca LP, Wilmington, DE), a pyrophosphate analog, inhibits CMV replication through the same mechanism as ganciclovir, it does not require phosphorylation to be activated. Foscarnet is administered intravenously at a dose of 60 mg/kg every 8 hours or 90 mg/kg every 12 hours for induction and 90 to 120 mg/kg once daily for maintenance therapy. Elimination occurs primarily through renal excretion, which necessitates dose adjustment in cases of renal insufficiency. In well-hydrated patients with no history of renal impairment, doses of foscarnet as high as 120 mg/kg/day may be tolerated with little or no rise in serum creatinine.[168] Foscarnet has a tedious administration schedule, requiring a 2-hour infusion time, using an infusion pump and simultaneous hydration.

Foscarnet is similar in efficacy to intravenous ganciclovir for treatment of CMV retinitis.[50] A difference has been demonstrated between treatment groups with regard to patient survival, however, with a significantly longer median survival in patients being treated initially with foscarnet,[50] possibly related to the fact that foscarnet has anti-HIV activity as well.[179] Subsequently, another clinical trial failed to show a difference in mortality between patients treated with ganciclovir and those treated with foscarnet.[168] The factors accounting for these different results are unknown.

Foscarnet therapy has been associated with side effects that may require discontinuation of drug administration; they include renal toxicity, nausea, neurologic changes, and penile ulceration.[50,180] Substantial renal toxicity may occur with concomitant administration of potentially nephrotoxic drugs, such as amphotericin B. Overall, foscarnet seems to be less well-tolerated than ganciclovir, and its side effects are more difficult to manage.[50]

Cidofovir

In contrast to ganciclovir, cidofovir (Vistide®, Gilead Sciences, Foster City, CA), a nucleotide analog, requires only diphosphorylation, which is mediated by cellular kinases; it does not require the action of virus-encoded enzymes.[181–184] Cidofovir exhibits higher anti-CMV activity in vitro than either ganciclovir or foscarnet, perhaps as a result of its extended intracellular half-life.

Due to its unique pharmacokinetic properties, intravenous cidofovir can be given on an intermittent treatment schedule, obviating the need for an indwelling catheter. Cidofovir is administered intravenously at a dose of 5 mg/kg once weekly for induction and 5 mg/kg once every 2 weeks for maintenance therapy. Its main route of elimination is renal, thus requiring dose adjustment in cases of renal insufficiency. To reduce the risk of renal toxicity that is known to occur with cidofovir treatment, concomitant administration of probenecid, with hydration, is given routinely to all patients on the day of cidofovir infusion.

Studies have shown cidofovir to be effective for control of both untreated CMV retinitis and lesions that have reactivated after treatment with other anti-CMV drugs.[165,167] In a clinical trial comparing cidofovir to a regimen that included oral ganciclovir and the ganciclovir implant for treatment of newly diagnosed or reactivated CMV retinitis lesions, no difference in outcomes were identified, although the study was terminated before fully enrolled, limiting the power to identify small differences in efficacy.[185]

Cidofovir-associated renal toxicity manifests as increased proteinuria and serum creatinine, especially in patients with pre-existing renal impairment or a tendency toward dehydration. Substantial renal toxicity may occur with concomitant administration of potentially nephrotoxic drugs, such as amphotericin B. Many patients become intolerant of probenecid, because of side effects that include nausea, headache, fever, and rash.

Intravenous cidofovir has also been associated with local ocular side effects. Anterior uveitis, characterized by an intense anterior chamber cellular and fibrinous reaction, occurs in 25% to 45% of treated patients.[186,187] Although inflammation can be suppressed with topical corticosteroids, even if cidofovir treatment is continued, the anterior uveitis can lead to permanent sequelae, including posterior synechiae.[186,187] Cidofovir has also been associated with an increased risk of IRU after immune reconstitution has been achieved.[145] Hypotony occurs in approximately 10% of cidofovir-treated patients, and may be severe and permanent.[186]

Fomivirsen

The most recently developed anti-CMV drug, fomivirsen (Vitravene®, Novartis Ophthalmics, Inc., Duluth, GA; Isis Pharmaceuticals, Carlsbad, CA), has not been available commercially since January 2004. It is an antisense phosphorothioate oligonucleotide that binds to mRNA transcribed from the major immediate-early region 2 of CMV,[188,189] which encodes two major polypeptides responsible for regulation of virus gene expression, thus inhibiting a critical step in CMV replication.[189,190] Fomivirsen has been shown in vitro to be 30- to 40-fold more potent than ganciclovir against CMV.[189] Fomivirsen was developed for intravitreous injection, and was reported to be effective for treatment of both newly diagnosed CMV retinitis and lesions that were active despite treatment with other anti-CMV agents.[171,172] Its associated side effects included anterior chamber and vitreous humor inflammatory reactions and elevated intraocular pressure, both of which could be controlled with medical therapy; retinal pigment epitheliopathy, cataracts, and CME are other reported complications.[173]

Drug resistance

Mutations in the CMV UL97 gene, which encodes the phosphotransferase involved in the first phosphorylation of ganciclovir, confer resistance to ganciclovir, while mutations in the CMV UL54 gene, which encodes DNA polymerase, can confer resistance to ganciclovir, foscarnet, and cidofovir.[191–195] Genotypic resistance testing may be useful in cases of disease progression despite ganciclovir treatment, to determine whether switching to a different anti-CMV agent is likely to be more effective.

Resistance is not an "all-or-none" phenomenon; phenotypic resistance to ganciclovir, as determined by in vitro testing of virus cultures, may be "low-level," indicating probably mutations in the UL97 gene, or "high-level," indicating UL54 mutations.[196,197] In some cases, higher drug levels, achieved either by increased systemic doses, or by placement of drug directly into the eye, may overcome resistance in vivo, and again bring disease under control.

Drug resistance generally develops during therapy, as mutant strains emerge in response to drug exposure. The risk of resistance increases with the duration of ganciclovir,[198,199] foscarnet,[200,201] and cidofovir[200] therapy.

Some investigators have shown good agreement between mutations in the UL97 gene from paired blood and vitreous humor specimens in populations-based studies,[202] suggesting that resistance-conferring mutations occur systemically and are widely distributed in the body; others have demonstrated that mutations can differ between isolates from blood and eye, or between isolates from the two eyes of individual patients with bilateral CMV retinitis,[196,203] suggesting that isolated resistance-conferring mutations may arise in the eye. Local emergence of such mutations within the eye may be a consequence of chronic, subtherapeutic drug delivery to the eye in some patients.

Clinically, the identification of resistance to anti-CMV drugs is associated with adverse outcomes, including increased risk for progression,[201,204–206] contralateral eye involvement,[199,205,206] and extraocular disease.[205] The routine application of testing for drug resistance is limited not only by the expense of testing, but also by the inability to isolate virus from blood or urine in some cases, and the lack of ocular specimens for most patients.

Local therapy

In response to concerns about the toxicity and limited efficacy of systemically administered anti-CMV drugs, local therapies have been developed, in which drugs are delivered directly into the eye.[207]

Intravitreous injections

The first techniques for local therapy involved injection of intravenous drug formulations directly into the eye, thereby increasing drug concentrations at the site of disease without added systemic toxicity. Ganciclovir is generally used at a dose of 2000 μg in 0.1 ml twice weekly for 3 weeks for induction and 2000 μg in 0.1 ml once weekly for maintenance.[208] Foscarnet doses for intravitreous injection are 2400 μg in 0.1 ml twice weekly for induction and 2400 μg in 0.1 ml once a week for maintenance.[209] Injections are performed through the superonasal, superotemporal, or inferotemporal pars plana, 4 mm posterior to the limbus, using a 30-gauge needle, after application of a topical anesthetic agent and disinfection with topical povidone-iodine 5%.

Uncontrolled case series[34,208–212] and single case reports[213–218] have demonstrated the ability of repeated ganciclovir or foscarnet injections to suppress lesion activity for extended periods of time. Although one series showed a significant difference in median time to progression between eyes treated with intravitreous ganciclovir (42 weeks) and those treated with intravenous ganciclovir (21 weeks),[208] the relative risks and benefits of this approach versus systemic therapies have never been evaluated in randomized trials.

Repeated injections are generally well tolerated, but they are inconvenient for the patient, and carry an additional risk of endophthalmitis,[34,208,211,215,219] retinal detachment,[34,210,219] vitreous hemorrhage,[212] and cataract formation.[207] Injections may also cause an immediate rise in intraocular pressure with the potential for occlusion of large retinal vessels and the optic disc vascular network. The retinal circulation appears to be more easily obstructed in CMV-infected eyes.[210] Repeated injections of ganciclovir or foscarnet do not appear to be associated with a high risk of drug-related complications. In a rabbit model, however, it has been shown by electron microscopy that multiple intravitreous injections of ganciclovir may result in vacuolization of photoreceptor inner segments.[220] One case of retinal necrosis resulting from the inadvertent injection of 400 mg of ganciclovir in 0.1 ml has been reported.[221]

Intravitreous injections of cidofovir have been studied extensively.[222–227] Although effective, published data have shown a substantial risk of severe toxicity leading to uveitis[223–226] and hypotony.[223,224,226] Because there appears to be a narrow therapeutic index associated with intravitreous cidofovir therapy, it is generally not used clinically.

Ganciclovir implant

The ganciclovir implant consists of 4.5 mg of ganciclovir in a 2.5 mm pellet that is completely coated with drug-permeable polyvinyl alcohol and then partially coated by drug-impermeable ethyl vinyl acetate, to allow sustained release of drug at a rate of approximately 1 μg/hour. The ganciclovir implant is inserted through a 5–6 mm sclerotomy at the pars plana, then secured with scleral sutures.

Studies have shown the median time to progression of CMV retinitis with the ganciclovir implant is about three times longer than with intravenous ganciclovir (approximately 7 to 8 months).[228–231] The mean vitreous humor concentration of ganciclovir achieved with the ganciclovir implant is 4.1 μg/ml,[228] compared to approximately 1 μg/ml after intravenous administration of ganciclovir at induction doses[232]; it is assumed that retinal tissue concentrations parallel those in the vitreous humor. The protracted time to progression corresponds roughly to the life of the ganciclovir implant, making replacement at approximately 7- to 8-month intervals a necessity in individuals who have not experienced immune reconstitution.[233] Timed ganciclovir implant exchange has been shown to provide good and lasting control of CMV retinitis.[233,234]

Patients may experience mild-to-moderate visual blurring and slight discomfort for 4 to 6 weeks after the implantation procedure. Serious complications of implantation or exchange are uncommon, but include retinal detachment,[228,231,235,236] endophthalmitis,[237] and vitreous hemorrhage.[207,228,230,231,235] Endophthalmitis occurs in approximately 0.5% of cases.[237] Vitreous hemorrhages and cataracts tend to be more frequent following multiple procedures.[234,238] The frequency of retinal detachment after placement of the ganciclovir implant is significantly increased in the short-term, as would be expected with any retinovitreous surgical procedure.[235] The benefit of better suppression of lesion activity, with a subsequent reduced risk of retinal detachment, appears to outweigh the effect of the surgical procedure over the long-term, however; studies have demonstrated that the long-term risk of retinal detachment was similar in patients treated with the ganciclovir implant versus those treated with systemic anti-CMV therapies.[235,239]

The long-term effects of having a ganciclovir implant in the eye among those individuals whose survival has increased as a result of HAART have not been well studied. Potential problems include fibrovascular proliferation at the sclerotomy site, pellet separation, or extrusion of the ganciclovir implant.

Response to treatment

Resolution of CMV retinitis lesions with effective anti-CMV therapy is characterized clinically by loss of satellite lesions, disappearance of venous sheathing, resolution of exudative retinal detachments, if present, and the formation of a more stable and harder-appearing lesion border that eventually evolves into a clinically inactive scar. Occasional "hard" opacities associated with scar formation must be distinguished from the granular opacity of active disease.[240]

Treatment strategies

Because multiple drugs and routes of administration are available, therapy can be individualized on the basis of a patient's potential for immune reconstitution and the availability of HAART; on the anatomic location and extent of his or her retinal lesions; on the presence of extraocular CMV disease; and on issues related to quality of life.[238,241]

People with AIDS

HIV-infected individuals for whom HAART is not available or for whom HAART fails to induce immune reconstitution are treated according to the traditional approach of induction followed by maintenance therapy. The main goals of therapy will be to prevent or slow the progression of retinitis; to prevent development of CMV retinitis in the contralateral eye of people who present with unilateral disease; and to suppress extraocular CMV disease. During maintenance therapy, there is clearly a dose effect, with slower rates of progression in patients treated with higher doses of drug[242]; however, this benefit must be weighed against potential adverse effects of drug at higher doses.

Although induction doses have traditionally been given for a set duration of 2 or 3 weeks,[50,102] some clinicians will continue to administer initial high doses until lesion opacity has completely resolved, indicating inactivity, especially if lesions are adjacent to the optic disc[104] or fovea. Patients receiving extended induction must be monitored closely for evidence of drug toxicity.

Management of progression

In the setting of severe immunosuppression, lesions will eventually reactivate despite long-term maintenance therapy; causes include further waning of immunity over time; inadequate drug levels, either because of dosing issues or poor drug delivery to the eye; or the development of anti-CMV drug resistance, especially later in the course of treatment.[102]

The median time to first progression has been reported to be approximately 50 days for either ganciclovir or foscarnet.[169] In HIV-infected individuals treated with either intravenous ganciclovir or foscarnet, risk factors for earlier reactivation and progression include smaller area of retinitis at diagnosis, greater border opacity, lower CD4+ T-lymphocyte counts, and positive CMV blood cultures[114,166]; with respect to the rate of lesion enlargement, independent risk factors include a smaller area involved, a shorter distance between the optic disc and the closest lesion border, and the presence of satellite lesions.[114] Times to progression become increasingly shorter with subsequent reactivations[169]; after many reactivations, it may be impossible to achieve inactivity, resulting in a clinical picture known as "smoldering disease" (Fig. 91-10). In such cases, slowing of border advancement may be the best that can be achieved with treatment.[106]

Suppression of disease reactivation during maintenance therapy is managed by "re-induction," using a variety of strategies. The most common approach is to increase the dose of the same drug that was used for maintenance until clinical inactivity is again achieved; this strategy seems to be effective particularly in the setting of a first reactivation.[46] When anti-CMV drug resistance

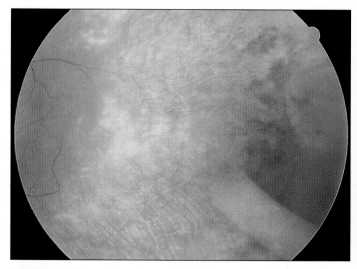

Fig. 91-10 A focus of poorly controlled cytomegalovirus retinitis characterized by minimal opacification of the lesion border. This type of lesion has been referred to as "smoldering retinitis."

is suspected to be a contributing cause, switching to a different drug may be more appropriate. Supplementation of systemic therapy with intravitreous injections, as discussed below, or treatment with a combination of drugs are other re-induction options.

Combination drug therapies

Ganciclovir and foscarnet are synergistic against CMV in vitro.[243,244] The combination of these drugs is associated with longer times to progression than either agent alone,[168,245,246] but the cost and impact on quality of life must be considered.[168] Synergistic or additive combination therapies may also involve the use of a systemic agent with local therapy.

Role of local therapy

Local therapy may be indicated in those patients who cannot receive systemic therapy, either because of adverse effects or impaired quality of life. In general, though, local therapy is not used alone in individuals for whom immune reconstitution is not anticipated. Contralateral eye involvement has been reported in 11% to 54.5% of patients treated with local therapy alone,[208,212,219,228] while clinically apparent extraocular CMV disease occurs in 10% to 30% of patients treated with local therapy alone.[208,212,228,231] To prevent these occurrences, local treatment should be combined with some form of systemic therapy. For example, the combination of a ganciclovir implant with oral ganciclovir offers the advantage of high intraocular drug levels, while protecting against disease elsewhere, which does not appear to require equally high drug levels. Furthermore, the combination of a ganciclovir implant with oral ganciclovir was significantly more effective for preventing CMV retinitis progression than the ganciclovir implant alone in one study.[235]

Survival is also an issue of concern if local therapy is used alone. In an early assessment of survival after development of CMV retinitis,[49] individuals treated with ganciclovir lived longer than untreated patients, although the study was not randomized. The survival benefit was attributed to treatment of extraocular, potentially life-threatening CMV disease. Thus, one might expect individuals treated with local therapy alone to have shorter survival times. Nevertheless, one series failed to report a survival advantage for patients treated with systemic ganciclovir when compared to patients treated with intravitreous ganciclovir alone,[208] and another series found a median survival time of approximately 13 months for people receiving weekly intravitreous ganciclovir maintenance therapy,[219] which is not lower than the survival figure published by the Studies of the Ocular Complications of AIDS Research Group in a large clinical trial,[50] although the number of patients and the study designs differed greatly.

In deciding whether to use supplemental local therapy alone for re-induction, one must consider the circumstances surrounding reactivation of disease. For example, local therapy may be appropriate if there is evidence that resistance mutations have arisen in the eye. Also, Tufail and associates[75] found that reactivation of CMV retinitis is preceded by increased CMV blood levels in some, but not all patients. Those individuals with rising CMV blood levels may have reactivation of extraocular CMV infection as well, and would probably benefit from a re-induction strategy that includes increased systemic drug doses. In contrast, those individuals whose reactivation of CMV retinitis lesions is not associated with detectable CMV blood levels (suggesting that reactivation is attributable to poor local drug delivery or local emergence of resistance mutations) might do well with local supplementation alone for re-induction. When used as a supplemental therapy, the ganciclovir implant seems to be effective at controlling recurrent CMV retinitis,[230] but its efficacy may be reduced in patients previously treated with intravenous ganciclovir for more than 6 months.[236]

There has been concern regarding efficacy and potential toxicity of local therapy in eyes filled with silicone oil. Time to progression of CMV retinitis does not seem to be affected when an implant is inserted into an eye with silicone oil.[247] Enhanced retinal toxicity of intravitreous ganciclovir has been reported in rabbit eyes filled with silicone oil,[248] and clinicians generally reduce the dose of both ganciclovir and foscarnet in half when injecting into eyes with silicone oil.

The effect of HAART

The availability of HAART has allowed clinicians to reconsider the approach to treatment of CMV retinitis in those patients for whom immune reconstitution is anticipated. HAART may induce complete inactivity of CMV retinitis without concurrent specific anti-CMV therapy because of improved host immunity.[110,116,117] Because of a delay in immune reconstitution after initiation of HAART, however, treatment should still be contemplated in every case of newly diagnosed CMV retinitis. Because of the potential for prolonged survival with immune reconstitution, aggressive anti-CMV therapy should be initiated to inactivate lesions, thereby preventing additional vision loss that might occur before immune reconstitution is achieved, and to limit the size of lesions, thus reducing the risk of subsequent retinal detachment. Valganciclovir is currently the most widely used treatment in this situation.[176]

The ganciclovir implant is generally avoided if immune reconstitution is anticipated, because of its potential for local, long-term complications.[237] It may be indicated, however, if zone 1 is involved, because the high dose that is achieved within the eye may be more effective at preventing early vision loss.

Discontinuation of specific anti-CMV maintenance therapy may be possible in selected patients who experience immune reconstitution on HAART, although there is as yet no consensus as to the most appropriate time to do so. In general, such a decision is based upon a rise in CD4+ T-lymphocyte counts, a drop in HIV RNA blood levels, the duration of HAART, and the duration of inactivity of CMV retinitis.[249-256]

Development of resistance to antiretroviral drugs may cause reactivation; in most cases, CD4+ T-lymphocyte counts will have fallen and HIV blood levels will be high.[70] Reactivation of CMV retinitis in such a setting should prompt a change in HAART to achieve immune reconstitution again, if possible.

A low CD4+ T-lymphocyte count remains a substantial risk factor for progression of CMV retinitis in the HAART era.[256a]

Nevertheless, even among patients who are considered to have failed HAART on the basis of CD4[+] T-lymphocyte counts <50 cells/mm³, the incidence of retinitis progression is substantially lower than the incidence reported in the pre-HAART era (0.58 events/person-year vs. 3.0 events/person-year, respectively),[256a] suggesting a benefit of HAART on host defences against CMV that is not reflected in the routine laboratory tests of immune status.

Many investigators have emphasized the CD4[+] T-lymphocyte count alone as a measure for assessing risk of CMV retinitis reactivation in people taking HAART.[251,252,257] In contrast, Lin and associates[258] suggested that the CD4[+] T-lymphocyte count may be a less useful predictor of recurrent CMV retinitis than HIV blood levels among people on HAART; in their study, the minimal HIV blood level was a much stronger predictor of outcome in such people. Other investigators have reported an absence of CMV-specific immunity despite high CD4[+] T-lymphocyte counts in some patients with multiple recurrences of CMV retinitis.[259] Thus, patients should undergo periodic indirect ophthalmoscopy after withdrawal of specific anti-CMV agents to rule out reactivation, which may be asymptomatic.[70] Even with apparent immune reconstitution (CD4[+] T-lymphocyte count >200 cells/mm³), there continues to be a low incidence of disease progression (0.02 events/person-year), second eye involvement (0.02 events/person-year), and retinal detachments (0.02 events/person-year).[256a,259a]

Treatment of other immunosuppressed hosts

In iatrogenically immunosuppressed patients, reduction or discontinuation of immunosuppression alone may allow for spontaneous resolution of CMV retinitis.[4,109] Otherwise, CMV retinitis is generally treated according to the same principles used to treat people with AIDS. CMV retinitis in people without HIV infection may respond more favorably to antiviral therapy, with a 2 to 5 months recurrence-free interval in one study.[260]

Treatment of children

There is little literature available that describes treatment of CMV retinitis in the setting of congenital CMV infection. Intravenous ganciclovir, administered for 6 weeks, has been used to treat newborns with symptomatic congenital CMV infection involving the central nervous system.[261] Some investigators recommend the use of intravenous ganciclovir 6 mg/kg every 12 hours, with twice-weekly complete blood counts, for treatment of infants who present with severe CMV end-organ disease, including life- or sight-threatening disease.[262] Such treatment has been shown to inactivate CMV retinitis lesions in such infants.

In children with AIDS, both ganciclovir and foscarnet, either alone or in combination, have been reported to treat CMV retinitis successfully.[263,264] The ganciclovir implant has been used effectively to treat bilateral CMV retinitis that was unresponsive to combined intravenous ganciclovir and foscarnet in a child with AIDS.[265] Older children who are immuno-

suppressed for other reasons also seem to benefit from ganciclovir or foscarnet therapy.[263,266]

PREVENTION

Anti-CMV drugs can be used for prophylaxis against development of CMV retinitis in severely immunosuppressed individuals. In people with advanced AIDS, oral ganciclovir 1000 mg three times daily and valaciclovir 2000 mg four times daily have been associated with significantly reduced risk of developing CMV disease, including CMV retinitis.[27,267] Prophylaxis is not used routinely in HIV-infected individuals who achieve immune reconstitution with HAART.

ACKNOWLEDGMENT

Emmett T. Cunningham MD, PhD, MPH and Jay S. Pepose MD, PhD contributed to earlier editions of this chapter.

REFERENCES

1. Sissons JG, Carmichael AJ, McKinney N et al. Human cytomegalovirus and immunopathology. Springer Semin Immunopathol 2002; 24:169–185.
2. Drew WL, Mintz L, Miner RC et al. Prevalence of cytomegalovirus infection in homosexual men. J Infect Dis 1981; 143:188–192.
3. Horwitz CA, Henle W, Henle G et al. Heterophil-negative infectious mononucleosis and mononucleosis-like illnesses. Laboratory confirmation of 43 cases. Am J Med 1977; 63:947–957.
4. Pollard RB, Egbert PR, Gallagher JG et al. Cytomegalovirus retinitis in immunosuppressed hosts. I. Natural history and effects of treatment with adenine arabinoside. Ann Intern Med 1980; 93:655–664.
5. Egbert PR, Pollard RB, Gallagher JG et al. Cytomegalovirus retinitis in immunosuppressed hosts. II. Ocular manifestations. Ann Intern Med 1980; 93:664–670.
6. Murray HW, Knox DL, Green WR et al. Cytomegalovirus retinitis in adults. A manifestation of disseminated viral infection. Am J Med 1977; 63:574–584.
7. Quinn TC, Piot P, McCormick JB et al. Serologic and immunologic studies in patients with AIDS in North America and Africa. The potential role of infectious agents as cofactors in human immunodeficiency virus infection. JAMA 1987; 257:2617–2621.
8. Stagno S, Reynolds DW, Huang ES et al. Congenital cytomegalovirus infection. N Engl J Med 1977; 296:1254–1258.
9. Pass R. Epidemiology and transmission of cytomegalovirus. J Infect Dis 1985; 152:243–248.
10. Stagno S, Pass RF, Dworsky ME et al. Maternal cytomegalovirus infection and perinatal transmission. Clin Obstet Gynecol 1982; 25:563–576.
11. Gaytant MA, Steegers EA, Semmekrot BA et al. Congenital cytomegalovirus infection: review of the epidemiology and outcome. Obstet Gynecol Surv 2002; 57:245–256.
12. Stagno S, Whitley RJ. Herpesvirus infections of pregnancy. Part I: Cytomegalovirus and Epstein–Barr virus infections. N Engl J Med 1985; 313:1270–1274.
13. de Jong MD, Galasso GJ, Gazzard B et al. Summary of the II International Symposium on Cytomegalovirus. Antiviral Res 1998; 39:141–162.
14. Stagno S, Pass R, Cloud G et al. Primary cytomegalovirus infection in pregnancy. Incidence, transmission to the fetus, and clinical outcome. JAMA 1986; 256:1904–1908.
15. Istas AS, Demmler GJ, Dobbins JG et al. Surveillance for congenital cytomegalovirus disease: a report from the National Congenital Cytomegalovirus Disease Registry. Clin Infect Dis 1995; 20:665–670.
16. Boppana SB, Pass RF, Britt WJ et al. Symptomatic congenital cytomegalovirus infection: neonatal morbidity and mortality. Pediatr Infect Dis J 1992; 11:93–99.
17. Raynor BD. Cytomegalovirus infection in pregnancy. Semin Perinatol 1993; 17:394–402.
18. Fowler K, Stagno S, Pass R et al. The outcome of congenital cytomegalovirus infection in relation to maternal antibody status. N Engl J Med 1992; 326:663–667.

19. Stagno S, Reynolds DW, Amos CS et al. Auditory and visual defects resulting from symptomatic and subclinical congenital cytomegaloviral and toxoplasma infections. Pediatrics 1977; 59:669–678.

20. Conboy TJ, Pass RF, Stagno S et al. Early clinical manifestations and intellectual outcome in children with symptomatic congenital cytomegalovirus infection. J Pediatr 1987; 111:343–348.

21. Boppana S, Amos C, Britt WJ et al. Late onset and reactivation of chorioretinitis in children with congenital cytomegalovirus infection. Pediatr Infect Dis J 1994; 13:1139–1142.

22. Trincado DE, Rawlinson WD. Congenital and perinatal infections with cytomegalovirus. J Paediatr Child Health 2001; 37:187–192.

23. Joint United Nations Programme on HIV/AIDS (UNAIDS). 2004 Report on the Global AIDS Epidemic: Executive Summary. Online. Available: http://www.unaids.org/bangkok2004/GAR2004_html/ExecSummary_en /ExecSumm_00_en.htm 10 Jul 2004.

24. Dennehy PJ, Warman R, Flynn JT et al. Ocular manifestations in pediatric patients with acquired immunodeficiency syndrome. Arch Ophthalmol 1989; 107:978–982.

25. Baumal CR, Levin AV, Kavalec CC et al. Screening for cytomegalovirus retinitis in children. Arch Pediatr Adolesc Med 1996; 150:1186–1192.

26. Kestelyn P, Lepage P, Karita E et al. Ocular manifestations of infection with the human immunodeficiency virus in an African pediatric population. Ocul Immunol Inflamm 2000; 8:263–273.

27. Spector SA, McKinley GF, Lalezari JP et al. Oral ganciclovir for the prevention of cytomegalovirus disease in persons with AIDS. Roche Cooperative Oral Ganciclovir Study Group. N Engl J Med 1996; 334:1491–1497.

28. Gallant JE, Moore RD, Richman DD et al. Incidence and natural history of cytomegalovirus disease in patients with advanced human immunodeficiency virus disease treated with zidovudine. The Zidovudine Epidemiology Study Group. J Infect Dis 1992; 166:1223–1227.

29. Peters BS, Beck EJ, Anderson S et al. Cytomegalovirus infection in AIDS. Patterns of disease, response to therapy and trends in survival. J Infect 1991; 23:129–137.

30. Hoover DR, Peng Y, Saah A et al. Occurrence of cytomegalovirus retinitis after human immunodeficiency virus immunosuppression. Arch Ophthalmol 1996; 114:821–827.

31. Holland GN, Pepose JS, Pettit TH et al. Acquired immune deficiency syndrome. Ocular manifestations. Ophthalmology 1983; 90:859–873.

32. Pepose JS, Holland GN, Nestor MS et al. Acquired immune deficiency syndrome. Pathogenic mechanisms of ocular disease. Ophthalmology 1985; 92:472–484.

33. Henderly DE, Freeman WR, Causey DM et al. Cytomegalovirus retinitis and response to therapy with ganciclovir. Ophthalmology 1987; 94:425–434.

34. Heinemann MH. Long-term intravitreal ganciclovir therapy for cytomegalovirus retinopathy. Arch Ophthalmol 1989; 107:1767–1772.

35. Jabs DA, Green WR, Fox R et al. Ocular manifestations of acquired immune deficiency syndrome. Ophthalmology 1989; 96:1092–1099.

36. Pertel P, Hirschtick R, Phair J et al. Risk of developing cytomegalovirus retinitis in persons infected with the human immunodeficiency virus. J Acquir Immune Defic Syndr 1992; 5:1069–1074.

37. Kuppermann BD, Petty JG, Richman DD et al. Correlation between CD4+ counts and prevalence of cytomegalovirus retinitis and human immunodeficiency virus-related noninfectious retinal vasculopathy in patients with acquired immunodeficiency syndrome. Am J Ophthalmol 1993; 115:575–582.

38. Lowder CY, Butler CP, Dodds EM et al. CD8+ T lymphocytes and cytomegalovirus retinitis in patients with the acquired immunodeficiency syndrome. Am J Ophthalmol 1995; 120:283–290.

39. Muccioli C, Belfort Junior R, Lottenberg C et al. Ophthalmological manifestations in AIDS: evaluation of 445 patients in one year. Rev Assoc Med Bras 1994; 40:155–158.

40. Kestelyn P, Van de Perre P, Rouvroy D et al. A prospective study of the ophthalmologic findings in the acquired immune deficiency syndrome in Africa. Am J Ophthalmol 1985; 100:230–238.

41. Kestelyn P. The epidemiology of CMV retinitis in Africa. Ocul Immunol Inflamm 1999; 7:173–177.

42. Beare NA, Kublin JG, Lewis DK et al. Ocular disease in patients with tuberculosis and HIV presenting with fever in Africa. Br J Ophthalmol 2002; 86:1076–1079.

43. Cochereau I, Mlika-Cabanne N, Godinaud P et al. AIDS related eye disease in Burundi, Africa. Br J Ophthalmol 1999; 83:339–342.

44. Jaffar S, Ariyoshi K, Frith P et al. Retinal manifestations of HIV-1 and HIV-2 infections among hospital patients in The Gambia, west Africa. Trop Med Int Health 1999; 4:487–492.

45. Biswas J, Madhavan HN, George AE et al. Ocular lesions associated with HIV infection in India: a series of 100 consecutive patients evaluated at a referral center. Am J Ophthalmol 2000; 129:9–15.

46. Gross JG, Bozzette SA, Mathews WC et al. Longitudinal study of cytomegalovirus retinitis in acquired immune deficiency syndrome. Ophthalmology 1990; 97:681–686.

47. Jabs DA, Enger C, Bartlett JG. Cytomegalovirus retinitis and acquired immunodeficiency syndrome. Arch Ophthalmol 1989; 107:75–80.

48. Palestine AG, Rodrigues MM, Macher AM et al. Ophthalmic involvement in acquired immunodeficiency syndrome. Ophthalmology 1984; 91: 1092–1099.

49. Holland GN, Sison RF, Jatulis DE et al. Survival of patients with the acquired immune deficiency syndrome after development of cytomegalovirus retinopathy. UCLA CMV Retinopathy Study Group. Ophthalmology 1990; 97:204–211.

50. Studies of Ocular Complications of AIDS Research Group in collaboration with the AIDS Clinical Trials Group. Mortality in patients with the acquired immunodeficiency syndrome treated with either foscarnet or ganciclovir for cytomegalovirus retinitis. N Engl J Med 1992; 326: 213–220.

51. Jabs DA, Bartlett JG. AIDS and ophthalmology: a period of transition. Am J Ophthalmol 1997; 124:227–233.

52. Collier AC, Coombs RW, Schoenfeld DA et al. Treatment of human immunodeficiency virus infection with saquinavir, zidovudine, and zalcitabine. AIDS Clinical Trials Group. N Engl J Med 1996; 334:1011–1017.

53. Walsh JC, Jones CD, Barnes EA et al. Increasing survival in AIDS patients with cytomegalovirus retinitis treated with combination antiretroviral therapy including HIV protease inhibitors. AIDS 1998; 12:613–618.

54. Palella FJ, Delaney KM, Moorman AC et al. Declining morbidity and mortality among patients with advanced human immunodeficiency virus infection. N Engl J Med 1998; 338:853–860.

55. Doan S, Cochereau I, Guvenisik N et al. Cytomegalovirus retinitis in HIV-infected patients with and without highly active antiretroviral therapy. Am J Ophthalmol 1999; 128:250–251.

56. Holtzer CD, Jacobson MA, Hadley WK et al. Decline in the rate of specific opportunistic infections at San Francisco General Hospital, 1994–1997. AIDS 1998; 12:1931–1933.

57. Komanduri KV, Viswanathan MN, Wieder ED et al. Restoration of cytomegalovirus-specific CD4+ T-lymphocyte responses after ganciclovir and highly active antiretroviral therapy in individuals infected with HIV-1. Nat Med 1998; 4:953–956.

58. Jacobson MA, Schrier R, McCune JM et al. Cytomegalovirus (CMV)-specific CD4+ T lymphocyte immune function in long-term survivors of AIDS-related CMV end-organ disease who are receiving potent antiretroviral therapy. J Infect Dis 2001; 183:1399–1404.

59. Torriani FJ, Freeman WR, Macdonald JC et al. CMV retinitis recurs after stopping treatment in virological and immunological failures of potent antiretroviral therapy. AIDS 2000; 14:173–180.

60. Nussenblatt RB, Lane HC. Human immunodeficiency virus disease: changing patterns of intraocular inflammation. Am J Ophthalmol 1998; 125:374–382.

61. Valdez H, Connick E, Smith KY et al. Limited immune restoration after 3 years' suppression of HIV-1 replication in patients with moderately advanced disease. AIDS 2002; 16:1859–1866.

62. Lucas GM, Chaisson RE, Moore RD. Highly active antiretroviral therapy in a large urban clinic: risk factors for virologic failure and adverse drug reactions. Ann Intern Med 1999; 131:81–87.

63. Fatkenheuer G, Theisen A, Rockstroh J et al. Virological treatment failure of protease inhibitor therapy in an unselected cohort of HIV-infected patients. AIDS 1997; 11:F113–116.

64. Davis MG, Kenney SC, Kamine J et al. Immediate-early gene region of human cytomegalovirus transactivates the promoter of human immunodeficiency virus. Proc Natl Acad Sci USA 1987; 84:8642–8646.

65. Skolnik PR, Kosloff BR, Hirsch MS. Bidirectional interactions between human immunodeficiency virus type 1 and cytomegalovirus. J Infect Dis 1988; 157:508–514.

66. Jabs DA. Ocular manifestations of HIV infection. Trans Am Ophthalmol Soc 1995; 93:623–683.

67. Hodge WG, Boivin JF, Shapiro SH et al. Clinical risk factors for cytomegalovirus retinitis in patients with AIDS. Ophthalmology 2004; 111:1326–1333.

68. Oka S, Nagata Y, Fujino Y et al. CD8+ T lymphocyte counts as an adjunctive predictor of cytomegalovirus retinitis in patients with acquired immunodeficiency syndrome. Intern Med 1997; 36:461–465.

69. Holland GN, Vaudaux JD, Jeng SM et al. Characteristics of newly diagnosed, untreated cytomegalovirus retinitis in patients with AIDS. I. Findings prior to the HAART era (1988–1994). (submitted).

70. Holland GN, Vaudaux JD, Shiramizu KM et al. Characteristics of newly diagnosed, untreated cytomegalovirus retinitis in patients with AIDS. II. Findings in the HAART era (1997–2000). (submitted).

71. Jacobson MA, Zegans M, Pavan PR et al. Cytomegalovirus retinitis after initiation of highly active antiretroviral therapy. Lancet 1997; 349:1443–1445.

72. Zurlo JJ, O'Neill D, Polis MA et al. Lack of clinical utility of cytomegalovirus blood and urine cultures in patients with HIV infection. Ann Intern Med 1993; 118:12–17.

73. Salmon D, Lacassin F, Harzic M et al. Predictive value of cytomegalovirus viraemia for the occurrence of CMV organ involvement in AIDS. J Med Virol 1990; 32:160–163.

74. Rasmussen L, Morris S, Zipeto D et al. Quantitation of human cytomegalovirus DNA from peripheral blood cells of human immunodeficiency virus-infected patients could predict cytomegalovirus retinitis. J Infect Dis 1995; 171:177–182.

75. Tufail A, Moe AA, Miller MJ et al. Quantitative cytomegalovirus DNA level in the blood and its relationship to cytomegalovirus retinitis in patients with acquired immune deficiency syndrome. Ophthalmology 1999; 106:133–141.

76. Shepp DH, Match ME, Ashraf AB et al. Cytomegalovirus glycoprotein B groups associated with retinitis in AIDS. J Infect Dis 1996; 174:184–187.

77. Shimakawa M, Kono C, Nagai T et al. CMV retinitis after renal transplantation. Transplant Proc 2002; 34:1790–1792.

78. Ciardella AP, Barile G, Langton K et al. Cytomegalovirus retinitis and FK 506. Am J Ophthalmol 2003; 136:386–389.

79. Paul AA, Leeper HF, Friberg TR. CMV retinitis and the use of FK 506. Transplant Proc 1991; 23:3042–3043.

80. Fishburne BC, Mitrani AA, Davis JL. Cytomegalovirus retinitis after cardiac transplantation. Am J Ophthalmol 1998; 125:104–106.

81. Ng P, McCluskey P, McCaughan G et al. Ocular complications of heart, lung, and liver transplantation. Br J Ophthalmol 1998; 82:423–428.

82. Quinlan MF, Salmon JF. Ophthalmic complications after heart transplantation. J Heart Lung Transplant 1993; 12:252–255.

83. Das T, Gupta A, Sakhuja V et al. Ocular complications in renal allograft recipients. Nephrol Dial Transplant 1991; 6:649–655.

84. Coskuncan NM, Jabs DA, Dunn JP et al. The eye in bone marrow transplantation. VI. Retinal complications. Arch Ophthalmol 1994; 112:372–379.

85. Suh DW, Ruttum MS, Stuckenschneider BJ et al. Ocular findings after bone marrow transplantation in a pediatric population. Ophthalmology 1999; 106:1564–1570.

86. Crippa F, Corey L, Chuang EL et al. Virological, clinical, and ophthalmologic features of cytomegalovirus retinitis after hematopoietic stem cell transplantation. Clin Infect Dis 2001; 32:214–219.

87. Griffiths PD, Clark DA, Emery VC. Betaherpesviruses in transplant recipients. J Antimicrob Chemother 2000; 45 Suppl T3:29–34.

88. Rao NA, Zhang J, Ishimoto S. Role of retinal vascular endothelial cells in development of CMV retinitis. Trans Am Ophthalmol Soc 1998; 96:111–123.

89. Read RW, Zhang J, Ishimoto SI et al. Evaluation of the role of human retinal vascular endothelial cells in the pathogenesis of CMV retinitis. Ocul Immunol Inflamm 1999; 7:139–146.

90. Glasgow BJ, Weisberger AK. A quantitative and cartographic study of retinal microvasculopathy in acquired immunodeficiency syndrome. Am J Ophthalmol 1994; 118:46–56.

91. Glasgow BJ. Evidence for breaches of the retinal vasculature in acquired immune deficiency syndrome angiopathy. A fluorescent microsphere study. Ophthalmology 1997; 104:753–760.

92. Rodrigues MM, Palestine A, Nussenblatt R et al. Unilateral cytomegalovirus retinochoroiditis and bilateral cytoid bodies in a bisexual man with the acquired immunodeficiency syndrome. Ophthalmology 1983; 90:1577–1582.

93. Newman NM, Mandel MR, Gullett J et al. Clinical and histologic findings in opportunistic ocular infections. Part of a new syndrome of acquired immunodeficiency. Arch Ophthalmol 1983; 101:396–401.

94. Jensen OA, Gerstoft J, Thomsen HK et al. Cytomegalovirus retinitis in the acquired immunodeficiency syndrome (AIDS). Light-microscopical, ultrastructural and immunohistochemical examination of a case. Acta Ophthalmol (Copenh) 1984; 62:1–9.

95. Freeman WR, Chen A, Henderly DE et al. Prevalence and significance of acquired immunodeficiency syndrome-related retinal microvasculopathy. Am J Ophthalmol 1989; 107:229–235.

96. Holland GN, Gottlieb MS, Foos RY. Retinal cotton-wool patches in patients with acquired immunodeficiency syndrome. N Engl J Med 1982; 307:1704.

97. Gonzalez CR, Wiley CA, Arevalo JF et al. Polymerase chain reaction detection of cytomegalovirus and human immunodeficiency virus-1 in the retina of patients with acquired immune deficiency syndrome with and without cotton-wool spots. Retina 1996; 16:305–311.

98. Skolnik PR, Pomerantz RJ, de la Monte SM et al. Dual infection of retina with human immunodeficiency virus type 1 and cytomegalovirus. Am J Ophthalmol 1989; 107:361–372.

99. Qavi HB, Green MT, SeGall GK et al. Demonstration of HIV-1 and HHV-6 in AIDS-associated retinitis. Curr Eye Res 1989; 8:379–387.

100. Rummelt V, Rummelt C, Jahn G et al. Triple retinal infection with human immunodeficiency virus type 1, cytomegalovirus, and herpes simplex virus type 1. Light and electron microscopy, immunohistochemistry, and in situ hybridization. Ophthalmology 1994; 101:270–279.

101. Studies of Ocular Complications of AIDS Research Group in collaboration with the AIDS Clinical Trials Group. Foscarnet–Ganciclovir Cytomegalovirus Retinitis Trial: 5. Clinical features of cytomegalovirus retinitis at diagnosis. Am J Ophthalmol 1997; 124:141–157.

102. Holland GN, Tufail A, Jordan MC. Cytomegalovirus diseases. In: Pepose JS, Holland GN, Wilhelmus KR, eds. Ocular Infection & Immunity. St Louis: Mosby, 1996; 1088–1129.

103. Gross JG, Sadun AA, Wiley CA et al. Severe visual loss related to isolated peripapillary retinal and optic nerve head cytomegalovirus infection. Am J Ophthalmol 1989; 108:691–698.

104. Patel SS, Rutzen AR, Marx JL et al. Cytomegalovirus papillitis in patients with acquired immune deficiency syndrome. Visual prognosis of patients treated with ganciclovir and/or foscarnet. Ophthalmology 1996; 103:1476–1482.

105. Holland GN, Buhles WC Jr, Mastre B et al. A controlled retrospective study of ganciclovir treatment for cytomegalovirus retinopathy. Use of a standardized system for the assessment of disease outcome. UCLA CMV Retinopathy Study Group. Arch Ophthalmol 1989; 107:1759–1766.

106. Holland GN, Shuler JD. Progression rates of cytomegalovirus retinopathy in ganciclovir-treated and untreated patients. Arch Ophthalmol 1992; 110:1435–1442.

107. Spaide RF, Vitale AT, Toth IR et al. Frosted branch angiitis associated with cytomegalovirus retinitis. Am J Ophthalmol 1992; 113:522–528.

108. Geier SA, Nasemann J, Klauss V et al. Frosted branch angiitis associated with cytomegalovirus retinitis. Am J Ophthalmol 1992; 114:514–516.

109. Meredith TA, Aaberg TM, Reeser FH. Rhegmatogenous retinal detachment complicating cytomegalovirus retinitis. Am J Ophthalmol 1979; 87:793–796.

110. Reed JB, Schwab IR, Gordon J et al. Regression of cytomegalovirus retinitis associated with protease-inhibitor treatment in patients with AIDS. Am J Ophthalmol 1997; 124:199–205.

111. Henderly DE, Freeman WR, Smith RE et al. Cytomegalovirus retinitis as the initial manifestation of the acquired immune deficiency syndrome. Am J Ophthalmol 1987; 103:316–320.

112. Sison RF, Holland GN, MacArthur LJ et al. Cytomegalovirus retinopathy as the initial manifestation of the acquired immunodeficiency syndrome. Am J Ophthalmol 1991; 112:243–249.

113. Hoover DR, Saah AJ, Bacellar H et al. Clinical manifestations of AIDS in the era of pneumocystis prophylaxis. Multicenter AIDS Cohort Study. N Engl J Med 1993; 329:1922–1926.

114. Holbrook JT, Davis MD, Hubbard LD et al. Risk factors for advancement of cytomegalovirus retinitis in patients with acquired immunodeficiency syndrome. Studies of Ocular Complications of AIDS Research Group. Arch Ophthalmol 2000; 118:1196–1204.

115. Luckie AP, Ai E. A foveal-sparing pattern of cytomegalovirus retinitis in the acquired immunodeficiency syndrome. Aust NZ J Ophthalmol 1996; 24:53–59.

116. Whitcup SM, Cunningham ET Jr, Polis MA et al. Spontaneous and sustained resolution of CMV retinitis in patients receiving highly active antiretroviral therapy. Br J Ophthalmol 1998; 82:845–846.

117. Whitcup SM, Fortin E, Nussenblatt RB et al. Therapeutic effect of combination antiretroviral therapy on cytomegalovirus retinitis. JAMA 1997; 277:1519–1520.

118. Freeman WR, Henderly DE, Wan WL et al. Prevalence, pathophysiology, and treatment of rhegmatogenous retinal detachment in treated cytomegalovirus retinitis. Am J Ophthalmol 1987; 103:527–536.

119. Roarty JD, Fisher EJ, Nussbaum JJ. Long-term visual morbidity of cytomegalovirus retinitis in patients with acquired immune deficiency syndrome. Ophthalmology 1993; 100:1685–1688.

120. Studies of Ocular Complications of AIDS (SOCA) Research Group in collaboration with the AIDS Clinical Trials Group (ACTG). Rhegmatogenous retinal detachment in patients with cytomegalovirus retinitis: the Foscarnet–Ganciclovir Cytomegalovirus Retinitis Trial. Am J Ophthalmol 1997; 124:61–70.

121. Orellana J, Teich SA, Lieberman RM et al. Treatment of retinal detachments in patients with the acquired immune deficiency syndrome. Ophthalmology 1991; 98:939–943.

122. Freeman WR, Quiceno JI, Crapotta JA et al. Surgical repair of rhegmatogenous retinal detachment in immunosuppressed patients with cytomegalovirus retinitis. Ophthalmology 1992; 99:466–474.

123. Irvine AR. Treatment of retinal detachment due to cytomegalovirus retinitis in patients with AIDS. Trans Am Ophthalmol Soc 1991; 89:349–363.

124. Jabs DA, Enger C, Haller J et al. Retinal detachments in patients with cytomegalovirus retinitis. Arch Ophthalmol 1991; 109:794–799.

125. Freeman WR, Friedberg DN, Berry C et al. Risk factors for development

of rhegmatogenous retinal detachment in patients with cytomegalovirus retinitis. Am J Ophthalmol 1993; 116:713–720.

126. Sidikaro Y, Silver L, Holland GN et al. Rhegmatogenous retinal detachments in patients with AIDS and necrotizing retinal infections. Ophthalmology 1991; 98:129–135.

127. Gangan PA, Besen G, Munguia D et al. Macular serous exudation in patients with acquired immunodeficiency syndrome and cytomegalovirus retinitis. Am J Ophthalmol 1994; 118:212–219.

128. Karavellas MP, Lowder CY, Macdonald C et al. Immune recovery vitritis associated with inactive cytomegalovirus retinitis: a new syndrome. Arch Ophthalmol 1998; 116:169–175.

129. Zegans ME, Walton RC, Holland GN et al. Transient vitreous inflammatory reactions associated with combination antiretroviral therapy in patients with AIDS and cytomegalovirus retinitis. Am J Ophthalmol 1998; 125:292–300.

130. Holland GN. Immune recovery uveitis. Ocul Immunol Inflamm 1999; 7:215–221.

131. Kuppermann BD, Holland GN. Immune recovery uveitis. Am J Ophthalmol 2000; 130:103–106.

132. Mutimer HP, Akatsuka Y, Manley T et al. Association between immune recovery uveitis and a diverse intraocular cytomegalovirus-specific cytotoxic T cell response. J Infect Dis 2002; 186:701–705.

133. Karavellas MP, Song M, Macdonald JC et al. Long-term posterior and anterior segment complications of immune recovery uveitis associated with cytomegalovirus retinitis. Am J Ophthalmol 2000; 130:57–64.

134. Nguyen QD, Kempen JH, Bolton SG et al. Immune recovery uveitis in patients with AIDS and cytomegalovirus retinitis after highly active antiretroviral therapy. Am J Ophthalmol 2000; 129:634–639.

135. Cassoux N, Lumbroso L, Bodaghi B et al. Cystoid macular oedema and cytomegalovirus retinitis in patients with HIV disease treated with highly active antiretroviral therapy. Br J Ophthalmol 1999; 83:47–49.

136. Postelmans L, Payen MC, De Wit S et al. Neovascularization of the optic disc after highly active antiretroviral therapy in an AIDS patient with cytomegalovirus retinitis – a new immune recovery-related ocular disorder? Ocul Immunol Inflamm 1999; 7:237–240.

137. Sanislo SR, Lowder CY, Kaiser PK. Optic nerve head neovascularization in a patient with inactive cytomegalovirus retinitis and immune recovery. Am J Ophthalmol 1998; 126:318–320.

138. Wright ME, Suzman DL, Csaky KG et al. Extensive retinal neovascularization as a late finding in human immunodeficiency virus-infected patients with immune recovery uveitis. Clin Infect Dis 2003; 36:1063–1066.

139. Canzano JC, Reed JB, Morse LS. Vitreomacular traction syndrome following highly active antiretroviral therapy in AIDS patients with cytomegalovirus retinitis. Retina 1998; 18:443–447.

140. Karavellas MP, Azen SP, MacDonald JC et al. Immune recovery vitritis and uveitis in AIDS: clinical predictors, sequelae, and treatment outcomes. Retina 2001; 21:1–9.

141. Goldberg DE, Freeman WR. Uveitic angle closure glaucoma in a patient with inactive cytomegalovirus retinitis and immune recovery uveitis. Ophthalmic Surg Lasers 2002; 33:421–425.

142. Karavellas MP, Plummer DJ, Macdonald JC et al. Incidence of immune recovery vitritis in cytomegalovirus retinitis patients following institution of successful highly active antiretroviral therapy. J Infect Dis 1999; 179:697–700.

143. Robinson MR, Reed G, Csaky KG et al. Immune-recovery uveitis in patients with cytomegalovirus retinitis taking highly active antiretroviral therapy. Am J Ophthalmol 2000; 130:49–56.

144. Arevalo JF, Mendoza AJ, Ferretti Y. Immune recovery uveitis in AIDS patients with cytomegalovirus retinitis treated with highly active antiretroviral therapy in Venezuela. Retina 2003; 23:495–502.

145. Song MK, Azen SP, Buley A et al. Effect of anti-cytomegalovirus therapy on the incidence of immune recovery uveitis in AIDS patients with healed cytomegalovirus retinitis. Am J Ophthalmol 2003; 136:696–702.

146. Silverstein BE, Smith JH, Sykes SO et al. Cystoid macular edema associated with cytomegalovirus retinitis in patients with the acquired immunodeficiency syndrome. Am J Ophthalmol 1998; 125:411–415.

147. Weinberg DV, Moorthy RS. Cystoid macular edema due to cytomegalovirus retinitis in a patient with acquired immune deficiency syndrome. Retina 1996; 16:343–344.

148. Conway MD, Tong P, Olk RJ. Branch retinal artery occlusion (BRAO) combined with branch retinal vein occlusion (BRVO) and optic disc neovascularization associated with HIV and CMV retinitis. Int Ophthalmol 1995–1996; 19:249–252.

149. Lee S, Ai E. Disc neovascularization in patients with AIDS and cytomegalovirus retinitis. Retina 1991; 11:305–308.

150. McCann JD, Margolis TP, Wong MG et al. A sensitive and specific polymerase chain reaction-based assay for the diagnosis of cytomegalovirus retinitis. Am J Ophthalmol 1995; 120:219–226.

151. Holland GN, Gottlieb MS, Yee RD et al. Ocular disorders associated with a new severe acquired cellular immunodeficiency syndrome. Am J Ophthalmol 1982; 93:393–402.

152. Elkins BS, Holland GN, Opremcak EM et al. Ocular toxoplasmosis misdiagnosed as cytomegalovirus retinopathy in immunocompromised patients. Ophthalmology 1994; 101:499–507.

153. Gagliuso DJ, Teich SA, Friedman AH et al. Ocular toxoplasmosis in AIDS patients. Trans Am Ophthalmol Soc 1990; 88:63–86.

154. Cunningham ET, Jr., Short GA, Irvine AR et al. Acquired immunodeficiency syndrome – associated herpes simplex virus retinitis. Clinical description and use of a polymerase chain reaction-based assay as a diagnostic tool. Arch Ophthalmol 1996; 114:834–840.

155. Engstrom RE, Jr., Holland GN, Margolis TP et al. The progressive outer retinal necrosis syndrome. A variant of necrotizing herpetic retinopathy in patients with AIDS. Ophthalmology 1994; 101:1488–1502.

156. Holland GN. Standard diagnostic criteria for the acute retinal necrosis syndrome. Executive Committee of the American Uveitis Society. Am J Ophthalmol 1994; 117:663–667.

157. Jabs DA, Newman C, De Bustros S et al. Treatment of cytomegalovirus retinitis with ganciclovir. Ophthalmology 1987; 94:824–830.

158. Holland GN, Sidikaro Y, Kreiger AE et al. Treatment of cytomegalovirus retinopathy with ganciclovir. Ophthalmology 1987; 94:815–823.

159. Jacobson MA, O'Donnell JJ, Brodie HR et al. Randomized prospective trial of ganciclovir maintenance therapy for cytomegalovirus retinitis. J Med Virol 1988; 25:339–349.

160. Jacobson MA, O'Donnell JJ, Mills J. Foscarnet treatment of cytomegalovirus retinitis in patients with the acquired immunodeficiency syndrome. Antimicrob Agents Chemother 1989; 33:736–741.

161. Palestine AG, Polis MA, De Smet MD et al. A randomized, controlled trial of foscarnet in the treatment of cytomegalovirus retinitis in patients with AIDS. Ann Intern Med 1991; 115:665–673.

162. Drew WL, Ives D, Lalezari JP et al. Oral ganciclovir as maintenance treatment for cytomegalovirus retinitis in patients with AIDS. Syntex Cooperative Oral Ganciclovir Study Group. N Engl J Med 1995; 333:615–620.

163. Danner SA, Matheron S. Cytomegalovirus retinitis in AIDS patients: a comparative study of intravenous and oral ganciclovir as maintenance therapy. AIDS 1996; 10 Suppl 4:S7–11.

164. Squires KE. Oral ganciclovir for cytomegalovirus retinitis in patients with AIDS: results of two randomized studies. AIDS 1996; 10 Suppl 4:S13–18.

165. Lalezari JP, Stagg RJ, Kuppermann BD et al. Intravenous cidofovir for peripheral cytomegalovirus retinitis in patients with AIDS. A randomized, controlled trial. Ann Intern Med 1997; 126:257–263.

166. Studies of Ocular Complications of AIDS (SOCA) Research Group in collaboration with the AIDS Clinical Trials Group (ACTG). Cytomegalovirus (CMV) culture results, drug resistance, and clinical outcome in patients with AIDS and CMV retinitis treated with foscarnet or ganciclovir. J Infect Dis 1997; 176:50–58.

167. Studies of Ocular Complications of AIDS Research Group in collaboration with the AIDS Clinical Trials Group. Parenteral cidofovir for cytomegalovirus retinitis in patients with AIDS: the HPMPC peripheral cytomegalovirus retinitis trial. A randomized, controlled trial. Ann Intern Med 1997; 126:264–274.

168. Studies of Ocular Complications of AIDS Research Group in collaboration with the AIDS Clinical Trials Group. Combination foscarnet and ganciclovir therapy vs monotherapy for the treatment of relapsed cytomegalovirus retinitis in patients with AIDS. The Cytomegalovirus Retreatment Trial. Arch Ophthalmol 1996; 114:23–33.

169. Studies of Ocular Complications of AIDS Research Group in collaboration with the AIDS Clinical Trials Group. Foscarnet–Ganciclovir Cytomegalovirus Retinitis Trial. 4. Visual outcomes. Ophthalmology 1994; 101:1250–1261.

170. The Oral Ganciclovir European and Australian Cooperative Study Group. Intravenous versus oral ganciclovir: European/Australian comparative study of efficacy and safety in the prevention of cytomegalovirus retinitis recurrence in patients with AIDS. AIDS 1995; 9:471–477.

171. The Vitravene Study Group. A randomized controlled clinical trial of intravitreous fomivirsen for treatment of newly diagnosed peripheral cytomegalovirus retinitis in patients with AIDS. Am J Ophthalmol 2002; 133:467–474.

172. The Vitravene Study Group. Randomized dose-comparison studies of intravitreous fomivirsen for treatment of cytomegalovirus retinitis that has reactivated or is persistently active despite other therapies in patients with AIDS. Am J Ophthalmol 2002; 133:475–483.

173. The Vitravene Study Group. Safety of intravitreous fomivirsen for treatment of cytomegalovirus retinitis in patients with AIDS. Am J Ophthalmol 2002; 133:484–498.

174. Holland GN, Tufail A. New therapies for cytomegalovirus retinitis. N Engl J Med 1995; 333:658–659.

175. Martin DF, Sierra-Madero J, Walmsley S et al. A controlled trial of valganciclovir as induction therapy for cytomegalovirus retinitis. N Engl J Med 2002; 346:1119–1126.

176. Lalezari J, Lindley J, Walmsley S et al. A safety study of oral valganciclovir maintenance treatment of cytomegalovirus retinitis. J Acquir Immune Defic Syndr 2002; 30:392–400.

177. Hochster H, Dieterich D, Bozzette S et al. Toxicity of combined ganciclovir and zidovudine for cytomegalovirus disease associated with AIDS. An AIDS Clinical Trials Group Study. Ann Intern Med 1990; 113: 111–117.

178. Tufail A, Weisz JM, Holland GN. Endogenous bacterial endophthalmitis as a complication of intravenous therapy for cytomegalovirus retinopathy. Arch Ophthalmol 1996; 114:879–880.

179. Devianne-Garrigue I, Pellegrin I, Denisi R et al. Foscarnet decreases HIV-1 plasma load. J Acquir Immune Defic Syndr Hum Retrovirol 1998; 18:46–50.

180. Studies of Ocular Complications of AIDS Research Group in collaboration with the AIDS Clinical Trials Group. Morbidity and toxic effects associated with ganciclovir or foscarnet therapy in a randomized cytomegalovirus retinitis trial. Arch Intern Med 1995; 155:65–74.

181. Ho HT, Woods KL, Bronson JJ et al. Intracellular metabolism of the antiherpes agent (S)-1-[3-hydroxy-2-(phosphonylmethoxy)propyl]cytosine. Mol Pharmacol 1992; 41:197–202.

182. Jacobson MA. Treatment of cytomegalovirus retinitis in patients with the acquired immunodeficiency syndrome. N Engl J Med 1997; 337:105–114.

183. Littler E, Stuart AD, Chee MS. Human cytomegalovirus UL97 open reading frame encodes a protein that phosphorylates the antiviral nucleoside analogue ganciclovir. Nature 1992; 358:160–162.

184. Sullivan V, Talarico CL, Stanat SC et al. A protein kinase homologue controls phosphorylation of ganciclovir in human cytomegalovirus-infected cells. Nature 1992; 358:162–164.

185. Studies of Ocular Complications of AIDS Research Group in collaboration with the AIDS Clinical Trials Group. The ganciclovir implant plus oral ganciclovir versus parenteral cidofovir for the treatment of cytomegalovirus retinitis in patients with acquired immunodeficiency syndrome: The Ganciclovir Cidofovir Cytomegalovirus Retinitis Trial. Am J Ophthalmol 2001; 131:457–467.

186. Davis JL, Taskintuna I, Freeman WR et al. Iritis and hypotony after treatment with intravenous cidofovir for cytomegalovirus retinitis. Arch Ophthalmol 1997; 115:733–737.

187. Akler ME, Johnson DW, Burman WJ et al. Anterior uveitis and hypotony after intravenous cidofovir for the treatment of cytomegalovirus retinitis. Ophthalmology 1998; 105:651–657.

188. Azad RF, Brown-Driver V, Buckheit RW Jr et al. Antiviral activity of a phosphorothioate oligonucleotide complementary to human cytomegalovirus RNA when used in combination with antiviral nucleoside analogs. Antiviral Res 1995; 28:101–111.

189. Azad RF, Driver VB, Tanaka K et al. Antiviral activity of a phosphorothioate oligonucleotide complementary to RNA of the human cytomegalovirus major immediate-early region. Antimicrob Agents Chemother 1993; 37:1945–1954.

190. Anderson KP, Fox MC, Brown-Driver V et al. Inhibition of human cytomegalovirus immediate-early gene expression by an antisense oligonucleotide complementary to immediate-early RNA. Antimicrob Agents Chemother 1996; 40:2004–2011.

191. Chou S, Erice A, Jordan MC et al. Analysis of the UL97 phosphotransferase coding sequence in clinical cytomegalovirus isolates and identification of mutations conferring ganciclovir resistance. J Infect Dis 1995; 171:576–583.

192. Wolf DG, Smith IL, Lee DJ et al. Mutations in human cytomegalovirus UL97 gene confer clinical resistance to ganciclovir and can be detected directly in patient plasma. J Clin Invest 1995; 95:257–263.

193. Chou S, Guentzel S, Michels KR et al. Frequency of UL97 phosphotransferase mutations related to ganciclovir resistance in clinical cytomegalovirus isolates. J Infect Dis 1995; 172:239–242.

194. Baldanti F, Underwood MR, Stanat SC et al. Single amino acid changes in the DNA polymerase confer foscarnet resistance and slow-growth phenotype, while mutations in the UL97-encoded phosphotransferase confer ganciclovir resistance in three double-resistant human cytomegalovirus strains recovered from patients with AIDS. J Virol 1996; 70:1390–1395.

195. Erice A. Resistance of human cytomegalovirus to antiviral drugs. Clin Microbiol Rev 1999; 12:286–297.

196. Liu W, Kuppermann BD, Martin DF et al. Mutations in the cytomegalovirus UL97 gene associated with ganciclovir-resistant retinitis. J Infect Dis 1998; 177:1176–1181.

197. Smith IL, Cherrington JM, Jiles RE et al. High-level resistance of cytomegalovirus to ganciclovir is associated with alterations in both the UL97 and DNA polymerase genes. J Infect Dis 1997; 176:69–77.

198. Drew WL, Miner RC, Busch DF et al. Prevalence of resistance in patients receiving ganciclovir for serious cytomegalovirus infection. J Infect Dis 1991; 163:716–719.

199. Jabs DA, Enger C, Dunn JP et al. Cytomegalovirus retinitis and viral resistance: ganciclovir resistance. CMV Retinitis and Viral Resistance Study Group. J Infect Dis 1998; 177:770–773.

200. Jabs DA, Enger C, Forman M et al. Incidence of foscarnet resistance and cidofovir resistance in patients treated for cytomegalovirus retinitis. The Cytomegalovirus Retinitis and Viral Resistance Study Group. Antimicrob Agents Chemother 1998; 42:2240–2244.

201. Weinberg A, Jabs DA, Chou S et al. Mutations conferring foscarnet resistance in a cohort of patients with acquired immunodeficiency syndrome and cytomegalovirus retinitis. J Infect Dis 2003; 187:777–784.

202. Hu H, Jabs DA, Forman MS et al. Comparison of cytomegalovirus (CMV) UL97 gene sequences in the blood and vitreous of patients with acquired immunodeficiency syndrome and CMV retinitis. J Infect Dis 2002; 185:861–867.

203. Kuo IC, Imai Y, Shum C et al. Genotypic analysis of cytomegalovirus retinitis poorly responsive to intravenous ganciclovir but responsive to the ganciclovir implant. Am J Ophthalmol 2003; 135:20–25.

204. Dunn JP, MacCumber MW, Forman MS et al. Viral sensitivity testing in patients with cytomegalovirus retinitis clinically resistant to foscarnet or ganciclovir. Am J Ophthalmol 1995; 119:587–596.

205. Jabs DA, Martin BK, Forman MS et al. Longitudinal observations on mutations conferring ganciclovir resistance in patients with acquired immunodeficiency syndrome and cytomegalovirus retinitis: The Cytomegalovirus and Viral Resistance Study Group Report Number 8. Am J Ophthalmol 2001; 132:700–710.

206. Jabs DA, Martin BK, Forman MS et al. Cytomegalovirus resistance to ganciclovir and clinical outcomes of patients with cytomegalovirus retinitis. Am J Ophthalmol 2003; 135:26–34.

207. Engstrom RE Jr, Holland GN. Local therapy for cytomegalovirus retinopathy. Am J Ophthalmol 1995; 120:376–385.

208. Young S, Morlet N, Besen G et al. High-dose (2000-microgram) intravitreous ganciclovir in the treatment of cytomegalovirus retinitis. Ophthalmology 1998; 105:1404–1410.

209. Diaz-Llopis M, Espana E, Munoz G et al. High dose intravitreal foscarnet in the treatment of cytomegalovirus retinitis in AIDS. Br J Ophthalmol 1994; 78:120–124.

210. Ussery FM, Gibson SR, Conklin RH et al. Intravitreal ganciclovir in the treatment of AIDS-associated cytomegalovirus retinitis. Ophthalmology 1988; 95:640–648.

211. Cantrill HL, Henry K, Melroe NH et al. Treatment of cytomegalovirus retinitis with intravitreal ganciclovir. Long-term results. Ophthalmology 1989; 96:367–374.

212. Cochereau-Massin I, Lehoang P, Lautier-Frau M et al. Efficacy and tolerance of intravitreal ganciclovir in cytomegalovirus retinitis in acquired immune deficiency syndrome. Ophthalmology 1991; 98:1348–1353.

213. Henry K, Cantrill HL, Fletcher C et al. Use of intravitreal ganciclovir (dihydroxy propoxymethyl guanine) for cytomegalovirus retinitis in a patient with AIDS. Am J Ophthalmol 1987; 103:17–23.

214. Buchi ER, Fitting PL, Michel AE. Long-term intravitreal ganciclovir for cytomegalovirus retinitis in a patient with AIDS. Case report. Arch Ophthalmol 1988; 106:1349–1350.

215. Heinemann MH. *Staphylococcus epidermidis* endophthalmitis complicating intravitreal antiviral therapy of cytomegalovirus retinitis. Case report. Arch Ophthalmol 1989; 107:643–644.

216. Desatnik HR, Foster RE, Lowder CY. Treatment of clinically resistant cytomegalovirus retinitis with combined intravitreal injections of ganciclovir and foscarnet. Am J Ophthalmol 1996; 122:121–123.

217. Diaz-Llopis M, Chipont E, Sanchez S et al. Intravitreal foscarnet for cytomegalovirus retinitis in a patient with acquired immunodeficiency syndrome. Am J Ophthalmol 1992; 114:742–747.

218. Velez G, Roy CE, Whitcup SM et al. High-dose intravitreal ganciclovir and foscarnet for cytomegalovirus retinitis. Am J Ophthalmol 2001; 131:396–397.

219. Hodge WG, Lalonde RG, Sampalis J et al. Once-weekly intraocular injections of ganciclovir for maintenance therapy of cytomegalovirus retinitis: clinical and ocular outcome. J Infect Dis 1996; 174:393–396.

220. Yoshizumi MO, Lee D, Vinci V et al. Ocular toxicity of multiple intravitreal DHPG injections. Graefes Arch Clin Exp Ophthalmol 1990; 228: 350–355.

221. Saran BR, Maguire AM. Retinal toxicity of high dose intravitreal ganciclovir. Retina 1994; 14:248–252.

222. Kirsch LS, Arevalo JF, De Clercq E et al. Phase I/II study of intravitreal cidofovir for the treatment of cytomegalovirus retinitis in patients with the acquired immunodeficiency syndrome. Am J Ophthalmol 1995; 119: 466–476.

223. Kirsch LS, Arevalo JF, Chavez de la Paz E et al. Intravitreal cidofovir

(HPMPC) treatment of cytomegalovirus retinitis in patients with acquired immune deficiency syndrome. Ophthalmology 1995; 102:533–542.

224. Rahhal FM, Arevalo JF, Munguia D et al. Intravitreal cidofovir for the maintenance treatment of cytomegalovirus retinitis. Ophthalmology 1996; 103:1073–1083.

225. Chavez-de la Paz E, Arevalo JF, Kirsch LS et al. Anterior nongranulomatous uveitis after intravitreal HPMPC (cidofovir) for the treatment of cytomegalovirus retinitis. Analysis and prevention. Ophthalmology 1997; 104:539–544.

226. Taskintuna I, Rahhal FM, Arevalo JF et al. Low-dose intravitreal cidofovir (HPMPC) therapy of cytomegalovirus retinitis in patients with acquired immune deficiency syndrome. Ophthalmology 1997; 104: 1049–1057.

227. Banker AS, Arevalo JF, Munguia D et al. Intraocular pressure and aqueous humor dynamics in patients with AIDS treated with intravitreal cidofovir (HPMPC) for cytomegalovirus retinitis. Am J Ophthalmol 1997; 124: 168–180.

228. Martin DF, Parks DJ, Mellow SD et al. Treatment of cytomegalovirus retinitis with an intraocular sustained-release ganciclovir implant. A randomized controlled clinical trial. Arch Ophthalmol 1994; 112:1531–1539.

229. Sanborn GE, Anand R, Torti RE et al. Sustained-release ganciclovir therapy for treatment of cytomegalovirus retinitis. Use of an intravitreal device. Arch Ophthalmol 1992; 110:188–195.

230. Marx JL, Kapusta MA, Patel SS et al. Use of the ganciclovir implant in the treatment of recurrent cytomegalovirus retinitis. Arch Ophthalmol 1996; 114:815–820.

231. Musch DC, Martin DF, Gordon JF et al. Treatment of cytomegalovirus retinitis with a sustained-release ganciclovir implant. The Ganciclovir Implant Study Group. N Engl J Med 1997; 337:83–90.

232. Kuppermann BD, Quiceno JI, Flores-Aguilar M et al. Intravitreal ganciclovir concentration after intravenous administration in AIDS patients with cytomegalovirus retinitis: implications for therapy. J Infect Dis 1993; 168:1506–1509.

233. Martin DF, Ferris FL, Parks DJ et al. Ganciclovir implant exchange. Timing, surgical procedure, and complications. Arch Ophthalmol 1997; 115:1389–1394.

234. Morley MG, Duker JS, Ashton P et al. Replacing ganciclovir implants. Ophthalmology 1995; 102:388–392.

235. Martin DF, Kuppermann BD, Wolitz RA et al. Oral ganciclovir for patients with cytomegalovirus retinitis treated with a ganciclovir implant. Roche Ganciclovir Study Group. N Engl J Med 1999; 340:1063–1070.

236. Roth DB, Feuer WJ, Blenke AJ et al. Treatment of recurrent cytomegalovirus retinitis with the ganciclovir implant. Am J Ophthalmol 1999; 127:276–282.

237. Shane TS, Martin DF. Endophthalmitis after ganciclovir implant in patients with AIDS and cytomegalovirus retinitis. Am J Ophthalmol 2003; 136: 649–654.

238. Martin DF, Dunn JP, Davis JL et al. Use of the ganciclovir implant for the treatment of cytomegalovirus retinitis in the era of potent antiretroviral therapy: recommendations of the International AIDS Society – USA panel. Am J Ophthalmol 1999; 127:329–339.

239. Kempen JH, Jabs DA, Dunn JP et al. Retinal detachment risk in cytomegalovirus retinitis related to the acquired immunodeficiency syndrome. Arch Ophthalmol 2001; 119:33–40.

240. Keefe KS, Freeman WR, Peterson TJ et al. Atypical healing of cytomegalovirus retinitis. Significance of persistent border opacification. Ophthalmology 1992; 99:1377–1384.

241. Whitley RJ, Jacobson MA, Friedberg DN et al. Guidelines for the treatment of cytomegalovirus diseases in patients with AIDS in the era of potent antiretroviral therapy: recommendations of an international panel. International AIDS Society – USA. Arch Intern Med 1998; 158:957–969.

242. Holland GN, Levinson RD, Jacobson MA. Dose-related difference in progression rates of cytomegalovirus retinopathy during foscarnet maintenance therapy. AIDS Clinical Trials Group Protocol 915 Team. Am J Ophthalmol 1995; 119:576–586.

243. Freitas VR, Fraser-Smith EB, Matthews TR. Increased efficacy of ganciclovir in combination with foscarnet against cytomegalovirus and herpes simplex virus type 2 in vitro and in vivo. Antiviral Res 1989; 12:205–212.

244. Manischewitz JF, Quinnan GV Jr, Lane HC et al. Synergistic effect of ganciclovir and foscarnet on cytomegalovirus replication in vitro. Antimicrob Agents Chemother 1990; 34:373–375.

245. Kuppermann BD, Flores-Aguilar M, Quiceno JI et al. Combination ganciclovir and foscarnet in the treatment of clinically resistant cytomegalovirus retinitis in patients with acquired immunodeficiency syndrome. Arch Ophthalmol 1993; 111:1359–1366.

246. Weinberg DV, Murphy R, Naughton K. Combined daily therapy with intravenous ganciclovir and foscarnet for patients with recurrent cytomegalovirus retinitis. Am J Ophthalmol 1994; 117:776–782.

247. McGuire DE, McAulife P, Heinemann MH et al. Efficacy of the ganciclovir implant in the setting of silicone oil vitreous substitute. Retina 2000; 20:520–523.

248. Hegazy HM, Kivilcim M, Peyman GA et al. Evaluation of toxicity of intravitreal ceftazidime, vancomycin, and ganciclovir in a silicone oil-filled eye. Retina 1999; 19:553–557.

249. Vrabec TR, Baldassano VF, Whitcup SM. Discontinuation of maintenance therapy in patients with quiescent cytomegalovirus retinitis and elevated CD4+ counts. Ophthalmology 1998; 105:1259–1264.

250. Jabs DA, Bolton SG, Dunn JP et al. Discontinuing anticytomegalovirus therapy in patients with immune reconstitution after combination antiretroviral therapy. Am J Ophthalmol 1998; 126:817–822.

251. Macdonald JC, Torriani FJ, Morse LS et al. Lack of reactivation of cytomegalovirus (CMV) retinitis after stopping CMV maintenance therapy in AIDS patients with sustained elevations in CD4 T cells in response to highly active antiretroviral therapy. J Infect Dis 1998; 177:1182–1187.

252. Whitcup SM, Fortin E, Lindblad AS et al. Discontinuation of anticytomegalovirus therapy in patients with HIV infection and cytomegalovirus retinitis. JAMA 1999; 282:1633–1637.

253. Curi AL, Muralha A, Muralha L et al. Suspension of anticytomegalovirus maintenance therapy following immune recovery due to highly active antiretroviral therapy. Br J Ophthalmol 2001; 85:471–473.

254. Tural C, Romeu J, Sirera G et al. Long-lasting remission of cytomegalovirus retinitis without maintenance therapy in human immunodeficiency virus-infected patients. J Infect Dis 1998; 177:1080–1083.

255. Postelmans L, Gerard M, Sommereijns B et al. Discontinuation of maintenance therapy for CMV retinitis in AIDS patients on highly active antiretroviral therapy. Ocul Immunol Inflamm 1999; 7:199–203.

256. Holland GN. Discussion of Macdonald JC, Karavellas MP, Torriani FJ et al. Highly active antiretroviral therapy-related immune recovery in AIDS patients with cytomegalovirus retinitis. Ophthalmology 2000; 107:877–883.

256a. Jabs DA, Van Natta ML, Thorne JE et al. Course of cytomegalovirus retinitis in the era of highly active antiretroviral therapy: 1. Retinitis progression. Ophthalmology 2004; 111:2224–2231.

257. Jabs DA, Van Natta ML, Kempen JH et al. Characteristics of patients with cytomegalovirus retinitis in the era of highly active antiretroviral therapy. Am J Ophthalmol 2002; 133:48–61.

258. Lin DY, Warren JF, Lazzeroni LC et al. Cytomegalovirus retinitis after initiation of highly active antiretroviral therapy in HIV infected patients: natural history and clinical predictors. Retina 2002; 22:268–277.

259. Johnson SC, Benson CA, Johnson DW et al. Recurrences of cytomegalovirus retinitis in a human immunodeficiency virus-infected patient, despite potent antiretroviral therapy and apparent immune reconstitution. Clin Infect Dis 2001; 32:815–819.

259a. Jabs DA, Van Natta ML, Thorne JE et al. Course of cytomegalovirus retinitis in the era of highly active antiretroviral therapy: 2. Second eye involvement and retinal detachment. Ophthalmology 2004; 111:2232–2239.

260. Palestine AG, Stevens G Jr, Lane HC et al. Treatment of cytomegalovirus retinitis with dihydroxy propoxymethyl guanine. Am J Ophthalmol 1986; 101:95–101.

261. Kimberlin DW, Lin CY, Sanchez PJ et al. Effect of ganciclovir therapy on hearing in symptomatic congenital cytomegalovirus disease involving the central nervous system: a randomized, controlled trial. J Pediatr 2003; 143:16–25.

262. Demmler GJ. Congenital cytomegalovirus infection treatment. Pediatr Infect Dis J 2003; 22:1005–1006.

263. Baumal CR, Levin AV, Read SE. Cytomegalovirus retinitis in immunosuppressed children. Am J Ophthalmol 1999; 127:550–558.

264. Walton RC, Whitcup SM, Mueller BU et al. Combined intravenous ganciclovir and foscarnet for children with recurrent cytomegalovirus retinitis. Ophthalmology 1995; 102:1865–1870.

265. Malley DS, Barone R, Heinemann MH. Treatment of bilateral cytomegalovirus retinitis with sustained-release ganciclovir implants in a child. Am J Ophthalmol 1996; 122:731–732.

266. Rosecan LR, Laskin OL, Kalman CM et al. Antiviral therapy with ganciclovir for cytomegalovirus retinitis and bilateral exudative retinal detachments in an immunocompromised child. Ophthalmology 1986; 93: 1401–1407.

267. Feinberg JE, Hurwitz S, Cooper D et al. A randomized, double-blind trial of valaciclovir prophylaxis for cytomegalovirus disease in patients with advanced human immunodeficiency virus infection. AIDS Clinical Trials Group Protocol 204/Glaxo Wellcome 123-014 International CMV Prophylaxis Study Group. J Infect Dis 1998; 177:48–56.

Chapter

92

Retinal Disease in HIV-infected Patients

Brian R. Kosobucki
William R. Freeman

Acquired immunodeficiency syndrome (AIDS) is a potentially fatal multisystem syndrome characterized by profound disruption of the immune system and a propensity for various opportunistic infections and neoplasms. It is characterized by the presence of opportunistic infections and specific neoplasms in persons infected with the human immunodeficiency virus (HIV), a retrovirus.[1-3] There is evidence that HIV existed in the United States in 1968[4] and in central Africa, albeit rarely, as long ago as 1959.[5]

Ocular involvement occurs in up to 73% of AIDS patients,[6,7] with the most common lesions being a retinal vasculopathy consisting of cotton-wool spots, retinal hemorrhages, and infectious retinopathy such as cytomegalovirus (CMV), herpetic, toxoplasmic, or luetic retinitis. Nonretinal lesions such as Kaposi's sarcoma of the conjunctiva are frequently seen as well.

EPIDEMIOLOGY OF HIV INFECTION AND AIDS

Through December 2002, a total of 886 575 persons with AIDS in the United States were reported to The Centers for Disease Control and Prevention (CDC); 57% of these persons (501 669 persons) have died. In 1996 the estimated number of persons diagnosed with an AIDS-defining opportunistic infection decreased for the first time since the HIV pandemic began in 1981, partly because of the use of highly active antiretroviral therapy (HAART). Improved survival and decreased morbidity of persons infected with HIV and treated with antiretroviral therapy have been repeatedly demonstrated.[8-10] As of December 2002, men who have sex with men or bisexuals accounted for 45% of cases of AIDS among adults and adolescents; injection drug users for 25%; men who have sex with men or bisexuals *and* injection drug use 6%, and 1% among recipients of blood transfusion, blood components, or tissue from HIV-infected donors. HIV also is spread heterosexually (approximately 12% of cases), both from female to male, and from male to female, the latter more efficiently.[8,11]

Through December 2001, 57 health care workers in the United States who have seroconverted after occupational exposure to HIV have been documented: 49 involved exposures to blood; one to visible bloody fluid; three to concentrated virus in the laboratory; and four to an unspecified fluid. An additional 137 health care workers, including six surgeons, have had pos-

sible occupational transmission of HIV infection.[12] The average risk of HIV transmission after percutaneous exposure to HIV-infected blood is approximately 0.3%.[13] The risk is lowered by double-gloving and is probably much lower in the ophthalmic setting, where needle-sticks from hollow needles filled with blood are less common.[14] There is also evidence that postexposure prophylaxis with antiretroviral therapy may be effective in preventing the transmission of HIV even after accidental needle-stick injury.[15] Institution of such treatment should begin as soon as possible after injury. To facilitate this, most health care institutions keep a starter package of these medications available in the operating room.

Currently, for percutaneous injuries, the U.S. Public Health Service recommends 4-week treatment with a basic 2-drug regimen if the exposure is less severe (solid needle and superficial injury) and the source patient has asymptomatic HIV infection or known low viral load (<1500 RNA copies/ml) [Class I patient]; an expanded 3-drug regimen is recommended if the exposure is severe (large-bore hollow needle, deep puncture, visible blood on device, or needle used in patient's artery or vein) or if the source patient has symptomatic HIV infection, AIDS, acute seroconversion, or known high viral load [Class II patient]. The basic 2-drug regimen includes zidovudine (AZT) 600 mg/day in two or three divided doses plus lamivudine (Epivir; 3TC) 150 mg twice a day. These drugs are also available as Combivir, which can be taken as one tablet twice a day. If resistance to AZT or 3TC is a concern, alternate basic regimens of lamivudine plus stavudine (Zerit; d4T) 40 mg twice a day or didanosine (Videx; ddI) 400 mg daily plus stavudine are recommended. The expanded 3-drug regimen adds either a protease inhibitor (PI) such as indinavir (Crixivan) 800 mg three times a day or nelfinavir (Viracept) 750 mg three times a day or 1250 mg twice a day or if PI resistance is a concern, efavirenz (Sustiva) 600 mg daily at bedtime or abacavir (Ziagen; ABC) 300 mg twice a day; Trizivir is a combination of ZDV, 3TC, and ABC that can be taken one tablet twice a day. Other drugs can be considered in the expanded regimen in consultation with an infectious disease specialist if other drug-resistance concerns exist. For mucous membrane or nonintact skin exposures, the basic 2-drug regimen is recommended for all small volume exposures (a few drops) and large volume (major blood splash) exposure in a Class I patient, with the

3-drug expanded regimen recommended for large volume exposure in a Class II patient. [13]

HIV VIROLOGY AND PATHOGENESIS

AIDS and the spectrum of HIV disease are caused by the human immunodeficiency virus (HIV) (formerly known as human T-cell lymphotrophic virus III [HTLV-III], lymphadenopathy-associated virus [LAV], and AIDS-related virus [ARV]).[16,17] HIV infection may damage or kill the CD4[+] lymphocyte, resulting in a reversal of the helper-to-suppressor T cell ratio.[18] The CD4[+]-to-CD8[+] ratio is about 1.0 to 2.0 in healthy people; AIDS patients typically have ratios well under 1.0. The reversal of the helper-to-suppressor T-cell ratio results in a cell-mediated immunoincompetence that predisposes to the occurrence of infection by select opportunistic pathogens and the development of characteristic neoplasms.

Our understanding of HIV infection has undergone immense changes in the mid-1990s. The concept of viral latency has been dispelled, with all stages of HIV infection characterized by a high rate of viral replication, including mutations in the HIV genome resulting in the emergence of viral variants. In the presence of selective pressure from antiretroviral agents, mutations that confer a decreased sensitivity to individual drugs are rapidly selected.[19–22] Changes in plasma HIV-1 RNA have been shown to predict the clinical progression of HIV-related disease.[23–29] The complex immunopathogenic mechanisms of HIV infection have been further elucidated.[18] Treatment also has evolved with the development of potent agents that target the protease enzyme in HIV,[30] especially with a three-drug combination that includes a protease inhibitor and two nucleoside analogs (HAART)[31,32]; this type of therapy has been designed to delay or prevent the emergence of drug resistance by minimizing viral replication. However, HIV may develop resistance to current therapies despite HAART in >75% of patients.[33] In addition, enfuvirtide (T-20), the first of a class of drugs that block the entry of the HIV virus into the host cell (fusion inhibitors) has been recently introduced.[34]

The clinical spectrum of HIV infection and disease is variable and includes asymptomatic persons, persons with various constitutional signs and symptoms, and AIDS. The "acute retroviral syndrome," or primary infection with HIV (the period of seroconversion), may be characterized by fever, pharyngitis, skin rash, arthralgias, malaise, mucosal ulcerations, and neurologic manifestations such as aseptic meningitis.[35] Patients infected with HIV also may present with a prodrome of generalized lymphadenopathy, fevers, night sweats, weight loss, and diarrhea of weeks' or months' duration and was formerly termed *AIDS-related complex* (ARC). It is currently believed that virtually all HIV-seropositive patients will progress to AIDS. Although highly active antiretroviral therapy often reduces plasma viremia of HIV-1 to undetectable levels, latent viral reservoirs of resting CD4[+] lymphocytes persist for years; Chun et al.[36] found integrated and unintegrated viral DNA in resting CD4[+] cells that was capable of producing infectious virus in patients receiving HAART. Wong et al.[37] found little sign of evolving resistance to

the antiretrovirals in these resting CD4[+] lymphocytes. Therefore, with the advent of HAART, long-term control of HIV infection may be possible.

Immune system abnormalities may lead to opportunistic infections and malignant tumor formation in AIDS patients. Opportunistic infections are responsible for the deaths of most AIDS patients. CMV, *Candida albicans*, *Pneumocystis carinii*, *Mycobacterium avium-intracellulare*, *Cryptococcus neoformans*, herpes simplex virus (HSV), *Cryptosporidium* spp., *Toxoplasma gondii*, and varicella-zoster virus (VZV) are among the most common pathogens encountered in AIDS.[3,38] CMV retinitis often is the initial sign of tissue-invasive systemic CMV infection in these patients.[39] Kaposi's sarcoma and non-Hodgkin's lymphoma are the two most common neoplasms seen in AIDS patients.

Precautions to be used in patient examination and treatment

In 1988 the CDC recommended universal precautions to prevent the occupational transmission of HIV and other bloodborne viruses in the health care setting.[40] Barrier precautions to prevent parenteral and mucocutaneous exposure to blood and other infectious body substances are essential. Water-impermeable footwear, a water-impermeable urology apron worn underneath a sterile surgical gown, an extra set of sterile sleeves, double latex gloves, and protective eyewear are effective methods of reducing the intraoperative exposure to blood.[41] Extra care must be exercised to avoid injury by needles or other sharp objects, that gloves be worn when handling any material infected or potentially infected with HIV, that gowns and protective eyewear are indicated if the possibility exists of spilling infected material, that contaminated articles be disposed of properly, and that good hand washing technique is essential after examination or before leaving patients' rooms.[40]

The CDC has given specific guidelines for ophthalmologic examinations in addition to the general recommendations given above. The use of gloves (especially if the skin of the examiner is compromised in any way) and good hand washing technique after procedures or examinations involving the eye are recommended because HIV may be present in tears. Sterilization of all instruments and equipment that come into contact with the eye in all patients is necessary using gas or steam autoclaving or a 5- to 10-minute soak in one of the following solutions: 3% hydrogen peroxide solution, 10% solution of sodium hypochlorite (common household bleach), or 70% ethanol or isopropanol. Instruments disinfected in this manner should be rinsed in water and dried before reuse.[42,43] Damage to tonometer tips has been reported with the use of 70% isopropanol; thus a 5- to 10-minute soak in 3% H_2O_2 or 1:10 dilution of household bleach may be preferable.[44] A MacKay–Marg tonometer with a disposable sleeve also may be used to check intraocular pressure.[43] It should be noted that there is no evidence of HIV transmission through contact with tears or instruments used to examine these patients.[42]

Contact lenses used in trial fittings on all patients should be disinfected by use of any commercially available cleaning method or solution (including heat disinfection, 3% H_2O_2, Boston cleaner or conditioner, Pliagel, Miraflow, and Softmate).[45] Inactivation of HIV by various disinfectants on surfaces has been reviewed.[46] Recommendations for prevention of HIV transmission in health care settings also have been published.[40,47] Guidelines for preventing transmission of HIV through transplantation of human tissue and organs (including corneal transplants) have been set forth.[48] Specific recommendations for postexposure management of needle-stick injuries or mucosal membrane exposures to secretions from patients with HIV infection have been published[49] and include the empiric use of three antiretroviral agents (see above).

OCULAR FINDINGS IN AIDS – AN OVERVIEW

HIV has been detected in the cornea,[50] conjunctival epithelium,[51] and in tears[52] but at very low titers. It is noteworthy that lymphocytes and macrophages are the cells most susceptible to HIV infection. The contribution of these cells to the detection of HIV in the retina is controversial, but there is no conclusive evidence that an HIV retinitis exists.[53]

Ocular manifestations of AIDS may be seen in up to 100% of patients. They are less common, but may be seen in patients with earlier, symptomatic HIV infection.[54] Most common are cotton-wool spots and other noninfectious retinopathies,[55] CMV retinitis, and conjunctival Kaposi's sarcoma, followed less frequently by herpes zoster ophthalmicus,[56,56A] retinal toxoplasmosis, choroidal *Pneumocystis carinii* infection, herpes simplex and herpes zoster retinitis (acute retinal necrosis [ARN]), and cryptococcal choroiditis.[6,57-65]

Iritis may occur in association with viral retinitis but especially with CMV; it is mild. Acute iritis may be associated with the use of oral rifabutin (used for the treatment and prophylaxis of mycobacterial infections)[66,67] or intravenous cidofovir used for CMV retinitis.

Choroidal infection with *Cryptococcus*, *Pneumocystis*, *M. tuberculosis*, *Aspergillus*, toxoplasmosis, histoplasmosis, and *M. avium-intracellulare* usually is associated with systemic infection.[68] *Histoplasma capsulatum* chorioretinitis and endophthalmitis,[69] paracoccidioidomycosis brasiliensis chorioretinitis,[70] keratitis sicca, cranial nerve paralysis, Roth's spots, papilledema,

perivasculitis, and fungal corneal ulcers are rare but have been reported.[71] Not all of these entities are clinically significant or even clinically apparent.[56,62,63,65,72,73]

It is of interest that *Toxoplasma* retinitis is relatively uncommon, and *Candida* retinitis is extremely rare in these patients despite the frequent occurrence of systemic toxoplasmosis (especially seen in the central nervous system) or mucosal infection (with *C. albicans*); invasive candidal infections occur only in the presence of other risk factors (e.g. injectable drug use, neutropenia, or the presence of central venous catheters).[57,62,74] Infective agents have not been reported to cause cotton-wool spots; these lesions should not be confused with *Candida* or other forms of fungal retinitis.[53]

NONINFECTIOUS RETINAL VASCULOPATHY

Noninfectious retinopathy refers to cotton-wool spots, retinal hemorrhages, and microvascular abnormalities that do not progress, enlarge, or cause visual symptoms. No infectious cause of these lesions has been demonstrated, and they appear to represent nonspecific retinal microvascular disease. A correlation between the number of cotton-wool spots and decreased cerebral blood flow (as shown by technetium 99m hexamethylpropyleneamine oxime single photon emission computed tomography) was shown in 25 patients with AIDS or symptomatic HIV infection.[75]

Cotton-wool spots are the most common ocular lesion seen in AIDS, occurring in 25% to 50% of patients[6,71] and in up to 75% of cases by autopsy examination.[63] In one study, up to 92% of AIDS patients were found to have evidence of retinovascular disease when examined using fluorescein angiography.[76] This high incidence of fluorescein angiographic abnormalities has not been confirmed by other groups.

Cotton-wool spots are nonspecific and may be seen in diabetes mellitus, hypertension, severe anemia, systemic lupus erythematosus, dermatomyositis, and leukemia.[77,78] Cotton-wool spots seen by ophthalmoscopy are a result of microinfarction of the nerve fiber layer of the retina. In AIDS these lesions usually are confined to the posterior pole near the optic disc[76] (Fig. 92-1).

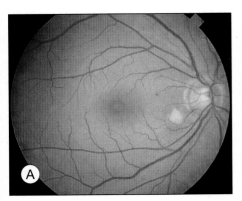 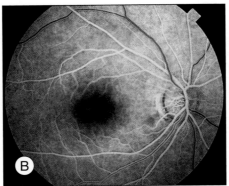 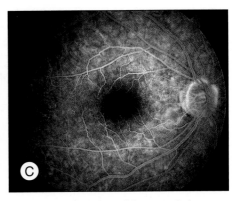

Fig. 92-1 A, Retinal cotton-wool spot seen inferotemporal to the disc. B, Early fluorescein angiogram shows blockage and possible nonperfusion. C, Late angiogram shows staining presumably from damaged retinal microvasculature.

Histopathologic study of retinal cotton-wool spots in AIDS patients has demonstrated that these lesions have pathologic features identical to those seen in cotton-wool spots of other cause. Histologically, a cytoid body is present, representing a swollen, interrupted axon. Localized edema and multiple cytoid bodies together make up the cotton-wool spots. Cotton-wool spots probably represent local areas of axoplasmic debris accumulation in the nerve fiber layer resulting from interruption of axoplasmic flow. Ischemia is the most common cause of focal interruption of axonal flow in the retinal nerve fiber layer that results in a cotton-wool spot. Any factor that causes focal interruption of axonal flow leads to similar accumulations.[78] Similar to the cotton-wool spots seen in other systemic diseases, this lesion in AIDS demonstrates no associated inflammation, no cells in the vitreous, and no vascular leakage on fluorescein angiography (Fig. 92-2). Studies of cotton-wool spots have not conclusively demonstrated that they are directly caused by HIV or CMV infection. Cotton-wool spots should not be confused with Candida or fungal retinitis, since these ocular infections are unusual in AIDS patients. Attempts to isolate organisms from cotton-wool spots in the hope of explaining their cause in AIDS as infectious have been unsuccessful, and the cause of this lesion in AIDS remains elusive.[6,63,79–81] Investigators have suggested that deposition of immune complexes may be responsible for the formation of cotton-wool spots. It is known that AIDS patients have high levels of circulating immune complexes, but the significance and nature of these are unclear.[82]

Cotton-wool spots have been speculated to be harbingers of CMV retinitis or perhaps sites of susceptibility to CMV infection, but substantiation of these ideas is lacking. Histopathologic studies of eyes at autopsy have failed to show clear evidence of a viral cause of cotton-wool spots.[53,83,84] The relationship between noninfectious retinal disease and HIV-related CNS dysfunction also is unknown.

We have reported that noninfectious retinopathy is not seen in HIV-seronegative men and is rare in ARC, but it is very common in patients with AIDS even in the absence of active opportunistic ophthalmic infection.[54] It is striking that this lesion may be seen in 50% to 75% of AIDS patients, and studies using multiple examinations indicate that the more frequently these patients are examined, the higher the incidence may be.[6,54] Cotton-wool spots probably are ophthalmoscopically visible for 6 to 12 weeks, and owing to the transient nature of the lesion and its apparent noninfectious cause, treatment is not indicated at this time. The time to regression of cotton-wool spots has been shown to be 6 to 12 weeks.[86]

In a cross-sectional study, the median CD4+ count (per microliter [μl]) in patients with cotton-wool spots was 14 cells (range, 0 to 160) and was 8 cells (range, 0 to 42) in patients with CMV retinitis.[87] In the absence of other systemic vascular disease, such as hypertension or diabetes mellitus, AIDS must be considered in the differential diagnosis of cotton-wool spots owing to their very high prevalence in these patients. Whether these lesions are an early manifestation of AIDS remains to be elucidated, but they may be apparent in HIV-infected persons before the onset of opportunistic infections.[54]

Morphologic studies have shown that the number of retrobulbar optic nerve fibers in patients with AIDS is decreased compared with the number of optic nerve fibers in normal control eyes as a result of axonal degeneration and an associated decrease in the number of optic nerve axons.[88–90] Infarctions of the nerve fiber layer develop in most patients with AIDS, and the number of such infarctions increases over time.[6,55,79] Visual dysfunction associated with multiple nerve fiber layer infarctions may be manifested by defects in color-vision and contrast-sensitivity testing in patients with AIDS; this is consistent with dysfunction of the macula or optic nerve.[91] Interestingly, in vivo studies of the retinal nerve fiber layer have shown both broad and slitlike defects, suggesting that retinal nerve fiber loss and optic nerve fiber loss are related to subclinical vision loss in HIV patients without infectious retinitis.[92] Electroretinographic studies of HIV patients without retinitis also have shown retinal dysfunction.[93]

Retinal hemorrhages

Retinal hemorrhages are seen in AIDS in association with CMV retinitis, cotton-wool spots, and as an isolated finding. These lesions have been reported in up to 30%[57,76] of AIDS patients, and autopsy evidence of retinal hemorrhages has been reported to be as high as 40%. Retinal hemorrhages usually take the form of flame-shaped lesions in the posterior pole, dot-blot hemorrhages, or as punctate intraretinal hemorrhages peripherally (Fig. 92-3). Occasionally the hemorrhage is manifested as Roth's spots (hemorrhage with a white central area).[57,76] The pattern of retinal hemorrhages changes over time. The hemorrhages do not appear to be related to a bleeding diathesis or coagulopathy, but rather seem to be a manifestation of AIDS itself.[6] Vision loss from retinal hemorrhage has not been described, and treatment is conservative if the lesions are not associated with CMV retinitis or septicemia. Retinal vasculitis has been reported in an occasional AIDS patient in the absence of CMV retinitis.[57,94] This has been a rare finding in prospective studies,[54]

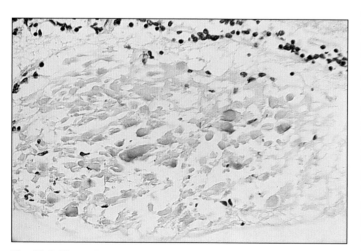

Fig. 92-2 Photomicrograph of retinal cotton-wool spot shows cytoid bodies and swelling of the nerve fiber layer of the retina. Retinal cellular elements are seen at the top of the photograph.

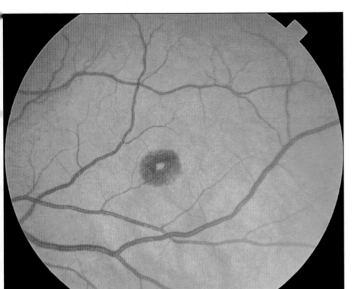

Fig. 92-3 White, centered retinal hemorrhage (Roth's spot) seen in an HIV-infected patient. These lesions do not progress.

with the exception of Africa, where the incidence of retinal vasculitis is relatively high and, interestingly, CMV retinitis less common.[58] It should be noted that CMV retinitis is commonly associated with a retinal vasculitis; however, retinal infiltrate and other signs of CMV retinitis also are present.[39,95–98] In the African series, three of 11 AIDS patients and two of nine ARC patients demonstrated retinal vascular sheathing in the peripheral retina. Interestingly, the three patients with AIDS manifested isolated retinal perivasculitis, whereas the two patients with ARC showed vasculitis in association with retinal hemorrhage or capillary changes.

Microvascular abnormalities

Microvascular changes are common in AIDS patients and may be detected in many patients by fluorescein angiography. Microvascular pathologic findings in AIDS, as demonstrated by fluorescein angiography, include microaneurysms, telangiectasias, focal areas of nonperfusion, and capillary loss.[71,76] These changes are similar to the changes seen in diabetes mellitus. The histologic findings of periodic acid–Schiff (PAS)-positive thickening of blood vessels and precapillary arteriolar closure also correlate with the findings in diabetes mellitus. Similar microangiopathy is seen in immune complex disease, such as systemic lupus erythematosus, and rheologic disorders,[99] such as leukemia. Because HIV infection may result in similar situations (immune complex formation and rheologic abnormalities from hypergammaglobulinemia), retinal microvascular disease may be a manifestation of these disorders.[76]

Branch or central retinal vein occlusion, branch retinal artery occlusion, and ischemic maculopathy have been reported in HIV patients without infectious retinitis. The incidence is unknown. It is possible that the cause may be related to lupus anticoagulant and other clotting abnormalities seen in HIV-infected patients.[100–102] Abnormalities of retinal blood flow have

also been reported in HIV patients and may contribute to the pathogenesis of microvascular abnormalities.[103–106]

INFECTIOUS RETINOPATHY

Cytomegalovirus retinitis: pathogenesis, diagnosis, and clinical manifestations

Cytomegalovirus infection is a major cause of morbidity and mortality in AIDS. CMV retinitis has been reported to occur in 15% to 40% of AIDS patients with the rate declining since the arrival of highly active antiretroviral therapy (HAART).[39,57,96,107,108] In contrast to the noninfectious lesions of AIDS, CMV retinitis demands aggressive treatment to prevent severe visual loss.[6,108A,109] Patients with active CMV disease may have systemic symptoms of fever, arthralgia, and pneumonitis, or leukopenia, retinitis, or hepatitis; blood cultures and urine specimens may be positive for CMV. CMV infects the retina, as well as the CNS, reticuloendothelial system, kidneys, adrenals, lungs, and gastrointestinal system.[109–111] CMV retinitis often is the presenting sign of systemic CMV infection, and all patients should be thoroughly evaluated for systemic disease.

The clinical presentation of CMV retinitis in AIDS is similar in many respects to CMV retinitis found in iatrogenically immunosuppressed patients and infants with cytomegalic inclusion disease.[112–114] Correlation of the clinical and typical pathologic findings at autopsy has been demonstrated.[115] Specifically, it is known that CMV is a neurotropic virus with a tendency to infect neural tissues and the retina. Necrosis of the retina in AIDS-associated CMV retinitis is typical, with pathognomonic cytomegaly and minimal inflammatory cells present in the lesions. Choroidal involvement is rare, and whether vascular endothelium is involved is unclear. These lesions also may appear as noncontiguous patches rather than the more commonly seen contiguous spreading lesion. Antigens to CMV have been found by immunofluorescence, immunoperoxidase staining, and DNA hybridization techniques.[116,117] The most distinctive anterior segment finding is the presence of fine stellate keratic precipitates on the corneal endothelium.[118] Retinal vascular nonperfusion and retinal neovascularization resulting from CMV retinitis and choroiditis also have been reported.[119]

CMV is a slowly progressive necrotizing retinitis that may affect the posterior pole, the periphery, or both, and may be unilateral or bilateral. Involved retinal areas appear as white intraretinal lesions, areas of infiltrate, and often necrosis along the vascular arcades in the posterior pole. In addition, prominent retinal hemorrhages often are present within the necrotic area or along its leading edge (Fig. 92-4). Peripherally, CMV retinitis occurs commonly; it tends to have a less intense white appearance with areas of granular, white retinitis that may or may not demonstrate associated retinal hemorrhage (Fig. 92-5). As the retinitis progresses, an area of atrophic, avascular retina may remain with underlying retinal pigment epithelial atrophy or hyperplasia.[6,39,120] Peripheral CMV retinitis is common in AIDS patients who initially may report only floaters with or without a visual field deficit. Peripheral CMV retinitis has only recently received attention in the literature,[39] and in

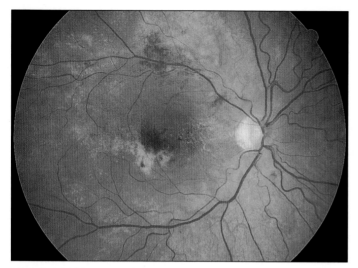

Fig. 92-4 CMV retinitis with hemorrhagic areas are seen superior to the fovea and a more dense area just below the fovea. Borders are opaque and associated with variable amounts of hemorrhage.

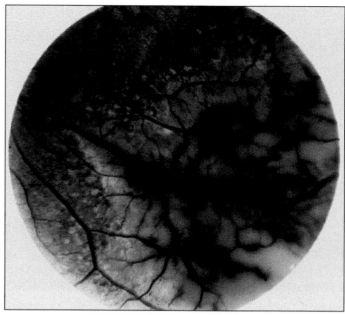

Fig. 92-6 Fluorescein angiogram of CMV retinitis lesion shows lack of perfusion and blockage, as well as staining and leakage of fluorescein from damaged retinal vessels.

prospective studies of AIDS patients examined with indirect ophthalmoscopy it may be the most common form of retinitis seen.[96] Wide-angle fundus photography and fluorescein angiography may be of benefit if the diagnosis is uncertain. These techniques may be used to document progression of retinitis, and fluorescein leakage in areas of retinitis may be helpful in confirming the diagnosis (Fig. 92-6).

Reactivation of CMV retinitis is characterized by reopacification of the border of the lesion followed by advancement. Smoldering retinitis (Fig. 92-7) and subtle reactivation may be difficult to recognize without prior fundus photographs. Several studies have shown that wide-angle fundus photographs are a more sensitive indicator of retinitis progression than is clinical examination by indirect ophthalmoscopy.[95,121,122]

Several investigators have shown that untreated CMV retinitis is inexorably progressive in AIDS patients.[6,57,114,116,124,125] As in our experience, untreated CMV becomes bilateral in the vast majority of patients.

In an observational study of 26 patients treated for CMV retinitis, vision scores decreased with greater abnormalities found on ophthalmologic examination. Visual symptoms were most strongly related to findings in the worse eye. Visual function and global vision scores were moderately correlated with findings from visual testing and examination and less strongly related to general health perceptions. Patients reported considerable

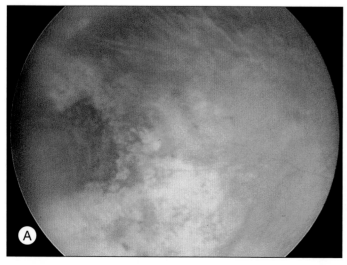

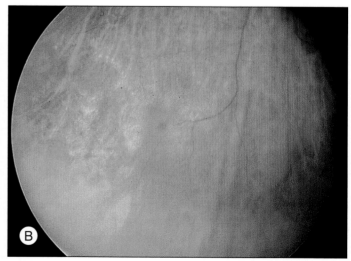

Fig. 92-5 A, Peripheral CMV retinitis without retinal hemorrhage is characterized by white areas of retinal necrosis. B, After healing, CMV retinitis leaves behind a glial scar without opacification (not same eye as in "A"). Often only minimal pigmentary changes are seen.

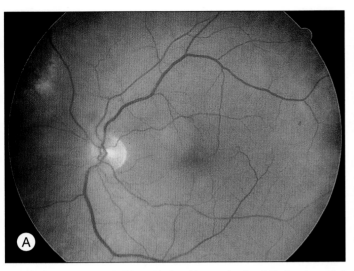 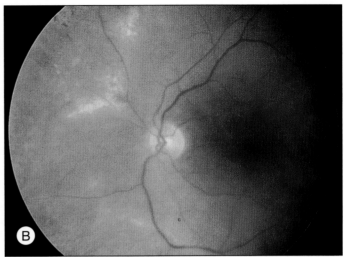

Fig. 92-7 Smoldering CMV retinitis is a low grade of retinitis border activity that is associated with slow progression of retinitis. It may be difficult to diagnose without fundus photographs. A, Low grade CMV lesion. B, Lesion has progressed slowly over 2 months.

impairment, including blurred vision (42%), difficulty reading (40%), difficulty driving (44%), treatment interference with social activities (40%), and substantial trouble with vision (50%).[125] Treatment of AIDS-related CMV retinitis minimizes loss of vision and may protect previously uninfected eyes, prolonging visual independence.[126]

Recurrent CMV retinitis exhibiting a foveal-sparing pattern within 1500 mm of the foveola has been described and occurs primarily in patients with recurrent CMV retinitis resistant to treatment ("clinically resistant"), particularly that which has arisen temporally. Despite its foveolar proximity and ultimate significant loss of function, the pattern of progression allows for preservation of useful foveal vision for longer periods than would have been expected.[127]

Other manifestations of CMV retinitis include retinal edema, attenuated vessels, perivascular sheathing, and exudative retinal detachment[128] (Fig. 92-8). In addition, vitreitis and anterior uveitis are often seen,[112,115] and optic atrophy may occur as a late manifestation resulting from widespread retinal destruction. CMV occasionally may be demonstrated in vitreous biopsy specimens in these patients.[116] The yield may be higher in the presence of marked vitreitis because CMV is a cell-associated virus. Other causes of retinitis, including herpes simplex retinitis,[113,129] toxoplasmosis,[74] Candida, Behçet's disease, syphilis, acute retinal necrosis,[129A,130,131] and subacute sclerosing panencephalitis,[61] usually can be distinguished from CMV on clinical grounds, although this may not be the case in retinitis caused by other members of the herpesvirus family.[129A] CMV has a very characteristic clinical appearance,[6,71,94] but the lesions in CMV retinitis vary from patient to patient,[96] and it is important to maintain a high index of suspicion for the above infections, especially in light of frequent superinfection of AIDS patients with multiple organisms.

CMV retinitis is a reflection of underlying active systemic CMV infection. In almost all cases it is a blinding disease if not controlled. If untreated, CMV retinitis portends a poor prog-

nosis for vision and life. Large-dose trials (20 mg/kg/day) of vidarabine had limited success in treating CMV retinitis in patients immunosuppressed for transplantation, but vidarabine was associated with significant gastrointestinal, hematologic, and neurologic side effects.[132] Interferon-alpha and acyclovir also were largely unsuccessful, but the use of ganciclovir (dihydroxypropoxy methyl guanine,9-[[2-hydroxy-1-(hydroxymethyl) ethoxy] methyl] guanine, DHPG, or BW759U), foscarnet, and cidofovir have been successful in the control, but not cure, of CMV retinitis.

Thus, in the face of changing mental status, development of focal signs on neurologic examination, or other symptoms consistent with subacute encephalitis in AIDS patients, a comprehensive ophthalmologic examination is indicated, and an increased index of suspicion of CMV infection of the CNS and possible

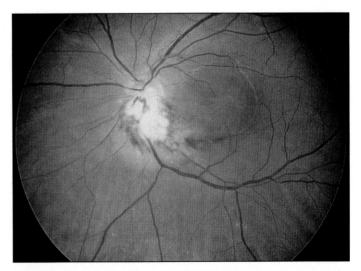

Fig. 92-8 CMV affecting the perifoveal area or the optic nerve can result in an exudative retinal detachment often involving the macula. If there has not been actual involvement of a vital structure, treatment may result in improvement of central vision.

CMV retinitis is warranted. There is also evidence that patients with CMV retinitis, especially peripapillary disease, have a much higher incidence of CMV encephalitis.[133]

CMV infection of the brain, optic nerves, and retinas from 47 consecutive autopsies of patients with AIDS was examined.[133] Immunocytochemistry demonstrated CMV infection in 11 (23%) brains, two (2%) of 94 optic nerves, and 38 (40%) of 94 retinas. Ten (91%) of 11 patients with CMV encephalitis had concurrent retinitis. While 10 (42%) of 24 patients with CMV retinitis had CMV encephalitis, when the retinitis included the peripapillary region, 75% had encephalitis. The optic nerve parenchyma usually was not infected histologically despite extensive peripapillary retinitis. The strength of these associations suggests that CMV retinitis defines a group of patients with AIDS at risk for development of CMV encephalitis (relative risk, 9.5%), especially when the retinitis involves the peripapillary region (relative risk, 13%). Furthermore, in patients with AIDS without CMV retinitis, central nervous system symptoms are unlikely to be attributable to CMV encephalitis.[133]

The development of CMV encephalitis has been reported in two patients with AIDS who were receiving ganciclovir maintenance therapy for CMV retinitis, suggesting that the currently recommended therapeutic protocols with ganciclovir may not be effective in the prevention and treatment of CMV encephalitis in patients with AIDS.[134] The pathologic correlation between ocular and cerebral lesions in patients with AIDS has been reviewed.[135]

CMV retinitis is less frequent in children with AIDS with reported rates of approximately 5–6%, though rates of extraocular CMV are higher than in adults. CMV retinitis has been reported in young children with high absolute CD4 counts, though these counts are low relative to the child's age. Older children tend to have low absolute CD4 counts similar to adults. There is a higher incidence of bilateral and posterior pole disease in children, however this is likely due in part to delays in diagnosis in children from lack of subjective vision complaints.[136–138]

SCREENING TECHNIQUES FOR RETINAL AND SYSTEMIC CYTOMEGALOVIRUS INFECTION

Screening for CMV retinitis is a difficult problem. Many patients who are CMV viremic or viruric many not have end organ disease, and studies employing quantitative CMV polymerase chain reaction (PCR) in plasma or CMV antigenemia have not been able to definitively predict the development of CMV retinitis.[139] Currently no laboratory marker exists that reliably predicts the occurrence of clinical CMV retinitis, although studies for the detection and quantitation of CMV antigens and nucleic acids in plasma or whole blood are ongoing.[140,141]

Urine is culture positive for CMV in over 50% of homosexual men and the majority of AIDS patients; thus urine culture may not be of diagnostic value. Serology in AIDS patients is nonspecific, and documentation of rising CMV titers is unusual.[6,116,142]

Studies of newly diagnosed CMV retinitis patients indicate that many are CMV culture negative in the blood. Positive blood cultures for CMV, fever, and weight loss are associated with more extensive CMV retinitis at the time of diagnosis.[143] The results of virologic blood assays for CMV also have been associated with clinical outcome in patients with CMV retinitis.[144] A positive blood culture for CMV has been associated with early CMV retinitis progression and death; however, urine cultures for CMV are not predictive of retinitis progression.

Positive CMV antigenemia has been reported to be more sensitive than conventional cell culture. Thus assays for the detection of CMV antigenemia may be a simple and rapid means of identifying those patients with unilateral retinitis at highest risk of developing CMV retinitis of the fellow eye or of visceral CMV disease if intravitreal injections or implants are used as the sole treatment for CMV retinitis.[145]

The presence of CMV DNA in serum analyzed by PCR was a good predictive marker of CMV retinitis in HIV-seropositive subjects in one study. A positive PCR result supports the clinical diagnosis and may be useful for monitoring response to antiviral treatment.[146] By prospective monitoring for increases in plasma CMV DNA copy number, it may be possible to identify HIV-seropositive patients who are at imminent risk for development of symptomatic CMV retinitis.[147]

The influence of cytomegaloviral load on response to ganciclovir, time to recurrence, and survival based on CMV viral load in the blood of AIDS patients has been reported to be an important factor in the pathogenesis of retinitis. Quantification of CMV could be used to select patients for controlled clinical trials and to optimize individual anti-CMV induction therapy.[148]

It is also reasonable and practical to use the CD4+ cell count as a threshold below which to screen patients, since the risk of CMV retinitis increases at CD4+ cell counts below 50/mm^3.[87] The incidence and prevalence of CMV retinitis in a cohort study of patients with CD4+ cell counts below $0.10 \times 10/l$ (100/µl) revealed a 25% chance for the development of CMV retinitis by 4 years of follow-up. Among those subjects in whom CMV retinitis developed, about 19% had retinitis before a CD4+ cell count of less than $0.05 \times 10/l$ (< 50/µl) was observed, and 81% had CMV retinitis after the CD4+ cell count reached this threshold.[149] In the HAART era, some patients may develop CMV retinitis with CD4 counts above 100/ml, probably because of incomplete restoration of the immune repertoire against CMV.[150] Development of CMV retinitis also was correlated in one study with CMV viruria in patients with CD4+ cells <100/µl of blood.[151]

A variant of the Amsler grid has been proposed for use as a screen for central CMV retinitis within a 22-degree radius (3 disc diameter) of the fovea.[152] This technique may detect up to two thirds of cases of CMV retinitis. A new technique, entoptic perimetry, which employs patient visualization of moving particles on a computer monitor, appears to have a very high sensitivity and specificity (over 90%) in detecting CMV retinitis within the central 30-degree radius of fixation[92] (Fig. 92-9).

Techniques for detection of CMV DNA based on PCR are increasingly being applied to ocular fluids; however, the clinical

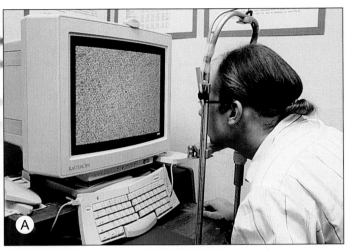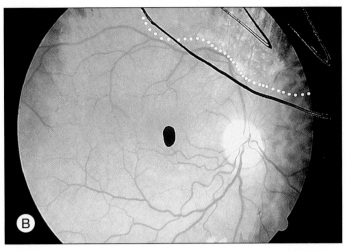

Fig. 92-9 Entoptic perimetry can allow detection of CMV retinitis lesions. A, The patient is asked to view particle motion programmed on a monitor. B, An overlay of the CMV lesion (dotted white border) and the patient's own sketch of the scotoma seen (black line).

significance of such findings can sometimes be unclear. The application of PCR-based methods to ocular fluids made a useful contribution to the treatment of the patients.[153]

This appears to be a sensitive and specific diagnostic assay that could assist in the diagnosis of CMV retinitis.[154] PCR detection of CMV DNA has been reported to be a more sensitive method than analysis of locally produced antibodies by calculating a Goldman–Witmer coefficient to determine local ocular antibody production.[155] There is also an immune predisposition to the development of CMV retinitis in patients with AIDS.[156]

Corneal endothelial deposits were studied in six patients with AIDS who had CMV retinitis and abnormal endothelial deposits in at least one eye. There were multiple, diffuse, fine, refractile, stellate-shaped deposits on the corneal endothelium in all affected eyes. The deposits were best seen with retro-illumination. Two of six patients examined with specular microscopy showed severe abnormalities, which included marked areas of polymegathism and decreased endothelial cell counts. Examination of one eye obtained postmortem disclosed chains of dendritic macrophages and fibrin adherent to the apical surface of the corneal endothelium. There was no evidence of direct infection of the corneal endothelium by CMV. Deposits on the corneal endothelium in patients with CMV retinitis most likely result from an anterior uveitis. A preponderance of macrophages observed by histopathologic examination may be related to the inability of immunodeficient patients to mount a normal T-cell response.[157]

TREATMENT OF CYTOMEGALOVIRUS RETINITIS

The treatment of CMV retinitis has recently been reviewed.[158–160] Treatment may be systemic, local, or a combination of the two. There are currently five medications approved by the U.S. Food and Drug Administration (FDA) for the treatment of CMV retinitis: ganciclovir, valganciclovir, cidofovir, foscarnet, and fomivirsen.

Systemic vs. local therapy

CMV retinitis may be treated systemically or intravitreally. However, systemic treatment is associated with less spread of CMV retinitis from one eye to the other.[161] In addition, local treatment including the sustained release ganciclovir implant has been shown to be associated with higher risk of the development of systemic CMV.[161–161C]

Systemic CMV may cause gastrointestinal disease, with colitis being the most common manifestation as well as esophagitis. CMV pneumonia or adrenalitis is less common. Systemic CMV diagnosis may be difficult and usually requires histopathologic evidence of CMV infection. In fact, CMV encephalitis is extremely difficult to diagnose, and clinically the diagnosis is rarely made. We have studied the brains of patients with CMV retinitis at autopsy and have found that CMV encephalitis was present in 42% patients with retinitis, but the converse (CMV encephalitis in patients without retinitis) is quite rare; 91% of patients with CMV encephalitis had retinitis. Thus a negative retinal examination may be very useful in determining whether CNS changes in an HIV-positive patient are due to CMV encephalitis.[133] The cumulative incidence of systemic CMV disease that becomes clinically apparent is approximately 25%.[162] Therefore, although systemic CMV disease may not be clinically apparent at the time of diagnosis of CMV retinitis, some experts believe that initial systemic therapy may be warranted despite the inconvenience, expense, and potential toxicities.

Intravenous ganciclovir

Ganciclovir is a nucleoside analog of 2-deoxyguanosine, similar to acyclovir.[163] Despite its structural similarities with acyclovir, ganciclovir is much more active in vitro against CMV than acyclovir.[164] Ganciclovir inhibits all herpes-viruses, including CMV, by preventing DNA elongation. The active form of ganciclovir is the triphosphate form, as with acyclovir. CMV lacks the virally specified thymidine kinase (TK) that converts ganciclovir (or acyclovir) to its monophosphate form.[165] TK-altered strains resistant to acyclovir are as sensitive to ganciclovir as the unaltered parent strains.[166,167] Thus ganciclovir is phosphorylated to its triphosphate form much more efficiently than acyclovir, which accounts for the greater activity of ganciclovir against CMV.[166]

The majority of AIDS patients treated with ganciclovir respond within 2 to 4 weeks with decreased retinal opacification and stabilization of the retinitis[96,120] (Fig. 92-10). Improved quality of life has been reported in AIDS patients treated with ganciclovir for CMV retinitis.[96] Ganciclovir is commercially available as an intravenous and oral formulation (and also is included in an intraocular device), and indefinite maintenance therapy is necessary as long as the patient remains in immune failure with a CD4 count below 50/μl. An intravenous loading dose of 5 mg/kg every 12 hours for 14 to 21 days should be followed by maintenance doses of 5 mg/kg/day. At many institutions patients are instructed to administer the infusion at home through a permanently implanted IV catheter. If the drug is discontinued, retinitis often recurs within 10 to 21 days, continuing its progression at the borders of healed areas.[96] Recurrences have been common, even during maintenance therapy, being reported 3 weeks to 5 months after institution of therapy and occurring in 30% to 40% of patients.[96] Many investigators have found that discontinuation or delay of ganciclovir therapy results in nearly 100% recurrence of retinitis, at which time reinstitution of the loading dose regimen often is necessary.[165,168,169] Multiple series in patients with AIDS and CMV retinitis have shown response rates of 80% to 100%, with 60% to 80% of patients achieving a remission with ganciclovir therapy.[39,109,120,169–174]

The treatment of CMV retinitis usually includes an induction phase followed by a maintenance phase to prevent relapse. Before the advent of HAART, relapse occurred almost universally, given a sufficiently long period after induction courses of ganciclovir. Therapy therefore continued for a lifetime. The median time to relapse in patients treated with just an induction dose is 3 to 4 weeks.[169] CMV retinitis also will relapse despite all types of maintenance therapy, with a cumulative rate of relapse by 1 year of 18% to 50%.[174A]

Most clinicians use a 14-day induction course of intravenous ganciclovir consisting of 5 mg/kg/day every 12 hours and indefinite maintenance of 5 mg/kg/day. Lower doses and every-other-day dosing schedules have been associated with high rates of early relapse. Since treatment may be lifelong if the patient's CD4 count cannot be elevated with anti-HIV therapy (see HIV disease in the HAART era, p. 1648), usually a permanent or semipermanent indwelling venous catheter is placed at the onset of therapy if intravenous therapy is chosen as maintenance therapy. Ganciclovir requires modification of dosing in the presence of renal insufficiency.

Side effects of ganciclovir include granulocytopenia, neurologic dysfunction, abnormal liver function tests, and rarely, thrombocytopenia. The most serious toxicity is granulocytopenia, which may occur in up to one-third of patients when defined as less than 500 neutrophils per microliter.[169] Granulocytopenia is generally reversible, and this adverse effect is exacerbated when used with AZT.[175] The use of colony-stimulating factors rGM-CSF (recombinant granulocyte–macrophage colony-stimulating factor) and rG-CSF (recombinant granulocyte colony-stimulating factor) for reversing or preventing neutropenia may be useful.

The prevalence of CMV resistance to ganciclovir is unknown, but ever-increasing induction regimens may be necessary to control CMV retinitis. In one series, CMV-resistant strains were isolated from five of 72 patients treated and from five of 13 patients who shed the virus while receiving the drug.[176] Strains of CMV that have developed resistance to ganciclovir have remained susceptible to foscarnet.[177] Because of the question of ganciclovir resistance, a trial of combined vs. alternating foscarnet–ganciclovir maintenance therapy has been reported to be effective.[178]

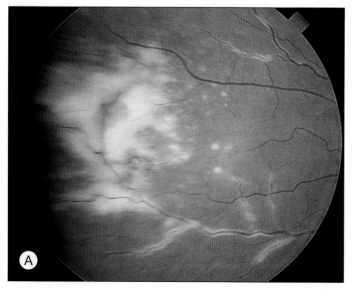 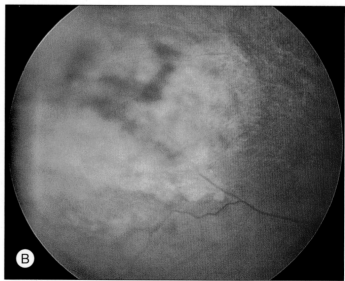

Fig. 92-10 A, Active peripheral CMV retinitis with secondary retinal vasculitis. B, The area is healed after intravenous ganciclovir therapy. Note absence of border opacification. Also seen are pigmentary changes characteristic of healed CMV.

Visual acuity depends on the location of the involved retina, and involvement of the fovea or optic nerve may result in decreased visual acuity even if there has been a response to therapy. In addition, in most published studies, there has been a bias introduced in that more immediately vision-threatening lesions tend to be treated earlier than peripheral lesions. Ganciclovir has been shown to be effective in preserving visual acuity. For example, 73% of eyes maintained a visual acuity of 20/40 or better when treated with ganciclovir.[179]

Ganciclovir also is effective in the treatment of systemic CMV infections, such as those of the gastrointestinal tract, but has less effect on CMV pneumonia.[109] CMV gastrointestinal infection usually results in colitis with severe diarrhea and weight loss, or in esophagitis with severe dysphagia and weight loss; ganciclovir treatment ameliorated these problems, although relapse is common in gastrointestinal CMV infection. Poor blood oxygenation and infiltrates on chest radiographs characterize CMV pneumonia. Initial study of ganciclovir treatment of CMV pneumonia has shown poor response to therapy.[109]

Oral ganciclovir

Oral ganciclovir (FDA approved, 1994) can be used for maintenance therapy of CMV retinitis after it has been healed with intravenous ganciclovir therapy. Studies using this drug regimen have shown efficacy, but it is clear that oral ganciclovir is less effective than intravenous ganciclovir for many patients.

Additional work has been reported involving the use of oral ganciclovir to prevent CMV retinitis in patients with $CD4^+$ cell counts below $100/\mu l$. For primary prevention of CMV disease, oral ganciclovir has been shown to have efficacy in one study[180] but not in a second study.[181]

Perhaps the most common use of oral ganciclovir is in patients being treated with intravitreal therapy (injections of cidofovir or ganciclovir implant) in whom it is desired to prevent systemic CMV disease. The efficacy of oral ganciclovir used in this manner is not completely known, but control of retinitis is excellent with intravitreal therapies, and many internists prefer to have some systemic anti-CMV coverage. Such use of oral ganciclovir also may reduce the incidence of CMV in the fellow eye if it is not involved.[180,182,183]

Recently oral ganciclovir for prophylaxis or treatment of CMV retinitis has been replaced by oral valganciclovir, which provides much higher blood levels.

Valganciclovir

Valganciclovir, the valine ester of ganciclovir, is an orally administered formulation of ganciclovir that earned FDA approval in the United States in February 2001. The valine ester confers enhanced permeability and absorption of the molecule through the cell membranes of the gut. Once in the blood stream, the valine ester is cleaved from the molecule by esterases, rendering plasma levels of ganciclovir comparable to those achieved with intravenous ganciclovir administration. The drug is transported by the intestinal peptide transporter PEPT1 and also recognized by the renal PEPT2.[184] A single-dose randomized crossover pharmacokinetic study reported the absolute ganciclovir bioavailability after oral valganciclovir administration is 60.9% compared to 5.6% bioavailability of oral ganciclovir.[185] A randomized crossover dose-ranging study determined that plasma levels of ganciclovir after an 875 mg dose of valganciclovir are similar to the plasma levels achieved with a dose of 5 mg/kg of intravenous ganciclovir (AUC 24.8 mg/ml*h vs. 26 mg/ml*h). The authors suggested the 900 mg dose of valganciclovir would approximate the AUC value of the 5 mg/kg dose of IV ganciclovir. In addition the study reported that the ganciclovir bioavailability after oral valganciclovir was increased when dosed with food (AUC_{fasted} 19.0 mg/ml*h vs. AUC_{fed} 24.8 mg/ml*h, $P = <0.001$).[186]

Valganciclovir has been studied for induction therapy for CMV retinitis. Martin et al. (Valganciclovir Study Group) reported a multicenter randomized, controlled clinical trial comparing oral valganciclovir 900 mg twice a day for three weeks induction therapy followed by 900 mg daily for 1 week maintenance therapy with intravenous ganciclovir 5 mg/kg twice a day for 3 weeks induction therapy followed by 5 mg/kg once daily for one week maintenance therapy. After 4 weeks both groups received continued maintenance therapy with 900 mg valganciclovir daily. Eighty patients with newly diagnosed CMV retinitis were randomized to each group in a 1:1 ratio. Patients were excluded if they had a history of treated CMV retinitis, had received systemic anti-CMV therapy for more than 3 weeks, or had received any systemic anti-CMV therapy within 3 months of randomization, though eligible patient may have received up to 3 months of prophylaxis with oral ganciclovir. Other exclusion criteria included the presence of severe diarrhea, absolute neutrophil count below 750 cells/mm^3, platelet count below 75 000/mm^3, and estimated creatinine clearance below 70 ml/min. Primary endpoint was photographically determined progression of CMV retinitis within 4 weeks after the initiation of treatment. In the valganciclovir group 9.9% of patients had progression of CMV retinitis within the first 4 weeks compared to 10.0% of patients assigned to IV ganciclovir. This 0.1 percentage point difference was not significant (95% CI, –9.7 to 10.0). Secondary end points included the achievement of a prospectively defined successful response to induction therapy and the time to progression of CMV retinitis. Seventy-seven percent of patients receiving IV ganciclovir and 71.9% of patients receiving oral valganciclovir achieved a satisfactory response to induction therapy. This 5.2 percentage point difference was not significant (95% CI, –20.4 to 10.1). The median times to progression of retinitis were 125 days in the IV ganciclovir group and 160 days in the oral valganciclovir group. The relative risk of progression of retinitis in the valganciclovir group compared to the ganciclovir group was 0.90 (95 CI, 0.58–1.38). Diarrhea was the most common adverse effect during the study and occurred more frequently in the valganciclovir group compared to the ganciclovir group (19% vs. 10%, $P = 0.11$). Neutropenia occurred with similar frequency in each group, 13% with valganciclovir and 14% with ganciclovir. Catheter related side effects were seen more frequently in the IV ganciclovir group than in the valganciclovir group (9% vs. 4%).[187] No clinical trials have been published specifically comparing efficacy of valganciclovir for maintenance therapy of CMV retinitis.

Lalezari et al. (Roche Valganciclovir Study Group) reported a large safety study of valganciclovir. The adverse event profile was similar to that reported from previous studies of intravenous and oral ganciclovir. Adverse events of note were diarrhea (38%), nausea (23%), fever (18%), neutropenia (absolute neutrophil count <500 cells/mm^3) (10%), and anemia (hemoglobin <8.0 g/dl) (12%), thrombocytopenia (platelet count <25 000 cells/mm^3) (2%). During the study, 16% of patients received granuloctye-colony stimulating factor or granuloctye/macrophage-colony stimulating factor and 7% of patients received erythropoietin.[188]

The authors reported the frequency of adverse event for patients taking valganciclovir and other AIDS medicines. Of note, there was no increased frequency of pancreatitis in patients also on didanosine though there is a known interaction with valganciclovir causing higher levels of didanosine. Several adverse events were reported 10% more frequently in patients taking valganciclovir with other AIDS medicines compared with valganciclovir alone. Valganciclovir and zidovudine combined (42 patients) had higher incidence of anemia (36% vs. 11%). Patients taking valganciclovir plus didanosine (66 patients) reported more diarrhea (47% vs. 30%), vomiting (26% vs. 11%), and abdominal pain (20% vs. 4%). Concomitant use of valganciclovir with hydroxyurea (35 patients) resulted in more neutropenia (37% vs. 14%), anemia (26 vs. 14%), weight loss (20% vs. 8%), peripheral neuropathy (17% vs. 5%), thrombocytopenia (14% vs. 3%), and cellulitis (11% vs. 1%). Finally, patients taking both valganciclovir and amphotericin B (15 patients) reported more headache (40% vs. 14%), sinusitis (33% vs. 8%), and pruritus (20% vs. 4%).[188]

In summary oral valganciclovir offers the obvious advantage of extreme effectiveness against CMV retinitis without the difficulties and inconveniences of intravenous administration. Furthermore, because valganciclovir is converted to ganciclovir in the blood stream, its pharmacologic safety profile, including side effects, is no different than that of intravenously administered ganciclovir. Thus oral valganciclovir is an effective and safe alternative to intravenous ganciclovir for the treatment of CMV retinitis. Recently (2004) oral ganciclovir has become unavailable but is now supplanted by valganciclovir (Roche personal communication 2/3/2004).

Foscarnet

The second drug for the treatment of CMV retinitis in patients with AIDS was licensed by the Food and Drug Administration (FDA) in 1993. Foscarnet is a pyrophosphate analog with broad antiviral activity via inhibition of viral polymerases, such inhibition not being dependent on activation or phosphorylation by viral or cellular enzymes. Foscarnet inhibits DNA chain elongation by preventing pyrophosphate exchange.[189]

Foscarnet inhibits the DNA polymerase of CMV and other herpesviruses (HSV-1, HSV-2, VZV, and Epstein–Barr virus [EBV]) and the replication of HIV in vitro and in vivo.[190] Both herpesvirus and HIV replication may be inhibited by thera-

peutically achievable concentrations of foscarnet. Since the drug is not metabolized and is excreted by the kidney, the dosage must be adjusted for renal insufficiency. Foscarnet also has been used successfully to treat HIV-infected patients with acyclovir-resistant HSV and VZV infections, in addition to CMV retinitis. It may be particularly useful for patients who develop herpetic retinitis (ARN) while taking oral acyclovir to suppress cutaneous disease.

Foscarnet acts directly on the viral polymerase of all herpesviruses and on the reverse transcriptase of HIV-1. Resistance of CMV to foscarnet is associated with mutations in the genes of these polymerases. Cross-resistance to antiviral drugs is likely to be an increasing problem, since patients with AIDS are living longer as a result of HAART and of the drugs used in the prophylaxis of various opportunistic infections, as well as because of the experience gained in the management of HIV-related problems.

Foscarnet has been shown to be useful against ganciclovir-resistant herpesviruses, such as CMV, because a mutation in a DNA polymerase gene conferring resistance to ganciclovir and acyclovir differs from the region conferring resistance to foscarnet.[191] Foscarnet also is an effective inhibitor of the HIV reverse transcriptase enzyme and acts in a dose-dependent manner. AZT and foscarnet have synergistic activity in vitro against HIV, and in vivo, foscarnet has activity against HIV as measured by surrogate markers.[192]

The use of foscarnet salvage therapy in patients with CMV retinitis who are intolerant of or resistant to ganciclovir was studied in AIDS patients with CMV retinitis who had documented hematologic intolerance or resistance to ganciclovir therapy. This study showed that in patients intolerant of ganciclovir, salvage foscarnet therapy resulted in a longer time to retinitis progression than reported previously in historic controls who terminated ganciclovir therapy. In patients who exhibited clinical resistance to ganciclovir, foscarnet appeared to have efficacy in controlling retinitis. No significant differences in either efficacy or toxicity were observed in the range of foscarnet maintenance doses studied.[193]

A large, randomized, multicenter, blinded clinical trial (the Foscarnet–Ganciclovir Cytomegalovirus Retinitis Trial) compared ganciclovir with foscarnet in the treatment of CMV retinitis in patients with AIDS. There were 234 patients enrolled and treated by a common protocol at 12 centers. No difference was reported between the treatment groups in the rate of progression of retinitis; however, the median survival was 8.5 months in the ganciclovir group and 12.6 months in the foscarnet group. Excess mortality was reported in a subset of patients in the foscarnet group whose renal function was compromised at entry. Differences in mortality could not be explained entirely on the basis of less antiretroviral therapy in the ganciclovir group, which suggests beneficial interactions between foscarnet and antiretroviral nucleosides. These results indicate that, for patients with AIDS and CMV retinitis, treatment with foscarnet initially offers a survival advantage over treatment with ganciclovir, although foscarnet was not as well tolerated as ganciclovir.[194]

A marginally prolonged survival seen in patients treated with foscarnet compared with those treated with ganciclovir may have been due to a direct effect on HIV replication. Both drugs had a suppressive effect on circulating p24 antigen, which was predictive of improved survival. The inhibitory effect on CMV replication also may have a beneficial effect on limiting HIV replication.[195]

A randomized, controlled, comparative trial of foscarnet and ganciclovir demonstrated that they equally controlled CMV retinitis but that foscarnet was associated with a longer survival, possibly as a result of its antiretroviral effect. However, foscarnet was less well tolerated than ganciclovir, primarily because of the nature of its side effects. Since foscarnet and ganciclovir have different side effects, initial treatment of CMV retinitis should be individualized.[196]

Since neutropenia was a frequent dose-limiting adverse effect of ganciclovir and precluded the use of AZT, it is tempting to view the advent of colony-stimulating factors such as G-CSF or GM-CSF with some optimism so that it may be possible to use ganciclovir more commonly with AZT.[174]

The most frequently reported major adverse effect associated with foscarnet administration is nephrotoxicity, with dose-limiting toxicity occurring frequently and cases of acute renal failure having been observed. Symptomatic hypocalcemia has been reported and may be responsible for arrhythmias and seizures, and the risk is increased by concurrent administration of intravenous pentamidine. Disturbances of other divalent cations and electrolytes occur and may cause hypercalcemia and hyperphosphatemia or hypophosphatemia. Decreases of ionized calcium have occurred transiently at the usual doses of foscarnet. Bone marrow suppression with neutropenia, anemia, and thrombocytopenia can be seen with foscarnet administration. Neutropenia was reported to be less common with foscarnet than with ganciclovir (14% vs. 34%).[194]

Practical guidelines for the use of foscarnet include administration through an infusion pump to avoid the potential consequences of overdose or too rapid infusion, adequate hydration of patients with saline loading[197] to reduce the risk of nephrotoxicity, avoidance of administration of other potentially nephrotoxic agents, and monitoring of renal function two or three times per week during induction therapy and once per week during maintenance therapy, with the dosage being recalculated on the basis of patient weight and serum creatinine. The toxicities of foscarnet have little overlap with those of AZT, and both can be used concomitantly. Foscarnet has identical pharmacokinetics when given either twice or three times daily.[198] Studies of foscarnet doses have suggested that patients receiving high maintenance doses (120 mg/kg/day) have slower rates of retinitis progression.[199,200]

Foscarnet is active against HIV, and studies have shown that it raises the CD4+ count transiently and decreases viral antigenemia (p24 antigen).[190] Because of its efficacy against CMV and HIV, it would appear to be a potentially effective agent for treating HIV-infected patients; however, it is currently only available for intravenous administration, and its use is associated with substantial toxicity (see above).[192,201–203]

Several factors have been shown to influence the time to progression of CMV retinitis among HIV-infected patients being treated with foscarnet. In a multivariate Cox model, only the area under the concentration-time curve (AUC) and the status of the baseline CMV blood culture significantly affected the time to progression of the retinitis. These results suggest that the AUC produced by a dose of foscarnet has a wide interindividual range. The AUC of foscarnet significantly altered time to progression of the retinitis. However, patients with positive baseline CMV blood cultures had a significantly more shallow dose-response curve. This indicates that the added risk of nephrotoxicity, which is present with aggressive foscarnet dosing, might be best borne by the subgroup of patients with a positive CMV blood culture at baseline.[204] Nephrotoxicity is seen with both foscarnet and cidofovir.

Cidofovir

Cidofovir, (S)-1-[3-hydroxy-2-(phosphonylmethoxy)propyl]-cytosine, formerly known as HPMPC, was the first antiviral nucleotide analog available for the treatment of CMV retinitis. Because cidofovir does not require viral activation, it has two advantages over the nucleoside analogs such as ganciclovir and acyclovir. Cidofovir is active in uninfected cells, may act preemptively, and may retain activity against ganciclovir-resistant strains. Preclinical studies showed the major toxicity of cidofovir to be dose-, schedule-, and species-dependent nephrotoxicity. The concomitant administration of probenecid protects animal models against cidofovir-induced nephrotoxicity. Four treatment modifications are indicated clinically to reduce the incidence of cidofovir-related nephrotoxicity: dose reduction or interruption for changes in renal function; concomitant administration of probenecid; administration of 1 liter of normal saline 1 hour before infusion; and extension of the dosing interval.[205]

The treatment of CMV retinitis with intravenous cidofovir was demonstrated to be effective in slowing the progression of peripheral CMV retinitis in patients with previously untreated CMV retinitis and AIDS.[206,207] Intravenous cidofovir also has been used for long-term suppression of CMV retinitis. Biweekly therapy (after induction therapy) was reported to have a time to progression of CMV retinitis of 120 days in one randomized, controlled trial[206] and 2.5 months in another randomized, controlled trial.[206A] Treatment and subsequent maintenance of CMV retinitis with 20 μg of intravitreously injected cidofovir, given at 5- to 6-week intervals, also is safe and highly effective.[208]

Treatment with parenteral cidofovir is complicated by nephrotoxicity, which can be reduced with saline hydration and concomitant administration of probenecid. Despite these additional treatments, the long-term reports from the HPMPC Peripheral Cytomegalovirus Retinitis Trial showed a rate of proteinuria of 1.22 per patient-year and a rate of elevated serum creatinine of 0.41 per patient-year. Over the course of the study 90% of patients with proteinuria showed resolution within a mean of 20 days and 80% of patients with elevated serum creatinine had normalization of creatinine levels within a mean of 28 days. In addition, no patients required dialysis. This study also reported that the rate of discontinuation of cidofovir related to probenecid reactions was 0.35 per person-year.[206A] Thus many patients may have difficulty tolerating cidofovir for a prolonged time.

Neutropenia has also been reported with cidofovir. One short-term study found that 15% of patients experienced neutropenia and a long-term study showed a rate of neutropenia to be 0.30 per person-year.[206,206A]

Unfortunately parenteral cidofovir has also been found to have ocular toxicity, including a high incidence of iritis (up to 50%), including recurrent iritis, and a risk of profound ocular hypotony with vision loss, similar to the iritis and hypotony seen with intravitreal injections of cidofovir.[209–212] It has been estimated in one study that cidofovir-related iritis developed in half of patients within approximately 4 months.[209] The long-term reports from the HPMPC Peripheral Cytomegalovirus Retinitis Trial showed a rate of cidofovir-associated uveitis of 0.20 per person-year and a rate of significant ocular hypotony of 0.16 per patient-year.[206A] Thus in the setting of iritis in HIV-infected patients, use of systemic cidofovir or rifabutin should be considered potential causes of iritis, and these drugs may need to be discontinued.

Nephrotoxicity may be cumulative in some patients and appears to be related to toxicity in the proximal tubule. This "secretory toxicity" also may be responsible for the hypotony and iritis that the drug causes when given intravenously or intravitreously. The ciliary body and the proximal tubule of the kidney have many similarities in terms of the mechanism involved in the secretion of fluids across epithelia. Oral administration of probenecid before and after the intravenous infusion appears to help ameliorate the nephrotoxicity of the drug, but the ocular side effects of iritis and hypotony occur despite concomitant probenecid administration.

CYTOMEGALOVIRUS RESISTANCE

The prevalence of resistance at diagnosis of CMV to ganciclovir or foscarnet was determined before the initiation of therapy in a prospective study in an AIDS clinic. Cultures of blood and urine samples for CMV were obtained, and testing of all positive isolates for sensitivity to ganciclovir and foscarnet was performed. No blood culture isolates were resistant to ganciclovir, and only one urine culture isolate (2% of patients) was resistant to ganciclovir; 3% of blood culture isolates and 4% of urine culture isolates (2% and 2% of patients, respectively) were resistant to foscarnet. Overall, 4% of patients had either a blood or urine culture isolate resistant to foscarnet. Resistance to ganciclovir or foscarnet at the time of diagnosis of CMV retinitis was uncommon in this study.[213]

However, many patients taking chronic maintenance therapy for CMV retinitis develop resistant virus. Development of in vitro resistance of CMV to ganciclovir and foscarnet and disease progression has been shown in several small studies,[176,214,215] and mechanisms of resistance to ganciclovir have been described.[216] In the study by Drew et al.[217] of 13 culture-positive patients treated for more than 3 months, five excreted CMV resistant to ganciclovir in the urine. In one prospective, randomized study of 207 patients with newly diagnosed CMV retinitis,

drug-resistant CMV occurred in four of nine ganciclovir-treated patients and in none of five foscarnet-treated patients.[144] In patients with CMV retinitis and AIDS treated with either oral or intravenous ganciclovir, isolates of CMV after a median exposure of 75 and 165 days, respectively, showed increasing resistance in vitro.[218] Jabs et al. reported that the cumulative incidence of ganciclovir resistance at 9 months was 27.5%.[215] Similar incidence rates of resistance occur for foscarnet and cidofovir.[219] In addition the incidence of resistance to valganciclovir appears to be similar to that for ganciclovir.[220]

Resistance to an anti-CMV drug can be described as phenotypic, expressed as an inhibitory concentration 50% greater than a certain threshold (IC_{50}). This is determined typically via plaque reduction assays, DNA hybridization assays, or antigen-reduction assays that requires large amounts of viable virus often requiring culturing.[217,218,221,231,234–238] For ganciclovir this IC_{50} level for what is termed low level resistance is typically 6.0 µM and 30 µM for high-level resistance.[213,215–217,221–230] Foscarnet and cidofovir IC_{50} resistance levels are typically 400–600 µM and 2–4 µM respectively.[216,217,231–234] Genotypic resistance is defined by the presence of a mutation in the CMV genome conferring resistance to a particular drug. PCR amplification techniques allow fast detection of resistance conferring mutations in the viral genome, requiring only small amounts of viral nucleic acids and can use nonviable virus.[234,239–241] Low-level ganciclovir resistance is typically associated with mutations in the CMV *UL97* gene. *UL97* codes for a phosphotransferase that catalyzes the first step of ganciclovir activation to the triphosphate form. High level ganciclovir resistance is typically caused by mutations in both the CMV *UL97* and *UL54* genes. *UL54* codes for the cytomegalovirus DNA polymerase.[216,223–230] Mutations in the *UL54* gene are also responsible for foscarnet and cidofovir resistance.[216,224,226,228,229,233,234,242–245] Strong correlation between phenotypic and genotypic resistance has been reported for ganciclovir and foscarnet.[230,234]

CMV UL54 DNA polymerase mutations conferring cidofovir resistance are typically seen with high-level ganciclovir resistance. UL54 mutations responsible for foscarnet resistance are usually distinct from those causing ganciclovir-cidofovir resistance. However, low-grade ganciclovir–foscarnet cross resistance has been reported plus Chou et al. reported a DNA polymerase mutation causing resistance to ganciclovir, cidofovir, and foscarnet.[215,216,224,226,228,229,233,242,245]

There is evidence that CMV blood specimens reflect events within the eye based on agreement found for mutations and polymorphisms between CMV DNA isolated from vitreous and blood samples.[246] In addition, studies have shown that the presence of resistant CMV in blood or urine correlates with worse ocular outcomes including higher rates of disease progression, larger retinal areas involved, and higher rates of contralateral disease in addition to higher rates of extraocular CMV.[215,223,247,248] Resistance to antiviral therapy as a potential cause of progression of CMV retinitis in patients with AIDS was investigated by conducting viral sensitivity testing in patients with clinically resistant retinitis who had positive results of blood or urine CMV cultures. Foscarnet-resistant CMV was isolated from two patients, one who was being treated with foscarnet. Ganciclovir-resistant CMV was isolated from four patients, three of whom were being treated with ganciclovir. Foscarnet- and ganciclovir-resistant CMV occurred with previous ganciclovir therapy in one patient. Clinical improvement occurred in three patients, whose change in therapy was made on the basis of viral sensitivity testing. In general, prolonged therapy with one drug was associated with a progressive increase in the ID_{50} for that drug.[247]

Treatment strategies in resistant CMV

When clinically resistant retinitis appears, many clinicians employ an alternative antiviral agent systemically; intravenous cidofovir or foscarnet are alternatives. Unfortunately as mentioned above, there can be cross-resistance between CMV isolates resistant to ganciclovir and resistant to cidofovir and/or foscarnet; this must be borne in mind in such patients. However, resistance may be step-wise as low level ganciclovir resistance is not associated with resistance to either cidofovir or to foscarnet.[215,216,224,226,228,229,233,234,242–245,249] Unfortunately, the probability of developing foscarnet or cidofovir resistance while taking these drugs appears similar to the rates of development of resistance to ganciclovir.[219] For this reason, clinicians often employ intravitreal therapies including the ganciclovir intraocular device when systemic therapy begins to fail. Intravitreal therapies appear to be more effective in such circumstances, largely because they deliver higher doses of anti-CMV medication to the retina.[249] In such circumstances, it is recommended to continue to treat the patient with some form of systemic therapy, often oral valganciclovir, to help prevent systemic CMV infection or infection of the fellow eye. Studies have shown that treatment with the ganciclovir implant alone is associated with a higher risk of contralateral CMV retinitis and extraocular CMV.[161A,248,250]

Combination therapies

Ganciclovir–foscarnet

Several studies have shown that combinations of foscarnet and ganciclovir are more effective in the treatment of recurrent or resistant retinitis than is continued monotherapy.[108A,78,251] Such combination intravenous therapy also has been shown to be safe and effective in children with CMV retinitis.[253] Unfortunately, combination intravenous therapy with these two drugs necessitates multiple intravenous infusions daily and has a marked negative effect on patients' lifestyle. Combination of IV foscarnet and oral valganciclovir has supplanted this combination intravenous therapy.

Since the clinical efficacy of long-term chemosuppressive or maintenance therapy has been reported to correlate with total weekly maintenance dose for both ganciclovir and foscarnet, and since toxicity is dose-limiting in up to 20% of patients receiving either drug chronically, it may be beneficial in long-term maintenance therapy to combine these two drugs. This strategy may result in a greater net antiviral effect with more efficacy and less toxicity than seen with either drug alone, because the toxicity profiles of each drug are quite different.

The combination of foscarnet and ganciclovir in patients with AIDS and CMV retinitis who have relapsed has been shown to be more effective than either agent given alone[178]; however, combination therapy was associated with the greatest negative impact of treatment on quality of life measures.

To determine the best therapeutic systemic regimen for treatment of relapsed CMV retinitis, a multicenter, randomized, controlled clinical trial of 279 patients with AIDS and either persistently active or relapsed CMV retinitis was reported. Patients were randomized to one of three therapeutic regimens: induction with foscarnet sodium at 90 mg/kg intravenously every 12 hours for 2 weeks, followed by maintenance at a dosage of 120 mg/kg per day (foscarnet group); induction with ganciclovir sodium at 5 mg/kg intravenously every 12 hours for 2 weeks followed by maintenance at 10 mg/kg per day (ganciclovir group); or continuation of previous maintenance therapy plus induction with the other drug (either ganciclovir or foscarnet) for 2 weeks followed by maintenance therapy with both drugs, ganciclovir sodium at 5 mg/kg per day and foscarnet sodium at 90 mg/kg per day (combination therapy group). The mortality rate was similar among the three groups. Median survival times were as follows: foscarnet group, 8.4 months; ganciclovir group, 9.0 months; and combination therapy group, 8.6 months ($P = 0.89$). Comparison of retinitis progression revealed that combination therapy was the most effective regimen for controlling the retinitis. The median times to retinitis progression were as follows: foscarnet group, 1.3 months; ganciclovir group, 2.0 months; and combination therapy group, 4.3 months ($P < 0.001$). Although no difference could be detected in visual acuity outcomes, visual field loss and retinal area involvement on fundus photographs both paralleled the progression results, with the most favorable results in the combination therapy group. The rates of visual field loss were as follows: foscarnet group, 28 degrees per month; ganciclovir group, 18 degrees per month; combination therapy group, 16 degrees per month ($P = 0.009$). The rates of increase of retinal area involved by CMV were as follows: foscarnet group, 2.47% per month; ganciclovir group, 1.40% per month; and combination therapy group, 1.19% per month ($P = 0.04$). Although side effects were similar among the three treatment groups, combination therapy was associated with the greatest negative impact of treatment on quality-of-life measures. This study suggests that for patients with AIDS and CMV retinitis whose retinitis has relapsed and who can tolerate both drugs, combination therapy appears to be the most effective therapy for controlling CMV retinitis.[178]

Small series suggest that combined intravitreal injections of ganciclovir and foscarnet may be effective in treating CMV retinitis when the infection is clinically resistant to either intravitreal drug alone.[254]

SUMMARY OF INITIAL SYSTEMIC CMV RETINITIS TREATMENT

The initial treatment of CMV retinitis is usually oral valganciclovir 900 mg twice a day for induction therapy of approximately 3 weeks followed by 900 mg daily for maintenance therapy. Intravenous ganciclovir can be used if a patient has a contraindication to oral treatment such as malabsorption. The dose for intravenous ganciclovir is 5 mg/kg twice a day for induction therapy for 2–3 weeks followed by maintenance therapy at 5 mg/kg daily or 6 mg/kg 5 days/week. Induction therapy with intravenous foscarnet is dosed at 90 mg/kg twice a day for approximately 2 weeks followed by maintenance therapy at 120 mg/kg daily. Intravenous cidofovir for induction therapy is dosed at 5 mg/kg weekly for approximately 3 weeks followed by maintenance therapy dosed at 3–5 mg/kg every 2 weeks.

INTRAOCULAR THERAPY OF VIRAL RETINITIS

Ganciclovir

Because of the difficulties associated with systemic ganciclovir, foscarnet, and cidofovir, interest in local administration has increased. Obviously, intraocular (or periocular) treatment will not affect the systemic CMV infection, but in some patients, especially those with systemic toxicity resulting from the drug, local administration may have certain advantages. In rabbits, intravitreal ganciclovir injections of up to 400 μg produced no ophthalmoscopic, histologic, or electroretinographic changes. However, multiple injections have been associated with retinal toxicity in animals; this does not appear to be the case in humans.[255,256] The median inhibitory dose of ganciclovir to inhibit CMV replication is less than 2 mg/ml. Similar inhibitory doses for HSV, VZV, and EBV have been shown.[257]

The intravitreous and plasma ganciclovir and foscarnet concentrations after intravenous administration in AIDS patients with CMV retinitis and retinal detachment were shown to result in borderline or progressively subtherapeutic concentrations, suggesting that local therapy may be more effective than systemic therapy.[249]

Multiple intraocular injections of ganciclovir have been successful in controlling CMV retinitis in at least one patient who was treated over 3 months with a total of 28 intravitreal injections totaling 200 mg.[96] No evidence of retinal toxicity was noted, and the estimated half-life of the drug in the human vitreous was 13 hours.

In 40 patients with primary CMV retinitis involving 57 eyes, all had received one 14-day course of intravenous ganciclovir and all were free of other end-organ CMV disease. All affected eyes received weekly intravitreal injections of 400 μg of ganciclovir for maintenance therapy. Median survival of patients was at least 13 months. Fifteen patients had 19 new opportunistic infections during the observation period, but none developed new nonocular CMV disease. Active retinitis recurred in 68.4% of the eyes while receiving maintenance therapy, with a median time to progression of 14.7 weeks. CMV retinitis occurred in 30.4% of the previously uninvolved eyes (follow-up 3.1 years). Bacterial endophthalmitis complicated treatment in one eye, and retinal detachment developed in five eyes. Thus the long-term treatment of CMV retinitis with weekly intraocular injections of ganciclovir was associated with survival and ocular outcomes similar to those reported with systemic ganciclovir.[258]

Intravitreal ganciclovir also was shown to be an effective alternative to systemic ganciclovir in patients with severe neutropenia and in patients who choose to continue receiving systemic zidovudine or didanosine.[259] Injections of high-dose intravitreal ganciclovir using a 2 mg dose revealed that weekly 2 mg injections appear to offer superior control of retinitis for periods of months or longer.[260] Extremely high doses of intravitreal ganciclovir (40 mg) have been shown to be extremely toxic.[261] Highly concentrated ganciclovir solution for intravitreal injection also reduced repeated amaurosis and ocular pain and was reported by patients to have improved their comfort and quality of life, thus increasing their compliance to treatment and reducing side effects, as compared with usual protocols.[262]

Foscarnet

Intravitreal foscarnet at a dose of 2.4 mg per injection given one or two times weekly also appears to be a safe and effective treatment method for CMV retinitis. However, resistance to this treatment regimen may develop.[263] High-dose intravitreal foscarnet for CMV retinitis was shown to be a safe, effective, and useful alternative in patients with intolerance to intravenous therapy.[264]

Ganciclovir intraocular device

An intraocular sustained-release ganciclovir delivery implant that releases drug into the vitreous is commercially available.[265] These surgically implanted, time-release implants have been shown to be more effective than intravenous ganciclovir alone in delaying the progression of CMV retinitis.[161A,248,250,266,267]

Insertion of the device requires a pars plana incision and a partial vitrectomy. The implant is sewn into the pars plana behind the lens.[265] Insertion of the ganciclovir intraocular device (GIOD) requires trimming the strut of the device so that it is nearly flush with the drug pellet. A 5.5 mm incision can be made 4 mm posterior to the limbus with a microvitreoretinal blade or similar instrument (Fig. 92-11). Cautery may be necessary, but bleeding oftentimes is minimal. A unimanual bipolar intraocular cautery can be used to coagulate bleeding choroid. It is important to ensure that the incision is full thickness, since the device can be inserted inadvertently under the pars plana. A suture is placed through the preplaced hole (the surgeon must make the hole) in the strut of the device; 8-0 Prolene can be used. The device is anchored in the middle of the wound, and running or interrupted sutures can be used to close the wound. Some surgeons incorporate the running suture and anchoring suture into one suture. Astigmatism can result from overzealous wound closure; this is usually transient. This procedure can be performed in an outpatient setting under local anesthesia.

Despite the relative ease of insertion, it has become clear that the risk of retinal detachment in the first 2 months after insertion is substantially higher than if other methods are used to control retinitis, though in the long term there is no statistical difference in retinal detachment rate.[161A,266,268–271] In addition, the risk of postoperative endophthalmitis appears to be a

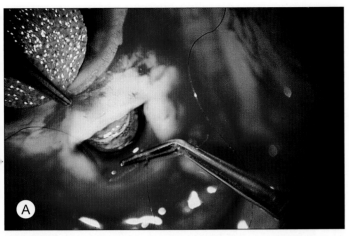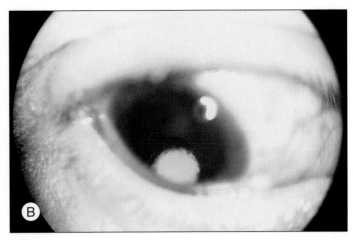

Fig. 92-11 A, Insertion of ganciclovir intraocular device. B, The device can be seen inferotemporally through a dilated pupil.

real one, with incidences on the order of 1% or sometimes higher.[272] The intravitreal levels attained by this drug are over twice those after intravenous administration, and this appears to be associated with a lower incidence of resistance and progression of retinitis. This is particularly true in newly diagnosed cases, but failure can occur in up to 25% of such cases within the first 2 months. In a study of 91 implants in 70 eyes, GIOD was effective as an adjunct to continued systemic therapy in those patients with recurrent CMV retinitis.[267] Intraocular sustained-release implants have been used to treat acute CMV disease and to prevent recurrence.[162,266] In this later, unpublished study, median time to progression for patients treated with intraocular sustained-release implants was 216 days vs. 104 days for those treated with intravenous ganciclovir ($P < 0.00001$). The median time to retinitis progression with the ganciclovir implant is 7 months in newly diagnosed cases; it is less in cases with resistant retinitis. Pathology studies of eyes having undergone implantation with the GIOD have shown no evidence of intraocular toxicity.[168] Adverse events associated with implantation of the GIOD include a risk of early retinal detachment that appears to be higher than would be associated with other therapies, as well as vision reduction in the postoperative period. In addition, vitreous hemorrhage and endophthalmitis appear to have an increased incidence with the implant. It is not certain whether implants should be exchanged at the 7-month time period or whether retinitis should be allowed to reactivate before replacing the implant. A longer acting implant, which would release ganciclovir for up to 2 years, was developed but never commercialized.

Intravitreal cidofovir

Another form of intraocular therapy is intravitreal cidofovir (HPMPC), which is injected every 6 weeks. This work was initiated after discovery of long-acting properties of the drug in the eye. In animal models of retinitis, the duration of a single injection of cidofovir was approximately 10 times that of intravitreal ganciclovir.[273] The safety and efficacy of intravitreal

cidofovir for CMV retinitis in humans were reported in a phase I/II unmasked, consecutive case series in a single-center institutional referral practice. Eligible patients with AIDS had active CMV retinitis in at least one eye, despite adequate intravenous therapy with ganciclovir or foscarnet, were intolerant to intravenous therapy, were noncompliant with intravenous therapy, or refused intravenous therapy. In a preliminary safety study (group 1), 10 eyes of nine patients received 14 injections of cidofovir while being treated concurrently with intravenous ganciclovir. In a dose-escalating efficacy study (group 2), eight eyes of seven patients received 11 injections of cidofovir as sole treatment for CMV retinitis. The primary outcome was time to retinitis progression. In the group 1 eyes receiving 20 µg of cidofovir, the median time to retinitis progression was between 49 and 92 days (mean, 78 days). In group 2 eyes treated with 20 µg of cidofovir, the median time to retinitis progression was 64 days (mean, 63 days). Hypotony occurred in the two eyes treated with a 100 µg dose of cidofovir and in one of three eyes receiving a 40 µg dose. No adverse effects resulted from the remaining 20 µg cidofovir injections. Cidofovir was found to be safe and effective for the local treatment of CMV retinitis, providing a long duration of antiviral effect[274] (Fig. 92-12).

It was then shown that injections of 20 µg of intravitreal HPMPC resulted in complete suppression of CMV replication with no advancement of retinitis borders when given every 6 weeks.[208,211,275-279] Pharmacologic studies have shown that after intravitreal injection, the phosphorylated metabolites of cidofovir remain in retinal cells for prolonged periods, with an estimated intracellular half-life of 3 days.[280] This medication must be given with oral probenecid. Probenecid 2 g is given orally 2 hours before, and 1 g 2 hours and 8 hours after injection. The infrequent administration of this probenecid regimen (once every 6 weeks) has not resulted in a significant incidence of allergic reaction.

Two types of adverse events may occur after intravitreal cidofovir injection: iritis and hypotony. The incidence of these is not dissimilar to what is seen after intravenous administration. The

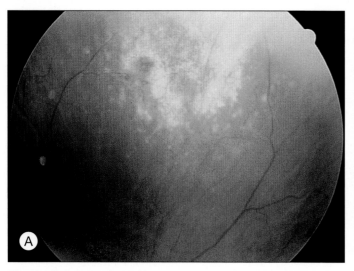
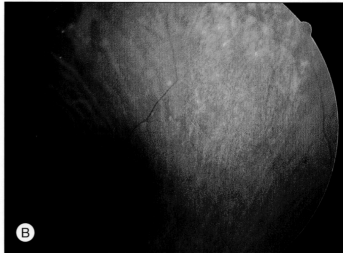

Fig. 92-12 A, Active CMV retinitis with no systemic treatment. The eye was injected with a single injection of cidofovir 20 µg via the pars plana. B, The retinitis remains healed 53 days later, with no other therapy.

incidence of iritis can be reduced from 70% to 18% if oral probenecid is used, and it is now recommended universally. Iritis can be managed with topical steroids and cycloplegia; however, it may lead to cataract and synechiae in the long term. The other complication of concern is lowering of intraocular pressure (IOP). A mild, asymptomatic 20% reduction in IOP is seen almost universally after cidofovir injection, and this appears to be of no concern. The mechanism of this has been defined by ultrasound biomicroscopy, which has disclosed that severe hypotony after cidofovir injections is associated with ciliary body atrophy.[275] Reduction in aqueous flow has been demonstrated by aqueous fluorophotometry. This effect on secretory epithelia also is probably responsible for the nephrotoxicity of the drug when given intravenously. Indeed, probenecid also is given before and after each intravenous infusion to prevent uptake by the proximal tubule of the kidney and associated nephrotoxicity. Profound hypotony with vision loss occurs in approximately 1% of injections. It has been possible to replicate the hypotony effect of cidofovir in the guinea pig eye, and it is hoped that this animal model will allow evaluation of other derivatives of this compound that may have larger therapeutic indices.[277,281]

A retrospective, cohort study described iritis and hypotony after treatment with intravenous cidofovir for CMV retinitis in association with intraocular inflammation.[209] Eleven cases of iritis (26%) occurred among 43 patients. In six cases the iritis was bilateral. Patients who experienced iritis were more likely to have been previously treated for CMV retinitis ($P = 0.03$), to be diabetic ($P = 0.05$), or to be receiving protease inhibitors ($P < 0.001$). Four patients and 15 control subjects had also taken rifabutin ($P = 0.70$). The onset of iritis occurred at a mean ($\pm$SD) of 4.9 $\pm$ 1.8 days after a cidofovir dose and after a mean ($\pm$SD) of 4.2 $\pm$ 1.6 doses of cidofovir. Six eyes of four patients had hypotony. Five eyes of five patients had a persistent decrease in visual acuity of at least two Snellen lines. Acute intraocular inflammation may occur with or without

hypotony after intravenous cidofovir therapy, similar to the reactions seen after intravitreous administration. Although the manifestations may be severe, they are manageable with topical corticosteroid therapy in most cases. Cidofovir therapy can be continued in some patients if medical necessity warrants, but inflammation may recur or permanent hypotony develop.

A lower cidofovir dose (10 µg) has been used to investigate methods of reducing the toxicity of intravitreal cidofovir. This dose is effective in healing retinitis in 75% of patients, but the response in 25% is inadequate. The 10 µg dose, however, is not associated with a significant incidence of iritis or IOP lowering. Cidofovir should be diluted in a sterile manner by a pharmacist. It can be diluted in normal saline and frozen for extended periods in single-dose vials.

The efficacy and safety of multiple intravitreal cidofovir (HPMPC) injections given every 5 to 6 weeks for the maintenance treatment of CMV retinitis with 20 µg intravitreally injected was shown to be highly effective, with only rare episodes of reactivation and progression.[211]

A correlation between intraocular pressure and CD4+ T-lymphocyte counts in patients with HIV with and without CMV retinitis has been described.[282] Intraocular pressure was measured with calibrated Goldmann applanation tonometers in two groups of patients. Group A included 84 HIV patients (120 eyes) with CMV retinitis, and group B included 110 HIV patients (183 eyes) without CMV retinitis; 33 patients without HIV (66 eyes) were included as a control group. Step-wise regression analysis of IOP included correlation with CMV retinitis (presence, extent, and activity), CD4+ T-lymphocyte count, age, and gender. The mean IOP was 9.8 mmHg in group A, 12.6 mmHg in group B, and 16.1 mmHg in the control group. All three groups were statistically different from each other when intraocular pressure was compared ($P < 0.0001$). Step-wise regression showed that low CD4+ T-lymphocyte count and extent of CMV retinitis both correlated to low IOP. These results demonstrate that IOP is lower than normal in patients with HIV and that decreased CD4$^+$ T-lymphocyte count is the major factor associated with low IOP, accounting for 20% of the effect. The extent of CMV retinitis accounts for 8% of the effect. The incidence of a previously reported mild anterior nongranulomatous uveitis associated with intravitreal injections of cidofovir was seen in 26% of patients after first-time HPMPC injection. Concomitant use of probenecid appeared to decrease the frequency of the iritis from 71% to 18% in patients with AIDS and CMV retinitis after the first intravitreal injection of HPMPC. Topical corticosteroid administration after injection (before iritis) was ineffective in preventing iritis; treatment with topical corticosteroids and cycloplegics resulted in resolution of all iritis cases.[281]

Fomivirsen

Fomivirsen, formerly called ISIS 2922,[283] was approved by the FDA in August 1998 for the treatment of CMV retinitis in AIDS patients intolerant of or who have a contraindication to other CMV regimens or who were insufficiently responsive to previous treatments for CMV retinitis. Fomivirsen is the first of a class of antisense oligonucleotides. This compound possesses potent anti-CMV activity, but does not target the CMV viral DNA polymerase. Fomivirsen is a 21-base synthetic phosphorothioate oligonucleotide designed to be complementary to CMV mRNA that encodes for the major immediate early region (IE2) proteins of CMV. Binding to this location results in specific inhibition of gene expression that is critical to production of essential viral proteins. The nucleotide sequence of fomivirsen (5'-GCG TTT GCT CTT CTT CTT GCG-3') appears to be unique for mRNA produced by CMV; it is not complementary to any known mRNA sequence in humans. Fomivirsen inhibits CMV in vitro over a range of concentrations form 0.03 ± 0.02 μM (EC50 in human RPE cells) to 0.34 ± 0.25 μM (EC50 in human fibroblast cells).[284–290]

Following intravitreal administration, the rate of vitreous clearance of fomivirsen is first-order with a half-life of approximately 55 hours in humans. Preclinical studies showed that fomivirsen distributes to the retina and is metabolized by exonuclease digestion. Measurable concentrations of drug are not detected in the systemic circulation after intravitreal injection making the interaction of fomivirsen with systemic drugs unlikely. In addition, the coadministration of fomivirsen with antiretrovirals and other anti-CMV medications is acceptable, the only warning being against administration within 2–4 weeks of cidofovir treatment because of the risk of ocular inflammation.[291] Preclinical studies of fomivirsen by Freeman and associates suggested that this type of antiviral antisense compound does inhibit viral replication; however, it did cause changes in the RPE and intraocular inflammation at doses only moderately higher than the dose needed to treat retinitis by the intravitreal route.[283,292]

Recently the Vitravene Study Group published the data from the clinical trials involving fomivirsen. Two prospective randomized open-label controlled clinical trials (USA/Brazilian and EuroCanadian Studies) compared two fomivirsen regimens for the treatment of reactivated CMV retinitis or CMV retinitis

that was persistently active despite other anti-CMV treatments. The more intense schedule (regimen A) included 61 patients (67 eyes) and consisted of three weekly 330 μg (0.05 ml) intravitreal injections for induction, then 330 μg every 2 weeks for maintenance therapy. The less intense schedule (regimen B) included 32 patients (39 eyes) and utilized a 330 μg injection for induction on day 1 and day 15, then 330 μg injections every 4 weeks for maintenance therapy. The study end point was time to progression based on masked evaluation of serial fundus photos. Eligibility criteria included AIDS patients with active CMV retinitis who had failed prior treatment with ganciclovir, foscarnet, or cidofovir.[293]

In the USA/Brazilian study, median time to progression was 106 days (interpolated median 88.6 days) for regimen A; 267 days (interpolated median 111.3 days) for regimen B ($P = 0.2179$ Wilcoxon rank sum test; 0.2950 log rank). In the EuroCanadian study the median time to progression was not determinable for regimen A; only four patients progressed (25th percentile 91 days). The median time to progression for regimen B was 403 days (interpolated median 182 days).[293]

A smaller study that evaluated fomivirsen for newly diagnosed CMV retinitis was also conducted. This prospective, randomized treatment intervention clinical trial compared immediate treatment with 165 μg fomivirsen (18 patients) to deferral (10 patients) until CMV retinitis progressed. Patients were randomized to treatment vs. deferral in a 2:1 ratio. The primary endpoint was time to first CMV retinitis progression based on masked fundus photo assessment. Treatment involved three weekly 165 μg intravitreal injections for induction then 165 μg injections every 2 weeks for maintenance therapy for at least 18 weeks. Treatment patients received regular exams until progression; deferral patients received weekly exams and were offered fomivirsen treatment at the time of progression. Baseline CD4 count was not significantly different between the two groups ($P = 0.188$).[290]

Median time to progression in treatment group was 71 days (95% CI 28 days–ND); in deferral group 13 days (95% CI 9–15 days) ($P = 0.0001$ Wilcoxon rank sum test). Progression occurred in 44% of treatment patients and in 70% of deferral patients. Despite the efficacy shown in this study the FDA did not approve fomivirsen for first line therapy based on the small sample size.[290]

The safety and toxicity of fomivirsen was also reported by the Vitravene study group. The most often reported adverse events were anterior chamber inflammation and increased IOP. For inflammation: 165 μg dose: 0.72 events/patient-year; 330 μg dose (less intense regimen): 1.28 events/patient-year; 330 μg injection (more intense regimen): 2.17 events/patient-year. In the USA/Brazilian study, 18 inflammatory events occurred in 14 patients; 15 events had treatment information reported: topical steroids were given to 11 patients with time to resolution ranging from 7–80 days (median 28 days).[294]

For IOP above 24 mmHg: 165 μg dose: 0.56 events/patient-year; 330 μg dose (less intense regimen): 0.36 events/patient-year; 330 μg dose (more intense regimen): 1.39 events/patient-year. Intraocular pressure rises were equally divided between mild (25–30 mmHg), moderate (31–40 mmHg), and severe (41–50 mmHg). In the USA/Brazilian study, of 21 episodes (median IOP 32.5 mmHg) 19 were treated with topical medicines; in all cases IOP returned to normal within 14 days.[294]

Retinal pigment epitheliopathy occurred in 5/10 patients in the trial for newly diagnosed CMV retinitis with the 330 mg dose; this prompted a change to the reported 165 µg dose used for the remainder of the study. No episodes of retinal pigment epitheliopathy were reported with the 165 µg dose. In the retreatment studies, retinal pigment epitheliopathy developed in 6/83 (0.21 events/patient-year) patients receiving the 330 µg more intense regimen. No patients developed retinal pigment epitheliopathy in the 330 µg less intense regimen.[294]

Confirmed visual field defect reported in two patients at the 165 µg dose (0.16 events/patient-year); with the 330 µg dose, only one patient in 330 µg less intense regimen developed a confirmed visual field defect (0.05 events/patient-year). Cataract incidence at the 165 µg dose was 0.08 events/patient-year (1 patient); for the 330 µg dose (both regimens) the incidence was 0.46 events/patient-year.[294]

The Vitravene Study Group did not statistically analyze adverse events between the two doses and long-term toxicity of fomivirsen is not known. The impact of retinal pigment epithelial toxicity on visual function is unclear because routine ERG or visual fields were not performed. It is also unclear if the toxicity is related to the dose administered or the cumulative dose. The short follow-up of these studies may preclude true estimate of problem. For the two doses, there has been no comparative study for efficacy of the 165 µg dose vs. the 330 µg dose. In addition, one is unable to analyze effects of oral GCV and HAART on time to progression or treatment failure with fomivirsen. As with other local therapeutic options for CMV retinitis, it is prudent to combine fomivirsen with oral ganciclovir or valganciclovir because for CMV retinitis, the estimated rate of contralateral eye disease is 50% and the rate of visceral disease is 31% at 6 months.[295]

Independent of the randomized clinical trials there have been reports of Vitravene induced peripheral retinal toxicity and serious inflammation with vision loss. In clinical practice fomivirsen has been used as a fourth line drug for CMV retinitis resistant to other therapy. The approved dose of fomivirsen is 330 µg intravitreally every two weeks for induction therapy for two doses followed by 330 µg intravitreally every month for maintenance therapy.[296,297]

INVESTIGATIONAL AGENTS FOR CMV RETINITIS

Maribavir

Maribavir (1263W94), currently in phase II trials, is a benzimidazole compound with in vitro activity against CMV. It does not require intracellular activation and has demonstrated activity against clinical isolates resistant to ganciclovir or foscarnet. The mechanism of action of maribavir is mediated through inhibition of the CMV UL97 gene product. The drug inhibits viral DNA synthesis through blocking of terminal DNA processing. UL97 is involved in the monophosphorylation of ganciclovir

and is essential for viral growth. Maribavir has no effect on the metabolism of HIV protease inhibitors. UL97 mutants that are compromised in their ability to phosphorylate ganciclovir are fully susceptible to maribavir. In vitro IC_{50} of maribavir was 0.12 µM compared to ganciclovir at 0.53 µM.[298–302]

Two phase I single dose escalation studies showed that maribavir in doses from 50 to 1600 mg orally can be given safely to healthy and HIV-infected patients. Maribavir was rapidly absorbed with peak concentrations occurring within 1–3 hours of the dose and plasma elimination half-life of 3–5 hours, unrelated to dose. Pharmacokinetics were dose proportional over the range tested, the drug was highly metabolized via N-dealkylation by CYP3A4 (40% recovered in the urine as metabolite with less than 2% recovered as parent drug), and maribavir was highly protein bound (98.5%). The consumption of a high-fat meal decreased the peak concentration and $AUC_{0\text{-infinity}}$ by 30%.[303]

The Phase I dose escalation study of maribavir was a multiple dose, randomized, paralleled study that evaluated pharmacokinetics, anti-CMV activity, and safety in HIV males with asymptomatic CMV shedding in urine and semen. AIDS patients over 18 years old with life expectancy >6 months and stable on HIV and prophylactic medicines for at least 1 month were included. The patients were divided into two groups: the main group included patients with semen CMV >5000 PFU/ml plus a positive CMV urine culture within 30 days (efficacy, safety, and pharmacokinetics were evaluated). No detectable CMV was needed for satellite group (safety and pharmacokinetics were evaluated) but these patients also had to have CD4 count less than 150 cells/mm³.[304]

Similar to the single dose escalation studies, maribavir pharmacokinetics were dose proportional over the dose range tested and were predictable based on the single dose data. Median semen concentration increased with increased dose, from 1.67 µg/ml at 100 mg TID to 11.85 µg/ml at 900 mg BID.[304]

Ninety-two CMV isolates were obtained for CMV sensitivity from day 1, day 28, and day 56 (plus 1 on day 11) from patients in the three times a day cohorts (58 semen, 34 urine). Median IC_{50} of maribavir for the isolates was 0.27 µM (range 0.05–0.88 µM). No significant differences for IC_{50} between day 1 and day 28 or day 56. The median IC_{50} for wild-type strain AD169 was 0.55 µM.[304]

Resistance testing IC_{50} increased when mixtures containing 25% resistant virus were added. Thus emergence of resistant variants comprising as little as 25% of the viral population would have been detected by the assays of the isolates. However in order to assess risk of developing resistance, the IC_{50} for isolates would need to be assessed from patients receiving maribavir for >90 days.[304]

Analysis of adverse events showed that 60/62 treatment patients and 10/16 patients receiving placebo experienced at least one adverse event. Most were neurological (taste problems, headache) or GI (diarrhea, nausea). Events reported by more than 10% of patients in both groups (treatment vs. placebo) were: taste problems 81% vs. 19%; headache 21% vs. 19%; diarrhea 26% vs. 13%; nausea 23% vs. 13%; rash 19% vs. 6%; pruritus 19% vs. 6%; fever 11% vs. 0; fatigue 10% vs. 13%;

vomiting 8 vs. 13%; upper respiratory symptoms 3 vs. 13%. Diarrhea and taste problems were dose related. Two serious nonocular events occurred in the placebo group (cholecystitis, pulmonary embolism). Clinical laboratory values were not statistically different between treatment and placebo groups and there were no dose-related trends in labs. Decreases in lymphocytes and increases in total protein consistent with HIV status and a modest decrease in Hgb consistent with phlebotomy requirements occurred (Hgb increased to screening values by the 4-week post-study visit).[304]

Biron et al. showed a strain of CMV resistant to maribavir isolated in vitro selection under drug pressure had a mutation in UL97 kinase.[298] In addition, Komazin et al. isolated strains of CMV resistant to maribavir. Sequencing identified a single coding mutation in ORF UL27 (Leu335Pro) as responsible for resistance to maribavir. Thus UL27 is directly or indirectly involved in the mechanism of action of maribavir. This also suggests that UL27 could play a role in CMV DNA synthesis or egress of CMV particles from the nucleus.[305,306] It has been shown that maribavir prevents nuclear egress of CMV particles.[298,307]

Tomeglovir

Tomeglovir is a 4-sulphonamide substituted naphthalene derivative with good activity in vitro against laboratory adapted and clinical strains of CMV (IC_{50} 1.17 μM vs. 5.77 μM ganciclovir). Tomeglovir is also active against ganciclovir resistant strains. Preclinical studies showed a significant decrease in mortality at all dosages in CMV-infected immunodeficient mice treated with tomeglovir. Preclinical pharmacokinetics showed that absorption from the gastrointestinal tract in dogs was approximately 65% with a rapid half-life (approximately 1 hour).[301,308] The major metabolite of tomeglovir is a monodesmethyl derivative, which also has significant anti-HCMV activity. This metabolite is present at higher free concentrations in plasma than the parent compound. Metabolism occurs via the CYP3A4 system, although the effects of tomeglovir on the metabolism of HIV protease inhibitors has not been formally reported. Drug-resistant strains of CMV generated by in vitro passage in the presence of tomeglovir, contained mutations in the *UL89* and *UL104* genes suggesting that this novel nonnucleoside class of compounds inhibits CMV by preventing cleavage of the polygenic concatameric viral DNA into unit length genomes.[301,309]

Safety and tolerability studies of single oral doses (up to 2000 mg) of tomeglovir in healthy male volunteers have been performed without significant adverse events being observed.[301,310]

RHEGMATOGENOUS RETINAL DETACHMENT IN CMV RETINITIS

Retinal detachment is a common cause of vision loss in patients with CMV retinitis. In the pre-HAART era, the incidence rate of retinal detachment in patients with CMV retinitis was approximately 33% per eye per year.[169,179,271,311–314] The incidence of retinal detachment in immunosuppressed patients

with CMV retinitis was believed to be higher in patients treated with anti-CMV therapies, specifically ganciclovir.[315–317] These retinal detachments were characterized by multiple peripheral breaks in areas of healed atrophic retinitis; and in some patients severe proliferative vitreoretinopathy resulted[318] (Fig. 92-13). Detachment occurred from weeks to months after institution of intravenous ganciclovir therapy and was frequently bilateral. Retinal detachment may also complicate the course of CMV retinitis.

However, it now appears that rhegmatogenous retinal detachment is associated with healed or active CMV retinitis due to breaks in the necrotic retina.[319] Results of a multicenter, prospective, randomized, controlled clinical trial analyzing incidence and risk factors for rhegmatogenous retinal detachment in a population of patients with newly diagnosed CMV retinitis treated with foscarnet vs. ganciclovir revealed that retinal detachment in patients with CMV retinitis is unrelated to the type of intravenous therapy used or to refractive error. The median time to retinal detachment in an involved eye with CMV retinitis and free of retinal detachment at baseline was 18.2 months.[313]

Studies have confirmed that the risk factors for retinal detachment in eyes with CMV retinitis include the extent of peripheral CMV disease, as well as retinitis activity and involvement of the anterior retina near the vitreous base.[207,271,312,314,320] This is logical, considering that in most cases the causative retinal breaks are within or at the border of healed CMV retinitis lesions. In addition, any intervention that violates the vitreous (e.g. vitreous biopsy or insertion of the ganciclovir implant) would be expected to accelerate the development of vitreous detachment or liquefaction, which would increase the risk of retinal detachment.[95,313,319] It has been reported that the risk of retinal detachment is higher in the first 2 months after GIOD insertion than if other methods are used to control the retinitis, though in the long term there is no statistical difference in retinal detachment rate between these methods of retinitis control.[161A,266,268–271]

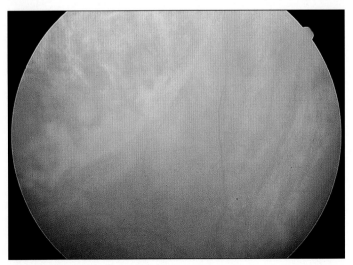

Fig. 92-13 Retinal breaks are seen just peripheral to the area of border opacification; the retina is detached.

With the advent of HAART therapy the incidence of CMV retinitis related retinal detachment has decreased by 60%. The success of HAART in the reduction of retinal detachment risk may be related to the improved immune control over CMV replication, thus protecting against progression of disease to larger lesion sizes. In addition it is suggested that increased inflammation seen in the retina of patients treated with HAART may cause a strong adhesion between the RPE and the neurosensory retina. The altered pattern of inflammation with HAART-mediated immune improvement may also change the course of vitreous detachment, a key step in the development of CMV related detachments, thus altering the retinal detachment risk.[95,179,271,266,321]

Patients with AIDS and CMV retinitis are surviving longer as a result of the use of HAART and improved treatment of opportunistic infections. As a result, though the incidence rate of retinal detachment is lower, the overall prevalence of retinal detachment may become an increasingly common cause of visual morbidity in these patients. In the pre-HAART era, the incidence and outcome of retinal detachment complicating CMV retinitis were studied at two London AIDS centers. Patients with CMV retinitis were identified prospectively and underwent standard treatment. Retinal detachments were diagnosed during regular follow-up. If retinal reattachment surgery was performed, a standard procedure of vitrectomy and internal tamponade with silicone oil was employed. Of 147 patients with CMV retinitis, 41 (28%) developed retinal detachments (47 eyes); 43 detachments were rhegmatogenous and four were exudative. Retinal reattachment surgery was performed in 15 eyes of nine patients with rhegmatogenous detachments. Of these, visual acuity remained stable or improved in 12 eyes (80%) in the immediate postoperative period. At the last clinic visit, eight eyes (53%) maintained a visual acuity of 6/60 or better. The visual results of surgery are good in selected patients,

bearing in mind the progressive nature of the underlying disease and poor life expectancy.[322]

Vitrectomy with silicone oil tamponade also was studied in eyes with retinal detachments related to CMV retinitis or acute retinal necrosis.[323] Anatomic reattachment was achieved in all eyes, and preservation of ambulatory vision was achieved in most eyes. Visual acuity was limited by concomitant optic nerve disease in some eyes. The authors noted that surgical repair employing silicone oil produces excellent results and that prognosis for vision is strongly related to preoperative visual acuity.

Treatment of retinal detachment consists of vitrectomy, posterior hyaloid removal, and intraocular tamponade with silicone oil or long-acting gas.[324] Retinal reattachment surgery in 29 eyes of 24 patients with AIDS and retinal detachment associated with CMV retinitis was described by Freeman et al.[319] In this study the total retinal reattachment rate was 76%, and the macular attachment rate was 90% after one operation. The mean postoperative visual acuity (best corrected) was 20/60, but in some patients visual acuity decreased because of progressive CMV retinitis. Prophylactic laser photocoagulation of fellow eyes did not appear to prevent retinal detachment (Fig. 92-14).

The repair of retinal detachment in eyes with viral retinitis is complex and is performed using a combination of pars plana vitrectomy, internal tamponade (usually with silicone oil or a long-acting gas such as perfluoropropane), and endolaser often combined with scleral buckling.[319] Pneumatic retinopexy can cause retinal traction and seldom is useful in these eyes. The most common causes of rhegmatogenous retinal detachment in AIDS patients with viral retinitis are acute retinal necrosis syndrome and previously treated CMV retinitis. In these eyes proliferative vitreoretinopathy occasionally is established at the time of detachment or has the potential to occur as a result of multiple retinal breaks and necrosis combined with intraocular inflammation. Scleral buckling alone often is unsuccessful in

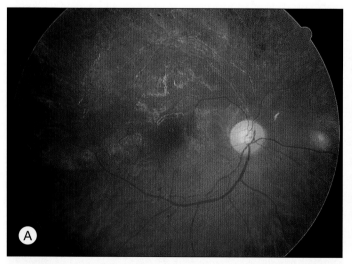
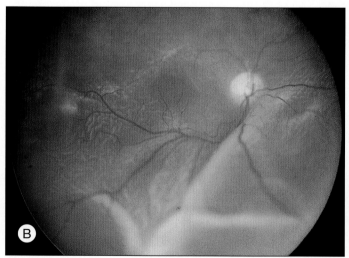

Fig. 92-14 A, Preoperatively the macula has been shallowly detached, associated with a rhegmatogenous CMV-related retinal detachment. B, Postoperatively the retina is reattached; silicone oil is in place, and the visual acuity is 20/40. Good visual recovery may be possible even with macula-off detachments because the detachment may be shallow as the vitreous is well formed; the retina may not be completely detached from the macula, and the macular detachments may be shallow.

these cases because of the numerous areas of retinal necrosis and break formation. Initially, retinal detachment in these eyes may appear exudative, but this probably is due to the relatively young age of these patients and the relatively intact vitreous. Retinal breaks are often not apparent until the time of vitrectomy, and the configurations of the retinal detachments are atypical because of peripheral retinal scarring and adhesion to the pigment epithelium and choroid. Thus in these eyes rhegmatogenous retinal detachments may not extend to the ora serrata. In eyes with CMV retinitis, we have favored an approach using complete delamination of the posterior hyaloid combined with endodrainage and permanent tamponade with silicone oil, although we have had good success with intraocular long-acting gases in cases of more limited retinitis and retinal detachment. We have had a very high surgical success rate with this approach. Patients with AIDS and CMV retinitis appear to be surviving longer, and survival after retinal reattachment surgery has been increased to 6 months to 2 years.[319]

To determine if scleral buckling is of any benefit in surgical repair of CMV-associated retinal detachment if combined with vitrectomy, silicone oil, and inferior midperipheral endolaser, 22 consecutive eyes with CMV-associated retinal detachments were repaired with vitrectomy and endolaser to all breaks and to the inferior midperipheral retina using silicone oil without scleral buckling. Results were compared with another series of 56 consecutive eyes undergoing vitrectomy, silicone oil injection, endolaser to all breaks, and 360 degrees encircling scleral buckling. Total retinal reattachment rates were 84% for group 1 and 86% for group 2. Rates of macular reattachment were 91% for group 1 and 91% for group 2. Mean best postoperative refracted visual acuity was 20/66 for group 1 and 20/67 for group 2. Median best postoperative refracted visual acuity was 20/74 for group 1 and 20/80 for group 2. These differences between the two groups were not statistically significant. Mean postoperative refractive error was +3.95 for group 1 and +4.92 for group 2. Patients who underwent surgery with the macula attached had a better postoperative visual outcome. Thus, scleral buckling may not be necessary in CMV-related retinal detachment if repaired with vitrectomy, silicone oil, and inferior midperipheral endolaser.[325] Elimination of scleral buckling may reduce intraoperative time, patient morbidity, and the risk of an accidental needle stick. Patients with macula-on retinal detachments also should be considered for surgery before macular detachment occurs.[326]

The long-term visual results of CMV retinal detachment surgery are still in question, however, and visual acuity may be limited by factors such as refractive problems resulting from silicone oil and cataract[318,327–331] (Fig. 92-15). In addition posterior capsule fibrosis is very common if subsequent cataract surgery is performed in the presence of silicone oil. Methods to reduce visual acuity loss from cataract include judicious use of gas tamponade with scleral buckling instead of silicone oil and removal of silicone oil prior to or at the time of cataract surgery. Posterior capsule fibrosis can be treated with Nd:YAG capsulotomy, though success is higher if the silicone oil has been previously removed.[328]

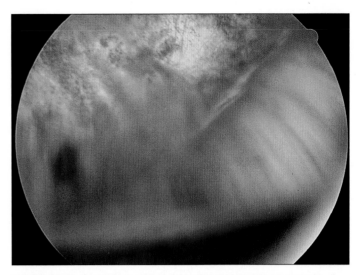

Fig. 92-15 Postoperatively, inferior retinal redetachment posterior to scleral buckle with use of silicone oil. The detachment has been walled off by laser that was applied intraoperatively. Inferior laser photocoagulation may obviate the need for encircling scleral buckling in CMV-related retinal detachments.

The general operative approach to these eyes is by pars plana vitrectomy, and the surgeon should leave the lens intact whenever possible. After the vitreous gel is removed, all epiretinal membranes are segmented and traction is removed, allowing the retina to become mobile. In some cases the peripheral vitreous gel is adherent to the necrotic peripheral retina and cannot be removed without causing further retinal damage. The use of a soft-tipped extrusion needle may allow the surgeon to remove the posterior hyaloid over broad areas of the retina. A posterior retinotomy is made, and, if an endoretinal biopsy is to be performed, it is done at the location of the posterior retinotomy that will be used for internal drainage.[319,324] A pneumohydraulic exchange is made through the retinotomy site, attaching the retina and filling the eye with air using a constant-pressure, sterile, air-delivery pump. Retinopexy is placed around all breaks in eyes to be treated with a long-acting gas. The peripheral retina may be encircled with either a small buckle or a band to relieve vitreous base traction, which may become a problem later in these inflamed eyes. In eyes with widespread retinal necrosis, most surgeons use silicone oil because it permanently tamponades all retinal breaks, including future sites of retinal necrosis and break formation.

In the HAART era, PVR may be seen in CMV detachment. This may be due to immune recovery uveitis causing a propensity to intraocular inflammation.[332]

The role of prophylactic laser photocoagulation in preventing retinal detachment in patients with viral retinitis is currently under investigation. The management of CMV-related rhegmatogenous retinal detachments has been reviewed.[333] Certainly, it may be useful in acute retinal necrosis (ARN) because rhegmatogenous retinal detachment develops in a large number of patients with ARN. Similar considerations apply in bilateral healed CMV retinitis. The difficulty in both diseases is that all areas of retinal involvement must be surrounded with three rows of argon laser treatment. It is often impossible to carry out treatment to the ora serrata, however, and fluid may leak anteriorly and cause retinal detachment despite treatment. The widespread availability of the indirect laser ophthalmoscopic delivery system should solve this problem. In addition, subretinal fluid may break through a wall of laser treatment if the mass of detached retina and subretinal fluid is relatively large. For this reason most surgeons advocate placement of a panretinal type of pattern within the area of healing retinitis as well.[333A–E]

HIV DISEASE/CMV RETINITIS IN THE HAART ERA

Since the advent of HAART many patient have had dramatic restoration of immune system function. Patients with extremely low CD4+ cell counts (including patients with CMV retinitis) have sustained elevations of CD4+ cell counts–in some cases, above 100/mm³. This also may be associated with a sustained drop in the plasma HIV viral load to low or undetectable levels. This suppression of plasma viremia may be prolonged; however, the HIV genome may still be found.[37,334] As mentioned earlier, with the prevalent use of HAART, the incidence of CMV retinitis has decreased approximately 75%.[335–339] For patients with CMV retinitis on HAART the risk of vision loss is lower,[311,335] the risk of retinal detachment is approximately 60% less,[271,335] and long term survival is much higher.[335,339–343]

In fact, for patients who have healed CMV retinitis and respond to HAART, discontinuation of maintenance therapy for CMV disease has been shown to be safe in a subset of patients.[335,344–350] This subset is characterized by CD4+ counts >50/µL, low viral loads, and other clinical factors. Patients with CD4+ counts >100 cells/µl and quiescent retinitis also showed prolonged, relapse-free intervals during HAART.[351] We have found that some of these patients may discontinue anti-CMV therapy without reactivation of retinitis (Fig. 92-16). These data suggest that HAART therapy also is permitting at least partial immune reconstitution in some patients. Thus a trial of withdrawal of CMV therapy may be indicated in some patients with good response to HAART therapy and well-healed CMV retinitis. Patients should have a sustained CD4+ count elevation of over 100 cells/mm³ for at least 3 to 6 months before discon-

tinuing anti-CMV treatment and should be carefully monitored for reactivation. Reactivation of CMV retinitis may occur after successful HAART therapy when the CD4+ count diminishes.[352] In addition, some patients may develop CMV retinitis on HAART with CD4 counts above 100/µl, probably because of incomplete restoration of the immune repertoire against CMV.[150]

The effects of HAART on the natural history of other AIDS-related opportunistic disorders have been summarized[353,354] and reflect the improvement or resolution of changes in the natural history of these disorders with inflammatory syndromes. Unusual clinical manifestations of CMV disease, such as pneumonia, adenitis, and pseudotumoral colitis, have been attributed to the effect of HAART on CMV infection.[111] The development of CMV retinitis relatively soon after initiation of HAART has been described.[356]

The addition of an HIV-1 protease inhibitor in the treatment of AIDS may lead to complete regression of CMV retinitis without specific anticytomegalovirus therapy. This effect may be related to reduced HIV-1 viral loads, a possible direct drug effect, an increase in CD4+ T lymphocyte counts, or other associated changes in immune status.[357] Stabilization of CMV retinitis has been reported to occur with treatment consisting of only AZT (without any other antiretroviral therapy). This has been attributed to enhancement of cell-mediated immunity, leading to suppression of CMV replication or suppression of interaction between HIV and CMV in the retina.[358,359]

Immune recovery uveitis

In conjunction with the dramatic improvements in the immune system reported in some patients on HAART therapy, a new syndrome has been described: "immune recovery vitreitis" or "immune recovery uveitis"[111,356,360–366] Immune recovery uveitis appears to occur in eyes with healed CMV lesions in patients with immune reconstitution on HAART. The incidence rate of this phenomenon has varied with reports from 0.11 to 0.83 per person-year in HAART responders with CMV retinitis.[367,368] Jabs et al reported the frequency of IRU at 15.5% of 200 prevalent cases of CMV retinitis.[369] Arevelo reported IRU in 37.5% of 32 patients.[370] Eyes in which CMV retinitis lesions involve large surface areas of retina seem to be at higher risk for the development of IRU.[371] Previous treatment with cidofovir may

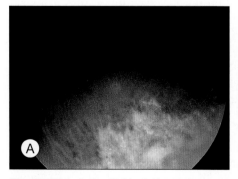 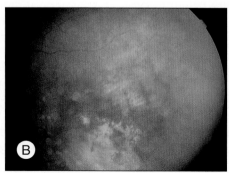 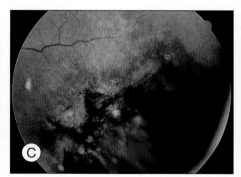

Fig. 92-16 A, Active CMV retinitis required treatment with systemic ganciclovir. B, The patient was subsequently treated with highly active antiretroviral therapy, with increase in CD4+ cell count to over 100 cells/mm³. The retinitis had remained healed. C, The patient's systemic anti-CMV therapy was withdrawn, and the retinitis has remained healed for over 6 months. The CD4+ cell count remains over 100.

also be a risk factor.[372] Patients with IRU exhibit signs of inflammation such as iritis, vitreitis, macular edema, and epiretinal membrane formation[373-376] (Fig. 92-17). Cataract, vitreomacular traction, proliferative vitreoretinopathy, optic disc and retinal neovascularization, panuveitis with hypopyon, and uveitic angle closure glaucoma with posterior synechia have also been reported in IRU.[376-383] Vision loss from these inflammatory sequelae may range from mild to moderate and is usually associated with macular edema and associated macular surface changes or cataract in most cases.[350,367,368]

The pathophysiology of immune recovery uveitis is not well understood. One hypothesis is that once the CMV retinitis is healed and the immune system is reconstituted, the patient can mount an inflammatory response to residual CMV antigens in retinal glial cells in or adjacent to the necrotic CMV lesion. Another hypothesis is that control of CMV retinitis is incomplete in certain individuals with continued subclinical virus or viral protein production that stimulates the immune system. It has been reported that CMV antigens persist in cells of all retinal layers at the borders of clinically healed CMV lesions and in CMV infected retinal glial cells after treatment with ganciclovir.[384-386] In addition Whitcup et al. reported persistence of CMV in blood of patients after the start of potent antiretroviral therapy despite apparently having clinically healed CMV disease.[350,384] Multimer et al. reported the presence of a broad complement of CD8[+] T cells in the vitreous of a patient with IRU suggesting a role of T-cell infiltration to residual CMV antigens or exposed autoantigens.[387] However, Siqueira et al. did not detect CMV DNA by PCR in the aqueous, vitreous, and blood leukocytes of five IRU patients.[388] Song et al. reported that continued maintenance therapy with ganciclovir (IV, oral, implant) or foscarnet did not affect the rate of development of IRU.[372] However, we have reported in a small prospective study of patients with IRU and macular edema that treatment with valganciclovir 450 mg twice a day was associated with a decrease in macular edema and mild increase in visual acuity.[389]

Periocular steroids may be used successfully to treat this disorder, but ophthalmologists should be aware of the systemic immunologic parameters, such as CD4[+] cell counts. It appears that if the CD4[+] cell count is elevated above 60/mm^3, treatment of immune recovery vitreitis can be carried out without reactivation of retinitis (Fig. 92-13).[360,377] Recently, one case of reactivated CMV retinitis has been reported after treatment of IRU with periocular steroids.[390]

OTHER CMV COMPLICATIONS

Central visual loss in AIDS patients with CMV retinitis occurs in two forms: direct macular tissue destruction and secondary involvement as part of rhegmatogenous retinal detachment. We treated 32 patients (35 eyes) with macular exudation that caused reversible visual loss and initially manifested as neurosensory retinal detachment and lipid exudates. Of 35 eyes, 25 showed papillary or peripapillary active retinitis and 10 showed retinitis 1500 to 3000 microns from the fovea. Of 23 eyes with reduced vision that were followed up until healing of the retinitis and resolution of subretinal fluid and lipid exudates, 22 (96%) showed visual improvement with anti-CMV treatment. Our findings suggest that macular exudation is a reversible cause of visual loss in patients with CMV retinitis.[128]

Cystoid macular edema can occur in the setting of resolving CMV retinitis in patients with immunodeficiency other than AIDS. This entity is distinct from serous macular exudation, which can occur in patients with AIDS with active CMV retinitis involving the posterior pole. The disparity between patients with and without AIDS in the development of CME may be important in understanding the pathogenesis of CME.[392] Cystoid macular edema is also seen in patients with healed CMV who develop immune recovery uveitis.[373,374]

Anterior segment findings were described in a study that evaluated 21 AIDS patients with CMV retinitis. Nineteen (90%) of these patients exhibited corneal endothelial deposits concurrent with CMV retinitis. The endothelial deposits were microscopic, opaque, linear flecks arranged in a reticular-like fashion. Of 42 eyes evaluated, 32 (76%) demonstrated active CMV retinitis. Corneal endothelial deposits were noted in 26 (81%) of the 32 eyes with retinitis. These corneal endothelial deposits were absent in the eyes that did not have CMV retinitis. Meticulous examination of the retina of an HIV-positive or AIDS patient who presents with reticularly arranged, linear, flecked corneal endothelial deposits should be performed to ensure that the diagnosis of CMV retinitis can be ruled out.[118]

HERPETIC RETINITIS

Acute retinal necrosis

Acute retinal necrosis (ARN) has been reported in AIDS patients.[393] It is a devastating disease characterized by the acute onset of a fulminant panuveitis with confluent, well-demarcated areas of retinitis, plus prominent anterior uveitis, occlusive retinal and choroidal vasculitis, vitreitis, and papillitis.[58,129A,391-396] In most cases the cause of the clinical syndrome of ARN is

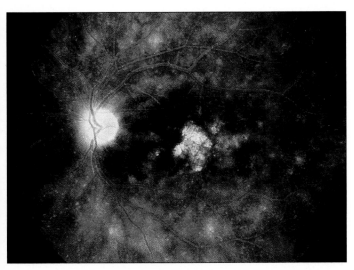

Fig. 92-17 Macular edema in a patient with immune-recovery vitreitis.

varicella zoster but HSV can also cause ARN. The retinitis is characterized by deep retinal whitening, minimal hemorrhage, and a rapid progression. In some cases, ARN in AIDS patients may be preceded by VZV optic neuropathy.[397] A history of preceding cutaneous zoster infection may be helpful in making the diagnosis in such cases.[398,399] In addition, the CD4 count is usually above 60/μl.[398] The diagnosis of ARN is clinical based on criteria established by the American Uveitis Society that do not include immune status of the patient.[400]

No evidence of retinal vascular abnormalities may be present either clinically or angiographically early in the course of ARN.[401] Retinal detachment is a common sequella, with multiple retinal breaks evident within areas of retinal necrosis. Retinal atrophy, often accompanied by proliferative vitreoretinopathy, is a common end-stage finding, and there may be associated anterior uveitis, scleritis, and ocular hypotension.[129A]

Large numbers of herpesvirus particles in retinal tissue affected with ARN have been demonstrated by electron microscopy using endoretinal biopsy techniques. Virus may be detectable only during the acute phase of the disease.[129A] Necrotic retinal tissue or retina reduced to thin glial remnants may not demonstrate virus. The difficulty in growing virus from these specimens is consistent with the hypothesis of VZV as the causative agent, since VZV is difficult to isolate and grow in vitro. However, one patient suffered from concurrent herpes simplex encephalitis, indicating this as the causative virus. It should be noted that EBV is difficult to culture with conventional tissue cultures, and certainly this virus has not been ruled out as a cause of ARN. CMV initially was believed to be the presumed infectious agent of ARN, but subsequent studies have not confirmed this.[402]

Amplification of the herpetic viral genome DNA by PCR in aqueous and vitreous humor was compared with Goldmann–Witmer coefficients against herpetic antigens in five patients with ARN and in two patients with CMV retinitis, using vitreous samples to determine the specificity of these diagnostic methods. The VZV genome DNA was amplified by PCR in four of the five patients with ARN, and CMV genome DNA was enhanced in both patients with CMV retinitis. Four patients who exhibited the VZV genome showed marked increase of the Goldmann–Witmer coefficient against VZV. Conversely, the two patients with CMV retinitis showed no remarkable changes among the antigens. This study concluded that the amplification of the viral genome DNA in the samples by PCR is specific in both diseases and that the increased level of local antibody production also is specific in VZV retinitis. In CMV retinitis, however, antibody production against CMV does not show an increase of the Goldmann–Witmer coefficient.[403]

Studies employing endoretinal biopsy and PCR techniques have enabled definitive identification and culture of the causative virus, which has important diagnostic and therapeutic implications. Recent studies have suggested that combination antiviral therapy given intravenously (usually acyclovir or ganciclovir in combination with foscarnet), if given promptly, can arrest the disease and salvage vision.[251] Retinal detachment in VZV retinitis is common (up to two-thirds of patients) and may

be associated with PVR or retinal shortening. Repair with vitrectomy and silicone oil after relief of traction with membrane segmentation and sometimes retinotomy may result in useful vision.[251,405] Prophylactic barrier laser around lesions should be considered to lower the risk of retinal detachment in ARN.

HSV is sensitive to acyclovir, but VZV and CMV are relatively resistant to that agent. Ganciclovir has good efficacy against all herpesviruses but has a lower therapeutic index and must be given indefinitely because it acts as a virostatic agent. Determination of a specific viral cause early in the course of the disease when large numbers of viral particles are present is therefore imperative. Both HSV and VZV may be sensitive to acyclovir. However, VZV requires higher serum concentrations than HSV. Treatment for ARN in AIDS patients is usually based on established treatment for non-HIV infected patient. Acyclovir IV 500 mg/m^2 or 10 mg/kg every 8 hours is effective followed by oral famciclovir 500 mg TID, acyclovir 800 mg 5 times a day or valacyclovir 1000 mg TID for maintenance therapy.[103] Duration of maintenance therapy is controversial with reports of contralateral ARN infection decades later.[406] This may support lifetime maintenance therapy especially in immunosuppressed AIDS patients. Valacyclovir 1000 mg TID has been reported effective for initial treatment of ARN in a small series of immunocompetent individuals.[406A] Intravenous Foscarnet may be used in acyclovir resistant cases.[407–412A] Corticosteroids have been used to decrease vitreitis in immunocompetent patients with ARN, but steroids are usually contraindicated in HIV patients with advanced immunosuppression.[103,398]

Progressive outer retinal necrosis

Progressive outer retinal necrosis (PORN) is another variant of herpetic retinitis in AIDS patients and is nearly always caused by VZV though HSV-1 has been reported to cause PORN syndrome.[413] The incidence of PORN has decreased during the HAART era.[103,414] It has been described in association with VZV as the onset of retinitis either succeeded or was coincident with an eruption of dermatomal zoster.[415] Most patients with this syndrome have had low CD4$^+$ cell counts (i.e. below 50/mm^3). In contrast to ARN, PORN syndrome is an extremely rapid progressive necrotizing retinitis characterized by early patchy multifocal deep outer retinal lesions (Fig. 92-18) with late diffuse thickening of the retina, absence of vascular inflammation and minimal to no vitreous inflammation.[416] Lesions may begin in the peripheral retina or the macula. Similar to ARN, optic neuropathy may precede or occur early in the course of disease.[397] Perivascular clearing of the retinal opacification is characteristic of PORN syndrome[420] (Fig. 92-19). Severe vision loss develops as a result of a widespread retinal necrosis and from retinal detachment, the latter reported in up to 70% of patients in early studies.[416–419] VZV was cultured from two chorioretinal specimens, and VZV antigen was detected in the vitreal aspirate from one. VZV antigen was found in the outer retinas of two enucleation specimens by immunocytochemistry; electron microscopic evidence of a herpesvirus was demonstrated in two enucleation specimens.[412A,420]

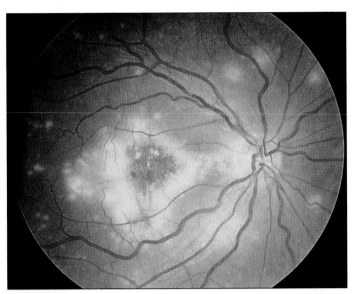

Fig. 92-18 Deep, round retinal lesions seen superior to the optic disc are characteristic of varicella zoster retinitis in AIDS patients, also termed progressive outer retinal necrosis (PORN) syndrome.

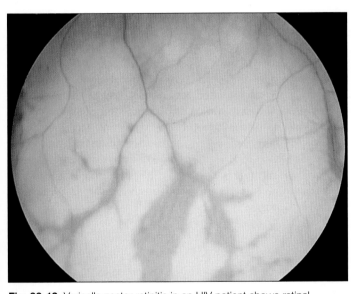

Fig. 92-19 Varicella zoster retinitis in an HIV patient shows retinal opacification and perivascular "clearing." The perivascular edema and necrosis is cleared first; the tissue is not spared.

Therapy of PORN often requires immediate high dose antizoster or -HSV therapy. The earliest reports of treatment of PORN with single intravenous antivirals, primarily acyclovir showed poor visual results.[416,418] Engstrom et al reported final vision of NLP in 67% of 63 eyes within 4 weeks.[416] Moorthy et al. reported final vision of NLP in 49% of 39 eyes after 6 months with some evidence that combined therapy with ganciclovir and foscarnet was more effective than acyclovir or either ganciclovir or foscarnet alone.[418] Poor outcomes with IV acyclovir were possibly due to development of HSV or VZV resistance to acyclovir in patients who developed PORN while on prophylactic anti-HSV therapy with acyclovir. Recent studies have shown improved visual outcomes employing combination intravenous and intravitreal antiviral treatment.[417,421–423] Scott et al. reported final vision of 20/80 or better in 5 of 11 eyes (45%) with only two of 11 eyes (18%) progressing to NLP vision utilizing a regimen of intravitreal ganciclovir and foscarnet plus IV foscarnet and IV ganciclovir or oral valganciclovir. In addition, the authors' data suggested that laser demarcation may be beneficial to decrease the rate of retinal detachment.[417] Occasionally a patient with PORN may have CNS involvement[424] which may cause a CNS infarction due to zoster cerebral arteritis. Thus a CNS evaluation may be indicated as well.

HSV and VZV resistance

Mutations in either the viral (HSV) thymidine kinase (TK) or polymerase may lead to acyclovir resistance. Acyclovir-resistant HSV has been recovered in patients with AIDS who have received long-term suppressive therapy with the drug. Foscarnet has been used in patients with AIDS and acyclovir-resistant HSV infection[407–412A] and has been shown to be superior to vidarabine.[411] The efficacy of foscarnet in these patients is due to its antiviral activity through inhibition of viral DNA polymerase, and it does not require phosphorylation by viral-induced TK, as in most TK-deficient or TK-altered strains of HSV. Resistance of HSV and VZV to foscarnet has developed in HIV-infected patients after several courses of therapy with foscarnet.[249] The mechanisms of resistance probably involve altered DNA polymerase. Therefore, with TK-deficient, acyclovir-resistant HSV or VZV, foscarnet is useful, but when acyclovir resistance is due to mutations in the viral DNA polymerase, there may be cross-resistance to foscarnet.

NONVIRAL INTRAOCULAR INFECTIONS IN AIDS PATIENTS

Nonviral intraocular infections have been reported in AIDS patients. Autopsy study has documented infections with *M. avium-intracellulare*,[57,425] *T. gondii*, *P. carinii*, syphilis,[60,65] *C. neoformans*,[72,425] and *H. capsulatum*.[426] *Mycobacterium avium-intracellulare* infections were not clinically apparent. Our group and others have seen fungal and bacterial ocular infections that resulted in severe visual loss in several AIDS patients.[427] Many of the opportunistic infections seen in patients with AIDS can be prevented with appropriate prophylactic agents.[428]

Pneumocystis carinii choroidopathy

In 1987 Macher and associates[429] described a patient with AIDS with disseminated pneumocystosis, and choroidal *P. carinii* was found at autopsy; no clinical correlation was reported.

In 1989 Rao and colleagues[64] reported the histopathologic findings in an autopsy series of three patients with AIDS who clinically demonstrated yellow choroidal infiltrates while receiving aerosolized pentamidine for *P. carinii* pneumonia (PCP) prophylaxis. In two cases a presumptive diagnosis of disseminated pneumocystosis was made by ophthalmologic examination. Histopathologically, the choroidal infiltrates were eosinophilic, acellular, vacuolated, and frothy, with the infiltrates within the choroidal vessels and choriocapillaris. Both Gomori's methenamine-silver stain and electron microscopy demonstrated organisms.

In 1989 Freeman et al.[430] described a woman with AIDS with multifocal, slowly enlarging, round-to-oval lesions in the choroid. Fluorescein angiography revealed early hypofluorescence with late staining of the lesions, which appeared deep to the retinal circulation, without evidence of retinal involvement or inflammation (Fig. 92-20). A transscleral choroidal biopsy revealed, by electron microscopy, cystic structures characteristic of *P. carinii* within necrotic choroid.

A multicenter study of *Pneumocystis* choroidopathy in 1991 reported 21 patients with AIDS and presumed *P. carinii* choroidopathy.[431] The lesions were characteristically yellow to pale yellow, appeared in the choroid, and were found in the posterior pole. They enlarged slowly before systemic anti-*Pneumocystis* therapy and eventually resolved. Of 21 patients, 18 were receiving topical therapy with aerosolized pentamidine. One patient did not have a history of PCP but was taking aerosolized pentamidine. There was little evidence of retinal destruction by visual acuity and visual field testing. The choroidal infiltrates were not associated with vitreous inflammation unless another infectious retinitis was present. Resolution of choroiditis took from 6 weeks to 4 months after systemic therapy. Survival after the diagnosis ranged from 2 to 36 weeks. The true incidence of *P. carinii* choroidopathy is unknown.

The CDC recommends double strength SMZ-TMP for primary prophylaxis of PCP when CD4 count is below 200/μl, with alternatives including dapsone, dapsone plus pyrimethamine and leucovorin, aerosolized pentamidine administered by the Respirgard II nebulizer, and atovaquone.[428]

PCP is the most common AIDS-defining opportunistic infection, occurring in up to 80% of HIV-infected persons.[432] Choroidal *P. carinii* infection appears to have been more common when the prophylactic use of nonsystemically absorbed aerosolized pentamidine for PCP was widespread. The choroidal lesions of *P. carinii* appear as pale, cream- or orange-colored, space-occupying lesions from several hundred to several thousand microns in size and they rarely are symptomatic or lead to a decrease in visual acuity. The lesions may be unilateral[430] or bilateral.[64,429–431,433–436]

Indications for specific treatment of *P. carinii* choroidopathy remain uncertain, but *P. carinii* choroidopathy appears to be a potential marker for disseminated pneumocystosis. In one patient treated with oral trimethoprim-sulfamethoxazole, as well as inhaled pentamidine, for PCP, the choroidal lesions did not increase in size over 2 months.[430] Another patient who was receiving aerosolized pentamidine had presumed *P. carinii* choroidopathy that improved during 14 weeks of oral trimethoprim-sulfamethoxazole.[436] Resolution of the choroidal lesions during 3 weeks in two patients (one treated with intravenous trimethoprim-sulfamethoxazole [Septra], the other with intravenous pentamidine) was described by Dugel et al.,[433] but a much slower response with intravenous pentamidine was seen in a study by Koser.[435] Intravenous pentamidine was used to treat three patients with *Pneumocystis* choroidopathy, and all choroidal lesions decreased in size. The choroiditis was exacerbated in two patients, however, after the maintenance dose of intravenous pentamidine was given less frequently.[434] The need for maintenance systemic therapy for choroidopathy has not been established.

Although the diagnosis of disseminated pneumocystosis may be suggested by the characteristic appearance of *P. carinii* choroidopathy, and isolated retinal disease may rarely be the earliest clinical manifestation of disseminated pneumocystosis, it is unclear from the literature whether early treatment with systemic therapy would alter the course of disease.

The incidence of *P. carinii* choroiditis has decreased, probably because of more widespread use of systemic PCP prophylaxis such as trimethoprim-sulfamethoxazole and protease inhibitor therapy as a part of HAART.[428,437]

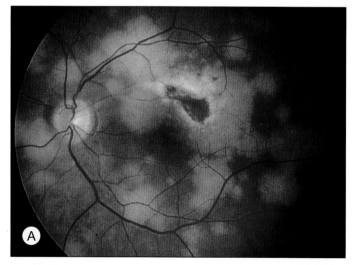
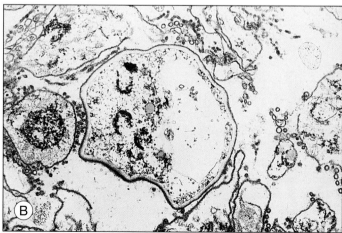

Fig. 92-20 A, Pneumocystis choroiditis. The round lesions are associated with minimal inflammation. Overlying the lesions in the superior portion of the macula is a typical CMV retinitis lesion. B, Electron micrograph of *Pneumocystis carinii* organisms seen after choroidal biopsy.

Ocular toxoplasmosis

Ocular toxoplasmosis in AIDS has been described.[74,437A,438,439] Toxoplasmosis is a common CNS opportunistic infection in patients with AIDS. Ocular toxoplasmosis is much less common, with reported incidence of 3% in HIV infected patients in France.[440] U.S. incidence is likely less with more widespread use of HAART plus primary toxoplasmosis prophylaxis with SMZ-TMP.[103] Eight patients with presumed ocular toxoplasmic retinochoroiditis were described in 1988 by Holland et al.[74] In two cases the diagnosis was confirmed histologically. Lesions were unilateral ($n = 3$) or bilateral ($n = 5$) and multifocal, with vitreous inflammation noted clinically, but histopathologic examination revealed only scant retinal inflammation in areas of necrosis. Therapy resulted in remission, but reactivation and progression of disease occurred in two of three patients when therapy was stopped. Three patients had retinal tears or detachment as a result of severe retinal necrosis. The ocular lesions were the first manifestation of toxoplasmosis in four of five patients with disseminated disease, although all patients had pre-existing HIV infection, and in four the diagnosis of AIDS had not been made. In four of five patients with no evidence of nonocular infection, evidence of *Toxoplasma* was demonstrated in the CNS (encephalitis or brain abscess). No patient had evidence of pre-existing chorioretinal scars, and all had IgG antibodies to *T. gondii* at the time of diagnosis. Ocular disease was believed to be either secondary to reactivation of *Toxoplasma* or to newly acquired or newly disseminated disease to the eye from nonocular sites of disease (Fig. 92-21).

An AIDS patient with diffuse unilateral disease that resembled ARN was described in 1986; histopathologic study revealed trophozoites in the inner retinal layers.[437A] A patient described by Heinemann et al.[438] in 1986 had a preexisting scar in the retina of one eye, but extensive diffuse disease bilaterally. Retinal toxoplasmosis infection in AIDS patients may present as a focal necrotizing nonhemorrhagic retinitis. It does not heal sponta-

neously and may simulate ARN, CMV, or luetic retinitis.[103,441] Prominent vitreous and anterior chamber reaction, relative absence of retinal hemorrhage, and thick, densely opaque yellow-white lesions with smooth nongranular borders suggest toxoplasmosis.[441] Endoretinal biopsy or PCR techniques may be useful if diagnosis is difficult.[103,441–443]

Toxoplasmosis in AIDS patients can present different clinically compared to infection in immunocompetent individuals. Ocular toxoplasmosis in HIV may spread as a contiguous retinitis or be multifocal.[442] AIDS patients more often have extensive areas of retinal necrosis plus multiple areas of active infection.[74,440,441,444–447] Reports of small partial thickness lesions in AIDS likely represent an earlier stage of infection.[74,446,448] Histopathologic studies show absent to scant inflammatory cells in the infected retina of immunocompromised patients.[74,449] AIDS patients can develop ocular toxoplasmosis in the absence of preexisting chorioretinal scars. This combined with common evidence of systemic toxoplasmosis at diagnosis suggests that acquired disease is more common than reactivation of congenital disease.[103] For immunocompetent individuals, current evidence also suggests that most patients with ocular toxoplasmosis were infected postnatally, even though the risk of ocular toxoplasmosis is higher from congenital infection.[448,450] (Fig. 92-21). Ocular toxoplasmosis in AIDS patients has also been reported to cause miliary disease, optic neuritis, panophthalmitis, and acute unilateral iridocyclitis without retinal lesions.[442,443,447,451,452]

Ocular, as well as disseminated, toxoplasmosis in patients with AIDS is treated with standard antitoxoplasma regimens used in immunocompetent patients such as sulfadiazine (4 to 6 g/day) or clindamycin in sulfa allergic patients plus pyrimethamine/leucovorin, with apparent response rates of 80%.[74,440,441,453–455] Other treatments for patients unable to tolerate sulfa drugs such as azithromycin or atovaquone have been primarily studied for CNS toxoplasmosis in AIDS patients and ocular toxoplasmosis in immunocompetent patients.[456–460] One patient with

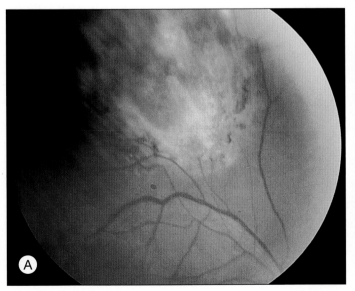
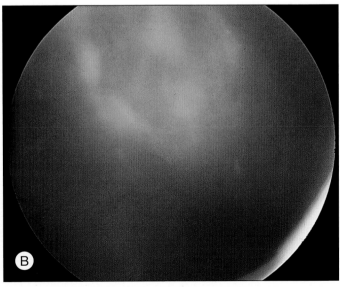

Fig. 92-21 A, Toxoplasmosis retinitis in an HIV patient who was healed after antitoxoplasmosis therapy with clindamycin. B, Systemic treatment for toxoplasmosis was withdrawn 6 months later, and the retinitis reactivated.

AIDS and toxoplasmic retinochoroiditis was treated with atovaquone because of intolerance to standard therapy and had an excellent clinical response.[460A] Atovaquone was originally synthesized as an antimalarial and has been shown to have activity against both *P. carinii* and *T. gondii*. Atovaquone has been approved for the treatment of PCP.[461] Though azithromycin and atovaquone are active against toxoplasma tissue cysts in animal models,[462,463] human studies of azithromycin and atovaquone have not shown reductions in disease recurrences.[457,458,460A]

Ocular toxoplasmosis in patients with AIDS frequently recurs when medical therapy is terminated,[74] so maintenance therapy generally is given. Corticosteroids may be given as adjunctive therapy for intracranial toxoplasmosis to reduce cerebral edema, although this is unproved; systemic corticosteroids are sometimes given to reduce inflammation in ocular disease, although these should be administered cautiously in HIV-infected patients. In addition, resolution of ocular toxoplasmosis in AIDS patients has been seen without corticosteroid therapy.[74] This is supported by histological studies showing little to no inflammation in the necrotic retina of immunocompromised patients.[74,449]

Primary prophylaxis against Toxoplasma encephalitis is recommended for seropositive patients with a CD4 count below 100/µl. Double-strength TMP-SMZ daily is currently recommended. For patients unable to tolerate TMP-SMZ, dapsone-pyrimethamine-leucovorin is the recommended alternative, or atovaquone with or without pyrimethamine-leucovorin can be considered.[428] Toxoplasma retinitis is becoming less common, probably because of more widespread use of antitoxoplasmosis medications, such as trimethoprim-sulfamethoxazole, to prevent CNS disease.[437] Currently the CDC recommends consideration of discontinuing maintenance therapy (sulfadiazine plus pyrimethamine/leucovorin with clindamycin used in sulfa allergic patients) for toxoplasma encephalitis if a patient maintains a CD4 count above 200/µl for greater than 6 months. However, recently Stout et al reported a case of ocular toxoplasmosis in a patient who stopped chronic maintenance therapy after successful treatment of toxoplasma encephalitis.[464]

Fungal diseases
Candida albicans
Since one of the risk factors for acquisition of HIV is intravenous drug use and candidemia is associated with intravenous drug use, it is surprising that *Candida* endophthalmitis is not seen more frequently in this patient population. However, focal retinal and chorioretinal lesions and endophthalmitis resulting from *Candida* spp. have been rarely described in patients with AIDS.[60,439,465,466] Traditional therapy for candida endophthalmitis has been systemic amphotericin B.[466,467] However limited vitreous penetration has resulted in treatment failures plus adverse effects including nephrotoxicity affect its use.[466,468,469] Fluconazole has been shown in animal models to have high vitreous penetration after systemic administration.[470,471] Trials comparing oral fluconazole to IV amphotericin B for systemic candidemia in immunocompetent patients suggested equivalent efficacy with fluconazole less toxic.[472,473] Vitrectomy and intravitreal amphotericin B can be helpful in cases failing systemic therapy.[466]

Cryptococcus neoformans
Cryptococcal infections may occur in 5% to 10% of patients with AIDS[474] and are associated with both direct and indirect ocular complications. Cryptococcal infection is a common occurrence in AIDS, resulting in meningitis and secondary ocular involvement (see CNS manifestations). Chorioretinitis, endophthalmitis, or both, caused by direct intraocular invasion of the organism have been described in immunosuppressed transplant patients.[475,476] Visual loss caused by cryptococcal infection has been demonstrated to result from invasion of the visual pathways, including the optic nerve, tract, and chiasm.[477] We have seen a patient who progressed to loss of light perception bilaterally with amaurotic pupils and optic atrophy. India ink stain and culture of the cerebrospinal fluid were positive for *Cryptococcus*. MRI was consistent with neural invasion by *Cryptococcus*. Cryptococcal endophthalmitis was recently reviewed in 27 patients, three of whom had AIDS.[478] The most common findings were choroiditis with or without associated retinitis with vitritis commonly associated with chorioretinal disease. Of the 27 patients, 25 had extraocular manifestations of cryptococcal infection, with 22 having symptomatic CNS involvement. Eye disease did, however, precede CNS disease in six of 22 patients.

The treatment of cryptococcal disease in patients with AIDS usually consists of an "induction" phase followed by a "maintenance" phase. Amphotericin B is most commonly used for induction, although a combination of fluconazole and 5-flucytosine has been employed successfully in some cases; maintenance therapy is usually prolonged and most commonly consists of oral fluconazole (200 to 400 mg/day).

Two cases of optic neuropathy in patients with AIDS and cryptococcal meningitis were described in 1989.[59] Visual loss occurred as a complication of known cryptococcal meningitis and was believed to be due to perineuritic adhesive arachnoiditis. Additional cases of intraocular infections resulting from C. neoformans were previously described by others.[72,425] However, C. neoformans infection usually is subclinical in AIDS patients. In one of the reported cases[425] C. neoformans was found in the meninges at autopsy. An afferent optic nerve defect was reported in another patient in the pre-AIDS era.[475] Ophthalmologic complications of cryptococcal meningitis were seen infrequently before the description of AIDS but have included optic atrophy, choroiditis, and retinitis.[479]

Histoplasmosis
Histoplasmosis was initially reported in patients with AIDS in 1982, and since then more than 100 systemic cases have been reported.[480] In 1987 the CDC expanded the case definition of AIDS to include extrapulmonary histoplasmosis in a person who is HIV-seropositive. The severe immunologic defect in AIDS predisposes to disseminated disease in nearly all cases.

Macher et al.,[426] in 1985, described a patient with histoplasmic chorioretinitis. The treatment of histoplasmosis in patients with AIDS usually consists of an induction phase with amphotericin B followed by a lifelong maintenance phase with either amphotericin B or itraconazole.[481]

Disseminated bilateral chorioretinitis resulting from *H. capsulatum* in a patient with AIDS was described in 1985.[426] Infection presents as perivascular retinal lesions or chorioretinitis with minimal inflammation. Histoplasmal infection of the retina or choroid is extremely rare in the HIV-infected population.

Gonzales et al. reported bilateral endogenous endophthalmitis in an HIV positive patient presenting with severe subretinal exudation, choroidal granulomas, and intraretinal hemorrhage leading to bilateral exudative retinal detachments. Vitreous cultures grew *H. capsulatum* var. *capsulatum*. Treatment involved systemic and bilateral intravitreal amphoteracin B plus vitrectomy/scleral buckle in one eye.[482]

Aspergillosis
Endogenous endophthalmitis caused by *Aspergillus fumigatus* rarely has been described in AIDS.[483] One case of disseminated, invasive aspergillosis with ocular involvement noted at autopsy was described in 13 patients with pulmonary aspergillosis; no clinical correlation of ocular findings was reported.[483] The patient had underlying factors of neutropenia and corticosteroid use in addition to "cytomegalovirus" and "*Pneumocystis carinii* pneumonia."[483] Ocular aspergillosis is very rare in the HIV population.

Coccidioidomycosis
To our knowledge, no cases of ocular coccidioidomycosis have been described in patients with AIDS. In a retrospective review of 77 patients with HIV infection and coccidioidomycosis, no case of endogenous endophthalmitis secondary to coccidioidomycosis was described, although disseminated disease (including meningitis) was described in a majority of patients.[484] Ocular vasculitic complications of coccidioidal meningitis in apparently non-HIV seropositive patients have included hemianopsia and photophobia,[485] endophthalmitis,[485A,486,487] and uveitis.[489] Other unusual mycotic infections causing endophthalmitis, some in association with chorioretinitis, but not necessarily HIV-seropositive patients, are reviewed by McDonnell and Green.[490]

Paracoccidioidomycosis
Severe CNS plus ocular infection with *Paracoccidioides brasiliensis* that simulated CNS and ocular toxoplasmosis has been reported in a pregnant HIV positive patient. The infection caused severe iridocyclitis, vitreitis, plus a granulomatous chorioretinal lesion also involving the optic nerve that ultimately progressed to retinal detachment, no light perception vision, and enucleation despite treatment.[491]

Advances in antifungal therapy
Fungal endophthalmitis traditionally has been treated with intravenous amphoteracin B.[467] Limitation of vitreous penetration plus systemic toxicity limit its effectiveness.[468,492–494] Flucytosine and fluconazole have higher vitreous penetration but are limited by lack of broad coverage against many of the organisms typically seen in fungal endophthalmitis.[471,493–495] As a result, vitrectomy and intravitreal amphoteracin B is usually recommended

in serious fungal endophthalmitis or cases unresponsive to systemic therapy.[494,496] However, the value of intravitreal amphoteracin has not been proven and toxicity concerns exist.[494,497]

New generation triazole antifungal medications voriconazole, posaconazole, and ravuconazole have been developed and possess increased efficacy against a broad spectrum of fungal organisms. Voriconazole has been shown to have mean aqueous and vitreous minimum inhibitory concentrations for 90% of isolates (MIC_{90}) for a wide spectrum of yeast and molds, including *Candida* and *Aspergillus* spp. after oral administration.[494] Voriconazole and posaconazole have also been reported to successfully treat fungal endophthalmitis that was unresponsive to traditional antifungal agents.[498–501] Animal studies have shown that intravitreal injection of voriconazole at doses up to 25 μg/ml does not cause retinal toxicity by ERG or histologic examination.[502] Voriconazole and posaconazole have been shown to have efficacy against candida albicans isolates from HIV patients.[503,504]

Bacterial and mycobacterial retinitis
Syphilis
Concurrent infection with HIV and *Treponema pallidum* has been suggested to be more aggressive than syphilis in the non-HIV infected host.[505] Ophthalmic manifestations of syphilis usually occur during or shortly after the secondary stage. Syphilitic uveitis and chorioretinitis in HIV-infected patients have been described. Nine patients with ocular syphilis and concurrent HIV infection were described by McLeish and colleagues in 1990.[506] They found iridocyclitis in three of 15 eyes, vitreitis in one eye, retinitis or neuroretinitis in five eyes, papillitis in two eyes, optic perineuritis in two eyes, and retrobulbar neuritis in two eyes. Three of nine patients with AIDS had the worst initial visual acuities. Six of nine had concomitant neurosyphilis. Benzathine benzylpenicillin, the only treatment in three of the patients, led to relapses in all three. Seven of nine patients treated with high-dose intravenous penicillin responded dramatically to therapy with no evidence of relapse.[506]

Concurrent ocular syphilis and neurosyphilis reported in two patients with HIV infection, in addition to a review of 13 other HIV-infected patients with ocular syphilis, revealed that 11 of the 13 HIV-infected patients with ocular syphilis had neurosyphilis.[507] The authors stress that neuro-ophthalmic syphilis may be the presenting feature of HIV infection and that ocular syphilis is strongly associated with concurrent neurosyphilis in patients that are HIV-seropositive (Fig. 92-22).

A case of secondary syphilis with ocular syphilis in an HIV-seropositive patient underlines the importance of testing for syphilis in all patients with HIV infection.[508] A case of recurrent syphilitic uveitis in an HIV-seropositive male who was treated with penicillin G benzathine demonstrates the inadequacy of this agent alone in the treatment of secondary syphilis in HIV-infected hosts.[509]

Ocular syphilis, including uveitis, optic neuritis, and retinitis, was reported in three HIV-seropositive males without AIDS, all of whom had cutaneous manifestations of secondary syphilis

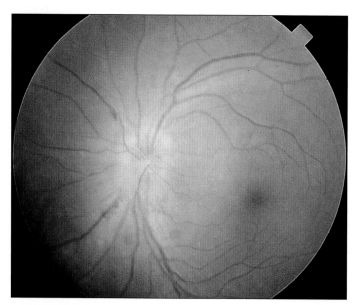

Fig. 92-22 Papillitis and vitreitis from syphilis in an HIV-positive patient. Intravenous penicillin resolved the findings.

(one had a negative serum VDRL early in the course) and an abnormal cerebrospinal fluid (CSF).[510] The authors also demonstrate that spontaneous improvement or response to corticosteroids in two of the cases suggest that the ocular disease may be noninfectious.

A case of unilateral retrobulbar neuritis in a patient with AIDS was first described in 1986 (the patient was seen in 1984),[511] and a case of bilateral optic neuritis secondary to syphilitic retrobulbar neuritis in conjunction with AIDS was described in 1987.[512]

Necrotizing retinitis has been reported in a patient with ARC and syphilis.[513] In some cases the appearance of luetic retinitis as a focal expanding white lesion may simulate CMV retinitis, ARN, or toxoplasmic retinitis. Marked inflammation of the vitreous and anterior chamber usually accompanies syphilitic retinal disease with posterior synechiae and keratic precipitates may be seen.[506,513–515]

The medical treatment of early syphilis in patients with and without HIV infection was recently shown to have no important differences in clinical response or neurologic events in a large randomized trial involving 101 HIV-infected patients.[516] For primary or secondary syphilis, intramuscular penicillin may be used. For retinitis, treatment for neurosyphilis with intravenous penicillin should be used,[103,506,517] although some will use ceftriaxone. With regard to diagnosis, false negative serum rapid plasma reagin (RPR) and Venereal Disease Research Laboratories (VDRL) are common in HIV-infected individuals. Thus more specific diagnostic tests are recommended in this population (i.e. Fluorescent treponemal antibody, absorbed [FTA-ABS]).[103,506]

Other bacterial infections

We have documented two cases of endogenous *Staphylococcus epidermidis* endophthalmitis in AIDS patients. This organism is a common cause of postoperative bacterial endophthalmitis, but neither of the patients we reported had undergone an operative procedure. Endogenous *S. epidermidis* intraocular infection should be considered in the differential diagnosis of opportunistic ocular infections in AIDS. Diagnosis of this infection may be confirmed if both tissue Gram stain and culture are positive. Both these patients had severe visual loss as a result of this infection despite response to antibiotics administered subconjunctivally and intravenously. One case was manifest as an inflammatory choroidal mass and the other as a diffuse uveitis. In both cases intraocular tissue (choroid and vitreous) demonstrated the organism on stain and culture. Endogenous bacterial retinitis in two patients with AIDS was described in 1989.[427] In these patients a slowly progressive, multifocal retinitis was described. One patient showed Gram-positive bacteria on electron microscopy of histiocytes in the retina, and the other patient had a documented staphylococcal bacteremia. Both responded to antibiotics.

Mycobacterial retinitis

Ocular infection with tuberculosis in AIDS patients is uncommon with multifocal choroidopathy the most common presentation.[514] A case of presumed choroidal tuberculosis in a patient with disseminated tuberculosis and AIDS was reported in 1989.[518] In this case a low-grade vitreitis and small, yellow-white choroidal infiltrates, which coalesced into larger, slightly elevated nodules, were noted. Additional cases have been described as part of a disseminated infection.[519–520] Chorioretinitis caused by *M. tuberculosis* was found in one patient by PCR of the aqueous humor.[521] Anterior uveitis or vitreitis can also be seen in patients with apparently healed choroidal lesions from previously treated tuberculosis.[103] Ocular infections with *M. avium-intracellulare* have been demonstrated in autopsies of patients with disseminated infection, but clinically significant *M. avium-intracellulare* infection of the posterior segment is likely to be extremely rare. The advent of a highly active class of antimicrobials (macrolides, such as clarithromycin or azithromycin) effective against *M. avium-intracellulare* has made this disseminated disease less prevalent.[522,523]

We have seen one case of *Nocardia asteroides* choroiditis in a patient with disseminated nocardiosis (L. Rickman, unpublished).

NEOPLASMS

Primary ocular lymphoma

HIV-associated primary lymphoma of the retina or retina/choroid, which has been infrequently reported,[524] shows confluent, yellowish white retinochoroidal infiltrates with perivascular sheathing (Fig. 92-23). HIV-associated primary lymphoma of the retina with or without CNS involvement is extremely rare.[525]

No cases of intraocular Kaposi's sarcoma have been reported.

CENTRAL NERVOUS SYSTEM MANIFESTATIONS OF AIDS

Central nervous system lesions in AIDS patients are common, occurring in up to 40% by clinical evaluation[526] and up to 87%

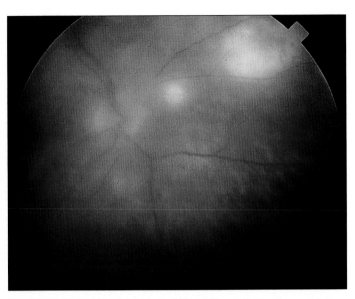

Fig. 92-23 Retinal lymphoma in an HIV-positive patient can present as an atypical retinitis. Diagnosis was made by endoretinal biopsy.

if autopsy examination is performed.[527] In addition, CNS abnormalities may be found in clinically asymptomatic HIV-seropositive patients.[528] Many of these lesions may cause visual symptoms, and knowledge of their pathophysiology may shed important light on the cause of retinal lesions. Viral syndromes such as subacute encephalopathy or AIDS-related dementia caused by CMV,[529] HIV, or multiple CNS viral infections (see below) appear in up to 17% of patients with CNS involvement. Aseptic meningitis is seen in 7%, herpes simplex encephalitis in 3%, and progressive multifocal leukoencephalopathy in 2% of patients; viral myelitis and varicella-zoster encephalitis have been reported. Nonviral infections are responsible for 50% of CNS abnormalities, with toxoplasmosis and cryptococcal infections being the most common, followed less frequently by *Candida*, mycobacterial, and other infections. Neoplasms of the CNS include primary CNS lymphomas (5%), systemic lymphomas with CNS involvement (4%), and Kaposi's sarcoma with metastatic involvement of the CNS (1%). Intraocular neoplasms have been reported in AIDS patients. Cranial nerve and peripheral nerve complications occur in up to 16% of neurologic patients with AIDS. Hemorrhage and infarction have been reported. Neuro-ophthalmologic manifestations of HIV disease have included papilledema, papillitis, optic atrophy, retrobulbar neuritis, visual field defects, cortical blindness, visual allesthesia, ocular motor nerve palsies, and pupillary abnormalities.[530]

Toxoplasmosis is one of the most common CNS infections. Patients with toxoplasmosis may present with focal deficits, lethargy, confusion, seizures, visual field defects, and ophthalmoplegia.[526] Treatment with pyrimethamine and sulfadiazine may relieve symptoms, but mortality approaches 70%; however, in half of these patients the cause of death was related to systemic complications.

Cryptococcal infection is the fourth most common opportunistic infection encountered in AIDS, ranging in incidence

from 7.5% to nearly 15% of patients. Cryptococcal meningitis is associated with secondary ocular abnormalities in nearly 40% of patients. These include diplopia, ptosis, amblyopia, nystagmus, ophthalmoplegia, anisocoria, papilledema, neuroretinitis, and optic atrophy.[479] Direct intraocular invasion by the organism resulting in chorioretinitis or endophthalmitis has been described in immunosuppressed patients without AIDS.

Brainstem ocular motility defects resulting from HIV infection as an initial manifestation of AIDS are rare[530] but were described in three patients, one of whom had concurrent infection with *T. pallidum*. A patient with AIDS and a third cranial nerve palsy as a result of presumptive CNS toxoplasmosis was described in 1987.[531]

INVASIVE DIAGNOSTIC TECHNIQUES FOR RETINAL DISEASE

In difficult cases, biopsy of the vitreous, choroid, or retina may allow for diagnosis. Vitreous biopsy may yield a diagnosis if a moderate to heavy cellular infiltrate is present. Most modern vitrectomy machines use sterile, disposable tubing and cassettes so that vitreous washings obtained are sterile. These washings may be filtered or centrifuged for appropriate stains, cultures, and cytologic study.

An alternative method may be used to obtain undiluted vitreous at the time of pars plana vitrectomy. After the infusion cannula can be visualized within the eye, the cannula is connected to a sterile, constant-air infusion pump, and a vitrectomy is carried out under air. In phakic eyes, a minus-power contact lens is used to visualize the retina under air. In this way the entire volume of the vitreous cavity may be removed in an undiluted form for study.

Appropriate processing of vitreous obtained as part of a diagnosis is mandatory, and the testing performed should reflect the differential diagnosis. Where infection is suspect, plating of undiluted vitreous on appropriate culture media for aerobic bacteria (chocolate and blood agar, brain–heart media), anaerobic bacteria (thioglycolate media and cooked meat broth), media for acid-fast bacilli, and fungal culture media is imperative and should be done in the operating room. Smears of the undiluted gel should be stained for these etiologic agents, and cytologic smears also should be obtained. In addition, histopathologic stains are useful in ruling out intraocular neoplasms, particularly intraocular lymphoma. Other important diagnostic aids include the use of cytospin preparations that concentrate the cells in vitreous washings, and the use of cell blocks, should enough cellular material be present in a vitreous specimen. The choice of fixatives should be considered carefully. In general, the use of electron microscopic fixatives such as glutaraldehyde may destroy the antigenicity of proteins, rendering immunostaining impossible. Buffered paraformaldehyde will preserve many antigens, although in some cases, frozen, nonfixed tissue is required. In situ hybridization may work on fixed or fresh tissue and can be valuable in determining the presence of pathogenic DNA.[532] A refinement of this procedure, the polymerase chain reaction, promises to become an important diagnostic tool.

PCR allows for the amplification of small segments of DNA and may be able to detect as little as one pathogenic genome. It is important to have a list of diagnostic possibilities in mind and to discuss these with the appropriate laboratory personnel before submitting vitreous or other ocular specimens for diagnostic studies.[324]

PCR techniques also may be useful in analyzing aqueous or vitreous specimens in difficult cases. Nonfixed fluids are best; they can be frozen for later evaluation or processed fresh. In cases of active retinitis, the test is very sensitive, although it may be somewhat nonspecific because it may detect CMV in the blood in the absence of retinal infection. PCR techniques are improving and becoming quantitative, and they likely will become more useful in the future.[533]

Choroidal biopsies may be indicated when infiltrative processes of the choroid are seen clinically. Fungal, bacterial, protozoal, or parasitic disease may cause metastatic focal or diffuse infiltrative lesions in the choroid.[534] Tuberculous disease and neoplastic disorders, including lymphoma, also may produce such lesions. All such diseases respond temporarily, if at all, to steroid therapy, and in many cases the diagnosis cannot be made by study of vitreous cells. Before undertaking this diagnostic procedure, prior arrangements for appropriate histologic examination of all materials obtained must be made, since the amount of material that can be obtained is usually small. Any cultures to be taken should be performed by direct plating of the tissue onto the appropriate media in the operating room, as outlined above.

Thorough preoperative examination of the posterior segment is necessary. The choroidal lesion to be biopsied must be well localized. Echography can be used to gain further information regarding the consistency of the lesion and the presence of subretinal or suprachoroidal fluid. It can also be useful in determining if an intraocular lesion has extraocular extension. It is best to select a site distant from the macular area; a nasal area of involvement is best.

In the operating room, the conjunctiva is removed from the limbus 360 degrees, and all four rectus muscles are isolated. Tenon's capsule is cleaned from the quadrant to be biopsied, and the margins of the lesion are marked. It is advantageous to choose a site where a serous or exudative retinal detachment is present overlying the lesion in question because this provides an added margin of safety. A half-thickness scleral dissection is performed 5 to 10 mm^2 and fashioned into a "trap door." Preplaced 5-0 polyester sutures can be used to allow the trap door to be closed quickly. A smaller area of underlying sclera is closed by diathermy to prevent bleeding, and then an area 3 to 4 mm on each side is resected. Care is taken to remove choroid and not retina. The trap door is then closed with 5-0 polyester sutures, and the area of resection is examined with the indirect ophthalmoscope. Some sclera should be visible if a full-thickness choroidal biopsy was performed. Retinal incarceration in the biopsy site is a potential source of problems and may have to be addressed using internal pars plana surgical techniques. Vitreous in the biopsy implies retinal incarceration or a retinal break that must be repaired using pars plana vitrectomy tech-

niques. Using this technique, embolic bacterial endophthalmitis, *Pneumocystis* choroidopathy, and other pathologic entities may be diagnosed. Because of the potential to damage the retina or perforate the eye, in some cases it may be preferable to perform a pars plana vitrectomy before choroidal biopsy. This will allow maintenance of intraocular pressure, as well as rapid internal access to the retina should complications arise.

Endoretinal biopsy is an exciting new technique that has been reported to be of value in the diagnosis of viral retinitis. Freeman et al.[129A] first reported this technique in 1986 when we proved that the cause of two cases of ARN was a member of the herpesvirus family. We pursued this technique in patients with CMV retinitis. After healing of retinitis with ganciclovir, rhegmatogenous retinal detachment developed in a large number of these patients as a result of numerous breaks in areas of necrotic and healed retina. We showed in several eyes that persistent infection was present, as viral particles were seen. At this time we do not recommend endoretinal biopsy for all cases of viral retinitis. Rather, we treat such cases with the appropriate antiviral drug and wait for a response. Such a response may not indicate a specific viral cause, however, because some antiviral drugs are broad-spectrum. For example, acyclovir is active against both HSV and VZV, although higher doses are necessary (intravenous treatment) in treating the latter infection. Similarly, ganciclovir is active against both of these viruses and against human CMV as well. Both drugs demonstrate activity against EBV, although ganciclovir is more active. Problems arise because ganciclovir is a much more toxic drug than acyclovir and can be administered only intravenously. In certain cases it is helpful to obtain an etiologic diagnosis. In addition, we have seen several cases of atypical retinitis in immunosuppressed patients. In these patients, apparently healed retinitis consistent with CMV was seen after treatment with antiretroviral drugs that may stimulate the immune system of AIDS patients. In these cases the typical, slowly progressive course of necrotizing retinitis was not seen, thus casting the diagnosis in doubt.

As new antiviral and immunostimulating drugs become available, viral retinitis may not take on the so-called classic clinical appearance, and aggressive diagnostic techniques may become more important. Currently we obtain endoretinal biopsies at the time of pars plana vitrectomy to repair rhegmatogenous retinal detachments in these patients. During these procedures, undiluted vitreous specimens are taken for viral cultures, and in some cases in situ nucleic acid hybridization studies are done. The retinal biopsy (described below) is divided into three small pieces, and each is placed on a small wedge of sterile paper or on an agar sandwich in the operating room using the operating microscope. Tissue is fixed in glutaraldehyde for electron microscopy, as well as in buffered formalin for light microscopy and some immunologic studies. The third piece of tissue may be frozen for further immunologic studies or cultured for virus. It is important to remember that the choice of fixative and tissue preparation technique is critically important; if an incorrect choice is made, it may not be possible to arrive at a diagnosis. Even when obtaining an endoretinal biopsy, the vitreous should also be examined because vitreous biopsy in cases of infectious retinitis may be positive for the causative organism.[116] One can also perform endoretinal biopsy in nondetached retinas. The preliminary results in animals have been encouraging, and refinement of these techniques in the future may shed light on a variety of retinal disorders.

In eyes undergoing endoretinal biopsy a pars plana vitrectomy with complete removal of the hyaloid is performed. The biopsy site also is used for internal drainage. To determine the etiologic diagnosis, it is important to make this location at the junction of healed and normal or active retinitis. Vessels are cauterized only posterior to the biopsy site. We prefer to use the pointed 20-gauge intraocular unimanual bipolar cautery. Low power must be used, and major vessels posterior to the biopsy site are cauterized. Using motorized vertical cutting scissors, a rectangular strip of retina is excised, which crosses the site of active retinitis or the leading border. The strip may be 2 mm wide and 3 to 5 mm long. It is chosen from an area of necrotic or gliotic nonfunctional retina so that no visual loss occurs. Removal of the tissue from the eye through the 20-gauge sclerotomy with a forceps may crush and mutilate the tissue, so, instead, we prefer to guide the tissue toward the sclerotomy with a pick or pick forceps. The tissue is released, and the instrument is then removed from the eye while the infusion bottle is elevated to the high position. In this way the tissue is hydraulically directed into the sclerotomy site and plugs it. The tissue is gently teased out of the sclerotomy with a 0.12 mm forceps and spread over the cornea, removing all folds.

Any ocular tissue, but particularly small endoretinal biopsy specimens, must be processed with care.[535] The surgeon must decide in advance on the location of the area to be biopsied and the fixatives and numbers of specimens to be processed. We have developed a mount that allows more facile mounting of retinal biopsy specimens.[536] The agar–albumin sandwich technique allows the small piece of retinal tissue to be floated onto a slab of clear agar and then "glued" to it with liquid agar that has been warmed in a microwave. When the tissue is draped on the agar, it can be readily identified and not lost during processing. Multiple sections of the tissue can then be cut for processing and immunostaining. The technique also works well for electron microscopy and other morphologic studies.

NEW DEVELOPMENTS IN THE TREATMENT OF HIV INFECTION AND AIDS

Management and prophylaxis of opportunistic infections that occur in AIDS are often successful, but the underlying immunodeficiency remains despite these treatments.[428,522,523] Thus great attention has turned to the control of HIV infection in the hope of improving the function of the immune system. Each step in the process of viral replication is a potential target for antiviral therapy. As anti-HIV therapy improves, amelioration of immunosuppression may be therapeutic for intraocular infections. Unfortunately, retinal opportunistic infections develop in most HIV-infected patients despite treatment with antiretroviral agents.

HIV-RNA viral load has been shown to be a superior predictor of clinical outcome over CD4+ counts,[26] and treatment guidelines for HIV infection now routinely include measurement of RNA viral load.[537] Based on the pathogenesis of HIV infection,[538] several therapeutic principles have been proposed for therapy of HIV infection. To limit the development of multiple viral strains, antiretroviral therapy should be initiated early in HIV infection. A combination of antiretroviral agents suppresses the development of mutations and should be routinely employed.[539,540] Although immune reconstitution is desirable, destruction of immune function may be permanent. In summary, current standard-of-care consists of an attempt to suppress viral replication completely. Antiretroviral drug resistance testing based on both phenotypic and genotypic assays has been reviewed recently.[541] These tests have become important tools in a variety of situations for the management of HIV infection though expert interpretation is recommended.

ANTIRETROVIRAL THERAPY

Various steps in the replicative cycle of HIV may be targeted for intervention. Currently available for clinical use are the antiretroviral nucleoside/nucleotide and non-nucleoside reverse transcriptase inhibitors, protease inhibitors, and a fusion inhibitor.[34,542,543] Many other antiretroviral agents are undergoing preclinical and clinical studies.[545,546] None of the drugs currently available has been shown to eradicate HIV infection, but when used in combination, they may decrease viral replication, improve immunologic status, delay infectious complications, and prolong life.

Three prominent groups have released clinical guidelines for the use of antiretroviral therapy: The US Department of Health and Human Services,[547] the International AIDS Society,[537] and the British HIV Association.[548] Several reviews of antiretroviral therapy have recently been published.[34,542,543]

Reverse transcriptase inhibitors

Reverse transcriptase converts viral RNA into proviral DNA before its incorporation into the host cell chromosome. This occurs at an early essential step in HIV replication. Drugs that inhibit this process prevent infection of susceptible cells but have little effect on cells already infected with HIV.[542] There are two classes of reverse transcriptase inhibitors: nucleoside/nucleotides and non-nucleosides.

Nucleoside/nucleotide reverse transcriptase inhibitors (NRTIs)

There are currently eight NRTIs approved by the U.S. FDA for the treatment of HIV infection: abacavir, didanosine, emtricitabine, lamivudine, stavudine, tenofovir, zalcitabine, and zidovudine. All NRTIs are substrates for reverse transcriptase and must be phosphorylated by host cell enzymes in the cytoplasm to become active. Once incorporated into the proviral DNA the NRTI's lack of a 3′-hydroxyl group terminates chain elongation. These drugs are most important as components of three- and four-drug regimens for HIV treatment.[542]

Ophthalmic adverse effects of certain NRTIs have been reported. Macular edema has been described in one patient treated with zidovudine (AZT).[549] Atrophy of the retinal pigment epithelium has been described with didanosine in children with HIV infection,[550] and it has been suggested that children be followed with indirect ophthalmoscopy every 4 to 6 months.[551] One case of optic neuritis associated with didanosine has also been reported.[549]

Nonnucleoside reverse transcriptase inhibitors (NNRTIs)

Three NNRTIs are approved by the U.S. FDA for the treatment of HIV: delavirdine, efavirenz, and nevirapine.

These agents are structurally unrelated to the nucleoside analogs and inhibit only HIV-1 reverse transcriptase. Unlike the nucleoside analogs, the NNRTIs interfere with the reverse transcriptase by noncompetitively binding downstream from the active catalytic site, inducing conformational changes in this site. The NNRTIs also do not undergo phosphorylation. These agents are useful in combination with other antiretroviral agents, most commonly a protease inhibitor and a nucleoside reverse transcriptase inhibitor.[542] The development of resistance when used alone makes monotherapy with the NNRTIs undesirable.[537]

Protease inhibitors

Eight protease inhibitors are approved by the U.S. FDA for the treatment of HIV: amprenavir, atazanavir, fosamprenavir, indinavir, lopinavir + ritonavir, nelfinavir, ritonavir, and saquinavir.

Protease inhibitors are the most potent antiretroviral agents available to date. These agents have been shown to produce rapid decreases in plasma HIV-RNA and increases in CD4+ lymphocyte counts; these effects are much more robust than those of the nucleoside analogs. The HIV-1 protease is an essential enzyme for the production of infectious HIV virions and functions by processing polypeptide precursors into active viral enzymes and structural proteins. Protease inhibitors reversibly bind to the active site of HIV protease and prevent cleavage of protein precursors that are essential for the maturation of HIV and the replication and infection of new cells. In vitro resistance may develop to these agents, especially when used as monotherapy; therefore they are always used in combination therapy.[542]

Fusion inhibitors

Recently, the U.S. FDA approved enfuvirtide (T-20), the first of a new class of antiretrovirals that block HIV virus entry into cells.[34]

HIV-1 virus infection starts with initial attachment and subsequent entry of the virus into host cells. Virus entry begins with interaction of the external viral envelope glycoprotein, gp120, with host CD4+ and chemokine receptor sites. After further structural changes in gp120, conformational changes in the HIV envelope glycoprotein 41 (gp41) result in the creation of a fusion pore in the CD4+ cell allowing passage of the HIV capsid.[34]

Enfuvirtide is a synthetic peptide that binds to the HR1 domain of gp41 ultimately interfering with the conformational changes required for the transition of gp41 into a fusion-active state. Clinical trials with enfuvirtide suggest that it be used in combination with other antiretrovirals for dependable suppression of viral load. Enfuvirtide is administered as repeated subcutaneous injections and currently does not have a bioavailable oral formulation.[34]

Recent reviews of available antiretroviral drugs has been published.[34,542,543]

Combination antiretroviral therapy

Combination antiretroviral therapy, the standard of care in treating patients with HIV infection, is used to delay resistance of HIV. Initial studies with various combinations of both nucleoside analogs and other antiretroviral agents demonstrated that combination therapy delays the emergence of resistant virus.[552,553] Drug combinations that reduce plasma HIV RNA and raise CD4+ cell counts are associated with increased survival.[10,32,554,555] The significance of the development of resistance of HIV to antiretroviral therapy has become more evident. Patients who have received multiple and/or sequential nucleoside drug combinations have developed HIV resistance, and even patients who receive drug combinations, including the highly active protease inhibitors, may develop drug resistance. Combination antiretroviral therapy without the administration of specific anti-CMV therapy in patients with CMV retinitis has been reported to prevent or delay the progression of retinitis.[556]

Investigational antiretroviral agents

Many antiretroviral agents based on interference with well defined stages in the replicative cycle of HIV-1 are currently in preclinical or clinical development.[545,546]

Compounds that bind to the viral envelope protein gp120 inhibit virus adsorption. Viral entry is inhibited by agents that block viral coreceptors CXCR4 and CCR5. NCp7 zinc finger-targeted agents block viral assembly and disassembly. Proviral DNA integration is inhibited by drugs that target HIV integrase. Finally HIV mRNA transcription is blocked by agents that inhibit the transcription (transactivation) process.[545,546]

In addition to compounds affecting new targets of the HIV-1 replicative cycle, new agents in the currently approved drug classes are also under clinical development. New nucleoside/nucleotide reverse transcriptase inhibitors, non-nucleoside reverse transcriptase inhibitors, protease inhibitors, and virus-cell fusion inhibitors are in development which offer improved metabolic properties and increased activity.[545,546]

Colony-stimulating factors

Currently, several recombinant growth factors are commercially available, including rG-CSF (filgrastim; Neupogen), rGM-CSF (sargramostim; Leukine), and EPO,[557] or epoetin alfa (Epogen, Procrit). Studies with HIV-related disease have concentrated on several potential uses, including augmentation of neutrophil cytotoxicity toward HIV-infected cells, reversing neutropenia (associated with HIV, antiretroviral therapy, or therapies directed against opportunistic infections such as ganciclovir for CMV), or dose escalation of cytotoxic therapy in

HIV-associated neoplasms. Administration of GM-CSF caused a progressive increase in total leukocyte count in 16 neutropenic patients with HIV infection.[558] There is a theoretical concern that stimulation of monocytes and macrophages that harbor HIV may be detrimental. No consistent role for these agents has been established in HIV-infected patients, and they remain expensive and must be delivered parenterally.

Anemia is the most common hematologic abnormality of HIV infection,[101] and treatment with AZT is associated with anemia.[559] Results of a randomized, double-blind, placebo-controlled trial of r-HuEPO (recombinant human erythropoietin) in moderately anemic patients with AIDS who were receiving AZT revealed that r-HuEPO was safe and effective for patients with less than 500 IU/l of endogenous EPO[942].

NEW DEVELOPMENTS IN HIV

Novel herpesvirus DNA sequences were detected in tissue from patients with Kaposi's sarcoma (KS) in 1994.[560] This virus, human herpesvirus 8 (HHV-8) also has been cultured and found in tissues from patients with KS (both HIV seropositive and seronegative).[561]

Drug interactions

Polypharmacy for patients infected with HIV infection is common, and therefore the potential for drug–drug interactions exist. The cytochrome P-450 enzyme system is one major pathway for the metabolism of drugs, and many drugs used in patients with HIV infection can significantly inhibit or induce these enzymes. The protease inhibitors are very potent inhibitors of CYP 3A, and clinically significant drug interactions can occur when these drugs are used with the commonly prescribed azole class of antifungals or macrolide antibiotics. Induction of these enzymes may also clinically reduce effective concentrations of the rifamycins. Ophthalmologists should be keenly aware of the potential for drug–drug interactions.[34,542,543,562]

SYNOPSIS

The common retinal manifestations of AIDS include noninfectious and infectious retinopathy. Chemotherapeutic agents have been developed to treat all known causes of infectious retinopathy and have been shown to be successful in clinical trials, although they are not without complications. The results of treatment of CMV retinitis with foscarnet, ganciclovir, valganciclovir, or cidofovir are very encouraging, but systemic toxicity and the availability of only one convenient oral preparation, valganciclovir, are serious problems, as is the development of rhegmatogenous retinal detachment after healing of retinitis. The vitreoretinal surgeon is commonly involved with AIDS patients in two scenarios. Retinal detachment can now be successfully repaired in a high percentage of cases of CMV retinitis eyes with a good visual outcome. Second, in some cases a tissue diagnosis is required because of the possibility of other forms of viral retinitis; this should be kept in mind when treating these patients, as well as the possibility of endogenous bacterial or fungal endophthalmitis. Implantation of ganciclovir implants can successfully control retinitis but may be associated with retinal detachment, endophthalmitis, and vitreous hemorrhage. Noninfectious, AIDS-associated retinopathy, manifested by retinal cotton-wool spots and hemorrhage, is extremely common. The presence of these lesions may suggest the diagnosis of AIDS in the appropriate clinical setting. Although the pathogenesis of these lesions remains obscure, the lesions do not cause visual loss and should not be confused with infectious retinitis. The advent of highly active antiretroviral therapy has changed the short-term natural history of opportunistic infections of patients infected with HIV and is associated with a new ocular inflammatory syndrome, immune recovery uveitis.

REFERENCES

1. Review of draft for revision of HIV infection classification system and expansion of AIDS surveillance case definition. MMWR Morb Mortal Wkly Rep 1991; 40:787.
2. Revision of the CDC surveillance case definition for acquired immunodeficiency syndrome. Council of State and Territorial Epidemiologists; AIDS Program, Center for Infectious Diseases. MMWR Morb Mortal Wkly Rep 1987; 36 Suppl 1:1S–15S.
3. Revision of the case definition of acquired immunodeficiency syndrome for national reporting – United States. MMWR Morb Mortal Wkly Rep 1985; 34:373–375.
4. Deeks SG, Smith M, Holodniy M et al. HIV-1 protease inhibitors: a review for clinicians. JAMA 1997; 277:145–153.
5. Zhu T, Korber BT, Nahmias AJ et al. An African HIV-1 sequence from 1959 and implications for the origin of the epidemic. Nature 1998; 391:594–597.
6. Freeman WR, Lerner CW, Mines JA et al. A prospective study of the ophthalmologic findings in the acquired immune deficiency syndrome. Am J Ophthalmol 1984; 97:133–142.
7. Jabs DA, Green R, Fox R et al. Ocular manifestations of acquired immune deficiency syndrome. Ophthalmology 1989; 96:1092–1099.
8. Centers for Disease Control and Prevention. Cases of HIV infection and AIDS in the United States, 2002, HIV/AIDS surveillance report, Vol. 14. Online. Available: http://www. cdc.gov/hiv/stats/hasr1402.htm.
9. Hogg RS, Health KV, Yi B et al. Improved survival among HIV-infected individuals following initiation of antiretroviral therapy. JAMA 1998; 279:450–454.
10. Palella FJ, Delaney KM, Moorman AC et al. Declining morbidity and mortality among patients with advanced human immunodeficiency virus infection. N Engl J Med 1998; 338:853–860.
11. Padian NS, Shiboski SC, Jewell NP. Female-to-male transmission of human immunodeficiency virus. JAMA 1991; 266:1664–1667.
12. Centers for Disease Control and Prevention. Surveillance of healthcare personnel with HIV/AIDS, as of December 2002. Online. Available: http://www.cdc.gov/ncidod/hip/BLOOD/hivpersonnel.htm.
13. U.S. Public Health Service. Updated U.S. public health service guidelines for the management of occupational exposures to HBV, HCV, and HIV and recommendations for postexposure prophylaxis. MMWR Recomm Rep 2001; 50(RR-11):1–52 .
14. Marcus R. Surveillance of health care workers exposed to blood from patients infected with the human immunodeficiency virus. N Engl J Med 1988; 319:1118–1123.
15. Cardo DM, Culver DH, Ciesielski CA et al. A case-control study of HIV seroconversion in health care workers after percutaneous exposure. N Engl J Med 1997; 137:1485–1490.
16. Gallo RC, Salahuddin SZ, Popovic M et al. Frequent detection and isolation of cytopathic retroviruses (HTLV-III) from patients with AIDS and at risk for AIDS. Science 1984; 224:500–503.
17. Levy JA, Hoffman AD, Kramer SM. Isolation of lymphocytopathic retroviruses from San Francisco patients with AIDS. Science 1984; 225:840–842.
18. Fauci AS. Immunopathogenic mechanisms of HIV infection. Ann Intern Med 1996; 124:654–663.
19. Feinberg MB. Changing the natural history of HIV disease. Lancet 1996; 348:239–246.
20. Havlir DV, Richman DD. Viral dynamics of HIV: implications for drug development and therapeutic strategies. Ann Intern Med 1996; 124:984–994.

21. Ho DD, Neumann AU, Perelson AS et al. Rapid turnover of plasma virions and CD4 lymphocytes in HIV-1 infection. Nature 1995; 373:123–126.

22. Perelson AS, Newmann AU, Markowitz M et al. HIV-1 dynamics in vivo: virion clearance rate, infected cell life-span, and viral generation time. Science 1996; 271:1582–1586.

23. Coombs RW, Welles SL, Hooper C et al. Association of plasma human immunodeficiency virus type 1 RNA level with risk of clinical progression in patients with advanced infection. J Infect Dis 1996; 174:704–712.

24. Hughes MD, Johnson VA, Hirsch MS. Monitoring plasma HIV-1 RNA levels in addition to CD4+ lymphocyte count improves assessment of antiretroviral therapeutic response. Ann Intern Med 1997; 127:929–938.

25. Mellors JW, Kingsley LA, Rinaldo CR Jr et al. Quantitation of HIV-1 RNA in plasma predicts outcome after seroconversion. Ann Intern Med 1995; 122:573–579.

26. Mellors JW, Rinaldo CR Jr, Gupta P et al. Prognosis in HIV-1 infection predicted by the quantity of virus in plasma. Science 1996; 272:1167–1170.

27. Mellors JW, Munoz A, Giorgi JV et al. Plasma viral load and CD4+ lymphocytes as prognostic markers of HIV-1 infection. Ann Intern Med 1997; 126:946–954.

28. O'Brien WA, Hartigan PM, Martin D et al. Changes in plasma HIV-1 RNA and CD4+ lymphocyte counts and the risk of progression to AIDS. N Engl J Med 1996; 334:426–431.

29. Welles SL, Jackson JB, Yen-Lieberman B et al. Prognostic value of plasma human immunodeficiency virus type 1 (HIV-1) RNA levels in patients with advanced HIV-1 disease and with little or no zidovudine therapy. J Infect Dis 1996; 174:696–703.

30. McDonald CK, Kuritzkes DR. Human immunodeficiency virus type 1 protease inhibitors. Arch Intern Med 1997; 157:951–959.

31. Gulick RM, Mellor JW, Havlir D et al. Treatment with indinavir, zidovudine, and lamivudine in adults with human immunodeficiency virus infection and prior antiretroviral therapy. N Engl J Med 1997; 337: 734–739.

32. Hammer SM, Squires KE, Hughes MD et al. A controlled trial of two nucleoside analogues plus indinavir in persons with human immunodeficiency virus infection and CD4 cell counts of 200 per cubic millimeter or less. N Engl J Med 1997; 337:725–733.

33. Ledergerber B, Egger M, Opravil M et al. Clinical progression and virological failure on highly active antiretroviral therapy in HIV-1 patients: a prospective cohort study. Swiss HIV Cohort Study. Lancet 1999; 353: 863–881.

34. Cervia JS, Smith MA. Enfuvirtide (T-20): a novel human immunodeficiency virus type 1 fusion inhibitor. Clin Infect Dis 2003; 37:1102–1106.

35. Pedersen C, Lindhardt BO, Jensen BL et al. Clinical course of primary HIV infection: consequences for subsequent course of infection. Br Med J 1989; 299:154–157.

36. Chun T, Stuyver L, Mezell S et al. Presence of an inducible HIV-1 latent reservoir during highly active antiretroviral therapy. Proc Natl Acad Sci USA 1997; 94:13193–13197.

37. Wong JK, Hezareh M, Gunthard HF et al. Recovery of replication-competent HIV despite prolonged suppression of plasma viremia. Science 1997; 278:1291–1295.

38. Update: acquired immunodeficiency syndrome – United States. MMWR Morb Mortal Wkly Rep 1986; 35:757–766.

39. Henderly DE, Freeman WR, Smith RE et al. Cytomegalovirus retinitis as the initial manifestation of the acquired immune deficiency syndrome. Am J Ophthalmol 1987; 103:316–320.

40. Update: universal precautions for prevention of transmission of human immunodeficiency virus, hepatitis B virus, and other bloodborne pathogens in health-care settings. MMWR Morb Mortal Wkly Rep 1988; 37:377–388.

41. Schecter WP. HIV infection: risk to the surgeon. Resident Staff Phys 1990; 36:23–27.

42. Leads from the MMWR. Recommendations for preventing possible HTLV-III/LAV virus from tears. JAMA 1985; 254:1429.

43. Update: acquired immunodeficiency syndrome – United States. MMWR Morb Mortal Wkly Rep 1985; 35:17–21.

44. Key CB, Whitman J. Alcohol soaking damages applanation tonometer heads. Arch Ophthalmol 1986; 104:800.

45. Vogt M, Ho DD, Bakar S et al. Safe disinfection of contact lenses after contamination with HTLV-III. Ophthalmology 1986; 93:771–774.

46. Sattar SA, Springthorpe VS. Survival and disinfectant inactivation of the human immunodeficiency virus: a critical review. Rev Infect Dis 1991; 13:430–447.

47. Recommendations for prevention of HIV transmission in health-care settings. MMWR Morb Mortal Wkly Rep 1987; 36 Suppl 2:S1–S18.

48. Centers for Disease Control and Prevention, Department of Health and Human Services. Guidelines for preventing transmission of human immunodeficiency virus through transplantation of human tissue and organs. MMWR Morb Mortal Wkly Rep 1994; 43:1–17.

49. Centers for Disease Control and Prevention. Update: provisional Public Health Service recommendations for chemoprophylaxis after occupational exposure to HIV. MMWR Morb Mortal Wkly Rep 1996; 45: 468–472.

50. Ablashi DV, Sturzenegger S, Hunter EA et al. Presence of HTLV-III in tears and cells from the eyes of AIDS patients. J Exp Pathol 1987; 3:693–703.

51. Fujikawa LS, Salahuddin SZ, Ablashi D et al. Human T-cell leukemia/lymphotropic virus type III in the conjunctival epithelium of a patient with AIDS. Am J Ophthalmol 1985; 100:507–509.

52. Fujikawa LS, Salahuddin SZ, Palestine AG et al. Isolation of human T-cell leukemia/lymphotropic virus type III (HTLV-III) from the tears of a patient with acquired immunodeficiency syndrome (AIDS). Lancet 1985; 2:529.

53. Faber DW, Wiley CA, Bergeron-Lynn G et al. Role of human immunodeficiency virus and cytomegalovirus in the pathogenesis of retinitis and retinal vasculopathy in AIDS patients. Invest Ophthalmol Vis Sci 1992; 33:2345–2353.

54. Freeman WR, Chen A, Henderly D et al. Prognostic and systemic significance of non-infectious AIDS associated retinopathy. Invest Ophthalmol Vis Sci 1987; 28(suppl):9.

55. Freeman WR, Chen A, Henderly DE et al. Prevalence and significance of acquired immunodeficiency syndrome-related retinal microvasculopathy. Am J Ophthalmol 1989; 107:229–235.

56. Cole EL, Meisler DM, Calabrese LH et al. Herpes zoster ophthalmicus and acquired immune deficiency syndrome. Arch Ophthalmol 1984; 102:1027–1029.

56A. Sandor EV, Millman A, Croxson TS et al. Herpes zoster ophthalmicus in patients at risk for the acquired immune deficiency syndrome (AIDS). Am J Ophthalmol 1986; 101:153–155.

57. Holland GN, Pepose JS, Pettit TH et al. Acquired immune deficiency syndrome, ocular manifestations. Ophthalmology 1983; 90:859–873.

58. Kestelyn P, Van de Perre P, Rouvroy D et al. A prospective study of the ophthalmologic findings in the acquired immune deficiency syndrome in Africa. Am J Ophthalmol 1985; 100:230–238.

59. Lipson BK, Freeman WR, Beniz J et al. Optic neuropathy associated with cryptococcal arachnoiditis in AIDS patients. Am J Ophthalmol 1989; 107:523–527.

60. Morinelli EN, Dugel PU, Riffenburgh R et al. Infectious multifocal choroiditis in patients with acquired immune deficiency syndrome. Ophthalmology 1993; 100:1014–1021.

61. Nelson DA, Weiner A, Yanoff M et al. Retinal lesions in subacute sclerosing panencephalitis. Arch Ophthalmol 1970; 84:613–621.

62. Pepose JS, Hilborne LH, Cancilla PA et al. Concurrent herpes simplex and cytomegalovirus retinitis and encephalitis in the acquired immune deficiency syndrome (AIDS). Ophthalmology 1984; 91:1669–1677.

63. Pepose JS, Nestor MS, Holland GN et al. An analysis of retinal cotton-wool spots and cytomegalovirus retinitis in the acquired immunodeficiency syndrome. Am J Ophthalmol 1983; 95:118–119.

64. Rao NA, Zimmerman PL, Boyer D et al. A clinical, histopathologic, and electron microscopic study of *Pneumocystis carinii* choroiditis. Am J Ophthalmol 1989; 107:218–228.

65. Weiss A, Margo CE, Ledord DK et al. Toxoplasmic retinochoroiditis as an initial manifestation of the acquired immune deficiency syndrome. Am J Ophthalmol 1986; 101:248–249.

66. Arevalo JF, Russack V, Freeman WR. New ophthalmic manifestations of presumed rifabutin-related uveitis. Ophthalmic Surg Lasers 1997; 28:321–324.

67. Chaknis MJ, Brooks SE, Mitchell KT et al. Inflammatory opacities of the vitreous in rifabutin-associated uveitis. Am J Ophthalmol 1996; 122: 580–582.

68. Glasgow BJ, Engstrom RE Jr, Holland GN et al. Bilateral endogenous Fusarium endophthalmitis associated with acquired immunodeficiency syndrome. Arch Ophthalmol 1996; 114:873–877.

69. Gonzales CA, Scott IU, Chaudhry NA et al. Endogenous endophthalmitis caused by *Histoplasma capsulatum* var. *capsulatum*: a case report and literature review. Ophthalmology 2000; 107:725–729.

70. Finamor LP, Muccioli C, Martins MC et al. Ocular and central nervous system paracoccidioidomycosis in a pregnant woman with acquired immunodeficiency syndrome. Am J Ophthalmol 2002; 134:456–459.

71. Rosenberg PR, Uliss AE, Friedland GH et al. Acquired immunodeficiency syndrome: ophthalmic manifestations in ambulatory patients. Ophthalmology 1983; 90:874–878.

72. Newman NM, Mandel MR, Gullett J et al. Clinical and histologic findings in opportunistic ocular infections: part of new syndrome of acquired immunodeficiency. Arch Ophthalmol 1983; 101:396.

73. Santos C, Parker J, Dawson C et al. Bilateral fungal corneal ulcers in a patient with AIDS-related complex. Am J Ophthalmol 1985; 102: 118–119.

74. Holland GN, Engstrom RE, Glasgow BJ et al. Ocular toxoplasmosis in patients with the acquired immunodeficiency syndrome. Am J Ophthalmol 1988; 106:653–667.

75. Geier SA, Schielke E, Klauss V et al. Retinal microvasculopathy and reduced cerebral blood flow in patients with acquired immunodeficiency syndrome. Am J Ophthalmol 1992; 113:100–101.

76. Newsome DA, Green W, Miller ED et al. Microvascular aspects of acquired immune deficiency syndrome retinopathy. Am J Ophthalmol 1984; 98:590–601.

77. Aronson AJ, Ordonez NG, Diddie KR et al. Immune-complex deposition in the eye in systemic lupus erythematosus. Arch Intern Med 1979; 139:1312–1313.

78. Yanoff M, Fine BS. Ocular pathology, 2nd edn. Philadelphia: Harper & Row, 1982.

79. Freeman WR, O'Connor GR. Acquired immune deficiency syndrome retinopathy, Pneumocystis, and cotton-wool spots. Am J Ophthalmol 1984; 98:235–237.

80. Kwok S, O'Donnell JJ, Wood IS. Retinal cotton-wool spots in a patient with Pneumocystis carinii infection. N Engl J Med 1982; 307:184–185.

81. O'Donnell JJ, Goodner EK, Shiba AH. A prospective study of eye disease in AIDS. Invest Ophthalmol Vis Sci 1986; 27(suppl):122.

82. Seligmann M, Chess L, Fahey JL et al. AIDS – an immunologic reevaluation. N Engl J Med 1984; 311:1286–1292.

83. Gonzalez CR, Wiley CA, Arevalo JF et al. Polymerase chain reaction detection of cytomegalovirus and human immunodeficiency virus-1 in the retina of patients with acquired immune deficiency syndrome with and without cotton-wool spots. Retina 1996; 16:305–311.

84. Honrubia FM, Ferrer E, Torron C et al. Study of the retinal fiber layer in patients with acquired immunodeficiency syndrome. Ger J Ophthalmol 1994; 3:1–4.

85. Update: universal precautions for prevention of transmission of human immunodeficiency virus, hepatitis B virus, and other bloodborne pathogens in health-care settings. MMWR Morb Mortal Wkly Rep 1988; 37:377–388.

86. Mansour AM, Rodenko G, Dutt R. Half-life of cotton wool spots in the acquired immunodeficiency syndrome. Int J STD AIDS 1990; 1:132–133.

87. Kuppermann BD, Petty JG, Richman DD et al. Cross-sectional prevalence of CMV retinitis in AIDS patients: correlation with CD4 counts. Invest Ophthalmol Vis Sci 1992; 33:750.

88. Sadun AA, Pepose JS, Madigan MC et al. AIDS-related optic neuropathy: a histological, virological and ultrastructural study. Graefes Arch Clin Exp Ophthalmol 1995; 233:387–398.

89. Sadun AA, Tenhula WN, Heller KB. Optic nerve pathology associated with AIDS: ultrastructural changes. ARVO Abstracts (supplement to Invest Ophthalmol Vis Sci). Philadelphia: JB Lippincott, 1990.

90. Tenhula WN, Sadun AA, Heller KB et al. Optic nerve axon losses in AIDS. Morphometric comparisons. ARVO Abstracts. Invest Ophthalmol Vis Sci 1990; 31(suppl):1793.

91. Quiceno JI, Capparelli E, Sadun AA et al. Visual dysfunction without retinitis in patients with acquired immunodeficiency syndrome. Am J Ophthalmol 1992; 113:8–13.

92. Plummer DJ, Arevalo JF, Fram N et al. Effectiveness of entoptic perimetry for locating peripheral scotomas caused by cytomegalovirus retinitis. Arch Ophthalmol 1996; 114:828–831.

93. Latkany PA, Holopigian K, Lorenzo-Latkany M et al. Electroretinographic and psychophysical findings during early and late stages of human immunodeficiency virus infection and cytomegalovirus retinitis. Ophthalmology 1997; 104:445–453.

94. Holland GN, Gottlieb MS, Foos RY. Retinal cotton-wool patches in acquired immunodeficiency syndrome. N Engl J Med 1982; 307:1702.

95. Freeman WR, Henderly DE, Wan WL et al. Prevalence, pathophysiology, and treatment of rhegmatogenous retinal detachment in treated cytomegalovirus retinitis. Am J Ophthalmol 1987; 103:527–536.

96. Henderly DE, Freeman WR, Causey DM et al. Cytomegalovirus retinitis and response to therapy with ganciclovir. Ophthalmology 1987; 94:425–434.

97. Murray HW, Knox DL, Green WR et al. Cytomegalovirus retinitis in adults: a manifestation of disseminated viral infection. Am J Med 1977; 63:574.

98. Spaide RF, Vitale AT, Toth IR et al. Frosted branch angiitis associated with cytomegalovirus retinitis. Am J Ophthalmol 1992; 113:522–528.

99. Engstrom RE, Holland GN, Hardy WD et al. Hemorheologic abnormalities in patients with human immunodeficiency virus infection and ophthalmic microvasculopathy. Am J Ophthalmol 1990; 109:153–161.

100. Conway MD, Tong P, Olk RJ. Branch retinal artery occlusion (BRAO) combined with branch retinal vein occlusion (BRVO) and optic disc neovascularization associated with HIV and CMV retinitis. Int Ophthalmol 1995–1996; 19:249–252.

101. Hambleton J. Hematologic complications of HIV infection. Oncology 1996; 10:671–680.

102. Cunningham ET Jr, Levinson RD, Jampol LM et al. Ischemic maculopathy in patients with acquired immunodeficiency syndrome. Am J Ophthalmol 2001; 132:727–733.

103. Levinson RD, Dunn JP, Holland GN. Ophthalmic disorders associated with selected primary and acquired immunodeficiency diseases. In: Duane's clinical ophthalmology, Chapter 40. CD-ROM. Hagerstown: Harper and Row, 2004.

104. Dejaco-Ruhswurm I, Kiss B, Rainer G et al. Ocular blood flow in patients infected with human immunodeficiency virus. Am J Ophthalmol 2001; 132:719–725.

105. Lim MC, Cumberland WG, Minassian SL et al. Decreased macular leukocyte velocity in HIV-infected individuals. Am J Ophthalmol 2001; 132:710–718.

106. Yung CW, Harris A, Massicotte S et al. Retinal blood flow indices in patients infected with human immunodeficiency virus. Br J Ophthalmol 1996; 80:723–727.

107. Palestine AG, Rodrigues MM, Macher AM et al. Ophthalmic involvement in acquired immune deficiency syndrome. Ophthalmology 1984; 91:1092–1099.

108. Jabs DA, Bartlett JG. AIDS and ophthalmology: a period of transition. Am J Ophthalmol 1997; 124:227–233.

108A. Studies of Ocular Complications of AIDS Research Group in collaboration with the AIDS Clinical Trials Group: Foscarnet–ganciclovir cytomegalovirus retinitis trial 4 – visual outcomes. Ophthalmology 1994; 101:1250–1261.

109. Collaborative DHPG Treatment Study Group. Treatment of serious cytomegalovirus infections with 9-(1,3-dihydroxy-2-propoxymethyl) guanine in patients with AIDS and other immunodeficiencies. N Engl J Med 1986; 314:801–805.

110. Felsenstein D, D'Amico DJ, Hirsch MS et al. Treatment of cytomegalovirus retinitis with 9-[2-hydroxy-1(hydroxy)methyl) ethoxymethyl] guanine. Ann Intern Med 1985; 103:377.

111. Gilquin J, Piketty C, Thomas V et al. Acute CMV infection in AIDS patients receiving combination therapy including protease inhibitors. Program and Abstracts of the Fourth Conference on Retroviruses and Opportunistic Infections. Washington DC, 1997: abstract 354.

112. Chumbley LC, Robertson DM, Smith TF et al. Adult cytomegalovirus inclusion retino-uveitis. Am J Ophthalmol 1975; 80:807.

113. Cogan DG. Immunosuppression and eye disease. Am J Ophthalmol 1977; 83:777–788.

114. Egbert PR, Pollard RB, Gallagher JG et al. Cytomegalovirus retinitis in immunosuppressed hosts. II. Ocular manifestations. Ann Intern Med 1980; 93:664.

115. DeVenecia G, Zu Rhein GM, Pratt MV et al. Cytomegalic inclusion retinitis in an adult, a clinical, histopathologic, and ultrastructural study. Arch Ophthalmol 1971; 86:44.

116. Friedman AH, Orellana J, Freeman WR et al. Cytomegalovirus retinitis: a manifestation of the acquired immune deficiency syndrome (AIDS). Br J Ophthalmol 1983; 67:372–380.

117. Kennedy PGE, Newsome DA, Hess J et al. Cytomegalovirus but not human T lymphotropic virus type III/lymphadenopathy associated virus detected by in-situ hybridization in retinal lesions in patients with the acquired immune deficiency syndrome. Br Med J 1986; 293:162–164.

118. Brody JM, Butrus SI, Laby DM et al. Anterior segment findings in AIDS patients with cytomegalovirus retinitis. Graefes Arch Clin Exp Ophthalmol 1995; 233:374–376.

119. Saran BR, Pomilla PV. Retinal vascular nonperfusion and retinal neovascularization as a consequence of cytomegalovirus retinitis and cryptococcal chorioiditis. Retina 1996; 16:510–512.

120. Palestine AG, Stevens G, Lane HC et al. Treatment of cytomegalovirus retinitis with dihydroxy propoxymethyl guanine. Am J Ophthalmol 1986; 101:95–101.

121. Studies of Ocular Complications of AIDS Research Group in collaboration with the AIDS Clinical Trials Group. Assessment of cytomegalovirus retinitis – clinical evaluation vs. centralized grading of fundus photographs. Arch Ophthalmol 1996; 114:791–805.

122. Studies of Ocular Complications of AIDS Research Group in collaboration with the AIDS Clinical Trials Group. Clinical vs. photographic assessment of treatment of cytomegalovirus retinitis. Foscarnet–ganciclovir cytomegalovirus retinitis trial report 8. Arch Ophthalmol 1996; 114:848–855.

123. Update: universal precautions for prevention of transmission of human immunodeficiency virus, hepatitis B virus, and other bloodborne pathogens in health-care settings. MMWR Morb Mortal Wkly Rep 1988; 37:377–388.

124. Roarty JD, Fisher EJ, Nussbaum JJ. Long-term visual morbidity of cytomegalovirus retinitis in patients with acquired immune deficiency syndrome. Ophthalmology 1993; 100:1685–1688.

125. Wu AW, Coleson LC, Holbrook J, Jabs DA, for Studies of Ocular Complications of AIDS Research Group. Measuring visual function and quality of life in patients with cytomegalovirus retinitis: development of a questionnaire. Arch Ophthalmol 1996; 114:841–847.

126. Bloom PA, Sandy CJ, Migdal CS et al. Visual prognosis of AIDS patients with cytomegalovirus retinitis. Eye 1995; 9:697–702.

127. Luckie AP, Ai E. A foveal-sparing pattern of cytomegalovirus retinitis in the acquired immunodeficiency syndrome. Aust NZ J Ophthalmol 1996; 24:53–59.

128. Gangan PA, Besen G, Munguia D et al. Macular serous exudation in patients with acquired immunodeficiency syndrome and cytomegalovirus retinitis. Am J Ophthalmol 1994; 118:212–219.

129. Minkler DS, Mcleon EB, Shaw CM et al. Herpes virus hominis encephalitis and retinitis. Arch Ophthalmol 1976; 94:89–95.

129A. Freeman WR, Thomas EL, Rao NA et al. Demonstration of herpes group virus in the acute retinal necrosis syndrome. Am J Ophthalmol 1986; 102:701–709.

130. Price JW Jr, Schlaegel TJ Jr. Bilateral acute retinal necrosis. Am J Ophthalmol 1980; 89:419–424.

131. Young SJ, Bird AC. Bilateral acute retinal necrosis. Br J Ophthalmol 1978; 62:581–590.

132. Pollard RB, Egbert PR, Gallagher JG et al. Cytomegalovirus retinitis in immunosuppressed hosts. I. Natural history and effects of treatment with adenine arabinoside. Ann Intern Med 1980; 93:655.

133. Bylsma SS, Achim CL, Wiley CA et al. The predictive value of cytomegalovirus retinitis for cytomegalovirus encephalitis in acquired immunodeficiency syndrome. Arch Ophthalmol 1995; 113:89–95.

134. Mastroianni CM, Ciardi M, Folgori F et al. Cytomegalovirus encephalitis in two patients with AIDS receiving ganciclovir for cytomegalovirus retinitis. J Infect 1994; 29:331–337.

135. Leger F, Vital C, Vital A et al. Pathologic correlations between ocular and cerebral lesions in 36 AIDS patients. Clin Neuropathol 1997; 16:45–48.

136. Livingston PG, Kerr NC, Sullivan JL. Ocular disease in children with vertically acquired human immunodeficiency virus infection. J AAPOS 1998; 2:177–181.

137. Du LT, Coats DK, Kline MW et al. Incidence of presumed cytomegalovirus in HIV-infected pediatric patients. J AAPOS 1999; 3:245–249.

138. Baumal CR, Levin AV, Read SE. Cytomegalovirus retinitis in immuno-suppressed children. Am J Ophthalmol 1999; 127:550–558.

139. Rasmussen L, Zipeto D, Wolitz RA et al. Risk for retinitis in patients with AIDS can be assessed by quantitation of threshold levels of cytomegalovirus DNA burden in blood. J Infect Dis 1997; 176:1146–1155.

140. Brice A, Crumpacker C, Britt W et al. Quantitation of cytomegalovirus (CMV) load in blood fraction of patients with AIDS: a comparative study of different laboratory methods (abstract 166). Abstracts of the Third Conference on Retroviruses and Opportunistic Infections. Alexandria, Va: Infectious Diseases Society of America, 1996.

141. Shinkai M, Bozzette SA, Powderly W et al. Utility of urine and leukocyte cultures and plasma DNA polymerase chain reaction for identification of AIDS patients at risk for developing human cytomegalovirus disease. J Infect Dis 1977; 175:302–308.

142. Zurlo JJ, O'Neill D, Polis MA et al. Lack of clinical utility of cytomegalovirus blood and urine cultures in patients with HIV infection. Ann Intern Med 1993; 118:12–17.

143. Studies of Ocular Complications of AIDS Research Group in collaboration with the AIDS Clinical Trials Group. Foscarnet–ganciclovir cytomegalovirus retinitis trial 5 – clinical features of cytomegalovirus retinitis at diagnosis. Am J Ophthalmol 1997; 124:141–157.

144. Studies of Ocular Complications of AIDS Research Group in collaboration with the AIDS Clinical Trials Group. Cytomegalovirus (CMV) culture results, drug resistance, and clinical outcome in patients with AIDS and CMV retinitis treated with foscarnet or ganciclovir. J Infect Dis 1997; 176:50–58.

145. Pannuti CS, Kallas EG, Muccioli C et al. Cytomegalovirus antigenemia in acquired immunodeficiency syndrome patients with untreated cytomegalovirus retinitis. Am J Ophthalmol 1996; 122:847–852.

146. Hansen KK, Ricksten A, Hofmann B et al. Detection of cytomegalovirus DNA in serum correlates with clinical cytomegalovirus retinitis in AIDS. J Infect Dis 1994; 170:1271–1274.

147. Rasmussen L, Morris S, Zipeto D et al. Quantitation of human cytomegalovirus DNA from peripheral blood cells of human immuno-deficiency virus-infected patients could predict cytomegalovirus retinitis. J Infect Dis 1995; 171:177–182.

148. Bowen EF, Wilson P, Cope A et al. Cytomegalovirus retinitis in AIDS patients: influence of cytomegaloviral load on response to ganciclovir, time to recurrence and survival. AIDS 1996; 10:1515–1520.

149. Hoover DR, Peng Y, Saah A et al. Occurrence of cytomegalovirus retinitis after human immunodeficiency virus immunosuppression. Arch Ophthalmol 1996; 114:821–827.

150. Song MK, Schrier RD, Smith IL. Paradoxical activity of CMV retinitis in patients receiving highly active antiretroviral therapy. Retina 2002; 22:262–267.

151. MacGregor RR, Pakola SJ, Graziani AL et al. Evidence of active cytomegalovirus infection in clinically stable HIV-infected individuals with CD4+ lymphocyte counts below 100/microliters of blood: features and relation to risk of subsequent CMV retinitis. J Acquir Immune Defic Syndr 1995; 10:324–330.

152. Teich SA, Saltzman BR. Evaluation of a new self-screening chart for cytomegalovirus retinitis in patients with AIDS. J Acquir Immune Defic Syndr 1996; 13:336–342.

153. Mitchell SM, Fox JD. Aqueous and vitreous humor samples for the diagnosis of cytomegalovirus retinitis. Am J Ophthalmol 1995; 120:252–253.

154. McCann JD, Margolis TP, Wong MG et al. A sensitive and specific poly-merase chain reaction-based assay for the diagnosis of cytomegalovirus retinitis. Am J Ophthalmol 1995; 120:219–226.

155. Doornenbal P, Seerp BP, Quinot G et al. Diagnostic assays in CMV retinitis: detection of herpesvirus by simultaneous application of the polymerase chain reaction and local antibody analysis in ocular fluid. Br J Ophthalmol 1996; 80:235–246.

156. Schrier RD, Freeman WR, Wiley CA et al. Immune predispositions for cytomegalovirus retinitis in AIDS. The HNRC Group. J Clin Invest 1995; 95:1741–1746.

157. Walter KA, Coulter VL, Palay DA et al. Corneal endothelial deposits in patients with cytomegalovirus retinitis. Am J Ophthalmol 1996; 121:391–396.

158. Dunn JP, Martin DF. Treatment of cytomegalovirus (CMV) retinitis in the era of highly active antiretroviral therapy. Medscape from WebMD Ophthalmology. 30 Sep 2003. Online. Available (with account): http://medscape.com/viewprogram/663.

159. Nichols WG, Boeckh M. Recent advances in the therapy and prevention of CMV infections. J Clin Virol 2000; 16:25–40.

160. See RF, Rao NA. Cytomegalovirus retinitis in the era of combined highly active antiretroviral therapy. Ophthalmol Clin North Am 2002; 15:529–536, viii.

161. Stalder N, Sudre P, Olmari M et al. Cytomegalovirus retinitis: decreased risk of bilaterality with increased use of systemic treatment. Swiss HIV Cohort Study Group. Clin Infect Dis 1997; 24:620–624.

161A. Musch DC, Martin DF, Gordon JF et al. Treatment of cytomegalovirus retinitis with a sustained-release ganciclovir implant. N Engl J Med 1997; 337:83–90.

161B. Martin DF, Kuppermann BD, Wolitz RA et al. Oral ganciclovir for patients with cytomegalovirus retinitis treated with a ganciclovir implant. Roche Ganciclovir Study Group. N Engl J Med 1999; 340:1063–1070.

161C. Jabs DA, Martin BK, Forman MS. Cytomegalovirus resistance to ganci-clovir and clinical outcomes of patients with cytomegalovirus retinitis. Ophthalmol 2003; 135:26–34.

162. Chiron Ganciclovir Implant Study Group. A randomized, controlled, multicenter clinical trial of sustained-release intraocular ganciclovir implant in AIDS patients with CMV retinitis (abstract 1215). Program and abstracts of the Thirty-fifth Interscience Conference on Antimicrobial Agents and Chemotherapy (San Francisco). American Society for Micro-biology. Washington, DC; 1995.

163. Bach MC, Bagwell SP, Knapp NP et al. 9-(1,3-dihydroxy-2-propoxy-methyl) guanine for cytomegalovirus infections in patients with the acquired immunodeficiency syndrome. Ann Intern Med 1985; 103:381.

164. Sha BE, Benson CA, Deutsch TA et al. Suppression of cytomegalovirus retinitis in persons with AIDS with high-dose intravenous acyclovir. J Infect Dis 1991; 164:777–780.

165. Biron KK, Stanat SC, Sorrell JB et al. Metabolic activation of the nucleoside analog 9-[[2-hydroxy-1-(hydroxymethyl) ethoxy]methyl] guanine in human diploid fibroblasts infected with human cytomegalovirus. Proc Natl Acad Sci USA 1985; 82:2473–2477.

166. Field AK, Daview ME, Dewitt C et al. 9-[[2-hydroxy-1-(hydroxymethyl)ethoxy]methyl] guanine: a selective inhibitor of herpes group virus replication. Proc Natl Acad Sci USA 1983; 80:4139–4143.

167. Smith KO, Galloway KS, Kennel WL et al. A new nucleoside analog 9-[[2-hydroxy-1-(hydroxymethyl) ethoxy]methyl] guanine highly active in vitro against herpes simplex virus types 1 and 2. Antimicrob Agents Chemother 1982; 22:55–61.

168. Anand R, Font RL, Fish RH et al. Pathology of cytomegalovirus retinitis treated with sustained release intravitreal ganciclovir. Ophthalmology 1993; 100:1032–1039.

169. Jabs DA, Enger C, Bartlett JG. Cytomegalovirus retinitis and acquired immunodeficiency syndrome. Arch Ophthalmol 1989; 107:75–80.

170. Holland GN, Sidikaro Y, Kreiger AE et al. Treatment of cytomegalovirus retinopathy with ganciclovir. Ophthalmology 1987; 94:815–823.

171. Jacobson MA, O'Donnell JJ, Porteous D et al. Retinal and gastrointestinal disease due to cytomegalovirus in patients with the acquired immune deficiency syndrome: prevalence, natural history, and response to ganciclovir therapy. Q J Med 1988; 67:473–486.

172. Laskin OL, Cederberg DM, Mills J et al. Ganciclovir for the treatment and suppression of serious infections caused by cytomegalovirus. Am J Med 1987; 83:201.

173. Orellana J, Teich SA, Friedman AH et al. Combined short- and long-term therapy for the treatment of cytomegalovirus retinitis using ganciclovir (BW B759U). Ophthalmology 1987; 94:831–838.

174. Studies of Ocular Complications of AIDS Research Group in collaboration with the AIDS Clinical Trials Group: Mortality in patients with the acquired immunodeficiency syndrome treated with either foscarnet or ganciclovir for cytomegalovirus retinitis. N Engl J Med 1992; 326:213–220.

174A. Jabs DA. Ganciclovir treatment of cytomegalovirus retinitis in patients with AIDS. In: Spector SA, ed. Ganciclovir therapy for cytomegalovirus infection. New York: Marcel Dekker, 1991.

175. Hoechst H, Dieterich D, Bozzette S et al. Toxicity of combined ganciclovir and zidovudine for cytomegalovirus disease associated with AIDS. Ann Intern Med 1990; 113:111–117.

176. Drew WL, Miner RC, Mehalko S et al. CMV resistance in patients receiving ganciclovir. Twenty-ninth Interscience Conference on Antimicrobial Agents and Chemotherapy. Houston, Sept 17–20, 1989: abstract 61.

177. Biron KK, Stanat SC, Reardon J et al. Ganciclovir-resistant clinical isolates of CMV: antiviral susceptibility profiles and mode of resistance studies. Paper presented at the Second International Cytomegalovirus Workshop. San Diego, March 27–30, 1989:abstract 65.

178. Studies of Ocular Complications of AIDS Research Group in collaboration with the AIDS Clinical Trials Group: Combination foscarnet and ganciclovir therapy vs. monotherapy for the treatment of relapsed cytomegalovirus retinitis in patients with AIDS: the cytomegalovirus retreatment trial. Arch Ophthalmol 1996; 114:23–33.

179. Gross JG, Bozzette SA, Mathews WC et al. Longitudinal study of cytomegalovirus retinitis in acquired immune deficiency syndrome. Ophthalmology 1990; 97:681–686.

180. Spector SA, McKinley GF, Lalezari JP et al. Oral ganciclovir for the prevention of cytomegalovirus disease in persons with AIDS. N Engl J Med 1996; 334:1491–1497.

181. Brosgart CL, Louis TA, Hillman DW et al. A randomized, placebo-controlled trial of the safety and efficacy of oral ganciclovir for prophylaxis of cytomegalovirus disease in HIV-infected individuals. Terry Beirn Community Programs for Clinical Research on AIDS. AIDS 1998; 12:269–277.

182. Oral Ganciclovir European and Australian Cooperative Study Group. Intravenous vs. oral ganciclovir: European/Australian comparative study of efficacy and safety in the prevention of cytomegalovirus retinitis recurrence in patients with AIDS. The Oral Ganciclovir European and Australian Cooperative Study Group. AIDS 1995; 9:471–477.

183. Squires KE. Oral ganciclovir for cytomegalovirus retinitis in patients with AIDS: results of two randomized studies. AIDS 1996; 10 (suppl 4):13–18.

184. Sugawara M, Huang W, Fei YJ. Transport of valganciclovir, a ganciclovir prodrug, via peptide transporters PEPT1 and PEPT2. J Pharm Sci 2000; 89:781–789.

185. Jung D, Dorr A. Single-dose pharmacokinetics of valganciclovir in HIV- and CMV-seropositive subjects. J Clin Pharmacol 1999; 39:800–804.

186. Brown F, Banken L, Saywell K et al. Pharmacokinetics of valganciclovir and ganciclovir following multiple oral dosages of valganciclovir in HIV- and CMV-seropositive volunteers. Clin Pharmacokinet 1999; 37:167–176.

187. Martin DF, Sierra-Madero J, Walmsley S et al. A controlled trial of valganciclovir as induction therapy for cytomegalovirus retinitis. N Engl J Med 2002; 346:1119–1126.

188. Lalezari J, Lindley J, Walmsley S et al. A safety study of oral valganciclovir maintenance treatment of cytomegalovirus retinitis. J Acquir Immune Defic Syndr 2002; 30:392–400.

189. Crumpacker CS. Mechanism of action of foscarnet against viral polymerases. Am J Med 1992; 92(suppl 2A):3–7.

190. Bergdahl S, Sonnerbor A, Larsson A et al. Declining levels of HIV p24 antigen in serum during treatment with foscarnet. Lancet 1988; 1:1052.

191. Crumpacker CS, Kowalsky PN, Oliver SA et al. Resistance of herpes simplex virus to 9-[[2-(hydroxymethyl) ethoxy]methyl] guanine (2-NDG); physical mapping of drug synergism within the viral DNA polymerase locus. Proc Natl Acad Sci USA 1984; 81:1556–1560.

192. Jacobson MA, Crowe S, Levy J et al. Effect of foscarnet therapy on infection with human immunodeficiency virus in patients with AIDS. J Infect Dis 1988; 158:862–865.

193. Jacobson MA, Wulfsohn M, Feinberg JE et al. Phase II dose-ranging trial of foscarnet salvage therapy for cytomegalovirus retinitis in AIDS patients intolerant of or resistant to ganciclovir (ACTG protocol 093). AIDS Clinical Trials Group of the National Institute of Allergy and Infectious Diseases. AIDS 1994; 8:451–459.

194. Studies of Ocular Complications of AIDS Research Group in collaboration with the AIDS Clinical Trials Group. Morbidity and toxic effects associated with ganciclovir or foscarnet therapy in a randomized cytomegalovirus retinitis trial. Arch Intern Med 1995; 155:65–74.

195. Studies of Ocular Complications of AIDS Research Group in collaboration with the AIDS Clinical Trials Group. Antiviral effects of foscarnet and ganciclovir therapy on human immunodeficiency virus p24 antigen in patients with AIDS and cytomegalovirus retinitis. J Infect Dis 1995; 172:613–621.

196. Jabs DA. Controversies in the treatment of cytomegalovirus retinitis: foscarnet vs. ganciclovir. Infect Agents Dis 1995; 4:131–142.

197. Deray G, Martinez F, Katlama C et al. Foscarnet nephrotoxicity: mechanism, incidence, and prevention. Am J Nephrol 1989; 9:316–321.

198. Castelli F, Tomasoni L, Zeroli C et al. Comparison of pharmacokinetics and dynamics of two dosage regimens of foscarnet in AIDS patients with cytomegalovirus retinitis. Eur J Clin Pharmacol 1997; 52:397–401.

199. Holland GN, Levinson RD, Jacobson MA. Dose-related difference in progression rates of cytomegalovirus retinopathy during foscarnet maintenance therapy. AIDS Clinical Trials Group Protocol 915 Team. Am J Ophthalmol 1995; 119:576–586.

200. Berthe P, Baudouin C, Garraffo R et al. Toxicologic and pharmacokinetic analysis of intravitreal injections of foscarnet, either alone or in combination with ganciclovir. Invest Ophthalmol Vis Sci 1994; 35:1038–1045.

201. Lehoang P, Girard B, Robinet M et al. Foscarnet in the treatment of cytomegalovirus retinitis in acquired immune deficiency syndrome. Ophthalmology 1989; 96:865–874.

202. Oberg BO. Antiviral effects of phosphonoformate (PFA, foscarnet sodium). Pharmacol Ther 1989; 40:213–285.

203. Palestine AG, Polis MA, De Smet MD et al. A randomized controlled trial of foscarnet in the treatment of cytomegalovirus retinitis in patients with AIDS. Ann Intern Med 1991; 115:665–673.

204. Drusano GL, Aweeka F, Gambertoglio J et al. Relationship between foscarnet exposure, baseline cytomegalovirus (CMV) blood culture, and the time to progression of CMV retinitis in HIV-positive patients. AIDS 1996; 10:1113–1119.

205. Lalezari JP. Cidofovir: a new therapy for cytomegalovirus retinitis. J Acquir Immune Defic Syndr 1997; 14 (suppl 1):22–26.

206. Lalezari JP, Stagg RJ, Kuppermann BD et al. Intravenous cidofovir for peripheral cytomegalovirus retinitis in patients with AIDS: a randomized, controlled trial. Ann Intern Med 1997; 126:257–263.

206a. The Studies of Ocular Complications of AIDS Research Group in collaboration with the AIDS Clinical Trials Group. Long-term follow-up of patients with AIDS treated with parenteral cidofovir for cytomegalovirus: the HPMPC Peripheral Cytomegalovirus Retinitis Trial. AIDS 2000; 14:1571–1581.

207. Studies of Ocular Complications of AIDS Research Group in collaboration with the AIDS Clinical Trials Group. Parenteral cidofovir for cytomegalovirus retinitis in patients with AIDS: the HPMPC peripheral cytomegalovirus retinitis trial – a randomized, controlled trial. Ann Intern Med 1997; 126:264–274.

208. Rahhal FM, Arevalo JF, Chavez de la Paz E et al. Treatment of cytomegalovirus retinitis with intravitreous cidofovir in patients with AIDS: a preliminary report. Ann Intern Med 1996; 125:98–103.

209. Davis JL, Taskintuna I, Freeman WR et al. Iritis and hypotony after treatment with intravenous cidofovir for cytomegalovirus retinitis. Arch Ophthalmol 1997; 115:733–737.

210. Kirsch LS, Arevalo JF, Chavez de la Paz E et al. Intravitreal cidofovir (HPMPC) treatment of cytomegalovirus retinitis in patients with acquired immune deficiency syndrome. Ophthalmology 1995; 102:533–543.

211. Rahhal FM, Arevalo JF, Munguia D, et al: Intravitreal cidofovir for the maintenance treatment of cytomegalovirus retinitis. Ophthalmology 1996; 103:1078–1083.

212. Palau LA, Tufty GT, Pankey GA. Recurrent iritis after intravenous administration of cidofovir. Clin Infect Dis 1997; 25:337–338.

213. Jabs DA, Dunn JP, Enger C et al. Cytomegalovirus retinitis and viral resistance: prevalence of resistance at diagnosis, 1994. Cytomegalovirus Retinitis and Viral Resistance Study Group. Arch Ophthalmol 1996; 114:809–814.

214. Crumpacker CSE. Drug resistance in cytomegalovirus: current knowledge and implications for patient management. J Acquir Immune Defic Syndr 1996; 12(suppl 1):6–7.

215. Jabs DA, Enger C, Dunn JP et al. Cytomegalovirus retinitis and viral resistance: 4. Ganciclovir resistance. J Infect Dis 1998; 177:770–773.

216. Smith KL, Cherrington JM, Jiles RE et al. High-level resistance of cytomegalovirus to ganciclovir is associated with alterations in both the UL97 and DNA polymerase genes. J Infect Dis 1997; 176:69–77.

217. Drew WL, Miner RC, Busch DF et al. Prevalence of resistance in patients receiving ganciclovir for serious cytomegalovirus infection. J Infect Dis 1991; 163:716–719.

218. Drew WL, Stempton MJ, Andrews J et al. Cytomegalovirus (CMV) resistance in patients with CMV retinitis and AIDS treated with oral or intravenous ganciclovir. J Infect Dis 1999; 179:1352–1355.

219. Jabs DA, Enger C, Forman M et al. Incidence of foscarnet resistance and cidofovir resistance in patients treated for cytomegalovirus retinitis. The Cytomegalovirus Retinitis and Viral Resistance Study Group. Antimicrob Agents Chemother 1998; 42:2240–2241.

220. Boivin G, Gilbert C, Gaudreau A et al. Rate of emergence of cytomegalovirus (CMV) mutations in leukocytes of patients with acquired immunodeficiency syndrome who are receiving valganciclovir as induction and maintenance therapy for CMV retinitis. J Infect Dis 2001; 184:1598–1602.

221. Drew WL, Miner RC, Saleh E et al. Antiviral susceptibility of cytomegalovirus: criteria for detecting resistance to antivirals. Clin Diagn Virol 1993; 1:179–185.

222. Enger C, Jabs DA, Dunn JP et al. Viral resistance and CMV retinitis: design and methods of a prospective study. Ophthalmic Epidemiol 1997; 4:41–48.

223. Jabs DA, Martin BK, Forman MS et al. Longitudinal observations on mutations conferring ganciclovir resistance in patients with acquired immunodeficiency syndrome and cytomegalovirus retinitis: the cytomegalovirus and viral resistance study group report number 8. Am J Ophthalmol 2001; 132:700–710.

224. Sullivan V, Biron KK, Talarico C et al. A point mutation in the human cytomegalovirus DNA polymerase gene confers resistance to ganciclovir and phosphonylmethoxyalkyl derivatives. Antimicrob Agents Chemother 1993; 37:19–25.

225. Chou S, Guentzel S, Michels KR et al. Frequency of UL97 phosphotransferase mutations related to ganciclovir resistance in clinical cytomegalovirus isolates. J Infect Dis 1995; 172:239–242.

226. Lurain NS, Thompson KD, Holmes EW et al. Point mutations in the DNA polymerase gene of human cytomegalovirus that result in resistance to antiviral agents. J Virol 1992; 66:7146–7152.

227. Erice A, Gil-Roda C, Perez JL et al. Antiviral susceptibilities and analysis of UL97 and DNA polymerase sequences of clinical cytomegalovirus isolates from immunocompromised patients. J Infect Dis 1999; 175:1087–1092.

228. Chou S, Marousek G, Guentzel S et al. Evolution of mutations conferring multidrug resistance during prophylaxis and therapy for cytomegalovirus disease. J Infect Dis 1997; 176:786–789.

229. Cihlar T, Fuller MD, Cherrington JM. Characterization of drug resistance-associated mutations in the human cytomegalovirus DNA polymerase gene by using recombinant mutant viruses generated from overlapping DNA fragments. J Virol 1998; 72:5927–5936.

230. Jabs DA, Martin BK, Forman MS et al. Mutations conferring ganciclovir resistance in a cohort of patients with AIDS and cytomegalovirus retinitis. J Infect Dis 2001; 183:333–337.

231. Cherrington JM, Fuller MD, Lamy PD et al. In vitro antiviral susceptibilities of isolates from cytomegalovirus retinitis patients receiving first- or second-line cidofovir therapy: relationship to clinical outcome. J Infect Dis 1998; 178:1821–1825.

232. Landry ML, Stanat S, Biron K et al. A standardized plaque reduction assay for determination of drug susceptibilities of cytomegalovirus clinical isolates. Antimicrob Agents Chemother 2000; 44:688–692.

233. Chou S, Miner RC, Drew WL. A deletion mutation in region V of the cytomegalovirus DNA polymerase sequence confers multidrug resistance. J Infect Dis 2000; 182:1765–1768.

234. Weinberg A, Jabs DA, Chou S et al. Mutations conferring foscarnet resistance in a cohort of patients with acquired immunodeficiency syndrome and cytomegalovirus retinitis. J Infect Dis 2003; 187:777–784.

235. Danker WM, Scholl D, Stanat SC et al. Rapid antiviral DNA–DNA hybridization assay for human cytomegalovirus. J Virol Methods 1990; 28:293–298.

236. Gerna G, Sarasini A, Percivalle E et al. Rapid screening for resistance to ganciclovir and foscarnet of primary isolates of human cytomegalovirus from culture-positive blood samples. J Clin Microbiol 1995; 33:738–741.

237. McSharry JM, Lurain NS, Drusano GJ et al. Flow cytometric determination of ganciclovir susceptibilities of human cytomegalovirus clinical isolates. J Clin Microbiol 1998; 958–964.

238. Tatarowicz WA, Lurain NS, Thompson KD. In situ ELISA for the evaluation of antiviral compounds effective against human cytomegalovirus. J Virol Methods 1991; 35:207–215.

239. Boivin G, Gilbert C, Morissette M et al. A case of ganciclovir-resistant cytomegalovirus (CMV) retinitis in a patient with AIDS: longitudinal molecular analysis of the CMV viral load and viral mutations in blood compartments. AIDS 1997; 11:867–873.

240. Spector SA, Hsia K, Wolf D et al. Molecular detection of human cytomegalovirus and determination of genotypic ganciclovir resistance in clinical specimens. Clin Infect Dis 1995; 21 (Suppl 2):S170–S173.

241. Erice A. Resistance of human cytomegalovirus to antiviral drugs. Clin Microbiol Rev 1999; 12:286–297.

242. Chou S, Lurain NS, Weinberg A et al. Interstrain variation in the human cytomegalovirus DNA polymerase sequence and its effect on the genotypic diagnosis of antiviral drug resistance. Antimicrob Agents Chemother 1999; 43:1500–1502.

243. Chou S, Marousek G, Parenti DM et al. Mutation in region III of the DNA polymerase gene conferring foscarnet resistance in cytomegalovirus isolates from 3 subjects receiving prolonged antiviral therapy. J Infect Dis 1998; 178:526–530.

244. Gilbert C, Bestman-Smith J, Boivin G. Resistance of herpesvirus to antiviral drugs: clinical impacts and molecular mechanisms. Drug Resist Updat 2002; 5:88–114.

245. Chou S, Lurain NS, Thompson KD et al. Viral DNA polymerase mutations associated with drug resistance in human cytomegalovirus. J Infect Dis 2003; 188:32–39.

246. Hu H, Jabs DA, Forman MS et al. Comparison of cytomegalovirus (CMV) UL97 gene sequences in the blood and vitreous of patients with acquired immunodeficiency syndrome and CMV retinitis. J Infect Dis 2002; 185:861–867.

247. Dunn JP, MacCumber MW, Forman MS et al. Viral sensitivity testing in patients with cytomegalovirus retinitis clinically resistant to foscarnet or ganciclovir. Am J Ophthalmol 1995; 119:587–596.

248. Jabs DA, Martin BK, Forman MS et al. Cytomegalovirus resistance to ganciclovir and clinical outcomes of patients with cytomegalovirus retinitis. Am J Ophthalmol 2003; 135:26–34.

249. Arevalo JF, Gonzalez C, Capparelli EV et al. Intravitreous and plasma concentrations of ganciclovir and foscarnet after intravenous therapy in patients with AIDS and cytomegalovirus. J Infect Dis 1995; 172:951–956.

250. Martin DF, Kuppermann BD, Wolitz RA et al. Oral ganciclovir for patients with cytomegalovirus retinitis treated with a ganciclovir implant. Roche ganciclovir study group. N Engl J Med 1999; 340:1063–1070.

251. Kuppermann BD, Flores-Aguilar M, Quiceno J et al. Combination ganciclovir and foscarnet therapy in the treatment of clinically resistant cytomegalovirus retinitis in patients with the acquired immune deficiency syndrome. Am J Ophthalmol 1993; 111:1359–1366.

252. Update: acquired immunodeficiency syndrome – United States. MMWR Morb Mortal Wkly Rep 1985; 35:17–21.

253. Walton RC, Whitcup SM, Mueller BU et al. Combined intravenous ganciclovir and foscarnet for children with recurrent cytomegalovirus retinitis. Ophthalmology 1995; 102:1865–1870.

254. Desatnik HR, Foster RE, Lowder CY. Treatment of clinically resistant cytomegalovirus retinitis with combined intravitreal injections of ganciclovir and foscarnet. Am J Ophthalmol 1996; 122:121–123.

255. Heinemann MH. Long-term intravitreal ganciclovir therapy for cytomegalovirus retinopathy. Arch Ophthalmol 1989; 107:1767–1772.

256. Yoshizumi M, Lee D, Vinci S et al. Ocular toxicity of multiple intravitreal DHPG injections. Graefes Arch Clin Exp Ophthalmol 1990; 228:350–355.

257. Pulido J, Peyman GA, Legar TI et al. Intravitreal toxicity of hydroxyacyclovir (BW-B759U), new antiviral agent. Arch Ophthalmol 1985; 103:840–841.

258. Hodge WG, Lalonde RG, Sampalis J et al. Once-weekly intraocular injections of ganciclovir for maintenance therapy of cytomegalovirus retinitis: clinical and ocular outcome. J Infect Dis 1996; 174:393–396.

259. Montero MC, Pastor M, Buenestado C et al. Intravitreal ganciclovir for cytomegalovirus retinitis in patients with AIDS. Ann Pharmacother 1996; 30:717–723.

260. Young S, Morlet N, Besen G et al. High-dose (2000-microgram) intravitreous ganciclovir in the treatment of cytomegalovirus retinitis. Ophthalmology 1998; 105:1404–1410.

261. Saran BR, Maguire AM. Retinal toxicity of high dose intravitreal ganciclovir. Retina 1994; 14:248–252.

262. Baudouin C, Chassain C, Caujolle et al. Treatment of cytomegalovirus retinitis in AIDS patients using intravitreal injections of highly concentrated ganciclovir. Ophthalmologica 1996; 210:329–335.

263. Tognon MS, Turrini B, Masiero G et al. Intravitreal and systemic foscarnet in the treatment of AIDS-related CMV retinitis. Eur J Ophthalmol 1996; 6:179–182.

264. Diaz-Llopis M, Espana E, Munoz G et al. High dose intravitreal foscarnet in the treatment of cytomegalovirus retinitis in AIDS. Br J Ophthalmol 1994; 78:120–124.

265. Sandorn GE, Anand R, Torti RE et al. Sustained-release ganciclovir therapy for treatment of cytomegalovirus retinitis: use of an intravitreal device. Arch Ophthalmol 1992; 110:188–195.

266. Martin DF, Parks DJ, Mellow SD et al. Treatment of cytomegalovirus retinitis with an intraocular sustained-release ganciclovir implant: a randomized controlled clinical trial [see comments]. Arch Ophthalmol 1994; 112:1531–1539.

267. Marx JL, Kapusta MA, Patel SS et al. Use of the ganciclovir implant in the treatment of recurrent cytomegalovirus retinitis. Arch Ophthalmol 1996; 114:815–820.

268. Martin D, Kupperman B, Wolitz R et al. Combined oral ganciclovir (GCV) and intravitreal GCV implant for the treatment of patients with cytomegalovirus (CMV) retinitis: a randomized, controlled study. In: 37th Interscience Conference of Antimicrobial Agents and Chemotherapy, Toronto, Ontario, Canada, December 28–October 1, 1997. Abstract LB-9.

269. Martin DF, Ferris FL, Brothers RJ et al. Retinal detachment in eyes treated with a ganciclovir implant [Letter]. Arch Ophthalmol 1995; 113:1355.

270. Martin DF, Dunn JP, Davis JL et al. Use of the ganciclovir implant for the treatment of cytomegalovirus retinitis in the era of potent antiretroviral therapy: recommendations of the International AIDS Society – USA panel. Am J Ophthalmol 1999; 127:329–339.

271. Kempen JH, Jabs DA, Dunn JP et al. Retinal detachment risk in cytomegalovirus retinitis related to the acquired immunodeficiency syndrome. Arch Ophthalmol 2001; 119:33–40.

272. Shane TS, Martin DF. Endophthalmitis after ganciclovir implant in patients with AIDS and cytomegalovirus retinitis. Am J Ophthalmol 2003; 136:649–654.

273. Flores-Aguilar M, Huang JS, Wiley CA et al. Long-acting therapy of viral retinitis with (S)-1-(3-hydroxy-2-phosphonylmethoxypropyl)cytosine. J Infect Dis 1994; 169:642–647.

274. Kirsch LS, Arevalo JF, De Clercq E et al. Phase I/II study of intravitreal cidofovir for the treatment of cytomegalovirus retinitis in patients with the acquired immunodeficiency syndrome. Am J Ophthalmol 1995; 119:466–476.

275. Banker AS, Arevalo JF, Munguia D et al. Intraocular pressure and aqueous humor dynamics in patients with AIDS treated with intravitreal cidofovir (HPMPC) for cytomegalovirus retinitis. Am J Ophthalmol 1997; 124:168–180.

276. Besen B, Flores-Aguilar M, Assil KK et al. Long-term therapy for herpes retinitis in an animal model with high-concentrated liposome-encapsulated HPMPC. Arch Ophthalmol 1995; 113:661–668.

277. Kirsch LS, Arevalo JF, Chavez de la Paz E et al. Intravitreal cidofovir (HPMPC) treatment of cytomegalovirus retinitis in patients with acquired immune deficiency syndrome [published erratum appears in Ophthalmology 102:702, 1995]. Ophthalmology 1995; 102:533–542; discussion 542–543.

278. Kuppermann BD, Assil KK, Vuong C et al. Liposome-encapsulated (S)-1-(3-hydroxy-2-phosphonylmethoxypropyl) cytosine for long-acting therapy of viral retinitis. J Infect Dis 1996; 173:18–23.

279. Taskintuna I, Rahhal FM, Arevalo JF et al. Low-dose intravitreal cidofovir (HPMPC) therapy of cytomegalovirus retinitis in patients with acquired immune deficiency syndrome. Ophthalmology 1997; 104:1049–1057.

280. Cundyc KC, Lynch G, Shaw JP et al. Distribution and metabolism of intravitreal cidofovir and cyclic HPMPC in rabbits. Curr Eye Res 1996; 15:569–576.

281. Chavez-de la Paz E, Arevalo JF, Kirsch LS et al. Anterior nongranulomatous uveitis after intravitreal HPMPC (cidofovir) for the treatment of cytomegalovirus retinitis: analysis and prevention. Ophthalmology 1997; 104:539–544.

282. Arevalo JF, Munguia D, Faber D et al. Correlation between intraocular pressure and CD4+ T-lymphocyte counts in patients with human immunodeficiency virus with and without cytomegalovirus retinitis. Am J Ophthalmol 1996; 122:91–96.

283. Flores-Aguilar M, Besen G, Vuong C et al. Evaluation of retinal toxicity and efficacy of anti-cytomegalovirus and anti-herpes simplex virus antiviral phosphorothioate oligonucleotides ISIS 2922 and ISIS 4015. J Infect Dis 1997; 175:1308–1316.

284. Azad RF, Driver VB, Tanaka K et al. Antiviral activity of a phosphorothioate oligonucleotide complementary to RNA of the human cytomegalovirus major immediate-early region. Antimicrob Agents Chemother 1993; 37:1945–1954.

285. Crooke ST. Proof of mechanism of antisense drugs. Antisense Nucleic Acid Drug Dev 1996; 6:145–147.

286. Zamecnik PC, Stephenson ML. Inhibition of Rous sarcoma virus replication and cell transformation by a specific oligodeoxynucleotide. Proc Natl Acad Sci USA 1978; 75:280–284.

287. Azad RF, Brown-Driver V, Buckheit RJ et al. Antiviral activity of a phosphorothioate oligonucleotide complementary to human cytomegalo-virus RNA when used in combination with antiviral nucleoside analogs. Antiviral Res 1995; 28:101–111.

288. Anderson KP, Fox MC, Brown-Driver V et al. Inhibition of human cytomegalovirus immediate-early gene expression by an antisense oligonucleotide complementary to immediate-early RNA. Antimicrob Agents Chemother 1996; 40:2004–2011.

289. Detrick B, Nagineni CN, Grillone LR et al. Inhibition of human cytomegalovirus replication in a human retinal epithelial cell model by antisense oligonucleotides. Invest Ophthalmol Vis Sci 2001; 42:163–169.

290. The Vitravene Study Group. A randomized controlled clinical trial of intravitreous fomivirsen for treatment of newly diagnosed peripheral cytomegalovirus retinitis in patients with AIDS. Am J Ophthalmol 2002; 133:467–474.

291. Geary RS, Henry SP, Grillone LR. Fomivirsen: clinical pharmacology and potential drug interactions. Clin Pharmacokinet 2002; 41:255–260.

292. Freeman WR. Retinal toxic effects associated with intravitreal fomivirsen. Arch Ophthalmol 2001; 119:458.

293. The Vitravene Study Group. Randomized dose-comparison studies of intravitreous fomivirsen for treatment of cytomegalovirus retinitis that has reactivated or is persistently active despite other therapies in patients with AIDS. Am J Ophthalmol 2002; 133:475–483.

294. The Vitravene Study Group. Safety of intravitreous fomivirsen for treatment of cytomegalovirus retinitis patients with AIDS. Am J Ophthalmol 2002; 133:484–498.

295. Jabs DA, Griffiths PD. Fomivirsen for the treatment of cytomegalovirus retinitis. Am J Ophthalmol 2002; 133:552–556.

296. Amin HI, Ai E. Retinal toxic effects associated with intravitreal fomivirsen. Arch Ophthalmol 2000; 118:426–427.

297. Uwaydat SH, Li HK. Pigmentary retinopathy associated with intravitreal fomivirsen. Arch Ophthalmol 2002; 120:854–857.

298. Biron KK, Harvey RG, Chamberlain SS. Potent and selective inhibition of human cytomegalovirus replication by 1263W94, a benzimidazole L-riboside with a unique mode of action. Antimicrob Agents Chemother 2002; 46:2365–2372.

299. Chulay JK, Biron K, Want L et al. Development of novel benzimidazole riboside compounds for treatment of cytomegalovirus disease. In: Mills J, Volberding P, Corey L, eds. Antiviral therapy 5: new directions for clinical applications and research. New York: Kluwer Academic/Plenum Publishers, 1999; 129–134.

300. Koszalka GW, Johnson NW, Good SS et al. Preclinical and toxicology studies of 1263W94, a potent and selective inhibitor of human cytomegalovirus replication. Antimicrob Agents Chemother 2002; 46:2373–2380.

301. Emery VC, Hassan-Walker AF. Focus on new drugs in development against human cytomegalovirus. Drugs 2002; 62:1853–1858.

302. De Clercq E. Antiviral drugs: current state of the art. J Clin Virol 2001; 22:73–89.

303. Wang LH, Peck RW, Yin Y et al. Phase I safety and pharmacokinetic trials of 1263W94, a novel oral anti-human cytomegalovirus agent, in healthy and human immunodeficiency virus-infected subjects. Antimicrob Agents Chemother 2003;47:1334–1342.

304. Lalezari JP, Aberg JA, Wang LH et al. Phase I dose escalation trial evaluating the pharmacokinetics, anti-human cytomegalovirus (HCMV) activity, and safety of 1263W94 in human immunodeficiency virus-infected men with asymptomatic HCMV shedding. Antimicrob Agents Chemother 2002; 46:2969–2976.

305. Komazin G, Ptak RG, Emmer BT et al. Resistance of human cytomegalovirus to the benzimidazole L-ribonucleoside maribavir maps to UL27. J Virol 2003; 77:11499–11506.

306. Komazin G, Ptak RG, Emmer BT et al. Resistance of human cytomegalovirus to D- and L-ribosyl benzimidazoles as a tool to identify potential targets for antiviral drugs. Nucleosides Nucleotides Nucleic Acids 2003; 22:1725–1727.

307. Krosky PM, Baek M, Coen DM. The human cytomegalovirus UL97 protein kinase, an antiviral target, is required at the stage of nuclear egress. J Virol 2003; 77:905–914.

308. Kern A, Blombach M, Schmeer K et al. In vivo metabolism in rat and dog of BAY 38-4766 – a novel non-nucleosidic inhibitor of human cytomegalovirus replication [abstract no. 943]. Proceedings of the 39th ICAAC; 1999 Sep 26–29; San Francisco.

309. Hallenberger S, Trappe J, Buerger I et al. Mechanism of antiviral action of BAY 38-4766 – a novel non-nucleosidic inhibitor of human cytomegalovirus replication [abstract no. 941]. Proceedings of the 39th ICAAC; 1999 Sep 26–29; San Francisco.

310. Nagelschmitz J, Moeller JG, Stass H et al. Safety, tolerability and pharmacokinetics of single oral doses of BAY 38-4766 – a novel, non-nucleosidic inhibitor of human cytomegalovirus (HCMV) replication – in healthy male subjects [abstract no. 945]. Proceedings of the 39th ICAAC; 1999 Sep 26–29; San Francisco.

311. Kempen JH, Jabs DA, Wilson LA et al. Risk of vision loss in patients with cytomegalovirus retinitis and the acquired immunodeficiency syndrome. Arch Ophthalmol 2003; 121:466–476.

312. Freeman WR, Friedberg DN, Berry C et al. Risk factors for development of rhegmatogenous retinal detachment in patients with cytomegalovirus retinitis. Am J Ophthalmol 1993; 116:713–720.

313. Studies of Ocular Complications of AIDS (SOCA) Research Group in Collaboration with the AIDS Clinical Trials Group (ACTG). Rhegmatogenous retinal detachment in patients with cytomegalovirus retinitis. Foscarnet–ganciclovir Cytomegalovirus Retinitis Trial. Am J Ophthalmol 1997; 124:61–70.

314. Jabs DA, Enger C, Haller J et al. Retinal detachment in patients with cytomegalovirus retinitis. Arch Ophthalmol 1991; 109:794–799.

315. Broughton WL, Cupples HP, Parver LM. Bilateral retinal detachment following cytomegalovirus retinitis. Arch Ophthalmol 1978; 96:618–624.

316. Freeman WR, Henderly DE, Wan WL. Rhegmatogenous retinal detachment in treated cytomegalovirus retinitis: prevalence, pathophysiology, and treatment. Am J Ophthalmol 1987; 103:527–536.

317. Sidikaro Y, Silver L, Holland GN et al. Rhegmatogenous retinal detachments in patients with AIDS and necrotizing retinal infections. Ophthalmology 1991; 98:129–135.

318. Irvine AR. Treatment of retinal detachment due to cytomegalovirus retinitis in patients with AIDS. Trans Am Ophthalmol Soc 1991; 89: 349–363.

319. Freeman WR, Quiceno JI, Crapotta JA et al. Surgical repair of rhegmatogenous retinal detachment in immunosuppressed patients with cytomegalovirus retinitis. Ophthalmology 1992; 99:466–474.

320. Holland GN, Buhles WC, Mastre B et al. A controlled retrospective study of ganciclovir treatment for cytomegalovirus retinopathy: use of a standardized system for the assessment of disease outcome. Arch Ophthalmol 1989; 107:1759–1766.

321. Freeman WR. Retinal detachment in cytomegalovirus retinitis: should our approach be changed? Retina 1999; 19:27–33.

322. Sandy CJ, Bloom PA, Graham EM et al. Retinal detachment in AIDS-related cytomegalovirus retinitis. Eye 1995; 9:277–281.

323. Regillo CD, Vander JF, Duker JS et al. Repair of retinitis-related retinal detachments with silicone oil in patients with acquired immunodeficiency syndrome. Am J Ophthalmol 1992; 113:21–27.

324. Freeman WR. Application of vitreoretinal surgery to inflammatory and infectious diseases of the posterior segment. Int Ophthalmol Clin 1992; 32:15–33.

325. Nasemann JE, Mutsch A, Wiltfang R et al. Early pars plana vitrectomy without buckling procedure in cytomegalovirus retinitis-induced retinal detachment. Retina 1995; 15:111–116.

326. Garcia RF, Flores-Aguilar M, Quiceno JI et al. Results of rhegmatogenous retinal detachment repair in cytomegalovirus retinitis with and without scleral buckling. Ophthalmology 1995; 102:236–245.

327. Davis JL, Chuang EL. Management of retinal detachment associated with CMV retinitis in AIDS patients. Eye 1992; 6:28–34.

328. Tanna AP, Kempen JH, Dunn JP. Incidence and management of cataract after retinal detachment repair with silicone oil in immune compromised patients with cytomegalovirus retinitis. Am J Ophthalmol 2003; 136:1009–1015.

329. Irvine AR, Lonn L, Schwartz D et al. Retinal detachment in AIDS: long-term results after repair with silicone oil. Br J Ophthalmol 1997; 81: 180–183.

330. Meldrum ML, Aaberg TM, Patel A et al. Cataract extraction after silicone oil repair of retinal detachments due to necrotizing retinitis. Arch Ophthalmol 1996; 114:885–892.

331. Azen SP, Scott IU, Flynn HW Jr et al. Silicone oil in the repair of complex retinal detachments. A prospective observational multicenter study. Ophthalmology 1998; 105:1587–1597.

332. Karavellas MP, Song M, MacDonald JC et al. Long-term posterior and anterior segment complications of immune recovery uveitis associated with cytomegalovirus retinitis. Am J Ophthalmol 2000; 130:57–64.

333. Baumal CR, Reichel E. Management of cytomegalovirus-related rhegmatogenous retinal detachments. Ophthalmic Surg Lasers 1998; 29:916–925.

333A. Althaus C, Loeffler KU, Schimkat M et al. Prophylactic argon laser coagulation for rhegmatogenous retinal detachment in AIDS patients with cytomegalovirus retinitis. Graefes Arch Clin Exp Ophthalmol 1998; 236:359–364.

333B. Vrabec TR. Laser photocoagulation repair of macula-sparing cytomegalovirus-related retinal detachment. Ophthalmology 1997; 104:2062–2067.

333C. Davis JL, Hummer J, Feuer WJ. Laser photocoagulation for retinal detachment and retinal tears in cytomegalovirus retinitis. Ophthalmology 1997; 104:2053–2060; discussion 2060–2061.

333D. McCluskey P, Grigg J, Playfair TJ. Retinal detachments in patients with AIDS and CMV retinopathy: a role for laser photocoagulation. Br J Ophthalmol 1995; 79:153–156.

333E. Meffert SA, Ai E. Laser photocoagulation prophylaxis for CMV retinal detachments. Ophthalmology 1998; 105:1353–1355.

334. Finzi D, Hermankova M, Pierson T et al. Identification of a reservoir for HIV-1 in patients on highly active antiretroviral therapy. Science 1997; 278:1295–1300.

335. Kempen JH, Martin BK, Wu AW et al. The effect of cytomegalovirus retinitis on the quality of life of patients with AIDS in the era of highly active antiretroviral therapy. Ophthalmology 2003; 110:987–995.

336. Palella FJ Jr, Delaney KM, Moorman AC et al. Declining morbidity and mortality among patients with advanced human immunodeficiency virus infection. HIV Outpatient Study Investigators. N Engl J Med 1998; 338:853–860.

337. Varani S, Spezzacatena P, Manfredi R et al. The incidence of cytomegalovirus (CMV) antigenemia and CMV disease is reduced by highly active antiretroviral therapy. Eur J Epidemiol 2000; 16:433–437.

338. Baril L, Jouan M, Agher R et al. Impact of highly active antiretroviral therapy on onset of *Mycobacterium avium* complex infection and cytomegalovirus disease in patients with AIDS. AIDS 2000; 14:2593–2596.

339. Deayton JR, Wilson P, Sabin CA et al. Changes in the natural history of cytomegalovirus retinitis following the introduction of highly active antiretroviral therapy. AIDS 2000; 14:1163–1170.

340. Walsh JC, Jones CD, Barnes EA et al. Increasing survival in AIDS patients with cytomegalovirus retinitis treated with combination antiretroviral therapy including HIV protease inhibitors. AIDS 1998; 12: 613–618.

341. Binquet C, Saillour F, Bernard N et al. Prognostic factors of survival of HIV-infected patients with cytomegalovirus disease: Aquitaine Cohort, 1986–1997. Groupe d'Epidemiologic Clinique du SIDA en Aquitaine (GECSA). Eur J Epidemiol 2000; 16:425–432.

342. Casado JL, Perez-Elias MJ, Marti-Belda P et al. Improved outcome of cytomegalovirus retinitis in AIDS patients after introduction of protease inhibitors. J Acquir Immune Defic Syndr Hum Retrovirol 1998; 19:130–134.

343. Lee V, Subak-Sharpe I, Shah S et al. Changing trends in cytomegalovirus retinitis with triple therapy. Eye 1999; 13:59–64.

344. MacDonald JC, Torriani FJ, Morse LS et al. Lack of reactivation of cytomegalovirus (CMV) retinitis after stopping CMV maintenance therapy in AIDS patients with sustained elevations in CD4 T cells in response to highly active antiretroviral therapy. J Infect Dis 1998; 177:1182–1187.

345. Jabs DA, Bolton SG, Dunn JP et al. Discontinuing anticytomegalovirus therapy in patients with immune reconstitution after combination antiretroviral therapy. Am J Ophthalmol 1998; 126:817–822.

346. MacDonald JC, Karavellas MP, Torriani FJ et al. Highly active antiretroviral therapy-related immune recovery in AIDS patients with cytomegalovirus retinitis. Ophthalmology 2000; 107:877–881.

347. Mezzaroma I, Carlesimo M, Pinter E et al. Clinical and immunologic response without decrease in virus load in patients with AIDS after 24 months of highly active antiretroviral therapy. Clin Infect Dis 1999; 29:1423–1430.

348. Jouan M, Saves M, Tubiana R et al. Discontinuation of maintenance therapy for cytomegalovirus retinitis in HIV-infected patients receiving highly active antiretroviral therapy. AIDS 2001; 15:23–31.

349. Curi AL, Muralha A, Muralha L et al. Suspension of anticytomegalovirus maintenance therapy following immune recovery due to highly active antiretroviral therapy. Br J Ophthalmol 2001; 85:471–473.

350. Whitcup SM, Fortin E, Lindblad AS et al. Discontinuation of anticytomegalovirus therapy in patients with HIV infection cytomegalovirus. JAMA 1999; 282:1633–1671.

351. Vrabec TR, Baldassano VF, Whitcup SM. Discontinuation of maintenance therapy in patients with quiescent cytomegalovirus retinitis and elevated CD4+ counts. Ophthalmology 1998; 105:1259–1264.

352. Song MK, Karavellas MP, MacDonald JC et al. Characterization of reactivation of cytomegalovirus retinitis in patients healed after treatment with highly active antiretroviral therapy. Retina 2000; 20:151–155.

353. Sepkowitz KA. Effect of HAART on natural history of AIDS-related opportunistic disorders. Lancet 1998; 351:228–230.

354. Michelet C, Arvieux C, Francois C et al. Opportunistic infections occurring during highly active antiretroviral treatment. AIDS 1998; 12: 1815–1822.

355. Update: acquired immunodeficiency syndrome – United States. MMWR Morb Mortal Wkly Rep 1985; 35:17–21.

356. Jacobson MA, Zegans M, Pavan PR et al. Cytomegalovirus retinitis after initiation of highly active antiretroviral therapy. Lancet 1997; 349: 1443–1445.

357. Reed JB, Schwab IR, Gordon J et al. Regression of cytomegalovirus retinitis associated with protease-inhibitor treatment in patients with AIDS. Am J Ophthalmol 1997; 124:199–205.

358. D'Amico DJ, Skolnik PR, Kosloff BR et al. Resolution of cytomegalovirus retinitis with zidovudine therapy. Arch Ophthalmol 1988; 106:1168–1169.

359. Guyer DR, Jabs DA, Brant AM et al. Regression of cytomegalovirus retinitis with zidovudine: a clinicopathologic correlation. Arch Ophthalmol 1989; 107:868–874.

360. Karavellas MP, Lower CY, Macdonald JC et al. Immune recovery vitreitis associated with inactive cytomegalovirus retinitis: a new syndrome. Arch Ophthalmol 1998; 116:169–175.

361. Michelet C, Arvieux C, Aubert V et al. Viral ocular involvement after initiation of antiprotease inhibitor therapy. Forty-sixth Conference on Retroviruses and Opportunistic Infections 1997; program and abstracts 122: abstract 315.

362. Neussenblatt RB, Lane HC. Human immunodeficiency virus disease: changing patterns of intraocular inflammation. Am J Ophthalmol 1998; 125:374–382.

363. Holland GN. Pieces of a puzzle: toward better understanding of intra-ocular inflammation associated with human immunodeficiency virus infection. Am J Ophthalmol 1998; 125:383–385.

364. Jabs DA. Cytomegalovirus retinitis and the evolving AIDS epidemic. Retina 1998; 18:395–398.

365. Zegans ME, Walton RC, Holland GN et al. Transient vitreous inflammatory reactions associated with combination antiretroviral therapy in patients with AIDS and cytomegalovirus retinitis. Am J Ophthalmol 1998; 125:292–300.

366. Holland GN. Immune recovery uveitis. Ocul Immunol Inflamm 1999; 7:215–221.

367. Karavellas MP, Plummer DJ, Macdonald JC et al. Incidence of immune recovery vitreitis in cytomegalovirus retinitis patients following institution of successful highly active antiretroviral therapy. J Infect Dis 1999; 179:697–700.

368. Nguyen QD, Kempen JH, Bolton SG et al. Immune recovery uveitis in patients with AIDS and cytomegalovirus retinitis after highly active antiretroviral therapy. Am J Ophthalmol 2000; 129:634–639.

369. Jabs DA, Van Natta ML, Kempen JH et al. Characteristics of patients with cytomegalovirus retinitis in the era of highly active antiretroviral therapy. Am J Ophthalmol 2002; 133:48–61.

370. Arevalo JF, Mendoza AJ, Ferretti Y. Immune recovery uveitis in AIDS patients with cytomegalovirus retinitis treated with highly active antiretroviral therapy in Venezuela. Retina 2003; 23:495–502.

371. Karavellas MP, Azen SP, Macdonald JC et al. Immune recovery vitreitis in AIDS: clinical predictors, sequella, and treatment outcomes. Retina 2001; 21:1–9.

372. Song M, Azen SP, Buley A et al. Effect of anti-cytomegalovirus therapy on the incidence of immune recovery uveitis in AIDS patients with healed cytomegalovirus retinitis. Am J Ophthalmol 2003; 136: 696–702.

373. Newsome R, Casswell T, O'Moore E et al. Cystoid macular oedema in patients with AIDS and cytomegalovirus retinitis on highly active antiretroviral therapy. Br J Ophthalmol 1998; 82:456–457.

374. Silverstein BE, Smith JH, Sykes SO et al. Cystoid macular edema associated with cytomegalovirus retinitis in patients with acquired immunodeficiency syndrome. Am J Ophthalmol 1998; 125:412–415.

375. Whitcup SM. Cytomegalovirus retinitis in the era of highly active antiretroviral therapy. JAMA 2000; 283:653–657.

376. Karavellas MP, Song MK, Macdonald JC et al. Long-term posterior and anterior segment complications of immune recovery uveitis associated with cytomegalovirus retinitis. Am J Ophthalmol 2000; 130:57–64.

377. Sanislo SR, Lowder CY, Kaiser PK. Optic nerve head neovascularization in a patient with inactive cytomegalovirus retinitis and immune recovery. Am J Ophthalmol 1998; 126:318–320.

378. Canzano JC, Reed JB, Morse LS. Vitreomacular traction syndrome following highly active antiretroviral therapy in AIDS patients with cytomegalovirus retinitis. Retina 1998; 18:443–447.

379. Robinson MR, Csaky KG, Lee SS et al. Fibrovascular changes misdiagnosed as cytomegalovirus retinitis reactivation in a patient with immune recovery. Clin Infect Dis 2004; 38:139–141.

380. Wright ME, Suzman DL, Csaky KG et al. Extensive retinal neovascularization as a late finding in human immunodeficiency virus-infected patients with immune recovery uveitis. Clin Infect Dis 2003; 36:1063–1066.

381. Biswas J, Choudhry S, Kumarasamy et al. Immune recovery vitreitis presenting as panuveitis following therapy with protease inhibitors. Indian J Ophthalmol 2000; 48:313–315.

382. Goldberg DE, Freeman WR. Uveitic angle closure glaucoma in a patient with inactive cytomegalovirus and immune recovery uveitis. Ophthalmic Surg Lasers 2002; 33:421–425.

383. Goldberg DE, Wang H, Azen SP et al. Long term visual outcome of patients with cytomegalovirus retinitis treated with highly active antiretroviral therapy. Br J Ophthalmol 2003; 87:853–855.

384. Kuppermann BD, Holland GN. Immune recovery uveitis. Am J Ophthalmol 2000; 130:103–106.

385. Pepose JS, Newman C, Bach MC et al. Pathologic features of cytomegalovirus retinopathy after treatment with the antiviral agent ganciclovir. Ophthalmology 1987; 94:414–424.

386. Burd EM, Pulido JS, Puro DG et al. Maintenance of replicative intermediates in ganciclovir-treated human cytomegalovirus-infected retinal glia. Arch Ophthalmol 1996; 114:856–861.

387. Multimer HP, Akatsuka Y, Manley T et al. Association between immune recovery uveitis and a diverse intraocular cytomegalovirus-specific cytotoxic T cell response. J Infect Dis 2002; 186:701–705.

388. Siqueira RC, Cunha A, Orefice F et al. PCR with the aqueous humor, blood leukocytes and vitreous of patients affected by cytomegalovirus retinitis and immune recovery uveitis. Ophthalmologica 2004; 218: 43–48.

389. Kosobucki BR, Goldberg DE, Bessho K et al. Valganciclovir therapy for immune recovery uveitis complicated by macular edema. Am J Ophthalmol 2004; 137:636–638.

390. D'Alessandro L, Bottaro E. Reactivation of CMV retinitis after treatment with subtenon corticosteroids for immune recovery uveitis in patients with AIDS. Scand J Infect Dis 2002; 34:780–782.

391. Update: acquired immunodeficiency syndrome – United States. MMWR Morb Mortal Wkly Rep 1986; 35:757–766.

392. Maguire AM, Nichols CW, Crooks GW. Visual loss in cytomegalovirus retinitis caused by cystoid macular edema in patients without the acquired immune deficiency. Ophthalmology 1996; 103:601–605.

393. Omerod LD, Larkin JA, Margo CA et al. Rapidly progressive herpetic retinal necrosis: a blinding disease characteristic of advanced AIDS. [see commentary by C.L. Lowder, pp. 46–47]. Clin Infect Dis 1998; 26:34–45.

394. Forster DJ, Dugel PU, Frangieh GT et al. Rapidly progressive outer retinal necrosis in the acquired immunodeficiency syndrome. Am J Ophthalmol 1990; 110:341–348.

395. Hellinger WC, Bolling JP, Smith TF et al. Varicella-zoster virus retinitis in a patient with AIDS-related complex: case report and brief review of the acute retinal necrosis syndrome. Clin Infect Dis 1993; 16:208–212.

396. Duker JS, Blumenkranz MS. Diagnosis and management of the acute retinal necrosis (ARN) syndrome. Surv Ophthalmol 1991; 35:327–343.

397. Friedlander S, Rahhal FM, Ericson L et al. Optic neuropathy preceding acute retinal necrosis in acquired immunodeficiency syndrome. Arch Ophthalmol 1996; 114:1481–1485.

398. Culbertson WW, Atherton SS. Acute retinal necrosis and similar retinitis syndromes. Int Ophthalmol Clin 1993; 33:129–143.

399. Sellitti TP, Huang AJ, Schiffman J et al. Association of herpes zoster ophthalmicus with acquired immunodeficiency syndrome and acute retinal necrosis. Am J Ophthalmol 1993; 116:297–301.

400. Holland GN. Standard diagnostic criteria for the acute retinal necrosis syndrome. Executive Committee of the American Uveitis Society. Am J Ophthalmol 1994; 117:663–667.

401. Gorman BD, Nadel AJ, Coles RS. Acute retinal necrosis. Ophthalmology 1982; 89:809.

402. Rungger-Brandle E, Roux L, Leuenberger PM. Bilateral acute retinal necrosis (BARN): identification of the presumed infectious agent. Ophthalmology 1984; 91:1648.

403. Abe T, Tsuchida K, Tamai M. A comparative study of the polymerase chain reaction and local antibody production in acute retinal necrosis syndrome and cytomegalovirus retinitis. Graefes Arch Clin Exp Ophthalmol 1996; 234:419–424.

404. Update: universal precautions for prevention of transmission of human immunodeficiency virus, hepatitis B virus, and other bloodborne pathogens in health-care settings. MMWR Morb Mortal Wkly Rep 1988; 37:377–388.

405. Weinberg DV, Lyon AT. Repair of retinal detachments due to herpes varicella-zoster virus retinitis in patients with acquired immune deficiency syndrome. Ophthalmology 1997; 104:279–282.

406. Schlingemann RO, Bruinenberg M, Wertheim-Van Dillen P et al. Twenty years' delay of fellow eye involvement in herpes simplex virus type 2-associated bilateral acute retinal necrosis syndrome. Am J Ophthalmol 1996; 122:891–892.

406a. Aslanides IM, De Souza S, Wong DTW et al. Oral valacyclovir in the treatment of acute retinal necrosis syndrome. Retina 2002; 22:352–354.

407. Causey DM, Rarick MU. Foscarnet treatment of acyclovir-resistant herpes simplex proctitis in an AIDS patient. Proceedings of the Fourth International Conference on AIDS. Stockholm. 1988; abstract 3589.

408. Chatis PA, Miller CH, Schrager LE et al. Successful treatment with foscarnet of an acyclovir-resistant mucocutaneous infection with herpes simplex virus in a patient with the acquired immunodeficiency syndrome. N Engl J Med 1989; 320:297–300.

409. Erlich KS, Jacobson MA, Koehler JE et al. Foscarnet therapy of severe acyclovir-resistant herpes simplex virus infections in patients with the acquired immunodeficiency syndrome. Ann Intern Med 1989; 110:71–73.

410. Safrin S, Assaykeen T, Follansbee S et al. Foscarnet therapy for acyclovir-resistant mucocutaneous herpes simplex virus infection in 26 AIDS patients: preliminary data. J Infect Dis 1990; 161:1078–1084.

411. Safrin S, Crumpacker CS, Chatis P et al. A controlled trial comparing foscarnet with vidarabine for acyclovir-resistant mucocutaneous herpes simplex in the acquired immunodeficiency syndrome. N Engl J Med 1991; 325:551–555.

412. Youle MM, Hawkins DA, Collins P et al. Acyclovir-resistant herpes in AIDS treated with foscarnet [Letter]. Lancet 1988; 2:341–342.

412a. Safrin S, Berger TG, Gilson I, at al. Foscarnet therapy in five patients with AIDS and acyclovir-resistant varicella-zoster virus infection. Ann Intern Med 1991; 115:19–21.

413. Kashiwase M, Sata T, Yamauchi Y et al. Progressive outer retinal necrosis caused by herpes simplex virus type 1 in a patient with acquired immunodeficiency syndrome. Ophthalmology 2000; 107:790–794.

414. Dunn JP. Viral retinitis. Ophthalmol Clin North Am 1999; 12:109.

415. Pavesio CE, Mitchell SM, Barton K et al. Progressive outer retinal necrosis (PORN) in AIDS patients: a different appearance of varicella-zoster retinitis. Eye 1995; 9:271–276.

416. Engstrom RJ, Holland GN, Margolis TP et al. The progressive outer retinal necrosis syndrome. A variant of necrotizing herpetic retinopathy in patients with AIDS. Ophthalmology 1994; 101:1488–1502.

417. Scott IU, Luu KM, Davis JL. Intravitreal antivirals in the management of patients with acquired immunodeficiency syndrome with progressive outer retinal necrosis. Arch Ophthalmol 2002; 120:1219–1222.

418. Moorthy RS, Weinberg DV, Teich SA et al. Management of varicella zoster virus retinitis in AIDS. Br J Ophthalmol 1997; 81:189–194.

419. Ciulla TA, Rutledge BK, Morley MG et al. The progressive outer retinal necrosis syndrome: successful treatment with combination antiviral therapy. Ophthalmic Surg Lasers 1998; 29:198–206.

420. Margolis TP, Lowder CY, Holland GN et al. Varicella-zoster virus retinitis in patients with the acquired immunodeficiency syndrome. Am J Ophthalmol 1991; 112:119–131.

421. Spaide RF, Martin DF, Teich SA et al. Successful treatment of progressive outer retinal necrosis syndrome. Retina 1996; 16:479–487.

422. Meffert SA, Kertes PJ, Lim P et al. Successful treatment of progressive outer retinal necrosis using high-dose intravitreal ganciclovir. Retina 1997; 17:560–562.

423. Perez-Blasquez E, Traspas R, Marin IM et al. Intravitreal ganciclovir treatment in progressive outer retinal necrosis. Am J Ophthalmol 1997; 124:418–421.

424. Kuppermann BD, Quiceno JI, Wiley C et al. Clinical and histopathologic study of varicella zoster virus retinitis in patients with the acquired immunodeficiency syndrome. Am J Ophthalmol 1994; 118:589–600.

425. Pepose JS, Holland GN, Nestor MS et al. Acquired immune deficiency syndrome: pathogenic mechanisms of ocular disease. Ophthalmology 1985; 92:472–484.

426. Macher A, Rodrigues MM, Kaplan W et al. Disseminated bilateral chorioretinitis due to histoplasma capsulatum in a patient with the acquired immunodeficiency syndrome. Ophthalmology 1985; 92:1159–1164.

427. Davis JL, Nussenblatt RB, Bachman DM et al. Endogenous bacterial retinitis in AIDS. Am J Ophthalmol 1989; 107:613–623.

428. Kaplan JE, Masur H, Holmes KK. Guidelines for preventing opportunistic infections among HIV-infected persons – 2002. Recommendations of the U.S. Public Health Service and the Infectious Disease Society of America. MMWR Recomm Rep 2002; 51 (RR–8):1–52.

429. Macher AM, Bardenstein DS, Zimmerman LE. Pneumocystis carinii choroiditis in a male homosexual with AIDS and disseminated pulmonary and extrapulmonary P. carinii infection. N Engl J Med 1987; 236:1092.

430. Freeman WR, Gross JG, Labelle J et al. Pneumocystis carinii choroidopathy: a new clinical entity. Arch Ophthalmol 1989; 107:863–867.

431. Shami MJ, Freeman WR, Friedberg D et al. A multicenter study of Pneumocystis choroidopathy. Am J Ophthalmol 1991; 112:15–22.

432. Glatt AE, Chirqwin K, Landesman SH. Current concepatients: treatment of infections associated with human immunodeficiency virus. N Engl J Med 1988; 318:1439–1448.

433. Dugel PU, Rao NA, Forster DJ et al. Pneumocystis carinii choroiditis after long-term aerosolized pentamidine therapy. Am J Ophthalmol 1990; 110:113–117.

434. Foster RE, Lowder CY, Meisler DM et al. Presumed Pneumocystis carinii choroiditis: unifocal presentation, regression with intravenous pentamidine, and choroiditis recurrence. Ophthalmology 1991; 98:1360–1365.

435. Koser MW, Jampol LM, MacDonell K. Treatment of Pneumocystis carinii choroidopathy. Arch Ophthalmol 1990; 108:1214–1215.

436. Sneed SR, Blodi CF, Berger BB et al. Pneumocystis carinii choroiditis in patients receiving inhaled pentamidine. N Engl J Med 1989; 322:936–937.

437. Centers for Disease Control and Prevention. HIV/AIDS surveillance report 1999; 11:2–38.

437a. Parke DW II, Font RL. Diffuse toxoplasmic retinochoroiditis in a patient with AIDS. Arch Ophthalmol 1986; 104:571–575.

438. Heinemann MH, Gold JMW, Maisel J. Bilateral toxoplasma retinochoroiditis in a patient with acquired immune deficiency syndrome. Retina 1986; 6:224.

439. Schuman JS, Friedman AH. Retinal manifestations of the acquired immune deficiency syndrome (AIDS): cytomegalovirus, Candida albicans, cryptococcus, toxoplasmosis, and Pneumocystis carinii. Trans Ophthalmol Soc UK 1983; 103:177.

440. Cochereau-Massin I, LeHoang P, Lautier-Frau M et al. Ocular toxoplasmosis in human immunodeficiency virus-infected patients. Am J Ophthalmol 1992; 114:130–135.

441. Elkins BS, Holland GN, Opremcak EM et al. Ocular toxoplasmosis misdiagnosed as cytomegalovirus retinopathy in immunocompromised patients. Ophthalmology 1994; 101:499–507.

442. Berger BB, Egwuagu CE, Freeman WR et al. Miliary toxoplasmic retinitis in acquired immunodeficiency syndrome. Arch Ophthalmol 1993; 111:373–376.

443. Cano-Parra JL, Diaz-Llopis ML, Cordoba JL et al. Acute iridocyclitis in a patient with AIDS diagnosed as toxoplasmosis by PCR. Ocul Immunol Inflamm 2000; 8:127–130.

444. Fardeau C, Romand S, Rao NA et al. Diagnosis of toxoplasmic retinochoroiditis with atypical clinical features. Am J Ophthalmol 2002; 134:196–203.

445. Moshfeghi DM, Dodds EM, Couto CA et al. Diagnostic approaches to severe, atypical toxoplasmosis mimicking acute retinal necrosis. Ophthalmology 2004; 111:716–725.

446. Holland GN. Ocular toxoplasmosis in the immunocompromised host. Int Ophthalmol 1989; 13:399–402.

447. Moorthy RS, Smith RE, Rao NA. Progressive ocular toxoplasmosis in patients with acquired immunodeficiency syndrome. Am J Ophthalmol 1993; 115:742–747.

448. Holland GN. Ocular toxoplasmosis: a global reassessment. Part II: Disease manifestations and management. Am J Ophthalmol 2004; 137:1–17.

449. Nicholson DH, Wolchok EB. Ocular toxoplasmosis in an adult receiving long-term corticosteroid therapy. Arch Ophthalmol 1976; 94:248–254.

450. Holland GN. Ocular toxoplasmosis: a global reassessment. Part I: Epidemiology and course of disease. Am J Ophthalmol 2003; 136:973–988.

451. Grossniklaus HE, Specht CS, Allaire G et al. Toxoplasma gondii retinochoroiditis and optic neuritis in acquired immune deficiency syndrome. Report of a case. Ophthalmology 1990; 97:1342–1346.

452. Rehder JR, Burnier MBJ, Pavesio CE et al. Acute unilateral toxoplasmic iridocyclitis in an AIDS patient. Am J Ophthalmol 1988; 106:740–741.

453. Gagliuso DJ, Teich SA, Friedman AH et al. Ocular toxoplasmosis in AIDS patients. Trans Am Ophthalmol Soc 1990; 88:63–86.

454. Tate GW Jr, Martin RG. Clindamycin in the treatment of human ocular toxoplasmosis. Can J Ophthalmol 1977; 12:188–195.

455. Lakhanpal V, Schocket SS, Nirankari VS. Clindamycin in the treatment of toxoplasmic retinochoroiditis. Am J Ophthalmol 1983; 95:605–613.

456. Jacobson JM, Hafner R, Remington J et al. Dose-escalation, phase I/II study of azithromycin and pyrimethamine for the treatment of toxoplasmic encephalitis in AIDS. AIDS 2001; 15:583–589.

457. Bosch-Driessen LH, Verbraak FD, Suttorp-Schulten MSA et al. A prospective, randomized trial of pyrimethamine and azithromycin vs pyrimethamine and sulfadiazine for the treatment of ocular toxoplasmosis. Am J Ophthalmol 2002; 134:34–40.

458. Pearson PA, Piracha AR, Sen H et al. Atovaquone for the treatment of toxoplasma retinochoroiditis in immunocompetent patients. Ophthalmology 1999; 106:148–153.

459. Kovacs JA. Efficacy of atovaquone in treatment of toxoplasmosis in patients with AIDS. The NIAID-Clinical Center Intramural AIDS Program. Lancet 1992; 340:637–638.

460. Spencer CM, Goa KL. Atovaquone. A review of its pharmacological properties and therapeutic efficacy in opportunistic infections. Drugs 1995; 50:176–196.

460a. Lopez JS, de Smet MD, Masur H et al. Orally administered 566C80 for treatment of ocular toxoplasmosis in a patient with the acquired immunodeficiency syndrome. Am J Ophthalmol 1992; 113:331–333.

461. Hughes WT. A new drug (566C80) for the treatment of Pneumocystis carinii pneumonia. Ann Intern Med 1992; 116:953–954.

462. Araujo FG, Huskinson J, Remington JS. Remarkable in vitro and in vivo activities of the hydroxynaphthoquinone 566C80 against tachyzoites and tissue cysts of Toxoplasma gondii. Antimicrob Agents Chemother 1991; 35:293–299.

463. Huskinson-Mark J, Araujo FG, Remington JS. Evaluation of the effect of drugs on the cyst form of *Toxoplasma gondii*. J Infect Dis 1991; 164:170–171.

464. Stout JE, Lai JC, Giner J et al. Reactivation of retinal toxoplasmosis despite evidence of immune response to highly active antiretroviral therapy. Clin Infect Dis 2002; 35:e37–e39.

465. Friedman AH. The retinal lesions of the acquired immune deficiency syndrome. Trans Am Ophthalmol Soc 1984; 82:447–491.

466. Miailhes P, Labetoulle M, Naas T et al. Unusual etiology of visual loss in an HIV-infected patient due to endogenous endophthalmitis. Clin Microbiol Infect 2001; 7:641–645.

467. Edwards JE, Foos RY, Montomerie JZ et al. Ocular manifestations of candida septicemia: review of seventy-six cases of hematogenous candida endophthalmitis. Medicine (Baltimore) 1974; 53:47–75.

468. Fischer JE. Penetration of amphoteracin B into the human eye. J Infect Dis 1983; 147:164–165.

469. Schmid S, Martenet A, Oelz O. Candidal endophthalmitis: clinical presentation, treatment and outcome in 23 patients. Infection 1991; 19:21–24.

470. Savani DV, Perfect JR, Cobo LM et al. Penetration of new azole compound into the eye and efficacy in experimental candida endophthalmitis. Antimicrob Agents Chemother 1987; 31:6–10.

471. O'Day DM, Foulds G, Williams TE et al. Ocular uptake of fluconazole following oral administration. Arch Ophthalmol 1990; 108:1006–1008.

472. Rex JH, Bennet JE, Sugar AM et al. A randomized trial comparing fluconazole with amphoteracin B for the treatment of candidemia in patients without neutropenia. N Engl J Med 1994; 331:1325–1330.

473. Anaissie EJ, Darouiche RO, Abi-Said D et al. Management of invasive candidal infections: results of a prospective, randomized, multicenter study of fluconazole vs. amphotericin B and review of the literature. Clin Infect Dis 1996; 23:964–972.

474. Panther LA, Sande MA. Cryptococcal meningitis in AIDS. In: Sande MA, Volberding PA, eds. The medical management of AIDS, 2nd edn. Philadelphia: WB Saunders, 1997.

475. Shields JA, Wright DM, Augsburger JJ et al. Cryptococcal chorioretinitis. Am J Ophthalmol 1980; 89:210.

476. O'Dowd GJ, Frable WJ. Cryptococcal endophthalmitis: diagnostic vitreous aspiration cytology. Am J Clin Pathol 1983; 79:382–385.

477. Kupfer C, McCrane E. A possible cause of decreased vision in cryptococcal meningitis. Invest Ophthalmol Vis Sci 1974; 13:801–804.

478. Crump JRC, Elner SG, Elner VM et al. Cryptococcal endophthalmitis: case report and review. Clin Infect Dis 1992; 14:1069–1073.

479. Okun E, Butler WT. Ophthalmologic complications of cryptococcal meningitis. Arch Ophthalmol 1964; 71:52–57.

480. Wheat LJ, Connolly-Stringfield PA, Baker RL et al. Disseminated histoplasmosis in the acquired immune deficiency syndrome: clinical findings, diagnosis and treatment, and review of the literature. Medicine (Baltimore) 1990; 69:361–374.

481. Wheat J, Hafner R, Wulfsohn M et al. Prevention of relapse of histoplasmosis with itraconazole in patients with the acquired immunodeficiency syndrome. Ann Intern Med 1993; 118:610–616.

482. Gonzales CA, Scott IU, Chaudhry NA et al. Endogenous endophthalmitis caused by *Histoplasma capsulatum* var. *capsulatum*: a case report and literature review. Ophthalmology 2000; 107:725–729.

483. Denning DW, Follansbee SE, Scolaro M et al. Pulmonary aspergillosis in the acquired immunodeficiency syndrome. N Engl J Med 1991; 324:654–662.

484. Fish DG, Ampel NM, Galgiani JN et al. Coccidioidomycosis during human immunodeficiency virus infection: a review of 77 patients. Medicine (Baltimore) 1990; 69:384–391.

485. Williams PL, Johnson R, Pappagianis D et al. Vasculitic and encephalitic complications associated with *Coccidioides immitis* infection of the central nervous system in humans: report of 10 cases and review. Clin Infect Dis 1992; 14:673–682.

485A. Glasgow BJ, Brown HH, Foos RV. Miliary retinitis in coccidioidomycosis. Am J Ophthalmol 1987; 104:24.

486. Blumenkranz MS, Stevens DS. Endogenous coccidioidal endophthalmitis. Ophthalmology 1980; 87:974.

487. Cutler JE, Binder PS, Paul TO. Metastatic coccidioidal endophthalmitis. Arch Ophthalmol 1978; 96:689.

489. Bell R, Font RL. Granulomatous anterior uveitis caused by *Coccidioides immitis*. Am J Ophthalmol 1972; 74:93.

490. McDonnell PJ, Green WR, Endophthalmitis. In: Mandell GL, Gordon RG, Bennett JE, eds. Principles and practice of infectious diseases, 4th edn. New York: Churchill Livingstone, 1995.

491. Finamor LP, Muccioli C, Martins MC et al. Ocular and central nervous system paracoccidioidomycosis in a pregnant woman with acquired immunodeficiency syndrome. Am J Ophthalmol 2002; 134:456–459.

492. Green WR, Bennett JE, Goos BD. Ocular penetration of amphoteracin B: a case report of postsurgical Cephalosporum endophthalmitis. Arch Ophthalmol 1965; 73:769–775.

493. O'Day DM, Head WS, Robinson RD et al. Intraocular penetration of systemically administered antifungal agents [published correction appears in Curr Eye Res 1986;5:547]. Curr Eye Res 1985; 4:131–134.

494. Hariprasad SM, Mieler WF, Holz ER et al. Determination of vitreous, aqueous, and plasma concentration of orally administered voriconazole in humans. Arch Ophthalmol 2004; 122:42–47.

495. Marco F, Pfaller MA, Messer SA et al. Antifungal activity of a new triazole, voriconazole (UK-109,496), compared with three other antifungal agents tested against clinical isolates of filamentous fungi. Med Mycol 1998; 36:433–436.

496. Brod RD, Flynn HW, Miller D. Endogenous fungal endophthalmitis. In: Duane's clinical ophthalmology, Chapter 11. CD-ROM. Hagerstown: Harper and Row, 2004.

497. Axelrod AJ, Peyman GA, Apple DJ. Toxicity of intravitreal injection of amphoteracin B. Am J Ophthalmol 1973; 76:578–583.

498. Garbino J, Ondrusova A, Baligvo E et al. Successful treatment of *Paecilomyces lilacinus* endophthalmitis with voriconazole [published correction appears on Scand J Infect Dis 2003; 35:79]. Scand J Infect Dis 2002; 34:701–703.

499. Reis A, Sundmacher R, Tinelnot K et al. Successful treatment of ocular invasive mould infection (fusariosis) with the new antifungal agent voriconazole [Letter]. Br J Ophthalmol 2000; 84; 932–933.

500. Sponsel WE, Graybill JR, Nevarez HL et al. Ocular and systemic posaconazole (SCH-56592) treatment of invasive *Fusarium solani* keratitis and endophthalmitis. Br J Ophthalmol 2002; 86:829–830.

501. Kim JE, Perkins SL, Harris GJ. Voriconazole treatment of fungal scleritis and epibulbar abscess resulting from scleral buckle infection. Arch Ophthalmol 2003; 121:735–737.

502. Hua G, Pennesi M, Shah K et al. Safety of intravitreal voriconazole: electroretinographic and histopathologic studies. Trans Am Ophthalmol Soc 2003; 101:183–189; discussion 189.

503. Ruhnke M, Schmidt-Westhausen A, Trautmann M. In vitro activities of voriconazole (UK-109,496) against fluconazole-susceptible and -resistant *Candida albicans* isolates from oral cavities of patients with human immunodeficiency virus infection. Antimicrob Agents Chemother 1997; 41:575–577.

504. Pizzo G, Barchiesi F, Falconi Di Francesco L et al. Genotyping and antifungal susceptibility of human subgingival *Candida albicans* isolates. Arch Oral Biol 2002; 47:189–196.

505. Musher DM, Hamill RJ, Baughn RE. Effect of immunodeficiency virus (HIV) infection on the course of syphilis and on the response to treatment. Ann Intern Med 1990; 113:872–881.

506. McLeish WM, Pulido JS, Holland S et al. The ocular manifestations of syphilis in the human immunodeficiency virus type 1-infected host. Ophthalmology 1990; 97:196–203.

507. Levy JH, Liss RA, Maguire AM. Neurosyphilis and ocular syphilis in patients with concurrent human immunodeficiency virus infection. Retina 1989; 9:175–180.

508. Joyce PW, Haye KR, Ellis ME. Syphilitic retinitis in a homosexual man with concurrent HIV infection. Genitourin Med 1989; 65:244–247.

509. Richards BW, Hessburg TJ, Nussbaum JN. Recurrent syphilitic uveitis. N Engl J Med 1989; 320:62.

510. Passo MS, Rosenbaum, JT. Ocular syphilis in patients with human immunodeficiency virus infection. Am J Ophthalmol 1988; 106:1–6.

511. Zaidman GW. Neurosyphilis and retrobulbar neuritis in a patient with AIDS. Ann Ophthalmol 1986; 18:260–261.

512. Zambrano W, Perez GM, Smith JL. Acute syphilitic blindness in AIDS. J Clin Neuro Ophthalmol 1987; 7:1–5.

513. Stoumbos VD, Klein ML. Syphilitic retinitis in a patient with acquired immunodeficiency syndrome-related complex. Am J Ophthalmol 1987; 103:103–104.

514. Holland GH, Levinson RD. Ocular infections associated with the acquired immunodeficiency syndrome. In: Duane's clinical ophthalmology, Chapter 82. CD-ROM. Hagerstown: Harper and Row, 1994.

515. Gass JDM, Braunstein RA, Chenoweth RG. Acute syphilitic posterior placoid chorioretinitis. Ophthalmology 1990; 97:1288–1297.

516. Rolfs RT, Joesoef MR, Hendershot EF et al. A randomized trial of enhanced therapy of early syphilis in patients with and without human immunodeficiency virus infection. N Engl J Med 1997; 337:307–314.

517. Shalaby IA, Dunn JP, Semba RD et al. Syphilitic uveitis in human immunodeficiency virus-infected patients. Arch Ophthalmol 1997; 115:469–473.

518. Blodi BA, Johnson MW, McLeish SM et al. Presumed choroidal tuberculosis in a human immunodeficiency virus-infected host. Am J Ophthalmol 1989; 108:605–607.

519. Goxatto JO, Master C, Puente S et al. Nonreactive tuberculosis in a patient with acquired immune deficiency syndrome. Am J Ophthalmol 1986; 102:660.

520. Lai L, Chen S, Kuo Y et al. Presumed choroidal atypical tuberculosis superinfected with cytomegalovirus retinitis in an acquired immuno-deficiency syndrome patient: a case report. Jpn J Ophthalmol 2002; 46:463–468.

521. Recillas-Gispert C, Ortega-Larrocea G, Arrelanes-Garcia L et al. Chorio-retinitis secondary to *Mycobacterium tuberculosis* in acquired immune deficiency syndrome. Retina 1997; 17:437–439.

522. USPHS/IDSA Prevention of Opportunistic Infections Working Group: Preface to the 1997 USPHS/IDSA guidelines for the prevention of opportunistic infections in persons infected with the human immuno-deficiency virus. Clin Infect Dis 1997; 25(suppl 3):299–312.

523. USPHS/IDSA Prevention of Opportunistic Infections Working Group: 1997 USPHS/IDSA guidelines for the prevention of opportunistic infections in persons infected with the human immunodeficiency virus: disease-specific recommendations. Clin Infect Dis 1997; 25(suppl 3): 313–335.

524. Schanzer MC, Font RL, O'Malley RE. Primary ocular malignant lym-phoma associated with the acquired immune deficiency syndrome. Ophthalmology 1991; 98:88–91.

525. Matzkin DC, Slamovits TL, Rosenbaum PS. Simultaneous intraocular and orbital non-Hodgkin lymphoma in the acquired immune deficiency syndrome. Ophthalmology 1994; 101:850–855.

526. Levy JA, Shimabukuro J, Hollander H et al. Isolation of AIDS-associated retroviruses from cerebrospinal fluid and brain of patients with neuro-logical symptoms. Lancet 1985; 2:586–588.

527. Jordan BD, Navia BA, Petito C et al. Neurological syndromes complic-ating AIDS. Front Radiat Ther Oncol 1985; 19:82–87.

528. Collier AC, Marra C, Coombs RW et al. Central nervous system manifes-tations in human immunodeficiency virus infection without AIDS. J Acquir Immune Defic Syndr 1992; 5:229–241.

529. Arribas JR, Storch GA, Clifford DB et al. Cytomegalovirus encephalitis. Ann Intern Med 1996; 125:577–587.

530. Hamed LM, Schatz NJ, Galetta SL. Brainstem ocular motility defects and AIDS. Am J Ophthalmol 1988; 106:437–442.

531. Antoworth MV, Beck RW. Third nerve palsy as a presenting sign of acquired immunodeficiency syndrome. J Clin Neuro Ophthalmol 1987; 7:125.

532. Freeman WR, Wiley CA. In situ nucleic acid hybridization. Surv Ophthalmol 1988; 34:187–192.

533. Verbraak FD, Galema M, van den Horn GH et al. Serological and polymerase chain reaction-based analysis of aqueous humour samples in patients with AIDS and necrotizing retinitis. AIDS 1996; 10:1091–1099.

534. de Smet MD. Differential diagnosis of retinitis and choroiditis in patients with acquired immunodeficiency syndrome. Am J Med 1992; 92:17S–21S.

535. Freeman WR, Stern WH, Gross JG et al. Pathologic observations made by retinal biopsy. Retina 1990; 10:195–204.

536. Schneiderman TE, Faber DW, Gross JG et al. The agar–albumin sand-wich technique for processing retinal biopsy specimens. Am J Ophthal-mol 1989; 108:567–571.

537. Yeni PG, Hammer SM, Carpenter CC et al. Antiretroviral treatment for adult HIV infection in 2002: updated recommendations of the Inter-national AIDS Society – USA Panel. [Erratum in: JAMA 2003; 11:32]. JAMA 2002; 288:222–235.

538. Wei X, Ghosh SK, Taylor ME et al. Viral dynamics in human immuno-deficiency virus type 1 infection, Nature 1995; 373:117–122.

539. Bartlett JA, Benoit SL, Johnson VA et al. Lamivudine plus zidovudine compared with zalcitabine plus zidovudine in patients with HIV infection: a randomized, double-blind, placebo-controlled trial. Ann Intern Med 1996; 125:161–172.

540. The Delta Coordinating Committee. Delta: a randomised, double-blind, controlled trial comparing combinations of zidovudine plus didanosine or zalcitabine with zidovudine alone in HIV-infected individuals. Lancet 1996; 348:283–291.

541. Hirsch MS, Brun-Vezinet F, Clotet B et al. Antiretroviral drug resistance testing in adults infected with human immunodeficiency virus type I: 2003 recommendations of an International AIDS Society – USA Panel. Clin Infect Dis 2003; 37:113–128.

542. Raffanti S, Haas DW. Antimicrobial agents (continued): antiretroviral agents. In: Hardman JG, Limbird LE, Gilman AG, eds. Goodman & Gilman's the pharmacologic basis of therapeutics, 10th edn. New York: McGraw-Hill, 2001; 1349–1380.

543. Preston SL, Piliero PJ, Drusano GL. Pharmacodynamics and clinical use of anti-HIV drugs. Infect Dis Clin North Am 2003; 17:651–674.

544. Update: universal precautions for prevention of transmission of human immunodeficiency virus, hepatitis B virus, and other bloodborne pathogens in health-care settings. MMWR Morb Mortal Wkly Rep 1988; 37:377–388.

545. De Clercq E. New developments in anti-HIV chemotherapy. Biochim Biophys Acta 2002; 1587:258–275.

546. Albrecht MA, Wilkin TJ, Coakley EPG et al. Advanced in antiretroviral therapy. Top HIV Med 2003; 11:97–127.

547. Fauci AS, Bartlett JG et al. Panel on Clinical Practices for the Treatment of HIV Infection. Guidelines for the use of antiretroviral agents in HIV-1-infected adults and adolescents. March 23, 2004. Online. Available: http://aidsinfo.nih.gov//guidelines/.

548. Pozniak A, Gazzard B, Anderson J et al. British HIV Association (BHIVA) guidelines for the treatment of HIV-infected adults with antiretroviral therapy. HIV Med 2003; 4 (Suppl 1):S1–S41.

549. Lafeuillade A, Aubert L, Chaffanjon P et al. Optic neuritis associated with dideoxyinosine. Lancet 1991; 337:615.

550. Whitcup SM, Butler KM, Caruso R et al. Retinal toxicity in human immunodeficiency virus-infected children treated with 2,3-dideoxyinosine. Am J Ophthalmol 1992; 113:1–7.

551. Whitcup SM, Butler KM, Pizzo PA et al. Retinal lesions in children treated with dideoxyinosine [Letter]. N Engl J Med 1992; 326:1226–1227.

552. Fauci AS. Combination therapy for HIV infection: getting closer. Ann Intern Med 1992; 116:85–86.

553. Meng TC, Fischl MA, Boota AM et al. Combination therapy with zidovu-dine and dideoxycytidine in patients with advanced human immuno-deficiency virus infection: a phase I/II study. Ann Intern Med 116:13–20.

554. Eron JJ, Benoit SL, Jensek J et al. Treatment with lamivudine, zidovu-dine, or both in HIV-positive patients with 200 to 500 CD4+ cells per cubic millimeter. N Engl J Med 1995; 333:1662–1669.

555. Katzenstein DA, Hammer SM, Hughes M et al. The relation of virologic and immunologic markers to clinical outcomes after nucleoside therapy in adults with 200 to 500 CD4+ cells per cubic millimeter: NIAID spon-sored AIDS Clinical Trials Group Study 175, a virology substudy. N Engl J Med 1996; 335:1091–1098.

556. Whitcup SM, Fortin E, Nussenblatt RB et al. Therapeutic effect of combination antiretroviral therapy of cytomegalovirus retinitis [Letter]. JAMA 1997; 1277:1519–1520.

557. Fischl MA, Galpin J, Levine JD et al. Recombinant human erythropoietin for patients with AIDS treated with zidovudine. N Engl J Med 1990; 322:1488–1493.

558. Groopman JE, Mitsuyasu RT, DeLeo MJ et al. Effect of recombinant human granulocyte-macrophage colony-stimulating factor on myelopoiesis in the acquired immunodeficiency syndrome. N Engl J Med 1987; 317:593–598.

559. Richman DD, Fischl MA, Grieco MH et al. The toxicity of azidothymi-dine (AZT) in the treatment of AIDS and AIDS-related complex. N Engl J Med 1987; 317:192–197.

560. Chang Y, Cesarman E, Pessin MS et al. Identification of herpesvirus-like sequences in AIDS–associated Kaposi's sarcoma. Science 1994; 266:1865–1869.

561. Moore PS, Chang Y. Detection of herpesvirus-like DNA sequences in Kaposi's sarcoma in patients with and those without HIV infection. N Engl J Med 1996; 332:1168–1172.

562. Drugs for HIV infection. Med Lett 1997; 39:111–116.

Chapter
93

Acute Retinal Necrosis Syndrome

Jay S. Pepose
Russell N. Van Gelder

DEFINITION

In 1971 Urayama and co-workers[1] first reported six cases of an apparently new syndrome characterized by acute necrotizing retinitis, vitreitis, retinal arteritis (Figs 93-1 to 93-3), choroiditis, and late-onset rhegmatogenous retinal detachment. Young & Bird[2] described two similar cases in 1978 and gave the syndrome the acronym BARN (bilateral acute necrosis syndrome). With the subsequent recognition of unilateral and asynchronous bilateral cases, the disease has been termed simply acute retinal necrosis syndrome, or ARN syndrome. ARN syndrome is characterized by the initial onset of episcleritis or scleritis, periorbital pain, and anterior uveitis, which may be granulomatous or stellate in appearance. This is followed by decreased vision resulting from vitreous opacification, necrotizing retinitis, and, in some cases, optic neuritis or neuropathy. The retinitis appears as deep, multifocal, yellow-white patches, typically beginning in the peripheral fundus (Figs 93-1 and 93-4) and then becoming concentrically confluent and spreading toward the posterior pole (Figs 93-2 and 93-5); the macula is frequently spared. An active vasculitis is present, with perivascular hemorrhages, sheathing, and terminal obliteration of arterioles by thrombi. The phase of active retinitis usually lasts 4 to 6 weeks, during which time an exudative retinal detachment may occur.[3-8]

With resolution, pigmentation of the peripheral lesions begins at their posterior margins, leaving a scalloped appearance (Fig. 93-6), frequently accompanied by retinal breaks at the junction of normal and necrotic retina. Giant retinal pigment epithelial tears may develop.[9] A rhegmatogenous retinal detachment has been observed in approximately 75% of untreated eyes, generally within 1 to 2 months of the onset of the disease. Earlier exudative and rhegmatogenous detachments have been noted, particularly in cases associated with herpes simplex virus (HSV).[3,6,8,10] Vitreous inflammation may lead to organization and proliferative vitreoretinopathy,[11] adding a traction component to the retinal detachment (Fig. 93-7). Vision may suddenly decrease as a result of anterior ischemic optic neuropathy. Macular pucker may also occur.

Computed tomography[12-14] and ultrasonography[14] have revealed enlargement of the optic nerve sheath in ARN cases associated with prominent optic disc edema. Even in ARN patients who are not immunocompromised and who have no clinical evidence of encephalitis, magnetic resonance imaging of selected cases has shown lesions of the lateral geniculate, optic tracts, and chiasm,[15] suggesting viral spread through the central nervous system by axoplasmic transport from retinal ganglion cells.

The contralateral eye is involved in approximately 36% of ARN cases, usually within 6 weeks of the onset of disease in the first eye.[9,16] However, the second eye can be affected as late as 34 years after involvement of the first eye,[17] and the fellow eye has become involved even after aciclovir treatment for ARN in the first eye.[18] Mild forms of ARN syndrome, characterized by patchy, peripheral retinal opacification, have been reported. These mild cases did not become rapidly confluent or lead to detachment.[19] It is unclear whether this atypical presentation is a result of intense aciclovir and corticosteroid therapy or a reflection of a wide range of disease severity. In addition, less involved forms of ARN have been reported after primary varicella, without concomitant therapy.[20]

PATIENT POPULATION

ARN syndrome occurs most commonly in otherwise healthy patients of either sex and of any age; in general, patients are not immunocompromised or systemically ill. However, ARN patients may demonstrate subclinical immune dysfunction. In one review of 216 patients with ARN, impaired cellular immunity was noted in 16%.[21] Skin testing of patients with ARN revealed anergy in five of seven tested cases and abnormal lymphocyte proliferative indices in one-third.[22] The significance of cutaneous anergy is unclear, however, since patients with zoster infections frequently demonstrate anergy.[23] Specific human leukocyte antigen (HLA) haplotypes may increase the relative risk of developing ARN syndrome, such as the HLA-DQw7 antigen and phenotype Bw62, DR4 in white patients in the USA[24] and HLA-Aw33, B44, and DRw6 in Japanese patients.[25] Pleocytosis of the cerebrospinal fluid frequently accompanies the syndrome,[9,13,26] and intrathecal production of antibodies against herpesviruses has been demonstrated in selected cases.[4] Some patients present with ARN before, after, or at the same time as they show skin manifestations of varicella-zoster infection[27,28] (e.g., primary varicella, herpes zoster ophthalmicus, or the Ramsay Hunt syndrome). Unilateral ARN has also been noted after herpes simplex keratitis.[29] Diffuse cerebral atrophy and labyrinthine deafness have been reported following ARN,[30] and some investigators

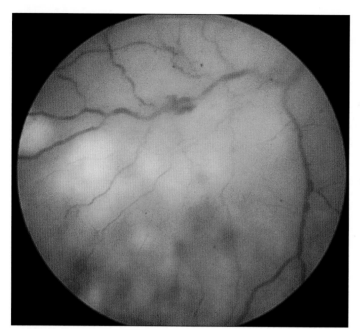

Fig. 93-1 Typical fundus appearance of early acute retinal necrosis syndrome demonstrating necrotizing peripheral retinitis, intraretinal hemorrhage, and vitreitis.

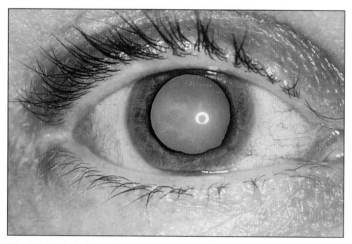

Fig. 93-2 Marked vitreitis associated with acute retinal necrosis syndrome. Episcleritis and keratic precipitates are also often seen early in the syndrome.

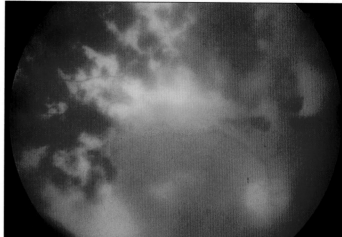

Fig. 93-3 Fundus appearance late in acute retinal necrosis syndrome. Dense vitreitis, confluent retinal necrosis, and intraretinal hemorrhage are encroaching on the posterior pole.

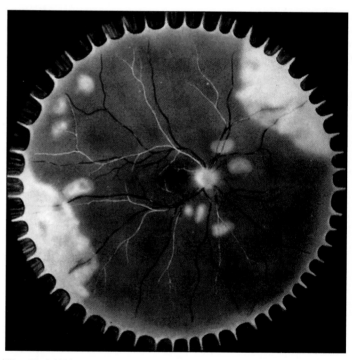

Fig. 93-4 White patches of retinal necrosis are seen in the periphery with isolated areas of necrosis more posterior early in the course of acute retinal necrosis.

have suggested that ARN should be considered as one of the uveomeningeal syndromes.[14]

Acute necrotizing retinitis that is clinically identical to ARN or shares many features with ARN has been reported in immunocompromised patients. ARN was first described in immunocompromised patients in 1985[31]; one case series has described 26 cases of ARN in acquired immunodeficiency syndrome (AIDS) patients, noting a generally fulminant course.[32] The cause of the retinitis in these immunocompromised patients may be particularly diverse or multifactorial. For example, an AIDS patient died after an ARN-like syndrome with concurrent encephalitis, and herpes simplex viral antigens were localized in the central nervous system at postmortem examination.[33] In contrast, several immunocompromised patients have presented with ARN in association with skin manifestations of zoster.[34] Although ARN syndrome was initially defined as manifesting in otherwise healthy patients, many authorities have broadened the diagnostic criteria to include immunocompromised hosts.[34-37] It is the evolution of clinical signs and symptoms, and not the specific pathogen or immune status of the patient, that serves as the sole basis by which ARN syndrome has been defined (see Differential Diagnosis, below).

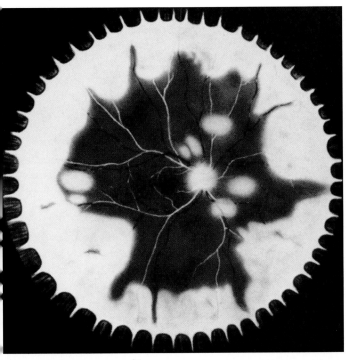

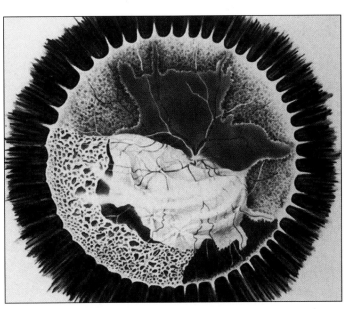

Fig. 93-7 Retinal breaks and the onset of proliferative vitreoretinopathy can lead to a combined tractional–rhegematogenous retinal detachment 1 to 2 months after the onset of the acute retinal necrosis syndrome. (Reproduced from Clarkson JG, Blumenkranz MS, Culbertson WW et al. Ophthalmology 1984; 91:1665–1668.)

Fig. 93-5 The peripheral retinitis becomes confluent for 360 degrees and is accompanied by an obliterative vasculitis and papillitis.

blind eye enucleated early in the course of the disease, and specific varicella-zoster antigens were identified in retinal tissue by immunocytologic staining[38] (Fig. 93-8). Varicella-zoster virus was identified by electron microscopy in necrotic retinal tissue (Fig. 93-9) in two other cases of ARN.[39] Varicella-zoster DNA in intraocular fluids of ARN cases has been confirmed by polymerase chain reaction (PCR),[40] and Witmer quotients of paired serum to intraocular fluid antibody levels have been diagnostic of varicella-zoster in numerous cases.[41,42] Varicella-zoster antigens have been demonstrated in vitreous aspirates of patients with ARN syndrome.[43]

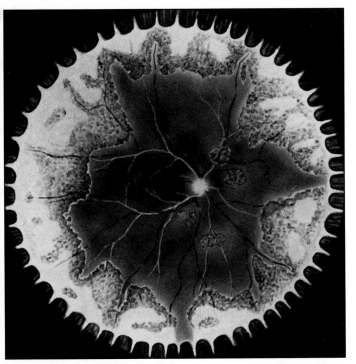

Fig. 93-6 During the resolution of active retinitis, the lesions become pigmented, starting at their posterior margins, leaving a scalloped border between necrotic and normal-appearing retina.

ETIOLOGY

Considerable evidence points to multiple members of the herpesvirus family in the etiology of ARN syndrome. Varicella-zoster virus was isolated in tissue culture from the vitreous of a

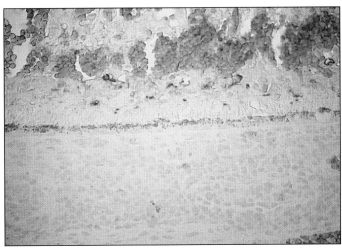

Fig. 93-8 Varicella-zoster antigens (brown) are seen in cells scattered in all layers of a necrotic retina.

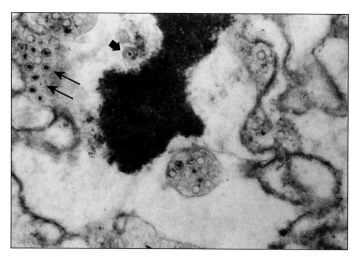

Fig. 93-9 Ultrasctructural studies of necrotic retina reveal multiple 100 nm nucleocapsids (double arrows) and enveloped virions typical of a herpes-type virus. (Courtesy of MS Blumenkranz.)

Restriction endonuclease patterns of the ARN virus isolate were similar to those of typical varicella-zoster strains and showed similar sensitivities to a panel of antiviral drugs.[44] Although strain heterogeneity has been observed in the varicella-zoster viruses associated with ARN syndrome,[45] these data do not support the notion that the ARN virus represents a mutant strain of varicella-zoster virus with significant alterations in either the viral thymidine kinase or DNA polymerase genes. It therefore remains enigmatic why an "old virus" should give rise to a "new" syndrome.

Some reports have suggested that other members of the herpesvirus family may cause ARN. A number of studies have implicated HSV because of concurrent herpes simplex skin lesions,[46] the detection of herpes simplex antigens on vitreous cells,[7] the presence of immune complexes containing herpes simplex antigens in aqueous or serum,[47] the documentation of intraocular antibody synthesis directed against HSV,[42] diagnostic changes in serum antibody levels to herpes simplex, PCR detection of herpes simplex,[48] or the culture of herpes simplex from vitreous humor.[3,8,38] Several cases have been described of ARN caused by reactivation of HSV type 2.[40,48,49] Interestingly, patients with HSV type 2 appear to be much younger (mean 21 years) than those with either HSV type 1 or varicella-zoster (mean age 40 years).[42,50,51] The proportion of ARN syndrome patients with disease caused by HSV-2 may be higher in Japan than in the USA, perhaps coincident with changing epidemiologic distributions of HSV-1 versus HSV-2 in this population.[52,53] Patients with ARN syndrome caused by herpes simplex type 1 appear to have a higher risk of encephalitis or meningitis than those with disease caused by varicella-zoster.[50,54-58] In one study of a case of ARN,[59] cytomegalovirus (CMV) was cultured and CMV antigens were demonstrated in retinal tissue, but megalic cells or electron-dense cytoplasmic inclusions, which have uniformly typified CMV infection of the retina, were not identified. In another case PCR yielded positive results for CMV in one immunocompetent individual whose vitreous was negative for

varicella-zoster and HSV types 1 and 2.[60] Epstein–Barr virus has also been postulated in some cases of ARN syndrome,[61] but definitive linkage of this nearly ubiquitous virus to disease remains problematic.

PATHOLOGIC FEATURES

Studies of blind eyes enucleated early in the course of ARN have demonstrated retinal necrosis, hemorrhage, and considerable vitreous debris. The retinal necrosis is full-thickness, and an underlying choroiditis is present that may be granulomatous (Fig. 93-10). Varicella-zoster virus DNA and antigens have been identified in lymphoid cells within choroidal infiltrates in an eye enucleated in the late stage of disease.[62] Eosinophilic intranuclear inclusions within cells of all layers of retina and retinal pigment epithelium were the first clues suggesting a possible viral etiology by a member of the herpes group.[39] There is histologic evidence of retinal arteritis (Fig. 93-11), although no virus particles have been detected in vascular endothelium. Deposits of immune complexes containing varicella-zoster viral antigens have been demonstrated in retinal vessel walls by immunocytologic methods and may play a role in the vasculitis seen during active stages. The perivasculitis is not restricted to retinal vessels alone and can involve the extraocular muscles (Fig. 93-12). Immune complexes with herpes simplex have also been identified in intraocular fluids in ARN cases.

Ultrastructural studies of retinal tissue have revealed 180 mm virions containing icosahedral capsids, consistent with particles of the herpes group[39] (Fig. 93-8). The optic nerve may be largely necrotic and heavily infiltrated with plasma cells, but no virus particles or antigens have been seen in the optic nerve. It is possible that the absence of viral antigens or particles reflects more the time point in the course of the disease when enucleation was performed in these rare cases than conclusive evidence regarding acute optic nerve infection. The multifocal, deep retinitis observed early in the course of ARN is compatible with either

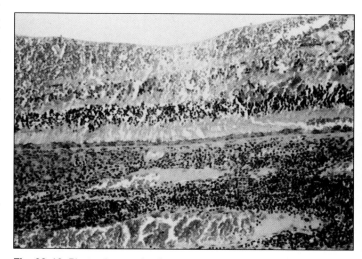

Fig. 93-10 Photomicrograph of a case of acute retinal necrosis shows full-thickness retinal necrosis with an underlying granulomatous choroiditis. (Courtesy of Robert Y. Foos.)

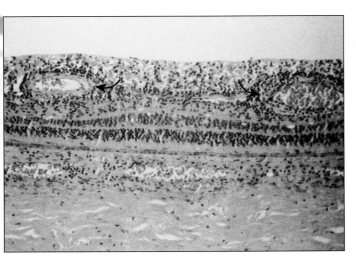

Fig. 93-11 Histologic evidence of retinal vasculitis (arrows) in acute retinal necrosis. (Courtesy of Robert Y. Foos.)

bloodborne spread of virus or transmission to the eye through a bilateral nerve pathway. An animal model of ARN using herpes simplex virus suggests that spread to the contralateral eye occurs by retrograde axonal transport between the suprachiasmatic nucleus of the hypothalamus and the contralateral retina.[63]

Retinal necrosis in ARN is probably the result of multiple factors, including a direct lytic viral infection of retina, immune complex disease mediating an obliterative arteritis, choroidal inflammation and occlusion, T-cell-mediated inflammation, and vitreous inflammation. All these elements contribute and lead to a combined traction–rhegmatogenous retinal detachment.

DIFFERENTIAL DIAGNOSIS

The American Uveitis Society released its criteria for diagnosis of ARN syndrome in 1994.[37] Under this definition, diagnosis of ARN syndrome is dependent solely on the observed clinical findings and their progression. Neither the identification of an etiologic agent nor knowledge of the patient's immune status is required to render a diagnosis of ARN syndrome. The diagnostic criteria are divided into mandatory and supporting categories and are summarized in Table 93-1. By this definition, retinal lesions presumptively caused by herpesviruses (but not part of other well-recognized syndromes such as CMV retinitis or progressive outer retinal necrosis: see below) are covered under the umbrella term *necrotizing herpetic retinopathy*.

The differential diagnosis of ARN includes CMV retinopathy, syphilitic retinitis, toxoplasmosis (particularly in immunocompromised hosts), large-cell lymphoma, and acute multifocal hemorrhagic retinal vasculitis. A more extensive differential diagnosis includes toxocariasis, fungal or bacterial retinitis, pars planitis, Behçet's disease, sarcoidosis, commotio retinae, central retinal artery or ophthalmic artery occlusion, ischemic ocular syndrome, collagen-vascular disease, intraocular leukemia/lymphoma (including T-cell-mediated[64]), and retinoblastoma.

ARN syndrome is readily distinguished from a separate form of varicella-zoster retinitis reported in human immunodeficiency

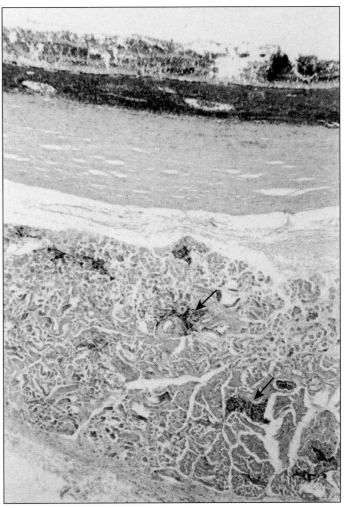

Fig. 93-12 Foci of perivascular inflammation (arrows) are seen in the inferior oblique muscle in a case of acute retinal necrosis. (Courtesy of Robert Y. Foos.)

virus (HIV)-infected patients, sometimes referred to as progressive outer retinal necrosis syndrome or PORN.[47,65] This latter entity shares an etiologic agent with some cases of ARN but is otherwise completely distinct. It is characterized by multifocal, patchy choroidal, and deep posterior retinal opacification that may initially be parafoveal. Additional features differentiating this syndrome from ARN include the absence of vitreous or anterior chamber inflammation or signs of active vasculitis. PORN progresses rapidly from the posterior pole to involve the entire retina, resulting in widespread retinal necrosis and atrophy. Despite a common etiologic agent, varicella-zoster retinitis should not be referred to as ARN syndrome. Indeed, the two diseases may even affect different eyes of the same patient.[66]

Although ARN syndrome is a clinical diagnosis established on the basis of a constellation of evolving signs and symptoms, which may be pathognomonic in many cases, in atypical or difficult diagnostic cases ancillary clinical history or laboratory tests can support the diagnosis. It is important to assess the patient's level of immunocompetence, since knowledge of seropositivity to HIV and syphilis may help to establish the appropriate specific

Table 93-1 American Uveitis Society criteria for diagnosis of acute retinal necrosis syndrome[37]

Required clinical criteria	Supporting clinical criteria
One or more foci of retinal necrosis with discrete borders, located in peripheral retina	Optic neuropathy/atrophy
Rapid progression of disease in the absence of therapy	Scleritis
Circumferential spread of disease	Pain
Evidence of occlusive vasculopathy and arteriolar involvement	
A prominent inflammatory reaction in the vitreous and anterior chamber	

diagnosis. Diagnostic vitrectomy is appropriate in cases of uncertain diagnosis. The most sensitive and specific method for the detection of herpesviruses in vitreous specimens is PCR. PCR assays are capable of detecting a single varicella-zoster virion from vitreous biopsy.[67] Simultaneous PCR for multiple herpesviruses has been used to screen for an etiologic agent in atypical cases of ARN and has implicated both CMV[67] and HSV[40] as potentially causative. PCR can be performed in multiplex for varicella-zoster virus, HSV, CMV, and toxoplasmosis.[68] Sensitivity for each, even in multiplex testing, is at least 10 genomes per microliter. With application of quantitative PCR (qPCR), accurate estimates of pathogen load can be achieved.[69,70] These data suggest significant heterogeneity in the pathogen load among individual cases of disease. The great sensitivity of PCR can be problematic, however; assays that yield false-positive results, likely through amplification of latent virus in host tissue, have been reported.[67] False-negative results can also occur. Consensus has not yet been reached regarding the negative predictive value of a negative PCR test for viral DNA. PCR requires meticulous technical performance and confirmation by probe hybridization to avoid specificity problems and is best performed by a laboratory with considerable experience with this method. In cases in which PCR is negative but clinical suspicion is high, endoretinal biopsy may be appropriate. Taking the biopsy from the transition zone between normal and necrotic retina during the acute phase of the disease greatly increases its diagnostic yield. Obtaining paired serum and intraocular fluid specimens and applying a modified Witmer quotient is of diagnostic value even in the early stages of ARN syndrome and develops increasing sensitivity with time.[41,71] In contrast, quantitative antiviral antibody levels in acute and chronic sera from ARN patients are consistent with a specific etiologic diagnosis in a minority of cases and have been falsely negative in cases in which vitreous cultures were positive for herpesviruses.

TREATMENT AND PROGNOSIS

Treatment of ARN syndrome is complex and must be individualized in response to the many pathogenic and temporal facets of the disorder, as well as to the specific vitreoretinal pathologic findings at hand. Cases of ARN associated with mild or minimal inflammation have been reported in which ARN did not progress to extensive retinal necrosis, traction, or detachment.[19,20] Controlled, randomized, prospective treatment studies on ARN have not been conducted, so current recommendations are based solely on anecdotal data. Early studies indicated that the natural history of classic ARN syndrome carries a generally poor prognosis in untreated eyes,[9] with only 28% of affected eyes obtaining a final vision better than 20/200 because of rhegmatogenous retinal detachment (75% of affected eyes), optic nerve dysfunction, or macular abnormality. The advent of antiviral therapy, vitrectomy techniques,[72] and prophylactic laser photocoagulation has decreased this level of vision loss to less than one-third of cases in recent years.[12] In one series of cases that were detected early and treated aggressively with aciclovir and laser photocoagulation, the outcome for 13 eyes of 12 patients showed 20/40 or better vision in 46% of eyes and 20/400 or better in 92%.[73]

In light of the characterization and the determination of antiviral sensitivities of the varicella-zoster isolate, aciclovir has been used in an effort to limit the direct cytopathic effect of virus on retinal tissue. Based on the dose required for a 50% reduction of virus plaques in tissue culture (ED_{50}), oral administration of aciclovir results in subtherapeutic serum levels; in contrast, intravenous aciclovir (13 mg/kg every 8 h) results in an intravitreal aciclovir level[4] over three times the ARN ED_{50}. After intravenous administration of aciclovir to ARN patients (1500 mg/m² per day in three divided doses), retinal lesions were first noted to regress 3.9 days after the beginning of therapy; new lesions did not develop, and existing lesions did not progress.[18] Intravenous therapy for 5 to 10 days may be followed by oral aciclovir at the zoster dosage (800 mg orally five times daily, assuming normal renal function) for up to 6 weeks after the onset of infection, and longer in immunocompromised patients. Valaciclovir (1 g orally three times daily) or famciclovir[74,75] (500 mg orally three times daily) may also be used following intravenous aciclovir administration. Side-effects of aciclovir include decreased renal function, gastrointestinal irritation, phlebitis, central nervous system dysfunction, and hypersensitivity reactions. Aciclovir has potent antiviral action against varicella-zoster virus, HSV types 1 and 2 (both of which have been implicated in ARN), and Epstein–Barr virus, but it has low activity against CMV. Valganciclovir is active against varicella-zoster virus, HSV, and CMV, but at present is only US Food and Drug Administration-approved for CMV retinitis. Although outpatient use of oral valaciclovir for treatment of ARN syndrome has been reported,[76] there is little literature on the efficacy of this treatment. Given the risk of encephalitis, particularly in patients with HSV-1-associated disease, close monitoring of patient's mental status is warranted.

Recent studies have suggested an adjunctive role for intravitreal antiviral medication in the treatment of ARN syndrome. In one small series, three patients treated with intravitreal ganciclovir as well as intravenous foscarnet, ganciclovir, or aciclovir led to excellent outcomes,[77] while in another three patients responded to intravitreal antiviral treatment despite progression on intravenous aciclovir.[78] A similar approach has been employed for progressive outer retinal necrosis.[79,80] Early administration of intravitreal antivirals also provides an opportunity for vitreous sampling (akin to the "tap and inject" for endophthalmitis), allowing for PCR-based identification of the causative virus.

Acute decreases in vision in ARN patients can result from ischemic optic neuropathy and have led to trials of anticoagulants such as aspirin, along with high-dose oral steroids early after initiation of antiviral therapy. Systemic corticosteroids may also limit intraocular inflammation and the vitreous reaction, but are generally only begun after 24 to 48 h of intravenous acyclovir. Virus particles or antigens have not been observed in the optic nerve in ARN, and it appears that the optic nerve dysfunction is caused by ischemia from swollen vascular endothelial cells, thrombotic arteriolar occlusion, and infiltration of the optic nerve by inflammatory cells. Hyperaggregation of platelets has been reported in six of seven patients with bilateral ARN studied, as determined by adenosine 5-diphosphate aggregation testing and partial prothrombin times.[81] Optic nerve dysfunction has been reported in ARN patients despite anticoagulation therapy or antiplatelet therapy. Studies have employed optic nerve sheath fenestration in conjunction with aciclovir therapy in a small group of ARN patients with optic neuropathy and disc edema, with reported improvement in final vision in six of eight eyes.[14] Better results were obtained in the subgroup that underwent decompression within 12 days of the onset of the optic neuropathy.

The second eye becomes involved in 36% of ARN patients, usually within 6 weeks of the first eye's involvement.[18] However, bilateral ARN has been reported up to 34 years after the first eye was affected,[17] raising a question as to the benefit of long-term antiviral prophylaxis. Risk of second-eye involvement may also be dependent on the etiologic agent causing disease. Additionally, rare cases of reactivation in the originally affected eye have been reported.[82] Whereas oral aciclovir may not result in high serum levels because of low absorption through the gastrointestinal tract, newly developed prodrugs of aciclovir such as valaciclovir have high systemic absorption and may be used for prophylaxis against involvement of the second eye.[3,83]

Retinal tears at the junction of normal and necrotic retina, as well as subsequent proliferative retinopathy creating a compli-cated combined traction–rhegmatogenous retinal detachment, pose a difficult problem in the management of ARN. Whereas Peyman et al.[7,16] obtained good results in selected patients with intravenous and intravitreal aciclovir in conjunction with prophylactic vitrectomy and scleral buckles in an uncontrolled study of active ARN cases that had not yet developed detachment, others have not been able to prevent retinal detachment by similar management.[84] In a study of 13 eyes of 12 ARN patients, the incidence of retinal detachment despite intravenous aciclovir therapy was 84%, suggesting that antiviral therapy alone does not effectively preclude retinal detachment. Several investigations have demonstrated the benefit of prophylactic laser photocoagulation posterior to areas of active retinitis.[26,39,73,85] Although laser treatment cannot stop the progression of the viral retinitis and may need to be repeated in cases with rapid progression, the overall incidence of retinal detachment appears lower in these treated series. When detachments did occur after prophylactic laser treatment, they were more commonly localized to the peripheral retina. With the use of modern microsurgical techniques, including intravitreal silicone oil, air–fluid exchange, demarcating laser photocoagulation, and a long-acting gas tamponade, a high percentage of retinas can be anatomically reattached. However, patients must be carefully selected, and it must be kept in mind that patients with known optic atrophy or minimal vision because of macular pucker or dysfunction before detachment are unlikely to obtain improved visual function despite anatomically successful retinal reattachment.

ARN syndrome remains a relatively new, visually devastating disorder of multifactorial pathogenesis. Its successful management appears to depend on further advances in antiviral chemotherapy, control of the ischemic vasculopathy, and prevention of proliferative vitreoretinopathy.

REFERENCES

1. Urayama A, Yamada N, Sasaki T et al. Unilateral acute uveitis with retinal periarteritis and detachment. Jpn J Clin Ophthalmol 1971; 25:607–619.
2. Young NJ Bird AC. Bilateral acute retinal necrosis. Br J Ophthalmol 1978; 62:581–590.
3. Duker JS, Nielsen JC, Eagle RC et al. Rapidly progressive acute retinal necrosis secondary to herpes simplex virus, type 1. Ophthalmology 1990; 97:1638–1643.
4. el Azazi M, Samuelsson A, Linde A et al. Intrathecal antibody production against viruses of the herpesvirus family in acute retinal necrosis syndrome. Am J Ophthalmol 1991; 112:76–82.
5. Lewis ML, Culbertson WW, Post JD et al. Herpes simplex virus type 1. A cause of the acute retinal necrosis syndrome. Ophthalmology 1989; 96:875–878.
6. Margolis T, Irvine AR, Hoyt WF et al. Acute retinal necrosis syndrome presenting with papillitis and arcuate neuroretinitis. Ophthalmology 1988; 95:937–940.
7. Peyman GA, Goldberg MF, Uninsky E et al. Vitrectomy and intravitreal antiviral drug therapy in acute retinal necrosis syndrome. Report of two cases. Arch Ophthalmol 1984; 102:1618–1621.
8. Watanabe J, Ashida M, Funaki A et al. [A case of acute retinal necrosis syndrome caused by herpes simplex virus type 1.] Nippon Ganka Gakkai Zasshi 1989; 93:65–71.
9. Fox GM, Blumenkranz M. Giant retinal pigment epithelial tears in acute retinal necrosis. Am J Ophthalmol 1993; 116:302–306.
10. Matsuo T, Date S, Tsuji T et al. Immune complex containing herpesvirus antigen in a patient with acute retinal necrosis. Am J Ophthalmol 1986; 101:368–371.
11. Ahmadieh H, Soheilian M, Azarmina M et al. Surgical management of retinal detachment secondary to acute retinal necrosis: clinical features, surgical techniques, and long-term results. Jpn J Ophthalmol 2003; 47:484–491.

12. Litoff D, Catalano RA. Herpes zoster optic neuritis in human immuno-deficiency virus infection. Arch Ophthalmol 1990; 108:782–783.

13. Sergott RC, Anand R, Belmont JB et al. Acute retinal necrosis neuropathy. Clinical profile and surgical therapy. Arch Ophthalmol 1989; 107:692–696.

14. Sergott RC, Belmont JB, Savino PJ et al. Optic nerve involvement in the acute retinal necrosis syndrome. Arch Ophthalmol 1985; 103:1160–1162.

15. Farrell TA, Wolf MD, Folk JC et al. Magnetic resonance imaging in a patient with herpes zoster keratouveitis and contralateral acute retinal necrosis. Am J Ophthalmol 1991; 112:735–736.

16. Carney MD, Peyman GA, Goldberg MF et al. Acute retinal necrosis. Retina 1986; 6:85–94.

17. Falcone PM, Brockhurst RJ. Delayed onset of bilateral acute retinal necrosis syndrome: a 34-year interval. Ann Ophthalmol 1993; 25:373–374.

18. Blumenkranz MS, Culbertson WW, Clarkson JG et al. Treatment of the acute retinal necrosis syndrome with intravenous aciclovir. Ophthalmology 1986; 93:296–300.

19. Matsuo T, Nakayama T, Koyama T et al. A proposed mild type of acute retinal necrosis syndrome. Am J Ophthalmol 1988; 105:579–583.

20. Kelly SP, Rosenthal AR. Chickenpox chorioretinitis. Br J Ophthalmol 1990; 74:698–699.

21. Rochat C, Herbort CP. [Acute retinal necrosis syndrome. Lausanne cases, review of the literature and new physiopathogenetic hypothesis.] Klin Monatsbl Augenheilkd 1994; 204:440–449.

22. Rochat C, Polla BS, Herbort CP. Immunological profiles in patients with acute retinal necrosis. Graefes Arch Clin Exp Ophthalmol 1996; 234:547–552.

23. Pepose JS. Skin test with varicella-zoster virus antigen for ophthalmic herpes zoster. Am J Ophthalmol 1984; 98:825–827.

24. Holland GN, Cornell PJ, Park MS et al. An association between acute retinal necrosis syndrome and HLA-DQw7 and phenotype Bw62, DR4. Am J Ophthalmol 1989; 108:370–374.

25. Ichikaw T, Sakai J, Usui M. HLA antigens of patients with Kirisawa's uveitis and herpetic keratitis. Atarashii Ganka 1989; 6:107–114.

26. Sternberg P Jr, Han DP, Yeo JH et al. Photocoagulation to prevent retinal detachment in acute retinal necrosis. Ophthalmology 1988; 95:1389–1393.

27. Browning DJ, Blumenkranz MS, Culbertson WW et al. Association of varicella zoster dermatitis with acute retinal necrosis syndrome. Ophthalmology 1987; 94:602–606.

28. Yeo JH, Pepose JS, Stewart JA et al. Acute retinal necrosis syndrome following herpes zoster dermatitis. Ophthalmology 1986; 93:1418–1422.

29. Sado K, Kimura T, Hotta Y et al. Acute retinal necrosis syndrome associated with herpes simplex keratitis. Retina 1994; 14:260–263.

30. Severin M, Neubauer H. Bilateral acute vascular retinal necrosis. Ophthalmologica 1981; 182:199–203.

31. Neetens A, Stevens W, Taelman R et al. Immune deficiency and necrotising retinopathy. Bull Soc Belge Ophtalmol 1985; 215:73–86.

32. Batisse D, Eliaszewicz M, Zazoun L et al. Acute retinal necrosis in the course of AIDS: study of 26 cases. Aids 1996; 10:55–60.

33. Freeman WR, Thomas EL, Rao NA et al. Demonstration of herpes group virus in acute retinal necrosis syndrome. Am J Ophthalmol 1986; 102:701–709.

34. Jabs DA, Schachat AP, Liss R et al. Presumed varicella zoster retinitis in immunocompromised patients. Retina 1987; 7:9–13.

35. Chambers RB, Derick RJ, Davidorf FH et al. Varicella-zoster retinitis in human immunodeficiency virus infection. Case report. Arch Ophthalmol 1989; 107:960–961.

36. Freeman WR, Wiley CA, Gross JG et al. Endoretinal biopsy in immuno-suppressed and healthy patients with retinitis. Indications, utility, and techniques. Ophthalmology 1989; 96:1559–1565.

37. Holland GN. Standard diagnostic criteria for the acute retinal necrosis syndrome. Executive Committee of the American Uveitis Society. Am J Ophthalmol 1994; 117:663–667.

38. Culbertson WW, Blumenkranz MS, Pepose JS et al. Varicella zoster virus is a cause of the acute retinal necrosis syndrome. Ophthalmology 1986; 93:559–569.

39. Culbertson WW, Blumenkranz MS, Haines H et al. The acute retinal necrosis syndrome. Part 2: histopathology and etiology. Ophthalmology 1982; 89:1317–1325.

40. Cunningham ET Jr, Short GA, Irvine AR et al. Acquired immunodeficiency syndrome-associated herpes simplex virus retinitis. Clinical description and use of a polymerase chain reaction-based assay as a diagnostic tool. Arch Ophthalmol 1996; 114:834–840.

41. Pepose JS, Flowers B, Stewart JA et al. Herpesvirus antibody levels in the etiologic diagnosis of the acute retinal necrosis syndrome. Am J Ophthalmol 1992; 113:248–256.

42. Van Gelder RN, Willig JL, Holland GN et al. Herpes simplex virus type 2 as a cause of acute retinal necrosis syndrome in young patients. Ophthalmology 2001; 108:869–876.

43. Soushi S, Ozawa H, Matsuhashi M et al. Demonstration of varicella-zoster virus antigens in the vitreous aspirates of patients with acute retinal necrosis syndrome. Ophthalmology 1988; 95:1394–1398.

44. Pepose JS, Biron K. Antiviral sensitivities of the acute retinal necrosis syndrome virus. Curr Eye Res 1987; 6:201–205.

45. Abe T, Sato M, Tamai M. Variable R1 region in varicella zoster virus in fulminant type of acute retinal necrosis syndrome. Br J Ophthalmol 2000; 84:193–198.

46. Ludwig IH, Zegarra H, Zakov ZN. The acute retinal necrosis syndrome. Possible herpes simplex retinitis. Ophthalmology 1984; 91:1659–1664.

47. Margolis TP, Lowder CY, Holland GN et al. Varicella-zoster virus retinitis in patients with the acquired immunodeficiency syndrome. Am J Ophthalmol 1991; 112:119–131.

48. Rahhal FM, Siegel LM, Russak V et al. Clinicopathologic correlations in acute retinal necrosis caused by herpes simplex virus type 2. Arch Ophthalmol 1996; 114:1416–1419.

49. Thompson WS, Culbertson WW, Smiddy WE et al. Acute retinal necrosis caused by reactivation of herpes simplex virus type 2. Am J Ophthalmol 1994; 118:205–211.

50. Ganatra JB, Chandler D, Santos C et al. Viral causes of the acute retinal necrosis syndrome. Am J Ophthalmol 2000; 129:166–172.

51. Tan JCH, Byles D, Stanford MR et al. Acute retinal necrosis in children caused by herpes simplex virus. Retina 2001; 21:344–347.

52. Hashido M, Lee FK, Nahmias AJ et al. An epidemiologic study of herpes simplex virus type 1 and 2 infection in Japan based on type-specific serological assays. Epidemiol Infect 1998; 120:179–186.

53. Itoh N, Matsumura N, Ogi A et al. High prevalence of herpes simplex virus type 2 in acute retinal necrosis syndrome associated with herpes simplex virus in Japan. Am J Ophthalmol 2000; 129:404–405.

54. Gain P, Chiquet C, Thuret G et al. Herpes simplex virus type 1 encephalitis associated with acute retinal necrosis syndrome in an immunocompetent patient. Acta Ophthalmol Scand 2002; 80:546–549.

55. Gaynor BD, Wade NK, Cunningham ET Jr. Herpes simplex virus type 1 associated acute retinal necrosis following encephalitis. Retina 2001; 21:688–690.

56. Kim C, Yoon YH. Unilateral acute retinal necrosis occurring 2 years after herpes simplex type 1 encephalitis. Ophthalm Surg Lasers 2002; 33:250–252.

57. Maertzdorf J, Van der Lelij A, Baarsma GS et al. Herpes simplex virus type 1 (HSV-1)-induced retinitis following herpes simplex encephalitis: indications for brain-to-eye transmission of HSV-1. Ann Neurol 2000; 48:936–939.

58. Tada Y, Negoro K, Morimatsu M et al. Findings in a patient with herpes simplex viral meningitis associated with acute retinal necrosis syndrome. AJNR Am J Neuroradiol 2001; 22:1300–1302.

59. Rungger-Brandle E, Roux L, Leuenberger PM. Bilateral acute retinal necrosis (BARN). Identification of the presumed infectious agent. Ophthalmology 1984; 91:1648–1658.

60. Silverstein BE, Conrad D, Margolis TP et al. Cytomegalovirus-associated acute retinal necrosis syndrome. Am J Ophthalmol 1997; 123:257–258.

61. Kramer S, Brummer C, Zierhut M. Epstein–Barr virus associated acute retinal necrosis. Br J Ophthalmol 2001; 85:114.

62. Rummelt V, Wenkel H, Rummelt C et al. Detection of varicella zoster virus DNA and viral antigen in the late stage of bilateral acute retinal necrosis syndrome. Arch Ophthalmol 1992; 110:1132–1136.

63. Vann VR, Atherton SS. Neural spread of herpes simplex virus after anterior chamber inoculation. Invest Ophthalmol Vis Sci 1991; 32:2462–2472.

64. Levy-Clarke GA, Buggage RR, Shen D et al. Human T-cell lymphotropic virus type-1 associated T-cell leukemia/lymphoma masquerading as necrotizing retinal vasculitis. Ophthalmology 2002; 109:1717–1722.

65. Forster DJ, Dugel PU, Frangieh GT et al. Rapidly progressive outer retinal necrosis in the acquired immunodeficiency syndrome. Am J Ophthalmol 1990; 110:341–348.

66. Gariano RF, Berreen JP, Cooney EL. Progressive outer retinal necrosis and acute retinal necrosis in fellow eyes of a patient with acquired immunodeficiency syndrome. Am J Ophthalmol 2001; 132:421–423.

67. Short GA, Margolis TP, Kuppermann BD et al. A polymerase chain reaction-based assay for diagnosing varicella-zoster virus retinitis in patients with acquired immunodeficiency syndrome. Am J Ophthalmol 1997; 123:157–164.

68. Dabil H, Boley ML, Schmitz TM et al. Validation of a diagnostic multiplex polymerase chain reaction assay for infectious posterior uveitis. Arch Ophthalmol 2001; 119:1315–1322.

69. Asano S, Yoshikawa T, Kimura H et al. Monitoring herpesvirus DNA in three cases of acute retinal necrosis by real-time PCR. J Clin Virol 2004; 29:206–209.

70. Dworkin LL, Gibler TM, Van Gelder RN. Real-time quantitative polymerase chain reaction diagnosis of infectious posterior uveitis. Arch Ophthalmol 2002; 120:1534–1539.

71. Luyendijk L, van der Horn GJ, Visser OH et al. Detection of locally produced antibodies to herpes viruses in the aqueous of patients with acquired immune deficiency syndrome (AIDS) or acute retinal necrosis syndrome (ARN). Curr Eye Res 1990; 9 (Suppl.):7–11.

72. Blumenkranz M, Clarkson J, Culbertson WW et al. Vitrectomy for retinal detachment associated with acute retinal necrosis. Am J Ophthalmol 1988; 106:426–429.

73. Crapotta JA, Freeman WR, Feldman RM et al. Visual outcome in acute retinal necrosis, Retina 1993; 13:208–213.

74. Figueroa MS, Garabito I, Gutierrez C et al. Famciclovir for the treatment of acute retinal necrosis (ARN) syndrome. Am J Ophthalmol 1997; 123:255–257.

75. Klein JL, Sandy C, Migdal CS et al. Famciclovir in AIDS-related acute retinal necrosis. Aids 1996; 10:1300–1301.

76. Aslanides IM, De Souza S, Wong DT et al. Oral valaciclovir in the treatment of acute retinal necrosis syndrome. Retina 2002; 22:352–354.

77. Chau Tran TH, Cassoux N, Bodaghi B et al. Successful treatment with combination of systemic antiviral drugs and intravitreal ganciclovir injections in the management of severe necrotizing herpetic retinitis. Ocul Immunol Inflamm 2003; 11:141–144.

78. Luu KK, Scott IU, Chaudhry NA et al. Intravitreal antiviral injections as adjunctive therapy in the management of immunocompetent patients with necrotizing herpetic retinopathy. Am J Ophthalmol 2000; 129:811–813.

79. Roig-Melo EA, Macky TA, Heredia-Elizondo ML et al. Progressive outer retinal necrosis syndrome: successful treatment with a new combination of antiviral drugs. Eur J Ophthalmol 2001; 11:200–202.

80. Scott IU, Luu KM, Davis JL. Intravitreal antivirals in the management of patients with acquired immunodeficiency syndrome with progressive outer retinal necrosis. Arch Ophthalmol 2002; 120:1219–1222.

81. Ando F, Kato M, Goto S et al. Platelet function in bilateral acute retinal necrosis. Am J Ophthalmol 1983; 96:27–32.

82. Matsuo T, Nakayama T, Baba T. Same eye recurrence of acute retinal necrosis syndrome. Am J Ophthalmol 2001; 131:659–661.

83. Pepose JS. The potential impact of the varicella vaccine and new antivirals on ocular disease related to varicella-zoster virus. Am J Ophthalmol 1997; 123:243–251.

84. Blumenkranz M, Clarkson J, Culbertson WW et al. Visual results and complications after retinal reattachment in the acute retinal necrosis syndrome. The influence of operative technique. Retina 1989; 9:170–174.

85. Han DP, Lewis H, Williams GA et al. Laser photocoagulation in the acute retinal necrosis syndrome. Arch Ophthalmol 1987; 105:1051–1054.

Endogenous Fungal Infections of the Retina and Choroid

Gary N. Holland

Fungi, a large and diverse group of eukaryotic organisms, are widespread in nature. Among the thousands of fungal species, a relatively small number cause serious primary and opportunistic human diseases. The eye is one of the organs susceptible to infection. Exogenous fungal infections of the eye are a well-recognized complication of trauma and surgery, and fungi may infect the eye by extension from periocular and orbital sites. Endogenous fungal infections of the retina and choroid can occur in disseminated fungal diseases, posing diagnostic challenges and difficult management problems.[1] Candidiasis is the most common endogenous infection of the eye. Other intraocular fungal infections are less common, but can be equally severe.

CANDIDIASIS

Candida species are usually commensal yeasts of low virulence for healthy persons. They can be found in the normal flora of the respiratory, gastrointestinal, and female genital tracts. With altered host defenses, however, they may cause serious disease of nearly all organ systems. Candidiasis is associated with high rates of morbidity and mortality,[2] and it is currently recommended that all patients with candidemia (both neutropenic and nonneutropenic patients) be treated with antifungal agents.[3]

Candidal chorioretinitis is the most common fungal infection of the retina and choroid, and is one of the most common of all endogenous infections of the eye. *Candida albicans* has been known as a potential cause of chorioretinitis for many decades but was diagnosed rarely, and usually at autopsy, before the 1970s, when it was recognized as an iatrogenic problem and one that is associated with intravenous drug abuse. It is now a well-characterized disorder that should be familiar to all ophthalmologists.

C. *albicans* remains the most common species of *Candida* to be isolated from blood of patients at tertiary care centers (45% of adults, 49% of children), but other species of *Candida* have become increasingly common causes of candidemia.[2] *Candida albicans* is the most common species that causes chorioretinitis,[4] but a variety of other species cause intraocular infections as well, including C. *tropicalis*, C. *parapsilosis*, C. *glabrata* (formerly *Torulopsis glabrata*),[5,6] and C. *guilliermondii*. Of the species other than C. *albicans*, C. *tropicalis* is the most common cause

of intraocular infection.[4,7] In an autopsy study by Griffin and associates,[8] 12 of 15 eyes with candidal chorioretinitis were infected with C. *albicans*, while only two were infected with C. *tropicalis*, and only one with C. *parapsilosis*. In a study of 38 patients with candidemia, 72% of cases were due to C. *albicans*, but of the resulting 11 cases of chorioretinitis, 10 (91%) were due to C. *albicans*;[9] the remaining case was due to C. *tropicalis*. In contrast, McDonnell and associates[10] found in a retrospective autopsy survey that ocular involvement was more common among patients with disseminated C. *tropicalis* infections than among patients with disseminated C. *albicans* infections. Although disseminated C. *tropicalis* infection is seen more commonly in immunocompromised hosts, few cases of endophthalmitis caused by this species have been reported.[9] Animal studies indicate that C. *albicans* may have a greater propensity for the eye than do other species.[11,12]

C. *krusei*, although much less virulent than C. *albicans*, has emerged as an important nosocomial pathogen in immunocompromised patients[13,14] and has been reported to be a cause of intraocular infection. The increased rate of C. *krusei* infections has been attributed to suppression of more virulent *Candida* species by antifungal prophylaxis;[15] it has also been associated with the use of antibacterial prophylaxis.[15] Because there have been so few outbreaks of infection with this organism, it is hard to generalize about risk factors.

Clinical features

The typical focus of candidal chorioretinitis is a white, circumscribed lesion, less than 1 mm in diameter, with an overlying haze of vitreous inflammatory cells (Figs 94-1 to 94-3). Early choroidal and deep retinal lesions may be difficult to appreciate on ophthalmoscopy and may be more easily identified on fluorescein angiography as hypofluorescent areas with late staining.[16] There may be vascular sheathing of retinal vessels in the area surrounding the lesions.

Symptoms may include decreased vision (due to macular lesions or vitreous involvement) or discomfort from associated anterior uveitis. Iridocyclitis is a frequent finding; the severity of the anterior chamber reaction varies, and hypopyon may be present.

By the time symptoms are noticed, at least two-thirds of patients have bilateral disease and more than half have vitreous

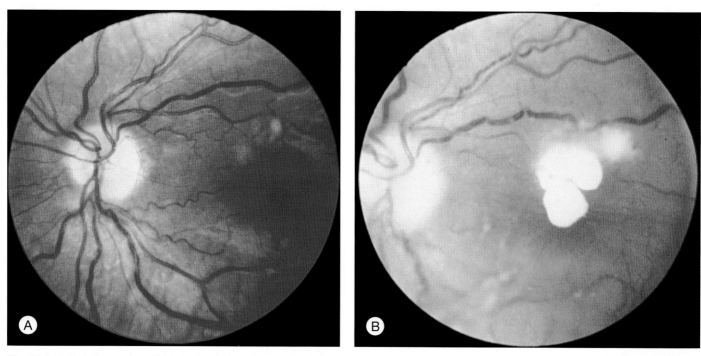

Fig. 94-1 A, Early focus of candidal chorioretinitis in the superior macula of the left eye of a patient with bacterial septicemia after abdominal surgery. B, The same eye 1 month later, showing expansion of the lesion with vitreous invasion. Perivascular inflammatory material is present. The patient had not received antifungal therapy. (Reproduced from Griffin JR, Pettit TH, Fishman LS, Foos RY. Blood-borne *Candida* endophthalmitis. A clinical and pathologic study of 21 cases. Arch Ophthalmol 1973; 89:450–456.)

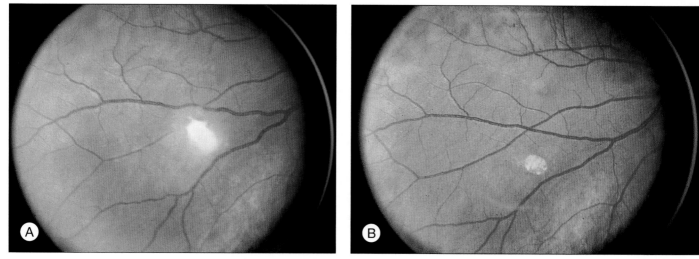

Fig. 94-2 A, A focus of early candidal chorioretinitis. B, The same eye after successful treatment with intravenous amphotericin B. A hypopigmented scar remains. (Courtesy of J. Robert Griffin, MD, and Thomas H. Pettit, MD.)

involvement.[8,17] At least half of patients have multiple lesions when first examined.[8,17] Occasionally lesions are associated with retinal hemorrhage and resemble a classic Roth spot.[17]

The clinical manifestations of intraocular infection with species other than C. *albicans* are similar to those caused by C. *albicans*.[7,13]

Diagnosis can usually be made clinically. If a vitrectomy is performed, specimens should be concentrated by centrifugation or filtration for culture.[18,19] Cultures of vitreous humor

aspirates alone may be negative because organisms become sequestered in inflammatory masses.

Risk factors

Fungi reach the eye hematogenously. A number of predisposing conditions have been associated with candidemia and intraocular fungal infection. Hospitalized patients who get candidal chorioretinitis frequently have a history of recent major surgery, bacterial sepsis, systemic antibiotic use, indwelling intravenous

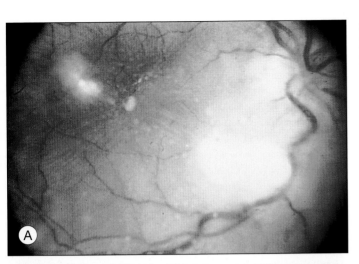

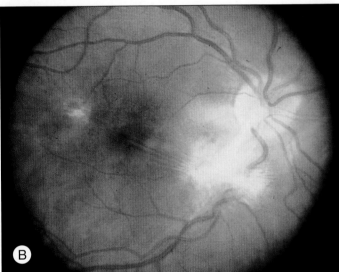

Fig. 94-3 A, Large candidal chorioretinitis lesion with vitreous humor invasion inferotemporal to the optic disc in the right eye. B, The same eye after successful treatment with amphotericin B. The healed lesion has resulted in retinal traction. (Courtesy of J. Robert Griffin, MD, and Thomas H. Pettit, MD.)

catheters, debilitating diseases, or a combination of these factors.[8,10,17,20,21] Surgical procedures are most frequently those involving the gastrointestinal system. In a study of six consecutive hospitalized patients who developed candidal chorioretinitis, Griffin and associates[8] found that all had had surgery and intravenous catheters and that five had had bacterial sepsis. In all patients, *Candida* species were cultured from their intravenous catheter tips on removal. Candidemia developed 6 to 58 days after catheter insertion, and visual symptoms developed 3 to 15 days after positive blood cultures were obtained. The same investigators found that nine of 15 patients with candidal chorioretinitis who were studied at autopsy had gastrointestinal perforations and that 11 of 15 had *Pseudomonas* species or *Escherichia coli* sepsis.[8] In a review of 14 unpublished and 62 previously published cases, Edwards and associates[17] found that frequent predisposing factors for candidal chorioretinitis included systemic antibiotic use (in at least 84% of cases) and

major surgery (in at least 63% of cases, with 60% of the procedures involving the gastrointestinal tract). At least 88% of patients had received some sort of intravenous infusion, and at least 46% had indwelling catheters. A number of coexisting, debilitating diseases were seen relatively frequently in these patients, including diabetes mellitus (13%), malignancies (21%), liver disease (8%), and alcoholism (8%). Among 23 patients receiving intravenous hyperalimentation who were studied by Montgomerie & Edwards,[22] candidal chorioretinitis developed in five patients (22%).

Candidal chorioretinitis is a frequently reported complication of intravenous drug abuse.[18,23-29] Fungal organisms are most likely introduced into the drug from contaminated drug paraphernalia or additives, and injected directly into the blood stream. Vitreous humor opacities frequently are the most prominent finding of candidal endophthalmitis in intravenous drug abusers, possibly because they are less likely to be examined early in the course of the disease.[18,26] Even in the absence of typical chorioretinal lesions, fungal infection should be suspected in any patient with unexplained uveitis and a history of intravenous drug abuse.

Candidal chorioretinitis is the most common intraocular fungal infection of newborns.[30-32] Disseminated candidiasis in infants results in respiratory deterioration, abdominal distention, guaiac-positive stools, carbohydrate intolerance, meningitis, erythematous rash, temperature instability, and hypotension.[30] Baley and associates[33] reported a series of eight infants with disseminated candidiasis seen over a 1-year period. All infants were of low birth weight and had evidence of sepsis. All had indwelling catheters and were receiving antibiotics. These infants made up 4% of all newborns weighing less than 1500 g during that period. Retinal and vitreous humor infections developed in four of the eight infants. In a similar series, the mean onset of signs or symptoms was 33 days after birth.[30] Low birth weight has been associated with candidal chorioretinitis by other investigators as well, although it may also occur in full-term, normal-birth-weight infants who require prolonged hospitalization.[32] Newborn and preterm infants have been shown to have a deficiency in the candidacidal ability of leukocytes, which may enhance the severity of *Candida* spp. endophthalmitis.[34]

Another group in which candidal chorioretinitis has been reported is postpartum women.[21,36] In view of the infrequency with which it is reported, it is probably very uncommon. Candidal endophthalmitis has also been reported after induced abortion.[35]

Several predisposing factors for candidal chorioretinitis are probably interrelated. *Candida* spp. are frequently present in the normal gastrointestinal tract. Surgical manipulation may allow seeding of the blood stream from this site. Patients undergoing gastrointestinal procedures are frequently given antibiotics to prevent infection from contaminated bowel contents, but these antibiotics may allow an overgrowth of fungi in the gastrointestinal tract, thereby increasing the risk of candidemia. Antibiotics have also been shown to enhance in vitro growth of *Candida* spp.[17]

There has been conflicting information regarding factors leading to the development of chorioretinitis in patients with candidemia. In a study of 38 patients with candidemia, Parke and associates[9] found a trend, although not statistically significant, toward increased frequency of eye infections in patients receiving hyperalimentation and hemodialysis. There was no relation between development of candidal chorioretinitis and age, sex, pre-existing diagnoses, use of antibiotics, immunosuppressive drugs, corticosteroids, white blood cell counts, or positive fungal cultures from other sites, when compared to patients who had candidemia but who did not develop eye disease.[9] Brooks[37] also found no predictive factors other than a possible increased risk of ocular infection with multiple positive blood cultures. In contrast, Donahue and associates[5] found that development of intraocular infection in patients with candidemia was associated with multiple positive blood cultures, C. *albicans* as the species, and immunosuppression.

Host defenses against *Candida* spp. infections involve a complex interaction between cellular and humoral immune mechanisms, but the influence of immunosuppression on the development of candidal chorioretinitis remains poorly understood. It is commonly stated that disseminated candidiasis may result from immunodeficiency, and deep organ infections have frequently been reported in patients receiving immunosuppressive drugs for malignancy or after organ transplantation. Neutrophils from such patients have impaired candidacidal activity.[11] Immunodeficiency, however, has not been among the prominent predisposing factors for intraocular candidal infections in many reported cases. Patients with debilitating diseases such as diabetes mellitus, which can be expected to alter host defenses, are at risk for candidal chorioretinitis, but primary and acquired immunodeficiency states are not common among patients with ocular candidal infections. Persons with a specific T-lymphocyte defect against *Candida* spp. may develop a disorder known as chronic mucocutaneous candidiasis. These patients develop severe skin and mucous membrane infections, which can include ulcerative candidal blepharitis and candidal keratoconjunctivitis.[11] This condition does not, however, result in candidemia or systemic candidiasis. Patients with the acquired immunodeficiency syndrome (AIDS) also develop severe mucocutaneous candidiasis, but candidal chorioretinitis is not among the common ophthalmic manifestations of the disorder.[38] Few cases of AIDS-related candidal chorioretinitis or endophthalmitis have been reported; they have occurred in patients with the same risk factors that are associated with intraocular candidal infections in immunocompetent patients, such as intravenous drug use and indwelling catheters.[39,40]

Previous use of immunosuppressive drugs or corticosteroids has also not been a prominent feature of patients who develop candidal chorioretinitis. Among 38 patients with candidemia studied by Parke and associates,[9] none who developed candidal endophthalmitis had received immunosuppressive drugs and only one had received systemic corticosteroids. In contrast, of those who did not develop eye disease, 29% had received systemic corticosteroids and 18% had received immunosuppressive drugs.[9] Only one of six patients with candidal chorioretinitis observed by Griffin and associates[8] had received systemic corticosteroids. In the review by Edwards and associates[17] of 76 cases of candidal chorioretinitis, only six patients (8%) were known to have received immunosuppressive drugs; only 41 (54%) were known to have received corticosteroids, and in many cases their use followed the development of infection. In vitro studies show that hydrocortisone does not alter neutrophilic fungicidal activity.[11]

Immunosuppression itself is probably not sufficient for the development of intraocular infection because it does not increase the risk of fungi entering the blood stream; however, in situations that result in a breakdown of mucocutaneous barriers with subsequent candidemia, immunosuppression appears to increase the risk and severity of ocular infection.

Prevalence

During a 5-year study at the University of California, Los Angeles that was reported in the early 1970s, 82 patients had blood cultures positive for *Candida* spp. Of patients with candidemia, 30% had clinical or autopsy evidence of ocular candidal infection.[41] In a similar study conducted in the late 1970s and early 1980s, Parke and associates[9] found that 11 of 38 patients (29%) with candidemia developed candidal chorioretinitis. All patients with more than three consecutive positive blood cultures developed ocular disease. In the mid-1980s, Brooks[37] found that 28% of patients with candidemia developed retinal lesions suggestive of ocular infection.

Using strict criteria for diagnosis in a prospective study of 118 patients with candidemia, Donahue and associates,[5] in the early 1990s, found that only 9% had chorioretinitis when examined within 72 h of a positive blood culture, and no patient had endophthalmitis. Nonspecific findings (cottonwool spots, retinal hemorrhages, and Roth spots) were present in 20% of patients. The authors could not rule out the possibility that these lesions were early manifestations of candidal retinitis, but none was associated with inflammatory changes that one would expect with infection. This observation raises the possibility that many of the presumed candidal lesions described in previous series were actually noninfectious lesions attributable to other conditions, such as anemia, hypertension, or coagulopathies, that might occur in debilitated patients. The lower rate of ocular infection in this series may also be attributed to the fact that patients were apparently receiving antifungal therapy.

In recent years, the prevalence of fungal endophthalmitis is believed to have been diminished by the practice of administering antifungal therapy to all patients on the basis of positive blood cultures alone.[42,43] By the late 1990s, the prevalence of candidal chorioretinitis and endophthalmitis was reported to be in the range of 2% to 3% by several groups of investigators.[43–46] In a study of 107 patients with fungemia,[43] 100 of whom were already receiving antifungal agents, only three (2.8%) had evidence of fungal chorioretinitis. All patients had risk factors for candidemia other than intravenous drug use; the types of factor were similar to those seen in previously reported series that had higher rates of ocular involvement. All three patients with ocular involvement had C. *albicans* infections, although at least five species of *Candida* were found in the total population.

The relationship between candidemia and retinal infections has been reviewed in detail by Rodriguez-Adrian and associates.[45] Because of the current, low prevalence of endogenous candidal infections of the eye among individuals with positive blood cultures, some clinicians have questioned the need to examine the fundi of all such individuals. It is critical, however, that infections be identified at an early stage, because of the serious consequences of candidal endophthalmitis. It is still, therefore, recommended that all patients with candidemia have ophthalmoscopic examinations. Also, examinations should be repeated 1 week later, even if patients have no ocular lesions initially, as there may be a delay between positive blood cultures and the development of lesions. Furthermore, nonspecific retinal lesions may evolve into typical foci of infection on follow-up examinations.[45]

Histopathology

On histologic examination, *Candida* spp. organisms can be recognized as budding yeasts having a characteristic "pseudohyphate" appearance (Figs 94-4 to 94-6). Most lesions contain relatively few organisms, surrounded by an intense inflammatory reaction consisting of a combination of suppurative and granulomatous inflammation. Lesions therefore may be atypical in patients with neutropenia.[47] Autopsy studies have shown that most early lesions are found in the inner choroid. Organisms may then break through Bruch membrane, form subretinal abscesses, and eventually spread to involve the retina[8,17] (Fig. 94-5). Lesions are contained entirely within the retina in only 16% of cases. The inner limiting lamina provides no barrier to expansion of infection; organisms migrate inward from the retina early during the course of infection to form vitreous abscesses (Fig. 94-6).

At autopsy 80% of cases have multiple lesions;[8,17] 64% of cases in one series had more than five lesions.[17] In all cases, grossly visible lesions were present posterior to the equator, and the majority of patients had macular lesions. Vitreous humor infection may occasionally extend anteriorly to involve the ciliary body.[17] Despite the intense anterior chamber reaction that can be seen in patients with candidal chorioretinitis, infection of the iris and ciliary body is rare.

Relationship between ocular and nonocular infections

It is frequently difficult for clinicians to distinguish candidemia from candidiasis (parenchymal infection of one or more internal organs). Serologic tests for anti-*Candida* spp. antibodies have proved unreliable for making this distinction. An ophthalmoscopic examination, on the other hand, can easily identify the presence of a tissue-invasive infection of the eye.

The exact relationship between candidal chorioretinitis and systemic candidiasis is not known, but several studies suggest that ocular lesions are common in patients with systemic infections and, conversely, that ocular lesions are strongly predictive of nonocular disease. Among patients with disseminated candidal infections, 82% may have a chorioretinal infection among the sites of disease.[9,41] Conversely, clinical and autopsy studies have

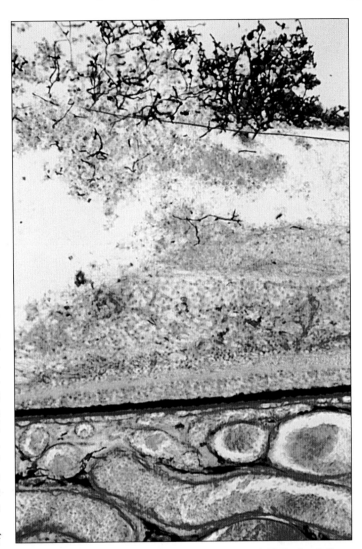

Fig. 94-4 Histologic section showing a focus of candidal chorioretinitis. Pseudohyphae are seen in the choroid, retina, and vitreous (hematoxylin & eosin). (Courtesy of Robert Y. Foos, MD, and Thomas H. Pettit, MD.)

shown that 78% to 88% of patients with candidal chorioretinitis have tissue-invasive infection of other organs as well.[8,9,17,41] The kidneys and the heart are the most common sites of nonocular tissue-invasive infections. Other organs and tissues infected by *Candida* spp. include brain and meninges, lungs, trachea, skeletal muscles, the gastrointestinal tract, liver, adrenals, thyroid, pancreas, breast, lymph nodes, and vascular walls.[17] Among patients with candidiasis, those with ocular lesions are likely to have infection in a greater number of organ systems than those without eye lesions.[10] Patients may not have developed signs of nonocular disease when visual symptoms occur.

Most studies of the relationship between ocular and nonocular disease have been performed in hospitalized patients with a variety of iatrogenic risk factors for candidiasis. The association between candidal chorioretinitis and tissue-invasive infections of other organs in intravenous drug abusers is less well understood. In one study, 15 (39%) of 38 drug abusers with systemic *C. albicans* infections had ocular disease.[23,24] Joints and skin may be sites of nonocular candidal infection in these patients;[24]

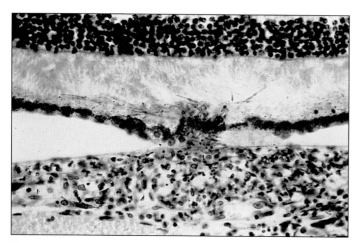

Fig. 94-5 Focal candidal chorioiditis with extension of pseudohyphae through the Bruch membrane and retinal pigment epithelium into the subretinal space. Inflammation is primarily granulomatous with scattered acute inflammatory cells (hematoxylin & eosin). (Reproduced from Griffin JR, Pettit TH, Fishman LS, Foos RY. Blood-borne *Candida* endophthalmitis. A clinical and pathologic study of 21 cases. Arch Ophthalmol 1973; 89:450–456.)

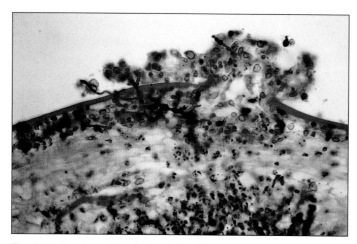

Fig. 94-6 Focal candidal chorioretinitis with extension of pseudohyphae through the internal limiting lamina into the vitreous humor (periodic acid–Schiff). (Courtesy of Robert Y. Foos, MD, and Thomas H. Pettit, MD.)

frequently, however, there are no clinical signs of nonocular disease.

ASPERGILLOSIS

Aspergillus spp. is a ubiquitous mold frequently found in decaying vegetable matter. It can also be a commensal organism, found in body secretions and within body orifices of healthy persons. It can colonize and invade traumatized tissue, and opportunistic, disseminated, tissue-invasive infection can occur in persons with compromised host defenses.

People at greatest risk of ocular infection are intravenous drug abusers and those with a variety of debilitating diseases, including organ transplant recipients, persons with endocarditis, and cancer patients.[19,48–53] Individuals with chronic pulmonary disease (espe-

cially if they are being treated with corticosteroids) constitute a large proportion of patients.[54] *Aspergillus* spp. is the second most common fungus to infect the retina and choroid after *C. albicans*.[55,56] It is reported to occur in 0.5% of bone marrow transplant recipients examined clinically (two of 397 patients; two of six cases of intraocular fungal infection)[57] and 7% of liver transplant patients at autopsy.[58] Rare cases involving immunocompetent patients without known history of intravenous drug use or other predisposing factors have also been reported.[59,60] *A. fumigatus* and *A. flavus* are the most commonly isolated species from patients with intraocular infection.[52–54]

Any organ can be involved in disseminated infection, but the lung is the most common site of tissue-invasive disease. In an autopsy series of patients who had undergone liver transplantation, the eye was the second most common site of infection in patients with invasive aspergillosis.[58] In many cases, ocular infection was not diagnosed until autopsy.

Studies in rabbits indicate that *C. albicans* has greater pathogenicity for the eye than do *A. fumigatus* and *Cryptococcus neoformans*, which may explain the lower prevalence of human intraocular infection with the latter pathogens.[12] In contrast, on the basis of human series, it has been argued that the risk of intraocular *Aspergillus* spp. infection with disseminated aspergillosis is greater than the risk of intraocular *Candida* spp. infection with disseminated candidiasis.[58]

Intraocular infection may be the presenting manifestation of disseminated aspergillosis,[53] and, in fact, intravenous drug users may develop no other signs of disseminated disease.[19,53] Despite disseminated infection, patients frequently have negative serologic tests and blood cultures for *Aspergillus* spp.[54,58]

Endogenous infection of the eye may be unilateral or bilateral. On fundus examination, yellow subretinal and retinal infiltrates can be seen, although in early infection the infiltration may be minimal.[51] *Aspergillus* spp. endophthalmitis is frequently characterized by rapid, severe vision loss, intensive inflammation, and retinal hemorrhage.[54,56,60] Infection usually occurs in the posterior pole,[54,56,58] and macular lesions are common.[54,56] In one autopsy series, the retina and vitreous body were involved more often than the choroid.[58]

With severe disease, septate, dichotomously branching hyphae can be found throughout the eye, including tissues of the anterior segment. Invasion of vessels with production of thrombosis and tissue infarction is a characteristic feature of *Aspergillus* spp. infections.[10] Occlusion of choroidal vessels can lead to exudative retinal detachment, while occlusion of retinal vessels may result in retinal necrosis.[49] Retinal necrosis may also be a direct result of fungal invasion of retinal tissue.

In a review of published cases of *Aspergillus* spp. endophthalmitis, Hunt & Glasgow[58] identified features that help to distinguish them from cases of candidal choriretinitis and endophthalmitis. As with *Candida* spp. infections, the posterior pole is usually involved, but lesions caused by *Aspergillus* spp. are usually larger and more likely to be hemorrhagic; there may also be broad areas of ischemic infarction, which is not seen with candidal infections. In another comparative study, Rao & Hidayat[61] showed that *Aspergillus* spp. appear to grow preferentially along the subretinal space and commonly invade retinal and choroidal vessels, while neither finding is characteristic of *Candida* spp. infections, which accounts for the differences in the clinical features of these two disorders.

PSEUDALLESCHERIASIS

Pseudallescheria boydii (formerly *Petriellidium boydii*) is a ubiquitous organism. The anamorph of the same fungus (i.e., the form that reproduces by asexual spores only) is known as *Scedosporium* (*Monosporium*) *apiospermum*. The most common form of disease is maduromycosis, a localized infection that follows traumatic implantation into soft tissues. Disseminated disease can occur in immunosuppressed or otherwise debilitated patients.[1,50,62,63]

Although endogenous *P. boydii* endophthalmitis has been reported rarely,[50,62,63] it should be included in the differential diagnosis of endogenous *Aspergillus* spp. infection. *P. boydii* infection occurs in similar clinical settings, and organisms are indistinguishable histopathologically from *Aspergillus* spp.

All reported cases of endogenous *P. boydii* infection of the eye have been characterized by severe endophthalmitis. Retinal infection can result in extensive, confluent exudative lesions at the retinovitreous interface.[63] In most cases, eyes have been enucleated or patients have died.

SCEDOSPORIOSIS

Disease caused by *Scedosporium prolificans* (*inflatum*) is nearly identical to that caused by *P. boydii*, although the fungus, which is found in soil, may have a somewhat more limited distribution in nature.[64] *S. prolificans* can colonize various body sites, including the ear canal and respiratory tract, in healthy individuals, and can cause localized musculoskeletal infections after trauma.[64-66] Disseminated disease occurs most often in immunocompromised individuals, particularly those with neutropenia.[64-67] Several cases of ocular involvement have been reported.[64,66-68] In some, infection was confirmed at autopsy, but few reports provide details about ophthalmic findings. Large (4 to 6 disc diameters) chorioretinal inflammatory lesions can develop.[66,68] Multiple smaller retinal lesions have also been reported,[64,67] although infection was not confirmed in these cases; the patients had leukemia, and thus, the findings might have been cottonwool spots or other noninfectious lesions.

S. prolificans appears to be resistant to nearly all antifungal agents (see Treatment section), and prognosis for survival with disseminated infections is poor.

CRYPTOCOCCOSIS

Cryptococcus neoformans is a yeast that is worldwide in distribution. It is frequently found in high concentrations in pigeon feces. Application of India ink to the organism reveals its characteristic broad capsule, which does not stain. Infection is acquired through the respiratory tract. It is also an opportunistic infection that can cause severe disseminated disease in immunosuppressed or debilitated patients. The fungus has a predilection for the central nervous system and is the most common cause of fungal meningitis; severe headache may be the first manifestation of an occult cryptococcal meningitis.

Meningitis and ocular cryptococcosis may occur in previously healthy persons,[69-71] but is more frequently seen in patients who are immunocompromised.[72,73] Development of ocular infection can occur many months after the onset of meningitis.[69-71] Conversely, there have been several reports of patients with solitary retinovitreous lesions containing *C. neoformans* that developed without or before the onset of clinically apparent meningitis.[74-76]

C. neoformans can produce a variety of intraocular lesions. It infects all tissues of the eye, including iris, ciliary body, vitreous body, retina, and choroid.[70] Retinal infection can result in necrosis over a series of weeks.[76] In most cases the fungus probably reaches the eye hematogenously, and intravascular organisms can be found within ocular tissues.[38,72,77] The frequent association of ocular cryptococcosis with meningitis, and the finding of yeast cells in the subarachnoid space around the optic nerve,[71] have led to the conclusion that ocular infection may be the result of direct extension from intracranial sites of disease as well.[70,73]

The most frequent presentation of ocular cryptococcosis is a multifocal chorioretinitis.[69-71] One or more discrete, yellow-white fundus lesions of various sizes, some as large as several disc diameters, may be present. Associated findings may include mutton-fat keratic precipitates, vascular sheathing, exudative retinal detachment, and variable amounts of vitreous inflammatory material.[69,76] Choroidal infection may occur without retinal involvement.[72] Shields and associates[71] hypothesized that infection usually begins in the choroid, with subsequent extension to other tissues. Infection of the retina without choroidal involvement, however, has also been reported, as noted above.[73,75] Inflammatory reactions associated with cryptococcal infection can vary from little to marked granulomatous and acute inflammation.[70,71,77]

Cryptococcosis is the most common fungal infection of the eye in patients with AIDS, although it remains an uncommon disease.[40,78-80] In an autopsy series of 235 patients with AIDS,[77] seven (3%) had cryptococcal infections of the choroid, accounting for 39% of all choroid infections. In five of these seven cases, cryptococcosis was the cause of death. In a series of 80 African patients with AIDS and *C. neoformans* infections,[80a] only one was confirmed as having an intraocular cryptococcal infection. Several cases have been diagnosed on the basis of lesion response to antifungal therapy in patients who have systemic cryptococcosis, although histopathologic confirmation of ocular infection was not obtained.[78-80] Some lesions have been described as multifocal and choroidal in location;[78,80] others appear to be primarily retinal, associated with hemorrhage.[79] Cryptococcal infection of the retina and choroid has also been found as an incidental finding at autopsy.[38] Early infections are characterized by invasion of vessels by the organism; lack of associated tissue inflammation is a typical finding. Early cryptococcal choroiditis can present with symptoms of intermittent blurring.[77] Intraocular infection can progress to severe endophthalmitis and can occur without meningeal infection or clinically apparent systemic cryptococcosis.[76]

HISTOPLASMOSIS

Histoplasma capsulatum is a dimorphic mold found predominantly in soil of the central and eastern USA. Infection is acquired through the respiratory tract and usually results in an asymptomatic, self-limited infection. A heavy inoculation can result in cavitary lung lesions that may be mistaken for tuberculosis. In those unusual patients who develop disseminated infection, the fungus has a predilection for the reticuloendothelial system, producing lymphadenopathy and hepatosplenomegaly. In tissue, the yeast form of the organism is frequently found intracellularly.

Ocular infection may result in multifocal choroidal lesions with little vitreous humor or anterior segment inflammation.[81] Individuals with such lesions may be asymptomatic. The lesions resolve completely or result in atrophic scars. Such lesions rarely come to the attention of ophthalmologists, but may be the basis for the presumed ocular histoplasmosis syndrome (POHS), which has been linked to *H. capsulatum* epidemiologically; POHS and its complications are discussed in Chapter 98.

There have been occasional reports of severe, active *H. capsulatum* infection of the eye with findings unrelated to POHS.[82-88] Such infections are associated with disseminated infection involving extraocular sites; immunosuppression, through drug therapy or disease, has been a prominent feature in these cases.[83,85-88] Many reported patients have succumbed to their disseminated disease.[85,87] There can be various forms of intraocular disease. Goldstein & Buettner[83] described a patient with a long history of relapsing histoplasmosis who eventually developed focal peripheral retinitis, destructive granulomatous iridocyclitis, and a dense vitreous inflammatory reaction. Examination of the enucleated eye revealed yeast-laden macrophages and extracellular fungi in the iris, ciliary body, and retina; the choroid was not involved.

Klintworth and associates[85] reported macular drusen-like changes that were found on autopsy examination to be associated with choroidal granulomata; organisms were found in the choroid and outer sensory retina. In contrast, autopsy examination of several patients who died of disseminated histoplasmosis revealed *H. capsulatum* in the choroid but no substantial inflammation or granuloma formation.[86,87] Specht and associates[88] reported multiple "creamy white retinal and subretinal infiltrates" up to one-fourth disc diameter in size, with distinct borders, in a patient with AIDS and histoplasmosis. Gonzales and associates[84] described a patient with AIDS whose infection progressed to endophthalmitis with tractional retinal detachments.

Organisms are frequently found in association with the vasculature. Scholz and associates[87] found yeast in cytoplasm of hyperplastic endothelial cells of choroidal arteries, veins, and choriocapillaries. Perivascular and intravascular aggregates of yeast can be found in the retinas of patients with AIDS and histoplasmosis.[86,88]

COCCIDIOIDOMYCOSIS

Coccidioides immitis is a dimorphic fungus found in soil of semiarid regions of the western hemisphere. Coccidioidomycosis is endemic to the San Joaquin valley of central California, in parts of Arizona, New Mexico, and west Texas, and in parts of Central and South America. Infection follows inhalation of the highly infectious, dustborne arthrospores. Infection is most common in winter months, and has been increasing in some areas, possibly because of factors that promote dust formation, including changes of climate and new construction.[89]

Infection is usually asymptomatic or results in a self-limited influenza-like respiratory illness characterized by fever, malaise, and cough. Between 5% and 10% of patients subsequently develop hypersensitivity reactions, including erythema nodosum, erythema multiforme, arthralgias, phlyctenular conjunctivitis and, possibly, episcleritis and scleritis.[90] Less than 1% of patients develop disseminated disease, which can include infection of the skin, liver, brain and meninges, heart, gastrointestinal tract, adrenals, kidney, and bladder. Blacks, Filipinos, pregnant women in their third trimesters, and immunocompromised individuals have an increased risk of disseminated disease.[91] Most patients are apparently healthy before development of disseminated coccidioidomycosis.

Ocular involvement in disseminated disease has been reported infrequently. The true prevalence is unknown, but a prospective study of patients referred for antimicrobial therapy for disseminated disease suggests that intraocular infection may be more common than heretofore realized.[92] Of 10 patients observed over a 12-month period, four developed evidence of choroidal infection. Uveal tissue is the usual site of intraocular disease; fungi may infect the iris, ciliary body, or choroid. Iridocyclitis is characterized by severe granulomatous inflammation with iris nodules and mutton-fat keratic precipitates. It can occur without posterior segment involvement,[90] but in some cases it can progress to endophthalmitis and loss of the eye.

The typical posterior infection is a multifocal choroiditis with numerous scattered, discrete, yellow-white lesions less than one disc diameter in size[93,94] (Fig. 94-7). Larger coccidioidal fundus lesions have been reported, but have not been confirmed histologically. Vascular sheathing, retinal hemorrhage, serous retinal detachment, and vitreous haze may occur in the acute phase of infection. Histopathologic examination of choroidal lesions reveals lymphocytes, plasma cells, macrophages, and multinucleated giant cells. These granulomata may contain numerous organisms, where *C. immitis* develops into a thick-walled spherule with endosporulation. Lesions usually occur posteriorly in the middle vascular layers of the choroid.[93] Bruch's membrane may be damaged focally.[94]

Patients with disseminated coccidioidomycosis and fundus lesions are sometimes reported to have "chorioretinitis," although there has been little evidence to suggest that the retina is frequently involved in the infectious process. Histopathologic examination has revealed mild degenerative changes and scant inflammation of the retina, but no organisms.[90,94] In contrast, Glasgow and associates[93] have reported a 12-year-old girl with disseminated coccidioidomycosis who was found at autopsy to

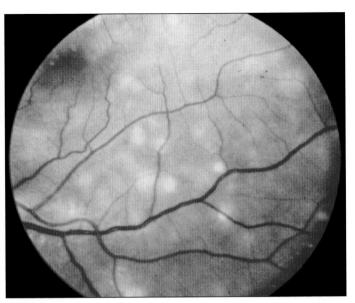

Fig. 94-7 Multifocal choroidal lesions of intraocular coccidioidomycosis. (Reproduced from Zakka KA, Foos RY, Brown WJ. Intraocular coccidioidomycosis. Surv Ophthalmol 1978; 22:313–321.[94])

have small white fluffy retinal lesions; microscopic examination revealed both choroidal and retinal granulomata containing coccidioidal spherules. The retinal and choroidal lesions were not contiguous, indicating independent sites of dissemination. Retinal granulomata were found in the inner, vascularized layers of the retina, primarily the inner nuclear and inner plexiform layers. The relation between granulomata and the choroidal and retinal vasculature indicates that fungi reached the eye hematogenously. Punched-out chorioretinal scars seen in patients with disseminated coccidioidomycosis may be sites of old healed intraocular infection.[92] The optic nerve is another reported site of infection.[94]

Ocular disease has been reported most frequently in patients with severe, life-threatening disseminated coccidioidomycosis. Ocular infection has also been confirmed in patients with no clinical evidence of nonocular disease, however.

SPOROTRICHOSIS

Sporothrix schenckii is a saprophytic, dimorphic fungus that is widespread in nature. It can result in cutaneous lesions after introduction by trauma and can occasionally result in disseminated disease. The yeast forms are found in infected tissue. Infection is most common in persons with environmental exposures, such as laborers who have contact with soil and vegetable matter; human-to-human or animal-to-human transmission does not occur.

Sporotrichosis, which occurs worldwide, is characterized by chronic granulomatous, subcutaneous lesions with abscess, ulcer, and pustule formation, and by spread along lymphatics. Such lesions may develop on the eyelids and adnexae. Disseminated infections occur less frequently, and intraocular infections, which frequently result in phthisis bulbi, are rare. Cassady & Foerster[95] reported a 50-year-old man with a chronic unilateral nongranu-

lomatous uveitis who eventually developed fulminant endophthalmitis. Examination of his enucleated eye revealed *S. schenckii* infection and massive inflammation of the choroid and retina; necrotic retinal tissue contained organisms. Font & Jakobiec[96] reported a 42-year-old man with progressive, necrotizing retinitis in one eye. Examination of the enucleated eye revealed *S. schenckii* in necrotic retina and subretinal exudative material. Granulomatous inflammation, but no organisms, was found in choroidal tissue. Neither of these patients had evidence of disseminated infection elsewhere in the body. Both had a history of alcohol abuse, and one was also diabetic, which suggests that debilitation of the host may increase the risk of this rare ocular infection. More recently, Curi and associates[97] described the successful treatment of an 18-year-old immunocompetent man with disseminated sporotrichosis who had cutaneous lesions, vitreous opacities, and a large retina granuloma in one eye. He retained good vision. Kurosawa and associates[98] reported *S. schenckii* endophthalmitis in a patient with AIDS. There were severe anterior segment inflammation and inflammatory deposits on the retinal surface, although there was no retinal necrosis.

BLASTOMYCOSIS

Blastomyces dermatitidis is also a saprophytic, dimorphic fungus with epidemiologic features similar to those described above for *S. schenckii*. Infection is most commonly reported in the southeastern USA, but also occurs elsewhere in North America, as well as in Central America and Africa. Blastomycosis is also a chronic granulomatous disease that can manifest as cutaneous lesions after trauma or as disseminated disease. Pulmonary lesions, mimicking tuberculosis or neoplasia, can occur, and may be a source of disseminated disease. Metastatic subcutaneous abscesses, bone and joint infection, and genitourinary lesions are frequent sites of dissemination. Palpebral lesions occur in blastomycosis, but intraocular infection is rare. Reported cases typically occur in patients with systemic disease. Ocular findings can include severe anterior segment inflammation, one or more choroidal lesions, and perivascular infiltrates.[99–101] Lesions occur primarily in the posterior segment but can progress to endophthalmitis and panophthalmitis.[102]

Font and associates[103] reported a 73-year-old man who had unilateral panophthalmitis. Examination of the enucleated eye revealed necrotic retina with acute inflammation; many organisms were present in retinal tissue, especially in areas adjacent to retinal vessels. Inflammation surrounded the choriocapillaris, and isolated organisms were present in choroidal giant cells. There were no systemic manifestations of the disease. Safneck and associates[104] reported a similar case in which there was no evidence of active, nonocular infection.

Lewis and associates[100] reported the successful resolution of a single choroidal lesion, with retention of excellent vision, after treatment with systemic amphotericin B. Gottlieb and associates[105] described two additional cases and reviewed previous cases in the literature. Both of their patients had systemic illnesses consistent with blastomycosis, including skin lesions. Ocular infection was characterized by choroidal lesions of various sizes (one case unilateral, one case bilateral), with involvement of the overlying retina in one case. In both cases, infection resolved with treatment.

PNEUMOCYSTOSIS

Pneumocystis carinii has been reported to cause endogenous infections of the choroid in severely immunocompromised individuals with AIDS. Although it has been reclassified as a fungus, *P. carinii* had traditionally been considered a protozoan, and has been treated with antibacterial and antiparasitic drugs. It is described in Chapter 91.

TREATMENT

As discussed above, the risk of endogenous candidal infections of the eye has been reduced by the treatment of patients with candidemia using antifungal agents. In one randomized study, there was no apparent difference in the frequency of ocular involvement between patients without neutropenia who received amphotericin B and those who received fluconazole.[106]

Antifungal therapy should be administered to all individuals with endogenous fungal infections of the eye. Only rarely, when there are no other predisposing factors, will removal of the source of fungemia, such as an infected catheter tip in a patient with candidiasis, lead to resolution of early chorioretinitis lesions without antifungal therapy.[107] In most cases, failure to treat results in severe endophthalmitis and blindness. As would be expected, earlier treatment of candidal endophthalmitis has been shown to be associated with better visual outcomes.[108]

Corticosteroid therapy may cause transient improvement in intraocular fungal infections because of its effect on inflammation. Ultimately, however, it is deleterious and therefore should be avoided.

There are several commercially available antifungal drugs. Knowledge of the infecting species of fungus is predictive of drug susceptibility and is used as a guide to therapy. Choice of drugs is not routinely based on laboratory susceptibility testing of fungal isolates.[109] When available, however, it may be helpful in dealing with infections due to species of *Candida* other than *albicans*.

Amphotericin B

Amphotericin B remains the drug of choice for most severe endogenous fungal infections, despite its considerable systemic toxicity. The drug is a polyene antibiotic that alters the permeability of fungal cell membranes by binding irreversibly to ergosterol, the main sterol in fungal cell membranes.[110] It is either fungistatic or fungicidal, depending on its concentration and the sensitivity of the organism. Experimental evidence has also shown that amphotericin B has an immunopotentiating action that may increase its antifungal effect.[111,112] The discussions that follow refer to the original deoxycholate (DOC) formulation, unless otherwise stated.

Before treatment with amphotericin B is begun, patients are given a test dose, usually 1 mg of drug in 20 ml of 5% dextrose in water, infused intravenously over 20 to 30 min, to determine tolerance to the drug. The test dose may be associated with fever, chills, hypotension, and dyspnea. In the absence of severe side-effects, amphotericin B therapy is begun with the administration of 0.7 mg/kg of drug in 500 ml of 5% dextrose in water infused intravenously over 2 to 6 h. If this dose is tolerated, the daily dosage is increased to 1.0 mg/kg of drug.[1,109,110] Total daily dosage rarely exceeds 40 to 50 mg of drug. Drug tolerance may be increased by the concurrent administration of 25 to 50 mg of hydrocortisone sodium succinate. The patient also may be given aspirin, diphenhydramine, and meperidine hydrochloride for chills and fever and prochlorperazine for nausea.[111] The use of amphotericin B may be limited by a variety of side-effects, including anaphylaxis, thrombocytopenia, flushing, generalized pain, convulsions, chills, fever, phlebitis, headaches, anemia, and anorexia. The most serious side-effect of treatment, however, is decreased renal function; 80% of patients develop azotemia.[110] The drug is not excreted by the kidney, however, and dosages need not be reduced in patients with pre-existing renal disease.[110,112]

Amphotericin B has been shown to be effective therapy in cases of intraocular *Candida* spp.,[8] *Aspergillus* spp.,[53] *Coccidioides* spp.,[92] and *Blastomyces* spp.[100] infections of the eye. It may cause clearing of vitreous haze and signs of resolution of candidal chorioretinitis lesions as early as day 7 of therapy.[8]

The length of treatment and the total dosage are based on the extent of disease and its response to therapy. An autopsy study showed that five of six patients receiving less than 200 mg of amphotericin B still had active candidal lesions of the choroid and retina at death, while only one of seven patients who received more than 1000 mg had active infection.[17] On the basis of clinical experience, Griffin and associates[8] reported that a total amphotericin B dose of 1000 mg was effective for treatment of candidal chorioretinitis in most cases in which there had been no invasion of the vitreous humor by organisms. Even higher doses have been associated with treatment failures, however. Patients therefore must be observed closely after termination of therapy.

Intravenously administered amphotericin B penetrates poorly into the vitreous humor, although in animal models there is evidence of increased penetration into eyes with intraocular inflammation.[113] Although successful treatment of infections that extend into the vitreous body using intravenous amphotericin B alone has been reported,[114] there is a substantial risk of treatment failure with this approach. Subconjunctivally administered amphotericin B also penetrates the eye poorly and is toxic to the tissues of the ocular surface.[113]

Because of the poor intraocular penetration of intravenous amphotericin B, intravitreal injection of the drug is used for treatment of some patients. A single intravitreal injection of 5 μg of amphotericin B may cure candidal chorioretinitis, in some cases with no apparent toxicity.[29] The drug should be given slowly in the central vitreous space, as a bolus of even very small doses near the retina may result in retinal necrosis.[115] On the basis of animal experimentation, Axelrod and associates[115] concluded that a 10 μg intravitreal injection of amphotericin B can be given safely and achieves levels effective against most ocular fungal pathogens. Stern and associates,[29] however, have expressed doubt that the levels achieved are effective against many fungi other than *C. albicans*. The frequency with which intravitreous injections can be given safely has not been determined. Animal studies indicate that drug clearance is more rapid after vitrectomy.[116]

Brod and associates[108] described the successful treatment of candidal chorioretinitis in eight patients using intravitreous amphotericin B, but no intravenous amphotericin B. Some investigators question the wisdom of treating intraocular infections with local therapy only. Although none of the patients reported by Brod and associates[108] had positive blood cultures or evidence of systemic candidiasis, only 50% to 60% of patients with candidiasis will have candidemia, and nonocular sites of infection may be clinically inapparent when ocular disease is diagnosed. Because candidal chorioretinitis is frequently associated with tissue-invasive infection of other organs, intravitreous therapy should still be considered an adjunct to, rather than a substitute for, intravenous therapy in most cases. Five of the cases reported by Brod and associates[108] did receive oral antifungal agents (ketoconazole or flucytosine) as well.

Severe nephrotoxicity with oliguria and anuria is common in neonates receiving amphotericin B; although doses up to 1 mg/kg per day have been used, it has been recommended that daily dosage in neonates not exceed 0.5 mg/kg to reduce renal toxicity.[117]

Rifampin, which has no antifungal activity itself, lowers the concentration of amphotericin B required to inhibit *Aspergillus* spp., *Histoplasma* spp., and *Candida* spp. in vitro. In one reported case, the addition of rifampin to intravenous amphotericin B therapy resulted in rapid resolution of candidal endophthalmitis.[118]

To address issues of toxicity, lipid-associated formulations of amphotericin B (amphotericin B lipid complex; liposomal amphotericin B) have been developed,[3] but experience with their use for intraocular infections is limited. In a rabbit model, liposomal amphotericin B achieved higher intraocular concentrations than either amphotericin B lipid complex or free amphotericin B after repeated intravitreous injections into eyes with experimentally induced uveitis.[119] Following intravitreous injection into rabbit eyes with experimental *C. albicans* endophthalmitis in another study, liposomal amphotericin B was less toxic, but was also less effective at controlling infection, than the same amount of free amphotericin B.[120] Case reports have described both successful[121] and unsuccessful[122] treatment of human candidal endophthalmitis with intravenous amphotericin B lipid complex.

Flucytosine

The systemic toxicity of amphotericin B has led to a search for other effective antifungal drugs for the treatment of intraocular infections. Flucytosine (5-fluorocytosine) is a fluorinated pyrimidine that has been used for the treatment of disseminated fungal infections.[110] It is converted in fungal cells by the enzyme cytosine deaminase to fluorouracil, which inhibits thymidylate synthetase and thereby interferes with nucleic acid synthesis.

Conversion to fluorouracil does not take place in other cells of the body, which accounts for its selective effect and relatively low toxicity. Potential side-effects include anemia, thrombocytopenia, leukopenia, nausea, vomiting, diarrhea, and (rarely) intestinal perforations. Reversible elevation of hepatic enzymes occurs infrequently. The drug is well absorbed orally and is usually given in a dosage of 100 to 150 mg/kg per day, divided into four doses given every 6 h.

Cases of candidal chorioretinitis have been cured by the use of flucytosine alone.[16] As many as 50% of candidal organisms may be resistant to flucytosine, however, and resistance to the drug can develop during therapy.[11] In a rabbit model of candidal endophthalmitis, flucytosine was significantly less effective than amphotericin B or fluconazole.[123] The majority of *Sporothix* spp. and *Aspergillus* spp., and all *Blastomyces dermatitidis*, *Histoplasma capsulatum*, and *Coccidioides immitis* organisms, are resistant as well.

It is recommended that flucytosine be used only in combination with other antifungal drugs for the treatment of fungal infections.[110] The combination of flucytosine with amphotericin B appears to be synergistic against candidal and cryptococcal infections,[124] possibly owing to the increased penetration of flucytosine through cell membranes damaged by amphotericin B. There also appears to be synergism in cases in which organisms are resistant to flucytosine alone.[11] This combination of drugs has been used successfully to treat candidal chorioretinitis and cryptococcal chorioretinitis in adults,[25,71] as well as neonatal candidal chorioretinitis.[33,125] Synergism between flucytosine and amphotericin B does not appear to occur in the treatment of histoplasmosis, blastomycosis, or coccidioidomycosis.[112]

Azole compounds

Since the mid-1990s, attention has been focused on the use of azole compounds as alternatives to amphotericin B for treatment of disseminated fungal infections. The pharmacology and use of azoles have been reviewed by Como & Dismukes.[126] The group includes the imidazoles (miconazole, ketoconazole) and the triazoles (fluconazole, itraconazole, voriconazole). The azoles inhibit ergosterol synthesis, thereby reducing the activity of membrane-associated enzymes, increasing cell membrane permeability, and inhibiting cell growth.[126] These agents are active against *Candida albicans*, *Cryptococcus neoformans*, *Coccidioides immitis*, *H. capsulatum*, *B. dermatitidis* (except miconazole), and *Sporothrix schenckii*. The azoles (with the exception of voriconazole) are not active against many species of *Candida* other than *C. albicans*, including *C. krusei* and *C. glabrata*;[126] amphotericin B with or without flucytosine remains the treatment of choice for infections caused by these species.[13,15] Azoles are also not recommended for treatment of *Aspergillus* spp. infections.[54]

Initial use of azoles for treatment of ocular infections was based on pharmacokinetics[127] and experience with extraocular fungal infections. Fluconazole has been the most useful of the azole compounds because it is tolerated well and has good intraocular penetration. Fluconazole can be given intravenously but is well absorbed orally. It has low affinity for plasma proteins. In animal studies, fluconazole penetrates ocular tissues well, achieving levels in the retina/choroid that are equal to serum levels, and aqueous and vitreous humor levels ≥ 70% of serum levels.[128,129] In a single case report, human vitreous humor drug level after 6 weeks of oral fluconazole therapy was similar to the plasma level.[130] Intravitreous injection of fluconazole is probably not necessary because of its good intraocular penetration.

In a small, prospective, randomized study of 40 patients with various forms of candidiasis,[131] fluconazole and the combination of amphotericin B and flucytosine were equally effective for curing infections, but the median time until elimination of fungi was longer for those treated with fluconazole. It was not specifically stated whether any patients had endophthalmitis.

The treatment of intraocular fungal infections with fluconazole has been described in several case reports and small uncontrolled case series.[55,74,130,132–137] It has been reported to be effective for treatment of infections of *Candida albicans*,[55,130,135,136] *C. tropicalis*,[55] *Coccidiodes immitis*,[136] and *Cryptococcus neoformans*,[74,132,137] although infection was not confirmed in all cases. Ackler and associates[133] reviewed the case histories of six newly described patients and 21 previously reported patients with intraocular candidal infections (a total of 38 infected eyes), who had received at least 2 weeks of therapy with oral fluconazole. The drug was used as sole therapy in 13 patients with endogenous infections (15 eyes); infection resolved without recurrence in all eyes. (A 16th eye, in a patient with exogenous infection after surgery, was not cured of infection.) Successful treatments were associated with total doses of 4000 to 19 800 mg of fluconazole over periods ranging up to 65 days. Patients had a variety of risk factors for candidemia, and had a spectrum of ophthalmic findings ranging from isolated retinal lesions to chorioretinitis with vitreitis; apparently only five patients had vitreous reactions. Although the series did provide evidence that fluconazole may be effective in some patients, it was not obvious from the report that the less severely involved eyes, such as those that had cottonwool spots, truly represented candidal infections.

The daily dose of oral fluconazole is 100 mg to 200 mg; patients are given a loading dose on the first day of twice the daily dose (200 mg to 400 mg). The higher doses have generally been preferred for intraocular infections. Published reports have even described loading doses on the first day as high as 800 mg, with subsequent daily doses as high as 400 mg for treatment of endogenous fungal endophthalmitis. The drug can be given once daily, although splitting of the daily total into two doses has been used. Therapy has generally been administered for at least 2 months in successfully treated cases.[133] Fluconazole is well tolerated, with dose-related gastrointestinal symptoms as its only frequent side-effect;[126] rare complications include agranulocytosis, exfoliative skin disorders, hepatotoxicity, and thrombocytopenia.

Indications for the use of fluconazole as a sole agent for the treatment of endogenous fungal endophthalmitis remain to be defined precisely. There is a growing consensus that use of oral fluconazole for treatment of endogenous candidal infections of the eye is appropriate in some cases, such as extramacular infections restricted to the choroid and retina.[138] Studies suggest that it may also be an appropriate "step-down" agent after initial treatment with amphotericin B,[133] and it is an important alternative for patients whose use of amphotericin B is limited by toxicity.

Animal studies have not necessarily supported the use of fluconazole in place of amphotericin B for ocular infections.[127,139] In one study,[139] fluconazole was just as effective as amphotericin B for treating rabbits with candidiasis through day 17 of therapy but was less effective than amphotericin B by day 24. In fact, ocular lesions appeared to be worse by that day in rabbits treated with fluconazole. Possible explanations include the fact that fluconazole is fungistatic only and that the rate at which resistance develops may be high. Until additional experience is gained, azole compounds as sole therapy should be used with caution and under close observation.

Resistant strains have emerged with use of fluconazole,[126] and treatment failures with fluconazole alone have been reported.[140,141] Vitrectomy, in addition to systemic administration of fluconazole, may be effective when drug therapy alone has failed.[55] Some investigators advocate the use of both fluconazole and flucytosine,[138] but experience with this combination to treat intraocular infections is limited. This combination was not more effective than fluconazole alone in a rabbit model of candidal endophthalmitis,[123] although the dose of fluconazole was higher (based on a comparison of pharmacokinetic parameters) than would generally be used to treat human infections.

Ketoconazole and miconazole have a limited role, if any, in the management of endogenous fungal infections of the eye. Miconazole, which is available for intravenous administration, is effective against *Candida* spp. and *Coccidioides immitis* in vitro. It has been effective against candidal chorioretinitis when 2400 mg or more is administered daily.[6,25] It may be less effective for treatment of candidal and cryptococcal infections of the eye than is amphotericin B, however.[142] Also, the reactivation of systemic coccidioidomycosis is higher after miconazole therapy than after amphotericin B therapy.[111] A combination of miconazole and flucytosine has been used successfully to treat candidal chorioretinitis.[25] The use of miconazole is limited by its frequent side-effects, which include nausea, vomiting, anemia, thrombocytosis, hyponatremia, various central nervous system toxicities, and anaphylactoid reactions. Miconazole may decrease the effectiveness of amphotericin B when the drugs are used in combination.[112] Intravitreous injection of miconazole has been used to treat endogenous *Pseudallescheria boydii* infection of the eye that was resistant to amphotericin B.[63]

Ketoconazole is well absorbed orally but has poor intraocular penetration. Sensitivities of various fungi, including *Cryptococcus neoformans*, *Coccidioides immitis*, *H. capsulatum*, and *B. dermatitidis*, vary. *Candida* spp., *Aspergillus* spp., and *Sporothix* spp. appear to be less sensitive. Ketoconazole and flucytosine have synergistic activity against *Cryptococcus neoformans*[124] and have been used successfully in the treatment of candidal chorioretinitis.[20] A combination of ketoconazole and amphotericin B has been reported to be successful in the treatment of some endogenous fungal infections.[23] Nevertheless, this combination has shown no additive effect in the treatment of cryptococcal meningitis,[124] and exposure of *Candida albicans* to ketoconazole may result in its resistance to amphotericin B.[143] It is therefore recommended that this combination of agents should not be used.

Itraconazole is more active than the other azole drugs against *Aspergillus* spp., and among the azoles it is preferred for treatment of chronic, nonocular forms of blastomycosis, coccidioidomycosis, and histoplasmosis because of its efficacy and tolerance.[126] Itraconazole penetrates into the eye poorly, however, and amphotericin B remains the treatment of choice for ocular involvement with these infections. Itraconazole may have some efficacy against *Scedosporium prolificans*, which is resistant to most antifungal agents.[64]

Voriconazole is a newer triazole compound that is used for the treatment of invasive aspergillosis and other serious fungal infections, including scedosporiosis, that are refractory to other antifungal agents.[109,144] Voriconazole is also active against *Candida* spp., including species such as *C. krusei* and *C. glabrata*, that are resistant to other azole compounds.[109] By early 2005, there had been little experience in the use of voriconazole for treating ocular fungal infections, but there was substantial interest in its potential application for endogenous fungal endophthalmitis, because of its high bioavailability and good intraocular penetration after oral administration. In one study, voriconazole levels within the vitreous humor of noninflamed human eyes were above in vitro mean inhibitory concentrations (90%) for a variety of fungi that cause endogenous fungal endophthalmitis, including *Candida albicans*, *C. parapsilosis*, *C. tropicalis*, *Cryptococcus neoformans*, *Aspergillus fumigatus*, *A. flavus*, *Blastomyces dermatitidis*, *Coccidioides immitis*, *Histoplasma capsulatum*, and *Scediosporium apiospermum*.[145] Studies using a rodent model suggested that intravitreous injections of 100 μg of voriconazole in human beings may also be safe.[145a]

The potential value of voriconazole treatment of candidal endophthalmitis in patients who have failed treatment with fluconazole has been demonstrated in a small case series.[145b] Patients treated with voriconazole can experience transient visual disturbances, including a sensation of increased light intensity, blurring, photophobia, and color alterations. These problems are usually apparent within the first week of treatment, and resolve within 30 minutes of dosing, without apparent sequellae.

Other antifungal drugs

Caspofungin is an echinocandin antifungal agent that inhibits formation of β(1,3)-D-glucans in the fungal cell wall.[110] It is active against most *Candida* spp., *Aspergillus* spp., and *H. capsulatum*, but *Cryptococcus* sp. and *Pseudallescheria boydii* are resistant.[110,146] Azole-resistant isolates of *Candida albicans* remain susceptible to caspofungin.[110] Although there is interest in the use of caspofungin for a variety of fungal infections, by early 2005 there had been little published data about its role in the treatment of intraocular infections. In one small case series, caspofungin was used in conjunction with intravenous or oral voriconazole, but its specific contribution to resolution of infection was not determined.[145b]

Vitrectomy

Pars plana vitrectomy may be a useful adjunctive therapy for intraocular fungal infections in some cases.[28] Vitrectomy is indicated if there is severe vitreous humor involvement (especially if there is a dense focal inflammation or abscess formation, extensive membrane formation, or retinal traction) or if there is progression of disease despite medical therapy. The procedure will debulk organisms from the vitreous cavity that may receive relatively little medication administered systemically; it will limit vitreoretinal traction that might occur after resolution of infection; and it will allow diffusion of intravitreously administered drug. Early vitrectomy on patients with candidal endophthalmitis has been reported to result in better visual outcomes.[26]

The need for vitrectomy in all cases has been questioned by some investigators, however.[114] It is argued that an intact vitreous body will more effectively limit the spread of infection. A vitreous inflammatory reaction by itself is not a sufficient criterion for vitrectomy.

Outcomes of treatment

If treated early, while organisms remain within the choroid or retina, candidal lesions can resolve without functional deficit. When healed, chorioretinal lesions result in a well-demarcated, hypopigmented scar (Fig. 94-2). If lesions are confined within the retina, they may leave only a translucent gliotic scar without pigmentary changes, which makes them difficult to appreciate ophthalmoscopically. If organisms have invaded the vitreous body, healing results in fibrosis that may produce tractional changes of the retina[8] (Fig. 94-3). Choroidal neovascularization can occur after resolution of infection, as a late, vision-threatening complication of candidal chorioretinitis; this complication may be more common than heretofore recognized.[147]

Treatment of *Aspergillus* spp. endophthalmitis is generally less successful than treatment of candidal endophthalmitis.[56] In various series, the majority of eyes with *Aspergillus* spp. endophthalmitis have been enucleated or left with poor vision.[55,56] In a few patients, however, early, aggressive therapy with vitrectomy and intravitreous injection of amphotericin B has been successful;[54,137] vision can improve in cases without macular involvement.

P. boydii is frequently resistant to amphotericin B and may be resistant to fluconazole. Treatment with miconazole or ketoconazole has been recommended,[1,62] but results of aggressive therapy for *P. boydii* endophthalmitis have generally been poor. *Scedosporium prolificans* appears to be even more resistant to treatment.[64]

Cryptococcal chorioretinitis can respond to fluconazole,[80a] although treatment results are generally poor, regardless of the therapy given.[74]

CONCLUSIONS

Fungal infections of the retina and choroid remain among the most devastating of ophthalmic disorders. Although uncommon, fungal infection should be considered in the differential diagnosis of chronic progressive intraocular inflammation, especially in patients at risk for fungemia, whether or not there is evidence of nonocular sites of disease. Patients with AIDS represent a population at risk for disseminated fungal disease, but reports of intraocular fungal infections in this group remain uncommon.

Candida spp. remain the most common cause of endogenous fungal chorioretinitis. The limited number of case reports describing other endogenous fungal infections, and the fact that infection of the eye is often discovered only at autopsy or in the terminal phases of disseminated disease, have made it difficult to assess their clinical findings, natural history, and response to treatment accurately. Unlike C. *albicans*, other intraocular fungal infections may be insensitive indicators of disseminated disease.

Successful management of endogenous fungal infections requires early and accurate diagnosis by clinicians who are aware of their manifestations and familiar with the conditions that predispose patients to their development. Although there have been no prospectively designed, randomized studies of treatment for endogenous fungal infections of the eye, a general approach to treatment has evolved on the basis of clinical experience.[3,56,109,138,148] With regard to candidal infections, early lesions that do not yet involve the vitreous body may be treated with oral fluconazole and close monitoring for evidence of progression. More severe infections are treated with intravenous amphotericin B, with or without flucytosine. If there is a focus of infection within the vitreous body, an intravitreous injection of amphotericin B should be considered, possibly in conjunction with pars plana vitrectomy, especially if the vitreous inflammatory reaction is severe. Amphotericin B remains the treatment of choice for most other infections, although there are some exceptions, as noted above. A continuing challenge is the need to develop more effective and less toxic treatments.

ACKNOWLEDGMENTS

Thomas H. Pettit, MD and Marc O. Yoshizumi, MD, of the Department of Ophthalmology, David Geffen School of Medicine at UCLA, provided assistance during preparation of the first edition of this chapter. John E. Edwards, Jr., MD, of the Department of Medicine, David Geffen School of Medicine at UCLA and Chief of the Infectious Disease Service, Harbor-UCLA Medical Center, Torrance, CA, provided valuable suggestions in the preparation of this chapter.

REFERENCES

1. Pettit TH, Edwards JE, Purdy EP et al. Endogenous fungal endophthalmitis. In: Pepose JS, Holland GN, Wilhelmus KR, eds. Ocular infection and immunity. St. Louis, MO: Mosby YearBook; 1996:1262–1285.
2. Pappas PG, Rex JH, Lee J et al. A prospective observational study of candidemia: epidemiology, therapy, and influences on mortality in hospitalized adult and pediatric patients. Clin Infect Dis 2003; 37:634–643.
3. Rex JH, Walsh TJ, Sobel JD et al. Practice guidelines for the treatment of candidiasis. Infectious Diseases Society of America. Clin Infect Dis 2000; 30:662–678.
4. Joshi N, Hamory BH. Endophthalmitis caused by non-*albicans* species of *Candida*. Rev Infect Dis 1991; 13:281–287.
5. Donahue SP, Greven CM, Zuravleff JJ et al. Intraocular candidiasis in patients with candidemia. Clinical implications derived from a prospective multicenter study. Ophthalmology 1994; 101:1302–1309.
6. Fitzsimons RB, Nicholls MD, Billson FA et al. Fungal retinitis: a case of *Torulopsis glabrata* infection treated with miconazole. Br J Ophthalmol 1980; 64:672–675.
7. Cohen M, Montgomerie JZ. Hematogenous endophthalmitis due to *Candida tropicalis*: report of two cases and review. Clin Infect Dis 1993; 17:270–272.
8. Griffin JR, Pettit TH, Fishman LS et al. Blood-borne *Candida* endophthalmitis. A clinical and pathologic study of 21 cases. Arch Ophthalmol 1973; 89:450–456.
9. Parke DW, Jones DB, Gentry LO. Endogenous endophthalmitis among patients with candidemia. Ophthalmology 1982; 89:789–796.
10. McDonnell PJ, McDonnell JM, Brown RH et al. Ocular involvement in patients with fungal infections. Ophthalmology 1985; 92:706–709.
11. Edwards JE, Jr., Lehrer RI, Stiehm ER et al. Severe candidal infections: clinical perspective, immune defense mechanisms, and current concepts of therapy. Ann Intern Med 1978; 89:91–106.
12. Fujita NK, Hockey LJ et al. Comparative ocular pathogenicity of *Cryptococcus neoformans*, *Candida glabrata*, and *Aspergillus fumigatus* in the rabbit. Invest Ophthalmol Vis Sci 1982; 22:410–414.
13. McQuillen DP, Zingman BS, Meunier F et al. Invasive infections due to *Candida krusei*: report of ten cases of fungemia that include three cases of endophthalmitis. Clin Infect Dis 1992; 14:472–478.
14. Samaranayake YH, Samaranayake LP. *Candida krusei*: biology, epidemiology, pathogenicity and clinical manifestations of an emerging pathogen. J Med Microbiol 1994; 41:295–310.
15. Wingard JR, Merz WG, Rinaldi MG et al. Increase in *Candida krusei* infection among patients with bone marrow transplantation and neutropenia treated prophylactically with fluconazole. N Engl J Med 1991; 325:1274–1277.
16. Robertson DM, Riley FC, Hermans PE. Endogenous *Candida* oculomycosis. Report of two patients treated with flucytosine. Arch Ophthalmol 1974; 91:33–38.
17. Edwards JE Jr, Foos RY, Montgomerie JZ et al. Ocular manifestations of *Candida* septicemia: review of seventy-six cases of hematogenous *Candida* endophthalmitis. Medicine (Baltimore) 1974; 53:47–75.
18. Aguilar GL, Blumenkrantz MS, Egbert PR et al. *Candida* endophthalmitis after intravenous drug abuse. Arch Ophthalmol 1979; 97:96–100.
19. Doft BH, Clarkson JG, Rebell G et al. Endogenous *Aspergillus* endophthalmitis in drug abusers. Arch Ophthalmol 1980; 98:859–862.
20. Graham E, Chignell AH, Eykyn S. *Candida* endophthalmitis: a complication of prolonged intravenous therapy and antibiotic treatment. J Infect 1986; 13:167–173.
21. Michelson PE, Stark W, Reeser F et al. Endogenous *Candida* endophthalmitis. Report of 13 cases and 16 from the literature. Int Ophthalmol Clin 1971; 11:125–147.
22. Montgomerie JZ, Edwards JE Jr. Association of infection due to *Candida albicans* with intravenous hyperalimentation. J Infect Dis 1978; 137:197–201.
23. Drouhet E, Dupont B. Laboratory and clinical assessment of ketoconazole in deep-seated mycoses. Am J Med 1983; 74 (Suppl. 1B):30–47.
24. Dupont B, Drouhet E. Cutaneous, ocular, and osteoarticular candidiasis in heroin addicts: new clinical and therapeutic aspects in 38 patients. J Infect Dis 1985; 152:577–591.
25. Gallo J, Playfair J, Gregory-Roberts J et al. Fungal endophthalmitis in narcotic abusers. Medical and surgical therapy in 10 patients. Med J Aust 1985; 142:386–388.
26. Martinez-Vazquez C, Fernandez-Ulloa J, Bordon J et al. *Candida albicans* endophthalmitis in brown heroin addicts: response to early vitrectomy preceded and followed by antifungal therapy. Clin Infect Dis 1998; 27:1130–1133.
27. Servant JB, Dutton GN, Ong-Tone L et al. Candidal endophthalmitis in Glaswegian heroin addicts: report of an epidemic. Trans Ophthalmol Soc UK 1985; 104:297–308.
28. Snip RC, Michels RG. Pars plana vitrectomy in the management of endogenous *Candida* endophthalmitis. Am J Ophthalmol 1976; 82:699–704.
29. Stern GA, Fetkenhour CL, O'Grady RB. Intravitreal amphotericin B treatment of *Candida* endophthamitis. Arch Ophthalmol 1977; 95:89–93.
30. Baley JE, Kliegman RM, Fanaroff AA. Disseminated fungal infections in very low-birth-weight infants: clinical manifestations and epidemiology. Pediatrics 1984; 73:144–152.
31. Hill HR, Mitchell TG, Matsen JM et al. Recovery from disseminated candidiasis in a premature neonate. Pediatrics 1974; 53:748–752.
32. Palmer EA. Endogenous *Candida* endophthalmitis in infants. Am J Ophthalmol 1980; 89:388–395.
33. Baley JE, Annable WL, Kliegman RM. *Candida* endophthalmitis in the premature infant. J Pediatr 1981; 98:458–461.

34. Xanthou M, Valassi-Adam E, Kintsonidou E et al. Phagocytosis and killing ability of *Candida albicans* by blood leucocytes of healthy term and preterm babies. Arch Dis Child 1975; 50:72–75.

35. Chen SJ, Chung YM, Liu JH. Endogenous *Candida* endophthalmitis after induced abortion. Am J Ophthalmol 1998; 125:873–875.

36. Cantrill HL, Rodman WP, Ramsay RC et al. Postpartum *Candida* endophthalmitis. JAMA 1980; 243:1163–1165.

37. Brooks RG. Prospective study of *Candida* endophthalmitis in hospitalized patients with candidemia. Arch Intern Med 1989; 149:2226–2228.

38. Pepose JS, Holland GN, Nestor MS et al. Acquired immune deficiency syndrome. Pathogenic mechanisms of ocular disease. Ophthalmology 1985; 92:472–484.

39. Heinemann MH, Bloom AF, Horowitz J. *Candida albicans* endophthalmitis in a patient with AIDS. Case report. Arch Ophthalmol 1987; 105:1172–1173.

40. Schuman JS, Friedman AH. Retinal manifestations of the acquired immune deficiency syndrome (AIDS): cytomegalovirus, *Candida albicans*, *Cryptococcus*, toxoplasmosis and *Pneumocystis carinii*. Trans Ophthalmol Soc UK 1983; 103:177–190.

41. Griffin JR, Foos RY, Pettit TH. Relationship between *Candida* endophthalmitis, candidemia, and disseminated candidiasis. Twenty-second concilium ophthalmologicum. Paris, Masson: 1974.

42. Donahue SP, Hein E, Sinatra RB. Ocular involvement in children with candidemia. Am J Ophthalmol 2003; 135:886–887.

43. Scherer WJ, Lee K. Implications of early systemic therapy on the incidence of endogenous fungal endophthalmitis. Ophthalmology 1997; 104:1593–1598.

44. Feman SS, Nichols JC, Chung SM et al. Endophthalmitis in patients with disseminated fungal disease. Trans Am Ophthalmol Soc 2002; 100:67–70.

45. Rodriguez-Adrian LJ, King RT, Tamayo-Derat LG et al. Retinal lesions as clues to disseminated bacterial and candidal infections: frequency, natural history, and etiology. Medicine (Baltimore) 2003; 82:187–202.

46. Schelenz S, Gransden WR. Candidaemia in a London teaching hospital: analysis of 128 cases over a 7-year period. Mycoses 2003; 46:390–396.

47. Henderson DK, Hockey LJ, Vukalcic LJ et al. Effect of immunosuppression on the development of experimental hematogenous *Candida* endophthalmitis. Infect Immun 1980; 27:628–631.

48. Demicco DD, Reichman RC, Violette EJ et al. Disseminated aspergillosis presenting with endophthalmitis. A case report and a review of the literature. Cancer 1984; 53:1995–2001.

49. Jampol LM, Dyckman S, Maniates V et al. Retinal and choroidal infarction from *Aspergillus*: clinical diagnosis and clinicopathologic correlations. Trans Am Ophthalmol Soc 1988; 86:422–440.

50. McGuire TW, Bullock JD, Bullock JD Jr et al. Fungal endophthalmitis. An experimental study with a review of 17 human ocular cases. Arch Ophthalmol 1991; 109:1289–1296.

51. Naidoff MA, Green WR. Endogenous *Aspergillus* endophthalmitis occurring after kidney transplant. Am J Ophthalmol 1975; 79:502–509.

52. Riddell IJ, McNeil SA, Johnson TM et al. Endogenous *Aspergillus* endophthalmitis: report of 3 cases and review of the literature. Medicine (Baltimore) 2002; 81:311–320.

53. Roney P, Barr CC, Chun CH et al. Endogenous *Aspergillus* endophthalmitis. Rev Infect Dis 1986; 8:955–958.

54. Weishaar PD, Flynn HW Jr, Murray TG et al. Endogenous *Aspergillus* endophthalmitis. Clinical features and treatment outcomes. Ophthalmology 1998; 105:57–65.

55. Christmas NJ, Smiddy WE. Vitrectomy and systemic fluconazole for treatment of endogenous fungal endophthalmitis. Ophthalm Surg Lasers 1996; 27:1012–1018.

56. Essman TF, Flynn HW Jr, Smiddy WE et al. Treatment outcomes in a 10-year study of endogenous fungal endophthalmitis. Ophthalm Surg Lasers 1997; 28:185–194.

57. Coskuncan NM, Jabs DA, Dunn JP et al. The eye in bone marrow transplantation. VI. Retinal complications. Arch Ophthalmol 1994; 112:372–379.

58. Hunt KE, Glasgow BJ. *Aspergillus* endophthalmitis. An unrecognized endemic disease in orthotopic liver transplantation. Ophthalmology 1996; 103:757–767.

59. Smith JR, Chee SP. Endogenous *Aspergillus* endophthalmitis occurring in a child with normal immune function. Eye 2000; 14:670–671.

60. Valluri S, Moorthy RS, Liggett PE et al. Endogenous *Aspergillus* endophthalmitis in an immunocompetent individual. Int Ophthalmol 1993; 17:131–135.

61. Rao NA, Hidayat AA. Endogenous mycotic endophthalmitis: variations in clinical and histopathologic changes in candidiasis compared with aspergillosis. Am J Ophthalmol 2001; 132:244–251.

62. Pfeifer JD, Grand MG, Thomas MA et al. Endogenous *Pseudallescheria boydii* endophthalmitis. Clinicopathologic findings in two cases [published erratum of serious dosage error appears in Arch Ophthalmol 1992; 110:449]. Arch Ophthalmol 1991; 109:1714–1717.

63. Stern RM, Zakov ZN, Meisler DM et al. Endogenous *Pseudoallescheria boydii* endophthalmitis. A clinicopathologic report. Cleve Clin Q 1986; 53:197–203.

64. Wood GM, McCormack JG, Muir DB et al. Clinical features of human infection with *Scedosporium inflatum*. Clin Infect Dis 1992; 14:1027–1033.

65. Berenguer J, Rodriguez-Tudela JL, Richard C et al. Deep infections caused by *Scedosporium prolificans*. A report on 16 cases in Spain and a review of the literature. *Scedosporium Prolificans* Spanish Study Group. Medicine (Baltimore) 1997; 76:256–265.

66. Marin J, Sanz MA, Sanz GF et al. Disseminated *Scedosporium inflatum* infection in a patient with acute myeloblastic leukemia. Eur J Clin Microbiol Infect Dis 1991; 10:759–761.

67. Nielsen K, Lang H, Shum AC et al. Disseminated *Scedosporium prolificans* infection in an immunocompromised adolescent. Pediatr Infect Dis J 1993; 12:882–884.

68. Maertens J, Lagrou K, Deweerdt H et al. Disseminated infection by *Scedosporium prolificans*: an emerging fatality among haematology patients. Case report and review. Ann Hematol 2000; 79:340–344.

69. Henderly DE, Liggett PE, Rao NA. Cryptococcal chorioretinitis and endophthalmitis. Retina 1987; 7:75–79.

70. Hiles DA, Font RL. Bilateral intraocular cryptococcosis with unilateral spontaneous regression. Report of a case and review of the literature. Am J Ophthalmol 1968; 65:98–108.

71. Shields JA, Wright DM, Augsburger JJ et al. Cryptococcal chorioretinitis. Am J Ophthalmol 1980; 89:210–217.

72. Avendano J, Tanishima T, Kuwabara T. Ocular cryptococcosis. Am J Ophthalmol 1978; 86:110–113.

73. Khodadoust AA, Payne JW. Cryptococcal (torular) retinitis. A clinicopathologic case report. Am J Ophthalmol 1969; 67:745–750.

74. Crump JR, Elner SG, Elner VM et al. Cryptococcal endophthalmitis: case report and review. Clin Infect Dis 1992; 14:1069–1073.

75. Hiss PW, Shields JA, Augsburger JJ. Solitary retinovitreal abscess as the initial manifestation of cryptococcosis. Ophthalmology 1988; 95:162–165.

76. Sheu SJ, Chen YC, Kuo NW et al. Endogenous cryptococcal endophthalmitis. Ophthalmology 1998; 105:377–381.

77. Morinelli EN, Dugel PU, Riffenburgh R et al. Infectious multifocal choroiditis in patients with acquired immune deficiency syndrome. Ophthalmology 1993; 100:1014–1021.

78. Carney MD, Combs JL, Waschler W. Cryptococcal choroiditis. Retina 1990; 10:27–32.

79. Denning DW, Armstrong RW, Fishman M et al. Endophthalmitis in a patient with disseminated cryptococcosis and AIDS who was treated with itraconazole. Rev Infect Dis 1991; 13:1126–1130.

80. Winward KE, Hamed LM, Glaser JS. The spectrum of optic nerve disease in human immunodeficiency virus infection. Am J Ophthalmol 1989; 107:373–380.

80a. Kestelyn P, Taelman H, Bogaerts J et al. Opthalmic manifestations of infections with *Cryptococcus neoformans* in patients with the acquired immunodeficiency syndrome. Am J Ophthalmol 1993; 116:721–727.

81. Katz BJ, Scott WE, Folk JC. Acute histoplasmosis choroiditis in 2 immunocompetent brothers. Arch Ophthalmol 1997; 115:1470–1472.

82. Carroll DM, Franklin RM. Vitreous biopsy in uveitis of unknown cause. Retina 1981; 1:245–251.

83. Goldstein BG, Buettner H. Histoplasmic endophthalmitis. A clinicopathologic correlation. Arch Ophthalmol 1983; 101:774–777.

84. Gonzales CA, Scott IU, Chaudhry NA et al. Endogenous endophthalmitis caused by *Histoplasma capsulatum* var. *capsulatum*: a case report and literature review. Ophthalmology 2000; 107:725–729.

85. Klintworth GK, Hollingsworth AS, Lusman PA et al. Granulomatous choroiditis in a case of disseminated histoplasmosis. Histologic demonstration of *Histoplasma capsulatum* in choroidal lesions. Arch Ophthalmol 1973; 90:45–48.

86. Macher A, Rodrigues MM, Kaplan W et al. Disseminated bilateral chorioretinitis due to *Histoplasma capsulatum* in a patient with the acquired immunodeficiency syndrome. Ophthalmology 1985; 92:1159–1164.

87. Scholz R, Green WR, Kutys R et al. *Histoplasma capsulatum* in the eye. Ophthalmology 1984; 91:1100–1104.

88. Specht CS, Mitchell KT, Bauman AE et al. Ocular histoplasmosis with retinitis in a patient with acquired immune deficiency syndrome. Ophthalmology 1991; 98:1356–1359.

89. Increase in coccidioidomycosis – Arizona, 1998–2001. MMWR Morb Mortal Wkly Rep 2003; 52:109–112.

90. Rodenbiker HT, Ganley JP. Ocular coccidioidomycosis. Surv Ophthalmol 1980; 24:263–290.

91. Rosenstein NE, Emery KW, Werner SB et al. Risk factors for severe pulmonary and disseminated coccidioidomycosis: Kern County, California, 1995–1996. Clin Infect Dis 2001; 32:708–715.

92. Blumenkranz MS, Stevens DA. Endogenous coccidioidal endophthalmitis. Ophthalmology 1980; 87:974–984.

93. Glasgow BJ, Brown HH, Foos RY. Miliary retinitis in coccidioidomycosis. Am J Ophthalmol 1987; 104:24–27.

94. Zakka KA, Foos RY, Brown WJ. Intraocular coccidioidomycosis. Surv Ophthalmol 1978; 22:313–321.

95. Cassady JR, Foerster HC. *Sporotrichum schenckii* endophthalmitis. Arch Ophthalmol 1971; 85:71–74.

96. Font RL, Jakobiec FA. Granulomatous necrotizing retinochoroiditis caused by *Sporotrichum schenkii*. Report of a case including immunofluorescence and electron microscopical studies. Arch Ophthalmol 1976; 94:1513–1519.

97. Curi AL, Felix S, Azevedo KM et al. Retinal granuloma caused by *Sporothrix schenckii*. Am J Ophthalmol 2003; 136:205–207.

98. Kurosawa A, Pollock SC, Collins MP et al. *Sporothrix schenckii* endophthalmitis in a patient with human immunodeficiency virus infection. Arch Ophthalmol 1988; 106:376–380.

99. Bond WI, Sanders CV, Joffe L et al. Presumed blastomycosis endophthalmitis. Ann Ophthalmol 1982; 14:1183–1188.

100. Lewis H, Aaberg TM, Fary DR et al. Latent disseminated blastomycosis with choroidal involvement. Arch Ophthalmol 1988; 106:527–530.

101. Sinskey RM, Anderson WB. Miliary blastomycosis with metastatic spread to posterior uvea of both eyes. Arch Ophthalmol 1955; 54:602–604.

102. Li S, Perlman JI, Edward DP et al. Unilateral *Blastomyces dermatitidis* endophthalmitis and orbital cellulitis. A case report and literature review. Ophthalmology 1998; 105:1466–1470.

103. Font RL, Spaulding AG, Green WR. Endogenous mycotic panophthalmitis caused by *Blastomyces dermatitidis*. Report of a case and a review of the literature. Arch Ophthalmol 1967; 77:217–222.

104. Safneck JR, Hogg GR, Napier LB. Endophthalmitis due to *Blastomyces dermatitidis*. Case report and review of the literature. Ophthalmology 1990; 97:212–216.

105. Gottlieb JL, McAllister IL, Guttman FA et al. Choroidal blastomycosis. A report of two cases. Retina 1995; 15:248–252.

106. Rex JH, Bennett JE, Sugar AM et al. A randomized trial comparing fluconazole with amphotericin B for the treatment of candidemia in patients without neutropenia. Candidemia Study Group and the National Institute. N Engl J Med 1994; 331:1325–1330.

107. Dellon AL, Stark WJ, Chretien PB. Spontaneous resolution of endogenous *Candida* endophthalmitis complicating intravenous hyperalimentation. Am J Ophthalmol 1975; 79:648–654.

108. Brod RD, Flynn HW Jr, Clarkson JG et al. Endogenous *Candida* endophthalmitis. Management without intravenous amphotericin B. Ophthalmology 1990; 97:666–672.

109. Pappas PG, Rex JH, Sobel JD et al. Guidelines for treatment of candidiasis. Clin Infect Dis 2004; 38:161–189.

110. Bennett JE. Antimicrobial agents (continued): Antifungal Agents. In: Hardman JG, Limbird LE, eds. Goodman and Gilman's The Pharmacological Basis of Therapeutics, 10th edn. New York: McGraw-Hill; 2001:1295–1312.

111. Medoff G, Brajtburg J, Kobayashi GS et al. Antifungal agents useful in therapy of systemic fungal infections. Annu Rev Pharmacol Toxicol 1983; 23:303–330.

112. Medoff G, Kobayashi GS. Strategies in the treatment of systemic fungal infections. N Engl J Med 1980; 302:145–155.

113. Green WR, Bennett JE, Goos RD. Ocular penetration of amphotericin B: a report of laboratory studies and a case report of postsurgical *Cephalosporium* endophthalmitis. Arch Ophthalmol 1965; 73:769–775.

114. Kinyoun JL. Treatment of *Candida* endophthalmitis. Retina 1982; 2:215–222.

115. Axelrod AJ, Peyman GA, Apple DJ. Toxicity of intravitreal injection of amphotericin B. Am J Ophthalmol 1973; 76:578–583.

116. Doft BH, Weiskopf J, Nilsson-Ehle I et al. Amphotericin clearance in vitrectomized versus nonvitrectomized eyes. Ophthalmology 1985; 92:1601–1605.

117. Baley JE, Kliegman RM, Fanaroff AA. Disseminated fungal infections in very low-birth-weight infants: therapeutic toxicity. Pediatrics 1984; 73:153–157.

118. Lou P, Kazdan J, Bannatyne RM et al. Successful treatment of *Candida* endophthalmitis with a synergistic combination of amphotericin B and rifampin. Am J Ophthalmol 1977; 83:12–15.

119. Goldblum D, Rohrer K, Frueh BE et al. Ocular distribution of intravenously administered lipid formulations of amphotericin B in a rabbit model. Antimicrob Agents Chemother 2002; 46:3719–3723.

120. Liu KR, Peyman GA, Khoobehi B. Efficacy of liposome-bound amphotericin B for the treatment of experimental fungal endophthalmitis in rabbits. Invest Ophthalmol Vis Sci 1989; 30:1527–1534.

121. Darling K, Singh J, Wilks D. Successful treatment of *Candida glabrata* endophthalmitis with amphotericin B lipid complex (ABLC). J Infect 2000; 40:92–94.

122. Virata SR, Kylstra JA, Brown JC et al. Worsening of endogenous *Candida albicans* endophthalmitis during therapy with intravenous lipid complex amphotericin B. Clin Infect Dis 1999; 28:1177–1178.

123. Louie A, Liu W, Miller DA et al. Efficacies of high-dose fluconazole plus amphotericin B and high-dose fluconazole plus 5-fluorocytosine versus amphotericin B, fluconazole, and 5-fluorocytosine monotherapies in treatment of experimental endocarditis, endophthalmitis, and pyelonephritis due to *Candida albicans*. Antimicrob Agents Chemother 1999; 43:2831–2840.

124. Craven PC, Graybill JR. Combination of oral flucytosine and ketoconazole as therapy for experimental cryptococcal meningitis. J Infect Dis 1984; 149:584–590.

125. Johnson DE, Thompson TR, Green TP et al. Systemic candidiasis in very low-birth-weight infants (less than 1500 grams). Pediatrics 1984; 73:138–143.

126. Como JA, Dismukes WE. Oral azole drugs as systemic antifungal therapy. N Engl J Med 1994; 330:263–272.

127. Savani DV, Perfect JR, Cobo LM et al. Penetration of new azole compounds into the eye and efficacy in experimental *Candida* endophthalmitis. Antimicrob Agents Chemother 1987; 31:6–10.

128. Mian UK, Mayers M, Garg Y et al. Comparison of fluconazole pharmacokinetics in serum, aqueous humor, vitreous humor, and cerebrospinal fluid following a single dose and at steady state. J Ocul Pharmacol Ther 1998; 14:459–471.

129. O'Day DM, Foulds G, Williams TE et al. Ocular uptake of fluconazole following oral administration. Arch Ophthalmol 1990; 108:1006–1008.

130. Urbak SF, Degn T. Fluconazole in the treatment of *Candida albicans* endophthalmitis. Acta Ophthalmol (Copenh) 1992; 70:528–529.

131. Kujath P, Lerch K, Kochendorfer P et al. Comparative study of the efficacy of fluconazole versus amphotericin B/flucytosine in surgical patients with systemic mycoses. Infection 1993; 21:376–382.

132. Agarwal A, Gupta A, Sakhuja V et al. Retinitis following disseminated cryptococcosis in a renal allograft recipient. Efficacy of oral fluconazole. Acta Ophthalmol (Copenh) 1991; 69:402–405.

133. Ackler ME, Vellend H, McNeely DM et al. Use of fluconazole in the treatment of candidal endophthalmitis. Clin Infect Dis 1995; 20:657–664.

134. Cruciani M, Di Perri G, Concia E et al. Fluconazole and fungal ocular infection. J Antimicrob Chemother 1990; 25:718–720.

135. del Palacio A, Cuetara MS, Ferro M et al. Fluconazole in the management of endophthalmitis in disseminated candidosis of heroin addicts. Mycoses 1993; 36:193–199.

136. Luttrull JK, Wan WL, Kubak BM et al. Treatment of ocular fungal infections with oral fluconazole. Am J Ophthalmol 1995; 119:477–481.

137. Urbak SF, Degn T. Fluconazole in the management of fungal ocular infections. Ophthalmologica 1994; 208:147–156.

138. Edwards JE Jr, Bodey GP, Bowden RA et al. International conference for the development of a consensus on the management and prevention of severe candidal infections. Clin Infect Dis 1997; 25:43–59.

139. Filler SG, Crislip MA, Mayer CL et al. Comparison of fluconazole and amphotericin B for treatment of disseminated candidiasis and endophthalmitis in rabbits. Antimicrob Agents Chemother 1991; 35:288–292.

140. Nomura J, Ruskin J. Failure of therapy with fluconazole for candidal endophthalmitis. Clin Infect Dis 1993; 17:888–889.

141. Ohnishi Y, Tawara A, Murata T et al. Postmortem findings two weeks after oral treatment for metastatic *Candida* endophthalmitis with fluconazole. Ophthalmologica 1999; 213:341–344.

142. Blumenkranz MS, Stevens DA. Therapy of endogenous fungal endophthalmitis: miconazole or amphotericin B for coccidioidal and candidal infection. Arch Ophthalmol 1980; 98:1216–1220.

143. Sud IJ, Feingold DS. Effect of ketoconazole on the fungicidal action of amphotericin B in *Candida albicans*. Antimicrob Agents Chemother 1983; 23:185–187.

144. Ostrosky-Zeichner L, Oude Lashof AM, Kullberg BJ et al. Voriconazole salvage treatment of invasive candidiasis. Eur J Clin Microbiol Infect Dis 2003; 22:651–655.

145. Hariprasad SM, Mieler WF, Holz ER et al. Determination of vitreous, aqueous, and plasma concentration of orally administered voriconazole in humans. Arch Ophthalmol 2004; 122:42–47.

145a.Gao H, Pennesi ME, Shah K et al. Intravitreal voriconazole: an electroretinographic and histopathologic study. Arch Ophthalmol 2004; 122:1687–1692.

145b.Breit SM, Hariprasad SM, Mieler WF et al. Management of endogenous fungal endophthalmitis with voriconazole and caspofungin. Am J Ophthalmol 2005; 139:135–140.

146. Cornely OA, Schmitz K, Aisenbrey S. The first echinocandin: caspofungin. Mycoses 2002; 45 (Suppl. 3):56–60.

147. Jampol LM, Sung J, Walker JD et al. Choroidal neovascularization secondary to *Candida albicans* chorioretinitis. Am J Ophthalmol 1996; 121:643–649.

148. Barza M. Treatment options for candidal endophthalmitis [editorial]. Clin Infect Dis 1998; 27:1134–1136.

Pars Planitis

Pravin U. Dugel
Derek Y. Kunimoto
Ronald E. Smith

Pars planitis is a common inflammatory syndrome of young adults and children. The clinical pattern for this uveitic syndrome has evolved over the years under a variety of names: *cyclitis*, used by Fuchs[1] in 1908 and by Duke-Elder[2] in 1941; *peripheral uveitis* by Schepens[3] in 1950; *peripheral cyclitis* by Brockhurst et al.[4] in 1960; *pars planitis* by Welch et al.[5] in 1960; *chronic cyclitis* by Hogan & Kimura[6] in 1961; *vitritis* by Gass[7] in 1968; and finally *intermediate uveitis* by the International Uveitis Study Group[8] in 1987. This terminology is confusing and reflects our ignorance about the cause of this condition.

Over the past 35 years the pars planitis syndrome has been increasingly recognized as a distinct clinical entity. It should be considered in any patient who has a generally quiet external eye and cells and debris concentrated in the vitreous cavity, but especially in patients with an exudate, or "snowbank," over the pars plana inferiorly.[9]

EPIDEMIOLOGY

Pars planitis has been better defined over the past 25 years, and it is now apparent that this is a relatively common form of uveitis, especially in children and young adults,[4, 5, 10-15] although it can occur at any age; both sexes are equally affected.

Approximately 80% of patients ultimately develop bilateral disease.[10] There are no known hereditary or environmental etiologic factors, but pars planitis has been described in several kindreds, with various family members affected.[11,16,17] It has occasionally been associated with other systemic diseases, the most common being multiple sclerosis,[10,18,19] and a pars planitis-like clinical picture can be also seen in patients with sarcoid.[9,10]

Most investigators agree that there are no distinct geographic or racial characteristics in pars planitis. However, in 1965, Hogan and associates[20] specifically pointed out the absence of African American patients among their group of 56 children with pars planitis, and Smith and associates[10] had just one African American in their series of 100 patients reported in 1973. Five years later, however (in 1978), Schlaegel[21] stated that he was not able to demonstrate a statistically significant difference in the distribution of pars planitis between the African American and white populations. Althaus & Sundmacher[22] were unable to find a major study of pars planitis patients from Japan or China, and they also emphasized that Hogan and associates[20] stated specifically

that they had not seen a case of pars planitis in Chinese or Japanese patients. Recently, an epidemiologic study was reported from a large community hospital in Mexico City,[23] which showed that pars planitis accounts for approximately 11% of all cases of uveitis. Forty-nine percent of the patients were between 10 and 14 years old, and there was a 71% male predominance. Ninety percent of the patients had bilateral involvement. This study indicates that the epidemiology of pars planitis in Mexico may be similar to that in the USA and Europe, as opposed to Asia and Africa.

Pars planitis is a relatively common form of uveitis. In a 1987 review of 600 patients with uveitis seen at the Doheny Eye Institute,[24] pars planitis was found in 15.4% of all patients with the diagnosis of uveitis. The classic pars planitis syndrome was found in 10% (characteristic pars plana exudate, in addition to the other frequently associated findings, including a relatively quiet anterior segment, marked vitreous cells, vitreous "snowballs" inferiorly, retinal periphlebitis, and frequent occurrence of cystoid macular edema (CME)). A variant form of pars planitis (discussed later) was found in 5.4% of these 600 cases. Pars planitis occurred more frequently in this series than had been reported in previous series; Schlaegel[25] reported it in 7.6% of cases in 1973, and Perkins & Folk[26] reported it in 4.6% in 1984.

Althaus & Sundmacher[22] studied the incidence of pars planitis from a mixed-patient population of private practitioners in hospital-based clinics, rather than from a uveitis referral center. Pars planitis was diagnosed in 25% of patients in this group. The male-to-female ratio was 2:1, and the average age at time of diagnosis was 9.3 years. Significantly, despite this difference in the clinical setting, the epidemiologic results were remarkably similar to those previously published.

Although pars planitis has been better characterized over the past 25 years, it remains a frequently underdiagnosed cause of uveitis, especially in young adults.

CLINICAL FINDINGS

The major symptoms are floaters and hazy vision resulting from cells in the vitreous or if the macula is affected with CME. There is usually no pain, redness, or photophobia and rarely any sign of severe iridocyclitis. However, the first episode of pars planitis may be associated with a more severe and symptomatic iridocyclitis. Subsequent episodes have a more characteristic chronic course.

One eye only is usually symptomatic, although the fellow eye (even if asymptomatic) often has signs of disease, including cells in the vitreous cavity, a few cells in the aqueous, and possibly even low-grade CME. Occasionally, patients present with vitreous hemorrhage. This may be the case if there is neovascularization of the pars plana exudate, or snowbank. In one series, 14% of 118 patients experienced vitreous hemorrhage.[27] Children were more likely to experience vitreous hemorrhage (28%) than adults (6%), and vitreous hemorrhage was the presenting feature of pars planitis in eight of 40 children (20%) and one of 78 adults (1%).

Although the external eye is usually quiet, there may well be small white keratic precipitates but usually no more than 1+ flare or cells in the anterior chamber. As a rule the pupil dilates well, but a few synechiae may form. Most of the signs are in the vitreous cavity, where there are numerous snowball opacities, cells, and debris; these are best seen with a direct ophthalmoscope or slit lamp. Posterior vitreous detachments are common. The snowball opacities are, for the most part, preretinal and concentrated inferiorly.

The retina may have a patchy peripheral periphlebitis. There may also be peripapillary retinal edema and CME, which is the most common cause of decreased vision[9,10,28] (Fig. 95-1). Exudate over the pars plana in the form of an inferiorly located snowbank is the hallmark of the disease (Fig. 95-2). However, this may not be present in all cases.[29] Although some evidence of all these signs is usually found in the symptomatic eye, similar signs may also be present in the asymptomatic eye at the time of the initial examination. Therefore a careful examination of the fellow eye should always be performed in cases of clinically symptomatic uveitis in any eye.

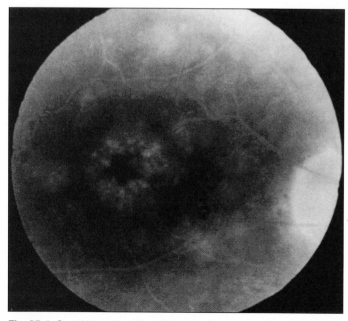

Fig. 95-1 Cystoid macular edema is the most common cause of decreased vision in pars planitis (late-phase angiogram).

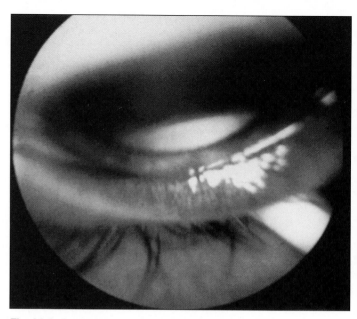

Fig. 95-2 Exudate over the pars plana, seen here during scleral depression, is the most characteristic clinical feature of pars planitis.

COURSE AND PROGNOSIS

Brockhurst and associates[4] divided their pars planitis patients into five groups depending on severity of the disease, with 28% having a benign course, 46% with a chronic, smoldering form, 12% who developed choroidal and retinal detachments without retinal breaks, 6% who underwent a malignant course with development of organizing membranes and exudate in the vitreous cavity, and 8% who developed occlusion of peripheral retinal veins with posterior progression and eventual optic atrophy. The complications of peripheral anterior and posterior synechiae, glaucoma, posterior capsule cataracts, and macular degeneration occurred most frequently in the most severe forms of pars planitis.

Welch et al.[5] described seven patients with exudates over the inferior pars plana and occasional obliteration of vessels of the ora serrata; 22 other patients had a more chronic, diffuse inflammatory form in which these authors discerned clouding of the vitreous base as evidence of old chorioretinitis. CME occurred in 82% of the patients in this latter group.

Kimura & Hogan[26] and Smith et al.[10] classified patients in their studies into those with mild, moderate, and severe forms of pars planitis (chronic cyclitis) on the basis of the amount of vitreous cells and debris seen on examination. They also described three characteristic patterns that the disease seemed to follow. Kimura & Hogan[12] reviewed 136 cases, 71 of which were bilateral; 43% were the mild form, 46% moderate, and 11% severe. Of the patients with pars planitis for more than 1 year, 51% had visual acuity of better than or equal to 20/30. The authors found that a decrease in visual acuity correlated well with severity of disease at onset and with duration. Of their patients, 44% had loss of vision to 20/200 or worse because of complications of the pars planitis.

In the review by Smith et al.[10] of 100 cases, 73% had bilateral disease at onset; 19% exhibited a mild form of inflammation, 42% had moderate inflammation, and 39% had severe inflammation. Follow-up ranged from 4 to 26 years (mean, 10.5 years). Of those with a mild form at initial examination, 6% cleared, 30% remained the same, and 64% worsened on follow-up. Of those with the moderate form, 41% improved, 44% remained the same, and 8% worsened, and in 7% the authors were unsure whether or how the inflammation had changed. Of those with a severe form, 83% improved, 12% remained the same, and 2% worsened, and in 3% the authors were unsure if the inflammation had changed.

Chester et al.[13] examined 51 patients, 41 (80%) of whom had bilateral involvement. In their study, in which follow-up ranged from 1 month to 20 years (average, 20 years), vision was 20/40 or better at onset in 74% of the patients; 86% of these had no further loss of vision.

In the long-term follow-up study by Smith et al.,[10] when the interim history of the 182 eyes in this series was analyzed, it became apparent that the pars planitis ran three patterns of disease: (1) a self-limiting course characterized by gradual improvement without a single episode of exacerbation of the low-grade activity; 10% of eyes fell into this category; (2) a prolonged course without exacerbations; 59% of the eyes were in this category; (3) a chronic, smoldering course with one or more episodes of exacerbation of the inflammation; 31% of the eyes were in this category. The actual natural course of chronic cyclitis was difficult to assess in this report (and in other series as well) because almost 95% of the patients had received some type of corticosteroid therapy.[10] Despite this limitation, however, the trends of a self-limited, benign course (pattern 1), a prolonged smoldering course (pattern 2), and a course with multiple exacerbations (pattern 3) emerge. Regardless of the type of course, most of the eyes improved or remained unchanged in terms of visual acuity. The prognosis for good vision related primarily to less severe inflammation and absence of CME rather than to duration. Although cataracts were the most common complication related to duration of disease, cataract surgery was well tolerated, and good visual acuity was usually restored if the macula was in good condition.[9,10,30] Resultant CME and degeneration, on the other hand, were irreversible. In the study of 173 eyes, with a minimum of 4 years' duration of disease, the visual prognosis was found to be ultimately very good, with a majority of patients maintaining vision of 20/50 or better; 73% maintained driving vision, while legal blindness (20/200 or worse) resulted in only 6%. The major cause of vision less than 20/40 was macular damage.

Most series reporting the course and complications of pars planitis have originated in uveitis referral centers, and this raises the issue of a selection bias. A recent study from the Leicester Royal Infirmary, UK,[31] reviewed all cases known to have originated in one English county. This was thought to be more representative of a general ophthalmology practice. Of 86 eyes of 48 patients, with a mean follow-up of 48 months, the principal threat to sight was CME (31%). Other complications included vitreous hemorrhage (8%), disc swelling (5%), periphlebitis (21%), and cataract (5%). Most patients required no treatment other than observation, and the overall visual outcome was good in 85% of patients. Sixty-three percent of eyes had vision of 6/9 or better. As with studies originating from uveitis referral centers, CME and snowbanking were significantly associated with worse visual outcome, whereas the other previously mentioned complications were not.

Boke[32] classified pars planitis on the basis of clinical presentation. The diffuse inflammatory type was characterized by dust-like opacities in the vitreous, most prominent inferiorly. Although snowball-like precipitates within the vitreous may be present and eventually overlay the ora serrata region of the retina, as well as the pars plana at the ciliary body, massive snowbank-like exudates were not seen. Slezak[33] has further divided this category into a serous form and an infiltrative form. While the former leaves the pars plana entirely uninvolved, the latter demonstrates small gray or yellow spots within the pars plana. Both types may progress to the exudative type.

The exudative type is characterized by a heavy and confluent exudate over the pars plana and ora serrata, and the exudates and snowball-like precipitates in the vitreous space are more severe than in the diffuse type. The heavy exudates covering the extreme periphery of the fundus may radiate in a finger-like manner toward the center of the vitreous cavity. If there is posterior vitreous detachment, the exudates may be present along the posterior surface of the vitreous or the peripheral retina, but they rarely reach the posterior surface of the lens. The vasoproliferative type is characterized by vascular changes. Marked sheathing, perivascular cuffing, and partial occlusion of the peripheral retinal vessels may be observed in both the diffuse inflammatory type and the exudative type. However, in the vasoproliferative type, these findings occur early in the course of the disease and may be particularly severe. Fine, new vessels may grow within the vitreous space (intrabasal) or outside the vitreous space (juxtabasal).

The significance of pars planitis in childhood uveitis deserves special emphasis. A 1996 study found that pars planitis occurred in 15.3% of patients seen at a referral center for childhood uveitis.[34] The mean age of onset was 9.9 years.

The authors emphasized the difficulty in diagnosis of uveitis in children and particularly in distinguishing various forms of childhood uveitis, such as juvenile rheumatoid arthritis, idiopathic uveitis, and pars planitis. The most frequent complication of pars planitis was maculopathy, which occurred in 55% of patients. The final visual acuity was less than 20/200 in 10.5% of patients with pars planitis. Most disturbing and unexpected in this study was the prevalence of poor vision at the time of first referral. Of all patients with childhood uveitis, 26% of eyes had visual acuity of less than 20/200 when the patients were first referred to this tertiary care center. In 26 of 37 eyes with a follow-up of at least 6 months, irreversible damage to the eye had already occurred, and vision could not be improved. The authors concluded that increased awareness by pediatricians, rheumatologists, and ophthalmologists of the seriousness of ocular complications of uveitis in childhood should lead to earlier diagnosis and more effective treatment regimens in the future.[34]

PATHOGENESIS AND PATHOLOGY

The cause of pars planitis remains unknown; no organisms have been observed in the few pathologic specimens available, and extensive laboratory studies in many patients have been inconclusive.[4,5,10,12,35]

Histopathologic studies have been done only on eyes with advanced pars planitis, and no eyes have been examined histologically in the acute phase of the disease. Brockhurst et al.[14] noted the presence of a cyclitic membrane with focal areas of choroiditis involving the peripheral choroid in two eyes they examined microscopically. Other studies have shown only minimal inflammatory reaction in the uvea, consisting of mild perivascular lymphoid infiltration.[36] Kimura & Hogan[12] reported a case that showed a fibrous exudate involving the vitreous base and covering the ciliary body; the peripheral retinal vessels showed thickened, hyalinized walls. Green et al.[35] examined seven enucleated eyes with long-standing pars planitis. These showed "primarily collapsed vitreous with fibrous organization at the vitreous base, mild chronic inflammatory cells in the vitreous, preretinal membranes, and signs of retinal inflammation, including phlebitis, periphlebitis, and edema of the optic nerve head and macula. By contrast, there was minimal inflammation of the uveal tract or none."[35] These authors also analyzed vitreous aspirates that had been obtained during earlier stages of the disease to remove vitreous opacities or preretinal membranes. Examination of these aspirates showed that "proliferating cells in the collapsed vitreous base are fibrous astrocytes producing new collagen ... and that the fluff balls [snowballs] in the vitreous are composed of intact and degenerative macrophages."[35]

Wetzig and associates[37] studied an eye that had previously undergone pars plana lensectomy or vitrectomy and retinal detachment repair. They described a thick layer of fibrous-like tissue covering the base of the ciliary body and pars plana. This consisted of a moderate amount of lymphocytic infiltration. Other manifestations of chronic inflammation may have been due to the previous surgical intervention. Eichenbaum and associates[38] have described an autopsy eye that had chronic nongranulomatous inflammation of the vitreous base, chronic inflammatory cell infiltrate of the ciliary body, occasional pigment-laden macrophages, retinal perivasculitis, and a fibrovascular membrane over the epithelium of the pars plana. Yoser et al.[39] reported an evisceration specimen that demonstrated organization of the vitreous space with the presence of tractional retinal detachment and a vitreous snowbank composed of organized collagen, fibroblasts, nonpigmented ciliary epithelium, and lymphocytic infiltration. Multiple blood vessels were seen within the fibrous tissue. The pars plana region revealed a proliferation of nonpigmented ciliary epithelium, neovascularization, and lymphocytic infiltration; the peripheral choroid also showed focal lymphocytic infiltration. The retinal pigment epithelium at the periphery showed focal hyperplasia, and extensive gliosis with focal perivascular lymphocytic infiltration was noted in the detached retina. Electron microscopic study revealed high endothelial venules in the region of the pars plana. The authors suggested that such endothelial cells may play a role in the lymphocytic traffic by attachment and migration through the vessel wall into the extra-cellular milieu. The presence of such endothelial cells within the fibrous organization at the pars plana may suggest a role for these cells in the inflammatory process, as well as in the recruitment of cells at the site of the pars plana exudate. The authors also speculated that the beneficial effects of cryotherapy may be due to the destruction of such endothelial cells.

Various theories based on known immunopathologic data obtained from pars planitis patients have been advanced. Pars planitis may represent an immune-mediated response, but the antigenic stimulus remains speculative. Rahi & Addison[40] have proposed a theory of autoimmunity to outer retinal layers as the cause of pars planitis. Animal models with pars plana snowbank exudates have been described: Hultsch[41] produced these findings in owl monkeys by multiple intravitreal injections of hyaluronic acid. Zimmerman & Silverstein[42] used injections of crystalline egg albumin into the vitreous to produce uveitis and snowball opacities in rabbits.

Gartner[43] examined eyes that had been enucleated for retinal or uveal tumors and found many vitreous cortex cells throughout the vitreous base, which were especially prominent in the inferior vitreous. He also described the presence of other cellular remnants in various stages of involution and attributed these to remnants of the primary vitreous. Fragments of basement membrane were also present in the vitreous of a 9-month-old infant's eye that he examined histologically. These basement membrane fragments may represent remnants of the former hyaloid system, and he postulated that these breakdown products may be the antigenic stimulus in pars planitis.

Kaplan et al.[44,45] analyzed the type of inflammatory cells present in the vitreous of two pars planitis patients who had undergone vitrectomy. These patients had a small number of T lymphocytes in the vitreous, compared with a large number of B lymphocytes. Another patient, who underwent anterior chamber paracentesis, showed a marked decrease in the number of T cells and a marked increase in the number of macrophages in the aqueous when compared with those in the peripheral blood. Belfort et al.[46] have made similar observations. Kaplan et al.[45] postulated that "intraocular T-cell immunoregulation of B-cell function may be defective in some stages of chronic idiopathic uveitis," including pars planitis.

Toledo de Abreu[47] and Nussenblatt[48] and their colleagues found decreased helper-to-suppressor T-cell ratios in the aqueous and peripheral blood of uveitis patients, including patients with pars planitis. Although these are interesting findings, their significance remains unknown.

Yokoyama et al.[49] have also studied cellular and humoral imprints in pars planitis patients, but with inconclusive results. Aaberg[50] observed that peripheral neovascularization in the area of the pars plana exudate may be important in the inflammatory process. He recommended ablative procedures to eliminate neovascularization in this area and possibly also to eliminate the associated ischemic peripheral retinal tissue. Elimination of neovascular tissue, in his experience, seems to reduce pars plana exudate accumulation and shorten the chronic phase of the disease.

Khodadoust et al.[51] suggested an autoimmune etiology based on the appearance of rows of keratic precipitates, suggestive of an immune line on the corneal endothelium. This hypothesis was challenged, however, in a letter by Tessler.[52]

Davis and colleagues[53] have suggested a two-stage process for the pathophysiology of pars planitis. The first stage is postulated to be immunologically mediated; the second, a nonspecific breakdown of intraocular regulatory mechanisms resulting in chronic eye disease. The authors further postulated that if pars planitis is indeed under immunologic control throughout its course, it may not necessarily be autoimmune. Rather than a self-antigen, the target antigen could be an exogenous viral or bacterial antigen. Ocular borreliosis of Lyme disease has been thought to cause a syndrome much like pars planitis.[54] Although animal models of experimental autoimmune uveitis have demonstrated that the eye can be a target of pathologic immune reactions, a relevant model of pars planitis has not been found. The immunization of primates with interphotoreceptor retinoid-binding protein (IRBP) produces some of the features of intermediate uveitis, such as prominent vascular leakage, but the retinal and choroidal inflammatory infiltrates are quite different.[55] Snowball-like opacities of the vitreous over the pars plana were induced by repeated injections of hyaluronic acid in owl monkeys,[41] and similar vitreitis and snowball opacities have been found to develop when albumin is injected into the vitreous cavity.[42] This study suggests that these clinical findings may be a nonantigen-specific response of the eye. Davis et al.[53] postulate that the immunology of intermediate uveitis involves an escape from regulatory control of helper T cells directed against a vitreoretinal antigen or antigens that remain to be identified. The clinical manifestations of pars planitis represent subsequent nonspecific retinal and vitreous inflammation. Certain patients may have a genetic susceptibility to the initiating event, as perhaps demonstrated by human leukocyte antigen (HLA) association.[56] Other pathogenetic mechanisms, such as anterior chamber-associated immune deviation[57] and antiretinal autoantibodies,[58] may also have a role in the pathogenesis of pars planitis.

Nussenblatt et al.[59] also suggested that pars planitis might somehow be related to demyelination; certainly some forms of uveitis are associated with multiple sclerosis.

The association of pars planitis with systemic manifestation has received much recent attention. HLA-DR15 serotyping has identified a subset of patients with pars planitis who may have a systemic association as well as distinct clinical features.[60] Thirteen of 18 patients (72%) were positive for HLA-DR15. The frequency was significantly higher than for controlled subjects. Each of four patients tested carried the specific allele DR B1 *1501, which has been associated with multiple sclerosis. In the HLA-DR15-positive group were four patients (31%) with coexisting multiple sclerosis or optic neuritis, one patient with coexisting narcolepsy, and three patients (23%) with a family history of multiple sclerosis. Retinal periphlebitis, especially if bilateral, was frequently associated with HLA-DR15-positive pars planitis (61%). In this study, 46% of HLA-15-positive patients demonstrated no snowbank formation; conversely, snowbank formations were seen in HLA-DR15-negative pars planitis. Therefore the finding of snowbank formation is not specific for HLA-DR15-positive pars planitis.

Other recent studies have associated pars planitis with HLA class II alleles DR15,[61,62] DR51,[61] and DR17.[61] HLA-A28 has also been associated with pars planitis and an increased prevalence of arthralgias and hypocomplementemia.[63] Not surprisingly, familial associations with pars planitis and other inheritable systemic and ocular conditions have been described. A report has described pars planitis in two sisters, one of whom had evidence of demyelinating disease at presentation,[64] and another report has described a family with dominantly inherited optic atrophy in which the father and one of two sons have also had pars planitis.[65]

For the first time, a potential pathogenic association between a purifiable protein and active pars planitis has been described.[66] The levels of a 36 kDa protein (p-36) were found to be six to eight times higher in 81% of patients with active pars planitis than in controls. Furthermore, the levels of this protein correlated with disease activity. The biologic function of this circulating protein is not known. The authors concluded that, although it is possible that high levels of this protein and active pars planitis may simply be the consequence of inflammation and tissue damage, this is unlikely because patients with ocular tissue damage from other causes, such as proliferative diabetic retinopathy after panretinal photocoagulation or glaucoma after a cyclodestructive procedure, do not have high levels of this protein.[66] Therefore the authors suggest that the 36 kDa circulating protein may have an etiologic role in pars planitis. This 36 kDa protein has been cloned and sequenced.[67] The DNA-deduced amino acid sequence revealed a high degree of similarity with nup100, a yeast nucleopore complex protein; the entire primary amino acid sequence of p-36 is 96.8% similar to the carboxy-terminal domain of nup100, and the overall amino acid identity is 88%. The authors suggest that p-36 is a nucleoporin-like protein and therefore referred to this protein as nup36. Southern blot analysis of human genomic DNA gave a simple hybridization pattern, suggesting that the p-36 gene is most likely present as a single copy per haploid genome and has a multiple gene structure; that is, it is encoded by a gene with few introns.[67] Protein nup36 may be an evolutionarily conserved nuclear pore complex-like protein present in increased levels in the circulation of patients with active pars planitis. If this association is confirmed by future studies, then measuring blood levels of nup36 may not only aid in the diagnosis of pars planitis, but also may be of value in monitoring disease activity and in guiding treatment.

COMPLICATIONS OF CHRONIC CYCLITIS

In a series of 100 patients, with a follow-up ranging from 4 years to more than 20 years (median and mean, 10.5 years), the complications of 182 eyes were studied.[30] The most common complication was cataract formation, which occurred in 42% of the eyes, then CME changes in the macula in 28%, followed in order of decreasing incidence by band keratopathy, glaucoma, retinal detachment, retinoschisis, vitreous hemorrhage, "retinitis pigmentosa" changes, and dragged disc vessels.

The major causes of visual morbidity in pars planitis at the time of the initial examination were macular edema (60% of the eyes) and vitreous opacities (39% of the eyes). At the time of the final examination, an average of 10 years later, macular disease accounted for 74% of patients with vision less than 20/40, while only 9% of patients with similar decreased vision had loss resulting from vitreous opacity (Table 95-1). However, 20% of patients had cataracts or had undergone lens extractions. Macular edema and resultant macular degeneration are therefore the most frequent and serious complications of pars planitis.[30,35,68]

Clinically, early macular edema appears as a loss of the foveal reflex with a wet appearance to the posterior pole and numerous glistening highlights reflected from the irregularly thickened, edematous retina. Cystoid macular changes similar to those associated with the Irvine–Gass postcataract syndrome and other forms of severe uveitis frequently ensue in the later stages of chronic edema. Fluorescein angiography reveals early leakage from small parafoveal capillaries into adjacent retinal tissue during the late stages of the fluorescein passage (Fig. 95-1). Often, abnormal leakage from multiple areas is seen throughout the fundus, including the far periphery.[7,68] Serous elevations of the neuroepithelium or pigment epithelium are rarely encountered. Involvement of the peripapillary retina frequently gives the appearance of papilledema. It is not surprising that CME is a common finding in pars planitis, since it is seen in many clinical situations associated with breakdown of the blood–retinal barriers.[69,70]

If macular edema persists for several months, chronic macular changes develop, with resultant permanent impairment of central vision; the degree of impairment reflects the severity of the changes. Alterations in the pigment epithelium, with dispersion, clumping, and patchy loss of pigment, are the clinical findings in such maculae. Fluorescein leakage is not invariably present in these cases, but multiple pigment epithelium window defects are observed. The macular changes in chronic cyclitis are not unique to this syndrome but, rather, are the final common pathway of late macular edema seen in a variety of ocular syndromes.

Heavy vitreous reaction and the presence[71] and extent[28] of the pars plana exudate seem to be evidence of severity of the disease process and appear to predispose to the development of macular edema. However, many eyes with minimal vitreous reaction develop symptomatic macular edema, demonstrating that the severity of vitreous reaction alone is not a reliable forecast for the development of macular disease.

Of importance to the clinician managing patients with chronic cyclitis is the finding that vitreous opacities were responsible for the visual loss in only 9% of all eyes with visual acuity of 6/12 (20/40) or less 10 years after the onset of disease (Table 95-1). This compares to 74% of visually impaired eyes that had poor acuity caused by macular changes. Vitreous cells, floaters, and opacities gradually disappear or become less important clinically over time, whereas macular edema may lead to chronic, permanent macular changes even when the disease process is inactive. Furthermore, the uniformly good functional results in eyes that did not develop macular complications implicate macular disease as the most important factor in determining the prognosis.[10,28,71]

Cataract formation is a frequent complication of any chronic inflammatory process, including pars planitis.[4,5,36] Eyes with increased evidence of vitreous disease and a prolonged course tend to develop more cataracts. However, the role of corticosteroids must not be overlooked. In several cases the development and progression of lens opacities appear to be related to the use of these drugs. Despite their frequent appearance, however, most cataracts did not affect visual function.[30] The opacities were considered dense enough to have caused visual acuity of 6/12 (20/40) or less in only 6% of eyes initially, and in 19% of eyes at the final examination (Table 95-1). Surgery was performed on 20 eyes, usually without complications and with visual results dependent on macular function.[10,30]

The use of an intraocular lens in patients with pars planitis and subsequent chronic iridocyclitis remains controversial. One report concluded that, given the confines of a limited study, it is probably safe to place an intraocular lens in patients with uveitis.[71] However, it has been pointed out that nearly a third of patients in whom an intraocular lens is implanted may have a poor visual outcome.[73] Until a large and definitive study is concluded, a general rule of thumb may be only to consider an intraocular lens implantation if uveitis has been quiescent with or without medication for several weeks or months. We suggest the use of an all-polymethyl-methacrylate (PMMA) lens in uveitis patients and discourage the use of a silicone lens, which, in our experience, tends to lead to poor vision as a result of pigmentary deposition on the lens itself. The newer acrylic lenses may provide another alternative, although experience is limited.

Glaucoma is probably not a complication of the disease per se, but rather the result of vigorous corticosteroid therapy or of a surgical procedure such as cataract extraction.[2] Corticosteroid therapy was probably responsible for increased intraocular pressure in 11 of the 15 affected eyes in this series; cataract extraction caused glaucoma in two other eyes.

Retinal detachment occurred less frequently in our series (22%)[30] than the 51% reported by Brockhurst and associates.[4,74] The retina specialization of the latter group and the patients referred probably account for the marked difference in the incidence of this complication. The repair and prognosis of such detachments have been well described.[74] Vitreous traction secondary to long-standing vitreous inflammation, band formation, and subsequent retinal hole formation probably account for most retinal detachments.[74]

Table 95-1 Causes of decreased visual acuity of 6/12 (20/40) or less at first and final examinations

	No. of eyes	Macular disease	Lens opacities	Vitreous opacities
First examination	70	42 (60%)	4 (6%)	27 (39%)
Final examination	69	51 (74%)	13 (19%)	6 (9%)

Reproduced from Smith RE, Godfrey WA, Kimura SJ. Chronic cyclitis. I. Course and visual prognosis. Trans Am Acad Ophthalmol Otolaryngol 1973; 77:760–768.[10]

Vitreous hemorrhage in chronic cyclitis has been described as a complication occurring in 3% to 14% of patients.[15,27,30] Neovascularization of the inferiorly situated exudate in the ora serrata region has been proposed as the possible cause of such hemorrhage.[15,49] Vitreous hemorrhages usually clear with no complications.

Retinal vessels leaving the disc margin with displacement of the macula occurred in two of our patients, probably as a result of peripheral vitreous traction bands.[30] Chronic cyclitis must be considered, along with retrolental fibroplasia, ocular *Toxocara canis*, Coats disease, and familial exudative vitreoretinopathy, in the differential diagnosis of heterotopia of the macula.

Bone-spicule pigmentation, resembling retinitis pigmentosa, which has been reported as an unusual complication of chronic cyclitis, developed in two eyes in our series.[2] The extensive reaction in the pigment epithelium in such cases suggests a diffuse inflammatory process as a possible cause of chronic cyclitis. Electroretinograms were normal.

SNOWBANKS AND THE DIAGNOSIS OF PARS PLANITIS: SIGNIFICANCE OF PARS PLANA EXUDATE

The diagnosis of pars planitis is established on the basis of the characteristic clinical findings outlined earlier, which usually include the presence of a pars plana exudate or snowbank inferiorly (Fig. 95-2). An important and frequently asked question is: does this diagnosis require the presence of a pars plana exudate (snowbank)? Although many cases present with bilateral exudates, some cases may have a classic pars plana exudate in one eye but only vitreous cells in the other eye (24% of cases).[71] Even more difficult to assess are cases wherein the findings are very similar to those seen in the classically described pars planitis (e.g., with minimal or no anterior chamber reaction, the presence of cells in the vitreous with vitreous snowballs, and peripheral periphlebitis), but without any evidence of a pars plana exudate on scleral depression. In our studies reported by Henderly et al.,[71,75] groups of patients were identified who had a pars plana exudate in one eye but only vitreous inflammatory cells, debris, and other clinical signs of pars planitis in the other eye. The second eye certainly could be assumed to be undergoing the same pathologic process and was therefore considered a case of "pars planitis," albeit without a snowbank.

The presence[71] or extent[28] of a snowbank and pars planitis was associated with more advanced or more severe vitreous inflammatory disease and the presence of CME. Although the differences between eyes with snowbanks and those without snowbanks were not statistically significant, probably because of the small sample size, there was a trend toward milder vitritis, better visual acuity, less CME, fewer vitreous snowballs, and less periphlebitis in eyes without a snowbank.[71] The presence of a pars plana exudate correlated with more severe vitritis and more CME. The findings therefore suggested that the presence of a snowbank in pars planitis is associated with more advanced or more severe ocular inflammatory disease. However, this was not always the case, since many eyes with pars plana exudate

had excellent vision and no CME.[71] Eyes with pars planitis but lacking the characteristic snowbank may suffer from a mild or early form of the disease that may or may not progress eventually to the snowbank phase. Since some eyes obviously have the pars planitis syndrome but do not have an exudate over the pars plana, an extension of this argument contends that some patients will have many of the signs of pars planitis but without a pars plana exudate in either eye.[75] We believe that these may indeed be cases of pars planitis and may be a milder or earlier form of the disease that may or may not eventually progress to development of the classic snowbank. These pars planitis "variants"[75] show slightly less severe clinical findings of the same basic disease process.

DIFFERENTIAL DIAGNOSIS

Pars planitis falls into the category of "vitreitis" in terms of approaching the differential diagnosis. Among the variety of conditions in which vitreous cells and opacities may be prominent, clinical features are listed in Box 94-1.

CME after cataract extraction (the Irvine–Gass syndrome) is the condition most often associated with cells and opacities in the vitreous. A slightly irritated eye is not unusual in these cases, but no other postoperative ocular inflammation is expected. The possibility that the cells reach the vitreous cavity from an active source of retinitis must also be considered in the differential diagnosis, and toxoplasmic retinochoroiditis must always be ruled out.

Vitreous cells are sometimes a secondary feature of vasculitis associated with Behçet's disease or with a collagen-vascular disease. Sarcoid (with or without significant anterior disease) may, in fact, show no sign of disease other than cells in the vitreous cavity. In masquerade syndromes caused by choroidal malignant melanoma or diffuse ocular reticulum cell sarcoma, vitreous cells may be present in eyes that are otherwise quiet, although other retinal and choroidal changes of reticulum cell sarcoma or melanoma are usually present.

Box 95-1 Eye conditions associated with cells in the vitreous cavity

Pars planitis (chronic cyclitis, peripheral uveitis)
Postcataract extraction with cystoid macular edema (Irvine–Gass syndrome)
Sarcoidosis
Amyloidosis
Active retinitis
Active retinal vasculitis
Trauma (recent)
Spillover from iridocyclitis
Masquerade syndrome (e.g., reticulum cell sarcoma)
Retinal detachment or tear
Whipple's disease
Lyme disease

Reproduced from Smith RE and Nozik R. Uveitis: a clinical approach to diagnosis and management. Baltimore: Williams & Wilkins; 1983.[9]

If the predominant clinical signs are cells and opacities in the vitreous cavity, and if there is no significant anterior chamber disease or retinitis, the cause of the vitreitis can usually be assigned to one of the syndromes listed in Box 94-1. However, cells may spill back into the vitreous cavity from any acute, severe iridocyclitis. It is not uncommon, for example, for patients with acute iridocyclitis associated with ankylosing spondylitis to have significant numbers of cells in the vitreous cavity.

If a snowbank exudate is present in a relatively quiet eye, with associated vitreous cells and perivenous sheathing, there is very little doubt of the diagnosis of pars planitis. In less characteristic cases, the mild peripheral uveitis associated with systemic diseases such as multiple sclerosis, in which mild peripheral uveitis occurs in as many as 20% of cases,[18] must be considered. Sarcoidosis must be ruled out, but many of these patients have an associated granulomatous iridocyclitis, which is uncommon in patients with pars planitis. The peripheral form of ocular toxocariasis is usually unilateral, and the peripheral granulomatous type of exudate is usually not located inferiorly. Toxocariasis is also found in younger patients than is pars planitis.

Behçet's syndrome has a more severe occlusion of the retinal vessels than does pars planitis with vasculitis and reduced vision. In Behçet's syndrome, there is no exudation of the pars plana, and there is often a characteristic recurrent hypopyon not found in pars planitis. Although vitreous cells occur in many types of ocular inflammation associated with retinitis – toxoplasmic retinochoroiditis, candidal retinochoroiditis, and cytomegalic inclusion disease retinitis are classic examples – these diseases have obvious retinal involvement and sometimes affect only one eye. There should be no serious problem with differentiating pars planitis from any form of retinitis.

In Fuchs' heterochromic cyclitis, which is primarily an iridocyclitis, a few cells are present in the vitreous cavity, and there may be some CME. However, this disease is unilateral, and there is a characteristic loss of the architectural structure of the iris on the side with definite or incipient heterochromia, none of which is a feature of pars planitis.

In a case report, a 21-year-old woman with bilateral mild vitreitis, retinal vasculitis, and exudates over the pars plana, who was thought to have pars planitis, was found to have cat-scratch disease caused by *Rochalimaea* species.[76] These are Gram-negative bacilli that have been found to be positive in 88% of patients with cat-scratch disease. The diagnosis is based on clinical findings, history of exposure to cats, and a positive serologic indirect immunofluorescent antibody test for *Rochalimaea* species. The patient was treated with 500 mg of oral ciprofloxacin hydrochloride twice daily for 14 days and improved. Therefore cat-scratch disease should also be considered in the differential diagnosis of pars planitis.[76]

Lyme disease, which has been suspected of having protean ophthalmic manifestations, is reported to cause iridocyclitis and vitreitis and therefore must be considered in the differential diagnosis of pars planitis.[54] However, since the majority of patients with Lyme disease may be unaware of the bite of the tiny tick, and since many patients do not have a history of erythema migrans, and since the variability of serologic testing can often result in seronegative Lyme disease, various other criteria have been used in establishing the diagnosis.

Polymerase chain reaction for *Borrelia burgdorferi* infection on vitreous fluid has been described in establishing the diagnosis of Lyme disease in a patient whose serum enzyme-linked immunosorbent assay (ELISA), Venereal Disease Research Laboratory (VDRL), and Mantoux tests were nonreactive and the serum immunoglobulin G immunoblot for Lyme disease showed faint reactivity.[77]

The US Centers for Disease Control and Prevention made Lyme disease reportable in 1982, and the current definition of a case of Lyme disease consists of any of the following:

- a patient who develops erythema migrans within 30 days of exposure in an endemic area
- a patient exposed to an endemic area who does not have erythema migrans but who does have signs of involvement of one organ system and a positive laboratory test
- a patient with a history of exposure but with erythema migrans as well as involvement of two organ systems
- a patient without exposure in an endemic area, but with erythema migrans and a positive serology

DIAGNOSTIC TESTS

There are no specific laboratory studies that establish the diagnosis of pars planitis. Rather, certain studies are important to rule out specific conditions that mimic the pars planitis pattern of clinical disease: serum lysozyme, angiotensin-converting enzyme, and chest radiographic studies help rule out sarcoidosis; tuberculin skin test and radiographic examination for tuberculosis; fluorescent treponemal antibody absorption test (FTA-ABS) or monoclonal antibody-*Treponema pallidum* for syphilis; and Lyme ELISA and indirect immunofluorescence antibody for Lyme disease. A fluorescein angiogram is probably the most important laboratory study to be performed, since the presence of CME is a guide to therapy. Electrophysiologic testing has been a useful adjunct in some clinicians' experience, but we do not use it.[78]

Ultrasound biomicroscopy is a relatively new diagnostic tool that functions at 50 MHz and has an axial resolution approximately 10 times that of standard ultrasound, with a depth of penetration of 5 mm. A 17-year-old boy whose conventional ultrasonography showed multiple vitreous membrane and in whom the pars plana and peripheral retina could not be imaged was found to have pars planitis on the basis of ultrasound biomicroscopy, which showed a homogeneous mass of medium reflectivity in the inferior pars plana and adjacent retina, believed to be snowbanking.[79] This was subsequently confirmed by a lensectomy and vitrectomy procedure.

TREATMENT

Various therapeutic regimens have been employed in patients with pars planitis. Although corticosteroids have been the mainstay of therapy and have been recommended even in early reports of this entity,[12,20] no controlled clinical trials have been performed to document the clinical impressions.

The use of immunosuppressive and cytotoxic agents has been reported by some investigators. A limited amount of success has been ascribed to the use of these potentially dangerous drugs.[80–82] In a series of six patients treated with tacrolimus (FK506) who were refractory to ciclosporin, five of six showed a visual acuity improvement of two or more Snellen lines. Five of six patients had side-effects, including abdominal pain, tremor, and paresthesias, but none required discontinuation of the medication.[83] A larger series of 28 patients refractory to conventional therapy examined the efficacy of chlorambucil.[84] Chlorambucil was discontinued in 25% of patients because of side-effects, including amenorrhea, gastrointestinal intolerance, infection, and progressive leukemia. Nineteen patients (68%) showed positive clinical response, and 43% had a visual acuity improvement. Systemic prednisone was successfully discontinued in 68% of patients and 50% (14 patients) were free of inflammation off systemic medication. The authors conclude that there exist effective alternative treatments, but that these are best reserved for intractable cases that fail to respond to corticosteroids.

Cryotherapy to the pars plana and peripheral retina has been performed, but the results are inconclusive, especially with reference to its effect on existing macular edema.[15,50]

In a retrospective review of therapy of 173 patients with pars planitis, Godfrey et al.[85] reported the findings in patients who had: (1) no therapy; (2) topical steroids only; (3) systemic steroids; or (4) periocular corticosteroids. Although the findings were inconclusive, the clinical impression was that corticosteroid therapy, especially when given by the periocular route, had a definite place in the management of patients with pars planitis if CME were present. However, corticosteroid therapy in these 173 eyes was associated with several complications, as noted in Table 95-2. These complications included not only glaucoma and cataract, but also a cushingoid appearance and other systemic side-effects of periocularly administered corticosteroids.

In a more recent study of the role of corticosteroids in pars planitis, Stoessel et al.[28] studied 40 eyes of 22 patients followed for an average of 36 months. Of these eyes, 21 (52.5%) had macular edema. The extent of pars plana exudate correlated with the presence of macular edema, as did peripheral venous sheathing and retinoschisis. The 21 eyes with severe disease and vision of less than 20/40 were treated with sub-Tenon's steroids or oral corticosteroids, or both; vision improved in 81% of these eyes and stabilized in 19%. No treated eyes worsened. Of the 19 untreated eyes, no eyes improved, whereas 68% were stable, and 32% worsened. Although the usual criticisms of a nonrandomized study could be leveled at this recent report, it was a prospective study, and the results showed an impressive trend of improved visual outcome in the steroid-treated eyes. Certainly, a controlled, randomized, prospective study seems to be warranted to determine whether this apparent visual improvement in steroid-treated eyes with pars planitis is truly significant. However, we agree with the authors of the Yale study[28] that a randomized controlled trial may never be done in pars planitis, given the history of the disease and the history of steroid therapy. All studies do point to a role for posterior sub-Tenon's steroids in eyes with pars planitis and visual loss to 20/40 or worse as a result of macular edema or severe vitreous inflammation.

This notion has been further supported by a study examining the effects of posterior sub-Tenon's injection of triamcinolone acetonide in patients with pars planitis.[86] Twenty consecutive patients were treated, with a median follow-up of 23.5 months. Snellen visual acuity improved by at least two lines in 12 (67%) of 18 patients who were examined after initial injection. Median time to improvement was 3 weeks. Patients with visual improvement had a median age of 29.0 years, compared with 41.5 years for nonresponders. There was a weak association between response to treatment and a history of not smoking, after correction for patient age. The increase in intraocular pressure occurred in six patients (30%), with onset at a median of 3 weeks after initial injection. The median interval to peak increase in intraocular pressure was 14 weeks after injection.[86]

In conclusion, factors associated with visual improvement are younger age and possibly a history of not smoking. Although sub-Tenon's steroid injections are effective, the higher than expected incidence of increased intraocular pressure is a concern. A previous study[29] has found that provocative testing with topical corticosteroids may not ensure that a patient will not develop

Table 95-2 Complications of corticosteroid therapy (173 eyes)		
Complications	No. of eyes	Percentage of eyes
Cataract*	76	44
Glaucoma	11	6
Cushingoid appearance	8	20
Other systemic effects of steroids†	4	10

*Relation to corticosteroid therapy is often unclear.
†Percentage of eyes treated in which complication occurred equals 100 multiplied by the number of eyes being treated in which this complication was noted and divided by the total number of eyes being treated with higher-dose corticosteroids.

glaucoma from repository corticosteroid injection. However, we continue to ask patients to use topical steroids four times a day for 2 weeks to see if the pressure rises. If not, we proceed with a sub-Tenon's steroid injection, taking care not to allow the steroid to migrate anteriorly. Posterior sub-Tenon's injections of corticosteroids are less likely to produce glaucoma than anterior sub-Tenon's injections.[29] The ophthalmologist should monitor intraocular pressure very closely for several months after a sub-Tenon's steroid injection and, during the informed consent, warn the patient that increased intraocular pressure may be a side-effect. This procedure may be relatively contraindicated in patients with concurrent glaucoma or patients who are known to be steroid responders.

Orbital floor steroid injection in the treatment of pars planitis has been described as an alternative to sub-Tenon's steroid injection to reduce the risk of globe perforation.[87] The therapeutic response in all cases of uveitis was 48%. However, any particular injection was not predictive of the response to subsequent or even preceding injections. This may be due to the variability of dispersion of steroids from the region of the orbital floor.[87] Systemic steroids may be helpful in some eyes with severe inflammation.

Four-step approach to therapy

For practical day-to-day management of pars planitis patients, we use a four-step approach to therapy, similar to that described by Kaplan.[88] In patients whose visual acuity has dropped to 20/40 or worse, or in those whose visual acuity is better than 20/40 but who have severe floaters, corticosteroid therapy is used. In patients with unilateral involvement, treatment with periocular injections is preferred. This consists of monthly sub-Tenon's injections of a long-acting corticosteroid, usually 40 mg methylprednisolone acetate. In patients unable to tolerate the injections, or in patients with bilateral involvement, oral prednisone is used. We start with a dose of 60 mg/day for 2 weeks, with a slow taper of 10 mg/week until the least amount of oral corticosteroid necessary to suppress the inflammation is achieved. High-dose pulsed intravenous corticosteroids may also be useful in desperate cases.

Patients who fail to respond to oral steroids or to sub-Tenon's corticosteroid injections may be treated with cryotherapy to the area of the snowbank[15,50,89]; retreatment may be necessary. Complications such as retinal detachment need to be considered. Cryotherapy is believed to decrease peripheral exudation and snowbanking by eliminating peripheral neovascularization.[90] If cryotherapy fails, a therapeutic pars plana vitrectomy is performed to remove inflammatory debris in the hope that this may reduce morbidity resulting from chronic macular edema.[88] If the inflammation continues to progress, the final step is the use of systemic antimetabolites.[91,92] Cyclophosphamide[93,94] and chlorambucil[80,95] have been used, but ciclosporin also appears to be effective with less systemic toxicity.[96] The choice of which antimetabolite to use is best determined by the experience of the internist or oncologist who has been consulted to help manage the therapy of the pars planitis patient who has not responded to all other forms of treatment.

Dugel and associates[97] studied 11 eyes of nine patients who underwent a standard three-port pars plana vitrectomy for CME and intraocular inflammation unresponsive to corticosteroids. Preoperative follow-up ranged from 20 to 144 months and averaged 70 months. Postoperative follow-up ranged from 3 to 108 months and averaged 21 months. Seven eyes (64%) improved four or more lines of Snellen acuity within 4 weeks. Two eyes (18%) remained unchanged, and two eyes (18%) worsened. CME improved by clinical examination and fluorescein angiography in nine eyes (82%) and by clinical examination alone in two eyes (18%). No intraoperative complications were noted. Postoperative complications consisted of cataract formation in one eye (9%), glaucoma in two eyes (18%), and epiretinal membrane formation in one eye (9%). However, of the six eyes with pars planitis, only three (50%) were among those that were classified as having improved. Therefore the role of pars plana vitrectomy for intraocular inflammation-related CME unresponsive to corticosteroids remains unclear.

The role of vitreoretinal surgery in pars planitis for indications other than CME has also been studied.[98] Forty-two eyes of 37 patients who underwent a pars plana vitrectomy for persistent floaters in the vitreous, persistent exacerbations of pars planitis, progressive visual loss, hypotony in the presence of cyclitic membranes, traction, or rhegmatogenous retinal detachment, and failure of intensive topical, periocular, and systemic corticosteroid therapy were evaluated. Overall, 75% of patients reached visual acuities of above 20/200; 80% of patients were satisfied with their results. The authors concluded that the best final visual results were achieved in eyes with the best preoperative visual acuity, shorter preoperative duration of pars planitis, and anatomic structural integrity.[98] After vitrectomy, recurrent exacerbations decreased, and corticosteroids were either discontinued or given at a low dose. The authors advocated vitrectomy for pars planitis if visual loss is progressive or prolonged or if topical, periocular, and systemic corticotherapy fails.[98]

Pars plana vitrectomy appears to be beneficial in pars planitis patients with nonclearing vitreous hemorrhage. In a small series, six eyes had a preoperative visual acuity of 20/200 or less. Postoperatively, five eyes improved to a final visual acuity (follow up 2 to 9 years) of 20/30 or better, and one eye improved to 20/100.[99]

In another small series, visual outcomes after pars plana vitrectomy for epiretinal membranes associated with pars planitis were studied.[100] All seven eyes were treated with varying forms of corticosteroids prior to surgery. Five eyes improved by three Snellen lines, one eye improved by one line, and one eye worsened by two lines. Six of seven eyes had progressive cataract development, four of which underwent cataract extraction. The authors concluded that removal of epiretinal membranes associated with pars planitis can be safely performed.

SUMMARY

Pars planitis is a disease whose cause remains unknown; neither histopathologic nor immunopathologic findings have established its pathogenesis. Although no treatment strategies have been proved effective, periocular or oral corticosteroids are recommended as initial therapy in patients with decreased vision and CME. Fortunately, many patients have a mild form of the disease and have a favorable prognosis despite years of active inflammation within the vitreous cavity.

ACKNOWLEDGMENT

This research was supported in part by the Heed Foundation Fellowship Award and the Ronald G. Michels Vitreoretinal Surgery Fellowship Award (Pravin U. Dugel, MD).

REFERENCES

1. Fuchs E. Textbook of ophthalmology (translated by A Duane). Philadelphia: JB Lippincott; 1908.
2. Duke-Elder WS. Textbook of ophthalmology, vol. 3. Diseases of the inner eye. St. Louis: Mosby; 1941.
3. Schepens CL. Examination of the ora serrata region: its clinical significance. Acta XVI Concilium Ophthalmologicum (Britannia). London: British Medical Association; 1950.
4. Brockhurst RJ, Schepens CL, Okamura ID. Uveitis. II. Peripheral uveitis: clinical description, complications, and differential diagnosis. Am J Ophthalmol 1960; 49:1257–1266.
5. Welch RB, Maumenee AE, Wahlen HE. Peripheral posterior segment inflammation, vitreous opacities, and edema of the posterior pole: pars planitis. Arch Ophthalmol 1960; 64:540–549.
6. Hogan MJ, Kimura SJ. Cyclitis and peripheral chorioretinitis. Arch Ophthalmol 1961; 66:667–677.
7. Gass JDM. Fluorescein angiography in endogenous intraocular inflammation. In: Aronson SB, ed. Clinical methods in uveitis. St. Louis: Mosby; 1968.
8. Bloch-Michel E, Nussenblatt RB. International Uveitis Study Group recommendations for the evaluation of intraocular inflammatory disease. Am J Ophthalmol 1987; 103:234–235.
9. Smith RE, Nozik R. Uveitis: a clinical approach to diagnosis and management. Baltimore: Williams & Wilkins; 1983.
10. Smith RE, Godfrey WA, Kimura SJ. Chronic cyclitis. I. Course and visual prognosis. Trans Am Acad Ophthalmol Otolaryngol 1973; 77:760–768.
10a. Kanski JJ. Care of children with anterior uveitis. Trans Ophthalmol Soc UK 1981; 101:387–390.
11. Culbertson WW, Giles CL, West C et al. Familial pars planitis. Retina 1983; 3:179–181.
12. Kimura SJ, Hogan MJ. Chronic cyclitis. Arch Ophthalmol 1964; 71:193–201.
13. Chester GH, Blach RK, Cleary PE. Inflammation in the region of the vitreous base: pars planitis. Trans Ophthalmol Soc UK 1976; 96:151–157.
14. Brockhurst RJ, Schepens CL, Okamura ID. Uveitis. III. Peripheral uveitis: pathogenesis, etiology, and treatment. Am J Ophthalmol 1961; 51:19–26.
15. Aaberg TM, Cesarz T, Flickinger RR. Treatment of peripheral uveoretinitis by cryotherapy. Am J Ophthalmol 1973; 75:685–688.
16. Augsburger JJ, Annesley WH Jr, Sergott RC et al. Familial pars planitis. Ann Ophthalmol 1981; 13:553–557.
17. Giles CL, Tanton JH. Peripheral uveitis in three children of one family. J Pediatr Ophthalmol Strabismus 1980; 17:297–299.
18. Breger BC, Leopold IH. The incidence of uveitis in multiple sclerosis. Am J Ophthalmol 1966; 62:540–545.
19. Giles CL. Peripheral uveitis in patients with multiple sclerosis. Am J Ophthalmol 1970; 70:17–19.
20. Hogan MJ, Kimura SJ, O'Connor GR. Peripheral retinitis and chronic cyclitis in children. Trans Ophthalmol Soc UK 1965; 85:39–52.
21. Schlaegel TF Jr. Ocular toxoplasmosis and pars planitis. New York: Grune & Stratton; 1978.
22. Althaus C, Sundmacher R. Intermediate uveitis: epidemiology, age and sex distribution. Dev Ophthalmol 1992; 23:9–14.
23. Ortega-Larrocea G, Arellanes-Garcia L. Pars planitis: epidemiology and clinical outcome in a large community hospital in Mexico City. Int Ophthalmol 1995; 19:117–120.
24. Henderly DE, Genstler AJ, Smith RE et al. Changing patterns of uveitis. Am J Ophthalmol 1987; 103:131–136.
25. Schlaegel TF Jr. Differential diagnosis of uveitis. Ophthalmol Digest 1973; 35:34–38.
26. Perkins ES, Folk J. Uveitis in London and Iowa. Ophthalmologica 1984; 189:36–40.
27. Lauer AK, Smith JR, Robertson JE et al. Vitreous hemorrhage is a common complication of pediatric pars planitis. Ophthalmology 2002; 109:95–98.
28. Stoessel KM, Thompson JT, Puklin JE. Pars planitis: clinical manifestations and response to steroids. Ophthalmology (in press).
29. Herschler J. Increased intraocular pressure induced by repository cortical steroids. Am J Ophthalmol 1976; 82:90–93.
30. Smith RE, Godfrey WA, Kimura SJ. Complications of chronic cyclitis. Am J Ophthalmol 1976; 82:277–282.
31. Deane JS, Rosenthal AR. Course and complications of intermediate uveitis. Acta Ophthalmol Scand 1997; 75:82–84.
32. Boke W. Clinical picture of intermediate uveitis. Dev Ophthalmol 1992; 23:20–27.
33. Slezak H. Zur Klinik, Pathogenese, und Differential diagnose der peripheren Uveitis. Graefes Arch Clin Exp Ophthalmol 1967; 174:9–33.
34. Tugal-Tutkun I, Havrlikova K, Power WJ et al. Changing patterns in uveitis of childhood. Ophthalmology 1996; 103:375–383.
35. Green WR, Kincaid MC, Michels RG et al. Pars planitis. Trans Ophthalmol Soc UK 1981; 101:361–367.
36. Muller-Hermelink HK. Recent topics in the pathology of uveitis. In: Kraus-Mackiw E, O'Connor GR, eds. Uveitis: pathophysiology and therapy. New York: Thieme-Stratton; 1983.
37. Wetzig RP, Chen CC, Nussenblatt RB et al. Clinical and immunopathological studies of pars planitis in a family. Br J Ophthalmol 1988; 75:5–10.
38. Eichenbaum JW, Friedman AH, Mamelok AE. A clinical and histopathological review of intermediate uveitis ("pars planitis"). Bull NY Acad Med 1988; 64:164–174.
39. Yoser SL, Forster DJ, Rao NA. Pathology of intermediate uveitis. Dev Ophthalmol 1992; 23:60–70.
40. Rahi AH, Addison DJ. Autoimmunity and the outer retina. Trans Ophthalmol Soc UK 1984; 103:428–437.
41. Hultsch E. Peripheral uveitis in the owl monkey: experimental model. Mod Probl Ophthalmol 1977; 18:247–251.
42. Zimmerman LE, Silverstein AM. Experimental ocular hypersensitivity: histopathologic changes observed in rabbits receiving a single injection of antigen into the vitreous. Am J Ophthalmol 1959; 48:447–465.
43. Gartner J. The vitreous base of the human eye and "pars planitis": electron microscopic observations. Mod Probl Ophthalmol 1972; 10:250–255.
44. Kaplan HJ, Aaberg TM, Keller RH. Recurrent clinical uveitis: cell surface markers on vitreous lymphocytes. Arch Ophthalmol 1982; 100:585–587.
45. Kaplan HJ, Waldrep JC, Nicholson JKA et al. Immunologic analysis of intraocular mononuclear cell infiltrates in uveitis. Arch Ophthalmol 1984; 102:572–575.
46. Belfort R Jr, Moura NC, Mendes NF. T and B lymphocytes in the aqueous humor of patients with uveitis. Arch Ophthalmol 1982; 100:465–467.
47. Toledo de Abreu M, Belfort R Jr, Matheus PC et al. T-lymphocyte subsets in the aqueous humor and peripheral blood of patients with acute untreated uveitis. Am J Ophthalmol 1984; 98:62–65.
48. Nussenblatt RB, Salinas-Carmona M, Leake W et al. T lymphocyte subsets in uveitis. Am J Ophthalmol 1983; 95:614–621.
49. Yokoyama MM, Matsui Y, Yamashiroya HM et al. Humoral and cellular immunity studies in patients with Vogt–Koyanagi–Harada syndrome and pars planitis. Invest Ophthalmol Vis Sci 1981; 20:364–370.
50. Aaberg TM. The enigma of pars planitis. Am J Ophthalmol 1987; 103:828–830.
51. Khodadoust AA, Karnama Y, Stoessel KM et al. Pars planitis and autoimmune endotheliopathy. Am J Ophthalmol 1986; 102:633–639.
52. Tessler HH. Pars planitis and autoimmune endotheliopathy. Am J Ophthalmol 1987; 103:599–600 (letter).
53. Davis JL, Chan CC, Nussenblatt RB. Immunology of intermediate uveitis. Dev Ophthalmol 1992; 23:71–85.
54. Winward KE, Smith JL, Culbertson WW et al. Ocular Lyme borreliosis. Am J Ophthalmol 1989; 108:651–657.
55. Hirose S, Kuwabara T, Nussenblatt RB et al. Uveitis induced in primates by interphotoreceptor retinoid-binding protein. Arch Ophthalmol 1986; 104:1698–1702.
56. Arocker-Mettinger E, Georgiew L, Grabner G et al. Intermediate uveitis: do HLA antigens play a role? Dev Ophthalmol 1992; 23:15–19.
57. Streilein JW. Role of anterior chamber-associated immune deviation in the pathogenesis of uveitis. Dev Ophthalmol 1992; 23:86–93.
58. Nolle B. Antiretinal autoantibodies in intermediate uveitis. Dev Ophthalmol 1992; 23:94–98.
59. Nussenblatt MJ, Masciulli L, Yarian DL et al. Pars planitis – a demyelinating disease? Arch Ophthalmol 1981; 99:697.
60. Tang WM, Pulido JS, Eckels DD et al. The association of HLA-DR15 and intermediate uveitis. Am J Ophthalmol 1997; 123:70–75.
61. Oruc S, Duffy BF, Mohanakumar T et al. The association of HLA class II with pars planitis. Am J Ophthalmol 2001; 131:657–659.
62. Raja SC, Jabs DA, Dunn JP et al. Pars planitis. Clinical features and class II HLA associations. Ophthalmology 1999; 106:594–599.

63. Martin T, Weber N, Schmitt C et al. Association of intermediate uveitis with HLA-A27: definition of a new systemic syndrome? Graefes Arch Clin Exp Ophthalmol 1995; 233:269–274.

64. Lee AG. Familial pars planitis. Ophthalm Genet 1995; 16:17–19.

65. Haimovici R, Lightman SL, Bird AC. Familial pars planitis and dominant optic atrophy. Ophthalm Genet 1997; 18:43–45.

66. Bora NS, Bora PS, Kaplan HJ. Identification, quantitation, and purification of a 36 kDa circulating protein associated with active pars planitis. Invest Ophthalmol Vis Sci 1996; 37:1870–1876.

67. Bora NS, Bora PS, Tandhasetti MT et al. Molecular cloning, sequencing, and expression of the 36 kDa protein present in pars planitis. Sequence homology with yeast nucleopore complex protein. Invest Ophthalmol Vis Sci 1996; 37:1877–1883.

68. Maumenee AE. Clinical entities in "uveitis": an approach to the study of intraocular inflammation. Am J Ophthalmol 1970; 69:1–27.

69. Cunha-Vaz JG, Travassos A. Breakdown of the blood–retinal barriers and cystoid macular edema. Surv Ophthalmol 1984; 28:485–492.

70. Mahlberg PA, Cunha-Vaz JG, Tessler HH. Vitreous fluorophotometry in pars planitis. Am J Ophthalmol 1983; 95:189–196.

71. Henderly DE, Haymond RS, Rao NA et al. The significance of the pars plana exudate in pars planitis. Am J Ophthalmol 1987; 103:669–671.

72. Tessler HH, Farber FM. Intraocular lens implantation versus no intraocular lens implantation in patients with chronic iridocyclitis and pars planitis. Ophthalmology 1993; 100:1206–1209.

73. Anderson AW. IOLs in uveitis patients. Ophthalmology 1994; 101:625–626 (letter).

74. Brockhurst RJ, Schepens CL. Uveitis. IV. Peripheral uveitis: the complication of retinal detachment. Arch Ophthalmol 1968; 80:747–753.

75. Henderly DE, Genstler AJ, Rao NA et al. Pars planitis. Trans Ophthalmol Soc UK 1986; 105:227–232.

76. Soheilian M, Markomichelakis N, Foster CS. Intermediate uveitis and retinal vasculitis as manifestations of cat scratch disease. Am J Ophthalmol 1996; 122:582–584.

77. Hilton E, Smith C, Sood S. Ocular Lyme borreliosis diagnosed by polymerase chain reaction on vitreous fluid. Ann Intern Med 1996; 125:424–425.

78. Cantrill HL, Ramsay RC, Knobloch WH et al. Electrophysiologic changes in chronic pars planitis. Am J Ophthalmol 1981; 91:505–512.

79. Garcia-Feijoo J, Martin-Carbjo M, Benitez del Castillo JM et al. Ultrasound biomicroscopy in pars planitis. Am J Ophthalmol 1996; 121:214–215.

80. Godfrey WA, Epstein WV, O'Connor GR et al. The use of chlorambucil in intractable idiopathic uveitis. Am J Ophthalmol 1974; 78:415–428.

81. Newell FW, Krill AE, Thomson A. The treatment of uveitis with six-mercaptopurine. Am J Ophthalmol 1966; 61:1250–1255.

82. Wakefield D, McCluskey P, Penny R. Intravenous pulse methylprednisolone therapy in severe inflammatory eye disease. Arch Ophthalmol 1986; 104:847–851.

83. Sloper CML, Powell RJ, Dua HS. Tacrolimus (FK506) in the treatment of posterior uveitis refractory to cyclosporine. Ophthalmology 1999; 106:723–728.

84. Miserocchi E, Baltatzis S, Ekong A et al. Efficacy and safety of chlorambucil in intractable noninfectious uveitis. The Massachusetts eye and ear infirmary experience. Ophthalmology 2002; 109:137–142.

85. Godfrey WA, Smith RE, Kimura SJ. Chronic cyclitis: cortico-steroid therapy. Trans Am Ophthalmol Soc 1976; 74:178–188.

86. Helm CJ, Holland GN. The effects of posterior subtenon injection of triamcinolone acetonide in patients with intermediate uveitis. Am J Ophthalmol 1995; 120:55–64.

87. Riordan-Eva P, Lightman S. Orbital floor steroid injections in the treatment of uveitis. I. Eye 1994; 8:66–69.

88. Kaplan HJ. Intermediate uveitis (pars planitis, chronic cyclitis) – a four-step approach to treatment. In: Saari KM, ed. Uveitis update. Amsterdam: Excerpta Medica; 1984.

89. Aaberg TM, Cesarz TJ, Flickinger RR Jr. Treatment of pars planitis. I. Cryotherapy. Surv Ophthalmol 1977; 22:120–125.

90. Josephberg RG, Kanter ED, Jaffee RM. A fluorescein angiographic study of patients with pars planitis and peripheral exudation (snowbanking) before and after cryopexy. Ophthalmology 1994; 101:1262–1266.

91. Newell FW, Krill AE. Treatment of uveitis with azathioprine (Imuran). Trans Ophthalmol Soc UK 1967; 87:499–511.

92. Wong VG. Immunosuppressive therapy of ocular inflammatory diseases. Arch Ophthalmol 1969; 81:628–637.

93. Buckley CE III, Gills JP Jr. Cyclophosphamide therapy of peripheral uveitis. Arch Intern Med 1969; 124:29–35.

94. Gills JP Jr, Buckley CE III. Oral cyclophosphamide in the treatment of uveitis. Trans Am Acad Ophthalmol Otolaryngol 1970; 74:505–508.

95. Nozik RA, Godfrey WA, Epstein WV et al. Immunosuppressive treatment of uveitis. Mod Probl Ophthalmol 1976; 16:305–308.

96. Nussenblatt RB, Palestine AG, Chan CC. Cyclosporin A therapy in the treatment of intraocular inflammatory disease resistant to systemic corticosteroids and cytotoxic agents. Am J Ophthalmol 1983; 96:275–282.

97. Dugel PU, Rao NA, Ozler S et al. Pars plana vitrectomy for intraocular inflammation related to cystoid macular edema unresponsive to corticosteroids: a preliminary study. Ophthalmology 1992; 99:1535–1541.

98. Schonfeld CL, Weissschadel S, Heidenkummer HP et al. Vitreoretinal surgery in intermediate uveitis. Germ J Ophthalmol 1995; 4:37–42.

99. Potter MJ, Myckatyn SO, Maberley AL et al. Vitrectomy for pars planitis complicated by vitreous hemorrhage: visual outcome and long-term follow-up. Am J Ophthalmol 2001; 131:514–515.

100. Dev S, Mieler WF, Pulido JS et al. Visual outcomes after pars plana vitrectomy for epiretinal membranes associated with pars planitis. Ophthalmology 1999; 106:1086–1090.

Chapter

96

Retinal Syphilis and Tuberculosis

David L. Knox

Ocular syphilis and tuberculosis, rare disorders in North America in the 21st century, were commonly diagnosed in the 1920s to 1940s for several reasons. First, many patients had these infections, and second, ophthalmologists' thinking at that time was so influenced by the prevalence of syphilis and tuberculosis that these infections were considered first and often diagnosed with no supportive evidence.

Fewer people in the 1970s and 1980s were diagnosed as having ocular syphilis or tuberculosis, primarily because fewer people in the community at large were infected. Penicillin and other antibiotics rapidly and effectively treat syphilis in most patients, who complete courses of therapy without interrupting work or social lives. This is in marked contrast to the multiple, painful injections of ars-phenamine (Salvarsan) or tryparsamide in the preantibiotic era. Identification of sexual contacts reduces the pool of available spirochetes. Congenital syphilis became extremely rare in North America, Europe, and Japan, because of routine serologic testing of women at the first prenatal visit to their obstetrician or clinic. However, it continues to occur in North America because of failure of women to attend prenatal clinics.[1]

The same set of events occurred with tuberculosis. Treatment is easier and less time-consuming, and antituberculous agents are so effective that fairly healthy patients rapidly become sputum-negative, leave hospital, and return to work and family. Isolation and early treatment of patients have reduced the pool of these organisms. Testing of dairy herds, destruction of infected animals, and pasteurization of milk have virtually removed bovine tuberculosis from North America.

With all these advantages, it is theoretically possible to rid the world of syphilis and tuberculosis in the same way that smallpox has been eradicated. Unfortunately, the nature of these infections and human behavior continue to provide a steady trickle of patients with these ocular diseases.

The number of patients with syphilis decreased both because of specific treatment and because treatment of gonorrhea also treated latent syphilis. The sexual revolution made possible for heterosexuals by contraceptive technology was paralleled by an increase in the sexual activity of male homosexuals. Anal sex facilitated the spread of syphilis because rectal chancres are both painless and invisible. Until the early 1990s, patients I saw with ocular syphilis and most of the those reported in the then-current world literature were homosexual males. The pattern has changed again, and both male and female heterosexuals are being diagnosed with syphilis, frequently compounded by positive human immunodeficiency virus (HIV) status. The painless character of chancres increases their capacity to transfer HIV.

In the 1990s the acquired immunodeficiency syndrome (AIDS) epidemic caused a major modification in homosexual behavior, resulting in longer-lasting monogamous relationships, use of condoms, and avoidance of 15-min anonymous encounters. New antiviral therapies for HIV and cytomegalovirus infections and antibiotics for concurrent infections have so prolonged life that many male homosexuals assume that prolonged life is a cure and return to highly promiscuous activity, with an attendant rise in the incidence of new cases. Bisexual behaviors of males infecting wives and shared intravenous drug paraphernalia continue to create new cases of AIDS.

Tuberculosis should be considered strongly in the following clinical circumstances:

1. Middle-aged or older alcoholics who are homeless, living alone on little or no income. These patients are often brought to hospital by police, subacutely ill, with pneumonia that is tuberculous, diagnosed by smear or culture of sputum.
2. Immigrants from South-east Asia, India, Africa, the Caribbean, and Central America. It is unclear how these people passed through medical screening in embassies around the world, since many present with advanced disease soon after their arrival in North America. Some become ill months to years after arrival.
3. HIV-positive individuals, with or without AIDS, who are residents of jails or prisons.[2] Drug use and forced or consensual homosexual activity has infected many with HIV. Airborne droplets from other prisoners with tuberculosis often contain virulent, multiple drug-resistant strains.
4. Health-care professionals who have been exposed to a patient with active disease before the diagnosis is made may be infected with large doses of virulent organisms that overwhelm their usual state of good health.
5. People who have been exposed in the past to active tuberculosis in family members or co-workers. A negative skin test soon after exposure needs to be repeated during

assessment for an active, enigmatic inflammation. A negative chest X-ray does not rule out tuberculosis. Many of these patients have been told that they do not have tuberculosis. Special diligence is needed to uncover significant historical facts. An explanation for ocular disease in this group is based on the concept that the eye has been sensitized immunologically by *Mycobacterium tuberculosis* organisms or protein-polysaccharide products of these organisms, which persist in foci remote from the eye. In these foci, products are released or antibodies generated which circulate to the eye, where they stimulate a sterile inflammatory reaction.

6. The final group comprises patients with a negative chest X-ray, a markedly positive skin test, and some type of extrapulmonary tuberculosis, such as scrofula or adrenal disease. Reported cases of tuberculosis with microorganisms demonstrated histopathologically in the eye have documented this set of events.[3-5] I rail and complain when I hear that some physician has declared that a patient's ocular problem could not be tuberculosis because the chest film was normal. I have wondered if cheeses made from unpasteurized cow's or goat's milk by villagers in developing countries could be a source of these infections.

LABORATORY TESTING

Good tests are available for both syphilis and tuberculosis. Serologic testing for syphilis begins with the rapid plasma reagin (RPR), which is usually positive in high titers in patients with active disease. If patients are treated early, titers subside, and some become negative. Currently the most sensitive test is the fluorescent treponemal antibody absorption test (FTA-ABS), which can remain positive for years after successful treatment. False positives occur because of infection with the spirochete of Lyme disease, *Borrelia burgdorferi*, and benign oral spirochetes.

Identification of *Treponema* spirochetes by dark-field examination of chancres or spinal fluid was a mainstay of diagnosis for many years. Examination of aqueous had a transient appeal[6] and was not sustained by a second group of investigators.[7]

Tuberculosis testing can be done in four ways: (1) skin testing; (2) radiography; (3) microbiologic; and (4) histopathologic studies. Tuberculin skin testing has a long history. In the past it was necessary to use skin test material within 5 days of diluting pellets of dried antigenic material. Many false-negative results were obtained because a bottle of skin test material stayed in a refrigerator for months before the second test was performed. Current skin test antigens maintain their activity because detergent added to the solution prevents antigen from being absorbed by the glass wall of the bottle. Antigens are prepared in 2, 5, 10, and 200 test units per 0.1 ml, the usual intradermal test volume. If one wishes to give two test units from a five-test unit solution, 0.04 ml can be given. Skin tests are measured 48 h after intradermal injection. It is important to record in millimeters the diameter of both erythema and induration and to determine whether there is vesiculation of the center. Tine testing methodology seems to be reliable, also requiring a reading 48 h

after placement, with the patient recording the size of the induration on a card.

A positive skin test indicates that the patient at some time in the past has been infected with *M. tuberculosis* or bacille Calmette-Guérin (BCG), given as a preventive immunization in many European countries, Russia, the Mediterranean area, and India. Atypical mycobacteria may also cause a positive tuberculin skin test.

In one sense, any degree of erythema and induration is a positive test. The decision to initiate a treatment regimen varies greatly, even in North America. For some, the fact that a patient's skin test converts from negative to positive is an indication for a year of chemotherapy. For others, a positive skin test with less than 10 mm of induration and erythema, and with no radiographic, culture, or tissue evidence, is not a reason for treatment. A reaction of 10 to 20 mm is an indication for treatment or for more careful monitoring of the patient without treatment. Over 25 mm deserves careful consideration for treatment, as does ocular inflammation that cannot be explained by any other means.[8]

Chest X-rays may show classic evidence of tuberculosis or be negative in those who have renal, adrenal, bone, or cervical lymph node (scrofula) involvement. A positive mycobacterium culture of sputum or urine is an indication for treatment, as is the finding of acid-fast organisms in a tissue that has been biopsied.[3]

Polymerase chain reaction

Laboratory diagnostic technology continuously evolves. Time-tested standards of biopsy with histopathology and special stains, cultures from tissues and body fluids and definition of antibodies by serologic techniques have been supplemented or unwisely totally replaced by polymerase chain reaction (PCR) technology which some writers more properly call "nucleic acid amplification."[9-11]

PCR methodology, developed in the 1980s, seeks to identify the presence of specific nucleic acids, from microorganisms in tissues or body fluids, from specific tissues or fluids as used in criminal identification testing, in the subclassification and definition of evolution of microorganisms.[12] The techniques are complicated and dependent upon specific primers, amplifiers, and templates necessary to replicate by repeated incubation and cooling, nucleic acids characteristic of sought-after micro organisms. While this technology produces high-sensitivity identification of miniscule amounts of genetic fragments, it also increases the risks of contamination, creating false positives and low levels of specificity.[13] These techniques are expensive and not useful for broad screening of enigmatic inflammations. Positive and negative control tissues and body fluids are expensive and time-consuming, but absolutely essential for significant diagnoses.[13] Small laboratories, infrequently doing tests for infrequent infections, are at great risk for giving unsubstantiated diagnoses.

The specific areas of vulnerability in PCR technology begin with laboratories having a low level of technical competence and a high level of "rookie errors," creating "home brew" assays in which technicians design and create their own primers and amplifiers. Artifacts, contamination with the desired nucleic acid, and poor design are likely to produce false positives. Commercially available kits have the same risks. In sequencing for primers, risks occur because homologous nucleic acids can be elicited from other organisms, "normal" tissues, or from tissues affected by other pathologic processes.[14] *M. tuberculosis*, because of lipid in its capsule, is a notoriously difficult organism from which to extract a stable specific nucleic acid.[9] Clinicians, investigators, reporting authors, and editorial reviewers should confirm that laboratories providing results are complying with clinical laboratory requirements established by CLIA. This is especially pertinent when unexpected results occur. Further risks occur because of contamination by the presence of nucleic acids on templates, poor preparation of templates, and airborne sources.[13] It must also be stated that identification of nucleic acid from an organism is not evidence that the organism is present in sufficient numbers with enough virulence or host reaction to cause inflammation or disease in a given patient.[15]

At this writing, authors and editorial reviewers are accepting PCR findings as the only evidence of specific infection. Corroborating evidence of the disease by older technology should be presented in published articles. Clinicians should demand controls by laboratories, explore alternate etiologic diagnoses, and establish support by standard methods of clinical science.[14]

TREATMENT

For over 60 years, penicillin has been the primary treatment for syphilis. Authorities differ as to the appropriate dose and schedule: 2.4 million units intramuscularly 10 days apart is sufficient to treat most patients with primary or secondary syphilis. Most believe that tertiary, ocular, and neurosyphilis should be treated with 10 million units intravenously daily for 10 days.[16] Rarely has a strain of syphilis or a patient not responded to penicillin, but it has happened.[17]

For patients whose allergy to penicillin prevents its use, oral tetracycline or erythromycin works well. In patients with secondary or tertiary syphilis, some specialists advise a short period of treatment with oral corticosteroids before and during penicillin therapy to prevent the Jarisch–Herxheimer reaction, which is a toxic fever with shaking chills, as a reaction to penicillin causing the sudden death of spirochetes.[18]

Patients should be reported to public health authorities so that sexual contacts can be interviewed, tested, and treated, if necessary.

Two uncontrolled therapeutic trials have been conducted in which no treatment for syphilis was given – one in Norway early in the 20th century,[19] before the development of antibiotics, and the other in Tuskeegee, Alabama, that was never completed because of justifiable unfavorable publicity. Progressive disease never developed in 25% of untreated patients.

Treatment for tuberculosis is more complex than for syphilis.[20,21] The organism has a slower metabolism, more variation in sensitivity, resistance to antimicrobial agents and a chronic and relapsing course. The easiest chemotherapy is isoniazid 300 mg every morning or 100 mg three times a day for patients who have evidence of prior infection, no sign of active disease, and are considered to have an allergic reaction to tubercle bacilli. If there is evidence of more active disease, it is necessary to give other agents such as *para*-aminosalicylic acid, streptomycin, rifampin, or ethambutol, all of which should be given with the assistance of specialists experienced in the management of these drugs and new agents which are constantly being developed.

Ethambutol is first given in doses of 20 to 25 mg/kg of body weight per day for several weeks, and then tapered to 15 mg/kg of body weight per day. An optic neuropathy can occur at the disc, in the orbital optic nerve, or chiasm, at any dose, but the

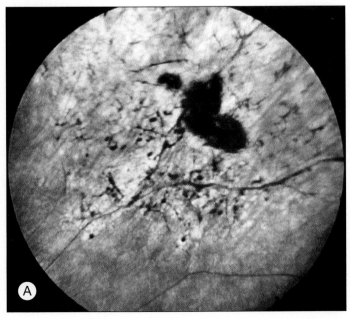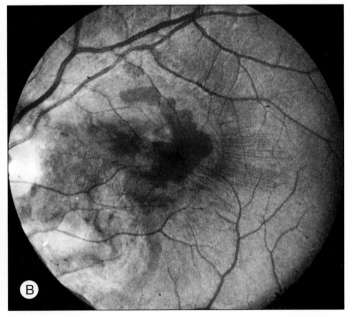

Fig. 96-1 A, Syphilitic peripheral pigmentation in a 22-year-old woman. B, Peripapillary exudation in the same eye.

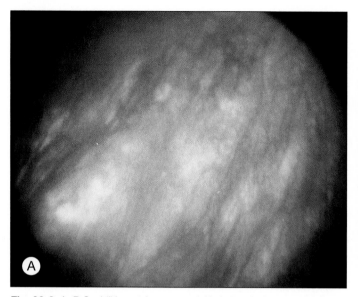

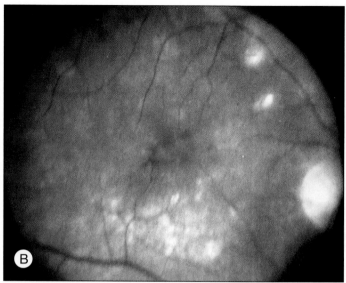

Fig. 96-2 A, B Syphilitic patchy neuroretinitis in two homosexual males.

risk is higher if the patient is receiving greater than 20 mg/kg per day for more than 3 weeks.[22] Isoniazid has caused optic neuropathy. This can be reduced or prevented by instituting a vitamin-rich diet or by giving supplemental multivitamins, specifically pyridoxine.

Treatment programs must be conducted with the knowledge that some strains are resistant to certain agents. Special attention must be given to the problems of patients with multiple-drug-resistant strains of tuberculosis. These first appeared in New York state prisons, are now being seen in other states, and often complicated by active AIDS.[2] The infections are highly virulent and difficult to manage. What to do about them is not clear at this writing.

OCULAR SYNDROMES

Congenital syphilis is associated with a pigmentary retinopathy that may be segmental or generalized and is morphologically difficult to distinguish from retinitis pigmentosa (Fig. 96-lA). It can be seen after a bout of classic interstitial keratitis or in eyes that have had no previous symptomatic episode of inflammation. In one patient, a peripapillary edema and exudation occurred in one eye at age 14 and in the other eye at age 21 (Fig. 96-lB). In this patient the pigmentary changes shown in Fig. 96-lA, were seen. When asked if anyone in the family had had syphilis, the patient replied that she suspected her mother, and when the mother confirmed this, the patient commented, "It is nice to have something on Mommy."

Acquired syphilis most commonly produces a patchy, diffuse neuroretinitis (Fig. 96-2) that may have areas of hemorrhage (Fig. 96-3). There is reduced acuity and irregular contraction of visual fields, which have progressed over weeks to months, sometimes to very small central islands. Aqueous and vitreous flare and cells are seen. Serum and spinal fluid antibodies are found. If neuroretinitis is treated early, acuity improves and visual fields expand.[23,24]

Aqueous and vitreous cells and flare resorb, with the retinopathy abating. Optic atrophy and narrow arteries may remain. Figs 96-4 and 96-5 demonstrate dramatic evidence of dilated vessels and perivascular and punctate intraretinal leakage in a patient with neuroretinal syphilis and positive HIV status.

In some instances intense patches of chorioretinal infiltrates are seen next to pigmented scarring[25] (Fig. 96-6).

Most of these morphologic variations of ocular syphilis were beautifully described and illustrated by paintings in Josef Igersheimer's text, *Syphilis und Auge.*[26]

Forster's choroiditis is a rare but extremely dramatic manifestation of late syphilis. The first and only patient I have ever seen came to our emergency room when I was a first-year

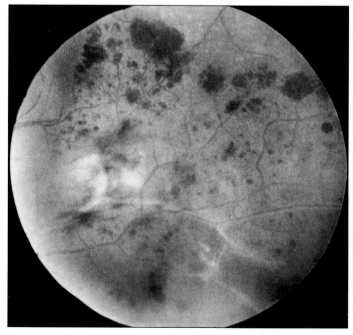

Fig. 96-3 Syphilitic hemorrhagic retinitis.

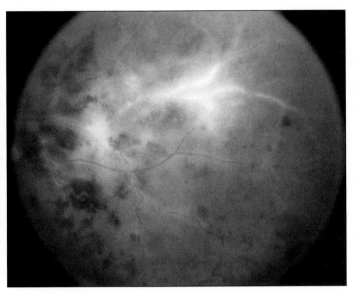

Fig. 96-4 Retinal vasculitis with intraretinal and subretinal hemorrhage in a 25-year-old man with syphilis and acquired immunodeficiency syndrome (AIDS). (Courtesy of Robert Liss, MD.)

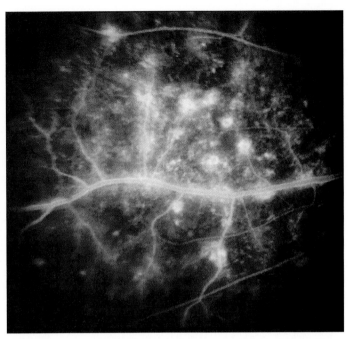

Fig. 96-5 Fluorescein angiogram in a 28-year-old African student with both syphilis and positive human immunodeficiency virus (HIV) status.

resident in 1959. I took the patient upstairs to Dr. Alan C. Woods, who took the patient into his darkroom, adjusted his aphakic spectacles, and, with his direct ophthalmoscope, studied the patient for 5 min. He then asked the patient, "When did you have syphilis?" "Ten years ago, sir," replied the patient. Fig. 96-7 is a painting by Annette S. Burgess that was reproduced from the last edition of Woods' *Endogenous Inflammations of the Uveal Tract*.[8] Unfortunately, this looks like fungal chorioretinopathy.

Late and indolent ocular syphilis produces two morphologic variations. Probably more common is the diffuse, irregular pigmentation usually found along major vessels, as shown in Fig. 96-8. Another variation is the slowly progressive and late mixed atrophic and hyperpigmentary retinopathy, as shown in Fig. 96-9. This patient had been forced to serve in a military

brothel in Greece in 1943. The retinopathy progressed despite penicillin therapy. She was intellectually intact at age 79 in 1996. The same entity was described by Igersheimer.[26]

Papillitis is an infrequent but real manifestation of secondary syphilis. Old posterior synechiae and aqueous inflammatory cells were present in the fellow eye of a 55-year-old male public bath attendant (Fig. 96-10). He had a patchy erythematous macular skin rash on his forearms and palms. Computed tomography (CT) scan of his head was negative, but medical workup included a serologic test for syphilis, which was positive. Treatment with penicillin resolved his papillitis and skin rash.

It was Alan Woods' opinion that some cases of ocular and general syphilis could be explained by direct spirochetal

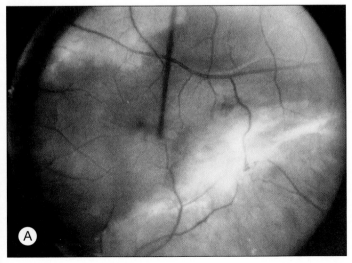

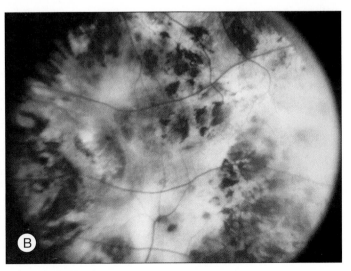

Fig. 96-6 A, Syphilitic deep retinal infiltrate in a 23-year-old woman. B, Scarring and hyperpigmentation in the same patient.

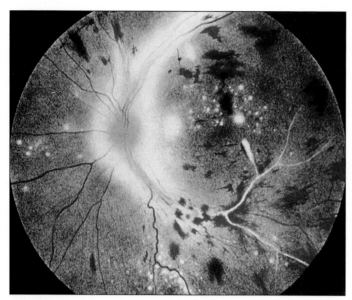

Fig. 96-7 Forster's choroiditis. (Painting by Annette S. Burgess, reproduced with permission from Woods AC. Endogenous inflammations of the uveal tract. Baltimore: Williams & Wilkins; 1961.[8])

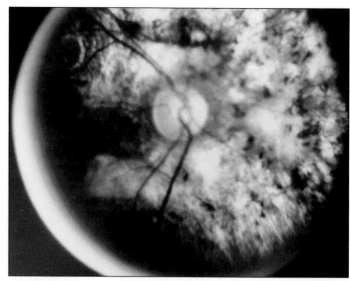

Fig. 96-9 Syphilitic, slowly progressive scarring with depigmentation, hyperpigmentation, and hard white exudates.

invasion of the tissue. Other manifestations were more logically explained by a systemic allergic reaction to tissues sensitized either directly by the spirochete, which was no longer present, or to some peculiar cross-reaction. Clearly, syphilitic interstitial keratitis is an example of a reaction in tissue where no organisms have ever been demonstrated.

TUBERCULOSIS

I have written this chapter based on personal experience in a North American university hospital referral practice from 1962 to 2003. What I have seen therefore is not totally applicable to the rest of the world or to the spectrum of disease that was

seen before the development of chemotherapy for tuberculosis. Two major reviews of ocular tuberculosis have been written by the same team of authors. Their elaboration and references should be consulted for more specifics than space allows here.[20,21] Review of articles abstracted in MedLine reveals that the same morphologic entities are still being seen over the entire world, most commonly in India, but also in Japan, Spain, the USA, and other countries. Chronic iridocyclitis, usually bilateral in a patient with a past history of active tuberculosis or with exposure to a person with tuberculosis, and a markedly positive skin test are the most common reasons I have used for instituting chemotherapy in patients with tuberculosis. Chronic iridocyclitis is characterized by the indolent onset of blurred vision with mild or no

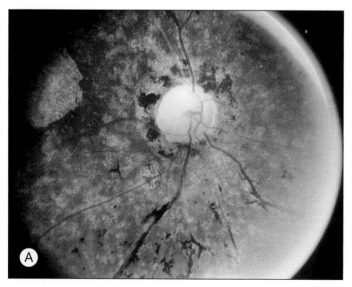

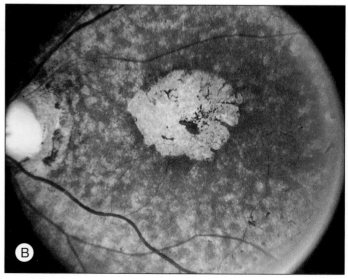

Fig. 96-8 Syphilitic pseudoretinitis pigmentosa with perivascular diffuse pigmentation and macular loss of pigment epithelium.

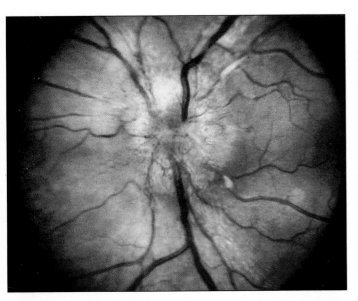

Fig. 96-10 Syphilitic papillitis.

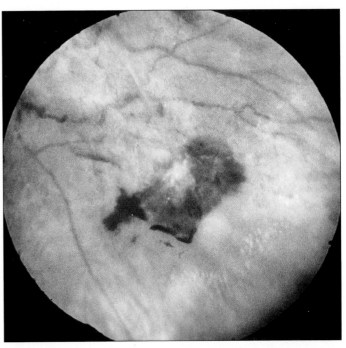

Fig. 96-12 Tuberculous retinal periphlebitis and hemorrhagic retinitis in a 50-year-old man.

discomfort and slight photophobia. Acuity may be reduced and slight redness is seen. Slit-lamp examination reveals mutton-fat keratitic precipitates (often large), aqueous flare and cells, a slightly thick iris, posterior synechiae, and vitreous cells and flare. The retina and choroid may be boggy. The only time I have seen an iris nodule from tuberculosis was as a medical student in Houston, Texas in 1954. In North America we no longer have the large number of patients with chronic tuberculosis, where ebb and flow of disease produces the classic abnormalities described in the prechemotherapy days.

It is in patients with chronic iridocyclitis that I clearly follow Woods' guidelines in which, after searching for and finding no other cause for the inflammation, the patient with a positive skin test is given a 6- to 12-month course of antituberculosis therapy (usually isoniazid 300 mg every morning). It is surprising how often these patients clear completely or markedly

improve. Improvement does not occur rapidly, and to understand a patient's ocular inflammation one must employ concepts of circulating immune complexes, cross-reaction of sensitized tissue or sensitization of ocular tissue by transient acid-fast bacilli, and the continued assault on this tissue by circulating antibodies. Few eyes with chronic iridocyclitis have been demonstrated to contain acid-fast bacilli.

Theodore F. Schlaegel, who devoted most of his career to the study of patients with uveitis, advocated an isoniazid therapeutic trial test to develop evidence of ocular tuberculosis in a patient.[27] Schlaegel would give a patient isoniazid for 3 weeks, and if the patient did not improve, he then concluded that the

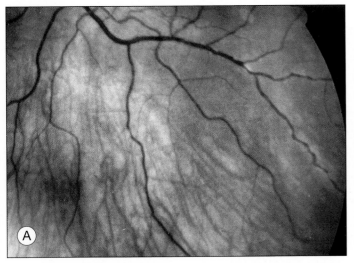
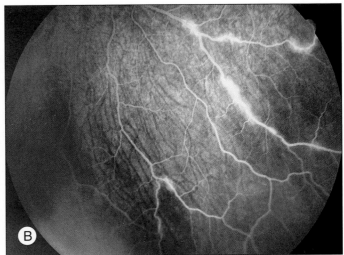

Fig. 96-11 A, Tuberculous periphlebitis in a young female nurse. B, Fluorescein leakage from affected vessels of A.

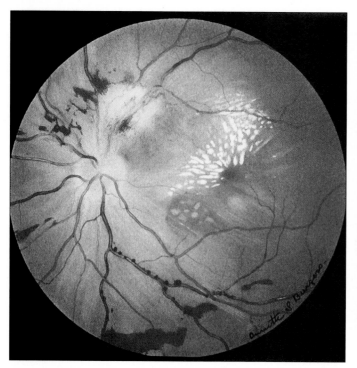

Fig. 96-13 Tuberculous retinal phlebitis. (Painting by Annette S. Burgess.)

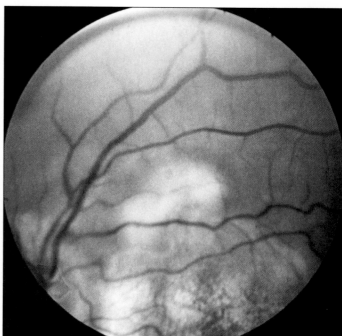

Fig. 96-14 Tuberculous choroiditis in a 24-year-old man.

disorder was not related to tuberculosis. If the patient improved, it was likely to be a tuberculous disorder. When Schlaegel was still active in academic circles and at meetings, I argued with him about this "test." My first point was that chronic irido-cyclitis did not necessarily imply that the organism was actively present in the eye and that more than 3 weeks were needed to document improvement. The second point was based on Schlaegel's concept that isoniazid was a drug specific for tuber-culosis. The euphoric effect of isoniazid was recognized in its first clinical trials. When patients began to feel better after 2 days of the drug, it was realized that this was too soon to be the result of stopping the metabolism and killing of microorganisms. The euphoric effect of isoniazid was studied further and became the starting point for a whole family of antidepression medications.

Periphlebitis of retinal vessels is, in my practice, the second most common ocular manifestation of tuberculosis.[18,28] Fig. 96-11A shows the characteristic accumulations of whitish material around retinal veins – perivenous clustering. Fig. 96-11B shows fluorescein leakage from these veins. I assume that the whitish material represents edema and inflammatory cells. When it subsides, the affected vein may have pigment along it and depigmentation of the pigment epithelium under the area of previous periphlebitis. Fig. 96-11 shows the fundus of a young female nurse who had worked with patients with tuber-culosis and had a markedly positive skin test. The eye improved with therapy.

Eales disease is a term applied to retinal periphlebitis asso-ciated with intraretinal hemorrhages.[29] A high percentage of patients with Eales disease are found to have evidence of currently or recently active tuberculosis. Fig. 96-12 is from a 50-year-old minister who complained of poor vision. Fundus

lesions were seen, and he was given oral corticosteroids. Four weeks later he complained of severe fatigue, and a chest film demonstrated hilar adenopathy. Thoracotomy revealed swollen lymph nodes which on histopathologic study were found to be loaded with acid-fast bacilli. Fig. 96-13 is a painting by Annette S. Burgess demonstrating the same phenomenon.

Choroiditis can occur focally or diffusely with either indolent or miliary tuberculosis.[30] Choroiditis is characterized by deep swelling that usually has a fuzzy yellow to white color with retinal edema over it and dilated retinal vessels (Fig. 96-14). Hyperemic choroidal congestion surrounds the area of choroiditis. In some instances focal choroiditis becomes a chorioretinitis and breaks through into the vitreous. Cases like these have occurred in patients with negative chest films and whose enucleated eyes have revealed acid-fast bacilli.[5,19] These are rare but strong arguments always to consider extrapul-monary tuberculosis.

Fig. 96-15 demonstrates the small multifocal lesions of miliary tuberculosis presenting as multifocal choroiditis. In this instance the patient also had AIDS. In the past this finding was rare, but HIV infection is changing many things.

"Serpigenous like choroiditis" in five Asian-Indians was blamed on their clinically active tuberculosis, with PCR support from aqueous or vitreous in four. Specific treatment for acid-fast disease was followed by improvement and resolution of active areas of choroiditis.[31] Intravesical urinary bladder instil-lation of BCG organisms for bladder cancer has been compli-cated by miliary chorioretinitis.[32]

Ethambutol optic neuropathy is the final aspect of posterior ocular disease associated with tuberculosis. The nerve head may be slightly swollen with dilated veins. Rarely at levels of

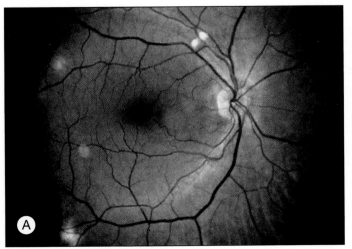 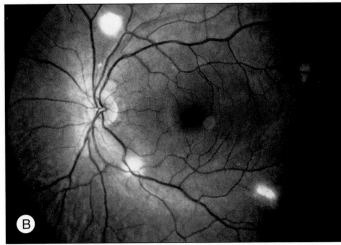

Fig. 96-15 A, B Miliary choroiditis in a patient with tuberculosis and acquired immunodeficiency syndrome (AIDS). (Courtesy of Douglas A. Jabs, MD.)

15 mg/kg body weight per day does rapid loss of vision occur because of optic neuropathy. Stopping the medication sometimes reverses the visual loss.

In summary, consideration of tuberculosis and syphilis will lead to diagnosis and effective therapy in infected patients. Making such diagnoses is exciting for the physician, and missing them is awful.[33]

REFERENCES

1. Mascola L, Pelosi R, Blount JH et al. Congenital syphilis. Why is it still occurring? JAMA 1984; 252:1719–1722.
2. Daley CL, Small PM, Schecter GF et al. An outbreak of tuberculosis with accelerated progression among persons infected with the human immunodeficiency virus. N Engl J Med 1992; 326:231–235.
3. Barondess MJ, Sponsel WE, Stevens TS et al. Tuberculous choroiditis diagnosed by chorioretinal biopsy. Am J Ophthalmol 1991; 11:460–461.
4. Darrell RW. Acute tuberculous panophthalmitis. Arch Ophthalmol 1967; 78:51–54.
5. Theobald GD. Acute tuberculous endophthalmitis. Trans Am Ophthalmol Soc 1957; 55:325–329.
6. Smith JL, Israel CW. The presence of spirochetes in late seronegative syphilis. JAMA 1967; 199:980–984.
7. Ryan SJ Jr, Nell EE, Hardy PH. A study of aqueous humor for the presence of spirochetes. Am J Ophthalmol 1972; 73:250–257.
8. Woods AC. Endogenous inflammations of the uveal tract. Baltimore: Williams & Wilkins; 1961.
9. Ortega-Larrocea G, Bobadilla-del-Valle M, Ponce-de-Leon A et al. Nested polymerase chain reaction of *Mycobacterium tuberculosis* DNA detection in aqueous and vitreous of patients with uveitis. Arch Medial Res 2003; 34:116–119.
10. van Gelder RN. Koch's postulates and the polymerase chain reaction. Ocular Immunol Inflamm 2002; 10:235–238.
11. van Gelder RN. CME review: polymerase chain reaction diagnostics for posterior segment disease. Retina 2003; 23:445–452.
12. Tarasevich IV, Shaginyan IA, Mediannikov OY. Problems and perspectives of molecular epidemiology of infectious diseases. Ann NY Acad Sci 2003; 990:751–756.
13. Fredricks D, Relman D. Sequence-based indentification of microbial pathogens: a reconsideration of Koch's postulates. Clin Microb Rev 1996; 9:18–33.
14. Trinker M, Hofler G, Sill H. False-positive diagnosis of tuberculosis with PCR. Lancet 1996; 348:1388.
15. Rich A. Pathogenesis of tuberculosis. Springfield, IL: Charles C Thomas; 1951:713.
16. Browning DJ. Posterior segment manifestations of active ocular syphilis, their response to a neurosyphilis regimen of penicillin therapy, and the influence of human immunodeficiency virus status on response. Ophthalmology 2000; 107:2015–2023.
17. Ryan SJ Jr, Hardy PH, Hardy JM et al. Persistence of virulent *Treponema pallidum* despite penicillin therapy. Am J Ophthalmol 1972; 73:258–261.
18. Duke-Elder S. System of ophthalmology, vol. 9. Diseases of the uveal tract. St Louis: Mosby; 1966.
19. Clark EG, Danbolt N. The Oslo study of the natural course of untreated syphilis: an epidemiologic investigation based on a restudy of the Boeck–Bruusgaard material. Clin North Am 1964; 48:613–623.
20. Dunn JP, Helm CJ, Davidson PT. Tuberculosis. In: Pepose JS, Holland GN, Wilhelmus KR, eds. Ocular infection and immunity. St Louis: Mosby; 1996.
21. Helm CJ, Holland GN. Ocular tuberculosis. Surv Ophthalmol 1993; 38:229–256.
22. Grant WM. Toxicology of the eye. Springfield, IL: Charles C Thomas; 1986.
23. Biswas J, Shome D. Choroidal tubercles in disseminated tuberculosis diagnosed by the polymerase chain reaction of aqueous humor. Ocular Immunol Inflamm 2002; 10:293–298.
24. Tamesis RR, Foster CS. Ocular syphilis. Ophthalmology 1990; 97:1281–1287.
25. Levy JH, Liss RA, Maguire AM. Neurosyphilis and ocular syphilis in patients with concurrent human immunodeficiency virus infection. Retina 1989; 9:175–180.
26. Igersheimer J. Syphilis und Auge. Berlin: Julius Springer; 1918.
27. Abrams J, Schlaegel TF. The role of the isoniazid therapeutic trial test in tuberculous uveitis. Am J Ophthalmol 1982; 94:511–515.
28. Fountain JA, Werner RB. Tuberculous retinal vasculitis. Retina 1984; 4:48–50.
29. Campinchi R ed. Uveitis: immunologic and allergic phenomena. (Translated by Golden B, Givoiset MM.) Springfield, IL: Charles C Thomas;1973.
30. Sharma PM, Singh R, Kumar A et al. Choroidal tuberculoma in miliary tuberculosis. Retina 2003; 23:101–104.
31. Gupta V, Gupta A, Arora S et al. Presumed tubercular serpiginouslike choroiditis. Ophthalmology 2003; 110:1744–1749.
32. Guex-Crosier Y, Chamot L, Zografos L. Chorioretinitis induced by intravesical bacillus Calmette–Guerin (BCG) instillations for urinary bladder carcinoma. Klin Monatsbl Augen Heilkd 2003; 220:193–195.
33. Gass JD, Braunstein RA, Chenoweth RG. Acute syphilitic posterior placoid chorioretinitis. Ophthalmology 1990; 97:1288–1297.

Chapter

97

Diffuse Unilateral Subacute Neuroretinitis

Janet L. Davis
J. Donald M. Gass
Karl R. Olsen

Diffuse unilateral subacute neuroretinitis (DUSN) is an infectious disease with protean manifestations caused by a single nematode that may wander in the subretinal space for years.[1–10] It most frequently affects otherwise healthy children or young adults and often causes profound loss of vision in one eye. Nematodes infesting both eyes[4] or two nematodes infesting the same eye[11] have been reported.

In approximately one-half of patients, particularly children, visual loss is insidious, and the patient comes to medical attention during the late stages of the disease. Those who have acute visual loss during its early stages usually present with mild to moderate vitreitis, mild optic disc edema, and recurrent crops of evanescent, multifocal, gray-white or yellow lesions at the level of the outer retina (Figs 97-1 to 97-4). These active lesions are typically clustered in only one segment of the fundus. The round, often glistening white worm, which is tapered at both ends, should be sought in the vicinity of the active lesions (Figs 97-1D, 97-2A and D to F, 97-3A, 97-4C, 97-5A and B, 97-6A and B). These active evanescent lesions disappear in 1 to 2 weeks. Less than 1% of these lesions are of sufficient intensity to cause a focal chorioretinal scar that simulates that seen in the presumed ocular histoplasmosis syndrome. During periods of inactivity of the worm, no white lesions may be evident, and the patient may be incorrectly diagnosed as having optic neuritis or, in the presence of some focal chorioretinal scars, diagnosis may be confused with multifocal choroiditis. In the absence of the white lesions there are no clues as to the location of the worm.

Other, less frequently encountered symptoms and signs during the early stages of the disease include ocular discomfort, congestion, iridocyclitis, retinal perivenous exudation, sheathing, hemorrhages, and subretinal hemorrhage, serous exudation, and evidence of subretinal neovascularization. Marked loss of visual acuity typically can be accompanied by minimal changes in the macular area and may be the result of toxic dysfunction of the retina and optic nerve induced by the nematode. Failure to recognize and to destroy the nematode with photocoagulation results in progressive optic atrophy, narrowing of the retinal arteries, marked focal as well as diffuse degenerative changes in the pigment epithelium and retina, and severe permanent loss of vision (Figs 97-3 and 97-4). Intraretinal migration of the pigment epithelium in a bone corpuscular pattern seldom occurs in

DUSN. The nematode may survive for 4 years or longer and may be found in the subretinal space long after the development of severe retinal and optic disc changes (Fig. 97-4).

DUSN is prevalent in the south-eastern USA, Caribbean area, and Latin America as far south as Brazil.[3,6,12] With greater awareness of the disease, it will probably prove to be recognized as being endemic in other tropical and subtropical areas of the world. There are case reports from Germany, Canada, and China, among others.[1,13,14] In the USA, DUSN is probably caused by at least two different nematodes, neither of which has been identified.[6] The smaller of the two, which measures between 400 and 1000 μm in length, with its diameter being approximately 1/20 of its length, is responsible for DUSN in patients in the south-eastern USA, Caribbean, and northern parts of South America (Figs 97-1 to 97-6). A larger nematode, 1500 to 2000 μm in length, is the cause of DUSN in patients in the northern midwestern USA (Fig. 97-7). It causes a sequence of fundus changes that is similar to those caused by the smaller nematode except for the late pigment epithelial degenerative changes, which are more coarsely mottled (Fig. 97-7).

DIAGNOSTIC EVALUATION

Indirect ophthalmoscopy is important in making the correct diagnosis and in locating the cluster of active gray-white outer retinal lesions. If the lesions are present, the nematode will usually be found biomicroscopically in their vicinity. In the absence of these lesions a tedious search of the entire fundus using a three-mirror contact lens can sometimes locate the worm.

Fluorescein angiography during the early stages of the disease shows leakage of dye from the optic nerve head. The active outer retinal lesions are hypofluorescent early and stain late with fluorescein (Fig. 97-2B and C). Perivenous leakage of dye may be evident. In more advanced stages of the disease, angiography shows widespread hyperfluorescence caused by window defects in the damaged pigment epithelium. Unfortunately, angiography is of no help in locating the nematode. Indocyanine green angiography shows widespread punctate hypofluorescence that does not directly correspond to the active lesions. Scanning laser ophthalmoscopy with blue light enhances contrast between the nematode and the ocular fundus and improves visualization as well as allowing videography of its movement.[15]

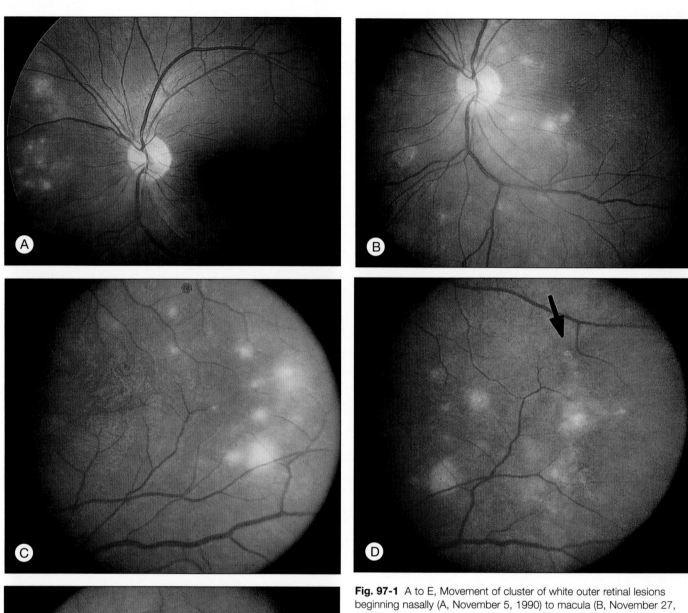

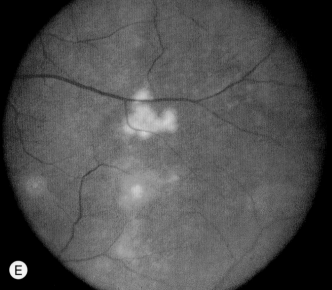

Fig. 97-1 A to E, Movement of cluster of white outer retinal lesions beginning nasally (A, November 5, 1990) to macula (B, November 27, 1990) and to supertemporal quadrant (C, December 4, 1990, and D, December 21, 1990). Worm (D, arrow) when first discovered and after treatment with laser (E). (Reproduced from Gass JD, Callanan DG, Bowman CB. Oral therapy in diffuse unilateral subacute neuroretinitis. Arch Ophthalmol 1992; 110:675–680. Copyright © (1992) American Medical Association. All rights reserved.[23])

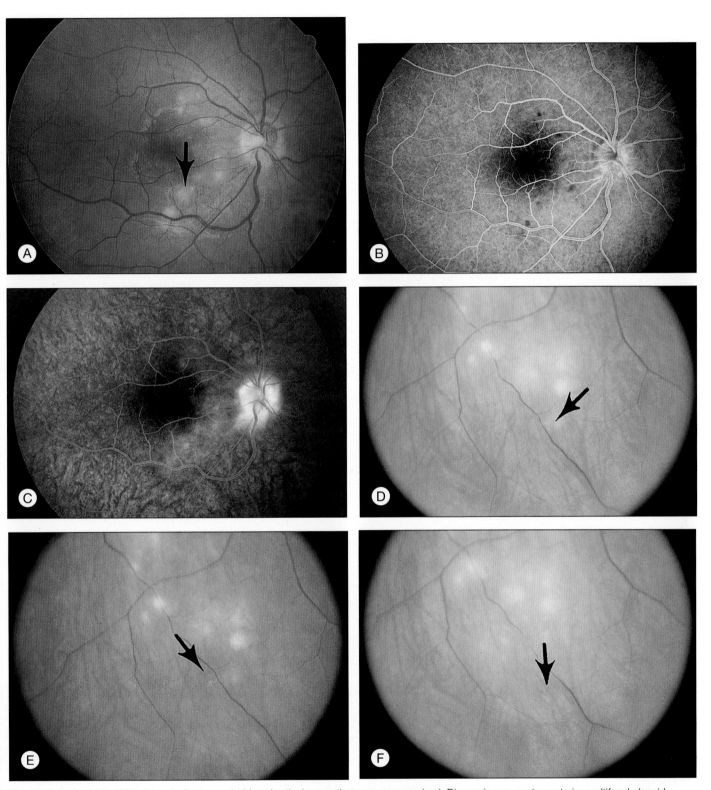

Fig. 97-2 A, April 23, 1993. Arrow indicates probable subretinal worm that was unrecognized. Diagnosis was acute posterior multifocal placoid pigment epitheliopathy. B and C, Angiography shows white lesions are hypofluorescent early and stain late. D to F, Movement of cluster of white spots and worm (arrows) inferiorly before discovery on May 4, 1993, at which time the worm was treated with photocoagulation. (Reproduced from Gass JD. Subretinal migration of a nematode in a patient with diffuse unilateral subacute neuroretinitis. Arch Ophthalmol 1996; 114:1526–1527. Copyright © (1996) American Medical Association. All rights reserved.[24])

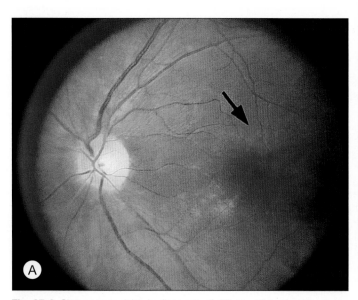
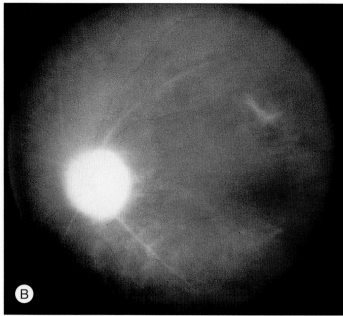

Fig. 97-3 Sixteen-year delay in diagnosis of diffuse unilateral subacute neuroretinitis. A and B, Arrow indicates worm, which was discovered by reviewing old photographs.

The electroretinogram (ERG) is typically subnormal in the affected eye during all stages of the disease, with the b-wave being more affected than the a-wave. Rarely the ERG is extinguished.[5,6] The ERG is normal in the unaffected eye. Eradication of the nematode resulted in improvement in multifocal ERG amplitudes in one case.[16] Visual field studies show a wide range of visual field defects that often cannot be explained on the basis of the visible fundus changes.

Serologic studies, stool examinations, and peripheral blood smears are of little value in making the diagnosis of DUSN.[5] Toxocaral and *Baylisascaris procyonis* antibody titers have been suggested as diagnostic tools to try to characterize which nematode is producing the disease.[17] No serologic test is currently available for *Ancylostoma*. Because of the possibility of commonly shared antigens by different nematodes, or seropositivity unrelated to the actual infesting nematode, interpretation of serologic testing is subject to some error.

PATHOLOGY AND PATHOGENESIS

Only one eye of a patient with clinical evidence of DUSN has been studied histopathologically.[7] The eye was enucleated 15 months after the onset of an ocular inflammation that was clinically suggestive of the early acute and subacute phases of DUSN. This occurred before recognition of the cause of this syndrome, and it is probable that the subretinal worm was lost while sectioning the eye during gross examination. Histopathologically the eye showed evidence of a nongranulomatous vitreitis, retinitis, and retinal and optic nerve perivasculitis with extensive degeneration of the peripheral retina, mild degeneration of the posterior retina, mild optic atrophy, mild degenerative changes in the retinal pigment epithelium (RPE), and a low-grade, patchy,

nongranulomatous choroiditis. No eosinophilia was present. Structural retinal and optic nerve damage appeared inadequate to explain the patient's light perception vision, suggesting that the pathogenesis of DUSN involves mechanical disruption and inflammation of the outer retina, as well as a more diffuse toxic reaction affecting both the inner and outer retinal tissues. This latter reaction is manifest initially by rapid loss of visual function and alteration of the ERG and later by evidence of loss of the ganglion cells (optic atrophy) and narrowing of the retinal vessels. The variability of the inflammatory signs and tissue damage seen in these patients may reflect differences in host immune response to the organism or the characteristics of the nematode itself.

ETIOLOGY

Authors have suggested *Dirofilaria*,[9] *Toxocara canis*,[18] *Ancylostoma caninum*,[8] and *Baylisascaris*[17] as possible causes of DUSN. Evidence that *T. canis* is not the cause includes the following: (1) there is a lack of consistent serologic evidence; (2) the infective second-stage larval form of *T. canis* is smaller than the small worm; (3) the clinical picture is unlike that associated with other forms of ocular toxocariasis; and (4) the worldwide prevalence of *T. canis* is not in keeping with the limited distribution of DUSN.[6]

A. caninum, a common hookworm parasite of dogs, is a suspect as the causative agent because it is a frequent cause of cutaneous larval migrans in the south-eastern USA, its infective third-stage larva measures approximately 650 μm, it can survive in host tissues for months to years without changing size or shape, and cutaneous larval migrans has immediately preceded the onset of DUSN in some patients.[8]

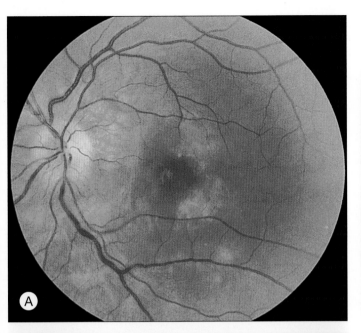

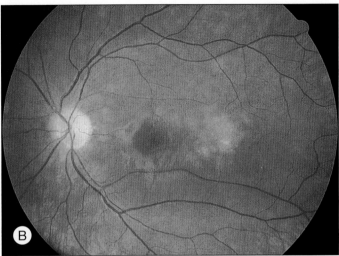

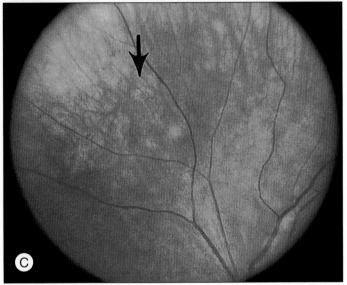

Fig. 97-4 A, Four-year delay in finding the worm, June 2, 1980. Note optic disc swelling and white lesions. B, Diagnosis of diffuse unilateral subacute neuroretinitis, but worm not found, May 4, 1982. C, Note optic atrophy, July 24, 1984. Worm (arrow) was found.

Scanning electron microscopic examination of the nematode illustrated in Fig. 97-5 and excised by means of an eye-wall biopsy was compatible with but not diagnostic for *A. caninum*.[8] Cunha de Souza & Nakashima extracted a subretinal nematode through a retinotomy after pars plana vitrectomy that was morphologically similar to third-stage toxocaral larva based on length of body and esophagus, and shape of tail and mouth.[18]

Baylisascaris procyonis, an intestinal nematode infecting raccoons and skunks, has been proposed as the larger nematode causing DUSN and there is suggestive evidence for this.[17,19] The infective larvae vary in size from 300 to 2000 μm and are an important cause of meningoencephalitis in other animals, as well as (rarely) in humans.[20] However, there is no central nervous system involvement in patients with DUSN and history of exposure to raccoons and skunks is uncommon.

DIFFERENTIAL DIAGNOSIS

DUSN can mimic many other diseases. Box 97-1 lists some of the disorders that may be confused with DUSN. This list is subdivided into the early and late stages of DUSN and is further subdivided according to which part of the eye is predominantly affected by the nematode and the host's response to it. It is important to realize that some of the features listed under early stages may be evident during the later stages of the disease because of the continued presence of the nematode.

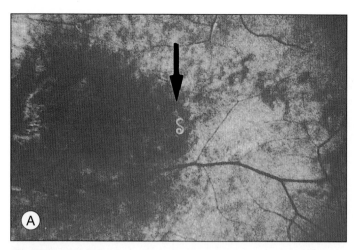

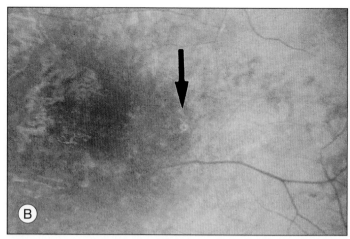

Fig. 97-5 A, B, Subretinal nematode (arrows) in S-shaped and coiled configuration.

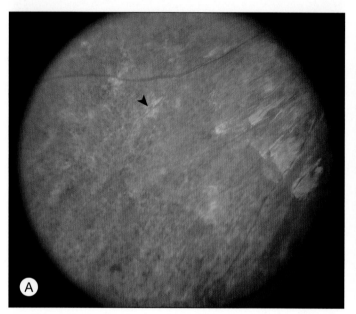

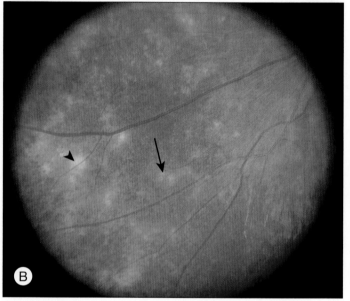

Fig. 97-6 A, Extensive retinal pigment epithelium changes are diffusely present in this 9-year-old boy with visual acuity of 20/200. Clinical and photographic examinations did not locate the nematode. B, Seventeen days later, white lesions are present and there is visible coiled nematode (arrow). Comparison of the two photographs suggests that a nematode in the S-shaped configuration, partially obscured by a branch retinal vein in A (arrowhead), was present in the same location as the largest white lesion in B (arrowhead).

In the early stages of DUSN, the deep gray-white lesions may mimic many other infectious and inflammatory conditions. Toxoplasmosis, cytomegalovirus, and bacterial or fungal abscesses may be distinguished by their usual involvement of the inner retina, their clinical course, and the prominent chorioretinal scarring left in the area of the retinitis. The acute lesions of DUSN involve only the outer retina and involve only one segment, usually 6 disc diameters or less of the fundus, resolve rapidly, and generally leave few or no changes in the RPE. Unlike DUSN, the active lesions in acute posterior multifocal placoid pigment epitheliopathy and serpiginous choroiditis are accompanied by loss of visual acuity only when the lesions involve the center of the fovea, and they always cause permanent visible alterations in the pigment epithelium. The white lesions in patients with Behçet's disease involve the inner retina, and the patient usually has other manifestations of the disorder, including aphthous ulcers, nondeforming arthritis, and erythema nodosum. The multiple evanescent white-dot syndrome (MEWDS) may be distinguished from DUSN by the following: a frequent history of an antecedent flu-like illness and photopsia; widely scattered, active, often subtle, gray-white outer retinal lesions; an enlarged blind spot; a peculiar wreathlike early-phase angiographic pattern of hyperfluorescent dots; a decrease in the ERG that does not necessarily selectively involve the b wave; and return of the fundus and visual function to normal in most patients within several months. Although the evanescent white

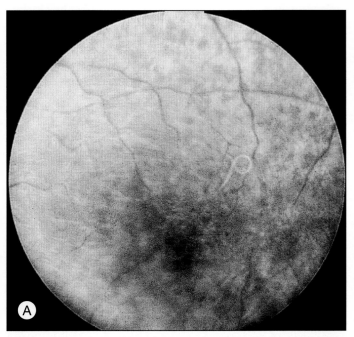

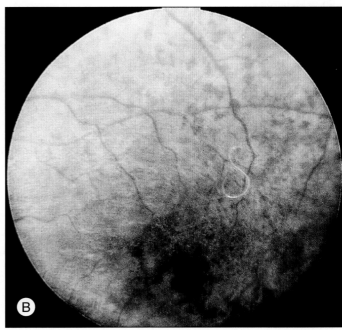

Fig. 97-7 A, B Large subretinal nematodes. (Reproduced from Gass JD, Braunstein RA. Further observations concerning the diffuse unilateral subacute neuroretinitis syndrome. Arch Ophthalmol 1983; 101:1689–1697. Copyright © (1983) American Medical Association. All rights reserved.[6])

Box 97-1 Differential diagnosis of diffuse unilateral subacute neuroretinitis

Early stage
Active retinal lesions
Toxoplasmosis
Cytomegaloviral disease
Fungal or bacterial retinal abscesses
Acute posterior multifocal placoid pigment epitheliopathy
Multiple evanescent white-dot syndrome
Serpiginous choroiditis
Behçet's disease
Pseudo-presumed ocular histoplasmosis syndrome

Perivasculitis
Sarcoidosis

Optic disc swelling
Acute neuroretinitis
Papilledema

Vitreitis
Pars planitis

Late stage
Retinal pigment epithelial atrophy
Presumed ocular histoplasmosis syndrome
Unilateral retinitis pigmentosa
Secondary to traumatic chorioretinopathy
Chorioretinal atrophy after ophthalmic artery occlusion

Optic atrophy
Secondary to optic neuritis
Compressive lesions
Ischemic optic neuropathy

---

lesions in both diseases look similar, those in DUSN block fluorescence early, whereas those in MEWDS typically do not.

Patients with DUSN occasionally may demonstrate severe perivenous candle-wax-dripping exudate or focal mounds of subretinal exudate identical to that seen in patients with sarcoidosis.[8]

After development of scattered focal chorioretinal scars, the fundus of patients with DUSN may be mistaken for the presumed ocular histoplasmosis syndrome (POHS). The frequent bilaterality of POHS, the normalcy of the RPE between the focal scars, the absence of vitreous inflammatory cells, and the lack of optic atrophy and retinal vessel narrowing differentiate POHS from DUSN. Patients with multifocal choroiditis and panuveitis syndrome can closely simulate DUSN if the disease is confined to one eye. Vitreitis, visual field loss unexplained by fundus changes, multiple white outer retinal active inflammatory lesions, multifocal chorioretinal scars, RPE changes in areas between the scars, and ERG abnormalities are all features common to both disorders.

The presence of bone-spicule migration of RPE into the retina and posterior subcapsular cataract, two common manifestations of retinitis pigmentosa, are rare in DUSN. In addition, retinitis pigmentosa is rarely unilateral. Trauma may cause either optic atrophy or diffuse pigmentary changes in the fundus, but rarely in the absence of a history or other evidence of trauma. The optic atrophy of DUSN may be mistaken for other causes of optic atrophy, particularly if the other features of DUSN are overlooked. Finally, eyes that have sustained occlusion of the ophthalmic artery may show signs similar to late-stage DUSN.

TREATMENT

Photocoagulation of the nematode using 200–500 μm, 0.2 to 0.5-s thermal laser application effectively destroys the worm and is the treatment of choice. It causes minimal or no post-treatment exacerbation of inflammation and is successful in causing prompt and permanent inactivation of the disease. Visual acuity often does not improve significantly unless the worm is killed soon after onset of visual loss. Locating the smaller nematode, which varies in size from 400 to 1000 μm

in length, may be difficult, time-consuming, require multiple patient visits, and is not always successful. The disappearance and reappearance of successive crops of white subretinal lesions in contiguous areas over a period of several weeks or months in one eye is strong presumptive evidence of persistent viability of the nematode.

Antihelminthic agents in patients with DUSN are usually ineffective in eradication of the nematode.[2,6] However, thiabendazole is effective in the treatment of some patients with a

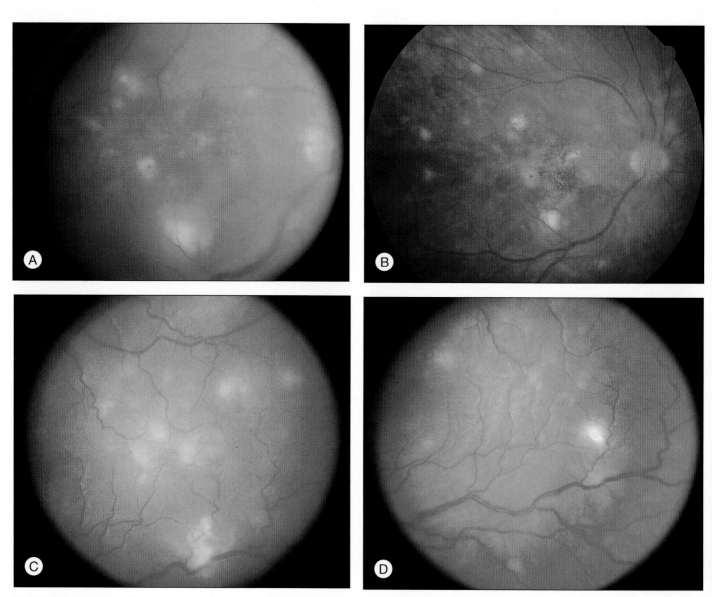

Fig. 97-8 A, Media opacification precluded an adequate clinical or photographic examination in this patient with severe vitreitis. B, Treatment with thiabendazole resulted in formation of a prominent white spot nasal to the optic nerve at 1 week (not shown) and complete clearing of the vitreous haze, shown here at 3.5 months after treatment. Vision remained 20/200. C, This 11-year-old Brazilian girl had recurrent attacks of severe hypopyon uveitis with crops of posterior lesions. Search for an intraocular nematode was unrevealing due to media haze. Note the acute white lesions, vitreous haze, and large inflammatory infiltrate temporal to the macula. D, Nine days after thiabendazole, there is marked clearing of the white lesions and vitreous haze. A new, prominent white spot is present adjacent to the inflammatory infiltrate and is presumed to be the site of the dead nematode. All inflammatory reactions ceased after treatment and vision remained 20/25.

moderate degree of vitreitis associated with a breakdown in the blood–retinal barrier (Fig. 97-8, A and B).[21,22] A new, intense focus of retinitis at the site of the dead or incapacitated nematode can sometimes be seen 4 to 7 days after the administration of thiabendazole and is taken as presumptive evidence of death of the nematode, especially if it occurs in the vicinity of a recent crop of active lesions (Fig. 97-8, C and D). Ivermectin, a drug treatment of filiarial diseases, and albendazole, an antiparasitic, have been used as less toxic alternatives to thiabendazole with equivocal results. Casella et al. reported that ivermectin failed to kill a nematode that was subsequently identified and destroyed with laser photocoagulation.[2] Another therapeutic strategy that has been successful in 3 patients with the typical course of DUSN, minimal vitreitis, and an occult worm is the use of moderately intense scatter photocoagulation in the vicinity of the white lesions to break down the blood–retinal barrier before the administration of thiabendazole[8] (Fig. 97-9, A, B, and C).

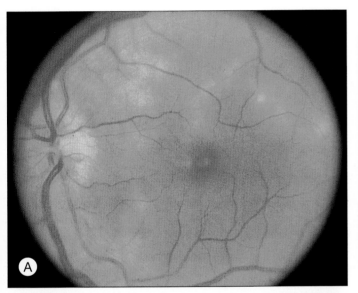

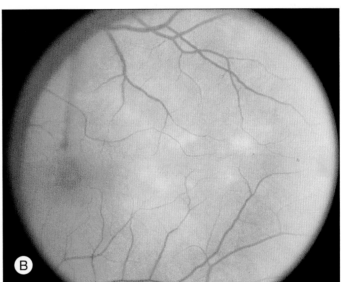

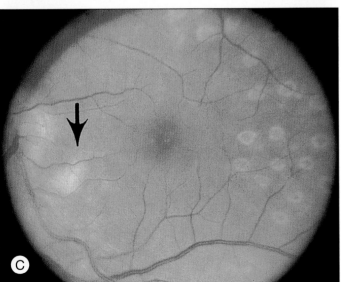

Fig. 97-9 A, Scatter laser treatment and thiabendazole treatment in a patient with mild vitreitis. Patient was seen on multiple occasions, and worm was not found, March 28, 1995. B, April 4, 1995. Note that the cluster of white lesions has moved to the temporal half of the macula. Scatter laser treatment was applied to this area, and tiabendazole was prescribed, C, April 17, 1995. Note that lesions in the area of laser have faded, and there is a new intense lesion (arrow) near the optic disc at the presumed site of the dead worm. The disease rapidly became inactive thereafter. (Reproduced with permission from Gass JDM, Callanan DG, Bowman CB. Oral therapy in diffuse unilateral subacute neuroretinitis. Arch Ophthalmol 1992; 110:675–680.[23])

REFERENCES

1. Cai J, Wei R, Zhu L et al. Diffuse unilateral subacute neuroretinitis in China. Arch Ophthalmol 2000; 118:721–722.

2. Casella AM, Farah ME, Belfort R Jr. Antihelminthic drugs in diffuse unilateral subacute neuroretinitis. Am J Ophthalmol 1998; 125:109–111.

3. de Souza EC, da Cunha SL, Gass JD. Diffuse unilateral subacute neuroretinitis in South America. Arch Ophthalmol 1992; 110:1261–1263.

4. de Souza EC, Abujamra S, Nakashima Y et al. Diffuse bilateral subacute neuroretinitis: first patient with documented nematodes in both eyes. Arch Ophthalmol 1999; 117:1349–1351.

5. Gass JD, Gilbert WR Jr, Guerry RK et al. Diffuse unilateral subacute neuroretinitis. Ophthalmology 1978; 85:521–545.

6. Gass JD, Braunstein RA. Further observations concerning the diffuse unilateral subacute neuroretinitis syndrome. Arch Ophthalmol 1983; 101:1689–1697.

7. Gass JDM, Scelfo R. Diffuse unilateral subacute neuroretinitis. J R Soc Med 1978; 71:95–111.

8. Gass JDM. Stereoscopic atlas of macular diseases: diagnosis and treatment, vol. 4. St. Louis: Mosby; 1997:622–628.

9. Parsons HE. Nematode chorioretinitis: report of a case, with photographs of a viable worm. Arch Ophthalmol 1952; 47:799–800.

10. Raymond LA, Gutierrez Y, Strong LE et al. Living retinal nematode (filarial-like) destroyed with photocoagulation. Ophthalmology 1978; 85:944–949.

11. Harto MA, Rodriguez-Salvador V, Avino JA et al. Diffuse unilateral subacute neuroretinitis in Europe. Eur J Ophthalmol 1999; 9:58–62.

12. Cialdini AP, de Souza EC, Avila MP. The first South American case of diffuse unilateral subacute neuroretinitis caused by a large nematode. Arch Ophthalmol 1999; 117:1431–1432.

13. Kuchle M, Knorr HL, Medenblik-Frysch S et al. Diffuse unilateral subacute neuroretinitis syndrome in a German most likely caused by the raccoon roundworm, *Baylisascaris procyonis*. Graefes Arch Clin Exp Ophthalmol 1993; 231:48–51.

14. Yuen VH, Chang TS, Hooper PL. Diffuse unilateral subacute neuroretinitis syndrome in Canada. Arch Ophthalmol 1996; 114:1279–1282.

15. Moraes LR, Cialdini AP, Avila MP et al. Identifying live nematodes in diffuse unilateral subacute neuroretinitis by using the scanning laser ophthalmoscope. Arch Ophthalmol 2002; 120:135–138.

16. Martidis A, Greenberg PB, Rogers AH et al. Multifocal electroretinography response after laser photocoagulation of a subretinal nematode. Am J Ophthalmol 2002; 133:417–419.

17. Kazacos KR, Raymond LA, Kazacos EA et al. The raccoon ascarid. A probable cause of human ocular larva migrans. Ophthalmology 1985; 92:1735–1744.

18. Cunha de Souza E, Nakashima Y. Diffuse unilateral subacute neuroretinitis. Report of transvitreal surgical removal of a subretinal nematode. Ophthalmology 1995; 102:1183–1186.

19. Kazacos KR, Vestre WA, Kazacos EA et al. Diffuse unilateral subacute neuroretinitis syndrome: probable cause. Arch Ophthalmol 1984; 102: 967–968.

20. Mets MB, Noble AG, Basti S et al. Eye findings of diffuse unilateral subacute neuroretinitis and multiple choroidal infiltrates associated with neural larva migrans due to *Baylisascaris procyonis*. Am J Ophthalmol 2003; 135:888–890.

21. Gass JD, Callanan DG, Bowman CB. Successful oral therapy for diffuse unilateral subacute neuroretinitis. Trans Am Ophthalmol Soc 1991; 89:97–112.

22. Maguire AM, Zarbin MA, Conner TB et al. Ocular penetration of thiabendazole. Arch Ophthalmol 1952; 108:1675.

23. Gass JDM, Callanan DG, Bowman CB. Oral therapy in diffuse unilateral subacute neuroretinitis. Arch Ophthalmol 1992; 110:675–680.

24. Gass JDM. Subretinal migration of a nematode in a patient with diffuse unilateral subacute neuroretinitis. Arch Ophthalmol 1996; 114:1526–1527.

Chapter

98

Scleral Inflammatory Disease

Albert T. Vitale
Maite Sainz de la Maza

INTRODUCTION

Inflammatory disease of the sclera is uncommon, ranging in severity from relatively benign superficial inflammation of the episclera to destructive involvement of the underlying tissue with frank necrosis. The distinction between episcleritis and scleritis is critical as the presentation, therapeutic approach, visual prognosis, ocular morbidity, and the association with potentially life-threatening underlying systemic disease vary considerably.[1,2] Episcleritis is an acute, self-limited condition of the episclera which rarely produces significant adverse ocular sequelae, is less frequently associated with systemic disease, and usually requires no more than systemic nonsteroidal anti-inflammatory drugs (NSAIDs) or topical corticosteroids if treatment is necessary.[3] In contrast, scleritis is a chronic, painful, potentially blinding disease involving both the episclera and sclera. The association of scleritis with systemic autoimmune diseases and the frequent occurrence of ocular complications, including keratitis, uveitis, and glaucoma with anterior disease and exudative retinal detachment, subretinal mass, and optic disc swelling with posterior scleritis, necessitates aggressive systemic therapy with NSAIDs, corticosteroids, and immunosuppressive agents, alone or in combination.[4–12] Posterior scleritis, in particular, is a source of diagnostic confusion due to its variable clinical features and obscure location and it carries a significant risk of visual loss.[13]

ANATOMIC AND STRUCTURAL CONSIDERATIONS

The sclera forms an incomplete shell covering approximately five-sixths of the eye, providing a protective outer coat and an attachment site for extraocular muscles, and it serves to stabilize intraocular pressure. It may be divided into three layers: (1) the outermost episclera; (2) the middle scleral stroma; and (3) the innermost lamina fusca, which merges with the suprachoroidal and supraciliary lamellae of the uveal tract. The sclera is opaque, relatively avascular, and acellular, and is comprised of 70% to 80% collagen by weight (predominantly type I, with smaller amounts of types III, V, and VI), moderate amounts of proteoglycan and glycoprotein, some elastin fibrils (2%), and few fibroblasts.[1,2,14] Tissue homeostasis is achieved by the functional and metabolic interdependence of these components. For example, matrix metalloproteinases (MMPs), which are constitutively expressed by scleral fibroblasts and induced by inflammation, are likely to play an important role in both in normal scleral connective tissue turnover as well as collagenolysis in necrotizing scleritis.[15]

The sclera is richly innervated by branches of the posterior ciliary nerves which perforate the sclera around the optic nerve. The posterior sclera is innervated by numerous short posterior ciliary nerves while the two long posterior ciliary nerves supply the anterior portion. Not surprisingly, scleritis is frequently accompanied by severe pain due to both stretching of the nerves from scleral edema and direct involvement.

The blood supply of the sclera is derived from the long posterior and anterior ciliary arteries which arborize within the episclera to form three vascular arcades. The most superficial vessels form the bulbar conjunctival plexus; the middle layer or the superficial episcleral plexus assumes a radial configuration within Tenon's capsule; and the deep vascular plexus lies adjacent to the sclera. Scleritis primarily involves this latter plexus while the overlying episcleral vessels are secondarily affected. With the exception of perforating vessels which traverse rather than supply the sclera, the stroma is poorly vascularized and derives its nutritional requirements by diffusion from the highly vascular episclera and, to a lesser degree, from the choroid.

EPIDEMIOLOGY AND CLASSIFICATION

A precise epidemiological description of scleral inflammatory disease is somewhat problematic given its relative rarity and the bias inherent in large retrospective series from tertiary centers from which these data are obtained. Nevertheless, certain generalizations can be made: Episcleritis is more frequent among young and middle-aged adults with a peak onset in the fourth decade while scleritis occurs more frequently among middle-aged and elderly individuals; both entities are extremely uncommon in children and have a female predominance and there are no known geographic, racial, or genetic associations with either disease. Scleral inflammatory disease is rare, comprising only 0.08% of 9600 referrals to two ophthalmology departments in Glasgow between 1966 and 1974[16] and 2.6% of 6,600 patients referred to the Immunology Service at the Massachusetts Eye and Ear Infirmary in Boston over an 11-year period.[2] Episcleritis is probably more common than the literature would suggest, given its self-limited course and frequent management by community ophthalmologists.

The classification scheme proposed by Watson & Hayreh[5] divides scleral inflammatory disease into two main categories, episcleritis and scleritis, depending on the anatomic site, extent of the inflammatory process, and the associated findings in the scleral vasculature (Table 98-1). Episcleritis is defined as inflammation and edema involving only the episcleral tissues and may be further classified as simple or nodular. Scleritis, defined as inflammation and edema involving the scleral and episcleral tissues with injection of both the superficial and deep episcleral vascular plexus, may be either anterior or posterior in location. Anterior scleritis is further subclassified into diffuse, nodular, necrotizing with inflammation (necrotizing), and necrotizing without inflammation (scleromalacia perforans). This classification has proven useful as it is uncommon for scleritis to progress from one subcategory to another during the course of the disease.[9] Nevertheless, transformation from diffuse to nodular or necrotizing disease may occur, and so careful examination at each recurrence is essential such that prompt and appropriate treatment may be initiated. In a recent study of the clinical features and treatment results of 134 patients with episcleritis and scleritis by Jabs and co-workers,[12] 94% maintained the same type of scleral inflammation throughout the course of their disease. Only two of 37 patients with episcleritis at initial presentation subsequently evolved into scleritis while six of 97 patients with scleritis progressed to another subtype throughout the follow-up period. One of the two patients with episcleritis who progressed to scleritis had rheumatoid arthritis while five of the six patients with scleritis whose disease changed from one subtype to another had an underlying systemic disease.

CLINICAL FEATURES

Presenting signs and symptoms

Episcleritis presents abruptly with mild to moderate ocular discomfort manifesting as burning, foreign-body sensation, epiphora, or mild photophobia. Unlike scleritis, tenderness to palpation of the globe is absent and frank pain is extremely uncommon. When it occurs, it is described as a slight ache localized to the eye. The cardinal signs are redness, ranging in intensity from a mild pinkish hue to a fiery red, with injection and dilation of the episcleral blood vessels, and edema of the episcleral tissues. Episcleritis may be bilateral, though not frequently simultaneous, in approximately one-third of cases: recurrence, not necessarily in the same location, is common over a period of years, decreasing in frequency after the first 3 to 4 years.[5]

Simple episcleritis, which may be sectorial or diffuse in nature, is more common than nodular episcleritis. In nodular episcleritis, inflammation is confined to a well-circumscribed area, forming a raised, red-pink, mobile nodule with scant surrounding congestion. In both cases, inflammation is limited to the episclera, resolving over a period of weeks, leaving the underlying sclera intact, in spite of recurrent disease. Vision is usually unaffected and extension of the inflammatory process to adjacent ocular structures is very uncommon.

In contradistinction, the presentation of scleritis is characterized by the insidious onset of moderate to severe penetrating ocular pain over a period of five to 10 days, frequently radiating to the forehead, jaw, or sinuses, with exquisite tenderness to palpation of the globe. Without treatment, pain may persist for several months. In some patients, such as those with necrotizing scleritis, pain may be so intense and chronic as to be totally debilitating, while in others, the severity of pain may be out of proportion with the clinical signs, leading to extensive and unnecessary neurological evaluation. As with episcleritis, epiphora and photophobia may be present. The principal signs of anterior scleritis are scleral edema and intense dilation of the deep episcleral vascular plexus producing redness and injection with a bluish to violaceous tinge. Scleral inflammation may be localized to one sector; most frequently to the interpalpebral zone, followed by the superior quadrants, or may involve the sclera diffusely. An exception is scleromalacia perforans (necrotizing scleritis without inflammation) which presents with neither pain nor redness. Simultaneous or sequential bilateral inflammation may occur in 34% to 50% of cases,[2,5,6] while recurrent disease is common over a period of many years, eventually waning in frequency after the first three to six years.[5] Visual acuity may be affected in anterior scleritis, and is frequently decreased in posterior scleritis, due to extension of the inflammatory process to adjacent ocular structures and the development of keratitis, uveitis, glaucoma, cataract, or posterior-segment pathology.

Ocular exam

An assessment of the level of inflammation in the episclera and sclera as a part of a general ocular exam is essential in distinguishing episcleritis from scleritis. This is best achieved by examining the episclera and sclera under conditions of daylight and with the slit lamp, employing diffuse, white light, the narrow slit beam, and red-free illumination. Examination in daylight is sometimes the only way to distinguish episcleritis from scleritis, as it does not distort the natural color of the sclera and renders the eye pink to red in the former and deep bluish-red or violaceous in the latter. If scleral necrosis is present, blue-gray to dark-brown areas corresponding to the underlying uvea may become visible through the translucent sclera. If tissue necrosis is progressive, the scleral area may become avascular, producing a central white

Table 98-1 Classification of scleral inflammatory disease[2,5,12]
A. Episcleritis (27.6–35%)
1. Simple (78.3–81.1%)
2. Nodular (17–21.7%)
B. Scleritis (65–72.4%)
1. Anterior (93–98%)
a. Diffuse (39.7–64.4%)
b. Nodular (22.2–44.5%)
c. Necrotizing (13.3–26%
with inflammation (9.6–23%)
without inflammation (3–4%)
2. Posterior (2–7.2%)

sequestrum surrounded by a well-demarcated black or dark-brown circle. The slough may be gradually replaced by granulation tissue, leaving the underlying uvea bare or covered by a thin layer of conjunctiva.[2]

Slit-lamp examination under conditions of diffuse illumination helps to localize the maximum level of congestion to the superficial episcleral plexus and identify the presence of nodules in episcleritis. In episcleritis, congested vessels follow the usual radial pattern and edema is confined to the episcleral tissue. This latter finding is confirmed by examination with the narrow slit beam, the anterior edge of which is displaced forward by underlying episcleral edema, while the posterior edge remains flat against the sclera, in its normal position. Topical application of 10% phenylephrine renders the eye white as its vasoconstrictor effect is greater on the superficial episcleral plexus with no significant effect on the deep episcleral vessels (Fig. 98-1). Red-free light is useful in delineating areas of maximal vascular congestion and to detect lymphocytic infiltrations of the episcleral tissue, which appear as yellow spots.[2]

In scleritis, slit-lamp examination with diffuse illumination helps to detect new and abnormal vessels and congestion of the deep episcleral plexus, a key finding in the differentiation from episcleritis. It also serves to confirm the macroscopic impression of avascular areas with sequestra or uveal show and to localize the presence of nodules, which, unlike those found in episcleritis, are nonmobile. The presence of primary scleral edema and that involving the overlying episcleral tissues is appreciated on narrow slit-beam examination in which both the anterior and posterior edges of the slit-lamp beam are displaced forward. The eye remains red following topical application of 10% phenylephrine as the deep episcleral plexus remains congested. Red-free light is helpful in revealing areas of maximal vascular congestion, avascularity, and new vascular channels.

The conjunctival, superficial episcleral and deep episcleral plexuses can also be imaged with videoangiography and high-speed, external, anterior-segment fluorescein and indocyanine green angiography (ICGA). The findings in anterior-segment fluorescein angiography (FA) in scleral inflammatory disease were initially described by Watson & Bovey[17] and have proven to be particularly helpful in the identification of early necrotizing scleritis. Most recently, Nieuwenhuizen and colleagues[18] have shown that combined, sequential anterior-segment FA and ICGA provides complementary information which may be useful in the differential diagnosis and monitoring of treatment of patients with scleritis as well as in detecting subclinical pathology.

Diffuse anterior scleritis

Diffuse anterior scleritis is the most benign and common presentation, comprising between 40% and 64% of patients with anterior scleritis and is the most likely subgroup to be confused with episcleritis[1,2,12] (Table 98-1). Slit-lamp examination discloses congestion of the superficial and deep episcleral plexus together with tortuosity, distortion, and loss of the normal radial vascular pattern and the appearance of new and abnormal vascular channels (Fig. 98-2). Both anterior-segment FA and ICG show rapid filling and short transit times with a structurally normal flow pattern.[18] However, an abnormal vascular pattern with anastamoses between the larger vessels in the superficial or deep episcleral plexuses with extensive leakage may be observed on FA following prolonged inflammation or recurrences.[17] These anastamoses may persist and remain permeable for a prolonged period of time, even in the absence of inflammation. There is no evidence of vascular closure. On ICG, there is no leakage except in regions of local vascular damage, which may signify accompanying deep inflammation.[18]

Clinical case

A 41-year-old woman with relapsing polychondritis replete with saddle-nose deformity, inflammation of auricular pinnae, and audiovestibular involvement presented with scleritis of 2 years' duration having been treated with high doses of steroids (prednisone 60 mg/day) for several months. Persistent diffuse scleritis was noted in both eyes in spite of the high doses of

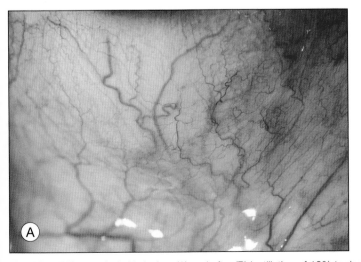
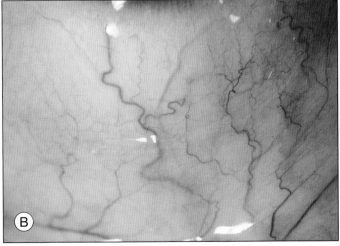

Fig. 98-1 Diffuse episcleritis before (A) and after (B) instillation of 10% topical phenylephrine.

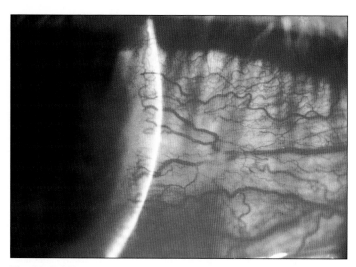

Fig. 98-2 Diffuse anterior scleritis. The globe is exquisitely tender to touch; congestion involves the superficial and deep episcleral plexus together with tortuosity, distortion, and loss of normal radial vascular architecture.

steroids, and so cyclophosphamide 1.5 mg/kg per day was commenced. Anterior-segment FA (Fig. 98-3 A and B) revealed increased transit time and hypoperfusion of both conjunctival and episcleral circulation (unexpected findings) while ICGA (Fig. 98-3 C and D) showed leakage in regions of vascular damage, signifying deep inflammation as well as an abnormal vascular pattern.

Of 30 patients with recurrent diffuse scleritis studied by Tuft & Watson, progression from diffuse to nodular or diffuse to necrotizing disease was observed in only 12 and three patients respectively.[9] In the same series, the incidence of visual loss (9%) was lowest among patients with diffuse scleritis for all subcategories of scleral inflammatory disease, whereas loss of visual acuity was recorded in 26% of 77 patients with diffuse anterior scleritis studied by Foster & Sainz de la Maza.[2] Decreased visual acuity was reported in 18% of 58 patients with diffuse anterior scleritis reported by Jabs and colleagues.[12] Between 45% and 62% of patients with diffuse anterior scleritis have an associated systemic disease, typically rheumatoid arthritis.[2,12]

Nodular anterior scleritis

Nodular scleritis is characterized by inflammation localized to deep red or violaceous scleral nodule(s) which are tender and immobile. Nodules are usually localized to the interpalpebral zone, approximately 3 to 4 mm from the limbus (Fig. 98-4). As with diffuse anterior scleritis, the onset of pain is gradual, reaching a peak over a 5- to 10-day period. Lack of mobility and detailed slit-lamp examination disclosing vascular congestion and tortuosity of both the superficial and deep episcleral plexuses overlying the nodule distinguish these nodules from those found in episcleritis. The normal radial pattern is disrupted and anastamotic shunts between arterial and venous channels may be seen. The findings on anterior-segment FA and ICG are similar to those found in diffuse anterior scleritis: rapid filling and short transit times with staining of the nodules in both studies.[18]

Progression to necrotizing scleritis was observed in approximately 20% of 54 patients with nodular anterior scleritis analyzed by Tuft & Watson.[9] Findings which may herald the progression to necrosis include the presence of avascular zones within the nodule which may slough, leaving bare choroid covered by a thin layer of conjunctiva, and circumferential involvement of the globe with nodular disease. In their study population, the incidence of visual loss for patients with nodular anterior scleritis was greater than that with diffuse anterior scleritis (26% versus 9%), whereas the converse was true (13% versus 26%) in the series reported by Foster & Sainz de la Maza.[2] An associated systemic disease is found in up to 45% of patients, the most common being connective tissue diseases, especially rheumatoid arthritis.[2,9,12]

Anterior scleritis with inflammation (necrotizing scleritis)

Necrotizing scleritis is the most destructive form of scleritis with a rate of ocular complications approaching 92% in a recent series reported by Jabs and colleagues.[12] Extension of the inflammatory process led to the development of anterior uveitis (69%), peripheral ulcerative keratitis (PUK) (41%), glaucoma (23%), and significant loss of visual acuity in 82% of the patients with necrotizing scleritis analyzed by Foster & Sainz de la Maza.[2] Furthermore, the presence of necrotizing scleritis is considered an ominous sign as it is highly associated with systemic connective tissue disease and/or a potentially lethal systemic vasculitic disease in 50% to 81% of patients.[2,12] Watson & Hayreh reported a 29% mortality among 207 patients within 5 years of the onset of necrotizing scleritis; many deaths were attributed to systemic vasculitic lesions.[5] In another study by Foster and colleagues,[19] seven of 20 patients with necrotizing scleritis had died within 8 years of the onset of ocular disease; again, mortality was due in large part to untoward vascular sequelae. Eleven of the 13 patients who remained alive received immunosuppressive therapy while none of the seven who died was treated systemically.

The principal findings on ocular exam are the presence of white avascular areas surrounded by edema of the sclera and acute congestion of the abnormal episcleral channels. The damaged sclera becomes thin and translucent, revealing the brown color of the underlying choroid (Fig. 98-5). If there is a sustained elevation in the intraocular pressure, staphyloma may form in areas of thinned sclera. Spontaneous perforation may occur but more often follows accidental or surgical trauma.

Anterior-segment FA shows hypoperfusion, venular occlusion, and new vessels which leak extensively.[17] In contrast to nodular scleritis, the transit time in necrotizing scleritis is markedly increased, even in the presence of ocular congestion. With severe inflammation, vaso-occlusive changes in the conjunctival vessels may also appear. ICGA also shows hypoperfusion, venular occlusion, increased transit time, and late leakage from new or damaged vessels in addition to providing detailed images of functioning vessels which might otherwise be obscured by edema or leakage of fluorescein dye.[18] Both FA and ICG are useful during the early treatment phases to confirm the presence or absence of vascular occlusion and to detect active vasculitis.

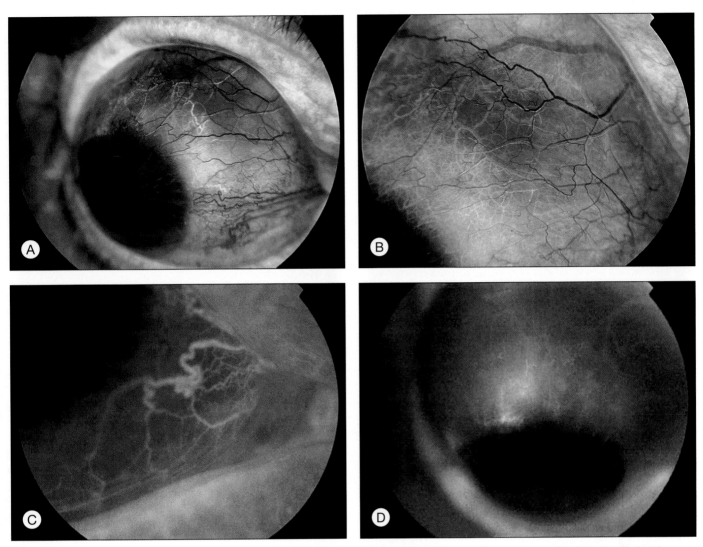

Fig. 98-3 Anterior-segment fluorescein angiography (A: 26 s; B: 41 s) shows increased transit time and hypoperfusion of both conjunctival and episcleral circulation (an unexpected finding). Indocyanine green angiography (C 1 min; D 17 min), shows leakage in regions of vascular damage (nasal and superior OD) signifying deep inflammation as well as an abnormal vascular pattern.

Necrotizing scleritis may also appear following various types of ocular surgery including cataract extraction, transscleral suture fixation of an intraocular lens, retinal detachment repair, non-penetrating and penetrating filtering procedures, strabismus correction, and pterygium excision.[20–23] The onset of surgically induced necrotizing scleritis, with or without PUK, is variable, ranging from several weeks to many months. Again, its presence may be indicative of an occult, potentially lethal systemic autoimmune vasculitic disease or may herald the recurrence of vasculitis in a patient with a previously diagnosed systemic autoimmune disease which had been in remission. With the exception of the use of adjunctive mitomycin C for pterygium surgery, an associated systemic autoimmune condition was seen in 60% to 90% of cases of surgically induced necrotizing scleritis.

Necrotizing scleritis without inflammation (scleromalacia perforans)

Scleromalacia perforans is a rare, bilateral condition, occurring predominantly among elderly females with a history of severe,

progressive, long-standing rheumatoid arthritis with extra-articular manifestations. In fact, rheumatoid arthritis was the only associated systemic disease found in 46% and 67% of patients with scleromalacia perforans studied by Watson & Hazleman[1] and Sainz de la Maza et al.[24] respectively. Ocular complications, including keratitis, uveitis, glaucoma, cataract, and macular edema, are not infrequent, resulting in visual loss in about a third of patients.[2]

In contrast to necrotizing scleritis with inflammation, the eye is not painful. The condition is characterized by the appearance of yellow to grayish patches on the sclera that gradually develop a necrotic slough or sequestrum which eventually separates from the underlying sclera, leaving bare choroid, covered by a thin layer of fibrous tissue or conjunctiva (Fig. 98-6). Progression can be prevented if treatment is instituted early. An initial characteristic finding on slit-lamp examination is a reduction in the number and size of vessels in the episclera surrounding the sequestrum, giving porcelain-like appearance. These vessels anastomose with each other and sometimes cross the abnormal area to join with perilimbal vessels. The necrotic process in scleromalacia perforans

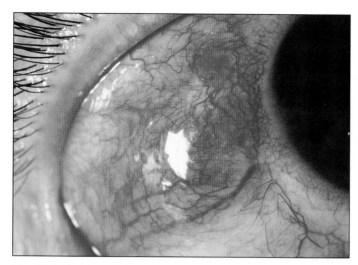

Fig. 98-4 Nodular anterior scleritis. Nodules are tender and immobile, typically localized to the interpalpebral zone.

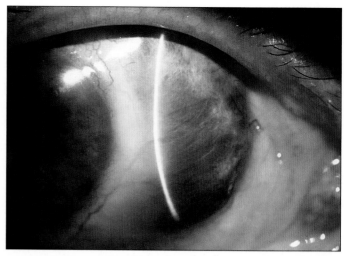

Fig. 98-6 Scleromalacia perforans in a patient with rheumatoid arthritis. There is a profound degree of scleral loss with uveal protrusion under the stretched conjunctiva.

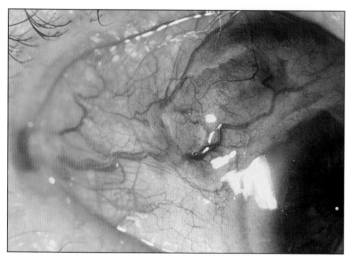

Fig. 98-5 Necrotizing scleritis. There is full-thickness scleral loss with uveal prolapse covered by a thin layer of conjunctival epithelium.

appears to be caused by arteriolar obliteration as evidenced by FA, as opposed to venular nonperfusion, which is more prominent in necrotizing scleritis.[7] The initial color changes in sclera from porcelain white to yellow are often noted by the patient while looking in the mirror, by the patient's family, rheumatologist, or on routine ocular exam. The areas of exposed choroid are conspicuous, appearing blue-black in color. Staphyloma do not develop unless the intraocular pressure is persistently elevated. While spontaneous perforation is rare, these eyes are quite susceptible to traumatic rupture.

Posterior scleritis

Posterior scleritis is defined as inflammation of the sclera posterior of the ora serrata which frequently extends to involve secondarily contiguous ocular structures, including the choroid, retina, optic nerve, extraocular muscles, and orbital tissues.[4,8,13,14,25,26] As with anterior scleritis, it is classified into diffuse, nodular,

and necrotizing variants[1] and may present either in association with anterior inflammatory disease in up to 60% of patients[11] or as an isolated condition. In the latter scenario, the diagnosis may be overlooked, contributing, in part, to the relative rarity of posterior scleritis, comprising between 2% and 7.2% of patients with scleritis in several large series[1,2,12] (Table 98-1). The spectrum of systemic disease associations is similar to that seen with anterior scleritis, albeit at a slightly reduced frequency, occurring in approximately 29% of patients.[11] While posterior scleritis may involve both eyes, it most commonly presents as unilateral recurrent disease among middle-aged women. Posterior scleritis among children is exceedingly rare, but may represent a distinct subgroup of patients, differing from the adult variety on the basis of gender (male), the lack of systemic disease association, and the paucity of ocular findings more typically seen in adults.[27]

Pain and visual loss are the predominant presenting symptoms of posterior scleritis. As with anterior scleritis, pain is characteristically severe and radiating, but may be attenuated in patients who are already on treatment for a systemic connective tissue disease. Visual loss may be mild and correctable with the addition of a convex lens, reflecting transient hyperopia induced by a reduction in the axial length secondary to posterior scleral thickening. On the other hand, moderate to profound uncorrectable visual loss, occurring in 17% to 84% of patients,[2,9,12] may be due to a variety of presenting signs, including choroidal folds and retinal striae, annular ciliochoroidal detachment, disc and macular edema, and fundus or orbital mass lesions. These complications may be reversible, with a good visual prognosis, provided there is early diagnosis and prompt, appropriate treatment at onset. Redness is a common presenting sign, especially when associated with anterior scleritis, but may be subtle or absent in posterior scleritis presenting in isolation. In fact, up to 15% of patients have no physical signs of posterior scleritis.[11] Proptosis, lid swelling, and painful limitation of ocular versions are not infrequent and may reflect extension of the inflammatory process to the extraocular muscles and/or orbit.

Funduscopic findings which support the diagnosis of posterior scleritis include optic disc swelling, exudative retinal detachment, choroidal folds, and, less commonly, focal subretinal mass-like lesions. While careful ocular examination is usually sufficient to make the diagnosis and differentiate the various types of anterior scleritis, high-quality ultrasonography is an essential investigation in the diagnosis of posterior scleritis as it demonstrates scleral and choroidal thickening and the presence of edema in Tenon's space, the so-called "T" sign[28-30] (Fig. 98-7). The combination of both A- and B-scan modalities provides the most useful results in distinguishing not only diffuse form nodular posterior scleritis but also posterior scleritis in general from orbital, choroidal, and retinal pathology that may mimic it clinically.[2] While not as sensitive as ultrasonography in detecting changes in eye-wall thickness, computed tomography (CT) is essential in excluding orbital inflammatory disease, tumors, thyroid eye disease, and sinus disease, and in identifying patients with posterior scleritis with extension of the inflammatory process into adjacent ocular structures.[31] Magnetic resonance scanning with gadolinium is able to distinguish scleral from choroidal thickening, which may be of value in patients with choroidal detachments.[32] Likewise, FA may highlight choroidal folds, reveal neurosensory retinal and pigment epithelial detachments, disc edema, and cystoid macular edema, and serve to clarify the differential diagnosis.

Given the highly varied spectrum of signs and symptoms, the differential diagnosis of posterior scleritis is broad and potentially confusing, and is probably best considered in the context of several patterns of presentation.[2,8,11] Foster & Sainz de la Maza[2] have suggested three such patterns: (1) presentations dominated by signs of proptosis, chemosis, lid swelling, and limitation of extraocular motility suggestive of an orbital process; (2) orbital, choroidal, and retinal pathology producing signs of a circumscribed fundus mass lesion or choroidal folds; and (3) serous detachments of the choroid, ciliary body, and neurosensory retina, optic disc swelling, and macular edema (Tables 98-2 to 98-4).

Acute diffuse idiopathic orbital inflammatory disease, orbital tumors, and thyroid ophthalmopathy may present not only with proptosis, conjunctival chemosis, lid swelling and limited extraocular versions, but also with choroidal folds and disc edema. Differentiation from posterior scleritis which has extended to involve adjacent orbital structures requires careful history and examination together with the findings on ultrasonography, CT, and magnetic resonance imaging (Table 98-2). In addition, these entities, together with sphenoid sinusitis and demyelinating optic neuropathy, may also present with acute painful visual loss and must be considered in the differential diagnosis of posterior scleritis.

Nodular posterior scleritis may present as a circumscribed subretinal mass lesion which must be distinguished from primary and secondary choroidal neoplasms (Table 98-3). Choroidal melanoma is distinguished clinically from the rather uniform color of the pigment epithelium overlying a scleral mass in posterior scleritis by the typical presence of hyperpigmentation or hypopigmentation (amelanotic melanoma) of the lesion, overlying orange lipofuscin pigment, and the infrequent finding of choroidal folds.[33] Furthermore, ultrasonography may reveal findings characteristic of choroidal melanoma, including low internal reflectivity, choroidal excavation, acoustic hollowness and orbital shadowing, together with the absence of retrobulbar edema. Circumscribed choroidal hemangiomas are usually pinkish-orange in color, display uniformly high internal reflectivity and the absence of choroidal excavation or retrobulbar edema on ultrasound, and show early hyperfluorescence of large irregular choroidal vessels prior to filling of the retinal vessels with progressive leakage on FA. Metastatic tumors to the choroid may present as a unilateral choroidal mass lesion with or without overlying subretinal fluid or choroidal folds but are typically yellowish or amelanotic and have associated hyperplastic pigment epithelial mottling. Again, ultrasonography reveals a choroidal mass with moderate to high internal reflectivity and the absence of retrobulbar edema, choroidal excavation, acoustic hollowness, or orbital shadowing – findings typically seen with posterior scleritis and choroidal melanoma respectively.

Choroidal folds, while a prominent finding in posterior scleritis, are found variably among patients with primary or secondary choroidal tumors, orbital tumors, idiopathic orbital inflammation, and thyroid ophthalmopathy (Fig. 98-8). Other entities which may present with choroidal folds include ocular hypotony, papilledema, and choroidal neovascularization, as well as following scleral buckling surgery for retinal detachment.

Differential diagnostic considerations in patients with posterior scleritis presenting with annular ciliochoroidal detachment and/or serous detachment of the neurosensory retina include uveal effusion syndrome, Vogt–Koyanagi–Harada (VKH) syndrome, and idiopathic central serous chorioretinopathy (Table 98-4). Choroidal detachment, often with accompanying serous retinal detachment, may also be seen in choroidal melanoma, metastatic choroidal tumors, and as a complication of hypotony following intraocular surgery or retinal detachment. Uveal effusion syndrome is distinct from posterior scleritis in that it usually presents bilaterally, is unaccompanied by pain or anterior scleritis, uveitis is absent, and there is a characteristic hyperpigmented pattern

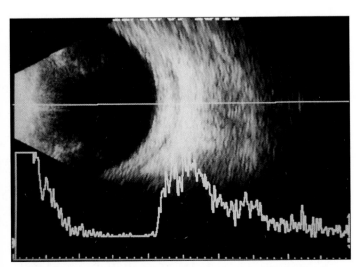

Fig. 98-7 B-scan showing diffuse posterior scleritis with scleral and choroidal thickening and the presence of edema in Tenon's space, the so-called "T" sign.

Table 98-2 Differential diagnosis of posterior scleritis: proptosis, chemosis, lid swelling, and limitation of ocular movements

Parameter	Posterior scleritis	Orbital tumor	Acute diffuse idiopathic orbital inflammation	Thyroid ophthalmopathy
Sex predilection	Female	–	–	Female
Age predilection	Middle-aged and elderly	–	–	Middle-aged and elderly
Laterality	Unilateral	Unilateral	Unilateral	Bilateral
Onset	Gradual	Gradual	Acute	Gradual
Pain	Variable	±	Variable	–
Tenderness	+	–	+	–
Anterior scleritis	+	–	–	–
Visual loss	+	±	±	Variable
Fundus mass	Variable	±	±	–
Color of the mass	Orange	Orange	Orange	–
Proptosis	±	+	+	+
Motility disturbance	±	+	+	–
Conjunctival chemosis	±	+	+	–
Lid edema	±	+	+	–
Pigment epithelium	Yellowish nodules	Normal	Normal	Normal
Disc edema	+	±	±	±
Uveitis	+	–	±	–
Choroidal folds	+	±	±	±
Serous retinal detachment	+	–	±	–
Fluorescein angiography (other than choroidal folds)	Multiple small leaks	Normal	Normal	Normal
Ultrasound	Scleral and choroid thickening: retrobulbar edema (high reflectivity)		Orbital mass (low reflectivity) and/or EOM enlargement	EOM enlargement
Computed tomography scan	Scleral and choroid thickening	Orbital mass with sinus involvement or involvement/bone erosion	Orbital mass without sinus involvement or bone erosion, EOM enlargement	EOM enlargement
Biopsy indication	No biopsy	Biopsy	Biopsy	No biopsy
Response to steroids	Good	Absent	Very good	Variable

EOM, extraocular muscle.
Reproduced with permission from Foster CS, Sainz de la Maza M. The sclera. New York: Springer-Verlag; 1994.[2]

(leopard spots) to the retinal pigment epithelium (RPE) with clear subretinal fluid.[34] FA shows slow choroidal perfusion with prolonged choroidal hyperfluorescence and, much less commonly, focal leaks from the RPE.[35] Despite the fact that both entities may share similar ultrasonographic findings, the presence of nanophthalmos or retrobulbar edema may serve to distinguish uveal effusion syndrome and posterior scleritis respectively. Finally,

unlike posterior scleritis, uveal effusion syndrome is unresponsive to systemic steroids.

Posterior scleritis and VKH may both present with exudative macular detachment, ciliochoroidal detachment, anterior and posterior uveitis, disc edema, turbid subretinal fluid, and multifocal, pinpoint leaks at the level of the RPE on FA. However, VKH is typically a bilateral disease, with patients having accompanying

Table 98-3 Differential diagnosis of posterior scleritis: subretinal mass

Parameter	Posterior scleritis	Choroidal melanoma	Metastatic uveal carcinoma	Choroidal hemangioma
Sex predilection	Female	–	–	–
Age predilection	Middle-aged and elderly	Elderly	Middle-aged and elderly	Middle-aged and elderly
Laterality	Unilateral	Unilateral	Unilateral	Unilateral
Onset	Gradual	Gradual	Gradual	Gradual
Pain	Variable	–	–	–
Tenderness	+	–	+	–
Anterior scleritis	+	–	–	–
Visual loss	+	Variable	Variable	Variable
Color of the mass	Orange	Hyper- or hypopigmented	Hypopigmented	Pinkish-orange
Overlying retina	Yellow deposits	Orange pigment	Dark mottling	Cystoid edema
Proptosis	±	–	–	–
Motility disturbance	±	–	–	–
Conjunctival chemosis	±	–	–	–
Lid edema	±	–	–	–
Disc edema	+	–	–	–
Uveitis	+	–	–	–
Choroidal folds	+	±	±	–
Serous retinal detachment/ subretinal fluid	+/cloudy	+/clear	+/clear	+/clear
Fluorescein angiography (other than choroidal folds)	Small leaks, intrinsic vasculature	Small leaks	Small leaks	Small leaks. Early fluorescence prior to filling retinal vessels
Ultrasound	Scleral and choroid thickening (high reflectivity); retrobulbar edema	Choroidal mass (low reflectivity); no retrobulbar edema	Choroidal mass (moderate reflectivity); no retrobulbar edema	Choroidal mass (high reflectivity); no retrobulbar edema
Response to steroids	Good	Absent	Absent	Absent

Reproduced with permission from Foster CS, Sainz de la Maza M. The sclera. New York: Springer-Verlag; 1994.[2]

integumentary findings (vitiligo, poliosis, and alopecia), neuromeningeal symptoms (tinnitus, dysacusus, ataxia, confusion, and focal neurological defects), and distinctive ethnicity (oriental, darkly pigmented individuals). Ultrasonographic analysis may reveal diffuse choroidal thickening and exudative retinal detachment in both entities; however, in VKH, the choroidal thickening is of low internal reflectivity and retrobulbar edema is absent. Exudative macular detachment, and, less commonly, bullous serous retinal detachment are well-described features of idiopathic central serous chorioretinopathy; however, unlike posterior scleritis, neither the ocular findings of uveitis, anterior scleritis, and disc edema, nor the ultrasonographic features of sclerochoroidal thickening or retrobulbar edema are characteristic of this entity.[34] Systemic steroids are well known to exacerbate the course of idiopathic central serous chorioretinopathy whereas they hasten the resolution of serous retinal detachments in posterior scleritis.

In addition to posterior scleritis, disc and macular edema are seen among a lengthy list of infectious and inflammatory uveitides and may complicate intraocular surgery.[25] A thorough ophthalmic and medical history, review of systems, directed laboratory, and ancillary imaging studies are essential in differentiating posterior scleritis from these entities.

Finally, as with anterior scleritis, masquerade syndromes should be considered in the differential diagnosis, especially in

Table 98-4 Differential diagnosis of posterior scleritis: serous detachment of choroid, ciliary body, and retina

Parameter	Posterior scleritis	Uveal effusion syndrome	Vogt–Koyanagi–Harada syndrome	Idiopathic central serous chorioretinopathy
Sex predilection	Female	Male	–	Male
Age predilection	Middle-aged and elderly	Middle-aged	Young and middle-aged	Middle-aged
Race predilection	–	–	Oriental and pigmented	Caucasian
Laterality	Unilateral	Bilateral	Bilateral	Unilateral
Pain	Variable	–	– (Photophobia)	–
Anterior scleritis	+	–	–	–
Uveitis	+	–	+	–
Disc edema	+	+	+	–
Pigment epithelium	Yellowish nodules	"Leopard spots"	Depigmented or hyperpigmented lines	Serous detachments of pigment epithelium
Serous retinal detachment	+	+	+	+
Serous ciliochoroid detachment	+	+	±	–
Subretinal fluid	Cloudy	Clear	Cloudy	Clear
Fluorescein angiography	Multiple small leaks	Slow choroidal perfusion; occasional leaks	Multiple small leaks; late-staining subretinal fluid	Serous detachments of pigment epithelium
Ultrasound	Scleral and choroidal thickening (high reflectivity); retrobulbar edema	Choroid thickened; serous ciliochoroid, and retinal detachment	Choroid thickened (low internal reflectivity detachment serous retinal	Serous retinal detachment
Miscellaneous	Collagen vascular disease association	High protein level in cerebrospinal fluid (50% of cases)	Headaches, fever dysacusus, vitiligo, meningism (50% of cases)	Anxiety

Reproduced with permission from Foster CS, Sainz de la Maza M. The sclera. New York: Springer-Verlag; 1994.[2]

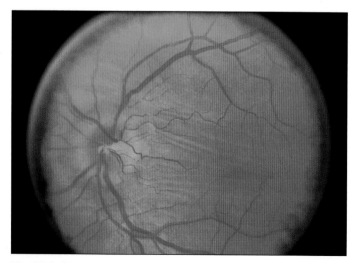

Fig. 98-8 Choroidal folds in a patient with posterior scleritis.

atypical cases of posterior scleritis or those responding incompletely to appropriate therapy. In addition to the primary and metastatic choroidal neoplasms already mentioned, primary ocular–entral nervous system lymphoma may mimic posterior scleritis[36] while mucosal-associated lymphoid tissue (MALT) lymphoma has been reported to masquerade as anterior scleritis.[37]

OCULAR COMPLICATIONS

Ocular complications directly attributable to episcleritis are uncommon. Occasionally, small, localized, nonprogressive, superficial and mid stromal inflammatory cell infiltration of the cornea adjacent to the episcleral edema and/or mild anterior-chamber cell and flare may be seen, usually resolving with or without treatment or untoward sequelae. Unfortunately, cataract and glaucoma arising in patients with episcleritis are more often related to the injudicious and thoughtless use of topical steroids than to the ocular inflammatory disease itself.

In contrast, ocular complications associated with scleritis are common, being present in approximately 50% of patients with anterior scleritis, 85.7% with posterior scleritis, and in 91.7% of patients with necrotizing scleritis, as recently reported by Jabs and colleagues.[12] In this series, decreased visual acuity was observed in 15.9% of patients with scleritis overall and appeared to be more strongly associated with the severity of inflammation and the presence of an underlying systemic disease rather than attributable to any single ocular complication or to the subtype of scleritis per se.

Corneal complications localized to the peripheral cornea are the most common ocular complications among patients with diffuse and necrotizing scleritis. Three patterns of peripheral cornea involvement have been described which are related to the type and severity of scleral inflammatory disease: (1) peripheral corneal thinning; (2) stromal keratitis; and (3) PUK.[38] Peripheral corneal thinning is the most benign form and is frequently associated with diffuse anterior scleritis. It is most often found in middle-aged and elderly patients with long-standing rheumatoid arthritis, although it may occur in young individuals with no underlying systemic condition. The peripheral cornea becomes grayish and thinned in one or more areas, ultimately extending circumferentially over a period of several years. The epithelium remains intact throughout; however, vascularization, lipid deposition, and progressive opacification and thinning may eventually involve the edematous stroma. Vision is usually unaffected unless the peripheral gutter deepens, producing astigmatism. While trauma may precipitate rupture of the thinned cornea, spontaneous perforation is rare.

Stromal keratitis, appearing as multiple white or gray nummular, mid stromal opacities, may arise with extension of diffuse nodular or necrotizing scleritis into the cornea. The keratitis is usually located in the corneal periphery, in the quadrant adjacent to the area of scleral inflammation; however, the central cornea may become involved. If treatment of scleritis is delayed, the stromal infiltrates may coalesce, resulting in large areas of diffuse corneal opacification, eventuating in an appearance akin to the sclera itself ("sclerosing" changes). Vessels may involve the superficial corneal stroma but are more typically far behind the advancing edge of the opacity. Crystalline deposits ("candy floss") may appear as a result of lipid accumulation in the stromal opacities.[5] While these opacities may disappear completely with prompt and aggressive treatment of scleritis, partial regression with permanent corneal changes more often results and may require penetrating keratoplasty if the central visual axis is involved.

PUK is the most severe corneal complication and is usually seen in association with necrotizing scleritis. It begins as a localized gray, edematous, infiltrated area adjacent to a sector of scleral inflammation which breaks down within a few days, leaving only a few layers of stroma and/or Descemet's membrane, with well-demarcated edges. An intrastromal yellow-white blood cell infiltrate may be easily visualized along the advancing edge of the ulcer, which progresses circumferentially rather than centrally.

If treatment is delayed, spontaneous corneal perforation may occur. The presence of PUK and/or necrotizing scleritis portends the presence of potentially lethal systemic vasculitic disease requiring aggressive systemic immunosuppressive therapy.[39]

Uveitis may arise by extension of both anterior and posterior scleral inflammatory disease and their concurrence should be considered a grave sign. At least one episode of mild to moderate anterior uveitis was noted in 42% of 172 patients with scleritis reported by Sainz de la Maza and colleagues.[40] In this study, the presence of anterior uveitis was highly associated with both necrotizing anterior scleritis and with posterior scleritis. Patients with scleritis-associated uveitis were more prone to have visual loss (49%), necrotizing scleritis (37%), PUK (22%), and glaucoma (19%). Posterior uveitis was uniformly present in patients with posterior scleritis. As posterior uveitis is uncommonly associated with anterior scleritis alone, the presence of posterior uveitis in a patient with anterior scleral inflammation should prompt a careful examination for posterior scleritis.[1]

Glaucoma in patients with scleritis, especially that associated with uveitis, is an ominous sign.[41] Elevated intraocular pressure is caused by accompanying scleral edema and uveal inflammation.[42] It is essential to monitor the intraocular pressure, perform gonioscopy, and examine the optic nerve regularly in patients with scleritis as glaucoma may arise by angle-closure, open-angle, and neovascular mechanisms. The reported frequency of elevated intraocular pressure in patients with scleritis varies between 9% and 22%.[1,2,6,12,42]

Cataract in patients with scleritis may be promoted by the presence of chronic anterior uveitis, particularly in association with necrotizing scleritis, long-term steroid treatment, or both. The development of posterior subcapsular cataract in two groups of patients receiving long-term treatment with systemic or local steroids was greater in those patients with scleritis (36%) as compared to those without scleritis (11.5%).[6] The frequency of cataract in patients with necrotizing scleritis ranges from 16.7% to 20%.[2,9,12]

In addition to uveitis, glaucoma, and cataract, patients with both anterior and posterior scleritis may develop hypotony. Ciliary-body hyposecretion with concomitant reduction of intraocular pressure may result from severe posterior-segment inflammation and/or anterior scleritis overlying a large area of the ciliary body. Retinal detachment, both rhegmatogenous and exudative, may produce hypotony which resolves with reattachment of the retina. Prompt and aggressive medical treatment of scleritis and intraocular inflammation usually results in restoration of ciliary-body function, resolution of serous detachment in patients with posterior scleritis, and normalization of intraocular pressure.

ASSOCIATED CONDITIONS

Noninfectious

Episcleritis, while most commonly idiopathic, may be associated with a wide variety of underlying systemic conditions in up to 36% of patients, including atopy, psoriasis, rheumatoid arthritis, inflammatory bowel disease, systemic lupus erythematosus (SLE), myositis, relapsing polychondritis, erythema nodosum,

Wegener's granulomatosis, and Cogan's syndrome[3] (Box 98-1). Nearly 30% of patients with episcleritis recently reported by Jabs and co-workers had an associated systemic rheumatic disease.[12] Other conditions associated with episcleritis include infectious entities such as herpes zoster, syphilis, and Lyme disease,[43] local ocular disease, most notably ocular rosacea, metabolic abnormalities such as hyperuricemia and gout, and drug reactions to pamidronate[44] and alendronate.[43–45] While episcleritis in childhood is rare, especially in children less than 5 years of age, in older children it is frequently associated with rheumatic disease.[46]

An associated systemic disease is present in approximately 40% to 57% of patients with scleritis; 30% to 48% have an associated connective tissue or vasculitic disease, 5% to 10% an infectious etiology, and 2% have atopy, rosacea, or gout.[1,2,5,6,9,10,12,47,48]

Box 98-1 Associated conditions in episcleritis and scleritis

Noninfectious

Connective tissue diseases
Rheumatoid arthritis
Systemic lupus erythematosus
Relapsing polychondritis
Seronegative spondyloarthropathies
Ankylosing spondylitis
Psoriatic arthritis
Reiter's syndrome
Arthritis and inflammatory bowel disease

Vasculitides
Wegener's granulomatosis
Polyarteritis nodosa
Allergic angiitis of Churg–Strauss
Cogan syndrome
Takayasu disease
Adamantiades–Behçet's disease
Giant-cell arteritis

Other diseases
Sarcoidosis
Porphyria
Waldenström macroglobulinemia

Infectious–multisystem diseases
Herpes zoster
Syphilis
Lyme disease
Tuberculosis
Nocardia
Streptococcus pneumoniae
Bartonellosis
Brucellosis
Toxoplasmosis
Acanthameba keratitis
Pseudomonas

Miscellaneous
Atopy
Rosacea
Gout
Foreign-body granuloma
Chemical injury
Postsurgical
Drugs (pamidronate, alendronate)

(Box 98-1). Furthermore, the frequency and severity of associated systemic diseases are related to the subtype of scleritis, occurring in 13% to 62% of patients with diffuse anterior scleritis, 28% to 45% of those with nodular anterior disease, in up to 95% of individuals with necrotizing scleritis, and in 19% to 45% of patients with posterior scleritis.[2,9,11,12] Rheumatoid arthritis is by far the most common systemic association, followed by Wegener's granulomatosis, relapsing polychondritis, SLE, and arthritis with inflammatory bowel disease.[12,24,47] Necrotizing scleritis is most frequently associated with increasing severity of disease in patients with Wegener's granulomatosis, rheumatoid arthritis, polyarteritis nodosa, or relapsing polychondritis, while it is less likely to be seen in those with SLE or the seronegative spondyloarthropathies. As with anterior scleritis, rheumatoid arthritis is the most common systemic disease association in posterior scleritis, followed by other connective tissue diseases (SLE, psoriatic arthritis) and systemic vasculitides (Wegener's granulomatosis, polyarteritis nodosa, relapsing polychondritis); however, one must also consider infectious etiologies (Lyme disease, toxoplasmosis, herpes zoster) and neoplastic masquerade syndromes.[11,49–54]

Scleritis with concomitant connective tissue or vasculitic disease carries a guarded systemic and ocular prognosis depending in large part on the severity of the underlying disease. Mortality from vasculitic complications in patients with Wegener's granulomatosis and polyarteritis nodosa is high in untreated patients[55,56] while ocular morbidity with visual loss is more likely due to the more frequent occurrence of necrotizing scleritis and PUK in patients with systemic vasculitic diseases.[10] For example, necrotizing scleritis associated with Wegener's granulomatosis can be relentlessly destructive, leading to blindness and loss of the eye despite aggressive treatment. On the other hand, scleritis associated with the seronegative spondyloarthropathies or with SLE is usually a more benign and self-limiting condition, while that associated with rheumatoid arthritis is of intermediate severity.

While in most cases the presence of an associated medical condition is apparent prior to the diagnosis of scleral inflammatory disease; scleritis was the initial manifestation of a connective tissue or vasculitic disease in approximately 15% of patients studied by Foster & Sainz de la Maza.[2] Indeed, among 107 patients with scleritis and an associated systemic disease recently reported by Akpek and colleagues,[48] approximately 78% had a previously diagnosed disease, 14% were diagnosed as a result of initial evaluation, and 8% developed a systemic disease during follow-up. The rate of occurrence of a rheumatic disease among patients with no apparent systemic disease at initial presentation was 4% per person-year. Patients with systemic vasculitis were more likely to be diagnosed by the initial evaluation and less likely to have been previously diagnosed than other rheumatic diseases.

Other noninfectious diseases may be associated with scleritis (Box 98-1). An unusual case of anterior scleritis in an 8-year-old boy with a complex systemic vasculitic presentation[57] and that of posterior scleritis with annular ciliochoroidal detachment in a 42-year-old male patient, both of whom had biopsy-proven sarcoidosis,[58] have been described. Bilateral necrotizing scleritis and diffuse anterior scleritis have been reported in association with congenital porphyria[59] and with Waldenström's macroglobulinemia[60] respectively. The latter association was thought to be coincidental.

Infectious–multisystem diseases

Infectious scleritis, either endogenous or exogenous, may be caused by the direct invasion of a microorganism or by the immune response to an infectious pathogen. Historical details that raise the index of suspicion of an infectious etiology include antecedent ocular trauma or surgery, especially a scleral buckling procedure, cataract extraction, or pterygium excision, and systemic immunosuppression.[61] All classes of microorganisms, including bacteria, viruses, parasites, and fungi, can infect the sclera and produce a clinical picture identical to that seen with immune-related disease (Box 98-1). Bacterial causes of scleritis include *Pseudomonas, Streptococcus, Staphylococcus, Mycobacterium*, and *Treponema*. Bacterial scleritis may result from extension of an adjacent keratitis. An inflammatory microangiopathy in the sclera may arise by the induction of immune-mediated responses in the vessel wall, such as the formation and deposition of immune complexes containing bacterial products.[62] Pseudomonal scleritis is a potentially devastating infection arising in tissue compromised by trauma or disease, particularly in eyes with prior pterygium surgery with the use of adjunctive Mitomycin C, and may respond to the addition of combination therapy with intravenous ceftazadime and aminoglycosides to topical therapy.[63] Tuberculosis, once considered a common cause of scleritis, is now rare, usually arising in the setting of endogenous systemic infection, appearing in the form of single or multiple scleral nodules. Severe scleral and conjunctival infection with the atypical, or nontuberculous, *Mycobacterium chelonae* has been reported following vitrectomy.[64] *Nocardia* sclerokeratitis has been reported in association with contact lens wear.[65,66] While brucellosis as a cause of uveitis is well established,[67] its association with episcleritis has recently been reported.[68,69]

Both anterior and posterior scleritis may be the presenting feature of syphilis.[70] More recently, posterior scleritis has been associated with another spirochetal infection, *Borrelia burgdorferi* (Lyme disease).[52]

Herpes zoster is probably the most common cause of infectious or late immune-related episcleral and/or scleral inflammation of viral etiology, occurring in as many as 8% of patients with herpes zoster ophthalmicus.[71] Indeed, posterior scleritis presenting with annular choroidal detachment as a complication of herpes zoster ophthalmicus has been recently reported[54] as well as that of recurrent nodular scleritis thought to be caused by reactivation of a varicella-zoster virus infection.[72] In addition, herpes-zoster virus sclerokeratitis and anterior uveitis have been observed in a child following varicella vaccination.[73]

Fungal scleritis, such as that caused by *Aspergillus*, is typically seen after ocular trauma but has also been reported following pterygium surgery.[74]

Protozoal infections with *Acanthamoeba*,[75] *Microsporidium*,[76] and *Toxoplasma gondii*[53] have also been identified as the causative agents in patients with severe sclerokeratitis, sclerouveitis with retinal detachment, and posterior scleritis respectively.

Miscellaneous conditions infrequently associated with scleritis include gout, atopy, rosacea, foreign-body granuloma, chemical injury, following various types of ocular surgery as previously discussed and drug reactions to pamidronate[44] and alendronate[43–45] (Box 98-1).

DIAGNOSTIC EVALUATION

A comprehensive medical, ophthalmic history, and review of systems together with a complete ocular and physical exam are the cornerstones to the diagnosis and management of patients with scleral inflammatory disease. Based on the foregoing discussion, it should be apparent that this approach is essential in determining the type, location, and severity of disease, the presence of associated systemic conditions, the formulation of differential diagnostic causes of scleral inflammation, and in the selection of appropriate laboratory investigations and imaging studies.

Given its benign, self-limited course, the first episode of episcleritis unaccompanied by significant positives on history and review of systems does not usually require complementary studies. Selective investigations should be performed in patients with a history of autoimmune disease, gout, or rosacea, while a more extensive workup may be indicated in those with prolonged or recurrent attacks.

The presence of scleritis always requires complementary investigations which are tailored to the patients' clinical presentation and guided by the history, review of systems, ocular and systemic examinations. More extensive workups are indicated with increasing disease severity, particularly in nodular, necrotizing, and posterior uveitis. Studies that are typically ordered as a part of the initial evaluation in patients with scleritis include chest X-ray, urine analysis, and serum chemistries (which might reveal evidence of renal dysfunction in systemic vasculitides), FTA-abs (syphilis), and antineutrophil cytoplasmic antibody (ANCA) testing. Further testing in the appropriate clinical context might include: rheumatoid factor or human leukocyte antigen (HLA)-B27 in the presence of polyarthritis or spondyloarthropathy, Lyme serology in an individual with a history of a tick bite from an endemic area, antinuclear antibodies in those where SLE was suggested on history and physical exam, radiographic imaging of the sinus in the presence of sinus symptomatology, and ultrasound examination in patients suspected of having posterior scleritis.

ANCAs are specific markers for a group of related systemic vasculitides, including Wegener's granulomatosis, microscopic polyarteritis nodosa, Churg–Strauss syndrome, and pauci-immunoglomerulonephritis. Specifically, ANCAs are antibodies directed against cytoplasmic azurophilic granules of neutrophils and monocytes, of which two classes have been described based on the pattern seen on immunofluorescence. The cytoplasmic pattern, or c-ANCA, is both sensitive and specific for Wegener's granulomatosis while the perinuclear pattern, or p-ANCA, is associated with microscopic polyarteritis nodosa, relapsing polychondritis, and renal vasculitis.

While in most cases cytoplasmic ANCA titers are diagnostic of scleritis associated with Wegener's granulomatosis,[77] there appears to be a distinct subset of patients with scleritis who have positive c-ANCA titers but no clinical evidence for systemic vasculitis on initial evaluation, that have recalcitrant disease, and typically require systemic immunosuppressive drug therapy.[48] Finally, cytoplasmic ANCA titers were predictive of disease relapse in a group of eight patients with scleritis alone or in combination with PUK, as reported by Power and colleagues.[78] Clinical remission was achieved in all eight using immunosuppressive therapy with c-ANCA levels reverting to normal in half of these patients. Subsequently, five patients suffered a relapse after treatment withdrawal, four of whom had c-ANCA levels that had failed to normalize.

Scleral biopsy may be indicated in selected cases, particularly in the diagnosis of infectious scleritis, the detection of foreign bodies, or when a masquerade syndrome is suspected. This procedure must be undertaken with great caution in patients with active scleritis as perforation at the site of the biopsy and/or exacerbation of inflammatory scleritis with further tissue loss are potential complications.

PATHOGENESIS

While the prevailing consensus is that scleritis is an immune-mediated disease leading to vessel and tissue damage, its precise pathogenesis remains enigmatic. The development of scleritis probably involves the interaction of genetically controlled mechanisms with environmental factors, such as infectious agents, or endogenous substances, which gives rise to a putative auto-immune process. Evidence in support of this hypothesis includes histopathological and immunofluorescence detection of an immune complex inflammatory microangiopathy with complement activation and neutrophil enzyme release (type III hypersensitivity reaction) in affected scleral biopsy specimens.[79] While scleritis is frequently associated with systemic autoimmune diseases associated with circulating immune complexes (SLE, rheumatoid arthritis, and polyarteritis nodosa), the specific antigens associated with scleral vessel and tissue damage have yet to be identified. The role of cellular immune dysfunction (type IV or delayed-type hypersensitivity reactions) in the pathogenesis of scleritis is further suggested by histopathological findings of chronic granulomatous inflammatory infiltrates (with a predominance of macrophages and T lymphocytes) in scleral biopsy specimens, possibly in response to antigens in the scleral tissue, such as type II collagen, or to antigens in the scleral blood vessels.[79] Indeed, immunopathological findings in a patient with posterior scleritis were compatible with a delayed-type hypersensitivity (autoimmune) reaction, replete with a predominance of T cells, many of which were CD4+ lymphocytes, infiltrating the scleral fibers.[80] Increased expression of leukocyte adhesion molecules such as intercellular adhesion molecule-1 (ICAM-1) and LFA-1 on the sclera and conjunctiva may also play a pathogenetic role in scleritis.[81] Dissolution of scleral collagen certainly develops as a consequence of the release of various proteases from inflammatory cells and the activation of MMP by proinflammatory cytokines such as tumor necrosis factor-alpha.[15,82] Finally, the favorable response of scleritis to immunosuppressive agents indirectly implicates underlying immune-mediated mechanisms as centrally pathogenetic.

THERAPY

An initial episode of episcleritis may or may not require treatment in asymptomatic patients with a negative review of systems given its favorable natural history. Simple episcleritis may be observed or treated supportively with cool compresses and iced lubrication as the vast majority will resolve without sequelae. Topical NSAIDs appear to be ineffective based on the results of a randomized double-masked placebo-controlled clinical trial.[83] While topical steroids may hasten the resolution of redness, their routine use in the treatment of episcleritis is to be discouraged as a rebound effect (more frequent and severe inflammation) is often encountered upon discontinuation of the steroids, effectively prolonging the duration of the disease, and so placing the patient at increased risk for the development of cataract and glaucoma.[1,2]

Patients with nodular episcleritis, persistent or recurrent disease, or whose professional or personal situation demands treatment are best managed with oral NSAIDs initially. Commonly prescribed NSAIDs, including the familiar cyclo-oxygenase (COX-1) inhibitors and the newer, selective inhibitors of COX-2 (celecoxib and rofecoxib) are listed in Table 98-5. While COX-2 inhibitors have not been subject to clinical trials in the treatment of episcleritis or scleritis, anecdotal experience suggests that they are at least as effective as nonselective COX-1 agents. Patients who do not respond to one NSAID may respond to another. Naturally, individuals should be advised as to the potential side-effects of these medications, including gastrointestinal upset and bleeding, photosensitivity skin rashes, renal and hepatotoxicity, and possible drug interactions. The paucity of gastrointestinal and anticoagulant side-effects with the use of COX-2 inhibitors is an immense advantage of these agents.

Table 98-5 Nonsteroidal anti-inflammatory drugs available for treatment of episcleritis and scleritis

Trade name	Generic name	Dosage
Indocin	Indometacin	75 mg SR b.i.d.
Ansaid	Flurbiprofen	100 mg t.i.d.
Naprosyn	Naproxen	250 to 500 mg b.i.d.
Voltaren	Diclofenac	75 mg b.i.d.
Orudis	Ketoprofen	100 mg t.i.d.
Dolobid	Diflunisal	500 mg b.i.d.
Tolectin	Tolmetin	400 mg t.i.d.
Meclomen	Meclofenamate	100 mg q.i.d.
Naflon	Fenoprofen	600 mg t.i.d.
Butazolidin	Phenylbutazone	100 mg t.i.d.
Feldene	Piroxicam	20 mg q.i.d.
Motrin	Ibuprofen	800 mg t.i.d.
Celebrex	Celecoxib	100 to 200 mg b.i.d.
Vioxx	Rofecoxib	25 mg q.d.

SR, slow-release.

Treatment of episcleritis associated with gout, atopy, herpes, or rosacea should be directed toward the specific underlying disease. Patients with specific connective tissue disease and episcleritis may require no more than NSAIDs. For example, patients with dermatologic or episcleral involvement with SLE may respond beautifully to oral hydroxychloroquine 200 mg b.i.d. while those with simple or nodular episcleritis associated with rheumatoid arthritis usually respond to one systemic NSAID or another. Indeed, only 16.7% of the 37 patients with episcleritis reported by Jabs and colleagues[12] needed more than topical steroids to control their disease, and these patients required oral NSAIDS alone.

Scleritis, on the other hand, almost always requires treatment with systemic medications. Of the 97 patients with scleritis studied by Jabs and associates,[12] 30.4% required oral NSAIDS while nearly 60% needed oral corticosteroids or immunosuppressive drugs to control their disease, including 90% and 100% of patients with necrotizing or posterior scleritis respectively. Important considerations in the formulation of a therapeutic plan include accurate classification of scleritis type and identification of concomitant local or systemic disease, the exclusion of possible infectious etiologies, and the potential for medication-related toxicity and/or possible drug interactions.

The first line of treatment for patients with diffuse or nodular scleritis not associated with an underlying systemic vasculitis (Wegener's granulomatosis, polyarteritis nodosa, relapsing polychondritis, etc.) is oral NSAIDs, with or without the use of topical corticosteroids.[84] A treatment response is usually evident within 2 to 3 weeks of commencing therapy, and, as previously mentioned, sequential trials of various NSAIDs may be necessary in order to find the agent which is most effective. Patients who respond to NSAIDs are treated for a minimum of 1 year before attempting to taper and discontinue the medication. The selective COX-2 inhibitors celecoxib and rofecoxib are advantageous in cases where adverse side-effects (gastrointestinal upset) or drug interactions (mainly with anticoagulants) might otherwise limit treatment. Patients with associated conditions such as gout, rosacea, or atopy require specific treatment of the underlying disease.

Therapeutic failure with oral NSAIDs necessitates the addition or substitution of systemic corticosteroids, commencing at high doses (prednisone 1 to 1.5 mg/kg per day), with subsequent taper and discontinuation as soon as is possible while maintaining clinical remission with or without continued NSAIDs. Typically, a slow and steady taper (10 mg per week) is commenced once scleral inflammation has been controlled (usually within 7 to 14 days) until a dose of 20 mg/day of prednisone is reached. The dose may then be further reduced by smaller decrements (2.5 to 5 mg per week) or an alternate dosage schedule may be employed in patients in whom a more protracted taper is anticipated in an effort to reduce steroid-associated side-effects.[85] Alternatively, intravenous high-dose methylprednisolone (1 g/day on three occasions within the first week followed by a reduced dose weekly thereafter), alone or in conjunction with other immunosuppressive agents, has been shown to be safe and effective in the induction of disease remission in patients with severe scleritis, obviating many of the potential side-effects associated with prolonged, high-dose oral corticosteroid therapy.[86]

Periocular injections of corticosteroids have been reported to be effective, both adjunctively and as primary therapy, in the treatment of various forms of scleritis,[87–90] but have not been widely employed due to concerns surrounding the potential exacerbation of scleral melting and/or scleral perforation. Most recently, Zamir and associates[90] reported complete resolution of inflammation in 11 of 12 eyes, with partial resolution in the other eye, among 10 patients with nonnecrotizing anterior scleritis treated with subconjunctival triamcinolone acetonide. One eye developed a conjunctival hemorrhage and another developed elevated intraocular pressure; however, none developed necrotizing scleritis over a 15-month period. While these data suggest that there may be a role for periocular steroid therapy in selected cases of anterior scleritis, further study with long-term follow-up is necessary to assess more fully the safety and efficacy of this therapeutic approach.

Immunosuppressive therapy is indicated in patients with severe scleritis who have failed to respond to high-dose oral or intravenous corticosteroids or in whom unacceptably high doses of systemic corticosteroids are necessary to achieve inflammatory control. In the latter case, the addition of immunosuppressive therapy is said to be "steroid-sparing," allowing lower doses of each medication to be used in an effort to achieve inflammatory quiescence while minimizing the side-effects of either agent used as monotherapy at higher doses. Immunosuppressive medications that have been used in the treatment of scleritis include cyclophosphamide, chlorambucil, azathioprine, methotrexate, ciclosporin, mycophenolate mofetil, daclizumab, and tumor necrosis factor inhibitors etanercept and infliximab. Typically these drugs are commenced together with oral corticosteroids, as a response to therapy may take up to 3 weeks, with the latter being tapered and discontinued as described above.

The scleritis associated with an underlying systemic vasculitis (such as Wegener's granulomatosis, polyarteritis nodosa, relapsing polychondritis) may present as diffuse, nodular, or necrotizing disease and requires systemic immunosuppressive therapy at the outset. This therapy is not only directed in an effort to control scleral inflammation, but is necessary for the treatment of the underlying systemic vasculitis which, if left untreated, carries a significantly high mortality, especially for patients with Wegener's granulomatosis and polyarteritis nodosa. Complete remission was induced in 93% of patients with Wegener's granulomatosis treated with cyclophosphamide and mortality was reduced to 7% over a mean follow-up of 51 months.[55] Likewise, the 5-year mortality for patients with polyarteritis nodosa treated with cyclophosphamide was reduced from 53% to 20%.[56] Based on these and similar data for the treatment of systemic vasculitides, cyclophosphamide is considered the first-line agent in treating patients with diffuse, nodular, or necrotizing scleritis associated with Wegener's granulomatosis or polyarteritis nodosa. A similar therapeutic attitude could be extended to patients with necrotizing scleritis associated with rheumatoid arthritis and relapsing polychondritis. The 5-year mortality from extraocular vasculitic lesions is approximately 50% in patients with rheumatoid arthritis who developed necrotizing scleritis and were not treated with immunosuppressive agents.[5,6,19] Cyclophosphamide was the only effective immunosuppressive agent in the treatment of three patients with necrotizing scleritis associated with relapsing polychondritis, a notoriously difficult disease to treat.[51] Finally, as previously mentioned, a positive c-ANCA in patients with no apparent clinical evidence of systemic vasculitic disease may be a marker for scleritis which is recalcitrant to therapy with both NSAIDs and corticosteroids alone and may require immunosuppressive therapy.

Certainly, immunosuppressive drugs, supplemented with corticosteroids, should be the initial choice in patients with non-infectious necrotizing scleritis in whom an underlying systemic vasculitic or connective tissue disease coexists in a high percentage of cases.[12,48,84] Indeed, this strategy was successful in controlling scleral inflammation in 74% of patients with necrotizing scleritis reported by Sainz de la Maza and colleagues.[84] Cyclophosphamide is probably the single most effective agent for necrotizing disease and may be administered as a single daily oral morning dose (1 to 3 mg/kg per day), or as intermittent, pulsed, intravenous therapy (1 g/m^2 body surface area, in 250 ml of normal saline, piggy-backed on to the second half of 1 l 0.5% dextrose in water, infused over a 2-h period, every 3 to 6 weeks). The latter approach is usually reserved for patients with very severe or recurrent disease in which a rapid induction is desired and is subsequently followed by maintenance oral therapy. Prehydration and copious oral intake of fluids (3 l/day) should be encouraged to minimize the risk of hemorrhagic cystitis associated with the use of cyclophosphamide.

Several other immunosuppressive drug additions or substitutions, to be discussed below, may be needed to achieve an effective and well-tolerated therapeutic regimen in patients with necrotizing scleritis. The responsibility for the details of the management of patients requiring immunomodulatory therapy must lie with a clinician who, by virtue of training and experience, is thoroughly familiar with the use of these agents and in the recognition and treatment of potentially serious adverse side-effects that may arise. A "hand-in-glove" collaboration between the ophthalmologist and chemotherapist (an oncologist, hematologist, or rheumatologist) works most effectively for patients requiring these medications.

Patients with diffuse or nodular scleritis, not associated with underlying systemic vasculitic disease, who have failed therapy with NSAIDs and/or systemic corticosteroids, may be treated with a variety of other immunomodulatory agents. Methotrexate (7.5 to 15 mg orally or 15 mg intramuscularly or subcutaneously once weekly), together with folic acid (1 mg/day) is probably the best initial choice as it is both efficacious and steroid-sparing in the treatment of scleritis and because of its favorable side-effect profile and lower oncogenic potential as compared to cytotoxic drugs (cyclophosphamide and chlorambucil). Oral azathioprine (1 to 2 mg/kg daily), although less effective as monotherapy than other immunosuppressive agents in controlling severe scleritis, is most frequently used in conjunction with systemic corticosteroids as a steroid-sparing agent and is

generally well tolerated. Similarly, oral mycofenolate mofetil (1 g twice daily)[91,92] may be most useful as a steroid-sparing agent in patients with controlled scleral disease rather than as adjunctive therapy in patients with severe active scleritis requiring additional immunosuppressive therapy. Oral cyclosporine (2.5 to 5 mg/kg daily)[93,94] has been shown to be effective in severe scleritis in patients who have been refractory to other immunomodulatory drugs. Daclizumab, a humanized immunoglobulin G monoclonal antibody that specifically binds CD25 of the human interleukin-2 receptor that is expressed on activated T lymphocytes, has been shown, in preliminary reports, to be safe and of benefit in the treatment of patients with refractory scleritis.[95] Finally, a recent case series reported nine patients with uveitis and seven patients with scleritis treated with the tumor necrosis factor inhibitors etanercept or infliximab.[96] While scleral inflammation remained quiescent in three of these seven patients, overall, five patients developed inflammatory eye disease for the first time while taking a tumor necrosis factor inhibitor, including three patients with scleritis. While the tumor necrosis factor inhibitors have proven invaluable in the management of the articular manifestations of rheumatologic diseases, their efficacy in the treatment of ocular inflammatory disease awaits further study.

Patients with infectious scleritis should be treated with appropriate and specific antimicrobial therapy, for example, quadruple therapy with the combination of isoniazid, rifampicin, pyrazinamide, and ethambutol for 6 months in cases of tuberculosis scleritis; neurosyphilis dosing regimens with penicillin G, 18 to 24 million units per day, administered as 3 to 4 million units intravenously every 4 h or continuous infusion for 10 to 14 days for syphilitic posterior scleritis;[97] intravenous ceftriaxone with steroids to treat posterior scleritis associated with Lyme disease;[52] and systemic aciclovir for scleritis due to herpes zoster.[98]

Surgery is rarely necessary in the management of scleritis except in instances of necrotizing scleritis that has progressed to the point of impending or actual perforation of the globe. The primary goal of surgery is to preserve the integrity of the globe by reinforcing areas of thinned or necrotic sclera. Scleral patch graft materials include sclera from fresh or frozen donor globes, glycerin-preserved scleral tissue, fascia lata, and autologous pretibial periosteum. Sainz de la Maza and colleagues reported their experience with 15 scleral homografts for scleral necrosis among 12 eyes of 12 patients, 10 of whom had systemic autoimmune disease and eight of whom were treated with immunosuppressive therapy.[99] All scleral grafts remained stable among patients treated with immunosuppressive therapy except two; one developed graft necrosis within 10 months of the discontinuation of chemotherapy while the other developed endophthalmitis secondary to microbial keratitis. The immunological process that produced scleral necrosis will initially invariably result in the destruction of any grafted material unless the destructive inflammatory process is interrupted with systemic immunosuppressive therapy prior to surgery. Finally, the eventual outcome of patients with infectious scleritis may be improved by surgical intervention including cryotherapy, penetrating and lamellar corneoscleral grafts, and tectonic penetrating keratoplasty.[100]

REFERENCES

1. Watson PG, Hazleman BL. The sclera and systemic disorders. London: WB Saunders; 1976.
2. Foster CS, Sainz de la Maza M. The sclera. New York: Springer-Verlag; 1994.
3. Akpek EK, Uy HS, Christen W et al. Severity of episcleritis and systemic disease association. Ophthalmology 1999; 106:729–731.
4. Calthorpe CM, Watson PG, McCartney AC. Posterior scleritis: a clinical and histological survey. Eye 1988; 2:267–277.
5. Watson PG, Hayreh SS. Scleritis and episcleritis. Br J Ophthalmol 1976; 60:163–191.
6. McGavin DD, Williamson J, Forrester JV et al. Episcleritis and scleritis. A study of their clinical manifestations and association with rheumatoid arthritis. Br J Ophthalmol 1976; 60:192–226.
7. Watson PG. Doyne Memorial Lecture, 1982. The nature and the treatment of scleral inflammation. Trans Ophthalmol Soc UK 1982; 102:257–281.
8. Benson WE. Posterior scleritis. Surv Ophthalmol 1988; 32:297–316.
9. Tuft SJ, Watson PG. Progression of scleral disease. Ophthalmology 1991; 98:467–471.
10. Sainz de la Maza M, Foster CS, Jabbur NS. Scleritis associated with systemic vasculitic diseases. Ophthalmology 1995; 102:687–692.
11. McCluskey PJ, Watson PG, Lightman S et al. Posterior scleritis: clinical features, systemic associations, and outcome in a large series of patients. Ophthalmology 1999; 106:2380–2386.
12. Jabs DA, Mudun A, Dunn JP et al. Episcleritis and scleritis: clinical features and treatment results. Am J Ophthalmol 2000; 130:469–476.
13. Benson WE, Shields JA, Tasman W et al. Posterior scleritis. A cause of diagnostic confusion. Arch Ophthalmol 1979; 97:1482–1486.
14. McCluskey P. Scleritis. London: BMJ Books; 2001.
15. Di Girolamo N, Lloyd A, McCluskey P et al. Increased expression of matrix metalloproteinases in vivo in scleritis tissue and in vitro in cultured human scleral fibroblasts. Am J Pathol 1997; 150:653–666.
16. Williamson J. Incidence of eye disease in cases of connective tissue disease. Trans Ophthalmol Soc UK 1974; 94:742–752.
17. Watson PG, Bovey E. Anterior segment fluorescein angiography in the diagnosis of scleral inflammation. Ophthalmology 1985; 92:1–11.
18. Nieuwenhuizen J, Watson PG, Jager MJ et al. The value of combining anterior segment fluorescein angiography with indocyanine green angiography in scleral inflammation. Ophthalmology 2003; 110:1653–1666.
19. Foster CS, Forstot SL, Wilson LA. Mortality rate in rheumatoid arthritis patients developing necrotizing scleritis or peripheral ulcerative keratitis. Effects of systemic immunosuppression. Ophthalmology 1984; 91:1253–1263.
20. O'Donoghue E, Lightman S, Tuft S et al. Surgically induced necrotising sclerokeratitis (SINS) – precipitating factors and response to treatment. Br J Ophthalmol 1992; 76:17–21.
21. Sainz de la Maza M, Foster CS. Necrotizing scleritis after ocular surgery. A clinicopathologic study. Ophthalmology 1991; 98:1720–1726.
22. Glasser DB, Bellor J. Necrotizing scleritis of scleral flaps after transscleral suture fixation of an intraocular lens. Am J Ophthalmol 1992; 113:529–532.
23. Scott JA, Clearkin LG. Surgically induced diffuse scleritis following cataract surgery. Eye 1994; 8:292–297.
24. Sainz de la Maza M, Foster CS, Jabbur NS. Scleritis associated with rheumatoid arthritis and with other systemic immune-mediated diseases. Ophthalmology 1994; 101:1281–1286; discussion 1287–1288.
25. Cleary PE, Watson PG, McGill JI et al. Visual loss due to posterior segment disease in scleritis. Trans Ophthalmol Soc UK 1975; 95:297–300.
26. Singh G, Guthoff R, Foster CS. Observations on long-term follow-up of posterior scleritis. Am J Ophthalmol 1986; 101:570–575.
27. Wald KJ, Spaide R, Patalano VJ et al. Posterior scleritis in children. Am J Ophthalmol 1992; 113:281–286.
28. Cappaert WE, Purnell EW, Frank KE. Use of B-sector scan ultrasound in the diagnosis of benign choroidal folds. Am J Ophthalmol 1977; 84:375–379.
29. Rochels R, Reis G. [Echography in posterior scleritis (author's translation).] Klin Monatsbl Augenheilkd 1980; 177:611–613.
30. Heiligenhaus A, Schilling M, Lung E et al. Ultrasound biomicroscopy in scleritis. Ophthalmology 1998; 105:527–534.
31. Chaques VJ, Lam S, Tessler HH et al. Computed tomography and magnetic resonance imaging in the diagnosis of posterior scleritis. Ann Ophthalmol 1993; 25:89–94.
32. Liew SC, McCluskey PJ, Parker G et al. Bilateral uveal effusion associated with scleral thickening due to amyloidosis. Arch Ophthalmol 2000; 118:1293–1295.
33. Cangemi FE, Trempe CL, Walsh JB. Choroidal folds. Am J Ophthalmol 1978; 86:380–387.
34. Wilson RS, Hanna C, Morris MD. Idiopathic chorioretinal effusion: an analysis of extracellular fluids. Ann Ophthalmol 1977; 9:647–653.
35. Gass JD, Jallow S. Idiopathic serous detachment of the choroid, ciliary body, and retina (uveal effusion syndrome). Ophthalmology 1982; 89:1018–1032.

36. Hunyor AP, Harper CA, O'Day J et al. Ocular–central nervous system lymphoma mimicking posterior scleritis with exudative retinal detachment. Ophthalmology 2000; 107:1955–1959.
37. Hoang-Xuan T, Bodaghi B, Toublanc M et al. Scleritis and mucosal-associated lymphoid tissue lymphoma: a new masquerade syndrome. Ophthalmology 1996; 103:631–635.
38. Sainz de la Maza M, Foster CS, Jabbur NS et al. Ocular characteristics and disease associations in scleritis-associated peripheral keratopathy. Arch Ophthalmol 2002; 120:15–19.
39. Messmer EM, Foster CS. Destructive corneal and scleral disease associated with rheumatoid arthritis. Medical and surgical management. Cornea 1995; 14:408–417.
40. Sainz de la Maza M, Foster CS, Jabbur NS. Scleritis-associated uveitis. Ophthalmology 1997; 104:58–63.
41. Fraunfelder FT, Watson PG. Evaluation of eyes enucleated for scleritis. Br J Ophthalmol 1976; 60:227–230.
42. Wilhelmus KR, Grierson I, Watson PG. Histopathologic and clinical associations of scleritis and glaucoma. Am J Ophthalmol 1981; 91:697–705.
43. Flach AJ, Lavoie PE. Episcleritis, conjunctivitis, and keratitis as ocular manifestations of Lyme disease. Ophthalmology 1990; 97:973–975.
44. Macarol V, Fraunfelder FT. Pamidronate disodium and possible ocular adverse drug reactions. Am J Ophthalmol 1994; 118:220–224.
45. Mbekeani JN, Slamovits TL, Schwartz BH et al. Ocular inflammation associated with alendronate therapy. Arch Ophthalmol 1999; 117:837–838.
46. Read RW, Weiss AH, Sherry DD. Episcleritis in childhood. Ophthalmology 1999; 106:2377–2379.
47. Sainz de la Maza M, Jabbur NS, Foster CS. Severity of scleritis and episcleritis. Ophthalmology 1994; 101:389–396.
48. Akpek EK, Thorne, JE, Qazi FA et al. Evaluation of patients with scleritis for systemic disease. Ophthalmology 2004; 111:501–506.
49. Altan-Yaycioglu R, Akova YA, Kart H et al. Posterior scleritis in psoriatic arthritis. Retina 2003; 23:717–719.
50. Akova YA, Jabbur NS, Foster CS. Ocular presentation of polyarteritis nodosa. Clinical course and management with steroid and cytotoxic therapy. Ophthalmology 1993; 100:1775–1781.
51. Hoang-Xaun T, Foster CS, Rice BA. Scleritis in relapsing polychondritis. Response to therapy. Ophthalmology 1990; 97:892–898.
52. Krist D, Wenkel H. Posterior scleritis associated with Borrelia burgdorferi (Lyme disease) infection. Ophthalmology 2002; 109:143–145.
53. Schuman JS, Weinberg RS, Ferry AP et al. Toxoplasmic scleritis. Ophthalmology 1988; 95:1399–1403.
54. Tranos PG, Ong T, Nolan W et al. Posterior scleritis presenting with annular choroidal detachment as a complication of herpes zoster ophthalmicus. Retina 2003; 23:716–717.
55. Fauci AS HB, Katz P, Wolff SM. Wegener's granulomatosis: prospective clinical and therapeutic experience with 85 patients for 21 years. Ann Intern Med 1983; 98:76–85.
56. Leib ES RC, Paulus HE. Immunosuppressive and corticosteroid therapy of polyarteritis nodosa. Am J Med 1979; 67:941–947.
57. Fernandes SR, Singsen BH, Hoffman GS. Sarcoidosis and systemic vasculitis. Semin Arthr Rheum 2000; 30:33–46.
58. Dodds EM, Lowder CY, Barnhorst DA et al. Posterior scleritis with annular ciliochoroidal detachment. Am J Ophthalmol 1995; 120:677–679.
59. Venkatesh P, Garg SP, Kumaran E et al. Congenital porphyria with necrotizing scleritis in a 9-year-old child. Clin Exp Ophthalmol 2000; 28:314–318.
60. Rosenbaum JT, Becker MD. The tyranny of the anecdote: Waldenstrom's macroglobulinemia and scleritis. Ocul Immunol Inflamm 2000; 8:111–113.
61. Hwang YS, Chen YF, Lai CC et al. Infectious scleritis after use of immunomodulators. Arch Ophthalmol 2002; 120:1093–1094.
62. Fong LP SdlMM, Rice BA et al. Immunopathology of scleritis. Ophthalmology 1991; 98:472–479.
63. Helm CJ, Holland GN, Webster RG Jr et al. Combination intravenous ceftazidime and aminoglycosides in the treatment of pseudomonal scleritis. Ophthalmology 1997; 104:838–843.
64. Margo CE, Pavan PR. Mycobacterium chelonae conjunctivitis and scleritis following vitrectomy. Arch Ophthalmol 2000; 118:1125–1128.
65. Knox CM, Whitcher JP, Cevellos V et al. Nocardia scleritis. Am J Ophthalmol 1997; 123:713–714.
66. Sridhar MS, Cohen EJ, Rapuano CJ et al. Nocardia asteroides sclerokeratitis in a contact lens wearer. Clao J 2002; 28:66–68.
67. Walker J, Sharma OP, Rao NA. Brucellosis and uveitis. Am J Ophthalmol 1992; 114:374–375.
68. Bourcier T, Cassoux N, Karmochkine M et al. [Episcleritis and brucellosis. A propos of a case.] J Fr Ophthalmol 1998; 21:126–127.
69. Gungor K, Bekir NA, Namiduru M. Recurrent episcleritis associated with brucellosis. Acta Ophthalmol Scand 2001; 79:76–78.
70. Casey R, Flowers CW Jr, Jones DD et al. Anterior nodular scleritis secondary to syphilis. Arch Ophthalmol 1996; 114:1015–1016.

71. Womack LW, Liesegang TJ. Complications of herpes zoster ophthalmicus. Arch Ophthalmol 1983; 101:42–45.

72. Livir-Rallatos C, El-Shabrawi Y, Zatirakis P et al. Recurrent nodular scleritis associated with varicella zoster virus. Am J Ophthalmol 1998; 126:594–597.

73. Naseri A, Good WV, Cunningham ET Jr. Herpes zoster virus sclerokeratitis and anterior uveitis in a child following varicella vaccination. Am J Ophthalmol 2003; 135:415–417.

74. Margo CE, Polack FM, Hood CI et al. *Aspergillus* panophthalmitis complicating treatment of pterygium. Cornea 1988; 7:285–289.

75. Lee GA, Gray TB, Dart JK et al. Acanthamoeba sclerokeratitis: treatment with systemic immunosuppression. Ophthalmology 2002; 109:1178–1182.

76. Mietz H, Franzen C, Hoppe T et al. Microsporidia-induced sclerouveitis with retinal detachment. Arch Ophthalmol 2002; 120:864–865.

77. Soukiasian SH, Foster CS, Niles JL et al. Diagnostic value of anti-neutrophil cytoplasmic antibodies in scleritis associated with Wegener's granulomatosis. Ophthalmology 1992; 99:125–132.

78. Power WJ, Rodriguez A, Neves RA et al. Disease relapse in patients with ocular manifestations of Wegener granulomatosis. Ophthalmology 1995; 102:154–160.

79. Fong LP, Sainz de la Maza M, Rice BA et al. Immunopathology of scleritis. Ophthalmology 1991; 98:472–479.

80. Bernauer W, Buchi ER, Daicker B. Immunopathological findings in posterior scleritis. Int Ophthalmol 1994; 18:229–231.

81. Sangwan VS, Merchant A, Sainz de la Maza M et al. Leukocyte adhesion molecule expression in scleritis. Arch Ophthalmol 1998; 116:1476–1480.

82. Di Girolamo N, Visvanathan K, Lloyd A et al. Expression of TNF-alpha by human plasma cells in chronic inflammation. J Leukoc Biol 1997; 61:667–678.

83. Lyons CJ, Hakin KN, Watson PG. Topical flurbiprofen: an effective treatment for episcleritis? Eye 1990; 4:521–525.

84. Sainz de la Maza M, Jabbur NS, Foster CS. An analysis of therapeutic decision for scleritis. Ophthalmology 1993; 100:1372–1376.

85. Fauci AS. Alternate-day corticosteroid therapy. Am J Med 1978; 64:729–731.

86. McCluskey P, Wakefield D. Intravenous pulse methylprednisolone in scleritis. Arch Ophthalmol 1987; 105:793–797.

87. Hakin KN, Ham J, Lightman SL. Use of orbital floor steroids in the management of patients with uniocular non-necrotising scleritis. Br J Ophthalmol 1991; 75:337–339.

88. Tu EY, Culbertson WW, Pflugfelder SC et al. Therapy of nonnecrotizing anterior scleritis with subconjunctival corticosteroid injection. Ophthalmology 1995; 102:718–724.

89. Croasdale CR, Brightbill FS. Subconjunctival corticosteroid injections for nonnecrotizing anterior scleritis. Arch Ophthalmol 1999; 117:966–968.

90. Zamir E, Read RW, Smith RE et al. A prospective evaluation of subconjunctival injection of triamcinolone acetonide for resistant anterior scleritis. Ophthalmology 2002; 109:798–805; discussion 805–807.

91. Larkin G, Lightman S. Mycophenolate mofetil. A useful immunosuppressive in inflammatory eye disease. Ophthalmology 1999; 106:370–374.

92. Sen HN SE, Al-Khatib SQ, Djalilian AR et al. Mycophenolate mofetil for the treatment of scleritis. Ophthalmology 2003; 110:1750–1755.

93. Wakefield D, McCluskey P. Cyclosporin therapy for severe scleritis. Br J Ophthalmol 1989; 73:743–746.

94. McCarthy JM, Dubord PJ, Chalmers A et al. Cyclosporine A for the treatment of necrotizing scleritis and corneal melting in patients with rheumatoid arthritis. J Rheumatol 1992; 19:1358–1361.

95. Papaliodis GN, Chu D, Foster CS. Treatment of ocular inflammatory disorders with daclizumab. Ophthalmology 2003; 110:786–789.

96. Smith JR, Levinson RD, Holland GN et al. Differential efficacy of tumor necrosis factor inhibition in the management of inflammatory eye disease and associated rheumatic disease. Arthr Rheum 2001; 45:252–257.

97. Prevention CfDCa. Sexually transmitted diseases treatment guidelines. MMWR 2002; 51:1–80.

98. Aylward GW, Claoue CM, Marsh RJ et al. Influence of oral acyclovir on ocular complications of herpes zoster ophthalmicus. Eye 1994; 8:70–74.

99. Sainz de la Maza M, Tauber J, Foster CS. Scleral grafting for necrotizing scleritis. Ophthalmology 1989; 96:306–310.

100. Reynolds MG, Alfonso E. Treatment of infectious scleritis and keratoscleritis. Am J Ophthalmol 1991; 112:543–547.

Ocular Histoplasmosis

Barbara S. Hawkins
Judith Alexander
Sharon D. Solomon
Andrew P. Schachat

The first description of an ocular abnormality associated with histoplasmosis was published by Reid et al.[1] in 1942 on the basis of their observations of a patient dying of acute disseminated histoplasmosis. Other investigators later reported activation of atrophic chorioretinal lesions coincident with histoplasmin skin testing.[2–4]

In 1959, Woods & Wahlen[4] described a clinical syndrome observed among 62 patients with granulomatous uveitis. They reported that these patients were more likely to react positively to histoplasmin skin testing than patients with nongranulomatous lesions and the normal population. Nineteen of the 62 patients "showed a peculiar and consistent pattern of ocular lesions" that included both discrete atrophic, sparsely pigmented or unpigmented, peripheral lesions (frequently referred to today as "histo spots") and later cystic lesions in the macula. All 19 patients reacted to histoplasmin; nine of the 19 had pulmonary calcifications but did not react to tuberculin. Woods & Wahlen concluded that earlier benign systemic histoplasmosis was responsible for the ocular findings in these 19 patients.[4] A few years later, Schlaegel & Kenney[5] demonstrated that atrophic lesions around the optic nerve were part of the clinical picture.

CLINICAL FEATURES OF OCULAR HISTOPLASMOSIS

A clinical diagnosis of ocular histoplasmosis is based on observation of the following lesions in the fundus of one or both eyes in the absence of inflammation of the vitreous or anterior segment:[6,7]

- Discrete, focal, atrophic choroidal scars in the macula or the periphery, smaller in size than the optic disc, that appear "punched out" of the inner layers of the choroid (histo spots) (Fig. 99-1).
- Peripapillary chorioretinal scarring ("peripapillary atrophy") (Fig. 99-2).
- Choroidal neovascularization (CNV) or hemorrhagic retinal detachment in the macula, often visible by ophthalmoscopy and on color photographs as a gray-green lacy net ("active disciform lesion") (Figs 99-3 to 99-5).
- Fibrovascular disciform macular scar from resolution of CNV or hemorrhagic retinal detachment ("disciform scar" or "inactive disciform lesion"); (Fig. 99-5B).

Most often both eyes have typical lesions, although the appearance may not be symmetric at initial presentation. The clinical condition is known as the *ocular histoplasmosis syndrome* (OHS) or, often, *ocular histoplasmosis*, the term used throughout the remainder of this chapter. When lesions of the first type are present, typically together with peripapillary atrophy, a person is said to have "histo spots only"; when either an active or inactive disciform lesion is also present, a person is said to have "disciform (or neovascular) histo." Because of the possibility of activating an inactive lesion by histoplasmin skin testing, there is a difference of opinion among ophthalmologists regarding the need to confirm the etiology of typical choroidal lesions when the fundus appearance is consistent with ocular histoplasmosis.

The early granulomatous stage of ocular histoplasmosis is rarely seen clinically.[6] The initial focal scars are probably too small to be seen with the ophthalmoscope. Gass[6] has postulated that lymphocytic infiltration of the surrounding tissue produces enlargement of the lesion over a period of years and thus allows it to become clinically detectable.

RELATIONSHIP OF THE OCULAR SYNDROME TO SYSTEMIC INFECTION

The etiology of ocular histoplasmosis is believed to begin with infection with *Histoplasma capsulatum*, via the respiratory tract, early in life. Although the relationship of the ocular disorder to infection by the organism *H. capsulatum* had not been demonstrated to satisfy Koch's postulates completely,[8,9] continuing experimental work with primates[10,11] may eventually satisfy this requirement.

Geographic distribution of *Histoplasma capsulatum* in the USA

As described by Comstock et al.,[12] the major portion of the region of the USA in which histoplasmosis is endemic is "a triangular area with its apices near Omaha, Nebraska, Columbus, Ohio, and Natchez, Mississippi." It includes most of the Ohio and Mississippi river valleys. In a large portion of this histo belt, 60% or more of the young adult, lifelong residents react positively to histoplasmin skin testing.[13]

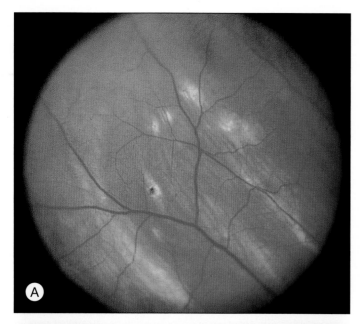

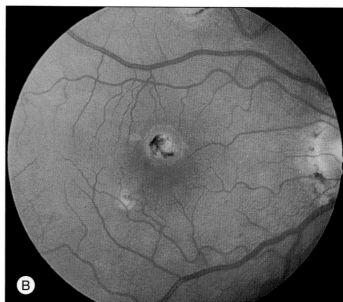

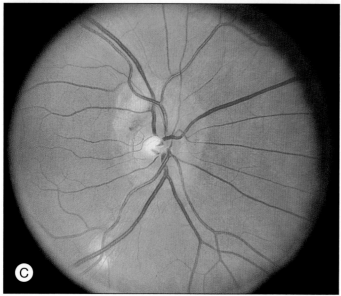

Fig. 99-1 Chorioretinal scars (i.e., "histo spots") characteristic of ocular histoplasmosis. A, Peripheral histo spots. B, Macular histo spots. Larger lesion with pigment proliferation may represent spontaneously regressed choroidal neovascularization (CNV). C, Histo spots and peripapillary scarring. The peripapillary lesion superotemporal and within the peripapillary scarring probably represents spontaneously regressed CNV.

Clinical presentation

Histoplasmosis has been classified by Goodwin et al.[14] as presented in Box 99-1. The usual histoplasmosis infection is a mild case with flu-like respiratory symptoms. Most patients do not seek medical care. Studies in Tennessee by Zeidberg et al.[15] demonstrated that almost 90% of children 13 years of age had positive reactions to histoplasmin skin tests. A great deal of variation has been observed in the distribution of positive reactors by neighborhood of residence.[12,16]

The fatal cases of histoplasmosis reported early during its recorded history were all instances of disseminated infection, which is associated with deficiencies in the immune system of the host. In such cases the disease has been reported to invade almost every organ and tissue in the body. Histoplasmosis is a common opportunistic infection among patients who have the acquired immunodeficiency syndrome (AIDS).

Epidemic histoplasmosis demonstrates somewhat more pronounced symptoms than endemic illness. Furthermore, the initial symptoms in epidemic disease may be atypical.[17–21] Epidemics of histoplasmosis have usually been associated with excavations,[22–25] demolition or renovation of old buildings,[26–29] cleaning or destruction of chicken coops or other fowl habitats,[17,27,30–32] or visits to caves that are inhabited by bats.[33–35]

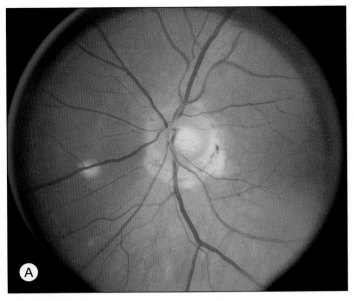
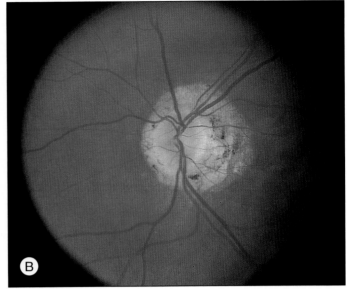

Fig. 99-2 Two examples of peripapillary scarring.

Causal or coincidental relationship?

Five observations support a causal relationship between *Histoplasma capsulatum* and the ocular histoplasmosis syndrome:

1. Cases of ocular histoplasmosis frequently present to ophthalmologists in the endemic area of the USA and rarely to those outside the area.[36]
2. Almost all patients diagnosed as having ocular histoplasmosis in the USA have lived some or all of their lives in an endemic area.[37,38]
3. Positive reactions to histoplasmin skin testing are more common among patients who have disciform lesions of ocular histoplasmosis than among controls.[38–40]
4. Activation of apparently inactive lesions of ocular histoplasmosis coincident with histoplasmin skin testing has been reported.[2–4,40–42]
5. DNA from *H. capsulatum* has been isolated from the enucleated eye of a man with chronic choroidal lesions of ocular histoplasmosis.[43]

Arguments have been put forward to refute the relationship between *H. capsulatum* and the ocular syndrome. Notably, patients with eye lesions indistinguishable from those of ocular histoplasmosis have been identified in the UK and in continental Europe among people who have never visited or lived in an endemic area.[44–48] *H. capsulatum* has not been identified in the UK, and only a small proportion of Europeans are positive reactors to histoplasmin skin testing.[49] However, it is possible that infection with some other organism endemic to the UK and continental Europe sometimes results in an ocular syndrome similar to ocular histoplasmosis.[46] Amphotericin B, which is used in the treatment of acute systemic histoplasmosis, has not proved effective for the treatment of the ocular disorder.[50] However, because the vision-threatening eye lesions are believed to develop years after the initial infection, this finding is not surprising.

EPIDEMIOLOGY OF OCULAR HISTOPLASMOSIS

Prevalence

Prevalence rates of ocular histoplasmosis from population-based studies in the USA are summarized in Table 99-1. In 1966, Asbury[39] reported an overall prevalence rate of 1.6% for asymptomatic histo spots among an institutionalized population in Ohio that consisted of 1417 adults and included blacks and whites, males and females. More than 50% of the 1417 residents reacted positively to a histoplasmin skin test. All of those with histo spots had either skin test or radiographic findings consistent with previous infection with *H. capsulatum*.

Two epidemiologic studies were carried out in western Maryland in the early 1970s. In Walkersville, 75% of residents 13 years old or older in the entire community had skin tests and eye examinations.[51] Among 842 people examined, 22 had histo spots and one of the 22 also had a disciform scar that was attributed to ocular histoplasmosis. Thus the prevalence rate of histo spots in the population was estimated to be 2.6%. The prevalence of disciform scars in the population was estimated to be 1.2 per 1000, or 0.1%; among those with atrophic lesions, the prevalence of disciform lesions was estimated to be 4.5%.

As part of a case-control study of the cause of ocular histoplasmosis in Washington county, Maryland, Ganley[38] examined the eyes of 252 county residents between the ages of 30 and 69 and performed histoplasmin skin tests and blood tests for complement-fixing antibodies using both yeast-phase and mycelial-phase *H. capsulatum* antigens. Among a random sample of 73 patients selected from the records of an ophthalmology practice in Washington county who were free of documented macular and paramacular scars, 2.7% had histo spots. Among a random sample of 57 county residents, 5.3% had such lesions. Ganley found no disciform lesions among the random samples selected from either the ophthalmology practice or the community.[38]

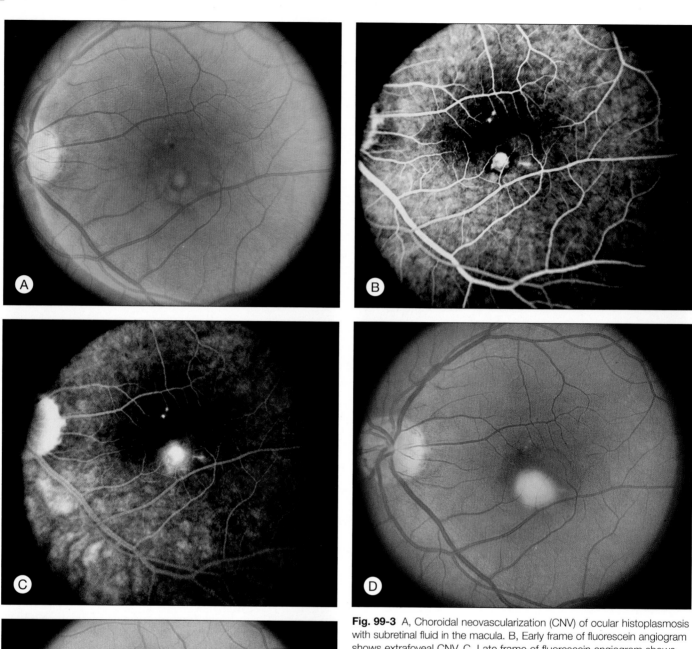

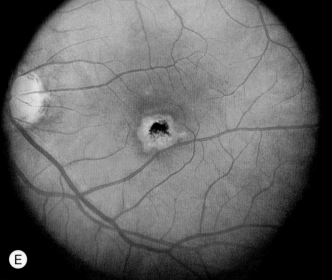

Fig. 99-3 A, Choroidal neovascularization (CNV) of ocular histoplasmosis with subretinal fluid in the macula. B, Early frame of fluorescein angiogram shows extrafoveal CNV. C, Late frame of fluorescein angiogram shows increased leakage of fluorescein dye. D, Color photograph taken 1 day after laser photocoagulation shows whitening of retina from treatment. E, Treatment scar 2 years after laser photocoagulation; no evidence of recurrent CNV.

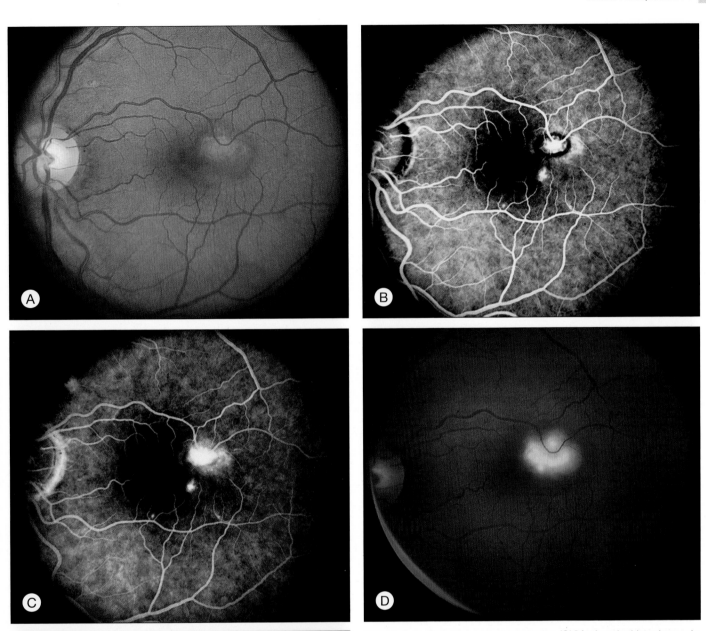

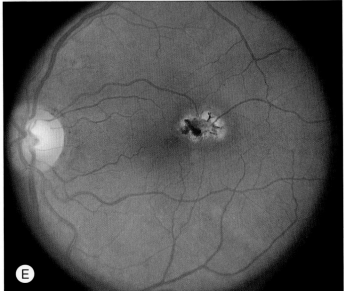

Fig. 99-4 A, Choroidal neovascularization (CNV) of ocular histoplasmosis with subretinal fluid in the macula. B, Extrafoveal CNV is visible on this early frame of a fluorescein angiogram. C, Late frame of fluorescein angiogram shows increased leakage of fluorescein dye from the CNV. D, Color photograph taken 1 day after laser photocoagulation shows whitening of retina from treatment. E, Atrophic treatment scar 2½ years after laser photocoagulation; no evidence of recurrent CNV.

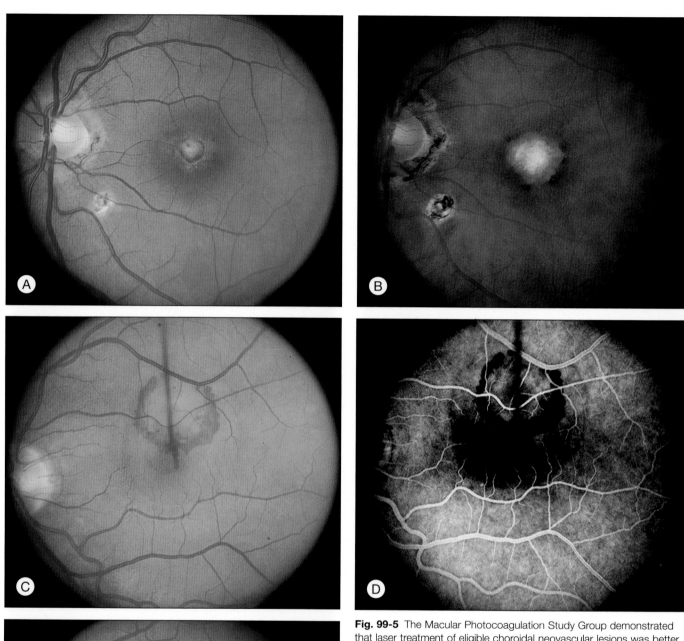

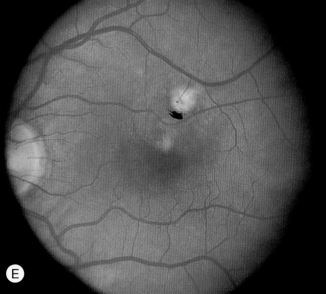

Fig. 99-5 The Macular Photocoagulation Study Group demonstrated that laser treatment of eligible choroidal neovascular lesions was better than no treatment with respect to delaying or preventing loss of visual acuity. However, some CNV regresses spontaneously. These two patients did not have laser treatment of their choroidal neovascularization (CNV), which involuted spontaneously. A, Juxtafoveal CNV in first patient. B, Disciform scar 4 years later. C, This patient had extrafoveal CNV with a rim of hemorrhage visible on the photograph. D, CNV, hemorrhage, and fluid are all visible on this early frame of a fluorescein angiogram. E, A small scar with pigment proliferation is visible 4 years later. Visual acuity returned to 20/20 3 months after enrollment and remained at 20/20 throughout the 5-year follow-up period.

Box 99-1 Classification of histoplasmosis

Normal Host

Mild exposure
Usual asymptomatic primary infection
Occasional symptomatic primary infection (young children)
Asymptomatic reinfection

Heavy exposure
Acute pulmonary histoplasmosis
Primary type
Reinfection type

Abnormal Host

Opportunistic infection
Disseminated histoplasmosis (immune defect)
Chronic pulmonary histoplasmosis (structural defect)

Excessive fibrotic response to healing pulmonary infection
Histoplasmoma
Mediastinal fibrosis or collagenosis

From Goodwin, RA, Shapiro, JL, Thurman, GH, Thurman, SS, and Des Prez, RM: Medicine 59:1-33, 1980.

Incidence

Little is known about the incidence of ocular histoplasmosis. An annual incidence rate of two new cases with neovascular disciform lesions per 100 000 population per year has been estimated from reports received during a 6-month period in Tennessee.[52] In 1983, 13 years after the original study in Walkersville, Maryland, 14 of 19 surviving residents who had histo spots in 1970 were re-examined. Of these 14 people, one was found to have experienced activation of an atrophic peripapillary lesion and loss of vision (K Todd, SL Fine, unpublished data), yielding a 13-year activation rate of 7.1%, or about 0.5%/year in this small group, but this case of activation had been described earlier.[53] Fifteen years after Ganley's case-control study in Washington county, Maryland, no cases with disciform lesions were found among 10 people examined who had histo spots only in 1970.[54]

Much higher incidence rates of development of disciform lesions in second eyes have been reported from follow-up of clinical case series. These rates are summarized in Table 99-2. Although development of new atrophic scars has been documented,[6,55] the population incidence rate of new cases with atrophic scars only is unknown.

Table 99-1 Observed prevalence rates of ocular histoplasmosis

Source	No. examined	Disciform lesion cases Rate (%)	Disciform lesion cases 95% CI[a]	Atrophic scar cases Rate (%)	Atrophic scar cases 95% CI[a]
Asbury[39]	1417	0.0	0.0–0.3	1.6	1.0–2.3
Smith & Ganley[53]	842	0.1	0.0–0.7	2.5	1.5–3.8
Ganley[38]	73[b]	0.0	0.0–5.1	2.7	0.3–9.9
	57[b]	0.0	0.0–6.5	5.3	1.1–15.4

[a]95% Confidence interval assuming Poisson distribution of cases.
[b]Participants 30 to 69 years of age.

Table 99-2 Annual incidence rates of neovascular lesions in second eyes

Source	No. of cases	Length of follow-up in years, mean (range)	No. of affected cases	Estimated annual incidence rate (%) (95% CI[a])
Macular Photocoagulation Study Group[55]	394	5 (4–5)	35	1.8 (1.3–2.6)
Lewis & Schiffman[98]	105	10 (1–21)	20	2.0 (0.2–6.9)
Watzke & Claussen[99]	40	13 (10–15)	9	1.7 (0.8–3.3)
Sawelson et al.[100]	25	2 (< 1–9)	6	12.0 (4.4–26.2)
Hawkins & Ganley[54]	8	15 (15–15)	0	0.0 (0.0–3.1)

[a]95% Confidence interval assuming Poisson distribution of cases.

Age

The median age of patients with vision-threatening disciform lesions has been reported by several investigators to be in the 30s and 40s (Table 99-3). Among new cases of ocular histoplasmosis presenting to ophthalmologists in Tennessee in 1980,[52] almost as many cases were in their 20s as in their 30s.

The median age of persons who have atrophic scars appears only slightly older than those of patients who have disciform lesions (Table 99-3). However, it should be noted that the age reported is the age at detection of histo spots by examination, not the age at which they developed in the eye. It is likely that atrophic scars appear earlier in life but are not detected except coincidentally during routine clinical examination or when a patient has visual symptoms. The median age of 36 reported by Smith et al.[56] is probably the most reliable estimate among the three listed in Table 99-3.

Gender and race

Cases of ocular histoplasmosis are about equally divided between males and females. Almost all the cases with disciform macular lesions of ocular histoplasmosis have been white. Only about one dozen cases of this form of ocular histoplasmosis have ever been reported in blacks,[57] although histo spots and positive skin tests have been reported to be roughly equal in prevalence among blacks and whites.[39,58] Schlaegel et al.[40] stated that, of 190 patients with ocular histoplasmosis examined, all had been white. In this context, "white" should be interpreted as white and of northern-European extraction. Gass & Wilkinson[59] reported that 100% of 130 cases of macular involvement were white despite the fact that over half of their clinic patients were black or Hispanic. Ganley & Smith found no blacks among cases of ocular histoplasmosis,[38,51] but both Washington county and Walkersville had few blacks in their populations.

Histocompatibility antigens

Several investigators have determined the prevalence of histocompatibility antigens among cases of ocular histoplasmosis, both with and without disciform lesions, in comparison to controls. Both human leukocyte antigen (HLA)-B7[60,61] and HLA-DRw2[62] were two to four times more common among disciform cases than among controls. HLA-DRw2 was twice as common among cases with histo spots only as among controls,[62] but there was less difference with respect to HLA-B7.[63] These findings suggest a genetic predisposition for development of histo spots and disciform macular lesions following infection with *H. capsulatum.*

Table 99-3 Age of cases of ocular histoplasmosis				
	Disciform lesion cases		Atrophic scar cases	
Source	No.	Median (range), years	No.	Median (range), years
Schlaegel & Weber[101]	155	34[a] (10–59)	–	–
Makley et al.[41]	79	37[b] (n/r)	–	–
Feman et al.[52]	98	40[b] (979)	–	–
Gass & Wilkinson[59]	81	41[b] (14–43)	–	–
Macular Photocoagulation Study Group[76]	288	41 (20–81)	–	–
Van Metre & Maumenee[37]	61	42 (17–66)	–	–
Macular Photocoagulation Study Group[85]	242	44(20–80)	–	–
Submacular Surgery Trials Group H Trial[81]				
First eye	167	46 (18–78)	–	–
Second eye	58	56 (29–79)	–	–
Ganley[38]	19	49(30–69)	15	49 (30–69)
Asbury[39]	–	–	22	55 (21–74)
Smith et al.[56]	–	–	21	36 (14–83)

[a]Interpolated from data in Schlaegel et al.[97]
[b]Mean age presented when median not reported (n/r).
–, Data not reported.

PATHOGENESIS

A number of theories of the pathogenesis of ocular histoplasmosis have been proposed. The most widely accepted theory is illustrated in Fig. 99-6.[6] The process is believed to begin with focal infection of the choroid at the time of the initial benign systemic infection. This focal infection may resolve as an atrophic scar that disrupts Bruch's membrane. Alternatively, the infection may affect the retinal pigment epithelium and the choriocapillaris and progress to serous and hemorrhagic retinal detachment that resolves as a fibrovascular disciform scar.

Allergic or other factors may promote CNV at the site of the atrophic scar. The resulting break in Bruch's membrane provides an opening through which neovascularization gains admittance to the retina.[64] The abnormal new blood vessels that compose the neovascular membrane are prone to rupture and hemorrhage. When hemorrhage occurs, the accumulation of blood and serous

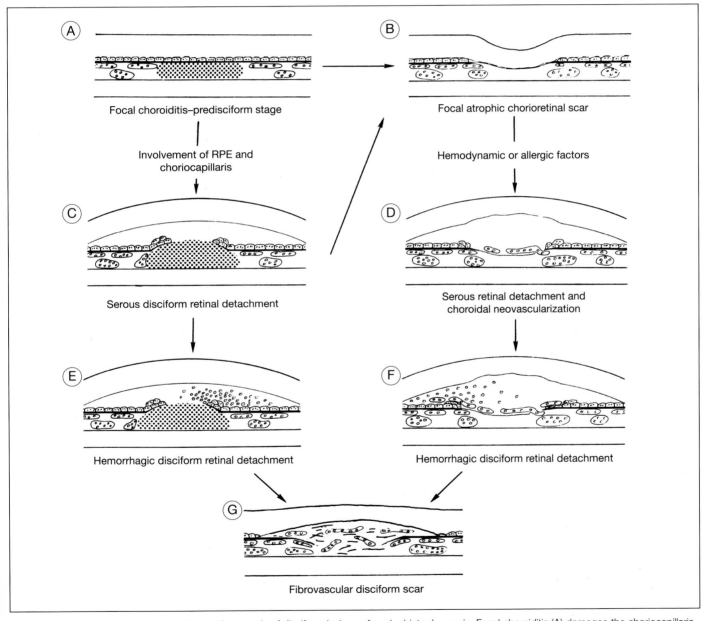

Fig. 99-6 Hypothesized mechanism of the pathogenesis of disciform lesions of ocular histoplasmosis. Focal choroiditis (A) damages the choriocapillaris, retinal pigment epithelium (RPE), and Bruch's membrane and produces an exudative detachment of the retina (B) or hemorrhage into the subretinal space (C). Any of these three stages may resolve, leaving either a focal area of atrophy of the retinal pigment epithelium, Bruch's membrane, and choroid (D) or, in the case of subretinal hemorrhage, a disciform scar (G). Either in the absence of further inflammation or under the influence of recurrent episodes of inflammation, the choroidal blood vessels surrounding an atrophic chorioretinal scar (D) may decompensate and cause serous exudation, choroidal neovascularization, and transient serous detachment of the retina (E). This process in turn may result in a hemorrhagic detachment of the retina (F) that resolves as a disciform scar (G). (Reproduced rom Gass JDM. Stereoscopic atlas of macular diseases, vol. 1, Diagnosis and treatment. St. Louis, MO: Mosby; 1987.[6])

fluid beneath the retinal pigment epithelium results in further disorganization of the layers of the retina. By either route, the final resolution of the active hemorrhagic or neovascular lesion is a fibrovascular scar.

The initiator for this abnormal growth of new blood vessels is unknown. The results from HLA typing suggest a possible genetic predisposition for progression from atrophic scars to disciform lesions in ocular histoplasmosis.[60–63] They also suggest that a genetic factor may account for development of clinically apparent histo spots in the eyes of some people infected with *H. capsulatum* but not others. Other hypotheses have attributed these phenomena to a larger initial inoculum of the fungus,[10,65] reinfection,[4,66] hypersensitivity,[4,38] and the presence of other factors that compromise the vascular system[38,67,68] or the immune system.[69]

ANIMAL MODELS

Histoplasmosis is known to occur in many species of animals.[70–74] Efforts to develop an animal model for ocular histoplasmosis have been hampered by two major factors: (1) nonprimates do not have a macula with its special anatomic, physiologic, and neurologic characteristics; and (2) decades are believed to elapse between initial infection with *H. capsulatum* and the development of characteristic symptomatic macular lesions. Thus the most promising animal models are primates, in which systemic infection and ocular lesions have been produced.[10,11]

EFFECT OF OCULAR HISTOPLASMOSIS ON VISION

The atrophic choroidal scars observed in ocular histoplasmosis usually have little, if any, observable effect on the patient's vision, although Rivers et al.[75] have reported visual symptoms that corresponded to atrophic scars in the macula preceding a clinical diagnosis of CNV. Active disciform lesions in the macula, which consist of CNV with associated hemorrhage and fluid accumulation, may cause a sudden decrease in central visual acuity or blurring and distortion of vision. Unfortunately, these lesions develop most often in the eyes of people who are in their most active and productive stage of life (Table 99-3). Anecdotal reports of recovery of central vision after large losses as a result of active lesions in the macular region have been confirmed in the Macular Photocoagulation Study (MPS)[55,76] and by other investigators.[77–79]

Among more than 70 million people who live in the histoplasmosis-endemic areas of the USA, as many as 2 million residents may have histo spots, and possibly 100 000 of them are thereby at risk of loss of vision.[80] Because histo spots are asymptomatic lesions, patients who have only histo spots usually do not come to medical attention unless CNV or some other problem produces distortion or loss of vision. It is not yet known to what extent people with histo spots alone are at excess risk of visual impairment or blindness resulting from development of disciform macular lesions. Cataracts, age-related macular degeneration, glaucoma, and other ocular conditions may also threaten their vision.[54]

Only two studies have addressed the public health importance of ocular histoplasmosis as a cause of visual impairment. Feman and colleagues[52] found that ocular histoplasmosis accounted for only 2.8% of blind eyes among applicants for aid to the blind in Tennessee. Hawkins & Ganley[54] found no statistically significant increase in the 15-year incidence of visual impairment or blindness among persons who had only histo spots initially in comparison to other residents of Washington county, Maryland.

The opinion of many ophthalmologists has been that people who have excellent vision in one eye function about as well as those who have excellent vision in both eyes. Only with the initiation of the Submacular Surgery Trials in 1997 has a systematic effort been made to collect data regarding perceptions of individuals with ocular histoplasmosis about their ability to function visually. In one of the Submacular Surgery Trials (Group H Trial) of submacular surgery versus observation for subfoveal CNV, participating patients were interviewed at baseline and at scheduled intervals thereafter for 2 to 4 years using a set of standardized questionnaires.[81] Findings from a vision-targeted instrument were of primary interest. Although best-corrected visual acuity of the better-seeing eye accounted for much of the variability in scores among these patients, a marked difference in scores was observed between patients with unilateral CNV and those with bilateral CNV, independent of visual acuity. Significantly impaired visual function was observed among both unilateral CNV cases and bilateral CNV cases at baseline. Deficits were similar to those seen with age-related macular degeneration.[81]

TREATMENT

In his 1977 monograph,[8] Schlaegel discussed a number of management approaches for patients who had ocular histoplasmosis. These approaches included avoidance of stress, avoidance of aspirin and the Valsalva maneuver, hyposensitization to histoplasmin, systemic and periocular steroid administration, immunosuppressive agents, and photocoagulation. Histoplasmin desensitization,[82] amphotericin B,[41,50] and other therapeutic and prophylactic interventions[83,84] have been tried by many ophthalmologists and discarded. Schlaegel suggested that the use of corticosteroids might abort activation of an inactive lesion.[8] No treatment is known to prevent inactive lesions from giving rise to exudative or hemorrhagic neovascular complexes that typically end in disciform macular scars.

Although never proved to yield better visual results than the natural course without treatment, highly respected ophthalmologists have considered the use of corticosteroids. For example, although Gass[6] stated that the medical treatment of ocular histoplasmosis is unsatisfactory and that steroids appeared to be of little practical value, he discussed their possible role in patients who have recent visual loss and patients who have CNV too close to the center of the foveal avascular zone. It is now known that patients who have ocular histoplasmosis and CNV in extrafoveal[85,86] and juxtafoveal[76,87] locations benefit from treatment with laser photocoagulation, even when CNV is located nasal to the fovea.[88,89] Therefore choroidal neovascular lesions that are "too close" to the center of the foveal avascular zone for laser treatment are those that are subfoveal. Gass suggested 40 to 100 mg of prednisone daily for several weeks.

Based on a small series of treated cases,[90] photodynamic therapy with verteporfin has been advocated for treating subfoveal CNV in eyes with ocular histoplasmosis. Although data are promising, a rigorous evaluation of the benefits and risks of this management approach will be necessary before this treatment option can be recommended for such eyes.

Several reports of results of surgical removal of subfoveal neovascular lesions from eyes with ocular histoplasmosis have been published in the past 10 years.[91–93] Early optimism based on short-term visual outcomes has been somewhat tempered by longer follow-up of surgically treated patients. In particular, rates of recurrence of CNV after surgery appear to exceed those observed after laser treatment of initially extrafoveal or juxtafoveal CNV.[94] The Submacular Surgery Trials group H trial was initiated in 1997 under the sponsorship of the National Eye Institute of the National Institutes of Health (US Department of Health and Human Services) to compare vision and quality-of-life outcomes between patients assigned to surgery and similar patients assigned to observation. Pre- and postsurgery photographs of an eye assigned to the surgery arm in the group H trial are displayed in Fig. 99-7. As discussed below, findings support a beneficial effect of surgery, at least for selected cases.

The only treatment unequivocally demonstrated to reduce the risk of visual loss after development of choroidal neovascular lesions in the macula in ocular histoplasmosis is laser photocoagulation of the CNV. The MPS group has demonstrated the effectiveness of laser treatment in two randomized clinical trials. Patients who have well-defined *extrafoveal* or *juxtafoveal* CNV should be treated with focal laser photocoagulation. It is not known whether patients with *subfoveal* CNV would have long-term benefit if treated with laser photocoagulation; a pilot trial showed no short-term benefit in comparison to observation.[95]

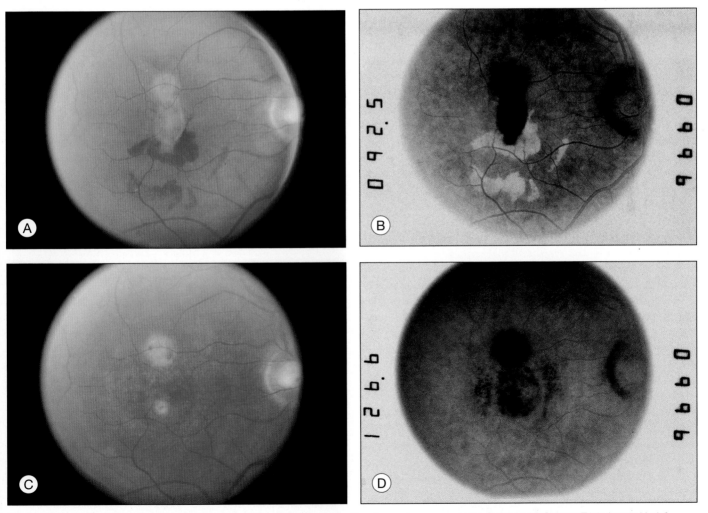

Fig. 99-7 Eye with subfoveal choroidal neovascularization (CNV) treated with submacular surgery in the Submacular Surgery Trials (group H trial). Color photograph (A) and early frame of fluorescein angiogram (B) shows subfoveal CNV in an eye with characteristic lesions of ocular histoplasmosis. Color photograph (C) and early frame of fluorescein angiogram (D) taken 6 months after submacular surgery show a well-demarcated postoperative disturbed area of the retinal pigment epithelium.

FINDINGS FROM RANDOMIZED CLINICAL TRIALS OF TREATMENT OF CNV

The MPS group initiated its first multicenter clinical trial of laser treatment for choroidal neovascular lesions secondary to ocular histoplasmosis in 1979. During a 4-year period, 262 patients with well-defined extrafoveal neovascular membranes were enrolled. The posterior border of these lesions could not be closer than 200 μm to the center of the foveal avascular zone; initial best-corrected visual acuity of the affected eye was 20/100 or better. Eligible eyes were randomly assigned to argon laser treatment or to no treatment. The eyes were re-examined twice each year, at which time best-corrected visual acuity was measured and color photographs were taken. Fluorescein angiograms were taken at time of study entry, 6 and 12 months after enrollment, and annually thereafter. Patient enrollment in this clinical trial was halted in 1983 after the MPS Data and Safety Monitoring Committee concluded that argon laser photocoagulation was beneficial in preventing or delaying large loss of visual acuity. From 18 months through 5 years, approximately 10% of eyes treated with laser photocoagulation versus approximately 40% of observed eyes had visual acuity that was six or more lines worse than at baseline.[86] (On the visual acuity charts used in the MPS, a loss of six lines of visual acuity is equivalent to quadrupling the minimum angle of resolution.) Five years after enrollment, median visual acuity had dropped from 20/25 at baseline to 20/40 in laser-treated eyes compared to 20/80 in observed eyes.[86] Persistence or recurrence of CNV was observed along the border of the laser treatment scar in 26% of eyes assigned to laser treatment; new areas of CNV not contiguous to the laser scar developed in another 7% of laser-treated eyes.[86]

The MPS group initiated a second trial of laser photocoagulation for neovascular disciform lesions secondary to ocular histoplasmosis in 1981. Patients who had neovascular lesions with the posterior border inside the foveal avascular zone but without subfoveal CNV were eligible for this clinical trial. In this trial, best-corrected visual acuity at entry was permitted to be as poor as 20/400 in the study eye. A total of 289 eyes were randomized between krypton laser treatment and no treatment before enrollment halted in 1986, again because the MPS Data and Safety Monitoring Committee concluded from the accumulating data that eyes treated with krypton laser were less likely to lose visual acuity than untreated eyes. The proportion of eyes that had lost six or more lines of visual acuity from baseline to the 18-month through the 5-year examination was close to 11% in eyes in the laser photocoagulation arm and about 30% of eyes in the observation arm.[87] Persistent or recurrent CNV contiguous with the laser treatment scar was observed in 33% of laser-treated eyes; new, noncontiguous areas of CNV developed in an additional 2% of eyes.[87]

Because of concerns regarding laser damage to the papillomacular bundle when CNV is peripapillary and nasal to the fovea, as well as to confirm findings from an earlier uncontrolled study,[88] a subgroup analysis was undertaken by the MPS group.[89] This analysis provided no evidence that laser treatment was contraindicated for neovascular lesions located nasal to the fovea.

Thus effective treatment is available for extrafoveal and juxtafoveal choroidal neovascular lesions of the condition.

From April 1997 through September 2001, patients with subfoveal CNV and visual acuity of 20/50 to 20/800 enrolled in the Submacular Surgery Trials group H trial of submacular surgery versus observation. Of the 225 patients who enrolled, 192 had ocular histoplasmosis and 33 had idiopathic CNV. By the 24-month examination, about 20% more eyes in the surgery arm than in the observation arm had visual acuity that was better than or about the same as baseline visual acuity.[96] This estimate of the effectiveness of surgery was smaller than the trial was designed to detect and was not statistically significant. Recurrence of CNV, and cataract in older patients, accounted for losses of visual acuity after initial gains following surgery. The 2-year benefit of surgery was almost exclusively confined to the prespecified subgroup of 92 eyes (47 in the surgery arm, 45 in the observation arm) with visual acuity worse than 20/100 at baseline. At the 24-month examination, 76% of surgery eyes versus 50% of observation eyes had visual acuity better than or nearly the same as baseline visual acuity, for a net benefit of 50% attributable to surgery. Furthermore, scores from vision-targeted quality-of-life interviews improved more after surgery than with observation.[97]

Recommendations to high-risk patients (i.e., those who have lost vision in one eye) include self-monitoring of reading vision and regular observation of an Amsler grid chart with each eye independently to detect, and to obtain laser treatment for, new patches of extrafoveal or juxtafoveal CNV that may arise, either in the eye that is already affected or in the fellow eye. For patients who present with subfoveal CNV and visual acuity worse than 20/100, submacular surgery should be considered. In addition, referral for counseling or other appropriate services should be considered when there is any evidence of depression associated with unilateral vision loss. Patients who lose vision in both eyes should be referred for low-vision rehabilitation.

REFERENCES

1. Reid JD, Scherer JH, Herbut PA et al. Systemic histoplasmosis diagnosed before death and produced experimentally in guinea pigs. J Lab Clin Med 1942; 27:419–434.
2. Krause AC, Hopkins WG. Ocular manifestation of histoplasmosis. Am J Ophthalmol 1951; 39:564–566.
3. Schlaegel TF. Granulomatous uveitis: an etiologic survey of 100 cases. Trans Am Acad Ophthalmol Otolaryngol 1958; 62:813–825.
4. Woods AC, Wahlen HE. The probable role of benign histoplasmosis in the etiology of granulomatous uveitis. Trans Am Ophthalmol Soc 1959; 57:318–343.
5. Schlaegel TF, Kenney D. Changes around the optic nerve head in presumed ocular histoplasmosis. Am J Ophthalmol 1966; 62:454–458.
6. Gass JDM. Stereoscopic atlas of macular diseases, vol. 1. Diagnosis and treatment. St. Louis, MO: Mosby; 1987.
7. Patz A, Fine SL. Presumed ocular histoplasmosis. In: Yanuzzi LA, Gitter KA, Schatz H, eds. The macula: a comprehensive text and atlas. Baltimore: Williams & Wilkins; 1979.
8. Schlaegel TF. Ocular histoplasmosis. New York: Grune & Stratton; 1977.
9. Wong VG, Kwon-Chung KJ, Hill WB. Koch's postulates and experimental ocular histoplasmosis. Int Ophthalmol Clin 1975; 15:139–145.
10. Smith RE. Natural history and reactivation studies of experimental ocular histoplasmosis in a primate model. Trans Am Ophthalmol Soc 1982; 80:695–757.
11. Jester JV, Smith RE. Subretinal neovascularization after experimental ocular histoplasmosis in a subhuman primate. Am J Ophthalmol 1985; 100:252–258.
12. Comstock GW, Vicens CN, Goodman NL et al. Differences in the distribution of sensitivity to histoplasmin and isolations of *Histoplasma capsulatum*. Am J Epidemiol 1968; 88:195–209.

13. Edwards LB, Acquaviva FA, Livesay VT et al. An atlas of sensitivity to tuberculin, PPD-B, and histoplasmin in the United States. Am Rev Respir Dis 1969; 99:1–132.
14. Goodwin RA, Shapiro JL, Thurman GH et al. Disseminated histoplasmosis: clinical and pathologic correlations. Medicine 1980; 95:1–33.
15. Zeidberg LD, Dillon A, Gass RS. Some factors in the epidemiology of histoplasmin sensitivity in Williamson county, Tennessee. Am J Public Health 1951; 41:80–89.
16. Zeidberg LD. The microdistribution of histoplasmin sensitivity in an endemic area. Public Health Monogr 1956; 39:190–197.
17. Burke DS, Churchill FE, Gaydos JC et al. Epidemic histoplasmosis in patients with undifferentiated fever. Mil Med 1982; 147:466–467.
18. Ryder KW, Jay SJ, Kiblawi SO et al. Serum angiotensin converting enzyme activity in patients with histoplasmosis. JAMA 1983; 249:1888–1889.
19. Weber TR, Grosfeld JL, Kleiman MB et al. Surgical implications of endemic histoplasmosis in children. J Pediatr Surg 1983; 18:486–491.
20. Weinberg GA, Kleiman MB, Grosfeld JL et al. Unusual manifestations of histoplasmosis in childhood. Pediatrics 1983; 72:99–105.
21. Wheat U, Stein L, Corya BC et al. Pericarditis as a manifestation of histoplasmosis during two large urban outbreaks. Medicine 1983; 62:110–119.
22. Brodsky AL, Gregg MB, Loewenstein MS et al. Outbreak of histoplasmosis associated with the 1970 Earth Day activities. Am J Med 1973; 54:333–342.
23. Schwarz J, Salfelder K, Viloria JE. Histoplasma capsulatum in vessels of the choroid. Ann Ophthalmol 1977; 9:633–636.
24. Schlech WF, Wheat U, Ho JL et al. Recurrent urban histoplasmosis, Indianapolis, Indiana, 1980–1981. Am J Epidemiol 1983; 118:301–312.
25. Waldman RJ, England AC, Tauxe R et al. A winter outbreak of acute histoplasmosis in northern Michigan. Am J Epidemiol 1983; 117:68–75.
26. Wilcox KR, Waisbren BA, Martin J. The Walworth, Wisconsin, epidemic of histoplasmosis. Ann Intern Med 1958; 49:388–418.
27. Younglove RM, Terry RM, Rose NJ et al. An outbreak of histoplasmosis in Illinois associated with starlings. Illinois Med J 1968; 134:259–263.
28. Larrabee WF, Ajello L, Kaufman L. An epidemic of histoplasmosis on the isthmus of Panama. Am J Trop Med Hyg 1978; 27:281–285.
29. Loosli CG, Grayston JT, Alexander ER et al. Epidemiological studies of pulmonary histoplasmosis in a farm family. Am J Hyg 1952; 55:392–401.
30. Bartlett PC, Vonbehren LA, Tewari RP et al. Bats in the belfry: an outbreak of histoplasmosis. Am J Public Health 1982; 72:1369–1372.
31. Morse DL, Gordon MA, Matte T et al. An outbreak of histoplasmosis in a prison. Am J Epidemiol 1985; 122:253–261.
32. Sorley DL, Levin ML, Warren JW et al. Bat-associated histoplasmosis in Maryland bridge workers. Am J Med 1979; 67:623–626.
33. Hasenclever HF, Shacklette MH, Young RV et al. The natural occurrence of Histoplasma capsulatum in a cave. 1. Epidemiologic aspects. Am J Epidemiol 1967; 86:238–245.
34. Johnson JE, Kabler JD, Gourley MF et al. Cave-associated histoplasmosis – Costa Rica. MMWR 1988; 37:312–313.
35. McMurray DN, Russell LH. Contribution of bats to the maintenance of Histoplasma capsulatum in a cave microfocus. Am J Trop Med Hyg 1982; 31:527–531.
36. Ellis FD, Schlaegel TF. The geographic localization of presumed histoplasmic choroiditis. Am J Ophthalmol 1973; 75:953–956.
37. Van Metre TE, Maumenee AE. Specific ocular uveal lesions in patients with evidence of histoplasmosis. Arch Ophthalmol 1964; 71:314–324.
38. Ganley JP. Epidemiologic characteristics of presumed ocular histoplasmosis. Acta Ophthalmol 1973 (suppl. 119):1–63.
39. Asbury T. The status of presumed ocular histoplasmosis: including a report of a survey. Trans Am Ophthalmol Soc 1966; 64:371–400.
40. Schlaegel TF, Weber JC, Helveston E et al. Presumed histoplasmic choroiditis. Am J Ophthalmol 1967; 63:919–925.
41. Makley TA, Long JW, Suie T et al. Presumed histoplasmic chorioretinitis with special emphasis on the present modes of therapy. Trans Am Acad Ophthalmol Otolaryngol 1965; 69:443–457.
42. McCulloch C. Histoplasmosis. Trans Can Ophthalmol Soc 1963; 26:107–125.
43. Spencer WH, Chan C-C, Shen DF et al. Detection of Histoplasma capsulatum DNA in lesions of chronic ocular histoplasmosis syndrome. Arch Ophthalmol 2003; 121:1551–1555.
44. Braunstein RA, Rosen DA, Bird AC. Ocular histoplasmosis syndrome in the United Kingdom. Br J Ophthalmol 1974; 58:893–898.
45. Craandijk A. Focal macular choroidopathy. Doc Ophthalmol 1979; 48:1–99.
46. Bottoni FG, Deutman AF, Aandekerk AL. Presumed ocular histoplasmosis syndrome and linear streak lesions. Br J Ophthalmol 1989; 73:528–535.
47. Suttorp-Schulten MSA, Bollemeijer JG, Bos PJM et al. Presumed ocular histoplasmosis in the Netherlands – an area without histoplasmosis. Br J Ophthalmol 1997; 81:7–11.
48. Ongkosuwito JV, Kortbeek LM, Van der Lelij A et al. Aetiological study of the presumed ocular histoplasmosis syndrome in the Netherlands. Br J Ophthalmol 1999; 83:535–539.
49. Edwards PQ, Billings EL. Worldwide pattern of skin sensitivity to histoplasmin. Am J Trop Med Hyg 1971; 20:288–319.
50. Giles CL, Falls HF. Further evaluation of amphotericin-B therapy in presumptive histoplasmosis chorioretinitis. Am J Ophthalmol 1961; 51:588–598.
51. Smith RE, Ganley JP. An epidemiologic study of presumed ocular histoplasmosis. Trans Am Acad Ophthalmol Otolaryngol 1971; 75:994–1005.
52. Feman SS, Podgorski SF, Penn MK. Blindness from presumed ocular histoplasmosis in Tennessee. Ophthalmology 1982; 89:1295–1298.
53. Smith RE, Ganley JP. The natural history of non-disciform ocular histoplasmosis. Can J Ophthalmol 1977; 12:114–120.
54. Hawkins BS, Ganley JP. Risk of visual impairment attributable to ocular histoplasmosis. Arch Ophthalmol 1994; 112:655–666.
55. Macular Photocoagulation Study Group. Five-year follow-up of fellow eyes of individuals with ocular histoplasmosis and unilateral extrafoveal or juxtafoveal choroidal neovascularization. Arch Ophthalmol 1996; 114:677–688.
56. Smith RE, Ganley JP, Knox DL. Presumed ocular histoplasmosis. II. Patterns of peripheral and peripapillary scarring in persons with nonmacular disease. Arch Ophthalmol 1972; 87:251–257.
57. Baskin MA, Jampol LM, Huamonte FU et al. Macular lesions in blacks with the presumed ocular histoplasmosis syndrome. Am J Ophthalmol 1980; 89:77–83.
58. Edwards PQ, Palmer CE. Sensitivity to histoplasmin among negro and white residents of different communities in the USA. Bull WHO 1964; 30:575–585.
59. Gass JDM, Wilkinson CP. Follow-up study of presumed ocular histoplasmosis. Trans Am Acad Ophthalmol Otolaryngol 1972; 76:672–694.
60. Godfrey WA, Sabates R, Cross DE. Association of presumed ocular histoplasmosis with HLA-B7. Am J Ophthalmol 1978; 85:854–858.
61. Braley RE, Meredith TA, Aaberg TM et al. The prevalence of HLA-B7 in presumed ocular histoplasmosis. Am J Ophthalmol 1978; 85:859–861.
62. Meredith TA, Smith RE, Duquesnoy RJ. Association of HLA-DRw2 antigen with presumed ocular histoplasmosis. Am J Ophthalmol 1980; 89:70–76.
63. Meredith TA, Smith RE, Braley RE et al. The prevalence of HLA-B7 in presumed ocular histoplasmosis in patients with peripheral atrophic scars. Am J Ophthalmol 1978; 86:325–328.
64. Weingeist TA, Watzke RC. Ocular involvement by Histoplasma capsulatum. Int Ophthalmol Clin 1983; 23:33–47.
65. Smith RE, Macy JI, Parrett C et al. Variations in acute multifocal histoplasmic choroiditis in the primate. Invest Ophthalmol Vis Sci 1978; 17:1005–1018.
66. Davidorf FH. The role of T-lymphocytes in the reactivation of presumed ocular histoplasmosis scars. Int Ophthalmol Clin 1975; 15:111–124.
67. Gamble CN, Aronson SB, Brescia FB. Experimental uveitis. 1. The production of recurrent immunologic (Auer) uveitis and its relationship to increased uveal vascular permeability. Arch Ophthalmol 1970; 84:321–330.
68. Aronson SB, Fish MB, Pollycove M et al. Altered vascular permeability in ocular inflammatory disease. Arch Ophthalmol 1971; 85:455–466.
69. Kaplan HJ, Waldrep JC. Immunological basis of presumed ocular histoplasmosis. Int Ophthalmol Clin 1983; 23:19–31.
70. De Monbreun WA. The dog as a natural host for Histoplasma capsulatum: report of a case of histoplasmosis in this animal. Am J Trop Med 1939; 19:565–587.
71. Emmons CW, Morlan HB, Hill EL. Histoplasmosis in rats and skunks in Georgia. Public Health Rep 1949; 64:1423–1430.
72. Akun RS. Histoplasmosis in a cat. J Am Vet Med Assoc 1950; 117:43–44.
73. Menges RW. Histoplasmin sensitivity in animals. Public Health Monogr 1956; 39:210–215.
74. Menges RW, Furcolow ML, Hinton A. The role of animals in the epidemiology of histoplasmosis. Public Health Monogr 1956; 39:277–281.
75. Rivers MB, Pulido JS, Folk JC. Ill-defined choroidal neovascularization within ocular histoplasmosis scars. Retina 1992; 12:90–95.
76. Macular Photocoagulation Study Group. Krypton laser photocoagulation for neovascular lesions of ocular histoplasmosis: results of a randomized clinical trial. Arch Ophthalmol 1987; 105:1499–1507.
77. Orlando RG, Davidorf FH. Spontaneous recovery phenomenon in the presumed ocular histoplasmosis syndrome. Int Ophthalmol Clin 1983; 23:137–149.
78. Jost BF, Olk RJ, Burgess DR. Factors related to spontaneous visual recovery in the ocular histoplasmosis syndrome. Retina 1987; 7:1–8.
79. Campochiaro PA, Morgan KM, Conway BP et al. Spontaneous involution of subfoveal neovascularization. Am J Ophthalmol 1990; 109:668–675.
80. Gunby P. Ocular histoplasmosis. JAMA 1980; 43:626–627.
81. Submacular Surgery Trials Research Group. Health- and vision-related quality of life among patients with ocular histoplasmosis or idiopathic choroidal neovascularization at time of enrollment in a randomized trial of submacular surgery. SST report no. 5. Arch Ophthalmol 2005; 123:78–88.
82. Kaiser RJ, Torsch T, O'Connor PR. Prognostic criteria in macular histoplasmic choroiditis. Int Ophthalmol Clin 1975; 15:41–49.

83. Makley TA, Long JW, Suie T. Therapy of chorioretinitis presumed to be caused by histoplasmosis. Int Ophthalmol Clin 1975; 15:181–195.

84. Schlaegel TF. Corticosteroids in the treatment of ocular histoplasmosis. Int Ophthalmol Clin 1983; 23:111–123.

85. Macular Photocoagulation Study Group. Argon laser photocoagulation for ocular histoplasmosis: results of a randomized clinical trial. Arch Ophthalmol 1983; 101:1347–1357.

86. Macular Photocoagulation Study Group. Argon laser photocoagulation for neovascular maculopathy: five-year results from randomized clinical trials. Arch Ophthalmol 1991; 109:1109–1114.

87. Macular Photocoagulation Study Group. Laser photocoagulation for juxtafoveal choroidal neovascularization: five-year results from randomized clinical trials. Arch Ophthalmol 1994; 112:500–509.

88. Turcotte P, Maguire MG, Fine SL. Visual results after laser treatment for peripapillary choroidal neovascular membranes. Retina 1991; 11:295–300.

89. Macular Photocoagulation Study Group. Laser photocoagulation for neovascular lesions nasal to the fovea: results from clinical trials for lesions secondary to ocular histoplasmosis and idiopathic causes. Arch Ophthalmol 1995; 113:56–61.

90. Saperstein DA, Rosenfeld PJ, Bressler NM et al. Photodynamic therapy of subfoveal choroidal neovascularization with verteporfin in the ocular histoplasmosis syndrome. One-year results of an uncontrolled, prospective case series. Ophthalmology 2002; 109:1499–1505.

91. Thomas MA, Kaplan HJ. Surgical removal of subfoveal neovascularization in the presumed ocular histoplasmosis syndrome. Am J Ophthalmol 1991; 111:1–7.

92. Thomas MA, Grand MG, Williams DF et al. Surgical management of subfoveal choroidal neovascularization. Ophthalmology 1992; 99:952–968.

93. Thomas MA, Dickinson JD, Melberg NS et al. Visual results after surgical removal of subfoveal choroidal neovascular membranes. Ophthalmology 1994; 101:1384–1396.

94. Melberg NS, Thomas MA, Dickinson JD et al. Managing recurrent neovascularization after subfoveal surgery in presumed ocular histoplasmosis syndrome. Ophthalmology 1996; 108:1064–1068.

95. Fine SL, Wood WJ, Isernhagen RD et al. Laser treatment of subfoveal neovascular membranes of ocular histoplasmosis. Arch Ophthalmol 1993; 111:19–20.

96. Submacular Surgery Trials Research Group. Surgical removal vs observation for subfoveal choroidal neovascularization, either associated with the ocular histoplasmosis syndrome or idiopathic. I. Ophthalmic findings from a randomized clinical trial: Submacular Surgery Trials (SST) group H trial: SST report no. 9. Arch Ophthalmol 2004; 122:1597–1611.

97. Submacular Surgery Trials Research Group. Surgical removal vs observation for subfoveal choroidal neovascularization, either associated with the ocular histoplasmosis syndrome or idiopathic. II. Quality-of-life findings from a randomized clinical trial: SST group H trial: SST report no. 10. Arch Ophthalmol 2004; 122:1616–1628.

98. Lewis ML, Schiffman JC. Long-term follow-up of the second eye in ocular histoplasmosis. Ophthalmol Clin 1983; 23:125–135.

99. Watzke RC, Claussen RW. The long-term course of multifocal choroiditis (presumed ocular histoplasmosis). Am J Ophthalmol 1981; 91:750–760.

100. Sawelson H, Goldberg RE, Annesley WH et al. Presumed ocular histoplasmosis syndrome: the fellow eye. Arch Ophthalmol 1976; 94:221–224.

101. Schlaegel TF, Weber JC. Follow-up study of presumed ocular histoplasmic choroiditis. Am J Ophthalmol 1971; 71:1192–1195.

Chapter

100

Birdshot Retinochoroidopathy

Stephen J. Ryan
Narsing A. Rao

At the 1975 Wilmer meeting, Ryan & Maumenee[1] used the term *birdshot retinochoroidopathy* to describe a rare ocular disorder that is characterized by bilateral chronic intraocular inflammation and multiple, discrete, cream-colored foci of depigmentation scattered diffusely throughout the fundus. These hypopigmented lesions often have a vascular orientation. Exacerbations and remissions characterize the course of the disease, which may result in markedly reduced visual acuity. There is a strong association of this intraocular inflammation with human leukocyte antigen (HLA)-A29.2.[2-4]

In the absence of a known etiology, Ryan & Maumenee[1] used the descriptive term *birdshot retinochoroidopathy* to reflect the striking clinical appearance of the hypopigmented spots. Gass[5] described this entity as *vitiliginous chorioretinitis*. In his series of 11 cases, 2 patients developed multiple white patches on the forearms and legs after the onset of visual symptoms, and another patient had two children with vitiligo. This is the only report, however, in which this systemic association is noted. Numerous other descriptive terms, such as *salmon patch choroidopathy*, used by Aaberg,[6] have been applied to what is most likely the same disease. Priem & Oosterhuis[4] point out that the earliest report of birdshot choroidopathy in the literature is probably a case report by Franceschetti & Babel[7] in 1949, which described a 63-year-old woman with a pale optic disc and multiple white retinal and chorioretinal spots; they called the condition *choriorétinite en taches de bougie*, or candle-wax spots. Amalric & Cuq[8] subsequently described a similar picture but likened it to a rice grain pattern *(choriorétinopathie en grains de riz)*.

EPIDEMIOLOGY

Birdshot retinochoroidopathy is an uncommon intraocular inflammatory disorder representing about 1 to 2% of cases referred to specialized uveitis clinics.[9,10] It is noted more frequently in people of northern European extraction. It appears that there is no gender predilection. The intraocular inflammation occurs during the third to sixth decades, at an average age of 50 years.

CLINICAL DESCRIPTION

The most common presenting symptoms are blurred vision resulting from cystoid macular edema and floaters caused by vitreous cells and debris. Classically, eyes with birdshot retinochoroidopathy are remarkable for their "quiet" appearance and, specifically, their lack of conjunctival injection. A few eyes may have some cells and flare in the anterior chamber. All eyes have cellular infiltrates in the vitreous cavity, usually more marked in the posterior portion. The severity of the infiltrate varies among patients and also in the same patient from examination to examination, but in several cases the density of cells appeared to be most severe during the early stages of the disease. The characteristic spots of depigmentation, which are usually cream-colored, are the most distinctive sign of birdshot retinochoroidopathy. There is no associated hyperpigmentation or visible clumping of melanin. Moreover there are no apparent changes within the sensory retina or retinal pigment epithelium (RPE). The cream-colored spots are densest surrounding the optic nerve and nasally. The spots tend to be oval, with the longer diameter radiating from the optic nerve to the periphery (Figs 100-1 and 100-2). The largest diameter is usually less than one-quarter of a disc diameter in extent. Occasionally these spots become confluent.

In typical cases of birdshot retinochoroidopathy the depigmented spots are almost invariably bilateral and, in most cases, symmetric. In some eyes the borders of these lesions are indistinct, whereas in others the depigmented patches are sharply delineated (Fig. 100-3). In some instances these foci of depigmentation appear in a confluent, beadlike arrangement, paralleling the course of the choroidal veins and radiating toward the periphery of the fundus.

Retinal vascular abnormalities, such as hyperpermeability of capillaries with resultant cystoid macular edema (Fig. 100-4), diffuse narrowing of retinal arterioles, perivascular hemorrhages in the nerve fiber layers, and tortuosity of vessels, are common findings in birdshot retinochoroidopathy. Optic disc swelling may also be observed.[11]

Although the visual acuity of patients with birdshot retinochoroidopathy varies among patients, most tend to have good vision.[1] In a study by Priem & Oosterhuis,[4] 148 of 203 (73%) eyes had a visual acuity of 6/18 or better. Considering that the diagnosis of birdshot retinochoroidopathy was not made initially and the clinical syndrome was not described until 1975,[12] the significance of this good visual acuity at the time of diagnosis is even more impressive. Priem & Oosterhuis presented

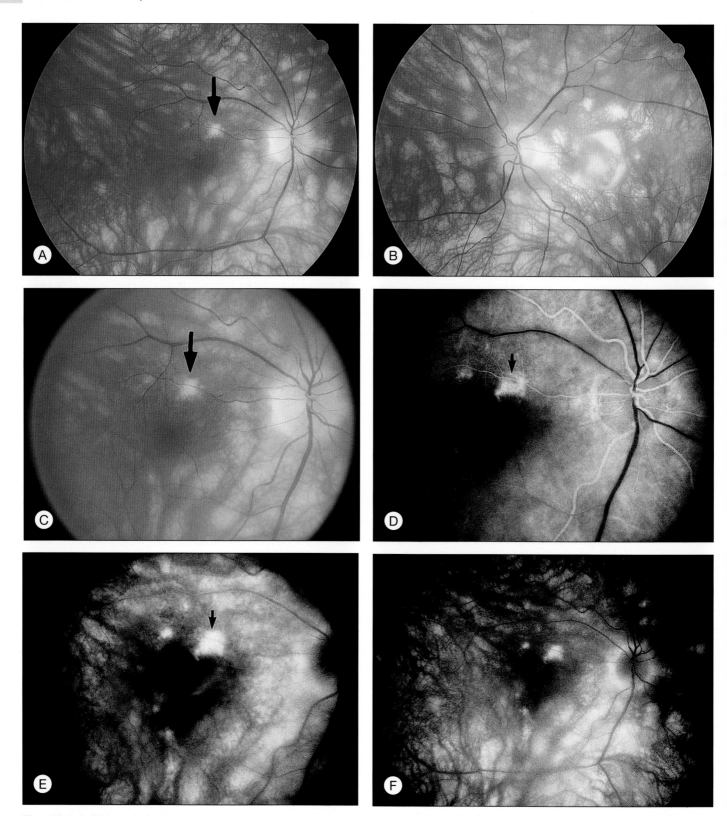

Fig. 100-1 A, Wide-angle fundus photograph (right eye) showing distribution and variability of spots. Spots located temporal to the vascular-free zone are discrete. The spot identified with an arrow demonstrated leaking of fluorescein in the pattern of subretinal neovascularization. B, Wide-angle fundus photograph (left eye) showing distribution of spots plus disciform lesion in the macula. C, Standard fundus photograph (right eye) showing a spot that leaked on angiography and that is the site of neovascularization (arrow). D, Fluorescein angiogram, early phase (right eye). Note that the spots are not remarkable. Hyperfluorescence corresponds to arrows in A and C. E, Fluorescein angiogram, late phase (right eye). Note hyperfluorescence of spot identified in A and D. F, Wide-angle fluorescein angiogram, late phase (right eye), showing more extensive staining of the birdshot spots.

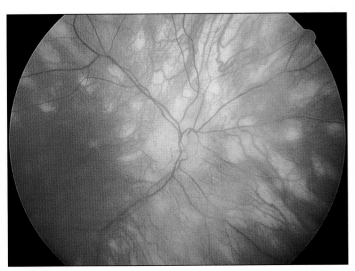

Fig. 100-2 Fundus photograph (right eye) showing depigmented spots around the optic disc.

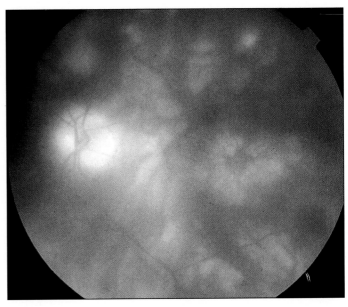

Fig. 100-4 Fluorescein angiogram (left eye), late phase, showing diffuse hyperfluorescence and cystoid macular edema.

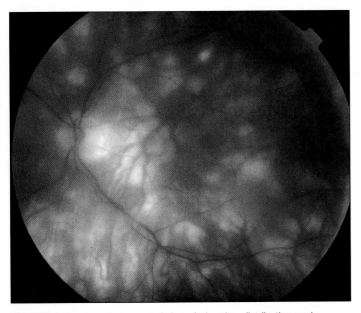

Fig. 100-3 Fundus photograph (left eye) showing distribution and variability of spots.

details of the anterior segment examination in 68 patients, of whom only 2 showed redness of one or both eyes.[4] Eight patients had bilateral fine keratic precipitates and 8 had very mild flare and cells in the anterior chamber of both eyes. In 80 patients, examination of the vitreous was recorded. Vitreous cells were seen in 76.1% of all eyes and opacities in 45.9%. In total, vitreous inflammation was present in 83% of all eyes examined.[4]

Rhegmatogenous retinal detachment has been reported to occur in birdshot retinochoroidopathy.[1,13–15] However, rhegmatogenous retinal detachment is a well-recognized complication of uveitis,[16] and it is not known whether the incidence is increased in patients with birdshot retinochoroidopathy. Priem & Oosterhuis[4] found only 2 of 79 patients for whom ocular

history was available to have had a rhegmatogenous retinal detachment; one other patient had undergone laser treatment for a peripheral retinal hole with operculum.

Several investigators[2,12,17,18] have reported subretinal neovascularization in eyes with birdshot retinochoroidopathy (see Fig. 100-1). In the review by Priem & Oosterhuis,[4] 15 of 203 eyes had retinal neovascularization, and 12 had a subretinal neovascular membrane. These investigators noted that retinal capillary closure was absent in all 15 eyes that had retinal neovascularization, suggesting that the growth of new vessels was not a response to ischemia. They further noted that Felder & Brockhurst[19] had reported retinal neovascularization in patients following episodes of uveitis and the absence of capillary nonperfusion. Henkind[20] considered local inflammation in the retinal vascular bed to be a sufficient stimulus for the growth of new vessels, which were more common in the peripapillary area than in the periphery. Priem & Oosterhuis,[4] however, noted peripapillary neovascularization in only 2 eyes, whereas peripheral retinal neovascularization was seen in 13 eyes. Although subretinal neovascularization is not a common finding in inflammatory conditions, it has been reported in association with inflammatory diseases such as Behçet's disease,[2] toxoplasmosis,[21] chronic nonspecific uveitis,[22] Harada's disease,[11,23] and presumed ocular histoplasmosis syndrome.[24] Subretinal neovascularization has been documented in a sufficient number of eyes with birdshot retinochoroidopathy to suggest that it is related to the disease per se and is not coincidental.

ASSOCIATED SYSTEMIC DISEASES

Several investigators have postulated the association of other diseases with birdshot retinochoroidopathy.[4,5] Through medical history and physical examination, Priem & Oosterhuis[4] found an incidence of vascular disease that was unusually high for the age group of their patients (range, 23 to 79 years; mean, 52.5 years). Of the 102 patients, 16 had hypertension, 5 had coronary artery disease, 2 had a history of cerebrovascular accident, and 3 had had central vein obstruction. They suggested that this surprisingly high incidence of vascular disease in this group of patients might indicate an association of vasculopathy and birdshot retinochoroidopathy. However, they concluded that the medical history and examination were not helpful in establishing an etiologic factor for birdshot retinochoroidopathy.

Gass[5] stressed the association of birdshot retinochoroidopathy with vitiligo. However, Priem & Oosterhuis[4] could find only 1 of 102 patients who was known to have depigmentation of the skin, and this occurred only after exposure to the sun. Moreover, Wagoner and associates[25] were able to find evidence of birdshot retinochoroidopathy in only 1 of 223 patients with vitiligo. Multifocal choroidal opacities similar to birdshot retinochoroidopathy have been described in sarcoidosis.[7,26-28] Priem & Oosterhuis[4] studied 38 patients by means of chest films, complete blood counts, calcium levels, angiotensin-converting enzyme, Kveim test, and, in several patients, biopsy of skin lesions and were able to identify one patient who had evidence of sarcoidosis. One other patient with sarcoidosis and simultaneous birdshot retinochoroidopathy has been reported in Japan.[29]

ETIOLOGY AND PATHOGENESIS

The etiology and pathogenesis of birdshot retinochoroidopathy are unknown. However, this inflammation is strongly associated with HLA-A29, suggesting a genetic predisposition to this retinochoroidopathy. Moreover, autoimmunity to retinal soluble protein (S-antigen) may play a role in the perpetuation of the intraocular inflammation or peptides of the S-antigen may bind to HLA-A29 leading to the autoimmunity.[30,31]

The association between birdshot retinochoroidopathy and the HLA-A29 gene has been calculated to have a relative risk of 224, the strongest association of all HLA-associated diseases.[32] Despite recent advances in defining individuals who are genetically susceptible to diseases such as birdshot retinochoroidopathy, it remains unclear how these associations between HLA antigens and specific diseases can be pathogenetically explained. Feltkamp[32] has suggested that major histocompatibility complex class I proteins (including HLA-A29) may play an important role in the destruction of virus-infected cells. Viral peptides may fit between two α-helices, which are situated on the α_1-α_2 domain of the class I molecule. He further suggests that, when such a molecule reaches the cell surface together with the viral peptide, it may contact certain cytotoxic T lymphocytes that have a receptor that fits in both the epitope of the peptide and the characteristic surface of the α-helices of the HLA molecule. The specific cytotoxic T cell then becomes stimulated, which leads to lysis of the peptide-presenting cell. The macrophages or B lymphocytes displaying HLA class II molecules may also play a comparable role in presentation of antigens to the helper T lymphocytes. Infectious agents such as viruses may thus be the initial triggers for many of the HLA-associated inflammatory diseases, such as birdshot retinochoroidopathy.[33]

Although depigmented choroid lesions are the most characteristic and prominent feature of birdshot retinochoroidopathy, the pathogenesis of such lesions is unknown. Ryan & Maumenee[1] believe that these depigmented spots may be related to previous accumulation of inflammatory cells beneath the RPE. Gass[5] reported that these patches are unlike most other infiltrative or atrophic hypopigmented fundus lesions in that they are neither elevated, as are nodular inflammatory infiltrates, nor depressed, as is atrophy of the choroid and retina. He postulates that they are caused by focal depigmentation of the choroidal melanocytes and believes they are analogous to vitiligo of the skin. However, a recent histopathologic study revealed focal aggregates of lymphocytes in the choroid.[34]

Priem & Oosterhuis[4] suggested that the lesions of birdshot retinochoroidopathy are located in the outer choroid and are associated with large choroidal vessels. Their hypothesis is based on the fact that large choroidal vessels are often clearly seen to cross over these lesions; that the lesions show a radial arrangement around the optic disc; that most eyes show macular sparing by the birdshot lesions, which is consistent with the distribution of large choroidal veins; and that lesions located more peripherally tend to be confluent and tend to form elongated yellow-white streaks that parallel choroidal vessels, suggestive of vascular sheathing. These streaks were most prominent inferonasal to the optic disc. Similar confluent lesions in the inferonasal quadrant have been reported by other investigators.[12,35] The relatively deep location of the lesions is thought to explain their indistinct appearance and lack of secondary RPE reaction, even in long-standing cases.

IMMUNOPATHOLOGY

Recently our histopathologic examination of an eye with birdshot retinochoroidopathy, presented by Dr. Brooks Crawford at the Verhoeff-Zimmerman Society meeting, revealed multiple focal aggregates of lymphocytes, primarily localized to middle layers of the choroid. The lymphoid infiltrates appeared to extend from the vessel walls in a comet shape (Fig. 100-5). The overlying RPE and choriocapillaris were not usually involved. Although the chronic inflammatory infiltration was primarily made up of nongranulomatous processes, occasional lesions displayed granulomatous changes containing epithelioid histiocytes. Our immunohistochemical analysis of the lymphoid infiltrates showed primarily T lymphocytes expressing CD-8, CD-20-positive B lymphocytes, CD-68-positive macrophages, and a few CD-4-positive T cells. Similar perivascular lymphoid infiltration was present in the retina (Fig. 100-6).

LABORATORY AND OTHER INVESTIGATIONS

HLA typing can be a valuable diagnostic tool; it has a sensitivity of 96% and a specificity of 93%.[32] Feltkamp[32] has used Bayes' theorem to determine the contribution of HLA typing in increasing the probability of a diagnosis of birdshot retinochoroidopathy. He calculates that a given probability of 70% rises to 97% if the patient is HLA-A29-positive. However,

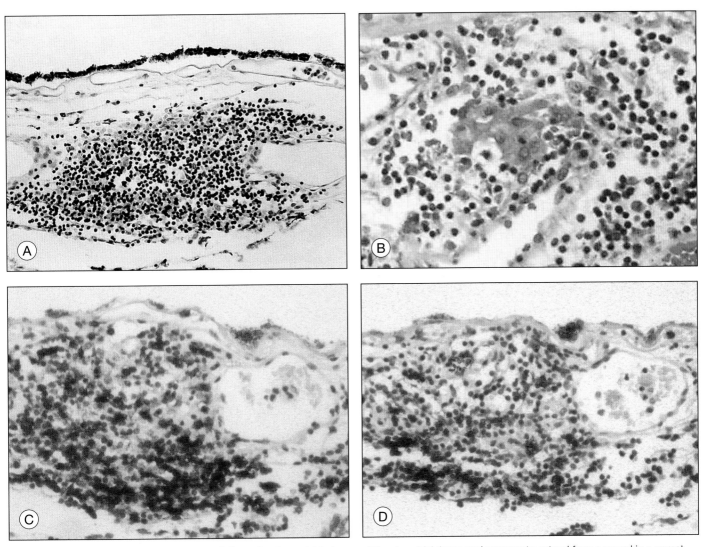

Fig. 100-5 A, Histologically, the inflammatory infiltrate involves middle layers of the choroidal tissue and appears to extend from a vessel in a comet shape. B, Focal granulomatous inflammation is present around a choroidal vessel. Immunohistochemically, the choroidal infiltrate consisted of mainly CD-8 T lymphocytes (C) and few CD-20-positive B lymphocytes (D).

if the patient is HLA-A29-negative, the probability drops from 70% to 8.5%. There is predominant linkage to the HLA-A29.2 subtype of HLA-A29.[36,37]

Fluorescein angiography of the choroidal spots in these patients characteristically reveals hypofluorescence in the early phase with slight diffuse hyperfluorescence in the late phase. Priem & Oosterhuis[4] believe that the late-phase mild hyperfluorescence of birdshot lesions is consistent with a deep-seated inflammatory focus that gradually accumulates fluorescein, and they suggest that this strengthens their hypothesis that the birdshot lesions are located in the outer choroid and are associated with large choroidal vessels. It is important to note that many of the depigmented lesions show neither early hypofluorescence nor late-phase hyperfluorescence; thus in many instances the lesions are more apparent by ophthalmoscopy than by angiography. The retinal circulation demonstrates marked leakage and accumulation of dye, as well as cystoid macular edema on fluorescein angiography. Priem & Oosterhuis[4] reported retinal vasculopathy to be a major feature of birdshot retinochoroidopathy. Cystoid macular edema was present in 127 (62.6%) of 203 eyes, and perivascular leakage was found in 81 (40%).

Indocyanine green angiography of birdshot lesions may show persistently hypofluorescent dark spots (Fig. 100-7), often located between large choroidal vessels.[38,39] Similar patterns are observed in Vogt–Koyanagi–Harada syndrome.

Kaplan & Aaberg[14] have emphasized that distinct electrophysiologic abnormalities appear to be associated with this condition. They performed electroretinography on 4 patients with birdshot retinochoroidopathy; in each case rod b-wave amplitudes and cone and rod b-wave implicit times were diminished. In these cases cone a- and b-wave amplitudes were borderline-low. Priem & Oosterhuis[4] studied visual evoked choroidal responses in 60 eyes and found 32 (53%) to have abnormal amplitude and another 13 to have increased latency. The electroretinogram (ERG) was abnormal in 18 of 84 eyes (21%), and the absence of oscillatory potentials was the only

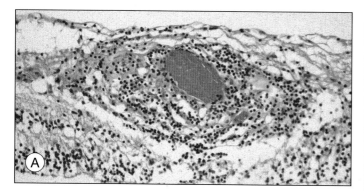

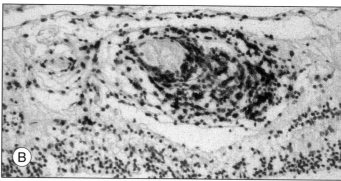

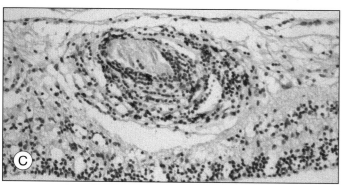

Fig. 100-6 A to C. The retinal vasculitis shows mononuclear cell infiltration (A). Immunohistochemically, most of the cells stained positive for CD-8 (B) and few stained for CD-20 (C).

abnormal finding in 4 eyes. Fourteen eyes were reported as borderline, and 46 eyes (54.7%) had abnormally low ERGs. Thus, of 84 eyes tested with the ERG, 60 demonstrated a subnormal light–dark ratio.[4] Priem et al.[40] thoroughly studied 16 patients using electrophysiologic and psychophysical methods. They report consistent changes, including an abnormal ERG with reduced amplitude and increased latency of the b wave. They also reported a normal fast but abnormal slow electro-oculogram oscillation and a marked disturbance in pattern

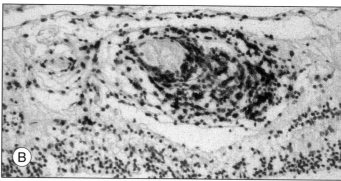

Fig. 100-7 Indocyanine green angiography reveals dark spots, which remained hypofluorescent.

visual evoked cortical potential (VECP). The a wave of the ERG and the flash VECP, in contrast, were well preserved. These laboratory tests suggested to these authors that inner retinal disease, as a result of retinal inflammation and vascular change, is presumably responsible for the electrophysiologic abnormalities.

DIFFERENTIAL DIAGNOSIS

The differential diagnosis of suspected cases of birdshot retinochoroidopathy includes a number of entities such as pars planitis, intraocular primary large B-cell lymphoma, syphilitic chorioretinitis, multiple evanescent white-dot syndrome, punctate inner choroidopathy, and other causes of multifocal choroiditis, including sarcoidosis.[27] Birdshot retinochoroidopathy can be distinguished from these entities on the bases of clinical course, the signs listed above, and most specifically, HLA-A29 testing.

THERAPY

Many patients described in the literature were treated with corticosteroids for various time periods. Several reported subjective improvement while taking these agents.[13,31] We have observed some patients whose visual acuity is exquisitely sensitive to steroids; this visual improvement after treatment with steroids reflects changes in the cystoid macular edema. There was no decrease in number or extent of depigmented foci. We use visual acuity, rather than presence or absence of floaters, as the gauge of treatment efficacy and to determine the appropriate dose or regimen of steroids for each patient and for the course of the disease. Initially, 40 to 60 mg of oral prednisone is given daily, and the steroids are eventually tapered after clinical response (i.e., improvement in the visual acuity). However, some patients may require prednisone 5 mg or less daily for several months.[41] Systemic prednisone can be supplemented with sub-Tenon's injections of depot corticosteroids.

Immunosuppressive agents, such as ciclosporin, and cytotoxic drugs, such as azathioprine and cyclophosphamide, may be used when corticosteroids alone cannot control the intraocular inflammation, or for those patients with medical problems or ophthalmic complications that may prevent the use of systemic or sub-Tenon's corticosteroids. Low-dose ciclosporin 2.5 mg/kg per day, alone or in combination with azathioprine 1.5 to 2 mg/kg per day, may improve or stabilize visual acuity.[10] Ciclosporin dosage can be decreased further by administering ketoconazole.[42] In recent years some clinicians have used fluorescein angiography, optical coherent tomography of macula, visual fields, indocyanine green angiography and ERG as adjuncts in determining when to initiate tapering of immunosuppressive therapy.[43]

COMPLICATIONS AND PROGNOSIS

To study the evolution of the birdshot lesions and the subsequent visual prognosis, Priem & Oosterhuis[4] reviewed 62 patients who had been followed for a period ranging from 1 month to 13 years. For those patients followed for 5 years or more, half of the eyes maintained a visual acuity of 6/18 or better. Visual acuity loss was due to cystoid macular edema, macular epiretinal membrane formation, macular hole, subretinal neovascular membrane, macular scar, and cataract. Chronic cystoid macular edema is the most common of these complications, occurring in about 63% of cases. Recent studies suggest that retinal functions, measured by ERG and visual fields, may deteriorate progressively over years, despite stable visual acuity.[43,44] In long-standing cases, optic atrophy (Fig. 100-8) and peripheral retinal pigmentary changes can occur.[45] Prolonged treatment with the above anti-inflammatory agents may be required to preserve the retinal functions and visual acuity.

Although vitreous hemorrhage and vitreous floaters were important causes of visual loss in the initial stages of the disease, they did not contribute to late visual loss in the group of patients followed for 5 years or more.[4] Improvement in visual acuity was seen in 13 eyes and reflected clearing of vitreous hemorrhage (3 eyes), cataract extraction (3 eyes), laser photocoagulation of subretinal neovascularization (3 eyes), and regression of inflammation (5 eyes). In this series, 5 patients initially had no clear evidence of birdshot spots in the fundus, presenting with papillitis, retinal vasculitis, and vitreitis of both eyes. Remarkably, the typical fundus picture of birdshot retinochoroidopathy was not evident until several years later, after the signs of acute inflammation had resolved.[4] Soubrane and associates[46] described 2 patients with bilateral recurrent vitreitis, retinal vasculitis, nonspecific and mild posterior uveitis, swollen optic discs, and leaking retinal capillaries as seen by fluorescein angiography. Fundus changes characteristic of birdshot retinochoroidopathy were visible only after 7 to 8 years of exacerbations and remissions of the vasculitis and vitreitis in these 2 patients. These

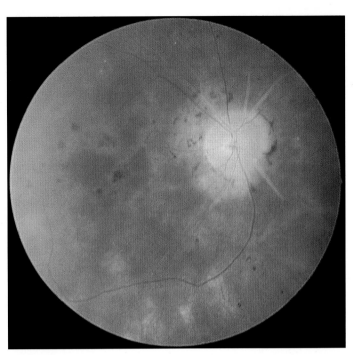

Fig. 100-8 Fundus photograph showing optic atrophy and sheathing of retinal vessels.

investigators have suggested that delay before onset of the retinochoroidal patches may result from variations in the rapidity and extent of involvement of the inflammatory process. These factors, in turn, may be determined by the individual's response to the disease itself.[46] Although the clinical appearance of the initial stages of birdshot retinochoroidopathy may be variable in a few patients,[4,46] Priem & Oosterhuis[4] have stated that the specificity of the funduscopic appearance, the consistency of its behavior, and its high association with the HLA-A29 gene suggest that birdshot retinochoroidopathy is indeed a single clinical entity, as opposed to being the final common pathway of various ocular disorders.

SUMMARY

Birdshot retinochoroidopathy is a relatively uncommon clinical entity characterized by scattered cream-colored or whitish depigmented areas in the fundus, cystoid macular edema, papilledema and chronic vitreitis, but with minimal or no anterior segment involvement. It is further characterized by a long-term course of exacerbations and remissions. The decreased visual acuity is primarily the result of cystoid macular edema. Although the definitive treatment for birdshot retinochoroidopathy is unknown, corticosteroids are used initially, as in pars planitis, that is, not for cells or floaters, but, rather, to improve visual acuity through reduction of macular edema. Low-dose ciclosporin may be useful in cases refractory to steroid therapy. The localization of the clinical changes, the protracted nature of the disease, and the finding of HLA-A29 antigen in virtually all patients strongly suggest that birdshot retinochoroidopathy is an ocular inflammatory disease with a genetic predisposition.

REFERENCES

1. Ryan SJ, Maumenee AE. Birdshot retinochoroidopathy. Am J Ophthalmol 1980; 89:31–45.
2. Nussenblatt RB, Mittal KK, Ryan S et al. Birdshot retinochoroidopathy associated with HLA-A29 antigen and immune responsiveness to retinal S-antigen. Am J Ophthalmol 1982; 94:147–158.
3. Priem HA, Kijlstra A, Noens L et al. HLA typing in birdshot chorioretinopathy. Am J Ophthalmol 1988; 105:182–185.
4. Priem HA, Oosterhuis JA. Birdshot chorioretinopathy: clinical characteristics and evolution. Br J Ophthalmol 1988; 72:646–659.
5. Gass JDM. Vitiliginous chorioretinitis. Arch Ophthalmol 1981; 99:1778–1787.
6. Aaberg TM. Diffuse inflammatory salmon patch choroidopathy syndrome. International Fluorescein Macula Symposium. Carmel, CA: 1979.
7. Franceschetti A, Babel J. La chorio-rétinite en "taches de bougie," manifestation de la maladie de Besnier-Boeck. Ophthalmologica 1949; 118:701–710.
8. Amalric P, Cuq G. Une forme très particulière de chorio-retinopathie en grains de riz. Bull Soc Ophtalmol Fr 1981; 81:131–134.
9. Henderly DE, Genstler AJ, Smith RE et al. Changing patterns of uveitis. Am J Ophthalmol 1987; 103:131–136.
10. Vitale AT, Rodriguez A, Foster CS. Low-dose cyclosporine therapy in the treatment of birdshot retinochoroidopathy. Ophthalmology 1994; 101:822–831.
11. Snyder DA, Tessler HH. Vogt–Koyanagi–Harada syndrome. Am J Ophthalmol 1980; 90:69–75.
12. Soubrane G, Coscas G, Binaghi M et al. Birdshot retinochoroidopathy and subretinal new vessels. Br J Ophthalmol 1983; 67:461–467.
13. Fuerst DJ, Tessler HH, Fishman GA et al. Birdshot retinochoroidopathy. Arch Ophthalmol 1984; 102:214–219.
14. Kaplan HJ, Aaberg TM. Birdshot retinochoroidopathy. Am J Ophthalmol 1980; 90:773–782.
15. Laroche L, Saraux H, Quentel G et al. Bird-shot chorio-retinopathy apres décollement de rétine: origine auto-immune probable. Bull Soc Ophtalmol Fr 1983; 83:1245–1247.
16. Brockhurst RJ, Schepens CL. Peripheral uveitis: the complication of retinal detachment. Arch Ophthalmol 1968; 80:747–753.
17. Brucker AJ, Deglin EA, Bene C et al. Subretinal choroidal neovascularization in birdshot retinochoroidopathy. Am J Ophthalmol 1985; 99:40–44.
18. Oosterhuis JA, Renger-van Dijk DH. Birdshot chorioretinopathy. In: Ryan SJ, Dawson AK, Little HL, eds. Retinal diseases. Orlando, FL: Grune & Stratton; 1985.
19. Felder KS, Brockhurst RJ. Neovascular fundus abnormalities in peripheral uveitis. Arch Ophthalmol 1982; 100:750–754.
20. Henkind P. Ocular neovascularization: the Krill memorial lecture. Am J Ophthalmol 1978; 85:287–301.
21. Cotliar AM, Friedman AH. Subretinal neovascularization in ocular toxoplasmosis. Br J Ophthalmol 1982; 66:524–529.
22. Augsburger JJ, Benson WE. Subretinal neovascularization in chronic uveitis. Graefes Arch Clin Exp Ophthalmol 1980; 215:43–51.
23. Moorthy RS, Inomata H, Rao NA. Vogt–Koyanagi–Harada syndrome. Surv Ophthalmol 1995; 39:265–292.
24. Cantrill HL, Burgess D. Peripapillary neovascular membranes in presumed ocular histoplasmosis. Am J Ophthalmol 1980; 89:192–203.
25. Wagoner MD, Albert DM, Lerner AB et al. New observations on vitiligo and ocular disease. Am J Ophthalmol 1983; 96:16–26.
26. Brod RD. Presumed sarcoid choroidopathy mimicking birdshot retinochoroidopathy. Am J Ophthalmol 1990; 109:357–358.
27. Read RW, Rao NA, Sharma OP. Sarcoid choroiditis initially diagnosed as birdshot choroidopathy. Sarcoidosis Vasc Diffuse Lung Dis 2000; 17:85–86.
28. Spalton DJ, Sanders MD. Fundus changes in histologically confirmed sarcoidosis. Br J Ophthalmol 1981; 65:348–358.
29. Yoshioka T, Yoshioka H, Tanaka F. Birdshot retinochoroidopathy as a new ocular sign of sarcoidosis. Nippon Ganka Gakkai Zasshi 1983; 87:283–288.
30. Boisgerault F, Khalil I, Tieng V et al. Definition of the HLA-A29 peptide ligand motif allows prediction of potential T-cell epitopes from the retinal soluble antigen, a candidate autoantigen in birdshot retinopathy. Proc Natl Acad Sci USA 1996; 93:3466–3470.
31. Oosterhuis JA, Baarsma GS, Polak BCP. Birdshot chorioretinopathy-vitiliginous chorioretinitis. Int Ophthalmol 1982; 5:137–144.
32. Feltkamp TEW. Ophthalmological significance of HLA-associated uveitis. Eye 1990; 4:839–884.
33. Zinkernagel RM. Major histocompatibility gene complex–disease associations may reflect T cell-mediated immunopathology. Eur J Clin Invest 1986; 16:101–105.
34. Gaudio PA, Kaye DB, Crawford JB. Histopathology of birdshot retinochoroidopathy. Br J Ophthalmol 2002; 86:1439–1441.
35. Salvanet-Bouccara A, Forestier F. Choriorétinopathie de type birdshot. J Fr Ophtalmol 1983; 6:671–676.
36. LeHoang P, Ozdemir N, Benhamou A et al. HLA–A 29.2 Subtype associated with birdshot retinochoroidopathy. Am J Ophthalmol 1992; 113:33–35.
37. Tabary T, LeHoang P, Betuel H et al. Susceptibility to birdshot chorioretinopathy is restricted to the HLA-A29.2 subtype. Tissue Antigens 1990; 36:177–179.
38. Fardeau C, Herbort CP, Kullmann N et al. Indocyanine green angiography in birdshot chorioretinopathy. Ophthalmology 1999; 106:1928–1934.
39. Stanga PE, Lim JI, Hamilton P. Indocyanine green angiography in chorioretinal diseases: indications and interpretation: an evidence-based update. Ophthalmology 2003; 110:15–21.
40. Priem HA, De Rouck A, De Laey JJ et al. Electrophysiologic studies in birdshot chorioretinopathy. Am J Ophthalmol 1988; 106:430–436.
41. Ladas JG, Arnold AC, Holland GN. Control of visual symptoms in two men with birdshot retinochoroidopathy using low-dose oral corticosteroid therapy. Am J Ophthalmol 1999; 128:116–118.
42. Silverstein BE, Wong IG. Reduction of cyclosporine dosage with ketoconazole in a patient with birdshot retinochoroidopathy. Am J Ophthalmol 1998; 125:106–108.
43. Zacks DN, Samson CM, Lowenstein J et al. Electroretinograms as an indicator of disease activity in birdshot retinochoroidopathy. Graefes Arch Clin Exp Ophthalmol 2002; 240:601–607.
44. Oh KT, Christmas NJ, Folk JC. Birdshot retinochoroiditis: long term follow-up of a chronically progressive disease. Am J Ophthalmol 2002; 133:622–629.
45. Willermain F, Greiner K, Forrester JV. Atypical end stage birdshot retinochoroidopathy. Ocul Immunol Inflamm 2003; 11:305–307.
46. Soubrane G, Bokobza R, Coscas G. Late-developing lesions in birdshot retinochoroidopathy, Am J Ophthalmol 1990; 109:204–210.

Chapter

101

Multifocal Choroiditis with Panuveitis, Diffuse Subretinal Fibrosis, and Punctate Inner Choroidopathy

James C. Folk
Jonathan D. Walker

Multifocal choroiditis with panuveitis (MCP), the diffuse subretinal fibrosis (DSF) syndrome, and punctate inner choroidopathy (PIC) are similar conditions characterized by inflammation at the level of the deep retina and choroid which causes chorioretinal scars. Affected individuals with MCP and DSF often have multiple episodes of recurrent inflammation. The etiologies and pathogenesis of each of these three conditions are unknown. It is unclear whether they are separate entities or various manifestations of one disease. Since the funduscopic appearance and clinical courses of the three conditions are similar, they may share the same underlying cause. Or perhaps this type of chorioretinal inflammation and scarring is a nonspecific response to a variety of etiologic agents. These three conditions are presented separately followed by a common differential diagnosis and treatment section.

MULTIFOCAL CHOROIDITIS WITH PANUVEITIS

In 1973, Nozik & Dorsch[1] described 2 patients with bilateral anterior uveitis and a distinctive ophthalmoscopic appearance that resembled the presumed ocular histoplasmosis syndrome (POHS). In 1984, Dreyer & Gass[2] reported a series of 28 patients with uveitis and lesions at the level of the RPE and choriocapillaris. They called the syndrome *multifocal choroiditis and panuveitis*. Subsequently, Deutsch & Tessler[3] described 28 patients with chorioretinal lesions and vitreous cells that they called *pseudo-POHS* because of the vitreous inflammation. However, most of Deutsch & Tessler's patients had additional findings suggesting systemic diseases such as sarcoidosis, syphilis, or tuberculosis. Morgan & Schatz[4] reported their findings on an additional 11 patients with clinical characteristics similar to the patients in the previously reported series and called the condition *recurrent multifocal choroiditis*. Most of the patients described in these reports represent a distinct clinical entity that is different from POHS and other secondary or idiopathic chorioretinal inflammatory disorders. We prefer the term *multifocal choroiditis with panuveitis* for this condition.

Clinical features

MCP is more common in females, with reported frequencies ranging from 75 to 100%.[2,4] Although most affected patients are in their 30s, the condition has been reported in patients aged 6 to 69 years. Most patients have never lived in areas endemic for histoplasmosis nor do they have affected family members. In Morgan & Schatz's series, 10 of 11 patients were moderately myopic.[4] MCP is bilateral in the majority of affected patients (79% in Dreyer & Gass's series), although frequently it presents asymmetrically, and many involved second eyes may be asymptomatic.[2,4]

Symptoms of MCP may include decreased central vision, central metamorphopsia, paracentral scotomata, floaters, photopsias, mild ocular discomfort, and photophobia. Visual acuity at initial presentation has ranged from 20/20 to light perception. Of 39 patients in two series, 22 (56%) presented with a visual acuity of 20/100 or worse in the more severely affected eye.[2,4]

Anterior uveitis is uncommon in MCP but may consist of mild to moderate (1+ to 3+) anterior chamber cells, nongranulomatous keratitic precipitates, and posterior synechiae. Dreyer & Gass[2] reported a 46% incidence of anterior uveitis in their series, a figure which seems high in the authors' experience. Wiechens & Nolle,[5] however, found abnormalities of the iris vasculature in all eyes with MCP using fluorescein angiography. The abnormalities included leakage at the pupillary margin, avascular zones, and neovascularization. Morgan & Schatz[4] observed vitreous inflammation in 45% of their patients, whereas Nozik & Dorsch[1] and Dreyer & Gass[2] noted vitreous cells in all of their patients. Vitreitis is usually mild to moderate in severity and can be asymmetric in bilateral cases. Once vitreous inflammation subsides, there is little residual vitreous debris.

The ophthalmic abnormalities seen in MCP primarily involve the retina and choroid. Acutely, several to several hundred yellow (sometimes gray) lesions are seen at the level of the RPE and choriocapillaris. Most lesions are 50 to 1000 μm in diameter but occasionally may be larger. The lesions usually are round or oval. Lesions are most commonly observed in the peripapillary region and in the midperiphery (Fig. 101-1). Reddy and co-authors[6] reported a preponderance of lesions in the nasal periphery. Lesions in MCP may be seen singly, in clusters, or arranged in a linear configuration, as seen in POHS.[1,2,7] Some active lesions may be associated with small amounts of subretinal fluid. As inflammation subsides, the lesions become deep, round, and atrophic with variable pigmentation that increases over time. New chorioretinal lesions may be seen in conjunction with old scars in patients who have recurrent episodes of inflammation.

Optic disc edema may be observed in MCP with active inflammation. With time, most patients develop peripapillary scarring similar to that seen in POHS. Optic disc pallor and narrowing of retinal vessels can be observed but are uncommon findings. Cystoid macular edema (CME) occurs in 10 to 20% of patients. Rarely, periphlebitis and retinal and optic disc neovascularization can also develop.[3] Macular and peripapillary choroidal neovascularization (CNV) develops in 25 to 39% of

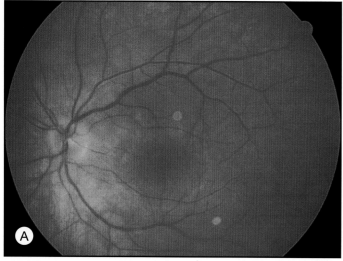

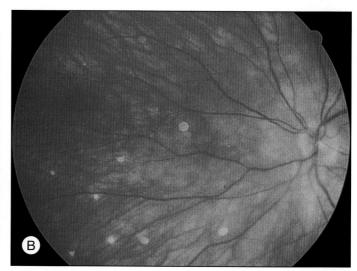

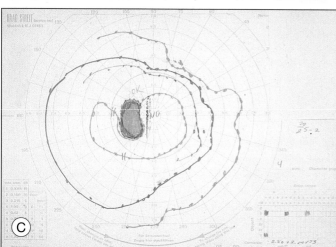

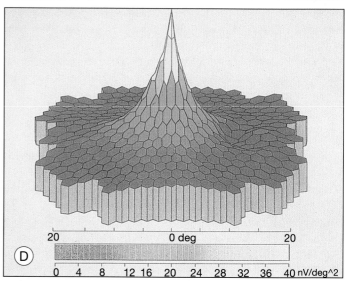

Fig. 101-1 Funduscopic photographs, visual fields, and multifocal electroretinograms (ERG) of a young woman with multifocal choroiditis with panuveitis (MCP) (left eye). A, The macula appeared normal in the left eye, but characteristic chorioretinal scar lesions could be seen in the midperiphery (B). Visual acuity was 20/20 (right eye) and 20/25 (left eye). C, Visual field testing revealed a normal blind spot in the right eye, but an enlarged blind spot in the left eye. D, A multifocal ERG demonstrated normal foveal function in the right eye but depressed foveal function in the left eye (E).

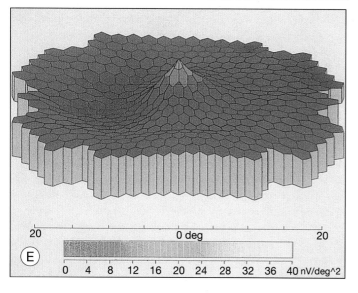

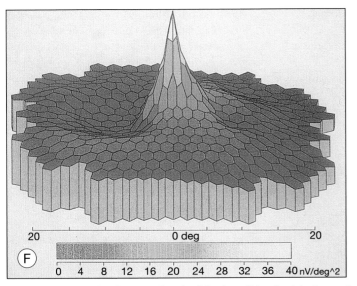

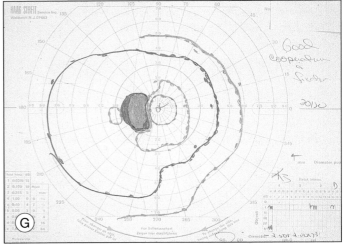

Fig. 101-1—cont'd F, Two months after injection of Kenalog into the posterior sub-Tenon's space of the left eye, visual acuity had improved to 20/20, and the multifocal ERG had improved but was still subnormal. G, The blind-spot enlargement did not change appreciably after Kenalog injection.

eyes with MCP and can be the presenting cause for decreased vision.[2,4,5]

Ancillary testing

Angiography
Very acute lesions are hypofluorescent early in the fluorescein angiogram and then gradually fill as the study progresses. Late in the angiogram the initially hypofluorescent lesions leak fluorescein. The leakage makes it difficult to determine whether CNV is present or not. Old scars typically act as window defects with early hyperfluorescence and late fading.

Indocyanine green
A number of authors, including Slakter et al.,[8] Bouchenaki et al.,[9] Vadala et al.,[10] and Cimino et al.,[11] have shown that indocyanine green (ICG) angiography often demonstrates many more lesions in eyes with MCP than are seen with fluorescein angiography or on clinical exam. The typical lesions are hypofluorescent round spots, 200 to 500 μm in diameter. Usually the lesions stay hypofluorescent throughout the angiogram. Severely involved areas with numerous spots often correspond to visual field defects. The authors believed that the hypofluorescent spots represented inflammatory products in the inner choroid but could not rule out ischemia as an etiology for their findings. The hypofluorescent spots observed on ICG angiography seemed to correlate with the degree of inflammation. Patients experienced a reduction in size and number of hypofluorescent spots associated with a decrease in vitreitis after oral prednisone therapy. Such hypofluorescent spots on ICG angiography may also be seen in other types of choroiditis.

Electrophysiologic testing
Dreyer & Gass[2] obtained electroretinograms (ERGs) on 29 eyes of 16 patients. They observed a normal or borderline ERG in 16 eyes (41%), moderately reduced ERG in 5 eyes (17%),

and severely reduced ERG in 6 eyes (21%). Oh et al.[12] observed abnormalities on multifocal ERG (MERG) testing in patients with MCP, which may prove more useful than full-field ERG in these patients (see Fig. 101-1). Unfortunately the MERG is so sensitive that it often becomes almost extinguished after a severe bout of MCP and may therefore not be useful to monitor the course of the disease.

Visual field testing
Visual field testing may demonstrate scotomata that correspond to chorioretinal lesions or associated serious detachments of the retina and RPE. In addition, large temporal field defects that do not correspond to visible fundus lesions are sometimes seen. Enlargement of the blind spot may be seen in MCP as one of the initial manifestations of the disease or with recurrent episodes of inflammation.[13,14] Of 32 patients with MCP seen at the University of Iowa between 1985 and 1992, 11 (34%) had enlargement of the blind spot in at least one eye that could not be explained by disc swelling or peripapillary chorioretinal scarring.[6,15] Some patients with enlarged blind spots had acute chorioretinal lesions clustered around the optic nerve, especially in the nasal periphery. Slakter and co-workers[8] found diffuse peripapillary hypofluorescence on ICG angiography in 5 patients with enlarged blind spots. Subsequent examinations demonstrated concurrent resolution of the peripapillary hypofluorescence and enlarged blind spots in 4 of the 5 patients.

DIFFUSE SUBRETINAL FIBROSIS SYNDROME

DSF syndrome is a rare syndrome that was described by Palestine and associates[16] in 1984. They reported their findings in 3 young women who had uveitis and subretinal fibrosis. Before this report, Doran & Hamilton[17] had described findings in 4 patients with uveitis and subretinal fibrosis and called the entity "disciform macular degeneration in young adults."

However, subretinal fibrosis in Doran & Hamilton's patients was preceded by CNV and therefore may have been caused by CNV rather than inflammation. Subsequent authors have reported widespread progressive subretinal fibrosis not preceded by CNV.[18] In 1986, Cantrill & Folk[19] described a series of 5 young patients who presented with multifocal choroiditis that progressed to subretinal fibrosis. Dreyer & Gass[2] described a similar case of subretinal fibrosis in a 19-year-old woman. Salvador and co-authors[20] reported multifocal choroiditis with progressive subretinal fibrosis in 2 young women with myopia in 1994. The majority of patients with DSF are women under the age of 45.

Clinical features

Acutely, most patients with DSF syndrome present with unilaterally decreased vision, floaters, scotomata or metamorphopsia, and occasional photopsia. Numerous small yellow lesions are seen at the level of the deep retina/retinal pigment epithelium (RPE)/choriocapillaris (Fig. 101-2). The lesions are typically clustered in the posterior pole while a few may extend out to the mid peripheral retina. Turbid fluid can accumulate around the lesions in the posterior pole and coalesce into a large yellow subneurosensory retinal detachment. Subretinal scarring can then develop quickly in the area of fluid. Associated anterior chamber reaction and/or vitreitis is usually mild. The condition is generally bilateral but initially asymmetric, with the second eye developing lesions up to 6 months after the first eye.

Histopathologic findings

Martin and co-workers[21] observed that the choriocapillaris was infiltrated by B lymphocytes and plasma cells in 2 patients with multifocal choroiditis and subretinal fibrosis. One patient had "multilaminated fibrous tissue" interposed between the RPE and Bruch's membrane. A third patient in Martin's series had a B-lymphocytic and plasmocytic infiltrate of the choroid but no

fibrosis. Gass et al.[22] examined 4 blind eyes of 3 elderly patients with DSF. In all eyes they observed extensive degeneration of the retina and RPE, fibrotic tissue interposed between the retina and Bruch's membrane posterior to the equator, lymphocytes, plasma cells, and giant cells around the fibrous tissue and along Bruch's membrane, and choroidal lymphocytic infiltration. Some eyes demonstrated focal destruction of the choriocapillaris, serosanguineous subretinal material, and vitreous hemorrhage.

Ancillary testing

Fluorescein angiography in the active phase of DSF syndrome demonstrates early hypofluorescence followed by late leakage in areas of the lesions and turbid subretinal fluid.[6,19,23] Leakage may be mild or severe, either due to the intense inflammation or perhaps an underlying CNV. Late staining is seen in zones of subretinal fibrosis.[24] Electrophysiologic testing has been performed in a few patients with variable results.[4,16,19,20]

PUNCTATE INNER CHOROIDOPATHY

Watzke and co-authors[25] initially described PIC in 1984. PIC affects young, healthy patients between the ages of 16 and 40. Over 90% of patients with PIC are women. Most affected patients are moderately myopic and typically have no history of preceding illness.[4,25–27] PIC is less common than MCP but more common than the rare DSF syndrome.

Clinical features

Patients with PIC have acute symptoms of blurred vision, central or paracentral scotomata, photopsias, and sometimes peripheral visual field loss. Although most patients have lesions in both eyes at initial presentation, often only one eye is symptomatic. Scotomata can usually be traced to one prominent lesion, a cluster of smaller lesions, or a serous detachment of

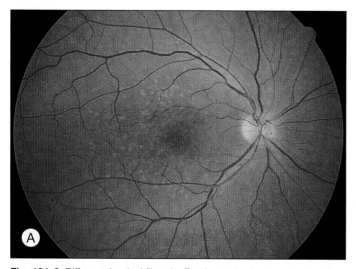 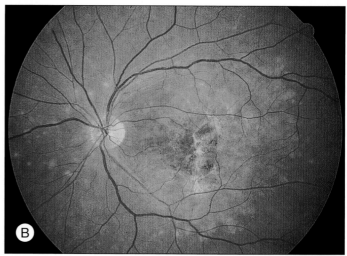

Fig. 101-2 Diffuse subretinal fibrosis. Funduscopic photographs and fluorescein angiography of a young woman with diffuse subretinal fibrosis syndrome. On initial presentation, visual acuity was 20/15 (right eye) and 20/1000 (left eye). Small, discrete white lesions at the level of the deep retina and/or RPE could be seen in the right eye (A), whereas extensive scarring and subretinal fibrosis were already present in the left eye (B).

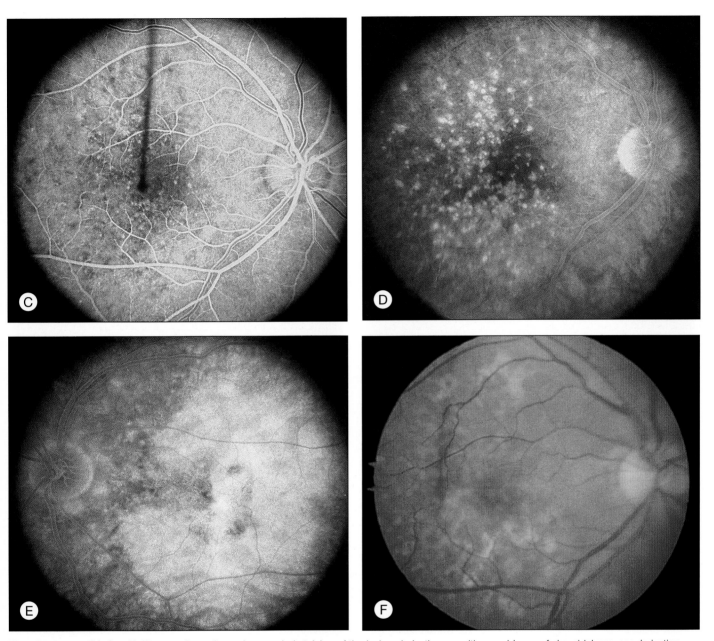

Fig. 101-2—cont'd C to E, Fluorescein angiography revealed staining of the lesions in both eyes with no evidence of choroidal neovascularization (CNV). The patient has had repeated bouts of inflammation around the scars in the right eye. These episodes have been treated with combinations of superior sub-Tenon Kenalog and oral prednisone, ciclosporin, and azathioprine (Imuran). Six years later the visual acuity remains 20/20 (right eye) and count fingers (left eye). F, Some subretinal fibrosis has developed in the right eye despite the aggressive treatment. No signs of CNV were ever seen in either eye.

the retina. Blurred central vision can result from clustering of lesions in the macula or from CNV. Initial visual acuity is usually good in both eyes but can be decreased in eyes with central lesions.

The acute lesions are yellow spots with indistinct borders that measure 100 to 300 μm in diameter. The spots are located at the level of the RPE and inner choroid. Some spots, or clusters of spots, may be associated with small amounts of overlying subretinal fluid or even a serous retinal detachment. Adjacent small lesions sometimes coalesce to form larger lesions. The number of lesions in the macula can be variable. Most of the lesions in PIC can be found in the posterior pole or near midperiphery, but typically not in the far periphery. The optic nerve is occasionally mildly hyperemic and edematous. Patients with PIC have no cells or other signs of inflammation in the vitreous or anterior chamber.

Ancillary testing

Fluorescein angiography of acute lesions usually demonstrates mild hyperfluorescence in the early phase with increasing hyperfluorescence and, sometimes, leakage in the late phases. Aside from the abnormal fluorescence seen at the sites of lesions seen clinically, no other abnormalities are evident on fluorescein angiography to suggest widespread RPE or choroidal dysfunction. Fluorescein angiography may also show CNV emanating from scars in eyes with PIC.

Tiffin et al.[28] observed ICG hypofluorescence corresponding to clinically visible subretinal lesions. Interestingly, some choroidal vessels were observed to have localized points of hyperfluorescence along vessel walls. These authors hypothesized that the hypofluorescent spots were indicative of choroidal hypoperfusion and that the localized points of choroidal vessel hyperfluorescence might be indicative of choroidal vasculitis. They observed that both types of abnormalities seen on ICG angiography improved over a 3-month period.

Visual fields

Patients can generally draw a central or paracentral scotoma on an Amsler grid. Some patients have an enlarged blind spot only, while others have large areas of temporal visual field loss corresponding to numerous nasal chorioretinal scars. Such patients often appear to have mild but diffuse RPE atrophy corresponding to the visual field defect and located between the more visible scars.

DIFFERENTIAL DIAGNOSIS

A number of diseases can manifest as multifocal inflammation in the retina and choroid. The most useful diagnostic tool is a complete history and physical exam. An exhaustive questionnaire such as that found in the Basic Clinical Science Course of the American Academy of Ophthalmology is a very helpful and efficient way of screening for significant systemic symptoms.[29] Any patient with a recent debilitating illness must be assumed to have an infection or systemic inflammatory disease until proven otherwise. A patient with a history of human immunodeficiency virus (HIV) exposure or intravenous drug use will probably have an infection. Although some patients with idiopathic white-dot syndromes may have had an antecedent viral illness, in general they are healthy. It is important to try and sort out whether the patient's history is consistent with a self-limited illness as opposed to a more ominous process. If the patient's history suggests problems in other areas, such as a rash or arthritis, arrangements should be made to have the symptomatic region evaluated as soon as possible.

The next step in assembling a differential diagnosis is the clinical exam. Although a general physical exam is outside the scope of most ophthalmic practitioners, it is easy at least to judge the patient's overall level of health based on his or her appearance. A patient who appears acutely ill needs a thorough systemic evaluation before one can comfortably diagnosis an idiopathic disease. The ophthalmic examination may also provide clues. Most of these entities do not cause severe vision loss, at least at first, unless there is a large subfoveal lesion. Also, the white-dot syndromes do not generally result in marked inflammation. An eye that is red with a lot of anterior segment inflammation and synechia and/or a significant amount of vitreous inflammation is likely to have a different diagnosis even if the fundus has scattered "white dots." The appearance of the lesions themselves is also helpful. The lesions in the diseases covered in this chapter may appear fuzzy yellow when active but they do not generally have evidence of full-thickness severe inflammation. A patient with lesions that are white and inflamed with fuzzy borders or that extend into the anterior retina is not likely to have one of the white-dot syndromes.

The laboratory evaluation will depend largely on the suspicion for systemic disease and the appearance of the fundus. A complete blood count will help rule out the presence of a hematological or infectious process or a rare leukemia. Some physicians will also use an erythrocyte sedimentation rate as a screening tool to look for evidence of unexpected systemic inflammatory activity. Other tests that are routinely done include both a treponemal and nontreponemal test for syphilis and titers for Lyme disease, even though the yield is quite low without a supportive history. The small risk of missing a potentially treatable infectious etiology provides the impetus for most physicians to continue to order these tests, although often more time is then spent evaluating false positives than in identifying true disease.

Another test that is often done is a skin test for tuberculosis, although it is unlikely that a patient would present with multifocal choroiditis due to tuberculosis without any suggestive symptoms. This information is certainly useful, however, if oral corticosteroids or systemic immunosuppression is being considered.

A number of other infectious diseases may be considered, depending on the clinical situation. Multifocal inflammation has been reported with cytomegalovirus, herpes simplex virus, herpes zoster virus, and others. Testing may include titers for these viruses and other entities such as *Bartonella henselae* or *Toxoplasmosa gondii*, depending on the clinical situation. Because people in the general population may have positive titers, one should decide in advance if the clinical suspicion warrants the use of these tests and they should not be used routinely in all patients in whom a white-dot syndrome is being considered. Rarely, blood cultures may be necessary to diagnose a septic choroiditis patient who is usually ill.

Tests for sarcoidosis are extremely important because this disease will often manifest as a multifocal choroiditis. Lardenoye et al.[30] reported lesions characteristic of MCP located primarily in the peripheral retina. Twenty-five percent of patients in this series were diagnosed with sarcoidosis, and another 29% had elevated angiotensin-converting enzyme levels. Hershey et al.[31] also found an association of numerous small lesions in the far peripheral retina and sarcoidosis, especially in elderly white women (Fig. 101-3). Screening tests include an angiotensin-converting enzyme test and a chest X-ray. If the suspicion is high one can also consider a gallium scan, chest computed tomography, or biopsy of involved areas such as the

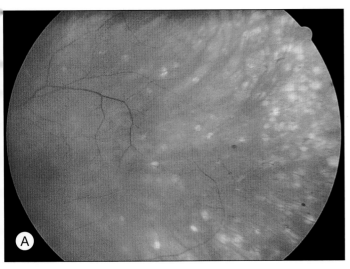
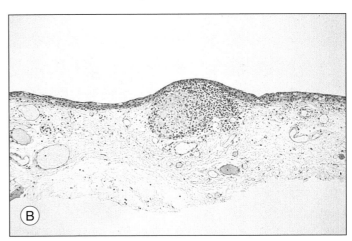

Fig. 101-3 Sarcoidosis presenting as multifocal choroiditis. A, Small, punched-out chorioretinal lesions can be seen in the peripheral retina. B, Conjunctival biopsy reveals a sarcoid granuloma.

conjunctiva.[31] In fact, there may be many cases of MCP that are really localized ocular sarcoid but are never diagnosed because of a paucity of systemic manifestations. In patients with chronic inflammation it is worthwhile periodically retesting for this disease.

Other conditions, both systemic and ocular, may be associated with findings similar to those seen in MCP. Box 101-1 lists entities that have been reported to cause or mimic multifocal inflammation in the retina and choroid. This list is not so much a specific differential diagnosis of the diseases discussed in this chapter but rather an overview of the possibilities that one should consider in a patient who seems to have scattered patches of inflammation in the fundus. Usually the clinical appearance and history are sufficient to allow differentiation. However, patients may present ambiguously and this list should be reviewed in suspicious cases to help rule out a more ominous systemic process.

An important "test" that should always be used is simply the clinical course of the patient over time. Any patient in whom the clinical picture becomes atypical or does not respond to treatment should be reassessed for the existence of a different problem. Most of the infectious etiologies will rapidly worsen without appropriate treatment. Intraocular lymphoma on the other hand may partially respond to treatment then recur. Appropriate studies, including neuroimaging, lumbar puncture, and vitreous biopsy should be considered in such patients (Fig. 101-4).

If a vitreous biopsy is being considered, it is important to take advantage of all available laboratory tests. This would include cytology to look for evidence of lymphoma and, if possible, flow cytometry to determine white blood cell populations. Cultures should be performed if an infectious etiology is suspected. The polymerase chain reaction has proven quite useful in identifying infectious agents that cannot be cultured.

Box 101-1 Diseases that may simulate multifocal choroiditis

Infectious
Viral
    Herpes simplex, herpes zoster, Epstein–Barr virus, cytomegalovirus, coxsackie virus

Bacterial
    Early metastatic endophthalmitis, septic choroiditis, syphilis, tuberculosis

Fungal
    Histoplasmosis, *Cryptococcus*, coccidioidomycosis, *Candida*

Protozoal
    Punctate outer retinal toxoplasmosis, *Pneumocystis carinii*

Helminthic
    Diffuse unilateral subacute neuroretinitis

Insect
    Ophthalmia nodosa, ophthalmomyiasis

Autoimmune
Systemic
    Familial juvenile systemic granulomatosis, tubulointerstitial nephritis and uveitis, inflammatory bowel disease, Reiter's syndrome, sarcoidosis, any disease that can cause multifocal choroidal vasculitis

Ocular
    Retinal pigment epitheliitis, multiple evanescent white-dot syndrome, acute posterior multifocal placoid pigment epitheliopathy, serpiginous choroiditis, birdshot chorioretinitis, presumed ocular histoplasmosis syndrome, sympathetic ophthalmia, Vogt–Koyanagi–Harada disease, relentless placoid chorioretinitis, acute multifocal inner retinitis

Masquerade
    Intraocular lymphoma, trauma, myopia, retinal dystrophies, multiple cottonwool spots from any cause, following retinal detachment surgery, scleral choroidal calcification

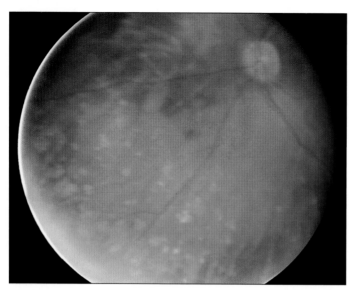

Fig 101-4 Fundus photograph of a 74-year-old woman who presented with ocular symptoms for the first time. Numerous round lesions are seen deep to the retina in the nasal midperiphery mimicking multifocal choroiditis. This patient had a vitrectomy, which showed intraocular lymphoma. Clues to correct diagnosis were advanced age when disease first manifested and yellow mound appearance to some of the spots.

Many times the performance of this test requires a specialized lab and preoperative consultation with someone experienced with this technique is important. Also, the technology is so sensitive that it may result in a false positive.[32] A related approach is to determine antibody levels to specific organisms in the eye and then compare this to serum titers in order to identify a localized response.[33]

Once a more ominous systemic process has been ruled out, the clinician should try to determine which of the reported white-dot syndromes the patient most closely resembles. It does at least help to attempt a specific diagnosis because it allows more precise prognostication and follow-up. A detailed discussion of the other eye white-dot syndromes is presented in the appropriate chapters. Specific points that allow differentiation of the entities covered in this chapter are discussed here.

The scars of MCP are similar to those of POHS. Unlike POHS, however, MCP is associated with anterior uveitis or vitreitis, a subnormal ERG in 50% of affected patients, and a female preponderance. Most patients with MCP are not from areas endemic for histoplasmosis and have negative skin tests for this organism. Enlarged blind spots are rare in histoplasmosis. Finally, unlike POHS, MCP patients are often seen with multiple acutely inflamed lesions that are causing symptoms and then evolve into scars while under observation. Parnell et al.[34] discuss a number of potential distinguishing features that are seen more frequently in MCP, such as RPE changes between scars, clustering of lesions, and subtle subretinal fibrosis.

MCP differs from birdshot retinochoroidopathy in that the lesions in MCP are generally punched-out scars with variable pigmentation rather than the larger, creamy yellow lesions without pigmentation that are seen in birdshot. MCP also typically occurs in younger patients, has a lower incidence of optic disc pallor, nyctalopia, and color vision deficits, and has a higher incidence of panuveitis and CNV than birdshot retinochoroidopathy. Birdshot retinochoroidopathy also has a high association with the human leukocyte antigen (HLA)-A29 phenotype.[35]

Unilateral MCP may sometimes be difficult to distinguish from early diffuse unilateral subacute neuroretinitis (DUSN), but the latter usually has more diffuse RPE atrophy and pigmentary changes, optic disc pallor, and retinal vascular narrowing. Multiple evanescent white-dot syndrome (MEWDS), like MCP, usually affects young women and may be associated with an enlarged blind spot. Unlike MCP, however, MEWDS lesions are typically located in the outer retina, not choroid, are transient, seldom cause significant permanent scarring, and do not usually recur. The macula in MEWDS patients typically exhibits an orange, granular appearance not seen in MCP. Finally CNV, common in MCP, rarely occurs in MEWDS.[36]

Ophthalmoscopic findings in PIC most closely resemble those seen in POHS, and neither is associated with anterior chamber or vitreous cells. However, PIC differs from POHS in several respects. PIC occurs primarily in young females with myopia, whereas POHS has no gender predilection. Patients with PIC often have acute symptoms of flickering lights or scotomata that correspond to acute, yellow lesions that then evolve into pigmented scars. Patients with POHS only develop symptoms due to CNV, and their scars do not change much with time. The majority of patients with PIC who have been tested have had negative serologies and skin tests for histoplasmosis.

Diagnosing DSF early is important because of the potential for rapid and severe vision loss. It usually presents with numerous clustered yellow lesions in the posterior pole often associated with subretinal fluid that may be turbid. The yellowish lesions may resemble MCP, acute posterior multifocal placoid pigment epitheliopathy (APMPPE), MEWDS, PIC, sarcoidosis, punctate outer retinal toxoplasmosis, POHS, syphilis, and tuberculosis. In the late stages, with widespread subretinal fibrosis and hemorrhage, the syndrome can mimic severe exudative age-related macular degeneration (AMD). Although patients with POHS, MCP, and PIC can develop subretinal fibrosis associated with CNV, the fibrosis is usually not as widespread as in the DSF syndrome. APMPPE, MEWDS, and acute macular neuroretinopathy (AMN) are self-limited conditions, do not develop subretinal fibrosis, and typically have a good visual prognosis. Patients with sarcoidosis usually have other systemic manifestations of the disease, which aids in this diagnosis. The medical history, serologic and skin testing, and chest X-ray can be used to differentiate toxoplasmosis, syphilis, and tuberculosis from DSF. Finally, patients with AMD often have a long history of visual loss, drusen, and CNV with hemorrhage before the subretinal fibrosis. DSF patients typically are younger than 45 years, whereas AMD patients typically are older than 55. Be especially concerned about the young patient who has already lost vision and has subretinal fibrosis in the first eye.

TREATMENT OVERVIEW

Once the diagnosis has been made the actual treatment becomes remarkably nonspecific. The only option is usually to suppress the immune system and deal with any secondary complications of the diseases such as CNV. First of all, there are no controlled trials that clearly define how aggressive to be with these patients. It is usually necessary to respond reactively and treat the patient as disease flare-ups occur. Each patient must be assessed individually. The clinical course determines the appropriate treatment. A patient with mild symptoms and no vision-threatening lesions may best be treated with observation. Patients with PIC tend to fall into this category. On the other hand, a patient with aggressive, recurrent disease may require long-term local or systemic immunosuppression. This is especially true with DSF where irreversible damage may occur if the inflammation is allowed to persist to the point of causing extensive fibrosis.

It is also important to be extremely flexible about the clinical variables used to determine the level of treatment. Simply looking for vitreous cell and measuring the central acuity may not allow a complete sense of disease activity. Often the scars do not change much even with flare-ups. The patient's history is the best place to start. Many of these patients become acute observers of their disease and will report subjective signs of activity such as peripheral photopsia or visual field changes, which may be very useful in determining further testing and treatment. Patients with long-standing disease can often become actively involved in the titration of their medication based on their symptoms.

More sophisticated testing of visual function is often mandatory. At the very least these patients should have periodic visual field testing. The visual field test may also help identify occult disease activity at times when patients may have symptoms without significant clinical evidence of active inflammation. It is even possible for some patients, especially with MCP, to develop irreversible peripheral field loss for which they may not be initially symptomatic. As a result, visual field testing should be considered even in the absence of clinically apparent inflammation. Other modalities such as a wide-field ERG or multifocal ERG may be useful to help determine the progression of disease. Fluorescein angiography, ICG angiography, and optical coherence tomography may also help identify subtle disease activity that can then be used to determine the need for treatment.

SPECIFIC TREATMENT AND PROGNOSIS

Clinical course of Multifocal Choroiditis with Panuveitis (MCP)

Most patients with MCP tend to have a few episodes of either mild central or peripheral visual loss that resolve either spontaneously or with subtenons Kenalog. Some of these patients may have chronic photopsia but retain excellent and stable vision. Most of these patients are not referred to large centers and are therefore not reported in the literature.

Perhaps about 25% of patients with MCP have a more chronic disorder with recurrent bouts of inflammation that occur in one

eye or both eyes, separately or simultaneously. The recurrent inflammation usually manifests as central or peripheral vision loss, vitreous cells, swelling around old scars, CME, or CNV. Occasionally new lesions appear that are not necessarily contiguous with old scars. The recurrent disease in these patients can usually be treated with repeated subtenons Kenalog or short courses of oral corticosteroids. Patients who remain with mild disease after 1 year of follow-up seldom degenerate into more severe disease thereafter.

Patients with more frequent recurrences may be treated with frequent depot steroids along with a low daily dose of prednisone. These patients should have periodic visual fields and maybe even ERG testing in addition to routine examinations to make sure they are not slowly losing visual ground. Dreyer & Gass[2] treated 18 of 28 patients with either oral or periocular steroids. Six patients had an improvement in vision; 2 patients had a halt in the rapid progression of visual loss; and 9 had no change in vision. In Morgan & Schatz's series of patients, visual improvement was noted in all 9 patients treated with steroids.[4] Brown et al.[24] observed an improvement in visual acuity and/or vitreitis in 57% of the 28 eyes they treated with oral prednisone or sub-Tenon's steroid injection. Nevertheless, 11 of the 28 eyes they treated with steroids had a final visual acuity of 20/200 or worse.

The patients reported from large referral centers have had more severe disease. For instance, Nussenblatt & Palestine[37] have found that the use of steroids was less helpful in their patients and that some patients require immunosuppressives to control their disease. Michel et al.[38] found that immunosuppressives were necessary to control disease in their 19 patients with MCP. These severe patients probably make up about 5 to 10% of all patients with MCP. They have chronic relapsing disease that requires a steroid-sparing agent or perhaps intraocular steroids.

CNV is the most common cause of visual loss in MCP and PIC and may or may not be related to acute exacerbations of inflammation. Flaxel et al.[39] found that oral corticosteroids could reduce leakage and stabilize vision. Unfortunately the CNV often recurs later. Thermal laser photocoagulation may be helpful for CNV not involving the fovea, but the recurrence rate is higher than in patients with PIC or POHS.[40] Surgical removal of subfoveal CNV in a number of uveitic conditions including MCP has been reported.[41,42] Thomas et al.[42] and Brindeau et al.[43] included 9 and 10 eyes with MCP respectively in their series of patients who underwent surgical removal of subfoveal CNV. Both groups had moderately good results. Their patients, who were followed for an average of 10 months postoperatively, had a mean improvement in visual acuity of 1.3 lines. Spaide et al.[44] reported moderate results using photodynamic therapy (PDT) in MCP patients with CNV. PDT coupled with subtenons or intraocular Kenalog seems especially promising in these patients, especially if the CNV is small (Fig.101-5).

The long-term visual prognosis in MCP is variable. The largest single series of patients with MCP followed for several years is that of Brown et al.,[24] who reported the visual findings in

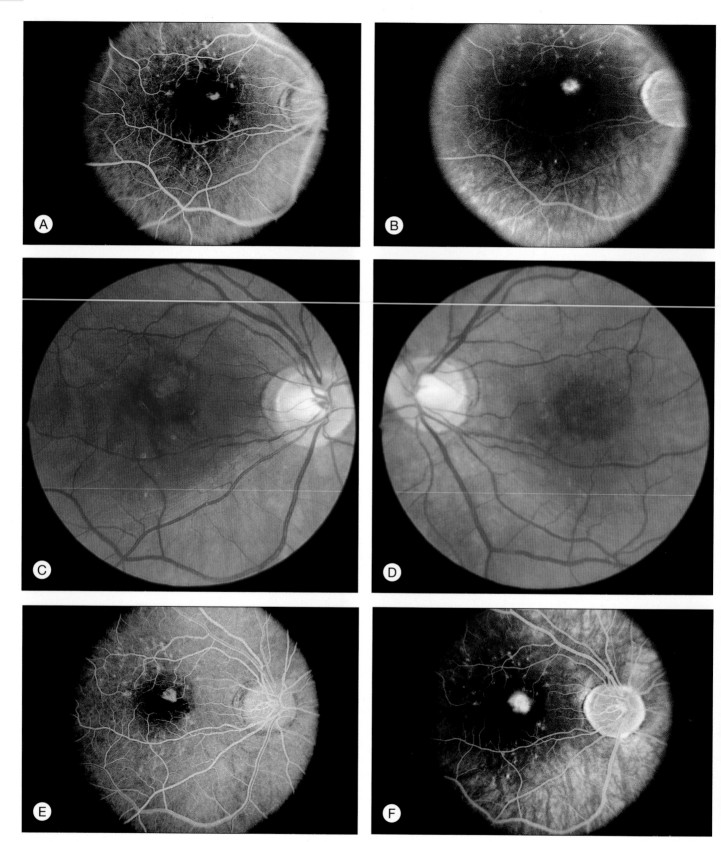

Fig. 101-5 Punctate inner choroidopathy with choroidal neovascularization (CNV) treated with subtenons Kenalog and Visudyne. A 31-year-old woman with high myopia developed scotomata and then inferior distortion temporal to fixation in right eye. Visual acuity was 20/25 in both eyes. A, B, Fluorescein angiogram shows punctate scars in the macula with late leakage supernasal to the fovea. The patient was given 40 mg of Kenalog in the superior subtenons. Two weeks later symptoms had worsened and visual acuity was 20/70 in the right eye. Color photos show pigmented CNV in the right eye (C) and punctate scars in the left eye (D). E, F, Fluorescein angiogram shows classic juxtafoveal CNV in the right eye. Visudyne treatment was given to the right eye. Three months later visual acuity was 20/20 in both eyes.

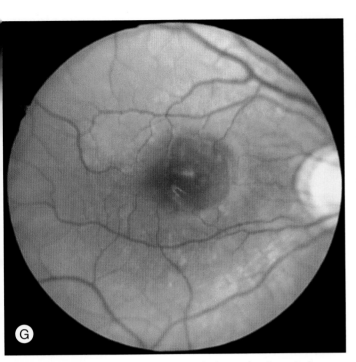

Fig. 101-5—cont'd G, Fundus photograph shows dry pigmented scar in the right eye.

41 patients (68 eyes) with MCP followed for a mean of 39 months. They found that 66% of 68 eyes had a visual acuity of 20/40 or better and that 39 of 41 patients (95%) had a visual acuity of 20/40 or better in at least one eye. Nine eyes (13%) had a visual acuity between 20/50 and 20/200. Fourteen eyes (21%) in 12 of the patients in Brown's series had a final visual acuity of 20/200 or worse, which could be attributed to subfoveal CNV (9 eyes), CME (3 eyes), foveal RPE atrophy (1 eye), and neovascular glaucoma secondary to refractory uveitis (1 eye). In other series, visual loss has been attributed to similar processes, with CNV being the most common cause of decreased vision.[2,4,25]

Clinical course

Over a few weeks the initially pale yellow spots evolve into deep, cylindrical, punched-out scars with loss of tissue in the inner choroid, RPE, and outer retina. Most lesions become more pigmented with time. As the lesions enlarge and become pigmented, it may appear that new lesions have developed. However, careful examination of serial photographs reveals that the larger scars can be traced back to smaller, fainter yellow lesions. New lesions can rarely develop but do so within 3 months of the onset of symptoms. The evolution from an acute inflammatory lesion to a scar may occur over 6 months or longer. Subretinal fibrosis is rarely seen in the absence of CNV.

Some patients have recurrent episodes of blurred central vision and photopsia months or years after the onset of disease. Typically, examination of these patients has not revealed any new chorioretinal lesions or signs of vitreous inflammation, and they do well without treatment.

Treatment

CNV is essentially the sole cause of vision loss in patients with PIC. It usually develops within the first 6 months of the onset of symptoms but can occur years later. Approximately 25% of eyes with PIC develop CNV. Most of the CNV in PIC is extrafoveal and responds well to laser photocoagulation. Subfoveal CNV seems to respond well to PDT coupled with subtenons or intraocular Kenalog (Fig. 101-5).

Prognosis

The visual prognosis of eyes with PIC that do not develop subfoveal CNV is good. About 75% of eyes retain vision of 20/25 or better. Eyes with foveal lesions or with central RPE atrophy due to adjacent lesions may have moderate visual loss in the 20/30 to 20/80 range. Eyes with subfoveal CNV often have a final visual acuity of 20/80 to 20/200 but this prognosis may be improving with PDT and steroid treatment.

Clinical course of Diffuse Subretinal Fibrosis (DSF)

Within a few days to weeks, swelling occurs around the numerous lesions in the posterior pole and turbid subretinal fluid accumulates in areas where the lesions are most numerous. Subsequently, over several months subretinal fibrosis develops around the lesions (Fig. 101-2). With time the focal areas of subretinal fibrosis coalesce to form diffuse sheets of fibrotic tissue underlying the retina. Fibrosis may occur around mid peripheral lesions and may worsen with recurrent episodes of inflammation. Choroidal neovascular membranes and subretinal hemorrhages have been observed in some cases. Optic disc edema has been reported.[20] The fibrotic stage of this condition is generally associated with profound visual loss, sometimes to the no-light-perception level.[22] Brown et al.[24] found that 7 of 10 eyes in 5 patients with DSF syndrome had visual acuity of 20/200 or worse after 2 years or more. In Brown's series, only 2 of 10 eyes retained a visual acuity of 20/40 or better.

Once extensive subretinal fibrosis develops in the posterior pole, vision is usually poor and treatment is of little or no benefit. Treatment therefore is dependent on early diagnosis and aggressive steroid and immunosuppressive treatment. Often the diagnosis of DSF syndrome is made when it manifests in the patient's second eye. In these cases high-dose oral corticosteroids or even intraocular Kenalog is warranted. Only a few patients have responded to either oral or periocular steroids alone during follow-up.[16,19] Therefore patients should also be evaluated and started on an immunosuppressive such as ciclosporin or azathioprine. Brown et al.[24] have followed 2 patients who have retained 20/40 vision or better in at least one eye on a regimen of prednisone, ciclosporin, and, in one case, azathioprine. An attempt to taper the immunosuppressives after 6 or 12 months can be tried but many patients need chronic therapy.

ETIOLOGY

The cause(s) of MCP, DSF syndrome, and PIC remain unknown, and therefore controversy persists regarding whether these conditions are separate entities or different manifestations of the same disease. Those who advocate that they are the same disease point out that all three of these disorders typically affect young, otherwise healthy women. They all cause scattered yellow lesions at the level of the RPE and inner choroid. All eventually develop POHS-like punched-out chorioretinal scars with pigmentation. Choroidal neovascular membranes or subretinal fibrosis can occur in all of these diseases.[36] Patients with any of these diseases can develop enlarged blind spots or other field defects that are much larger than would be expected from the number of visible scars. These field defects can be associated with abnormalities of outer retinal function seen on ERGs. Because of these common findings, some clinicians believe that these diseases are closely related and even propose that they, along with MEWDS, AMN, and idiopathic blind-spot enlargement be grouped under the term *acute zonal occult outer retinopathy (AZOOR)*.[45]

Others believe that these conditions are separate diseases because their differences outweigh their similarities. Patients with PIC develop all of the lesions at once or over a very short time, whereas patients with MCP and DSF syndrome have multiple bouts of recurrent inflammation and scarring. PIC is not associated with anterior chamber or vitreous cells, whereas vitreous inflammation and associated CME are prominent manifestations of both MCP and the DSF syndrome. Although subretinal fibrosis has been observed in both MCP and PIC, it is minimal compared to the DSF syndrome. Finally, it is difficult to believe that one etiology and disease can result in such a wide variety of fundus lesions and outcomes. Perhaps the similarities among the diseases are a consequence of the eye being able to respond to different insults in only a limited number of ways. Investigators have so far not been able to find any HLA antigen association with these diseases, which suggests they may be heterogeneous.[46] Also, field defects and outer retinal dysfunction may be common to a number of different uveitic diseases. The more important question is: why do some patients have very limited disease and are stable on follow-up, whereas others have numerous relapses and ultimately lose vision?

The clinical course of these disorders suggests an initial insult that may sensitize susceptible individuals to antigens within the photoreceptors, RPE, or choroid. Several different inciting agents have been hypothesized. Tiedeman[47] suggested a viral etiology for MCP when he found serologic evidence of active Epstein–Barr virus (EBV) infection in 10 patients with MCP but not in 8 control patients. A subsequent study by Spaide et al.[48] did not support this hypothesis. Moreover, patients with MCP do not have systemic signs of chronic EBV infection. In a series of 7 patients with MCP reported by Frau et al.,[49] analysis of serum and aqueous aspirates for herpes viruses supported recent infection with herpes zoster in 2 of 7 patients and herpes simplex in 2 of 7 patients. Rudich et al.[50] reported a patient whose disease was triggered by environmental mold exposure. Mutations in the nucleotide-binding region of NOD 2 have been found to be responsible for familial juvenile systemic granulomatosis whose eye findings are indistinguishable from MCP.[51, 52]

In the near future the blood, intraocular fluids, and ocular tissue specimens of patients with acute disease should be analyzed for antibody or cellular-mediated inflammation or DNA evidence of an infectious agent. EBV has been implicated, but proving this virus to be a cause of these diseases is difficult because it is so ubiquitous in humans. HLA testing of patients may provide information as far as which patients are susceptible to these diseases in general or which ones are prone to severe recurrent inflammation. New clues as to the pathogenesis include the presence of hypofluorescent lesions on ICG angiography, large field defects, and abnormal full-field or multifocal ERGs. Longer prospective studies are needed to determine how these findings are related and if they change over follow-up or with anti-inflammatory treatment. In addition, patients with other types of uveitis should undergo ICG angiography, perimetry, and electroretinography to determine if the abnormalities seen in the white-dot syndromes are present in other types of uveitis.

SUMMARY

1. Most patients with MCP have a benign course with minimal visual loss, although some of these patients will have chronic photopsia.

2. About 25% of patients with MCP will have recurrent disease. In almost all of these patients the recurrent disease will manifest within the first year of presentation. Most of these patients can be managed with subtenons Kenalog along with low-dose oral prednisone. About 5% of all patients with MCP will need an immunosuppressive agent.

3. Elderly white women with numerous small yellow lesions in the inferior retinal periphery resembling the lesions in MCP often have noncaseating granulomas on conjunctival biopsy or other evidence of sarcoidosis.

4. Patients with the DSF syndrome need immediate high-dose oral corticosteroid treatment or intraocular Kenalog. They should also be started on an immunosuppressive such as ciclosporin or azathioprine. These patients have numerous, small, indistinct, yellow lesions in the posterior pole that quickly coalesce into an area of yellow subretinal fluid. Severe subretinal fibrosis and visual loss follow quickly. Even prompt treatment is often ineffective, and the majority of these patients become legally blind.

5. Patients with PIC usually develop spots all at one time. They have no signs of vitreous or aqueous inflammation. Their visual prognosis is good, and no treatment is needed unless they develop CNV threatening central vision. CNV develops in about 25% of patients with PIC. Laser photocoagulation is effective for extrafoveal or juxtafoveal CNV, with a low recurrence rate.

6. PDT treatment with subtenons or intraocular Kenalog appears to improve vision in patients with PIC or MCP and subfoveal CNV. The CNV responds best when it is small and thin, so patients should be treated as soon as possible.

REFERENCES

1. Nozik RA, Dorsch W. A new chorioretinopathy associated with anterior uveitis. Am J Ophthalmol 1973; 76:758–762.

2. Dreyer RF, Gass JDM. Multifocal choroiditis and panuveitis: a syndrome that mimics ocular histoplasmosis. Arch Ophthalmol 1984; 102:1776–1784.

3. Deutsch TA, Tessler HH. Inflammatory pseudohistoplasmosis. Ann Ophthalmol 1985; 17:461–465.

4. Morgan CM, Schatz H. Recurrent multifocal choroiditis. Ophthalmology 1986; 93:1138–1147.

5. Wiechens B, Nolle B. Iris angiographic changes in multifocal chorioretinitis with panuveitis. Graefes Arch Clin Exp Ophthalmol 1999; 237:902–907.

6. Reddy CV, Brown J Jr, Folk JC et al. Enlarged blind spots in chorioretinal inflammatory disorders. Ophthalmology 1996; 101:606–617.

7. Spaide RF, Yannuzzi LA, Freund KB. Linear streaks in multifocal choroiditis and panuveitis. Retina 1991; 11:229–231.

8. Slakter JS, Giovannini A, Yannuzzi LA et al. Indocyanine green angiography of multifocal choroiditis. Ophthalmology 1997; 104:1813–1819.

9. Bouchenaki N, Cimino L, Auer C et al. Assessment and classification of choroidal vasculitis in posterior uveitis using indocyanine green angiography. Klin Monatsbl Augenheilkd 2002; 219:243–249.

10. Vadala M, Lodata G, Cillino S. Multifocal choroiditis: indocyanine green angiographic features. Ophthalmologica 2001; 215:16–21.

11. Cimino L, Auer C, Herbort CP. Sensitivity of indocyanine green angiography for the follow-up of active inflammatory choriocapillaropathies. Ocular Immuno Inflamm 2000; 8:275–283.

12. Oh KT, Folk JC, Maturi RK et al. Multifocal electroretinography in multifocal choroiditis and the multiple evanescent white dot syndrome. Retina 2001; 21:581–589.

13. Khorram KD, Jampol LM, Rosenberg MA. Blind spot enlargement as a manifestation of multifocal choroiditis. Arch Ophthalmol 1991; 109:1403–1407.

14. Singh K, de Frank MP, Shults WT et al. Acute idiopathic blind spot enlargement: a spectrum of disease. Ophthalmology 1991; 98:497–502.

15. Reddy CV, Folk JC. Multifocal choroiditis with panuveitis, diffuse subretinal fibrosis, and punctate inner choroidopathy. In: Ryan SJ, Schachat AP, Murphy RP, Patz A, eds. Retina, 2nd edn, vol. 2. Medical retina. St Louis: Mosby; 1994.

16. Palestine AG, Nussenblatt RB, Parver LM et al. Progressive subretinal fibrosis and uveitis. Br J Ophthalmol 1985; 68:667–673.

17. Doran RML, Hamilton AM. Disciform macular degeneration in young adults. Trans Ophthalmol Soc UK 1982; 102:471–480.

18. Kaiser PK, Gragoudas ES. The subretinal fibrosis and uveitis syndrome. Intern Ophthalmol Clin 1996; 36:145–152.

19. Cantrill HL, Folk JC. Multifocal choroiditis associated with progressive subretinal fibrosis. Am J Ophthalmol 1986; 101:170–180.

20. Salvador F, Garcia-Arumi J, Mateo C et al. Multifocal choroiditis with progressive subretinal fibrosis. Ophthalmologica 1994; 208:163–167.

21. Martin DF, Chan CC, de Smet MD et al. The role of chorioretinal biopsy in the management of posterior uveitis. Ophthalmology 1993; 100:705–714.

22. Gass JDM, Margo CE, Levy MH. Progressive subretinal fibrosis and blindness in patients with multifocal granulomatous chorioretinitis. Am J Ophthalmol 1996; 122:76–85.

23. Palestine AG, Nussenblatt RB, Chan CC et al. Histopathology of the subretinal fibrosis and uveitis syndrome. Ophthalmology 1984; 92:838–844.

24. Brown J Jr, Folk JC, Reddy CV et al. Visual prognosis of multifocal choroiditis, punctate inner choroidopathy, and diffuse subretinal fibrosis syndrome. Ophthalmology 1996; 103:1100–1105.

25. Watzke RC, Packer AJ, Folk JC et al. Punctate inner choroidopathy. Am J Ophthalmol 1984; 98:572–584.

26. Folk JC. Punctate inner choroidopathy. In: Ryan SJ, Schachat AP, Murphy RP et al., eds. Retina, 1st edn, vol. 2. Medical retina. St Louis: Mosby; 1989.

27. Folk JC, Pulido JS, Wolf MD. White dot chorioretinal inflammatory syndromes. In: Focal points: 1990 clinical modules for ophthalmologists, vol. 8, module 11. San Francisco: American Academy of Ophthalmology; 1990.

28. Tiffin PA, Maini R, Roxburgh ST et al. Indocyanine green angiography in a case of punctate inner choroidopathy. Br J Ophthalmol 80:90–91, 1996.

29. Basic and Clinical Science Course Section 9. Intraocular inflammation and uveitis. San Francisco, CA: American Academy of Ophthalmology; 2003: 118–121.

30. Lardenoye CW, Van der Lelij A, de Loos WS et al. Peripheral multifocal choroiditis: a distinct clinical entity. Ophthalmology 1997; 104:1820–1826.

31. Hershey JM, Pulido JS, Folberg R et al. Non-caseating conjunctival granulomas in patients with multifocal choroiditis and panuveitis. Ophthalmology 1994; 101:596–601.

32. Van Gelder RN. Koch's postulates and the polymerase chain reaction. Ocul Immuno Inflamm 2002; 10:235–238.

33. Bodaghi B, Rozenberg F, Cassoux N et al. Nonnecrotizing herpetic retinopathies masquerading as severe posterior uveitis. Ophthalmology 2003; 110:1737–1143.

34. Parnell JR, Jampol LM, Yannuzzi LA et al. Differentiation between presumed ocular histoplasmosis syndrome and multifocal choroiditis with panuveitis based on morphology of photographed fundus lesions and fluorescein angiography. Arch Ophthalmol 2001; 119:208–212.

35. Nussenblatt RB, Mittal KK, Ryan S et al. Birdshot retinochoroidopathy associated with HLA-A29 antigen and immune responsiveness to retinal S-antigen. Am J Ophthalmol 1982; 94:147–158.

36. Callanan D, Gass JDM. Multifocal choroiditis and choroidal neovascularization associated with the multiple evanescent white dot and acute idiopathic blind spot enlargement syndrome. Ophthalmology 1992; 99:1678–1675.

37. Nussenblatt RB, Palestine AG. White dot syndromes. In: Uveitis: fundamentals and clinical practice. Chicago, IL: Mosby; 1989.

38. Michel SS, Ekong A, Baltatzis S et al. Multifocal choroiditis and panuveitis: immunomodulatory therapy. Ophthalmology 2002; 109:378–383.

39. Flaxel CJ, Owens SL, Mulholland B et al. The use of corticosteroids for choroidal neovascularization in young patients. Eye 1998; 12:266–272.

40. Wolf MD, Folk JC. Choroidal neovascularization in inflammatory diseases of the choroid and retina. Invest Ophthalmol Vis Sci 1991; 32:689.

41. Olsen TW, Capone A Jr, Sternberg P Jr et al. Subfoveal choroidal neovascularization in punctate inner choroidopathy: surgical management and pathologic findings. Ophthalmology 1996; 103:2061–2069.

42. Thomas MA, Dickinson JD, Melberg NS et al. Visual results after surgical removal of subfoveal choroidal neovascular membranes. Ophthalmology 1994; 101:1384–1396.

43. Brindeau C, Glacet-Bernard A, Coscas F et al. Surgical removal of subfoveal choroidal neovascularization: visual outcome and prognostic value of fluorescein angiography and optical coherence tomography. Eur J Ophthalmol 2001; 11:287–295.

44. Spaide RF, Freund KB, Slakter J et al. Treatment of subfoveal choroidal neovascularization associated with multifocal choroiditis and panuveitis with photodynamic therapy. Retina 2002; 22:545–549.

45. Jacobson SG, Morales DS, Sun XK et al. Pattern of retinal dysfunction in acute zonal occult outer retinopathy. Ophthalmology 1995; 102:1187–1198.

46. Spaide RF, Skerry JE, Yannuzzi LA et al. Lack of HLA-DR2 specificity in multifocal choroiditis and panuveitis. Br J Ophthalmol 1990; 74:536–537.

47. Tiedeman JS. Epstein–Barr viral antibodies in multifocal choroiditis and panuveitis. Am J Ophthalmol 1987; 103:658–663.

48. Spaide RF, Sugin S, Yannuzzi LA et al. Epstein–Barr virus antibodies in multifocal choroiditis and panuveitis. Am J Ophthalmol 1991; 112:410–413.

49. Frau E, Dussaix E, Offret H et al. The possible role of herpes simplex virus in multifocal choroiditis and panuveitis. Int Ophthalmol 1990; 14:365–369.

50. Rudich R, Santilli J, Rockwell WJ. Indoor mold spore exposure: a possible factor in the etiology of multifocal choroiditis. Am J Ophthalmol 2003; 135:402–404.

51. Latkany PA, Jabs DA, Smith JR et al. Multifocal choroiditis in patients with familial juvenile systemic granulomatosis. Am J Ophthalmol 2002; 134:897–904.

52. Rosenbaum JT, Planck SR, Davey MP et al. With a mere nod, uveitis enters a new era. Am J Ophthalmol 2003; 136:729–732.

Chapter

102

Multiple Evanescent White-Dot Syndrome

Linda M. Tsai
Lee M. Jampol

Multiple evanescent white dot syndrome (MEWDS), originally described in 1984,[1] is an acute, multifocal, usually unilateral retinopathy affecting young adults. Multiple white dots are seen at the level of the deep retina or retinal pigment epithelium (RPE) (Figs 102-1 to 102-3). The white dots are mostly concentrated in the paramacular area, usually sparing the fovea itself, and are less prominent and numerous beyond the major vascular arcades.[1] Vitreal cells, retinal venous sheathing, and blurring of the disc margins (Fig. 102-4) are often seen. The macula usually shows granular orange or yellow dots, distinct from the larger white dots (Figs 102-3 to 102-6). Often patients complain of blurred vision, photopsias, and sometimes a temporal scotoma. Visual field testing often shows an enlarged blind spot. The white spots disappear completely after a number of weeks or months. They may be replaced by mild pigment mottling, or sometimes, scattered chorioretinal scarring resembling multifocal choroiditis.

CLINICAL FEATURES

In the initial 69 cases reported worldwide, no particular racial or regional predisposition for MEWDS was reported, with 43 cases from the USA, 18 cases from Europe, 6 cases from Japan (4 cases reported under the name *acute disseminated retinal pigment epitheliopathy*), and 2 cases from China. There was a strong female predominance (75%). Thirty-seven (54%) of the patients had right-eye involvement at some time, whereas 46 (66%) had left-eye involvement. Initial visual acuity ranged from 20/20 to 20/300 and, after an average duration of approximately 6 weeks, almost always returned to normal levels. Those affected were young, ranging from 14 to 57 years of age (average age, 26.8 years). Subsequent cases of MEWDS have been reported in children as young as 10 years old and in patients as old as 67 years old.[2,3] Most patients, however, cluster near the mean age of 26.8 years.

ANCILLARY TESTING

Angiography

Fluorescein angiographic findings (Figs 102-5B and 102-6) include early and late hyperfluorescence of the white dots; diffuse, but patchy, late staining at the level of the retinal

pigment epithelium (RPE) and retina; and disc capillary leakage. After resolution of the acute lesions, window defects may be noted in the macula and, less often, elsewhere.

Indocyanine green (ICG) angiography in patients with MEWDS shows no abnormalities of large choroidal vessels in the early phase, but hypofluorescent lesions are evident in the late phase, corresponding to the white dots[4] (Fig. 102-7). This suggests but does not prove that MEWDS may affect the choriocapillaris, as well as its well-known effect on the RPE and photoreceptors.[5,6] These lesions gradually disappear upon recovery,[6,7] but abnormalities on ICG have been reported to be present up to 9 months after the initial presentation, even after clinical symptoms have resolved.[8] Since ICG angiography definitely reveals lesions not seen clinically or by fluorescein angiography,[9] it has been recommended with some enthusiasm in the patients with MEWDS, mainly to help establish a diagnosis and provide some useful guidance for therapy.[10] This is due to the fact that signs are seen longer with ICG testing than in the clinical or fluoroscein exam.[11] It has been suggested that the blind-spot enlargement of MEWDS corresponds to multiple peripapillary lesions, sometimes only detected with ICG

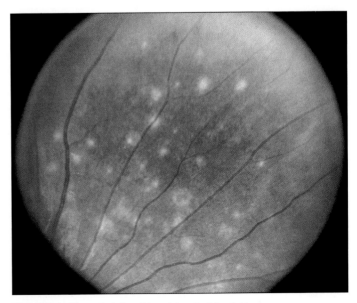

Fig. 102-1 Characteristic mid peripheral white dots.

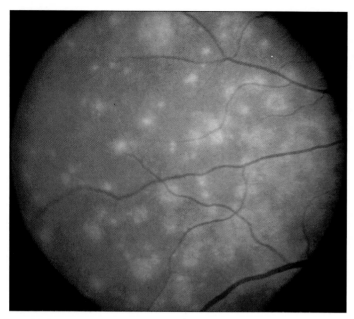

Fig. 102-2 Multiple confluent white dots at the level of the retinal pigment epithelium (RPE)–photoreceptor complex.

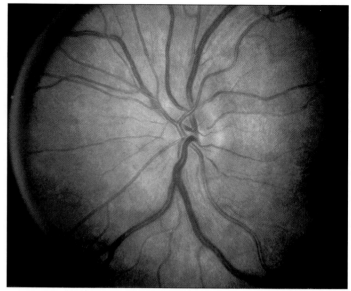

Fig. 102-4 Mild disc blurring is present.

angiography. In rare cases of MEWDS, a progressive geographic circumpapillary discoloration, appearing as a giant white spot, can be a presenting sign[12] and peripapillary scarring may occasionally be seen after the acute lesions have healed.[13]

Electrophysiologic testing

Electrophysiologic studies in patients with acute MEWDS[14] have found that the electroretinogram (ERG) shows reduced a-waves and reduced early receptor potential (ERP) amplitudes that would suggest a primary involvement of the outer segments of photoreceptors. Focal ERG studies reveal delayed recovery of oscillatory potential (OP), which implies some inner retinal

involvement.[15] Recent studies[16] have used foveal densitometry and color matching to show that, even with normal ERG findings, abnormalities exist during the active stage of MEWDS at the level of the cone photoreceptor outer segments. A transient metabolic disturbance at the level of the pigment epithelium–photoreceptor complex has been suggested. Multifocal electroretinogram (MERG) shows areas of depression which correspond to scotomata while full-field ERG shows a general depression. These abnormalities typically resolve with clinical symptoms after 6 weeks.[17] In addition, MERG shows supernormal amplitudes of the first-order kernel of N1 and P1-wave amplitudes at the beginning of the disease; these values decrease to normal or subnormal values by 2 weeks and may be helpful in detecting early stages of MEWDS and for follow up.[18]

CLINICAL COURSE

MEWDS is usually a self-limited disease, and recovery of visual function occurs over several weeks with a concurrent dramatic improvement of the ERG and ERP amplitudes.[1,14] Several cases of recurrent MEWDS have been reported, but determinants predisposing toward recurrence have not yet been identified.[19] Although usually unilateral, bilateral MEWDS has been reported. Bilateral involvement can be either simultaneous or sequential (seen as recurrence of MEWDS in the opposite eye). Bilateral cases may show asymmetric involvement, with only one symptomatic eye, or simultaneous symptoms.[20] There is also a chronic form of MEWDS with evidence of multiple recurrences over many years and involving both eyes.[21]

ETIOLOGY

The cause of MEWDS is unknown. Gass has used the term AZOOR (acute zonal occult outer retinopathy) complex to encompass the following entities: MEWDS, multifocal

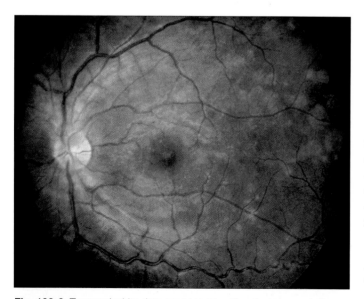

Fig. 102-3 Temporal white dots are seen as well as foveal granularity. Some retinal vascular sheathing is seen.

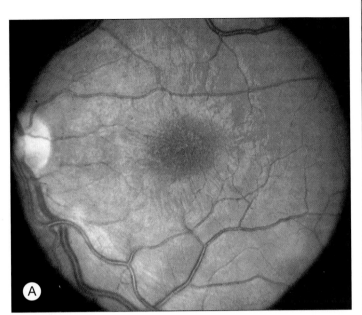

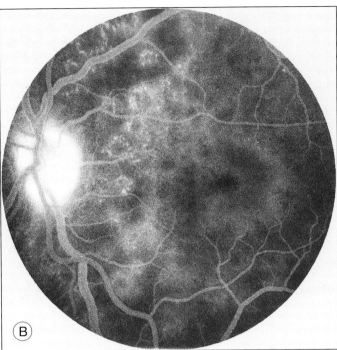

Fig. 102-5 A, Characteristic granular fovea. B, Fluorescein angiogram shows late staining of the disc and outer retina.

choroiditis, punctate inner choroidopathy (PIC), acute idiopathic blind-spot enlargement, acute macular neuroretinopathy, acute annular outer retinopathy, and AZOOR. Others have espoused similar opinions.[22,23] He suggests that these diseases represent parts of a spectrum of what is probably a single disease. Gass believes that these diseases may be of viral origin, with the virus entering the retina from the peripapillary area or at the ora serrata. He postulates that the virus gains access to the photoreceptor cells and spreads from cell to cell. He believes that the difference in clinical presentation results from genetic and immune system differences. In this case, a search for a virus or infectious agent as a trigger would be indicated.[24]

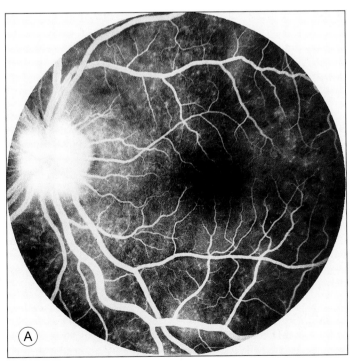

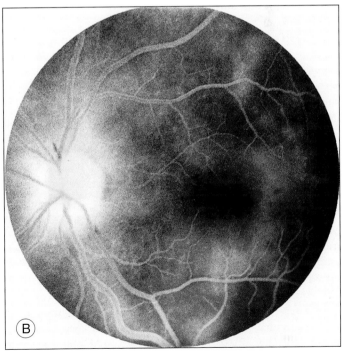

Fig. 102-6 A, Midphase angiogram shows small hyperfluorescent dots and early leakage at the level of the retinal pigment epithelium. B, Late phase shows disc leakage and extensive outer retinal leakage.

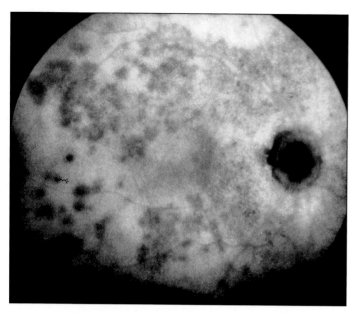

Fig. 102-7 Late-phase indocyanine green angiogram shows multiple hypofluorescent lesions, clustering in the posterior pole. (Courtesy of Michael Klein, MD.)

To date, there is no direct evidence supporting this hypothesis; no virus has been reproducibly isolated in patients with these various diseases.

At the present time, we do not have definite evidence for a viral or an immunologic cause for MEWDS. The response of a single patient with chronic relapsing MEWDS to cyclosporine therapy suggests an autoimmune component.[25] Laatikainen & Immonen[26] described an increased level of protein in the cerebrospinal fluid in MEWDS patients. The occurrence of MEWDS following varicella infection[27] and vaccination for hepatitis A[28] or hepatitis B[29] suggests environmental triggers. One case of MEWDS from China with no previous or concurrent illness exhibited increased serum immunoglobulin M (IgM) and IgG values.[30] Recovery of vision in 3 weeks was coincident with the return of the IgM value to normal values. Data from this case suggested that MEWDS might be associated with a viral syndrome, although tests for herpes zoster, herpes simplex, mumps, and measles were inconclusive. Any explanation of the etiology of MEWDS must explain the strong female predominance, the occurrence of occasional chronic relapsing cases, the occasional occurrence of MEWDS in patients with other white-spot syndromes and the excellent visual outcome in virtually every case. Kevin Becker at the National Institute on Aging in Baltimore, Maryland, has presented evidence supporting a hypothesis of the origin of many systemic inflammatory diseases of unknown etiology; this hypothesis seems to fit the white-spot syndromes, including MEWDS.[31] This theory states that these inflammatory/autoimmune diseases are discrete entities. The presentation of these diseases is based upon the interplay of genetics, the effects of the immune system, and environmental triggers. The key point in this hypothesis is that there exist in humans relatively common nondisease-specific genes at certain loci on the human chromosomes. These loci predispose to autoimmune disease, and these genes are probably associated with immune dysregulation. With specific environmental triggers and interplay with other genes (e.g., the human leukocyte antigen (HLA) complex), the patients then develop specific autoimmune/inflammatory diseases. Because of immune dysregulation, one or several of these autoimmune diseases may develop in these patients, and they may demonstrate overlapping patterns of disease.

Environmental triggers appear to play a key role (e.g., infections, vaccinations). The HLA locus may also be important. Of note, a preliminary study found the frequency of HLA-B51 haplotype to be 3.7 times more common in patients with MEWDS than a normal control white group.[32,33]

Our present suggestion is that a variety of relatively common susceptibility genes may be responsible for MEWDS. These predispose to immune dysregulation. Precipitated by environmental triggers, MEWDS may develop. If this theory is true, then patients with MEWDS may demonstrate a family or personal history of autoimmunity. We are presently investigating this by familial aggregation studies.[31] While the etiology of MEWDS is studied further, we believe that MEWDS is a distinct clinical entity that should not be confused with other white-spot syndromes.

DIFFERENTIAL DIAGNOSIS

The differential diagnosis of MEWDS includes acute posterior multifocal placoid pigment epitheliopathy (APMPPE), acute retinal pigment epitheliitis, birdshot retinochoroidopathy, multifocal choroiditis, sarcoidosis, diffuse unilateral subacute neuroretinitis, and, rarely, ocular infiltration by lymphoma. APMPPE can cause transient visual loss in young patients, with frequent recovery of visual function and resolution of the RPE placoid lesions. APMPPE, however, is usually bilateral. APMPPE lesions are considerably larger and block fluorescence early in the fluorescein angiogram, as opposed to early hyperfluorescence in MEWDS. Much more pigment disruption develops with APMPPE than with MEWDS.

Acute retinal pigment epitheliitis is similar to MEWDS in that it affects relatively young patients and causes acute visual loss followed by almost total recovery in 7 to 10 weeks. However, the macular lesions in this condition consist of dark spots surrounded by a halo of depigmentation at the level of the RPE. The lesions, as seen on fluorescein angiography, are hypofluorescent areas surrounded by hyperfluorescence. The ERG and cortical-evoked responses are normal.

Birdshot retinochoroidopathy manifests as multiple, cream-colored lesions at the level of RPE or deeper. It differs from MEWDS in that it is found in older patients, is usually bilateral, and usually demonstrates more vitreous reaction and retinal vascular leakage than MEWDS. Acute onset is not characteristic of birdshot retinochoroidopathy. HLA-A29 is very frequently noted (90%) in patients with birdshot disease.

Multifocal choroiditis mostly occurs in young, healthy women and causes acute loss of vision. It is an RPE-choroidal inflammatory disorder with multiple relapses. Multifocal choroiditis may respond to corticosteroid treatment, although recurrences are common and CNV may develop. Multifocal choroiditis frequently has photopsias and an enlarged blind spot,[34] similar to MEWDS, and MEWDS may have chorioretinal scarring similar to multifocal choroiditis. Acutely, white lesions may be seen. Multifocal choroidal scarring has been reported both before and after MEWDS.[35] Callahan & Gass[36] have suggested overlap between these two diseases. However, MERG results differ in these two diseases. In multifocal choroiditis, there is a diffuse loss of function with partial or no recovery after acute episodes; in MEWDS, although there is initially greater focal depression that corresponds to visual field defects, there is near-total recovery to baseline with resolution of the disease.[37]

Sarcoidosis and other forms of uveitis may occasionally present with deep, small, white lesions of the retina. The remainder of the clinical picture is usually distinguishable from MEWDS. Diffuse unilateral subacute neuroretinitis is another syndrome seen in young adults who present with loss of vision and sometimes white dots in the retina. The clinical course tends to be more prolonged than that of MEWDS, and a progressive loss of vision and visual field, with optic atrophy and retinal vessel narrowing, and diffuse and focal RPE degeneration are seen. This syndrome is caused by an intraocular nematode.

Some patients thought to have MEWDS have been reported to have primary intraocular lymphoma later. A misdiagnosis of the patient as having MEWDS delayed the correct diagnosis. Lymphoma should be considered in the differential, especially in patients over the age of 50.[38]

Acute idiopathic blind spot enlargement (AIBSE) is a syndrome described by Fletcher et al.[39] Young patients develop photopsias and demonstrate enlarged blind spots. It has many common features with MEWDS. Both may exhibit photopsias, scotomata, predominance among young women, occasional recurrences, and bilaterality, as well as a predictable resolution. The main difference between MEWDS and AIBSE is that AIBSE does not have the white spots found in MEWDS. The retinal findings of MEWDS may be very subtle and fleeting, with residual symptoms and signs that could easily be mistaken for AIBSE.[40] Aaberg[41] proposed that some fundus photographs and fluorescein angiograms published in the article by Fletcher et al.[39] suggest the clinical diagnosis of MEWDS. The presentation of 2 MEWDS patients with protracted enlargement of the blind spot several weeks after the resolution of fundus abnormalities supports the conclusion that AIBSE may be the same disease as MEWDS.[13] MEWDS patients with blind-spot enlargement, if their central vision is unimpaired, may seek care later when the evanescent white dots and vitreous inflammatory cells have already resolved. An additional case reported by Kimmel et al.[42] supports this theory.

In 1991, 10 cases of AIBSE were analyzed by Singh et al.[43] Only 3 of these patients were believed to have MEWDS. The others had acute macular neuroretinopathy or ocular histoplasmosis or had normal retinal appearances. The authors concluded that MEWDS is only one cause of AIBSE.[43] Recently, 27 additional cases of AISBE were reviewed by Volpe et al.[44] AIBSE has a predilection for peripapillary retina, suggesting a local etiologic factor. Recovery of visual fields occurs in MEWDS but does not occur with AIBSE. These authors concluded that MEWDS and AIBSE are distinct from acute macular neuroretinopathy (AMN), multifocal choroiditis, and AZOOR. The conclusions have been rebutted by Gass.[45]

MEWDS has also been associated with AMN,[46] suggesting a possible common etiology. Two patients were described: the first had AMN in one eye, and 5 years later developed MEWDS in the same eye; the second patient developed MEWDS and shortly thereafter showed AMN in the same eye. Similarities between AMN and MEWDS include the female predominance, young age, and possible level of involvement of the retina. The size, shape, color, and distribution of the lesions, however, are different. AMN lesions are red-orange, wedge-shaped, petaloid, oval, or round, and are confined to the central macular area. In AMN, the retina, and apparently not the RPE, is affected, in contrast to biomicroscopic and angiographic changes of deep retinal and RPE involvement seen in MEWDS.

Patients with MEWDS often present with signs and symptoms suggesting primary optic nerve disease, including disc edema (see Fig. 102-6), visual loss, afferent pupillary defect, enlarged blind spot, and other optic nerve field defects. Dodwell et al.[47] reported 5 cases that were initially misdiagnosed as primary optic nerve disease, as the white spots were subtle findings. Optic nerve involvement in MEWDS could theoretically contribute to the central visual loss, visual field loss, afferent pupillary defect, and even dyschromatopsia. MEWDS should be considered in the differential diagnosis of young, healthy patients who present with unilateral or bilateral optic nerve dysfunction.[48,49]

Rare instances of late CNV have been noted in patients with MEWDS.[27,50] Many disorders of the RPE are associated with CNV, and, since MEWDS is primarily a disease of the RPE and deep retina, it is not surprising that choroidal (including peripapillary) neovascularization may be associated with MEWDS. Some "idiopathic" cases of CNV may be MEWDS with resolution of other ocular changes before presentation. In a patient with concurrent Best disease, there was a severity of visual symptoms that may have been due to the additive affect of the two retinal pigment epithelium disorders.[51] There has been a reported case of a retinal tear associated with acute MEWDS. The speculation is that inflammatory changes accompanying MEWDS increased vitreal traction.[52]

Gass[45] in 1993 described a new clinical syndrome, AZOOR, characterized by: (1) acute loss of one or more zones of outer retinal function; (2) minimal or no fundus changes initially; (3) electroretinographic abnormalities; and (4) permanent visual field loss. He has suggested an overlap and possible similar etiology to AZOOR, MEWDS, AMN, multifocal choroiditis, and punctate inner choroidopathy. We believe that these entities can be distinguished and divided into the following groups: (1) AZOOR; (2) MEWDS; (3) multifocal choroiditis, punctate inner choroidopathy, and subretinal fibrosis; and (4) AMN. Each has a distinct clinical picture.[53]

The challenge of correctly diagnosing MEWDS lies in its variable, sometimes subtle, presentation and the rapid reversal of the visual loss with disappearance of the white dots. These factors may explain its recent discovery, and the scarcity of documented cases. Its uncertain association with other ophthalmic conditions such as AZOOR, AMN, and multifocal choroiditis requires further investigation.

REFERENCES

1. Jampol LM, Sieving PA, Pugh D et al. Multiple evanescent white dot syndrome. I. Clinical findings. Arch Ophthalmol 1984; 102:671–674.
2. Olitsky SE. Multiple evanescent white-dot syndrome in a 10-year-old child. J Pediatr Ophthalmol Strabismus 1998; 35:288–289.
3. Lim JI, Kokame GT, Douglas JP. Multiple evanescent white dot syndrome in older patients. Am J Ophthalmol 1999; 127:725–728.
4. Ie D, Glaser BM, Murphy RP et al. Indocyanine green angiography in multiple evanescent white-dot syndrome. Am J Ophthalmol 1994; 117:7–12.
5. Borruat FX, Auer,C, Piguet B. Choroidopathy in multiple evanescent white dot syndrome. Arch Ophthalmol 1995; 113:1569–1571.
6. Obana A, Kusumi M, Miki T. Indocyanine green angiographic aspects of multiple evanescent white dot syndrome. Retina 1996; 16:97–104.
7. Obana A, Kusumi M, Moriwaki M et al. [Two cases of multiple evanescent white dot syndrome examined with indocyanine green angiography.] Nippon Ganka Gakkai Zasshi 1995; 99:244–251.
8. Yen MT, Rosenfeld PJ. Persistent indocyanine green angiographic findings in multiple evanescent white dot syndrome. Ophthalmic Surg Lasers 2001; 32:156–158.
9. Herbort CP, Borruat FX, de Courten C et al. Angiographie au vert d'indocyanine dans les uvéites postérieures. Klin Monatsbl Augenheilkd 1996; 208:321–326.
10. Stanga PE, Lim JI, Hamilton P. Indocyanine green angiography in chorioretinal diseases: indications and interpretation: an evidence-based update. Ophthalmology 2003; 110:15–21; quiz 22–23.
11. Tsukamoto E, Yamada T, Kadoi C et al. Hypofluorescent spots on indocyanine green angiography at the recovery stage in multiple evanescent white dot syndrome. Ophthalmologica 1999; 213:336–338.
12. Luttrull JK, Marmor MF, Nanda M. Progressive confluent circumpapillary multiple evanescent white-dot syndrome. Am J Ophthalmol 1999; 128:378–380.
13. Daniele S, Daniele C, Ferri C. Association of peripapillary scars with lesions characteristic of multiple evanescent white-dot syndrome. Ophthalmologica 1995; 209:217–219.
14. Sieving PA, Fishman GA, Jampol LM et al. Multiple evanescent white dot syndrome. II. Electrophysiology of the photoreceptors during retinal pigment epithelial disease. Arch Ophthalmol 1984; 102:675–679.
15. Horiguchi M, Miyake Y, Nakamura M et al. Focal electroretinogram and visual field defect in multiple evanescent white-dot syndrome. Br J Ophthalmol 1993; 77:452–455.
16. Keunen JE, Van Norren D. Foveal densitometry in the multiple evanescent white-dot syndrome. Am J Ophthalmol 1988; 105:561–562.
17. Chen D, Martidis A, Baumal CR. Transient multifocal electroretinogram dysfunction in multiple evanescent white dot syndrome. Ophthalmic Surg Lasers 2002; 33:246–249.
18. Feigl B, Haas A, El-Shabrawi Y. Multifocal ERG in multiple evanescent white dot syndrome. Graefes Arch Clin Exp Ophthalmol 2002; 240:615–621.
19. Aaberg TM, Campo RV, Joffe L. Recurrences and bilaterality in multiple evanescent white-dot syndrome. Am J Ophthalmol 1985; 100:29–37.
20. Jost BF, Olk RJ, McGaughy A. Bilateral symptomatic multiple evanescent white-dot syndrome. Am J Ophthalmol 1986; 101:489–490.
21. Tsai L, Jampol LM, Pollock SC et al. Chronic recurrent multiple evanescent white dot syndrome. Retina 1994; 14:160–163.
22. Holz FG, Kim RY, Schwartz SD et al. Acute zonal occult outer retinopathy (AZOOR) associated with multifocal choroidopathy. Eye 1994; 8:77–83.
23. Jacobson SG, Morales DS, Sun XK et al. Pattern of retinal dysfunction in acute zonal occult outer retinopathy. Ophthalmology 1995; 102:1187–1198.
24. Gass JD. Are acute zonal occult outer retinopathy and the white spot syndromes (AZOOR complex) specific autoimmune diseases? Am J Ophthalmol 2003; 135:380–381.
25. Figueroa MS, Ciancas E, Mompean B et al. Treatment of multiple evanescent white dot syndrome with cyclosporine. Eur J Ophthalmol 2001; 11:86–88.
26. Laatikainen L, Immonen I. Multiple evanescent white dot syndrome. Graefes Arch Clin Exp Ophthalmol 1988; 226:37–40.
27. McCollum CJ, Kimble JA. Peripapillary subretinal neovascularization associated with multiple evanescent white-dot syndrome. Arch Ophthalmol 1992; 11:13–15.
28. Fine L, Fine A, Cunningham ET. Multiple evanescent white dot syndrome following hepatitis A vaccination. Arch Ophthalmol 2001; 119:1856–1858.
29. Baglivo E, Safran AB, Borruat FX. Multiple evanescent white dot syndrome after hepatitis B vaccine. Am J Ophthalmol 1996; 122:431–432.
30. Chung YM, Yeh TS, Liu JH. Increased serum IgM and IgG in the multiple evanescent white-dot syndrome. Am J Ophthalmol 1987; 104:187–188.
31. Jampol LM, Becker KG. White spot syndromes of the retina: a hypothesis based on the common genetic hypothesis of autoimmune/inflammatory disease. Am J Ophthalmol 2003; 135:376–379.
32. Desarnaulds AB, Borruat FX, Herbort CP et al. Le multiple evanescent white dot syndrome: une predisposition genetique? Klin Monatsbl Augenheilkd 1996; 208:301–302.
33. Borruat FX, Herbort CP, Spertini F et al. HLA typing in patients with multiple evanescent white dot syndrome (MEWDS). Ocular Immunol Inflamm 1998; 6:39–41.
34. Khorram KD, Jampol LM, Rosenberg MA. Blind spot enlargement as a manifestation of multifocal choroiditis. Arch Ophthalmol 1991; 109:1403–1407.
35. Bryan RG, Freund KB, Yannuzzi LA et al. Multiple evanescent white dot syndrome in patients with multifocal choroiditis. Retina 2002; 22:317–322.
36. Callahan D, Gass JDM. Multi-focal choroiditis and choroidal neovascularization associated with the multiple evanescent white dot syndrome and acute idiopathic blind spot enlargement syndrome. Ophthalmology 1992; 99:1678–1685.
37. Oh KT, Folk JC, Maturi RK et al. Multifocal electroretinography in multifocal choroiditis and the multiple evanescent white dot syndrome. Retina 2001; 21:581–589.
38. Shah GK, Kleiner RC, Augsburger JJ et al. Primary intraocular lymphoma seen with transient white fundus lesions simulating the multiple evanescent white dot syndrome. Arch Ophthalmol 2001; 119:617–620.
39. Fletcher WA, Imes RK, Goodman D et al. Acute idiopathic blind spot enlargement: a big blind spot syndrome without optic disc edema. Arch Ophthalmol 1988; 106:44–49.
40. Hamed LM, Glaser JS, Gass JDM et al. Protracted enlargement of the blind spot in multiple evanescent white dot syndrome. Arch Ophthalmol 1989; 107:194–198.
41. Aaberg TM. Multiple evanescent white dot syndrome. Arch Ophthalmol 1988; 106:1162–1163.
42. Kimmel AS, Folk JC, Thompson HS et al. The multiple evanescent white-dot syndrome with acute blind spot enlargement. Am J Ophthalmol 1989; 107:425–426.
43. Singh K, De Frank MP, Shults WT et al. Acute idiopathic blind spot enlargement. Ophthalmology 1991; 98:497–502.
44. Volpe NJ, Rizzo JF, Lessell S. Acute idiopathic blind spot enlargement syndrome: a review of 27 new cases. Arch Ophthalmol 2001; 119:59–63.
45. Gass JD. Acute zonal occult outer retinopathy. J Clin Neuroophthalmol 1993; 13:79–97.
46. Gass JDM, Hamed LM. Acute macular neuroretinopathy and multiple evanescent white dot syndrome occurring in the same patients. Arch Ophthalmol 1989; 107:189–193.
47. Dodwell CG, Jampol LM, Rosenberg M et al. Optic nerve involvement associated with the multiple evanescent white dot syndrome. Ophthalmology 1990; 97:862–868.
48. Fong KS, Fu ER. Multiple evanescent white dot syndrome – an uncommon cause for an enlarged blind spot. Ann Acad Med Singapore 1996; 25:866–868.
49. Reddy CV, Brown J Jr, Folk JC et al. Enlarged blind spots in chorioretinal inflammatory disorders. Ophthalmology 1996; 103:606–617.
50. Wyhinny GJ, Jackson JL, Jampol LM et al. Subretinal neovascularization following multiple evanescent white-dot syndrome. Arch Ophthalmol 1990; 108:1384–1385.
51. Park DW, Polk TD, Stone EM. Multiple evanescent white dot syndrome in a patient with Best disease. Arch Ophthalmol 1997; 115:1342–1433.
52. Ikeda N, Ikeda T, Nagata M et al. A retinal tear associated with multiple evanescent white dot syndrome. Retina 2002; 22:349–352.
53. Jampol LM, Wiredu A. MEWDS, MFC, PIC, AMN, AIBSE, and AZOOR: one disease or many? Retina 1995; 15:373–378.
54. Barile GR, Reppucci VS, Schiff VM et al. Circumpapillary chorioretinopathy in multiple evanescent white dot syndrome. Retina 1997; 17:75–77.
55. Borruat FX, Othenin-Girad P. Multiple evanescent white dot syndrome. Klin Monatsbl Augenheilkd 1991; 198:453–456.
56. Grand MG, Storch GA. Presumed parvovirus B19-associated retinal pigment epitheliopathy. Retina 2000; 20:199–202.
57. Hamed LA, Schatz NJ, Glaser JS et al. Acute idiopathic blind spot enlargement without optic disc edema. Arch Ophthalmol 1988; 106:1030–1031.
58. Ikeda N, Ikeda T, Nagata M et al. Location of lesions in multiple evanescent white dot syndrome and the cause of the hypofluorescent spots observed by indocyanine green angiography. Graefes Arch Clin Exp Ophthalmol 2001; 239:242–247.
59. Lefrancois A, Hamard H, Corbe C et al. A case of MEWDS: the multiple evanescent white-dot syndrome. J Fr Ophtalmol 1989; 12:103–109.

60. Leys A, Leys M, Jonckheere P et al. Multiple evanescent white dot syndrome (MEWDS). Bull Soc Belge Ophtalmol 1990; 236:97–108.

61. Lombardo J. Multiple evanescent white dot syndrome and acute zonal occult outer retinopathies. Optom Vis Sci 2003; 80:673–680.

62. Mamalis N, Daily MJ. Multiple evanescent white-dot syndrome: a report of eight cases. Ophthalmology 1987; 94:1209–1212.

63. Meyer RJ, Jampol LM. Recurrences and bilaterality in the multiple evanescent white-dot syndrome. Am J Ophthalmol 1986; 101:388–389.

64. Nakao K, Isashiki M. Multiple evanescent white dot syndrome. Jpn J Ophthalmol 1986; 30:376–384.

65. Oh KT, Christmas NJ, Russell SR. Late recurrence and choroidal neovascularization in multiple evanescent white dot syndrome. Retina 2001; 21:182–184.

66. Slusher MM, Weaver RG. Multiple evanescent white dot syndrome. Retina 1988; 8:132–135.

67. Takeda M, Kimura S, Tamiya M. Acute disseminated retinal pigment epitheliopathy. Folia Ophthalmol Jpn 1984; 35:2613–2620.

68. Tejada Palacios P, Pina Hurtado E, Mendez Romas MJ. Multiple evanescent white dot syndrome. Ann Ophthalmol 1993; 25:216–218.

69. van Neel GJ, Keunen JEE, van Norren D et al. Scanning laser densitometry in multiple evanescent white dot syndrome. Retina 1993; 13:29–35.

70. Quillen DA, Davis JB, Gottlieb JL et al. The white dot syndromes. Am J Ophthalmol 2004; 137:538–550.

Chapter

103

Sarcoidosis

Douglas A. Jabs
Quan Dong Nguyen

Sarcoidosis is a multisystem granulomatous disorder of unknown etiology characterized by intrathoracic involvement. Ocular involvement is common and occurs in approximately 15% to 25% of patients with sarcoidosis.[1,2] Posterior-segment manifestations may account for up to 28% of the lesions seen in patients with ocular sarcoid. Most large case series of patients with uveitis report that approximately 5% of patients with uveitis have biopsy-confirmed systemic sarcoidosis.[3-6]

GENERAL CONSIDERATIONS

Epidemiology

Sarcoidosis is worldwide in its distribution, but it is most frequently recognized in developed countries where adequate diagnostic facilities are available. All races are affected, but series in the USA generally show that the disease is more prevalent in blacks than in whites. Both sexes are affected, with the overall frequency showing a very slight excess of females (approximately 60%). Sarcoidosis is a disease of young adults, with almost three-fourths of cases occurring in those younger than 40 years of age. Children may be affected, but this is uncommon.[1,7-10] The clinical course of childhood sarcoidosis is often atypical; that is, there is less frequent pulmonary involvement and more frequent extrathoracic disease.[11,12] These children must be differentiated from children with juvenile rheumatoid arthritis and those with familial juvenile systemic granulomatosis[13-16] because of the similarity of ocular and articular involvement. Many cases of familial juvenile systemic granulomatosis are misdiagnosed as childhood sarcoidosis.[17]

Etiology and pathogenesis

The etiology of sarcoidosis is unknown. Multiple theories have been proposed, including a variety of infectious agents, allergy to pine pollen and peanut dust, chewing pine pitch, and hypersensitivity to chemicals such as beryllium or zirconium. To date, there is no conclusive evidence to implicate any of these as an etiologic agent. Familial studies and human leukocyte antigen (HLA) typing have suggested a possible genetic predisposition, but these studies are far from conclusive.[1] A cooperative multicenter study, A Case Control Etiologic Study of Sarcoidosis (ACCESS group), enrolled 736 biopsy-confirmed cases from 10 centers in the USA, suggested a genetic predisposition for

sarcoidosis, and presented evidence for the allelic variation at the HLA-DRB1 locus as a contributing factor to the disease.[18]

Patients with sarcoidosis are characterized by depression of delayed-type hypersensitivity, reflected by T-cell anergy, and skin tests that are often negative. Peripheral blood lymphocytes from patients with sarcoidosis show diminished responses to mitogens.

Bronchoalveolar lavage has enabled investigators to determine the immunologic events at the area of active disease in the lungs. These studies have shown entirely different results from peripheral blood lymphocytes. In the lungs, there is an excess of helper T lymphocytes ($CD4^+$). These activated helper T cells spontaneously secrete lymphokines, including interleukin-2 (IL-2), and will polyclonally activate B cells to produce immunoglobulins. These studies have been interpreted to show that an active T-cell-driven immunologic response occurs at the target organ site and eventually leads to granuloma formation.[19,20] Studies of bronchoalveolar lavage fluids have suggested that macrophages may also play a role in the pathogenesis of pulmonary sarcoidosis by inducing changes in the pulmonary microvasculature.[21]

Immunohistologic studies of biopsy tissue from patients with sarcoidosis have demonstrated the presence of cells of macrophage lineage and activated T cells in the granuloma. The vast majority of lymphocytes are T cells of the helper subset ($CD4^+$) and express activation markers, including class II antigens and the IL-2 receptor.[22-24]

Clinical features

The organs most frequently involved by sarcoidosis are the lungs, lymph nodes and spleen, skin, eyes, nervous system, and bones and joints[1,2,8,9,25] (Table 103-1).

Intrathoracic sarcoidosis

Several series have demonstrated that intrathoracic involvement is the most common manifestation of sarcoidosis and occurs in 90% of patients. An abnormality on chest radiograph examination is evident at the onset of sarcoidosis in almost all patients. Chest radiograph abnormalities have been classified according to a simple staging system, which closely correlates with the eventual outcome. Stage 0 is characterized by a normal chest radiograph. Stage 1 is characterized by bilateral hilar lymphadenopathy without pulmonary infiltration and is seen in 65% of patients

Table 103-1 Organ system involvement in sarcoidosis

Organ system	Frequency (%)
Intrathoracic	84–93
Hilar nodes	60–77
Lung parenchyma	40–56
Lymph nodes	23–37
Eyes	11–32
Skin	12–27
Erythema nodosum	4–31
Spleen	1–18
Bones	2–9
Parotid	5–8
Central nervous system	2–7

with pulmonary sarcoidosis. Stage 2 is characterized by hilar lymphadenopathy associated with pulmonary infiltration and is seen in 22% of patients with sarcoid. Stage 3 sarcoid is characterized by pulmonary infiltration with fibrosis but without bilateral hilar adenopathy and occurs in 13% of patients. The overall rates of radiographic resolution are 59%, 39%, and 38% for stage 1, 2, and 3 disease, respectively.[1]

Extrapulmonary lesions

Involvement of the reticuloendothelial system, particularly the extrapulmonary lymph nodes or spleen, or both, is common and occurs in 23% to 37% of patients with sarcoidosis. Biopsy of a palpable lymph node is often used for histologic confirmation of the diagnosis of sarcoidosis (see below). Skin lesions occur frequently in sarcoidosis and include erythema nodosum, lupus pernio, maculopapular rashes, cutaneous plaques, and subcutaneous nodules. Lupus pernio (dusky-purple infiltration of the skin of the nose) and sarcoid plaques are typically associated with chronic disease, whereas erythema nodosum is typically associated with acute disease.[26] Neurosarcoidosis occurs in 2% to 7% of patients with sarcoid. Facial palsy is the most frequent manifestation of neurosarcoidosis. Other presentations include other cranial nerve palsies, papilledema, peripheral neuropathy, meningitis, space-occupying cerebral lesions, cavernous sinus syndrome,[27] and endocrine disorders such as hypopituitarism or diabetes insipidus resulting from space-occupying lesions. Musculoskeletal involvement includes bone cysts in patients with chronic sarcoid, polyarthralgias and periarthritis in patients with acute sarcoid, and, less commonly, myopathy from granulomatous lesions within muscles.[1,2,10,25,27–30]

Laboratory evaluation

The single best test for the evaluation of patients with suspected sarcoidosis is the chest film, since it is abnormal in approxi-mately 90% of patients with sarcoid. Although the chest film is the best test for detecting the presence of sarcoidosis, it does not unequivocally establish the diagnosis.

Histologic confirmation (Table 103-2) is generally required to establish the diagnosis of sarcoid. Sites most often biopsied include the lungs, mediastinal lymph nodes, skin, peripheral lymph nodes, liver, and conjunctiva. Biopsy of clinically evident skin lesions or palpable lymph nodes is frequently performed because of the high yield and low morbidity. Fiberoptic bronchoscopy with transbronchial lung biopsy is positive in 80% of patients with intrapulmonary sarcoidosis. This procedure is routinely performed by pulmonary physicians and has a relatively low morbidity. The liver biopsy is often positive in patients with sarcoidosis, but the finding of granulomatous lesions on liver biopsy must be interpreted with caution, as they can be produced by other disorders. Other potential biopsy sites include peripheral lymph nodes and minor salivary glands.

The Kveim skin test was a simple, specific, outpatient skin test using human sarcoid tissue. It was positive in 78% of patients with sarcoidosis and was helpful in delineating multisystemic sarcoidosis from other granulomatous disorders. The antigen was a saline suspension of human sarcoid tissue prepared from the spleen of a patient suffering from active sarcoidosis. This material was injected intradermally, and the site inspected for nodule formation after 3 to 6 weeks. A palpable nodule was biopsied, and the finding of noncaseating granulomas on biopsy established the diagnosis of sarcoid.[1,31,32] Concerns about the injection of human tissue with its potential for disease transmission have essentially eliminated the use of the Kveim test. Conjunctival biopsies are positive in 25% to 57% of patients with histologically documented sarcoidosis. Variations in these reports are the result of whether clinically evident lesions are biopsied or whether a "blind" conjunctival biopsy is performed. In addition, the yield can be increased by techniques such as bilateral conjunctival biopsies and serial sectioning of the specimens.* Because of the very low morbidity involved, careful inspection of the conjunctiva for any visibly evident nodules and a conjunctival biopsy may be performed. Transconjunctival lacrimal gland biopsy can also be used for histologic diagnosis, but the procedure is not used routinely.[33,34]

Noninvasive tests

Multiple attempts have been made to find noninvasive tests that could be both sensitive and specific in the diagnosis of sarcoidosis. These have included measurement of serum calcium, urinary calcium, serum lysozyme, and serum immunoglobulins. Although all these may be abnormal in patients with sarcoid, they are nonspecific and nondiagnostic. The serum angiotensin-converting enzyme (ACE) level has been touted as a useful measurement in the diagnosis of sarcoidosis. The ACE level is frequently abnormal in patients with active sarcoidosis and appears to reflect the total-body granuloma content in such patients. As such, it may be useful in following patients with active sarcoid.[32,35,36] However, it is not diagnostic of sarcoidosis and appears to be of limited utility in the diagnostic dilemma of patients with possible sarcoid uveitis but a normal chest film.

Table 103-2 Yield of different biopsy sites in the diagnosis of sarcoidosis

Technique	Study	Positive/total	(%)
Liver biopsy	Branson & Park (1954)[90]	48/63	76
	Israel & Sones (1964)[32]	22/24	92
	Klatskin (1976)[91]	17/23	94
Scalene lymph node biopsy	Beahrs et al. (1957)[92]	20/34	59
	Rochlin & Enterline (1958)[93]	27/34	79
	Williams & Webb (1962)[72]	32/39	82
Scalene fat pad biopsy	Romer et al. (1973)[94]	115/142	81
	Rasmussen & Neukirch (1976)[95]	41/99	52
Mediastinoscopy	Carlens (1964)[96]	118/123	96
	Palva (1964)[71]	27/28	96
	Romer et al. (1973)[94]	47/48	98
Lung biopsy, transbronchial	Koerner et al. (1975)[97]	21/23	91
Bronchoscope	Koontz (1978)[98]	74/104	71
Conjunctival biopsy	Crick et al. (1961)[40]	20/79	25
	Bornstein et al. (1962)[73]	16/64	25
	Kahn et al. (1977)[99]	20/60	33
	Solomon et al. (1978)[100]	8/15	57
	Garver (unpublished, 1980)	10/21	48
	Nichols et al. (1980)[75]	30/55	55
	Karcioglu & Brear (1985)[74]	14/28	50
Minor salivary gland biopsy	Nessan & Jacoway (1979)[70]	44/75	58

Modified from Green WR. Inflammatory diseases and conditions of the eye. In: Spencer WH, ed. Ophthalmic pathology: an atlas and textbook, vol. 3. Philadelphia, PA: WB Saunders; 1986.[31]

Gallium scanning has also been suggested as a useful diagnostic test for sarcoidosis. Gallium is actively accumulated in sarcoid granulomas. The test is again nonspecific, and gallium uptake is seen in other diseases, including infection and lymphoma. It has been suggested that the combination of gallium scanning and an elevated ACE level is highly specific for sarcoidosis, but these studies have employed patients specifically chosen for very active sarcoid.[37] As such, these tests may be of less utility in a patient with presumed sarcoid uveitis and no obvious evidence of systemic sarcoidosis. The greatest use of these tests may be in following patients with active disease.[33,36]

In a study of 22 patients with sarcoid uveitis compared to 70 patients with uveitis secondary to other disorders, Power et al.[38] reported that the sensitivity and specificity of an elevated ACE alone in diagnosing sarcoidosis were 73% and 83%, respectively, and that the sensitivity and specificity of the gallium scan alone were 91% and 84%, respectively. Using the combination of a gallium scan and an elevated serum ACE, the specificity for diagnosing sarcoidosis was 100% and the sensitivity was 73%. The authors concluded that the combination of serum ACE level and whole-body gallium scan might be useful for diagnosing sarcoidosis in patients with uveitis. However, because of the study design inherent in investigating the values of these tests, their actual utility in patients with normal chest radiographs and without clinical evidence of sarcoid remains uncertain. Furthermore, because the reported prevalence of sarcoid uveitis is approxi-

mately 5% among patients with biopsy-confirmed systemic sarcoidosis,[3-6] routine screening of all patients with uveitis by both ACE levels and gallium scan may have a low positive predictive value and therefore may be misleading. Nevertheless, in selected patients in whom sarcoidosis is highly likely, these tests may be useful.

For following patients with active intrapulmonary sarcoid, pulmonary function tests, particularly forced vital capacity, forced expiratory volume, and diffusing capacity, are far more useful tests. Changes in the pulmonary function tests are often used to follow patients with sarcoidosis and to adjust the corticosteroid dosage.[8]

Jabs & Johns[7] reported that over 80% of patients with ocular sarcoid had their ocular lesions at the time of diagnosis of sarcoidosis, and Hunter & Foster[39] reported that only 3% of patients with uveitis were diagnosed as having sarcoid after the initial evaluation for a systemic disease revealed no diagnosable systemic disorder. Although patients who present with uveitis should be evaluated for sarcoid, repetitive workups appear to have limited value unless new symptoms arise.

Course and prognosis

There appear to be two distinct paradigms of sarcoidosis, acute and chronic, with differences in onset, natural history, course, prognosis, and response to treatment. Acute sarcoidosis tends to have an abrupt, explosive onset in young patients and to go into spontaneous remission within 2 years of onset. Acute iritis is often seen in acute sarcoidosis. The response to systemic corticosteroids is generally quite good, and the long-term complications are minimal. Löfgren's syndrome comprises erythema nodosum, bilateral hilar adenopathy, and acute iritis; it generally has a good long-term prognosis.[1,2,25]

Chronic sarcoidosis is defined as disease persistence of greater than 2 years' duration. The disease may have a more insidious onset and generally has intrapulmonary involvement with chronic pulmonary disease as a major source of morbidity. Corticosteroid therapy is generally required and may be prolonged. Chronic ocular disease, particularly chronic uveitis, may be a feature of chronic sarcoidosis.[1,2,7,8,25]

The overall mortality from sarcoidosis is 3% to 5%, but neurosarcoid is associated with a mortality of 10%.[40] Corticosteroids are the mainstay of treatment, although antimalarial agents can be used for patients with mucocutaneous lesions. Patients with hilar adenopathy without abnormalities of pulmonary function and without intrapulmonary infiltration may not need systemic corticosteroid treatment.

Ocular manifestations

Multiple studies have documented the common occurrence of ocular involvement in sarcoidosis and the various ocular manifestations of sarcoid. Frequency estimates vary and have ranged to as high as 50%.[40] However, most series are generally closer to 15% to 28%.[1,2,7,10,25,41] These differences undoubtedly relate to the patient population studied, definitions of ophthalmic involvement, and the nature of the evaluation conducted. Some studies have suggested that ocular involvement is more common in African Americans with sarcoid. Furthermore, high frequencies of ocular involvement are reported when keratoconjunctivitis sicca is sought carefully and included as evidence of lacrimal involvement in sarcoidosis.[40]

Sarcoidosis may affect most of the ocular structures, as well as the orbit and adnexa. Ocular lesions described in sarcoidosis include anterior uveitis, iris nodules, conjunctival nodules, scleral nodule[42] and corneal disease with either band keratopathy or interstitial keratitis; posterior-segment disease including chorioretinitis, periphlebitis, chorioretinal nodules, vitreous inflammation, and retinal neovascularization; and orbital disease, including involvement of the lacrimal gland, nasolacrimal duct, optic nerve, and orbital granulomas. The various ocular lesions along with the prevalence estimates are outlined in Table 103-3.

Anterior uveitis is the most common ocular lesion and occurs in approximately two-thirds of patients with ocular sarcoid. The uveitis may be an acute iridocyclitis or a chronic granulomatous uveitis. Acute iridocyclitis is most often seen in patients with acute sarcoid but can be seen in those with chronic sarcoid as well. The prognosis is worse for those with chronic disease, who may develop complications such as secondary glaucoma, band keratopathy, cataracts, macular edema, and visual loss. Iris nodules are occasionally seen in association with anterior uveitis in patients with sarcoidosis.

Conjunctival and corneal lesions in patients with sarcoidosis are less common. These are generally described as conjunctival

Table 103-3 Ocular manifestations of sarcoidosis

Ocular manifestation	Frequency in patients with ocular sarcoid (%)
Anterior-segment disease	
Anterior uveitis	66–70
Acute	15–32
Chronic	39–53
Iris nodules	11–16
Conjunctival lesions	7–47
Cornea	
Band keratopathy	5–14
Interstitial keratitis	1
Posterior-segment disease	14–28
Vitritis	3–25
Periphlebitis	10–17
Chorioretinitis	11
Choroidal nodules	4–5
Retinal neovascularization	1–5
Orbital and other disease	26
Lacrimal gland	7–60
Keratoconjunctivitis sicca	5–60
Enlargement	7–28
Orbital granuloma	1
Optic-nerve granuloma	<1–7

nodules, which on biopsy reveal the characteristic granuloma formation of sarcoidosis. Occasionally a nonspecific or phlyctenular keratoconjunctivitis is described in association with other mucocutaneous lesions of sarcoidosis. The cornea is infrequently involved but may develop band keratopathy either because of chronic uveitis or because of hypercalcemia. In addition, occasional cases of interstitial keratitis in association with sarcoidosis have been described.

The frequency of orbital, particularly lacrimal-gland, lesions varies widely among series and depends on the patient selection and investigations used. Clinical enlargement is present in less than one-third of patients with ocular sarcoid, but when sought, keratoconjunctivitis sicca may be present in a greater percentage.[7,10,25,40,41] Orbital granuloma, independent of the lacrimal gland, occurs infrequently.[43–45] Massive lacrimal gland enlargement simulating a lacrimal gland tumor may occur and require biopsy.

Posterior-segment disease

Posterior-segment lesions are reported to occur in approximately 14% to 28% of patients with ocular sarcoid.[7,10,25,40,41] The actual frequency may be higher, since most patients with posterior segment disease also have an anterior uveitis. Posterior lesions include vitreitis, chorioretinitis, periphlebitis, vascular occlusion, retinal neovascularization, and optic nerve head granulomas.

Vitreous infiltration within sarcoidosis can appear as cellular infiltration, a nonspecific vitreitis. However, more classically, the lesions demonstrate clumping and an accumulation of vitreous debris, called either "snowballs" or a "string of pearls" (Fig. 103-1).

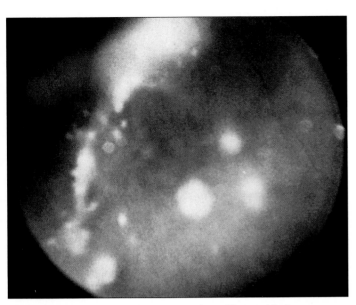

Fig. 103-1 Vitreous inflammation in a patient with sarcoidosis.

These lesions may be somewhat similar in appearance to those seen in pars planitis, although snowball formation is generally not seen in sarcoid uveitis. Sarcoid granulomata can also present in the optic nerve, peripheral retina, pars plana, and anterior choroid, and can be imaged by high-resolution ultrasound biomicroscopy as different forms of uveal thickening.[46]

Perivascular sheathing is the second most common finding and occurs in 10% to 17% of patients with ocular sarcoid. It is generally a mid peripheral periphlebitis without significant vascular

occlusion (Figs 103-2 and 103-3). However, several series have documented the occasional occurrence of occlusive retinal vascular disease, particularly branch retinal vein occlusion (Fig. 103-4). Central retinal vein occlusion is less common. Histologic studies have demonstrated vascular compromise by the granulomatous inflammatory material.[47,48] More severe forms of periphlebitis have been called "candle wax drippings." Sanders & Shilling[49] have described an "acute retinopathy of sarcoidosis" with extensive perivascular sheathing, vascular occlusion, and intraretinal hemorrhages. These cases were complicated by subsequent retinal neovascularization.

Deeper chorioretinal lesions have also been reported. These can vary in size from small "Dalen–Fuchs-like" granulomas to large choroidal nodules simulating a metastatic tumor. If located in the macular region, these lesions can cause severe visual loss. Corticosteroid therapy has been able to shrink these lesions.

Exudative retinal detachments are rarely seen in patients with sarcoid uveitis but do occur in those patients with large nodular chorioretinal granulomas. These detachments appear to be an overlying detachment of the neurosensory retina and may resolve with oral corticosteroid therapy.[35,50]

Rarely, visual loss can occur from epiretinal membrane formation and cystoid macular edema in patients with sarcoidosis. Once the inflammation has been controlled, pars plana vitrectomy with membrane peeling may have a beneficial effect on restoring vision, although development of cataract and membrane recurrence may require additional surgeries.[51,52] In one small uncontrolled case series, triamcinolone acetonide has been injected into the vitreous cavity to assist the visualization of the vitreous for the vitrectomy,[53] but the role of this approach is uncertain.

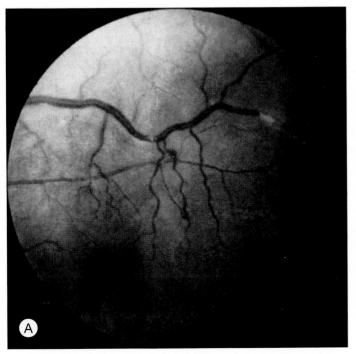

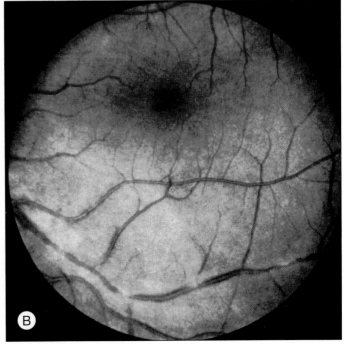

Fig. 103-2 A and B, Perivascular sheathing in a patient with sarcoidosis. (Reproduced from Green WR. Inflammatory diseases and conditions of the eye. In: Spencer WH, ed. Ophthalmic pathology: an atlas and textbook, vol. 3. Philadelphia, PA: WB Saunders; 1986.[31])

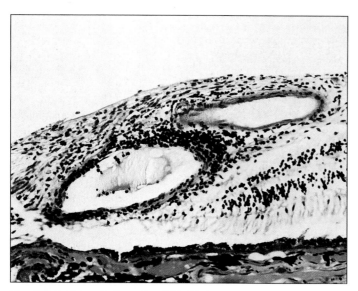

Fig. 103-3 Histopathology of periphlebitis in a patient with sarcoidosis (periodic acid-Schiff reaction; ×225). (Reproduced from Green WR. Inflammatory diseases and conditions of the eye. In: Spencer WH, ed. Ophthalmic pathology: an atlas and textbook, vol. 3. Philadelphia, PA: WB Saunders; 1986.[31])

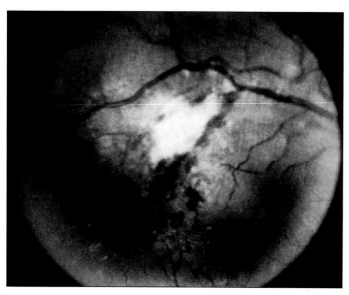

Fig. 103-4 Perifoveal branch vein occlusion in a patient with sarcoidosis.

Peripheral retinal neovascularization or neovascularization of the optic nerve head is present in less than 5% of patients with ocular sarcoid but can be associated with significant visual loss due to vitreous hemorrhage. Peripheral retinal neovascularization is generally seen in patients with a defined vaso-occlusive disorder such as a branch retinal vein occlusion. The peripheral neovascular lesions may even simulate a sea fan, similar to that seen in sickle-cell disease. Neovascularization of the disc may also develop after a branch or central vein occlusion. The rare occurrence of peripapillary choroidal neovascularization in the absence of uveitis or optic nerve disease has been reported, and reported to

be responsive to oral corticosteroids.[53] Doxanas and co-workers[55] described a patient with sarcoidosis and a steroid-responsive neovascularization of the optic nerve head without retinal nonperfusion (Fig. 103-5). Hoogstede & Cooper[48] have described one case of subretinal neovascularization, which they attributed to sarcoid uveitis. Duker et al.[56] reported the clinical features of proliferative sarcoid retinopathy in 11 eyes of seven patients. In these cases the new retinal vessels were associated with concomitant peripheral retinal capillary nonperfusion. The authors suggested that, in these patients, capillary nonperfusion secondary to microvascular shutdown, rather than a direct effect of inflammation, was the stimulus for the formation of retinal neovascularization.

It has been reported that, when posterior segment involvement is seen in patients with sarcoid uveitis, there is an increased frequency of central nervous system involvement. In a retrospective review of the literature, Gould & Kaufman[57] suggested that the prevalence of central nervous system involvement increased from 2% to 30% when fundus lesions were found. However, Spalton & Sanders[58] found no such association, leaving the issue in doubt.

Optic nerve involvement, particularly multiple granulomas of the optic nerve head, occur in 0.5% to 7.0% of patients with ocular sarcoid[7,10,25,31,58] (Fig. 103-6). Histologic descriptions have shown granuloma formation[31,59] (Fig. 103-7). Optic disc edema without granulomatous invasion of the optic nerve head may be seen in patients either with chronic uveitis or with papilledema[29] from CNS sarcoid. Occasionally, isolated sarcoid optic neuropathy (optic atrophy, optic neuritis, optic disc edema) may occur and may be the first manifestation of neurosarcoidosis.[60–63]

In addition to these conventionally observable lesions, Mizuno & Takahashi[64] have used cycloscopy to document the common occurrence of lesions in the ciliary processes of patients with intraocular sarcoidosis. In their series, nodules of the ciliary processes were seen in 41% of eyes, waxy exudates in 24%, and cyclitic membrane-like exudates in 3%. Only 20% of eyes with intraocular sarcoid had no observable lesions.

Course, treatment, and prognosis

Treatment of the anterior uveitis of sarcoidosis is generally with intensive topical corticosteroids. Chronic corticosteroid therapy may be required. In some patients with refractory anterior uveitis, the judicious use of oral corticosteroids may be necessary to suppress the inflammation. Patients with sarcoidosis generally respond to corticosteroid therapy, but chronic therapy may be necessary. Posterior-segment lesions in sarcoidosis generally require the use of systemic corticosteroids. Dosages are often in the range of prednisone 40 to 80 mg/day. Posterior-segment lesions such as perivascular sheathing and peripheral chorioretinal nodules that are not associated with visual loss may not mandate oral corticosteroid therapy. However, vascular occlusion, neovascularization, macular mass lesions, and optic disc lesions may produce profound visual loss and require corticosteroid therapy. Occasionally, corticosteroid-sparing agents, such as hydroxychloroquine, methotrexate, azathioprine, mycophenolate mofetil, or ciclosporin, may be useful in patients with corticosteroid-dependent sarcoidosis in whom corticosteroid side-effects are problematic.[65–68]

The development of secondary glaucoma in association with sarcoid uveitis appears to be a poor prognostic sign and is associated with severe visual loss. In one series,[7] most of these patients had a panuveitis with both anterior- and posterior-segment involve-ment associated with the development of secondary glaucoma, suggesting a more severe ocular disease. Treatment should be directed towards immediately suppressing the inflammation and minimizing any potential ocular complications.

Karma and co-workers[41] classified the course of ocular sarcoidosis as monophasic, relapsing, or chronic. The three different

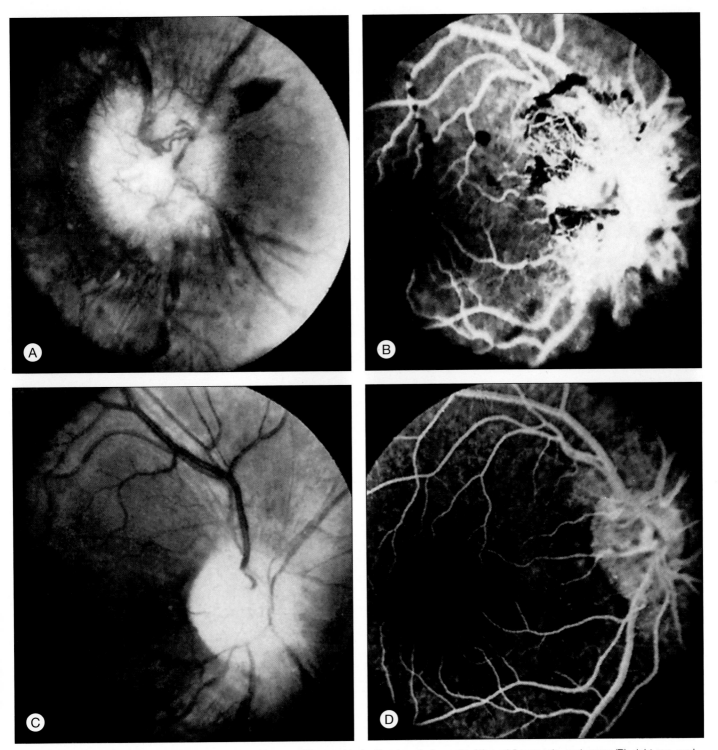

Fig. 103-5 Neovascularization of the optic nerve in a patient with sarcoidosis. Fundus photography (A), and fluorescein angiogram (B), right eye, and fundus photograph (E) and fluorescein angiogram (F), left eye, before steroid treatment. Fundus photograph (C) and fluorescein angiogram (D), right eye, and fundus photograph (G)

Continued

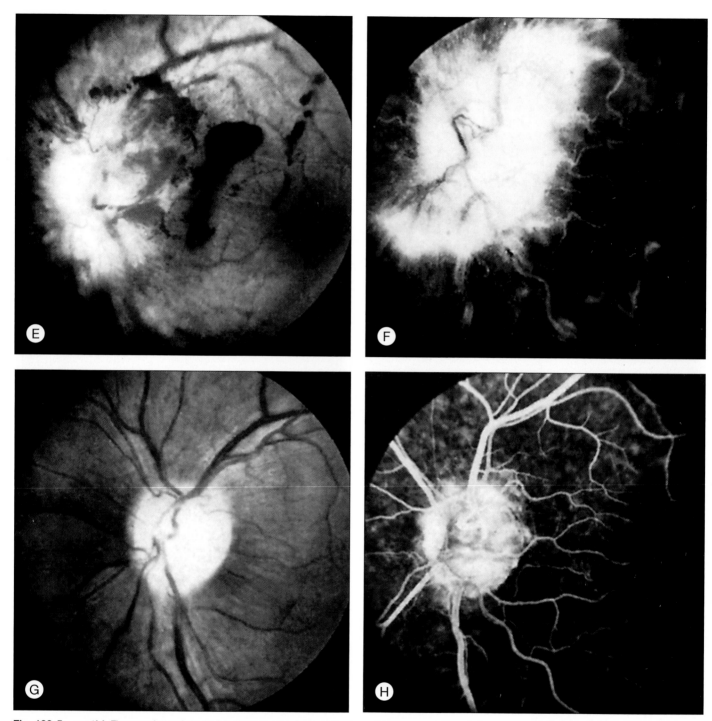

Fig. 103-5—cont'd Fluorescein angiogram (H), left eye, after treatment, demonstrating resolution of disc neovascularization. (Reproduced from Doxanas MT, Kelley JS, Prout TE. Sarcoidosis with neovascularization of the optic nerve head. Am J Ophthalmol 1980; 90:347–351.[55])

courses of uveitis correlated with the visual outcome. Patients with a monophasic uveitis retained 20/30 or better visual acuity in 88% of eyes, with relapsing uveitis in 72% of eyes, and with chronic uveitis in none of six eyes. Similarly, those with monophasic uveitis had a visual acuity of 20/70 or worse in 12% of eyes, with relapsing uveitis in 28% of eyes, and chronic uveitis in 67% of eyes. Hence the course of uveitis appears to correlate with the long-term visual outcome.

In a retrospective study of 60 patients with sarcoid-associated uveitis who were followed at a subspecialty eye care and referral center, Dana et al.[69] identified prognostic factors for visual outcomes in sarcoid uveitis. The factors most strongly associated with *both* a lack of visual acuity improvement and a final visual acuity worse than 20/40 were: (1) delay in presentation to a uveitis subspecialist of greater than 1 year; (2) development of glaucoma; and (3) presence of intermediate or posterior

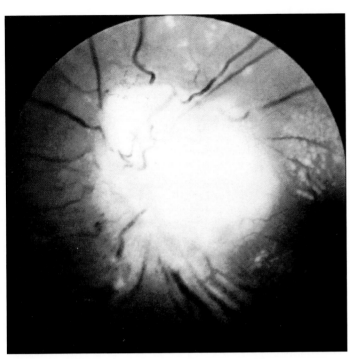

Fig. 103-6 Optic nerve mass in a patient with sarcoidosis. (Courtesy of Robert Nussenblatt.)

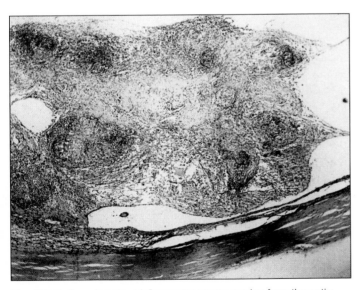

Fig. 103-7 Granulomatous inflammatory mass coming from the optic nerve head in a patient with sarcoidosis (hematoxylin & eosin; ×35). (Reproduced from Green WR. Inflammatory diseases and conditions of the eye. In: Spencer WH, ed. Ophthalmic pathology: an atlas and textbook, vol. 3. Philadelphia, PA: WB Saunders; 1986.[31])

uveitis. There was a substantial increase in the relative odds of both visual improvement and the likelihood of achieving a visual acuity of at least 20/40 among patients in whom systemic corticosteroids were used for treatment. Because patients with more severe disease are more likely to receive systemic corticosteroid therapy, this result strongly supports the use of systemic corticosteroids for selected patients with sarcoid uveitis.

REFERENCES

1. James DG. Sarcoidosis. In: Wyngaarden JB, Smith LH Jr, eds. Cecil textbook of medicine, 17th edn. Philadelphia: WB Saunders; 1985.
2. James DG, Neville E, Siltzbach LE. A worldwide review of sarcoidosis. Ann NY Acad Sci 1976; 278:321–334.
3. Henderly DE, Genstler AJ, Smith RE et al. Changing patterns of uveitis. Am J Ophthalmol 1987; 103:131–136.
4. Karma A. Ophthalmic changes in sarcoidosis. Acta Ophthalmol 1979; 141 (suppl):1.
5. Perkins ES, Folk J. Uveitis in London and Iowa. Ophthalmologica 1984; 189:36.
6. Rosenbaum JT. Uveitis: an internist's view. Arch Intern Med 1989; 149:1173.
7. Jabs DA, Johns CJ. Ocular involvement in chronic sarcoidosis. Am J Ophthalmol 1986; 102:297–301.
8. Johns CJ, Schonfeld A, Scott PP et al. Longitudinal study of chronic sarcoidosis with low-dose maintenance corticosteroid therapy: outcome and complications. Ann NY Acad Sci 1986; 465:702–712.
9. Mayock RL, Bertrand P, Morrison CE et al. Manifestations of sarcoidosis: analysis of 145 patients, with a review of nine series selected from the literature. Am J Med 1963; 35:67–89.
10. Obenauf CD, Shaw HE, Sydnor CF et al. Sarcoidosis and its ophthalmic manifestations. Am J Ophthalmol 1978; 86:648–655.
11. Rosenberg AM, Yee EH, MacKenzie JW. Arthritis in childhood sarcoidosis. J Rheumatol 1983; 10:987–990.
12. Seamone CD, Nozik RA. Sarcoidosis and the eye. Ophthalmol Clin North Am 1992; 5:567–576.
13. Bain JG, Riley W, Logothetis J. Optic nerve manifestations of sarcoidosis. Arch Neurol 1965; 3:307–309.
14. Jabs DA, Houk JL, Bias WB et al. Familial granulomatous synovitis, uveitis, and cranial neuropathies. Am J Med 1985; 78:801–804.
15. Rose CD, Eichenfield AH, Goldsmith DP et al. Early-onset sarcoidosis with arthritis: "juvenile systemic granulomatosis?" J Rheumatol 1990; 17:102–106.
16. Scerri L, Cook LJ, Jenkins EA et al. Familial juvenile systemic granulomatosis (Blau's syndrome). Clin Exp Dermatol 1996; 21:445–448.
17. Latkany PA, Jabs DA Smith JR et al. Multifocal choroiditis in patients with juvenile systemic granulomatosis. Am J Ophthalmol 2002; 134:897–904.
18. Rossman MD, Thompson B, Frederick M et al. HLS-DRBI*1101: a significant risk factor for sarcoidosis in blacks and whites. Am J Hum Genet 2003; 73:720–735.
19. Crystal RG, Roberts WC, Hunninghake GW et al. Pulmonary sarcoidosis: a disease characterized and perpetuated by activated lung T-lymphocytes. Ann Intern Med 1981; 94:73–94.
20. Hunninghake GW, Crystal RG. Pulmonary sarcoidosis: a disorder mediated by excess helper T-lymphocyte activity at sites of disease activity. N Engl J Med 1981; 305:429–434.
21. Meyer KS, Kaminski MJ, Calhoun WJ et al. Studies of bronchoalveolar lavage cells and fluids in pulmonary sarcoidosis. I. Enhanced capacity of bronchoalveolar lavage cells from patients with pulmonary sarcoidosis to induce angiogenesis in vivo. Am Rev Respir Dis 1989; 140:1446–1449.
22. Buechner SA, Winkelmann RK, Banks PM. T-cell subsets in cutaneous sarcoidosis Arch Dermatol 1983; 119:728–732.
23. Chan CC, Wetzig RP, Palestine AG et al. Immunohistopathology of ocular sarcoidosis. Arch Ophthalmol 1987; 105:1398–1402.
24. Semenzato G, Agostini C, Zambello R et al. Activated T cells with immunoregulatory functions at different sites of involvement in sarcoidosis. Ann NY Acad Sci 1986; 465:56–73.
25. James DG. Ocular sarcoidosis. Ann NY Acad Sci 1986; 465:551–563.
26. Mana J, Marcoval J, Graells J et al. Cutaneous involvement in sarcoidosis: relationship to systemic disease. Arch Dermatol 1997; 133:882–888.
27. Zarei M, Anderson JR, Higgins JN et al. Cavernous sinus syndrome as the only manifestation of sarcoidosis. J Postgrad Med 2002; 48:119–121.
28. Delaney P. Neurologic manifestations in sarcoidosis. Ann Intern Med 1977; 87:336–345.
29. James DG, Zatouroff MA, Trowell J et al. Papilloedema in sarcoidosis. Br J Ophthalmol 1967; 51:526–529.
30. Sugo A, Seyama K, Yaguchi T et al. [Cardiac sarcoidosis with myopathy and advanced A-V nodal block in a woman with a previous diagnosis of sarcoidosis.] Nippon Kyobu Shikkan Gakkai Zasshi 1995; 33:1111–1118.
31. Green WR. Inflammatory diseases and conditions of the eye. In: Spencer WH, ed. Ophthalmic pathology: an atlas and textbook. Philadelphia, PA: WB Saunders; 1986.
32. Israel HL, Sones M. Selection of biopsy procedures for sarcoidosis diagnosis. Arch Intern Med 1964; 113:147–152.
33. Weinreb RN. Diagnosing sarcoidosis by transconjunctival biopsy of the lacrimal gland. Am J Ophthalmol 1984; 97:573–576.
34. Weinreb RN, Tessler H. Laboratory diagnosis of ophthalmic sarcoidosis. Surv Ophthalmol 1984; 28:653–664.

35. Baarsma GS, La Hey EL, Glasius E et al. The predictive value of serum angiotensin-converting enzyme and lysozyme levels in the diagnosis of ocular sarcoidosis. Am J Ophthalmol 1987; 104:211–217.

36. Rohatgi PK, Ryan JW, Lindeman P. Value of serial measurement of serum angiotensin-converting enzyme in the management of sarcoidosis. Am J Med 1981; 70:44–50.

37. Nosal A, Schleissner LA, Mishkin FS et al. Angiotensin-1-converting enzyme and gallium scan in noninvasive evaluation of sarcoidosis. Ann Intern Med 1979; 90:328–331.

38. Power WJ, Neves RA, Rodriguez A et al. The value of combined serum angiotensin-converting enzyme and gallium scan in diagnosing ocular sarcoidosis. Ophthalmology 1995; 102:2007–2011.

39. Hunter DG, Foster CS. Isolated ocular sarcoidosis: late development of systemic manifestations in uveitis patients. Invest Ophthalmol Vis Sci 1991; 32:681 (abstract).

40. Crick RP, Hoyle C, Smellie H. The eyes in sarcoidosis. Br J Ophthalmol 1961; 45:461–481.

41. Karma A, Huhti E, Poukkula A. Course and outcome of ocular sarcoidosis. Am J Ophthalmol 1988; 106:467–472.

42. Qazi FA, Thorne JE, Jabs DA. Scleral nodule associated with sarcoidosis. Am J Ophthalmol 2003; 136:752–754.

43. Collison JMT, Miller NR, Green WR. Involvement of orbital tissues by sarcoid. Am J Ophthalmol 1986; 102:302–307.

44. Faller M, Purohit A, Kennel N et al. Systemic sarcoidosis initially presenting as an orbital tumour. Eur Respir J 1996; 8:474–476.

45. Khan JA, Hoover DL, Giangiacomo J et al. Orbital and childhood sarcoidosis. J Pediatr Ophthalmol Strabismus 1986; 23:190–194.

46. Gentile RC, Berinstein DM, Liebmann J et al. High-resolution ultrasound biomicroscopy of the pars plana and peripheral retina. Ophthalmology 1998; 105:478–484.

47. Gass JD, Olson CL. Sarcoidosis with optic nerve and retinal involvement. Arch Ophthalmol 1976; 94:945–950.

48. Hoogstede HA, Cooper AC. A case of macular subretinal neo-vascularization in chronic uveitis probably caused by sarcoidosis. Br J Ophthalmol 1982; 66:530–535.

49. Sanders MD, Shilling JS. Retinal, choroidal, and optic disc involvement in sarcoidosis. Trans Ophthalmol Soc UK 1976; 96:140–144.

50. Letocha CE, Shields JA, Goldberg RE. Retinal changes in sarcoidosis. Can J Ophthalmol 1975; 10:184–192.

51. Kiryu J, Kita M, Tanabe T et al. Pars plana vitrectomy for cystoid macular edema secondary to sarcoid uveitis. Ophthalmology 2001; 108:1140–1144.

52. Kiruy J, Kita M, Tanabe T et al. Pars plana vitrectomy for epiretinal membrane associated with sarcoidosis. Jpn J Ophthalmol 2003; 47:479–483.

53. Sonoda KH, Enaida H, Ueno A et al. Pars plana vitrectomy assisted by triamcinolone acetonide for refractory uveitis: a case series study. Br J Ophthalmol 2003; 87:1010–1014.

54. Cheung CM, Durrani OM, Stavrou P. Peripapillary choroidal neovascularization in sarcoidosis. Ocul Immunol Inflamm 2002; 10:69–73.

55. Doxanas MT, Kelley JS, Prout TE. Sarcoidosis with neovascularization of the optic nerve head. Am J Ophthalmol 1980; 90:347–351.

56. Duker JS, Brown GC, McNamara JA. Proliferative sarcoid retinopathy. Ophthalmology 1988; 95:1680–1686.

57. Gould H, Kaufman HE. Sarcoid of the fundus. Arch Ophthalmol 1961; 65:453–456.

58. Spalton DJ, Sanders MD. Fundus changes in histologically confirmed sarcoidosis. Br J Ophthalmol 1981; 65:348–358.

59. Kelley JS, Green WR. Sarcoidosis involving the optic nerve head. Arch Ophthalmol 1973; 89:486–488.

60. Galetta S, Schatz NJ, Glaser JS. Acute sarcoid optic neuropathy with spontaneous recovery. J Clin Neuroophthalmol 1989; 9:27–32.

61. Ing EB, Garrity JA, Cross SA et al. Sarcoid masquerading as optic nerve sheath meningioma. Mayo Clin Proc 1997; 72:38–43.

62. Katz B. Disc edema, transient obscurations of vision, and a temporal fossa mass. Surv Ophthalmol 1991; 36:133–139.

63. Mansour AM. Sarcoid optic disc edema and optociliary shunts. J Clin Neuroophthalmol 1986; 6:47–52.

64. Mizuno K, Takahashi J. Sarcoid cyclitis. Ophthalmology 1986; 93:511–517.

65. Gedalia A, Molina JF, Ellis GS et al. Low-dose methotrexate therapy for childhood sarcoidosis. J Pediatr 1997; 130:25–29.

66. Kaye I, Palazzo E, Grossin M et al. Low-dose methotrexate: an effective corticosteroid-sparing agent in the musculoskeletal manifestations of sarcoidosis. Br J Rheumatol 1995; 34:642–644.

67. Lower EE, Baughman RP. Prolonged use of methotrexate for sarcoidosis. Arch Intern Med 1995; 155:846–851.

68. Mathur A, Kremer JM. Immunopathology, rheumatic features, and therapy of sarcoidosis. Curr Opin Rheumatol 1992; 4:76–80.

69. Dana MR, Merayo-Lloves J, Schaumberg DA et al. Prognosticators for visual outcome in sarcoid uveitis. Ophthalmology 1996; 103:1846–1853.

Chapter

104

Acute Multifocal Placoid Pigment Epitheliopathy

Alan C. Bird

Gass[1] described a condition with acute onset in which there are multiple pale lesions at the level of the retinal pigment epithelium, and rapid loss of central vision. Spontaneous resolution follows within 2 to 3 weeks, leaving discrete pigment epithelial scars. The disorder almost invariably affects both eyes, and occurs characteristically between the ages of 20 and 50 years.

SYMPTOMS

The patients usually experience rapid onset of visual loss that may be central or paracentral, depending on the site of the pigment epithelial lesions. Typically spontaneous recovery occurs within 3 weeks of the onset of disease. In an early report, 80% of patients had recovery of visual acuity to levels of 6/12 (20/40) or better.[2] In a series of 30 patients followed up for at least 1 year, Gass[1] found that only two of 59 eyes failed to attain a visual acuity of better than 20/30 (6/9).

Fundus appearance

The characteristic change seen in the fundus consists of multifocal yellow-white lesions at the level of the retinal pigment epithelium of the posterior pole (Fig. 104-1A). These are usually round and discrete. Within 1 week the opacification of the pigment epithelium appears to resolve, and within an additional 2 weeks, a well-defined scar replaces the original lesion. After onset of the original posterior pole lesions, further lesions may be seen in the peripheral fundus; new lesions are identified for up to 3 weeks after the initial symptoms. Peripheral lesions tend to be oval or linear, with the long axis oriented radially. Occasionally, patients have a single central lesion rather than multiple lesions, and in severe disease there appears to be a continuous involvement of the pigment epithelium over large areas of the fundi.

FLUORESCEIN ANGIOGRAPHY

The fluorescein angiographic appearance of placoid pigment epitheliopathy as originally described is quite characteristic: the lesions appear dark during the initial dye transit (Fig. 104-1B) but become hyperfluorescent later in the study (Fig. 104-1C). Occasionally, large choroidal vessels can be seen in the depths of the lesion (Fig. 104-2), although this is not always apparent.

In large areas of confluent involvement, solitary choriocapillaris lobules may be seen to be perfused (Fig. 104-3). In many cases the filling phase of the choroid appears to be prolonged (Fig. 104-4).

CLINICAL VARIATION IN DISEASE

Soon after the original description of the disorder, patients were described who had the retinal pigment epithelial lesions characteristic of acute placoid pigment epitheliopathy, but who also had serous detachment of the posterior retina[3] (Figs 104-4 and 104-5A). This contrasted with the account of Gass,[1] in which serous detachment of the retina was not evident. There is clearly some doubt as to whether it is legitimate to use the term "placoid pigment epitheliopathy" to describe cases in which there is serous detachment, a feature that was not present in the original patients. If it could be shown that patients with and without serous detachment had identical basic pathologic changes, or shared etiologic factors, it would be legitimate to amalgamate the conditions with apparent disparate clinical presentations into a single nosologic entity. Evidence has accumulated since that time to suggest a common pathogenic mechanism in such cases (see below).

The difficulty in diagnosis has been illustrated by a series of patients who appeared to form a continuum of disease.[4] In all patients there were multifocal lesions at the level of the retinal pigment epithelium, and evidence of abnormal perfusion of the choriocapillaris was seen at some stage during the evolution of the disorder (see Pathogenesis). Some patients had the typical appearance of placoid pigment epitheliopathy as described by Gass,[1] while others had serous detachment of the posterior retina. Patients without serous detachment all had spontaneous resolution of the disease.

Of those patients with detachment, some had self-limited disease, while in others resolution only occurred after treatment with corticosteroids. In patients who required treatment, recurrence was common. The only feature at presentation that was predictive of the likely outcome was the presence of optic nerve head disease in all patients who required treatment; this was absent in most patients who experienced spontaneous resolution. Systemic symptoms, such as headache and dysacusis, were also more common in those who required treatment. It is clear

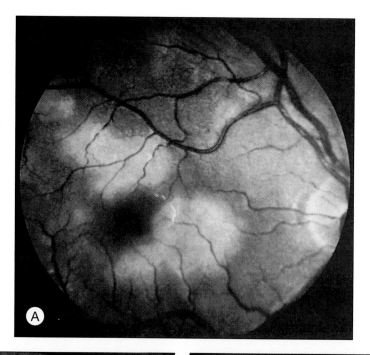

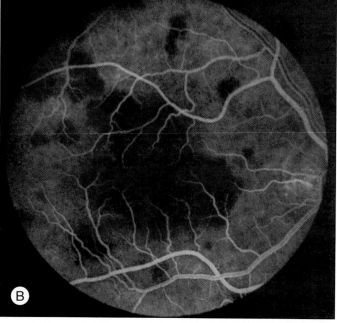

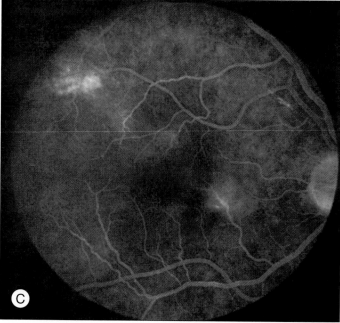

Fig. 104-1 A, Red-free photograph of multifocal opacification of retinal pigment epithelium (RPE) during the acute stage of placoid pigment epitheliopathy in a 36-year-old man. On fluorescein angiography the lesions are hypofluorescent early in the study (B), becoming hyperfluorescent late (C).

that these would fall into the category of Harada disease. The disorder in the others may represent a limited form of the same disease. However, the natural history, the lack of recurrence, and the lack of systemic symptoms are dissimilar from the pattern of disease usually associated with Harada disease, the natural history being more like that of placoid pigment epitheliopathy. Therefore, it is possible that the intermediate disorder represents a form of placoid pigment epitheliopathy that is associated with serous detachment.

Although it was initially believed that recurrent disease does not occur in placoid pigment epitheliopathy, recurrent attacks have been reported.[5-9] It is also evident that visual acuity may not recover well if the fovea is involved either in the initial attack or with recurrent disease.[10-14]

Pathogenesis

Gass[1] considered two possible explanations for the fluorescein angiographic appearance associated with the disorder: (1) that the choroid did not fill in the areas of swelling; or (2) that the swollen pigment epithelium obscured the choroidal fluorescence. In either case the late hyperfluorescence could have been caused by leakage of fluorescein from the perfused choroid into the

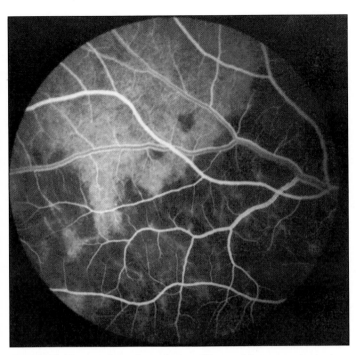

Fig. 104-2 Fluorescein angiography in a 19-year-old woman who had confluent disease in the posterior pole, showing hypofluorescence corresponding to the area of pigment epithelial pallor. Perfused major choroidal blood vessels can be seen in the depths of the lesion.

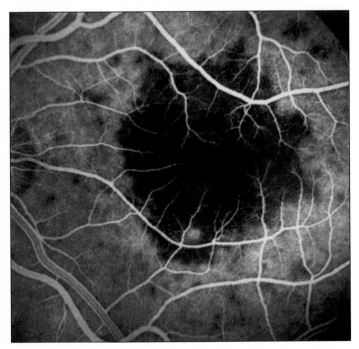

Fig. 104-3 A single hypofluorescent lesion at the macula in a 43-year-old man during the acute phase of disease. A choriocapillaris lobule appears to be perfused in the inferior part of the lesion, and perfusion of the surrounding choroid is slow.

diseased pigment epithelial cells. On the basis of evidence at that time it was not possible to distinguish between these alternatives with any confidence, but Gass favored primary pigment epithelial disease, possibly caused by infection, as the origin of

the disorder.[1] Other authors supported the theory that a virus is the causative agent.[15-17]

Van Buskirk and co-workers[18] were the first to report an ocular condition identical to acute posterior multifocal placoid pigment epitheliopathy occurring in a patient with manifest systemic vascular disease. This association, combined with prolonged choroidal filling shown by fluorescein angiography at some stage in the disorder (Figs 104-4 and 104-5), suggested to them that the ocular disease was caused by choroidal vascular obstruction. This view was supported by many authors who believed that the lesions represented focal infarcts of the retinal pigment epithelium caused by intrinsic choroidal vascular disease.

The most persuasive early evidence for abnormal choroidal perfusion was that reported by Deutman & Lion[19] who, using fluorescein angiography, demonstrated perfusion of major choroidal vessels underlying the placoid lesion (Fig. 104-2). They concluded that obscuration of the choroidal fluorescence could not fully account for the dark appearance during the dye transit, and suggested that the obstruction was at the level of the precapillary arterioles. However, some masking undoubtedly occurs, since large choroidal blood vessels cannot be seen in the depths of all lesions. The more recent findings using indocyanine green angiography support the concept that there is choroidal hypoperfusion.[20-25]

Choroidal ischemia

The concept of focal choroidal infarction would have been difficult to defend at a time when anatomic studies implied that the choriocapillaris was a continuous network of capillaries supplied by many arterioles.[26,27] However, Dollery and associates[28] showed that the choriocapillaris in pigs filled not as a continuous layer but as a series of dots that later enlarged to become uniform if the intraocular pressure were raised; they concluded that this pattern of filling indicated the presence of individual choriocapillaris units. Hayreh[29] demonstrated the lobular pattern of choriocapillaris filling in the posterior pole of normal animals. Other anatomic studies in normal eyes[30-32] have supported the conclusion that the lobules of the choriocapillaris in the submacular choroid are supplied by short, precapillary arterioles without functioning anastomosis between capillary units. This lobular arrangement is less well defined in the anterior choroid, in which there is a more direct capillary connection between the arteries and veins.[32]

The potential for choroidal ischemia was demonstrated in experimental occlusion of vessels at different levels. Hayreh & Baines[33,34] found that occlusion of the lateral short posterior ciliary arteries in the orbit resulted in nonperfusion of the temporal half of the choroid, with a watershed at the optic disc. The disturbance of blood supply was sufficient to produce infarcts of the pigment epithelium and outer retina that appeared as large oval patches in the posterior fundus or as triangular areas more peripherally; these areas stained with fluorescein late in the study and became atrophic during a period of 2 to 3 weeks. Within 2 weeks of the occlusion, the temporal choroid filled, but the filling was delayed and there was still some delay after 3 months. Their work demonstrated the presence of potential

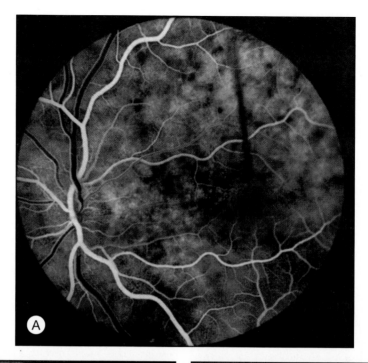

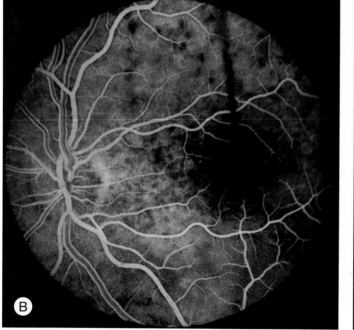

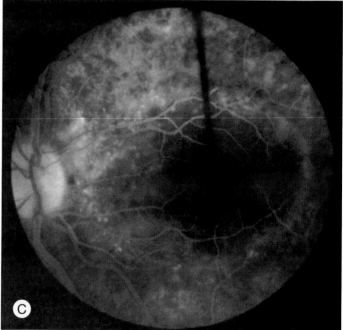

Fig. 104-4 A and B, Fluorescein angiograms of a 38-year-old woman who had posterior retinal detachment, showing a prolongation of choroid filling. C, In the late phase, fluorescein enters the subretinal space.

anastomotic channels that became functional after an acute arterial occlusion. Ernest et al.[30] have shown that this may occur more rapidly if the venous drainage of the choroid is also compromised.

Stern & Ernest[35] also identified changes in the retinal pigment epithelium and overlying retina after embolic occlusion of vessels within the choroid. Injection of embolic microspheres into the lateral short posterior ciliary arteries resulted in delayed choroidal filling, with spotty leakage through the retinal pigment epithe-

lium. Histological studies showed focal necrosis of the pigment epithelium and a concentration of microspheres at the posterior pole. Within 4 days, the entire choroid filled rapidly and simultaneously, and by 2 months the only detectable angiographic abnormality was hyperfluorescence corresponding to the small atrophic pigment epithelial defects. Retinal detachment accompanied these changes in the acute phase in animals with experimentally induced hypertension. The pattern of pigment epithelial infarction contrasted with that seen after occlusion of the short posterior ciliary arteries in that it was multifocal, but was seen only at the macula despite the widespread distribution of microspheres.

These experimental observations have their clinical counterparts. Amalric[36,37] and Foulds et al.[38] described triangular lesions of the retinal pigment epithelium in the peripheral fundus, and ascribed them to occlusion of a short ciliary artery.

Small multifocal infarcts similar to those reported by Stern & Ernest[35] are found in accelerated hypertension,[29,39–42] giant cell arteritis,[38,40] Goodpasture syndrome,[43] disseminated intravascular coagulopathy,[40,44] secondary syphilis[45] and, rarely, sickle-cell disease,[46] and are known or presumed to be caused by occlusion of the choroidal precapillary arterioles. In these conditions there is diffuse choroidal vascular disease that produces

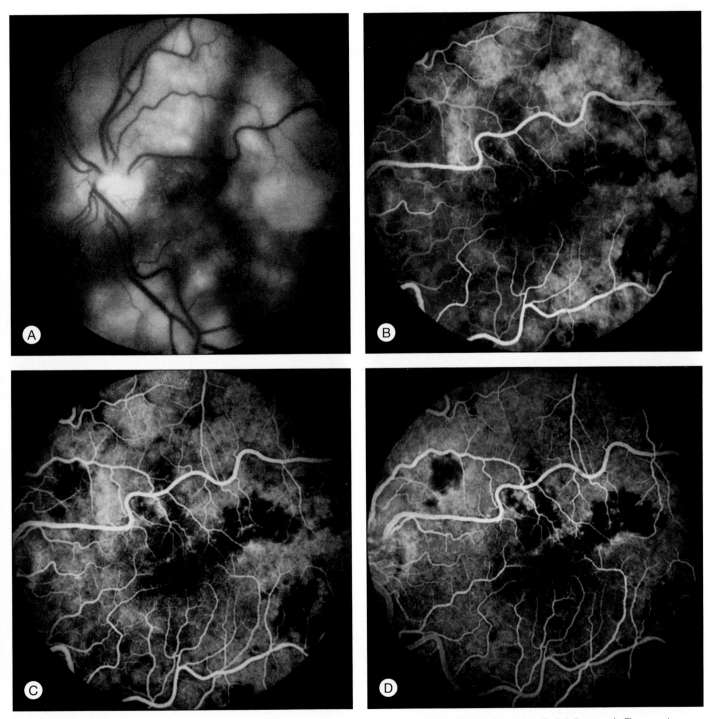

Fig. 104-5 A 42-year-old man presented with serous detachment of the posterior retina with multifocal pigment epithelial disease. A, Fluorescein angiography showed hyperfluorescence of the subretinal fluid in the late stage of the study. B and C, Within 5 days there was spontaneous reattachment of the retina, at which time angiography demonstrated slow choroidal filling and focal retinal pigment epithelial disturbance (D).

Continued

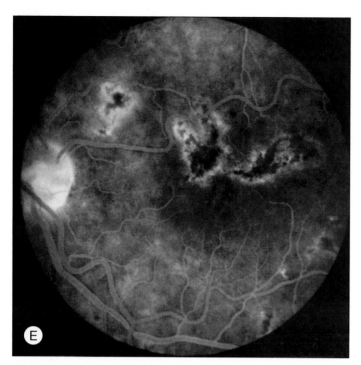

Fig. 104-5—cont'd E, Within an additional 7 days, focal pigment epithelial scars were evident.

clinical state in which choroidal hypoperfusion is sufficient to cause dysfunction of the pigment epithelium but not to induce atrophy. The evidence indicates that these patients have decreased choroidal perfusion, but the lack of focal scarring suggests that the overt manifestations are a product of ischemic dysfunction rather than of frank infarction of the retinal pigment epithelium. The likelihood of these patients having a common disorder is supported by one patient who had bullous retinal detachment initially, but who 1 week later had fundus changes indistinguishable from those of acute posterior multifocal placoid pigment epitheliopathy (Fig. 104-5). On recovery, the patient had well-defined retinal pigment epithelial scars in the posterior pole.

A small number of cases have been described with unilateral fundus changes,[7,50–52] but abnormal choroidal flow has been demonstrated by fluorescein angiography in the apparently normal fellow eye.[49] This is consistent with the previous finding that mild reduction of choroidal blood flow does not necessarily disrupt normal function.

Despite the variety of fundus appearances, there is sufficient evidence to indicate that the manifest disorders are produced by intrinsic choroidal vascular disease. The polymorphism may be caused by variations in the rapidity, completeness, and site and extent of the obstruction, which in turn may be determined by the nature of the basic disorder causing the obstruction.

ASSOCIATED FEATURES

Since the initial report, many associated ocular and systemic abnormalities have been described, including uveitis,[6,18,45,50,52–54] retinal vasculitis,[18,55] episcleritis,[7,50,52] cerebral vasculitis,[53,54,56] and erythema nodosum.[7,18,53] Headaches,[10,18,20,51,57] cerebrospinal fluid changes,[54,55,58,59] neurological deficit,[54,59] central diabetes insipidus,[60] and obstruction of cerebral blood vessels[18,54,59,61–65] have been described often enough to indicate that cerebrovascular inflammation associated with infarction is causally related to the ocular disorder. Cerebral infarction may occur during or several weeks after the retinal disease. Acute dysacusis and tinnitus have also been described in placoid pigment epitheliopathy,[66] making even more difficult the distinction of this disorder from Harada disease. The presence of ocular disease simulating placoid pigment epitheliopathy in patients with indicators of systemic vasculitis supports the general concept of the lesions being due to ischemia consequent upon arteriolar obstruction.[67–72]

ETIOLOGY

The precipitating causes of the choroidal perfusion abnormality have not yet been defined. In several cases there is good evidence that the disorder has followed a viral infection.[15]

Other reported associations include immunization,[67,73] streptococcal infection,[21,74] and Lyme disease.[75] The disorder has also been seen following treatment with antimicrobial medication, particularly ampicillin and sulfonamides.[3,12] In some instances the antimicrobial agent was prescribed for an upper respiratory tract infection, so two possible etiologic agents exist. On the other hand, in some cases the antibiotic was given for a distant bacterial

widespread arteriolar obstruction but only focal infarcts. It was noted by Gaudric and colleagues[40] that widespread perfusion defects could be demonstrated in eyes with normal fundus appearance, that those with retinal detachment had little pigment epithelial scarring, and that pigment epithelial infarction did not cause retinal detachment.

RELEVANCE TO PLACOID PIGMENT EPITHELIOPATHY

These observations are compatible with ischemia being the primary disorder in acute posterior multifocal placoid pigment epitheliopathy.[40]

In patients with small discrete lesions, the size of the swollen areas may be equivalent to a choriocapillaris lobule, and it is possible that these lesions are related to a single or collection of nonperfused lobules, as previously postulated by Hayreh & Baines,[29,33] even though angiography showed diffusely abnormal choroidal flow. The radial arrangement of lesions in the periphery is in accord with the putative organization of choroidal lobules.

The presence of a single confluent plaque of infarction (Fig. 104-3) could be ascribed to occlusion of a specific submacular vessel. However, the presence of such a vessel has been disputed,[2,27,29,47,48] and enlargement of the lesion in two cases, the diffuse abnormality of choroidal perfusion beyond the borders of the presumed infarct, and hyperfluorescence of the optic disc reflect the widespread nature of the disorder.[49]

The presence of serous detachments was the most obvious distinguishing feature in patients who sustained no pigment epithelial atrophy. This would correspond with the proposed infection,[3] in which case it is unlikely that the infective agent was responsible for the disorder. Many now believe that the choroidal vascular obstruction is immune-mediated, whether affecting the arteries or arterioles of the choroid, and can be precipitated by several agents.

Management

Since recovery of visual function is good in most patients, treatment does not appear to be indicated. If the disorder is on an immune basis, it is likely that the duration of the disease process could be shortened by corticosteroids. It seems justified to give steroids for a short time if the fovea is compromised and visual acuity is poor, although the effect of such treatment on the course of the disease is unproven. It is important that a potential precipitating agent be sought, since recurrent disease has been reported with the repeated intake of certain antimicrobial agents. If such an agent is unequivocally identified, further attacks may be prevented by avoiding the precipitating cause.

REFERENCES

1. Gass JDM. Acute posterior multifocal placoid pigment epitheliopathy. Arch Ophthalmol 1968; 80:177–185.
2. Heimann K. Zur Gefassentwicklung der macularen Aderhautzone. Klin Monatsbl Augenheilkd 1970; 157:636–642.
3. Bird AC, Hamilton AM. Placoid pigment epitheliopathy presenting with bilateral serous retinal detachment. Br J Ophthalmol 1972; 56:881–886.
4. Wright BE, Bird AC, Hamilton AM. Placoid pigment epitheliopathy and Harada's disease. Br J Ophthalmol 1978; 62:609–621.
5. Damato BE, Nanjiani M, Foulds WS. Acute posterior multifocal placoid pigment epitheliopathy; a follow up study. Trans Ophthalmol Soc UK 1983; 103:517–522.
6. Fitzpatrick PJ, Robertson DM. Acute posterior multifocal placoid pigment epitheliopathy. Arch Ophthalmol 1973; 89:373–376.
7. Gass JDM. Acute posterior multifocal placoid pigment epitheliopathy: a long term follow up. In: Fine SL, Owen SL, eds. Management of retinal vascular and macular disorders. Baltimore, MD: Williams & Wilkins; 1983:176–181.
8. Lewis RA, Martonyi CL. Acute posterior multifocal pigment epitheliopathy: a recurrence. Arch Ophthalmol 1975; 93:235–238.
9. Lyness AL, Bird AC. Recurrences of acute posterior multifocal placoid pigment epitheliopathy. Am J Ophthalmol 1984; 98:203–207.
10. Daniele S, Daniele C, Orcidi F et al. Progression of choroidal atrophy in acute posterior multifocal placoid pigment epitheliopathy. Ophthalmologica 1998; 212:66–72.
11. Foulds WS, Damato BE. Investigation and prognosis in the retinal pigment epitheliopathies. Aust NZ J Ophthalmol 1986; 14:301–311.
12. Jones BE, Jampol LM, Yannuzzi LA et al. Relentless placoid chorioretinitis: a new entity or an unusual variant of serpiginous chorioretinitis? Arch Ophthalmol 2000; 118:931–938.
13. Pagliarini S, Piguet B, Ffytche TJ et al. Foveal involvement and lack of visual recovery in APMPPE associated with uncommon features. Eye 1995; 9:42–47.
14. Saraux H, Pelosse B. Acute posterior multifocal placoid pigment epitheliopathy. A long-term follow-up. Ophthalmologica 1987; 194:161–163.
15. Azar P Jr, Gohd RS, Waltman D et al. Acute posterior multifocal placoid pigment epitheliopathy associated with an adenovirus type 5 infection. Am J Ophthalmol 1975; 80:1003–1005.
16. Fishman GA, Rabb MF, Kaplan J. Acute posterior multifocal placoid pigment epitheliopathy. Arch Ophthalmol 1974; 92:173–177.
17. Thomson SP, Roxburgh ST. Acute posterior multifocal placoid pigment epitheliopathy associated with adenovirus infection. Eye 2003; 17:542–544.
18. Van Buskirk EM, Lessell S, Friedman E. Pigmentary epitheliopathy and erythema nodosum. Arch Ophthalmol 1971; 85:369–372.
19. Deutman AF, Lion F. Choriocapillaris nonperfusion in acute multifocal placoid pigment epitheliopathy. Am J Ophthalmol 1977; 84:652–658.
20. Dhaliwal RS, Maguire AM, Flower RW et al. Acute posterior multifocal placoid pigment epitheliopathy. An indocyanine green angiographic study. Retina 1993; 13:317–325.
21. Howe LJ, Woon H, Graham EM et al. Choroidal hypoperfusion in acute posterior multifocal placoid pigment epitheliopathy. An indocyanine green angiography study. Ophthalmology 1995; 102:790–798.
22. Park D, Schatz H, McDonald HR et al. Indocyanine green angiography of acute multifocal posterior placoid pigment epitheliopathy. Ophthalmology 1995; 102:1877–1883.
23. Scheider A. Indozyaningrunangiographie mit einem infrarot-scanning-laser-ophthalmoskop. Erste klinische Erfahrungen. Ophthalmologe 1992; 89:27–33.
24. Schneider U, Inhoffen W, Gelisken F. Indocyanine green angiography in a case of unilateral recurrent posterior acute multifocal placoid pigment epitheliopathy. Ophthalmol Scand 2003; 81:72–75.
25. Stanga PE, Lim JI, Hamilton P. Indocyanine green angiography in chorioretinal diseases: indications and interpretation: an evidence-based update. Ophthalmology 2003; 110:15–21.
26. Ring HG, Fujino T. Observations on the anatomy and pathology of the choroidal vasculature. Arch Ophthalmol 1967; 78:431–444.
27. Wybar KC. Vascular anatomy of the choroid in relation to selective localization of ocular diseases. Br J Ophthalmol 1954; 38:513–527.
28. Dollery CT, Henkind P, Kohner EM et al. Effect of raised intraocular pressure on the retinal and choroidal circulation. Invest Ophthalmol 1968; 7:191–198.
29. Hayreh SS. Recent advances in fluorescein fundus angiography. Br J Ophthalmol 1974; 58:391–412.
30. Ernest JT, Stern WH, Archer DB. Submacular choroidal circulation. Am J Ophthalmol 1976; 81:574–582.
31. Torczynski E, Tso MOM. The architecture of the choriocapillaris of the posterior pole. Am J Ophthalmol 1976; 81:428–440.
32. Yoneya S, Tso MOM. Angioarchitecture of the human choroids. Arch Ophthalmol 1987; 105:681–687.
33. Hayreh SS, Baines JAB. Occlusion of the posterior ciliary artery. I. Effects on choroidal circulation. Br J Ophthalmol 1972; 56:719–735.
34. Hayreh SS, Baines JAB. Occlusion of the posterior ciliary artery. II. Chorioretinal lesions. Br J Ophthalmol 1972; 56:736–753.
35. Stern WH, Ernest JT. Microsphere occlusion of the choriocapillaris in rhesus monkeys. Am J Ophthalmol 1974; 78:438–448.
36. Amalric P. L'examen clinique des arteres ciliaires courtes posterieures. Note preliminaire. Bull Soc Ophthalmol Fr 1968; 68:562–567.
37. Amalric P. Acute choroidal ischaemia. Trans Ophthalmol Soc UK 1971; 91:305–324.
38. Foulds WS, Lee WR, Taylor WOG. Clinical and pathological aspects of choroidal ischaemia. Trans Ophthalmol Soc UK 1971; 91:325–343.
39. Friedman E, Smith TR, Kuwabara T et al. Choroidal vascular patterns in hypertension. Arch Ophthalmol 1964; 71:842–850.
40. Gaudric A, Coscas G, Bird AC. Choroidal ischemia. Am J Ophthalmol 1982; 94:489–498.
41. Gitter KA, Houser BP, Sarin LK et al. Toxemia of pregnancy: an angiographic interpretation of fundus changes. Arch Ophthalmol 1968; 80:449–454.
42. Klien BA. Ischemic infarcts of the choroid (Elschnig spots): a cause of retinal separation in hypertensive disease with renal insufficiency. A clinical and histopathologic study. Am J Ophthalmol 1968; 66:1069–1074.
43. Jampol LM, Lahav M, Albert DM et al. Ocular clinical findings and basement membrane changes in Goodpasture's syndrome. Am J Ophthalmol 1975; 79:452–463.
44. Cogan DG. Ocular involvement in disseminated intravascular coagulopathy. Arch Ophthalmol 1975; 93:1–8.
45. Gass JD, Braunstein RA, Chenoweth RG. Acute syphilitic posterior placoid chorioretinitis. Ophthalmology 1990; 97:1288–1297.
46. Condon PI, Serjeant GR, Ikeda H. Unusual chorioretinal degeneration in sickle cell disease: possible sequelae of posterior ciliary vessel occlusion. Br J Ophthalmol 1973; 57:81–88.
47. Shimizu K. Segmental nature of angioarchitecture of the choroid. In: Shimizu K, Oosterhuis JA, eds. Ophthalmology. Amsterdam: Excerpta Medica; 1979:215–219.
48. Weiter JJ, Ernest JT. Anatomy of the choroidal vasculature. Am J Ophthalmol 1974; 78:583–590.
49. Young NJA, Bird AC, Sehmi K. Pigment epithelial diseases with abnormal choroidal perfusion. Am J Ophthalmol 1980; 90:607–618.
50. Annesley WH, Tomer TL, Shields JA. Multifocal placoid pigment epitheliopathy. Am J Ophthalmol 1973; 76:511–518.
51. Ryan SJ, Maumenee AE. Acute posterior multifocal placoid pigment epitheliopathy. Am J Ophthalmol 1972; 74:1066–1074.
52. Savino PJ, Weinberg RJ, Yassin JG et al. Diverse manifestations of acute posterior multifocal placoid pigment epitheliopathy. Am J Ophthalmol 1974; 77:659–662.
53. Deutman AF, Oosterhuis JA, Boen-tan TN et al. Acute posterior multifocal placoid pigment epitheliopathy. Br J Ophthalmol 1972; 56:863–874.
54. Holt WS, Regan CDJ, Trempe C. Acute posterior multifocal placoid pigment epitheliopathy. Am J Ophthalmol 1976; 81:403–412.
55. Kirkham TH, Ffytche TJ, Sanders MD. Placoid pigment epitheliopathy with retinal vasculitis and papillitis. Br J Ophthalmol 1972; 56:875–880.
56. Stoll G, Reiners K, Schwartz A et al. Acute posterior multifocal placoid pigment epitheliopathy with cerebral involvement. J Neurol Neurosurg Psychiatry 1991; 54:77–79.

57. Reuscher A. Zur Pathogenese der sogenannten akuten hinteren multifokalen placoiden Pigmentepitheliopathie. Klin Monatsbl Augenheilkd 1974; 165:775–784.

58. Fishman GA, Baskin M, Jednock N. Spinal fluid pleocytosis in acute posterior multifocal placoid pigment epitheliopathy. Ann Ophthalmol 1977; 9:33–36.

59. Sigelman J, Behrens M, Hilal S. Acute posterior multifocal placoid pigment epitheliopathy associated with cerebral vasculitis and homonymous hemianopia. Am J Ophthalmol 1979; 88:919–924.

60. Watanabe A, Ishii R, Hirano K et al. Central diabetes insipidus caused by non-specific chronic inflammation of the hypothalamus: case report. Surg Neurol 1994; 42:70–73.

61. Althaus C, Unsold R, Figge C et al. Cerebral complications in acute posterior multifocal placoid pigment epitheliopathy. Germ J Ophthalmol 1993; 2:150–154.

62. Bewermeyer H, Nelles G, Huber M et al. Pontine infarction in acute posterior multifocal placoid pigment epitheliopathy. J Neurol 1993; 241:22–26.

63. Bodiguel E, Benhamou A, Le-Hoang P et al. Infarctus cerebral, epitheliopathie en plaques et sarcoidose. Rev Neurol Paris 1992; 148:746–751.

64. Comu S, Verstraeten T, Rinkoff JS et al. Neurological manifestations of acute posterior multifocal placoid pigment epitheliopathy. Stroke 1996; 27:996–1001.

65. O'Halloran HS, Berger JR, Lee WB et al. Acute multifocal placoid pigment epitheliopathy and central nervous system involvement: nine new cases and a review of the literature. Ophthalmology 2001; 108:861–868.

66. Clearkin LG, Hung SO. Acute posterior multifocal placoid pigment epiliopathy associated with transient hearing loss. Trans Ophthalmol Soc UK 1983; 103:562–564.

67. Bouchenaki N, Cimino L, Auer C et al. Assessment and classification of choroidal vasculitis in posterior uveitis using indocyanine green angiography. Klin Monatsbl Augenheilkd 2002; 219:243–249.

68. Chiquet C, Lumbroso L, Denis P et al. Acute posterior multifocal placoid pigment epitheliopathy associated with Wegener's granulomatosis. Retina 1999; 19:309–313.

69. Floegel I, Haas A, El-Shabrawi Y. Acute-multifocal placoid pigment epitheliopathy-like lesions as an early presentation of subacute sclerosing panencephalopathy. Am J Ophthalmol 2003; 135:103.

70. Matamoros N, Julia MR, Pallares L et al. Acute posterior multifocal placoid epitheliopathy and antineutrophil cytoplasmic antibodies. A frequent association? Med Clin (Barc) 2001; 117:238.

71. Matsuo T, Horikoshi T, Nagai C. Acute posterior multifocal placoid pigment epitheliopathy and scleritis in a patient with pANCA-positive systemic vasculitis. Am J Ophthalmol 2002; 133:566–568.

72. Uthman I, Najjar DM, Kanj SS et al. Anticardiolipin antibodies in acute multifocal posterior placoid pigment epitheliopathy. Ann Rheum Dis 2003; 62:687–688.

73. Brezin AP, Massin-Korobelnik P, Boudin M et al. Acute posterior multifocal placoid pigment epitheliopathy after hepatitis B vaccine. Arch Ophthalmol 1996; 113:297–300.

74. Lowder CY, Foster RE, Gordon SM et al. Acute posterior multifocal placoid pigment epitheliopathy after acute group A streptococcal infection. Am J Ophthalmol 1996; 22:115–117.

75. Bodine SR, Marino J, Camisa TJ et al. Multifocal choroiditis with evidence of Lyme disease. Ann Ophthalmol 1992; 24:169–173.

Chapter

105

Serpiginous Choroiditis

J. Michael Jumper
H. Richard McDonald
Robert N. Johnson
Everett Ai
Arthur D. Fu

Serpiginous choroiditis, also called geographic helicoid peripapillary choroidopathy or geographic choroiditis, is a rare, usually bilateral, chronically recurring inflammatory disease of unknown cause that primarily involves the choroid and retinal pigment epithelium (RPE).[1-8] Most patients affected by this disease are middle-aged or older,[7] but serpiginous choroiditis can occur in younger patients.[8] While the majority of patients reported with this disease are white, serpiginous choroiditis has been noted in blacks,[8] Asians,[9,10] and Hispanics.[11] There is a slight male predominance in the case series reported to date. Serpiginous choroiditis appears to be a purely ocular disease, with no systemic manifestations or association with drugs, trauma, or allergy.[4] There is no known familial propensity.

PRESENTATION

This condition is generally asymptomatic until the macula is affected.[1,3,8] Initially, patients may have only one eye affected, whereas the other eye shows no changes. Occasionally, patients are not even aware of decreased vision in one eye until the disease involves the fellow eye. Vision may become severely decreased depending on the degree of foveal involvement.[1,3] Intraocular pressure tends to be normal, and results of external and slit-lamp examinations are usually normal, although a nongranulomatous anterior-chamber inflammatory reaction is occasionally seen.[12] In addition, the vitreous contains cells in one-fourth to one-third of patients.

CLINICAL FINDINGS

The acute lesion is at the level of the RPE or inner choroid and has a grayish-yellow, fuzzy appearance[7] (Figs 105-1D and 105-2A). It is usually geographic in shape, with distinct borders that seem to glow (Fig. 105-3A) because of the light border that dramatically demarcates the leading edge of the lesion from normal tissue. Active lesions usually emanate from the optic nerve head with fingerlike polypoid extensions spreading outward in a serpentine fashion. Active lesions may occur in more than one area, and skipped areas (Fig. 105-4D) are not uncommon.[2] Within a few weeks the grayish lesion becomes pale and eventually atrophies (Fig. 105-2F). Fibrous scar tissue and loss of choroidal tissue (Fig. 105-5) can be seen in older lesions, along with marked pigment epithelial hyperplasia adjacent to areas of atrophy.[2]

The active, acute gray lesions extend outward, often in a serpentine fashion, beyond the older, chronic scars. An eye that has been severely affected may show lesions emanating from the optic nerve head with finger-like extensions spreading in a helicoid fashion out to the equator and affecting large parts of the fundus (Figs 105-4 and 105-6). Lesions may either skip or circumvent the central fovea (Fig. 105-4, A to D). Macular serpiginous choroiditis represents a variant of the disease in which the typical lesions are located initially or exclusively in the macular region[5,11] (Fig. 105-1D). These lesions may grow not only toward the disc (Fig. 105-2D), but also peripherally.[8] Individuals with macular serpiginous choroiditis may have a poorer visual prognosis, and accurate diagnosis and prompt treatment are paramount.

Choroidal neovascularization (CNV) may occur in association with serpiginous choroiditis lesions[1,13-15] (Fig. 105-1). Therefore it is essential to determine accurately the cause of recent visual loss in a patient with known serpiginous choroiditis. One must decide whether a new juxtafoveal or foveal lesion is caused by fresh inflammation, and therefore amenable to steroid treatment, or is caused by CNV,[13,14] and possibly amenable to laser therapy. CNV usually emanates from an older or subacute lesion rather than from an acute one. Hemorrhage and exudate do not occur in association with active inflammatory lesions but are common with CNV. Fluorescein and possibly indocyanine green (ICG) angiography helps to distinguish between these two entities.

Other associated findings include anterior uveitis, cystoid macular edema,[16] retinal vasculitis (most often phlebitis),[8,17] (Fig. 105-3D), branch vein occlusion,[1,17] sensory retinal detachment,[3] RPE detachment,[18] and optic disc and retinal neovascularization.[1,14,18] The optic nerve is otherwise usually normal.

Recurrent attacks are the rule and can occur weeks, months, or even years after the initial attack[5] (Fig. 105-2). The recurrent inflammatory episodes tend to involve larger and larger areas of the fundus (Figs 105-3, 105-4, and 105-6). Asymptomatic recurrence has been noted in up to one-third of patients.[8]

Disease pattern and level of activity in one eye do not generally correspond to changes in the fellow eye. One eye may have an acute macular lesion, whereas the other may have a peripapillary lesion.[5] Likewise, one eye may have CNV, whereas the other may have only acute inflammatory changes (Fig. 105-1).

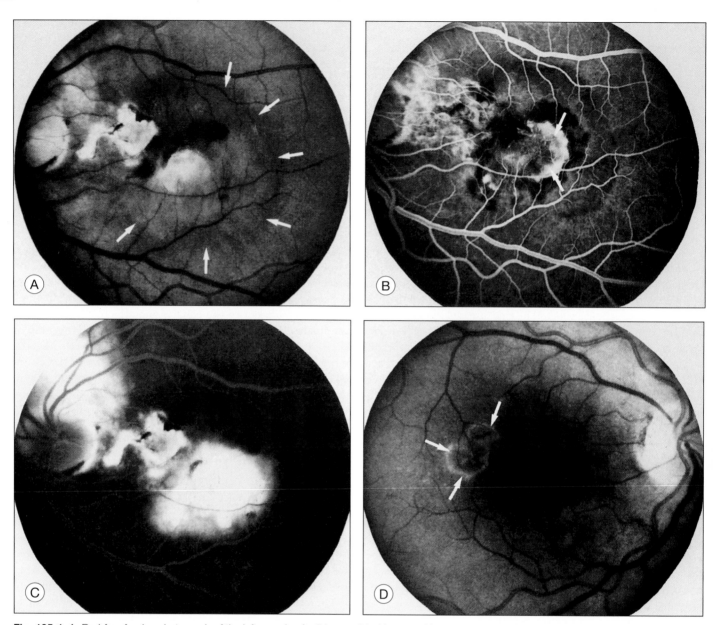

Fig. 105-1 A, Red-free fundus photograph of the left macula of a 54-year-old white man. Note sensory detachment of the macula (arrows), subretinal hemorrhage centrally, and a geographic scar in the papillomacular bundle. B, Arteriovenous-phase fluorescein angiogram of the left macula. Note the patch of subretinal neovascularization in the central macula (arrows). The geographic lesion is in the papillomacular bundle. C, Late arteriovenous-phase fluorescein angiogram of the left macula. Note staining of the geographic lesion in the papillomacular bundle and fuzzy fluorescence of the subretinal neovascularization in the macula, which is leaking fluorescein under the sensory retinal detachment of the macula. D, Red-free fundus photograph of the right macula. The small, active inflammatory geographic lesion just temporal to the macula has "glowing" acute inflammatory edges (arrows).

The visual fields usually correspond to the appearance of the lesions. Patients can usually draw scotomata corresponding exactly to the lesions in their fundi, making Amsler grid testing an excellent means of both monitoring and assessing treatment response in patients with serpiginous choroiditis.

Results of electrophysiologic tests are generally normal, although in extremely severe cases in which large areas of the fundus are affected, an abnormal electroretinogram or abnormal electro-oculogram may be recorded.[2]

Fluorescein angiography findings

The early phase of the fluorescein angiogram of an acute lesion usually shows hypofluorescence[7] (Figs 105-2 to 105-4). Later in the angiogram, the acute lesions fluoresce in a soft, fuzzy fashion, indicating acute inflammatory activity. The fluorescence usually starts from the edge of the lesion and spreads inward. The angiogram is quite typical, showing the total picture of "fingers" of affected tissue. This contrasts with the fluorescence of CNV, which shows lacy, irregular, and nodular hyperfluorescence in early-phase photos (Fig. 105-1B).

Old or acute lesions hypofluoresce because the choriocapillaris, and often the choroid, have been destroyed. Occasionally, large choroidal vessels can be seen coursing through old areas of inflammation (Fig. 105-5). Late hyperfluorescent staining of fibrous scar tissue within old lesions is also commonly seen.

Indocyanine green angiography findings

If the disease is acute, zones of active inflammation show marked hypofluorescence throughout all phases of the ICG angiography study (Fig. 105-7). This hypofluorescence could represent either an abnormality at the level of the choroidal vessels or increased intravascular resistance at the level of the choriocapillaris resulting from a relative deficit of choroidal perfusion. Although this suggests the presence of vascular occlusion in the choroid, it is unknown whether this change is primary or secondary to the inflammatory process. In addition, it is possible that the hypofluorescence of active lesions could result from a combination of choroidal nonperfusion and blockage by exudation or edema at the level of the outer retina, RPE, and choriocapillaris. There may also be localized areas of hyperfluorescence outside these areas. These latter lesions do not correspond to any clinically visible changes of the retina, RPE, or choroid and could represent areas

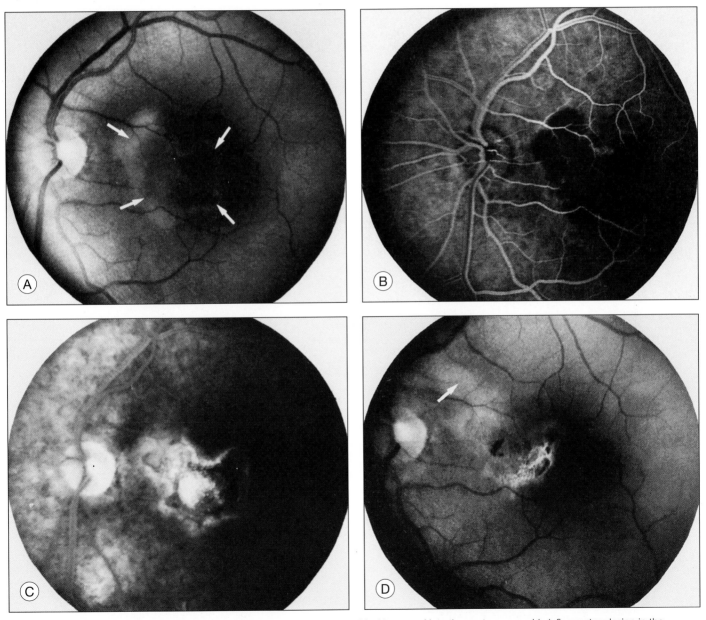

Fig. 105-2 A, Red-free fundus photograph of the left macula of a 50-year-old white man. Note the acute geographic inflammatory lesion in the macula and papillomacular bundle (arrows). B, Early arteriovenous-phase fluorescein angiogram of the left macula. Note hypofluorescence of the acute inflammatory lesion. C, Late-phase fluorescein angiogram of the left macula. Note staining of the acute inflammatory lesion. D, Red-free fundus photograph of the left macula 4 months later. Note the scarring of the older geographic lesion in the macula and the fresh inflammatory lesion (arrow) extending superonasal from the macula in the upper part of the papillomacular bundle.

Continued

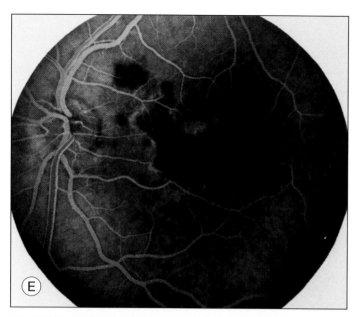

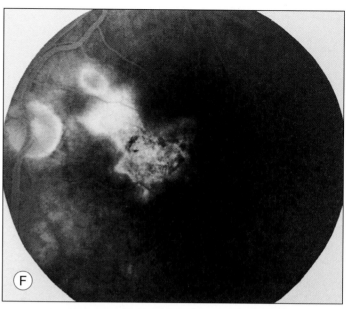

Fig. 105-2—cont'd E, Arteriovenous-phase fluorescein angiogram of the left macula. Note new acute lesions in the upper part of the papillomacular bundle. F, Late-phase fluorescein angiogram of the left macula. Note mild staining of the old inflammatory lesion in the macula and more intense fluorescent staining of the new inflammatory lesion in the upper part of the papillomacular bundle.

of subclinical choroidal inflammation.[19] In any event, ICG angiography usually reveals a larger zone of involvement than can be seen on fluorescein angiography. Giovannini and co-workers have proposed a classification system based on the combination of fluorescein angiography and ICG findings which includes a subclinical or choroidal stage consisting of ICG hypofluorescence without fluorescein angiography changes.[20]

DIFFERENTIAL DIAGNOSIS

A number of inflammatory diseases can mimic serpiginous choroiditis.[21] The condition that most resembles serpiginous choroiditis is acute multifocal posterior placoid pigment epitheliopathy (AMPPPE). Although AMPPPE can affect only one eye, with the fellow eye unaffected until a later date, in most instances both eyes are affected at the same time. In addition,

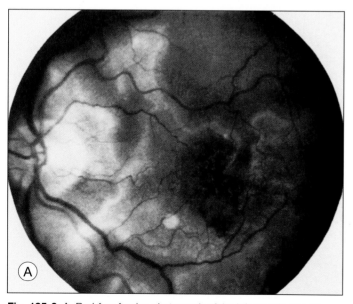

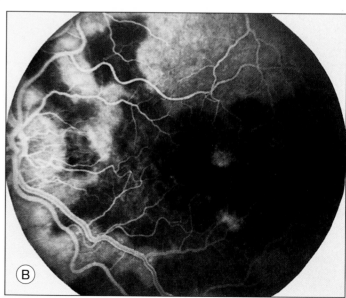

Fig. 105-3 A, Red-free fundus photograph of the left macula of a 51-year-old white man. An extensive acute geographic inflammatory lesion extends from the optic nerve head and involves much of the central, lower, and temporal macula, as well as the upper part of the papillomacular bundle. The only area seemingly not involved is the upper macula. B, Early arteriovenous-phase fluorescein angiogram of the left macula. Note hypofluorescence of the acute inflammatory lesion in the macula and papillomacular bundle.

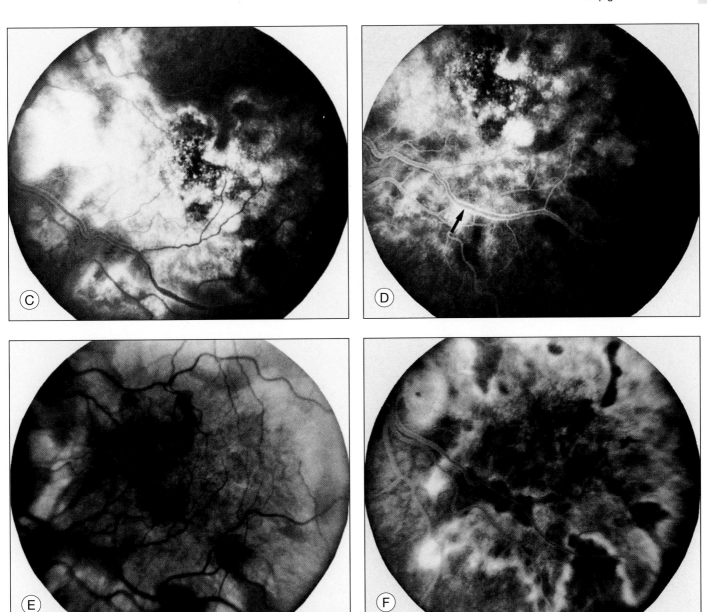

Fig. 105-3—cont'd C, Late-phase fluorescein angiogram of the left macula. Note staining of the geographic lesion in the macula. D, Note leakage of the retinal vein below the macula (phlebitis, arrow) overlying the acute inflammatory lesion. E, Red-free fundus photograph of the left macula 1 year later. The acute inflammatory geographic lesion in the upper part of the macula has extended to involve the entire macular area. Vision has been markedly reduced. F, Fluorescein angiogram of the left macula. There is extensive involvement of the entire macular and papillomacular bundle area.

AMPPPE does not usually recur; if it does, it is usually within the first few weeks or months of its initial presentation. Recurrences of AMPPPE do not happen over the course of years, as in serpiginous choroiditis. Finally, permanent vision loss in AMPPPE is unusual.

The shape of the lesion in serpiginous choroiditis is different from that in AMPPPE. In AMPPPE the lesions tend to be oval or irregularly round and somewhat separate from one another, only irregularly attaching. They are usually randomly distributed over the entire posterior pole. AMPPPE usually affects younger patients, whereas serpiginous choroiditis affects older individuals. A history of pre-existing viral upper respiratory tract infection

can often be elicited from patients with AMPPPE; this does not occur with serpiginous choroiditis. Severe choroidal scarring is rare with AMPPPE but is frequently seen with serpiginous choroiditis. Once the fovea is involved in serpiginous choroiditis, visual acuity rarely recovers. However, complete recovery is common with AMPPPE. Finally, whereas CNV has been seen with AMPPPE, it is quite rare.

Other conditions that can mimic serpiginous choroiditis include those that cause peripapillary CNV with scarring, such as ocular histoplasmosis, macular degeneration, or angioid streaks. Outer retinal toxoplasmosis may appear similar to serpiginous choroiditis. Other inflammatory conditions of the choroid, such as posterior

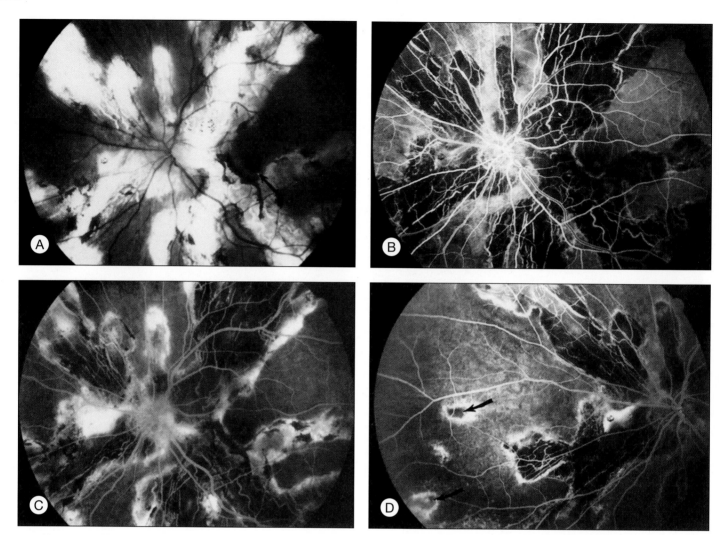

Fig. 105-4 A, Red-free fundus photograph of the left posterior pole of a 40-year-old white man. Large geographic areas of atrophy extend in a propeller-like fashion from the optic nerve head. The lesion just skips the left fovea (arrow). Note also the pigment epithelial hyperplasia. B, Early arteriovenous-phase fluorescein angiogram of the left posterior pole. Lesions show large choroidal vessels but no choriocapillaris; these are old lesions with absent choriocapillaris and pigment epithelium. C, Later arteriovenous-phase fluorescein angiogram of the left posterior pole. There is staining along the edges of the lesions. D, Late arteriovenous-phase fluorescein angiogram of the left nasal mid-periphery. Lesions extend out from the disc. Unattached lesions (arrows) show skipped areas.

scleritis,[22] recurrent multifocal choroiditis, or sarcoidosis,[23] can also imitate serpiginous choroiditis. Infiltrative lesions of the choroid, including non-Hodgkin's lymphoma,[24] metastatic tumor, or choroidal osteoma, can also imitate some aspects of serpiginous choroiditis. Finally, some end-stage hereditary retinal dystrophies may mimic the chorioretinal atrophic change seen in longstanding cases of serpiginous choroiditis.

PATHOLOGY OF SERPIGINOUS CHOROIDITIS

The etiology of serpiginous choroiditis is not known, although it is believed to be a chronic, recurring multifocal choroiditis (perhaps nongranulomatous)[3,15] that primarily affects the inner choroid and RPE and, secondarily, the retina. King et al.[25] reported that factor VIII–von Willebrand factor antigen levels are elevated

in serpiginous choroiditis, and this may indicate an occlusive vascular phenomenon involving the choroid.

Wu et al.[15] reported the clinicopathologic findings in an eye of a patient who had features typical of serpiginous choroiditis. There was a diffuse and focal infiltrate of lymphocytes in the choroid with a larger aggregate of lymphocytes at the margin of the lesions. There was a loss of overlying RPE and photoreceptor cells. Most of the margins of the lesions had a variable degree of hyperplastic RPE. Some had breaks in Bruch's membrane through which fibroglial tissue extended.[15]

TREATMENT

Treatment for serpiginous choroiditis includes therapy for the underlying inflammation as well as the vision-threatening side-

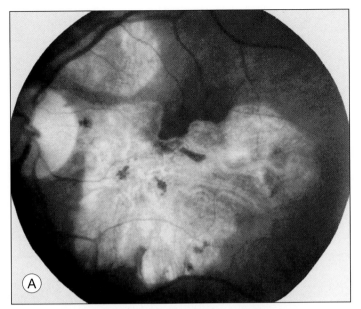

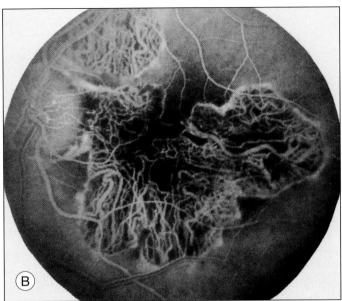

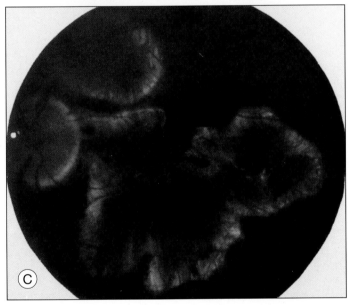

Fig. 105-5 A, Red-free fundus photograph of the left macula of a 51-year-old white man. The atrophic geographic lesion extends from the optic nerve head and involves the central, temporal, and lower parts of the macula. B, Arteriovenous-phase fluorescein angiogram. The choriocapillaris and pigment epithelium are gone, as evidenced by the visibility of large choroidal vessels within the lesion. C, Late-phase fluorescein angiogram of the left macula. Note staining along the edges of the geographic lesion.

effects such as CNV and cystoid macular edema. The rarity of serpiginous choroiditis makes proper study of treatment difficult. As current evidence suggests that this disease is immune-mediated, anti-inflammatory and immunosuppressive agents have been most commonly used. Reports on the efficacy of corticosteroids in the form of oral prednisone or periocular injection of triamcinolone acetonide are mixed. While some authors have observed a rapid resolution of inflammatory changes,[5] others have found little objective evidence that corticosteroids affect either early or long-term improvement over the natural history of this disease.[2,6] Intravitreal triamcinolone acetonide has been reported as therapy for other choroidal inflammatory diseases.[26] The potential role of this form of steroid delivery in serpiginous choroiditis is as yet unknown.

Clinicians have also used immunosuppressive chemotherapy, including antibiotics (cyclosporin), antimetabolites (azathioprine), and alkylating agents (cyclophosphamide, chlorambucil), typically in conjunction with corticosteroids. Conflicting data exist regarding the use of cyclosporin combined with oral prednisone but one long-term study suggests that disease control and remission after therapy is discontinued are possible.[27–29] An immunosuppressive regimen which included prednisone, cyclosporin, and azathioprine was reported to control inflammation rapidly and improve vision but in two of five patients there was immediate recurrence upon discontinuation of treatment.[30] Akpek and colleagues have used alkylating agents, either cyclophosphamide or chlorambucil, which led to drug-free remission in 7 of 9 patients.[31]

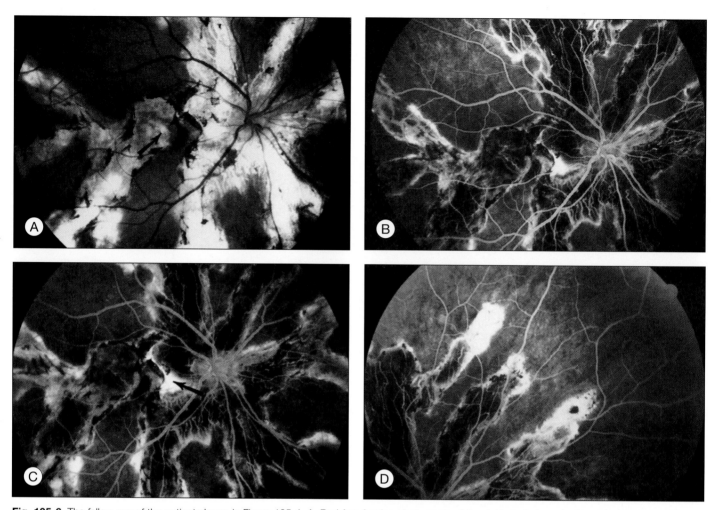

Fig. 105-6 The fellow eye of the patient shown in Figure 105-4. A, Red-free fundus photograph of the right posterior pole. Large lesions extend from the optic nerve head and involve the macula (arrow). This eye had a marked reduction in visual acuity. Note the scarring and pigment epithelial hyperplasia. B, Arteriovenous-phase fluorescein angiogram of the right posterior pole. Large choroidal vessels within lesions show that the choriocapillaries and pigment epithelium are gone. There is hyperfluorescence along the edges of the lesions. C, Late arteriovenous-phase fluorescein angiogram of the posterior pole, right fundus. There is early staining along the edges of the lesion and staining of the fibrous scar (arrow). D, Late arteriovenous-phase fluorescein angiogram of the right eye, superonasal area. Note the finger-like projections extending toward the mid-periphery.

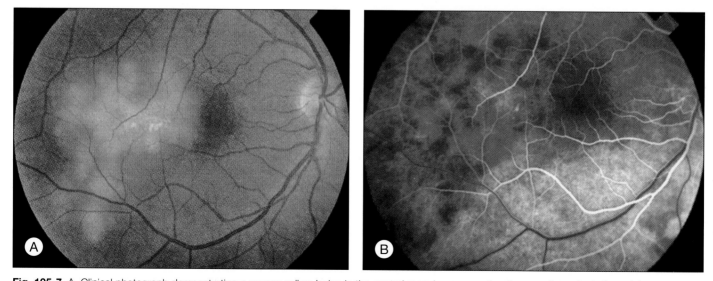

Fig. 105-7 A, Clinical photograph demonstrating a creamy yellow lesion in the central macula, representing the macular variant of serpiginous choroidopathy. B, Early-phase fluorescein study demonstrating hypofluorescence of the acute lesion. The margins of the lesion are not well demarcated.

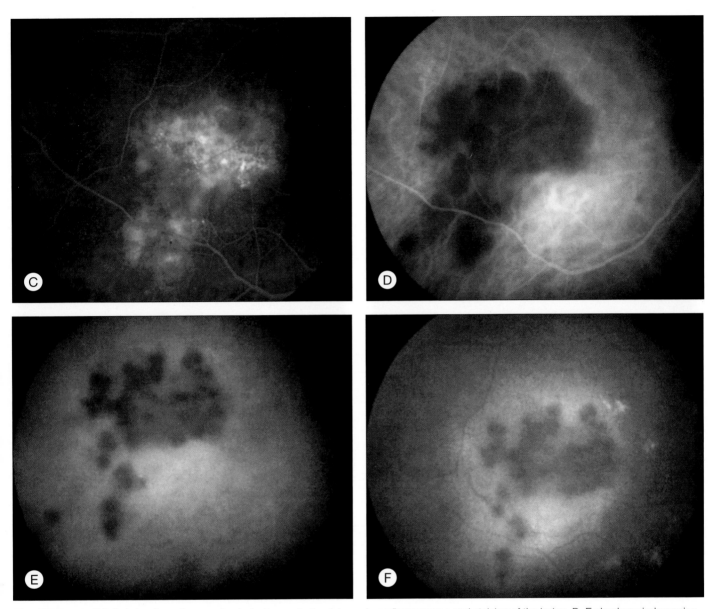

Fig. 105-7—cont'd C, Late-phase fluorescein study demonstrating intense hyperfluorescence and staining of the lesion. D, Early-phase indocyanine green (ICG) study demonstrating marked hypofluorescence of the lesion. Overlying retinal vessels are visualized, but all detail of the underlying choroidal vasculature is lost. E, Late-phase ICG study demonstrating persistent hypofluorescence and well-demarcated margins of the lesion. F, Very-late-phase ICG study demonstrating persistent hypofluorescence of the lesion and a halo of hyperfluorescence along its margin. Also note the focal, intense hyperfluorescent spots that may represent sites of subclinical choroidal inflammation. (Reproduced from Yannuzzi LA, Flower RW, Slakter S: Indocyanine green angiography. St. Louis, MO: Mosby; 1997.)

There are no reports of successful management of CNV associated with serpiginous choroiditis with anti-inflammatory agents. Thermal laser has been the main form of therapy for extrafoveal or juxtafoveal CNV.[1,13,14] Recurrence after laser has been reported.[11] Subfoveal CNV due to serpiginous choroiditis may be amenable to verteporfin photodynamic therapy but there are no reports describing results to date.

Patients with serpiginous choroiditis are instructed to perform frequent Amsler grid testing to monitor for the presence of recurrent disease or CNV. Because similar central vision changes can occur with either, patients are instructed to return for immediate examination and angiography when symptoms occur.

VISUAL PROGNOSIS

Significant loss of central and even peripheral vision can occur as a result of inflammatory disease and its sequelae. Frequencies of central vision loss have been reported to be as high as 50% of involved eyes.[7,8,32] This is especially true in patients with macular serpiginous choroiditis. In addition, CNV can occur in up to

25% of patients. Nevertheless, most patients with serpiginous choroiditis maintain central function in at least one eye.

ACKNOWLEDGMENT

This research was supported by the Pacific Vision Foundation, San Francisco, California.

REFERENCES

1. Blumenkranz MS, Gass JDM, Clarkson JG. Atypical serpiginous choroiditis. Arch Ophthalmol 1982; 100:1773–1775.
2. Chisholm IH, Gass JDM, Hutton WL. The late stage of serpiginous (geographic) choroiditis. Am J Ophthalmol 1976; 82:343–351.
3. Gass JDM. Stereoscopic atlas of macular diseases: diagnosis and treatment, 4th edn. St Louis: Mosby; 1997.
4. Hamilton AM, Bird AC. Geographical choroidopathy. Br J Ophthalmol 1974; 58:784–797.
5. Hardy RA, Schatz H. Macular geographic helicoid choroidopathy. Arch Ophthalmol 1987; 105:1237–1242.
6. Laatikainen L, Erkkila H. Serpiginous choroiditis. Br J Ophthalmol 1974; 58:777–783.
7. Schatz H, Maumenee AE, Patz A. Geographic helicoid peripapillary choroidopathy: clinical presentation and fluorescein angiographic findings. Trans Am Acad Ophthalmol Otolaryngol 1974; 78:747–761.
8. Weiss H, Annesley WH Jr, Shields JA et al. The clinical course of serpiginous choroidopathy. Am J Ophthalmol 1979; 87:133–142.
9. Fujisawa C, Fujiwara H, Hasegawa E et al. [The cases of serpiginous choroiditis (author's translation).] Nippon Ganka Gakkai Zasshi 1978; 82:135–143.
10. Gupta V, Agarwal A, Gupta A et al. Clinical characteristics of serpiginous choroidopathy in North India. Am J Ophthalmol 2002; 134:47–56.
11. Mansour AM, Jampol LM, Packo KH et al. Macular serpiginous choroiditis. Retina 1988; 8:125–131.
12. Masi RJ, O'Connor GR, Kimura SJ. Anterior uveitis in geographic or serpiginous choroiditis. Am J Ophthalmol 1978; 86:228–232.
13. Jampol LM, Orth D, Daily MJ et al. Subretinal neovascularization with geographic (serpiginous) choroiditis. Am J Ophthalmol 1979; 88:683–689.
14. Laatikainen L, Erkkila H. Subretinal and disc neovascularisation in serpiginous choroiditis. Br J Ophthalmol 1982; 66:326–331.
15. Wu JS, Lewis H, Fine SL et al. Clinicopathologic findings in a patient with serpiginous choroiditis and treated choroidal neovascularization. Retina 1989; 9:292–301.
16. Steinmetz RL, Fitzke FW, Bird AC. Treatment of cystoid macular edema with acetazolamide in a patient with serpiginous choroidopathy. Retina 1991; 11:412–415.
17. Friberg TR. Serpiginous choroiditis with branch vein occlusion and bilateral periphlebitis. Arch Ophthalmol 1988; 106:585–586.
18. Wojno T, Meredith TA. Unusual findings in serpiginous choroiditis. Am J Ophthalmol 1982; 94:650–655.
19. Morés JM, Slakter JS. Serpiginous choroidopathy. In: Yannuzzi LA, Flower RW, Slakter SJ, eds. Indocyanine green angiography. St Louis: Mosby; 1997.
20. Giovannini A, Mariotti C, Ripa E et al. Indocyanine green angiographic findings in serpiginous choroidopathy. Br J Ophthalmol 1996; 80:536–540.
21. Quillen DA, Davis JB, Gottlieb JL et al. The white dot syndromes. Am J Ophthalmol 2004; 137:538–550.
22. Sonika, Narang S, Kochhar S et al. Posterior scleritis mimicking macular serpiginous choroiditis. Ind J Ophthalmol 2003; 51:351–353.
23. Edelsten C, Stanford MR, Graham EM. Serpiginous choroiditis: an unusual presentation of ocular sarcoidosis. Br J Ophthalmol 1994; 78:70–71.
24. Rattray KM, Cole MD, Smith SR. Systemic non-Hodgkin's lymphoma presenting as a serpiginous choroidopathy: report of a case and review of the literature. Eye 2000; 14:706–710.
25. King DG, Grizzard WS, Sever RJ et al. Serpiginous choroidopathy associated with elevated factor VIII-von Willebrand factor antigen. Retina 1990; 10:97–101.
26. Martidis A, Duker JS, Puliafito CA. Intravitreal triamcinolone for refractory cystoid macular edema secondary to birdshot retinochoroidopathy. Arch Ophthalmol 2001; 119:1380–1383.
27. Araujo AA, Wells AP, Dick AD et al. Early treatment with cyclosporin in serpiginous choroidopathy maintains remission and good visual outcome. Br J Ophthalmol 2000; 84:979–982.
28. Laatikainen L, Tarkkanen A. Failure of cyclosporin A in serpiginous choroiditis. J Ocul Ther Surg 1984; 3:280–282.
29. Secchi AG, Tognon MS, Maselli C. Ciclosporin-A in the treatment of serpiginous choroiditis. Int Ophthalmol 1990; 14:395–399.
30. Hooper PL, Kaplan HJ. Triple agent immunosuppression in serpiginous choroiditis. Ophthalmology 1991; 98:944–951.
31. Akpek EK, Jabs DA, Tessler HH et al. Successful treatment of serpiginous choroiditis with alkylating agents. Ophthalmology 2002; 109:1506–1513.
32. Laatikainen L, Erkkila H. A follow-up study on serpiginous choroiditis. Acta Ophthalmol (Copenh) 1981; 59:707–718.

Sympathetic Ophthalmia
Narsing A. Rao

Sympathetic ophthalmia, also known as *sympathetic ophthalmitis* and *sympathetic uveitis*, is a rare bilateral, diffuse granulomatous uveitis that occurs a few days to several decades after penetrating accidental or surgical trauma to an eye. Both the traumatized eye, commonly referred to as the "exciting" eye, and the fellow eye, referred to as the "sympathizing" eye, are affected. Injury to and incarceration of uveal tissue has been a feature of nearly all cases of sympathetic ophthalmia. The clinical signs and symptoms are usually detected in the sympathizing eye within the first 3 months after trauma to the fellow eye.[1]

Mackenzie, in 1830, provided a comprehensive clinical description and first used the term *sympathetic ophthalmia* to describe this entity.[1,2] Fuchs,[3] in 1905, detailed the characteristic histologic features. The pathogenesis of sympathetic ophthalmia has, however, remained an enigma despite years of study, although the two most commonly held views were that it represented an autoimmune response or was infectious. There is now some experimental evidence implicating the development of an autoimmune delayed hypersensitivity reaction to melanocytes or retinal tissue antigen as a possible pathogenic mechanism.

INCIDENCE

Sympathetic ophthalmia is a relatively rare disease, although exact incidence figures are difficult to determine because the onset or diagnosis, or both, are often delayed for months to years after the initial injury; also, histologic confirmation of the diagnosis is made in only about one-third of the suspected cases but is established pathologically in others not suspected clinically.[4] In 1972, Liddy & Stuart[5] reported an incidence of 0.19% following penetrating injuries and 0.007% following intraocular surgery. Surgical procedures that may lead to sympathetic ophthalmia include cataract extraction, iridectomy, paracentesis, cyclodialysis, retinal detachment repair, keratectomy, freeing of iris adhesions, vitrectomy, evisceration, laser cyclocoagulation, and others.[6-9]

Although advances in modern surgical technique may be contributing to a lower incidence of sympathetic ophthalmia, this is probably being offset by more aggressive surgical management of severely traumatized eyes, which in the past would have been promptly enucleated. However, the incidence of sympathetic ophthalmia after vitrectomy alone has been reported to be 0.01%.[10] For these reasons, sympathetic ophthalmia should not be considered a disappearing disease.

Some studies of the sex incidence of sympathetic uveitis show a male preponderance, but this is believed to be a reflection of the higher incidence of accidental trauma in males. Indeed, when only cases of surgical trauma are considered, the ratio is equal. In Winter's[11] series of 257 cases, there was no difference in age incidence among the case studies. Other authors have reported relative peaks in childhood and early adult years, thought to reflect a higher incidence of accidental trauma in these ages, and an additional peak in the sixth and seventh decades, thought to represent an increased incidence of surgical procedures among persons in this age group.[12]

CLINICAL FINDINGS

The clinical onset of sympathetic ophthalmia is typically heralded by the development of a mild inflammation in the sympathizing eye and a worsening of inflammation in the exciting eye. Symptoms in the sympathizing eye include mild pain, photophobia, and increased lacrimation, blurring of vision, visual fatigue, or paresis of accommodation. The exciting eye may have a decrease in vision and an increase in photophobia. Moreover, both eyes may show ciliary injection, a partially dilated, poorly responsive pupil, a thickened iris, and clouding of the vitreous. The most ominous sign in the exciting eye is the development of keratic precipitates on the corneal endothelium.[1]

The clinical signs and symptoms in the sympathizing eye are variable and may be either insidious or fairly rapid in onset. They may present as mild anterior or posterior uveitis with slight tenderness of the globe, mild ciliary flush, cells and flare in the anterior chamber, mild vitreous haze, and keratic precipitates on the endothelium. Posterior segment findings in sympathetic ophthalmia include papillitis, generalized retinal edema, and small yellow-white deposits beneath the retinal pigment epithelium, so-called Dalen–Fuchs nodules. The peripheral fundus may show areas of choroiditis and, in some cases, exudative retinal detachments. Occasionally, multiple choroidal granulomas may be present (Fig. 106-1). Scleral involvement is rarely seen clinically, even though it is a common finding on microscopic examination of enucleated eyes.

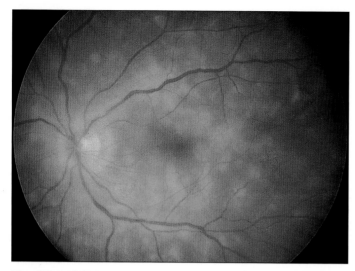

Fig. 106-1 Multiple choroidal granulomas in sympathetic ophthalmia.

The interval between the time of injury and the onset of inflammation in the sympathizing eye has been reported to be as short as 5 days and as long as 66 years after the trauma.[1,13] In general, however, sympathetic ophthalmia rarely occurs sooner than 2 weeks after trauma, with 80% of cases occurring within 3 months and 90% within 1 year of injury.[1] The peak incidence occurs between 4 and 8 weeks after trauma.

The diagnosis of sympathetic ophthalmia is a clinical one. No serologic or immunologic tests are available to aid in the diagnosis. However, fluorescein angiography may at times be quite helpful in establishing the clinical diagnosis. It typically shows multiple fluorescing dots at the level of the retinal pigment epithelium in the venous phase, and these dots persist (Fig. 106-2). Coalescence of the dye from these foci may occur if there are areas of exudative detachment. Vogt–Koyanagi–Harada disease is the other condition that has a similar angiographic picture. Less frequently there may be early focal obscurations of the background choroidal fluorescence, with later staining similar to the angiographic findings noted in acute posterior multifocal placoid pigment epitheliopathy. Numerous hypofluorescent dark dots may be visible during the intermediate phase of indocyanine green angiography. Some of these dots may become isofluorescent at the late phase.[14] In those severely traumatized eyes that later require enucleation, histopathologic examination may help to make or confirm the diagnosis.

COURSE AND COMPLICATIONS

Untreated sympathetic ophthalmia runs a long, variable, and complicated course marked initially by episodes of acute inflammation followed by quiescent periods that can last several months to several years. With time, the disease becomes chronically active, eventually producing irreversible ocular damage and leading to phthisis bulbi. The long-term complications of this ocular inflammation include development of cataracts, secondary glaucoma, exudative retinal detachments, chorioretinal scarring, choroidal neovascularization, subretinal fibrosis, and optic atrophy.[12,15,16]

PATHOLOGY

In sympathetic ophthalmia the pathologic alterations are similar in both the exciting and sympathizing eyes. They typically consist of a diffuse granulomatous inflammation made up of lymphocytic infiltration of the uveal tract with nests of epithelioid cells; pigment is often present within these epithelioid cells and also within giant cells (Fig. 106-3). In the majority of cases the inflammatory process does not involve the choriocapillaris or the retina. Absence of necrosis is another characteristic feature. Infiltration of the pars plana of the ciliary body occurs early in the course of the disease, and the inflammatory cells from this site may spill over into the vitreous cavity. Similar iris infiltration results in the clinical appearance of a thickened iris. The inflammation can spread over the anterior lens capsule surface and contribute to the formation of posterior synechiae. The choroid is diffusely involved and thickened by an infiltration of predominantly lymphocytes, some epithelioid cells, and a few giant cells; neutrophils are rarely seen. Plasma cells may be present, particularly in patients treated with corticosteroids. Eosinophils can also be found and are frequently concentrated in the inner choroid, particularly in heavily pigmented persons. Nodular clusters of epithelioid cells containing pigment are often seen lying between the retinal pigment epithelium and Bruch's membrane; these appear clinically as the drusen-like, yellow-white dots known as Dalen–Fuchs nodules (Fig. 106-4).

The retina is usually free of inflammatory infiltrates, except for collections of mononuclear cells around the vessels, occasional involvement in the areas overlying the Dalen–Fuchs nodules, and in the pars plana region. Other pathologic changes include scleral involvement with infiltrates around the emissary veins and extension of the granulomatous process into the optic nerve and surrounding meningeal sheaths.[2] Some of the eyes with typical histologic features of sympathetic ophthalmia but with breaks in the lens capsule may additionally show features of phacoanaphylaxis with zonal granulomatous inflammation around the lens material.[17] Even though typical features of sympathetic ophthalmia include nonnecrotizing granulomatous uveitis, there are cases exhibiting atypical features such as nongranulomatous choroiditis or chorioretinal adhesions with the inflammatory process involving choriocapillaris, similar to the histologic features of chronic Vogt–Koyanagi–Harada disease.[17,18] Immunohistochemical studies have revealed infiltration of predominantly T lymphocytes in the uveal tract. Both helper and suppressor/cytotoxic lymphocytes were observed.

ETIOLOGY

The exact cause of sympathetic ophthalmia is unknown. Clinical studies in the past have shown that the predominant predisposing factors are accidental penetrating trauma, which accounts for approximately 60 to 70% of cases, and perforating surgical trauma, which accounts for nearly 30%. A small percentage of cases are the result of contusion injuries with occult scleral rupture and perforating corneal ulcers. The common denominator in the overwhelming majority of cases

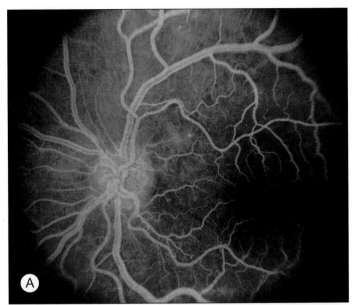
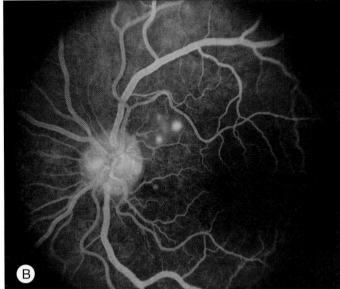
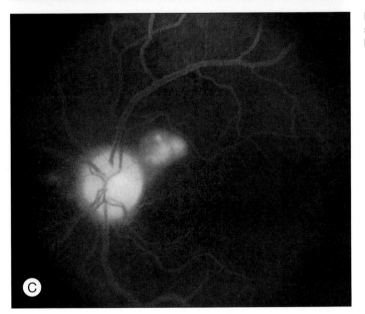

Fig. 106-2 A, Early arteriovenous phase of fluorescein angiography shows hyperfluorescent dots. B and C, Later phases exhibit increased hyperfluorescence and leakage.

is the presence of a penetrating injury in which wound healing is complicated by incarceration of the iris, ciliary body, or choroid.

Historically, the pathogenesis of sympathetic ophthalmia has been considered to be either infective or immunologic. No organisms have ever been isolated from cases of sympathetic ophthalmia, however, and an infective agent has not induced the disease in laboratory animals.

Several investigators propose an immunologic basis for sympathetic ophthalmia, in which an autosensitivity against an antigenic protein from the uvea[19] or retina is involved. Marak[20,21] and Wong and colleagues[22] demonstrated enhanced transformation of peripheral lymphocytes from patients with histologically confirmed sympathetic ophthalmia when exposed to homologous uveal–retinal extracts in tissue culture, suggesting that these patients have lymphocytes that are sensitized to some component(s) of uveal–retinal antigen.

When antigens extracted from the retina are injected into guinea pigs, an ocular inflammation develops in these animals that is very similar to sympathetic ophthalmia. The experimental studies suggest that sympathetic ophthalmia may result from altered T-cell response to one of the soluble proteins associated with the retinal photoreceptor membranes, called the retinal S antigen, or to other retinal or choroidal melanocyte antigens.[19,23,24]

There may be a genetic predisposition to the development of sympathetic ophthalmia. Human leukocyte antigen (HLA) association has been reported in sympathetic ophthalmia, and this association includes HLA-A11, HLA-B40, HLA-DR4/DRw53, and HLA-DR4/DQ w3 haplotypes.[25,26] Recent studies from

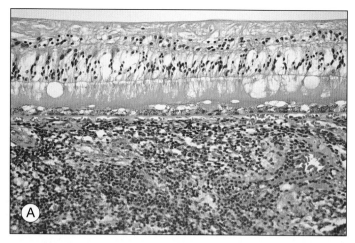 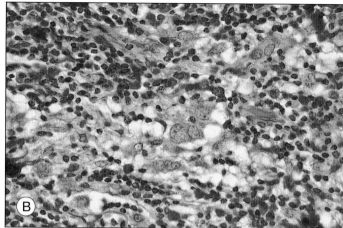

Fig. 106-3 A, Note granulomatous inflammation of the choroid with focal serous detachment of the retina (hematoxylin & eosin; ×130). B, Multinucleated giant cells have pigment in their cytoplasm (hematoxylin & eosin; ×565).

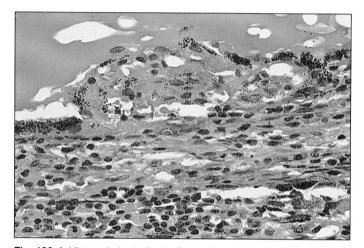

Fig. 106-4 Histopathologically, the Dalen–Fuchs nodule is characterized by focal collections of epithelioid cells at the level of Bruch's membrane (hematoxylin & eosin; ×250).

Japan and the UK reported a significant association of HLA-DRB1*04 and -DQB1*04 with sympathetic ophthalmia.[7,27] A similar association was seen in patients with Vogt–Koyanagi–Harada disease.

DIFFERENTIAL DIAGNOSIS

Sympathetic ophthalmia must be differentiated from several other conditions and disease entities. Certain bacterial and fungal infections can produce a granulomatous anterior or posterior uveitis, but these can usually be differentiated by history and by associated clinical findings. Infectious endophthalmitis must always be considered following any perforating trauma to the eye. Reactivation of a pre-existing uveitis by the injury, or the development of a posttraumatic iritis or iridocyclitis, can also occur.

Phacoanaphylaxis can closely simulate the clinical picture of sympathetic ophthalmia. Furthermore, an association appears to exist between phacoanaphylaxis and sympathetic ophthalmia.

Although unilaterality may be a clue, phacoanaphylaxis is not invariably unilateral. The incidence of phacoanaphylaxis in cases of sympathetic ophthalmia has been variously estimated at 4 to 25%. Unlike sympathetic ophthalmia, in bilateral phacoanaphylaxis the eye first involved is usually quiet by the time inflammation begins in the second eye. A careful slit-lamp examination should always be carried out to search for ruptured lens capsule and pieces of lens cortex in the anterior chamber. If this condition exists, a lens extraction can be curative, thereby avoiding an unnecessary enucleation.

Vogt–Koyanagi–Harada syndrome is an inflammatory uveo-meningeal disorder with bilateral diffuse granulomatous uveitis, exudative retinal detachments, alopecia, vitiligo, dysacusis, and fluctuating meningeal signs and symptoms. While vitiligo and alopecia are more common in Vogt–Koyanagi–Harada syndrome, they can also be seen in cases of sympathetic ophthalmia. A history of penetrating trauma is helpful in the differential diagnosis.

THERAPY

The only truly effective management of sympathetic ophthalmia is the prevention of its occurrence, which entails careful microsurgical wound toilet and prompt closure of all penetrating injuries. Of course, every attempt should be made to save any eye with a reasonable prognosis for useful vision, but in those eyes with barely discernible or no visual function, and with demonstrable disorganization of the ocular contents, enucleation within 2 weeks after injury has long been advised to preclude the development of sympathetic ophthalmia. At one time it was believed that the use of steroids following penetrating injury would in some instances prevent the development of sympathetic ophthalmia; this has not proved to be the case.

Enucleation of the exciting eye once sympathetic ophthalmia has commenced remains a topic of considerable controversy. Some studies[12,28] suggest that early enucleation of the exciting eye may improve the prognosis for the sympathizing eye; however, careful review of the data presented in these studies does not support this conclusion.[29] A review by Winter[11] of 257 cases of histologically proven sympathetic ophthalmia indicated no benefit to the sympathizing eye from enucleation of the exciting eye, whether performed briefly before, concomitant with, or subsequent to the development of sympathetic ophthalmia at various elapsed intervals following injury. Indeed, it is possible that the exciting eye may eventually provide the better visual acuity, and its enucleation would therefore deprive the patient of that visual potential.[29]

Although steroids have not been shown to be effective in the prevention of sympathetic ophthalmia, they do constitute the mainstay of its therapy. Large doses of steroids should be given early in the course of the disease and continued for at least 6 months after the apparent resolution of inflammation. For the first week, 100 to 200 mg of oral prednisone is given daily and then reduced to an every-other-day dosage; steroids are eventually tapered following clinical response of the uveitis. The systemic prednisone is supplemented with sub-Tenon's injection of depot steroids and topical drops. Mydriatic and cycloplegic agents are, of course, used adjunctively.

In a number of patients, medical problems or systemic or ophthalmologic complications may prevent the long-term use of high doses of steroids. In these patients, supplemental treatment with immunosuppressive agents (azathioprine, methotrexate, or chlorambucil) has been shown to suppress inflammation effectively, allow reduction of corticosteroid therapy to nontoxic levels, and, in some cases, induce an apparent remission of the disease.[30] Andrasch and associates[31] presented a regimen for the use of these immunosuppressive agents consisting of prednisone, 10 to 15 mg/day, combined with azathioprine, 2.0 to 2.5 mg/kg per day, or combined with chlorambucil, 6 to 8 mg orally once per day. They reported that a response to this regimen is usually noted within 4 weeks. Once remission is induced, the prednisone is reduced in 2.5-mg increments every 1 to 2 weeks until a maintenance dose of 2.5 mg/day is reached. Thereafter, slower tapering of the chemotherapy continues. It is suggested that if intolerance or adverse reactions to one chemotherapeutic agent are noted, the patient can be switched to another; this can usually be done with no problem. Of course, during the course of chemotherapy all patients should be closely monitored with the assistance of an oncologist or internist; marrow suppression, renal or hepatic toxicity, and the development of neoplasms can occur with prolonged use of these agents. Suppression of uveal inflammation with systemic ciclosporin therapy can be achieved, particularly in combination with systemic administration of corticosteroids. Ciclosporin is used 5 mg/kg in general. In light of serious side-effects, it is highly recommended that all of the chemotherapeutic agents and the immunosuppressive drugs be reserved for use only in those cases of severe uveitis where conventional treatment with prednisone is not feasible or is ineffective.

PROGNOSIS

Before the use of corticosteroids, the visual prognosis was generally poor. However, Makley & Azar[32] found that in patients treated with steroids a visual acuity of 20/60 or better was achieved in 64%. Exacerbations of sympathetic ophthalmia occurred in 60% of the patients, in some instances with long intervals between observed relapses. Chan et al.[33] reported visual acuity of 20/40 or better in 50% of patients treated with steroids and immunosuppressive agents. With prompt and aggressive corticosteroid therapy, and with immunosuppressive therapy in some, many eyes with sympathetic ophthalmia should, these days, retain useful vision.

In conclusion, sympathetic ophthalmia is a serious entity, often with many exacerbations and a relentlessly progressive course that frequently results in very poor vision. Long-term follow-up of these patients is essential. It is hoped that, with the use of large-dose steroid therapy early in the course of the disease, and supplementation with immunosuppressive agents when indicated, the prognosis in these patients need not be as grim as it has traditionally been.

REFERENCES

1. Duke-Elder S, Perkins ES. Diseases of the uveal tract. In: Duke-Elder S, ed. System of ophthalmology, vol. 9. St Louis: Mosby; 1966.
2. Albert DM, Diaz-Rohena R. A historical review of sympathetic ophthalmia and its epidemiology. Surv Ophthalmol 1989; 34:1–14.
3. Fuchs E. Über sympathisierende Entzündung (nebst Bemerkungenüber seröse traumatische Iritis). Graefes Arch Clin Exp Ophthalmol 1905; 61:365–456.
4. Goto H, Rao NA. Sympathetic ophthalmia and Vogt–Koyanagi–Harada syndrome. Int Ophthalmol Clin 1990; 30:279–285.
5. Liddy BSL, Stuart J. Sympathetic ophthalmia in Canada. Can J Ophthalmol 1972; 7:157–159.
6. Bechrakis NE, Muller-Stolzenburg NW, Helbig H et al. Sympathetic ophthalmia following laser cyclocoagulation. Arch Ophthalmol 1994; 112:80–48.
7. Kilmartin DJ, Dick AD, Forrester JV. Prospective surveillance of sympathetic ophthalmia in the UK and Republic of Ireland. Br J Ophthalmol 2000; 84:259–263.
8. Lakhanpal V, Dogra MR, Jacobson MS. Sympathetic ophthalmia associated with anterior chamber intraocular lens implantation. Ann Ophthalmol 1991; 23:139–143.
9. Lavine MR, Pou CR, Lash RH. The 1998 Wendell Hughes lecture. Evisceration: is sympathetic ophthalmia a concern in the new millennium? Ophthalm Plast Reconstr Surg 1999; 15:4–8.
10. Gass JDM. Sympathetic ophthalmia following vitrectomy. Am J Ophthalmol 1982; 93:552–558.
11. Winter FC. Sympathetic uveitis: a clinical and pathologic study of the visual result. Am J Ophthalmol 1955; 39:340–347.
12. Lubin JR, Albert DM, Weinstein M. Sixty-five years of sympathetic ophthalmia: a clinicopathologic review of 105 cases (1913–1978). Ophthalmology 1980; 87:109–121.
13. Zaharia MA, Lamarche J, Laurin M. Sympathetic uveitis 66 years after injury. Can J Ophthalmol 1984; 19:240–243.
14. Bernasconi O, Auer C, Zografos L et al. Indocyanine green angiographic findings in sympathetic ophthalmia. Graefes Arch Clin Exp Ophthalmol 1998; 236:635–638.
15. Bom S, Young S, Gregor Z et al. Surgery for choroidal neovascularization in sympathetic ophthalmia. Retina 2002; 22:109–111.
16. Wang RC, Zamir E, Dugel PU et al. Progressive subretinal fibrosis and blindness associated with multifocal granulomatous chorioretinitis: a variant of sympathetic ophthalmia. Ophthalmology 2002; 109:1527–1531.
17. Croxatto JO, Rao NA, McLean IW et al. Atypical histopathologic features in sympathetic ophthalmia: a study of a hundred cases. Int Ophthalmol 1982; 4:129–135.
18. Rao NA, Marak GE. Sympathetic ophthalmia simulating Vogt–Koyanagi–Harada's disease: a clinico-pathologic study of four cases. Jpn J Ophthalmol 1983; 27:506–511.
19. Sugita S, Sagawa K, Mochizuki M et al. Melanocyte lysis by cytotoxic T lymphocytes recognizing the MART-1 melanoma antigen in HLA-A2 patients with Vogt–Koyanagi–Harada disease. Int Immunol 1996; 8:799–803.
20. Marak GE Jr. Recent advances in sympathetic ophthalmia. Surv Ophthalmol 1979; 24:141–156.

21. Rao NA, Wacker WB, Marak GE Jr. Experimental allergic uveitis: clinico-pathologic features associated with varying doses of S antigen. Arch Ophthalmol 1979; 97:1954–1958.

22. Wong VG, Anderson R, O'Brien PJ. Sympathetic ophthalmia and lymphocyte transformation. Am J Ophthalmol 1971; 72:960–966.

23. Jakobiec FA, Marboe CC, Knowles DM et al. Human sympathetic ophthalmia: an analysis of the inflammatory infiltrate by hybridoma – monoclonal antibodies, immunochemistry, and correlative electron microscopy. Ophthalmology 1983; 90:76–95.

24. Rao NA, Robin J, Hartmann D et al. The role of the penetrating wound in the development of sympathetic ophthalmia: experimental observations. Arch Ophthalmol 1983; 101:102–104.

25. Azan P, Marak GE, Minckler DS et al. Histocompatibility antigens in sympathetic ophthalmia. Am J Ophthalmol 1984; 98:117–119.

26. Davis JL, Mittal KK, Freidlin V et al. HLA association and ancestry in Vogt–Koyanagi–Harada disease and sympathetic ophthalmia. Ophthalmology 1990; 97:1137–1142.

27. Shindo Y, Ohno S, Usui M et al. Immunogenetic study of sympathetic ophthalmia. Tissue Antigens 1997; 49:111–115.

28. Reynard M, Riffenburgh RS, Maes EF. Effect of corticosteroid treatment and enucleation on the visual prognosis of sympathetic ophthalmia. Am J Ophthalmol 1983; 96:290–294.

29. Marak GE Jr. Sympathetic ophthalmia. Ophthalmology 1982; 89:1291.

30. Tessler HH, Jennings T. High-dose short-term chlorambucil for intractable sympathetic ophthalmia and Behçet's disease. Br J Ophthalmol 1990; 74:353–357.

31. Andrasch RH, Pirofsky B, Burns RP. Immunosuppressive therapy for severe chronic uveitis. Arch Ophthalmol 1978; 96:247–251.

32. Makley TA Jr, Azar A. Sympathetic ophthalmia: a long-term follow-up. Arch Ophthalmol 1978; 96:257–262.

33. Chan CC, Roberg RG, Whitcup SM et al. 32 cases of sympathetic ophthalmia: a retrospective study at the National Eye Institute, Bethesda, MD, from 1982–1992. Arch Ophthalmol 1995; 113:597–600.

Chapter

107

Vogt–Koyanagi–Harada Disease

P. Kumar Rao
Narsing A. Rao

Vogt–Koyanagi–Harada (VKH) disease is a bilateral granulomatous uveitis often associated with exudative retinal detachment and with extraocular manifestations, such as pleocytosis in the cerebrospinal fluid and, in some cases, vitiligo, poliosis, alopecia, and dysacusis. In many patients, VKH presents with severe signs of panuveitis associated with multifocal serous retinal detachment, hyperemia of the optic disc, and meningeal irritations. The meningeal manifestations, which occur in the initial stage of the disease, consist of headache, meningismus, and, rarely, focal neurological signs. The auditory disturbances include tinnitus and hearing loss and, rarely, vertigo. The cutaneous manifestations that usually develop during the chronic phase of the disease include patchy alopecia, vitiligo, and poliosis of lashes, eyebrows, and scalp hair. The clinical course of VKH typically follows four stages: the prodromal, uveitic, chronic, and chronic recurrent stages.[1] During the prodromal stage of the disease, patients may develop a viral-like illness that lasts for 3 to 5 days. This is followed by the uveitic stage, during which patients exhibit the signs and symptoms of acute uveitis; this stage may last for several weeks. The next stage is the chronic (convalescent) stage; patients in this stage may develop integumentory and uveal depigmentation. The chronic stage may last for months to years depending on therapeutic intervention. In the chronic recurrent stage, patients may exhibit resolving chronic uveitis, interrupted by recurrent bouts of anterior uveitis.[1]

When a patient presents with the ocular and the extraocular manifestations, the diagnosis of VKH is made with certainty and such cases are considered "typical." However, extraocular manifestations such as dysacusis and cutaneous changes are relatively rare, and the dermatologic changes mainly occur late in the course of the disease.[1,2] Because of the variation in clinical presentations of VKH, the American Uveitis Society (AUS) in 1978 recommended the following diagnostic criteria: (1) the absence of any history of ocular trauma or surgery; and (2) the presence of at least three of the following four signs: (a) bilateral chronic iridocyclitis; (b) posterior uveitis, including exudative retinal detachment, forme fruste of exudative retinal detachment, disc hyperemia or edema and "sunset-glow" fundus; (c) neurologic signs of tinnitus, neck stiffness, cranial nerve, or central nervous system disorders, or cerebrospinal fluid pleocytosis; and (d) cutaneous findings of alopecia, poliosis, or vitiligo.[3]

Since VKH manifestations vary depending upon the clinical course, a given patient may not initially present with the features required for the diagnosis of VKH by AUS criteria. Read & Rao recently evaluated the utility of the existing AUS criteria in 71 consecutive patients with VKH who were diagnosed based on the clinical features and the course of the disease, combined with fluorescein angiography with or without utrasonography in selected cases.[4] Patients presenting in the acute, convalescent, and chronic recurrent stages met the AUS criteria for VKH diagnosis in 56%, 48%, and 58% of cases, respectively. The authors concluded that AUS criteria for diagnosis of VKH may not be adequate.[4] Taking into account the multisystem nature of VKH and allowing for the different ocular findings present in the early and late stages of the disease, the First International Workshop on VKH proposed revised diagnostic criteria to include clinical manifestations at various stages of disease.[5] These revised diagnostic criteria are summarized in Box 107-1.

HISTORICAL ASPECTS

Poliosis associated with ocular inflammation was described by Ali-ibn-Isa, an Arab physician who lived in the first century AD (cited by Pattison).[6] This association was reported by Schenkl in 1873,[7] by Hutchinson in 1892,[8] and by Vogt in 1906.[9] Einosuke Harada described a primary posterior uveitis with exudative retinal detachments in association with cerebrospinal fluid pleocytosis.[10] Three years later, in 1929, Koyanagi described six patients with bilateral chronic iridocyclitis, patchy depigmentation of the skin, patchy hair loss, and whitening of the hair, especially the eyelashes.[11] This constellation of findings was termed "uveitis with polosis, vitiligo, alopecia and dysacusis." Babel in 1932[12] and Bruno & McPherson in 1945[13] combined the findings of Vogt, Koyanagi, and Harada and suggested that these processes represent a continuum of the same disease, thereafter recognized as Vogt–Koyanagi–Harada syndrome. In the past, such a constellation of these signs and symptoms warranted the term "syndrome," but in recent years the entity has been well characterized; thereafter the First International Workshop on VKH, held in 1999, adopted the term Vogt–Koyanagi–Harada disease.[5]

EPIDEMIOLOGY

The incidence of VKH is variable. It appears to be more common in Japan, where it accounts for 6.8% to 9.2% of all uveitis referrals.[1]

Box 107-1 The revised diagnostic criteria proposed by the First International Workshop on Vogt–Koyanagi–Harada (VKH) disease*

A. Complete VKH disease
  1. Bilateral ocular involvement (a or b must be met, depending on the stage of disease when the patient is examined)
    a. Early manifestations of disease
      (1) There must be evidence of a diffuse choroiditis (with or without anterior uveitis, vitreous inflammatory reaction, or optic disc hyperemia), which may manifest as one of the following:
        (a) Focal areas of subretinal fluid, or
        (b) Bullous serous retinal detachments
      (2) With equivocal fundus findings, both of the following must be present as well:
        (a) Focal areas of delay in choroidal perfusion, multifocal areas of pinpoint leakage, large placoid areas of hyperfluorescence, pooling within subretinal fluid, and optic-nerve staining (listed in order of sequential appearance) by fluorescein angiography, and
        (b) Diffuse choroidal thickening, without evidence of posterior scleritis by ultrasonography
    b. Late manifestations of disease
      (1) History suggestive of prior presence of findings from 1a, and either both (2) and (3) below, or multiple signs from (3):
      (2) Ocular depigmentation (either of the following manifestations is sufficient):
        (a) Sunset-glow fundus, or
        (b) Sugiura's sign
      (3) Other ocular signs:
        (a) Nummular chorioretinal depigmented scars, or
        (b) Retinal pigment epithelium clumping and/or migration, or
        (c) Recurrent or chronic anterior uveitis
  2. Neurological/auditory findings (may have resolved by time of examination)
    a. Meningismus (malaise, fever, headache, nausea, abdominal pain, stiffness of the neck and back, or a combination of these factors; headache alone is not sufficient to meet the definition of meningismus, however), or
    b. Tinnitus, or
    c. Cerebrospinal fluid pleocytosis
  3. Integumentary finding (not preceding onset of central nervous system or ocular disease)
    a. Alopecia, or
    b. Poliosis, or
    c. Vitiligo
B. Incomplete VKH disease (point 1 and either 2 or 3 must be present)
  1. Bilateral ocular involvement as defined for complete VKH disease
  2. Neurologic/auditory findings as defined for complete VKH disease above, or
  3. Integumentary findings as defined for complete VKH disease above.
C. Probable VKH disease
  1. Bilateral ocular involvement as defined for complete VKH disease above.

*In all cases there should not be a history of penetrating ocular injury or surgery preceding the initial onset of uveitis and no clinical or laboratory evidence suggestive of other ocular disease criteria.
Modified from Read RW, Holland GN, Rao NA et al. Revised diagnostic criteria for Vogt–Koyanagi–Harada disease: report of an international committee on nomenclature. Am J Ophthalmol 2001; 131:647–652.[5]

In the USA, it accounts for 1% to 4% of all uveitis clinic referrals. VKH tends to affect more pigmented races, such as Asians, Hispanics, American Indians, and Asian Indians.[1,14] In the USA, there appears to be variability in the racial distribution of patients with VKH syndrome.[1,3,15,16] In northern California, VKH was seen mainly in Asians (41%), followed by whites (29%), Hispanics (16%), and blacks (14%).[16] In contrast, reports from southern California show that 78% of VKH patients were Hispanic while 3% were white, 10% were Asian, and 6% were black.[1] A series reported from the National Institutes of Health (NIH) showed that 50% VKH patients were white, 35% were black, and 13%

were Hispanic.[15] However, most of those patients reported in the NIH series had remote American Indian ancestry. Most studies report that women tend to be affected more frequently than men; however, Japanese investigators have not found such a female predilection.[14] Most patients are in their second to fifth decades of life, but children may also be affected.[1,17]

CLINICAL DESCRIPTION

Typical clinical features of VKH include bilateral panuveitis associated with exudative retinal detachment(s); meningismus associated with headache and pleocytosis of cerebrospinal fluid; tinnitus or hearing loss; and cutaneous changes, such as vitiligo, poliosis, and alopecia. However, all of these features are rarely seen during the initial presentation, and the clinical features vary depending upon the stage of the disease.

The prodromal stage

The prodromal stage may last only a few days and may be limited to headaches, nausea, dizziness, fever, orbital pain, and meningismus. Light sensitivity and tearing may occur 1 to 2 days following the above symptoms. Specific neurological signs may occur, but these are rare. These neurological signs include cranial nerve palsies and optic neuritis. Cerebrospinal fluid analysis usually reveals pleocytosis.

The uveitic stage

This stage follows the prodromal phase and presents with blurring of vision in both eyes. One eye may be affected first, followed a few days later by the second eye. Despite a delay in symptoms, careful examination will reveal bilateral posterior uveitis. This uveitis consists of thickening of the posterior choroid with elevation of the peripapillary retinochoroidal layer, multiple serous retinal detachments (Fig. 107-1), hyperemia, and edema of the optic nerve head. Alterations in the retinal pigment epithelium (RPE) associated with multifocal choroidal inflammation may be seen. This is most easily observed with fluorescein angiography, which reveals multiple focal areas of leakage at the level of RPE and subretinal fluid accumulation (Figs 107-2 and 107-3). The inflammation eventually becomes diffuse, extending into the

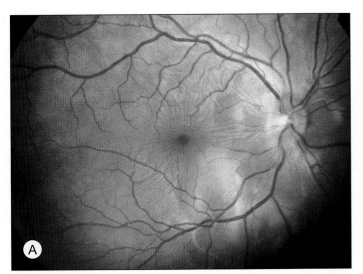
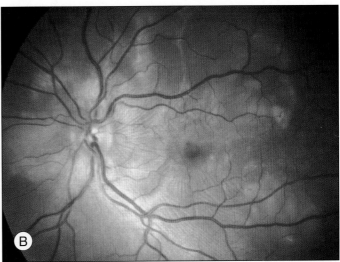

Fig. 107-1 Bilateral multiple serous retinal detachments in the uveitis stage of Vogt–Koyanagi–Harada disease.

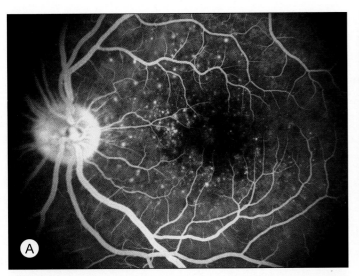
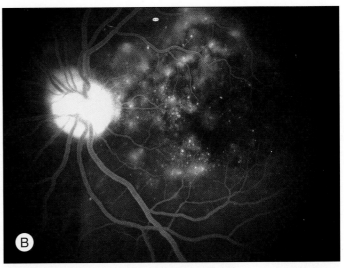

Fig. 107-2 A, Early anteriovenous phase of fluorescein angiogram exhibiting multiple hyperfluorescent dots at the retinal pigment epithelium level. B, Late phase of the angiogram shows increased fluorescence of the dots and staining of subretinal fluid. Note disc staining.

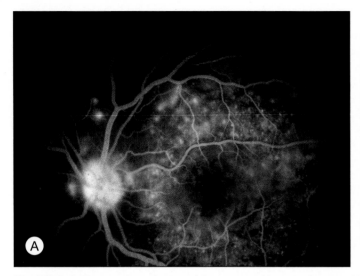

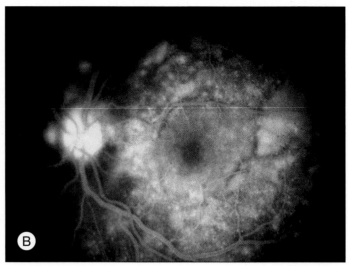

Fig. 107-3 A, Fluorescein angiogram of the acute uveitis stage shows multiple hyperfluorescent dots at the level of retinal pigment epithelium during the mid ateriovenous phase. B, Note staining of the subretinal fluid during the late phase of the angiogram.

anterior segment and revealing the presence of flare and cells in the anterior chamber. Less commonly, mutton-fat keratic precipitates, small nodules on the iris surface and papillary margin, may be seen.[1] The inflammatory infiltrate in the ciliary body and choroid may cause forward displacement of the lens iris diaphragm, leading to acute angle-closure glaucoma or annular choroidal detachment.[18,19]

The chronic stage

The chronic or convalescent stage occurs several weeks after the acute uveitic stage and is characterized by development of vitiligo, poliosis (Fig. 107-4), and depigmentation of the choroid (Fig. 107-5). Perilimbal vitiligo, also known as Sugiura's sign (Fig. 107-6), may develop at this stage; but this sign is mainly seen in Japanese patients.[1,5] Choroidal depigmentation occurs a few

months after the uveitic phase. This leads to the characteristic pale disc with a bright red-orange choroid known as "sunset-glow fundus."[5] The juxtapapillary area may show marked depigmentation. In Hispanics, the sunset-glow fundus may show foci of RPE changes in the form of hyperpigmentation or hypopigmentation.[1] At this stage small, yellow, well-circumscribed areas of chorioretinal atrophy may appear mainly in the inferior midperiphery of the fundus. This convalescent phase may last for several months.

The chronic recurrent stage

The chronic recurrent stage consists of a smoldering panuveitis with acute episodic exacerbations of granulomatous anterior uveitis. Recurrent posterior uveitis with exudative retinal detachment is uncommon. The anterior uveitis may be resistant to local and

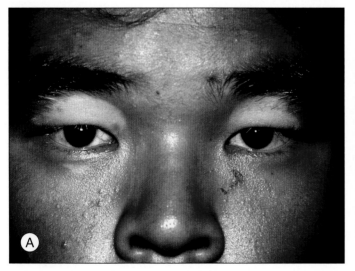

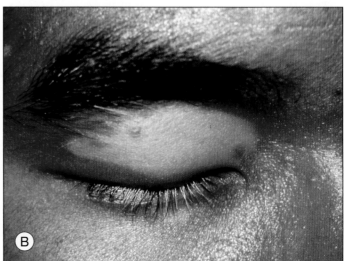

Fig. 107-4 Bilateral upper-eyelid vitiligo (A) and poliosis (B) developed during the chronic stage of Vogt–Koyanagi–Harada disease.

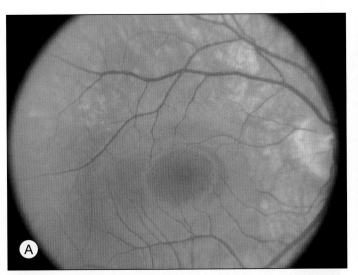

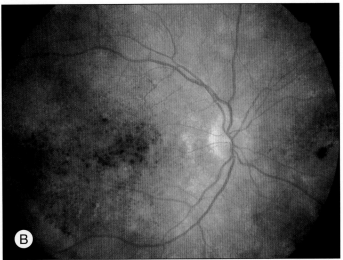

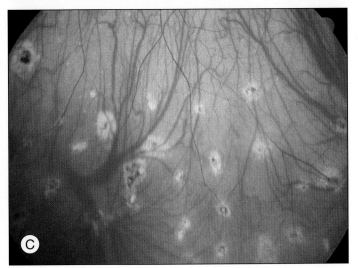

Fig. 107-5 Chronic stage of Vogt–Koyanagi–Harada disease revealing sunset-glow fundus in an Asian patient (A) and in a Hispanic woman (B). Note oval nonpigmented and pigmented retinal pigment epithelium atrophic lesions (C).

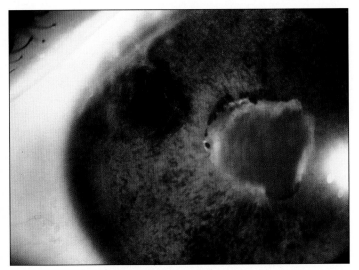

Fig. 107-6 Chronic stage of Vogt–Koyanagi–Harada disease shows extensive posterior synechiae, areas of depigmentation involving iris, and loss of pigment at the limbus (Sugiura's sign).

systemic corticosteroid therapy. Iris nodules may be seen during this phase (Fig. 107-7). These appear as round, whitish, well-circumscribed nodules on a background of atrophic iris stroma. The most visually debilitating complication of the chronic inflammation during this stage appears to be the development of subretinal neovascular membranes.[20] Posterior subcapsular cataract, as well as glaucoma, either angle-closure or open-angle, and posterior synechiae, may also be seen.[21,22] Linear pigmentary changes similar to those seen in the ocular histoplasmosis syndrome and arteriovenous anastomosis may be seen in occasional patients.[23]

Extraocular manifestations

Neurologic, auditory, and integumentory manifestations appear at various stages of the disease. Sensitivity of scalp hair occurs early in the prodromal phase; poliosis and vitiligo develop during the convalescent stage. Neurologic signs and symptoms are most common during the prodromal stage and include neck stiffness, headache, and confusion. Rarely, patients develop focal neurologic signs, hemiparesis, transverse myelitis, and ciliary ganglionitis.

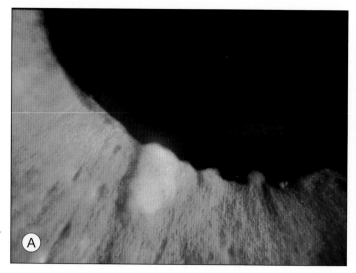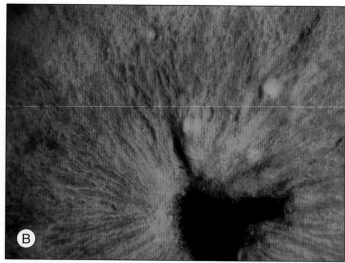

Fig. 107-7 A, Note the iris nodule at the papillary margin in a Hispanic male with chronic recurrent-stage Vogt–Koyanagi–Harada disease. B, Chronic recurrent stage of Vogt–Koyanagi–Harada disease showing multiple small nodules in the iris and extensive posterior synechiae.

However, more than 80% of patients develop cerebrospinal fluid lymphocytic pleocytosis that may persist for up to 8 weeks.[16]

Auditory manifestations may be detected in 75% of patients and may include dysacusis, tinnitus, and vertigo. Typically, cochlear hearing loss develops in the early stage of the disease, and the inner-ear dysfunction improves in 2 to 3 months. Vestibular dysfunction is uncommon in VKH disease.[1]

Integumentary changes include poliosis of the eyebrow, eyelashes, and scalp hair; vitiligo occurs during the convalescent stage and corresponds closely with fundus depigmentation, and sunset-glow fundus. The vitiligo is often distributed symmetrically, involving the facial regions, eyelids and trunk, and the skin over the sacrum.[18] Depending on race, 10% to 63% of patients with VKH may develop vitiligo.[1,2,16] The incidence of such cutaneous and other extraocular manifestations is relatively low in Hispanics, despite the fact that they have typical ocular and neurologic manifestations (Table 107-1).

Table 107-1 Variations in clinical features in Vogt–Koyanagi–Harada syndrome		
	Moorthy et al.[1] Hispanic (n = 51)	Non-Hispanic* (n = 14)
Meningismus	30 (59%)	8 (57%)
Dysacusis	4 (8%)	3 (21%)
Tinnitus	5 (10%)	4 (28%)
Vitiligo	4 (8%)	2 (14%)
Alopecia	7 (14%)	0 (0%)
Poliosis	2 (4%)	1 (7%)

*Seven were Asians, four were African Americans, two were Caucasians, and one was Native American.

PATHOLOGY

VKH is a nonnecrotizing diffuse granulomatous inflammation involving the uvea. The choroidal thickening is prominent in the juxtapapillary area and gradually decreases towards the anterior part of the uvea. Although a granulomatous process is the primary feature of the disease, the histopathologic changes vary depending on the stage of the disease.[24] At the uveitic stage, the granulomatous inflammation is present throughout the uvea. The uvea is thickened by diffuse infiltration of lymphocytes and macrophages, admixed with epithelioid cells and multinucleated giant cells. Occasional eosinophilic leukocytes may be noted in the uveal infiltrate. The neural retina is detached from the RPE, and the subretinal space contains proteinaceous fluid exudates (Fig. 107-8). In the choroid, the infiltrating lymphocytes and macrophages are seen in close proximity to the uveal melanocytes. The epithelioid and giant cells contain pigment granules. Although damaged choroidal melanocytes may not be detected, their pigment granules are engulfed by activated macrophages, and these histiocytes subsequently transform into epithelioid cells and multinucleated giant cells.

The peripapillary choroid is the predominant site for the granulomatous inflammatory infiltration; and a similar but less prominent inflammation is noted in the equatorial and anterior choroid. Moreover, the inflammation of the ciliary body and iris is essentially granulomatous. Granulomatous inflammation is also seen in the perivascular and perineural loose connective tissues in the sclera and is present at the sites of melanocytes. Dalen–Fuchs nodules, which represent focal aggregates of epithelioid histiocytes admixed with RPE, are located between Bruch's membrane and the RPE.[24] In severe cases, the choroidal lymphocytic infiltration extends into the choriocapillaris and Bruch's membrane and may involve the RPE.[13] Immunohistochemical techniques reveal that the choroidal infiltrates are composed predominantly of T lymphocytes. Class II major histocompatibility complex antigens are expressed on choroidal melanocytes and on the endothelium of the choriocapillaris.[25]

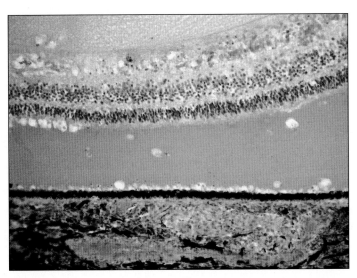

Fig. 107-8 Acute uveitic stage of Vogt–Koyanagi–Harada disease shows serous detachment of the retina, preservation of choriocapillaris from inflammatory cell infiltration, and thickening of choroid from granulomatous inflammatory cell infiltration (hematoxylin & eosin). (Courtesy of Prof. H. Inomata.)

In the convalescent stage, the choroidal melanocytes decrease in number and disappear (Fig. 107-9), resulting in the sunset glow appearance of the fundus.[24] The numerous focal yellowish oval or round lesions seen in the inferior peripheral fundus by ophthalmoscopy histologically display a focal loss of RPE cells and the formation of chorioretinal adhesions.[24] The choroidal inflammation tends to subside with the disappearance of the choroidal melanocytes; but a mild to moderate degree of lymphocytic infiltration remains in the ciliary body and iris.

In the long-standing chronic recurrent stage, the RPE and neural retina show degenerative changes (Fig. 107-10). The RPE may reveal hyperplasia and fibrous metaplasia with or without associated subretinal neovascularization.[24] The uveal tract may display granulomatous inflammation, most prominently in the anterior uvea. Chorioretinal adhesions with inflammatory cell involvement of choriocapillaris may be present.[24,26]

ETIOLOGY AND PATHOGENESIS

Histopathologic studies have shown inflammation with loss of melanocytes in the uveal tract and skin, and similar changes could be taking place at the site of melanocytes in the meninges of the central nervous system and in the inner ear. Although the exact cause for the inflammation directed at the melanocytes remains unknown, current evidence suggests that it involves an autoimmune process driven by T lymphocytes against an as yet unidentified antigen(s) associated with melanocytes.[1,27,28] The mechanism that triggers the autoimmune process is unknown, but sensitizations to melanocyte antigenic peptides by cutaneous injury or viral infection have been proposed as possible factors in some cases.[29] The antigenic peptides may include tyrosinase or tyrosinase-related proteins, an unidentified 75-kDa protein and S-100 protein.[30,31] However, experimental animal studies, as well as T-cell clones raised specific to tyrosinase family protein from the peripheral blood of patients with VKH, suggest that autoreactive T cells against tyrosinase and/or tyrosinase-related proteins may play a role in the development of VKH in a genetically susceptible individual.[31]

There is a strong association with the human leukocyte antigen (HLA) DR4 in Japanese patients with VKH, and these patients and individuals from Korea showed predominant alleles of DRB1 *0405 and HLA-DRB1 *0410.[32] However, in other racial groups, such as mestizo Hispanic individuals from Southern California,

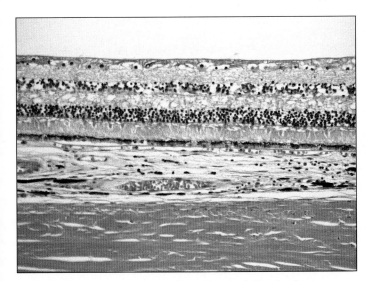

Fig. 107-9 Convalescent stage of Vogt–Koyanagi–Harada disease, exhibiting loss of choroidal melanocytes and infiltration of lymphocytes and plasma cells in the choroid. Note relatively intact retinal pigment epithelium and neurosensory retina (hematoxylin & eosin). (Courtesy of Prof. H. Inomata.)

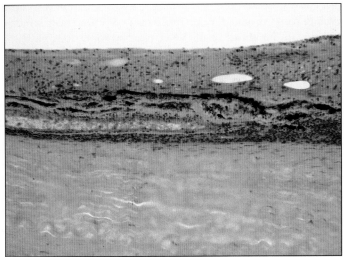

Fig. 107-10 Chronic recurrent stage of Vogt–Koyanagi–Harada disease shows choroidal inflammation, retinal pigment epithelium proliferation, and degeneration of overlying retina (hematoxylin & eosin). (Courtesy of Prof. H. Inomata.)

either HLA-DR1 or HLA-DR4 was found in 84% of patients with VKH disease.[33] Indeed, there was a higher relative risk with HLA-DR1 than HLA-DR4 (4.11 versus 1.96, respectively). Similar HLA-DR1 and HLA-DR4 subtypes were noted in 89% of Mexican mestizo patients.[23] All of these studies indicate that specific HLA genes may confer risk for development of VKH disease.

LABORATORY INVESTIGATIONS

In the vast majority of cases, the diagnosis of VKH is a clinical one when the patient presents with ocular and extraocular manifestations. However, when the disease presents without extraocular changes, fluorescein angiography, lumbar puncture, and ultrasonography have been found useful for substantiating the diagnosis. In recent years, indocyanine green (ICG) angiography and optical coherence tomography (OCT) have been used to diagnose and monitor resolution of the uveitis.

Fluorescein angiography in the acute stage reveals numerous punctate hyperfluorescent dots at the level of RPE. These dots enlarge and stain the surrounding subretinal fluid. The late phase of the angiogram shows multiple serous retinal detachments with pooling of dye in the subretinal space. Over 70% of patients show disc leakage.[1] Retinal vascular leakage is rarely noted. In the chronic and recurrent stages of VKH disease, the angiogram takes on a "moth-eaten" appearance, with multiple hyperfluorescent RPE window defects without progressive staining.

Although lumbar puncture is commonly performed in Japan and other countries to confirm the diagnosis of VKH disease, the procedure is rarely necessary in a typical case, particularly when history and clinical examination suggest VKH. However, this procedure is a useful adjunctive test in cases with atypical features. Ohno et al. found that more than 80% of patients with VKH disease had cerebrospinal fluid pleocytosis, consisting mostly of lymphocytes.[16] In their study, the pleocytosis was present in 80% of patients within 1 week and in 97% of patients within 3 weeks of the onset of uveitis. The cerebrospinal fluid pleocytosis, however, is transient and resolves within 8 weeks, even in patients who develop recurrences of intraocular inflammation. In our series of 65 VKH patients, only four patients underwent lumbar puncture, and all of those were found to have pleocytosis.[1] Indeed, history and clinical examination combined with fluorescein angiography and/or ultrasonography are often sufficient to establish the diagnosis of VKH disease.

In patients with inadequate pupillary dilation caused by posterior synechiae or dense vitritis that obscures the view of the fundus, ultrasonography may help establish the diagnosis.[34] The ultrasound findings include diffuse, low-to-medium reflective thickening of the posterior choroid, serous retinal detachment located in the posterior pole or inferiorly, vitreous opacities, and posterior thickening of the sclera. The choroidal thickening is most prominent in the peripapillary area and generally extends to the equatorial region, becoming progressively thinner away from the optic nerve. These findings are generally bilateral.[34] Ultrasound biomicroscopic examination during the uveitis stage may reveal shallow anterior-chamber, ciliochoroidal detachment and thickened ciliary body.[19]

In the uveitic stage, ICG may reveal delay in choriocapillaris and larger choroidal vessel perfusion. Multiple hypofluorescent spots are noted throughout the fundus and hyperfluorescent pinpoint changes are observed in areas of exudative retinal detachment. In the chronic recurrent stage of the disease, multiple hypofluorescent spots are present; these spots may persist when the fundus appearance and fluorescein angiogram may not yield diagnostic clues.[35] Recently OCT has been used to monitor resolution of serous retinal detachment in patients treated with corticosteroids. This imaging modality is useful for detecting cystoid macular edema, edema of the detached retina, and subretinal neovascular membranes.

DIFFERENTIAL DIAGNOSIS

The differential diagnosis of VKH includes sympathetic ophthalmia, uveal effusion syndrome, posterior scleritis, primary intraocular lymphoma, uveal lymphoid infiltration, acute posterior multifocal placuoid pigment epitheliopathy (APMPPE), and sarcoidosis.[1] Sympathetic ophthalmia can present with bilateral panuveitis associated with retinal detachment and meningismus. However, a history of penetrating ocular injury is the rule in this disorder. Extraocular manifestations, such as dysacusis, vitiligo, poliosis, and alopecia, can occur in sympathetic ophthalmia, but they are rare.[36]

Uveal effusion syndrome may clinically mimic VKH disease. Angiographically, the effusion syndrome may reveal numerous fluorescent blotches in the subretinal space during the serous detachment phase. The syndrome can involve both eyes, although not simultaneously. Unlike VKH disease, the effusion syndrome lacks intraocular inflammation. Posterior scleritis affects predominantly women and is often bilateral. Patients may present with pain, photophobia, and loss of vision, and the vitreous often reveals cells. Exudative macular detachment and choroidal folds may be noted. Usually patients with bilateral involvement have a history of rheumatoid disease. Ultrasonography can help to differentiate posterior scleritis from the VKH disease. The former reveals flattening of the posterior aspect of the globe, thickening of the posterior coats of the eye, retrobulbar edema, and high internal reflectivity of the thickened sclera. Other entities, such as uveal lymphoid infiltrates, sarcoidosis, and APMPPE, can be differentiated based on their clinical features, ultrasonography, and fluorescein angiography.

TREATMENT

Early and aggressive use of systemic corticosteroids followed by slow tapering over 3 to 6 months is the treatment of choice to suppress the intraocular inflammation and to prevent the development of complications related to the ocular inflammation.[1] Such treatment may prevent progression of the disease to the chronic recurrent stage and may also reduce the incidence and/or severity of extraocular manifestations, including the development of sunset-glow fundus. If the ocular inflammation relapses after tapering of systemic corticosteroids, the relapse may reflect a too-rapid tapering of the corticosteroids. Such recurrences become increasingly steroid-resistant, and cytotoxic/immuno-suppressive agents are usually required to control the inflammation. Patients with inflammatory cell infiltration in the anterior chamber require topical corticosteroids and cycloplegics to reduce ciliary spasm and prevent posterior synechiae formation.

High-dose oral corticosteroids, 80 to 100 mg per day of prednisone or 200 mg of intravenous methylprednisolone for 3 days, followed by oral administration of high-dose corticosteroids with a slow taper, are the mainstay of therapy for VKH disease.[37,38] The use of intravenous corticosteroids, up to 1 g/day for 3 days, followed by a slow taper has been recommended by some. However, Sasamoto et al. found a similar beneficial effect of decreased intraocular inflammation with either 1 g or 200 mg/day of intravenous corticosteroids.[38] Patients treated with 80 to 100 mg of oral corticosteroids also respond well to the treatment.[1] Similar to patients who receive those intravenous corticosteroid treatments, patients managed initially with the high-dose oral corticosteroids require gradual tapering of the corticosteroids over 6 months to prevent recurrences. Of course, as is always the case when corticosteroids are prescribed, careful attention to possible risks and side-effects is warranted.

Although the initial episode of uveitis can be managed successfully in the majority of cases with intravenous and/or oral corticosteroids, recurrences do not respond as well to systemic corticosteroid treatment.[1] Such patients may show some initial response to sub-Tenon's injections of triamcinolone, but they usually require immunosuppressive or cytotoxic agents, such as ciclosporin, azathioprine, cyclophosphamide, chlorambucil, mycophenolate mofetil (Cell Cept), and FK506. Ciclosporin 5 mg/kg per day is generally preferred when the intraocular inflammation is corticosteroid-resistant or when the patient experiences intolerable side-effects from the long-term use of corticosteroids. Administration of the immunosuppressive and cytotoxic agents requires a careful pretreatment evaluation and careful subsequent evaluations during the follow-up examinations for any side-effects associated with the therapy. Various immunosuppressive and cytotoxic agents used in the treatment of VKH are summarized in Table 107-2.

PROGNOSIS AND COMPLICATIONS

In general, those VKH patients who are treated with initial high-dose systemic corticosteroids followed by gradual tapering will usually have a fair visual prognosis; nearly two-thirds of these patients retain 20/40 or better visual acuity.[1,37] On average, most patients require treatment for 6 months. The complications of chronic recurrent VKH include cataract, glaucoma, choroidal neovascularization, subretinal fibrosis, and optic atrophy.[1,39,40]

A retrospective analysis of the records of 101 patients with VKH disease followed at the Doheny Eye Institute revealed the development of at least one complication in 51% of eyes.[40] Cataract occurred in 42%, glaucoma in 27%, choroidal neovascularization in 11% (Figs 107-11 and 107-12), and subretinal fibrosis in 6% (Fig. 107-13). The patients who developed these complications had a significantly longer median duration of disease and significantly more recurrences then did those patients

Table 107-2 Immunosuppressive/cytotoxic agents used in the treatment of Vogt–Koyanagi–Harada disease
1. Corticosteroids[1,37,38] 　(a) Oral prednisone 100 to 200 mg initially, followed by gradual taper over 3 to 6 months 　(b) Pulse dose of methylprednisolone 1 g/day for 3 days, followed by gradual tapering of oral prednisone over 3 to 6 months 　(c) Intravenous methylprednisolone 100 to 200 mg/day for 3 days, followed by gradual tapering of oral prednisone over 3 to 6 months
2. Immunosuppressive agents[1] 　(a) Cyclosporin 5 mg/kg per day 　(b) FK506 0.1 to 0.15 mg/kg per day
3. Cytotoxic agents[1] 　(a) Azathioprine 1 to 2.5 mg/kg per day 　(b) Mycophenolate mofetil 1 to 3 g/day 　(c) Cyclophosphamide 1 to 2 mg/kg per day 　(d) Chlorambucil 0.1 mg/kg per day; dose adjusted every 3 weeks to a maximum of 18 mg/day

who developed no complications. Moreover, eyes possessing a better visual acuity at presentation had better visual acuity at final follow-up, and patients who developed VKH at a more advanced age had a worse visual acuity.[40]

There is general agreement that cataract surgery should be delayed until the intraocular inflammation has subsided, at which time safe cataract extraction with posterior-chamber intraocular lens implantation can be successfully accomplished. Occasionally, patients with significant vitreous opacities and debris may require a combined procedure of pars plana vitrectomy and lensectomy.[22]

Glaucoma secondary to angle closure from peripheral anterior synechiae and posterior synechiae have been noted in the majority of patients with glaucoma.[21] Acute angle closure with elevated intraocular pressure has been reported as a presenting sign of VKH disease. Although sustained elevated intraocular pressure can be controlled by medical therapy alone, most patients require surgical intervention in the form of iridectomy, trabeculectomy with 5-fluorouracil, and Molteno or other implant procedures.

Chronic recurrent anterior uveitis and fundus pigmentary disturbances seem to predispose patients to the development of choroidal neovascularization.[20] These subretinal membranes present with white gliotic raised masses, which may be associated with subretinal hemorrhage. ICG angiography is useful for detecting the membranes, and photocoagulation may help with the management. Photodynamic therapy with verteporfin for subfoveal choroidal neovascularization has been attempted with some success.

SUMMARY

VKH is a bilateral granulomatous panuveitis that usually presents with serous retinal detachment, with signs of meningeal irritation, with or without extraocular manifestations such as poliosis,

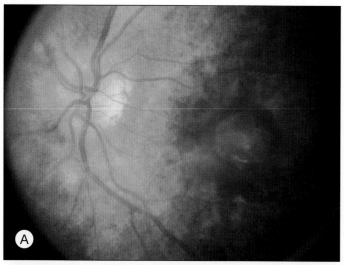

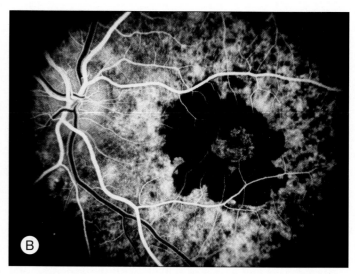

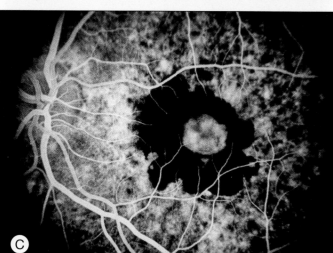

Fig. 107-11 A 28-year-old Hispanic female developed submacular choroidal neovascular membrane and hemorrhage during the chronic recurrent stage (A); the fluorescein angiogram shows typical neovascular membrane (B and C).

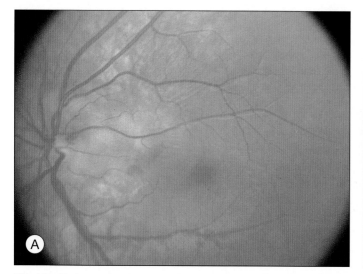

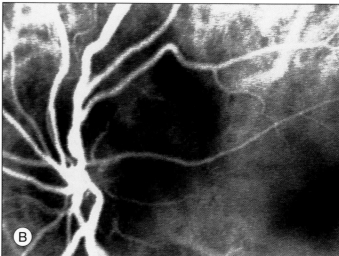

Fig. 107-12 A, Juxtapapillary area shows choroidal neovascularization with hemorrhage. B, Indocyanine green angiography delineates the neovascular membrane.

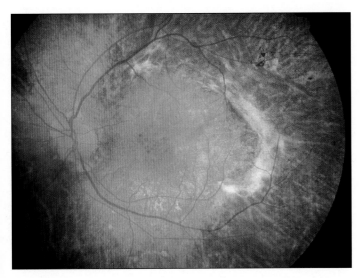

Fig. 107-13 The fundus showing subretinal fibrosis in a patient with chronic recurrent stage of Vogt–Koyanagi–Harada disease.

vitiligo, and auditory disturbances. In most cases, the diagnosis is a clinical one, but the diagnosis of atypical cases may require the use of fluorescein angiography, lumbar puncture, and ultrasonography. VKH is treated initially with high-dose systemic corticosteroids. Successful outcome requires a gradual tapering of the corticosteroids over a 3- to 6-month period. Complications of this disease include cataract, glaucoma, choroidal neovascularization, and subretinal fibrosis. The overall prognosis for adequately managed cases is fair, with nearly 60% to 70% of patients retaining vision of 20/40 or better.

REFERENCES

1. Moorthy RS, Inomata H, Rao NA. Vogt–Koyanagi–Harada syndrome. Surv Ophthalmol 1995; 39:265–292.
2. Beniz J, Forster DJ, Lean JS et al. Variations in clinical features of the Vogt–Koyanagi–Harada syndrome. Retina 1991; 11:275–280.
3. Snyder DA, Tessler HA. Vogt–Koyanagi–Harada syndrome. Am J Ophthalmol 1980; 90:69–75.
4. Read RW, Rao NA. Utility of existing Vogt–Koyanagi–Harada syndrome diagnostic criteria at initial evaluation of the individual patient: a retrospective analysis. Ocul Immunol Inflamm 2000; 8:227–234.
5. Read RW, Holland GN, Rao NA et al. Revised diagnostic criteria for Vogt–Koyanagi–Harada disease: report of an international committee on nomenclature. Am J Ophthalmol 2001; 131:647–652.
6. Pattison EM. Uveo-meningoencephalitic syndrome (Vogt–Koyanagi–Harada). Arch Neurol 1965; 12:197–205.
7. Schenkl A. Ein Fall von plötzlich aufgetretener Poliosis circumscripta der Wimpern. Arch Dermatol Syph 1873; 5:137–139.
8. Hutchinson J. A case of blanched eyelashes. Arch Surg 1892; 4:357.
9. Vogt A. Frühzeitiges Ergrauen der Zilien und Bemerkungen über den sogenannten plötzlichen Eintritt dieser Veränderung. Klin Monatsbl Augenheilkd 1906; 44:228–242.
10. Harada E. Beitrag zur klinischen Kenntnis von nichteitriger Choroiditis (choroiditis diffusa acuta). Acta Soc Ophthalmol Jpn 1926; 30:356–378.
11. Koyanagi Y. Dysakusis, Alopecia und Poliosis bei schwerer Uveitis nichttraumatischen Ursprungs. Klin Monatsbl Augenheilkd 1929; 82:194–211.
12. Babel J. Syndrome de Vogt–Koyanagi (Uveite bilaterale, poliosis, alopecie, vitiligo et dysacousie). Schweiz Med Wochenschr NR 1932; 44:1136–1140.
13. Bruno MG, McPherson SD Jr. Harada's disease. Am J Ophthalmol 1949; 32:513–522.
14. Shimizu K. Harada's, Behçet's, Vogt–Koyanagi syndromes – are they clinical entities? Trans Am Acad Ophthalmol Otolaryngol 1973; 77:OP281–OP290.
15. Nussenblatt RB. Clinical studies of Vogt–Koyanagi–Harada's disease at the National Eye Institute, NIH, USA. Jpn J Ophthalmol 1988; 32:330–333.
16. Ohno S, Char DH, Kimura SJ et al. Vogt–Koyanagi–Harada syndrome. Am J Ophthalmol 1977; 83:735–740.
17. Forster DJ, Green RL, Rao NA. Unilateral manifestation of the Vogt–Koyanagi–Harada syndrome in a 7-year-old child. Am J Ophthalmol 1991; 111:380–382.
18. Kawano Y, Tawara A, Nishioka Y et al. Ultrasound biomicroscopic analysis of transient shallow anterior chamber in Vogt–Koyanagi–Harada syndrome. Am J Ophthalmol 1996; 121:720–723.
19. Yamamoto N, Naito K. Annular choroidal detachment in patients with Vogt–Koyanagi–Harada disease. Graefes Arch Clin Exp Ophthalmol 2004; 242:355–358.
20. Moorthy RS, Chong LP, Smith RE et al. Subretinal neovascular membranes in Vogt–Koyanagi–Harada syndrome. Am J Ophthalmol 1993; 116:164–170.
21. Forster DJ, Rao NA, Hill RA et al. Incidence and management of glaucoma in Vogt–Koyanagi–Harada syndrome. Ophthalmogy 1993; 100:613–618.
22. Moorthy RS, Rajeev B, Smith RE et al. Incidence and management of cataracts in Vogt–Koyanagi–Harada syndrome. Am J Ophthalmol 1999; 118:197–204.
23. Arellanes-Garcia L, Bautista N, Mora P et al. HLA-DR is strongly associated with Vogt–Koyanagi–Harada disease in Mexican Mestizo patients. Ocul Immunol Inflamm 1998; 6:93–100.
24. Inomata H, Rao NA. Depigmented atrophic lesions in sunset glow fundi of Vogt–Koyanagi–Harada disease. Am J Ophthalmol 2001; 131:607–614.
25. Sakamoto T, Murata T, Inomata H. Class II major histocompatibility complex on melanocytes of Vogt–Koyanagi–Harada disease. Arch Ophthalmol 1991; 109:1270–1274.
26. Perry HD, Font RL. Clinical and histopathologic observations in severe Vogt–Koyanagi–Harada syndrome. Am J Ophthalmol 1997; 83:242–254.
27. Norose K, Yano A. Melanoma specific Th1 cytotoxic T lymphocyte lines in Vogt–Koyanagi–Harada disease. Br J Ophthalmol 1996; 80:1002–1008.
28. Sugita S, Sagawa K, Mochizuki M et al. Melanocyte lysis by cytotoxic T lymphocytes recognizing the MART-1 melanoma antigen in HLA-A2 patients with Vogt–Koyanagi–Harada disease. Int Immunol 1996; 8:799–803.
29. Rathinam SR, Namperumalsamy P, Nozik RA et al. Vogt–Koyanagi–Harada syndrome after cutaneous injury. Ophthalmology 1999; 106:635–638.
30. Gocho K, Kondo I, Yamaki K. Identification of autoreactive T cells in Vogt–Koyanagi–Harada disease. Invest Ophthalmol Vis Sci 2001; 42:2004–2009.
31. Hayakawa K, Ishikawa M, Yamaki K. Ultrastructural changes in rat eyes with experimental Vogt–Koyanagi–Harada disease. Jpn J Ophthalmol 2004; 48:222–227.
32. Shindo Y, Ohno S, Yamamoto T et al. Complete association of the HLA-DRB1*04 and DQ1*04 alleles with Vogt–Koyanagi–Harada's disease. Hum Immunol 1994; 39:169–176.
33. Weisz JM, Holland GN, Roer LN et al. Association between Vogt–Koyanagi–Harada syndrome and HLA-DR1 and -DR4 in Hispanic patients living in Southern California. Ophthalmology 1995; 102:1012–1015.
34. Forster DJ, Cano MR, Green RL et al. Echographic features of the Vogt–Koyanagi–Harada syndrome. Arch Ophthalmol 1990; 108:1421–1426.
35. Bouchenaki N, Herbort CP. The contribution of indocyanine green angiography to the appraisal and management of Vogt–Koyanagi–Harada disease. Ophthalmology 2001; 108:54–64.
36. Rao NA, Marak GE. Sympathetic ophthalmia simulating Vogt–Koyanagi–Harada's disease: a clinico-pathologic study of four cases. Jpn J Ophthalmol 1983; 27:506–511.
37. Rubsamen PE, Gass JDM. Vogt–Koyanagi–Harada syndrome. Clinical course, therapy, and long-term visual outcome. Arch Ophthalmol 1991; 109:682–687.
38. Sasamoto Y, Ohno S, Matsuda H. Studies on corticosteroid therapy in Vogt–Koyanagi–Harada disease. Ophthalmologica 1990; 201:162–167.
39. Kuo IC, Rechdouni A, Rao NA et al. Subretinal fibrosis in a patient with Vogt–Koyanagi–Harada syndrome. Ophthalmology 2000; 107:1721–1728.
40. Read RW, Rechodouni A, Butani N et al. Complications and prognostic factors in Vogt–Koyanagi–Harada disease. Am J Ophthalmol 2001; 131:599–606.

Drug Toxicity of the Posterior Segment

Robert A. Mittra
William F. Mieler

A variety of systemic medications can generate retinal toxicity. Fortunately, in the majority of cases the loss of visual function is minimal or reversible following discontinuation of the inciting drug. Nevertheless, permanent or progressive visual loss may occur in some instances. We present only those medications known to produce a well-described anomaly and have omitted those that have not been definitively proven to cause retinal abnormalities. The medications are grouped according to the type of retinal toxicity they produce (Box 108-1).

DISRUPTION OF THE RETINA AND RETINAL PIGMENT EPITHELIUM

Phenothiazines

Thioridazine

Blurred vision, dyschromatopsia (reddish or brownish discoloration of vision), and nyctalopia characterize acute toxicity with thioridazine.[1] In the earliest stages the fundus appearance may be normal or display only mild granular pigment stippling (Fig. 108-1). An intermediate stage is characterized by circumscribed nummular areas of retinal pigment epithelial (RPE) loss from the posterior pole to the midperiphery[2] (Fig. 108-2A). Fluorescein angiography (FA) reveals disruption of the choriocapillaris in these zones of pigment rarefaction (Fig. 108-2B). In late stages of thioridazine toxicity, widespread areas of depigmentation alternating with hyperpigmented plaques, vascular attenuation, and optic atrophy are seen[3] (Fig. 108-3).

Retinal toxicity from thioridazine is dependent more on the total daily dose than on the cumulative amount of drug received.[4] With higher daily doses, toxicity can occur rapidly, even within the first 2 weeks of therapy.[5] Toxicity is rare at dosages less than 800 mg/day. Nonetheless, a few cases have been reported with lower doses given over several years.[6-10] As a result, many now suggest that any patient taking thioridazine, regardless of the daily dose, be monitored for the development of visual symptoms or fundus changes.

In the initial stages of toxicity, visual field testing can reveal mild constriction, paracentral scotomas, or ring scotomas. Electroretinography (ERG) is either normal or shows decreased oscillatory potentials. In the later stages, both the rod and cone functions of the ERG, as well as the electro-oculography (EOG), are markedly abnormal.[11] If the drug is stopped early, ERG testing improves over the first year.[12] Histologic studies demonstrate that atrophy and disorganization of photoreceptor outer segments occurs primarily, with a secondary loss of the RPE and choriocapillaris.[3]

The early fundus changes associated with thioridazine often progress despite discontinuation of therapy.[2] It is unclear whether this degeneration represents continued toxicity of the drug or a delayed expansion of chorioretinal scarring to areas of subclinical, pre-existing damage.[12] Visual function, in contrast to fundus appearance, usually improves over the first year after a toxic reaction; this undoubtedly would not occur if thioridazine caused persistent toxicity.

The mechanism of thioridazine-mediated toxicity remains unknown. Many phenothiazines bind melanin granules of the RPE and uveal tissue, but not all commonly instigate retinal toxicity.[13-15] The compound NP-207 (piperidyl-chlorophenothiazine hydrochloride) has a remarkably similar chemical structure to thioridazine, including the same piperidyl side chain. NP-207 was never marketed because of the pronounced pigmentary retinopathy that developed during early clinical trials.[16] This piperidyl side chain is not present in other phenothiazines such as chlorpromazine, which exhibit much less retinal toxicity. Experimental studies demonstrate that phenothiazines both alter enzyme kinetics and inhibit oxidative phosphorylation with subsequent abnormalities in rhodopsin synthesis.[17-19] Other studies postulate that phenothiazine toxicity is due to the drug's effect on the dopamine receptors in the retina. Further study is necessary to determine whether these observed effects are involved in the pathogenesis of thioridazine toxicity.

A review of the daily and cumulative drug dosage is essential in patients taking thioridazine. Baseline fundus photography and possibly ERG testing may be helpful if future toxicity develops. Given the many antipsychotic medications available today, consideration of alternative agents may be discussed with the patient's psychiatrist. At the earliest sign of toxicity, thioridazine should be discontinued.

Chlorpromazine

Chlorpromazine is a piperazine similar to thioridazine but lacks the piperidyl side chain mentioned above. The compound binds strongly to melanin and can cause hyperpigmentation in the skin, conjunctiva, cornea, lens, and retina[20-24] (Fig. 108-4). Other ocular

Box 108-1 Patterns of retinal toxicity

Disruption of the retina and retinal pigment epithelium
Phenothiazines
Quinine sulfate
Thioridazine
Clofazimine
Chlorpromazine
Deferoxamine
Chloroquine derivatives
Corticosteroid preparations
Chloroquine
Cisplatin and BCNU (carmustine)
Hydroxychloroquine

Vascular damage
Quinine sulfate
Aminoglycoside antibiotics
Cisplatin and BCNU (carmustine)
Interferon
Ergot alkaloids
Talc
Phenylpropanolamine
Oral contraceptives

Cystoid macular edema
Epinephrine
Latanoprost
Nicotinic acid

Retinal folds
Sulfa antibiotics
Hydrochlorothiazide
Acetazolamide
Triamterene
Ethoxyzolamide
Metronidazole
Chlorthalidone

Crystalline retinopathy
Tamoxifen
Talc
Canthaxanthine
Nitrofurantoin
Methoxyflurane

Uveitis
Rifabutin
Cidofovir

Miscellaneous
Digoxin
Methanol

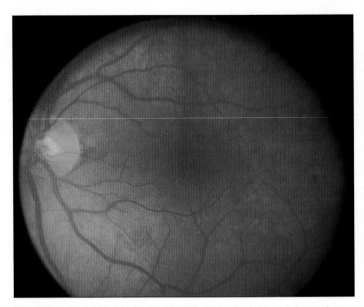

Fig. 108-1 Early thioridazine toxicity. Photograph shows mild granular pigment stippling of the temporal macular region.

Chloroquine derivatives
Chloroquine

Chloroquine was first used as an antimalarial drug in World War II. Currently it is prescribed for treatment of amebiasis, rheumatoid arthritis, systemic lupus erythematosus, and for prophylaxis against malaria. Retinal toxicity with degeneration of the RPE and neurosensory retina as a result of long-term daily use of chloroquine has been well described.[25-32] However, most cases of retinopathy have developed when a higher than currently recommended (3 mg/kg/day using lean body weight) dose was used.[33] A daily dose exceeding 250 mg with a total cumulative dose between 100 and 300 g is customarily needed to produce toxicity.[34] One study showed a 19% incidence of chloroquine retinopathy in patients taking a mean daily dose of 329 mg.[35] Conversely, with strict adherence to a low dose per diem, the incidence of retinal abnormalities is minimal even when cumulative doses reach over 1000 g.[36]

A paracentral scotoma may be the earliest manifestation of retinal toxicity and can precede the development of any ophthalmoscopic or ERG abnormality.[37] Subtle macular pigment stippling with a loss of the foveal light reflex (Fig. 108-6) usually appears on fundus examination before the development of a classic bull's-eye maculopathy, in which a ring of depigmentation surrounded by an area of hyperpigmentation is seen centered on the fovea (Fig. 108-7). Visual acuity decreases when the RPE abnormalities involve the center of the fovea. The peripheral retina can display pigment mottling, which may, in severe cases, develop into the appearance of primary tapetoretinal degeneration with narrowed retinal vessels, optic disc pallor, and eventual blindness (Fig. 108-8).

After the cessation of chloroquine treatment, early subtle macular changes can revert to normal. Although far advanced cases may progress despite discontinuation of the drug, most patients remain stable with long-term follow-up.[38,39] Chloroquine,

effects include oculogyric crisis, miosis, and blurred vision caused by paralysis of accommodation. Usual doses range from 40 to 75 mg/day, but dosages up to 800 mg/day are not uncommon.

Retinal toxicity from chlorpromazine is rare. When massive doses are given (e.g. 2400 mg/day for 12 months), pigmentary changes may occur in the retina with attenuation of retinal vessels and optic nerve pallor[23] (Fig. 108-5). Similar to thioridazine, the development and extent of toxicity are more closely related to daily dosage than total amount of drug taken.

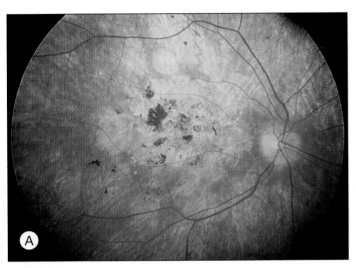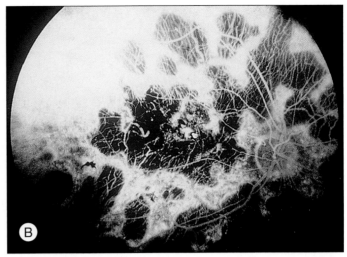

Fig. 108-2 Intermediate thioridazine toxicity. Photograph (A) and fluorescein angiogram (B) show central and peripheral nummular pigmentary changes with corresponding atrophy of the choriocapillaris.

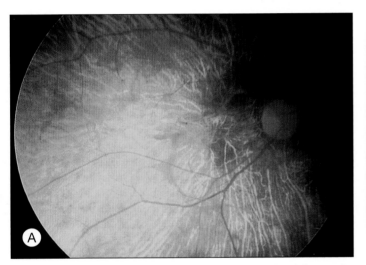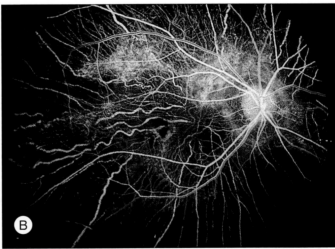

Fig. 108-3 End-stage thioridazine toxicity. Photograph (A) and fluorescein angiogram (B) show diffuse pigmentary and choriocapillaris atrophy, optic atrophy, and vascular attenuation.

however, is very slowly excreted from the body. It has been detected in the plasma, red blood cells, and urine of patients 5 years after their last known ingestion.[40] This prolonged presence may account for the rare cases of delayed onset of chloroquine retinopathy seen up to 7 years or longer after discontinuation.[41,42]

Fluorescein angiography can be helpful in the early demonstration of pigment abnormalities in the macula (see Figs 108-6 and 108-7). There is minimal evidence of damage to the choriocapillaris on FA in the areas of pigment disturbance. The ERG and EOG may be abnormal early, although the EOG is sometimes supernormal initially.[43] Histopathologic sections demonstrate loss of RPE pigmentation with an accumulation of pigment-laden cells in the outer retinal layers with damage and reduction of photoreceptors.[44] Electron microscopic studies reveal more widespread damage to the retina, especially the ganglion cell layer.[45]

The mechanism of chloroquine-mediated retinal toxicity is unknown. Like the phenothiazines, chloroquine is bound by melanin and concentrated in the RPE and uveal tissues.[46] Possible explanations include inhibition of critical enzymes and interference with the metabolic function of the RPE and photoreceptors.[41,47]

Hydroxychloroquine

Given the incidence of toxicity with chloroquine, most rheumatologists prefer hydroxychloroquine for the treatment of rheumatoid arthritis and systemic lupus erythematosus. Although it can produce a retinopathy identical to chloroquine, its occurrence is rare.[48–51] Only a few cases of toxicity have been well documented, involving decreased visual acuity, paracentral scotoma, and a bull's-eye maculopathy (Figs 108-9 and 108-10).[52–57] Many of these patients received above the recommended daily

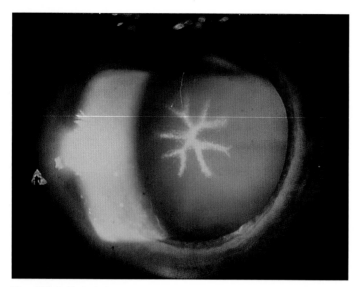

Fig. 108-4 Typical chlorpromazine-induced anterior stellate lens opacities.

dosage of 6.5 mg/kg/day, but the classic fundus findings have been reported at lower doses as well.[58-60]

Several authors have questioned the utility of screening given the low yield, high cost, and the difficulty in diagnosing the condition early enough to prevent damage.[61-64] Nevertheless, toxicity does occur, and if retinal and functional changes are detected early, severe visual impairment can be averted.[65,66] Use of static perimetry through the vertical meridian with a red test object may be the best method to detect an early paracentral scotoma.[37] These changes usually occur before visible retinal abnormalities and therefore should be performed on follow-up examinations. The red Amsler grid is also useful in detecting an early paracentral scotoma and may be substituted for static perimetry.[67] In addition, the grid can be given to patients so that they can monitor their visual function at home. Recent data suggest that multifocal electroretinographic evaluation may detect toxicity at its earliest stages.[68-72]

The American Academy of Ophthalmology guidelines for screening include a baseline examination performed at the commencement of therapy.[73] Screening exams during the first five years of therapy can be performed during routine ophthalmic examination (interval to be determined by age of the patient). If the dosage used is higher than 6.5 mg/kg/day for hydroxychloroquine (3 mg/kg/day for chloroquine), the patient is obese, has renal or liver dysfunction, has concomitant macular disease or is more than 60 years of age, screening should be performed at least annually. After five years of therapy, screening should be performed at least annually.[74] If ocular toxicity occurs,[75-78] and is recognized at an early stage, efforts should be made to communicate this directly to the prescribing physician so that alternatives can be discussed with the patient. In almost all cases, cessation of the drug should be suggested.

Quinine sulfate

Quinine sulfate was first used for the treatment of malaria in World War II, but it currently is prescribed for the management of nocturnal muscle cramps or "restless leg syndrome." The recommended daily dose is less than 2 g. Signs of systemic toxicity occur with doses greater than 4 g, and the fatal oral dose is 8 g. Ocular toxicity with quinine develops after an overdose, either by accidental ingestion or by attempted abortion or suicide. Rarely, chronic ingestion at low levels can result in ocular toxicity as well.[79] With an overdose, a syndrome known as *cinchonism* is rapidly produced, consisting of nausea, vomiting, headache, tremor, and sometimes hypotension and loss of consciousness. When patients awake they often are completely blind and have dilated, unreactive pupils.[80] In the acute stages of toxicity, fundus examination reveals mild venous dilation with minimal retinal edema and normal arterial caliber. The FA

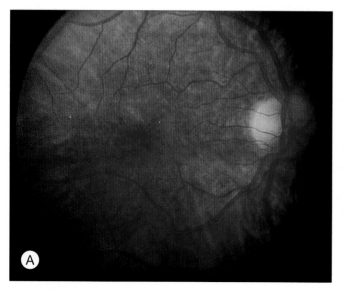

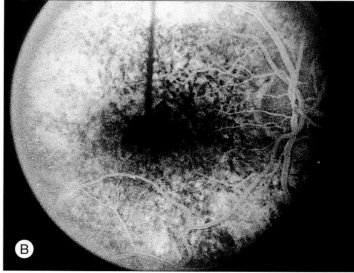

Fig. 108-5 Chlorpromazine toxicity. Photograph (A) and fluorescein angiogram (B) show granular pigment changes less severe than those seen with thioridazine.

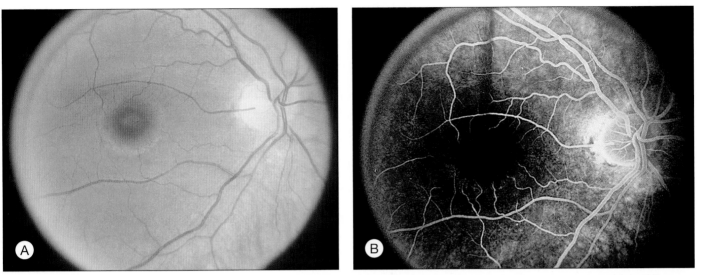

Fig. 108-6 Early chloroquine toxicity. Photograph (A) and fluorescein angiogram (B) show early perifoveal pigmentary changes. From Mieler WF. Focal points. American Academy of Ophthalmology, Dec 1997.

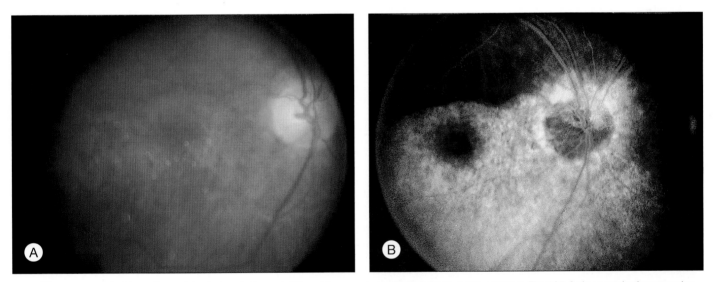

Fig. 108-7 Advanced chloroquine toxicity. Later photograph (A) and fluorescein angiogram (B) from the patient in Fig. 107-6 show marked progression with advanced widespread pigmentary changes. From Mieler WF. Focal points. American Academy of Ophthalmology, Dec 1997.

displays minimal abnormalities. ERG testing shows an acute slowing of the a-wave with increased depth, loss of oscillatory potentials, and a decreased b-wave. EOG and visual evoked potential (VEP) testing are also abnormal.

Over the next few days visual acuity returns, but the patient is left with a small central island of vision. There is a progressive attenuation of the retinal arterioles with the development of optic disc pallor over the next few weeks to months (Fig. 108-11). Early investigators believed the mechanism of quinine toxicity to be vascular in origin. This was based primarily on the fundus appearance several weeks after ingestion, which showed marked arteriolar attenuation and optic disc pallor.[80,81] More recent experimental and clinical studies have demon-

strated minimal involvement of the retinal vasculature in the early stages of quinine toxicity.[80-82] Furthermore, ERG and histologic studies show that the site of toxicity is likely the retinal ganglion, bipolar, and photoreceptor cells.[80,82] The exact mechanism of quinine toxicity is unidentified, but some have suggested that it may act as an acetylcholine antagonist and disrupt cholinergic transmission in the retina.[83]

Clofazimine

Clofazimine is a red phenazine dye that has been used to treat dapsone-resistant leprosy, psoriasis, pyoderma gangrenosum, discoid lupus, and more recently, *Mycobacterium avium*-complex infections in AIDS patients. With treatment over several months,

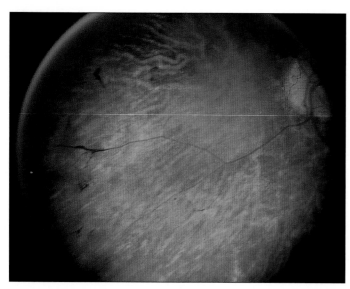

Fig. 108-8 Chloroquine retinopathy. Photograph shows bone-spicule pigmentary changes that can develop in advanced cases. The appearance is similar to end-stage retinitis pigmentosa.

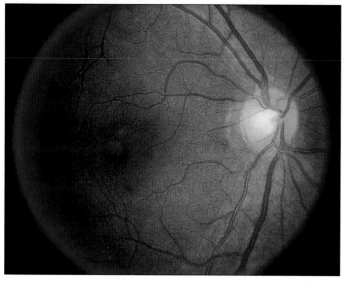

Fig. 108-9 Hydroxychloroquine toxicity. Photograph displays pigmentary changes in the central macula.

clofazimine crystals may accumulate in the cornea. Two cases of bull's-eye maculopathy with pigmentary retinopathy (Fig. 108-12) have been reported in AIDS patients with doses of 200 to 300 mg/day (total dose, 40 to 48 g).[84,85] Visual acuity was mildly affected, with reduced scotopic, photopic, and flicker ERG amplitudes. Cessation of treatment may result in the clearance of the corneal deposits but does not appear to affect the retinopathy.

DDI

A midperipheral pigmentary retinopathy has been noted in three children with AIDS receiving high dose therapy with the antiviral 2′,3′-dideoxyinosine.[86] The cases were associated with ERG and EOG changes. The retinal toxicity stabilized after discontinuation of the medication.

Deferoxamine

Intravenous (IV) and subcutaneous (SQ) administration of defer-oxamine has been used to treat patients who require repeated blood transfusions and subsequently develop complications of iron overload. High-dose IV and SQ therapy has produced visual loss, nyctalopia, peripheral and central field loss, and reduced ERG amplitudes and EOG ratios.[87,88] Fundi can be normal initially, or there may be a faint graying of the macula.[89] Pigmentary changes in the macula and periphery develop within a few weeks and are particularly highlighted by fluorescein angiography (Fig. 108-13).[90] Macular changes can resemble vitelliform maculopathy.[91] Return of visual function occurs with cessation of therapy. Deferoxamine chelates many metals other than iron, and it is possible that the mechanism of toxicity may involve the removal of copper from the RPE.[87] Histopathologic changes occur primarily in the RPE and include loss of microvilli from the apical surface, patchy depigmentation, vacuolation of the cytoplasm, swelling and calcification of mitochondria, and disorganization of the plasma membrane.[92]

Corticosteroid preparations

The vehicles of several common corticosteroid preparations have been shown to cause retinal necrosis when inadvertently injected into the eye[93,94] (Fig. 108-14). The corticosteroids themselves probably have a minimal toxic effect on the retina.[95] Celestone Soluspan, with its vehicle benzalkonium chloride, and Depo-Medrol, with myristyl gamma-picolinium chloride, caused the most extensive retinal damage in an experimental study comparing several depot steroids.[96] If one of these agents is inadvertently injected, immediate surgical removal should be instituted.

Cisplatin and BCNU (carmustine)

Cisplatin and BCNU are used for the treatment of malignant gliomas and metastatic breast cancer. Three different types of retinal toxicity have been reported with these agents. One type of change consists of a pigmentary retinopathy of the macula with markedly decreased visual acuity and frequently abnormal electrophysiologic testing. This pigmentary change has been reported after administration of combined intraarterial cisplatin and BCNU and with cisplatin alone for malignant glioma.[97,98] These findings probably are the result of platinum toxicity of the retina. Severe bilateral visual loss was reported after intravenous cisplatin in a patient that received four times the intended dose for treatment of lymphoma.[99] Later histology showed a splitting of the outer plexiform layer.

A second type of retinopathy has been described and consists of cotton-wool spots, intraretinal hemorrhages, macular exudate, and optic neuropathy with disc swelling. This was reported in the setting of high-dose chemotherapy with cisplatin, cyclophosphamide, carmustine, and autologous bone marrow transplantation for metastatic breast cancer.[100] The third type of change

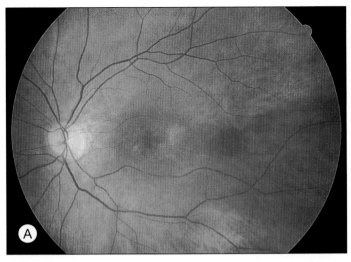

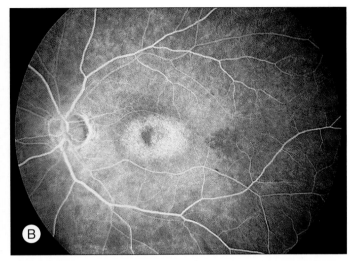

Fig. 108-10 Hydroxychloroquine toxicity. Photograph (A) and fluorescein angiogram (B) show a marked bull's-eye maculopathy.

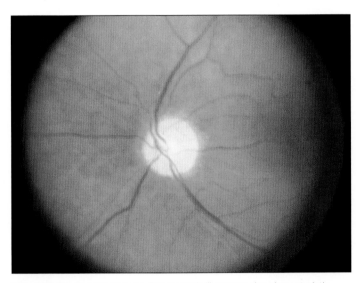

Fig. 108-11 Quinine toxicity. Photograph illustrates the characteristic optic nerve head pallor with diffuse arteriolar attenuation approximately 2 months after ingestion.

involves a vascular retinopathy or optic neuropathy, which can include arterial occlusion, vasculitis, and papillitis. This has been seen in approximately 65% of patients receiving intraarterial BCNU alone or combined with cisplatin for malignant glioma.[98] These fundus changes are associated with a profound visual loss that begins about 6 weeks after the start of therapy. Other ocular effects may include orbital pain, chemosis, secondary glaucoma, internal ophthalmoplegia, and cavernous sinus syndrome. Injection of medication above the ophthalmic artery can still result in toxicity.[101] The visual loss usually is progressive, and no treatment is known.

Potassium iodate

Overdose of potassium iodate, an iodized salt used for iodine supplementation in areas endemic for goiter, has been shown to cause profound visual loss and extensive fundus pigmentary abnormalities.[102] Fluorescein angiography reveals RPE window defects and ERG and VEP testing shows marked impairment of retinal function. Visual acuity may improve slowly over several months.

VASCULAR DAMAGE

Quinine sulfate
See Disruption of the retina and retinal pigment epithelium, p. 1839.

Cisplatin and BCNU (carmustine)
See Disruption of the retina and retinal pigment epithelium, p. 1839.

Talc
A characteristic retinopathy consisting of small, white, glistening crystals concentrated in the end arterioles of the posterior pole has been described in intravenous (IV) drug abusers[103–105] (Fig. 108-15). These addicts crush oral medications such as methylphenidate hydrochloride (Ritalin) or methadone HCl and then create an aqueous suspension by adding water and heating the mixture. The solution is subsequently drawn up into a syringe, with occasional attempts at filtering the mixture with cotton fibers, gauze, or cigarette filters. These oral medications contain talc (hydrous magnesium silicate) as inert filler material; after IV administration, talc particles embolize to the pulmonary vasculature, where the larger particles are trapped. After repeated injections over months to years, collateral vasculature develops, allowing the particles to enter the systemic circulation and embolize to other organs, including the eye. Even before shunt development, particles smaller than 7 μm can traverse the pulmonary capillary bed and enter the retinal circulation.[106]

Once a large number of talc particles lodge in the small arterioles of the retinal vasculature, a characteristic picture of an ischemic retinopathy begins to develop. Capillary nonperfusion,

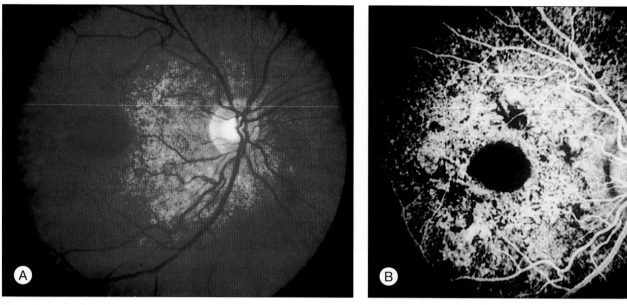

Fig. 108-12 Clofazimine toxicity. Photograph (A) and fluorescein angiogram (B) show moderate macular pigmentary changes in a bull's-eye pattern.

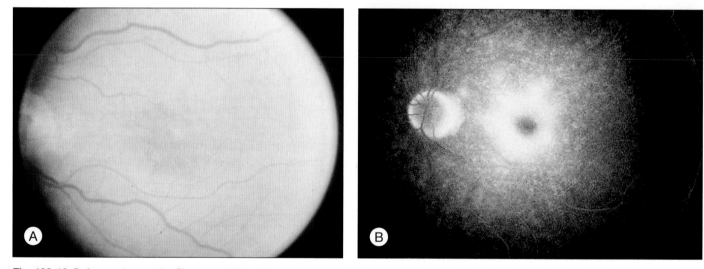

Fig. 108-13 Deferoxamine toxicity. Photograph (A) and fluorescein angiogram (B) show a diffuse pigmentary retinopathy with macular and retinal edema.

microaneurysm formation, cotton-wool spots, and venous loops can all be seen.[107] In severe cases optic disc and peripheral neovascularization and vitreous hemorrhage can develop[108,109] (Fig. 108-16). An experimental model of talc retinopathy in monkeys has demonstrated with light and electron microscopic techniques that the vascular abnormalities induced are very similar to other ischemic retinopathies seen in humans, such as sickle cell and hypertensive retinopathy.[110–112]

Once talc retinopathy is diagnosed, an attempt at educating the patient as to the cause of the disorder is indicated. Treatment of neovascularization and vitreous hemorrhage should be undertaken using laser photocoagulation and pars plana vitrectomy if

necessary in a manner similar to that used for sickle cell or proliferative diabetic retinopathy.

Oral contraceptives

Oral contraceptives have been implicated in some cases of central retinal vein occlusion, retinal and cilioretinal artery obstruction, and retinal edema occurring in young women.[113–119] The synthetic estrogen and progesterone contained in contraceptive pills are thought to adversely effect coagulation factors and induce a hypercoagulable state leading to thromboembolic complications. Most of the studies reporting ocular complications are from the 1960s and 1970s, when the estrogen concentrations used in "the

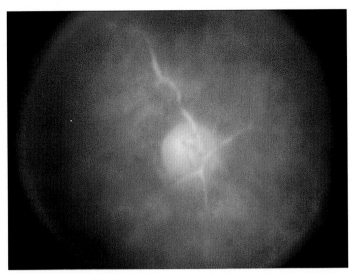

Fig. 108-14 Intraocular corticosteroid injection. Photograph shows end-stage retinopathy, with sclerotic vessels and diffuse pigmentary changes, after an inadvertent intraocular injection of corticosteroid.

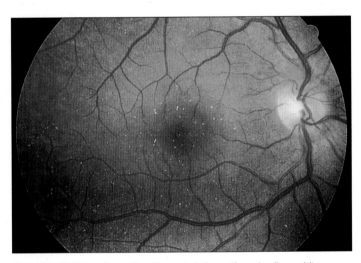

Fig. 108-15 Talc retinopathy. Characteristic perifoveal yellow-white glistening crystals.

pill" were much higher. More recent prospective studies have failed to show an increased incidence of ocular complications with the drug.[120,121]

Aminoglycoside antibiotics

Retinal toxicity from aminoglycoside antibiotics has been reported after inadvertent intraocular injection of massive doses, intravitreal injection for bacterial endophthalmitis, prophylactic intravitreal injection after pars plana vitrectomy, prophylactic subconjunctival injections after routine ocular surgery, and with the use of small amounts in the infusion fluid during cataract extraction.[122–126] Gentamicin is the most toxic antibiotic in the aminoglycoside family, followed by tobramycin and amikacin.[127] Massive doses result in early superficial and intraretinal hemorrhages, retinal edema, cotton-wool patches, arteriolar narrowing, and venous

beading (Fig. 108-17).[125] Fluorescein angiography reveals severe vascular nonperfusion in the acute stages. Visual loss is profound, and late rubeosis iridis, neovascular glaucoma, pigmentary retinopathy, and optic atrophy are common. Intra-vitreal injection of smaller doses thought to be safe for the eye (100 to 400 μg) can still cause toxicity with less severe fundus changes.[123–125] The major preservatives found in injectable gentamicin (methylparaben, propylparaben, sodium bisulfite, and edetate disodium) likely play an additive role in its ocular toxicity.

A number of factors appear to affect the extent of toxicity observed with similar doses of these medications. Peyman found that retinal toxicity could be enhanced with an intra-vitreal injection directed at the posterior pole with the bevel of the needle pointed toward the retina, and Zachary and Forster demonstrated that an increased rate of injection during intraocular administration could also increase the retinal toxicity observed.[128,129] One investigator stated that eyes that have undergone a previous pars plana vitrectomy are at greater risk for gentamicin toxicity, but an experimental model has shown no difference between eyes that had cataract extraction alone compared with those that underwent lensectomy and vitrectomy.[126,130] Finally, increased ocular pigmentation protects the rabbit retina from aminoglycoside toxicity and may explain some of the wide variability seen with intraocular exposure in humans.[131,132]

Although clinical aminoglycoside toxicity appears to affect the retinal vasculature primarily, pathologic studies have revealed that gentamicin in small doses causes the formation of abnormal lamellar lysosomal inclusions in the RPE, and larger doses cause increasing amounts of retinal necrosis, first of the outer then inner segments.[133–136] Histologically, vessel closure appears to result from granulocytic plugging.

Prevention of aminoglycoside toxicity can be accomplished by abandoning the use of these medications as routine prophylaxis following intraocular surgery, eliminating them from intra-ocular infusion fluids used in vitrectomy and cataract surgery, and using alternative medications for the treatment of bacterial endophthalmitis. Animal studies have demonstrated that thinned sclera alone without perforation can result in markedly elevated intraocular gentamicin levels after subconjunctival injection.[137] If inadvertent intraocular injection does occur, immediate pars plana vitrectomy with posterior segment lavage should be performed.[138,139] Since there is some evidence that gravity plays a role in the predilection of gentamicin-induced toxicity for the macula, the patient should be placed upright as soon as possible after surgery.[140]

Interferon

Interferon-α is used to treat Kaposi's sarcoma, hemangiomas of infancy, chronic hepatitis C, melanoma, renal cell carcinoma, in chemotherapy protocols for leukemia, lymphoma and hemangiomatosis, and experimentally for the treatment of choroidal neovascular membranes. Interferon therapy has been associated with the development of multiple cotton-wool spots associated with retinal hemorrhages[141–143] (Fig. 108-18). Optic disc edema, branch arterial and venous occlusion, central retinal venous obstruction and CME have been reported with the more severe

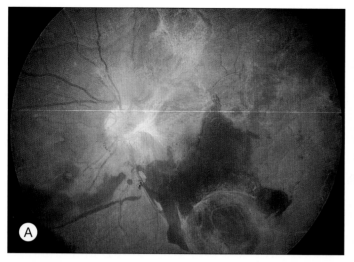
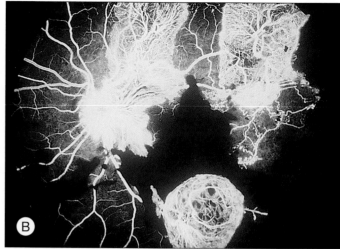

Fig. 108-16 Ischemic talc retinopathy. Photograph (A) and fluorescein angiogram (B) show widespread capillary dropout, neovascularization, and preretinal hemorrhage.

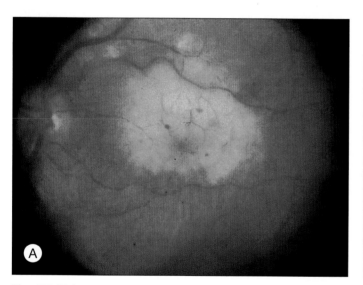
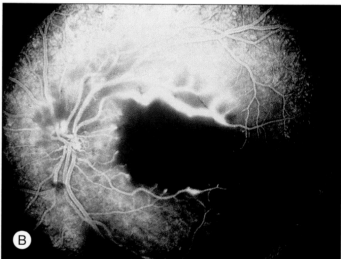

Fig. 108-17 Intraocular gentamicin injection. Photograph (A) and fluorescein angiogram (B) show acute macular necrosis.

findings observed in patients receiving high dose therapy.[144–146] Visual acuity usually is not affected if the fundus findings are limited to cotton-wool spots and intraretinal hemorrhage. Changes are noted within the first 4 to 8 weeks of therapy and are seen more frequently in diabetic and hypertensive patients.[147] Intravitreal injection of interferon-α-2b is well tolerated in the rabbit eye up to dosages of 1 million units; 2 million units causes a vitreous haze and intraretinal hemorrhages.[148] Interferon toxicity may be caused by an increase in immune complex deposition and activated complement C5a with leukocyte infiltration.

Miscellaneous agents

Ergot alkaloids in higher than recommended doses have been reported to cause retinal vasoconstriction,[149,150] and over-the-counter phenylpropanolamine used in appetite suppressants and decongestants has been implicated in one case of central retinal vein occlusion.[151]

CYSTOID MACULAR EDEMA

Epinephrine

The use of epinephrine compounds in glaucoma has decreased with the advent of newer, more efficacious agents. Topical epinephrine can cause macular edema in aphakic eyes, indistinguishable clinically and angiographically from postoperative aphakic cystoid macular edema (CME). In the largest controlled study, 28% of aphakic eyes treated with epinephrine and 13% of untreated aphakic eyes had macular edema, a difference that was statistically significant.[152] Most cases of CME resolve with cessation of epinephrine usage. This medication should be avoided in the treatment of the glaucomatous aphakic and pseudophakic eyes.

Nicotinic acid

High doses of niacin have been used to reduce serum lipid and cholesterol levels. Better-tolerated HMG-CoA reductase

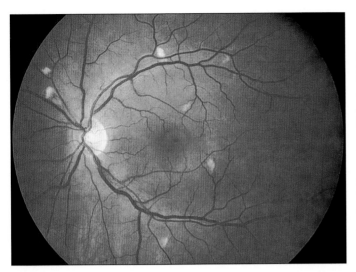

Fig. 108-18 Interferon microangiopathy. Multiple cotton-wool spots dispersed throughout the posterior pole.

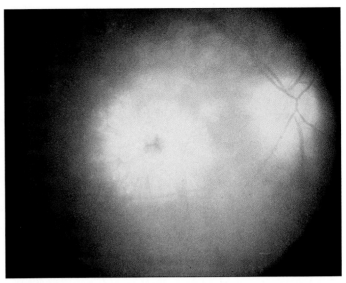

Fig. 108-19 Latanaprost-associated cystoid macular edema. Angiogram shows characteristic fluorescein filling of the cystic spaces.

inhibitor agents have largely curtailed its use. At doses greater than 1.5 g/day, a minority of patients will report blurred central vision, sometimes associated with a paracentral scotoma or metamorphopsia.[153] Fluorescein angiography fails to demonstrate vascular leakage despite the typical clinical appearance of CME.[154,155] This has led to speculation of a direct toxic effect on Müller cells, resulting in intracellular edema.[156] Optical coherence tomography reveals cystoid spaces in the inner nuclear and outer plexiform layers.[157] With cessation of treatment, the CME resolves, and vision generally returns to normal. Given the rarity of this condition, only patients who are taking high-dose niacin and who have visual symptoms should be evaluated.

Latanoprost

Latanoprost is a prostaglandin analog that is used for the control of a variety of forms of glaucoma. Although initial human and animal studies did not show an association between latanoprost and CME, recent case reports and studies have documented that approximately 2–5% of susceptible patients with glaucoma may develop CME and anterior uveitis, which resolves after discontinuation of the drug[158–166] (Fig. 108-19). This may be caused by the preservative used in the drug formulation.[167] Patients with CME who are taking latanoprost should undergo a trial off the medication before initiating further therapy for the edema. High-risk CME patients, such as those with a history of recent surgery or uveitis, should be managed with other agents.

RETINAL FOLDS

Sulfa antibiotics, acetazolamide, ethoxyzolamide, chlorthalidone, hydrochlorothiazide, triamterene, metronidazole

Several medications, most with a structure similar to sulfanilamide, as those above, can cause a syndrome of transient acute myopia and anterior chamber shallowing. This is thought to occur as a result of ciliary body swelling or choroidal effusion, or both,

with subsequent forward rotation of the lens-iris diaphragm.[168–170] Retinal folds in the macula are seen in young patients with this syndrome, but FA does not reveal retinal leakage (Fig. 108-20). The folds presumably develop as a result of vitreous traction on the macula that is caused by the forward shift of the lens and iris.

CRYSTALLINE RETINOPATHY

Tamoxifen

Tamoxifen is an antiestrogen agent used in the treatment of advanced breast carcinoma and as adjuvant therapy after surgical resection of early disease. Retinal toxicity consisting of decreased visual acuity and color vision with white intraretinal crystalline deposits, macular edema, and punctate retinal pigmentary changes can occur.[171] The intraretinal deposits appear to reside in the inner retina and are most numerous in paramacular areas (Fig. 108-21). Early reports involved patients who had received high doses (60 to 100 mg/day, total dosage >100 g) of the drug over 1 year.[172] More recent studies have demonstrated that chronic low-dose administration (10 to 20 mg/day) with as little as 7.7 g total, also can cause ocular toxicity.[173–176] Even asymptomatic patients may exhibit intraretinal crystalline formation.[177] Visual function and edema improve after discontinuation of the drug, but the refractile deposits remain.

Fluorescein angiography demonstrates late focal staining in the macula consistent with CME. Decreased photopic and scotopic a- and b-wave amplitude is noted on ERG testing.[178] Light microscopy reveals lesions confined to the nerve fiber and inner plexiform layers, which stain positive for glycosaminoglycans. Small (3 to 10 μ) intracellular and large (30 to 35 μ) extracellular lesions within axons are noted on electron microscopy.[179] The lesions appear to represent products of axonal degeneration similar to corpora amylacea.

Decreased vision with bilateral optic disc swelling and retinal hemorrhages has been reported in a patient just 3 weeks after

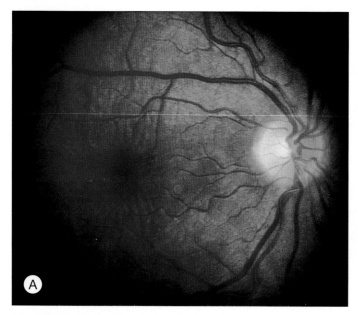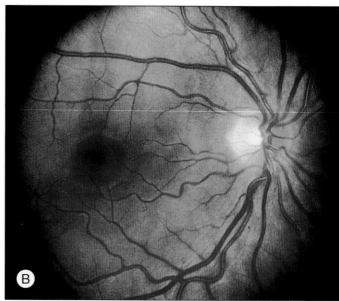

Fig. 108-20 Chlorthalidone-induced retinal folds. Photograph (A) shows perifoveal retinal folds associated with chlorthalidone therapy, which resolve after discontinuation of the drug (B).

commencement of therapy with tamoxifen. These findings resolved completely after the drug was stopped.[180] It is unclear whether the findings in this patient were related to the more commonly seen toxic effects. With current low-dose therapy (10 to 20 mg/day), retinal lesions are rare, and routine examination of asymptomatic patients is not indicated.[180,181] If a patient taking tamoxifen is noted to have intraretinal crystals, FA should be performed, primarily to rule out juxtafoveal telangiectasis, which can have similar-appearing lesions.[182] With confirmed evidence of toxicity causing a visual disturbance, the medication should be stopped.

Canthaxanthine

Canthaxanthine is a naturally occurring carotenoid. It is used as a food-coloring agent, for skin pigmentation in the treatment of vitiligo, and for the treatment of photosensitivity disorders such as erythropoietic protoporphyria, psoriasis, and photosensitive eczema. It also has been used over-the-counter in high doses as an oral tanning agent. Many reports have described a characteristic ring-shaped deposition of yellow-orange crystals in the superficial retina with high doses (usually a total dose greater than 19 g over 2 years)[183–185] (Fig. 108-22). The crystals appear more prominently in eyes with pre-existing retinal disease and with concurrent use of beta-carotene.[183,186]

Patients usually are asymptomatic, and FA usually is normal. There have been published reports of both normal and abnormal ERG, EOG, dark adaptation, and static threshold perimetry.[187–190] Although only clinically evident in the macula, the lipid-soluble crystals are found pathologically in the entire inner retina and ciliary body.[191] The crystals are, as would be expected, larger and more numerous surrounding the fovea. Canthaxanthine crystals are localized to the spongy degeneration of the inner neuropil and are associated with atrophy of the Müller cells. An experimental model of canthaxanthine-induced retinopathy also has demonstrated RPE cell vacuolization and disruption of phagolysosomes.[192]

With discontinuation of treatment, deposits may slowly clear over many years.[193,194] This slow reversal correlates with the detection of high plasma levels of canthaxanthine many months after discontinuation of the drug. Rarely, a fundus picture identical to canthaxanthine maculopathy can be seen in patients who have no known history of extradietary canthaxanthine.[195] A high dietary intake concurrent with pre-existing retinal disease is thought to partially explain this phenomenon.

Methoxyflurane

Methoxyflurane is an inhalational anesthetic, which, if used for extended periods, especially in patients with renal insufficiency, causes irreversible renal failure as a result of deposition of calcium oxalate crystals in the kidney. These crystals are also deposited elsewhere throughout the body. Fundus examination of these patients reveals numerous yellow-white punctate lesions in the posterior pole and periarterially[196,197] (Fig. 108-23). The deposits are located histologically in both the RPE and inner retina.[198,199]

Talc

See Vascular damage, p. 1845.

Nitrofurantoin

A single case of crystalline retinopathy following 19 years of nitrofurantoin (Macrodantin) use has been reported.[200]

UVEITIS

Rifabutin

Rifabutin is a semisynthetic rifamycin antibiotic that is used for the treatment and prevention of disseminated *Mycobacterium avium*-complex (MAC) infection in patients with AIDS.[201–210] A

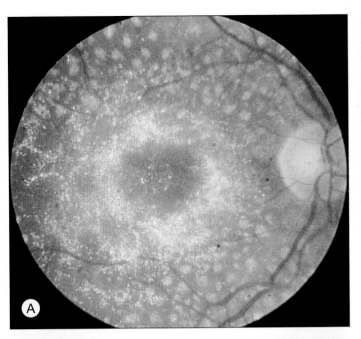

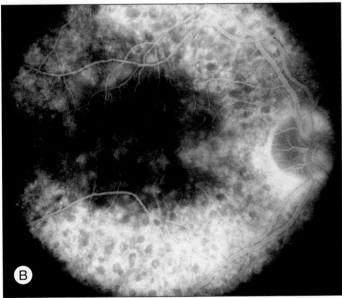

Fig. 108-21 Tamoxifen retinopathy. Characteristic yellow-white macular crystals.

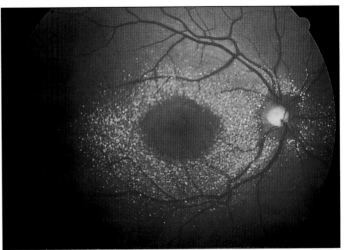

Fig. 108-22 Canthaxanthine retinopathy. Prominent perifoveal punctate yellow deposits in a doughnut-shaped ring surrounding the macula.

Rifabutin-associated uveitis can be treated successfully with topical corticosteroids or by decreasing or discontinuing the medication. Long-term use may result in ERG abnormalities.[215] Patients without systemic MAC infection who are taking rifabutin for prophylaxis and also are taking fluconazole or clarithromycin should be warned about the potential for uveitis and counseled as to its signs and symptoms.

Cidofovir

Cidofovir, also known as HPMPC, is a nucleotide analogue that inhibits viral DNA polymerase and is used for the treatment of cytomegalovirus (CMV) retinitis.[32,216–224] Cidofovir therapy, with both intravenous and intravitreous (20 μg) routes of administration, has been associated with an anterior uveitis, hypotony, and visual loss. These complications can be treated and sometimes prevented with the use of topical corticosteroids, cycloplegics, and oral probenecid. Cidofovir has been shown experimentally and clinically to cause a direct toxic effect to the ciliary body, with a resulting iritis and intraocular pressure decrease.[225,226] Although a 10 μg intravitreous dose had fewer side effects, it is also much less effective against CMV retinitis.[227] Investigations continue to try to determine the optimal dose and route of administration of cidofovir.

Latanoprost

See the drugs listed under Cystoid macular edema, p. 1848.

MISCELLANEOUS

Cardiac glycosides

Cardiac glycosides such as digoxin are used in the treatment of chronic heart failure and as antiarrhythmic agents. Although these drugs do not cause a characteristic fundus abnormality, ocular symptoms including blurred vision, scintillating scotomas, and xanthopsia (yellowing of vision) are common.[228,229] These changes probably are caused by direct toxicity to the photoreceptors. The visual symptoms are reversible with discontinuation of the drug.

small percentage of patients treated with higher doses of rifabutin (>450 mg/day) for systemic MAC infection, or lower doses (300 mg/day) for prophylaxis against MAC, can develop uveitis. The uveitis usually is bilateral and can be severe enough to cause a hypopyon that simulates infectious endophthalmitis. It can occur from 2 weeks to 14 months after initiation of the drug.[211] Concomitant use of clarithromycin and/or fluconazole, especially when lower doses of rifabutin are used, greatly increases the chance of a uveitic episode. Both systemic fluconazole and clarithromycin elevate rifabutin levels by inhibiting metabolism of the drug via the hepatic microsomal cytochrome P-450.[212] Although most cases have reported mainly an anterior uveitis, posterior vitreitis and retinal vasculitis have been described as well.[213,214]

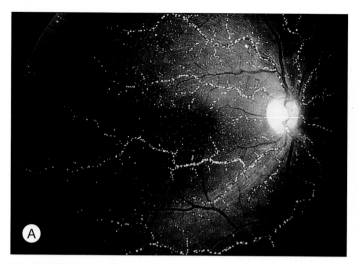

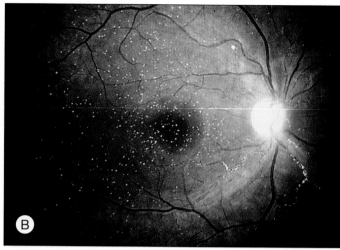

Fig. 108-23 Methoxyflurane crystals. A, Photograph displays periarterial crystals throughout the posterior pole in a patient chronically abusing methoxyflurane. B, Photograph of the same patient several months later demonstrates greater dispersion of the crystals. From Novak MA, Roth AS, Levine MR. Retina 1988; 8:230–236.

Methanol

Methanol occasionally is ingested by alcoholics. Visual blurring and field deficits are seen within 18 hours. Early fundus findings include optic nerve hyperemia and retinal edema, and late findings include optic atrophy[230–242] (Fig. 108-24). Nerve toxicity is mediated by formic acid, a breakdown product of methanol, which directly affects the inner retina and optic nerve.[230] The degree of systemic acidosis correlates well with the extent of visual dysfunction. Early hemodialysis is effective in removing methanol from the body, but if visual recovery is not evident by 6 days, it often remains permanently decreased.

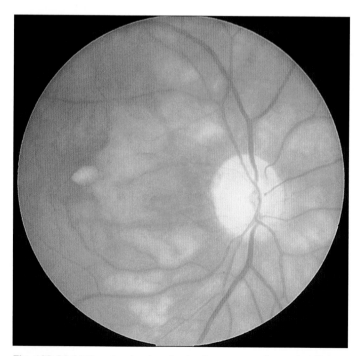

Fig. 108-24 Methanol poisoning. Acute changes revealing peripapillary retinal whitening and edema.

Vigabatrin

Vigabatrin is used for treatment of epilepsy, and has been associated with optic atrophy and visual field defecits.[233,235]

SUMMARY

Although there are thousands of systemic medications, only a small number of these agents produce retinal changes. Retinal toxicity can occur when agents are used at standard therapeutic levels, and when they are used for nonapproved indications. The mechanism by which toxicity develops is unknown in many cases. With several new drugs reaching the market annually, ophthalmologists need to maintain a high index of suspicion that patients' symptoms and clinical findings may be related to one or more of their medications.

REFERENCES

1. Weekley RD, Potts AM, Reboton J et al. Pigmentary retinopathy in patients receiving high doses of a new phenothiazine. Arch Ophthalmol 1960; 64:65–76.
2. Meredith TA, Aaberg TM, Willerson D. Progressive chorioretinopathy after receiving thioridazine. Arch Ophthalmol 1978; 96:1172–1176.
3. Hayreh MS, Hayreh SS, Baumbach GL et al. Methyl alcohol poisoning, III. Ocular toxicity. Arch Ophthalmol 1977; 95:1851–1858.
4. Connell MM, Poley BJ, McFarlane JR. Chorioretinopathy associated with thioridazine therapy. Arch Ophthalmol 1964; 71:816–821.
5. Henkind P, Rothfield NF. Ocular abnormalities in patients treated with synthetic antimalarial drugs. N Engl J Med 1963; 269:433–439.
6. Hamilton JD. Thioridazine retinopathy within the upper dosage limit (Letter). Psychosomatics 1985; 26:823–824.
7. Hobbs HE, Edeadie SP, Sommervile F. Ocular lesions after treatment with chloroquine. Br J Ophthalmol 1961; 45:284–297.
8. Hobbs HE, Sorsby A, Freedman A. Retinopathy following chloroquine therapy. Lancet 1959; 2:478–480.
9. Jacobs DS, Piliero PJ, Kuperwaser MG et al. Acute uveitis associated with rifabutin use in patients with human immunodeficiency virus infection. Am J Ophthalmol 1994; 118:716–722.
10. Tekell JI, Silva JA, Maas JA et al. Thioridazine-induced retinopathy. Am J Psychiat 1996; 153:1234–1235.
11. Miyata M, Imai H, Ishikawa et al. Changes in human electroretinography associated with thioridazine administration. Ophthalmologica 1980; 181:175–180.

12. Marmor MF. Is thioridazine retinopathy progressive? Relationship of pigmentary changes to visual function. Br J Ophthalmol 1990; 74: 739–742.

13. Potts AM. Further studies concerning accumulation of polycyclic compounds on uveal melanin. Invest Ophthalmol Vis Sci 1964; 3:399–404.

14. Potts AM. The concentration of phenothiazines in the eye of experimental animals. Invest Ophthalmol Vis Sci 1962; 1:522–530.

15. Potts AM. The reaction of uveal pigment in vitro with polycyclic compounds. Invest Ophthalmol Vis Sci 1964; 3:405–416.

16. Kinross-Wright JT. Clinical trial of a new phenothiazine compound NP-207. Psychiatr Res Rep Am Psychiatr Assoc 1956; 4:89–94.

17. Bonting SL, Caravaggio LL, Canady MR. Studies on sodium potassium-activated adenosine triphosphatase. X. Occurrence in retinal rods and relation to rhodopsin. Exp Eye Res 1964; 3:47–56.

18. Cerletti A, Meier-Ruge W. Toxicological studies on phenothiazine-induced retinopathy. Excerpt Med Internat Congr Ser 1968; 145:170–188.

19. Muirhead JF. Drug effects on retinal oxidation: retinal alcohol: NAD+ oxidoreductase. Invest Ophthalmol Vis Sci 1967; 6:635–641.

20. DeLong SL, Poley BJ, McFarlane JR. Ocular changes associated with long-term chlorpromazine therapy. Arch Ophthalmol 1965; 73:611–617.

21. Mathalone MBR. Eye and skin changes in psychiatric patients treated with chlorpromazine. Br J Ophthalmol 1967; 51:86–93.

22. Oshika T. Ocular adverse effects of neuropsychiatric agents: incidence and management. Drug Safety 1995; 12:256–263.

23. Siddal JR. The ocular toxic findings with prolonged and high dosage chlorpromazine intake. Arch Ophthalmol 1965; 74:460–464.

24. Wolf ME, Richer S, Berk MA et al. Cutaneous and ocular changes associated with the use of chlorpromazine. Int J Clin Pharmacol Ther Toxicol 1993; 31:365–367.

25. Cambiaggi A. Unusual ocular lesions in a case of systemic lupus erythematosus. Arch Ophthalmol 1957; 57:451–453.

26. Henkind P, Rothfield NF. Ocular abnormalities in patients treated with synthetic antimalarial drugs. N Engl J Med 1963; 269:433–439.

27. Hobbs HE, Edeadie SP, Sommervile F. Ocular lesions after treatment with chloroquine. Br J Ophthalmol 1961; 45:284–297.

28. Hobbs HE, Sorsby A, Freedman A. Retinopathy following chloroquine therapy. Lancet 1959; 2:478–480.

29. Marks JS. Chloroquine retinopathy: is there a safe daily dose? Ann Rheum Dis 1982; 41:52–58.

30. Nylander U. Ocular damage in chloroquine therapy. acta Ophthalmol 1967; 92:5–71.

31. Okun E, Gouras P, Bernstein H et al. Chloroquine retinopathy. Arch Ophthalmol 1963; 69:59–71.

32. Taskintuna I, Rahhal FM, Arevalo F et al. Low-dose intravitreal cidofovir (HPMPC) therapy of cytomegalovirus retinitis in patients with acquired immune deficiency syndrome. Ophthalmology 1997; 104:1049–1057.

33. Ochsendorf FR, Runne U. Chloroquine: consideration of maximum daily dose (3.5 mg/kg ideal weight) prevents retinopathy. Dermatology 1996; 192:382–383.

34. Tobin DR, Krohel GB, Rynes RL. Hydroxychloroquine: seven-year experience. Arch Ophthalmol 1982; 100:81–83.

35. Finbloom DS, Silver K, Newsome DA et al. Comparison of hydroxychloroquine and chloroquine use and the development of retinal toxicity. J Rheumatol 1985; 12:692–694.

36. Mackenzie AH, Scherbel AL. A decade of chloroquine maintenance therapy: rate of administration governs incidence of retinotoxicity. Arthritis Rheum 1968; 11:496.

37. Hart WM, Burde RM, Johnston GP et al. Static perimetry in chloroquine retinopathy: perifoveal patterns of visual field depression. Arch Ophthalmol 1984; 102:377–380.

38. Brinkley JR, Dubois EL, Ryan SJ. Long-term course of chloroquine retinopathy after cessation of medication. Am J Ophthalmol 1979; 88:1–11.

39. Carr RE, Henkind P, Rothfield N et al. Ocular toxicity of antimalarial drugs. Am J Ophthalmol 1968; 66:738.

40. Rubin M, Bernstein HN, Zvaifler NJ. Studies on the pharmacology of chloroquine. Arch Ophthalmol 1963; 70:80–87.

41. Ehrenfeld M, Nesher R, Merin S. Delayed-onset chloroquine retinopathy. Br J Ophthalmol 1986; 70:281–283.

42. Sassani JW, Brucker AJ, Cobbs W et al. Progressive chloroquine retinopathy. Ann Ophthalmol 1983; 15:19–22.

43. Heckenlively JR, Matin D, Levy J. Chloroquine retinopathy. Am J Ophthalmol 1980; 89:150.

44. Wetterholm DH, Winter FC. Histopathology of chloroquine retinal toxicity. Arch Ophthalmol 1964; 71:82–87.

45. Ramsey MS, Fine BS. Chloroquine toxicity in the human eye: histopathologic observation by electron microscopy. Am J Ophthalmol 1972; 73:229–235.

46. Bernstein H, Zvaifler N, Rubin M et al. The ocular deposition of chloroquine. Invest Ophthalmol 1963; 2:384–392.

47. Ivanina TA, Zueva MY, Lebedeva MM et al. Ultrastructural alterations in rat and cat retina and pigment epithelium induced by chloroquine. Graefes Arch Clin Exp Ophthalmol 1983; 22:32–38.

48. Coyle JT. Hydroxychloroquine retinopathy. Ophthalmology 2001; 108:243–244.

49. Grierson DJ. Hydroxychloroquine and visual screening in a rheumatology outpatient clinic. Ann Rheum Dis 1997; 56:188–190.

50. Levy GD, Munz SJ, Paschal J et al. Incidence of hydroxychloroquine retinopathy in 1207 patients in a large multicenter outpatient practice. Arthritis Rheum 1997; 40:1482–1486.

51. Rynes RI. Ophthalmologic considerations in using antimalarials in the United States. Lupus 1996; 5:73–74.

52. Falcone PM, Paolini L and Lou PL. Hydroxychloroquine toxicity despite normal dose therapy. Ann Ophthalmol 1993; 25:385–388.

53. Johnson MW, Vine AK. Hydroxychloroquine therapy in massive total doses without retinal toxicity. Am J Ophthalmol 1987; 104:139–144.

54. Mavrikakis M, Papazoglou S, Sfikakis PP et al. Retinal toxicity in long-term hydroxychloroquine treatment. Ann Rheum Dis 1996; 55:187–189.

55. Shearer, RV, Dubois, EL. Ocular changes induced by long-term hydroxychloroquine therapy. Am J Ophthalmol 1967; 64:245–252.

56. Weiner A, Sandberg MA, Gaudio AR et al. Hydroxychloroquine retinopathy. Am J Ophthalmol 1991; 112:528–534.

57. Weiser A, Sandberg MA, Gaadio AR et al. Hydroxychloroquine retinopathy. Am J Ophthalmol 1991; 121:582–584.

58. Falcone PM, Paolini L, Lou PL. Hydroxychloroquine toxicity despite normal dose therapy. Ann Ophthalmol 1993; 25:385–388.

59. Mavrikakis M, Papazoglou S, Sfikakis PP et al. Retinal toxicity in long-term hydroxychloroquine treatment. Ann Rheum Dis 1996; 55:187–189.

60. Weiser A, Sandberg MA, Gaadio AR et al. Hydroxychloroquine retinopathy. Am J Ophthalmol 1991; 121:582–584.

61. Easterbrook M, Bernstein H. Ophthalmic monitoring of patients taking antimalarials: preferred practice patterns. J Rheumatol 1997; 24:1390–1392.

62. Morsman CDG, Livesey SJ, Richards IM et al. Screening for hydroxychloroquine retinal toxicity: is it necessary? Eye 1990; 4:572–576.

63. Shipley M, Silman A. Should patients on hydroxychloroquine have their eyes examined regularly? Br J Rheumatol 1997; 30:514–515.

64. Silman A, Shipley M. Ophthalmological monitoring for hydroxychloroquine toxicity: a scientific review of available data. Br J Rheumatol 1997; 36:599–601.

65. Browning DJ. Hydroxychloroquine and chloroquine retinopathy: screening for drug toxicity. Am J Ophthalmol 2002; 133:649–656.

66. Easterbrook M. Hydroxychloroquine retinopathy. Ophthalmology 2001; 108:2158–2159.

67. Easterbrook M. The use of Amsler grids in early chloroquine retinopathy. Ophthalmology 1984; 91:1368–1372.

68. Maturi RK, Yu M, Weleber RG. Multifocal electroretinographic evaluation of long-term hydroxychloroquine users. Arch Ophthalmol 2004; 122:973–81.

69. Moschos MN, Moschos MM, Apostolopoulos M et al. Assessing hydroxychloroquine toxicity by the multifocal ERG. Doc Ophthalmol 2004; 108:47–53.

70. Neubauer AS, Stiefelmeyer S, Berninger T et al. The multifocal pattern electroretinogram in chloroquine retinopathy. Ophthalmic Res 2004; 36:106–13.

71. Penrose PJ, Tzekov RT, Sutter EE et al. Multifocal electroretinography evaluation for early detection of retinal dysfunction in patients taking hydroxychloroquine. Retina 2003; 23:503–12.

72. Tzekov RT, Serrato A, Marmor MF. ERG findings in patients using hydroxychloroquine. Doc Ophthalmol 2004; 108:87–97.

73. Marmor MF, Carr RE, Easterbrook M et al. Recommendations on screening for chloroquine and hydroxychloroquine retinopathy: a report by the American Academy of Ophthalmology. Ophthalmology 2002; 109:1377–1382.

74. Mavrikakis I, Sfikakis PP, Mavrikakis E et al. The incidence of irreversible retinal toxicity in patients treated with hydroxychloroquine: a reappraisal. Ophthalmology 2003; 110:1321–1326.

75. Johnson MW, Vine AK. Hydroxychloroquine therapy in massive total doses without retinal toxicity. Am J Ophthalmol 1987; 104:139–144.

76. Shearer RV, Dubois EL. Ocular changes induced by long-term hydroxychloroquine therapy. Am J Ophthalmol 1967; 64:245–252.

77. Weiner A, Sandberg MA, Gaudio AR et al. Hydroxychloroquine retinopathy. Am J Ophthalmol 1991; 112:528–534.

78. Maturi RK, Folk JC, Nichols B et al. Hydroxychloroquine retinopathy. Arch Ophthalmol 1999; 117:1262–1262.

79. Horgan SE, Williams RW. Chronic retinal toxicity due to quinine in Indian tonic water. Eye 1995; 9:637–663.

80. Brinton GS, Nortona EWD, Zahn JR et al. Ocular quinine toxicity. Am J Ophthalmol 1980; 90:403–410.

81. Bacon P, Spalton DJ, Smith SE. Blindness from quinine toxicity. Br J Ophthalmol 1988; 72:219–224.

82. Buchanan TAS, Lyness RW, Collins AD et al. An experimental study of quinine blindness. Eye 1987; 1:522–524.

83. Canning CR, Hague S. Ocular quinine toxicity. Br J Ophthalmol 1988; 72:23–26.

84. Craythorn JM, Swartz M, Creel DJ. Clofazimine-induced bull's-eye retinopathy. Retina 1986; 6:50–52.

85. Cunningham CA, Friedberg DN, Carr RE. Clofazimine-induced generalized retinal degeneration. Retina 1990; 10:131–134.

86. Whitcup SM, Butler KM, Caruso R et al. Retinal toxicity in human immunodeficiency virus-infected children treated with 2',3'-dideoxyinosine. Am J Ophthalmol 1992; 113:1–7.

87. Davies SC, Hungerford JL, Arden GB et al. Ocular toxicity of high-dose intravenous desferrioxamine. Lancet 1983; 2:181–184.

88. Mehta AM, Engstrom RE, Kreiger AE. Deferoxamine-associated retinopathy after subcutaneous injection. Am J Ophthalmol 1994; 118:260–262.

89. Gass JDM. Stereoscopic atlas of macular diseases: diagnosis and treatment, 4th edn. London: Mosby, 1997.

90. Haimovici R, D'Amico DJ, Gragoudas ES et al. Deferoxamine Retinopathy Study Group. The expanded clinical spectrum of deferoxamine retinopathy. Ophthalmology 2002; 109:164–171.

91. Gonzales CR, Lin AP, Engstrom RE et al. Bilateral vitelliform maculopathy and deferoxamine toxicity. Retina 2004; 24:464–467.

92. Rahi AHS, Hungerford JL, Ahmed AI. Ocular toxicity of desferrioxamine: light microscopic histochemical and ultrastructural findings. Br J Ophthalmol 1986; 70:373–381.

93. Hida T, Chandler D, Arena JE et al. Experimental and clinical observations of the intraocular toxicity of commercial corticosteroid preparations. Am J Ophthalmol 1986; 101:190–195.

94. Pendergast SD, Eliott D, Machemer R. Retinal toxic effects following inadvertent intraocular injection of celestone soluspan. Arch Ophthalmol 1995; 113:1230–1231.

95. McCuen BW II, Bessler M, Tano Y et al. The lack of toxicity of intravitreally administered triamcinolone acetonide. Am J Ophthalmol 1981; 91:785–788.

96. Piccolino FC, Pandolfo A, Polizzi A et al. Retinal toxicity from accidental intraocular injection of depomedrol. Retina 2002; 22:117–119.

97. Kupersmith MJ, Seiple WH, Holopigian K et al. Maculopathy caused by intra-arterially administered cisplatin and intravenously administered carmustine. Am J Ophthalmol 1992; 113:435–438.

98. Miller DF, Bay JW, Lederman RJ et al. Ocular and orbital toxicity following intracarotid injection of BCNU (carmustine) and cisplatinum for malignant gliomas. Ophthalmology 1985; 92:402–406.

99. Katz BJ, Ward JH, Digre KB et al. Persistent severe visual and electroretinographic abnormalities after intravenous Cisplatin therapy. J Neuroophthalmol 2003; 23:132–135.

100. Khawly JA, Rubin P, Petros W et al. Retinopathy and optic neuropathy in bone marrow transplantation for breast cancer. Ophthalmology 1996; 103:87–95.

101. Margo CE, Murtagh FR. Ocular and orbital toxicity after intra-carotid cisplatin therapy. Am J Ophthalmol 1993; 116:508–509.

102. Singalavaniga A, Ruangvaravate N, Dulayajinda D. Potassium iodate toxic retinopathy: a report of five cases. Retina 2000; 20:378–383.

103. Atlee WE. Talc and cornstarch emboli in eyes of drug users. JAMA 1972; 219:49.

104. Murphy SB, Jackson WB, Pare JAP. Talc retinopathy. Can J Ophthalmol 1978; 13:152–156.

105. Tse DT, Ober RR. Talc retinopathy. Am J Ophthalmol 1980; 90:624–640.

106. Schatz H, Drake M. Self-injected retinal emboli. Ophthalmology 1979; 86:468.

107. Friberg TR, Gragoudas ES, Regan CDJ. Talc emboli and macular ischemia in intravenous drug abuse. Arch Ophthalmol 1979; 97:1089.

108. Brucker AJ. Disk and peripheral retinal neovascularization secondary to talc and cornstarch emboli. Am J Ophthalmol 1979; 88:864.

109. Kresca LJ, Goldberg MF, Jampol LM. Talc emboli and retinal neovascularization in a drug abuser. Am J Ophthalmol 1979; 87:334.

110. Jampol LM, Setogawa T, Rednam KRV et al. Talc retinopathy in primates: a model of ischemic retinopathy. I. Clinical studies. Arch Ophthalmol 1981; 99:1273–1280.

111. Kaga N, Tso MOM, Jampol LM et al. Talc retinopathy in primates: a model of ischemic retinopathy. II. A histopathologic study. Arch Ophthalmol 1982; 100:1644–1648.

112. Kaga N, Tso MOM, Jampol LM. Talc retinopathy in primates: a model of ischemic retinopathy. III. An electron microscopic study. Arch Ophthalmol 1982; 100:1649–1657.

113. Gombos GM, Moreno DH, Bedrossian PB. Retinal vascular occlusion induced by oral contraceptives. Ann Ophthalmol 1975; 7:215–217.

114. Goren GB. Retinal edema secondary in oral contraceptives. Am J Ophthalmol 1967; 64:447–449.

115. Lyle TK, Wybar K. Retinal vasculitis. Br J Ophthalmol 1961; 45:778–788.

116. Perry HD, Mallen FJ. Cilioretinal artery occlusion associated with oral contraceptives. Am J Ophthalmol 1977; 84:56–58.

117. Stowe GC, Jakov AN, Albert DM. Central retinal vascular occlusion associated with oral contraceptives. Am J Ophthalmol 1978; 86:798–801.

118. Varga M. Recent experiences on the ophthalmological complications of oral contraceptives. Ann Ophthalmol 1976; 8:925–934.

119. Walsh FB, Clark DB, Thompson RS et al. Oral contraceptives and neuro-ophthalmologic interest. Arch Ophthalmol 1965; 74:628–640.

120. Garg SK, Chase P, Marshall G et al. Oral contraceptives and renal and retinal complications in young women with insulin-dependent diabetes mellitus. JAMA 1994; 271:1099–1102.

121. Petersson GJ, Fraunfelder FT, Meyer SM. Oral contraceptives. Ophthalmology 1981; 88:368–371.

122. Balian JV. Accidental intraocular tobramycin injection: a case report. Ophthalmic Surg 1983; 14:353–354.

123. Campochiaro PA, Conway BP. Aminoglycoside toxicity – a survey of retinal specialists: implications for ocular use. Arch Ophthalmol 1991; 109:946–950.

124. Campochiaro PA, Lim JI. Aminoglycoside toxicity in the treatment of endophthalmitis. Arch Ophthalmol 1994; 112:48–53.

125. McDonald HR, Schatz H, Allen AW et al. Retinal toxicity secondary to intraocular gentamicin. Ophthalmology 1986; 93:871–877.

126. Rosenbaum JD, Krumholz DM, Metz DM. Gentamicin retinal toxicity after cataract surgery in an eye that underwent vitrectomy. Ophthalmic Surg Laser 1997; 28:236–238.

127. D'Amico DJ, Caspers-Velu L, Libert J et al. Comparative toxicity of intravitreal aminoglycoside antibiotics. Am J Ophthalmol 1985; 100:264–275.

128. Peyman GA, Vastine DW, Crouch ER et al. Clinical use of intravitreal antibiotics to treat bacterial endophthalmitis. Trans Am Acad Ophthalmol Otolaryngol 1974; 78:862–875.

129. Zachary IG, Forster RK. Experimental intravitreal gentamicin. Am J Ophthalmol 1976; 82:604–611.

130. Talamo JH, D'Amico DJ, Hanninen LA et al. The influence of aphakia and vitrectomy on experimental retinal toxicity of aminoglycoside antibiotics. Am J Ophthalmol 1985; 100:840–847.

131. Kane A, Barza M, Baum J. Intravitreal injection of gentamicin in rabbits: effect of inflammation and pigmentation on half-life and ocular distribution. Invest Ophthalmol Vis Sci 1981; 20:593–597.

132. Zemel E, Loewenstein A, Lei B et al. Ocular pigmentation protects the rabbit retina from gentamicin-induced toxicity. Invest Ophthalmol Vis Sci 1995; 36:1875–1884.

133. Brown GC, Eagle RC, Shakin EP et al. Retinal toxicity of intravitreal gentamicin. Arch Ophthalmol 1990; 108:1740–1744.

134. Conway BP, Tabatabay CA, Campochiaro PA et al. Gentamicin toxicity in the primate retina. Arch Ophthalmol 1989; 107:107–112.

135. D'Amico DJ, Libert J, Kenyon KR et al. Retinal toxicity of intravitreal gentamicin: an electron microscopic study. Invest Ophthalmol Vis Sci 1984; 25:564–572.

136. Hines J, Vinores SA, Campochiaro PA. Evolution of morphologic changes after intravitreous injection of gentamicin. Curr Eye Res 1993; 12:521–529.

137. Loewenstein A, Zemel E, Vered Y et al. Retinal toxicity of gentamicin after subconjunctival injection performed adjacent to thinned sclera. Ophthalmology 2001; 108:759–754.

138. Burgansky Z, Rock T, Bartov E. Inadvertent intravitreal gentamicin injection. Eur J Ophthalmol 2002; 12:138–140.

139. Chu TG, Ferreira M, Ober RR. Immediate pars plana vitrectomy in the management of inadvertent intracameral injection of gentamicin: a rabbit experimental model. Retina 1994; 14:59–64.

140. Lim JI, Hutchinson A, Buggage, RR et al. The role of gravity in gentamicin-induced toxic effects in a rabbit model. Arch Ophthalmol 1994; 112:1363–1367.

141. Guyer DR, Tiedeman J, Yannuzzi LA et al. Interferon-associated retinopathy. Arch Ophthalmol 1993; 111:350–356.

142. Kawano T, Shegehira M, Uto H et al. Retinal complications during interferon therapy for chronic hepatitis C. Am J Gastroenterol 1996; 91:309–313.

143. Schulman JA, Liang C, Kooragayala LM et al. Posterior segment complications in patients with hepatitis C treated with interferon and ribavirin. Ophthalmology 2003; 110:437–442.

144. Hejny C, Sternberg P, Lawson DH et al. Retinopathy associated with high-dose interferon alfa-2b therapy. Am J Ophthalmol 2001; 131:782–787.

145. Kiratli H, Irkee M. Presumed interferon-associated bilateral macular arterial branch obstruction. Eye 2000; 14:920–922.

146. Tokai R, Ikeda T, Miyaura T et al. Interferon-associated retinopathy and cystoid macular edema. Arch Ophthalmol 2001; 119:1077–1079.

147. Wilson RL, Ross RD, Wilson LM et al. Interferon-associated retinopathy in a young, insulin-dependent diabetic patient. Retina 2000; 20:413–415.

148. Kertes PJ, Britton WA, Addison DJ et al. Toxicity of intravitreal interferon alpha-2b in the rabbit. Can J Ophthalmol 1995; 30:355–359.

149. Gupta DR, Strobos RJ. Bilateral papillitis associated with Cafergot therapy. Neurology 1972; 22:793.

150. Mindel JS, Rubenstein AE, Franklin B. Ocular ergotamine tartrate toxicity during treatment of Vacor-induced orthostatic hypotension. Am J Ophthalmol 1981; 92:492–496.

151. Gilmer G, Swartz M, Teske M et al. Over-the-counter phenylpropanolamine: a possible cause of central retinal vein occlusion. Arch Ophthalmol 1986; 104:642.

152. Thomas JV, Gragoudas ES, Blair NP et al. Correlation of epinephrine use and macular edema in aphakic glaucomatous eyes. Arch Ophthalmol 1978; 96:625–628.

153. Fraunfelder FW, Fraunfelder FT, Illingworth DR. Adverse ocular effects associated with niacin therapy. Br J Ophthalmol 1995; 79:54–56.

154. Gass JDM. Nicotinic acid maculopathy. Am J Ophthalmol 1973; 76:500–510.

155. Millay RH, Klein ML, Illingworth DR. Niacin maculopathy. Ophthalmology 1988; 95:930–936.

156. Jampol LM. Niacin maculopathy. Ophthalmology 1988; 95:1704–1705.

157. Spirn MJ, Warren FA, Guyer DR et al. Optical coherence tomography findings in nicotinic acid maculopathy. Am J Ophthalmol 2003; 135:913–914.

158. Furuichi M, Chiba T, Abe K et al. Cystoid macular edema associated with topical latanoprost in glaucomatous eyes with a normally functioning blood–ocular barrier. J Glaucoma 2001; 10:233–236.

159. Halpern DL, Pasquale LR. Cystoid macular edema in aphakia and pseudophakia after use of prostaglandin analogs. Semin Ophthalmol 2002; 17:181–186.

160. Hoyng PFJ, Rulo AH, Greve EL et al. Fluorescein angiographic evaluation of the effect of latanoprost treatment on blood–retinal barrier integrity: a review of studies conducted on pseudophakic glaucoma patients and on phakic and aphakic monkeys. Surv Ophthalmol 1997; 41(suppl 2):83–88.

161. Moroi S, Gottfredsdottir MS, Johnson MW et al. Anterior uveitis and cystoid macular edema associated with latanoprost. Am Acad Ophthalmol Abstracts 1997; 172.

162. Rowe JA, Hattenhauer MG, Herman DC. Adverse side effects associated with latanoprost. Am J Ophthalmol 1997; 124:683–685.

163. Lima MC, Paranhos A Jr, Salim S et al. Visually significant cystoid macular edema in pseudophakic and aphakic patients with glaucoma receiving latanoprost. J Glaucoma 2000; 9:317–321.

164. Schumer RA, Camras CB, Mandahl AK. Latanoprost and cystoid macular edema: is there a causal relation? Curr Opin Ophthalmol 2000; 11:94–100.

165. Wand M, Gaudio AR, Shields MB. Latanoprost and cystoid macular edema in high-risk aphakic or pseudophakic eyes. J Cataract Refract Surg 2001; 27:1397–1401.

166. Warwar RE, Bullock JD, Ballal D. Cystoid macular edema and anterior uveitis associated with latanoprost use. Ophthalmology 1998; 105:263–268.

167. Miyake K, Ibaraki N. Prostaglandins and cystoid macular edema. Surv Ophthalmol 2002; 47, Suppl 1:S203–218.

168. Grinbaum A, Ashkenazi I, Avni I et al. Transient myopia following metronidazole treatment for trichomonas vaginalis. JAMA 1992; 267:511–512.

169. Ryan EH, Jampol LM. Drug-induced acute transient myopia with retinal folds. Retina 1986; 6:220–223.

170. Soylev MF, Green RL, Feldon SE. Choroidal effusion as a mechanism for transient myopia induced by hydrochlorothiazide and triamterene. Am J Ophthalmol 1995; 120:395–397.

171. Alwitry A, Gardner I. Tamoxifen maculopathy. Arch Ophthalmol 2002; 120:1402.

172. Kaiser-Kupfer MI, Kupfer C, Rodrigues MM. Tamoxifen retinopathy. Cancer Treat Rep 1978; 62:315–320.

173. Chang T, Gonder JR, Ventresca MR. Low-dose tamoxifen retinopathy. Can J Ophthalmol 1992; 27:148–149.

174. Griffiths MFP. Tamoxifen retinopathy at low dosage. Am J Ophthalmol 1987; 104:185–186.

175. Pavlidis NA, Petris C, Briassoulis E et al. Clear evidence that long-term, low-dose tamoxifen treatment can induce ocular toxicity. Cancer 1992; 69:2961–2964.

176. Noureddin BN, Seoud M, Bashshur Z et al. Ocular toxicity in low-dose tamoxifen: a prospective study. Eye 1999; 13:729–733.

177. Heier JS, Dragoo RA, Enzenauer RW et al. Screening for ocular toxicity in asymptomatic patients treated with tamoxifen. Am J Ophthalmol 1994; 117:772–775.

178. McKeown CA, Swartz M, Blom J et al. Tamoxifen retinopathy. Br J Ophthalmol 1981; 65:177–179.

179. Kaiser-Kupfer MI, Kupfer C, Rodrigues MM. Tamoxifen retinopathy: a clinicopathologic report. Ophthalmology 1981; 88:89–93.

180. Ashford AR, Donev I, Tiwari RP et al. Reversible ocular toxicity related to tamoxifen therapy. Cancer 1988; 61:33–35.

181. Nayfield SG, Gorin MB. Tamoxifen-associated eye disease: a review. J Clin Oncol 1996; 14:1018–1026.

182. Kalina RE, Wells CG. Screening for ocular toxicity in asymptomatic patients with tamoxifen (Letter). Am J Ophthalmol 1995; 119:112–113.

183. Chang TS, Aylward W, Clarkson JG et al. Asymmetric canthaxanthine retinopathy. Am J Ophthalmol 1995; 119:801–802.

184. Espaillat A, Aiello LP, Arrigg PG et al. Canthaxanthine retinopathy. Arch Ophthalmol 1999; 117:412–413.

185. Lonn LI. Canthaxanthine retinopathy. Arch Ophthalmol 1987; 105:1590–1591.

186. Cortin P, Boudreault G, Rousseau AP et al. La retinopathie a la canthaxanthine. II. Facteurs predisposants. Can J Ophthalmol 1984; 19:215–219.

187. Boudreault G, Cortin P, Corriveau LA et al. La retinopathie a la canthaxanthine. I. Etude clinique de 51 consommateurs. Can J Ophthalmol 1983; 18: 325–328.

188. Harnois C, Cortin P, Samson J et al. Static perimetry in canthaxanthine maculopathy. Arch Ophthalmol 1988; 106:58–60.

189. Metge P, Mandirac-Bonnefoy C, Bellaube P. Thesaurismose retinienne a la canthaxanthine. Bull Mem Soc Fr Ophtalmol 1984; 95:547–549.

190. Weber U, Goerz G, Hennekes R. Carotenoid retinopathie. I. Morphologische und funktionell befunde. Klin Monatsbl Augenheilkd 1985; 186:351–354.

191. Daicker B, Schiedt K, Adnet JJ et al. Canthaxanthin retinopathy: an investigation by light and electron microscopy and physiochemical analysis. Graefes Arch Clin Exp Ophthalmol 1987; 225:189–197.

192. Scallon LJ, Burke JM, Mieler WF et al. Canthaxanthine-induced retinal pigment epithelial changes in the cat. Curr Eye Res 1988; 7:687–693.

193. Harnois C, Samson J, Malenfant M et al. Canthaxanthine retinopathy: anatomic and functional reversibility. Arch Ophthalmol 1989; 107:538–540.

194. Leyon H, Ros A, Nyberg S et al. Reversibility of canthaxanthin deposits within the retina. Acta Ophthalmol 1990; 68:607–611.

195. Oosterhuis JA, Remky H, Nijman NM et al. Canthaxanthine-retinopathie ohne canthaxanthine-einnahime. Klin Monatsbl Augenheilkd 1989; 194:110–116.

196. Bullock JD, Albert DM. Fleck retina: appearance secondary to oxalate crystals from methoxyflurane anesthesia. Arch Ophthalmol 1975; 93:26–31.

197. Novak MA, Roth AS, Levine MR. Calcium oxalate retinopathy associated with methoxyflurane abuse. Retina 1988; 8:230–236.

198. Albert DM, Bullock JD, Lahav M et al. Flecked retina secondary to oxalate crystals from methoxyflurane anesthesia: clinical and experimental studies. Trans Am Acad Ophthalmol Otolaryngol 1975; 79:817–826.

199. Wells CG, Johnson RJ, Qingli L et al. Retinal oxalosis: a clinicopathological report. Arch Ophthalmol 1989; 107:1638–1643.

200. Ibanez HE, Williams DF, Boniuk I. Crystalline retinopathy associated with long-term nitrofurantoin therapy. Arch Ophthalmol 1994; 112:304–305.

201. Arevalo JF, Russack V, Freeman WR. New ophthalmic manifestations of presumed rifabutin-related uveitis. Ophthalmic Surg Laser 1997; 28:321–324.

202. Becker K, Schimkat M, Jablonowski H et al. Anterior uveitis associated with rifabutin medication in AIDS patients. Infection 1996; 24:36–38.

203. Chaknis MJ, Brooks SE, Mitchell KT et al. Inflammatory opacities of the vitreous in rifabutin-associated uveitis. Am J Ophthalmol 1996; 122:580–582.

204. Jacobs DS, Piliero PJ, Kuperwaser MG, et al. Acute uveitis associated with rifabutin use in patients with human immunodeficiency virus infection. Am J Ophthalmol 1994; 118:716–722.

205. Karbassi M, Nikou S. Acute uveitis in patients with acquired immunodeficiency syndrome receiving prophylactic rifabutin. Arch Ophthalmol 1995; 113:699–701.

206. Kelleher P, Helbert M, Sweeney J et al. Uveitis associated with rifabutin and macrolide therapy for Mycobacterium avium-intracellulare infection in AIDS patients. Genitourin Med 1996; 72:419–421.

207. Nichols CW. Mycobacterium avium complex infection, rifabutin, and uveitis is there a connection? Clin Infect Dis 1996; 22:43–49.

208. Rifai A, Peyman GA, Daun M et al. Rifabutin-associated uveitis during prophylaxis for Mycobacterium avium complex infection. Arch Ophthalmol 1995; 113:707.

209. Saran BR, Maguire AM, Nichols C et al. Hypopyon uveitis in patients with acquired immunodeficiency syndrome: treatment for systemic Mycobacterium avium complex infection with rifabutin. Arch Ophthalmol 1994; 112:1159–1165.

210. Tseng AL, Walmsley SL. Rifabutin-associated uveitis, Ann Pharmacother 1995; 29:1149–1155.

211. Tseng AL, Walmsley SL. Rifabutin-associated uveitis, Ann Pharmacother 1995; 29:1149–1155.

212. Saran BR, Maguire AM, Nichols C et al. Hypopyon uveitis in patients with acquired immunodeficiency syndrome: treatment for systemic Mycobacterium avium complex infection with rifabutin. Arch Ophthalmol 1994; 112:1159–1165.

213. Arevalo JF, Russack V, Freeman WR. New ophthalmic manifestations of presumed rifabutin-related uveitis. Ophthalmic Surg Laser 1997; 28:321–324.

214. Chaknis MJ, Brooks SE, Mitchell KT et al. Inflammatory opacities of the vitreous in rifabutin-associated uveitis. Am J Ophthalmol 1996; 122:580–582.

215. Ponjavic V, Granse L, Bengtsson Stigmar E et al. Retinal dysfunction and anterior segment deposits in a patient treated with rifabutin. Acta Ophthalmol Scand 2002; 80:553–556.

216. Banker AS, Arevalo JF, Munguia D et al. Intraocular pressure and aqueous humor dynamics in patients with AIDS treated with intravitreal cidofovir (HPMPC) for cytomegalovirus retinitis. Am J Ophthalmol 1997; 124:168–180.

217. Davis JL, Taskintuna I, Freeman WR et al. Iritis and hypotony after treatment with intravitreal cidofovir for cytomegalovirus retinitis. Arch Ophthalmol 1997; 115:733–737.

218. Friedberg DN. Hypotony and visual loss with intravenous cidofovir treatment of cytomegalovirus retinitis. Arch Ophthalmol 1997; 115:801–802.

219. Jabs DA. Cidofovir. Arch Ophthalmol 1997; 115:785–786.

220. Kirsch LS, Arevalo JF, De Clereq E et al. Phase I/II study of intravitreal cidofovir for the treatment of cytomegalovirus retinitis in patients with the acquired immunodeficiency syndrome. Am J Ophthalmol 1995; 119:466–476.

221. Kirsch LS, Arevalo JF, de la Paz EC. Intravitreal cidofovir (HPMPC) treatment of cytomegalovirus retinitis in patients with acquired immune deficiency syndrome. Ophthalmology 1995; 102:533–543.

222. Lea AP, Bryson HM. Cidofovir. Drugs 1996; 52:225–230.

223. Rahal FM, Arevalo JF, Munguia D et al. Intravitreal cidofovir for the maintenance treatment of cytomegalovirus retinitis. Ophthalmology 1996; 103:1078–1083.

224. Taskintuna I, Banker AS, Rao NA et al. An animal model for cidofovir (HPMPC) toxicity: intraocular pressure and histopathologic effects. Exp Eye Res 1997; 64:795–806.

225. Banker AS, Arevalo JF, Munguia D et al. Intraocular pressure and aqueous humor dynamics in patients with AIDS treated with intravitreal cidofovir (HPMPC) for cytomegalovirus retinitis. Am J Ophthalmol 1997; 124:168–180.

226. Taskintuna I, Banker AS, Rao NA et al. An animal model for cidofovir (HPMPC) toxicity: intraocular pressure and histopathologic effects. Exp Eye Res 1997; 64:795–806.

227. Taskintuna I, Rahhal FM, Arevalo F et al. Low-dose intravitreal cidofovir (HPMPC) therapy of cytomegalovirus retinitis in patients with acquired immune deficiency syndrome. Ophthalmology 1997; 104:1049–1057.

228. Blair JR, Mieler WF. Retinal toxicity associated with commonly encountered systemic agents. Int Ophthalmol Clin 1995; 35:137–156.

229. Weleber RG, Shults WT. Digoxin retinal toxicity: clinical and electrophysiologic evaluation of a cone dysfunction syndrome. Arch Ophthalmol 1981; 99:1568–1572.

230. Treichel JL, Murray TG, Lewandowski MF et al. Retinal toxicity in methanol poisoning. Retina 2004; 24:309–312.

231. Lam RW, Remick RA. Pigmentary retinopathy associated with low-dose thioridazine treatment. Can Med Assoc J 1985; 132:737.

232. Baumbach GL, Cancilla PA, Martin-Amat G et al. Methyl alcohol poisoning IV. Alterations of the morphological findings of the retina and optic nerve. Arch Ophthalmol 1977; 95:1859–1865.

233. Eells JT, Makar AB, Noker PE et al. Methanol poisoning and formate oxidation in nitrous oxide-treated rats. J Pharmacol Exp Ther 1981; 217:57–61.

234. Frisen L, Malmgren K. Characterization of vigabatrin-associated optic atrophy. Acta Opthalmol Scand 2003; 81:466–473.

235. Gilger AP, Pons AM. Studies on the visual toxicity of methanol the role of acidosis in experimental methanol poisoning. Am J Ophthalmol 1955; 39:63–85.

236. Malmgren K, Ben-Menachem E, Frisen L. Vigabatrin visual toxicity: evolution and dose dependence. Epilepsia 2001; 42:609–615.

237. Hayreh MS, Hayreh SS, Baumbach GL et al. Methyl alcohol poisoning. III. Ocular toxicity. Arch Ophthalmol 1977; 95:1851–1858.

238. Ingemansson SO. Clinical observations on ten cases of methanol poisoning. Acta Ophthalmol 1984; 62:15–24.

239. Martin-Amat G, McMartin KE, Hayreh SS et al. Methanol poisoning, ocular toxicity produced by formate. Toxicol Appl Pharmacol 1978; 45:201-208

240. Martin Amat G, Tephly TR, McMartin KE et al. Methyl alcohol poisoning II Development of a model for ocular toxicity in methyl alcohol poisoning using the rhesus monkey. Arch Ophthalmol 1977; 95:1847–1850.

241. Mieler WF, Williams DF, Sneed SR et al. Systemic therapeutic agents and retinal toxicity. Semin Ophthalmol 1991; 6:45–64.

242. Murray IG, Burton TC, Rajani C et al. Methanol poisoning: a rodent model with structural and functional evidence for retinal involvement. Arch Ophthalmol 1991; 109:1012–1016.

Chapter 109

Retinal Injuries from Light: Mechanisms, Hazards, and Prevention

Martin A. Mainster
Patricia L. Turner

Light can alter ocular tissues photomechanically, photothermally, or photochemically.[1–5] Each mechanism has its clinical applications and hazards.

Several parameters are used to specify retinal light exposure. Power describes the rate at which optical energy is delivered to the retina (the temporal confinement of energy). Power is high or low if a given amount of energy is delivered quickly or slowly, respectively. Radiant exposure (energy density in joules/cm^2) describes the spatial confinement of optical energy (joules). Irradiance (power density in watts/cm^2) describes the spatial confinement of power (watts). Radiant exposure and irradiance are high when optical energy and power are concentrated in small areas of tissue. Radiant exposure is used to specify the dose of light in photodynamic therapy or experimental photic retinopathy. Retinal irradiance is proportional to retinal temperature rise during laser photocoagulation for a particular patient pigmentation and laser spot size, pulse duration, and wavelength.

Few ophthalmologists encounter patients with real or alleged retinal light injuries. Understanding the chorioretinal effects of light exposure is valuable for analyzing a possible victim's history, symptoms, and ocular findings, for managing chorioretinal problems, and for dealing with the social and legal issues that can ensue.

PHOTOMECHANICAL EFFECTS

Photomechanical mechanisms

Most accidental laser injuries are caused by photomechanical laser–tissue interactions.[6–9] Photomechanical interactions used in ophthalmic surgery include photodisruption, photofragmentation, and photovaporization.[5] Photodisruption occurs in Nd:YAG laser capsulotomy and lamellar keratectomy when infrared (IR) laser energy ionizes target tissue molecules, producing plasma and a rapidly expanding shock wave that dissects target tissue. Photofragmentation occurs in excimer laser photorefractive keratectomy when ultraviolet (UV) laser energy breaks bonds in corneal surface molecules and residual energy volatilizes molecular fragments. Photovaporization occurs in holmium laser sclerotomy and erbium laser phacolysis when rapid water vapor expansion excavates target tissues. Thermomechanical effects are not useful in retinal practice, but they can occur inadvertently when rapid chorioretinal heating from intense photocoagulation causes sudden tissue expansion and local blood vessel rupture.

Photomechanical retinal injuries

Q-switched lasers cause most photomechanical retinal laser injuries, typically producing thermomechanical chorioretinal distortion or photovaporization rather than photodisruption in exposures ranging in duration from hundreds of femtoseconds (10^{-15} s) to microseconds (10^{-6} s). Fewer than 15 accidental retinal laser injuries take place annually throughout the world.[8,10–15] Accidental laser injuries could be prevented if appropriate laser safety eyewear were used at all times. Unfortunately, most contemporary safety glasses or goggles reduce fine-detail vision, making it more difficult to perform critical visual tasks.

Dedicated Q-switched surgical lasers can produce high irradiances, but laser beams typically are confined to small, restricted regions, making accidents highly improbable. Typical industrial accidents occur when a laboratory Q-switched laser is misfired after a bystander has removed safety goggles to perform a critical visual task. Q-switched rangefinders and target designators are responsible for most military accidents.[7–9,16,17]

The most common initial clinical finding after an industrial or military Q-switched laser injury is a prominent vitreous and/or chorioretinal hemorrhage.[6–8,10,11,18] The size and density of blood vessels at the laser impact site determine how much bleeding occurs initially.[7] The structural integrity of adjacent tissues determines how effectively blood is tamponaded locally.[7] Large retinal areas can be rendered dysfunctional if blood spreads laterally in subhyaloid, subretinal, or sub-retinal pigment epithelium (RPE) spaces. Persistence of hemorrhage in subretinal space can cause permanent photoreceptor degeneration locally.[19] Macular holes can occur in severe injuries.[6,8,10,11,18] Retinal scars form and remodel at the laser impact site, often causing scarring of adjacent chorioretinal sites.

The severity of initial vision loss after a retinal laser injury depends on the distance of the laser impact site from the center of the fovea, the extent of chorioretinal disruption, and the amount of chorioretinal bleeding. Vision may improve over several days to months. Visual prognosis is excellent if retinal findings are minor or do not involve the fovea. Amsler grid findings should be consistent, stable, and well correlated with retinal findings in cooperative patients.

In actual laser accidents, (1) the laser source is usually known; (2) typical chorioretinal damage occurs; (3) an unambiguous temporal relationship exists between the laser incident and serious visual symptoms; (4) the severity of visual symptoms is commensurate with the extent of clinically detectable retinal damage; and (5) typical chorioretinal remodeling occurs after the injury.[20]

Most victims of definite laser injuries experience immediate severe vision loss in one eye, often preceded by a brilliant light flash. They sometimes hear a loud snap at the time of their exposure. Momentary pain may occur at the time of ocular laser injury, but only rarely. If pain does occur, it resolves promptly, just as in clinical retinal photocoagulation.

Noninjurious laser exposures and most laser injuries are painless, but rubbing an eye after a laser exposure can cause a transient, painful self-inflicted corneal abrasion. Individuals may attribute corneal pain to a real or perceived laser exposure, accounting for newspaper reports of painful vision losses in children after laser pointer exposures.[21,22] Actual retinal laser injuries do not cause chronic headache or head, neck, or jaw pain. Visually significant retinal laser injuries cause immediate visual problems. They produce retinal lesions that are ophthalmoscopically apparent and readily documented photographically and/or angiographically.

The ease of laser injury diagnosis is directly proportional to the severity of the laser injury. In ambiguous cases, subtle retinal findings are consistent with excellent visual prognosis and clinical outcomes. When a retinal laser injury is alleged and objective findings are absent or within normal limits, diagnosis of laser injury should be deferred pending a rigorous review of the patient's retinal findings, ophthalmic and systemic tests, clinical course, and past medical history. This review may take weeks to perform or even months if there is a complex past medical history. A guideline for this type of analysis is presented elsewhere.[20]

Pressure by patients or attorneys to reach quick conclusions in alleged but inapparent laser injuries should be resisted.[20,23] There can be a wide variety of psychiatric, financial, or other explanations for complaints of nonorganic origin.[24–35] Differentiation of those origins is challenging, but organic laser injuries do not cause chronic pain, and if a significant visual abnormality is present, it should be reproducible and consistent with a significant chorioretinal abnormality.

PHOTOTHERMAL EFFECTS

Photothermal mechanisms

Thermal injuries are usually produced by high retinal laser irradiances in brief exposures ranging from microseconds to seconds in duration. Melanin in the RPE and choroid absorbs laser light, converting light energy into heat energy, which briefly increases the temperature of exposed pigmented tissues.[36–39] Heat conduction then spreads this temperature rise from the heated pigmented tissues to adjacent tissues, damaging overlying neural retina and unexposed collateral retina and choroid.[36,38]

Elevated chorioretinal temperature denatures proteins and damages intracellular structures, interrupting enzymatic processes and producing local and remote[40,41] inflammation and cell damage.

Damaged neural retina at a photocoagulation site may lose its transparency for hours to days before its clarity returns. Opacified neural retina is visible ophthalmoscopically because it scatters white fundus illumination light back at the observer. Injured RPE and choroid undergo inflammation and scarring after thermal injury. Retinal burns increase in size over time due to postoperative scarring and collateral chorioretinal damage that is not apparent at treatment time.[38] The beneficial and harmful effects of photocoagulation derive from: (1) thermal vascular thrombosis, sclerosis, or leukostasis; (2) apoptosis of choroidal or retinal neovascularization; (3) upregulation or downregulation of chemical factors such as pigment epithelium-derived factor (PEDF), vascular endothelial growth factor (VEGF), and heat shock protein (HSP); and (4) alterations in inner and outer blood–retinal barriers that can briefly increase and subsequently decrease retinal edema.[42–49]

The extent of any chorioretinal thermal injury depends on the magnitude and duration of the temperature increase that the retina and choroid encounter (Arrhenius integral of their temperature history).[37,50,51] Some reciprocity exists between temperature elevation and exposure time. Thus, a long exposure to a low temperature rise may produce chorioretinal effects similar to that of a short exposure to a high temperature rise. Typical clinical photocoagulation with exposures a few tenths of a second in duration causes brief chorioretinal temperature elevations well in excess of 20°C[50,52] and chorioretinal lesions that are visible immediately. Conversely, 60 s transpupillary thermotherapy for choroidal neovascularization (CNV)[53] produces sustained temperature increases of only around 10°C and subvisible chorioretinal lesions.[43] Brief photocoagulation exposures less than a millisecond in duration can localize laser effects by producing temperature profiles similar to retinal irradiance profiles.[36,39]

Melanin in the RPE is the most effective chorioretinal light absorber.[38] Since melanin density is ordinarily highest in the RPE, initial temperature rise is highest at the photoreceptor–RPE junction in the center of retinal lesions where thermal source strength is highest.[36] For exposures longer than roughly a millisecond, heat conduction spreads temperature elevation laterally and axially.[36] Melanin absorption decreases with increasing wavelength, so the RPE temperature rise for a particular retinal irradiance is higher for shorter laser wavelengths such as argon green than for longer ones such as diode IR.[54,55]

Photothermal retinal injuries

Surgical lasers are potentially harmful as well as beneficial. Surgical Q-switched laser systems have numerous safeguards that restrict high optical irradiances to small, restricted spatial volumes. Conversely, laser beams from lower-power, longer-exposure, continuous-wave (CW) laser photocoagulators are potentially harmful throughout a treatment room.

Operating room injuries

Operating room laser accidents typically go unreported in the medical literature because of confidentiality clauses in legal settlements that prohibit the publication of real or purported injuries. Indirect ophthalmoscopic laser photocoagulators pose the greatest risk in ophthalmic operating rooms because their treatment beams and reflections are potentially hazardous for many meters. Bystanders should put on protective eyewear before a laser indirect ophthalmoscopic photocoagulator is switched from standby to treatment mode. In endoscopic laser photocoagulation, protective operating microscope filters should be properly in place and the endoscopic delivery probe should be inside the patient's eye before the photocoagulator is switched to its treatment mode. The retina is a poor reflector, but laser flashback does occur during endoscopic photocoagulation, and flashback is potentially hazardous to surgeons and assistants if protective filters are not installed properly prior to photocoagulation.

Slit-lamp photocoagulators

Operators of slit-lamp laser photocoagulators are protected from back-scattered laser light by fixed filters in their line of sight or filters switched into their field of view when the photocoagulator foot pedal is depressed.[37,42] Unprotected bystanders adjacent to the surgeon are potentially vulnerable to specular reflections from contact ophthalmoscopy lenses, even though the lenses have antireflective coatings.[1,56,57] In conventional argon laser photocoagulation, this hazard extends up to 2 m from a flat-surfaced, Goldmann-type contact lens.[56] We know of no injury ever caused by such a reflection, but bystanders in photocoagulation treatment areas should wear laser safety glasses or goggles.

Laser photocoagulator operators usually view an aiming beam without ocular protection. Aiming beam brightness can be adjusted, but aiming beam reflections from a contact lens can occasionally be dazzling to the operator, prompting concern about their potential hazardousness.[58] These reflections could be annoying and distracting with older argon laser systems, but they are below maximal permissible exposure standards and do not pose a hazard for photocoagulator operators.[59]

Laser pointers

Laser pointers sold in the USA are regulated by the Food and Drug Administration (FDA).[21,22,60] They must produce less than 5 mW (milliwatt) of power and have an attached warning label that cautions users not to stare into the laser beam. Staring deliberately at a laser pointer for more than 10 s is potentially harmful,[21,22] but most accidental or inadvertent laser pointer exposures are terminated in less than 0.25 s by normal aversion responses to uncomfortable, dazzling light.[21,60,61] Laser pointers are valuable presentation devices. Unfortunately, pranksters have used them to annoy and harass athletes, police officers, and motor vehicle operators.[21,22]

The falling cost of laser pointers has put them into the hands of adults and children who may be undeterred by warning labels. Fortunately, laser pointer injuries are rare and difficult to produce.[62–65] One injury occurred when an 11-year-old girl stared at a red laser pointer beam for more than 10 s to satisfy the curiosity of classmates who wanted to see if doing so would constrict her pupil.[62] Prominent foveolar pigment mottling occurred in her affected eye, along with an initial decrease in her visual acuity to 20/60. Her pigment mottling faded and visual acuity returned to normal over several months. There was no prior history of trauma or inflammation that might have produced similar findings. Acute UV-blue phototoxicity has an action spectrum that increases with decreasing wavelength, so it is highly unlikely to have caused the injury.[66–68] The injury probably represents threshold photocoagulation because the laser pointer exposure would have produced a multisecond localized chorioretinal temperature elevation of roughly 10°C, comparable to the temperature elevation in transpupillary thermotherapy for CNV.[43] Laser pointers should be kept away from infants and not sold as toys to children.[21,22]

PHOTOCHEMICAL EFFECTS

Photochemical mechanisms

Photochemical (actinic) retinal damage occurs with and without exogenous photosensitizers. Photosensitized molecules can react directly with target tissues in type 1 (free radical) reactions, or with molecular oxygen to produce singlet oxygen or superoxide which in turn reacts with target tissues in type 2 (photodynamic) reactions.[69–71] Photosensitized verteporfin is used to sclerose CNV in photodynamic therapy (PDT).

Photochemical retinal injury without exogenous photosensitizers is termed photic retinopathy or retinal phototoxicity. Photic retinopathy occurs when retinal defenses are overwhelmed by prolonged exposure to light levels that would be well tolerated if experienced only transiently. Phototoxicity is a retinal hazard, but it is also a response that is used in experimental studies of retinal degeneration and cell biology.[72–76] Photic retinopathy was first documented in 1966.[77] It is caused by prolonged light exposures, ranging in duration from seconds to hours, which produce retinal irradiances and temperature increases too low for photocoagulation.[68,78–81] Photic retinopathy is a cumulative process[77,82,83] that may be enhanced by increased oxygen tension[84,85] or body temperature.[77,80,86] Its extent depends on individual defense mechanisms and the location and area of exposed retina.[87–89] Retinal phototoxicity also depends on the duration, intensity, and spectrum of the light exposure.[68,81]

Optical radiation includes visible light between 400 and 700 nm and UV radiation at shorter wavelengths (UV-C from 100 to 280 nm, UV-B from 280 to 315 nm, and UV-A from 315 to 400 nm). In a normal human eye, the cornea absorbs UV radiation below 300 nm, protecting the retina from its potentially damaging effects.[90] The cornea is transparent between 300 and 400 nm, but the crystalline lens protects the retina by absorbing most of this radiation.[90] Other defense mechanisms that decrease retinal exposure to UV radiation and visible light include shadowing by the eyebrow, corneal reflection of light not incident perpendicular to its surface (Fresnel's law), and the aversion, squint, and blink responses.[61,91]

The retina has internal defenses against its oxygen-rich environment and light exposure,[67,69,92–95] including superoxide dismutase, catalase, glutathione peroxidase, vitamin E, vitamin C, lutein, and zeaxanthin.[72,88,93,96,97] Photoreceptors shed potentially damaged outer segments discs in a circadian rhythm.[98,99] Macular xanthophyll decreases photoreceptor and RPE exposure to blue light and may help quench activated oxygen species generated by light.[100] Xanthophyll is a carotenoid pigment present in inner and outer plexiform layers in the macula. Its density is highest in the fovea, declining rapidly with retinal eccentricity.[101] The role of RPE melanin as a photosensitizer or photoprotective agent remains under investigation.[102–106]

A photon's energy is inversely proportional to its wavelength. Thus, UV photons have more energy than blue light photons, and blue light photons have more energy than red light photons. Action spectra characterize the effectiveness of different wavelengths in producing photochemical effects.[107] Experimental studies have identified at least two classes of action spectra for photic retinopathy, a UV-blue and a blue-green type of acute retinal phototoxicity.[68,69,77,88,108]

Lengthy light exposures less than 12 h in duration usually cause acute retinal phototoxicity in aphakic animals with an action spectrum that increases with decreasing wavelength, as shown by A_λ (for aphakic) in Fig. 109-1.[1,68,69,108–115] This UV-blue type of retinal phototoxicity is sometimes termed class 2 or Ham-type photic retinopathy.[69] It is also referred to as "blue-light" damage because its action spectrum peaks around 440 nm when a crystalline lens blocks UVR and shorter-wavelength visable light, as shown in Fig. 109-1.[112–114] UV-blue-type acute retinal phototoxicity primarily affects the RPE. It is probably responsible for solar and operating microscope macular injuries.

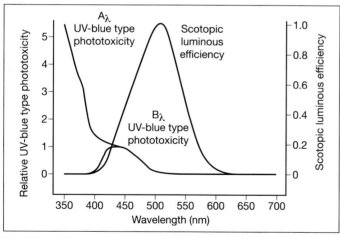

Fig. 109-1 At least two types of acute photic retinopathy have been identified in experimental studies: an ultraviolet (UV)-blue type and blue-green type of acute retinal phototoxicity. A_λ and B_λ describe how the action spectrum of the UV-blue type of phototoxicity varies with wavelength in aphakic and phakic eyes, respectively.[112] The action spectrum of the blue-green-type retinal phototoxicity is similar to the absorption spectrum of rhodopsin and scotopic luminous efficiency (sensitivity). Production of blue-green-type phototoxicity in experimental studies requires lower retinal irradiances in longer exposures than UV-blue-type phototoxicity.[69]

Prolonged exposures longer than 12 h in duration usually cause acute retinal phototoxicity with an action spectrum that peaks in the blue-green part of the spectrum, similar to scotopic luminous efficiency or the absorption spectrum of rhodopsin (Fig. 109-1).[69,77,108,109,112–114,116] This blue-green type of retinal phototoxicity is also referred to as white light, class 1 or Noell-type photic retinopathy. Blue-green-type retinal phototoxicity occurs at substantially lower retinal irradiances than UV-blue-type retinal phototoxicity, but very prolonged exposures are required to produce damage in a single irradiation.[69,108,109] Blue-green-type acute retinal phototoxicity affects both the neural retina and RPE. It may be responsible for reduced blue color contrast vision in long-time users of older argon blue-green photocoagulators, as discussed below.

Rhodopsin, its photoproducts and/or cytochrome-c oxidase in mitochondria probably mediate acute blue-green retinal phototoxicity.[76,77,81,117–120] Lipofuscin in RPE cells may mediate acute blue phototoxicity.[94,105,106,121–128,130] Photosensitive retinal ganglion cells which affect circadian rhythm have been discovered recently,[131–134] and it is possible that their photopigment melanopsin may be a mediator of retinal phototoxicity.

Photochemical retinal injuries
Acute solar exposure

Brief accidental solar observation must be safe or it would be potentially dangerous to look upwards on a bright day. The retinal image of the sun at its zenith is 160 μm in diameter,[52] smaller than the 350-μm-diameter foveola. Even at noontime on a clear day, direct solar observation with a 3-mm pupil diameter causes only a 4°C retinal temperature rise, far too low for photocoagulation.[52] Thus, most cases of solar maculopathy are due to retinal phototoxicity rather than retinal photocoagulation. Conversely, solar observation with a dilated 7-mm pupil produces a 22°C retinal temperature increase, well above the 10°C threshold for retinal photocoagulation.[36,52] Telescope-assisted solar observation can cause higher retinal temperature increases.[1,52] Solar eclipse observation is particularly hazardous because of possible pupil dilation.[1] Injuries have been reported after sungazing during severe hypoglycemia[135] and drug abuse.[136,137] There are many indirect methods for safely viewing solar eclipses.[1,138]

A typical solar injury is a yellowish foveolar lesion, as shown in Fig. 109-2.[139,140] The lesion fades over a week or two, sometimes followed by foveolar distortion or hole formation.[137,139,141,142] Fig. 109-3 shows the fovea of a 64-year-old woman who had gazed at the sun while taking psychotropic medications 24 years earlier. Common visual complaints after acute solar injury include afterimage, erythropsia, blurred vision, and central scotoma. Fluorescein angiography is typically normal, but minor foveal RPE transmission defects may occur in severe injuries. Post-injury visual acuity may be normal, but it is often decreased to the 20/40 to 20/200 range. Visual acuity usually returns to the 20/20 to 20/40 range over a 6-month interval.[139,143]

The severity of solar retinopathy depends on the type of exposure.[141,144] Damage is worst with prolonged solar obser-

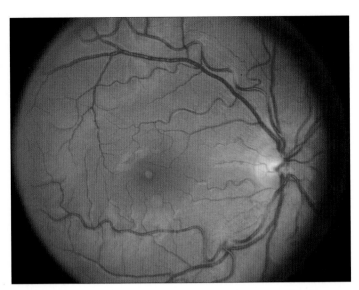

Fig. 109-2 Acute solar retinopathy typically produces a small white foveolar lesion, as seen in this 15-year-old girl with 20/200 visual acuity.

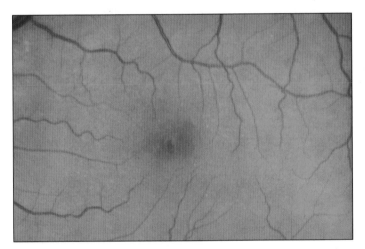

Fig. 109-3 Foveolar distortion is present in this 64-year-old woman who had stared at the sun during brief fluphenazine hydrochloride (Prolixin) therapy 24 years earlier. A similar lesion was present in her right eye. Her visual acuity was 20/50 in each eye.

vation and pharmacologically dilated pupils. Experimental photic retinopathy is enhanced by elevated body temperature,[77,80,86] so increased body temperature from a hot day, exercise, or infection could increase the risk of retinal phototoxicity, perhaps accounting for the age-old admonishment to protect children with viral fevers from bright sunlight. Higher chorioretinal pigmentation would increase local chorioretinal temperature rise associated with solar observation, perhaps further increasing the risk of damage.

High local irradiance from direct sungazing places the foveola at greatest risk for damage from solar observation. Some solar retinopathy victims deny direct sungazing,[145,146] however, and it is not clear why the foveola is more likely to be damaged than other retinal areas in the absence of direct sungazing. Indeed, the fovea is protected by relatively high xanthophyll concentrations.[101,147–149] One possible explanation for foveolar damage

without sungazing is fiberoptic transmission of shorter-wavelength photons by the Henle nerve fiber layer.[150] Henle fiberoptic transmission increases and xanthophyll protection decreases below 450 nm where UV-blue-type retinal phototoxicity increases.[150,151] Thus, Henle-layer fiberoptic transmission could increase relative foveolar irradiance by channeling blue-light photons from perifoveal regions to the center of the fovea.[150]

Foveomacular retinitis is a general term that has been applied to conditions producing foveolar abnormalities resembling acute solar retinopathy. These conditions include blunt ocular trauma and whiplash injury,[152–154] but similar findings have been reported in individuals with no prior history of photic or mechanical trauma.[155,156] Foveomacular retinitis was first reported in military personnel during World War II, but additional episodes were reported between 1966 and 1973.[157–160] Outbreaks have been ascribed to solar exposure,[158,161] an association supported by reports of solar retinopathy in three individuals who were sunbathing but not sungazing during a period of decreased atmospheric ozone.[145,146]

Reduced atmospheric ozone increases ocular exposure significantly only for wavelengths less than 310 nm, so decreased ozone protection should not affect the retina if the cornea and crystalline lens provided complete protection against UV radiation. That apparently is not the case, at least in young individuals. As noted earlier, the crystalline lens protects the retina from UV radiation between 300 and 400 nm. Crystalline lens transmittance is greater in young people, however, and a small fraction of UV-B radiation between 300 and 310 nm may penetrate the cornea and lens to reach their retinas.[90,162]

Welding arc exposure

Photokeratitis is a common welding injury, but maculopathy is quite rare. Welder's maculopathy was first reported during construction of the Paris subway in 1902.[1,163] It is caused by photic retinopathy because retinal temperature increase is too low for photocoagulation.[1,164] Welder's maculopathy has the same ophthalmoscopic appearance and clinical course as solar retinopathy.[164–167] CNV can occur after a welding arc injury.[168]

Victims of welding arc maculopathy are generally young people, at risk for retinal injury because of their occupational inexperience and clear ocular media. Visible light from a welding arc (especially 400-440 nm violet light) may be sufficient to cause photic retinopathy, but the potential 300- to 310-nm "window" in younger eyes discussed above may permit some hazardous UV radiation to penetrate the cornea and crystalline lens and reach the retina.[90,162] UV radiation may be responsible for a retinal injury caused by an intense flash from a short-circuiting high-tension electric circuit.[169]

Operating microscope maculopathy

Macular injuries were first attributed to operating microscopes in 1977.[170] Further warnings of potential light injury appeared in 1979.[171] The first cases of operating microscope maculopathy were reported in 1983.[172,173] Operating microscope injuries have been reported after cataract, vitreoretinal, kerato-refractive, and corneal transplant surgery.[174-180] Fiberoptic illuminators have produced similar lesions in vitreoretinal surgery.[86,181]

Typical operating microscope injuries are oval, 0.5 to 2 disc diameter lesions.[176,178] Their long axis often parallels the filament of the operating microscope's lamp.[182] Lesions are most common in the inferior macula because of microscope tilt and illumination positioning.[183,184] Lesions from fiberoptic illuminators can occur elsewhere,[185] as shown in Fig. 109-4.

Operating microscope injuries are probably mostly caused by the UV-blue type of acute photic retinopathy. The primary damage is located at the level of the RPE and photoreceptors.[83,186,187] Lesions sometimes have an overlying serous retinal detachment, as may also occur in PDT for CNV. The typical yellowish-white initial lesion appearance fades quickly, followed by local RPE atrophy and variable pigment mottling. Lesions may be easier to detect angiographically than ophthalmoscopically, as shown in Fig. 109-5. CNV may occur after an operating microscope injury,[188] as shown in Fig. 109-6.

Initial vision loss from an operating microscope injury is determined by the size, location, and severity of the retinal lesion. Patients under general rather than local anesthesia are at increased risk of injury because of their immobilization and possibly higher blood oxygen.[189] Higher body temperature and chorioretinal pigmentation potentially increase thermal enhancement of retinal phototoxicity. Photosensitizing systemic medications also increase the risk of injury,[190,191] including hydroxychloroquine, hydrochlorothiazide, furosemide, allopurinol, and the benzodiazepines (Valium, Librium, Halcyon).[192] Systemic diseases such as diabetes mellitus and hypertension may also increase the risk of injury.[182,193]

The risk of operating microscope maculopathy is reduced by using the lowest operating microscope intensities necessary, minimizing the duration of a patient's coaxial illumination exposure, and discontinuing systemic photosensitizing medications preoperatively whenever possible.[83,191,194-196] Other techniques that may be useful when appropriate include maintaining the patient's eye in downgaze,[191] tilting the operating microscope appropriately,[184] using corneal occluders,[197-199] and avoiding supplemental oxygen usage and/or elevated patient body temperature.

Operating microscopes produce little UV radiation,[196,200,201] so UV filters are of limited value. For example, an experimental human retinal injury was produced in a blind phakic eye despite UV and IR filters.[202] An IR-blocking filter for wavelengths longer than 700 nm theoretically decreases thermal enhancement of photic retinopathy without affecting tissue visualization.[194,203] A violet and blue light-blocking filter also theoretically reduces the risk of acute retinal phototoxicity,[204,205] but some blue light may be useful for tissue visualization.

Operating microscopes differ in the amount of violet and blue light they produce and thus their phototoxic risk.[196] Past operating microscope maculopathy rates were reported to be as high as 7%.[182] Injuries are less frequent now because of improved and faster cataract surgery techniques, but they can still occur in brief surgical procedures.[206] Some studies have found but others have failed to find an association between cataract surgery and progression of macular degeneration.[207-217]

Indocyanine green (ICG) is used for retinal angiography and as an internal limiting membrane (ILM) stain during macular hole and epiretinal membrane surgery. It has also been used during retinal photocoagulation to increase local vascular absorption[218] and produce photodynamic effects.[219] ICG

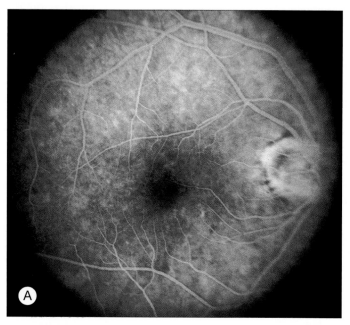
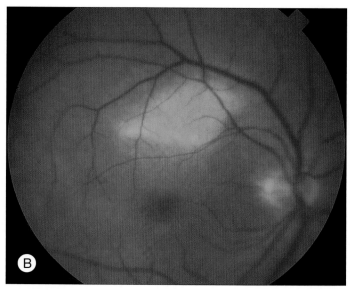

Fig. 109-4 An endoilluminator lesion is present in this patient after vitrectomy, scleral buckling, and anterior chamber intraocular lens explantation. A, The fluorescein angiogram was taken 1 day preoperatively. B, Fundus photograph taken 4 months postoperatively. The lesion spared the central macula. The patient's visual acuity was 20/70 preoperatively and 20/50 postoperatively. (Courtesy of Marc M. Whitacre, MD.)

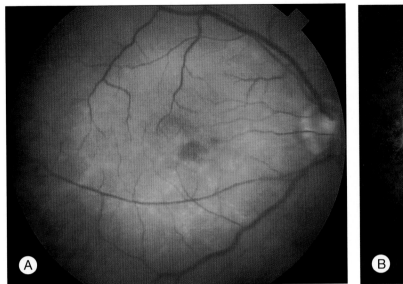
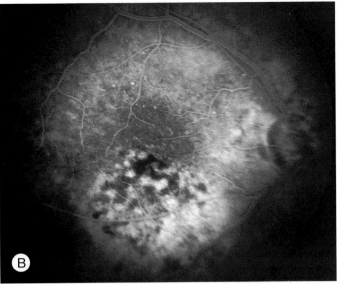

Fig. 109-5 An operating microscope lesion in a 67-year-old male with diabetes who had undergone an intraocular lens exchange operation 1 year earlier. An oval-shaped area of retinal pigment epithelial degeneration was not prominent ophthalmoscopically, as shown in the fundus photograph (A), but the lesion was quite apparent in the fluorescein angiogram taken on the same day (B).

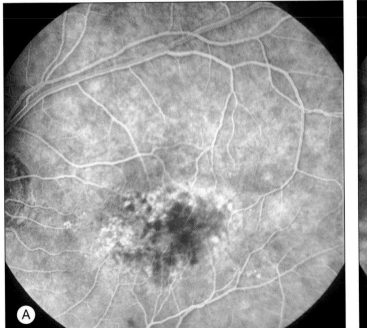
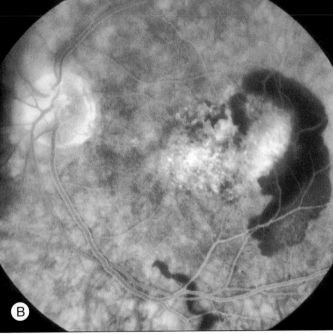

Fig. 109-6 Choroidal neovascularization (CNV) can occur after an operating microscope injury. This 65-year-old woman sustained an operating microscope injury during an intraocular lens exchange procedure 3 months before the fluorescein angiogram image (A) was taken. A, A prominent operating microscope lesion in the central and inferior macula. B, CNV with subretinal hemorrhage and exudation developed 2 months later.

fluorescence can persist for months after ICG-assisted vitreo-retinal surgery.[220–222] RPE damage[223,224] and visual field defects[225,226] have been reported after these procedures. The potential surgical benefit of staining the ILM with ICG during vitreoretinal surgery must be weighed against the potential risk of ICG retinal phototoxicity.[223,224,227–230]

Slit-lamp photocoagulators

Subtle defects in blue-color contrast sensitivity have been documented in long-term operators of argon blue-green laser photocoagulators.[231–233] The color contrast defects were believed to be due to the cumulative effect of viewing argon blue (488 nm) aiming beam reflections.[231–233] Blue light was eliminated from photocoagulator aiming beams in the early 1980s, and modern red aiming beams[234] pose no significant risk for retinal phototoxicity.

Ophthalmoscope and fundus camera exposure

Indirect ophthalmoscopes and fundus cameras produce dazzling exposures and transient erythropsia, but there is no evidence that they cause photochemical or thermal retinal injury in routine clinical use.[194,235,236] An indirect ophthalmoscope can produce photic retinopathy in an anesthetized primate when a particular retina area undergoes a prolonged exposure.[80] Deliberate attempts to produce similar lesions in human eyes about to undergo enucleation were not successful, at least in part because corneal edema developed before retinal damage occurred.[237] This finding is consistent with radiometric studies showing that fundus camera, indirect ophthalmoscope, and scanning laser ophthalmoscope irradiances are lower than experimentally determined damage thresholds.[194,235,236,238] Anterior segment slit-lamp photography has been reported to cause photic retinopathy under unusual circumstances.[239]

Ophthalmic instruments must provide adequate illumination for examining patients with hazy media. Illumination needed for such patients may be uncomfortable and perhaps even hazardous in rare circumstances for patients with clear media. Patient safety and comfort demand that examinations be performed with the lowest effective illumination levels. Filtering out light with wavelengths below 450 nm reduces the risk of acute UV-blue-type photic retinopathy, but blue light can be useful for detecting inner retinal abnormalities.[194,240–242] Filtering out wavelengths greater than 700 nm eliminates unnecessary IR radiation that could thermally enhance photochemical damage.[203]

Neonatal intensive care unit exposure

Neonatal intensive care unit (NICU) illumination can be quite bright.[243–245] Neonatal retinal irradiance depends on many factors, including the geometry and reflectance of NICU walls, the location and spectral output of room and accessory lighting, the duration of eyelid closure, pupillary size and reactivity, and neonatal eyelid and ocular media transmittance.[246–248] Infants have very clear ocular media which transmit short-wavelength blue light and UV radiation more effectively than adult ocular media.[90] Prospective studies have failed to document any relationship between NICU light exposure and retinopathy of prematurity.[249–253]

Commercial tanning-booth exposure

Modern commercial tanning booths produce high-intensity UV-A and some UV-B radiation.[254] Tanning for cosmetic reasons is ill-advised because it can cause skin damage, promote skin cancer, and induce photoallergic and phototoxic reactions to certain drugs.[255] Tanning-booth exposure can cause a photokeratitis similar to welding.[256] Macular injuries to two tanning-booth users were mentioned in one study, but not confirmed.[256] The crystalline lens and cornea protect the retina from most UV tanning-booth radiation, but tanning-booth users should always wear proper eye protection to reduce the risk of photokeratitis, cataractogenesis, and retinal phototoxicity.

ENVIRONMENTAL ISSUES

Light and macular degeneration

Retinal defenses against photic retinopathy decline with aging.[88,257–260] The relationship between environmental light exposure and age-related macular degeneration (ARMD) has been suspected for over 80 years,[88,261–264] but never proven conclusively. In 1920 a study found that ARMD was uncommon in cataract patients.[261] A later study found the incidence of ARMD to be decreased in nuclear but not cortical cataract patients.[265] Subsequent studies have shown, however, that cataract formation may be associated with an increased risk of ARMD.[214,217]

Macular disorders were prevalent among World War II prisoners in the South Pacific, where malnutrition was combined with high environmental light exposure and temperature.[266] The potential role of environmental light exposure in causing ARMD in susceptible individuals is also suggested by: (1) solar retinopathy without direct solar observation;[141,145,146,155] (2) the visual effects of bright repetitive environmental exposures[267] and laboratory UV exposures;[268] and (3) striking similarities in the retinal abnormalities caused by ARMD and repetitive experimental acute phototoxicity.[262,263,269,270]

It has been hard to establish that ARMD is related to environmental light exposure, largely because it is difficult retrospectively to determine an individual's lifelong environmental light exposure. The Chesapeake Bay Waterman study found that severe ARMD was associated with a higher estimated sunlight exposure over the previous two decades.[271,272] A similar relationship was found in the Beaver Dam eye study.[273,274] None the less, recent large case-control studies found no relationship between ARMD and sunlight exposure.[275–277]

Pseudophakia

Intraocular lenses (IOLs) were initially fabricated from polymethyl methacrylate (PMMA) that transmitted potentially phototoxic UV radiation below 400 nm to the retina. The danger of these clear PMMA IOLs was first recognized in 1978,[263,278] and most IOLs had UV-absorbing chromophores by 1986.[279] UV-only blocking IOLs transmit more blue light than a crystalline lens,[280] but they decrease the incidence of erythropsia,[281–284] blue-cone sensitivity loss in pseudophakes,[285] blood–retinal barrier disruption in pseudophakes,[286] and the risk of retinal phototoxicity in experimental animals.[287,288]

IOLs that adsorb blue light as well as UV radiation were introduced recently. They have been advocated as reducing the risk of ARMD, even though relationships between ARMD and either sunlight exposure or retinal phototoxicity remain unproven. Current UV+blue-absorbing IOLs theoretically reduce the risk of UV-blue-type phototoxicity, but they do not provide significant protection against blue-green-type phototoxicity. Thus, if environmental light exposure does play a role in ARMD, it remains prudent for pseudophakes to wear sunglasses in bright environments,[194,278] regardless of whether they have a UV-only-absorbing or a UV+blue-absorbing IOL. A significant problem with current UV+blue-absorbing IOLs is that they theoretically decrease scotopic vision significantly,[115] scotopic visual sensitivity decreases with age in older adults,[289–291] and the scotopic sensitivity of individuals with ARMD is worse than that of their peers of the same age.[291–294] Sunglasses can be taken off for optimal scotopic vision, but the blue-light-absorbing chromophores in IOLs cannot be removed for improved vision in dim environments.

Sunglasses

Sunglasses are worn for comfort, fashion, or to improve visual performance. There is growing evidence that environmental UV exposure plays a significant role in cataractogenesis.[295–297] Thus, UV-blocking sunglasses and other avoidance strategies may decrease the risk of cataract formation. Since environmental light exposure may play some role in macular aging in susceptible individuals, groups that might benefit from wearing sunglasses for retinal protection include: (1) young, lightly pigmented people, particularly if they are in warm climates; (2) individuals taking photosensitizing drugs for skin or other systemic diseases; (3) people suffering from malabsorption syndromes or other problems contributing to malnutrition; and (4) aphakes or pseudophakes. Sunglass wearers were found to have a decreased risk of soft drusen in the Pathologies Oculaires Liées à l'Age (POLA) study.[276]

Sunglass design is a trade-off between visual performance and ocular protection. There must be sufficient visible light transmission to permit effective perception of fine detail and color contrast,[91,298] but enough absorption or reflection of optical radiation to provide comfort and protection. Use of a brimmed hat would reduce overhead light exposure, although most of the eye's UV exposure comes from reflective terrain below or viewing the horizontal sky.[107,299] Sunglasses are not safe for direct solar observation.[138, 194]

Safety standards

Safety standards that affect laser users include the voluntary American National Standard Institute (ANSI) standards "Safe Use of Lasers" (ANSI Z136.1-2000)[300] and "Safe Use of Lasers in Health Care Facilities" (ANSI Z136.3-1996).[301] The ANSI Z136.1 standard is quite similar to the international standard IEC 60825-1.[302] ANSI standards are technically "voluntary," but regulatory groups use them in assessing the safety of medical laser facilities and litigants use them in evaluating purported injuries.[57,303]

Safety standards that affect laser manufacturers include the US FDA regulatory "Laser Performance Standard" (21 CFR1040). This standard requires manufacturers to equip laser devices with features such as emission indicators and keyed switches. There are also specific standards for ophthalmic devices such as slit lamps and endoilluminators.[304–306]

ANSI standards define four laser classes.[57,300] Class 1 lasers are considered to be incapable of causing damaging ocular exposures and do not require control measures. Their maximum power output in the visible spectrum ranges from 0.0004 mW or less for blue or green light to 0.024 mW or less for red light. Class 2, 3a, and 3b lasers produce laser power that is less than 1 mW, between 1 and 5 mW, and between 5 and 500 mW,

respectively. Most laser pointers sold in the USA are Class 3a devices. Class 4 lasers include potentially hazardous industrial, military, or medical lasers that generate more than 500 mW of laser power. Safety standards assign control measures to each laser class.[300,301]

Practical considerations

Control measures are designed to decrease the risk of laser accidents.[1,57,303] "Engineering" controls are protective measures built into laser systems such as housings, labels, and interlocks. "Administrative" and "procedural" controls are designed to assure the proper use of potentially hazardous laser systems. They include written protocols for: (1) operating, maintaining, and servicing laser systems; (2) assuring proper personnel education and training; and (3) using appropriate protective eyewear.

For an ophthalmic laser facility, the ANSI Z136.3-1996 standard recommends that: (1) a Laser Safety Officer be given local safety oversight responsibility; (2) a warning sign with the signal word "danger" be displayed on the outside of the closed treatment room door during any laser procedure; (3) personnel wear laser eye protection in the nominal hazard zone where diffuse reflections and stray beams could be hazardous; and (4) operators be trained in the safe use of their laser equipment.[301,303] From a practical perspective, the nominal hazard zone is the treatment or operating room in which a surgical laser is located. The laser safety office is responsible for assuring that: (1) protective eyewear is available and used regularly; (2) personnel using lasers are properly trained; and (3) laser safety measures are audited regularly.

Thresholds

A threshold for retinal light damage is the exposure needed for a 50% probability of a retinal effect.[39,89] The ANSI Z136.1-2000 and IEC 60825-1 standards reduce decades of experimental data on retinal laser effects into a set of formulae for calculating the maximum permissible exposure (MPE) for laser exposures of a particular wavelength, duration, spot size, and power.[1,112,113,300,302]

MPEs are used to design laser equipment, assess personnel risks, and analyze real or alleged laser accidents. In terms of laser energy delivered to the cornea, an MPE provides a safety margin for visible laser lesions of approximately 10× for a single 0.1-s laser exposure and 100× for multiple 300-ms micropulses in a 0.2-s repetitively pulsed laser exposure. MPEs can also be used as a rough benchmark for examining clinical treatment parameters. For example, laser parameters are 1.4× MPE for verteporfin photodynamic therapy,[307] 9.3× MPE for subvisible CNV transpupillary thermotherapy,[43,53] 37× MPE for conventional visible endpoint argon photocoagulation, 50 to 100× MPE for subvisible 300-ms diode IR repetitive pulse photocoagulation and over 200× MPE for 0.8-ms subvisible FD-YAG green[308] repetitive pulse photocoagulation.

CONCLUSION

Light can damage the retina by ablative, thermal, and photochemical mechanisms. Laser accidents can be prevented by appropriate protective eyewear. Actual laser injuries do not cause chronic pain. Any significant visual abnormalities from a purported laser injury should be well correlated with chorioretinal abnormalities. There are at least two classes of acute photic retinopathy, a UV-blue and blue-green type of retinal phototoxicity. The UV-blue type of retinal phototoxicity is probably responsible for solar, operating microscope and welder's maculopathy. There are countermeasures for each type of photic injury. Solar retinopathy can occur with or without sungazing. Infants and adolescents are at greatest risk for photic retinopathy because of their clear ocular media. The roles of photic retinopathy and chronic environmental light exposure in ARMD are suspected but still unproven. Further reduction in global atmospheric ozone could increase the incidence of photic retinopathy and perhaps ARMD.

REFERENCES

1. Sliney DH, Wolbarsht ML. Safety with lasers and other optical sources: a comprehensive handbook. New York: Plenum Press; 1980:1035.
2. Mainster MA. Finding your way in the photoforest: laser effects for clinicians. Ophthalmology 1984; 91:886–888.
3. Marshall J. Structural aspects of laser-induced damage and their functional implications. Health Phys 1989; 56:617–624.
4. Mainster MA. Photic retinal injury. In: Ryan SJ, ed. Retina. St Louis: Mosby-Year Book; 1989:749–757.
5. Mainster MA. Classification of ophthalmic photosurgery. Lasers Light Ophthalmol 1994; 6:65–67.
6. Thach AB. Laser injuries of the eye. Int Ophthalmol Clin 1999; 39:13–27.
7. Mainster MA. Retinal laser accidents: mechanisms, management and rehabilitation. J Laser Appl 2000; 12:3–9.
8. Barkana Y, Belkin M. Laser eye injuries. Surv Ophthalmol 2000; 44: 459–478.
9. Harris MD, Lincoln AE, Amoroso PJ et al. Laser eye injuries in military occupations. Aviat Space Environ Med 2003; 74:947–952.
10. Boldrey EE, Little HL, Flocks M et al. Retinal injury due to industrial laser burns. Ophthalmology 1981; 88:101–107.
11. Gabel VP, Birngruber R, Lorenz B et al. Clinical observations of six cases of laser injury to the eye. Health Phys 1989; 56:705–710.
12. Rockwell RJ Jr. Laser accidents: reviewing 30 years of incidents: what are the concerns – old and new? J Laser Appl 1994; 6:203–211.
13. Thach AB, Lopez PF, Snady-McCoy LC et al. Accidental Nd:YAG laser injuries to the macula. Am J Ophthalmol 1995; 119:767–773.
14. Ness JW, Hoxie SW. Database structure for the laser accident and incident registry (LAIR). SPIE Proc Laser Noncoherent Ocul Effects: Epidemiol Prev Treat 1997; 2974:2–7.
15. Stuck BE, Zwick H, Lund BJ et al. Accidental human retinal injuries by laser exposure: implications to laser safety. Int Laser Safety Conf Proc 1997; 3:576–585.
16. Mellerio J, Marshall J, Tengroth B et al. Battlefield laser weapons: an assessment of systems, hazards, injuries and ophthalmic resources required for treatment. Lasers Light Ophthalmol 1991; 4:41–67.
17. Tengroth B, Anderberg B. Blinding laser weapons. Lasers Light Ophthalmol 1991; 4:35–39.
18. Stuck BE, Zwick H, Molchany JW et al. Accidental human laser retinal injuries from military laser systems. SPIE Proc Laser-Inflict Eye Inj Epidemiol Prev Treat 1996; 2674:7–20.
19. Hochman MA, Seery CM, Zarbin MA. Pathophysiology and management of subretinal hemorrhage. Surv Ophthalmol 1997; 42:195–213.
20. Mainster MA, Stuck BE, Brown J Jr. Assessment of alleged retinal laser injuries. Arch Ophthalmol 2004; 122:1210–1217.
21. Mainster MA, Timberlake GT, Warren KA et al. Pointers on laser pointers. Ophthalmology 1997; 104:1213–1214.
22. Mainster MA. Blinded by the light – not! Arch Ophthalmol 1999; 117:1547–1548.
23. Mainster MA, Sliney DH, Marshall J et al. But is it really light damage? Ophthalmology 1997; 104:179–180.
24. Drews RC. Organic versus functional ocular problems. Int Ophthalmol Clin 1967; 7:665–696.
25. Kramer KK, La Piana FG, Appleton B. Ocular malingering and hysteria: diagnosis and management. Surv Ophthalmol 1979; 24:89–96.
26. Keltner JL, May WN, Johnson CA et al. The California syndrome. Functional visual complaints with potential economic impact. Ophthalmology 1985; 92:427–435.
27. Keltner JL. The California syndrome. A threat to all. Arch Ophthalmol 1988; 106:1053–1054.
28. Fahle M, Mohn G. Assessment of visual function in suspected ocular malingering. Br J Ophthalmol 1989; 73:651–654.
29. Bose S, Kupersmith MJ. Neuro-ophthalmologic presentations of functional visual disorders. Neurol Clin 1995; 13:321–339.
30. Barsky AJ, Borus JF. Somatization and medicalization in the era of managed care. JAMA 1995; 274:1931–1934.
31. Martin TJ. Threshold perimetry of each eye with both eyes open in patients with monocular functional (nonorganic) and organic vision loss. Am J Ophthalmol 1998; 125:857–864.
32. Barsky AJ, Borus JF. Functional somatic syndromes. Ann Intern Med 1999; 130:910–921.
33. Mojon DS, Schlapfer TE. Nonorganic disorders in ophthalmology: overview of diagnosis and therapy. Klin Monatsbl Augenheilkd 2001; 218:298–304.
34. Graf MH, Roesen J. Ocular malingering: a surprising visual acuity test. Arch Ophthalmol 2002; 120:756–760.
35. Scott JA, Egan RA. Prevalence of organic neuro-ophthalmologic disease in patients with functional visual loss. Am J Ophthalmol 2003; 135:670–675.
36. Mainster MA, White TJ, Tips JH et al. Retinal-temperature increases produced by intense light sources. J Opt Soc Am 1970; 60:264–270.
37. Mainster MA. Ophthalmic laser surgery: principles, technology, and technique. Trans New Orleans Acad Ophthalmol 1985; 33:81–101.
38. Mainster MA. Wavelength selection in macular photocoagulation. Tissue optics, thermal effects, and laser systems. Ophthalmology 1986; 93:952–958.
39. Mainster MA. Decreasing retinal photocoagulation damage: principles and techniques. Semin Ophthalmol 1999; 14:200–209.
40. Marshall J, Clover G, Rothery S. Some new findings on retinal irradiation by krypton and argon lasers. In: Birngruber R, Gabel VP, eds. Laser treatment and photocoagulation of the eye. The Hague: Junk; 1982:21–37.
41. Nonaka A, Kiryu J, Tsujikawa A et al. Inflammatory response after scatter laser photocoagulation in nonphotocoagulated retina. Invest Ophthalmol Vis Sci 2002; 43:1204–1209.
42. Mainster MA, Warren KA. Retinal photocoagulation. In: Guyer DR, Yannuzzi LA, Chang S et al., eds. Retina–vitreous–macula. New York: WB Saunders; 1999:61–68.
43. Mainster MA, Reichel E. Transpupillary thermotherapy for age-related macular degeneration: long- pulse photocoagulation, apoptosis, and heat shock proteins. Ophthalm Surg Lasers 2000; 31:359–373.
44. Stefansson E. The therapeutic effects of retinal laser treatment and vitrectomy. A theory based on oxygen and vascular physiology. Acta Ophthalmol Scand 2001; 79:435–440.
45. Desmettre T, Maurage CA, Mordon S. Heat shock protein hyperexpression on chorioretinal layers after transpupillary thermotherapy. Invest Ophthalmol Vis Sci 2001; 42:2976–2980.
46. Mori K, Gehlbach P, Ando A et al. Regression of ocular neovascularization in response to increased expression of pigment epithelium-derived factor. Invest Ophthalmol Vis Sci 2002; 43:2428–2434.
47. Ogata N, Wada M, Otsuji T et al. Expression of pigment epithelium-derived factor in normal adult rat eye and experimental choroidal neovascularization. Invest Ophthalmol Vis Sci 2002; 43:1168–1175.
48. Wilson AS, Hobbs BG, Shen WY et al. Argon laser photocoagulation-induced modification of gene expression in the retina. Invest Ophthalmol Vis Sci 2003; 44:1426–1434.
49. Desmettre T, Maurage CA, Mordon S. Transpupillary thermotherapy (TTT) with short duration laser exposures induce heat shock protein (HSP) hyperexpression on choroidoretinal layers. Lasers Surg Med 2003; 33:102–107.
50. Birngruber R. Thermal modeling in biological tissues. In: Hillenkamp F, Pratesi R, Sacchi CA, eds. Lasers in medicine and biology. New York: Plenum; 1980:77–97.
51. Sliney DH, Marshall J. Tissue specific damage to the retinal pigment epithelium: mechanisms and therapeutic implications. Lasers Light Ophthalmol 1992; 5:17–28.
52. White TJ, Mainster MA, Wilson PW et al. Chorioretinal temperature increases from solar observation. Bull Math Biophys 1971; 33:1–17.
53. Reichel E, Berrocal AM, Ip M et al. Transpupillary thermotherapy of occult subfoveal choroidal neovascularization in patients with age-related macular degeneration. Ophthalmology 1999; 106:1908–1914.
54. Mainster MA, White TJ, Allen RG. Spectral dependence of retinal damage produced by intense light sources. J Opt Soc Am 1970; 60:848–855.
55. Vogel A, Birngruber R. Temperature profiles in human retina and choroid during laser coagulation with different wavelengths ranging from 514 to 810 nm. Lasers Light Ophthalmol 1992; 5:9–16.

56. Jenkins DL. Hazard evaluation of the Coherent model 900 photocoagulator laser system, non-ionizing radiation protection specialty study no. 25-42-0310-79 (NTIS no. ADA 068713). Aberdeen Proving Ground, MD: US Army Environment Hygiene Agency; 1979.

57. Sliney DH, Mainster MA. Ophthalmic laser safety: tissue interactions, hazards and protection. Ophthalmol Clinics North Am 1998; 11:157–164.

58. Ward B. Mirror laser-treatment lenses: possible risks associated with lens design. Arch Ophthalmol 1986; 104:1585.

59. Sliney DH, Mainster MA. Potential laser hazards to the clinician during photocoagulation. Am J Ophthalmol 1987; 103:758–760.

60. Sliney DH, Dennis JE. Safety concerns about laser pointers. J Laser Applications 1994; 6:159–164.

61. Stamper DA, Lund DJ, Molchany JW et al. Human pupil and eyelid response to intense laser light: implications for protection. Percept Motor Skills 2002; 95:775–782.

62. Sell CH, Bryan JS. Maculopathy from handheld diode laser pointer [see comments]. Arch Ophthalmol 1999; 117:1557–1558.

63. Zamir E, Kaiserman I, Chowers I. Laser pointer maculopathy. Am J Ophthalmol 1999; 127:728–729.

64. Israeli D, Hod Y, Geyer O. Laser pointers: not to be taken lightly. Br J Ophthalmol 2000;84:555–556.

65. Robertson DM, Lim TH, Salomao DR et al. Laser pointers and the human eye: a clinicopathologic study. Arch Ophthalmol 2000; 118:1686–1691.

66. Ham WT Jr, Mueller HA, Ruffolo JJ Jr et al. Action spectrum for retinal injury from near-ultraviolet radiation in the aphakic monkey. Am J Ophthalmol 1982; 93:299–306.

67. Ham WT Jr, Mueller HA, Ruffolo JJ Jr et al. Basic mechanisms underlying the production of photochemical lesions in the mammalian retina. Curr Eye Res 1984; 3:165–174.

68. Ham WT Jr, Mueller HA, Sliney DH. Retinal sensitivity to damage from short wavelength light. Nature 1976; 260:153–155.

69. Mellerio J. Light effects on the retina. In: Albert DM, Jakobiec FA, eds. Principles and practice of ophthalmology. Philadelphia: WB Saunders; 1994:1326–1345.

70. Girotti AW. Photodynamic lipid peroxidation in biological systems. Photochem Photobiol 1990; 51:497–509.

71. Glickman RD. Phototoxicity to the retina: mechanisms of damage. Int J Toxicol 2002; 21:473–490.

72. Reme C, Reinboth J, Clausen M et al. Light damage revisited: converging evidence, diverging views? Graefes Arch Clin Exp Ophthalmol 1996; 234:2–11.

73. Reme CE, Hafezi F, Marti A et al. Light damage to the retinal pigment epithelium. In: Marmor MF, Wolfensberger TJ, eds. The retinal pigment epithelium: function and disease. New York: Oxford University Press; 1998.

74. Wenzel A, Grimm C, Marti A et al. c-fos controls the "private pathway" of light-induced apoptosis of retinal photoreceptors. J Neurosci 2000; 20:81–88.

75. Grimm C, Wenzel A, Hafezi F, Reme CE. Gene expression in the mouse retina: the effect of damaging light. Mol Vis 2000; 6:252–260.

76. Grimm C, Wenzel A, Williams T et al. Rhodopsin-mediated blue-light damage to the rat retina: effect of photoreversal of bleaching. Invest Ophthalmol Vis Sci 2001; 42:497–505.

77. Noell WK, Walker VS, Kang BS et al. Retinal damage by light in rats. Invest Ophthalmol 1966; 5:450–473.

78. Noell WK. Possible mechanisms of photoreceptor damage by light in mammalian eyes. Vision Res 1980; 20:1163–1171.

79. Kuwabara T, Gorn RA. Retinal damage by visible light. An electron microscopic study. Arch Ophthalmol 1968; 79:69–78.

80. Friedman E, Kuwabara T. The retinal pigment epithelium. IV. The damaging effects of radiant energy. Arch Ophthalmol 1968; 80:265–279.

81. Lawwill T. Three major pathologic processes caused by light in the primate retina: a search for mechanisms. Trans Am Ophthalmol Soc 1982; 80:517–579.

82. Griess GA, Blankenstein MF. Additivity and repair of actinic retinal lesions. Invest Ophthalmol Vis Sci 1981; 20:803–807.

83. Irvine AR, Wood I, Morris BW. Retinal damage from the illumination of the operating microscope. An experimental study in pseudophakic monkeys. Arch Ophthalmol 1984; 102:1358–1365.

84. Crockett RS, Lawwill T. Oxygen dependence of damage by 435 nm light in cultured retinal epithelium. Curr Eye Res 1984; 3:209–215.

85. Ruffolo JJ Jr, Ham WT Jr, Mueller HA et al. Photochemical lesions in the primate retina under conditions of elevated blood oxygen. Invest Ophthalmol Vis Sci 1984; 25:893–898.

86. Rinkoff J, Machemer R, Hida T et al. Temperature-dependent light damage to the retina. Am J Ophthalmol 1986; 102:452–462.

87. Sykes SM, Robison WG Jr, Waxler M et al. Damage to the monkey retina by broad-spectrum fluorescent light. Invest Ophthalmol Vis Sci 1981; 20:425–434.

88. Mainster MA. Light and macular degeneration: a biophysical and clinical perspective. Eye 1987; 1:304–310.

89. Sliney DH, Mellerio J, Gabel VP et al. What is the meaning of threshold in laser injury experiments? Implications for human exposure limits. Health Phys 2002; 82:335–347.

90. Boettner EA, Wolter JR. Transmission of the ocular media. Invest Ophthalmol 1962; 1:776–783.

91. Sliney DH. Eye protective techniques for bright light. Ophthalmology 1983; 90:937–944.

92. Feeney-Burns L, Ellersieck MR. Age-related changes in the ultrastructure of Bruch's membrane. Am J Ophthalmol 1985; 100:686–697.

93. Feeney L, Berman ER. Oxygen toxicity: membrane damage by free radicals. Invest Ophthalmol 1976; 15:789–792.

94. Boulton M, Rozanowska M, Rozanowski B. Retinal photodamage. J Photochem Photobiol B 2001; 64:144–161.

95. Ben-Shabat S, Parish CA, Hashimoto M et al. Fluorescent pigments of the retinal pigment epithelium and age-related macular degeneration. Bioorg Med Chem Lett 2001; 11:1533–1540.

96. Snodderly DM. Evidence for protection against age-related macular degeneration by carotenoids and antioxidant vitamins. Am J Clin Nutr 1995; 62:1448S–1461S.

97. Kennedy CJ, Rakoczy PE, Constable IJ. Lipofuscin of the retinal pigment epithelium: a review. Eye 1995; 9:763–771.

98. Young RW. Visual cells and the concept of renewal. Invest Ophthalmol Vis Sci 1976; 15:700–725.

99. Marshall J. Radiation and the ageing eye. Ophthalm Physiol Opt 1985; 5:241–263.

100. Kirschfeld K. Carotenoid pigments: their possible role in protecting against photooxidation in eyes and photoreceptor cells. Proc R Soc Lond B Biol Sci 1982; 216:71–85.

101. Snodderly DM, Auran JD, Delori FC. The macular pigment. II. Spatial distribution in primate retinas. Invest Ophthalmol Vis Sci 1984; 25:674–685.

102. Lawwill T. Effects of prolonged exposure of rabbit retina to low-intensity light. Invest Ophthalmol 1973; 12:45–51.

103. Hoppeler T, Hendrickson P, Dietrich C et al. Morphology and time-course of defined photochemical lesions in the rabbit retina. Curr Eye Res 1988; 7:849–860.

104. Gorgels TG, Van Norren D. Two spectral types of retinal light damage occur in albino as well as in pigmented rat: no essential role for melanin. Exp Eye Res 1998; 66:155–162.

105. Sparrow JR, Nakanishi K, Parish CA. The lipofuscin fluorophore A2E mediates blue light-induced damage to retinal pigmented epithelial cells. Invest Ophthalmol Vis Sci 2000; 41:1981–1989.

106. Rozanowska M, Korytowski W, Rozanowski B et al. Photoreactivity of aged human RPE melanosomes: a comparison with lipofuscin. Invest Ophthalmol Vis Sci 2002; 43:2088–2096.

107. Sliney DH. How light reaches the eye and its components. Int J Toxicol 2002; 21:501–509.

108. Kremers JJ, van Norren D. Two classes of photochemical damage of the retina. Lasers Light Ophthalmol 1988; 2:41–52.

109. Kremers JJ, van Norren D. Retinal damage in macaque after white light exposures lasting 10 minutes to 12 hours. Invest Ophthalmol Vis Sci 1989; 30:1032–1040.

110. van Norren D, Schellekens P. Blue light hazard in rat. Vision Res 1990; 30:1517–1520.

111. Rapp LM, Smith SC. Morphologic comparisons between rhodopsin-mediated and short-wavelength classes of retinal light damage. Invest Ophthalmol Vis Sci 1992; 33:3367–3377.

112. Threshold limit values for chemical substances physical agents: biological exposure indices. Cincinnati: American Conference of Governmental Industrial Hygienists; 1997.

113. Guidelines on limits of exposure to broad-band incoherent optical radiation (0.38 to 3 microM). International Commission on Non-Ionizing Radiation Protection. Health Phys 1997; 73:539–554.

114. Sliney DH, Bitran M. The ACGIH action spectra for hazard assessment: The TLVs. In: Matthes R, Sliney DH, eds. Measurements of optical radiation hazards. Oberschleissheim, Germany: International Commission on Non-Ionizing Radiation Protection (ICNIRP 6/98) and CIE (x016-1998); 1998:241–259.

115. Mainster MA, Sparrow JR. How much blue light should an IOL transmit? Br J Ophthalmol 2003; 87:1523–1529.

116. Williams TP, Howell WL. Action spectrum of retinal light-damage in albino rats. Invest Ophthalmol Vis Sci 1983; 24:285–287.

117. Pautler EL, Morita M, Beezley D. Hemoprotein(s) mediate blue light damage in the retinal pigment epithelium. Photochem Photobiol 1990; 51:599–605.

118. Gorgels TG, van Norren D. Ultraviolet and green light cause different types of damage in rat retina. Invest Ophthalmol Vis Sci 1995; 36:851–863.

119. Saari JC, Garwin GG, Van Hooser JP et al. Reduction of all-trans-retinal limits regeneration of visual pigment in mice. Vision Res 1998; 38: 1325–1333.

120. Grimm C, Reme CE, Rol PO et al. Blue light's effects on rhodopsin: photoreversal of bleaching in living rat eyes. Invest Ophthalmol Vis Sci 2000; 41:3984–3990.

121. Rozanowska M, Jarvis-Evans J, Korytowski W et al. Blue light-induced reactivity of retinal age pigment. In vitro generation of oxygen-reactive species. J Biol Chem 1995; 270:18825–18830.

122. Parish CA, Hashimoto M, Nakanishi K et al. Isolation and one-step preparation of A2E and iso-A2E, fluorophores from human retinal pigment epithelium. Proc Natl Acad Sci USA 1998; 95:14609–14613.

123. Schutt F, Davies S, Kopitz J et al. Photodamage to human RPE cells by A2-E, a retinoid component of lipofuscin. Invest Ophthalmol Vis Sci 2000; 41:2303–2308.

124. Suter M, Reme C, Grimm C et al. Age-related macular degeneration. The lipofusion component N-retinyl-N-retinylidene ethanolamine detaches proapoptotic proteins from mitochondria and induces apoptosis in mammalian retinal pigment epithelial cells. J Biol Chem 2000; 275:39625–39630.

125. Sparrow JR, Cai B. Blue light-induced apoptosis of A2E-containing RPE: involvement of caspase-3 and protection by Bcl-2. Invest Ophthalmol Vis Sci 2001; 42:1356–1362.

126. Sparrow JR, Zhou J, Ben-Shabat S et al. Involvement of oxidative mechanisms in blue-light-induced damage to A2E-laden RPE. Invest Ophthalmol Vis Sci 2002; 43:1222–1227.

127. Sparrow JR, Zhou J, Cai B. DNA is a target of the photodynamic effects elicited in A2E-laden RPE by blue-light illumination. Invest Ophthalmol Vis Sci 2003; 44:2245–2251.

128. Sparrow JR. Therapy for macular degeneration: insights from acne. Proc Natl Acad Sci USA 2003; 100:4353–4354.

129. Ben-Shabat S, Parish CA, Vollmer HR et al. Biosynthetic studies of A2E, a major fluorophore of retinal pigment epithelial lipofuscin. J Biol Chem 2002; 277:7183–7190.

130. Sparrow JR, Vollmer-Snarr HR, Zhou J et al. A2E-epoxides damage DNA in retinal pigment epithelial cells. Vitamin E and other antioxidants inhibit A2E-epoxide formation. J Biol Chem 2003; 278:18207–18213.

131. Provencio I, Jiang G, De Grip WJ et al. Melanopsin: an opsin in melanophores, brain, and eye. Proc Natl Acad Sci USA 1998; 95:340–345.

132. Van Gelder RN. Non-visual ocular photoreception. Ophthalm Genet 2001; 22:195–205.

133. Berson DM, Dunn FA, Takao M. Phototransduction by retinal ganglion cells that set the circadian clock. Science 2002; 295:1070–1073.

134. Menaker M. Circadian rhythms. Circadian photoreception. Science 2003; 299:213–214.

135. Aiello LP, Arrigg PG, Shah ST et al. Solar retinopathy associated with hypoglycemic insulin reaction. Arch Ophthalmol 1994; 112:982–983.

136. Schatz H, Mendelblatt F. Solar retinopathy from sun-gazing under the influence of LSD. Br J Ophthalmol 1973; 57:270–273.

137. Steinkamp PN, Watzke RC, Solomon JD. An unusual case of solar retinopathy. Arch Ophthalmol 2003; 121:1798–1799.

138. Mainster MA. Solar eclipse safety. Ophthalmology 1998; 105:9–10.

139. Gass JDM. Stereoscopic atlas of macular diseases, 3rd edn. St Louis: Mosby-Year Book; 1987.

140. Tso MO, La Piana FG. The human fovea after sungazing. Trans Am Acad Ophthalmol Otolaryngol 1975; 79:OP788–OP795.

141. Jacobs NA, Headon M, Rosen ES. Solar retinopathy in the Manchester area. Trans Ophthalmol Soc UK 1985; 104:625–628.

142. Yeh LK, Yang CS, Lee FL et al. Solar retinopathy: a case report. Zhonghua Yi Xue Za Zhi (Taipei) 1999; 62:886–890.

143. MacFaul PA. Visual prognosis after solar retinopathy. Br J Ophthalmol 1969; 53:534–541.

144. Dhir SP, Gupta A, Jain IS. Eclipse retinopathy. Br J Ophthalmol 1981; 65:42–45.

145. Gladstone GJ, Tasman W. Solar retinitis after minimal exposure. Arch Ophthalmol 1978; 96:1368–1369.

146. Yannuzzi LA, Fisher YL, Krueger A et al. Solar retinopathy: a photobiological and geophysical analysis. Trans Am Ophthalmol Soc 1987; 85:120–158.

147. Snodderly DM, Brown PK, Delori FC et al. The macular pigment. I. Absorbance spectra, localization, and discrimination from other yellow pigments in primate retinas. Invest Ophthalmol Vis Sci 1984; 25:660–673.

148. Chang Y, Lee FL, Chen SJ et al. Optical measurement of human retinal macular pigment and its spatial distribution with age. Med Phys 2002; 29:2621–2628.

149. Robson AG, Moreland JD, Pauleikhoff D et al. Macular pigment density and distribution: comparison of fundus autofluorescence with minimum motion photometry. Vision Res 2003; 43:1765–1775.

150. Mainster MA. Henle fibers may direct light toward the center of the fovea. Lasers Light Ophthalmol 1988; 2:79–86.

151. Werner JS, Donnelly SK, Kliegl R. Aging and human macular pigment density. Appended with translations from the work of Max Schultze and Ewald Hering. Vision Res 1987; 27:257–268.

152. Grey RH. Foveo-macular retinitis, solar retinopathy, and trauma. Br J Ophthalmol 1978; 62:543–546.

153. Kelley JS, Hoover RE, George T. Whiplash maculopathy. Arch Ophthalmol 1978; 96:834–835.

154. Abebe MT, De Laey JJ. Foveomacular retinitis as a result of ocular contusion. Bull Soc Belge Ophtalmol 1992; 243:171–175.

155. Kuming BS. Foveomacular retinitis. Br J Ophthalmol 1986; 70:816–818.

156. Jacobs NA. Foveomacular retinitis. Br J Ophthalmol 1987; 71:563.

157. Cordes FC. A type of foveomacular retinitis observed in the US Navy. Am J Ophthalmol 1944; 27:803–816.

158. Ritchey CL, Ewald RA. Sun gazing as the cause of foveomacular retinitis. Am J Ophthalmol 1970; 70:491–497.

159. Kerr LM, Little HL. Foveomacular retinitis. Arch Ophthalmol 1966; 76:498–504.

160. Marlor RL, Blais BR, Preston FR et al. Foveomacular retinitis, an important problem in military medicine: epidemiology. Invest Ophthalmol 1973; 12:5–16.

161. Wergel FLJ, Brenner EH. Solar retinopathy foveomacular retinitis. Ann Ophthalmol 1975; 7:495–503.

162. Sliney DH. Defining biologic exposures to light. In: Cronly-Dillon J, Rosen ES, Marshall J, ed. Hazards of light. New York: Pergamon Press; 1986.

163. Terrien F. De trouble visuel provoqué par l'électricité. Arch Ophthalmol 1902; 22:692–696.

164. Naidoff MA, Slinkey DH. Retinal injury from a welding arc. Am J Ophthalmol 1974; 77:663–668.

165. Uniat L, Olk RJ, Hanish SJ. Welding arc maculopathy. Am J Ophthalmol 1986; 102:394–395.

166. Wurdemann HV. The formation of a hole in the macula: light burn from exposure to electric welding. Am J Ophthalmol 1936; 19:457–460.

167. Fich M, Dahl H, Fledelius H et al. Maculopathy caused by welding arcs. A report of 3 cases. Acta Ophthalmol (Copenh) 1993; 71:402–404.

168. Kozielec GF, Smith CW. Welding arc-like injury with secondary subretinal neovascularization. Retina 1997; 17:558–559.

169. Gardner TW, Ai E, Chrobak M et al. Photic maculopathy secondary to short-circuiting of a high-tension electric current. Ophthalmology 1982; 89:865–868.

170. Henry MM, Henry LM. A possible cause of chronic cystic maculopathy. Ann Ophthalmol 1977; 9:455–457.

171. Calkins JL, Hochheimer BF. Retinal light exposure from operation microscopes. Arch Ophthalmol 1979; 97:2363–2367.

172. Macy JI, Baerveldt G. Pseudophakic serous maculopathy. Arch Ophthalmol 1983; 101:228–231.

173. McDonald HR, Irvine AR. Light-induced maculopathy from the operating microscope in extracapsular cataract extraction and intraocular lens implantation. Ophthalmology 1983; 90:945–951.

174. Boldrey EE, Ho BT, Griffith RD. Retinal burns occurring at cataract extraction. Ophthalmology 1984; 91:1297–1302.

175. Brod RD, Barron BA, Suelflow JA. Phototoxic retinal damage during refractive surgery. Am J Ophthalmol 1986; 102:121–123.

176. Fishman GA. Light-induced maculopathy from surgical microscopes during cataract surgery. In: Ernest JT, ed. The 1985 year book of ophthalmology. St Louis: Mosby-Year Book; 1985:177–180.

177. Khwarg SG, Geohegan M, Hanscom TA. Light-induced maculopathy from the operating microscope. Am J Ophthalmol 1984; 98:628–630.

178. Michels M, Sternberg P Jr. Operating microscope-induced retinal phototoxicity: pathophysiology, clinical manifestations and prevention. Surv Ophthalmol 1990; 34:237–252.

179. Robertson DM, Feldman RB. Photic retinopathy from the operating room microscope. Am J Ophthalmol 1986; 101:561–569.

180. Mares-Perlman JA, Brady WE, Klein BE et al. Diet and nuclear lens opacities. Am J Epidemiol 1995; 141:322–334.

181. Fuller D, Machemer R, Knighton RW. Retinal damage produced by intraocular fiber optic light. Am J Ophthalmol 1978; 85:519–537.

182. Khwarg SG, Linstone FA, Daniels SA et al. Incidence, risk factors, and morphology in operating microscope light retinopathy. Am J Ophthalmol 1987; 103:255–263.

183. Brod RD, Olsen KR, Ball SF et al. The site of operating microscope light-induced injury on the human retina. Am J Ophthalmol 1989; 107:390–397.

184. Pavilack MA, Brod RD. Site of potential operating microscope light-induced phototoxicity on the human retina during temporal approach eye surgery. Ophthalmology 2001; 108:381–385.

185. Michels M, Lewis H, Abrams GW et al. Macular phototoxicity caused by fiberoptic endoillumination during pars plana vitrectomy. Am J Ophthalmol 1992; 114:287–296.

186. Parver LM, Auker CR, Fine BS. Observations on monkey eyes exposed to light from an operating microscope. Ophthalmology 1983; 90:964–972.

187. Green WR, Robertson DM. Pathologic findings of photic retinopathy in the human eye. Am J Ophthalmol 1991; 112:520–527.

188. Leonardy NJ, Dabbs CK, Sternberg P Jr. Subretinal neovascularization after operating microscope burn. Am J Ophthalmol 1990; 109:224–225.

189. Jaffe GJ, Irvine AR, Wood IS et al. Retinal phototoxicity from the operating microscope. The role of inspired oxygen. Ophthalmology 1988; 95:1130–1141.

190. Mauget-Faysse M, Quaranta M, Francoz N et al. Incidental retinal phototoxicity associated with ingestion of photosensitizing drugs. Graefes Arch Clin Exp Ophthalmol 2001; 239:501–508.

191. Manzouri B, Egan CA, Hykin PG. Phototoxic maculopathy following uneventful cataract surgery in a predisposed patient. Br J Ophthalmol 2002; 86:705–706.

192. Ferguson J. Photosensitivity due to drugs. Photodermatol Photoimmunol Photomed 2002; 18:262–269.

193. Li S, Lam TT, Fu J et al. Systemic hypertension exaggerates retinal photic injury. Arch Ophthalmol 1995; 113:521–526.

194. Mainster MA, Ham WT Jr, Delori FC. Potential retinal hazards. Instrument and environmental light sources. Ophthalmology 1983; 90:927–932.

195. McIntyre DJ. Phototoxicity. The eclipse filter. Ophthalmology 1985; 92:364–365.

196. Sliney DH, Armstrong BC. Radiometric analysis of surgical microscope lights for hazards analyses. Appl Opt 1986; 25:1882–1889.

197. O'Brien DP, Francis IC. The corneal quilt: a protective device designed to reduce intraoperative retinal phototoxicity. Ophthalm Surg 1994; 25:191–194.

198. Kraff MC, Lieberman HL, Jampol LM et al. Effect of a pupillary light occluder on cystoid macular edema. J Cataract Refract Surg 1989; 15:658–660.

199. Nevyas HJ, Nevyas JY. Surgical corneal light occluder made of black HEMA. Ophthalm Surg 1985; 16:696–698.

200. Jampol LM, Kraff MC, Sanders DR et al. Near-UV radiation from the operating microscope and pseudophakic cystoid macular edema. Arch Ophthalmol 1985; 103:28–30.

201. Keates RH, Genstler DE. UV radiation. Ophthalm Surg 1982; 13:327.

202. Robertson DM, McLaren JW. Photic retinopathy from the operating room microscope. Study with filters. Arch Ophthalmol 1989; 107:373–375.

203. Michels M, Dawson WW, Feldman RB et al. Infrared. An unseen and unnecessary hazard in ophthalmic devices. Ophthalmology 1987; 94:143–148.

204. Keates RH, Armstrong PF. Use of a short wavelength filter in an operating microscope. Ophthalm Surg 1985; 16:40–41.

205. Landry RJ, Miller SA, Byrnes GA. Study of filtered light on potential retinal photic hazards with operation microscopes used for ocular surgery. Appl Opt 2002; 41:802–804.

206. Kleinmann G, Hoffman P, Schechtman E et al. Microscope-induced retinal phototoxicity in cataract surgery of short duration. Ophthalmology 2002; 109:334–338.

207. Oliver M. Posterior pole changes after cataract extraction in elderly subjects. Am J Ophthalmol 1966; 62:1145–1148.

208. Blair CJ, Ferguson J Jr. Exacerbation of senile macular degeneration following cataract extraction. Am J Ophthalmol 1979; 87:77–83.

209. van der Schaft TL, Mooy CM, de Bruijn WC et al. Increased prevalence of disciform macular degeneration after cataract extraction with implantation of an intraocular lens. Br J Ophthalmol 1994; 78:441–445.

210. Pollack A, Marcovich A, Bukelman A et al. Age-related macular degeneration after extracapsular cataract extraction with intraocular lens implantation. Ophthalmology 1996; 103:1546–1554.

211. Pollack A, Bukelman A, Zalish M et al. The course of age-related macular degeneration following bilateral cataract surgery. Ophthalm Surg Lasers 1998; 29:286–294.

212. Shuttleworth GN, Luhishi EA, Harrad RA. Do patients with age related maculopathy and cataract benefit from cataract surgery? Br J Ophthalmol 1998; 82:611–616.

213. Wong TY. Cataract surgery in patients with cataract and age related macular degeneration: do the benefits outweigh the risks? Br J Ophthalmol 2000; 84:1337–1338.

214. Klein R, Klein BE, Wong TY et al. The association of cataract and cataract surgery with the long-term incidence of age-related maculopathy: the Beaver Dam eye study. Arch Ophthalmol 2002; 120:1551–1558.

215. Armbrecht AM, Findlay C, Aspinall PA et al. Cataract surgery in patients with age-related macular degeneration: one-year outcomes. J Cataract Refract Surg 2003; 29:686–693.

216. Wang JJ, Klein R, Smith W et al. Cataract surgery and the 5-year incidence of late-stage age-related maculopathy: pooled findings from the Beaver Dam and Blue Mountains eye studies. Ophthalmology 2003; 110:1960–1967.

217. Freeman EE, Munoz B, West SK et al. Is there an association between cataract surgery and age-related macular degeneration? Data from three population-based studies. Am J Ophthalmol 2003; 135:849–856.

218. Reichel E, Puliafito CA, Duker JS et al. Indocyanine green dye-enhanced diode laser photocoagulation of poorly defined subfoveal choroidal neovascularization. Ophthalm Surg 1994; 25:195–201.

219. Costa RA, Farah ME, Freymuller E et al. Choriocapillaris photodynamic therapy using indocyanine green. Am J Ophthalmol 2001; 132:557–565.

220. Ciardella AP, Schiff W, Barile G et al. Persistent indocyanine green fluorescence after vitrectomy for macular hole. Am J Ophthalmol 2003; 136:174–177.

221. Tadayoni R, Paques M, Girmens JF et al. Persistence of fundus fluorescence after use of indocyanine green for macular surgery. Ophthalmology 2003; 110:604–608.

222. Machida S, Fujiwara T, Gotoh T et al. Observation of the ocular fundus by an infrared-sensitive video camera after vitreoretinal surgery assisted by indocyanine green. Retina 2003;2 :183–191.

223. Gandorfer A, Haritoglou C, Gass CA et al. Indocyanine green-assisted peeling of the internal limiting membrane may cause retinal damage. Am J Ophthalmol 2001; 132:431–433.

224. Engelbrecht NE, Freeman J, Sternberg P Jr. et al. Retinal pigment epithelial changes after macular hole surgery with indocyanine green-assisted internal limiting membrane peeling. Am J Ophthalmol 2002; 133:89–94.

225. Haritoglou C, Gandorfer A, Gass CA et al. Indocyanine green-assisted peeling of the internal limiting membrane in macular hole surgery affects visual outcome: a clinicopathologic correlation. Am J Ophthalmol 2002; 134:836–841.

226. Uemura A, Kanda S, Sakamoto Y et al. Visual field defects after uneventful vitrectomy for epiretinal membrane with indocyanine green-assisted internal limiting membrane peeling. Am J Ophthalmol 2003; 136:252–257.

227. Sippy BD, Engelbrecht NE, Hubbard GB et al. Indocyanine green effect on cultured human retinal pigment epithelial cells: implication for macular hole surgery. Am J Ophthalmol 2001; 132:433–435.

228. Gandorfer A, Haritoglou C, Kampik A. Retinal damage from indocyanine green in experimental macular surgery. Invest Ophthalmol Vis Sci 2003; 44:316–323.

229. Kampik A, Sternberg P. Indocyanine green in vitreomacular surgery – (why) is it a problem? Am J Ophthalmol 2003; 136:527–529.

230. Gass CA, Haritoglou C, Schaumberger M et al. Functional outcome of macular hole surgery with and without indocyanine green-assisted peeling of the internal limiting membrane. Graefes Arch Clin Exp Ophthalmol 2003; 241:716–720.

231. Arden GB, Berninger T, Hogg CR et al. A survey of color discrimination in German ophthalmologists. Changes associated with the use of lasers and operating microscopes. Ophthalmology 1991; 98:567–575.

232. Berninger TA, Canning CR, Gunduz K et al. Using argon laser blue light reduces ophthalmologists' color contrast sensitivity. Argon blue and surgeons' vision. Arch Ophthalmol 1989; 107:1453–1458.

233. Gunduz K, Arden GB. Changes in colour contrast sensitivity associated with operating argon lasers. Br J Ophthalmol 1989; 73:241–246.

234. Whitacre MM, Manoukian N, Mainster MA. Argon indirect ophthalmoscopic photocoagulation: reduced potential phototoxicity with a fixed safety filter. Br J Ophthalmol 1990; 74:233–234.

235. Delori FC, Parker JS, Mainster MA. Light levels in fundus photography and fluorescein angiography. Vision Res 1980; 20:1099–1104.

236. Delori FC, Pomerantz O, Mainster MA. Light levels in ophthalmic diagnostic instruments. Proc Soc Photo Optical Instrum Enginering 1980; 229:154–160.

237. Robertson DM, Erickson GJ. The effect of prolonged indirect ophthalmoscopy on the human eye. Am J Ophthalmol 1979; 87:652–661.

238. Klingbeil U. Safety aspects of laser scanning ophthalmoscopes. Health Phys 1986; 51:81–93.

239. Kohnen S. Light-induced damage of the retina through slit-lamp photography. Graefes Arch Clin Exp Ophthalmol 2000; 238:956–959.

240. Delori FC, Gragoudas ES, Francisco R et al. Monochromatic ophthalmoscopy and fundus photography. The normal fundus. Arch Ophthalmol 1977; 95:861–868.

241. Ducrey NM, Delori FC, Gragoudas ES. Monochromatic ophthalmoscopy and fundus photography. II. The pathological fundus. Arch Ophthalmol 1979; 97:288–293.

242. James RH, Bostrom RG, Remark D et al. Handheld ophthalmoscopes for hazard analysis: an analysis. Appl Opt 1988; 27:5072–5076.

243. Hamer RD, Dobson V, Mayer MJ. Absolute thresholds in human infants exposed to continuous illumination. Invest Ophthalmol Vis Sci 1984; 25:381–388.

244. Landry RJ, Scheidt PC, Hammond RW. Ambient light and phototherapy conditions of eight neonatal care units: a summary report. Pediatrics 1985; 75:434–436.

245. Abramov I, Hainline L. Light in the developing visual system. In: Marshall J, ed. The susceptible visual apparatus. London: Macmillan Press; 1991: 104–133.

246. Moseley MJ, Fielder AR. Light toxicity in the neonatal eye. Clin Vision Sci 1988; 3:75–82.

247. Robinson J, Bayliss SC, Fielder AR. Transmission of light across the adult and neonatal eyelid in vivo. Vision Res 1991; 31:1837–1840.

248. Robinson J, Moseley MJ, Thompson JR et al. Eyelid opening in preterm neonates. Arch Dis Child 1989; 64:943–948.

249. Ackerman B, Sherwonit E, Williams J. Reduced incidental light exposure: effect on the development of retinopathy of prematurity in low birth weight infants. Pediatrics 1989; 83:958–962.

250. Seiberth V, Linderkamp O, Knorz MC et al. A controlled clinical trial of light and retinopathy of prematurity. Am J Ophthalmol 1994; 118:492–495.

251. Mills MD. Light exposure is not associated with retinopathy of prematurity. Arch Ophthalmol 1998; 116:1517–1518.

252. Kennedy KA, Fielder AR, Hardy RJ et al. Reduced lighting does not improve medical outcomes in very low birth weight infants. J Pediatr 2001; 139:527–531.

253. Reynolds JD, Hardy RJ, Kennedy KA et al. Lack of efficacy of light reduction in preventing retinopathy of prematurity. Light Reduction in Retinopathy of Prematurity (LIGHT-ROP) Cooperative Group. N Engl J Med 1998; 338:1572–1576.

254. Watson AB. Artificial tanning and suntan salons. Med J Aust 1982; 1:430–431.

255. Bruyneel-Rapp F, Dorsey SB, Guin JD. The tanning salon: an area survey of equipment, procedures, and practices. J Am Acad Dermatol 1988; 18:1030–1038.

256. Walters BL, Kelley TM. Commercial tanning facilities: a new source of eye injury. Am J Emerg Med 1987; 5:386–389.

257. Robison WG, Kuwabara T, Bieri JG. The roles of vitamin E and unsaturated fatty acids in the visual process. Retina 1982; 2:263–281.

258. Hunyor AB. Solar retinopathy: its significance for the ageing eye and the younger pseudophakic patient. Aust NZ J Ophthalmol 1987; 15:371–375.

259. Beatty S, Koh H, Phil M et al. The role of oxidative stress in the pathogenesis of age-related macular degeneration. Surv Ophthalmol 2000; 45:115–134.

260. Bernstein PS, Zhao DY, Wintch SW et al. Resonance Raman measurement of macular carotenoids in normal subjects and in age-related macular degeneration patients. Ophthalmology 2002; 109:1780–1787.

261. van der Hoeve J. Eye lesions produced by light rich in ultraviolet rays: senile cataract, senile degeneration of the macula. Am J Ophthalmol 1920; 3:178–194.

262. Ts'o MO, La Piana FG, Appleton B. The human fovea after sungazing. Trans Am Acad Ophthalmol Otolaryngol 1974; 78:OP-677.

263. Mainster MA. Solar retinitis, photic maculopathy and the pseudophakic eye. J Am Intraocul Implant Soc 1978; 4:84–86.

264. Young RW. A theory of central retinal disease. In: Sears ML, ed. New directions in ophthalmic research. New Haven, CT: Yale University Press; 1981:237–270.

265. Sperduto RD, Hiller R, Seigel D. Lens opacities and senile maculopathy. Arch Ophthalmol 1981; 99:1004–1008.

266. Clarke CA, Sneddon IB. Nutritional neuropathy in prisoners-of-war internees from Hong Kong. Lancet 1946; 1:734–737.

267. Hecht S, Hendley CD, Ross S et al. The effect of exposure to sunlight on night vision. Am J Ophthalmol 1948; 31:1573–1580.

268. Wolf E. Effects of exposure to ultra-violet light on human dark adaptation. Proc Natl Acad Sci USA 1946; 32:219–226.

269. Marshall J. Ageing changes in human cones. Acta XXIII Concil Ophthalmol (Kyoto) 1978; 1:375–378.

270. Borges J, Li ZY, Tso MO. Effects of repeated photic exposures on the monkey macula. Arch Ophthalmol 1990; 108:727–733.

271. Taylor HR, West S, Munoz B et al. The long-term effects of visible light on the eye. Arch Ophthalmol 1992; 110:99–104.

272. West SK, Rosenthal FS, Bressler NM et al. Exposure to sunlight and other risk factors for age-related macular degeneration. Arch Ophthalmol 1989; 107:875–879.

273. Cruickshanks KJ, Klein R, Klein BE. Sunlight and age-related macular degeneration. The Beaver Dam eye study. Arch Ophthalmol 1993; 111:514–518.

274. Cruickshanks KJ, Klein R, Klein BE et al. Sunlight and the 5-year incidence of early age-related maculopathy: the Beaver Dam eye study. Arch Ophthalmol 2001; 119:246–250.

275. Darzins P, Mitchell P, Heller RF. Sun exposure and age-related macular degeneration. An Australian case–control study. Ophthalmology 1997; 104:770–776.

276. Delcourt C, Carriere I, Ponton-Sanchez A et al. Light exposure and the risk of age-related macular degeneration: the Pathologies Oculaires Liées a l'Age (POLA) study. Arch Ophthalmol 2001; 119:1463–1468.

277. McCarty CA, Mukesh BN, Fu CL et al. Risk factors for age-related maculopathy: the Visual Impairment Project. Arch Ophthalmol 2001; 119:1455–1462.

278. Mainster MA. Spectral transmittance of intraocular lenses and retinal damage from intense light sources. Am J Ophthalmol 1978; 85:167–170.

279. Mainster MA. The spectra, classification, and rationale of ultraviolet-protective intraocular lenses. Am J Ophthalmol 1986; 102:727–732.

280. Mantyjarvi M, Syrjakoski J, Tuppurainen K et al. Colour vision through intraocular lens. Acta Ophthalmol Scand 1997; 75:166–1669.

281. Kamel ID, Parker JA. Protection from ultraviolet exposure in aphakic erythropsia. Can J Ophthalmol 1973; 8:563–565.

282. Saraux H, Manent JP, Laroche L. Erythropsia in a patient with lens implant. Physiologic and electrophysiologic study. J Fr Ophtalmol 1984; 7:557–562.

283. Jordan DR, Valberg JD. Dyschromatopsia following cataract surgery. Can J Ophthalmol 1986; 21:140–143.

284. Bennett LW. Pseudophakic erythropsia. J Am Optom Assoc 1994; 65: 273–276.

285. Werner JS, Steele VG, Pfoff DS. Loss of human photoreceptor sensitivity associated with chronic exposure to ultraviolet radiation. Ophthalmology 1989; 96:1552–1558.

286. Miyake K, Ichihashi S, Shibuya Y et al. Blood–retinal barrier and autofluorescence of the posterior polar retina in long-standing pseudophakia. J Cataract Refract Surg 1999; 25:891–897.

287. Peyman GA, Zak R, Sloane H. Ultraviolet-absorbing pseudophakos: an efficacy study. J Am Intraocul Implant Soc 1983; 9:161–170.

288. Nilsson SE, Textorius O, Andersson BE et al. Clear PMMA versus yellow intraocular lens material. An electrophysiologic study on pigmented rabbits regarding "the blue light hazard." Prog Clin Biol Res 1989; 314:539–553.

289. Jackson GR, Owsley C, McGwin G Jr. Aging and dark adaptation. Vision Res 1999; 39:3975–3982.

290. Jackson GR, Owsley C. Scotopic sensitivity during adulthood. Vision Res 2000; 40:2467–2473.

291. Jackson GR, Owsley C, Curcio CA. Photoreceptor degeneration and dysfunction in aging and age-related maculopathy. Ageing Res Rev 2002; 1:381–396.

292. Sunness JS, Rubin GS, Applegate CA et al. Visual function abnormalities and prognosis in eyes with age-related geographic atrophy of the macula and good visual acuity. Ophthalmology 1997; 104:1677–1691.

293. Owsley C, Jackson GR, Cideciyan AV et al. Psychophysical evidence for rod vulnerability in age-related macular degeneration. Invest Ophthalmol Vis Sci 2000; 41:267–273.

294. Owsley C, Jackson GR, White M et al. Delays in rod-mediated dark adaptation in early age-related maculopathy. Ophthalmology 2001; 108:1196–202.

295. Taylor HR, West SK, Rosenthal FS et al. Effect of ultraviolet radiation on cataract formation. N Engl J Med 1988; 319:1429–1433.

296. West SK, Duncan DD, Munoz B et al. Sunlight exposure and risk of lens opacities in a population-based study: the Salisbury Eye Evaluation project. JAMA 1998; 280:714–718.

297. Delcourt C, Carriere I, Ponton-Sanchez A et al. Light exposure and the risk of cortical, nuclear, and posterior subcapsular cataracts: the Pathologies Oculaires Liées a l'Age (POLA) study. Arch Ophthalmol 2000; 118:385–392.

298. Rabin JC, Wiley RW, Levine RR et al. US Army sunglasses: issues and solutions. J Am Optom Assoc 1996; 7:215–222.

299. Sliney DH. Photoprotection of the eye – UV radiation and sunglasses. J Photochem Photobiol B 2001; 64:166–175.

300. American national standard for the safe use of lasers, ANSI Z136.1-2000. Washington, DC: American National Standards Institute, 2000.

301. American national standard for the safe use of lasers in health care facilities, ANSI Z136.3-1996. Washington, DC: American National Standards Institute, 1996.

302. Safety of laser products – Part 1: Equipment classification requirements and user's guide, IEC 60825-1. Geneva, Switzerland: International Electrotechnical Commission; 2001.

303. Sliney DH, Trokel SL. Medical lasers and their safe use. New York: Springer-Verlag, 1993.

304. Slit lamp guidance, 1.0. Washington, DC: Center for Devices and Radiological Health, United States Food and Drug Administration, 1998.

305. Ophthalmic instruments – slit-lamp microscopes, ISO 10939. Geneva, Switzerland: International Organization for Standardization, 1998.

306. Ophthalmic instruments – endoilluminators – fundamental requirements and test methods for optical radiation safety, ISO 15752. Geneva, Switzerland: International Organization for Standardization, 2000.

307. Photodynamic therapy of subfoveal choroidal neovascularization in age-related macular degeneration with verteporfin: one-year results of 2 randomized clinical trials – TAP report. Treatment of age-related macular degeneration with photodynamic therapy (TAP) study group. Arch Ophthalmol 1999; 117:1329–1345.

308. Framme C, Brinkmann R, Birngruber R et al. Autofluorescence imaging after selective RPE laser treatment in macular diseases and clinical outcome: a pilot study. Br J Ophthalmol 2002; 86:1099–1106.

Traumatic Chorioretinopathies

James S. Kelley

Surveys indicate that 1% of the US population will have an eye injury each year. Among the roughly 2.5 million trauma cases, 70 000 have significant temporary or permanent disability.[1–3] The population affected tends to be young, with the majority under 30 years of age.[3] This underscores the social and economic effect of these injuries.[4]

As a result of the shift toward outpatient surgery in ophthalmology, eye trauma will soon be the primary reason for ophthalmic-related hospitalizations in North America.[5–7] Ocular trauma as a cause of hospital admissions has a bimodal distribution, with the highest peak consisting of adolescents and young adults and another peak representing those 75 years or older.[8] Indeed, almost 50% of ocular trauma requiring medical attention occurs in children.[2,9] Most injuries to children (aged less than 16 years) occur during sports or play activities.[3,10] In adults, motor vehicle and industrial accidents, physical assaults, and sports injuries are frequently reported causes.[7,11,12] Patients tend to be males (72 to 90%), most being younger than 30 years of age.[13] Blunt injuries account for 51 to 66% of ocular injuries in both prospective and retrospective studies,[3,12] with the majority of retinal lesions being unilateral. Recent reports in the literature have implicated bungee cords, water balloons, golf balls, soccer balls, and paint balls as objects that can cause ocular morbidity and blindness.[14–17]

The chorioretinopathies considered in this chapter are divided into those due to remote injuries to areas of the body other than the eye and to those due to direct injury to the eye by blunt forces, leaving the sclera intact. Penetrating injuries are discussed in Chapter 138. Specific effects related to the vitreous base, dialysis, and tears are discussed in Chapter 137.

CHORIORETINOPATHIES FROM DIRECT OCULAR INJURIES

The force acting on the eye can cause effects at the site of impact, a coup injury, usually in the anterior segment. In addition, the force can act remotely in the opposite or posterior part of the eye by contrecoup injury. The contrecoup effect may be caused by shock waves acting at the interface of tissues of different densities. Direct blunt trauma also distorts the globe, compressing the eye in the axis of the force and signifi-

cantly stretching the tissues in the perpendicular plane. This stretching may contribute to indirect injury.[18]

Commotio retinae

Berlin,[19] in 1873, invoked the Latin term for retinal contusion, *commotio retinae*, to describe a transient whitening of the retina resulting from blunt ocular trauma. It can occur peripherally or within the posterior pole region, in which case it is referred to as *Berlin's edema*. Extensive posterior pole involvement may give rise to a cherry-red spot. Berlin was able to produce similar lesions in rabbit eyes using an elastic stick, and he suggested that extracellular edema was present.[19] In the posterior pole the mechanism of injury is contrecoup. Although a patient may report decreased vision, the lesion may take several hours to be visible ophthalmoscopically.

Commotio retinae consists of two variations, a milder condition, retinal concussion, and a more severe condition, retinal contusion. This clinical terminology is borrowed from descriptions of head trauma. The division into two entities, mild and severe, is traditional[20] and clinically useful. Further study may define the spectrum of blunt injuries more scientifically.

Retinal concussion

Retinal concussion may be regarded as one end of the spectrum of traumatic retinal opacification. The initial vision is better than 20/200, the gray-white change is less dramatic, and hemorrhages are less frequent. Most important, the clinical changes are reversible, with no visible late pigment scarring and good final acuity. Studies show no change in the blood–retinal barrier.[21]

On fluorescein angiography the areas of opaque retina block background choroidal fluorescence. The retinal vessels are unimpaired, with complete capillary filling. There is no leakage of dye into or under the retina[22] (Fig. 110-1). The retinal whitening clears spontaneously in a few days.[23–25] There may be a transient myopic shift due to ciliary body and crystalline lens changes.[26]

Retinal contusion

Like retinal concussion, contusion can occur anteriorly at the point of impact (coup) or posteriorly remote from impact (contrecoup). The retinal whitening is more intense; hemorrhages are more frequent, and visual loss is more common.

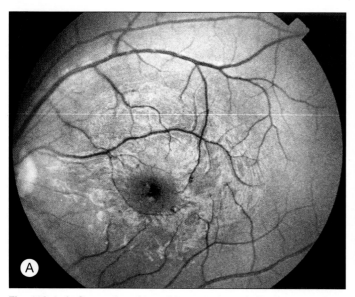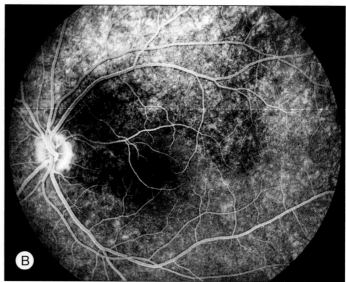

Fig. 110-1 A, Commotio retinae of the posterior pole (Berlin's edema) in association with fine superficial hemorrhages. B, Normal midtransit fluorescein angiogram pattern. No dye leakage is demonstrable.

If the macula is affected, central acuity is lost, usually permanently.[27,28]

Early hypofluorescence may still be present on fluorescein angiography. However, bright leakage at the level of the pigment epithelium, referred to as *acute pigment epithelial edema*,[27] occurs later (Fig. 110-2). Acute pigment epithelial damage leads to a permanent pigmented or mottled scar over a few weeks. If the hyperfluorescence involves the fovea, loss of visual function and central acuity is permanent.

The increasing number of histologic studies do not separate clearly into two categories. The functional and longitudinal data confirming the clinical classifications are not available. The studies are presented in a suggestive order of increasing severity.

Using owl monkeys, Sipperley and co-workers[29] were able to produce a picture of commotio retinae similar to that seen in humans. The opacity in the retina corresponded to areas of fragmented photoreceptor outer segments (Fig.110-3). There was no extracellular or intracellular edema of any retinal cells.

Blight & Hart[23] investigated the structural changes in the retina following blunt trauma to pig eyes. They demonstrated immediate fragmentation of the photoreceptor outer segments, loss of the apical processes of the retinal pigment epithelium (RPE), and intracellular edema of retinal glia. There were no long-term pigment changes as seen in retinal contusion.

Mansour and co-workers[30] studied commotio retinae in an eye enucleated 24 h after injury. They noted photoreceptor disruption similar to that reported in Sipperley's study.

In addition, there was loss of RPE apical processes, disruption of the RPE plasma membrane, and formation of microcytic spaces.

The majority of the elegant electron microscope photographs in these studies show only receptor damage. This may correspond to the reversible clinical condition, retinal concussion, in which there is no acute fluorescein leakage. Hints of RPE

damage would account for the leakage seen in the cases of retinal contusion. Gaps remain in our understanding of this fascinating condition. Vascular effects such as ischemic necrosis may play a role.[31]

No specific treatment has been beneficial in either retinal concussion or retinal contusion.

Traumatic macular hole

Postcontusion macular holes were first described by Knapp in 1869 and by Noyes in 1875.[32] The first description of an inner lamellar macular hole, by Fuchs in 1901,[33] was in the setting of blunt trauma. Macular cysts or holes were seen in 4% of boxers in one series.[34] The mechanism whereby blunt trauma causes a macular hole, according to Gass,[27] consists of one or a combination of the following: (1) contusion necrosis with cystoid degeneration; (2) subfoveal hemorrhage in conjunction with a choroidal rupture; and (3) anteroposterior vitreous traction. Frangieh and associates,[35] in 1981, reviewed 44 eyes of 39 patients with lamellar holes, full-thickness holes, or macular cysts and suggested that cystoid degeneration with cyst coalescence and subsequent hole formation is the most common cause of macular holes. They concluded that vitreoretinal traction with or without an operculum was infrequently associated with macular holes. Interestingly, the largest macular holes (up to 1.5 mm diameter) were full-thickness and associated with blunt trauma (average, 0.86 mm versus 0.66 mm in non-traumatic holes).[35] Surgical repair, including internal limiting membrane removal, is anatomically successful but final vision depends on the associated injuries.[36,37]

Vitreoretinal traction is thought to play a role in the syndrome of whiplash maculopathy, which occurs without direct eye involvement and following a flexion–extension type of head and neck injury. Visual acuity, even early in the course of whiplash maculopathy, is rarely worse than 20/50; a slight

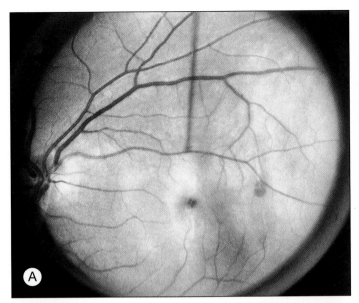

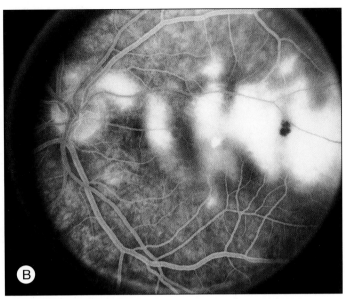

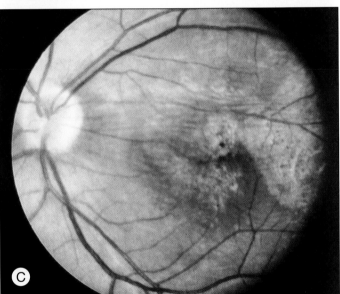

Fig. 110-2 A, Severe commotio retinae of the posterior pole (Berlin's edema) with dramatic whitening and a pseudo-cherry-red spot. B, The more severe contusion injury is associated with fluorescein leakage at the level of the retinal pigment epithelium without elevation of tissue. C, Late pigmentary changes accompany permanent visual loss in the more severe response to trauma.

grayish retinal haze, a craterlike depression of less than 100 mm diameter, and a slight RPE disturbance are evident[38] (Fig. 110-4). Occasionally, a wisp of vitreoretinal tissue extends anteriorly from the pitlike depression in the fovea.[39] Within a few days visual acuity improves to 20/20. The tiny foveal pit remains as a marker of previous trauma. No treatment is necessary for this condition. The most likely cause of whiplash maculopathy is vitreoretinal traction, as indicated by the appearance of a micro-operculum in reported cases. The susceptibility of the fovea to such an injury can be explained by a marked thinning of the inner limiting membrane and vitreous attachment plaques at the crest of the foveal clivus.[40,41]

Traumatic retinal pigment epithelial tears

Tears of the RPE were first reported in 1981 by Hoskin et al.[42] as a complication of serous detachments of the pigment epithelium in patients with age-related maculopathy.

Levin et al.[43] in 1991 reported 2 patients with RPE tears that developed after blunt trauma to the eye.

They hypothesized that this unusual phenomenon is caused by an acute tractional force oriented tangentially to the macular plane, the result of a rapid, spherically expansile deformation of the globe during trauma.

Chorioretinal rupture

Goldzieher,[44] in 1901, introduced the term *chorioretinitis plastica sclopetaria* to describe the appearance of direct choroidal and retinal rupture in the peripheral retina following trauma from a bullet wound in the orbital area. The abbreviated term, *chorioretinitis sclopetaria*, is now used. Fundus examination shows an exuberant fibroglial scar with sharp, serrated borders and pigment proliferation (Fig. 110-5). The projectile does not penetrate the globe but passes in close proximity to it, inducing a rupture of the retina and choroid with hemorrhage. The visual

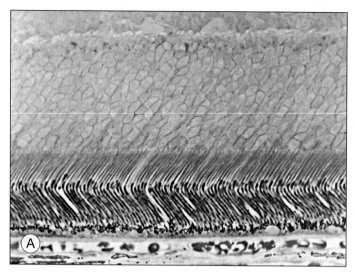 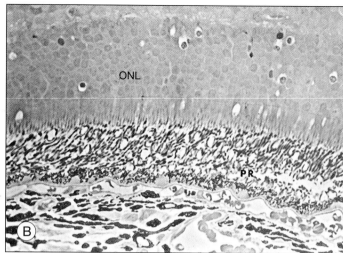

Fig. 110-3 A, Photomicrograph of normal owl monkey retina. B, Owl monkey retina 4 h after trauma from an air-rifle pellet. Note the disruption of the photoreceptor outer segments (PR) and pyknotic nuclei in the outer nuclear layer (ONL) (paraphenylenediamine; ×125). (From Sipperley JO, Quigley HA, Gass JDM. Traumatic retinopathy in primates: the explanation of commotio retinae. Arch Ophthalmol 1978; 96:2267–2273. Copyright © (1978) American Medical Association. All rights reserved.[29])

prognosis depends on the extent and location of intraocular injury, since coup or contrecoup macular injury may occur in addition to optic nerve injury caused by the missile itself.[45] Indocyanine green dye permits visualization of deeper choroids and may show ruptures not seen clinically.[45] Massive injury may even result in confluent peripheral retinal and macular chorioretinitis sclopetaria. Posterior chorioretinal rupture can occur, with permanent field defects and anastomosis between retina and choroid (Fig. 110-6). Surprisingly, retinal detachment is rare even without surgical intervention because firm chorioretinal adhesion develops at the edges of the lesion and acts as a spontaneous retinopexy.[46]

Dubovy et al.[47] in 1997 reported on the clinicopathologic features in the eye of a patient who sustained chorioretinitis sclopetaria from a gunshot wound to the orbit, with clinical follow-up of more than 20 years. These features included direct traumatic chorioretinal rupture followed by marked fibrovascular proliferation with variable replacement of choroid and retina with no retinal detachment. Posteriorly, indirect macular choroidal ruptures with hyperplasia and migration of the RPE into the retina and choroid, epiretinal membrane formation,

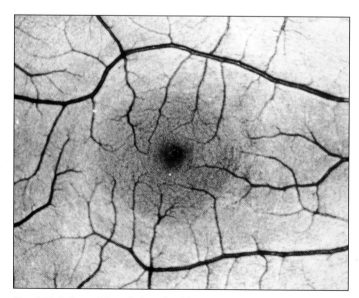

Fig. 110-4 A small foveal pit outlined by a gray ring correlates with immediate mild visual blur and a whiplash injury (×2).

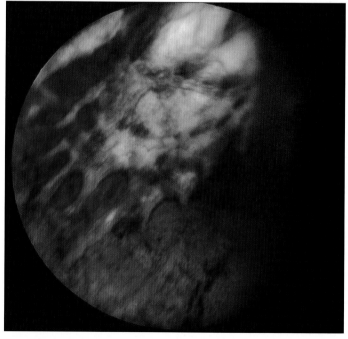

Fig. 110-5 Anterior chorioretinal rupture (chorioretinitis sclopetaria) with irregular tears surrounded by hemorrhage.

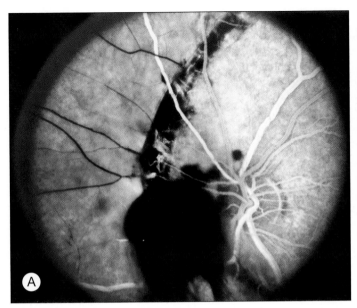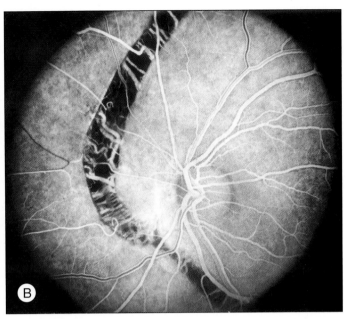

Fig. 110-6 A, Posterior chorioretinal rupture with full-thickness tear denoted by interruption of the nasal retinal vessels. B, Three months later the nasal circulation has been restored by anastomoses between the retina and choroid. Note that no retinal detachment has occurred.

loss of photoreceptors, and marked hemiatrophy of the optic nerve were present. This case followed the typical course of trauma, with hemorrhage and the subsequent exuberant proliferation of fibrous tissue.[47]

Choroidal rupture

Choroidal rupture is a common complication of compressive and contusional injuries of the eye. With blunt trauma the sclera is strong enough to resist rupturing and the retina is distensible enough to resist tearing. However, the relatively inelastic Bruch's membrane ruptures, along with the closely apposed RPE and choriocapillaris.[48–50] The risk of retinal detachment from this type of injury is very low. Direct choroidal ruptures due to direct contusion necrosis of the choroid are relatively uncommon and are found anterior to the equator, where they tend to be oriented parallel to the ora serrata. Indirect choroidal ruptures are more common and are crescent-shaped and concentric to the optic disc (Fig. 110-7A). Indirect choroidal ruptures result from compressive injury to the posterior pole of the eye,[48,49] with the crescent-shaped tears occurring concentric to the disc because of the tethering or stabilizing effect of the optic nerve.[50]

Between 5 and 10% of blunt ocular injuries lead to indirect choroidal rupture.[46] In the histopathologic report of Aguilar & Green,[48] 7 of 17 eyes (41%) without globe rupture had direct choroidal ruptures, and 17 (100%) had indirect choroidal ruptures. Of all eyes studied (including those with globe rupture), 78.7% had indirect choroidal ruptures, and 21.3% had direct ruptures.

Indirect choroidal ruptures are seen as crescent-shaped rents in the RPE–Bruch's membrane–choriocapillaris complex that are concentric to the disc margin and are often associated with intrachoroidal, subretinal, and intraretinal hemorrhage. The

associated hemorrhage, in addition to accompanying commotio retinae, may conceal the presence of the tears, which become visible only after the blood clears in 2 to 3 months. They are usually single but may be concentric and multiple (in 25%) and are seen temporal to the disc in 80%.[50,51] Less commonly, choroidal tears occur nasal to the disc, have a radial orientation, and assume an irregular configuration.[49,52] Occasionally they may not be readily evident ophthalmoscopically, and their presence is confirmed after fluorescein angiography. Indocyanine green angiography may show broader areas of pathology than visible clinically.[52] Visual acuity at presentation varies from 20/20 to 20/400 or less, depending on the location of the rupture; it is worse in eyes with ruptures under or near to the fovea.[50] When Bruch's membrane is weakened, as in angioid streaks, relatively trivial trauma has an exaggerated effect, causing widespread hemorrhage, the extension of established breaks, and the creation of new ones. Patients with angioid streaks therefore should take precautions to avoid trauma in sports activities.[53,54]

In histopathologic studies, Aguilar & Green[48] showed that the choroidal rupture is followed by bleeding, fibrovascular tissue proliferation, and RPE hyperplasia. The overlying retina is variably affected, from loss of the outer layers to discontinuity of the full thickness, and heals with a fibroglial response. In more severe trauma, fibrovascular scar tissue from the choroid may extend through the retina and into the vitreous cavity. Neovascularization is a consistent part of the process of scar formation, and in the majority of cases this neovascularization regresses without sequelae. In the series of Aguilar & Green, direct and indirect choroidal ruptures healed within 14 to 21 days after trauma.[48]

Choroidoretinal vascular anastomoses have been described by Goldberg[55] as an infrequent complication of choroidal ruptures involving contiguous choroid and retina. Gass and others have described the development of subretinal choroidal neovascularization arising from foci of choroidal rupture from 1 month to 4 years after injury[27,56,57] (Fig. 110-7B). Although the natural history of choroidal neovascularization complicating choroidal ruptures is unknown, there is probably a role for laser photocoagulation of fluorescein angiographically demonstrable lesions.[56,57] Gross et al.[58] in 1996 reported on 3 patients with traumatic choroidal rupture in whom subfoveal choroidal neovascularization developed. These patients underwent pars plana vitrectomy with surgical excision of the neovascular membrane. Visual results were excellent, with visual acuities improving to 20/30 or better in each patient. These cases underscore the need for long-term follow-up even in patients who experience the return of good macular function after blunt trauma.

Optic nerve avulsion

Optic nerve avulsion can result from blunt ocular trauma. In optic nerve avulsion (or anterior indirect traumatic optic neuropathy), the optic nerve is forcibly disinserted from the retina, choroid, and vitreous, resulting in retraction of the lamina cribrosa from the scleral rim.[59] Recent reports suggest that final visual outcome is dependent on initial postinjury visual acuity.[60] With clear media, the diagnosis of optic nerve avulsion is usually straightforward. Examination of the fundus reveals a hole or cavity where the optic disc has retracted from the sclera and into its dural sheath.[60] If the view of the optic disc is blocked by media opacity, the diagnosis is more difficult to make. Ultrasonography of the globe may show a posterior-wall defect implying avulsion.[61] Neuroimaging has been shown to be unreliable in the diagnosis of this injury.[60] However, computed tomography or magnetic resonance imaging can be useful in the diagnosis of associated ocular and orbital injuries. Because no medical or surgical treatment has proved helpful in cases of optic nerve avulsion, early diagnosis may spare the patient unnecessary intervention, such as high-dose corticosteroid treatment and optic canal decompression.

CHORIORETINOPATHIES FROM REMOTE INJURIES

Purtscher's retinopathy

In 1910 Otmar Purtscher, a Tyrolean ophthalmologist, described a syndrome of sudden blindness in 5 severely traumatized patients, with multiple areas of superficial retinal whitening located primarily in the posterior pole of both eyes.[62] Papillitis, scattered intraretinal hemorrhages, and a preretinal hemorrhage were also seen. A cherry-red spot of the macula is evident in some cases.[63] Purtscher called this condition *angiopathia retinae traumatica* and postulated that the white spots were lymphatic extravasations caused by a sudden increase in intracranial pressure related to head trauma.[62,64] Traumatic retinal angiopathy has come to be known as *Purtscher's retinopathy*, and the white patches are now recognized as cottonwool spots (Fig. 110-8). Similar fundus findings have since been seen in such diverse settings as compressive chest trauma, hydrostatic pressure syndrome,[65] posttraumatic fat embolism from long bone fractures, acute pancreatitis, lupus erythematosus, dermatomyositis, scleroderma, during childbirth (amniotic fluid embolism), and in the postpartum period.[66–68] Although usually bilateral in presentation, unilateral Purtscher's retinopathy has been

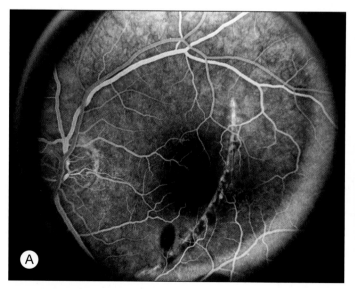

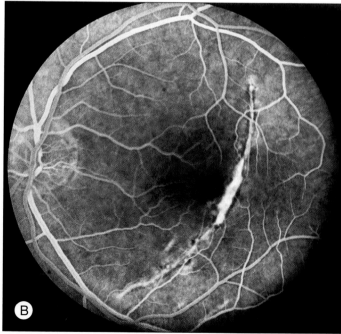

Fig. 110-7 A, Fluorescein angiogram of acute indirect choroidal rupture showing the classic crescent shape concentric to the optic disc and blockage from associated subretinal hemorrhage. No active leakage seen. B, Follow-up angiogram of the patient 4 months later. Increasing fluorescein leakage indicates choroidal neovascularization.

reported.[67,69] Some controversy exists as to whether the unilateral cases in fact represent markedly asymmetric involvement of bilateral disease.

Visual acuities in affected eyes range from 20/200 to finger-counting and may improve after several months to the 20/30 to 20/200 range. With resolution of the acute fundus abnormalities, nerve fiber layer dropout and optic disc atrophy with minimal gliosis may ensue (Fig. 110-8C). The very early fluorescein angiographic findings may show only arterial staining and leakage from the capillary bed, as reported in one patient seen within an hour of injury.[65] Other reports demonstrate later nonperfusion with closure of preterminal arterioles and venules, staining of vessel walls, and venous dilation and leakage.[67,68]

Several mechanisms have been proposed for the pathogenesis of Purtscher's retinopathy, including: (1) fat embolization in long bone fractures and acute pancreatitis (due to enzymatic digestion of omental fat);[67] (2) air embolization from compressive chest injuries;[67] (3) venous reflux with endothelial cell swelling and capillary engorgement of the upper body;[70] (4) severe angiospastic response following a sudden increase in venous pressure;[63] and (5) complement-induced granulocyte aggregation.[71]

Leukocyte aggregation by activated complement factor 5 (C5a) has been shown to occur in such diverse conditions as trauma, acute pancreatitis, and connective tissue disease and has been proposed as being the most likely mechanism.

Venous retinopathy

Incompetent or absent valves in the venous system of the head and neck allow direct transmission of intrathoracic or intra-abdominal pressures, as with the Valsalva maneuver, into the

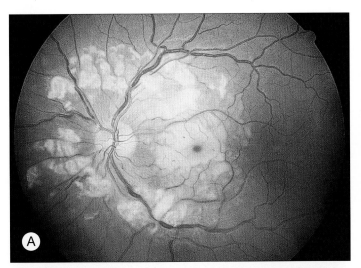

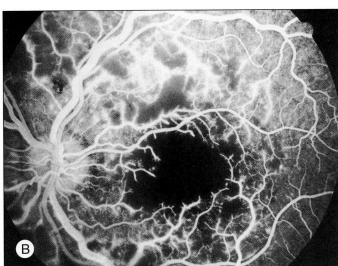

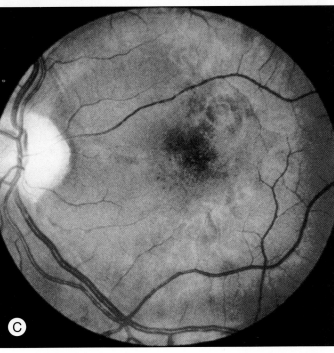

Fig. 110-8 A, Fundus photograph of the left eye of a 25-year-old man 2 days after a snowmobile injury. Large numbers of cottonwool spots with a pseudo-cherry-red spot and a few superficial retinal hemorrhages are evident. B, Late-transit fluorescein angiogram frame reveals paramacular capillary nonperfusion, obstructed arterioles, and perivenous staining. C, Fundus photograph of the patient 18 months after injury. Arcuate zones of nerve fiber layer atrophy are distal to previous cottonwool spots, and optic atrophy is evident. (Courtesy of Alan Cruess, MD.)

head and neck.[72] Sudden elevations of venous pressure may cause a decompensation in the retinal capillary bed, with sub-internal limiting membrane hemorrhages that infrequently may break through and become subhyaloid or intravitreal.[73] Valsalva retinopathy may occur in healthy young adults as a result of heavy lifting, natural childbirth, automobile airbag-related trauma, or even vigorous sexual activity[73-76] (Fig. 110-9). Vision almost invariably returns to normal after the blood clears, and no treatment is necessary.

Traumatic asphyxia, a rare clinical condition identified by a blue discoloration of the face and upper body, follows a severe compression injury of the chest. Associated soft retinal exudates have been documented, as in Purtscher's retinopathy. The dramatic skin changes of deoxygenated blood in dilated skin capillaries are almost certainly caused by sudden and massive venous reflux[72] (Fig. 110-10). Traumatic asphyxia differs clinically from Purtscher's retinopathy, mainly in its dramatic cutaneous manifestations.

Child-abuse syndromes

The presenting sign of child abuse involves the eye in 4 to 6% of cases. Diagnosis requires a high index of suspicion and knowledge of the manifestations of child abuse. The most common ocular manifestation is retinal hemorrhages (followed by periorbital ecchymosis and vitreoretinal damage).[77,78] Retinal hemorrhages occur in 11 to 23% of all physically abused children and in 50 to 80% of shaken babies[79-81] (Fig. 110-11). The term *whiplash-shaken-baby syndrome* was coined by Caffey[82] to describe the occurrence in infants of retinal hemorrhages, subdural or subarachnoid hemorrhages, and minimal or absent signs of external trauma. Although the term *shaken-baby syndrome* has become well-entrenched in the literature of child abuse, it is common for a history of shaking to be lacking. Shaking is

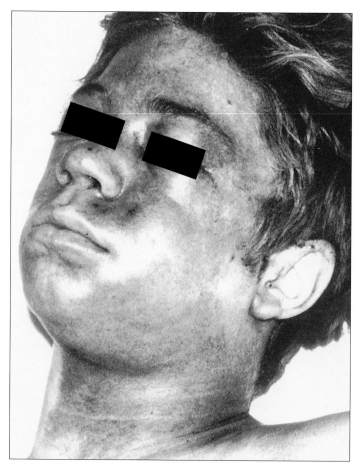

Fig. 110-10 Dramatic skin changes accompanying traumatic asphyxia, indicating a role for increased venous pressure in the pathogenesis of these disorders. (Courtesy of James Ravin, MD.)

often assumed on the basis of a cardinal triad of skeletal injuries (metaphyseal avulsions, rib fractures, and stripping of periosteum), computed tomography findings of intracranial bleeding, and retinal hemorrhages. The head constitutes 10% of the total volume and weight of an infant, and infants have poor neural control of the muscles of the neck. During shaking the head experiences severe accelerations and decelerations, with resulting shear and tensile strains in the infant's soft, poorly myelinated brain. When external signs of trauma are lacking, the ophthalmologist is often called on to establish the diagnosis. Retinal hemorrhages, on this setting, are suggestive of abuse but can also occur with accidental trauma and certain blood disorders.[83] This syndrome carries a 15% mortality rate and a 50% morbidity rate.

Less common retinal findings in child abuse include traumatic retinoschisis and retinal folds. These are due to contrecoup forces resulting from trauma, in addition to the peculiarities of sudden, oscillating vitreous traction in children with formed vitreous gel and firm attachments to the perimacular retina.[83-85]

Ophthalmologists must be familiar with the retinal manifestations of child abuse as part of a multidisciplinary approach to the diagnosis and management of these unfortunate children and to be able to testify as an expert witness.

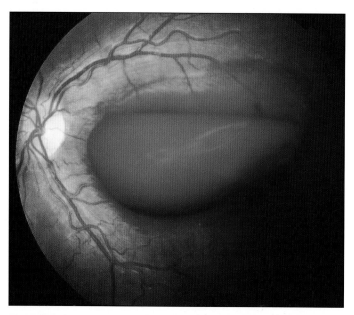

Fig. 110-9 Fundus photograph of subinternal limiting membrane hemorrhage in a 28-year-old man after power weight lifting competition.

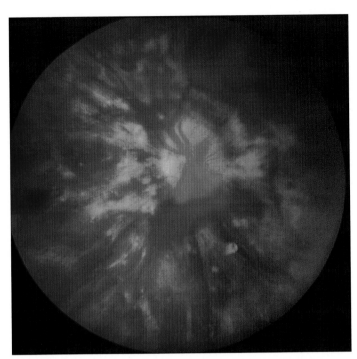

Fig. 110-11 Dense nerve fiber layer and preretinal hemorrhages in a battered child. Similar findings occur in the shaken-baby syndrome. (Courtesy of Jeffery Gross, MD.)

Lightning maculopathy

Lightning is an uncommon cause of ocular injury. Cataract, macular hole, and macular edema have been reported as complications of being struck by lightning. Handa & Jaffe[86] in 1994 reported on a case of maculopathy that they believed consisted of cystic macular edema masquerading as a macular hole. On initial presentation the patient's visual acuity measured 20/300 (right eye) and 20/30 (left eye). Ophthalmoscopy revealed bilateral macular cysts with negative Watzke–Allen tests. During the following 5 months the patient's visual acuity worsened as a result of progressive posterior subcapsular cataracts. The patient underwent uncomplicated cataract surgery on both eyes and at 14 months postinjury measured 20/20 on both eyes. The authors concluded that careful retinal examination is essential in the preoperative workup of patients with lightning-induced cataracts to inform them of their vision potential.

Retinal hemorrhage from epidural steroid injection

Chronic back pain is a highly prevalent cause of discomfort and debilitation among adult patients and is frequently managed by epidural injection of drugs. Kushner & Olson[87] in 1995 reported on four cases of retinal hemorrhages following epidural steroid injection for chronic back pain. The mechanism of action producing retinal hemorrhages in these cases is not clear, but it may be similar to the one that is generally accepted for Terson's syndrome. Presumably, an acute increase in cerebrospinal fluid pressure is transmitted through the optic nerve sheaths to the posterior retinal venous circulation.[88] Kushner &

Olsen concluded that retinal hemorrhage is an uncommon but significant complication of this therapy, and patients should be fully informed of this potential complication.[87]

SUMMARY

With trauma becoming the most common indication for ophthalmic-related hospitalizations, ophthalmologists must be familiar with its ocular manifestations to establish the correct diagnosis and institute proper management. This includes performing a complete ophthalmologic evaluation, including a dilated fundus examination. Direct and indirect ocular manifestations of trauma have medicolegal implications for children, who collectively account for half of all these patients.

No specific treatment has been shown to improve the visual outcome for most of these patients, but treatable late complications should be sought. Emphasis must be placed on the rehabilitation of individual patients, with ambulation training and low-vision aids. Ensuring the safety of an intact fellow eye must be a top priority. At a societal level, involvement of ophthalmologists in sponsoring eye-protection programs in schools, in the workplace, and in individual and team sports should be our mission. We need to educate the community on the socioeconomic impact of ocular injuries with the hope of limiting the occurrence of ocular trauma. Trauma registries can be helpful in collecting data not available to the individual physician.[89,90]

REFERENCES

1. Baker RS, Wilson MR, Flowers CW et al. Demographic factors in a population-based survey of hospitalized, work-related, ocular injury. Am J Ophthalmol 1996; 122:213–219.
2. Schein OD, Hibberd PL, Shingleton BJ et al. The spectrum and burden of ocular injury. Ophthalmology 1988; 95:300–305.
3. LaRoche GR, McIntyre L, Schertzer RM. Epidemiology of severe eye injuries in childhood. Ophthalmology 1988; 95:1603–1607.
4. McCarty CA, Fu CL, Taylor HR. Epidemiology of ocular trauma in Australia. Ophthalmology 1999; 106:1847–1852.
5. Steinberg P, Aaberg TM. The persistent challenge of ocular trauma. Am J Ophthalmol 1989; 4:421–424.
6. Tielsch JM, Parver LM. Determinants of hospital charges and length of stay for ocular trauma. Ophthalmology 1990; 97:231–237.
7. Tielsch JM, Parver L, Shankar B. Time trends in the incidence of hospitalized ocular trauma. Arch Ophthalmol 1989; 107:519–523.
8. Klopfer J, Tielsch JM, Vitale S et al. Ocular trauma in the United States: eye injuries resulting in hospitalization, 1984 through 1987. Arch Ophthalmol 1992; 110:838–842.
9. Rapoport I, Rommem M, Kinek M et al. Eye injuries in children in Israel: a nationwide collaborative study. Arch Ophthalmol 1990; 108:376–379.
10. Koval R, Teller J, Belkin M et al. The Israeli ocular injuries study: a nationwide collaborative study. Arch Ophthalmol 1988; 106:776–780.
11. Larrison WI, Hersh PS, Kunzweiler T et al. Sports-related ocular trauma. Ophthalmology 1990; 97:1265–1269.
12. Liggett PE, Pince KJ, Barlow W et al. Ocular trauma in an urban population: review of 1132 cases. Ophthalmology 1990; 97:581–584.
13. Feist RM, Farber MD. Ocular trauma epidemiology. Arch Ophthalmol 1989; 107:503–504.
14. Bullock JD, Ballal DR, Johnson DA et al. Ocular and orbital trauma from water balloon slingshots: a clinical, epidemiologic, and experimental study. Ophthalmology 1997; 104:878–887.
15. Cooney MJ, Pieramici DJ. Eye injuries caused by bungee cords. Ophthalmology 1997; 104:1644–1647.
16. Mieler WF, Nanda SK, Wolf MD et al. Golf-related ocular injuries. Arch Ophthalmol 1995; 113:1410–1413.
17. Capao FJA, Fernandes VL, Barros H et al. Soccer-related ocular injuries. Arch Ophthalmol 2003; 121:687–694.

18. Delori F, Pomerantzeff O, Cox MS. Deformation of the globe under high speed impact: its relation to contusion injuries. Invest Ophthalmol 1969; 8:290–301.

19. Berlin R. Zur sogenannten Commotio retinae. Klin Monatsbl Augenheilkd 1873; 11:42–79.

20. Duke-Elder S, McFaul PA. Electrical injuries. II. Nonmechanical injuries. In: Duke-Elder S, McFaul PA, eds. System of ophthalmology, vol. 14. St Louis: Mosby; 1972.

21. Pulido JS, Blair NP. The blood–retinal barrier in Berlin's edema. Retina 1987; 7:233–236.

22. Hart JCD, Frank HJ. Retinal opacification after blunt non-perforating concussional injuries to the globe: a clinical and retinal fluorescein angiographic study. Trans Ophthalmol Soc UK 1975; 95:94–100.

23. Blight R, Hart JCD. Structural changes in the outer retinal layers following blunt mechanical non-perforating trauma to the globe: an experimental study. Br J Ophthalmol 1977; 61:573–587.

24. Liem AT, Keunen JE, VanNorren D. Reversible cone photoreceptor injury in commotio retinae of the macula. Retina 1995; 15:58–61.

25. Greven CM, Collins AS, Slusher MM et al. Visual results, prognostic indicators and posterior segment findings following surgery for cataract/lens subluxation–dislocation secondary to ocular contusion injuries. Retina 2002; 22:575–580.

26. Ikeda N, Ikeda T, Nagata M et al. Pathogenesis of transient high myopia after blunt eye trauma. Ophthalmology 2002; 109:501–507.

27. Gass JDM. Stereoscopic atlas of macular diseases: diagnosis and treatment. St Louis: Mosby; 1987.

28. Williams DF, Mieler WF, Williams GA. Posterior segment manifestations of ocular trauma. Retina 1990; 10:35–44.

29. Sipperley JO, Quigley HA, Gass JDM. Traumatic retinopathy in primates: the explanation of commotio retinae. Arch Ophthalmol 1978; 96:2267–2273.

30. Mansour AM, Green WR, Hogge C. Histopathology of commotio retinae. Retina 1992; 12:24–48.

31. O'Rourke J, D'Amato D, Luthra C et al. Effects of eye trauma on the intraocular microcirculation: a clinical viewpoint. In: Freeman, HM, ed. Ocular trauma. New York: Appleton-Century-Crofts; 1979.

32. Wolter JR. Coup–contrecoup mechanism of ocular injuries. Am J Ophthalmol 1963; 56:785–796.

33. Fuchs E. Zur Veranderung der Macula lutea nach Contusion. Z Augenheilkd 1901; 6:181–186.

34. Giovinazzo VJ, Yannuzzi LA, Sorenson JA et al. The ocular complications of boxing. Ophthalmology 1987; 94:587–596.

35. Frangieh GT, Green WR, Engel HM. A histopathologic study of macular cysts and holes. Retina 1981; 1:311–336.

36. Kuhn F, Morris R, Mester V et al. Internal limiting membrane removal for traumatic macular holes. Ophthalm Surg Lasers 2001; 32:308–315.

37. Ismail R, Tanner V, Williamson TH. Optical coherence topography imaging of severe commotio retinae and associated macular hole. Available online at: www.bjophthalmol.com (accessed September 26, 2001).

38. Kelley JS, Hoover RE, George T. Whiplash maculopathy. Arch Ophthalmol 1978; 96:834–835.

39. Daily L. Further observations on foveolar splinter and macular wisps. Arch Ophthalmol 1973; 90:102–103.

40. Foos RY. Vitreoretinal juncture: topographical variations. Invest Ophthalmol 1972; 11:801–808.

41. Hart JCD, Raistrick ER. Indirect choroidal tears and late onset serosanguineous maculopathies. Graefes Clin Exp Ophthalmol 1982; 218:206–210.

42. Hoskin A, Bird AC, Sehmi K. Tears of detached retinal pigment epithelium. Br J Ophthalmol 1981; 65:417.

43. Levin AL, Seddon JM, Topping T. Retinal pigment epithelial tears associated with trauma. Am J Ophthalmol 1991; 112:396–400.

44. Goldzieher W. Beitrag zur Pathologie der orbitalen Schussverletzungen. Z Augenheilkd 1901; 6:277.

45. Maguluri S, Hartnett M. Radial choroidal ruptures in sclopetaria. J Am Coll Surg 2003; 197:689–690.

46. Benson WE, Shakin J, Sarin LK. Blunt trauma. In: Tasman W, Jaeger EA, eds. Clinical ophthalmology, vol. 3. Philadelphia: JB Lippincott; 1988.

47. Dubovy SR, Guyton DL, Grenn WR. Clinicopathologic correlation of chorioretinitis sclopetaria. Retina 1997; 17:510–520.

48. Aguilar JP, Green WR. Choroidal rupture: a histopathologic study of 47 eyes. Retina 1984; 4:269–275.

49. Hilton GF. Late serosanguineous detachment of the macula after traumatic choroidal rupture. Am J Ophthalmol 1975; 79:997–1000.

50. Wyszynski RE, Grossniklaus HE, Frank KE. Indirect choroidal rupture secondary to blunt ocular trauma: a review of eight eyes. Retina 1988; 8:237–243.

51. Hart JCD, Natsikos VE, Raistrick ER et al. Indirect choroidal tears at the posterior pole: a fluorescein angiographic and perimetric study. Br J Ophthalmol 1980; 64:59–67.

52. Kohno T, Miki T, Shiraki K et al. Indocyanine green angiographic features of choroidal rupture and choroidal vascular injury after contusion ocular injury. Am J Ophthalmol 2000; 129:38–46.

53. Archer DB, Canavan YM. Contusional eye injuries: retinal and choroidal lesions. Aust J Ophthalmol 1983; 11:251–264.

54. Levin DB, Bell DK. Traumatic retinal hemorrhages with angioid streaks. Arch Ophthalmol 1977; 95:1072.

55. Goldberg MF. Choroidoretinal vascular anastomoses after blunt trauma to the eye. Am J Ophthalmol 1976; 82:892–895.

56. Fuller B, Gitter KA. Traumatic choroidal rupture with late serous detachment of macula: report of successful argon laser treament. Arch Ophthalmol 1973; 89:354–355.

57. Smith RE, Kelley JS, Harbin TS. Late macular complications of choroidal ruptures. Am J Ophthalmol 1974; 77:650–658.

58. Gross JG, King LP, de Juan E et al. Subfoveal neovascular membrane removal in patients with traumatic choroidal rupture. Ophthalmology 1996; 103:579–585.

59. Sanborn GE, Gonder JR, Goldberg RE et al. Evulsion of the optic nerve: a clinicopathological study. Can J Ophthalmol 1984; 19:10–16.

60. Foster BS, March GA, Lucarelli MJ et al. Optic nerve avulsion. Arch Ophthalmol 1997; 115:623–630.

61. Tandon R, Vanathi M, Verma L et al. Traumatic optic nerve avulsion: role of ultrasonography. Eye 2003; 17:667–670.

62. Purtscher O. Noch unbekannte Befunde nach Schadeltrauma. Berl Dtsch Ophthal Ges 1910; 36:294–301.

63. Pratt MV, De Venecia G. Purtscher's retinopathy: a clinicopathological correlation. Surv Ophthalmol 1970; 14:417–423.

64. Purtscher O. Angiopathia retinae traumatica: Lymphorrhagien des Augengrundes. Graefes Arch Klin Exp Ophthalmol 1912; 82:347–371.

65. Kelley JS. Purtscher's retinopathy related to chest compression by safety belts: fluorescein angiographic findings. Am J Ophthalmol 1972; 74:278–283.

66. Blodi B, Johnson MW, Gass JDM et al. Purtscher's-like retinopathy after childbirth. Ophthalmology 1990; 97:1654–1659.

67. Burton TC. Unilateral Purtscher's retinopathy. Ophthalmology 1980; 87:1096–1105.

68. Patel M, Bains A, O'Hara JP et al. Purtscher retinopathy as the initial sign of thrombotic thrombocytopenic purpura/hemolytic uremic syndrome. Arch J Ophthalmol 2001; 119:1388–1390.

69. Fischbein F, Safir A. Monocular Purtscher's retinopathy: a fluorescein angiographic study. Arch Ophthalmol 1971; 85:480–484.

70. Shah GK, Penne R, Grand MG. Purtscher's retinopathy secondary to airbag injury. Retina 2001; 21:68–69.

71. Jacob HS, Craddock PR, Hammerschmidt DE et al. Complement-induced granulocyte aggregation: and unsuspected mechanism of disease. N Engl J Med 1980; 302:789–794.

72. Ravin JG, Meyer RF. Fluorescein angiographic findings in a case of traumatic asphyxia. Am J Ophthalmol 1973; 75:643–647.

73. Duane TD. Valsalva hemorrhagic retinopathy. Trans Am Ophthalmol Soc 1972; 70:298–311.

74. Friberg TR, Braunstein RA, Bressler NM. Sudden visual loss associated with sexual activity. Arch Ophthalmol 1995; 113:738–742.

75. Manche EF, Goldberg RA, Mondino BJ. Air bag-related ocular injuries. Ophthalm Surg Lasers 1997; 28:246–250.

76. Ladjimi A, Zaouali S, Messaoud R et al. Valsalva retinopathy induced by labour. Eur J Ophthalmol 2002; 12:336–338.

77. Buys YM, Levin AV, Enzenauer RW et al. Retinal findings after head trauma in infants and young children. Ophthalmology 1992; 99:1718–1723.

78. Levin AV. Ocular manifestations of child abuse. Ophthalmol Clin North Am 1990; 3:249–264.

79. Pierre-Kahn V, Roche O, Dureau P et al. Ophthalmic findings in suspected child abuse victims with subdural hematomas. Ophthalmology 2003; 110:1718–1723.

80. Reece RM, Sege R. Childhood head injuries: accidental or inflicted? Arch Pediatr Adolesc Med 2000; 154:11–15.

81. Morad Y, Kim YM, Armstrong DC et al. Correlation between retinal abnormalities and intracranial abnormalities in the shaken baby syndrome. Am J Ophthalmol 2002; 134:354–359.

82. Caffey J. The whiplash-shaken infant syndrome: manual shaking by the extremities with whiplash-induced intracranial and intraocular bleedings, linked with residual permanent brain damage and mental retardation. Pediatrics 1974; 54:396–403.

83. Rooms L, Fitzgerald N, McCain KL. Hemophagocytic lymphohistiocytosis masquerading as child abuse: presentation of three cases and review of central nervous system findings in hemophagocytic lymphohistiocytosis. Pediatrics 2003; 111:636–640.

84. Elner SG, Elner VM, Arnall M et al. Ocular and associated systemic findings in suspected child abuse: a necropsy study. Arch Ophthalmol 1990; 108:1094–1101.

85. Greenwald MJ, Weiss A, Oesterle CS et al. Traumatic retinoschisis in battered babies. Ophthalmology 1986; 93:618–625.

86. Handa JT, Jaffe GJ. Lightning maculopathy: a case report . Retina 1994; 14:169–172.

87. Kushner FH, Olsen JC. Retinal hemorrhage as a consequence of epidural steroid injection. Arch Ophthalmol 1995; 113:309–313.

88. Browning DJ. Acute retinal necrosis following epidural steroid injections. Am J Ophthalmol 2003; 136:192–194.

89. Pieramici DJ, Sternberg P Jr, Aaberg TM et al. A system for classifying mechanical injuries of the eye (globe). The Ocular Trauma Classification Group. Am J Ophthalmol 1998; 125:565–566.

90. Viestenz A, Kuchle M. Ocular contusion caused by elastic cords: a retrospective analysis using the Erlangen Ocular Contusion Registry. Clin Exp Ophthalmol 2002; 30:266–269.

Chapter

111

Optic Disc Pits and Associated Serous Macular Detachment

Alfredo A. Sadun

Optic disc pits are congenital excavations of the optic nerve head usually seen in association with other abnormalities of the optic nerve and peripapillary retina, including large optic nerve head size, large inferior colobomas of the optic disc, and retinal colobomas. These associations gave rise to the hypothesis that optic disc pits develop as a result of incomplete closure of the superior end of the embryonic fissure. Additionally, optic disc pits have been associated with posterior vitreous detachments and, in about half of all cases, with serous retinal detachment. The prevailing theory is that the associated subretinal (and probably intraretinal) fluid derives from liquefied vitreous that passes through the opening created by the optic disc pit.

OPTIC DISC ANOMALIES

A variety of congenital optic disc anomalies challenge the clinical acumen of ophthalmologists, internists, and pediatricians. Since some of these abnormalities are known by various names, it is worthwhile reviewing the general categories.

Megalopapilla

Megalopapilla is a rare anomaly of the optic disc that occasionally affects visual acuity. The optic disc may be unilaterally or bilaterally involved and appears pale owing to the thinning of the nerve fiber distribution across the large optic nerve head. Megalopapilla is often associated with large refractive errors and with midline congenital deformities.[1]

Aplasia

Aplasia of the optic nerve head is extremely rare, often overstated (careful examination would reveal remnants of the optic nerve), and probably represents an extreme form of optic nerve head hypoplasia. Optic nerve aplasia may be associated with the absence or gross maldevelopment of the globe.[1]

Hypoplasia

Optic disc hypoplasia is a congenital underdevelopment of the optic nerve head in which there is a reduced number of axons. The smaller optic nerve head can be appreciated ophthalmoscopically, as well as by ultrasound or even by neuroimaging (preferably magnetic resonance imaging). Hypoplastic optic discs are probably underdiagnosed and may vary considerably in

the extent to which they are "stunted."[2] Optic nerve hypoplasia may be associated with any level of visual acuity and with a variety of visual field defects.

Cavities in the optic nerve head

Excavated and colobomatous defects of the optic nerve head encompass a spectrum of abnormalities, including tilted discs, peripapillary staphyloma, morning-glory disc anomaly, colobomas, and congenital optic disc pits. Optic disc pits were regarded as atypical colobomas by Grear,[3] who reviewed the subject in 1942.

Optic disc pits should probably be considered one manifestation along a spectrum of cavitary optic disc anomalies. Slusher and co-workers[4] described a family of 35 members spanning five generations with an autosomal dominant pattern of congenital optic disc abnormalities. Remarkably, a myriad of morphologic variations of phenotype were expressed, including optic disc pits, morning-glory syndrome, and coloboma of the optic nerve. One gene defect can result in a variety of optic disc abnormalities; therefore the traditional classification schemes that describe varieties of cavitary optic disc anomalies should be reconsidered.

ANATOMY

A brief review of the anatomy and embryology of the optic nerve head permit an increased understanding of these abnormalities.

The retinal ganglion cells of each retina contribute approximately 1.2 million unmyelinated axons that converge at a point approximately 4 mm nasal to the foveola, through which they exit the globe, acquire a myelin sheath, and form the optic nerve. These axons project to various primary visual nuclei in the brain,[5] constitute a fiber tract rather than a nerve, and, as such, have histologic and functional similarities to brain tissue. The optic nerve is enclosed by three meningeal sheaths that are contiguous with the meningeal coverings of the brain. Before exiting the eye, however, the axons of the retinal ganglion cells must converge centripetally, make a sharp turn, traverse the lamina cribrosa, form nerve bundles enclosed by connective tissue septa, and then, once posterior to the lamina cribrosa, become ensheathed by myelin (Fig. 111-1).

Thus, the optic nerve head is remarkable in several respects. Axons deriving from the retina become part of the nerve, go

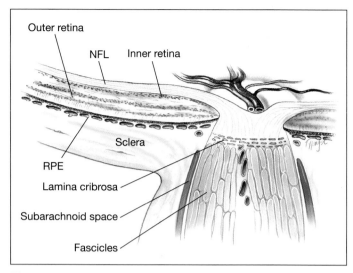

Fig. 111-1 Axial view of optic nerve head and surrounding tissues. Fibers from the retina collect at the optic disc, pass down through the lamina cribrosa, become myelinated, and form fascicles. Note the three parts of the optic nerve: I, anterior portion (retinal); II, midportion (prelaminar or choroidal); III, posterior portion (lamina cribrosa or scleral) at optic nerve head. NFL, Nerve fiber layer; RPE, retinal pigment epithelium.

from an unmyelinated to a myelinated state, traverse the sieve-like lamina cribrosa, are partitioned into groups by glial columns, and go from an area of high (intraocular) pressure to relatively low interstitial pressure. Not surprisingly, anomalies of structure at this critical juncture often lead to marked physiologic consequences.[6]

Gross anatomy

The optic nerve head is composed of three parts: retinal, choroidal, and scleral (see Fig. 111-1). The optic nerve head is slightly oval; its vertical axis averages about 1.5 mm in diameter.[7] The physiologic cup, a depression occupying the center of the optic disc, may vary in size from less than 10% to 80% of the disc diameter (expressed as decimal portions of one). This cup-to-disc ratio is usually very similar between fellow eyes. The central retinal artery and central retinal vein enter and exit the globe through the optic nerve head. The central artery may divide within the optic nerve head or more distally in the retina. The margins of the optic nerve head, usually viewed by an ophthalmoscope, border the retina, retinal pigment epithelium (RPE), Bruch's membrane, and the choroid and scleral canal. However, in about one-fourth of all eyes a juxtapapillary temporal crescent is noted. This is seen most often in myopic eyes but may also represent a congenital abnormality.

Histology

The most anterior component of the optic nerve head is the retinal nerve fiber or surface layer. It is composed of retinal ganglion cell nerve fibers that enter the optic nerve from all regions of the retina. Anterior to these nerve fibers is the inner limiting membrane of Elschnig, composed of astrocytes and continuous with the inner limiting membrane of the retina.[7]

Posterior to the surface layer is the prelaminar region or choroidal level of the optic nerve head (see Fig. 111-1). Here the 1.2 million axons form approximately 1000 fascicular bundles, which are separated by glial columns (astrocytic glia) that provide support as the unmyelinated axons bend 90 degrees to form the optic nerve. These astrocytic glia are continuous with collagenous, glial, and elastic tissues that surround the optic nerve and separate it from the choroid (border tissue of Elschnig).

The most posterior of the three layers of the optic nerve head is the lamina cribrosa or scleral lamina (see Fig. 111-1). The lamina cribrosa consists of a stack of fenestrated leaves of connective tissue continuous with the surrounding sclera.[7] These sieve-like plates are not in perfect alignment, so the fenestration of one plate may not be directly above or below the fenestration of the adjacent plate. This portion of the lamina cribrosa is relatively noncompliant and provides support for the axons that will form the optic nerve. This supportive sieve-like structure is lined with astrocytic glia, which may help provide a seal between the high intraocular pressure and the relatively low pressure of the posterior laminar interstitium.[6] A ring of astrocytic glial tissue further surrounds the posterior laminar optic nerve, forming a seal with the contiguous sclera. The bundles of nerve fibers within the pores of the lamina are avascular. They are nourished by capillaries within the intervening collagen beams.

Embryology

The retina, RPE, and optic nerve head all originate from layers of the optic cup. The sclera and choroid, however, derive from mesoderm that encircles the cup. Differentiation of the sclera and choroid proceeds posteriorly as the optic cup proceeds anteriorly, and in the period between 7 and 20 weeks of gestation the sclera surrounds the retina and optic nerve, forming the globe.

The optic vesicle invaginates; its inner part forms the neural retina, while its outer part forms the pigment epithelium. As it does so, a groove remains open inferiorly. This embryonic fissure permits mesodermal tissue to enter the optic cup to form the hyaloid artery. This fissure begins to close at approximately 5 weeks of gestation; failure of tissues to fuse properly results in many of the congenital colobomatous defects discussed.

At approximately 5½ weeks of gestation, axons deriving from retinal ganglion cells collect posteriorly and pass into the optic stalk; these fibers do not reach the optic chiasm until about 7 weeks of gestation. As the fibers penetrate the primitive epithelial papilla of the optic nerve head, they become sequestered centrally. Myelination of these fibers begins centrally (at the brain) and proceeds toward the eye, usually reaching the lamina cribrosa shortly after birth.[7]

Optic disc dysplasia

Congenital abnormalities of the vasculature, RPE, and glial tissues of the optic nerve head produce a wide spectrum of anomalies. The morning-glory syndrome consists of a unilaterally enlarged and severely distorted optic disc with a funnel-shaped excavation surrounded by a ring of elevated chorioretinal pigmentary tissue.

When an optic disc coloboma involves changes in the retina, RPE, Bruch's membrane, or sclera, it is believed to reflect a defect in closure of the fetal fissure. Such colobomas, when limited to the optic disc tissues, probably reflect defects in development of the primitive optic papilla.

OPTIC DISC PITS

In 1882, Wiethe[8] described abnormalities in both optic discs of a 62-year-old woman. His description of dark-gray depressions in the optic nerve heads was probably the first report of optic disc pits. Since Wiethe's initial description, excavations of the optic nerve head have variously been described as craters, holes, cavities, and, most recently, congenital pits of the optic nerve head.

Recent studies suggest that optic pits occur in approximately 1 in 10 000 eyes, although there is considerable variance among studies.[3,9] Men and women are equally affected. Approximately 10 to 15% of optic disc pits are bilateral. Most optic disc pits are nonfamilial; however there are a few reports with an autosomal dominant pattern of inheritance.[36] One such report describes a family for which several members had small iris colobomas, some in combination with the pit, providing insight as to the etiology.[10] About 70% of the pits are on the temporal side of the disc, and about 20% are situated centrally; the remainder are found inferiorly, superiorly, and nasally.[11]

Serous retinal detachments can be associated with optic disc pits. These may occur at any age but are most frequent in early adulthood. However, there have been reports of associated retinal detachment occurring as early as 6 years of age and in patients as old as in the ninth decade of life.[11] Some have suggested that the clinical course differs and leads to better visual acuity in children as spontaneous resolution is the rule.[12,13] More recently, through the analysis of stereoscopic transparencies, it has been proposed that the fluid that enters through the optic disc pit actually travels between the inner and outer layers of the retina to produce a retinal schisis.[14,15] Optical coherence tomography (OCT) has shown such inner retinal schises preceding outer-layer detachment.[16] Following this, detachment of the outer retinal layer may occur as a secondary process.[16] Although no histopathologic studies have confirmed this, the application of OCT has provided compelling evidence for at least two levels of retinal separation.[17] OCT has also been used to demonstrate a marked reduction in thickness of the retinal nerve fiber layer in the quadrant corresponding to the optic nerve pit.[18]

In the series of Brown et al.,[11] most optic disc pits were gray in color, although they varied from yellow to black. Their size can range from minute to large, occupying most of the surface of the optic disc.

Visual defects

The optic disc pit is most often associated with two types of visual field defects.[19] The first type is typified by arcuate scotomas that probably reflect the absence of the wedge of nerve fibers displaced by the optic disc pit. Larger pits may be associated with large Bjerrum-type scotomas or even altitudinal visual field defects. Nasal or temporal steps are often detectable; less frequently, paracentral scotomas and generalized constriction may be seen.[11] However, Walsh & Hoyt[20] reviewed several studies that demonstrated only an enlarged blind spot as a forme fruste of the visual field defect in association with optic pits.

The second type of visual field defect is that associated with serous detachment of the macula. In 1960 Kranenburg[21] described the association of optic nerve pits and central serous retinopathy. He found that 16 of his 24 patients with optic disc pits had serous detachments of the macula, with corresponding central scotomas or other central visual field changes.

Associated retinal changes

Optic nerve head pits that are centrally located are least likely to be associated with retinal changes. Optic disc pits along the rim of the optic disc are usually seen in association with peripapillary chorioretinal atrophy and RPE changes (Fig. 111-2). These peripapillary changes may develop over time with or without central serous retinal detachments. In following the development of a serous macular detachment, Walsh & Hoyt[20] described the appearance of what they termed an "occult hole" in the optic nerve head.

Serous detachment of the macula is now known as a common complication of the optic disc pit. The natural history of this complication has been well described by Sobol et al.[22] They followed 15 patients with optic disc pits and macular detachments for an average of 9 years and found that 80% lost vision to 20/200 or worse. The visual loss was generally complete within 6 months of presentation. Long-term macular changes included full-thickness or laminar (through the outer retina) retinal holes, RPE mottling, and general cystic changes of the macula.[22]

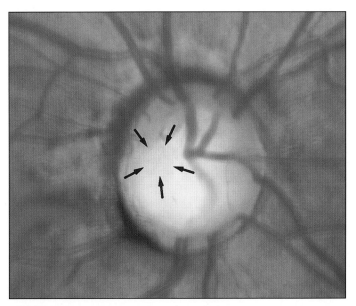

Fig. 111-2 Optic disc pits near the temporal margin are common and are most likely to lead to serous macular detachments.

Vascular telangiectasis has been reported in connection with intraschitic hemorrhage from a temporal optic disc pit.[23]

A gray fibroglial membrane appears to overlie the pit in many cases (Fig. 111-3). This membrane may be intact or may incompletely cover the pit. The fact that patients with serous macular detachments almost invariably have defects in their diaphanous membrane has prompted theories on how the optic nerve pit leads to the development of serous macular detachment.

MACULAR DETACHMENT

Several investigators have estimated that between 40 and 50% of patients with optic nerve pits have either an associated nonrhegmatogenous, serous retinal detachment or retinal changes suggestive of previous detachment.[11,24] The macular serous detachment (or retinoschisis) seen in association with optic disc pits appears most commonly when the pit is located in the temporal region of the optic disc and in larger pits. Conversely, small pits and those located more centrally are less likely to lead to serous retinal detachments.[11,21]

Appearance of maculopathy

In 1908, Reis[25] described a case of an optic nerve pit with associated maculopathy. However, this association was not taken seriously until Petersen,[26] in 1958, described several patients with what he called craterlike holes in the optic disc who also had a central serous chorioretinopathy. This relationship was firmly emphasized by Kranenburg[21] in 1960, who described 24 cases of optic disc pits. One-third of these patients had serous retinal detachments, and another third had macular changes that he interpreted as reflecting a previous episode of nonrhegmatogenous serous retinal detachment.

Most of the retinal detachments are temporal to the disc and confined between the superior and inferior vascular arcades. Infrequently, a serous retinal detachment is located outside the

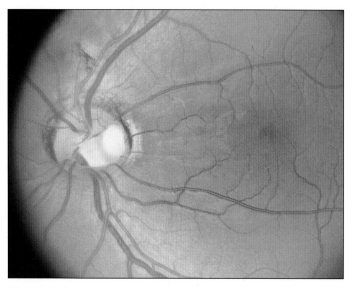

Fig. 111-3 Optic nerve pit. Note overlying gray fibroglial membrane.

arcades if the pit is situated on the nasal side of the optic disc. Often, the serous retinal detachment is contiguous with the optic disc, sometimes through a visible isthmus of subretinal fluid.

The serous macular detachments are generally low (less than 1.0 mm in height). The elevated retina often contains cystic regions that have been demonstrated on histologic examination to exist within the inner nuclear layer.[9] Occasionally the cystic areas rupture outward, producing a lamellar macular hole that, unlike idiopathic lamellar macular holes, retains an intact internal limiting membrane.

The variability of the retinal separation is also consistent with an alternative description of the maculopathy proposed by Lincoff and colleagues.[27] In a recent case report they provide clear optic coherence tomographs to show a schisis cavity between the inner and outer retina and a larger outer-layer retinal detachment. The two are connected by a hole in the outer layer near the fovea.[27]

Course of associated serous macular detachment

It is difficult to determine the time interval between the beginning of a serous macular detachment and the earliest visual changes, because the patient usually seeks evaluation after symptoms of blurred vision and metamorphopsia occur secondary to foveal involvement. However, Brown & Tasman[28] described one case in which the retinal detachment started at the temporal margin of the optic disc. This serous retinal detachment expanded slowly in a temporal direction until, after several months, it covered the entire macular area. They also described small yellow precipitates seen under the elevated retina late in the course of serous macular detachment.

In analyzing their 15 patients followed over an average of 9 years, Sobol et al.[22] found that most eyes with optic disc pits presented with visual acuities of about 20/40 to 20/60. However, each patient lost three or more lines of vision within the next 6 months. After 6 months, a few of these patients got worse and even fewer got better. Ultimately, only 20% of the patients maintained visual acuities of better than 20/200.[22] Generally, however, patients with optic disc pits present later in the course of their macular detachments when their visual acuities are already worse than 20/70.[29]

Theories of pathophysiology

By 1960 it was clear that serous macular detachments often occurred as complications of optic disc pits. Ferry[9] had the opportunity to examine histologically two eyes with optic disc pits associated with macular detachments. He suggested that progressive gliosis and "contraction of the retinal elements" contained in the pit produced a traction detachment of the macula. In 1964 Sugar[30] suggested that fluid from the vitreous cavity could enter the subretinal space through a macular hole. However, this is most unlikely because macular holes seen with optic pits are usually lamellar and are only infrequently seen in association with the serous detachment.

It has been reported that fluorescein angiographic examination reveals late hyperfluorescence of the optic disc pit.[24] It was therefore considered possible that blood vessels in this area leaked fluid, which then entered the subretinal space.[24] However, Brown et al.[11] reported that many patients with serous macular detachments had no leakage on their fluorescein angiogram.

Others have speculated that there may be a direct source of fluid from the choroid that penetrates through Bruch's membrane under the macular detachment; it was hypothesized that peripapillary chorioretinal atrophic changes permitted this leakage.[31] However, fluorescein angiographic findings do not support this theory. Moreover, many other diseases produce extensive chorioretinal atrophy that does not lead to serous macular detachment.[11]

A few investigators,[32] including Gass,[33] have suggested that cerebrospinal fluid may leak from the optic nerve subarachnoid space into the optic pit and from there into the subretinal space. However, intrathecal fluorescein injections in humans and in animals and histologic studies have failed to demonstrate any such connection.[9,34-36]

Currently, the most widely accepted explanation is that originally proposed by Sugar[37] in 1962 and later endorsed by Brockhurst[38] in 1975. Sugar proposed that fluid from the vitreous leaked through the optic disc pit to fill the subretinal space (Fig. 111-4). In corroboration of this theory, Brown et al.[11] demonstrated that more than three-fourths of patients with optic disc pits and associated serous macular detachments have posterior vitreous detachments. This would allow liquefied vitreous to be contiguous with the optic disc cavity. Moreover, most of the patients in their series who had pits without macular serous elevations did not have posterior vitreous detachments.[11] Additionally, Brown and his colleagues[35] demonstrated experimentally in dogs a direct connection between the posterior vitreous space and the subretinal space via a congenital optic disc pit. Irvine et al.[32] demonstrated in vivo that there is a continuity between the posterior vitreous cavity and the optic nerve subarachnoid space by observing bubbles percolating out of an optic nerve sheath window after pars plana vitrectomy and gas injection.

The most recent variation on these theories of pathophysiology is that proposed by Lincoff et al.,[27] who suggest that the primary communication from the optic disc pit is to the retina temporal to the optic disc.[14] Fluid slips under the inner retina, lifting it and the nerve fiber layer up and away from the outer retina (Fig. 111-4). This has been corroborated by OCT[17] and extended to show both this retinal schisis and an outer retinal detachment connected by a hole in the outer retinal layer.

Although the theory of direct vitreous fluid entry via the optic pit into the subretinal space is appealing, it does not explain why serous macular detachments tend to occur first in young adulthood. Brown & Tasman[28] suggest that posterior vitreous detachments may be a precipitating factor. Another possibility is that the impelling factor is macular traction, which occurs with age.

Prognosis

Although the optic nerve head pits, being congenital, are stationary, their associated retinal abnormalities may be progressive. The prognosis for return of vision after serous macular detachment is variable. Walsh & Hoyt[20] described a patient followed between the ages of 14 and 23 years who developed multiple serous macular detachments that remitted to near-normal vision after each episode. A more rigorous study was conducted by Brown et al.[11] in a group of 20 eyes with optic disc pits and serous macular detachments. These eyes were followed for 5 years, untreated. The mean visual acuity at the end of this time was about 20/80. The authors found very little correlation between the visual acuity at the time of detachment and the long-term visual outcome. They also noted that some detachments resolved spontaneously, whereas others persisted for years. Most patients still had some subretinal macular fluid present after 5 years. Other macular changes, as described above, also persisted. Recent long-term studies confirm the earlier impressions that untreated macular detachments caused by optic disc pits have an overall poor prognosis.[22]

Treatment

Several medical and surgical interventions have been attempted to help clear or prevent the serous macular detachment seen in association with optic disc pits. Systemic steroids, optic nerve sheath decompression, and scleral buckling procedures have not been demonstrated to be very effective.[38,39] However, several series have favorably compared the outcome of photocoagulated eyes with untreated eyes in the resolution of the serous macular detachment and in final visual outcome.[33,38-40] The argon laser procedure was used in most of these series to produce photocoagulation burns in one or several rows between the area of serous retinal detachment and the optic disc. Usually, the burns are only applied to areas of elevated retina. Brockhurst,[38] Gass,[40] and Theodossiadis[41] used similar

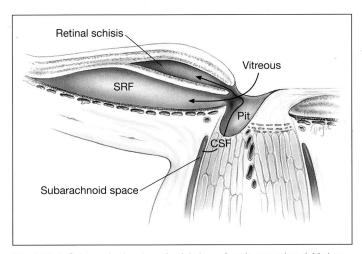

Fig. 111-4 Schematic drawing of axial view of optic nerve head. Various theories describe mechanisms by which fluid enters the subretinal space. Cerebrospinal fluid (CSF) could derive from the subarachnoid space. However, the more widely accepted explanation is that fluid in the vitreous space passes into the optic pit and from there directly into the subretinal space. An optic disc pit located near the margin of the optic nerve head is far more likely to permit fluid to leak subretinally. SRF, Subretinal fluid.

photocoagulation protocols, and all reported that their patients were likely to have good resolution of the serous detachment to a flat macula.

Combining their results, 15 of the 18 patients in these three series had reattachments of their maculas, as opposed to only 5 of 20 untreated patients in the series of Brown et al.[11] However, the difference in final visual outcome between the treated and untreated groups was less pronounced. The photocoagulated eyes in the three studies had ultimate visual acuities that averaged a little worse than 20/80. This does not compare favorably with the 20/80 final visual outcome in the series of Brown et al. In making a similar comparison, Brown & Tasman[28] concluded that photocoagulation therapy is effective for flattening the retinal detachment but not for improving final visual outcome.

Macular buckling procedure successfully treated cases of serous detachment in optic disc pit. In such cases, OCT showed a resultant closure of the connection between the pit and a retinal schisis with resolution of the schisis.[42] Multifocal electroretinography was performed in 10 patients with optic disc pit with serous macular detachment before and after treatment with macular buckling procedures.[43] Improvement was measured in all eyes at 12 months, though often this was not accompanied by an increase in visual acuity.[43] Silicon oil has been used successfully in cases of macular hole in association with the optic disc pit.[44]

More recent attempts to combine photocoagulation therapy with posterior vitrectomy and gas–fluid exchange have led to more encouraging long-term visual outcomes.[45] Bonnet[46] looked at 25 eyes with optic disc pits in 24 patients who presented with visual loss due to serous macular detachments. High-magnification biomicroscopy and fluorescein angiography of these eyes revealed evidence of vitreous traction on the retina and on the optic nerve head. Most particularly, Bonnet noted that none of the patients had posterior vitreous detachments at presentation and that in the 2 cases that subsequently developed a posterior vitreous detachment, reattachment of the macula occurred spontaneously. Fluorescein dye was seen to stain the optic nerve head, especially at the pit and temporal margin of the disc. This dye leakage was not seen in cases that underwent surgical peeling of the posterior vitreous face. Moreover, Bonnet observed a small hole in the roof of the optic pit in several cases and small bubbles of gas passing from the vitreous cavity to the subretinal space via the optic disc pit in a case that underwent vitrectomy and gas injection but not photocoagulation. Hence, Bonnet concluded that macular detachments in optic disc pits have a rhegmatogenous component (at the optic disc), that they are associated with vitreous traction, and that the subretinal fluid comes from the vitreous space via the optic disc pit.[46]

Cox and colleagues[47] looked at three treatment methods. They concluded that the combination of vitrectomy plus gas tamponade plus photocoagulation of the retina temporal to the disc was more effective than vitrectomy and gas or photocoagulation alone. They obtained short-term surgical success in all of their 8 eyes and long-term attachment in 4 out of 8 eyes

using the three-part combination therapy.[47] Others have also obtained good anatomic results in optic disc pit with macular detachment using the combination of vitrectomy, air–fluid exchange, and photocoagulation in patients whose final visual acuities averaged 20/60.[48] These and other precipitating events may combine with the mechanism described above, leading to macular detachment by vitreous fluid entry into the subretinal space via the optic disc pit.

REFERENCES

1. Sadun AA, Yanoff M. Pathology of the optic nerve. In: Duane TD, Jaeger EA, eds. Biomedical foundations of ophthalmology, vol. 3, Philadelphia: Harper & Row; 1986.
2. Nelson M, Lessell S, Sadun AA. Optic nerve hypoplasia and maternal diabetes mellitus. Arch Neurol 1986; 43:20–25.
3. Grear JN Jr. Pits, or crater-like holes in the optic disk. Arch Ophthalmol 1942; 28:467–483.
4. Slusher MM, Weaver RG, Greven CM et al. The spectrum of cavitary optic disc anomalies in a family. Ophthalmology 1989; 96:342–347.
5. Sadun AA, Schaecter JD. Tracing axons in the human brain: a method utilizing light and TEM techniques. J Electron Microsc Tech 1985; 2:175–186.
6. Sadun AA, Currie JN, Lessell S. Transient visual obscurations with elevated optic discs. Ann Neurol 1984; 16:489–494.
7. Hogan MJ, Alvarado JA, Weddell JE. Histology of the human eye: an atlas and textbook, Philadelphia, PA: WB Saunders; 1971.
8. Wiethe T. Ein Fall von angeborener Deformitat der Sehnervenpapille. Arch Augenheilkd 1882; 11:4–19.
9. Ferry AP. Macular detachment associated with congenital pit of the optic nerve head: pathologic findings in two cases simulating malignant melanoma of the choroid. Arch Ophthalmol 1963; 70:346–357.
10. Singerman LJ, Mittra RA. Hereditary optic pit and iris coloboma in three generations of a single family. Retina 2001; 21:273–275.
11. Brown GC, Shields JA, Goldberg RE. Congenital pits of the optic nerve head. II. Clinical studies in humans. Ophthalmology 1980; 87:51–65.
12. Brodsky MC. Congenital optic pit with serous maculopathy in childhood. J AAPOS 2003; 2:150.
13. Yuen CHW, Kaye SB. Spontaneous resolution of serous maculopathy associated with optic disc pit in a child: a case report. J AAPOS 2002; 6: 330–331.
14. Lincoff H, Lopez R, Kreissig I et al. Retinoschisis associated with optic nerve pits. Arch Ophthalmol 1988; 106:61–67.
15. Lincoff H, Yannuzzi L, Singerman L et al. Improvement in visual function after displacement of the retinal elevations emanating from optic pits. Arch Ophthalmol 1993; 111:1071–1079.
16. Lincoff H, Kreissig I. Optical coherence tomography of pneumatic displacement of optic disc pit maculopathy. Br J Ophthalmol 1998; 82:367–372.
17. Krivoy D, Gentile R, Liebmann JM et al. Imaging congenital optic disc pits and associated maculopathy using optic coherence tomography. Arch Ophthalmol 1996; 114:165–170.
18. Myer CH, Rodrigues EB, Schmidt JC. Congenital optic nerve head pit associated with reduced retinal nerve fibre thickness at the papillomacular bundle. Br J Ophthalmol 2003; 87:1300–1301.
19. Simpson DE. Optic nerve pit. J Am Optom Assoc 1987; 58:118–120.
20. Walsh FB, Hoyt WF. Clinical neuro-ophthalmology, 3rd edn. Baltimore, MD: Williams & Wilkins; 1969.
21. Kranenburg EW. Crater-like holes in the optic disc and central serous retinopathy. Arch Ophthalmol 1960; 64:912–924.
22. Sobol WM, Boldi CF, Folk JC et al. Long-term visual outcome in patients with optic nerve pit and serous retinal detachment of the macula. Ophthalmology 1990; 97:1539–1542.
23. Quinn SM, Charles SJ. Telangiectasis as a cause of intra-schitic haemorrhage in optic disc pit maculopathy. Acta Ophthalmol Scand 2004; 82:93–95.
24. Gordon R, Chatfield RK. Pits in the optic disc associated with macular degeneration. Br J Ophthalmol 1969; 53:481–489.
25. Reis W. Eine wenig bekannte typische Missbildung am Sehnerveneintritt: Umschriebene Grubenbildung auf der Papilla n. optici. Z Augenheilkd 1908; 19:505–528.
26. Petersen HP. Pits or crater-like holes in the optic disc. Acta Ophthalmol 1958; 36:345–443.
27. Lincoff H, Schiff W, Krivoy D et al. Optic coherence tomography of optic disk pit maculopathy. Am J Ophthalmol 1996; 122:264–266.
28. Brown GC, Tasman WS. Congenital anomalies of the optic disk. New York: Grune & Stratton; 1983.

29. Theodossiadis GP. Visual acuity in patients with optic nerve pit. Ophthalmology 1991; 98:563.

30. Sugar HS. An explanation for the acquired macular pathology associated with congenital pits of the optic disc. Am J Ophthalmol 1964; 57:833–835.

31. Wise G, Dollery C, Henkind P. The retinal circulation. New York: Harper & Row; 1971.

32. Irvine AR, Crawford JB, Sullivan JH. The pathogenesis of retinal detachment with morning glory disk and optic pit. Retina 1986; 6:146–150.

33. Gass JDM. Serous detachment of the macular secondary to congenital pit of the optic nerve head. Am J Ophthalmol 1969; 67:821–841.

34. Brown GC, Shields JA, Patty BE et al. Congenital pits of the optic nerve head. I. Experimental studies in collie dogs. Arch Ophthalmol 1979; 97: 1341–1344.

35. Brown GC, Shields JA, Patty BE et al. Congenital optic pits and serous retinal detachment. Trans Pa Acad Ophthalmol Otolaryngol 1979; 32:151–154.

36. Kalina RE, Conrad WC. Intrathecal fluorescein for serous macular detachment. Arch Ophthalmol 1976; 94:1421.

37. Sugar HS. Congenital pits in the optic disc with acquired macular pathology. Am J Ophthalmol 1962; 53:307–311.

38. Brockhurst RJ. Optic pits and posterior retinal detachment. Trans Am Ophthalmol Soc 1975; 73:264–291.

39. Mustonen E, Varonen T. Congenital pit of the optic nerve head associated with serous detachment of the macular. Acta Ophthalmol 1972; 50:689–698.

40. Gass JDM. Stereoscopic atlas of macular diseases. St Louis: Mosby; 1977.

41. Theodossiadis G. Evolution of congenital pit of the optic disk with macular detachment in photocoagulated and nonphotocoagulated eyes. Am J Ophthalmol 1977; 84:620–631.

42. Theodossiadis GP, Theodossiadis PG. Optical coherence tomography in optic disk pit maculopathy treated by the macular buckling procedure. Am J Ophthalmol 2001; 132:184–190.

43. Theodossiadis G. Theodossiadis P, Lalias J et al. Prepoperative and postoperative assessment by multifocal electroretinography in the management of optic disc pits with serous macular detachment. Ophthalmology 2002; 109:2295–2302.

44. Bechmann M, Mueller AJ, Gandorfer A et al. Macular hole surgery in an eye with an optic pit. Am J Ophthalmol 2001; 132:263–264.

45. Pahwa V. Optic pit and central serous detachment. Ind J Ophthalmol 1985; 33:175–176.

46. Bonnet M. Serous macular detachment associated with optic nerve pits. Graefes Arch Clin Exp Ophthalmol 1991; 229:526–532.

47. Cox MS, Witherspoon CD, Morris RE et al. Evolving techniques in the treatment of macular detachment caused by optic nerve pits. Ophthalmology 1988; 95:889–896.

48. Schatz H, McDonald HR. Treatment of sensory retinal detachment associated with optic nerve pit or coloboma. Ophthalmology 1988; 95:178–186.

Index